Fetal and Neonatal Neurology and Neurosurgery

FOURTH
EDITION

Dedicated to our fathers, Dr Maurice Levene and Mr Frank Chervenak, who continue to live through their sons' commitment to helping fetal and neonatal patients throughout the world

For Elsevier

Commissioning Editor: Ellen Green/Pauline Graham
Development Editor: Helen Leng
Project Manager: Kathryn Mason
Design Direction: Erik Bigland
Illustrations Manager: Merlyn Harvey
Illustrator: Lois Hague

Fetal and Neonatal Neurology and Neurosurgery

FOURTH EDITION

EDITED BY

MALCOLM I LEVENE MD FRCPCH FMedSc

Professor of Paediatrics, Leeds General Infirmary
Head of Academic Department of Paediatrics and Child Health
University of Leeds, UK

FRANK A CHERVENAK MD FACOG MMM

Given Foundation Professor and Chairman
Department of Obstetrics and Gynecology
New York Weill Cornell Medical Center
New York, USA

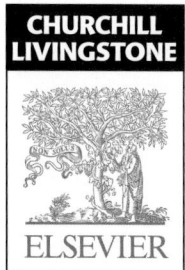

CHURCHILL LIVINGSTONE

ELSEVIER

EDINBURGH LONDON NEW YORK PHILADELPHIA ST LOUIS SYDNEY TORONTO 2009

CHURCHILL
LIVINGSTONE
ELSEVIER

First edition 1988
Second edition 1995
Third edition 2001
Fourth edition 2008

ISBN 9780443104077

BRITISH LIBRARY CATALOGUING IN PUBLICATION DATA
A catalogue record for this book is available from the British Library

LIBRARY OF CONGRESS CATALOGING IN PUBLICATION DATA
A catalog record for this book is available from the Library of Congress

Note
Knowledge and best practice in this field are constantly changing. As
new research and experience broaden our knowledge, changes in
practice, treatment and drug therapy may become necessary or
appropriate. Readers are advised to check the most current information
provided (i) on procedures featured or (ii) by the manufacturer of each
product to be administered, to verify the recommended dose or formula,
the method and duration of administration and contraindications. It is
the responsibility of the practitioner, relying on their own experience
and knowledge of the patient, to make diagnoses, to determine dosages
and the best treatment for each individual patient, and to take all
appropriate safety precautions. To the fullest extent of the law, neither
the publisher nor the editors assume any liability for any injury and/or
damage to persons or property arising out or related to any use of the
material contained in this book. *The Publisher*

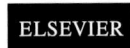
ELSEVIER your source for books,
journals and multimedia
in the health sciences
www.elsevierhealth.com

Working together to grow
libraries in developing countries
www.elsevier.com | www.bookaid.org | www.sabre.org

ELSEVIER   BOOK AID   Sabre Foundation
               International

The
publisher's
policy is to use
**paper manufactured
from sustainable forests**

Printed in China

Contents

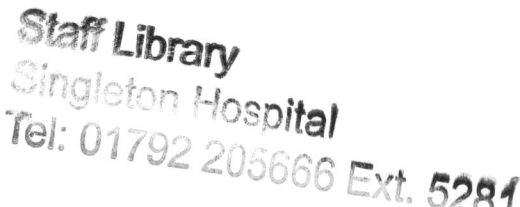

Preface to the fourth edition

Continuing progress in developmental neurobiology of the brain and clinical applications of this new knowledge together with the introduction of emerging technologies have enhanced the clinician's ability to investigate and manage disorders of the developing brain and nervous system. At the same time dilemmas, uncertainties and ethical constraints continue to emerge as a result of these opportunities. The fourth edition of our book is intended to cover the basic science as it merges into clinical science as well as indicating best evidence for the management of clinical disorders seen in perinatal practice.

In the seven years since our last edition, the field of perinatal medicine continues to progress apace with major recent developments, including 3D ultrasound technology for imaging fetal activity and structure, magnetic resonance as a valuable method for imaging the fetal brain as well as providing novel insight into newborn brain development and the emerging therapy of hypothermia for neonatal brain injury.

In 1988 when the first edition was published we intended to produce a book that covered the spectrum of brain development and its disorders from virtual conception to well into the first year of life and bring together international experts in the fields of basic science, fetal medicine, neonatal and pediatric medicine and neurosurgery. Judging by the widespread use of our book we believe that we have fulfilled our aims and hope that this, the latest edition written some 20 years after the first edition, will continue to inform and educate to the benefit of our fetal and neonatal patients now and in the future.

Malcolm Levene
Frank Chervenak

Preface to the first edition

Neurological disability is the most feared complication of pregnancy, labor and the early months of life. The earliest recognizable neural tissue develops approximately 18 days after fertilization and development of the central nervous system proceeds to maturity some six years later. The developing brain is an extremely vulnerable organ and is subject to a wide range of insults that may alter structure or function. Problems affecting the immature brain may come under the care of the obstetrician, neonatologist, general pediatrician or pediatric neurologist and neurosurgeon. Investigations may encompass a wide range of other specialists including radiologists, physicists, pharmacologists, microbiologists, physiologists, pathologists, biochemists and ophthalmologists. These major cross-specialty links make it difficult to consider the developing central nervous system (CNS) for what it is: a complex but continuous process rather than a series of loosely related parts.

The basic aim of this book is to consider the developmental neurology and pathology of the developing CNS from conception to the end of the first year of life. We have approached the subject as specialists representing obstetrics, pediatrics and neurosurgery but with a particular interest in the immature brain. We have attempted to break down the constraints of our respective specialty training to produce a book that crosses these divisions and brings together all the aspects of brain development and pathology during the critical stages of early development. We have been supported in this aim by our 55 contributors who represent a wide range of disciplines and the experience of 10 different countries within Europe, Australia and North America.

The book is presented in three parts: morphological development, methods of investigation and management. Part 1 is a comprehensive review of embryology and developmental anatomy of the CNS and provides the basic foundation necessary to understand much of the pathology that may occur. Part 2 incorporates methods of investigating the immature brain, both fetal and neonatal. The rapid advance in our understanding of cerebral pathology is directly related to the recent introduction of these methods. We have drawn upon the experience to discuss their role and limitations. Some of these methods are already used in routine clinical practice and others are state-of-the-art and unlikely to ever come into routine use but give important information on both structure and function. Part 3 involves the management of disorders of the developing brain and this is further subdivided into sections related to particular areas of clinical interest.

We hope that this book will provide all those involved in the management of the fetus and infant with the information necessary to understanding better the delicate mechanisms that exist within the CNS. Perhaps better understanding of these fragile tissues will, in the future, enable more effective treatment or prevention of neurological handicap.

M I L, M J B, J P
Leicester, 1988

Acknowledgments

As ever we are grateful to our publishers at Elsevier who have eased the labor pains and facilitated a beautiful birth of this, the fourth edition. We are particularly grateful to Ellen Green and Helen Leng.

A book of this size and scope depends on the support and enthusiasm of our contributors who number over 80 in over 20 different countries. We thank these international authorities for their selfless contributions.

List of contributors

Charles E Ahlfors MD
Formerly Department of Neonatology
California Pacific Medical Center
San Francisco, USA

Medhat Alberry MB BCh MSc
Clinical Research Fellow of Maternal and Fetal Medicine
University of Bristol
St Michael's Hospital
Bristol, UK

Claudine Amiel-Tison MD
Professor Emerita of Pediatrics
University of Paris V
Saint-Vincent de Paul Hospital
Paris, France

Kristian Aquilina FRCS
Specialist Registrar in Neurosurgery
Department of Neurosurgery
Frenchay Hospital
Bristol, UK

Birgit Arabin MD PhD
Professor
Department of Perinatology
Isala Clinics, Location Sophia
Zwolle, The Netherlands
Clara Angela Foundation
Institute of Research and Development
Witten, Germany

Robert H Ball MD
Associate Professor
Maternal-Fetal Medicine
St Mark's Hospital
Salt Lake City, USA

Laura Bennet PhD
Associate Professor
Department of Physiology
University of Auckland
Auckland, New Zealand

Guillaume Benoist MD
Service de Gynécologie Obstétrique
Centre Hospitalier Intercommunal de Poissy-St Germain
Poissy, France

Harm-Gerd K Blaas MD PhD
Consultant
National Center for Fetal Medicine
Department of Laboratory Medicine
Children's and Women's Health
St Olav's Hospital
Trondheim, Norway

Eve Blair PhD
Senior Research Fellow
Centre for Child Health Research
University of Western Australia
Telethon Institute for Child Health Research
West Perth, Australia

Isaac Blickstein MD
Professor of Obstetrics and Gynecology
Kaplan Medical Center, Rehovot
Hadassah-Hebrew University School of Medicine
Jerusalem, Israel

Geraldine B Boylan MSc PhD
Clinical Scientist & Lecturer in Paediatrics
Dept of Paediatrics & Child Health
Clinical Investigations Unit
Cork University Hospital
Cork, Ireland

Sally Brocksen PhD
Assistant Professor
Department of Sociology and Social Work
Appalachian State University, USA

Angels García Cazorla MD PhD
Pediatric Neurologist
Neurology Unit
Hospital Sant Joan de Deu
Barcelona, Spain

Frank A Chervenak MD
Given Foundation Professor and Chairman
Department of Obstetrics and Gynecology
New York Weill Cornell Medical Center
New York, USA

Roger V Clements BM BCh FRCS FRCOG MBAE
Consultant Obstetrician and Gynaecologist
Harley Street
London, UK

Luc Cornette MD PhD FRCPCH
Head of Neonatal Intensive Care Unit
AZ St Jan AV
Department of Paediatrics
Brugge, Belgium

Serena J Counsell
Honorary Lecturer
Robert Steiner MRI Unit
Imaging Sciences Department
Imperial College London
Hammersmith Hospital
London, UK

Laura A Crawley BSc MBChB MRCP MRCOphth
Registrar in Ophthalmology
North Thames Rotation
London

Vincent Degos MD
Inserm, U676
Université Paris 7
Faculté de Médecine Denis Diderot
IFR02 and IFR25
Paris, France

Sergio de la Fuente
Department of Obstetrics and Gynaecology
St Michael's Hospital
Bristol, UK

Linda S de Vries MD PhD
Professor of Neonatal Neurology
Department of Neonatology
Wilhelmina Children's Hospital UMC
Utrecht, The Netherlands

Maurice L Druzin MD
Professor
Department of Obstetrics & Gynecology
Stanford University Medical Center
Stanford, USA

Victor Dubowitz BSc MD PhD FRCP DCH
Professor of Paediatrics
Department of Paediatrics and Dubowitz Neuromuscular
Centre
Hammersmith Hospital, Imperial College School of
Medicine
London, UK

Sturla H Eik-Nes MD PhD
Professor of Obstetrics
National Center for Fetal Medicine
Department of Laboratory Medicine
Children's and Women's Health
St Olav's Hospital
Trondheim, Norway

Offer Erez MD
Perinatology Research Branch
NICHD, NIH, DHHS
Bethesda, Maryland and Detroit, Michigan
USA

Jimmy Espinoza MD
Perinatology Research Branch
NICHD, NIH, DHHS
Bethesda, Maryland and Detroit, Michigan
Department of Obstetrics and Gynecology
Wayne State University
Detroit, USA

Alistair Fielder FRCP FRCS FRCOphth
Professor of Ophthalmology
Department of Optometry & Visual Science
City University
London, UK

Peter D Gluckman MBChB DSc FRACP
Dean, Faculty of Medical and Health Sciences
The Liggins Institute
University of Auckland
Auckland, New Zealand

Julie Gosselin PhD OTR
Associate Professor
School of Rehabilitation
Faculty of Medicine
University of Montreal
Montréal (Québec), Canada

Francesca Gotsch MD
Perinatology Research Branch
NICHD, NIH, DHHS
Bethesda, Maryland and Detroit, Michigan
USA

Gorm Greisen MD Dr Med Sci
Professor of Paediatrics
Department of Neonatology
Rigshospitalet
Copenhagen, Denmark

Pierre Gressens
Inserm, U676
Université Paris 7
Faculté de Médecine Denis Diderot
IFR02 and IFR25
AP HP, Hôpital Robert Debré
Service de Neurologie Pédiatrique
Paris, France

Alistair J Gunn MBChB PhD FRACP
Associate Professor
Fetal Physiology and Neuroscience Group
Department of Physiology
University of Auckland
Auckland, New Zealand

Michael Harrison MD FACS FAAP
Professor of Surgery and Pediatrics
Co-Director, Fetal Treatment Program
Chief, Division of Pedriatric Surgery University of
California
San Francisco, USA

Sonia Hassan MD
Perinatology Research Branch
NICHD, NIH, DHHS
Bethesda, Maryland and Detroit, Michigan.
Department of Obstetrics and Gynecology
Wayne State University, Detroit, Michigan.
USA

Jane M Hawdon MA MBBS MRCP FRCPCH PhD
Consultant Neonatologist and Honorary Senior Lecturer
Institute for Women's Health
Elizabeth Garrett Anderson and Obstetric Hospital
University College London Hospitals NHS Foundation
Trust
London, UK

Lena Hellström-Westas
Neonatologist
Neonatal Intensive Care Unit
Department of Paediatrics
University Hospital
Lund, Sweden

Edgar Hernandez-Andrade MD PhD
Clinical Research Coordinator
Fetal and Perinatal Research Group
Maternal-Fetal Medicine Unit
Department of Obstetrics, Hospital Clinic
University of Barcelona, Spain

Anthony D Hockley FRCS LLM
Emeritus Consultant Neurosurgeon
Dept of Paediatric Neurosurgery
Birmingham Children's Hospital
Birmingham, UK

Petra S Hüppi
Professor of Pediatrics
Department of Pediatrics
Division of Child Development and Growth
University Children's Hospital Geneva
Switzerland

David Isaacs MB BChir MD MRCP FRACP
Clinical Professor, Paediatric Infectious Diseases
Department of Immunology
Children's Hospital Westmead
Westmead, Australia

Russell W Jennings MD
Director, Center for Advanced Care of Unborn Children
Department of Surgery, Harvard Medical School
The Fetal Treatment Center, Children's Hospital
Boston, USA

Juan Pedro Kusanovic MD
Perinatology Research Branch
NICHD, NIH, DHHS
Bethesda, Maryland and Detroit, Michigan
USA

Hugo Lagercrantz MD PhD
Professor of Neonatology
Karolinska Institute
Astrid Lindgren Children's Hospital
Stockholm, Sweden

Marc R Lebed
Medical Dispute Professional
Shell Beach, CA
USA

Hanmin Lee MD
Pediatric Surgeon
Department of Pediatric Surgery
UCSF Children's Hospital
San Francisco, USA

Vincent Lelièvre PhD
Associate Professor
Inserm, U676
Université Paris 7
Faculté de Médecine Denis Diderot
IFR02 and IFR25
Paris, France

Malcolm I Levene MD FRCPCH
Professor of Paediatrics
Leeds General Infirmary
Head of Academic Department of Paediatrics and Child
Health
University of Leeds
Leeds, UK

Jay McCauley
Medical Dispute Professional
Shell Beach, CA
USA

Laurence B McCullough PhD
Professor of Medicine and Medical Ethics
Center for Medical Ethics and Health Policy
Baylor College of Medicine
Houston, USA

Neil McIntosh Dsc FRCP FRCPCH
Professor of Child Life & Health
Department of Child Life & Health
University of Edinburgh
Edinburgh, UK

Eugenio Mercuri MD PhD
Lecturer in Paediatric Neurology
Department of Paediatrics and Dubowitz Neuromuscular
Centre
Hammersmith Hospital, Imperial College School of
Medicine
London, UK
Pediatric Neurology Unit, Catholic University, Rome, Italy

David A Miller MD
Associate Professor of Obstetrics
Gynecology and Pediatrics Division of Maternal-Fetal
Medicine
Keck School of Medicine
University of Southern California Children's Hospital
Medical Director CHLA-USC
Institute for Maternal Fetal Health
USC Perinatal Group
Los Angeles, USA

Aubrey Milunsky MBBCh DSc FRCP FACMG DCH
Professor of Human Genetics, Pediatrics, Pathology, and
Obstetrics & Gynecology
Director, Center for Human Genetics
Boston University School of Medicine
Boston, USA

Ana Monteagudo MD
Associate Professor of Obstetrics and Gynecology
Department of Obstetrics & Gynecology
New York University Medical Center
New York, USA

Gonzalo Moscoso MD PhD
Invited Professor Early Human Development
Faculty of Medicine
University of Granada
Granada, Spain

Jan G Nijhuis MD PhD
Head of Department of Obstetrics and Gynaecology
University Hospital Maastricht
The Netherlands

Dr Hiroshi Nishikawa MD FRCS
Consultant Plastic Surgeon
Birmingham Children's Hospital
Birmingham, UK

Jacky Nizard MD
Senior Lecturer
CHI Poissy-St-Germain
Université de Versailles Saint-Quentin-en-Yvelines
Poissy, France

KyongHon Pooh MD
Department of Neurosurgery
Kagawa National Children's Hospital
Kagawa, Japan

Ritsuko K Pooh MD PhD
Chief Director
CRIFM Clinical Research Institute of Fetal Medicine
Kagawa, Japan

Luca A Ramenghi MD
Consultant Neonatologist
Neonatal Department
Scientific Foundation IRCCS
Ospedale Maggiore Policlinico Mangiagalli
University of Milan
Italy

Janet M Rennie MA, MD, FRCP, FRCPCH, DCH
Consultant and Senior Lecturer in Neonatal Medicine
Elizabeth Garrett Anderson Obstetric Hospital
University College London Hospitals
London, UK

Thomas Ringstedt PhD
Research Fellow
Karolinska Institute
Astrid Lindgren Children's Hospital
Stockholm, Sweden

Roberto Romero MD
Chief, Perinatology Research Branch
NICHD, NIH, DHHS
Bethesda, Maryland and Detroit, Michigan
Center for Molecular Medicine and Genetics
Wayne State University, Detroit, Michigan
USA

Lewis Rosenbloom FRCP FRCPCH
Consultant Paediatric Neurologist
83 Waterloo Warehouse
Waterloo Road
Liverpool. UK

Barry S Schifrin MD
6345 Balboa Boulevard
Encino, USA

Nadav Schwartz MD
Fellow
Department of Obstetrics and Gynecology
New York University Medical Center
New York, USA

K S Sirimanna MS FRCS DLO(RCS) MSc FRCP
Consultant Audiological Physician and Honorary Senior
Lecturer
Great Ormond Street Hospital
London, UK

James F Smith Jr MD FACOG
Clinical Associate Professor
Department of Obstetrics and Gynecology
Stanford University
Stanford, USA

Thomas Snelling
Department of Immunology
Children's Hospital Westmead
Westmead, Australia

Guirish A Solanki MBBS FRCSI FRCS
Consultant Paediatric Neurosurgeon
Birmingham Children's Hospital
Birmingham, UK

Peter Soothill MBBS BSc MD MRCOG
Professor of Maternal & Fetal Medicine
Head of Obstetrics and Gynaecology
University of Bristol
St Michael's Hospital
Bristol, UK

Kimberlee A Sorem MD
Assistant Clinical Professor
Department of Obstetrics and Gynecology
Division of Maternal Fetal Medicine
Stanford University School of Medicine
Standford, USA

Fiona Stanley MD FFPHM FAFPHM MFCCH FRACP
FRACOG
Director, Telethon Institute for Child Health Research
University of Western Australia
West Perth, Australia

Horst Steiner MD PhD
Vice-Chairman and Head of Prenatal Medicine
Department of Obstetrics and Gynecology
Paracelsus Private Medical University
Salzburg, Austria

Terence Stephenson DM FRCP FRCPCH
Professor of Child Health
Dean Faculty of Medicine and Health Sciences
The Medical School
Queen's Medical Centre
Nottingham, UK

Mohnish Suri MD MRCP
Consultant Clinical Geneticist
Department of Clinical Genetics
Nottingham City Hospital
Nottingham, UK

Ilan E Timor-Tritsch MD
Director, Obstetrical and Gynecological Ultrasound
Department of Obstetrics and Gynecology
New York University Medical Center
New York, USA

Kim Van Naarden Braun PhD
Epidemiologist
National Center on Birth Defects and Developmental
Disabilities
Centers for Disease Control and Prevention
Atlanta, USA

Yves G Ville MD
Professeur Service de Gynécologie Obstétrique
Centre Hospitalier Intercommunal de Poissy-St Germain.
Poissy, France

Lan T Vu MD
Postdoctoral Research Fellow
University of California
San Francisco, USA

Jennifer A Westgate MBChB, MD, MRCOG, FRANZCOG
Associate Professor in Obstetrics and Gynaecology
University of Auckland
Faculty of Medical and Health Services
Auckland, New Zealand

Elspeth Whitby BSc MBChB FFDRCSI
Senior Lecturer and Honorary Consultant
Department of Radiology
Royal Hallamshire Hospital and University of Sheffield
Sheffield, UK

Andrew Whitelaw MD FRCPCH
Professor of Neonatal Medicine
Neonatal Intensive Care
Southmead Hospital
Westbury-on-Trym
Bristol, UK

Marshalyn Yeargin-Allsopp MD
Medical Epidemiologist
National Center on Birth Defects and Developmental
Disabilities
Centers for Disease Control and Prevention
Atlanta, USA

Bo Hyun Yoon MD PhD
Department of Obstetrics and Gynecology
Seoul National University College of Medicine
Seoul, Korea

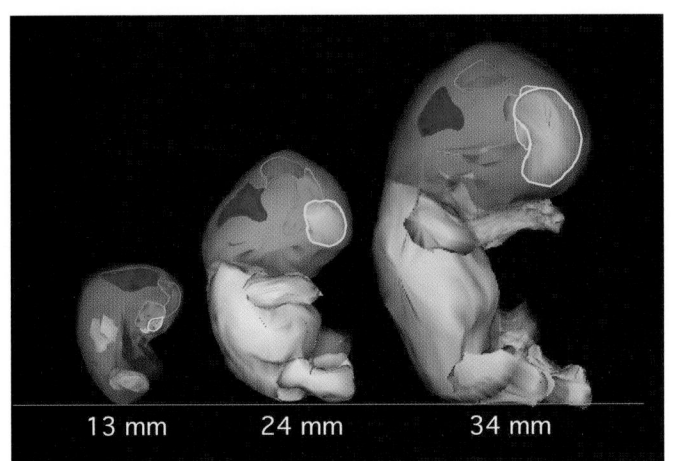

13 mm   24 mm   34 mm

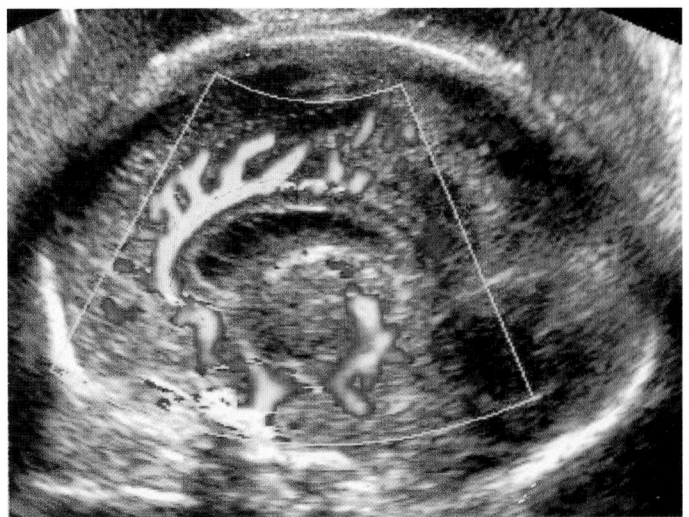

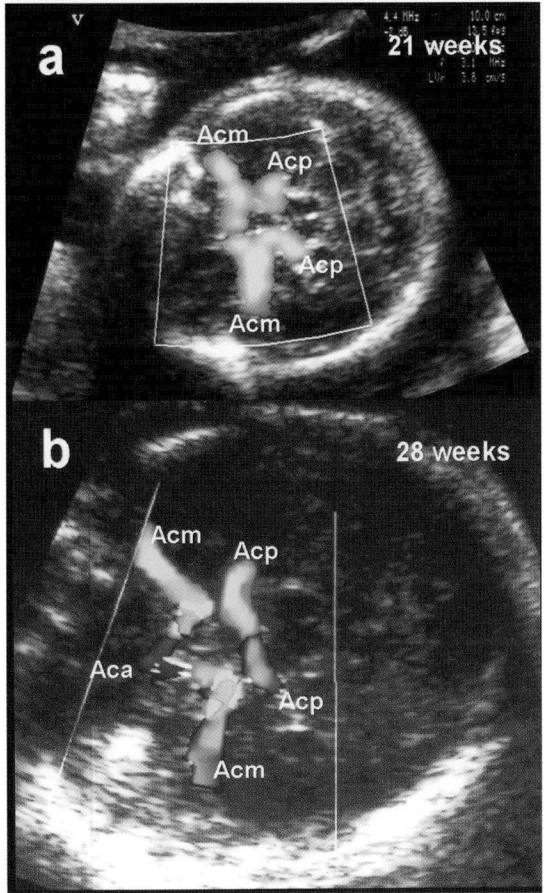

a   21 weeks

Acm

Acp

Acp

Acm

b   28 weeks

Acm

Acp

Aca

Acp

Acm

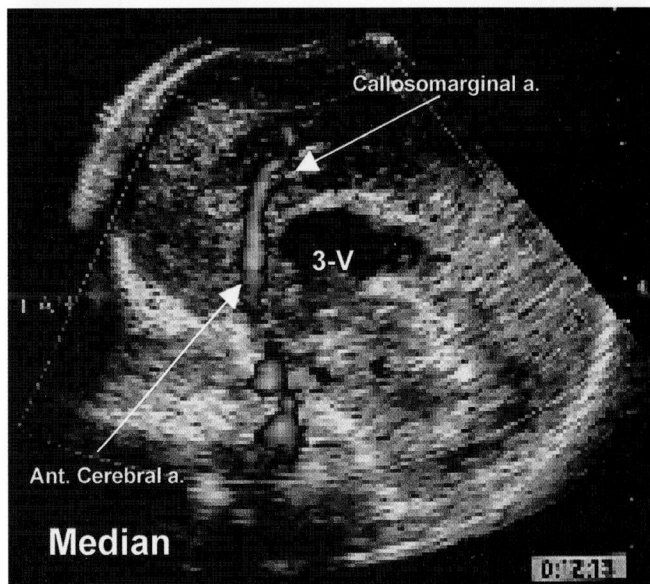

Callosomarginal a.

3-V

Ant. Cerebral a.

Median

CHAPTER

1

The molecular basis of brain development

Hugo Lagercrantz and Thomas Ringstedt

The development of the CNS proceeds through a series of milestones (Table 1.1). This includes patterning events like induction of the neuroectoderm and segmentation of the neural tube, and morphogenetic events like neurulation and cephalic folding. Cell proliferation, differentiation and migration are processes essential for the brain's development. Once formed and positioned, the new neurons send out axonal projections that, guided by molecular cues, reach their distant targets (axon guidance). The brain is then fine-tuned by weeding out the excess projecting neurons, and by strengthening wanted and functional synapses and neural circuits. The first steps are probably strictly genetically controlled, while the build-up of functional neuronal synapses and circuits is more influenced by environmental inputs. It is interesting to note that while the human brain has about 100 billion neurons and trillions of synapses, we only have a few thousand more genes (22000) than the nematode *Caenorhabditis elegans* (18000 genes), which only has 302 neurons. So how is the vastly higher complexity of the human brain accomplished? One solution to this problem is 'combination'. The human genome contains many, perhaps thousands, of genes that bind to and regulate the transcription of other genes. Several of these so-called transcription factors can be combined in a single cell like an alphabetic code. Time and space also matter. A single transcription factor can be used and re-used in different roles throughout development. Diffusible agents create gradients across the brain and the cells react to it in a dose-dependent manner. It is also possible that genes create a scaffold of, in part, repeated structures, which are then further developed or eliminated by the action of environmental influences (Edelman & Tononi 1996). Epigenetic mechanisms seem to act as interfaces between genetic control and environment (Richards 2006).

INDUCTION AND PATTERNING OF THE FETAL HUMAN BRAIN

During gastrulation, 'the most important event during life' (Wolpert 1997), the notochord is formed from the mesenchyme between the endoderm and ectoderm. This structure forms the cranial–caudal axis of the embryo. It induces the neural plate and subsequently the neural tube. It is also responsible for the differentiation of the motor neurons. The phenomenon of neural induction was discovered as early as 1924 by Hans Spemann and Hilde Mangold. They grafted a piece of a newly formed newt embryo to another newt embryo and obtained a two-headed embryo. The grafted tissue itself did not develop into a new head but chemically induced head development in the receiving embryo. Spemann and Mangold demonstrated this by transplanting tissue from an unpigmented to a pigmented newt. The resulting extra head was pigmented, i.e. induced in the receiving embryo. It was believed that the induction was transmitted by a chemical substance, which has been called Spemann's organizer (Wolpert 1997).

Later research has added complexity to our understanding of neural induction. It has been proposed that the neural tissue is formed by a default pathway and that blocking signals (bone morphogenic protein (BMP) inhibitors) are needed to retain the non-neuronal ectoderm bordering the neural plate. However, this is probably an oversimplification that might be correct for an embryo at a certain stage but not over time. Neural induction is more likely achieved through interplay between antineural signals (BMPs, Wnts), their inhibitors, and proneural signals (fibroblast growth factor (FGF)) (Stern 2005) (Fig. 1.1).

The embryo and neural plate are narrowed and elongated through a process where cells from the periphery migrate and intercalate at the midline, called convergent extension (Copp et al 2003a, 2003b). Neural folds are formed, elevate and eventually fuse to form the neural tube. During neural tube closure, a population of cells detach from the edges that are about to close, and migrate to different destinations in the body. These so-called neural-crest cells build up peripheral ganglia and many other tissues, including part of the skeleton (Jacobsson 1991, Wolpert 1997). The process of neural tube closure is called neurulation, and is influenced by convergent extension movements and by signals from the underlying notochord. This expresses the gene Sonic hedgehog (*SHH*) that is important for both morphogenesis and the subsequent differentiation of the neural tube. Particularly the 'ballooning' of the forebrain and the midbrain vesicles seems to depend on *SHH*. If the notochord is ablated the *SHH* levels drop and the normal formation of brain vesicles does not take place (Britto et al 2002). If *SHH* is knocked out the animal will develop a cyclopic eye. Mutation of this gene in the human results in holoprosencephaly.

The rostro–caudal axis of the embryo is formed with help of the *Hox* family of genes, a distinct branch of the homeobox containing genes (homeoboxes constitute a class of binding sites for transcription factors). Interestingly, in most investigated species, also mammals, their positions on the

Table 1.1 Milestones of CNS development weeks after conception

• Formation of the neural tube	3–4 w
• Prosencephaly	5–10 w
• Neuronal proliferation	8–18 w
• Synaptogenesis	20 w–
• Wiring, organization, myelination	30 w–

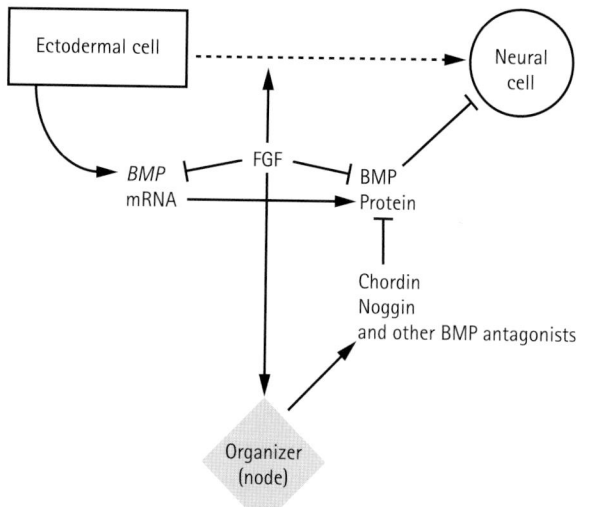

Figure 1.1 Mechanisms of neural induction. Ectodermal cells can develop to neural cells by a default pathway, but this is inhibited by a tonic BMP activity (BMP — bone morphogenic protein). FGF (fibroblast growth factor) represses BMP and in this way promotes neuronal differentiation. Chordin and noggin are secreted from the organizer and ensure the progression of neuronal differentiation (modified after Jessell & Sanes 2006).

chromosomes are collinear with their expression pattern on the body axis (Fig. 1.2). Their origin (and co-linear arrangement) goes back to the ancestor of all bilaterian animals, a marine wormlike creature that lived around 550 million years ago. In mammals the *Hox* genes exists in 4 sets, or clusters, that have arisen by genetic duplication during evolution (Lemons & McGinnis 2006). The combined expression of several *Hox* genes from different clusters determines the developmental potential of the body segments. This is achieved via the so called 'Hox code'; meaning that cells expressing many *Hox* genes develop posterior structures, while those expressing fewer *Hox* genes develop anterior structures (Krumlauf 1994). Knock-out of a *Hox* gene results in an anterior shift of the brain stem rhombomeres. Excess doses of retinoic acid, which affect the expression of more posterior *Hox* genes, disrupt the order of rhombomeres. This was discovered when vitamin A was used by pregnant

women for the treatment of severe acne in the 1980s. *Krox-20* is necessary for the development of the cranial nerves in the hindbrain.

More anterior (and evolutionary more recent) structures of the brain do not express *Hox* genes. Other homeobox containing genes are involved in specifying these areas. The engrailed family of genes and *Wnt1* are required for formation of the midbrain and cerebellum. *Otx1*, *Otx2*, *Emx1* and *Emx2* are expressed in the forebrain and midbrain regions. The *Otx* genes are necessary for forebrain (telencephalon) formation. Telencephalic development can proceed in the absence of *Emx2*, but results in schizencephaly.

Neurons of the future brain develop with an initial rostral character (Stern 2001). A rostro–caudal gradient created by *Wnt* gene expression in the paraxial mesoderm influences the neurons to adopt successively more caudal characters (Nordstrom et al 2002). Dorso–ventral differentiation is initially driven by signals from ventral and dorsal organizing centers. *SHH* derived from the notochord and floorplate is necessary for the creation of motorneurons. If this gene is knocked out all neurons will become sensory neurons. The floorplate expresses BMPs which influence neurons to adopt a dorsal character.

The opposing gradients of *SHH* and BMP are translated into regional expression of transcription factors from the homeodomain and the bHLH (basic helix-loop-helix) families (Jessell & Sanes 2000). Among these is the *Pax* gene family. The name is derived from the paired-box first identified in the fruit fly. Mutations of *Pax3* in the human result in Waardenburg syndrome and of *Pax6* in Peters anomaly (aniridia).

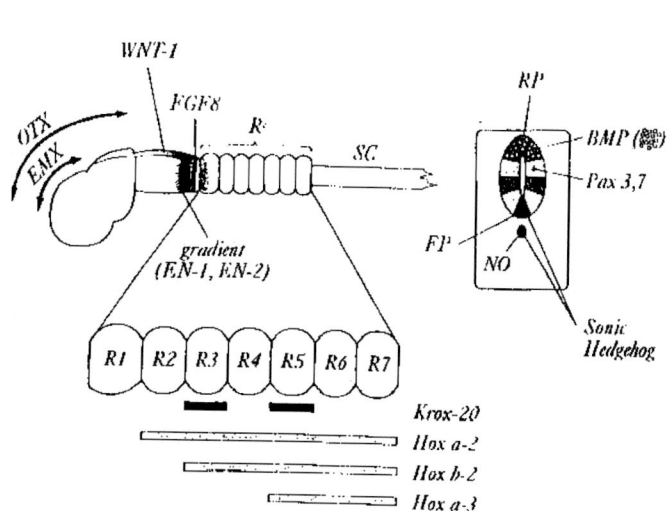

Figure 1.2 Some genes involved in the patterning of the rostro–caudal and dorso–ventral axis of the mammalian CNS. RP: roof plate, FP: floor plate, NO: notochord. R: rhombomeres, SC: spinal cord (from Lagercrantz et al 2001).

How do these early immature nerve cells know how to differentiate? The concentration of the inducing substance seems to be important. For example, high concentrations of the SHH protein induce the formation of most of the ventral cells of the neural plate, while lower levels specifically induce motor neurons. Thus, if undifferentiated cells are exposed to a high concentration of the substance they will become different types of cells than if they had been exposed to lower levels (Wolpert 1997).

The anterior pore of the neural tube closes at 24 days and the posterior pore after 28 days postconceptionally. Neural tube defects have a prevalence of about 1 in 1000. More than half of the expected cases can be prevented with folic acid. This seems to stimulate cellular methylation reactions and promote neural tube closure (Blom et al 2006).

NEURONAL PROLIFERATION

After formation of the neural tube and prosencephali, proliferation of new neurons takes place. New neurons originate from the ventricular zone (VZ) and the ganglionic eminences (GE) (Polleux et al 2002, Rakic & Caviness 1995). In these areas the neural stem or progenitor cells initially undergo symmetric division to expand the progenitor pool, i.e. two daughter cells with properties identical to each other and the mother cells are formed (Fig. 1.3). Division subsequently becomes asymmetric, yielding one progenitor cell capable of proliferation, and one daughter cell destined to differentiate. Artificially enhancing the β-catenin signaling pathway (the main *Wnt* signaling pathway) in the mouse brain forces the cells to undergo further cycles of symmetric divi-sion before asymmetric division begins. This results in an enhanced expansion of the progenitor pool and increased brain size, which therefore is forced to fold in gyri and sulci (Chenn & Walsh 2002). Thus, mutations affecting the decision to switch from symmetric to asymmetric division have likely been a driving force in the evolution of larger and more complex brains. The newly born cells will migrate radially (from VZ) or tangentially (from GE) to form the neocortex.

The pace of neuron production is dependent on the exit rate of cells from the proliferative zones (Caviness et al 1995). The rate of proliferation can be determined by labeling the dividing cells by the thymidine analogue BrdU, which, after it has incorporated in the DNA, can be detected with specific antibodies. By using this cumulative labeling, parameters such as the duration of the cell cycle or neurogenetic interval can be calculated. In the mouse there are 11 cell cycles over a 6-day period.

In the human fetus about 200 000 new neurons are formed every minute between the 8th and 18th week of gestation. The fact that most nerve cells are formed after the 8th and before the 18th gestational week was first established by Dobbing and Sands (1970), who analyzed DNA in aborted fetuses. This was also learnt in a tragic way: fetuses that were exposed to the first atomic bombs in Hiroshima and Nagasaki during this period of pregnancy became microcephalic, while fetuses that were younger or older at the time did not (Miller & Blot 1972).

Based on a series of very careful studies in monkeys whose DNA was pulse-labeled with ³H thymidine, Rakic postulated that there is no neurogenesis after birth in

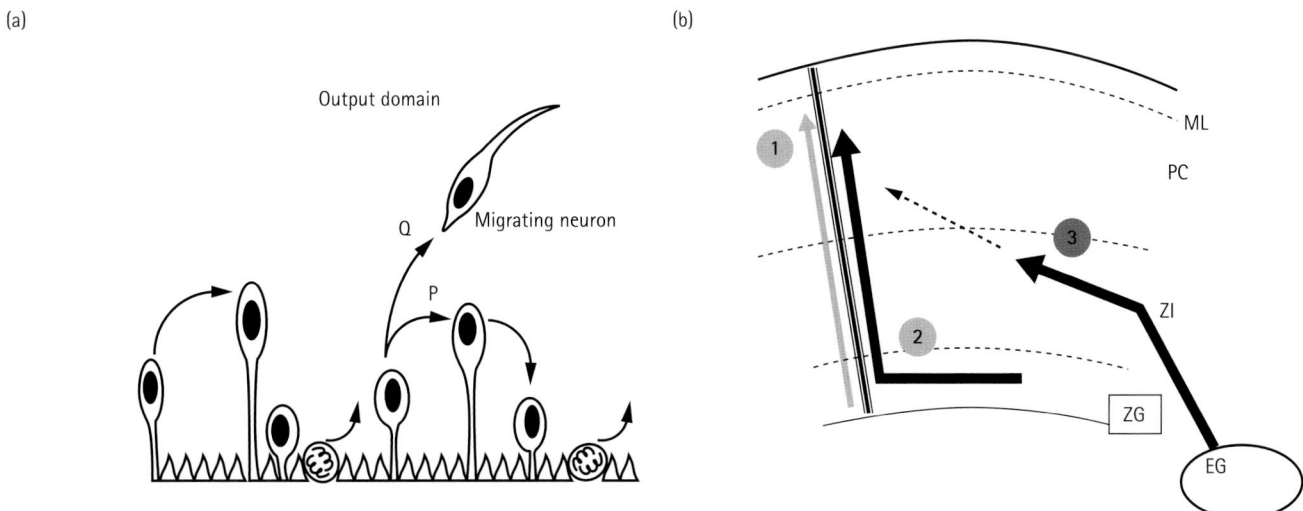

(a)

(b)

Figure 1.3 (a) Proliferation of neurons. A stem cell from the germinative zone divides into two daughter cells. One returns to the basement layer and begins a new cycle, while the other is differentiated to a neuron and starts migration (after Caviness et al 1995). (b) Radial migration along glia (1) from the germinative zone and tangential migration from ganglia eminence (from Gressens 1998).

primates (Rakic 1985, Rakic & Caviness 1995). This is contrary to the situation in other vertebrates such as fish and birds. Male canary birds generate new nerve cells in the singing center during the mating season. The number of syllables that they perform seems to be directly related to the number of neurons (Nottebohm & Arnold 1976). Later studies indicate that some new neurons can be formed even in the human adult. Terminally ill cancer patients were given radioactively labeled thymidine, and after their deaths the nuclei of about a few hundred hippocampal neurons were found to be labeled, implicating that they were newly formed neurons (Eriksson et al 1998). It is now accepted that neurogenesis occurs in the hippocampal dentate gyrus in adult mammals. Furthermore, increased hippocampal neurogenesis correlates with learning in rodents, but this may not be the case in primates. The long-lived belief that, despite the evidence presented by Rakic, there might be some remaining stem cells in the human neocortex capable of generating neurons, recently received a final blow. Above-ground testing of atomic bombs between the years 1955–1963 doubled the atmospheric level of ^{14}C. This has since decreased exponentially. The levels of ^{14}C incorporated into the DNA of neocortical nerve cells from patients born later than 1963 were investigated. It was found that the levels equaled atmospheric levels at the patients' births. Patients born before 1955 displayed the same low ^{14}C levels as the atmosphere before testing began (Spalding et al 2005).

MIGRATION

The neocortex is formed by postmitotic neurons that migrate from the proliferative zones (Fig. 1.3), either radially from the VZ (future projecting neurons) or tangentially from the GE (mainly GABAergic interneurons) (Polleux et al 2002, Rakic & Caviness 1995). The first arriving cells form the pre-plate. Among these are the Cajal–Retzius cells, which enter by tangential migration from the GE. Cells born later migrate into the pre-plate and split it into an outer marginal zone or future layer I, which contains the Cajal–Retzius cells, and an inner sub-plate. Radial migrating cells migrate along a fan-like scaffold of glial cells (radial glia). Newly born neurons that arrive in the cortical plate continue along the radial glia and migrate past those that arrived earlier. The neocortex therefore has an inside-out pattern, with the latest born cells in layer II and the first-born (excepting those in the subplate and the marginal zone) in layer VI. Integrin receptors guide the migrating neurons along the radial glia. Reelin, secreted by the Cajal–Retzius cells (and later by GABAergic cells in the cortical plate), is also essential in guiding the radial migrating cells (D'Arcangelo et al 1995). If reelin is not produced, as in the reeler mouse, the pre-plate is never split. Instead, the neurons line up below it in the order that they were born. Its mechanism of action is still debated. It is often assumed that it acts by inhibiting the migrating neurons, instructing them to leave the radial glia and obtain their final positions. Thus, reelin would act as a stop signal for the successive waves of cortical neurons. Remarkably, a recent report of transgenic mice with the Cajal–Retzius cells ablated, describes no major defects in cortical lamination. The authors speculate that the Cajal–Retzius cells also express other guidance factors for the migrating neurons that balance the effects of reelin. Removal of reelin would then result in signaling imbalance, while removal of the Cajal–Retzius cells themselves equally affects all signals, thus resulting in a null result (Yoshida et al 2006). Furthermore, the Cajal–Retzius cells are not the only source of reelin in the developing neocortex.

Neuronal migration can be affected by glutamate. N-methyl-D-aspartate (NMDA) antagonists were found to retard migration or result in the formation of heterotopias and the arrest of migrating neurons (Gressens 1998). Neurotrophic factors such as neurotrophin-4 (NT-4) and brain-derived neurotrophic factor (BDNF) can also affect neuronal migration (Behar et al 1997, Ringstedt et al 1998). Migration occurs mainly between embryonic day 12 and the first postnatal days in rodents, and between the 12th and 24th week of gestation in the human fetus. Severe disturbance of migration can be seen in the Zellweger cerebro-hepato-renal syndrome, which is a peroxisomal disease. Migration disorders are also involved in schizencephaly and lissencephaly (Evrard et al 1997).

The adult neocortex is subdivided into areas with distinct functions, cytoachitecture and projections. These are specified already during the period of progenitor proliferation and neuronal migration. Like in the spinal cord, signals from patterning centers are involved (Grove & Fukuchi-Shimogori 2003). FGF8 has been implicated as such a signal. Unlike in the spinal cord however, the signals from the patterning centers are not translated into clearly delineated areas of transcription factor expression. Instead transcription factors, like Emx2 and Pax6, are expressed as gradients across the developing neocortex. Transgenic overexpression of Emx2 in progenitor cells in mouse neocortex shifted primary sensory and motor areas rostro–caudally (Hamasaki et al 2004). Thus, the absolute levels of Emx2 in the cortical progenitor cells specify the future area identity in their progeny. Later during development, the incoming projections from thalamus likely fine-tune area identities in the neocortex.

AXONAL GUIDANCE

Neurons send out axonal projections that make contact with targets that can be very distant. How do they find their way to a specific target, which might be hidden by layers of intervening tissue? Navigating the interstates from New York to San Francisco is relatively easy compared to what the neurons of the developing nervous system must do in order to reach their goals, as it was expressed in *Science* (Travis 1994).

In 1892 the Spanish anatomist Ramon y Cajal discovered that the axons have special growth cones on their tips. These growth cones are like immune cells sniffing out chemical

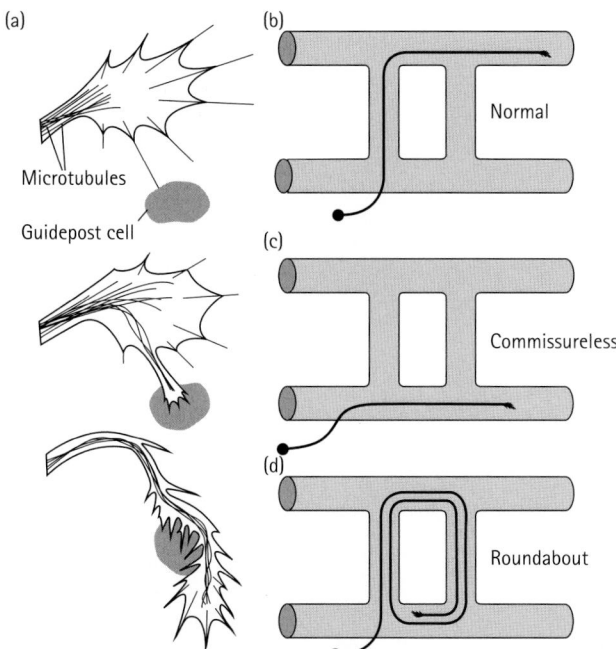

(a)

Microtubules

Guidepost cell

(b) Normal

(c) Commissureless

(d) Roundabout

Figure 1.4 (a) The growth is attracted or repelled by axonal guidance molecules. (b) Neurons normally cross the midline, but (c) if the commissureless guidance molecule is deleted in the *Drosophila* they do not. (d) Deletion of the round-about guidance protein results in this pattern of axonal migration.

scents released by different tissues (Fig. 1.4). The target can release diffusible substances that promote their own inner-vations. These are called chemo-attractants. Given that the distance between the target and the neuron sending out its axon can be quite long, mechanisms other than simple attraction are also involved. By analogy with the traveler crossing continental USA, the axon divides its path into several steps, maneuvering between choice points along more or less established routes.

The signals that guide a growing axon along its way can, based on their mode of action, be subdivided into four categories: chemo-attractive, chemo-repellent, contact-attractive and contact-repellent (Mueller 1999). While the chemo-attractive and chemo-repellent signals are diffusible molecules that act over distance, the contact-attractive and contact-repellent molecules are bound to cell membranes or to the extracellular matrix. Contact-repulsive signals are important in axonal guidance, because they can outline a permissive path for the advancing axons. The complicated task of navigating long distances through the CNS is eased by following routes established by pioneer axons, which reached their targets during early development, when the brain was smaller and its structure considerably less complex. Axons that grow along these routes are bundled together in fascicles. At the various choice points they have to de-fasciculate in order to change route. The regulation of fas-ciculation is therefore an important aspect of axon guidance,

and is often regulated by the same factors (Van Vactor 1998).

Certain structures in the brain are of particular importance to navigating axons (Cook et al 1998). An example of this is the floor-plate, an area with mainly non-neuronal cells in the ventral part of the developing spinal cord. The floor plate expresses several guidance cues. Among these is Netrin, which acts as a chemo-attractant on commissural neurons in the upper part of the spinal cord. Netrin is evolutionary conserved and is also found in the fruit fly. The midline of the fly's nervous system is, similarly to the spinal cord floor plate, an important landmark for axons. Axons are attracted towards the midline by Netrin. The midline also expresses the diffusible ligand Slit, which repulses axonal growth cones carrying the Slit receptor Robo (Kidd et al 1998). These are thereby prevented from entering the midline, and stay on the ipsilateral side (Robo is an abbreviation of round-about, as found along British roads). However, neurons with axons that are destined to cross the midline to reach target areas on the contra-lateral side face a problem. Expression of Robo is an obvious hindrance to entering the midline. If they do not express Robo, they can cross the midline, but nothing prevents them from re-crossing (which also happens in mutants lacking robo). This is solved with the help of a regu-latory gene, Commissureless. The crossing neurons express Robo, but also Commissureless, which prevents Robo from being transported to the growth cone. Upon entering the midline, Commissureless is downregulated, Robo is trans-ported to the growth cone, and the axon is repelled from the midline and cannot re-cross (Keleman et al 2005). The com-bined influences of Netrin, Slit, their receptors and Commis-sureless thus guide the axons across the midline and ensure that they do not re-cross it. Like Netrin, Slit and Robo are also found in mammals (including humans).

Other important families of axon guidance factors include the Semaphorins and the Ephrins. The Semaphorins have several members, both secreted and membrane-bound, divided in 7 classes. Semaphorins can signal both attraction and repulsion, and at least in some cases the same ligand can serve both functions. The Ephrins mediate contact-repulsion and contact-attraction via their receptors, the Eph tyrosine kinase receptors. These constitute the largest sub-group within the tyrosine kinase receptors. The Ephrins are membrane-bound like their receptors and have signaling activity of their own. Thus Ephrin–Eph interaction is bidirectional.

A growth cone is likely to carry receptors for several classes of axon guidance molecules. The inputs from these are integrated into a 'decision' (Stoeckli & Landmesser 1998). One way that this could be achieved is by intracellular sig-naling mechanisms affecting the growth cone's (Ca^{2+}) level. Growth cones have been demonstrated to turn either towards or away from a Netrin source depending on their intracel-lular (Ca^{2+}) levels (Zheng 2000). The (Ca^{2+}) level affects the small Rho-like GTPases RhoA, Cdc42 and Rac1, which act on the cytoskeleton. Many axonal guidance molecules have been shown to induce both attraction and repulsion, although this also might be influenced by the type of receptor involved (Bashaw & Goodman 1999).

Axon guidance factors also have other functions. As an example, Slit also affects cell migration. Axonal guidance and cell migration share common mechanisms. The migrating cell sends out a leading process that trails ahead of the cell soma and orients towards the target with help of a growth cone. Interestingly, blood vessels utilize the same molecules and receptors for guidance as axons. They can also follow nerve trajectories towards a distant target, sticking to their guide with the help of ephrins and Eph receptors.

NEUROTROPHIC FACTORS

In the 1950s Rita Levi-Montalcini together with Victor Hamburger studied the mechanism of neuronal survival in chicks (Fig. 1.5). Hamburger had previously shown that removal of a target organ also reduced the number of neurons innervating the organ. Levi-Montalcini and Levi had demonstrated that the neurons initially are formed and grow normally, but subsequently degenerate. To further study the effects of the target organ, Levi-Montalcini and Hamburger transplanted fragments of mouse tumors into the body wall of chick embryos. This increased innervation of internal organs in the chick embryo. By changing the experimental setup to in vitro co-cultures of chick sensory ganglia and mouse sarcoma tumors, they demonstrated that the mouse tumor produced a diffusible substance that promoted neuronal survival. Together with Stanley Cohen, Levi-Montalcini managed to isolate and purify this substance. It was named nerve growth factor (NGF). (See the fascinating autobiography by Rita Levi-Montalcini (Levi-Montalcini 1998)).

Molecules similar to NGF have since then been discovered. NGF, brain-derived neurotrophic factor (BDNF), neurotrophin 3 (NT-3) and neurotrophin 4 (NT-4) together make up the neurotrophin family (Bibel & Barde 2000). Other families of neurotrophic factors have subsequently been discovered, most importantly the glial-derived neurotrophic factor (GDNF) family (Airaksinen & Saarma 2002). This consists of GDNF, neurturin (NTN), artemin (ART) and persephin (PSP).

Levi-Montalcini described NGF as a survival factor for neurons innervating peripheral targets. During vertebrate development, the targets become contacted by an excess number of neurons. About half of these are later weeded out through the process of naturally occurring cell death (apoptosis). During this process the neurons have to compete for nerve growth factors (neurotrophic support) from the target. Thereby survival of the best-positioned neuronal projections is ensured. Knock-out of neurotrophin genes (in mice) results in clear size-reductions of ganglia innervating peripheral targets, thus reflecting the neurotrophins survival-promoting effect. Very little cell death is observed in the brains however (Snider 1994). This is something of a paradox, since the neurotrophins have been shown to promote brain neuronal survival in vitro and in lesioned animal models.

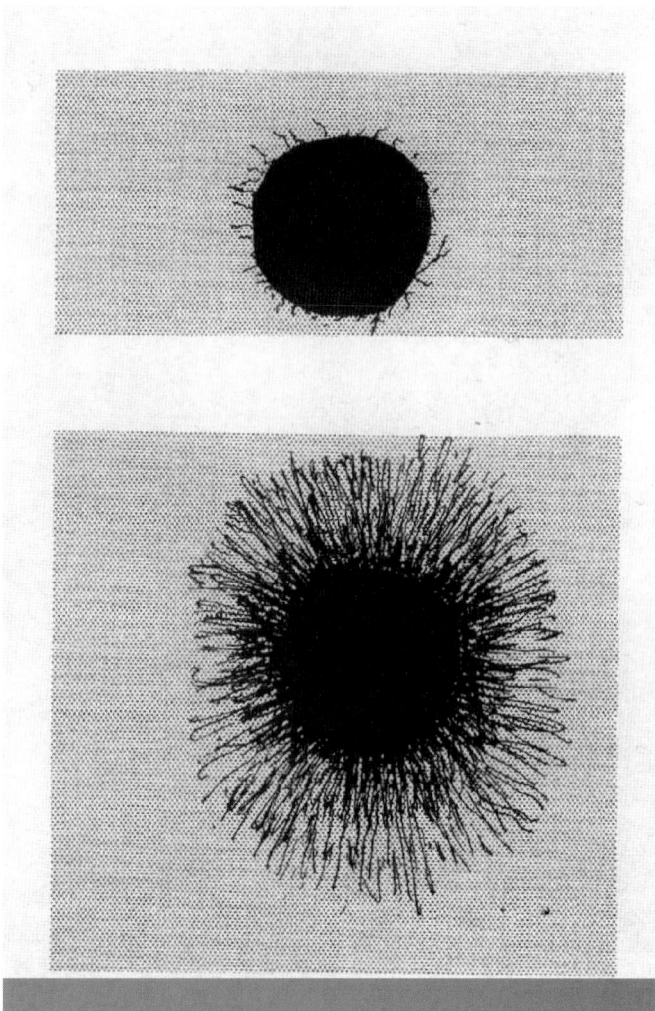

Figure 1.5 A ganglion cell does not develop any dendrites without the presence of nerve growth factor (published with permission from Rita Levi-Montalcini).

The explanation is probably that the knock-out animals can only be studied up to a couple of weeks after birth (they do not survive longer), and that brain neurons develop neurotrophin dependence after this period. Interestingly, neurotrophin homologues are not found in invertebrates. It has therefore been suggested that the plasticity inferred by a cell-extrinsic regulation of neuronal survival (as opposed to cell-intrinsic regulation) has co-evolved with higher neuronal complexity (Bibel & Barde 2000).

In addition to their first described role as target-derived neuronal survival factors, the neurotrophins are now known to affect neuronal differentiation, maturation, migration, axonal guidance and plasticity. In particular BDNF seems to be an important regulator of cell migration and plasticity in the brain. It is also a survival factor for Cajal–Retzius cells and a negative regulator of reelin expression (Ringstedt et al 1998). Throughout development and adulthood, BDNF and reelin frequently act on the same systems, although with opposing effects.

NEUROTRANSMITTERS

Although the development of the CNS scaffold mainly is determined by genetic information, the detailed wiring of the neuronal circuits is more self-generated, depending on the action of neurotransmitters and neuromodulators. They can promote, amplify, block, inhibit or attenuate the micro-electric signals which are passed on to them and through them, and thereby give rise to the signaling patterns between myriads of neuron that provide the physical networks of cerebral neurons. Catecholamines appear in the embryos of vertebrate and invertebrate animals even before neurons are differentiated. Possibly, they then function as morphogenetic or trophic factors. Some of the neural crest-derived neurons are noradrenergic during early development, but later become cholinergic through environmental influences.

A neuroreactive agent might be abundantly expressed during certain stages of development, but later remains in only a small proportion of the CNS synapses. This agent may play a transitory role during a critical window of development or remain mainly as an evolutionary residue with only minor functions, e.g. in mammals (Lagercrantz et al 2001).

It is interesting to note that if the synthesis of some of these neurotransmitters and modulators is blocked pharmacologically or knocked out by transgenic techniques, the apparent effect may be minimal. This illustrates the plasticity of the brain during early development. Other neuroactive agents seem to be able to take over.

Norepinephrine (noradrenaline) and acetylcholine are regarded as classic neurotransmitters and dominate in the peripheral nervous system. They appear at an early stage both evolutionary and during ontogenesis. Many of the neuropeptides were first identified in the gastrointestinal tract and probably also appear early during development. They act slowly since they have to be synthesized, packaged in the cell soma and carried to the terminals before they are released. The more developed and sophisticated mammalian brain requires more fast-switching neurotransmitters acting directly on ion channels, such as excitatory amino acids. These seem to dominate in the mature brain, whilst the monoamines and neuropeptides may act more as neuromodulators.

In the immature brain, synaptic transmission is weak, extremely plastic and mediated to a large extent by NMDA receptors. The AMPA (α-amino-3-hydroxy-5-methyl-4-isoxazolepropionic acid) receptors are more or less silent at resting membrane potentials (Fox et al 1999). During maturation many NMDA receptors are substituted by AMPA receptors. Dark-rearing newborn animals or blocking the activity with tetrodoxin results in preservation of the NMDA receptors. Dark-rearing also preserves the immature form of the NMDA receptors (that contains the NR2B subunit), and expression of NR2A is delayed. This subunit is essential for rapid synaptic transmission. Thus, NMDA

receptors are important for the experience-dependent synaptic traffic.

Another amino acid, γ-aminobutyric acid (GABA), is known as an inhibitory neurotransmitter in the mature brain. However, it is excitatory in the developing brain. This is due to the high Cl^- concentration in immature cells (Miles 1999). When GABA binds to and opens a chloride channel, the immature cell is excited since the high Cl^- concentration forces Cl^- out of the cell, depolarizing the cell. When the cell matures it starts to express the potassium-chloride co-transporter KCC2 that lowers its Cl^- concentration (Rivera et al 1999). This leads to a reversal of the effects of GABA: GABA-induced opening of Cl^- channels leads to an outflow of Cl^-, hyperpolarizing and inhibiting the cell. In this way GABA-switches from being an excitatory amino acid in the fetus to being inhibitory after birth.

SYNAPTOGENESIS

Five 'waves' of synaptogenesis have been identified in the primary visual cortex of the macaque monkey (Bourgeois 1997) (Fig. 1.6). Based on studies of the human occipital cortex (Zecevic 1998), a tentative timetable can be applied for humans.

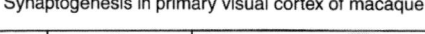

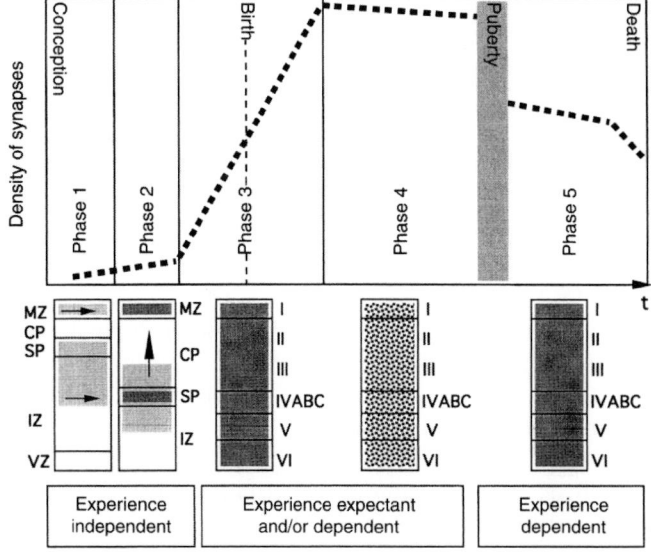

Figure 1.6 Changes in the relative densities of synapses expressed on a log scale. The figure is based on studies of the visual cortex of the macaque monkey, but can be extrapolated to the human. During phase 1 synapses appear first in the marginal zone (MZ), subplate (SP) and intermediate zone (IZ). During phase 2 they also appear in the cortical plate (CP) (from Bourgeois 1997).

- Phase 1: begins around 6–8 weeks of gestation, at the same time as the onset of neuron proliferation. Synaptogenesis is limited to lower structures such as the subplate.
- Phase 2: begins after 12–17 weeks and is relatively sparse. It occurs in the cortical plate. These early synapses form contacts on the neuronal dendritic shafts of the neurons.
- Phase 3: is much more rapid and is assumed to start around midgestation (20–24 wk) and persists up to 8 months after birth. The rate of this synaptogenesis has been estimated to be up to one million new synapses every second in the whole brain. It occurs simultaneously with the arborization of axons and dendrites.
- Phase 4: lasts until puberty and at a very high rate. There is also synapse elimination during this phase. Nearly 50% of the synapses have disappeared at about 1 year of age and even more synapses disappear until midpuberty (Huttenlocher & de Courten 1987).
- Phase 5: synaptogenesis continues up to 70 years of age, and there is a considerable loss of synapses during this phase.

The first two phases are unaffected by a lack of sensory stimulation, but the third phase might be partially dependent on sensory input. This was demonstrated in young macaques which were visually stimulated or deprived. Synaptogenesis during the third phase is partially intrinsic and partially dependent on sensory stimulation. Thus, it coincides with the critical periods. Many of the sensory, motor and cognitive skills function very early after birth when the synaptoarchitectony is still being laid down. Synaptogenesis during the fourth phase is even more dependent on experience. During this phase there is reorganization and fine tuning of neuronal circuits. When this phase has ended during puberty there seems to be a freezing of personality and the end of several basic learning capacities such as learning to speak a new language without an accent.

WIRING THE BRAIN

The wiring of the precise neural circuits seems to be dependent on neuronal activity, which could be stimulated by either sensory input or endogenously driven activity. Redundant numbers of neural pathways and circuits are formed in the fetal brain. About half of the neurons disappear before birth by apoptosis – naturally occurring cell death (as mentioned earlier). This was found in the 1930s by Hamburger, who observed that the number of neurons innervating the chicken wing decreases during maturation (Purves & Lichtman 1985).

The importance of sensory stimulation was discovered in the 1960s by Hubel and Wiesel. They found that surgically closing one eye during a critical period in kittens or young monkeys results in disruption of the corresponding ocular dominance columns (afferents to the visual cortex have their terminals segregated in eye-specific ocular dominance columns), and blindness in the eye once it was re-opened after the critical period (Hubel 1995). In kittens the critical period for ocular dominance plasticity is between 4 weeks and 4 months postnatal, in monkeys somewhat earlier.

A similar process also occurs before birth (Penn & Shatz 1999). Penn and Schatz studied the lateral geniculate in prenatal ferrets. The optic nerves from the eyes grow into the geniculate and fan out through all layers. During maturation these structures become organized and layers are formed. This process is dependent on spontaneous neuronal activity in the retina. Blocking this with tetrodoxin disturbs the segregation into layers.

The spontaneous activity begins at some focus of the retina and spreads from there in waves. This can be visualized in retina whole mounts from newborn ferrets by a fluorescence imaging technique. The activity seems to be generated by cholinergic amacrine cells, since it can be reversibly blocked by a nicotinic acetylcholine receptor antagonist (Feller et al 1996). Each wave lasts for several seconds, followed by a 1-min interval. Neighboring cells seem to fire in synchrony and this local retinal synchrony forms the basis for the layering of the geniculate bodies and the ocular dominance columns in the cortex. Schatz coined the expression: 'Cells that fire together wire together while those which don't won't' (Fig. 1.7).

However, later studies by Crowley and Katz (Crowley & Katz 1999) showed that ocular dominance columns can be formed without electrophysiological stimulation, and thus are genetically determined. They admit that visual stimulation is important for the refinement of the ocular dominance columns, and thus for vision. In concurrence with this, dark-rearing animals delays the critical period for ocular dominance plasticity. The neurotrophin BDNF might mediate the effects of visual experience in the development of ocular dominance columns. Transgenic overexpression of BDNF in mice postnatal neocortex shortens the critical period for ocular dominance plasticity, and accelerates maturation of the visual cortex (Huang et al 1999). Contrary to wild-type mice, dark-rearing the BDNF overexpressing mice does not delay the plasticity window (Gianfranceschi et al 2003). Thus, BDNF stimulation can replace the need for visual experience. This illustrates the interplay between environmental and internal stimuli, including gene activity, in the formation of neuronal circuits.

Proteins traditionally classified as immune proteins also seem to play a role in the wiring of the brain. Neurons can express major histocompatibility complex (MHC) proteins. This expression seems to be controlled by neuronal activity, particularly during development (Boulanger & Shatz 2004). They seem to be involved in the refinement of the neural circuits and are also required for long-term potentiation (LTP), and may therefore be involved in memory and learning. This may be of clinical interest since there is a genetic link between autism and the immune system.

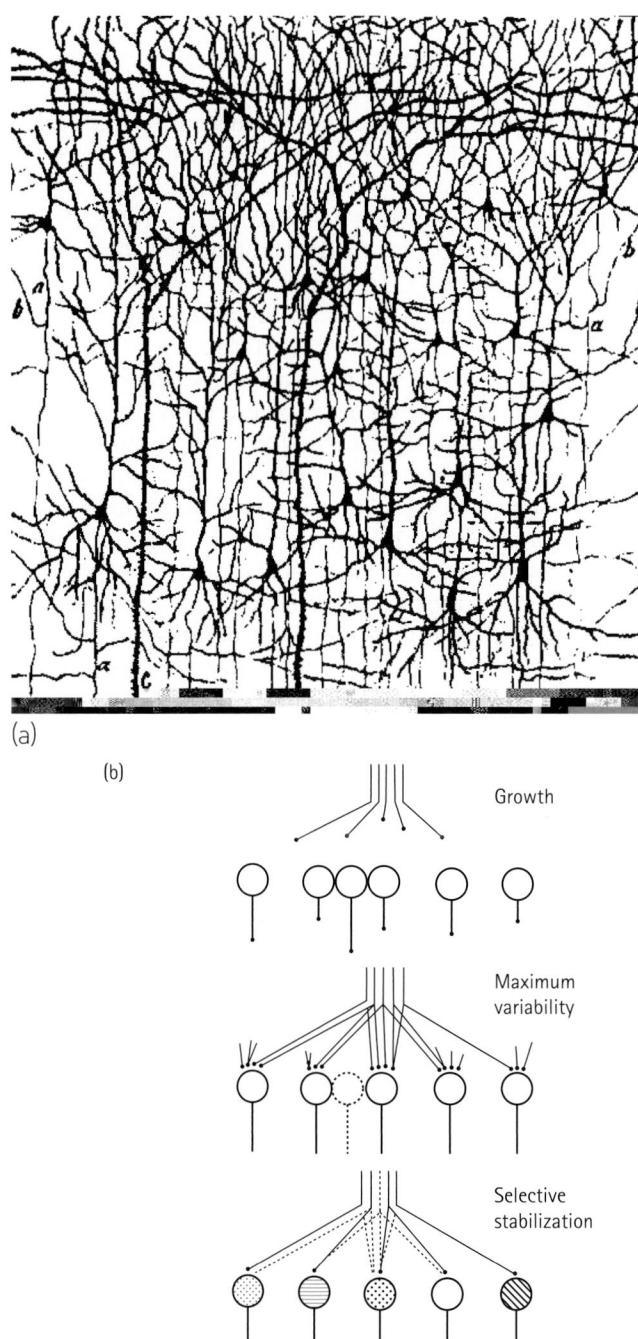

(a)

(b)

Growth

Maximum
variability

Selective
stabilization

Figure 1.7 (a) The immature brain is like a jungle (Edelman). (b) To organize the CNS useful pathways are selected, while redundant pathways disappear due to neuronal activity. 'Neurons which fire together wire together, while those which don't won't.'

MYELINATION

The unmyelinated nerves which dominate during fetal life have a conduction velocity of 0.5–1 m/s. By wrapping the axons in myelin, the conduction speed can increase up to 150 m/s since the propagation becomes saltatory by way of the nodes of Ranvier (Purves 2004).

Myelin is produced by oligodendroglia in the CNS and Schwann cells in the peripheral nervous system. Progenitors of oligodendroglia are formed in the ventricular-subventricular zone from around the 20th gestational week. These cells align the axons and their plasma membranes become myelin. In fetal life progenitor oligodendroglia dominate. These are very vulnerable to oxidative stress. Preterm birth before the 30th week seems to result in deficient myelination, particularly if the infant has suffered from intraventricular bleeding (Nagy et al 2003, Seghier et al 2006).

Most of the sensory and motor neurons seem to be myelinatated during early infancy. However, myelination of particularly the interneurons in the frontal and parietal lobes does not seem to occur until late adolescence. This may explain why the brain of the teenager is not yet mature with regard to executive functions and judgment. Myelination is crucial for rapid neuronal conduction between various areas, which may be involved in for example executive functions.

ORGANIZATION OF THE BRAIN

The fetal and the neonatal brain is not like a computer: It is rather a jungle, according to Edelman (Edelman & Tononi 1996). This metaphor is more appropriate. The characteristic feature of the developing brain is the redundancy of neurons and their connections. There are neuronal pathways connecting the retina with the auditory cortex and the cochlea with the visual cortex (Sur & Leamey 2001). Thus in theory the fetus can see the thunder and hear the lightning. Some children retain these neuronal pathways responsible for synesthesia, but normally they disappear, probably since they are found useless and are inactivated. In a similar way infants have the capacity to differentiate between sounds in all languages (universal grammar). However, already after 6 months this ability disappears and the infant can only recognize the sounds of its mother tongue (Kuhl 2004).

The organization of the brain starts from about midgestation and continues to adolescence, maybe even later. The brain scaffold is probably mainly constructed by the genes involved in the making of the brain. It was earlier believed that the brain is mainly hardwired by the genes. There seem to be a redundant production of neurons, dendrites and synapses. The brain seems to be organized by the selection of the most optimal pathways due to environmental and epigenetic mechanisms. The concept of selectionism (Fig. 1.7) has been proposed by Changeux (2002). In a similar way the concept of neuronal darwinism (Edelman & Tononi 1996) explains how the brain is constructed with regard to the limited number of genes encoding the formation of the brain. This theory consists of three tenets: The first is the proliferation of neurons, their arborization and synaptogenesis. There is a stochastic fluctuation of cell movements, cell process extension and cell deaths. In the next step a variety of functional circuits are carved out and strengthened. In the third tenet physiology and psychology are combined.

Maps are formed in the brain by sensory impressions and new impressions reinforce the neuronal wiring of certain maps. Neurotransmitters such as acetylcholine and dopamine have been proposed to be involved in this selection mechanism.

Recent studies indicate that epigenetic mechanisms may modulate the hardwiring. Maternal handling seems to affect gene expression. Rat pups which have been licked and

groomed extensively by their mothers seem to perform better in various behavioral tests as adults than more neglected pups (Fig. 1.8). This seems to be an environmental effect since the same results were obtained after rearing the pups by foster mothers (Meaney & Szyf 2005). The mechanism seems to be due to methylation/demethylation of the genome, thereby activating or silencing genes (Richards 2006). Thus there is an interaction between genetically controlled events and the environment.

SUMMARY

Brain development begins in the third conceptional week with induction of the neural plate through interplay between pro- and anti-neural signals. The neural tube is formed by neurulation. Co-linear arranged homeotic genes are responsible for compartmentalization of the rostro–caudal axis. The notochord which is formed under the neural tube expresses Sonic hedgehog proteins that induce the ballooning of the hemispheres, and differentiation of the motor neurons. Proliferation of neurons occurs between the 10th and 20th gestational weeks. The newly formed neurons migrate and start to branch and form synapses. This early phase of brain development is mainly genetically determined. However, this immature brain is like a jungle with a lot of redundant pathways. Spontaneous neuronal activity, environmental influences and epigenetic mechanisms are involved in the wiring and organization of the brain, which start during late gestation and continue throughout childhood (Fig. 1.9). Programmed cell death and elimination of synapses are important for this process, as are neurotrophic factors and neurotransmitters. Myelination seems to be the last step in brain maturation. It increases nerve conduction, which is of importance for the executive functions of the forebrain.

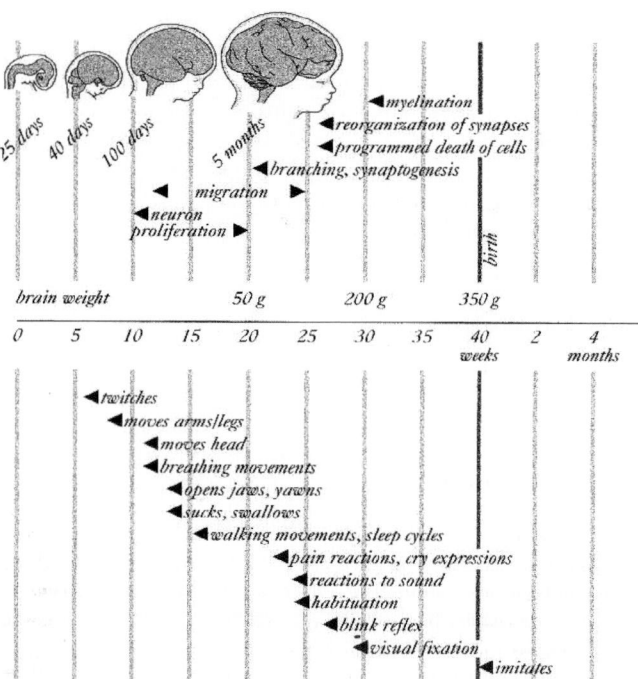

Figure 1.8 Overview of the morphological and functional development of the CNS.

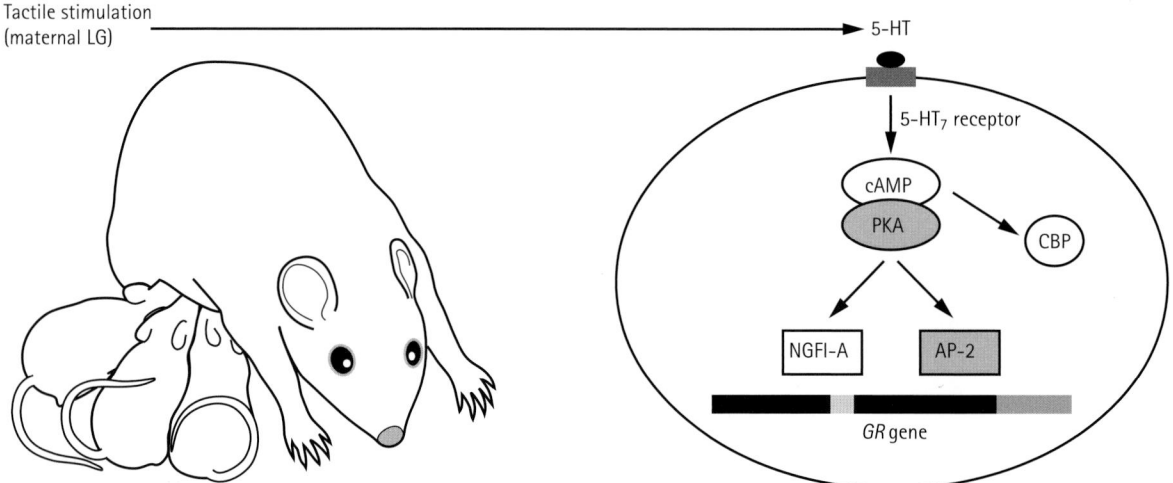

Figure 1.9 Epigenetic mechanisms affect the development of the brain. Increased maternal licking and grooming of rat pups increase serotonin (5-HT) turnover in the hippocampus. This results in an increased expression of NGF1-A (nerve growth factor) and AP-2 (adaptor protein) via cyclic AMP. This results in an increased expression of glucocorticoid receptors, which eliminate the influence of early experience on hyperphenylalaninemia (HPA) responses to stress (after Meaney & Szyf 2005).

REFERENCES

Airaksinen M S, Saarma M 2002 The GDNF family: signalling, biological functions and therapeutic value. Nat Rev Neurosci 3:383–394.

Bashaw G J, Goodman C S 1999 Chimeric axon guidance receptors: the cytoplasmic domains of slit and netrin receptors specify attraction versus repulsion. Cell 97:917–926.

Behar T N, Dugich-Djordjevic M M, Li Y X et al 1997 Neurotrophins stimulate chemotaxis of embryonic cortical neurons. Eur J Neurosci 9:2561–2570.

Bibel M, Barde Y A 2000 Neurotrophins: key regulators of cell fate and cell shape in the vertebrate nervous system. Genes Dev 14:2919–2937.

Blom H J, Shaw G M, den Heijer M, Finnell R H 2006 Neural tube defects and folate: case far from closed. Nat Rev Neurosci 7:724–731.

Boulanger L M, Shatz C J 2004 Immune signalling in neural development, synaptic plasticity and disease. Nat Rev Neurosci 5:521–531.

Bourgeois J P 1997 Synaptogenesis, heterochrony and epigenesis in the mammalian neocortex. Acta Paediatr Suppl 422:27–33.

Britto J, Tannahill D, Keynes R 2002 A critical role for sonic hedgehog signaling in the early expansion of the developing brain. Nat Neurosci 5:103–110.

Caviness V S Jr, Takahashi T, Nowakowski R S 1995 Numbers, time and neocortical neuronogenesis: a general developmental and evolutionary model. Trends Neurosci 18:379–383.

Changeux J-P 2002 Reflexions on the origin of the human brain. In: Lagercrantz H, Hanson M, Evrard P, Rodeck C et al (eds) The newborn brain. Cambridge University Press, Cambridge.

Chenn A, Walsh C A 2002 Regulation of cerebral cortical size by control of cell cycle exit in neural precursors. Science 297:365–369.

Cook G, Tannahill D, Keynes R 1998 Axon guidance to and from choice points. Curr Opin Neurobiol 8:64–72.

Copp A J, Greene N D, Murdoch J N 2003a Dishevelled: linking convergent extension with neural tube closure. Trends Neurosci 26: 453–455.

Copp A J, Greene N D, Murdoch J N 2003b The genetic basis of mammalian neurulation. Nat Rev Genet 4:784–793.

Crowley J C, Katz L C 1999 Development of ocular dominance columns in the absence of retinal input. Nat Neurosci 2:1125–1130.

D'Arcangelo G, Miao G G, Chen S C et al 1995 A protein related to extracellular matrix proteins deleted in the mouse mutant reeler. Nature 374:719–723.

Dobbing J, Sands J 1970 Timing of neuroblast multiplication in developing human brain. Nature 226:639–640.

Edelman G, Tononi G 1996 Selection and development: the brain as a complex system. Cambridge University Press, Cambridge.

Eriksson P S, Perfilieva E, Bjork-Eriksson T et al 1998 Neurogenesis in the adult human hippocampus. Nat Med 4:1313–1317.

Evrard P, Marret S, Gressens P 1997 Environmental and genetic determinants of neural migration and postmigratory survival. Acta Paediatr Suppl 422:20–26.

Feller M B, Wellis D P, Stellwagen D et al 1996 Requirement for cholinergic synaptic transmission in the propagation of spontaneous retinal waves. Science 272:1182–1187.

Fox K, Henley J, Isaac J 1999 Experience-dependent development of NMDA receptor transmission. Nat Neurosci 2:297–299.

Gianfranceschi L, Siciliano R, Walls J et al 2003 Visual cortex is rescued from the effects of dark rearing by overexpression of BDNF. Proc Natl Acad Sci U S A 100:12486–12491.

Gressens P 1998 Mechanisms of cerebral dysgenesis. Curr Opin Pediatr 10:556–560.

Grove E A, Fukuchi-Shimogori T 2003 Generating the cerebral cortical area map. Annu Rev Neurosci 26:355–380.

Hamasaki T, Leingartner A, Ringstedt T, O'Leary D D 2004 EMX2 regulates sizes and positioning of the primary sensory and motor areas in neocortex by direct specification of cortical progenitors. Neuron 43:359–372.

Huang Z J, Kirkwood A, Pizzorusso T et al 1999 BDNF regulates the maturation of inhibition and the critical period of plasticity in mouse visual cortex. Cell 98:739–755.

Hubel D 1995 Eye, brain and vision. Scientific American Library, New York.

Huttenlocher P R, de Courten C 1987 The development of synapses in striate cortex of man. Hum Neurobiol 6:1–9.

Jacobsson M 1991 Developmental neurobiology. Plenum, New York.

Jessell T M, Sanes J R 2000 Development. The decade of the developing brain. Curr Opin Neurobiol 10:599–611.

Keleman K, Ribeiro C, Dickson B J 2005 Comm function in commissural axon guidance: cell-autonomous sorting of Robo in vivo. Nat Neurosci 8:156–163.

Kidd T, Brose K, Mitchell K J et al 1998 Roundabout controls axon crossing of the CNS midline and defines a novel subfamily of evolutionarily conserved guidance receptors. Cell 92:205–215.

Krumlauf R 1994 HOX genes in vertebrate development. Cell 78:191–201.

Kuhl P K 2004 Early language acquisition: cracking the speech code. Nat Rev Neurosci 5:831–843.

Lagercrantz H, Hanson M, Evrard P, Rodeck C (eds) 2001 The newborn brain. Neurotransmitters and neuromodulators. Cambridge University Press, Cambridge.

Lemons D, McGinnis W 2006 Genomic evolution of HOX gene clusters. Science 313:1918–1922.

Levi-Montalcini R 1998 My life and my work. Basic Books, New York.

Meaney M J, Szyf M 2005 Maternal care as a model for experience-dependent chromatin plasticity? Trends Neurosci 28:456–463.

Miles R 1999 Neurobiology. A homeostatic switch. Nature 397:215–216.

Miller R W, Blot W J 1972 Small head size after in-utero exposure to atomic radiation. Lancet 2:784–787.

Mueller B K 1999 Growth cone guidance: first steps towards a deeper understanding. Annu Rev Neurosci 22:351–388.

Nagy Z, Westerberg H, Skare S et al 2003 Preterm children have disturbances of white matter at 11 years of age as shown by diffusion tensor imaging. Pediatr Res 54:672–679.

Nordstrom U, Jessell T M, Edlund T 2002 Progressive induction of caudal neural character by graded Wnt signaling. Nat Neurosci 5:525–532.

Nottebohm F, Arnold A P 1976 Sexual dimorphism in vocal control areas of the songbird brain. Science 194:211–213.

Penn A A, Shatz C J 1999 Brain waves and brain wiring: the role of endogenous and sensory-driven neural activity in development. Pediatr Res 45:447–458.

Polleux F, Whitford K L, Dijkhuizen P A et al 2002 Control of cortical interneuron migration by neurotrophins and PI3-kinase signaling. Development 129:3147–3160.

Purves D 2004 Neuroscience. Sunderland, Massachusetts.

Purves D, Lichtman J 1985 Principles of neuronal development, Sinauer, Sunderland, MA.

Rakic P 1985 Limits of neurogenesis in primates. Science 227:1054–1056.

Rakic P, Caviness V S, Jr 1995 Cortical development: view from neurological mutants two decades later. Neuron 14:1101–1104.

Richards E J 2006 Inherited epigenetic variation-revisiting soft inheritance. Nat Rev Genet 7:395–401.

Ringstedt T, Linnarsson S, Wagner J et al 1998 BDNF regulates reelin expression and Cajal–Retzius cell development in the cerebral cortex. Neuron 21:305–315.

Rivera C, Voipio J, Payne J A et al 1999 The K$^+$/Cl$^-$ co-transporter KCC2 renders GABA hyperpolarizing during neuronal maturation. Nature 397: 251–255.

Seghier M L, Lazeyras F, Hüppi P S 2006 Functional MRI of the newborn. Semin Fetal Neonatal Med 11:479–488.

Snider W D 1994 Functions of the neurotrophins during nervous system development: what the knockouts are teaching us. Cell 77:627–638.

Spalding K L, Bhardwaj R D, Buchholz B A et al 2005 Retrospective birth dating of cells in humans. Cell 122:133–143.

Stern C D 2001 Initial patterning of the central nervous system: how many organizers? Nat Rev Neurosci 2:92–98.

Stern C D 2005 Neural induction: old problem, new findings, yet more questions. Development 132:2007–2021.

Stoeckli E T, Landmesser L T 1998 Axon guidance at choice points. Curr Opin Neurobiol 8:73–79.

Sur M, Leamey C A 2001 Development and plasticity of cortical areas and networks. Nat Rev Neurosci 2:251–262.

Travis J 1994 Wiring the nervous system. Science 266:568–570.

Van Vactor D 1998 Adhesion and signaling in axonal fasciculation. Curr Opin Neurobiol 8:80–86.

Wolpert L 1997 Principles of development. Oxford University Press, Oxford.

Yoshida M, Assimacopoulos S, Jones K R, Grove E A 2006 Massive loss of Cajal–Retzius cells does not disrupt neocortical layer order. Development 133:537–545.

Zecevic N 1998 Synaptogenesis in layer I of the human cerebral cortex in the first half of gestation. Cereb Cortex 8:245–252.

Zheng J Q 2000 Turning of nerve growth cones induced by localized increases in intracellular calcium ions. Nature 403:89–93.

Early embryonic development of the brain

Gonzalo Moscoso

INTRODUCTION

The human brain is a unique organ that subordinates every organ system in the body. It generates the mind, a complex framework that tells us that 'we are' or that 'we exist,' and also that we are different from the surroundings. To the capacity of learning the brain adds the emotional component that comes into play at some point during development. Thus the individual can feel pleasure, pain, aggression or fear. The combination of intellectual and emotional reactions will determine behavior commonly, exteriorized as 'actions'. Today, humans can modify the environment in such a way that no other living creature has ever been capable of since the creation of the universe.

At present neuropathology, adult psychopathology and child psychiatry are actively revisiting developmental neurobiology in an effort to identify the origins of neurologic and psychological disorders. There are two main reasons for this effort. The first is the concept that factors affecting brain development, which could start operating early during pregnancy, may play a central role in the pathogenesis of neurologic and psychiatric illness. Based on good experimental evidence, an organic basis for schizophrenia and major depressive illness has been put forward by more than one team of researchers (Suddath et al 1990, Weinberger 1987, Weinberger et al 1982, 1987). The second reason is the development of new tools for research at molecular, cell and organ-system levels using genetically modified animal models, thereby providing the investigator with clearer variables to study the emergence of form and function of the CNS in health and disease, from the earliest stages of development until well after birth.

Brain development proceeds according to intrinsic and extrinsic influences. Intrinsic influences are given by the genetic code that modulates the development of form and symmetry and primes neural circuits for function. The extrinsic influences start in utero and will continue until the death of the individual. At organ level, brain development starts with the formation of the neural tube or neurulation, followed by neuronal migration and neuritic differentiation with synapse formation and controlled neural 'pruning' (Bourgeois et al 1989). The last two stages have become areas of great interest in recent years. More importantly, it is now well accepted that environmental influences condition brain development.

This chapter describes the development of the CNS at organ level from the start of embryonic life to the end of the first trimester of pregnancy. In addition, some data on gene expression during brain development observed in some animal models will be presented, suggesting that similar patterns of gene expression may operate in humans.

ORGANOGENESIS

In the human, as in higher vertebrates, the development of the CNS starts with the formation of the neural plate at about the 18/19th day postfertilization (Carnegie stage 8). The neural plate develops cranial to the primitive streak along the midsagittal line (Fig. 2.1). It is shortly followed by the emergence of two neural folds which fuse at the level of the first pair of somites during days 20 and 21 (Carnegie stages 9–10) (O'Rahilly & Müller 1999). As a result of this fusion the embryonic disk adopts a tubular shape, when the crown–rump length is about 3.3 mm (Fig. 2.2). Closing of the neural tube proceeds in a zip-up action from day 20 to day 25 when the anterior neuropore closes (Fig. 2.3); 2 days later the caudal neuropore closes at the level of somite 31 or where the second sacral segment will differentiate. In this fashion the neural tube becomes isolated from the amniotic environment. Observed at 17 days postfertilization, by the 25th day the notochord is already fully formed. The otocyst becomes apparent on the 26th day.

Observations in mutant mice lacking laminin α5 chain showed multiple developmental defects, including failed closure of the anterior neuropore (exencephaly) (Miner et al 1998). Therefore, absence of laminin, a non-collagen glycoprotein and normal constituent of the basal lamina, appears to play an important role during closure of the neural tube. From the initial stages of neural tube closing, a population of neural crest cells emerges at the level of the fusing neural crests and migrates, following chemical cues, along the lateral sides of the embryo's body to specific target organs. Their role during morphogenesis and organogenesis, however, is ample and complex and beyond the scope of this chapter.

In the early twenties, whilst studying early *Drosophila* embryos, Bridges and Morgan (1923) identified a cluster of homeotic selector genes, the *HOM* complex, which participate in modulating the development and orientation of specific body segments and limbs (Dolle et al 1989; Oliver et al 1989). Today, it is known that mammals and other vertebrates have homeoboxes containing tightly linked clusters or *HOM* complexes, for example, *Hox-1*, *Hox-2*, *Hox-3* and *Hox-5* genes that are expressed in early mouse embryos.

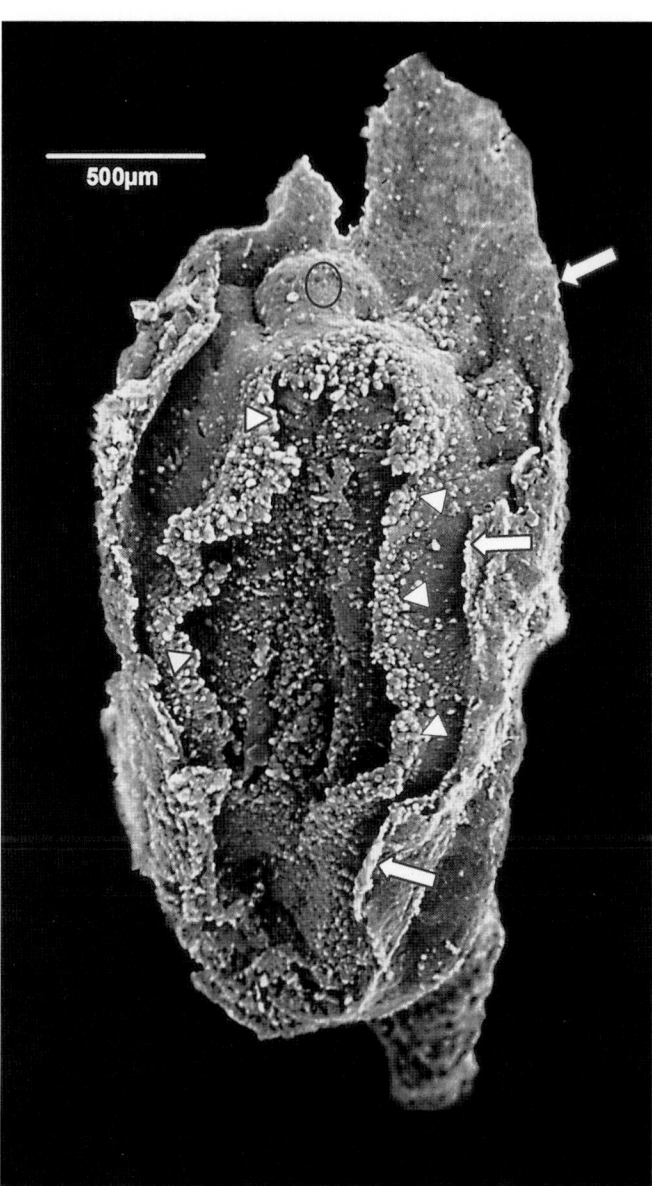

Figure 2.1 Human embryo at 19 days postfertilization (stage 8). There are prominent marginal lobulations at the cephalic end (circled). Some ectoderm has been removed (arrow heads) to reveal a midline triangular ridge and two flaking grooves. These formations are beneath the primitive streak. The amnion (arrows) has been partially removed to expose the embryonic disk. SEM × 180.

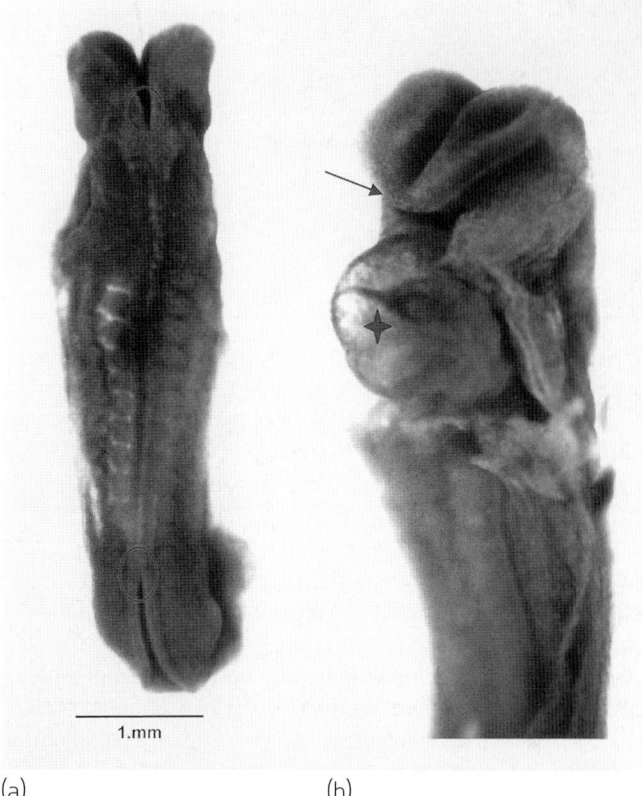

(a)   (b)

Figure 2.2 Human embryo at 23 days postfertilization (stage 11). (A) Posterior view. Note the tubular shape of the embryo's body. The anterior and caudal neuropores are open (circles). (B) Left lateral view. The cephalic end of the neural tube (arrow) and the cardiac loop (star) are very close to each other at this stage. This will facilitate neural crest cell migration to selected areas of the developing heart.

Similarly, *HOX* genes that modulate the development of the CNS also are expressed in early embryonic stages (Holland & Hogan 1988). This is discussed in detail in Chapter 1.

When examined at the appropriate time of development, the hindbrain of the chicken presents eight bulges known as rhombomeres limited by constrictions (Lumsden & Keynes 1989). In-situ hybridization has shown selective expression first of *Krox-20* gene in rhombomere 3 followed by expression in rhombomere 5. Downregulation occurred in the same order, and these observations indicate that segmentation

of the hindbrain occurs in an antero-posterior direction (Wilkinson et al 1989). Furthermore, histological examination of these levels showed a neuronal organization in these segments, directly related to cranial sensory ganglia and cranial nerve roots connecting branchial and pharyngeal arches. Thus, patterning of the body axis and of the CNS seems to be dependent on a specific set of *HOM* genes if normal development is to be achieved.

The Sonic hedgehog gene (p. 1) is also expressed during early embryogenesis and the peptides it generates will assist in the formation of the notochord and neural tube (neurulation). Later on, it will induce the differentiation of spinal motor neurons (Roelink et al 1994), midbrain dopaminergic neurons (Hynes et al 1994; Wang et al 1995) and dorsal forebrain dopaminergic neurons (Ericson et al 1995) (Fig. 2.4). Interestingly, the Sonic hedgehog gene has a protective effect on neurons when challenged with specific neurotoxins, i.e. MMP (Miao et al 1997), and contributes to determining the body axis (Tanabe & Jessel 1996).

The almost straight 'tubular' embryo at 22 days gradually folds into a 'C'-shape embryo already apparent at 29 ± 1

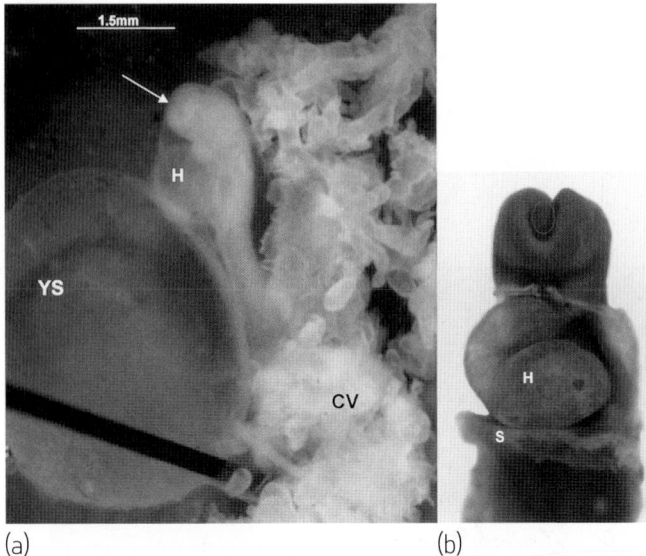

(a)   (b)

Figure 2.3 Human embryo at 25 days postfertilization (stage 11). (a) Left lateral view. Note the tubular shape of the embryo's body and the attached secondary yolk sac (YS). The cardiac loop is larger than the head. (b) Frontal view of the embryo in (a). The rostral neuropore (circle) is about to close. The cardiac loop shows a transverse (H) and an ascending segment (outflow portion). S = septum transversum.

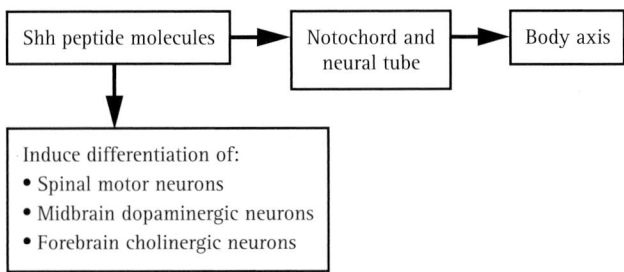

Figure 2.4 Neural development and the Sonic hedgehog gene.

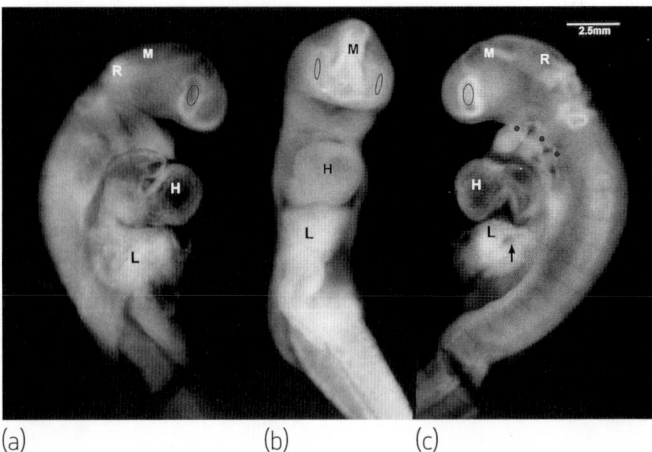

(a)   (b)   (c)

Figure 2.5 Human embryo at 29 days postfertilization (stage 13). On a frontal view (b), the telencephalic vesicles are clearly seen (open circles). These are also seen laterally in (a) and (c). The head is now larger than the cardiac loop. M = mesencephalon, R = rhombencephalon. The dots point to three pharyngeal arches. The black arrow in (c) points to the stomach containing some fluid seen by translucency. H = heart; L = rhombic lips.

Table 2.1 Neuromeres in the human embryo

Primary neuromeres		Secondary neuromeres	
Prosencephalon		Telencephalon	S10
		Diencephalon 1	
		Diencephalon 2	
		Parencephalon rostralis	S14
		Parencephalon caudalis	
		Synecephalon	S13
Mesencephalon		Mesencephalon 1	S12
		Mesencephalon 2	S9
		Isthmic neuromere	S13
Rhombomeres	Rh. A	Rhombomeres: Rh. 1	
		Rh. 2	
		Rh. 3	
	Rh. B	Rh. 4	S11
	Rh. C	Rh. 5	
		Rh. 7	
	Rh. D	Rh. 8	

S = Developmental stage.
Source: From R. O'Rahilly & F. Müller 1999 with permission.

days postfertilization (stage 12) (Fig. 2.5) and remains so through to the end of the embryonic period (8th week of gestation) when the body axis 'unfolds' slightly whilst the head stays bent forwards over the chest.

Following closure of the neuropores, the brain enters into a stage of rapid differential growth, and the gentle cervical flexure, already evident at stage 12, becomes more prominent at 35 days postfertilization (stage 15) when, on external examination, a midbrain flexure and the pontine flexure can be observed (Fig. 2.6a). However, a midsagittal histological section shows four bending points (Fig. 2.6b). The morphogenetic mechanisms, at gene, cell and tissue levels, determining and modulating the appearance and roles of these four 'bearing' points, have yet to be elucidated.

The appearance of flexures in the body of the embryo is associated with segmentation of the CNS. These become more apparent following closure of the neural tube. At 29 days postfertilization (stage 13), three brain vesicles or neuromeres can be clearly identified on close examination: the prosencephalon, the mesencephalon and the rhombencephalon (Fig. 2.5). The optic vesicle invaginates to form the optic cup. At 32 days postfertilization (stage 13), each segment will develop subsegments expected to emerge at given stages of development (Table 2.1).

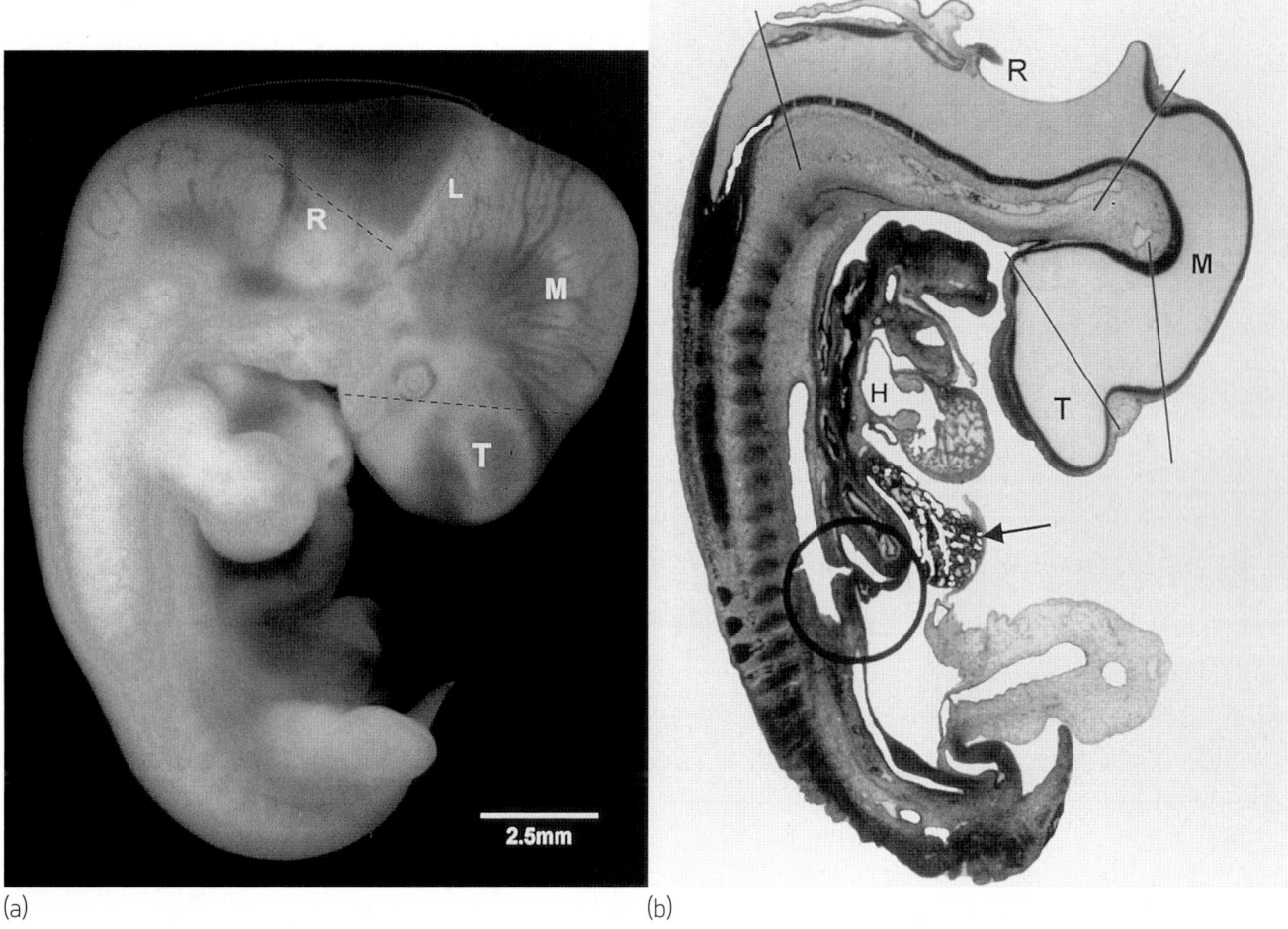

(a)   (b)

Figure 2.6 (a) Human embryo at 35 days postfertilization (stage 15). Note the pronounced flexion of the head over the chest. The telencephalic vesicles are approaching the level of pigmented eye (lower dashed line). The mesencephalon (M) is a predominant brain segment. The pontine flexure appears as a straight angle made up by the rhombic lips (L) and the floor of the fourth ventricle. The space (curved red dotted line) thus created contains water-clear fluid. Brain blood vessels appear to emerge at the level of the temporal region to spread radially. R = rhombencephalon. (b) Paramedial sagittal section of the human embryo in (a). There are four bending points (lines). Note the attenuated epidermal and neural tissue (R) making together a thin membrane covering the pontine flexure. The heart (H) shows unfused atrioventricular cushions. Liver (arrow). M = mesencephalon; T = telencephalic vesicle.

The prosencephalon or forebrain is the most anterior neuromere which presents two small telencephalic vesicles at 29 ± 1 days postfertilization (stage 13) (Fig. 2.5). By the end of the 38th day (stage 16), the telencephalic vesicles have gone past the level of the eye when observed on a lateral view (Fig. 2.7). Towards the end of the embryonic period (8 weeks gestation), the telencephalic vesicles can be recognized as developing brain hemispheres. Their outer surface appears smooth and will remain so for the first 12 weeks of gestation (Fig. 2.8). However, at 12 weeks, their medial sagittal aspect, facing the falx cerebri, shows emerging gyri, suggesting a faster growth on their medial aspect (Fig. 2.9).

At the histological level, the differential growth of the brain segments is accompanied by significant changes in the histological architecture of each segment and in the topology of the gray and white matter. Here it should be remembered that the anterior neuropore closes at the level where the rhombencephalon will develop. At this point, as the neural tube closes, neuroblasts start to differentiate from neuroepithelial cells generating first the periventricular germinal layer. From it, neurons will originate and migrate towards the pia, creating the second or mantle layer to become the gray matter. A third, outermost acellular layer of the brain will be formed by interconnecting neural fibers which later become the white matter. In the prospective brain hemispheres, the marginal layer or primordial plexiform lamina appears at 33 days (stage 15) according to O'Rahilly et al (1984). Although Marin-Padilla (1983) finds it at 42 postovulatory days (stage 18), this is followed, nev-

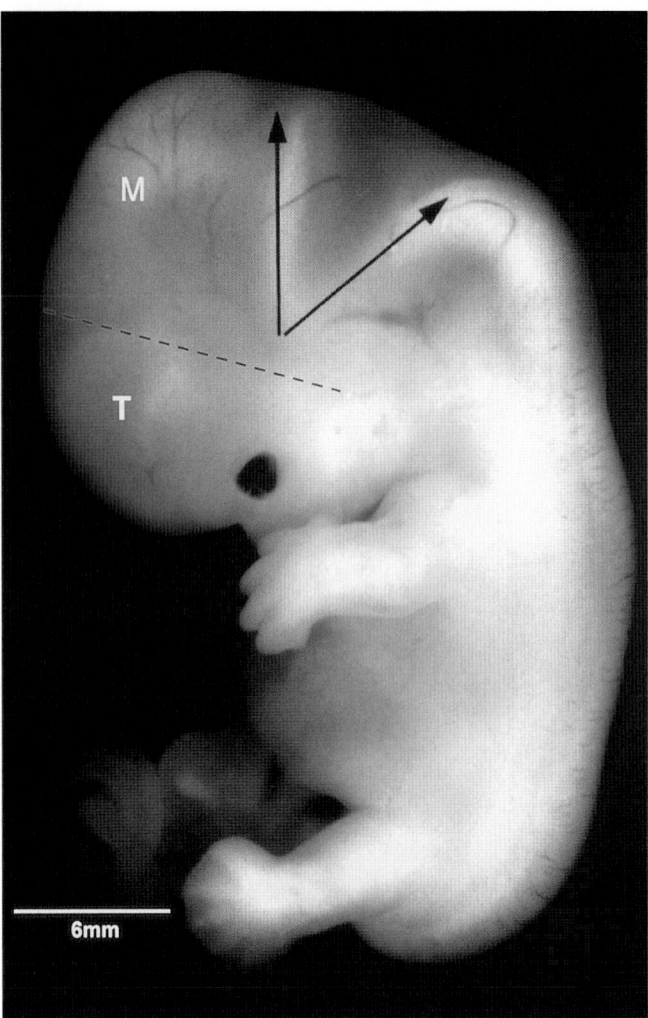

Figure 2.7 Human embryo at 46 days postfertilization (stage 18). The left telencephalic vesicle (T) is beyond the eye level. The mesencephalon (M) still predominates in size over the other brain segments. The pontine flexure (between the arrows) has an angle less than 90 degrees.

the perivascular spaces. Most of these islands disappear before 1 year of age.

Studies of gene expression in the hippocampus of some animal models show that morphogenesis and neuronal differentiation depends in part on the *LIM* homeobox gene *Lhx5* (Zhao et al 1999) encoding a transcription factor present in a region the earliest differentiated Cajal–Retzius (C-R) cells (Soriano et al 1994). These C-R cells guide neural migration during the development of the hippocampus (D'Arcangelo et al 1995; Nakahima et al 1997). In mutant mice, absence of *Lhx5* is associated with a malformed hippocampus, agenesis of the choroids plexus in both the lateral and third ventricles and absent callosal axons crossing the midline. Furthermore, several homeobox genes, including *Lhx2*, *Emx2* and *Otx1*, are needed during morphogenesis of the telencephalic choroid plexus (Pellegrine et al 1996; Porter et al 1997; Yoshida et al 1997). Absence of *Lhx5* in mutant mouse embryos is associated with poor expression of *Wnt5*, *Bmp4* and *Bmp7*, resulting in abnormal patterning of the midtelencephalic wall from which the hippocampus will differentiate (Zhao et al 1995). Moreover, there is rapidly accumulating evidence indicating that hippocampal cells maintain the capability for generating neurons from progenitor cells in the adult human brain (Roy et al 2000). Therefore, the hippocampus appears to hold a potential for neuron regeneration believed to be impossible once brain development is completed. The therapeutic potential, perhaps including memory improvement among others, is of much relevance (Gould et al 1999).

The mesencephalon or second neuromere, once prominent shortly after closure of the neural tube (Fig. 2.5), undergoes fewer changes than the other two primary neuromeres: the forebrain and the rhombencephalon. Its main contribution is in the formation of the cerebral aqueduct. It is also associated with the brain peduncles, the origin of the tegmentum and the substantia nigra appear to be derived from the basal plate or the mesencephalon.

A family of transcription factors containing the fork head (fkh) domain, a region-specific homeotic gene, has been identified in *Drosophila*. Deficient *fkh-5*, the homologue gene in mice, is responsible for dysgenesis in the caudal midbrain and hypothalamic mamillary body (Wehr et al 1997).

From the early stages in embryogenesis the rhomboencephalon shows increasing complexity. At 20 days postfertilization (stage 9) it reaches its peak of prominence; making up to 51–67% of the neural plate (Müller & O'Rahilly, 1983; O'Rahilly et al 1984). At 34 days postfertilization, the pontine flexure is a prominent feature made up by the rhombic lips at its cephalic end and by the developing floor of the fourth ventricle at its caudal end. The 'roof' of the pontine flexure is made up of attenuated neural and ectodermic layers (Fig. 2.5b). The pontine 'chamber' thus created at 34 days is a large space within the central neural system at this stage. It contains clear watery fluid (CSF). The pontine 'angle' decreases with continuing growth and becomes significantly

ertheless, by the appearance of the cortical plate at about 50 days postfertilization (stage 21). Neuronal migration is assisted by radial glias which extend from the ventricular walls to the pia mater. The glia processes are present at 12 weeks of gestation (Choi 1986) and can be demonstrated immunohistochemically using glial fibrillary acid protein (GFAP). In the ensuing months, the telencephalic vesicles will grow at spectacular speed to form the brain hemispheres. According to Mikhailets (quoted by Blinkov & Glezer 1968), half-way through pregnancy the brain has over 400% of the volume of the embryo's body but by the end of gestation the volume is only about 42%. The original germinal layer is a continuous and tightly packed subependymal sheet of undifferentiated cells lining the ventricles up until about the 30th week of gestation when it starts to thin out. Gradually it breaks into cell islands by the 36th week of gestation. These can still be observed after birth around

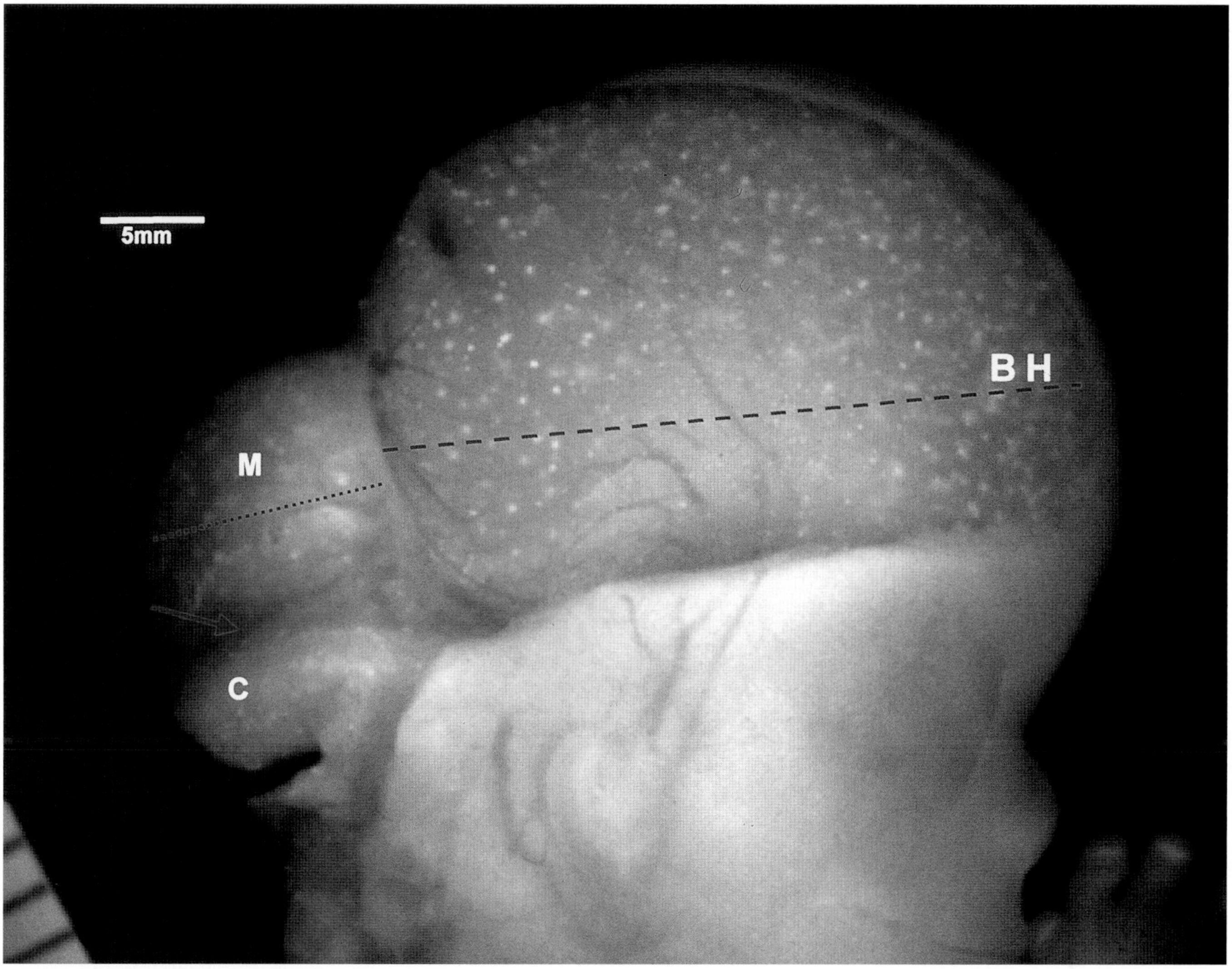

Figure 2.8 Human fetus at 10 weeks gestation. The outer surface of the right brain hemisphere appears smooth. The caudal end of the mesencephalon (M) is in contact with the tentorium (arrow). The right cerebellar hemisphere has a smooth surface.

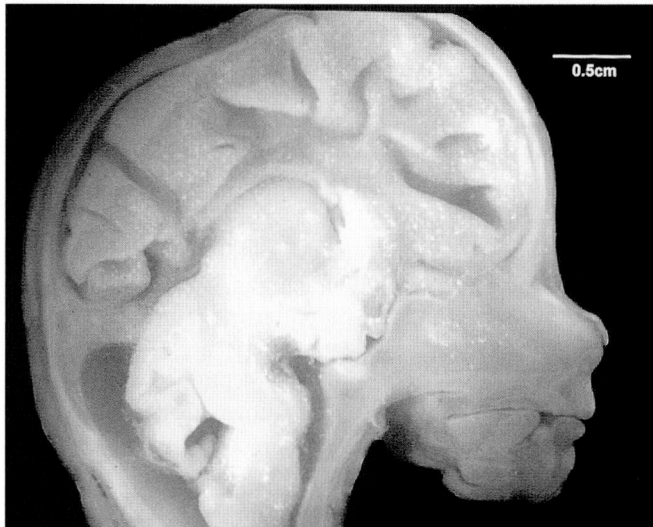

Figure 2.9 Fetal brain at 12 weeks gestation. Sagittal view of the developing left hemisphere of the brain facing the falx cerebri. Note the emerging gyri suggestive of a faster growth on this side when compared with its smooth parietal brain surface.

reduced to a few degrees by the end of the embryonic period.

The rhombic lips contribute significantly to the formation of the cerebellum whose rate of growth accelerates towards the end of the embryonic period. At this point, the rhombic lips resemble the roof-top of an oriental temple (Fig. 2.10a). As the embryo approaches the end of the first trimester, the cerebellar hemispheres showing a smooth outer surface are clearly defined, and the vermis is developing as a medial raphe (Fig. 2. 10b). Cerebellar foliation will not form until the 14th week. Precursors of Purkinje cells form a thin lamina separated from the granular layer by a clear zone named lamina dissecans (Rakic & Sidman 1970). The granular layer forms from germinal cells of rhombic lip. Cerebellar morphogenesis is slow and will be completed after the second year of life.

Proliferation, migration and differentiation are but a few cell attributes needed for normal organogenesis. Using posi-

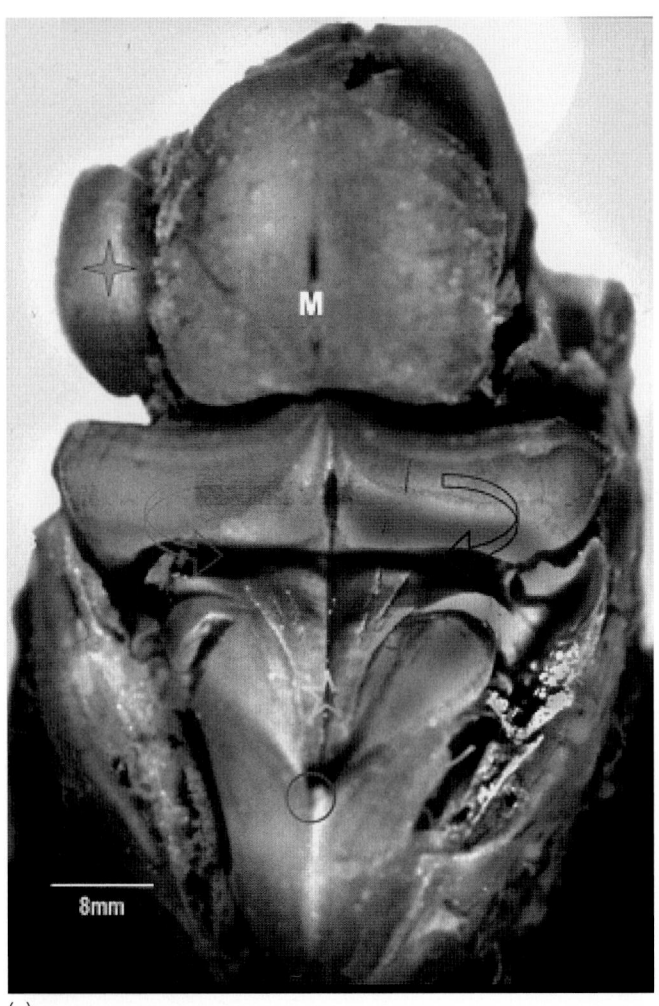

(a)

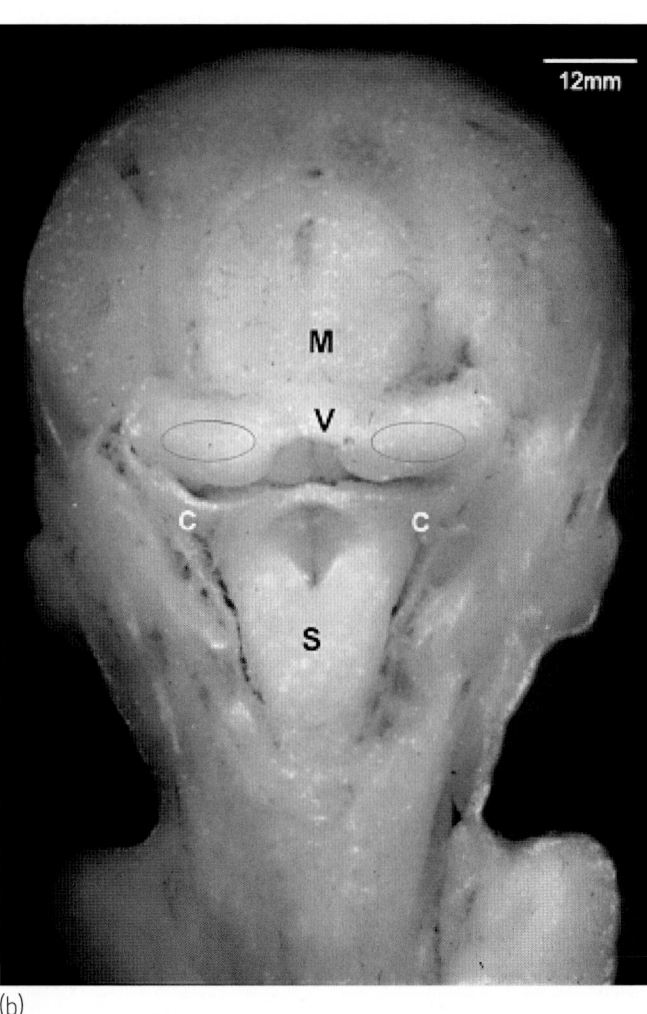

(b)

Figure 2.10 (a) Posterior view of the CNS of a human fetus at 8 weeks gestation. Note the prominent mesencephalon and the characteristic 'winged' shape of the rhombic lips. The curved arrows indicate their convergence during growth. The cerebellar vermix has not yet differentiated. The brain stem (circle) has a lily-like shape. The brain hemispheres (star) have not covered the mesencephalon. (b) A view of the posterior fossa of a human fetus at 11 weeks gestation. The rhombic lips (circles) have fused (V) in the midline. Thus the cerebellum can be recognized. The choroid plexus (C) crosses freely the fourth ventricle. M = mesencephalon; S = brain stem.

tional cloning techniques it has been demonstrated that the 30-zinc finger transcription factor Zfp423(OAZ) modulates the development of glial and neuronal precursors of midline structures in the brain. Mutation of Zfp423 results in malformation of the cerebellum resulting in lesions similar to those observed in Dandy–Walker malformation. Furthermore, loss of Zfp423 is associated with absent corpus callosum and with an abnormal external germinal layer due to a diminished proliferation of granule cell precursors (Alcaraz et al 2006).

The floor of the fourth ventricle in the brain stem appears as an unfolded lily (Fig. 2.10). Tanaka et al (1987) have identified a set of supra-ependymal cells and supra-ependymal fibers. Some of the latter appear to penetrate the ependymal layer but their role is unknown.

At 11 weeks gestation, the choroid plexus crosses freely the fourth ventricular space between the cerebellum and the floor of the fourth ventricle (Fig. 2.10b). During this time, the foramina of Luschka and Magendie communicate the fourth ventricle with the subarachnoidal space.

Cell communication and its pattern together with timing with reference to brain organogenesis are now gradually being unraveled. Tyrosine kinases, peptide growth factors for receptor tyrosine kinase, are known to play important roles during neuron migration, axon guidance and neuron cell differentiation (Fantl et al 1993, Schlessinger & Ukkrick 1992). Furthermore, neural cell activity has been documented shortly before the end of the first trimester. At this time brain cells are proliferating at a rate approaching 250000/min (Rakic 1995, Shatz 1996).

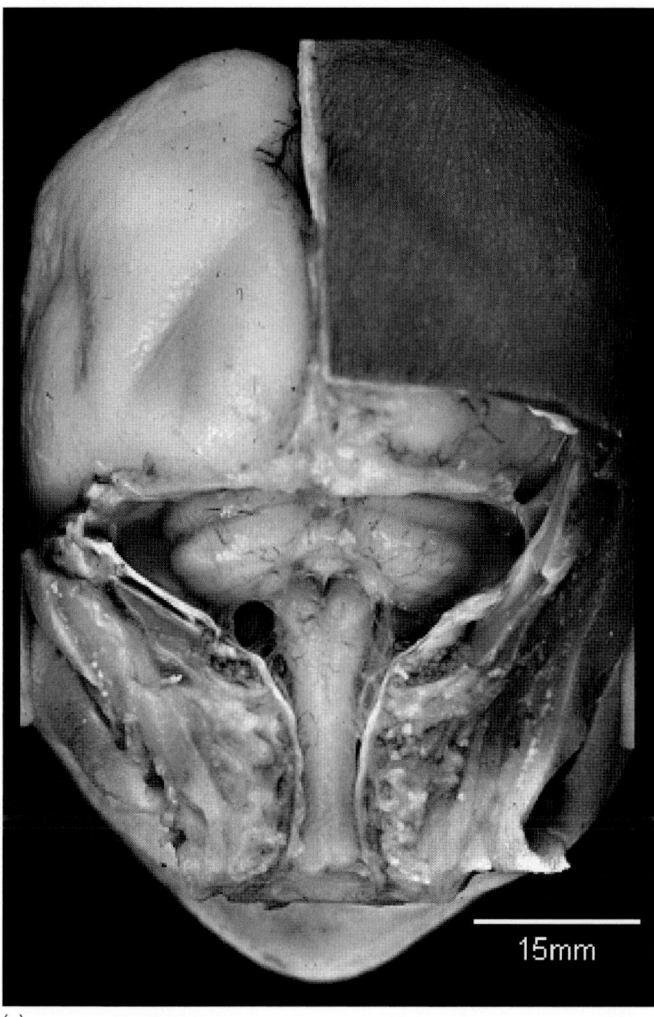

(c)

Figure 2.10 Continued

FUTURE PROSPECTS

The exact temporal and spatial distribution of differentiating cells during neurogenesis has been difficult to establish so far, and how organs are assembled in complex three dimensions has escaped plausible explanations. However, the advent of new methods such as genetic fate mapping, transgenic and gene targeting techniques, together with recent advances in genetic-inducible fate mapping may help in determining when and where specific cell types are generated; in other words the fundamentals or, at least, parts of tri/fourth (the time factor)-dimensional patterns of organogenesis at the molecular level may be unraveled (Carlen et al 2006, Joyner & Zervas 2006). Whilst much of the rapidly accumulating new knowledge on brain development appears to be oriented to the understanding of brain pathology after birth, the application of diagnostic ultrasound at ever earlier stages of gestation is making possible the accurate imaging of the developing human brain (Blaas 1999). This together with other tests based on the isolation of fetal cells from maternal blood may assist, in the not-too-distant future, in diagnosing and perhaps treating neurologic disorders.

REFERENCES

Alcaraz W A, Gold D A, Raponi E et al 2006 Zfp423 controls proliferation and differentiation of neural precursors in cerebellar vermis formation. Proc Natl Acad Sci USA 103:19424–19429.

Blaas H-G K 1999 The embryonic examination: ultrasound studies on the development of the human embryo. Thesis, Norwegian University of Science and Technology, Tapir Trykkeri,

Blinkov S M, Glezer I I (eds) 1968 The human brain in figures and tables. Plenum, New York, pp. 126–334.

Bourgeois J P, Jastreboff P J, Rakic P 1989 Synaptogenesis in visual cortex of normal and preterm monkeys: evidence for intrinsic regulation and synaptic overproduction. Proc Natl Acad Sci USA 86:4297–4301.

Bridges C B, Morgan T H 1923 The third chromosome group of mutant characters of *Drosophila melanogaster*. Carnegie Institute, Washington, p. 251.

Carlen M, Meletis K, Barnabe-Heider F, Frisen J 2006 Genetic visualisation of neurogenesis. Exp Cell Res 312:2851–2859.

Choi B H 1986 Glial fibrillary acid protein in radial glia of early human fetal cerebrum: a light and electron microscopy immunoperoxidase study. J Neuropathol Exp Neural 45:408–418.

D'Arcangelo G, Miao G G, Chen S C et al 1995 A protein related to extracellular matrix proteins deleted in the mouse mutant reeler. Nature 374:719–723.

Dolle P, Izpisua-Belmonte J C, Falkestein H 1989 Coordinate expression of the murine Hox-5 complex homeobox-containing genes during limb pattern formation. Nature 342:767–772.

Ericson J, Muhr J, Placzek M et al 1995 Sonic hedgehog induces differentiation of ventral forebrain neurons: a common signal for ventral patterning within the neural tube. Cell 81:747–756.

Fantl W J, Johnson D E, William L T 1993 Signalling by receptor tyrosine kinases. Annu Rev Biochem 62:453–481.

Gould E, Beylin A, Tanapat P et al 1999 Learning enhances adult neurogenesis in the adult hippocampal formation. Nature Neurosci 2:260–265.

Holland P W, Hogan B L 1988 Expression of homeo box genes during mouse development: a review. Genes Dev 2:773–782.

Hynes M A, Porter J A, Chiang C et al 1995 Induction of midbrain dopaminergic neurons by sonic hedgehog. Neuron 15:35–44.

Joyner A L, Zervas M 2006 Genetic inducible fate mapping in mouse: establishing genetic lineages and defining genetic neuroanatomy in the nervous system. Dev Dyn 235:2376–2385.

Lumsden A, Keynes R 1989 Segmental patterns of neuronal development in the chick hindbrain. Nature 337:424–428.

Marin-Padilla M 1983 Structural organization of the human cerebral cortex prior to the appearance of the cortical plate. Anat Embryol 168:21–40.

Miao N, Wang M, Ott J A et al 1997) Sonic hedgehog promotes the survival of specific CNS neuron

populations and protects these cells from toxic insult in vitro. J Neurosci 17:5891–5899.

Miner J H, Cunningham J, Sanes J R 1998 Roles for laminin in embryogenesis: exencephaly, syndactyly and placentopathy in mice lacking the laminin a5 chain. J Cell Biol 143:1713–1723.

Müller F, O'Rahilly R 1983 The first appearance of the major divisions of the human brain at stage 9. Anat Embryol 168:419–432.

Nakajima K, Mikoshiba K, Miyata T et al 1997 Disruption of hippocampal development in vivo by CR-50mAb against reelin. Proc Natl Acad Sci USA 94:8196–8201.

O'Rahilly R, Müller F (eds) 1999 The embryonic human brain: an atlas of developmental stages, 2nd edn. Wiley-Liss, New York.

O'Rahilly R, Müller F, Hutchins G M, Moore G W 1984 Computer ranking of the sequence of appearance of 100 features of the brain and related structures in staged human embryos during the first 5 weeks of development. Am J Anat 171:243–257.

Oliver G, Sidell N, Fiske W et al 1989 Complementary homeoprotein gradients in developing limb buds. Genes Dev 3:641–650.

Pellegrine M, Mansouri A, Simeoni A et al 1996 Dentate gyrus formation requires Emx2. Development 122:3898–3993.

Porter F D, Drago J, Xu Y et al 1997 Lhx2, a LIM Homeobox gene, is required for eye, forebrain and definitive erythrocyte development. Development 124:2935–2944.

Rakic P 1995 The development of the frontal lobe. A view from the rear of the brain. Adv Neurol 66: 1–6.

Rakic P, Sidman R L 1970 Histogenesis of cortical layers in human cerebellum, particularly the lamina dissecans. J Camp Neural 139:473–500.

Roelink H, Porter J A, Chiang C et al 1994 Floor plate and motor neuron induction by Vhh-1, a vertebrate homolog of hedgehog expressed by the notochord. Cell 76:761–775.

Roy N S, Wang S, Jian L 2000 In-vitro neurogenesis by progenitor cells isolated from the adult human hippocampus. Nat Med 6:271–277.

Schlessinger J, Ukkrich A 1992 Growth factor signalling by receptor tyrosine kinases. Neuron 9:383–391.

Shatz C J 1996 Emergence of order in visual system development. J Physiol 90:141–150.

Soriano E, Del Rio J A, Martinez H, Super O O 1994 Organization of the embryonic and early postnatal murine hippocampus. I. Immunocytochemical characterization of neuronal populations in the subplate and marginal zone. J Comp Neurol 342:571–595.

Suddath R L, Christison G W, Torrey F E et al 1990 Anatomical abnormalities in the brain of monozygotic twins discordant for schizophrenia. N Engl J Med 322:789–794.

Tanabe Y, Jessell T M 1996 Diversity and pattern in the developing spinal cord. Science 274:1115–1123.

Tanaka O, Otani H, Fujimoto K 1987 Fourth ventricular floor in human embryos: scanning electron microscopy observations. Am J Anat 178:193–203.

Wang M Z, Jin P, Bumcrot D A et al 1995 Induction of dopaminergic neuron phenotype in the midbrain by sonic hedgehog protein. Nature Med 1:1184–1188.

Wehr R, Mansouri A, de Maeyer T, Gruss P 1997 Fkh5-deficient mice shows dysgenesis in the caudal midbrain and hypothalamic mamillary body. Development 124:4447–4456.

Weinberger D R 1987 Implications of normal brain development for the pathogenesis of schizophrenia. Arch Gen Psychiatry 44:660–669.

Weinberger D R, Berman K G, Illowsky B P 1988 Physiological dysfunction of dorsolateral prefrontal cortex in schizophrenia. III. A new cohort and evidence for a monoaminergic mechanism. Arch Gen Psychiatry 45:609–615.

Weinberger D R, DeLisi L E, Perman G P et al 1982 Computed tomography in schizophreniform disorder and other acute psychiatric disorders. Arch Gen Psychiatry 39:778–783.

Wilkinson D G, Bhatt S, Chavrier P 1989 Segment specific expression of a zinc-finger gene in the developing nervous system of the mouse. Nature 337:461–464.

Yoshida M, Suda Y, Matsuo I et al 1997 Emx1 and Emx2 functions in development of the dorsal telencephalon. Development 124:101–111.

Zhao Y, Sheng H Z, Amini R et al 1999 Control of hippocampal morphogenesis and neuronal differentiation by the LIM Homeobox gene Lhx5. Science 284:1155–1158.

CHAPTER

3

Development of consciousness: fetal, neonatal and maternal interactions

Hugo Lagercrantz

Key Points

- Human consciousness cannot be established until the anatomical thalamocortical connections have been established. This occurs around the 24th gestational week
- The newborn infant full-term infant fulfills the following criteria of being conscious: he or she processes tactile, painful, olfactory and auditory stimuli at a cortical level (according to investigations with near-infrared spectroscopy); he or she is awake and aware if the body and the self and shows emotions. Furthermore the newborn can recognize faces and imitate face expression, habituate and show preference for human speech as compared with noise
- Thus the newborn has reached a minimal level of consciousness
- The fetus is probably not conscious, due to low PO_2 and sedation by endogenous neuromodulators
- The preterm infant may begin to develop minimal consciousness from the 24th gestational week

---

A simple definition of consciousness is sensory awareness of the body, the self and the world. The fetus may be aware of the body, for example, perceiving pain. The newborn may be aware of itself but it takes some time to develop voluntary control and self-regulation. According to Piaget (1954) the child below 2 years is a reflex sensory–motor organism and not aware of the world. It takes an even longer time for the child to fulfill the criteria described by Bergson (1920): 'To retain what no longer is, to anticipate what as yet is not — these are the primary functions of consciousness.' Using new brain imaging and functional techniques it is now possible to explore the neuronal correlates of consciousness in the fetus and the newborn. Although the knowledge of the developing brain has increased considerably thanks to these new techniques, surprisingly little is known about the development of the brain with regard to the emergence of consciousness.

NEURONS: THE ATOMS OF CONSCIOUSNESS

Neurons are the atoms of perception, memory, thought and action; thus, the atoms of consciousness (see Koch 2004). They differ from other cells, for example, the intestine or the skin, in that they are explicit. Although nearly all cells react to the environment, only the neurons make this information explicit and available for conscious thinking. The neurons of the immature fetal brain are round and have very few connections with other cells, which explains why they are less explicit. Cortical pyramidal neurons in the primary visual cortex of the human sprout increasingly more and from the 26th week (Purpura 1982). The neurons branch, acquire dendritic spines and connect with each other.

THE LOCALIZATION OF CONSCIOUSNESS

The exact anatomical localization of consciousness is not known, even in the adult. The thalamus is probably essential as the gateway to the neocortex (Koch 2004). Particularly, the parietal lobes seem to be important to shape mental images and gather information about the world around us and, possibly, within us (Baars et al 2003). If we consider verbal report ability as a hallmark of human consciousness (see Perner & Dienes 2002), the following areas seem to be involved: the anterior cingulate gyrus of the frontal lobe, left lateral frontal and posterior cortex, in areas involved with processing the meaning of words or sentences, and the right cerebellum (Posner & Rothbart 1998). Pyramidal cells from layers 2 and 3 in the dorsal lateral prefrontal and inferoparietal cortical structures are probably essential (Dehaene & Changeux 2004). Long-distance axons link most, if not all, the cortical and thalamic regions forming a neuronal workspace (Fig. 3.1). In this way one becomes conscious of sensory stimuli (Baars et al 2003, Changeux 2004). Koch also believes there are specific 'consciousness neurons'. An alternative view is that there is a 'dynamic core' consisting of correlated activities of a large number of neurons in the cortex, thalamus and the limbic system (Edelman & Tononi 2000).

DEVELOPMENTAL ANATOMY OF CONSCIOUSNESS

A primary requisite to be conscious is to be aware of sensory impressions, i.e. the neuronal pathways mediating this information must exist and function. Palmar cutaneous sensory receptors appear around the 10th week of gestational age in the human. Spinal reflexes evoked by stimulation of most body areas can be observed from the 14th week. Nociceptive reactions can be recorded from the 19th week (Rees & Rawson 2002).

The genesis of the cochlea starts around the fifth week after conception and the hair cells differentiate and grow from the 11th week until the 21st when they nearly have reached adult size.

The sensory cells in the nasal cavity and the nasal septum are probably in contact with amniotic fluid from the 22nd week of gestation (Schaal et al 2004).

The eyelids are closed until the 22nd week and the retina is very immature when the eyes open. Photoreceptors are relatively short and wide at birth. The fovea is also very immature.

(a)

(b)

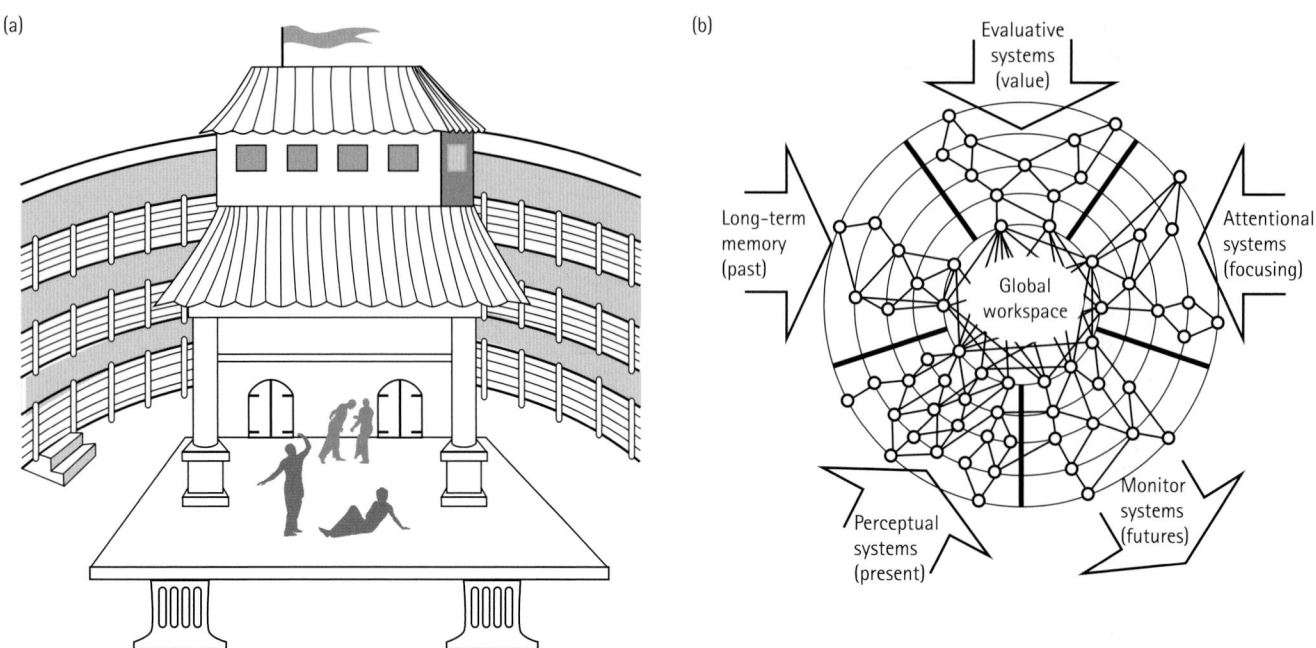

Figure 3.1 Consciousness has been proposed to be localized in a global workspace which receives inputs via long neurons from perceptual, attentional and evaluating systems and memory (Dehaene & Changeux 2004). A metaphor of the global workspace is a theater scene as proposed by Baars (1998). A number of events occur in the scene, behind the scene, among the auditorium, etc., but the conscious mind is focused on what is happening in the scene. The prefrontal cortex selects what is attended to and interprets it to a voluntary action. This is applicable only to a limited extent in the baby.

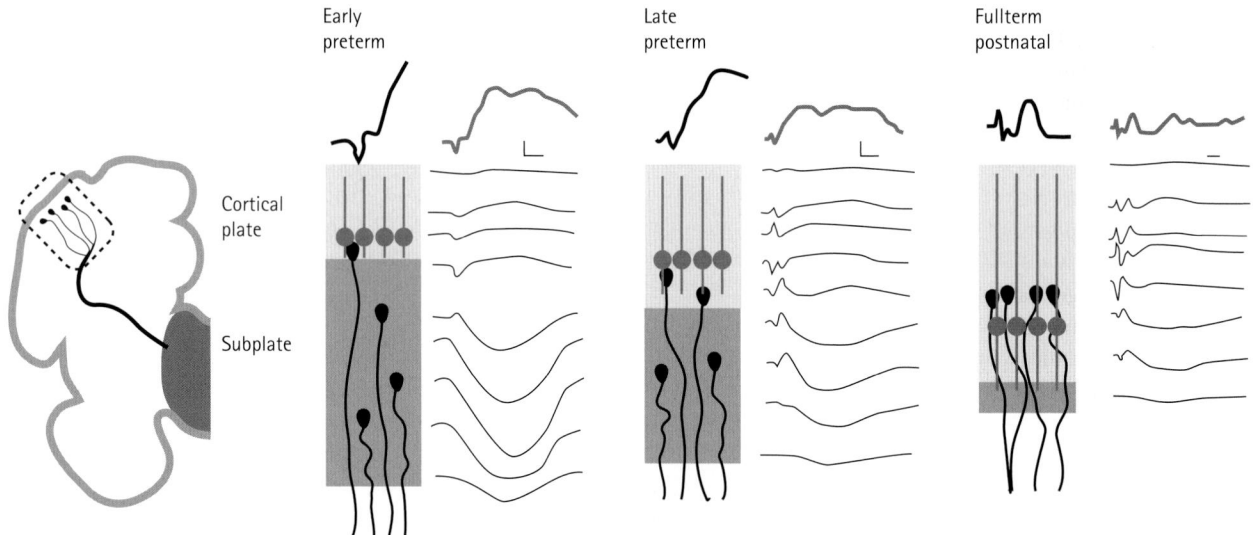

Figure 3.2 Maturation of the thalamo-cortical connections and the somatosensory evoked potentials (SEP) responses. This is essential to be able to process sensory inputs in the global workspace, i.e. being conscious. (Courtesy of S. Vanhatalo.)

To be conscious the various sensory modalities must become accessible to the cortex. All sensory impressions, except olfactory impressions, are relayed in the thalamus. Thalamic afferents to the cortex appear from about 12–16 weeks gestation, but these projections only reach the subplate, which is regarded as a 'waiting compartment' for afferents to the cortex (Fig. 3.2). At this stage only very long somatosensory evoked potentials (SEP) from the deep layers can be recorded at the scalp (Vanhatalo & Lauronen 2006). First, after about 24 weeks, there is an ingrowth of thalamocortical axons in the somatosensory, auditory, visual and frontal cortex (Kostovic & Rakic 1984). Thalamocortical pathways mediating pain perception do not seem to function before the 29–30 gestational weeks according to Lee et al (2005). At about this time there also seems to be some synchrony of the EEG rhythm of the two hemispheres (Vanhatalo & Kaila 2006).

The cerebral cortex, particularly the prefrontal area, matures late in the human. The neurons do not become completely myelinated until early adulthood, allowing rapid neuronal activity and mature executive, actions (Sowell et al 2004). However, subcortical structures are probably of greater importance for consciousness during early life. The fusiform area, for face recognition, and the amygdala, for emotions, etc., seem to function already in the newborn. These areas are of great importance for the social brain and probably also for consciousness (Johnson 2005). These sub-cortical structures should not necessarily be regarded as subordinate to the cortex, particularly not in the infant.

THE NEUROCHEMISTRY OF CONSCIOUSNESS

Excitatory amino acids generate synchronous oscillatory activity, which probably is essential for the maintenance of consciousness.

Gamma-aminobutyric acid (GABA) is the dominating excitatory neurotransmitter during fetal life. Around birth it becomes the main inhibitory neurotransmitter. This is due to the fact that the immature neurons are depolarized by GABA, while the mature neurons become hyperpolarized. This is caused by the expression of the K^+/Cl^- co-transporter KCC_2, which maintains a low intracellular Cl^- concentration. Glutamate and aspartate probably take over the role of GABA as the major excitatory amino acids after birth (see Vanhatalo & Kaila 2006).

Classic neurotransmitters like norepinephrine (noradrena-line) and acetylcholine may also be involved in the genera-tion of consciousness by stimulating wakefulness and awareness.

Noradrenergic neurons originating from the locus coeru-leus have been proposed to be involved in arousal. The norepinephrine turnover was found to be relatively low in the rat fetus, but surged after birth (Lagercrantz 1996). If we extrapolate to the human newborn baby this increased nor-epinephrine turnover may explain the arousal of the newborn baby, who is usually awake in the first 2 hours after birth (Fig. 3.3). Although increased norepinephrine turnover has not been demonstrated in the human brain, we know that enormously high levels of catecholamines are released after vaginal delivery and that there are strong indications that the central and peripheral catecholamine systems are acti-vated simultaneously (Lagercrantz 1996).

Acetylcholine also seems to be a more likely candidate as the neurotransmitter of consciousness (Changeux 2006). Cholinergic basal forebrain neurons send their axons to a much wider array of target structures, innervating the thala-mus, hippocampus, amygdala and cerebral cortex. The idea of acetylcholine as the transmitter of consciousness is cor-roborated by the finding of increased activity during awake-ness. Furthermore, in dementia, diseases like Parkinson and Alzheimer, associated with depressed consciousness, there is a selective loss of cholinergic neurons. Acetylcholine

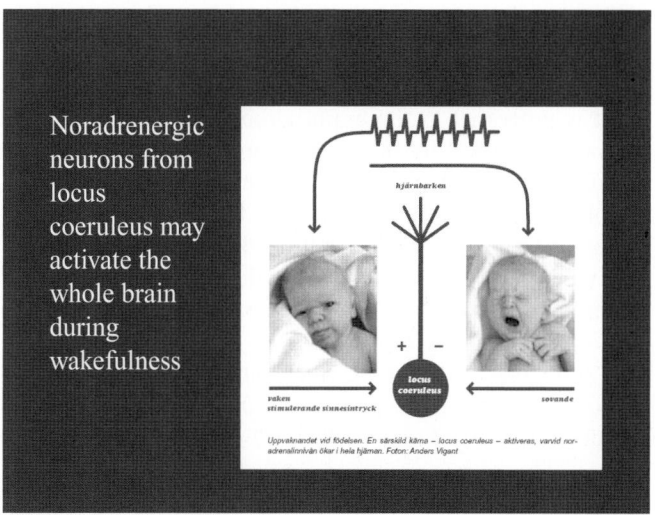

Noradrenergic neurons from locus coeruleus may activate the whole brain during wakefulness

Figure 3.3 The newborn is awakened and aroused at birth possibly due to activation of the locus coeruleus.

has been found to promote cortical processing of incoming stimuli. Newborn mice lacking the β_2 nicotinic acetylcholine receptor subunit showed impaired arousal response during hypoxia (Cohen et al 2005).

METHODS TO STUDY CONSCIOUSNESS IN THE FETUS AND THE INFANT

Functional magnetic resonance imaging (fMRI) has been used to study how the human fetus processes sensory input (Gowland & Fulford 2004). However, it is difficult since the fetus must be immobilized. Another technique is magneto-encephalography (MEG), which has been used by some research groups (Preissl et al 2004). The principle is to record magnetic signals corresponding to the electrical activity in the brain. It is completely passive and non-invasive with superior temporal resolution. However, it does not provide any anatomical information; this has to be obtained by combining MEG with ultrasound or other techniques. The method has been used to study auditory and visual evoked responses in the fetus (Huotilainen 2006).

Conventional EEG, amplitude integrated EEG, event-related potentials can be used to assess neonatal conscious-ness (see Ch. 12 and Fellman et al 2006). fMRI is considered as the leading technique to explore the function of the brain (Seghier et al 2006). However, the infant must be immobi-lized and usually asleep, which makes it difficult for studies of consciousness.

This is not necessary when using near-infrared spectro-scopy (NIRS). This method is non-invasive, relatively simple and is a useful method to assess how the neonatal brain processes various sensory signals (Meek 2002). NIRS is based on measuring the hemodynamic responses over the cortical areas. Near-infrared light which is transmitted by optodes placed on the skull is reflected by oxyhemoglobin and deoxyhemoglobin and measured. Changes in hemoglobin oxygenation and blood volume and flow can be computed by algorithms and used as indexes of neural activation. Using this method it is at least possible to study how sensory input is processed in the brain, although it only indirectly indicates whether the infant is aware or conscious of the stimuli. The spatial resolution is 1–2 cm and the temporal sampling resolution 0.01 s, which is better than fMRI. One limitation is that structures situated deeper than 2–3 cm under the skull cannot be studied with NIRS.

With this method positive responses to visual, auditory and olfactory stimulation have been documented (Bartocci et al 2000, Meek et al 1998). This method has also been used to study how the infant perceives human speech (Dehaene-Lamberts et al 2002).

COMPONENTS OF CONSCIOUSNESS

A catalog of conscious experiences or components of consciousness can be listed for the fetus and the neonate:

1. SENSORY EXPERIENCES AND PAIN

Tactile and painful stimuli (e.g. venepuncture) elicit specific hemodynamic responses in the somatosensory cortex (Fig. 3.4), implying conscious sensory perception already in the preterm neonates (Bartocci et al 2006, Slater et al 2006). The mean gestational age was 32 weeks (range 28–36) in the study by Bartocci et al (2006). A more pronounced response was seen in the youngest infants consistent with the finding that the pain threshold is lower in preterm infants. On the other hand there was a positive correlation between pain response and postnatal age, consistent with a postnatal decay of fetal inhibition. The latency between venepuncture and cortical activity was comparable to that of adults.

Higher responses to noxious stimulation were seen in awake infants (Slater et al 2006), confirming the idea of

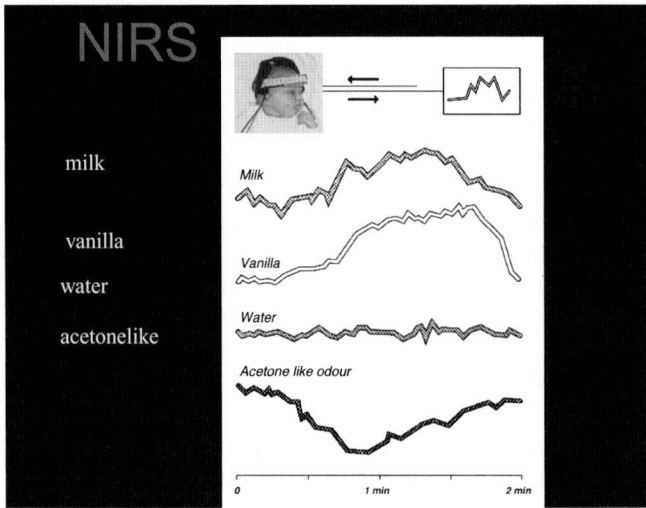

Figure 3.4 Recording of the responses to smell by near-infrared spectroscopy (NIRS) from the olfactory cortex. This shows that various smells are processed at a cortical level.

being conscious of the pain. The lateralization of pain processing, the latency and duration of these responses and their gradations across gestational age and postanatal age, and the neuroanatomical location of these responses suggest that preterm infants may be consciously processing the acute pain from venepuncture. However, it is less likely that fetuses and preterm infants below 25 weeks can be aware of pain (see Derbyshire 2006).

2. SMELL AND TASTE

Early infant behavior is influenced by olfactory cues, many originating from the intrauterine environment (Schaal et al 2004, Varendi et al 2002).

They seem to be more attractive to the smell of amniotic fluid than to other odors. Exposure to amniotic fluid and other maternal odors has a soothing effect in newborns. When babies were exposed to clothes with their own mother's odors they stopped crying. Infants also seemed to prefer tastes that they were exposed to during fetal life through their mother's diet (Schaal et al 2004). Odors were found to be processed in the orbito-frontal olfactory area by the use of NIRS (Bartocci et al 2000, 2001).

3. HEARING AND SEEING

Low-frequency sounds can be recorded from about the 16th week. However, the fetus does not react to sounds in general until the 20th week, when tachycardia can be elicited by noise (Counter 2002). External sound is reduced to about half of its strength when it reaches the fetal cochlea. However, it is plausible that the maternal voice is transmitted also by direct conduction. This may explain why newborn infants seem to be able to discriminate between the mother's and unfamiliar women's voices (Gray & Philbin 2004). The full-term infant can orient visually to auditory signals by turning the head and the eyes towards the sound. If an infant is shown, for example, an object at the same time as being presented with a sound, it will turn the eyes towards the sound, suggesting that hearing is more mature at birth. On the other hand, the preterm infant has difficulties orientating towards an auditory stimulus.

Fetal brain activity has been studied during visual stimulation. Bright light was shone at the maternal abdomen for short periods (8 s) repetitively and brain activity was monitored with fMRI. Activity could be recorded in the frontal eye fields but not in the primary visual cortex in the occipital region (Preissl et al 2004).

Visual acuity in the full-term newborn infants is only $1/40$ visual acuity but they can recognize faces and imitate (Johnson 2005).

4. WAKEFULNESS

The human fetus is mainly asleep, although it can be observed on ultrasound that it sometimes opens its eyes (see Mellor et al 2005). However, it may be awake without being conscious, like in some patients in vegetative states. The fetus is mainly asleep in REM sleep, which is characterized by rapid eye movements. Non-REM sleep increases successively during maturation.

It can be argued that one is conscious also during dream or REM sleep at least after birth. However, if we assume that awakefulness is required for being fully conscious, there are indications that the fetus is never awake and conscious. Rigatto et al (1986) recorded electrocortigram, eye and breathing movements in parallel with behavior in fetal sheep, which was monitored by video camera observations. No wakeful periods were discovered when analyzing videotape recordings of more than 5000 hours during 8 years. Furthermore, a number of inhibitory substances have been found in the placenta which suppress the fetus and promote sleep. The low partial oxygen level of the fetus (Mount Everest in utero) may also contribute to suppress the fetal brain. This may, for example, increase the endogenous levels of adenosine (Irestedt et al 1989), which inhibits neuronal activity.

The normal newborn infant is usually awake in the first 2 hours after birth. The eyes are wide open and the pupils are big. This awake state was probably missed a few decades before, because the babies received Crédé prophylaxis. After a couple of hours they usually fall asleep. The awakening of the newborn baby may be due to activation of the locus coeruleus. A surge of catecholamines occurs particularly after vaginal delivery (Lagercrantz & Slotkin 1986). There is probably a parallel activation of the cerebral noradrenergic system (Lagercrantz 1996).

Extremely preterm infants (<25 wk) have, mostly, closed eyes, indicating that they are asleep (McMillan et al 1987). By gentle stimulation they can be encouraged to open their eyes briefly. After 26 weeks of gestation longer periods of wakefulness can be observed (Fig. 3.5). It is now possible to briefly fix the sight of the mother. According to the EEG pattern, wakefulness can be seen first after 30 weeks. However, it is somewhat dubious to identify awakefulness only by EEG, since patients who have lost their autonomy may exhibit an EEG typical of awakefulness (see D'Allest et al 2002).

5. SELF-AWARENESS

According to classic studies, self-awareness does not appear until the end of the second year when the child recognizes itself in a mirror and says I. However, already a newborn baby appears to have some degree of self-awareness. It reacts differently to tactile stimulation by the mother as compared with self-stimulation, which it does not respond to (Rochat 2003).

6. SHOWING EMOTIONS

Emotions can be defined as external events perceived by the individual that result in bodily responses, particularly from the autonomic nervous system. By this definition the newborn certainly show emotions. They seem to be able to activate the same facial muscles as adults and express primary emotions such as joy, disgust, surprise and distress (Tronick 1989). They react with negative emotions to pain,

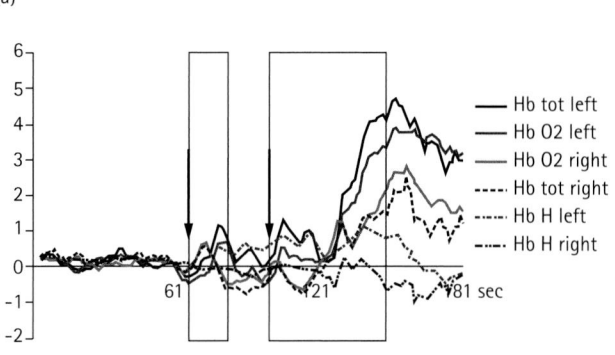

(a)

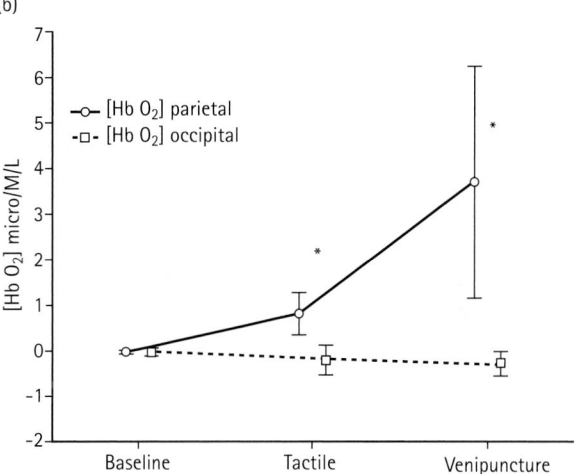

(b)

Figure 3.5 (a) Recording of NIRS over the sensorimotor area. (b) Responses to tactile and noxious (venepuncture) stimulation at the somatosensory area in preterm infants. No response was seen over the occipital area. (From Bartocci et al 2006.)

cold temperature, bad smells (Bartocci et al 2001) and tastes. They can also react with positive emotions to sensory stimulation, such as when breastfeeding and seeing their mother. Newborns also react with positive emotions when exposed to harmonic music, but with apnea when listening to disharmonic music or noise (Zentner & Kagan 1996).

7. IMITATION

Imitation is necessary for a higher level of consciousness. Newborn infants can imitate the grimaces of an adult, as established in a seminal study by Meltzoff et al (1977). It is probably not just a reflex response, because there is some latency.

8. FACE PROCESSING

The subcortical face-detection system seems to function at an early stage. Newborns react to figures showing faces with eyes and a mouth presented in high contrast. We do not know whether face processing functions in extremely preterm infants. There are separate routes for face detection and face identification. Blind sighted patients seem to detect faces at a subcortical level. Thus it is likely that the infant perception of faces is subcortical (Johnson 2005).

Infants, like adults, prefer attractive faces. They are sensitive to the presence of eyes in the face and dislike scrambled faces (Mehler et al 2002).

9. MEMORY

The most primitive form of memory, i.e. habituation, appears around the 22nd to 23rd gestational week in the human fetus. If the fetus is exposed to a repetitive stimulus like the vibration of an electric tooth brush it reacts by movements. However, after multiple stimuli it seems to remember the stimulus and no longer reacts. There are also reports demonstrating that infants can remember rhymes or musical jingles which they have been exposed to during fetal life (Hepper 1996). However, a real representative memory probably does not emerge until the second to fourth month, when babies can experience sensations and emotions and start to think about objects and events.

Working memory appears around 7 months, according to most textbooks of developmental psychology. However, even younger babies seem to remember, for example, a soother which suddenly disappears. There seems to be some kind of mental representation of faces and things at about 2 months. Thus the previously held view that out of sight is out of mind may not be true.

10. LANGUAGE

The newborn brain responds specifically to normal speech after a few hours of experience with speech signals outside the womb. Newborns were exposed to normal forward speech as compared with reversed backward speech. A significantly greater activity was found in the left hemisphere when the babies listened to normal speech (Dehaene-Lambertz et al 2002).

11. SELF-REGULATION

Infants less than 3 months are difficult to soothe if they are distressed by, for example, pain. Holding and rocking the infant may help. After 3 months the infant can be quietened by distraction, bringing attention to other stimuli (Posner & Rothbart 1998).

INTEGRATION OF THE COMPONENTS

It is plausible that the sensory signals are not integrated in the newborn brain to the same extent as later in life. Maybe there is an evolutionary parallel. For example, reptiles are not able to integrate the sight and the smell of a prey (Sjölander 1999). The snake is governed by sight to strike a prey, for example a mouse, but to start to swallow the head of its prey it must use its smell of the dead mouse. The snake has no concept of a mouse: no 'object constancy' according to Piaget (1954). A mouse disappearing behind an obstacle has simply disappeared; it does not exist for the reptile. Reptiles do not possess the ability that mammals have to combine sensing, vision and hearing.

Full-term human infants seem to be able to connect what they see with what they hear (Morrongillo et al 1998).

One well-known example of the ability to combine sensory sensations is that newborn infants feeling pain can be calmed by sucking sucrose (Zeifman et al 1996). To achieve an optimal effect a 4-week-old baby must also see its caregiver. This was not necessary in the 2-week-old baby, indicating that the integration of sensory inputs from different modalities has to mature.

MATERNAL INTERACTION

Self-consciousness is very dependent on social interaction. From an early age the child is not only begging for attention, it is pleading for existence itself (see Rochat 2003) by crying 'Watch me, watch me.' Already very preterm infants look longer on the mother's face than on objects. The caring philosophy Nidcap (neonatal individualized developmental care and assessment program) is based on the idea of promoting maternal–infant interaction.

The awakened newborn normal infant is looking at its parents with wide pupils, due to the catecholamine surge (Lagercrantz 1996). This is probably important for the parents to get the feeling of 'becoming parents'.

Infants seem to recognize their mothers at an early stage (by the second month). Already a newborn prefers to listen to its own mother's voice and prefers the smell of its mother compared with the smell of other women by 2 weeks after birth.

Already newborns imitate adults, coo and make hand gestures when spoken to (see Trevarthen & Aitken 1994). They raise the right hand more than the left. From about 2 months infants can communicate with their parents with a protoconversation. If the mother freezes her face the baby becomes desperate and waves with the hands to stimulate the attention of the mother. On the other hand the baby responds easily to smiling by imitation. The mother also adapts to the baby, for example, by talking with a high-pitched voice, so-called motherese (Kuhl 2004).

MINIMAL CONSCIOUSNESS

One must also be conscious about something, i.e. some kind of intentionality in Brentano's sense (Zelazo 2004). The newborn infant does not fulfill the criteria of being conscious as defined for the adult human. However, the newborn seems to be aware of pleasure such as pleasant smells and tastes and unpleasant stimuli like pain, although it is unreflective, present-oriented and makes no reference to the concept of self. According to Zelazo (2004), the infant has reached a minimal level of consciousness. In minimal consciousness one is conscious of what one sees, but not seeing what one sees. One cannot recall seeing what one saw.

This condition lasts until the end of the first year when the infant develops recursive consciousness: starting to label objects, i.e. a lamp or a dog. During the second year the

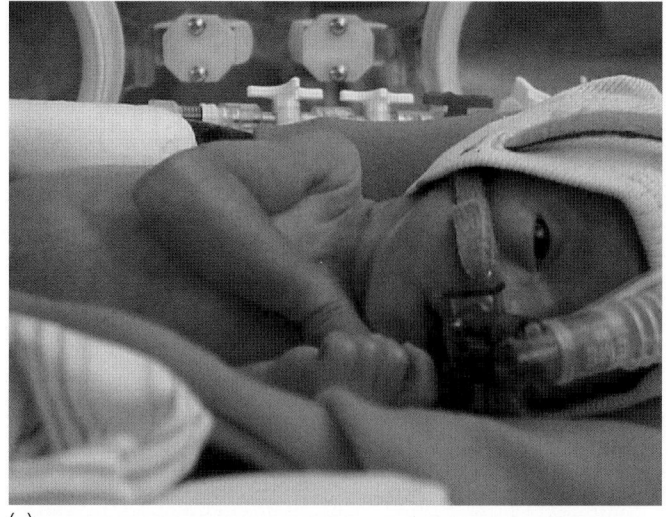

(a)

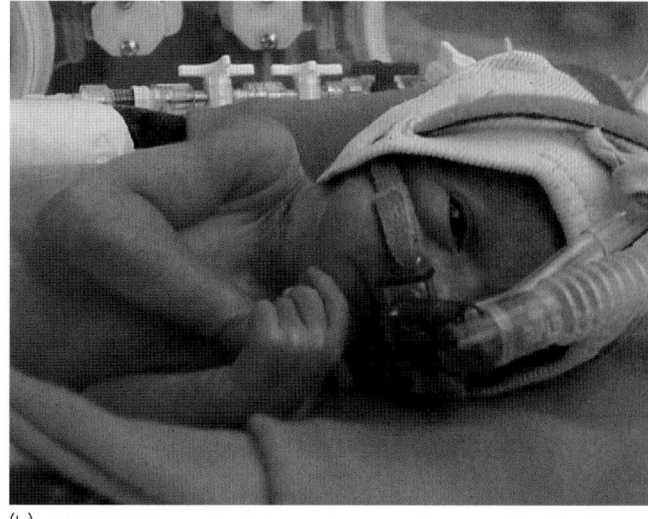

(b)

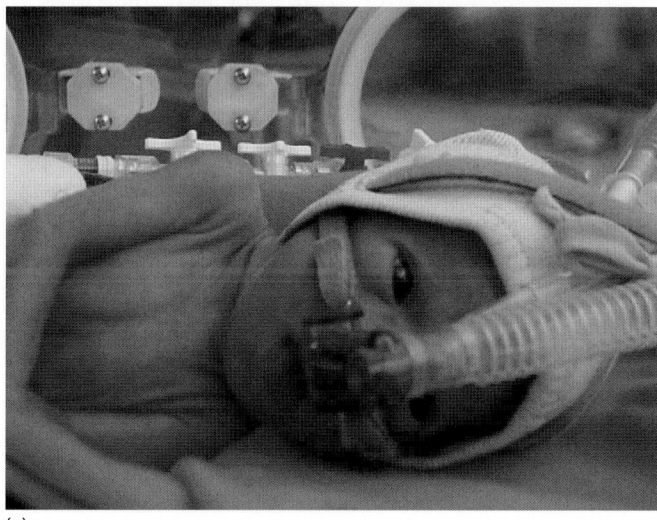

(c)

Figure 3.6 (a–c) A preterm infant at 26 weeks is awake for short periods and seems to fix the gaze for short moments towards his mother. He also seems to be able to move its arms for protection (self-awareness). (Photos by Ann-Sofie Gustafsson.)

child develops self-consciousness and during the third reflective consciousness.

This does not apply to the newborn infant who has only reached a minimal level of consciousness. The infant, of course, has not reached the highest level of consciousness of humankind: the ability to understand the thinking of others (see Changeux 2004). This level develops gradually around the age of 4 years. At this age the child can recognize false beliefs and understands what lying is. This is also of importance for the feeling of empathy.

However, some empathetic feelings can be observed in newborns. It is well known that if an infant in a room with newborn babies starts to cry all the other babies also cry. The crying babies are probably not aware why they are crying. But this type of imitation is probably important for the future development of empathy.

Even preterm infants, born from the 26th to 28th gestational week, seem to have reached a minimal level of consciousness. They react to tactile, auditory and visual stimulation as well as pain at a cortical level (as discussed

above). They awake for short periods, show avoidance reactions to harmful stimuli and seem to establish minimal eye contact with their mothers (Fig. 3.6).

However, the preterm infant born before 26 weeks (<800 g) does not fulfill these criteria of minimal consciousness, probably due to the fact that the thalamic connections have not yet penetrated the cortical plate. Nevertheless, the somatosensory cortex does not seem to be essential to perceive pain, even in adults. It is possible that the extremely preterm infant can be conscious of pain at a subcortical level.

ETHICAL CONSIDERATIONS

The moment of birth is the moral and legal point at which human life must be preserved, independent of gestational age, according to the Nuffield Council on bioethics (2006). A prerequisite is that the newborn 'encompasses the capacity to breathe either independently, or with a support of a ventilator.'

To use the onset of air breathing, even on a ventilator, as a moral and legal breaking point could be considered dubious in the near future. It may be possible to sustain life of new-borns below 23 weeks or exteriorized fetuses by oxygen-ation with fluid ventilation or extracorporal oxygenation of the blood (ECMO). To use air breathing as a hallmark will be as old-fashioned in the near future as to define death only as definitive heart arrest.

An alternative limit of viability could be when a fetus or a preterm infant has developed a brain to achieve a minimal level of consciousness. After about 24 weeks there is an ingrowth of thalamocortical axons in the somatosensory, auditory, visual and frontal cortex. Thus infants born before

24 weeks do not seem to have any anatomical ability to be conscious at a cortical level. However, we cannot exclude the possibility of some kind of consciousness at a subordi-nate level. Newborns below 23 weeks, anencephalic infants and some severely brain-damaged infants (e.g. neonatal encephalopathy grade III) are less likely to be conscious even at a minimal level and, therefore, it should be possible to withhold or withdraw treatment.

Thus instead of using the onset of breathing air as a crucial limit of viability I think it is now time to discuss the emer-gence of a minimal consciousness as an alternative threshold.

REFERENCES

Baars B J, Ramsoy T Z, Laurey S 2003 Brain, conscious experience and the observing self. Trends Neurosci 26:671–675.

Bartocci M, Bergqvist L L, Lagercrantz H, Anand K J S 2006 Pain activates cortical areas in the preterm newborn brain. Pain 122:109–117.

Bartocci M, Winberg J, Papendieck G et al 2001 Cerebral hemodynamic response to unpleasant odors in the preterm newborn measured by near-infrared spectroscopy. Pediatr Res Aa50:324–330.

Bartocci M, Winberg J, Ruggiero C et al 2000 Activation of olfactory cortex in newborn infants after odor stimulation: a functional near-infrared spectroscopy study. Pediatr Res 48:18–23.

Bergson H 1920 Mind-energy: lectures and essays. Kolt, New York.

Changeux J-P 2004 The physiology of the truth. Harvard University Press, Cambridge, MA.

Changeux J-P 2006 The Ferrier lecture 1998 The molecular biology of consciousness investigated with genetically modified mice. Phil Trans R Soc Lond B 1098:1–21.

Cohen G, Roux J-C, Grailhe R et al 2005 Perinatal exposure to nicotine causes deficits associated with a loss of nicotinic receptor function. PNAS 102:3817–3821.

Counter S A 2002 Fetal and neonatal development of the auditory system. In: Lagercrantz H, Hanson M, Evrard P, Rodeck C H (eds) The newborn brain. Neuroscience and applications. Cambridge University Press, Cambridge, UK, pp. 226–251.

D'Allest A M, André M 2002 Electroencephalography. In: Lagercrantz H, Hanson M, Evrard P, Rodeck C H (eds) The newborn brain. Neuroscience and applications. Cambridge University Press, Cambridge, UK, pp. 339–367.

Dehaene S, Changeuxx J-P 2004 Neural mechanisms for access of consciousness. In: Gazzaniga M S (ed.) The cognitive neurosciences III. MIT Press, Cambridge, MA, pp. 1145–1154.

Dehaene-Lamberts G, Dehaene S, Hertz-Pannier L 2002 Functional neuroimaging of speech perception in infants. Science 298:2013–2015.

Derbyshire S W G 2006 Can fetuses feel pain. BMJ 332:909–912.

Edelman G M, Tononi G A 2000. A universe of consciousness. How matter becomes imagination. Basic Books, New York.

Fellman V, Huotilainen M 2006 Cortical auditory event-related potentials in newborn infants. Semin Fetal Neonatal Med 11:452–458.

Gowland P, Fulford J 2004 Initial experience of performing fetal fMRI. Exp Neuro 190:S22–S27.

Gray L, Philbin M K 2004 Effects of the neonatal intensive care unit on auditory attention and distraction. Clin Perinatol 31:243–260.

Hepper PG 1996 Fetal memory: Does it exist? What does it do? Acta Paediatr Suppl 416:16–20.

Huotilainen M 2006 Magnetoencephalography of the newborn brain. Semin Fetal Neonatal Med 11:437–443.

Irestedt L, Dahlin I, Hertzberg T et al 1989 Adenosine concentration in umbilical cord blood of newborn infants after vaginal delivery and cesarean section. Pediatr Res 26:106–108.

Johnson M H 2005 Subcortical face processing. Nature Neurosci Rev 6:766–774.

Koch C 2004 The quest for consciousness: a neurobiological approach. Roberts, Englewood, CO, p. 429.

Kostovic I, Rakic P 1984 Development of prestriate visual projections in the monkey and human fetal cerebrum revealed by transient cholinesterase staining. Neurosci 4:25–42.

Kuhl P K 2004 Early language acquisition: cracking the speech code. Nat Rev Neurosci 2004 5(11):831–843.

Lagercrantz H 1996 Stress, arousal, and gene activation at birth. N Physiol Sc 11:214–218.

Lagercrantz H, Slotkin T 1986 The stress of being. Sci Am 254:100–107.

Lee S J et al 2005 Fetal pain. A systematic multidisciplinary review of the evidence. JAMA 294:947–954.

Lewis M 2003 The emergence of consciousness and its role in human development. Ann N Y Acad Sci 1001:104–133.

McMillen I C, Kok J S, Adamson T M et al 1987 Development of circadian sleep–wake rhythms in preterm and full-term infants. Pediatr Res 29:381–384.

Meek J 2002 Optical imaging of infants. Dev Sci 5:271–380.

Meek J H, Firbank M, Elwell C E et al 1998 Regional hemodynamic responses to visual stimulation in awake infants. Pediatr Res 43:840–843.

Mehler J, Dupoux W 2002 Naitre humain. Odile Jacob, Paris.

Mellor D, Diesch T J, Gunn A J, Bennet L 2005 The importance of 'awareness' for understanding fetal pain. Brain Res Rev 49:455–471.

Meltzoff A N, Moore M K 1977 Imitation of facial and manual gestures by human neonates. Science 198:75–78.

Morrongillo B A, Fenwick K D, Chana G 1998 Crossmodel learning in newborn infants. Infant Behav Dev 21:543–553.

Perner J, Dienes Z 2003 Developmental aspects of consciousness. Conscious Cogn 12:63–82.

Piaget J 1954 The construction of reality in the child. Basic Books, New York.

Posner M I, Rothbart M K 1998 Attention, self-regulation and consciousness. Phil Trans R Soc Lond B 353:1915–1927.

Preissl H, Lowery C L, Eswaran H 2004 Fetal magnetoencephalography: current progress and trends. Exp Neurol 190:S28–S36.

Purpura D P 1982 Normal and abnormal development of cerebral cortex in man. Neurosci Res Program Bull 4:569–577.

Rees S, Rawson J 2002 Development of the somatosensory system. In: Lagercrantz H, Hanson M, Evrard P, Rodeck C H (eds) The newborn brain. Neuroscience and applications. Cambridge University Press, Cambridge, UK, pp. 177–203.

Rigatto H, Moore M, Cates D 1986 Fetal breathing and behavior measured through a double-wall Plexiglas window in sheep. J Appl Physiol 66:106–114.

Rochat P 2003 Five levels of self-awareness as they unfold early in life. Conscious Cogn 12:717–731.

Schaal B, Hummel T, Soussignan R 2004 Olfaction in the fetal and premature infant: Functional status and clinical implications. Clin Perinatol 31:261–285.

Seghier M L, Lazeyras, Hüppi P 2006 Functional MRI of the newborn. Semin Fetal Neonatal Med 11: 479–488.

Sjölander S 1999 How animals handle reality. In: Rigler A, Stein A V, Pesche M (eds) Does representation need reality. Plenum, New York.

Slater R, Cantarella A, Gallella S et al 2006 Cortical pain responses in human infants. J Neurosci 26:3662–3666.

Sowell E R, Thomson P M, Leonard C M et al 2004 Longitudinal mapping of cortical thickness and brain growth in normal children. J Neurosci 24:8223–8231.

Trevarthen C, Aitken K J 1994 Brain development, infant communication, and empathy disorders. Intrinsic factors in child mental health. Dev Psychopathol 6:599–635.

Tronick EZ 1989 Emotions and emotional communication in infants. Am Psychol 44:112–119.

Vanhatalo S, Kaila K 2006 Development of neonatal EEG activity: From phenomenology to physiology. Semin Fetal Neonatal Med 11:471–478.

Vanhatalo S, Lauronen L 2006 Neonatal SEP — Back to bedside with basic science. Semin Fetal Neonatal Med 11:464–470.

Varendi H, Porter R H, Winberg J 2002 The effect of labor on olfactory exposure learning within the first postnatal hour. Behav Neurosci 116:206–211.

Zeifman D, Delaney S, Blass E M 1996 Sweet taste, looking and calm in 2- and 4-week-old infants: The eyes have it. Dev Psychol 32:1090–1099.

Zelazo P D 2004 The development of conscious control in childhood. Trends Cognitive Sci 8:12–17.

Zentner M R, Kagan J 1996 Perception of music by infants. Nature 383:29.

Ultrasound assessment of normal fetal brain development

Harm-Gerd K. Blaas and Sturla H. Eik-Nes

INTRODUCTION

The technical development of ultrasound equipment has made possible major advances in the imaging of the developing fetal brain. In the 1960s, with the help of the A-scan, the fetal head, the skull and the falx could be identified. Today, the use of high-frequency transvaginal transducers has improved the image quality to such an extent that a detailed anatomical description of the living embryo has become possible. The large hypoechogenic cavities of the embryonic brain have, naturally, attracted the attention of ultrasound examiners (Takeuchi 1994, Timor-Tritsch & Monteagudo 1991, Timor-Tritsch et al 1988, 1990, Warren et al 1989). Two-dimensional (2-D) measurements of the embryonic brain have been made to describe the normal development and dimensions of the cavities of the hemispheres, the diencephalon, the mesencephalon (Blaas et al 1994, 1995a) and the rhombencephalon (Blaas et al 1995b, 1998, Zalen-Sprock et al 1996). Three-dimensional (3-D) ultrasound allows the off-line analysis of a recorded ultrasound volume in any plane, making it possible to measure the diameters and volumes of interest more precisely as well as to make more precise diagnoses (Blaas & Eik-Nes 2002a, Blaas et al 1995a, 1998).

In this chapter we review the development of the brain as described by embryologists and anatomists and compare this with sonoanatomic descriptions. The anatomic descriptions are limited to details that are of interest for the understanding of ultrasound examinations. The most dramatic changes of size and shape take place in early pregnancy; therefore, the embryonic period is described week by week.

The ultrasound descriptions of the brain development until 12 weeks are based on longitudinal 2-D and 3-D studies (Blaas 1999b, Blaas et al 1994, 1995b, 1998). All statements of gestational age are based on the last menstrual period (LMP), expressed in completed weeks and completed days, assuming a regular cycle with ovulation at 2 weeks 0 days. Though the term 'trimester' is imprecise (Blaas 1999a), it is used in this review as a rough subdivision of the pregnancy.

CHOICE OF TRANSDUCER AND APPROACH

During 38 weeks, from the unicellular stage at 2 weeks LMP-based gestational age to the newborn at 40 weeks, the conceptus goes through extensive changes of size and appearance, and various ultrasound techniques and approaches are needed to image the brain in this period.

The very small size and the constantly changing anatomical appearance of the brain in the embryonic and early fetal period are well suited to the transvaginal approach with high-frequency transducers such as 7.5 MHz. Phased and annular array transducers may be used. Because of the symmetric focusing, annular array technology produces very thin ultrasound tomograms; such mechanical transducers make it possible to image the tiny embryonic brain structures so that features of clinical interest can be identified. 3-D ultrasound may be used to obtain new ultrasound images, in planes not available in the original scan plane, to present form and shape of an object of interest and to calculate volume. The basis and prerequisite for all 3-D imaging are clear 2-D tomograms.

The embryonic/early fetal brain with its large ventricles can easily be imaged by the transvaginal approach and is well suited to 3-D imaging. A study from 2000 showed that transvaginal ultrasound could be applied throughout the pregnancy for 3-D neurosonography of the fetal brain (Monteagudo et al 2000). The increasing size of the early fetus at the end of the first and the beginning of the second trimesters makes the transvaginal approach for the CNS examination more difficult in breech presentations. Then, lower frequencies, usually 5 MHz, for the transabdominal route have to be chosen. However, this will often lead to poor resolution of the images because of more acoustic noise and attenuation when the ultrasound beam has to pass the abdominal wall of the mother.

During mid-pregnancy, the transabdominal route with a 5 MHz transducer usually gives acceptable images of the growing fetal brain. In vertex presentations, the transvaginal approach makes it possible to obtain very detailed information of the neuroanatomy (Timor-Tritsch & Monteagudo 1996).

At the end of the pregnancy, the increasing ossification of the skull impairs the examination of the brain, especially when the head is positioned low down in the maternal pelvis. Low frequencies such as 3.5–5 MHz have to be used for the transabdominal approach. As always in vertex presentations, the transvaginal route improves the imaging (Timor-Tritsch & Monteagudo 1996), though it may be very difficult to obtain the classic standard scan planes for the neuroanatomic examination as is done in the newborn (Cremin et al 1983). Because of the relatively large size of the head, lower frequencies are appropriate. The access through the fetal fontanelle as an optic window can be difficult in the asynclitic position of the head.

FIRST TRIMESTER, <14 WEEKS

2 WEEKS 0 DAYS TO APPROXIMATELY 6 WEEKS 6 DAYS

Embryology

The first 5 postovulatory weeks of embryonic development are described by Carnegie stages 1 to 15. The embryo develops from the unicellular stage 1 through stages characterized by the bilaminar and trilaminar disc into a cylindric body by a folding process. This folding process takes place during week 5 (LMP-based) and is completed at stage 12. The primordium of the CNS, the neural tube, develops from this ectodermal neural plate after a transitional stage of neuroectodermal folding. The closure of the caudal neuropore, creating the ventricular system, takes place at Carnegie stage 12 (O'Rahilly & Müller 2006), i.e. ≈5 weeks 6 days. At Carnegie stages 14 (≈6 weeks, 4 days) and 15 (≈6 weeks 5 days) the forebrain divides into the telencephalon, with the cerebral hemispheres as small evaginations, and into the diencephalon (O'Rahilly & Müller 2006). Then, the ventricular system is divided into five brain regions on its cranial pole: the telencephalon (future hemispheres) and the diencephalon (future between-brain) derive from the prosencephalon (forebrain); the mesencephalon (midbrain) remains undivided, and the metencephalon (future cerebellum and pons) and the myelencephalon (medulla oblongata) derive from the rhombencephalon (hindbrain).

Ultrasound

The pregnancy becomes detectable after 4.5 weeks as a ring structure lying in the decidua. Not before the end of week 6 do the first brain structures become identifiable. The hypoechogenic oblong cavity of the rhombencephalon is found at the top of the embryonic head/body (Fig. 4.1a–c).

7 WEEKS 0–6 DAYS; CROWN–RUMP LENGTH (CRL) 9–14 MM

Embryology

No longitudinal fissure is found between the laterally bulging cerebral hemispheres at this Carnegie stage. At the end of the week, at Carnegie stage 17 (≈7 weeks 5 days), the interventricular foramen is delimited by the corpus striatum and the ventral thalamus. The cerebellar primordium grows and the isthmus rhombencephali is evident.

Ultrasound

The hypoechogenic brain cavities can be identified, including the separated cerebral hemispheres (Fig. 4.2a–c). The lateral ventricles are shaped like small round vesicles. The cavity of the diencephalon (future third ventricle) runs posteriorly. The medial telencephalon forms a continuous cavity between the lateral ventricles. In the sagittal plane, the height of the cavity of the diencephalon (future third ventricle) is slightly greater than that of the mesencephalon (future Sylvian aqueduct). Thus, the wide border between the cavities of the diencephalon and the mesencephalon is

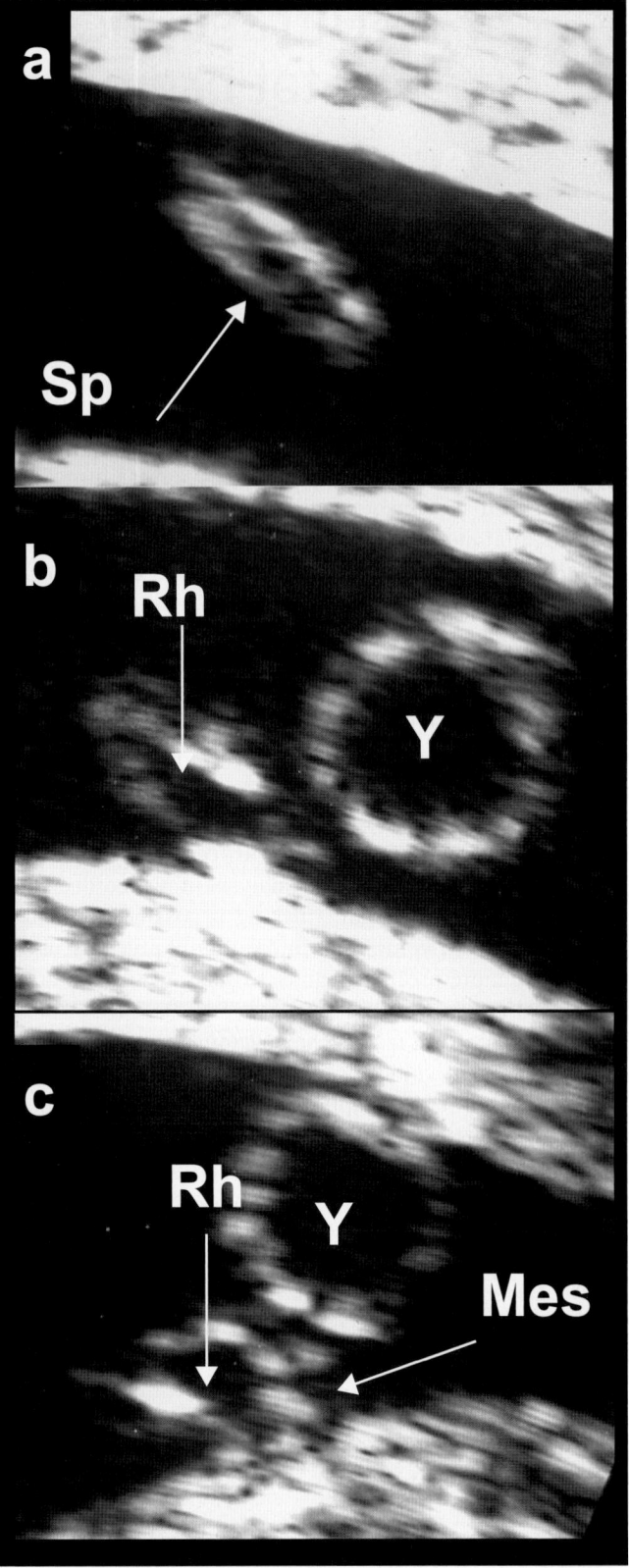

Figure 4.1 Ultrasound sections through a 7-week 0-day-old embryo. Crown–rump length 8 mm. (a) Coronal section through the spine (Sp). (b) Horizontal section through the head, the arrow points at the rhomboid cavity of the rhombencephalon (Rh); Y = yolk sac. (c) The section is tilted slightly anteriorly, in order to see the isthmus rhombencephali leading into the mesencephalic cavity (Mes); Y = yolk sac.

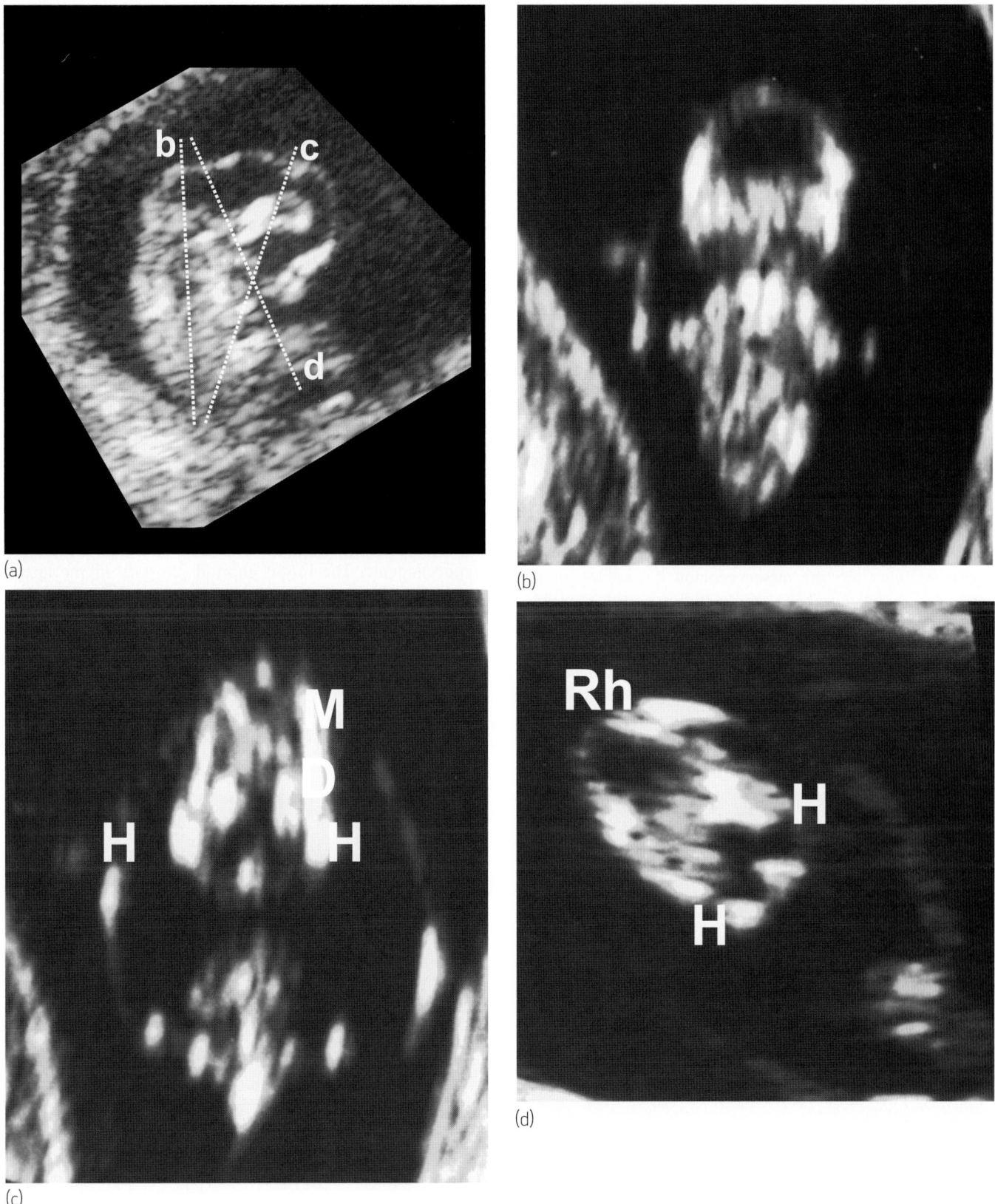

(a)

(b)

(c)

(d)

Figure 4.2 Images of an embryo at the end of week 7, Crown–rump length 13 mm. (a) Sagittal section, showing the continuum of the brain cavities from the shallow fourth ventricle in the top of the head, via the bent mesencephalic cavity (to the right) into the third ventricle (down to the left); the lines indicate the sections in parts (b–c). (b) Posterior coronal section, showing the typical 'hole in the head', which is the fourth ventricle. (c) Anterior coronal section through the mesencephalon (M), diencephalon (D) and hemispheres (H). (d) This section shows the rhombencephalic cavity (Rh) and the forebrain divided into two hemispheres (H).

indicated. The curved tube-like mesencephalic cavity lies anteriorly, its rostral part pointing caudally. It straightens considerably during the subsequent weeks. By week 8 it is regularly identified. The rather broad and shallow rhombencephalic cavity is always visible. It has a well-defined rhombic shape in the cranial pole of the embryo. The future spine appears as two parallel lines (Fig. 4.1a).

8 WEEKS 0–6 DAYS; CRL 15–22 MM
Embryology
Half of the diencephalon is covered by the hemispheres. The mesencephalon is on the top of the brain (O'Rahilly & Müller 1987). The choroid plexuses of the lateral ventricles and of the fourth ventricle develop at stage 18 (O'Rahilly & Müller 2006).

Ultrasound
The brain cavities are easily seen as large 'holes' in the embryonic head (Figs 4.2 and 4.3). The hemispheres enlarge, developing via thick round slices originating anterocaudally from the third ventricle into a crescent shape. The choroid plexus in the lateral ventricles becomes visible as tiny echogenic areas. The future foramina of Monro become more accentuated. The third ventricle is still wide, as is the mesencephalic cavity. At this time, the mesencephalon lies on top of the head. The rhombencephalic cavity (future fourth ventricle) has a pyramid-like shape with the central deepening of the pontine flexure as the peak of the pyramid. The first signs of the bilateral choroid plexuses are lateral echogenic areas originating near the branches of the medulla oblongata caudal to the lateral recesses. Within a short time, the choroid plex-

uses traverse the roof of the fourth ventricle, meeting at the midline and dividing the roof into two portions (Fig. 4.4; see Fig. 4.6a,b); about two-thirds are located rostrally and one-third caudally. In the sagittal section, the choroid plexuses are identified as an echogenic fold of the roof.

9 WEEKS 0–6 DAYS; CRL 23–31 MM
Embryology
The chondrocranium and the skeletogenous layer of the head become recognizable. At the end of the embryonic period, the falx cerebri starts to develop from the skeletogenous layer. The cerebral hemispheres nearly conceal the diencephalon. Fusion of the medial walls of the hemispheres does not occur during the embryonic period. The foramina of Monro reduce to dorso-ventral slits. The insula appears. The thalami are thickening. The cavity of the mesencephalon is still wide. The rhombic lips have developed into cerebellar hemispheres. The choroid plexuses of the fourth ventricle divide the roof into the pars membranacea superior and inferior.

Ultrasound
The lateral ventricles are always visible. Their size increases rapidly. They are best seen in the parasagittal plane, where the C-shape becomes apparent. The cortex is smooth and hypoechogenic. The bright choroid plexuses of the lateral ventricles are regularly detectable at 9 weeks 4 days (Fig. 4.5c). They show rapid growth, similar to the hemispheres, and soon fill most of the ventricular cavities.

In the 2-D image, the width of the diencephalic cavity narrows gradually while the width of the mesencephalon remains wide (Fig. 4.5a). The wall of the diencephalon,

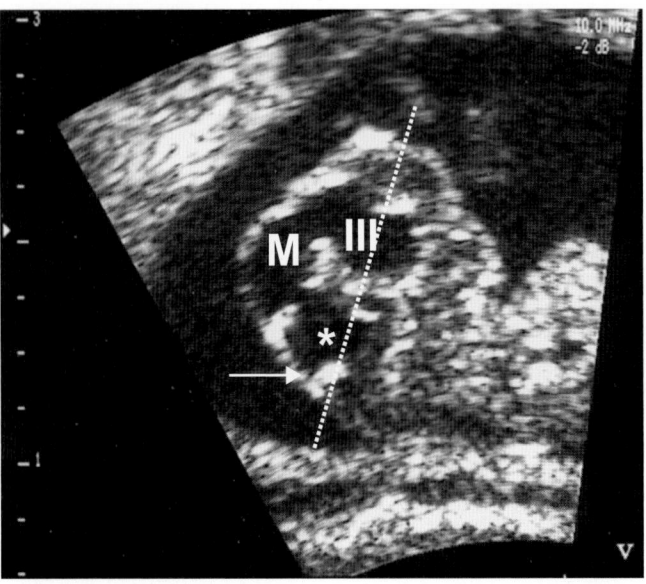

Figure 4.3 Sagittal section through an embryo, Crown–rump length 22 mm; the arrow points at the choroid plexus in the roof of the fourth ventricle (*); the pontine flexure is deep (cf. Fig. 4.2a). M = mesencephalic cavity, III = third ventricle.

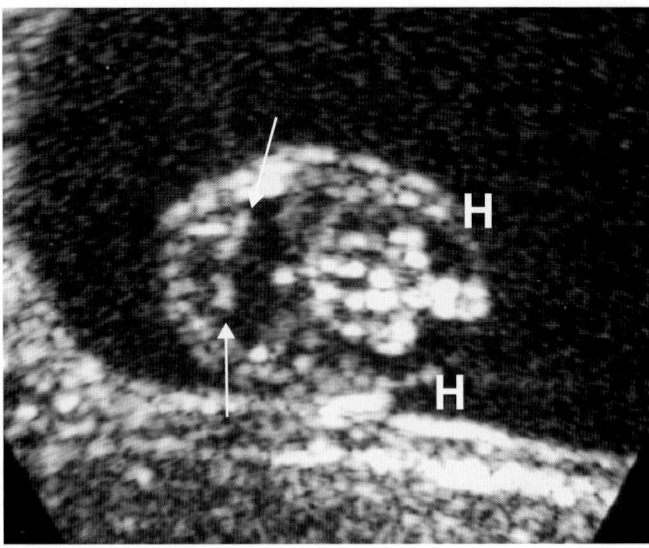

Figure 4.4 Section (stippled line in Fig. 4.3) through the head of a 9-week-old embryo, Crown–rump length 23 mm; the arrows point at the choroid plexuses of the fourth ventricle (cf. Fig. 4.2d); the echogenic choroid plexuses of the hemispheres (H) can be seen.

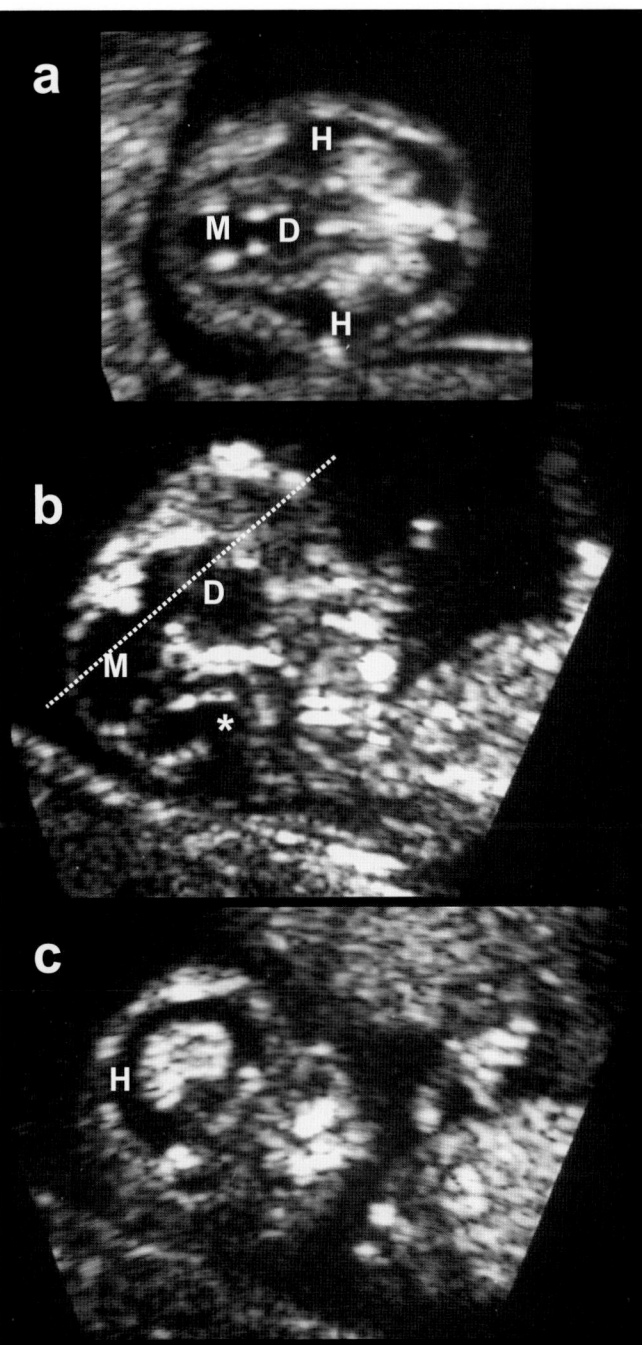

Figure 4.5 Ultrasound images of an embryo at the end of the embryonic period. Crown–rump length 31 mm. (a) Horizontal section through the mesencephalon, diencephalon and hemispheres (cf. part b, stippled line). (b) Sagittal section through the head, the stippled line indicates the section of part a; anterior to the fourth ventricle (*) lies the pons; D = diencephalon, M = mesencephalon. (c) Parasagittal section through a hemisphere (H); the cortex is thin, the echogenic choroid plexus lies in the hypoechogenic ventricle.

initially very thin, thickens considerably starting from week 8 to 9. The volume of the third ventricle decreases during week 9 and the cavity becomes narrow, especially at its upper anterior part due to the growing thalami. A distinct border ('isthmus prosencephali') has developed between the cavity of the mesencephalon and the third ventricle.

The cavity of the mesencephalon remains relatively large (Fig. 4.5a,b), especially the posterior part. The height and the width are about equal in size. The isthmus rhomben-cephali is always distinct.

During weeks 8 and 9, the rhombic fossa becomes deeper due to the progressive flexure of the pons (Figs 4.2a, 4.3 and 4.5b). The lateral corners of the rhombencephalic cavity, called the lateral recesses (Fig. 4.4), are easily identified at 7 and 8 weeks. During this period, the distance between these recesses increases (rhombencephalon width). Later, during weeks 9 and 10, the lateral recesses often become covered by the enlarging cerebellar hemispheres. Thus only the central part of the hypoechogenic fourth ventricle, which is divided by the choroid plexuses, is visible. The choroid plexuses of the fourth ventricle are bright landmarks dividing the ventricle into a rostral and a caudal compart-ment (Fig. 4.6a). There is a clear gap between the rhomben-cephalic and the mesencephalic cavity due to the growing cerebellum, which is easily detectable. The primordia of cerebellar hemispheres are clearly separated in the midline during the embryonic period. The isthmus rhombencephali is narrow; in most cases it is not visible in its complete length. The spine is still characterized by two echogenic parallel lines.

EARLY POSTEMBRYONIC PERIOD, 10 AND 11 WEEKS, CRL 32–54 MM

Anatomic development

A staging system for the fetal period is not available. Among the most noticeable external changes of the brain are the apparent union of the cerebellar hemispheres with the devel-opment of the upper vermis and the increasing concealment of the diencephalon and mesencephalon by the cerebral hemispheres. The cerebellum enlarges, drawing the roof of the fourth ventricle beneath its caudal border. The mesen-cephalic cavity is still wide.

Various 2-D measurements for the embryonic/fetal brain and brain cavities have been proposed (Day 1959, O'Rahilly & Müller 1990, Westergaard 1971), but no systematic stan-dardized measurements of the embryonic brain have been adopted. The development of the form of the brain compart-ments was demonstrated by 3-D reconstructions from his-tological slices as shown by Hochstetter (Hochstetter 1919, Kostovic 1990) using the technique described by Born (1883), or by 3-D casts from the lateral ventricles of aborted speci-mens (Day 1959, Westergaard 1971, Woollam 1952). Jenkins calculated the volumes of embryonic and fetal brain com-partments obtained from 3-D reconstructions of a few speci-mens from the Carnegie collection (Jenkins 1921).

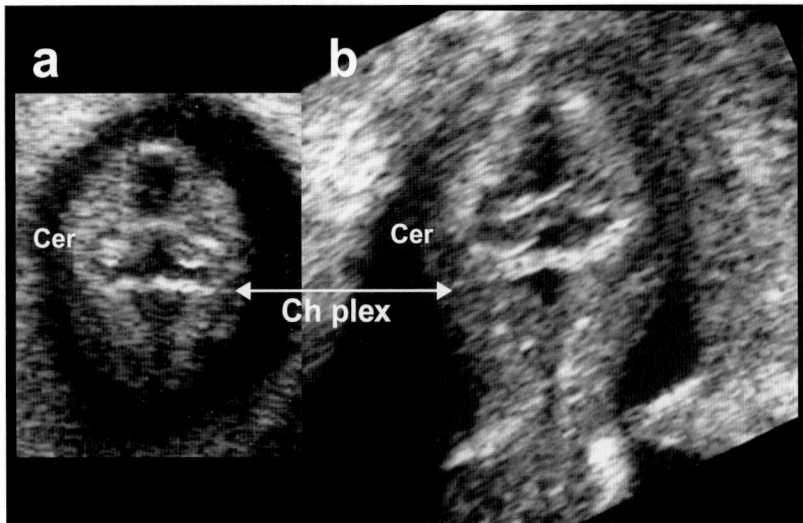

Figure 4.6 (a) Coronal section through the posterior head of a 9-week-old embryo. Crown–rump length (CRL) 25 mm; the choroid plexuses (Ch plex) divide the roof of the fourth ventricle into an area membranacea superior and inferior. (b) Coronal section through the posterior head of an 11-week-old fetus, CRL 45 mm; the choroid plexuses lie close to the caudal border of the cerebellar hemispheres; the double-headed arrow points at the echogenic choroid plexuses; Cer = cerebellum.

Ultrasound

The thick crescent lateral ventricles fill the anterior part of the head and conceal the diencephalic cavity. The thickness of the cortex is about 1 mm at the end of the first trimester. The diencephalon lies between the hemispheres, and the mesencephalon gradually moves towards the center of the head. The width of the third ventricle definitely becomes narrow towards the end of the first trimester. There is a gap between the mesencephalic and the rhombencephalic cavity which is filled with the growing cerebellum. The cerebellar hemispheres seem to meet in the midline during weeks 11 to 12. After 10 weeks 3 days, the choroid plexuses of the fourth ventricle can always be seen. The distance between the choroid plexuses and the cerebellum becomes shorter during weeks 9 to 11 (Fig. 4.6b). At the end of the first trimester the choroid plexuses are found close to the caudal border of the cerebellum. Successively, the ossification of the spine appears.

The reference points for measuring the head of the second trimester fetus (biparietal diameter (BPD), occipito-frontal diameter (OFD), and head circumference (HC)) such as the cavum septi pellucidi and thalami are not formed in the first trimester. The shape of the embryonic head and the position of the intracranial structures change significantly during the early development, as described in the embryologic literature (O'Rahilly & Müller 2006). At 7 weeks, at Carnegie stages 16 and 17, the horizontal plane through the embryonic head includes the rhombencephalon and the posterior part of the mesencephalon. This plane lies above the diencephalon and the hemispheres. The largest width is found at the height of the rhombic lips, the future cerebellum. The greatest length extends from the cervical flexure to the

anterior wall of the bent mesencephalon. Owing to the development of the brain, characterized by uneven growth of the brain compartments and by the 'deflection' of the brain, the greatest width alters its position during the embryonic and early fetal period. At the beginning of week 9, Carnegie stages 21 and 22, the plane for the measurement of the head size includes the hemispheres anteriorly, the diencephalon in the middle of the head, and the cerebellum posteriorly. At the end of the embryonic period, at Carnegie stage 23, the measurement plane comprises the hemispheres, the diencephalon and the upper part of the cerebellum. In the early fetal period, the future cranium becomes successively distinguishable. Thus, the terms BPD and OFD are basically not suitable for the embryonic period, and it would be more correct to use terms like 'width of the head' and 'antero-posterior diameter'. There is a sliding transition from the embryonic 'head width' to the fetal 'biparietal diameter,' therefore the historically oldest term BPD should be kept.

3-D MEASUREMENTS

Table 4.1 (Blaas & Eik-Nes 2002b) and Figure 4.7 (Blaas et al 1998) show volume calculations of the brain cavities of 34 7–10-week-old embryos/fetuses (Blaas et al 1998; Blaas & Eik-Nes 2002a, 2002b). These volume estimations of embryonic brains represent new insight into embryonic development with information that could not be obtained from aborted specimens. When we look at the 3-D images and volume estimations of the specimens in Figures 4.7 and 4.8, we clearly perceive the dynamic process that alters the appearance of the brain within a few weeks. The brain compartments change rapidly in their form, size and relation to one another; for example, the telencephalon develops from

Table 4.1 Mean (± 2 SD) volumes of embryonic body and cavities of the brain (N = 34). In the 3D segmentation process, the brain cavities were outlined at the inner surfaces of the ventricular walls. The choroid plexus were included in the measurements. CRL = crown–rump length. (Reprinted with permission from Cambridge Press (Blaas and Eik-Nes 2002))

CRL mm	Body (mm³)	Total brain (mm³)	Hemispheres (mm³)	Diencephalon (mm³)	Mesencephalon (mm³)	Rhombencephalon (mm³)
10	96 (209; 26)	5.2 (18.2; 0.1)	0.5 (2.7; 0.0)	1.7 (4.8; 0.2)	1.1 (3.3; 0.1)	7.3 (15.9; 2.0)
15	402 (611; 237)	25.6 (49.4; 9.5)	6.7 (15.1; 2.2)	4.4 (9.0; 1.5)	3.6 (7.1; 1.3)	13.4 (24.4; 5.7)
20	918 (1222; 657)	61.3 (96.1, 34.3)	25.9 (44.6; 13.4)	6.7 (12.1; 2.8)	6.6 (11.2; 3.2)	18.8 (31.6; 9.4)
25	1644 (2044; 1288)	112.4 (158.1; 74.4)	65.7 (98.7; 41.0)	7.5 (13.3; 3.4)	9.4 (14.7; 5.3)	22.6 (36.4; 12.0)
30	2581 (3076; 2129)	178.8 (235.3; 129.9)	133.4 (184.8; 92.6)	6.7 (12.1; 2.9)	11.5 (17.3; 6.9)	23.9 (38.1; 13.0)
35	3727 (4318; 3180)	260.5 (328.0; 200.7)	236.6 (310.4; 175.5)	4.5 (9.1; 1.5)	12.5 (18.6; 7.7)	22.7 (36.5; 12.1)

CRL 10 mm ≅ 7 weeks 2 days gestational age based on the last menstrual period
CRL 15 mm ≅ 8 weeks 0 days
CRL 20 mm ≅ 8 weeks 5 days
CRL 25 mm ≅ 9 weeks 2 days
CRL 30 mm ≅ 9 weeks 6 days
CRL 35 mm ≅ 10 weeks 2 days

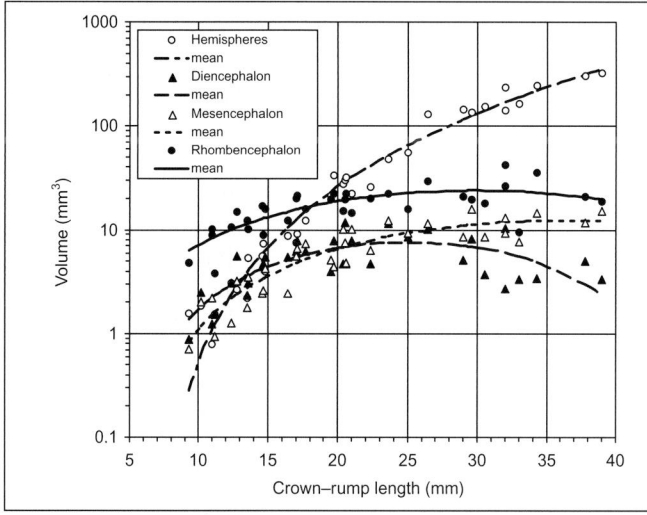

Figure 4.7 Measurements and mean volume of lateral ventricles, cavities of diencephalon, mesencephalon, and rhombencephalon. (Reprinted with permission from Elsevier Science, *The Lancet* (Blaas et al 1998)).

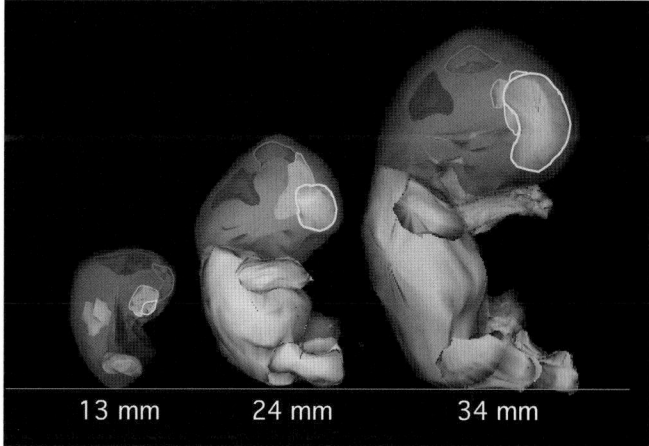

Figure 4.8 3D reconstructions of two embryos, 13 mm ≈ 7 weeks, 24 mm ≈ 9 weeks and one fetus, 34 mm ≈ 10 weeks. The cavities of the brain are colored: blue = rhombencephalon, red = mesencephalon, green = diencephalon, yellow = lateral ventricles.

two tiny balls into large crescent-shaped cavities, dominating the brain at the end of the first trimester. The cavity of the rhombencephalon alters too. Initially, at 7 weeks, it lies as a large, shallow and broad cavity in the top of the head. Later, it becomes deeper and shorter, as is also reflected by the change of the angle of the pontine flexure, and it is 'pushed' posteriorly. The ultrasound volume estimations of the brain (Table 4.1) correspond well with Jenkins' solid 3-D reconstructions of two embryos (Jenkins 1921). Jenkins calculated the volume of the brain to be 41 mm³ in an embryo with a CRL of 16 mm, and 126 mm³ in an embryo with a CRL of 25 mm.

The 2-D and 3-D ultrasound analyses of the embryonic brain compartments reflect, so to speak, the phylogenetic development of the brain: the 'old' rhombencephalon is large during the early phase, while the 'young' hemispheres are very small. During a few weeks, this correlation becomes reversed. Ultrasound also reveals another embryonic feature: the cavities of the diencephalon (third ventricle) and mesencephalon (Sylvian aqueduct) are relatively very large. The mean diameter of the mesencephalic cavity even has a similar diameter in the early postembryonic period, as it is found in children and adults (Flyger & Hjelmquist 1957).

LATE FIRST TRIMESTER, 12 AND 13 WEEKS, BPD ≫20–29 MM

Anatomic development

The lateral ventricle has an anterior and an inferior horn. From approximately 11 weeks on (CRL >40 mm), the posterior horn becomes visible (Westergaard 1971). The hippocampal formation and its subdivisions are identifiable in fetuses of CRL 70 mm (Lemire 1975). The massa intermedia is a tissue bridge of gray matter which develops between the dorsal thalami and crosses the third ventricle in most individuals (Lemire 1975). The development of the corpus callosum begins at about 12–13 weeks, thus creating one of the main landmarks for the ultrasound evaluation of the head, namely the cavum septi pellucidi. Whether the cavum septi pellucidi initially is an open pocket that is bridged by the corpus callosum, or is formed by necrosis within the massa commissuralis, is not certain (O'Rahilly & Müller 1994). The aqueduct is still relatively large and the corpus callosum is still limited to the rostral region (O'Rahilly & Müller 1994).

Ultrasound

The smooth hemispheres dominate the brain. The thickness of the cortex is between 1 and 2 mm. The lateral ventricles are large and filled by the echogenic choroid plexuses. The insula appears as a slight depression on the lateral surface. The third ventricle has become a narrow slit (Fig. 4.9). In early hydrocephaly, the massa intermedia may be detected in a dilated third ventricle (Blaas & Eik-Nes 1999). The cavity of the mesencephalon is still wide. The choroid plexuses of the fourth ventricle are 'pulled' to the lower border of the cerebellar hemispheres, the fourth ventricle is found covered by the cerebellum.

SECOND TRIMESTER

APPROXIMATELY 14 TO 27 WEEKS, BPD ≫30–74 MM

Anatomic development

The cavum septi pellucidi becomes a landmark in the horizontal imaging of the brain. Its width increases slowly from 3.4 mm at 19–20 weeks to 6.4 mm at 27–28 weeks (Jou et al 1998). The posterior horns of the lateral ventricles gradually become more elongated, as shown in casts from fetal ventricles (Kier 1977, Westergaard 1971). The hippocampus in the human temporal lobe projects into the temporal horn (Kier 1977). Sulci begin to appear on the surface of the cerebral hemisphere at about the middle of prenatal life (Dorovini-Zis & Dolman 1977, O'Rahilly & Müller 2006). Chi and coworkers have described the chronological development of the gyri and sulci (Chi et al 1976): together with the development of the corpus callosum, the corresponding callosal sulcus appears at the 14th week. The corpus callosum forms the roof of a cavity, which is the cavum septi pellucidi et Vergae. This cavity usually closes postnatally when the infant is 2 months old (Shaw & Alvord 1969). During 16 to 19 weeks the cingulate gyrus appears on the medial surface of the hemispheres. At the same time, the parieto-occipital fissure appears and delineates the primitive occipital lobe from the parietal lobe, while the calcarine fissure gradually indents the occipital horn of the lateral ventricle. By 27 weeks, the adjacent cuneus and lingual

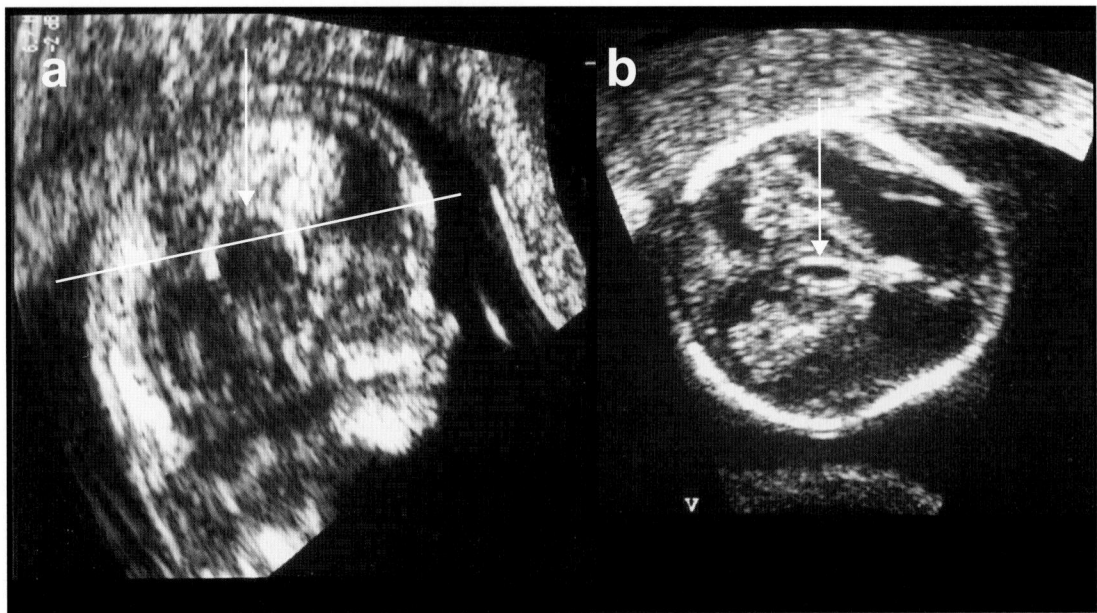

Figure 4.9 (a) Sagittal section through the head of a 13-week-old fetus; the third ventricle lies relatively high in the middle of the head (arrow). (b) Horizontal section as indicated in part a; the arrow points at the third ventricle, which should not be taken for the cavum septi pellucidi.

gyrus have become distinct. Between 20 and 23 weeks, the central sulcus and the superior temporal sulcus appear. Before the end of the second trimester, additional sulci become visible, such as the pre- and postcentral sulcus, the middle temporal sulcus, the interparietal sulcus, superior frontal sulcus, and lateral occipital sulcus. The cavity of the mesencephalon becomes gradually reduced, particularly because of the growth of the tectum (Kier 1977). The cerebellar development is not completed at the beginning of the second trimester: the midline fusion of the cerebellar primordia gives rise to the vermis, which progressively grows caudally and dorsally with the cerebellar hemispheres, but at a relatively slower rate (Lemire 1975; Müller & O'Rahilly 1990). Primary and secondary folia of the vermis and the cerebellar hemispheres appear during the first half of the second trimester (Lemire 1975).

Ultrasound

By scanning in different planes, it is possible to evaluate the shape of the brain and its ventricles (Figs 4.10 and 4.11). Recently, guidelines for the 'basic examination' of the CNS and for the 'fetal neurosonogram' have been published that show how horizontal, coronal and sagittal sections can be used to examine the CNS systematically (ISUOG Guidelines 2007).

Since ultrasound has been introduced, many biometric parameters and ratios have been proposed to evaluate the fetal brain and its ventricular system. Examples of such parameters are cerebro-frontal horn distance (Goldstein et al 1988), cerebro-atrial distance (Pilu et al 1989), posterior horn width, cerebro-posterior horn distance (Goldstein et al 1990), occipital horn height, thalamus-to-tip-of-occipital-horn distance, midline-to-edge of lateral ventricle (Monteagudo et al 1993) and many others. A variety of these parameters have been presented and discussed in a comprehensive outline by Monteagudo and coworkers (Monteagudo et al 1996). For the clinical practice simple measurements are preferable. The atrial width of the lateral ventricle (Fig. 4.10b) has shown to have a constant value throughout the second and third trimesters as shown by Cardoza and coworkers (7.6 ± 0.6 mm) and Pilu and coworkers (6.9 ± 1.3 mm) (Cardoza et al 1988, Pilu et al 1989). Therefore, atrial diameters above 10 mm should raise the suspicion of ventriculomegaly (Cardoza et al 1988). The surface of the cortices can be evaluated by tangential (oblique) sections (Fig. 4.11c), which is not easy, or by sections perpendicular to the surface of the brain. In a study involving 262 normal fetuses, the gestational age at which fissures and sulci were first detected was 14 weeks for the callosal sulcus, 18 weeks for the lateral sulcus, the parieto-occipital and calcarine fissures, and 26 weeks for the cingulate sulcus (Monteagudo & Timor-Tritsch 1997). The third ventricle is relatively well imaged in the early second trimester, but it narrows as gestation progresses, and develops into a virtual space between the thalami (Fig. 4.10a) (Timor-Tritsch & Monteagudo 1996).

The corpus callosum and the cavum septi pellucidi are easily depicted in the sagittal section (Figs 4.11a, 4.12 and 4.13a). The cerebral aqueduct of Sylvius develops into a narrow tube during the early second trimester. The lower cerebellar vermis may still be small until 16–18 weeks (Babcook et al 1996, Bromley et al 1994). There are no normative data on the size of the fetal fourth ventricle at 12–24 weeks of gestation. Bronshtein and colleagues noted that the lateral diameter of the fourth ventricle comprises less than half of the lateral cerebellar width, while the postero-anterior diameter of the fourth ventricle is less than two-thirds of the cerebellar postero-anterior diameter (Bronshtein et al 1998).

Measurements of the transverse diameter of the cerebellum have shown that the value of this parameter expressed in millimeters corresponded approximately to the gestational age expressed in weeks during the second trimester (Goldstein et al 1987; Hata et al 1989). Thus, the mean transverse diameter was found to be 14 mm at 15 weeks, increasing to 30–31 mm at 27 weeks (Goldstein et al 1987, Hill et al 1990). The depth of the cisterna magna is measured as the midline diameter from the inner table of the occiput to the posterior aspect of the cerebellum in the standard horizontal plane of the cerebellum. The mean depth of the cisterna magna in normal second and third trimester fetuses is 5 ± 3 mm, with a maximum of 10 mm (Mahony et al 1984). Typically one can find septa-like linear echoes extending approximately from the edges of the vermis towards the posterior wall of the posterior fossa (Fig. 4.14). These cisterna magna septa have been extensively described by Robinson and Goldstein, who suggest that they represent the walls of the Blake pouch, a phylogenetic vestigial structure observed during ontogeny, the remnants of which are probably present in the neonatal period (Robinson & Goldstein 2007). A persistent Blake pouch, because of a failure of fenestration of the Blake pouch and the foramen of Luschka, might lead to dilatation of the fourth ventricle and elevation of a normal vermis.

THREE-DIMENSIONAL ULTRASOUND

During the last ten years 3-D ultrasound has been increasingly used as a tool for neurosonography. A sagittal section through the brain is important for the evaluation of cerebral midline structures such as the corpus callosum and the vermis cerebelli. The lateral position of the fetal head in the second and especially third trimester makes it often difficult to obtain adequate imaging of these brain structures. However, 3-D sonography permits 'navigating' in the volume scan of fetal brains using the multiplanar mode and creating new ultrasound sections that were not obtainable in the original 2-D scan either by the transvaginal (Monteagudo et al 2000) or transabdominal approach (Correa et al 2006). The 3-D operator must bear in mind that the resolution in the range plane, which lies perpendicular to the axial ultrasound beam, is significantly poorer than in the azimuth

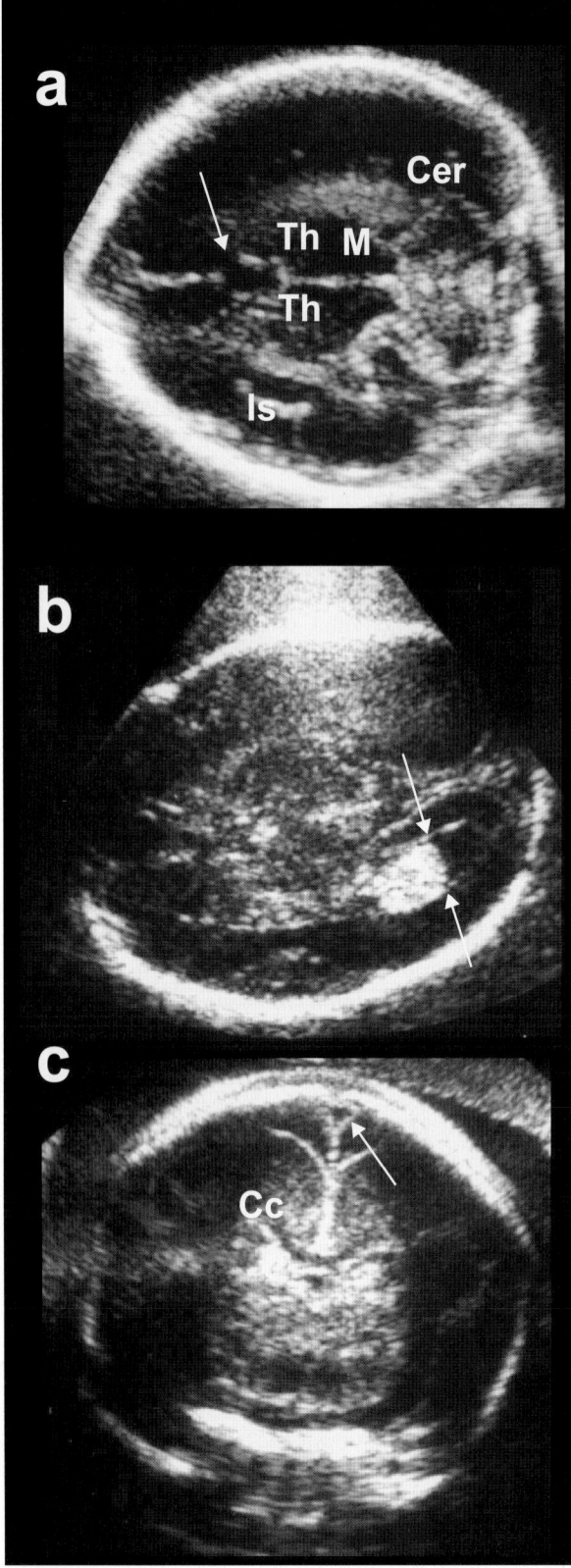

Figure 4.10 Ultrasound sections through the head of fetuses between 22 and 25 weeks. (a) Horizontal section through the cavum septi pellucidi (arrow), thalami (Th), mesencephalon (M) and cerebellum (Cer), Is = insula and lateral sulcus. (b) Horizontal section through the lateral ventricle with emphasis on the atrium; the arrows indicate where to measure the lateral ventricular atrium width. (c) Coronal section, showing the superior sagittal venous sinus (arrow) and the corpus callosum (Cc).

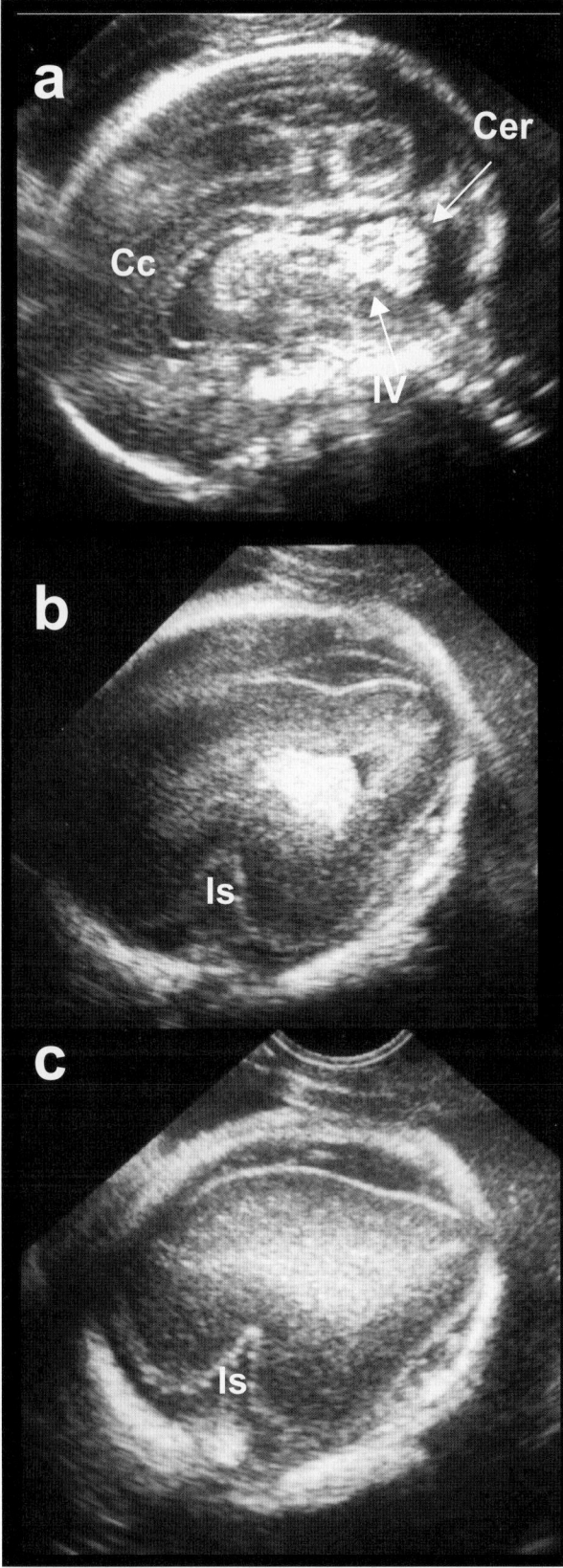

Figure 4.11 Ultrasound sections through the head of fetuses between 22 and 25 weeks. (a) Sagittal section through the corpus callosum (Cc), cavum septi pellucidi, diencephalon, mesencephalon, cerebellum (Cer) and fourth ventricle (IV). (b) Oblique section through the posterior of the lateral ventricle with its echogenic choroid plexus; Is = lateral sulcus. (c) Further oblique section through the smooth cortex and the lateral sulcus.

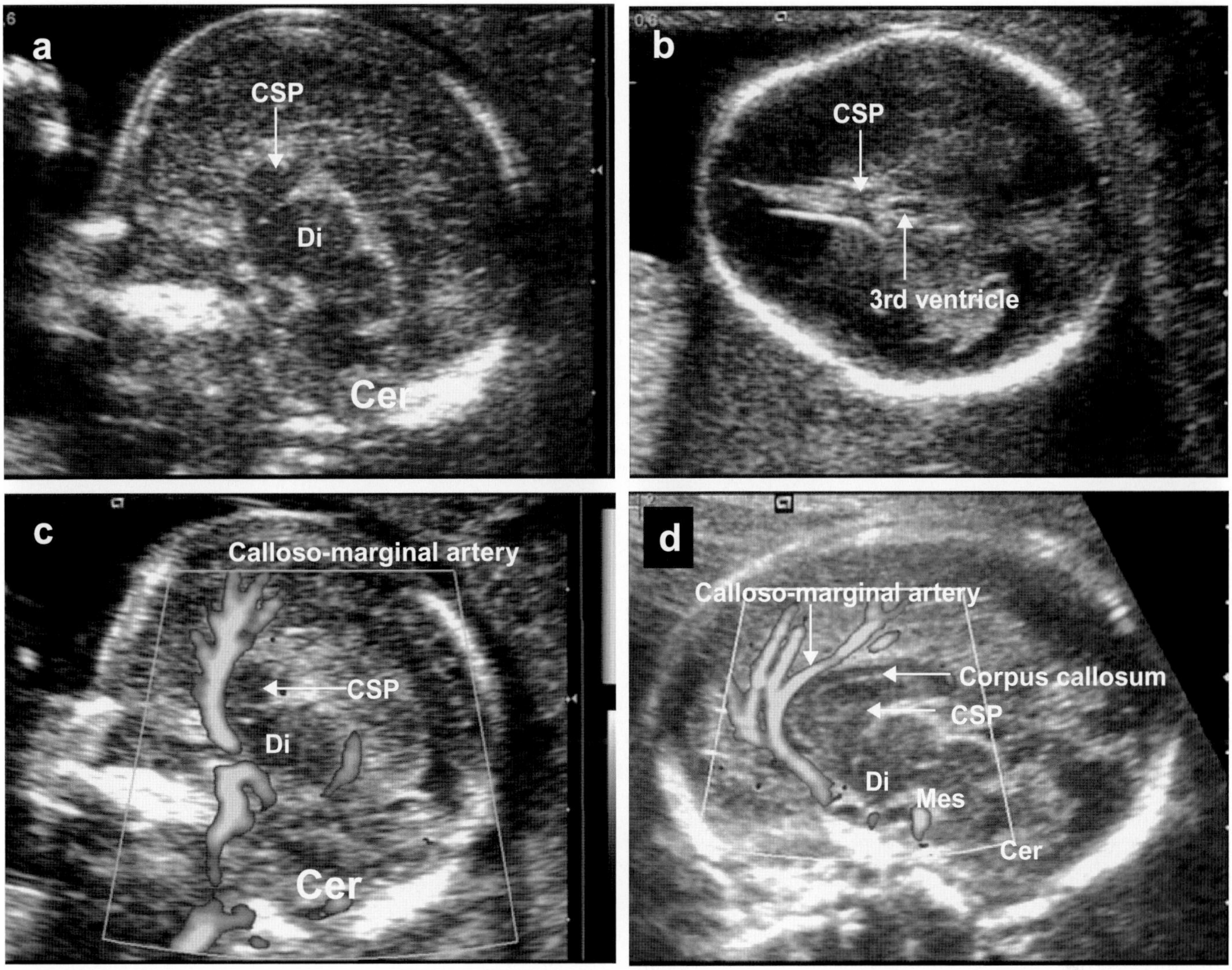

Figure 4.12 Ultrasound sections through the head of a 15-week-old fetus (a–c) and a 22-week-old fetus (d). (a) Sagittal section through the cavum septi pellucidi (CSP), diencephalon (Di) and cerebellum (Cer). (b) Horizontal section showing the area of the developing corpus callosum and CSP; the third ventricle is a narrow split. (c) Power Doppler of the anterior cerebral artery, its branches and its continuation into the calloso-marginal artery. (d) Sagittal section as in (c); the corpus callosum and CSP are well developed; Mes = mesencephalon.

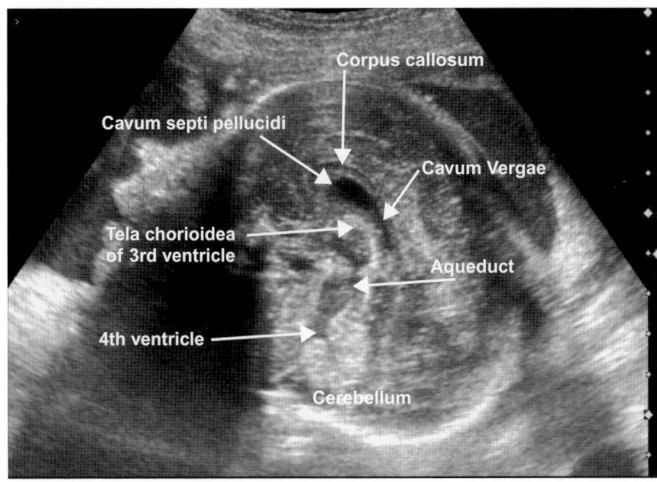

Figure 4.13 Sagittal image of the central brain, showing the rather large corpus callosum, the cavum septi pellucidi and cavum Vergae at 28 weeks (cf. Fig. 4.12). The roof of the third ventricle consists of the echogenic tela chorioidea. The sylvian aqueduct can be identified.

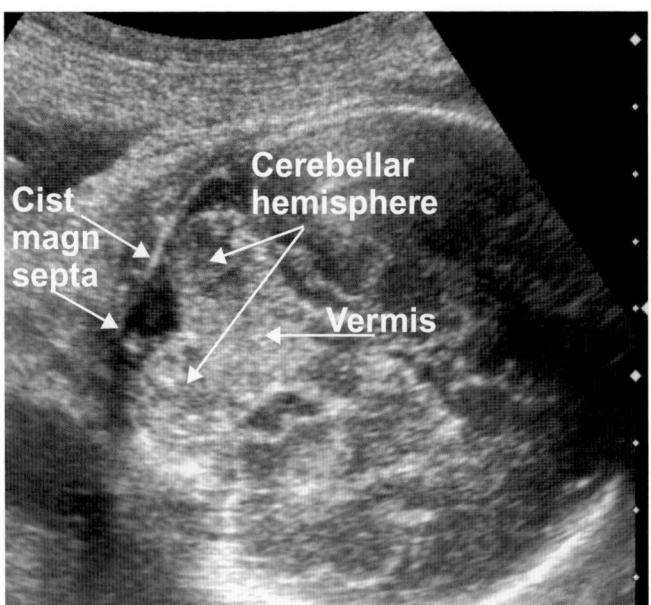

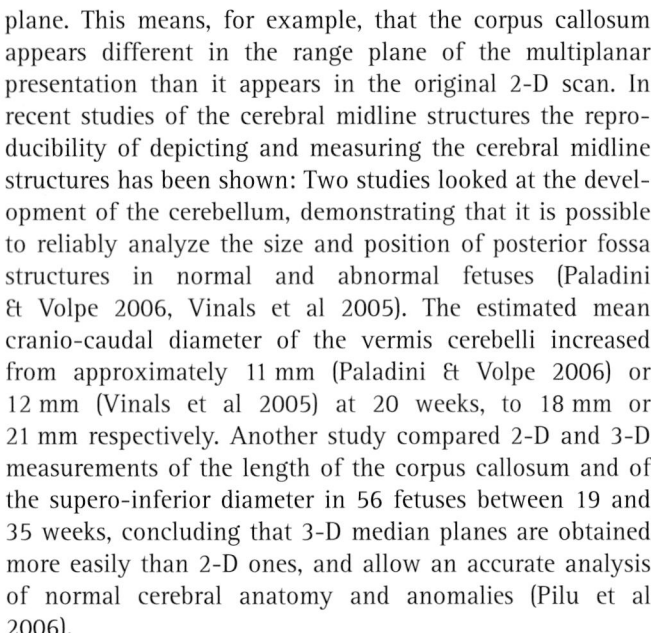

Figure 4.14 Horizontal section through hemispheres and vermis of the cerebellum at 28 weeks. The arrows point at the septa of the cisterna magna (Cist magn septa).

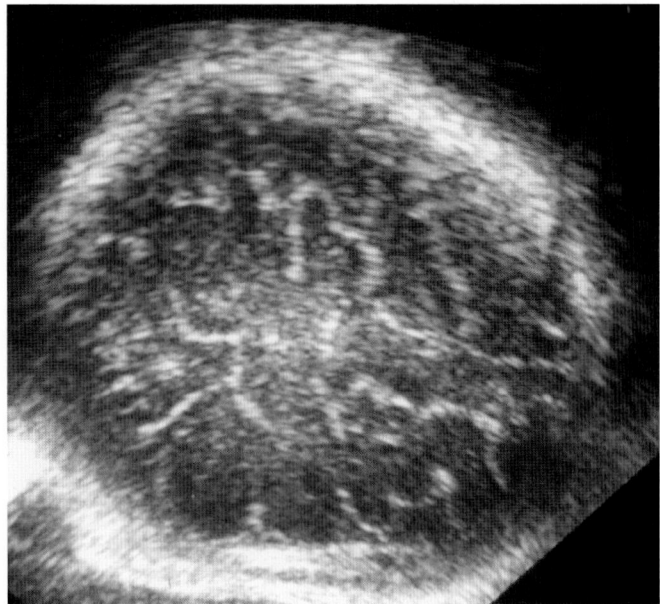

Figure 4.15 Oblique section of the cortex at 36 weeks showing numerous sulci (echogenic lines) and gyri.

plane. This means, for example, that the corpus callosum appears different in the range plane of the multiplanar presentation than it appears in the original 2-D scan. In recent studies of the cerebral midline structures the reproducibility of depicting and measuring the cerebral midline structures has been shown: Two studies looked at the development of the cerebellum, demonstrating that it is possible to reliably analyze the size and position of posterior fossa structures in normal and abnormal fetuses (Paladini & Volpe 2006, Vinals et al 2005). The estimated mean cranio-caudal diameter of the vermis cerebelli increased from approximately 11 mm (Paladini & Volpe 2006) or 12 mm (Vinals et al 2005) at 20 weeks, to 18 mm or 21 mm respectively. Another study compared 2-D and 3-D measurements of the length of the corpus callosum and of the supero-inferior diameter in 56 fetuses between 19 and 35 weeks, concluding that 3-D median planes are obtained more easily than 2-D ones, and allow an accurate analysis of normal cerebral anatomy and anomalies (Pilu et al 2006).

Volume reconstructions of fetal brain cavities during the second and third trimester have shown that it is possible to illustrate the development of the shape (Pooh et al 2000). When we look at the casts of the lateral ventricles from the first (Blaas et al 1995, 1998) to the third trimesters (Pooh et al 2000), we can see that the differentiation of the posterior and inferior horns of the ventricles develops at the end of the first and the beginning of the second trimester. Further, volume calculations of the total fetal brain reflect a nearly 10-fold increase between 18 and 34 weeks of pregnancy, representing 14–17% of the total estimated fetal weight (Roelfsema et al 2003).

THIRD TRIMESTER

APPROXIMATELY 28 WEEKS TO TERM, BIPARIETAL DIAMETER = 75 MM

Anatomic development

At 28 weeks, the appearance of the superior temporal sulcus is a constant feature (Dorovini-Zis & Dolman 1977). A great growth spurt occurs between the 28th and 30th weeks: numerous sulci and gyri develop, and the brain assumes a much more 'finished' appearance. After 30 weeks, the assessment of gestational age by looking at the external brain becomes more difficult (Dorovini-Zis & Dolman 1977). By the 40th week, tertiary sulci have made their appearance (Dorovini-Zis & Dolman 1977). The insula remains smooth until 28–29 weeks, after which the frontal, temporal and parietal opercula begin to override it (Chi et al 1976).

Ultrasound

The diameter of the cavum septi pellucidi decreases from 6.1 mm at 29–30 weeks to 5.5 mm at 41–42 weeks (Jou et al 1998). The transverse diameter of the cerebellum increases from 31–33 mm at 28 weeks to 52 mm at 40 weeks (Goldstein et al 1987, Hill et al 1990). In principle, it is possible to depict all hemispherical sulci by ultrasound. Still, the complexity of the cerebral surface makes the correlation of a sonographically described sulcus with the correct definition on the anatomical map difficult (Fig. 4.15). Therefore, usually only the main sulci may be identified, especially those on the median surfaces of the hemispheres, which are rather easily identifiable by sagittal and coronal sections (Timor-Tritsch & Monteagudo 1996). The increased ossification of the skull at the end of the pregnancy impedes the accessibility for the ultrasound imaging of the brain, such that the transfontanelle approach becomes essential.

VASCULATURE OF THE BRAIN

The blood supply of the brain originates from an anterior circulation through the internal carotid arteries, and a posterior circulation through the vertebral arteries via the common single basilar artery. These arterial circulations communicate with each other through the circulus arteriosus of Willis (Fig. 4.16a,b). The main components of the circulus arteriosus are present at Carnegie stage 16 and the circle is

complete at Carnegie stage 19 (O'Rahilly & Müller 2006). The middle cerebral artery (MCA) is the largest branch of the circle and runs laterally in the sylvian fissure as a direct continuation of the internal carotid artery. The two MCAs supply most of the cerebral cortex on the convexity of the hemispheres, and the deep parts of the cerebrum, such as

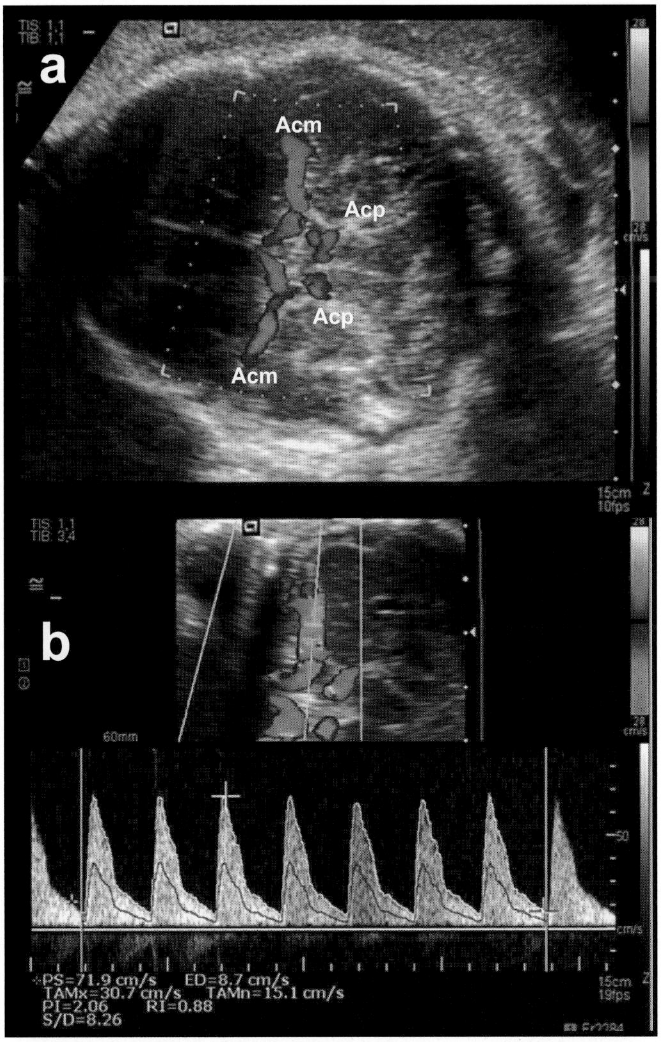

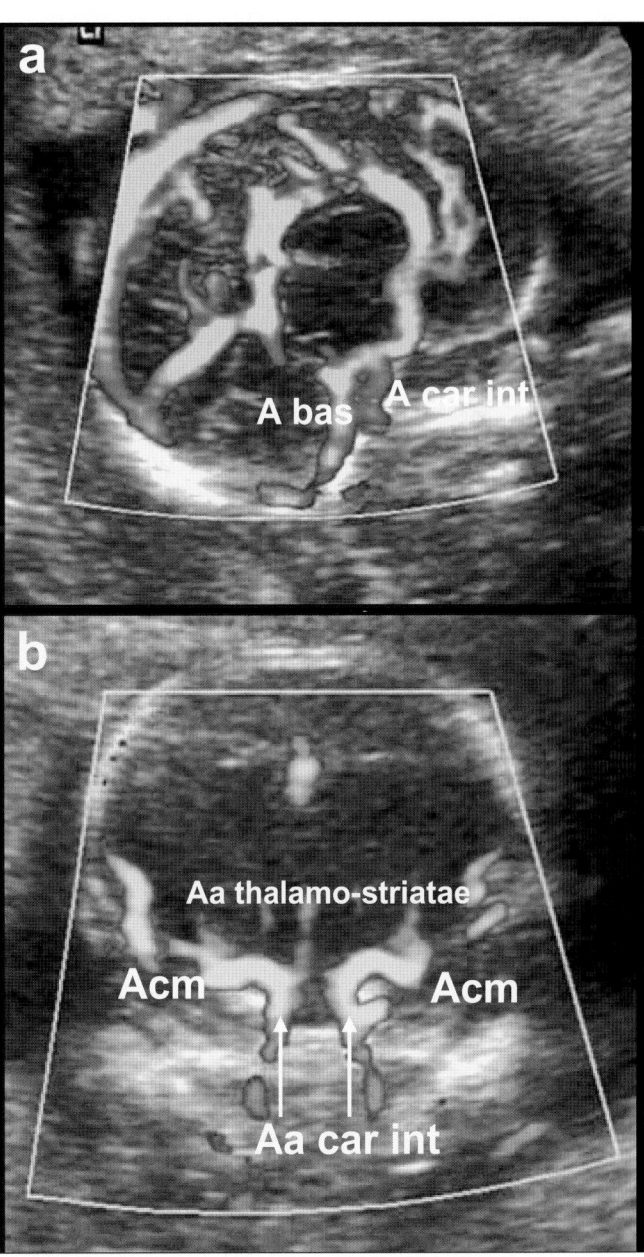

Figure 4.17 (a) Sagittal section through the brain of a 21-week-old fetus with serious growth retardation and brain-sparing effect; power Doppler image of numerous arteries and veins. (b) Power Doppler image of the same fetus in the coronal section, the thalamo-striatic arteries can be seen; A bas = arteria basalis; Acm = arteria cerebri media; A car int = arteria carotis interna.

Figure 4.16 (a) Color Doppler image of the circulus Willisii in a 27-week-old fetus with Rhesus isoimmunization at 27 weeks. (b) Flow velocimetry of the middle cerebral artery; the high peak velocity (72 cm/s) of the middle cerebral artery indicates anemia; Acm = arteria cerebri media; Acp = arteria cerebri posterior.

the basal ganglia and the internal capsule. The brain stem and cerebellum are supported from the vertebral arteries and their branches. The venous circulation drains the blood into dural sinuses, which meet in the confluence of the sinuses at the occipital pole. From here, the blood passes into the jugular veins. Pulsed Doppler (Fig. 4.17) and color Doppler (Fig. 4.16a) have been used to image and evaluate the cerebral arterial blood flow. One of the first studies on cerebral blood flow was measurements of the carotid arteries (Marsál et al 1984). Especially the fetal middle cerebral artery has been the object of Doppler measurements (Fig. 4.16b) and studied as a representative blood vessel of the cerebral circulation (Dubiel et al 1997, Maesel 1996, Mari 2000, Vyas et al 1990). At present there are two main areas in which the middle cerebral artery velocity waveform is useful in the diagnosis and surveillance of fetuses, namely the brain-sparing effect in growth-retarded fetuses and the increasing peak velocity in anemic fetuses. The increase in blood flow to the brain in growth-retarded fetuses was already shown by Doppler ultrasound of the middle cerebral artery 20 years ago (Mari & Deter 1992, Wijngaard et al 1989, Woo et al 1987). This effect has been called the 'brain-sparing effect' and is characterized by an increase of diastolic blood flow and thus a lower value of the pulsatility index. In 1995 Mari and colleagues showed that there was a significant correlation between high peak velocities of the middle cerebral artery (MCA PV) in anemic fetuses (Mari et al 1995). Later studies by Mari confirmed that MCA PV measurements could be used to predict normal blood count or different degrees of fetal anemia in the surveillance of fetuses at risk for anemia, and the timing of transfusions (Mari 2000; Mari et al 2005).

2-D and 3-D-power Doppler angiography (Fig. 4.17) has demonstrated that many vessels of both arterial and venous circulation can be imaged by this ultrasound application (Pooh & Aomo 1996, Pooh et al 2000). These authors showed clear power Doppler images of the main anterior and posterior arterial circulation as early as at the end of the first trimester (Pooh & Aomo 1996).

CONCLUSION

In the growing embryo, the brain is the first organ system to develop in such a way that it can be imaged with ultrasound technology at a level where the diagnosis of malformations can be made. Due to its nature, holoprosencephaly is probably the first condition that can be recognized with ultrasound in the developing embryo. At present, we are at the borderline of being able to diagnose holoprosencephaly when the embryo is 7–8 weeks. At 9 weeks, significant diagnoses such as holoprosencephaly (Blaas et al 2000b), spina bifida (Blaas et al 2000a), acrania (Blaas & Eik-Nes 1996), encephalocele (Blaas & Eik-Nes 1999a) and Meckel–Gruber syndrome (Blaas & Eik-Nes 1999b) have been made. These malformations may be imaged in greater detail during the subsequent few weeks of pregnancy. From 12 weeks and onwards, additional conditions such as Arnold–Chiari malformation (Blaas et al 2000a) and Dandy–Walker malformation (Achiron et al 1993) may be diagnosed. Later in pregnancy most of the structural maldevelopments of the CNS may be recognized and have been described. Thus, women at risk for having a fetus with brain anomalies may have early examination at the specific time when the diagnosis can be made.

To utilize the potential of ultrasound diagnosis in the embryonic/fetal period, it is important to have a basic knowledge of the normal development. It is also essential to establish the time when the various diagnoses can be made with adequate certainty, in order to offer women at risk an examination at the appropriate time.

We have come so far that the expected development of the ultrasound technology will probably not make it possible to make diagnosis of brain anomalies significantly earlier than at present, but will increase reliability. We may expect the rapidly developing 3-D technology, with the option of any-plane slicing, to help us establish diagnoses in the future. Such multiplane presentations of a diagnosis will contribute to increasing the diagnostic accuracy.

REFERENCES

Achiron R, Achiron A, Yagel S 1993 First trimester transvaginal sonographic diagnosis of Dandy–Walker malformation. J Clin Ultrasound 21: 62–64.

Babcook C J, Chong B W, Salamat M S et al 1996 Sonographic anatomy of the developing cerebellum: normal embryology can resemble pathology. Am J Roentgenol 166:427–433.

Blaas H-G K 1999a Editorial: The examination of the embryo and early fetus: how and by whom? Ultrasound Obstet Gynecol 14(3):153–158.

Blaas H-G K 1999b The embryonic examination. Ultrasound studies on the development of the human embryo. National Centre for Fetal Medicine,

Dept Ob & Gyn, Norwegian University of Science and Technology, Trondheim, pp. 1–178.

Blaas H-G K, Eik-Nes S H 2002a Three-dimensional ultrasonography of the embryonic brain. In: Levine M I, Chervenak F A, Whittle M (eds) Fetal and neonatal neurology and neurosurgery. Churchill Livingstone, London, Ch. 4, pp. 39–44.

Blaas H-G K, Eik-Nes S H 2002b The description of the early development of the human central nervous system using two- and three-dimensional ultrasound. In: Hanson M, Lagercrantz H (eds) The newborn brain — Neuroscience and clinical applications. Cambridge University Press, Cambridge, pp. 278–288.

Blaas H-G K, Eik-Nes S H, Isaksen C V 2000a The detection of spina bifida before 10 gestational weeks using 2D- and 3D ultrasound. Ultrasound Obstet Gynecol 16:25–29.

Blaas H-G K, Eik-Nes S H, Vainio T, Isaksen C V 2000b Alobar holoprosencephaly at 9 weeks gestational age visualized by two- and three-dimensional ultrasound. Ultrasound Obstet Gynecol 15:62–65.

Blaas H-G, Eik-Nes S H 1996 Ultrasound assessment of early brain development. In: Jurkovic D, Jauniaux E (eds) Ultrasound and early pregnancy. Parthenon, New York, pp. 3–18.

Blaas H-G, Eik-Nes S H 1999a Das Zentralnervensystem. Die normale Entwicklung und die Entwicklung von Anomalien — Ultraschalldiagnostik in der Frühschwangerschaft. Gynäkologe 32:181–191.

Blaas H-G, Eik-Nes S H 1999b First-trimester diagnosis of fetal malformations, Ch. 49. In: Rodeck C, Whittle M (eds) Fetal medicine: Basic science and clinical practice. Harcourt Brace, London, pp. 581–597.

Blaas H-G, Eik-Nes S H, Berg S, Torp H 1998 In-vivo three-dimensional ultrasound reconstructions of embryos and early fetuses. Lancet 352(9135): 1182–1186.

Blaas H-G, Eik-Nes S H, Kiserud T et al 1995a Three-dimensional imaging of the brain cavities in human embryos. Ultrasound Obstet Gynecol 5:228–232.

Blaas H-G, Eik-Nes S H, Kiserud T, Hellevik L R 1994 Early development of the forebrain and midbrain: a longitudinal ultrasound study from 7 to 12 weeks of gestation. Ultrasound Obstet Gynecol 4:183–192.

Blaas H-G, Eik-Nes S H, Kiserud T, Hellevik L R 1995b Early development of the hindbrain: a longitudinal ultrasound study from 7 to 12 weeks of gestation. Ultrasound Obstet Gynecol 5:151–160.

Bromley B, Nadel A S, Pauker S et al 1994 Closure of the cerebellar vermis: evaluation with second trimester US. Radiology 193:761–763.

Bronshtein M, Zimmer E Z, Blazer S 1998 Isolated large fourth ventricle in early pregnancy — a possible benign transient phenomenon. Prenat Diagn 18:997–1000.

Cardoza J D, Goldstein R B, Filly R A 1988 Exclusion of fetal ventriculomegaly with a single measurement: the width of the lateral ventricular atrium. Radiology 169:711–714.

Chi J G, Dooling E C, Gilles F H 1976 Gyral development of the human brain. Ann Neurol 1:86–93.

Correa F F, Lara C, Bellver J et al 2006 Examination of the fetal brain by transabdominal three-dimensional ultrasound: potential for routine neurosonographic studies. Ultrasound Obstet Gynecol 27:503–508.

Cremin B J, Chilton S J, Peacock W J 1983 Anatomical landmarks in anterior fontanelle ultrasonography. Br J Radiol 56:517–526.

Day R W 1959 Casts of foetal lateral ventricles. Brain 82:109–115.

Dorovini-Zis K, Dolman C L 1977 Gestational development of brain. Arch Pathol Lab Med 101:192–195.

Dubiel M, Gudmundsson S, Gunnarsson G, Marsál K 1997 Middle cerebral artery velocimetry as a predictor of hypoxemia in fetuses with increased resistance to blood flow in the umbilical artery. Early Hum Dev 47:177–184.

Flyger G, Hjelmquist U 1957 Normal variations in the caliber of the human cerebral aqueduct. Anat Record Philad 127:151–162.

Goldstein I, Reece A, Pilu G et al 1987 Cerebellar measurements with ultrasonography in the evaluation of fetal growth and development. Am J Obstet Gynecol 156:1065–1069.

Goldstein I, Reece E A, Pilu G et al 1988 Sonographic evaluation of the normal developmental anatomy of fetal cerebral ventricles: I. The frontal horn. Obstet Gynecol 72:588–592.

Goldstein I, Reece E A, Pilu G, Hobbins J C 1990 Sonographic evaluation of the normal development anatomy of fetal cerebral ventricles. IV. The posterior horn. Am J Perinat 7(1):79–83.

Hata K, Hata T, Senoh D et al 1989 Ultrasonographic measurement of the fetal transverse cerebellum in utero. Gynecol Obstet Invest 28:111–112.

Hill L M, Guzick D, Fries J et al 1990 The transverse cerebellar diameter in estimating gestational age in the large for gestational age fetus. Obstet Gynecol 75:983–992.

Hochstetter F 1919 Beiträge zur Entwicklungsgeschichte des menschlichen Gehirns. Franz Deuticke, Wien.

ISUOG Guidelines 2007 Sonographic examination of fetal central nervous system: guidelines for performing the 'basic examination' and the 'fetal neurosonogram'. Ultrasound Obstet Gynecol 29:109–116.

Jenkins G B 1921 Relative weight and volume of the component parts of the brain of the human embryo at different stages of development. Contributions to Embryology Carnegie Institution 13:41–60.

Jou H-J, Shyu M-K, Wu S-C et al 1998 Ultrasound measurement of the fetal cavum septi pellucidi. Ultrasound Obstet Gynecol 12:419–421.

Kier E L (ed.) 1977 The cerebral ventricles: a phylogenetic and ontogenetic study. Anatomy and pathology. Radiology of the skull and the brain. Mosby, Saint Louis.

Kostovic I 1990 Zentralnervensystem. In: Hinrichsen K V (ed.) Humanembryologie. Springer-Verlag, Berlin, pp. 381–448.

Lemire R J 1975 Deep cerebral nuclei. In: Lemire R J, Loeser J D, Leich R W, Alvord E C (eds) Abnormal development of the human nervous system. Harper & Row, Hagerstown, Maryland, pp. 169–195.

Maesel A 1996 Human fetal cerebral circulation. Dept Ob & Gyn, Malmö University Hospital Perinatal Doppler velocimetry and fetal pulse oximetry studies. Lund, Malmö, pp. 1–86.

Mahony B S, Callen P W, Filly R A, Hoddick W K 1984 The fetal cisterna magna. Radiology 153:773–776.

Mari G 2000 Noninvasive diagnosis by Doppler ultrasonography of fetal anemia due to maternal red-cell alloimmunization. N Engl J Med 342(1): 9–14.

Mari G, Adrignolo A, Abuhamad A Z et al 1995 Diagnosis of fetal anemia with Doppler ultrasound in the pregnancy complicated by maternal blood group immunization. Ultrasound Obstet Gynecol 5:400–405.

Mari G, Deter R L 1992 Middle cerebral artery flow velocity waveforms in normal and small-for-gestational-age fetuses. Am J Obstet Gynecol 166:1262–1270.

Mari G, Zimmermann R, Moise K J, Deter R L 2005 Correlation between middle cerebral artery peak systoloic velocity and fetal hemoglobin after 2 previous intrauterine transfusions. Am J Obstet Gynecol 193:1117–1120.

Marsál K, Lingman G, Giles W 1984 Evaluation of the carotid, aortic and umbilical blood velocity waveformes in the human fetus. 11th Annual Conf Soc Study of Fetal Physiology, Oxford.

Monteagudo A, Haratz-Rubinstein N, Timor-Tritsch I E 1996 Biometry of the fetal brain. Timor-Tritsch I E, Monteagudo A, Cohen H L (eds) Ultrasonography of the prenatal and neonatal brain. Appleton & Lange, Stamford, Connecticut.

Monteagudo A, Timor-Tritsch I E 1997 Development of fetal gyri, sulci and fissures: a transvaginal sonographic study. Ultrasound Obstet Gynecol 9:222–228.

Monteagudo A, Timor-Tritsch I E, Mayberry P 2000 Three-dimensional transvaginal neurosonography of the fetal brain: 'navigating' in the volume scan. Ultrasound Obstet Gynecol 16:307–313.

Monteagudo A, Timor-Tritsch I E, Moomjy M 1993 Nomograms of the fetal lateral ventricles using transvaginal sonography. J Ultrasound Med 5:265–269.

Müller F, O'Rahilly R 1990 The human brain at stages 21–23, with particular reference to the cerebral cortical plate and the development of the cerebellum. Anat Embryol 182:375–400.

O'Rahilly R, Müller F 1987 Developmental stages in human embryos. Carnegie Instn Publ, Washington, DC.

O'Rahilly R, Müller F 1990 Ventricular system and choroid plexuses of the human brain during the embryonic period proper. Am J Anat 189:285–302.

O'Rahilly R, Müller F 1994 The embryonic human brain. An atlas of developmental stages. Wiley-Liss, New York.

O'Rahilly R, Müller F 2006 The embryonic human brain. An atlas of developmental stages. Wiley, New York.

Paladini D, Volpe P 2006 Posterior fossa and vermian morphometry in the characterization of fetal cerebellar abnormalities: a prospective three-dimensional ultrasound study. Ultrasound Obstet Gynecol 27:482–489.

Pilu G, Reece E A, Goldstein I et al 1989 Sonographic evaluation of the normal developmental anatomy of the fetal cerebral ventricles: II. The atria. Obstet Gynecol 73:250–256.

Pilu G, Segata M, Ghi T et al 2006 Diagnosis of midline anomalies of the fetal brain with the three-dimensional median view. Ultrasound Obstet Gynecol 27:522–529.

Pooh R K, Aomo T 1996 Transvaginal power Doppler angiography of the fetal brain. Ultrasound Obstet Gynecol 8:417–421.

Pooh R K, Pooh K H, Nakagawa Y et al 2000 Clinical application of three-dimensional ultrasound in fetal brain assessment. Croat Med J 41:245–251.

Robinson A, Goldstein R 2007 The cisterna magna septa. J Ultrasound Med 26:83–95.

Roelfsema N M, Hop W C J, Boito S M E, Wladimiroff J W 2003 Three-dimensional sonographic measurement of normal fetal brain volume during the second half of pregnancy. Am J Obstet Gynecol 190:275–280.

Shaw C-M, Alvord E C 1969 Cava septi pellucidi et Vergæ: their normal and pathological states. Brain 92:213–224.

Takeuchi H 1994 Sonoembryology in the central nervous system. In: Kurjak A, Chervenak F A (eds) The fetus as a patient. Advances in diagnosis and therapy. Parthenon, New York, pp. 141–150.

Timor-Tritsch I E, Farine D, Rosen M G 1988 A close look at the embryonic development with the high frequency transvaginal transducer. Am J Obstet Gynecol 159:678–681.

Timor-Tritsch I E, Monteagudo A 1991 Transvaginal sonographic evaluation of the fetal central nervous system. Obstet Gynecol Clin North Am 18(4):713–748.

Timor-Tritsch I E, Monteagudo A 1996 Normal neurosonography of the prenatal brain. In: Timor-Tritsch I E, Monteagudo A, Cohen H L (eds) Ultrasonography of the prenatal and neonatal brain. Appleton & Lange, Stamford, Connecticut, pp. 11–88.

Timor-Tritsch I E, Peisner D B, Raju S 1990 Sonoembryology: an organ-oriented approach using a high-frequency vaginal probe. J Clin Ultrasound 18:286–298.

Vinals F, Munoz M, Naveas R et al 2005 The fetal cerebellar vermis: anatomy and biometric assessment using volume contrast imaging in the C-plane (VCI-C). Ultrasound Obstet Gynecol 26:622–627.

Vyas S, Nicolaides K H, Bower S, Campbell S 1990 Middle cerebral artery flow velocity waveforms in fetal hypoxaemia. Br J Obstet Gynaecol 97: 797–803.

Warren W B, Timor-Tritsch I E, Peisner D B et al 1989 Dating the pregnancy by sequential appearance of embryonic structures. Am J Obstet Gynecol 161:747–753.

Westergaard E 1971 The lateral cerebral ventricles of human foetuses with a crown-rump length of 26–178 mm. Acta Anat 79:409–421.

Wijngaard J A v d, Groenenberg I A, Wladimiroff J W, Hop W C 1989 Cerebral Doppler ultrasound of the human fetus. Br J Obstet Gynaecol 96: 845–849.

Woo J S, Liang S T, Lo R L, Chan F Y 1987 Middle cerebral artery Doppler flow velocimetry waveforms. Obstet Gynecol 70:613–616.

Woollam D 1952 Casts of the ventricles of the brain. Brain 75:259–267.

Zalen-Sprock R M v, Vugt J M G v, Geijn H P v 1996 First-trimester sonographic detection of neurodevelopmental abnormalities in some single-gene disorders. Prenat Diagn 16:199–202.

CHAPTER

5

Magnetic resonance imaging of the fetal central nervous system

Elspeth Whitby

Key Points

- Advanced MR imaging techniques are required for good-quality fetal MRI. T2-weighted single-shot fast spin echo is the main imaging sequence used but this requires supplementation by other sequences depending on the pathology
- Maternal and fetal comfort and safety are paramount and improve image quality
- Fetal MRI is an adjunct to antenatal ultrasound
- Fetal MRI provides detail on the developing brain not seen with ultrasound
- Knowledge of normal is essential for diagnostic accuracy
- Fetal MRI allows detailed study of normal and abnormal brain developments
- Fetal MR is an expanding and developing technique

INTRODUCTION

Imaging of the fetal central nervous system (CNS) has been undertaken for several decades predominantly using ultrasound.

Magnetic resonance (MR) imaging of the fetus was initially restricted by motion artifact (Fig. 5.1). This was overcome by the use of pancuronium bromide injected into the umbilical vessels or fetal musculature (Weinreb et al 1985). This restricted the procedure to patients undergoing fetal sedation for other therapeutic or interventional procedures and the in utero MR was performed whilst the paralysis lasted (about 2 hours). Another approach was to give the mother large doses of benzodiazepines to sedate her and the fetus (Williamson et al 1989). Again this was used for other diagnostic or therapeutic procedures and not routinely used for the purpose of fetal MR. The initial studies under such conditions allowed us to assess the scope and likely value of fetal MR, if movement artifacts could be overcome. These studies often used T1-weighted images.

THE SEQUENCES

The advent of ultrafast imaging techniques allowed a rapid increase in the use of MR to image the fetus. Single-shot fast spin echo (SSFSE) produces a slice every second, effectively freezing fetal motion and producing a heavily T2-weighted image (Stehling et al 1990) (Fig. 5.2). SSFSE or rapid acquisition recalled echo (RARE), as it was originally named by its developer Jurgen Hennig (Hennig et al 1986), uses a train of

180 degree pulses following an initial 90 degree pulse. The spin echoes collected after each 180-degree pulse are separately phase-encoded to collect all of k-space within a single T2-signal decay. The images tend to be very T2-weighted and were originally used to produce MR myelograms of the spine to highlight the cerebrospinal fluid.

The degree of T2 weighting achieved can be varied by locating the center of k-space at different times within the T2 decay by altering the way the phase encode gradients are applied. The echo spacing is important in determining filtering effects (blurring) on the image due to T2 decay. Motion during data collection can also cause complex artifacts in SSFSE. Ideally short echo spacing is used to minimize artifacts, although this requires increased bandwidth which affects the signal to noise ratio. Susceptibility artifacts are not prominent on SSFSE sequences, which make them insensitive for hemorrhage.

When performing multi-slice SSFSE, significant magnetization transfer effects may be seen between mobile and bound proton pools, which can give rise to variable contrast effects between slices. This technique obtains the information required for 20 slices within 20 seconds effectively freezing fetal motion (Fig. 5.2).

SAFETY

There have been concerns over the safety of imaging the fetus using magnetic resonance for two main reasons. The imaging technique is associated with acoustic noise and this is in the order of 98 dB and has the potential to damage hearing, although amniotic fluid may reduce the acoustic noise by 30–50 dB (Glover et al 1995). The most recent information comes from a prospective study that followed up children who had been imaged in utero in the third trimester. Thirty-five children who were between 1 and 3 years of age and 9 children who were between 8 and 9 years of age at assessment were studied. These children had all undergone clinical scans in utero at 1.5T and in some cases the study also included PRESS and STEAM spectroscopy sequences in addition to T2-weighted imaging. Detailed follow-up was obtained together with a detailed neurological examination at 3 months of age. In all but two cases findings were normal. The abnormalities in these two cases may or may not be related to the MR imaging. No problems were detected with hearing. Although in this study no harmful effects were detected, total safety of the MR technique can never be fully established.

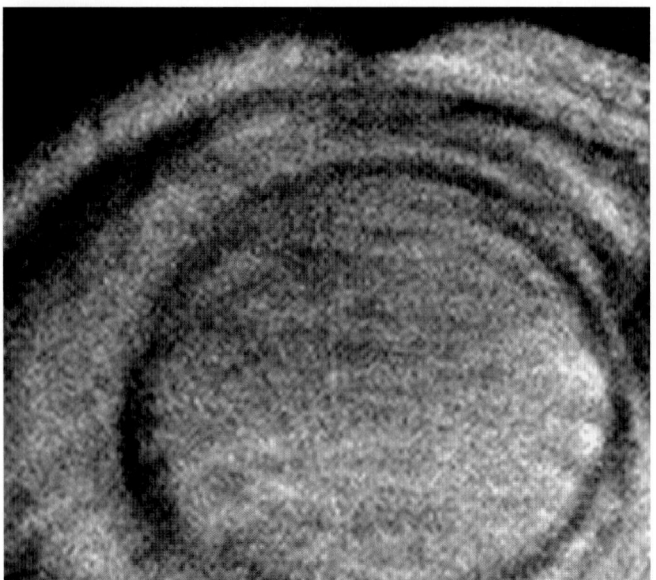

Figure 5.1 Axial section through the fetal brain obtained using standard MR T2 sequences. All detail is lost due to movement artifact.

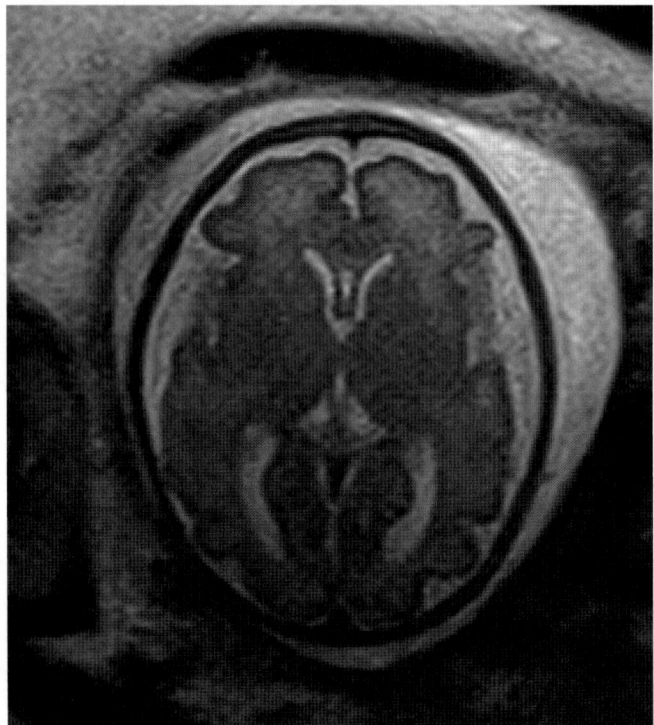

Figure 5.2 Axial section through the fetal brain obtained using ultrafast MR techniques. The brain detail is clearly seen.

There is also heat disposition within the body tissues. Guidelines are set out by the National Radiation Protection Board (NRPB) as to the amount of heat (termed specific absorption rate (SAR)) that can be generated whilst conducting the examination. The SAR is maximal at the surface of the maternal body so the risk to the fetus is minimal due to the efficient heat-dissipating action of the amniotic fluid. There have been no documented effects on follow-up studies (Baker et al 1994, Clements et al 2000, Kok et al 2004, Myers et al 1998) but further studies with larger numbers are required to prove this.

The medical devices agency advise that a decision to scan should be made at the time by the referring clinician, an MR radiologist and the patient, based on information about risks versus benefit. Pregnant women should not be exposed above the advised lower levels of restriction, i.e. not to fields above 2.5T. Currently it is advisable to keep the field strength to 1.5T, use low SAR, keep scan times as short as possible and avoid scanning in the first trimester. Intravenous contrast is not advised due to the dechelation of the gadolinium across the placenta and the recirculation of the gadolinium in the amniotic fluid, thus increasing its half-life (Rofsky et al 1994).

THE TECHNIQUE

Fast sequences that produce T2-weighted images are the work horse of in utero MR imaging. These are supplemented by T1-weighted images and in recent months diffusion-weighted imaging and spectroscopy (Girard et al 2006b) have been used successfully in fetal imaging.

In most centers neither sedation nor anesthesia is used. Some centers ask the mother to fast for several hours to help reduce fetal motion (Glenn & Barkovich 2006a, 2006b) and others use a breath-hold technique, particularly if the fetus is breech and they wish to image the CNS.

Imaging is performed on a 1.5T magnet. The mother lies on the table in the lateral decubitus position to reduce venous compression and enters the magnet feet-first to reduce the risk of claustrophobia. We use a four-channel phased-array body coil to obtain the images. Imaging usually takes 30 minutes. T2-weighted slices, 5 mm thick, are obtained in three orthogonal planes and supplemented with 3 mm thick T2-weighted slices and T1, DWI and spectroscopy as required for clinical need (Whitby et al 2001, 2004) (Fig. 5.3a–c). If the fetus is still increasing the number of acquisitions increases the image quality, especially if using thin slices (Fig. 5.4a, b).

Standard imaging parameters are given below:

SSFSE

TE 75 ms, TR 22 000 ms, inter-echo time 7.5 ms, echo train 132, phase matrix 175, read matrix 256, 1 average, 25 cm FOV, 20 slices, thickness 5 mm, no slice gap.

T1 RFFAST

TE 4.47 ms, TR 210 ms, flip angle 80, BW 41.67, phase matrix 140, read matrix 256, 1 average, 25 cm FOV, 20 slices, thickness 5 mm, no slice gap (Fig. 5.3a,b).

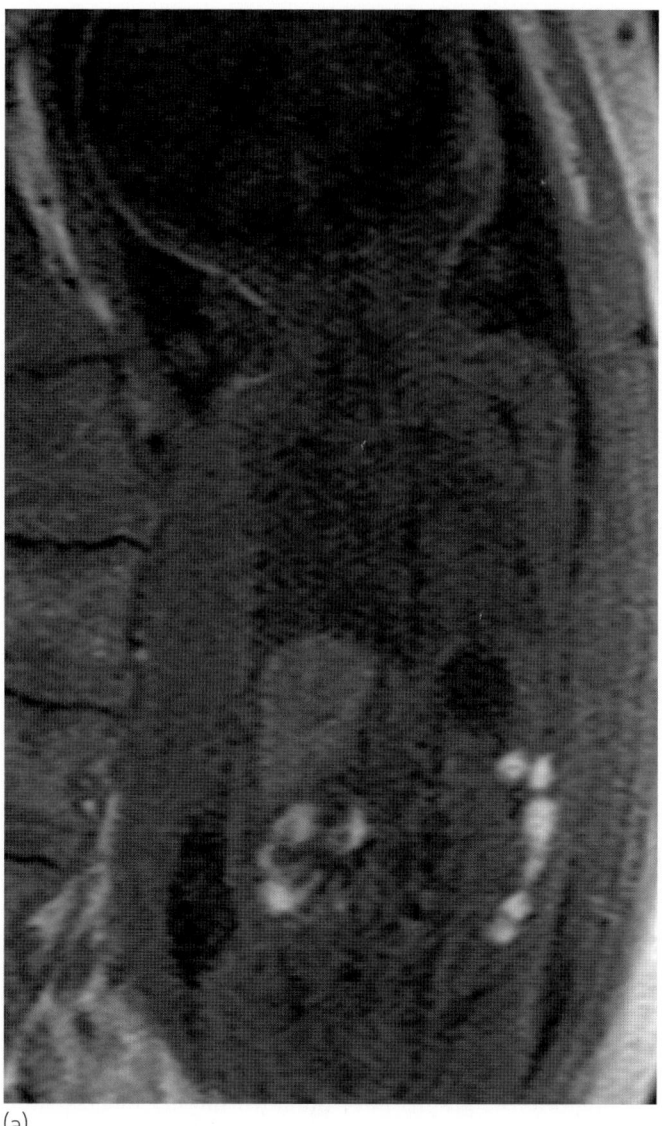

(a)

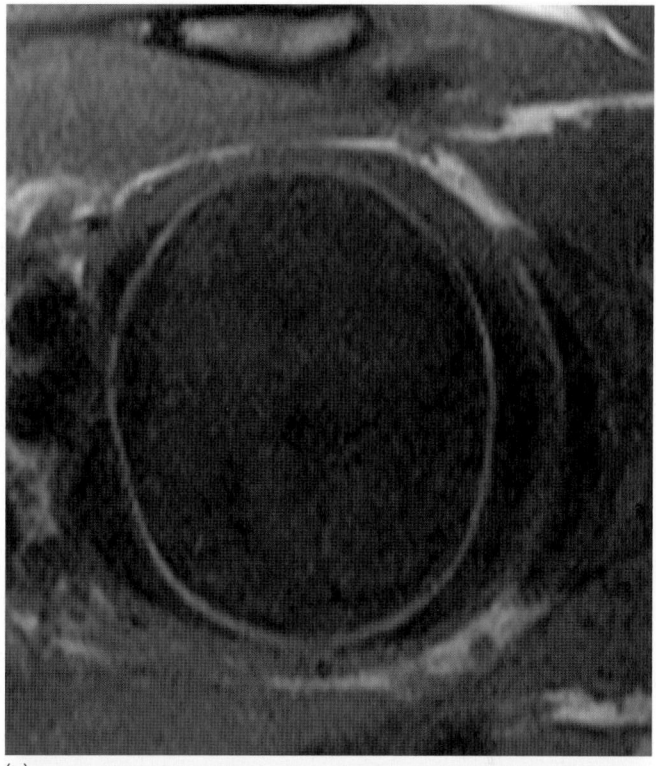

(b)

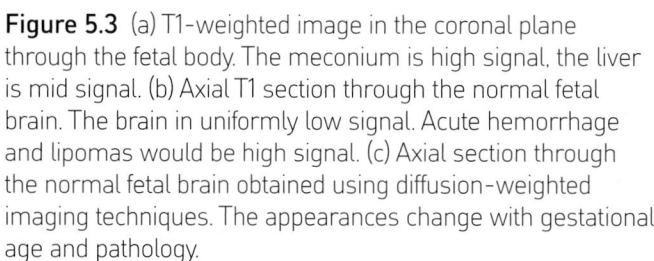

(c)

Figure 5.3 (a) T1-weighted image in the coronal plane through the fetal body. The meconium is high signal, the liver is mid signal. (b) Axial T1 section through the normal fetal brain. The brain in uniformly low signal. Acute hemorrhage and lipomas would be high signal. (c) Axial section through the normal fetal brain obtained using diffusion-weighted imaging techniques. The appearances change with gestational age and pathology.

EPI DIFFUSION

TE 114.5 ms, TR 3300, inter-echo time 885 μm, echo train 144, 2 averages, 30 cm FOV, 11 slices, thickness 5 mm, no slice gap, b values 400 and 700 ms/mm² (Fig. 5.3c).

CLINICAL APPLICATIONS

Fetal MR has several advantages over ultrasound including improved contrast resolution, ability to assess the developing parenchyma, and is not restricted by acoustic shadows so all the cerebral hemispheres are seen clearly. This also helps in visualization of the posterior fossa and its contents

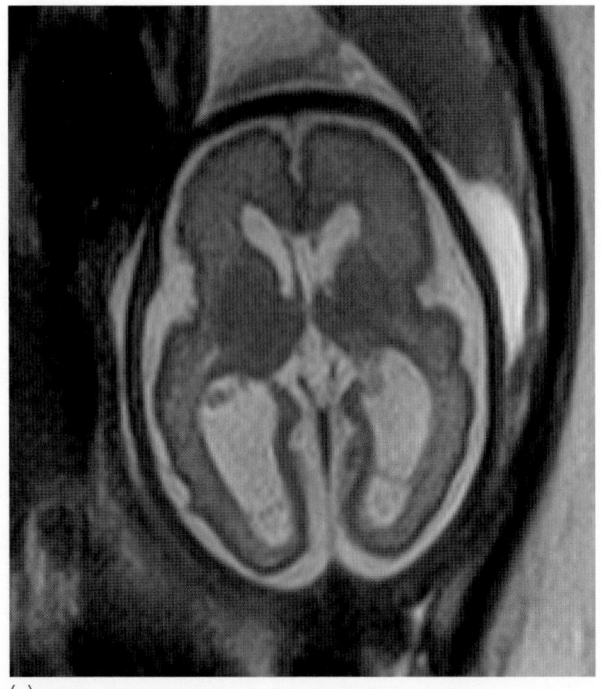

(a)

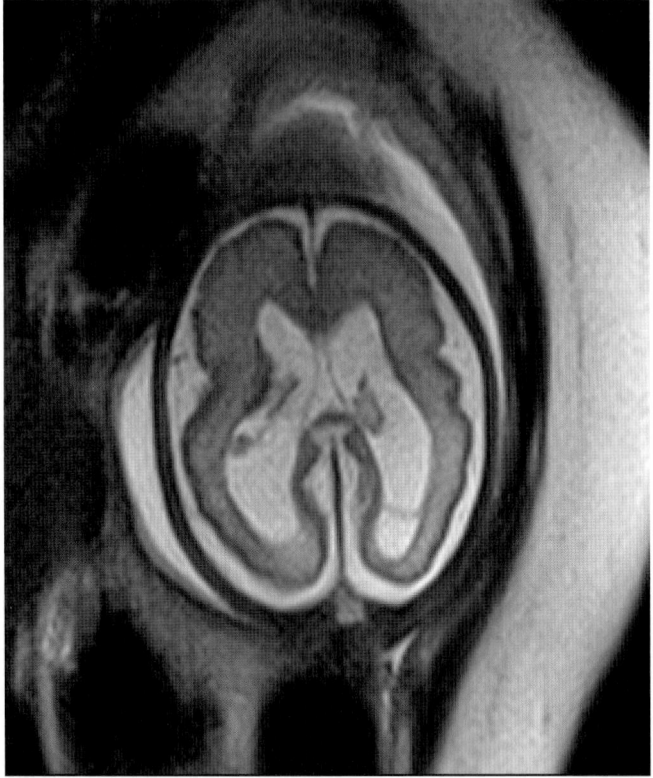

(b)

Figure 5.4 (a) Axial section through a normal fetal brain obtained with ultrafast techniques and a single acquisition in the MR sequence. (b) Axial section through the same fetal brain as in (a) but with an increase in the number of acquisitions. This increases the detail seen but only if the fetus is very still as it also increases the time required to obtain the image.

(Guibaud 2004). MR imaging is also independent of fetal position. Maternal habitus does affect the quality of the MR images but to a lesser extent than its effects on ultrasound images.

It is well established that fetal MR, compared with ultrasound imaging of the fetal CNS, can detect additional abnormalities in up to 50% of cases (Coakley et al 1999, Levine et al 1997, 1999a, Simon et al 2000, Whitby et al 2004). In all studies the ultrasound is the initial screening technique and referral to MR occurs after the initial abnormality is detected. Fetal MR will never become a screening tool. The abnormalities detected include both developmental and acquired, e.g. agenesis of the corpus callosum (d'Ercole et al 1998, Rickard et al 2006), ventriculomegaly (Morris et al 2007, Ouahba et al 2006, Salomon et al 2006, Valsky et al 2004), sulcation abnormalities, cerebellar hypoplasia, intraventricular and germinal matrix hemorrhages (Fukui et al 2001), periventricular leukomalacia (Breysem et al 2004, de Laveaucoupet et al 2001) abnormal cortical development (Fogliarini et al 2005b, Glenn et al 2005b) and heterotopias (Fogliarini et al 2005b).

The main limitations are fetal movement although if the same imaging sequences are done in groups together the fetus appears to settle as the noise becomes more repetitive. Maternal discomfort can be reduced by laying the mother in the lateral decubitus position (Whitby et al 2004). Maternal claustrophobia remains a problem.

NORMAL BRAIN DEVELOPMENT

For accurate interpretation of the images it is essential to have a good knowledge of normal fetal development at each gestational age. The acquisition of this knowledge has been limited by the restriction on imaging normal fetuses. The majority of groups have obtained normal images from patients who have been imaged for non-CNS malformations (Fogliarini et al 2005a, Garel et al 2003, Girard et al 2006a, 2006b), e.g. diaphragmatic hernias or patients where there has been a strong family history of abnormalities. The publication of a bench book of fetal MR development has greatly help image interpretation for any one starting in this area (Garel 2004a). Our knowledge in this area is expanding rapidly and there are now several reference articles on fetal brain development with respect to MR imaging (Fogliarini et al 2005a, 2005b, Garel 2004b, Girard et al 2006b) and relating the appearance to embryology, pathology and histology (Kostovic & Jovanov-Milosevic 2006, Rados et al 2006).

NEURONAL MIGRATION

In brief MR imaging of the fetal cerebral hemispheres is characterized by layers of differing signal intensity that represent the migrating neurons. These layers change in appearance and thickness with increasing gestational age and as sulcal and gyral development occurs (Brisse et al 1997, Girard & Raybaud 1992, Rados et al 2006). Knowledge

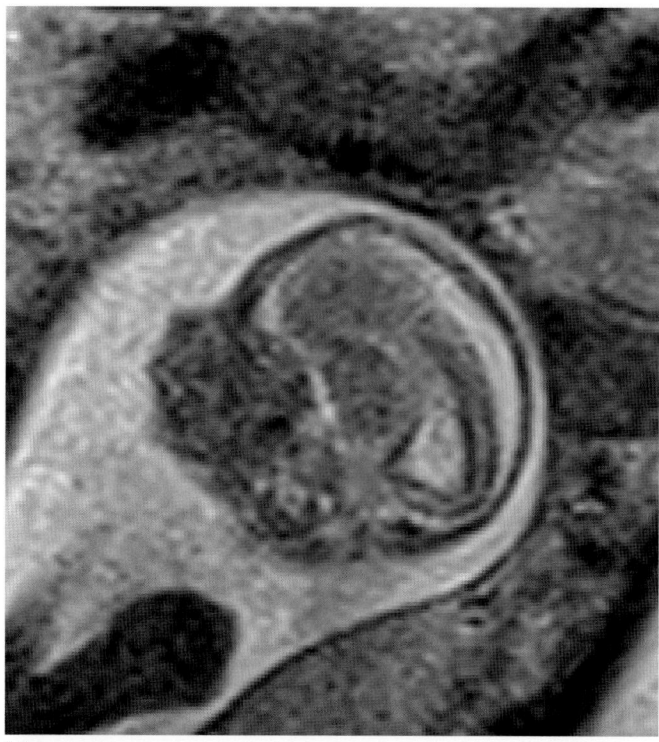

(a)

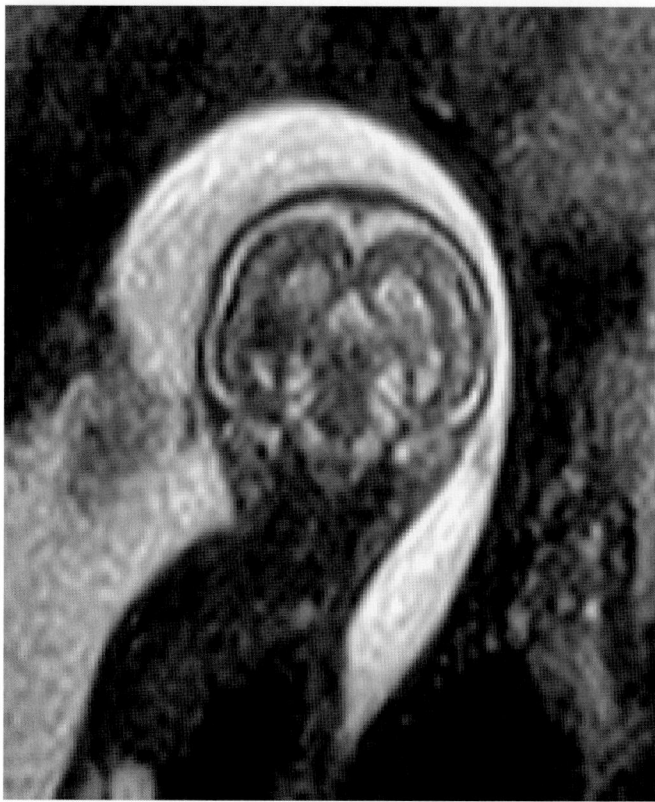

(b)

Figure 5.5 Normal fetal brain at 18 weeks gestation.

of these layers and the pattern of sulcal and gyral development are essential for accurate interpretation of the images obtained in clinical practice. Figures 5.5–5.7 show a normal developing brain at 18, 24 and 32 weeks gestation in sagittal or parasagittal and coronal planes.

Prior to 24 weeks there are five main layers:

1. The ventricular zone, this is of low signal intensity on T2 images.
2. The subventricular zone/deep intermediate zone that is of high signal intensity and fiber-rich histologically.
3. The subventricular cellular zone that is of intermediate signal intensity and blends with the intermediate zone.
4. The subplate of high signal intensity.
5. The cortical plate of low signal intensity that is seen as a 'pencil-thin' rim around the developing parenchyma.

The pathological studies done on dissected specimens and MR imaging have mainly used T1-weighted imaging techniques resulting in the layers having the opposite signal intensities (Kostovic & Jovanov-Milosevic 2006, Rados et al 2006). By 24–32 weeks the subplate has thickened as neuronal connections have started to develop and the ventricular zone has disappeared as the cells have migrated to the subplate. By 33–35 weeks the subplate thickness has decreased again.

Pathological studies such as these help us to understand the development of pathologies that occur at the different gestational ages.

SULCAL AND GYRAL DEVELOPMENT

Sulcal and gyral development follows a predefined pattern with the sequential development of primary, secondary and tertiary sulci with increasing gestational age (Garel et al 2003, Rados et al 2006).

The sulci are initially shallow and wide then, as development continues, they become progressively deeper and narrower. The sylvian fissure is the first to develop as a smooth indentation at 18 weeks, best seen on fetal MR at 20 weeks, it is wide open initially then the edges become 'square' in appearance by 23 weeks due to the development of the anterior and posterior operculum, finally the edges become opposed as in the neonatal brain (Garel 2004a) (Fig. 5.8a–c). The time lag between the neuropathological development of the cingulate gyrus and detection in utero using ultrasound is at least 8 weeks (Monteagudo & Timor-Tritsch 1997). Sulcal and gyral development is more easily detected using fetal MR than ultrasound. Studies have reported a 0–8 weeks lag in MR imaging visualization of the sulci compared with visualization on anatomical specimens (Fogliarini et al 2005a, 2005b, Levine & Barnes 1999). This is partly because pathologists count sulcal development from the first tiny indentation and this is not seen on 5 mm thick slices. With increasing technological advances and thinner slices it may be possible to detect early sulcal formation in utero.

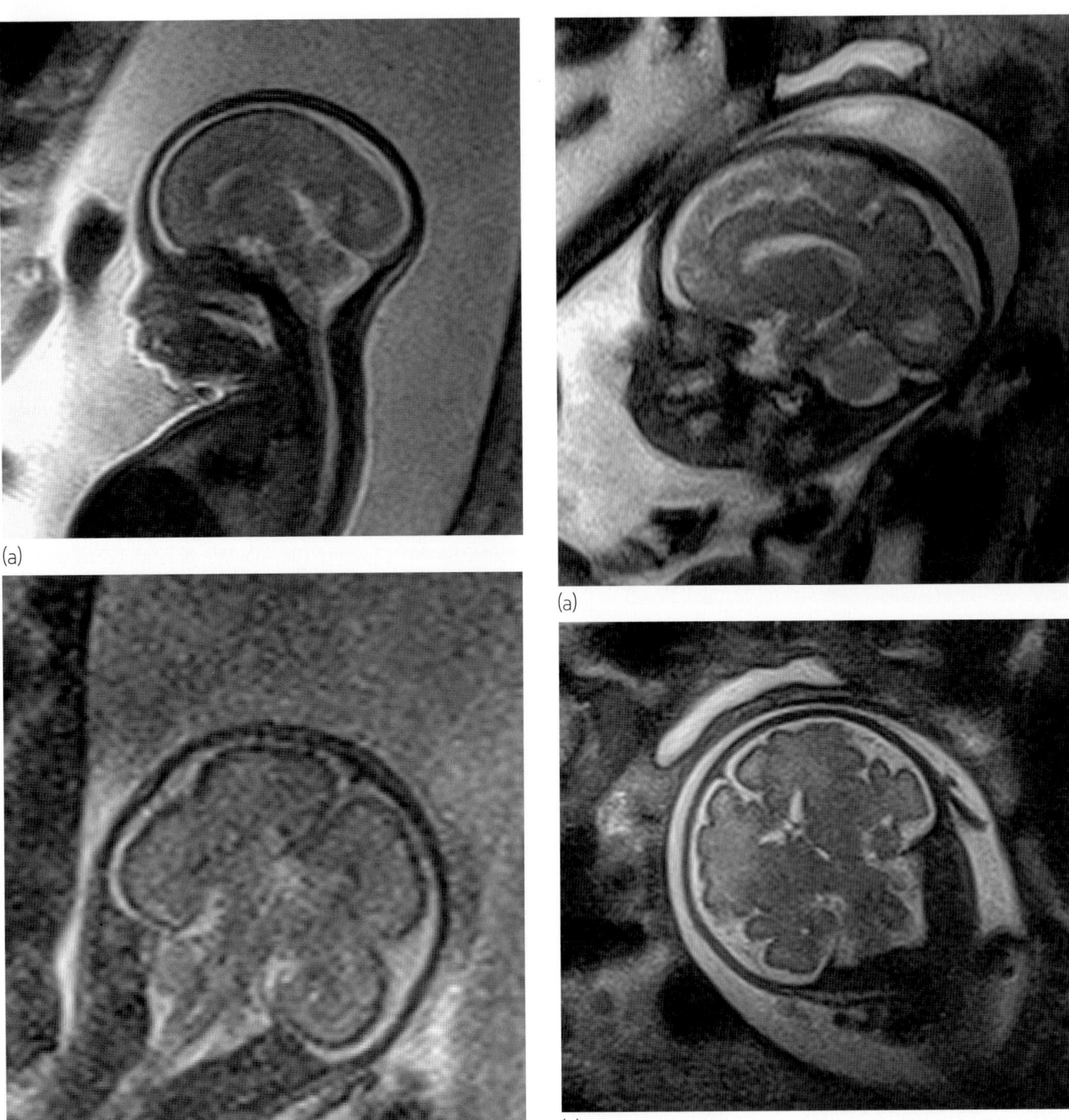

(a)

(b)

Figure 5.6 Normal fetal brain at 22 weeks gestation.

(a)

(b)

Figure 5.7 Normal fetal brain at 32 weeks gestation.

There is also some variation in the normal development between different fetuses and this has been reported as up to 2 weeks (Garel et al 2001). It is also reported to be delayed in twin pregnancies. Delay in the sulcation and gyration is an indication of abnormal development (Brunel et al 2004, Levine & Barnes 1999).

CORPUS CALLOSUM

This is fully developed by 20 weeks but we have seen cases where it appears to be partial at this stage and then has developed by 24 weeks, so care must be taken when imaging for corpus callosal abnormalities at this stage in the second trimester. The corpus callosum starts to develop at 8 weeks and can be seen best on the coronal views (Figs 5.5–5.8) supplemented by direct visualization of a dark band on the

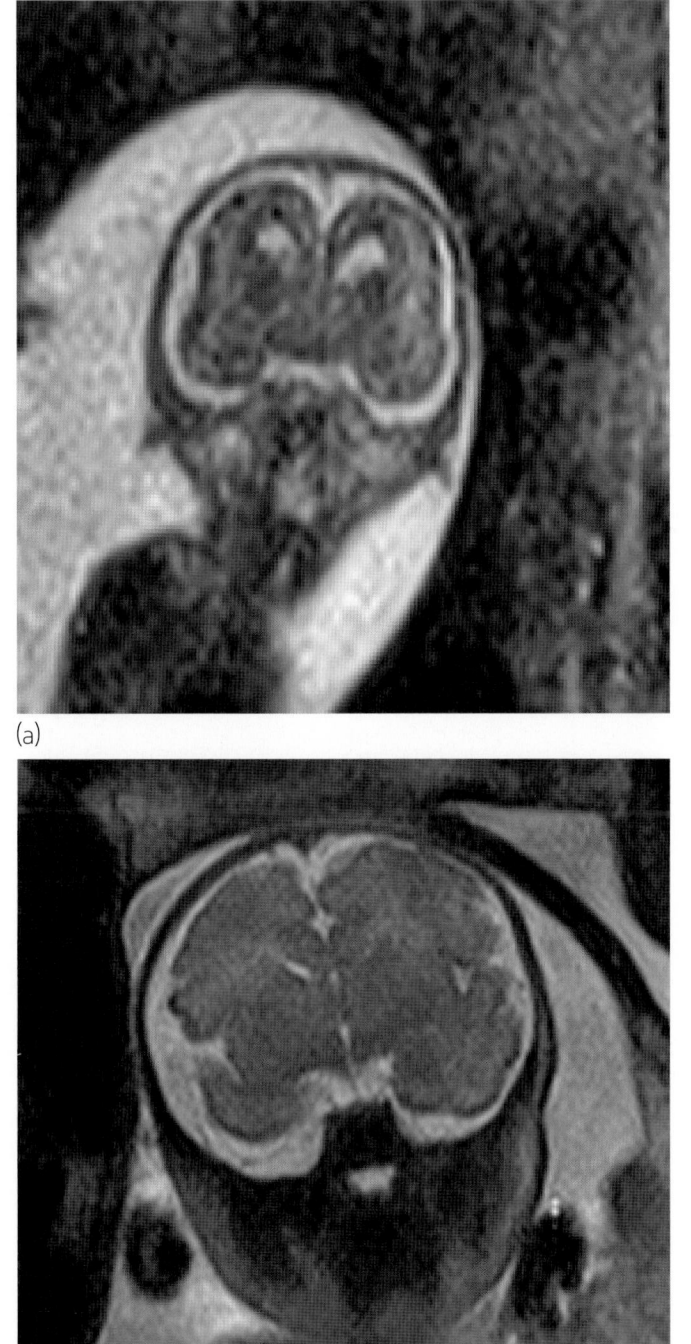

(a)

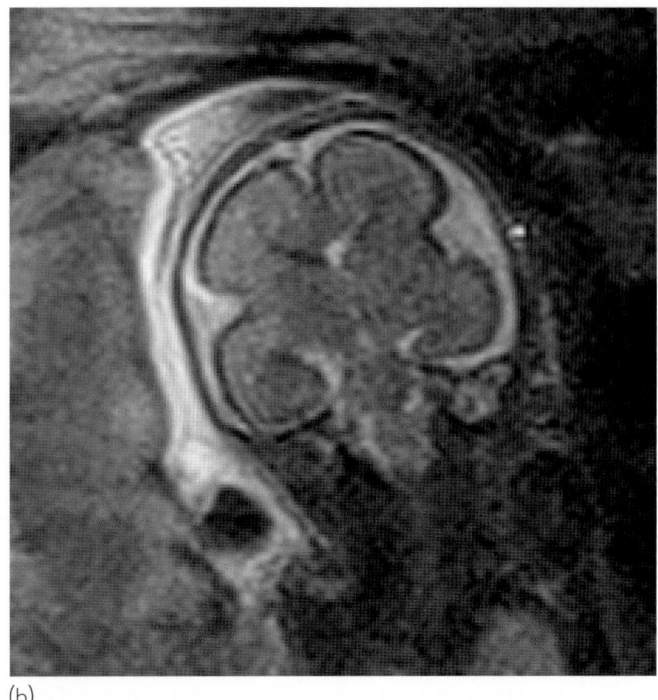

(b)

(c)

Figure 5.8 Changes in the appearance of the sylvian fissure at increasing gestational age. Initially an indentation (a) at 18 weeks, then the edges become 'squared' (b) at 24 weeks; finally the edges become almost opposed (c) at 32 weeks.

midline sagittal image. It is of uniform thickness throughout its length.

CEREBRAL VENTRICLES

A measurement of 10 mm at the level of the trigone is taken as the upper limit of normal both on sonographic imaging and MR imaging. There is a good correlation between ultrasound and MR measurement of the ventricles (Garel & Alberti 2006). The morphological appearance of the ventricles is also important and can be seen clearly on both ultrasound and MR images (Levine et al 2002). The surrounding parenchyma and overlying cortical development is more easily seen on MR imaging.

POSTERIOR FOSSA

Direct visualization of the size of the posterior fossa based on the point of insertion of the neck muscle in relation to the level of the torcula (they should correspond) is possible on the sagittal image. The cerebellar vermis is also clearly seen on

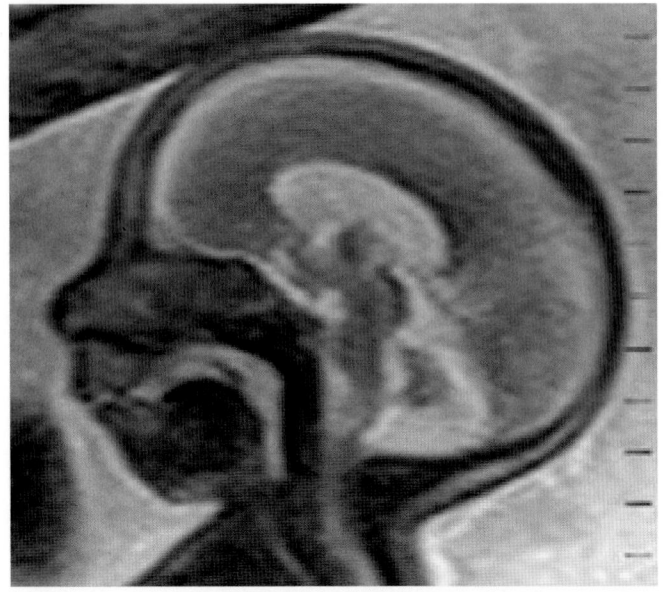

(a)

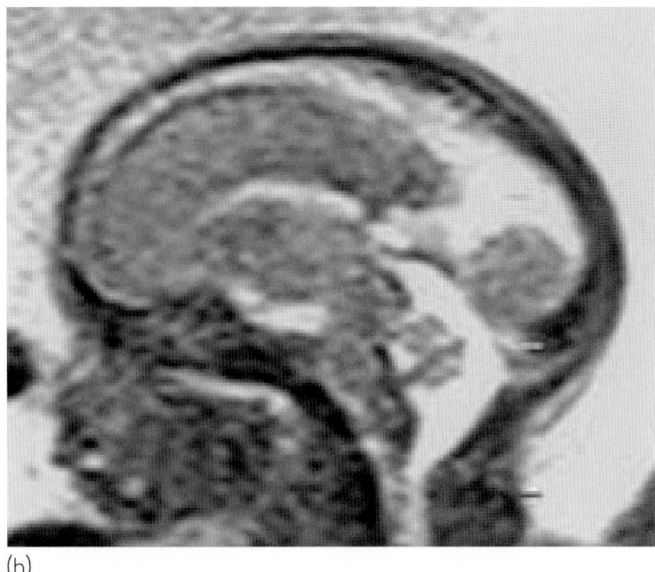

(b)

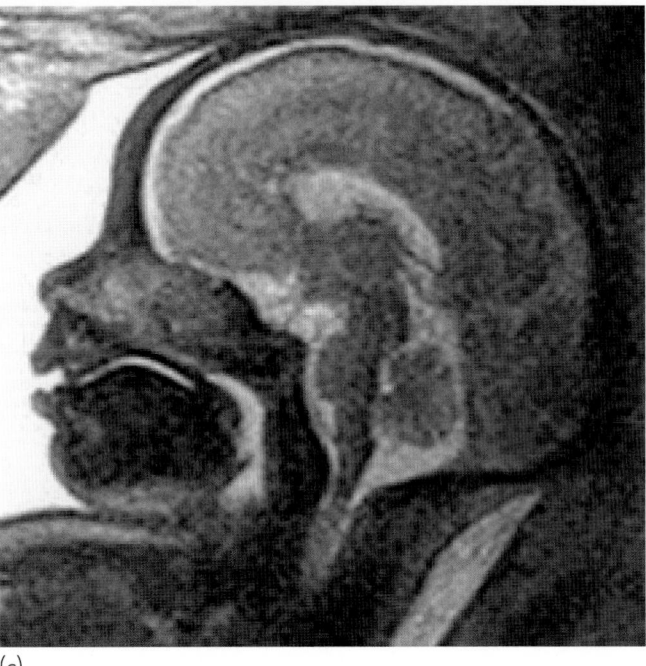

(c)

Figure 5.9 The developing posterior fossa is seen on the sagittal images with a proportionally smaller cerebellum in the earlier gestational ages that later fills the bony compartment. Images at (a) 20, (b) 26 and (c) 32 weeks gestation.

this view. The cerebellum is one of the first structures of the brain to start to develop but one of the last to finish. The cerebellar development appears to lag behind that of the bony posterior fossa. This results in an apparent large cisterna magna in the first and second trimester that disappears by the third trimester (Fig. 5.9a–c). The developing cerebellar hemispheres are best seen on the axial and coronal images.

FETAL MR MEASUREMENTS

MR measurements appear to correlate to ultrasound measurements in most cases but care should be taken to assess the plane in which the measurements were taken and the angulation of the probe/slice in each case (Garel & Alberti 2006).

Quantitative MR measurements have been undertaken and a recent report by Grossman et al, studied volumes and ratios rather than direct measurements of brain structures. The ventricular volume was constant throughout gestation but as expected the parenchymal volume increased and was strongly correlated with gestational age. It is suggested that the parenchymal to ventricular volume ratio is sensitive to pathology (Grossman et al 2006).

MR SPECTROSCOPY

This work is still in its infancy. A study of 48 normal patients has recently been published but further work is needed to establish the normal range at each gestational age and the likely role that spectroscopy will have in the clinical setting (Girard et al 2006b).

DIFFUSION-WEIGHTED IMAGING (DWI)

Initial work suggested that DWI may be useful in acquired pathologies but again there is little data on the normal appearance at each gestational age (Agid et al 2006, Prayer & Prayer 2003).

PATHOLOGIES

The range of pathologies in the fetal CNS detected on in utero imaging is vast and only the most common will be covered here.

DEVELOPMENTAL ABNORMALITIES

PRIMARY NEURULATION

Abnormalities at this stage of development result in anencephaly and cephaloceles. Anencephaly can be accurately diagnosed by sonographic techniques and few if any are referred for MR imaging. Cephaloceles are more complex and it is often difficult to accurately visualize the contents of the cephalocele with ultrasound. MR imaging allows detection of the cephalocele, depiction of the contents, e.g. fluid, fluid and parenchyma or fluid, parenchyma and ventricles (Figs 5.10 and 5.11). It also allows accurate localization of any defect, especially in the case of occipital lesions that may also involve the upper cervical spine (Fig. 5.12). These details are essential for accurate counseling as the prognosis depends on the site, size and contents. Sixty to eighty percent of babies with cephaloceles will develop normally if there is no brain tissue within the sac but if parenchymal tissue is seen in the sac this is reduced to 10–20%. Associated abnormalities also affect the prognosis, especially ventriculomegaly and other developmental abnormalities of the brain. Cephaloceles are often associated with other abnormalities including cardiac, renal and respiratory as well as CNS and chromosomal disorders (Cohen & Lemire 1982, Robson & Barnewolt 2004, Wininger & Donnenfeld 1994). Sonographic studies are as important as the in utero MR for complete evaluation in these cases. MR imaging also allows pediatric neurosurgeons to plan the postnatal care prior to delivery.

VENTRAL INDUCTION

Abnormal ventral induction results in holoprosencephaly due to abnormal expansion and cleavage. The severest form is alobar holoprosencephaly where there is virtually no attempt at cleavage of the forebrain, the thalami are fused and the lateral ventricles form a monoventricle (Fig. 5.13)

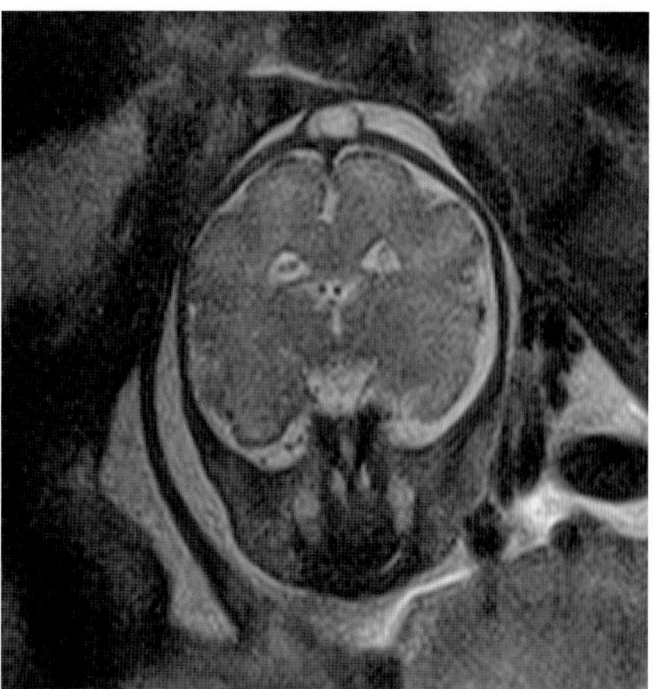

(a)

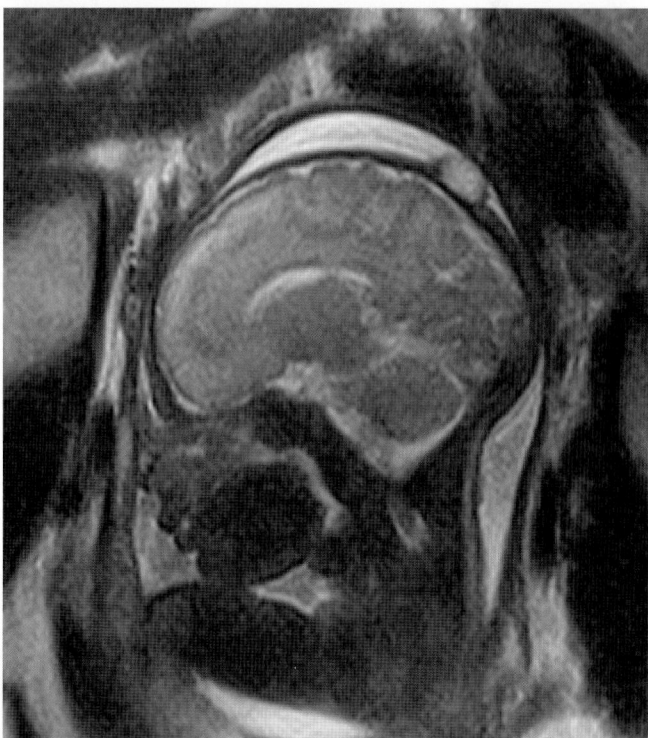

(b)

Figure 5.10 An atretic encephalocele where there is no defect in the skull and a small cystic structure on the external surface. Images obtained at 32 weeks gestation. (a) Coronal. (b) Sagittal.

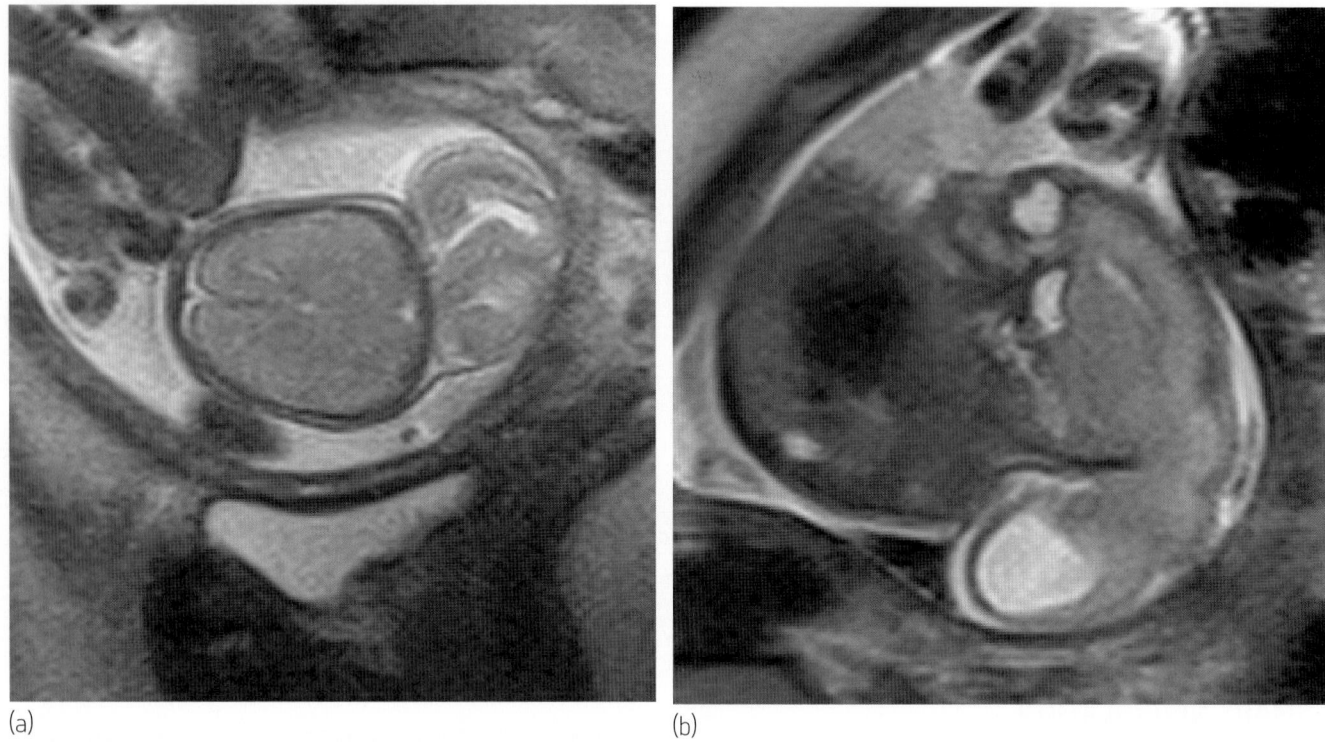

(a)   (b)

Figure 5.11 A large posterior encephalocele. The contents of the sac include most of the brain and the posterior horns of the lateral ventricles. (a) Sagittal section, (b) axial section at 22 weeks gestation.

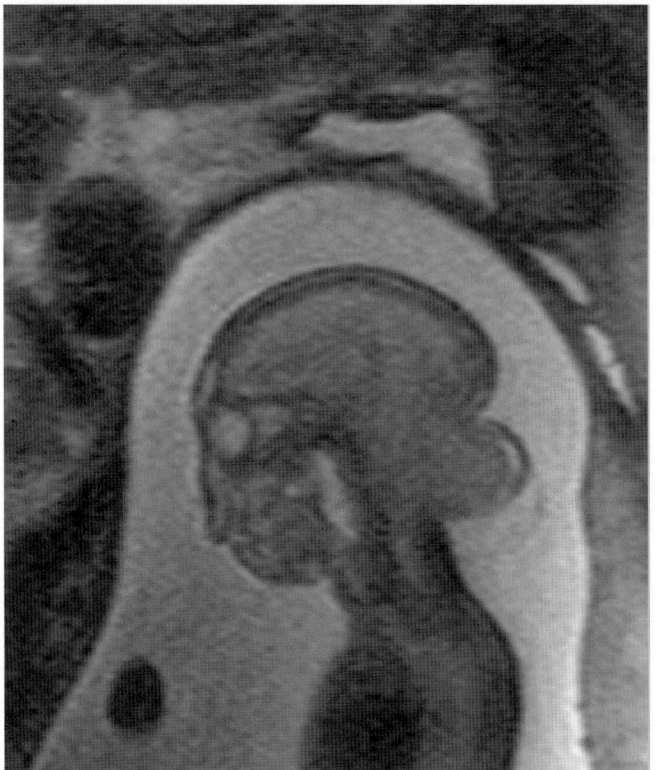

Figure 5.12 Iniencephaly where the defect extends into the upper cervical spine, 22 weeks gestation.

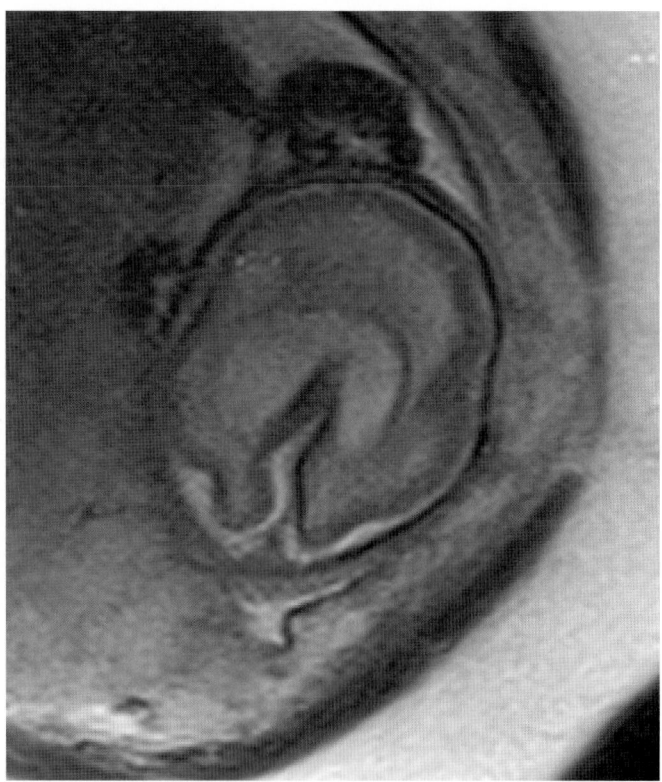

Figure 5.13 Alobar holoprosencephaly. Axial section at 24 weeks gestation. The thalami are fused and there is a single ventricle. There has been no attempt to form two cerebral hemispheres.

without the interhemispheric fissure and falx, and the third ventricle is absent. These fetuses are usually aborted or stillborn; long-term survival is not possible. The least severe form is lobar holoprosencephaly where the frontal horns of the lateral ventricles, the frontal lobes and anterior falx are poorly formed (DeMyer 1975) (Fig. 5.14). The septum pellucidum is always absent but these findings can be subtle and difficult to detect. Semilobar holoprosencephaly has features between the two extremes (Fig. 5.15). These disorders are best seen on the coronal images to assess the thalami which are partly fused. In all cases the fornix and septum pellucidum are absent. Although holoprosencephaly can occur sporadically it is seen in 1–2% of children of diabetic mothers and is associated with chromosomal abnormalities. MR imaging is essential in these cases to accurately define the severity of the abnormality which may be confused with severe ventriculomegaly or intracerebral cysts (Peebles 1998). Sonography is also important for the complete evaluation and detection of any associated abnormalities.

Isolated absence of the septum pellucidum is also possible and is increasingly being diagnosed with the development of higher-resolution ultrasound and fetal MR. The prognosis for this condition is not fully understood and absence of the septum pellucidum can also occur associated with optic nerve dysplasia (which cannot be confidently diagnosed antenatally at present) and ischemic lesions, e.g. schizencephaly (Barkovich & Norman 1989, Pilu et al 1993, 2005, Supprian et al 1999) (Fig. 5.16).

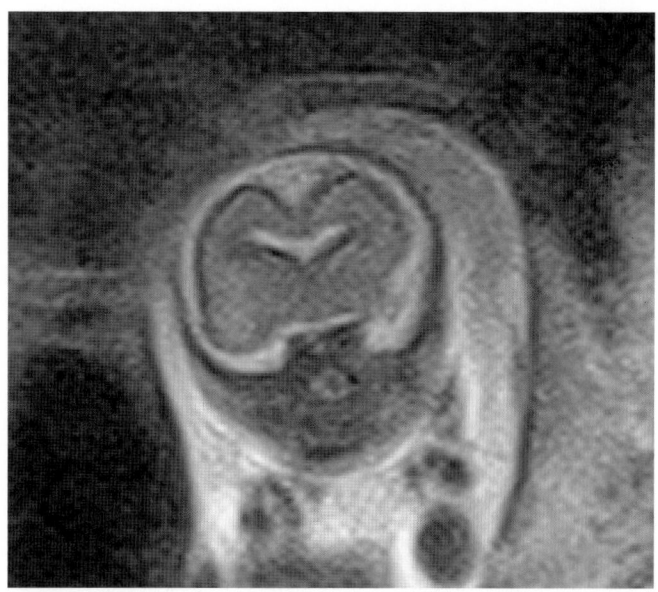

Figure 5.15 Semilobar holoprosencephaly at 24 weeks gestation.

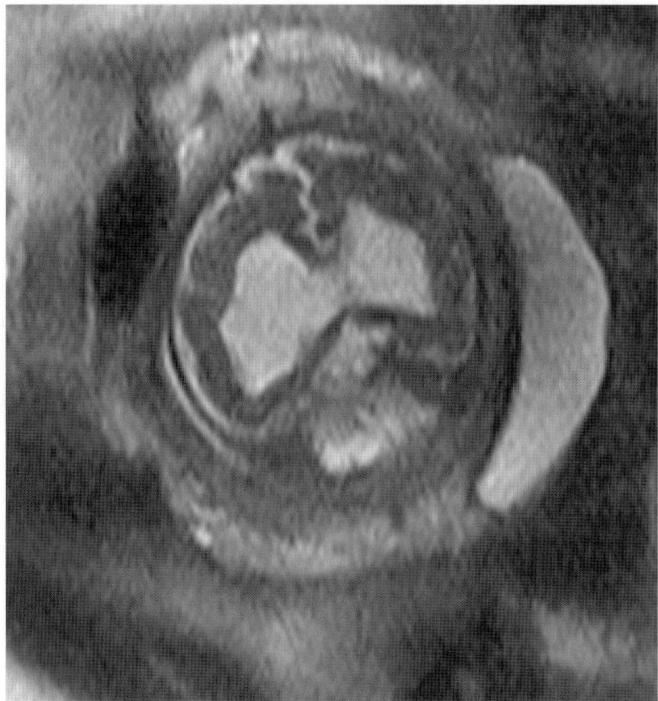

Figure 5.14 Lobar holoprosencephaly, 28 weeks gestational age.

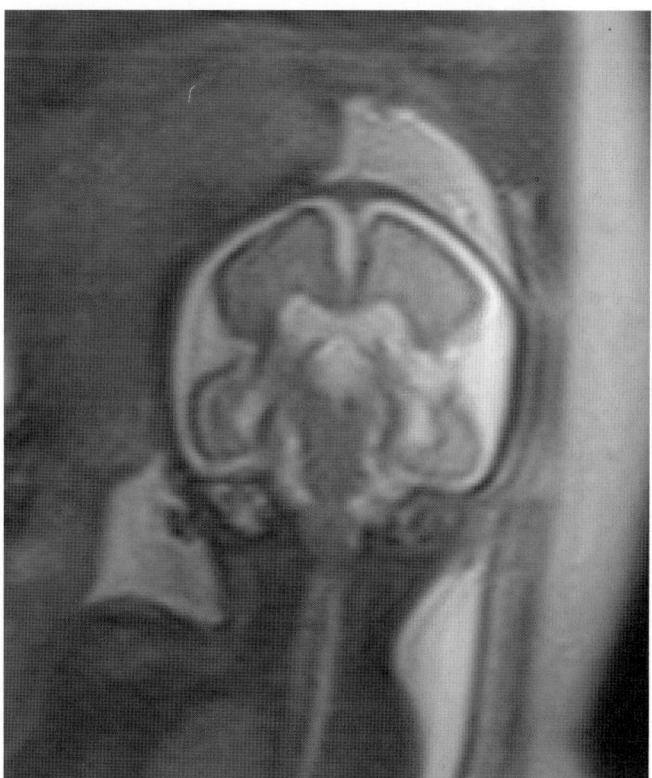

Figure 5.16 Schizencephaly and septo-optic dysplasia. There is absence of the septum pellucidum. There is open-lipped schizencephaly on the left and closed-lipped on the right. The developing cortex is seen as a darker rim and this lines the cleft. If the cleft was due to a destructive process after formation there would be a disruption of the developing cortex.

FAILURE OF COMMISSURATION

The largest commissure is the corpus callosum. Development starts with the genu at 11 weeks gestation followed by the body, isthmus and splenium and finally the rostrum at 18–20 weeks. Failure of development results in agenesis, partial agenesis and hypoplasia can also occur. Hypoplasia is associated with inherited metabolic diseases and may represent loss of neurons rather than underdevelopment. Agenesis characteristically results in straightening of the ventricular contours of the lateral ventricles, resulting in parallel ventricles that have widely spaced frontal horns. Other indirect signs include dilatation of the posterior horns (colpocephaly), high-riding third ventricle and radial deposition of the sulci on the internal aspects of the cerebral hemisphere (Fig. 5.17a–c). The sagittal image allows direct visualization of the corpus callosum both with ultrasound and fetal MR. The coronal and axial images are important to assess the indirect

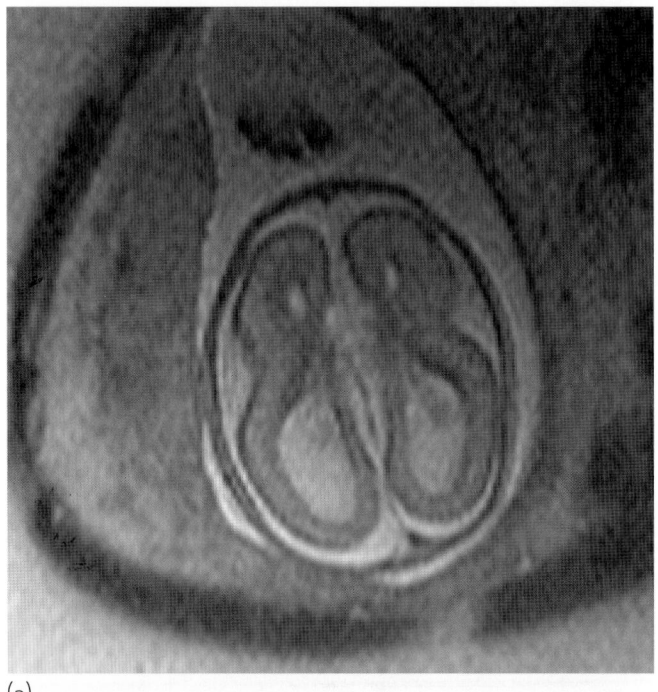

(a)

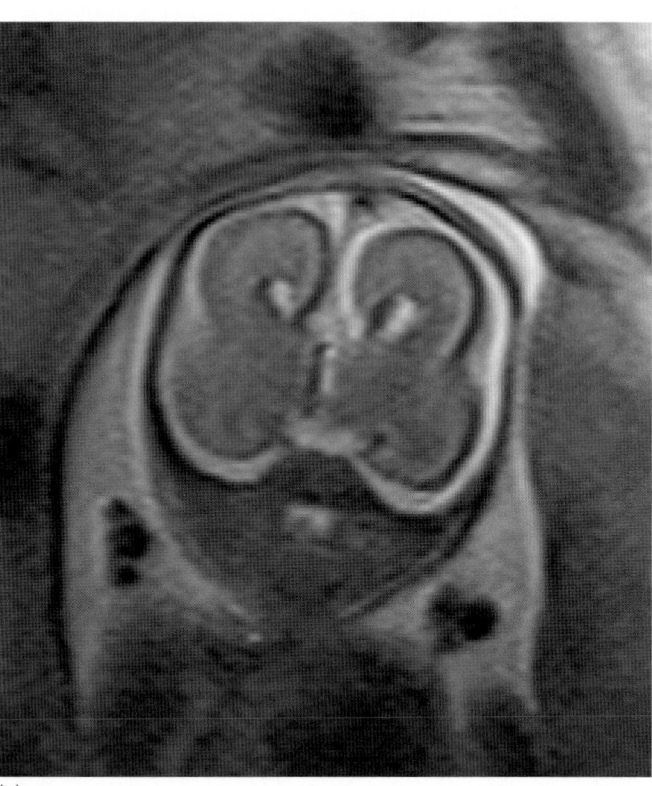

(b)

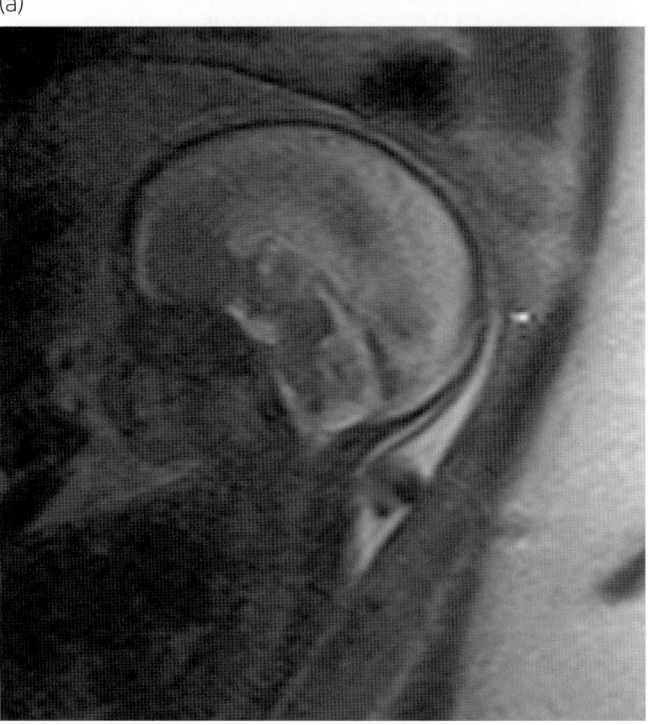

(c)

Figure 5.17 Agenesis of the corpus callosum. (a) Axial section. The ventricles are parallel. (b) Coronal section. Note the complete absence of the corpus callosum that should be seen as a 'bridge' joining to two hemispheres. (c) Sagittal section. The normal dark band of the corpus callosum is absent.

signs of agenesis. The coronal image allows visualization of the corpus callosum in cross section and are the images we find most helpful in partial agenesis but thin slices are essential. The role of fetal MR to detect or confirm agenesis of the corpus callosum probably remains the most controversial. Several studies have produced different detection rates between ultrasound and fetal MR (Glenn et al 2005a, Levine et al 1997, 1999b, Sonigo et al 1998, Whitby et al 2001, 2004) and there remains a group of experienced sonographers that believe ultrasound detects all cases if performed by experienced personnel (Timor-Tritsch 2006, Timor-Tritsch & Monteagudo 2003). In our experience there are cases where a prominent fornix and/or a prominent hippocampal commissure mimic the corpus callosum, making sonographic diagnosis extremely difficult (Fig. 5.18). There are also cases detected postnatally that have never been questioned antenatally. If there is any concern over the corpus callosum a fetal MR is advised. Fetal MR also detects the associated cortical malformations, usually gyration and migrational abnormalities that are extremely difficult to detect sonographically. Posterior fossa abnormalities are also associated with callosal agenesis including Arnold–Chiari malformations, Dandy–Walker variants, cerebellum and/or brain stem hypoplasia and cerebellar heterotopias (Adamsbaum et al 2005, Gupta & Lilford 1995). If the absence of the corpus callosum is due to destruction, there are often other hypoxic or ischemic lesions.

Lipomas of the corpus callosum are rare and usually associated with agenesis or hypogenesis. They appear as low signal mass on T2-weighted images, and high signal on T1 in the third trimester fetal MR is useful to detect any associated abnormalities.

ABNORMAL CORTICAL FORMATION

Many of the structural developmental abnormalities are associated with abnormalities of cortical malformation ranging form heterotopias to subtle sulci and gyral abnormalities.

Pathological and histological studies have shown that neurons migrate from the ganglionic eminence adjacent to the lateral ventricles outwards to the cortex. These are seen on fetal MR images as migrating bands of differing shades of gray (Rados et al 2006). The presence of the different bands and their thickness relate to the gestational age (Rados et al 2006). Indeed with an in-depth understanding the maturity of the fetus can be dated from these changes. Abnormalities in their appearance and thickness relate to developmental abnormalities. It has been reported, as mentioned above, that the appearance may be delayed compare to pathological studies. However, recent pathological studies have included MR imaging and a more detailed description of the imaging appearances and the relationship to histology is now available. Such work is essential to our understanding and interpretation of clinical images.

Abnormal migration results in a range of cortical abnormalities that are familiar to pediatric radiologist and neurologists. These include the following.

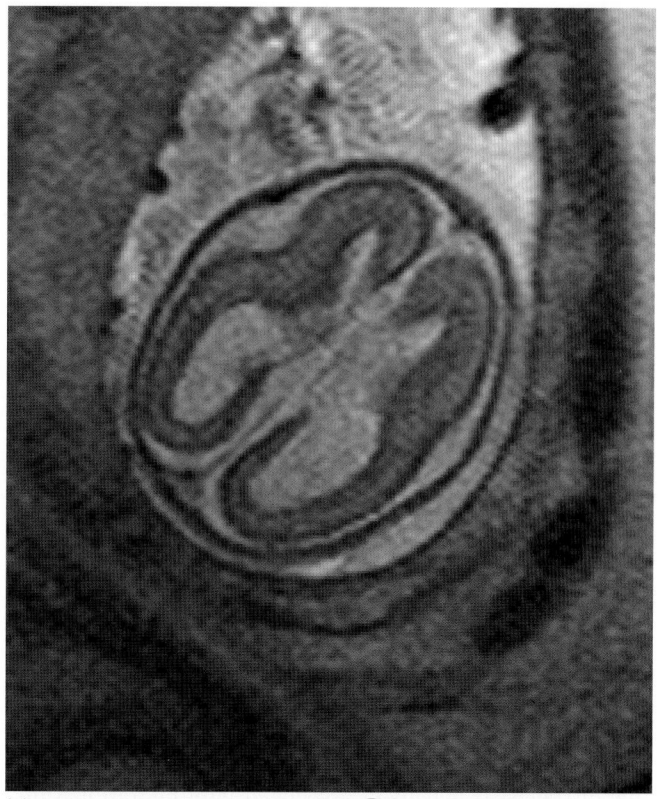

(a)

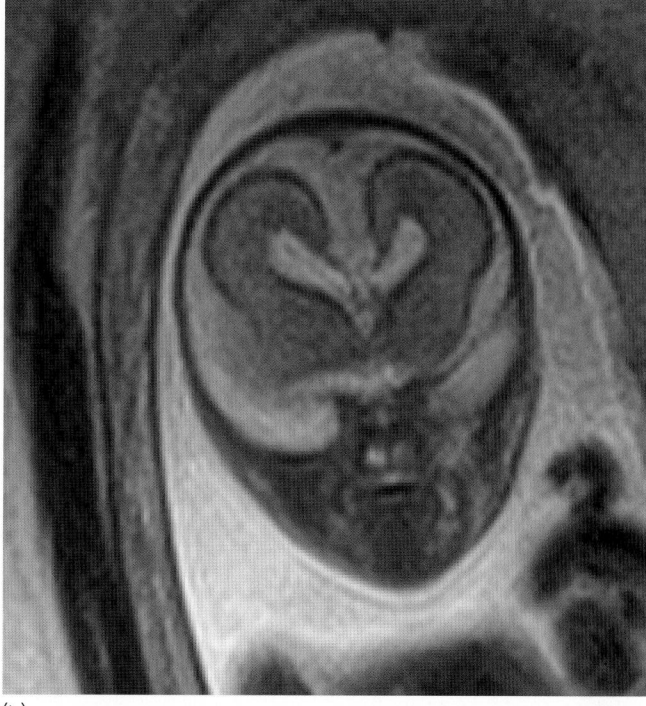

(b)

Figure 5.18 Axial and coronal sections of the fetal brain with agenesis of the corpus callosum. There is a prominent fornix and hippocampal commissure that mimic a thin septum pellucidum and corpus callosum respectively.

MICROCEPHALY

This is defined as a head circumference 2 standard deviations below the mean for gestational age. Most cases are sporadic although some can be familial and are usually due to poor growth and development (Martin 1970). If there is normal sulcal and gyral development it is termed radial micro brain; these cases are rare. It is usually associated with other abnormalities including lissencephaly, porencephaly, holoprosencephaly, ventriculomegaly and agenesis of the corpus callosum. Fetal MR allows direct measurement of the brain parenchyma rather than the skull, which is used for sonographic measurements. This makes the diagnosis and detection of microcephaly much more accurate (Raybaud et al 2003).

MEGALENCEPHALY

Here there is an increase in neuronal proliferation resulting in an increase in the size and weight of the brain. Hemimegalencephaly is when half of the brain is affected. This is often misdiagnosed as unilateral ventriculomegaly on ultrasound if it is subtle and only when the parenchymal changes are seen on fetal MR is the diagnosis made (Fig. 5.19). It occurs in a variety of syndromes thus having varying clinical manifestations including motor and cognitive disorders. It is usually associated with migrational disorders including heterotopias and polymicrogyria. These are best visualized with fetal MR.

POLYMICROGYRIA

Fetal MR is superior to ultrasound for the diagnosis of subtle heterotopias (Delle Urban et al 2004, Glenn et al 2005b, Kuzniecky 1994, Osborn et al 1988). Polymicrogyria may present with or without laminar necrosis. It occurs due to over folding of the laminar with or without fusion of the adjacent sulci. It occurs most frequently around the sylvian fissures (Fig. 5.20).

Lissencephaly

This can only be accurately detected with an in-depth knowledge of the sulcal and gyral formation and remains difficult to detect before the third trimester. The more recent pathological studies are increasing our understanding of normal development and thence making the diagnosis of lissencephaly at an earlier gestation more likely in the future. Lissencephaly may be widespread over the cortical surface or localized (Fig. 5.21). The affected children normally present with developmental delay and seizures.

Schizencephaly

This is a cleft in the parenchyma that has a gray-matter lining and extends from the ventricles to the subarachnoid space. There are two types – closed and open-lipped – depending on whether the gray matter from each side on the cleft is opposed or not (Barkovich & Norman 1989, Huang et al 2006, Lituania et al 1989, Smith et al 2005) (Fig. 5.17).

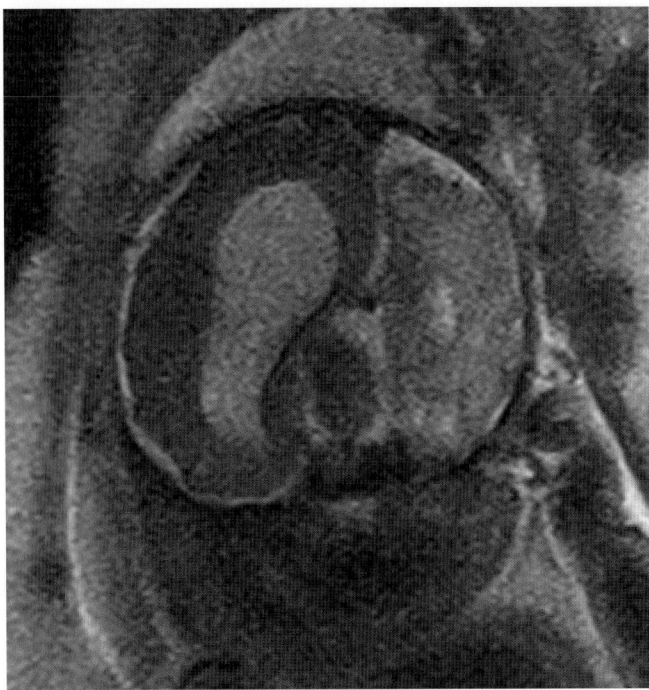

Figure 5.19 Hemimegalencephaly of the right cerebral hemisphere. All the structures are enlarged and the normal layering pattern of the developing cortex is replaced by thick irregular bands consistent with cortical heterotopias.

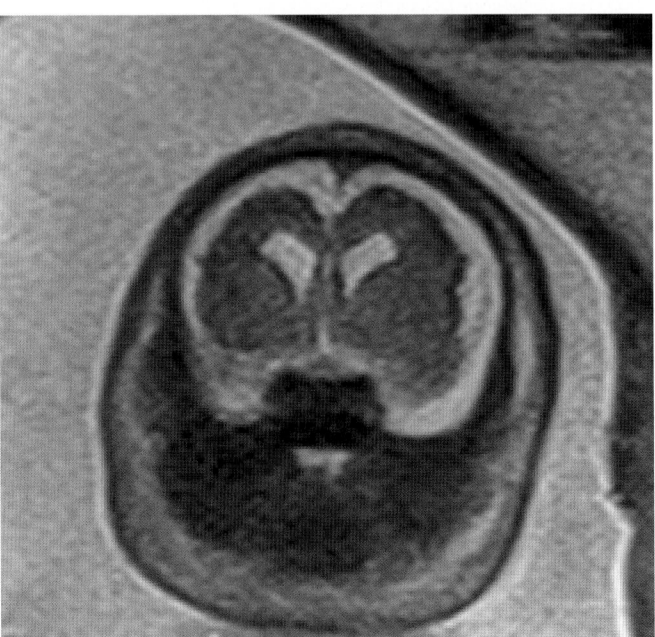

Figure 5.20 Polymicrogyria. The brain in small and the cortical margin thickened and irregular.

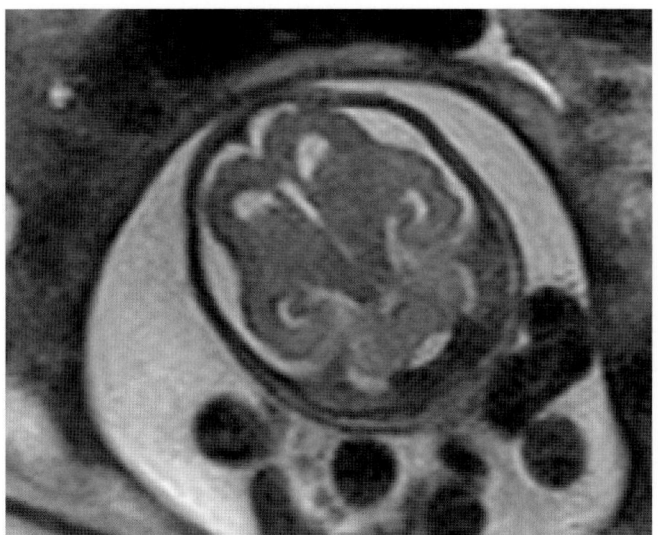

Figure 5.21 Microlissencephaly. The brain is small and poorly developed. The frontal and parietal lobes are not in proportion with the temporal lobes and the sulcal and gyral pattern is significantly delayed for gestational age of 27 weeks.

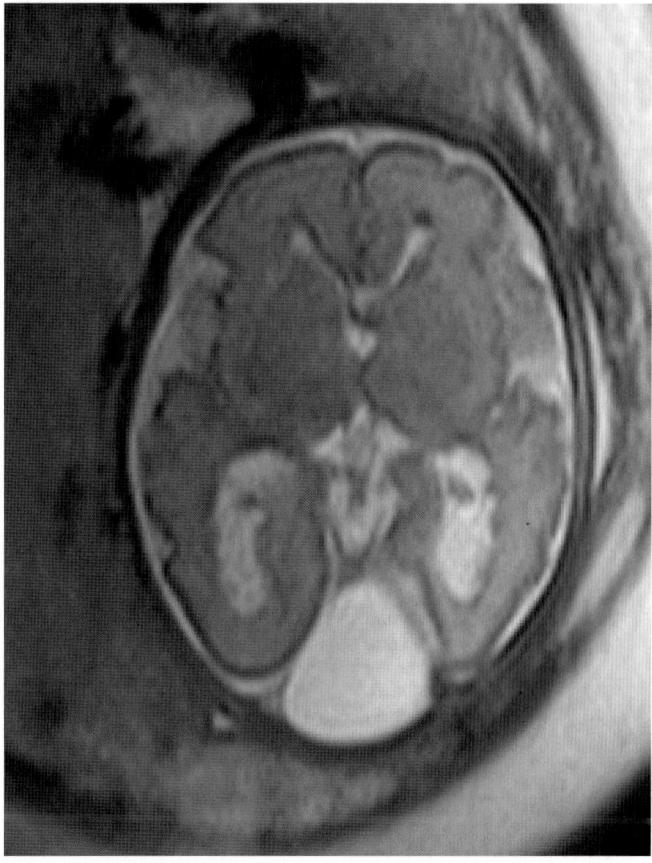

Figure 5.22 Axial section at 32 weeks gestation. There is a cyst between the posterior aspect of the two cerebral hemispheres. The internal walls of the lateral ventricles are irregular, consistent with nodular heterotopia.

HETEROTOPIAS

These are either subependymal or subcortical and are clusters of neurons that have failed to migrate to their correct place. They may be focal or diffuse, unilateral or bilateral. They may be an isolated finding but are often associated with other CNS abnormalities. They can be sporadic or genetic and may be inherited as dominant, recessive or X-linked patterns. Fetal MR shows many formats including bands of neurons in the parenchyma and nodules lining the ventricles (Fig. 5.22).

Several groups have detailed the use of fetal MR in cases with cortical migration/development abnormalities (Glenn et al 2005b, Kuzniecky 1994, Levine et al 1997, Osborn et al 1988, Raymond et al 1995).

VENTRICULOMEGALY

This is probably the main reason for referral for MR imaging of the fetus. Several groups have reported that MR imaging detects abnormalities not detectable by ultrasound in up to 50% of cases (Blaicher et al 2003; Breysem et al 2003; Girard et al 2003; Levine et al 1999a, 2002; Morris et al 2007; Whitby et al 2001, 2004). The abnormalities detected include agenesis of the corpus callosum, intraventricular bleeds, parenchymal abnormalities, e.g. periventricular leukomalacia, and associated abnormalities of cortical formation that cannot be identified sonographically. The detection rate is less in specific subgroups but even when isolated mild ventriculomegaly cases were selected for MR imaging additional major pathology was found in 12.2% of cases (Ouahba et al 2006) (Figs 5.23a,b).

Fetal MR also allows assessment of the ventricular walls (Fig. 5.22) and the surrounding parenchyma more easily than MR.

Severe ventriculomegaly may mimic hydranencephaly on ultrasound images, especially at later gestational ages when the calvarium is calcified and causes acoustic shadowing. Fetal MR clearly demonstrates the thin cortical rim in cases of severe ventriculomegaly (Fig. 5.24) and its absence in hydranencephaly (Fig. 5.25).

HYDRANENCEPHALY

This is due to a vascular insult that results in temporary or complete occlusion of the middle cerebral arteries and loss of most of the cerebral parenchyma. The remaining parenchyma is at the frontal and occipital regions and a rim that links the two areas like a 'basket handle' adjacent to the sagittal sinus (Fig. 5.25).

POSTERIOR FOSSA

Fetal MR is useful in identifying abnormalities of the posterior fossa which include Dandy–Walker malformations

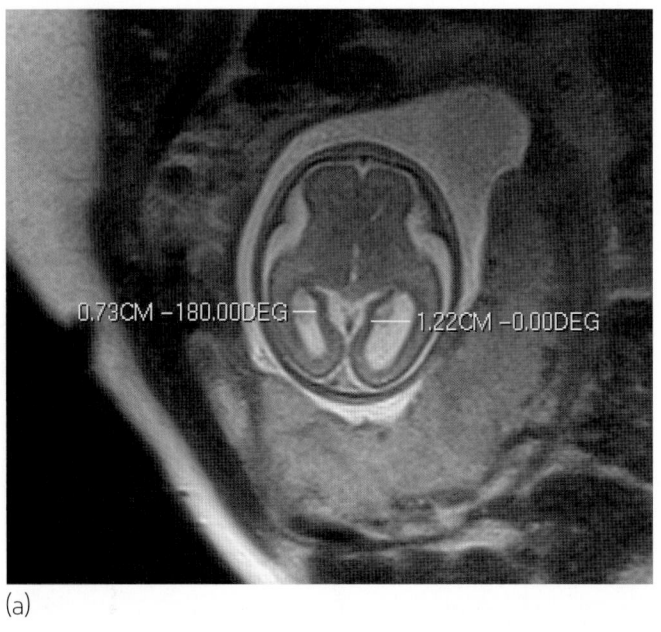

(a)

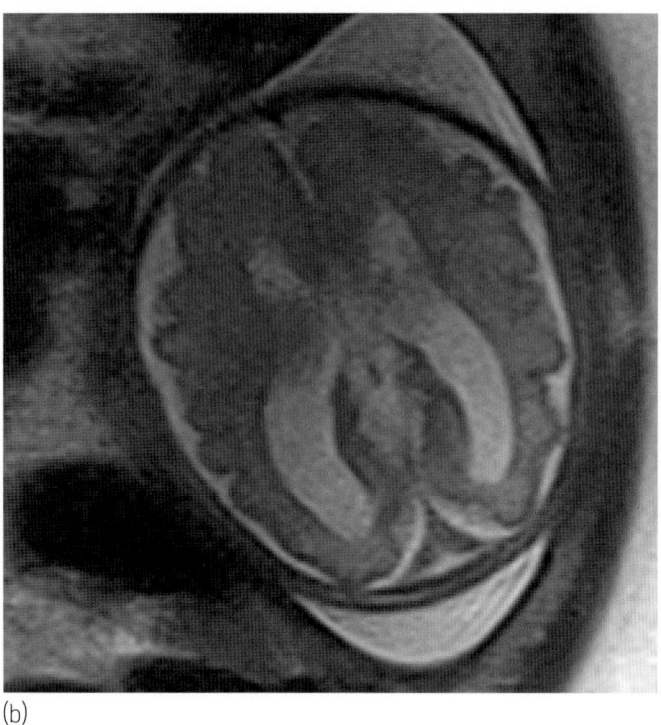

(b)

Figure 5.23 Isolated mild ventriculomegaly. (a) Unilateral at 22 weeks. (b) Bilateral at 32 weeks.

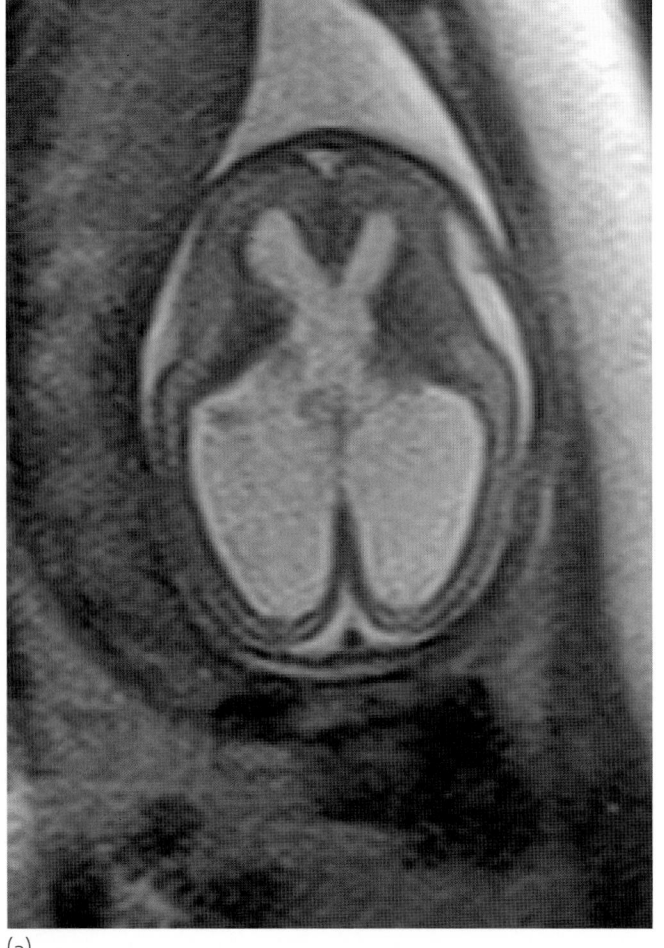

(a)

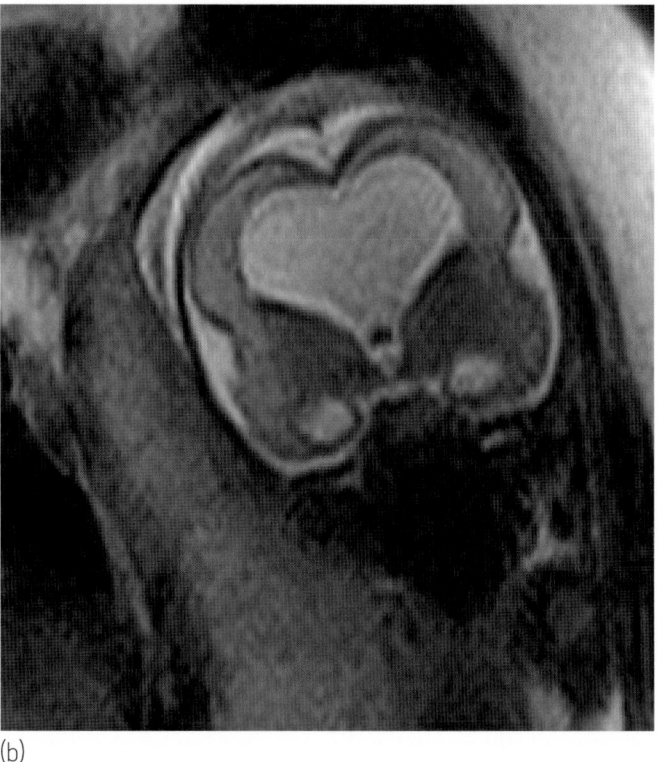

(b)

Figure 5.24 Severe bilateral ventriculomegaly at 23 weeks due to aqueduct stenosis. (a) Axial section. (b) Coronal section.

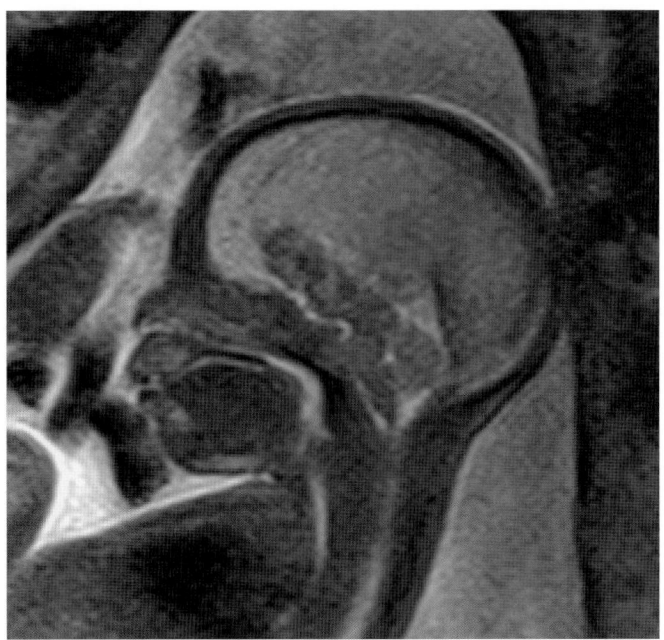

Figure 5.25 Sagittal section of a fetus with hydranencephaly. Note the absence of most of the supratentorial structures.

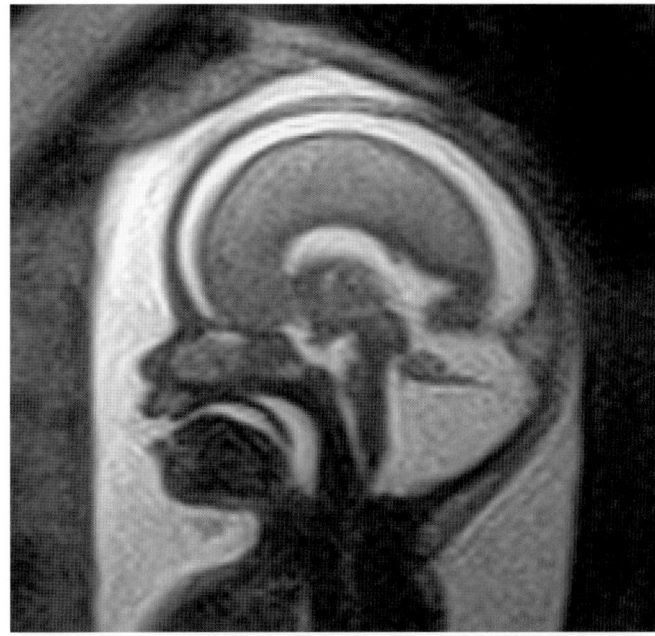

(a)

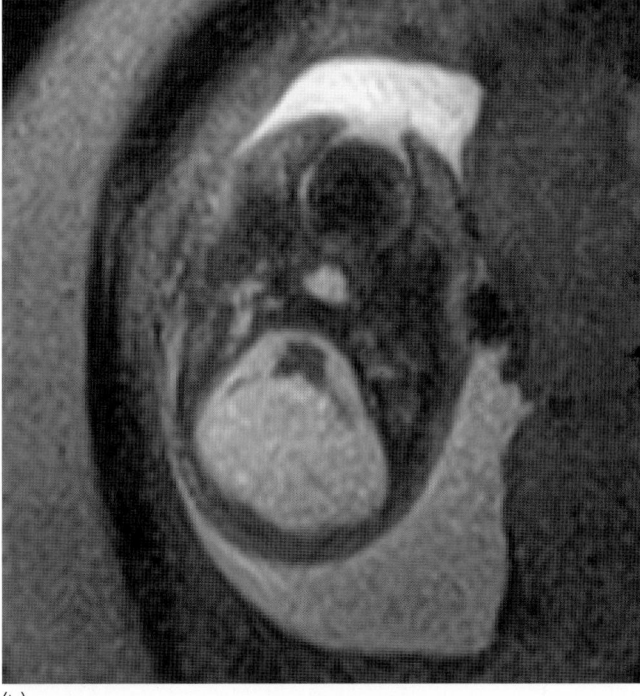

(b)

Figure 5.26 23 weeks gestation fetus with Dandy–Walker malformation. There is a large posterior fossa, and absence of the inferior cerebellar vermis. Ventriculomegaly may not occur in utero. (a) Sagittal section. (b) Axial section.

(Fig. 5.26a,b) and Dandy–Walker variant, megacisterna magna (Fig. 5.27), cerebellar hypoplasia (Fig. 5.28), arachnoid cyst, Walker–Warburg (Fig. 5.29) and Chiari malformations (Fig. 5.30) amongst others. Although sonographic techniques can accurately identify the severe forms of these abnormalities more subtle changes are difficult and again associated abnormalities involving cortical development are more accurately identified with fetal MR (Adamsbaum et al 2005, Guibaud 2004).

Fetal MR is helpful to fully define the cerebellum and the size of the posterior fossa allowing accurate identification of a mega cisterna magna or cerebellar hypoplasia. It is also useful to define the anatomical location of posterior fossa cysts. In cases of Dandy–Walker variants the outcome is dependent upon the presence of other abnormalities and the degree of vermian hypoplasia. Fetal MR is able to detect these abnormalities better than ultrasound.

Fetal MR has been shown to be superior to ultrasound in the identification and location of hemorrhagic lesions in the posterior fossa (Gorincour et al 2006). Acute hemorrhage is high signal on T1- and low signal on T2-weighted images. Dural arteriovenous fistulas are often of low flow and mimic cysts in the posterior fossa. They cause displacement and compression of the cerebellum which may mimic a Chiari malformation. Recent experience has shown that these resolve or at least become smaller with increasing gestational age and have a good prognosis (Jung et al 2006). Cerebellar capillary telangiectasia has been reported to be easily visualized with ultrasound and not seen with MR. It has been suggested that echo bright lesions on ultrasound in this region that are not visible with MR are characteristic

of capillary telangiectasia but further studies are required to confirm this (Guibaud et al 2003).

MONOCHORIONIC TWINS

Fetal MR is increasingly used in cases of twin-to-twin transfusion following death of a co-twin and/or intervention to prevent twin-to-twin transfusion syndrome. In these cases

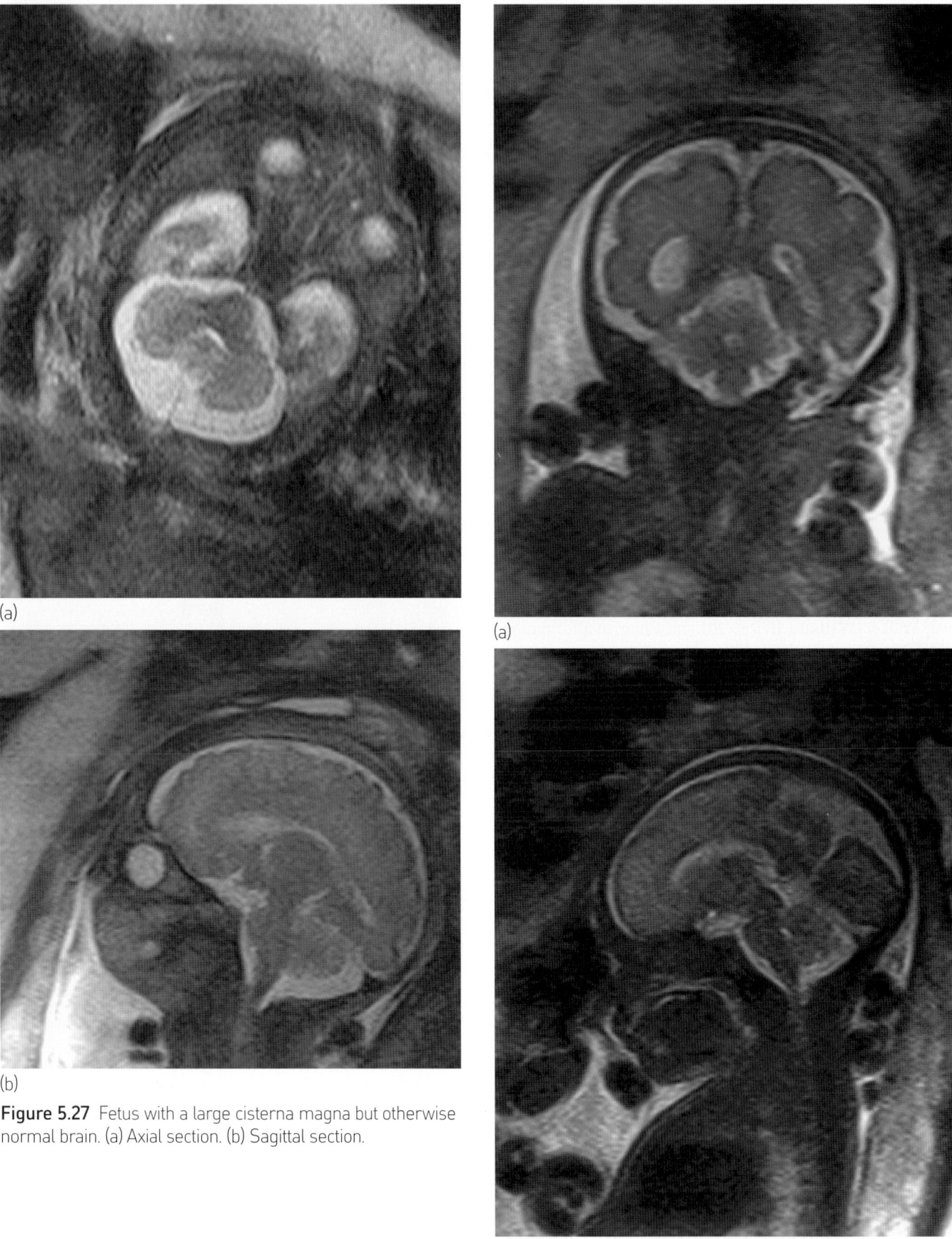

(a)

(b)

Figure 5.27 Fetus with a large cisterna magna but otherwise normal brain. (a) Axial section. (b) Sagittal section.

(a)

(b)

Figure 5.28 (a) Cerebellar hypoplasia affecting the left cerebellum only seen on the coronal view. (b) The sagittal view is normal as the cerebellar vermis is intact.

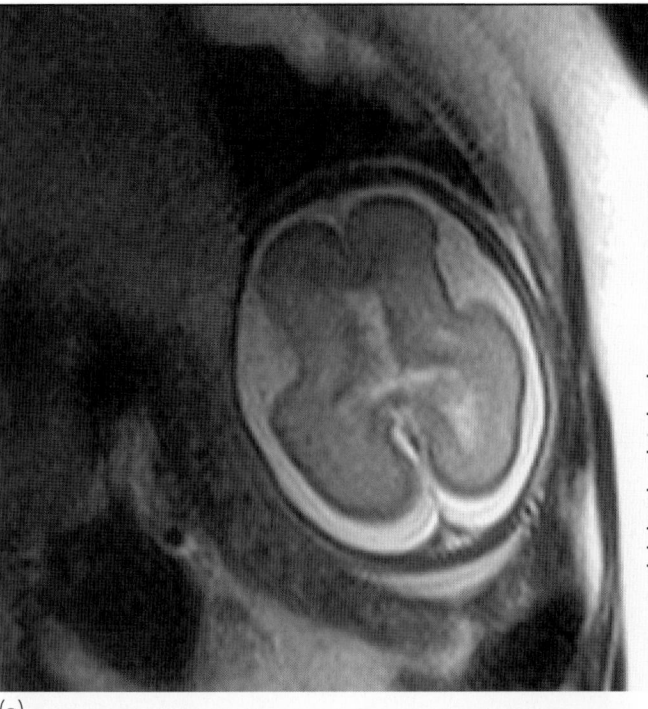

(a)

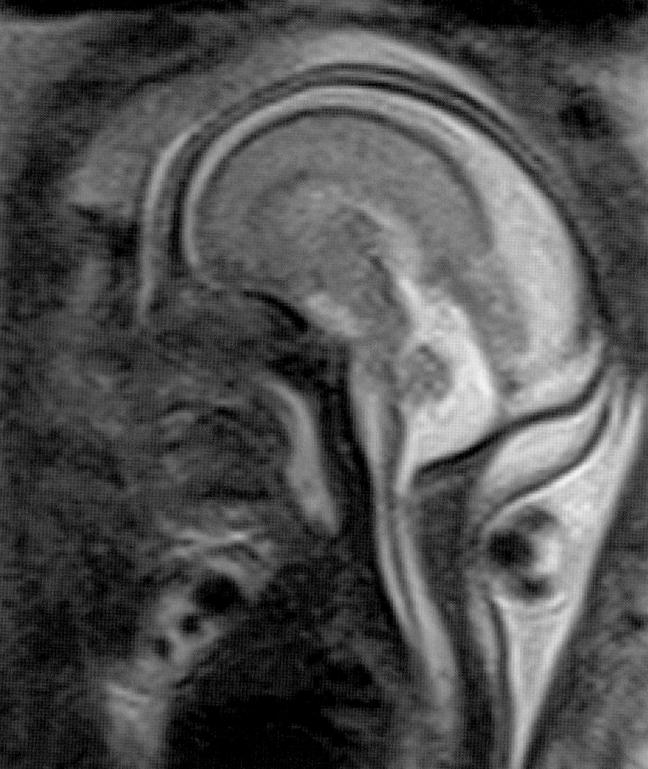

(b)

Figure 5.29 A fetus with Walker–Warburg syndrome. The cerebellum is small, there is increased extra-axial CSF space and there is a delay in the sulcal and gyral pattern for gestation age of 26 weeks.

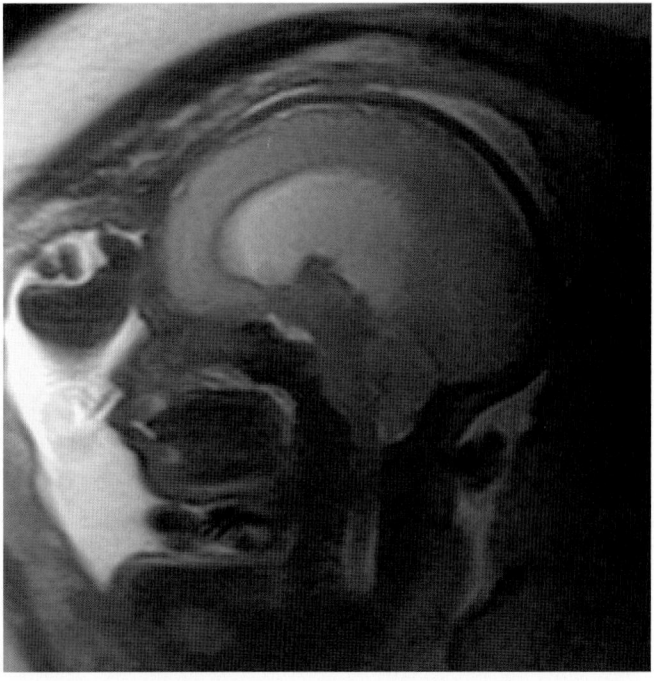

Figure 5.30 Chiari II malformation in the brain. The posterior fossa is small and the cerebellum has descended into the cervical spine.

most centers image 4 weeks after the event to detect any vascular damage (hypoperfusion or embolic) to the twins or in the cases of fetal demise of one twin assessment of the remaining viable twin (Hu et al 2006, Huisman et al 2005). Further development and understanding of diffusion-weighted imaging of the fetus will be useful to detect early parenchymal damage in such cases.

CONGENITAL INFECTIONS

Fetal MR is being increasingly used for cases with congenital infections although the majority are suspected sonographically and confirmed serologically. In these cases the fetal MR is performed to assess the effects on the developing brain and fully delineate the abnormalities. Calcifications are poorly seen on fetal MR but easily seen sonographically and the two modalities together provide the best means of obtaining accurate diagnostic information.

SPINAL ABNORMALITIES

Fetal MR has established itself as a valuable investigation for the fetal brain but its value in spinal imaging is still debated (Appasamy et al 2006, Miller et al 2006, Nakahara et al 1993, Simon 2004, von Koch et al 2005). Ultrasound shows the bony abnormalities more easily and accurately than MR which can demonstrate the neural tissue component more accurately (Appasamy et al 2006, von Koch et al 2005) (Fig. 5.31a–d). The two techniques are complementary. Fetal MR demonstrates the hindbrain abnormalities

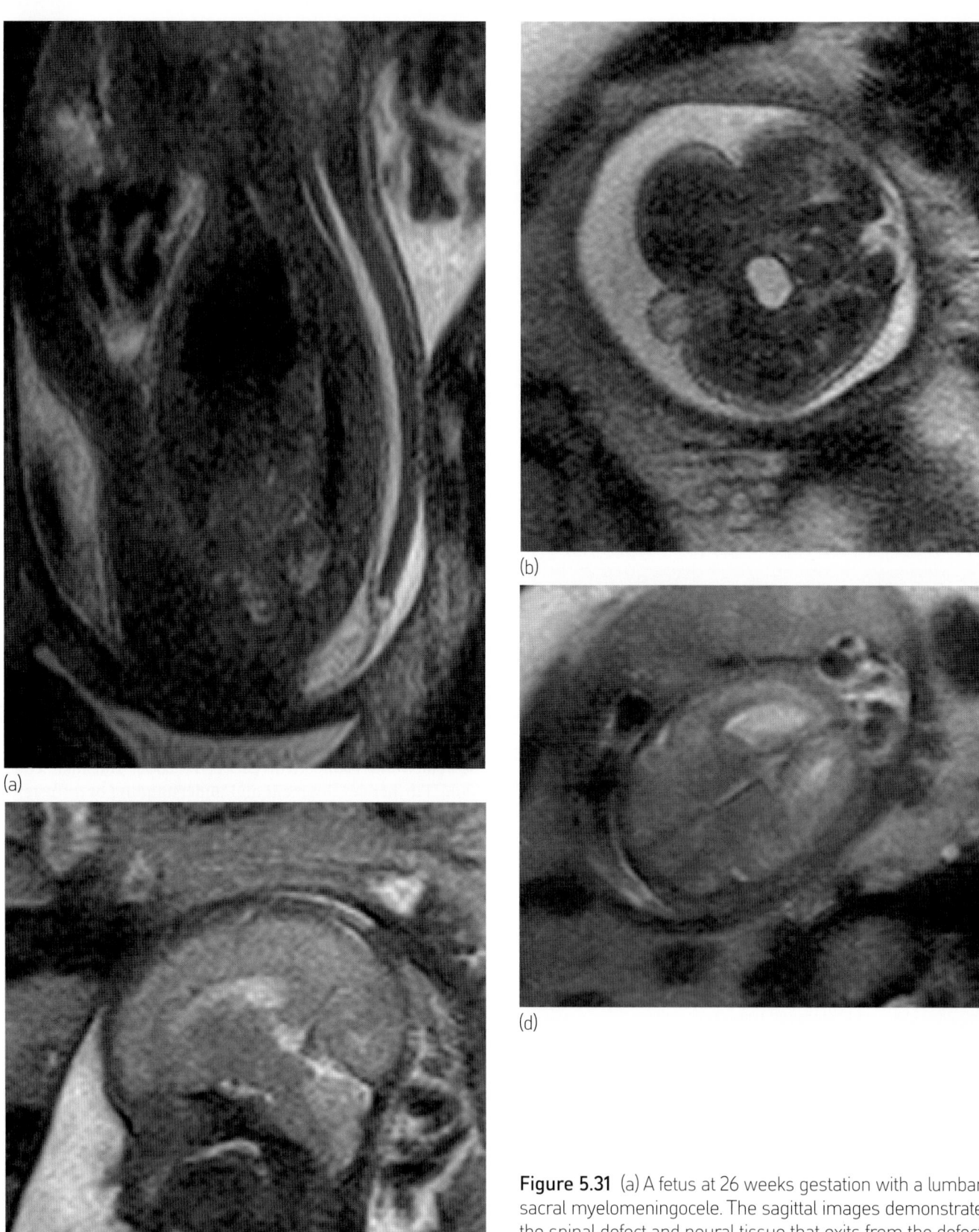

Figure 5.31 (a) A fetus at 26 weeks gestation with a lumbar sacral myelomeningocele. The sagittal images demonstrate the spinal defect and neural tissue that exits from the defect to form a placode on the wall of the meningocele. (b) An axial section through the defect in the spine demonstrates the neural tissue as a dark dot in the meningocele. (c) The fetus has an associated Chiari malformation and almost complete lack of extra-axial CSF space, best seen on the axial images (d).

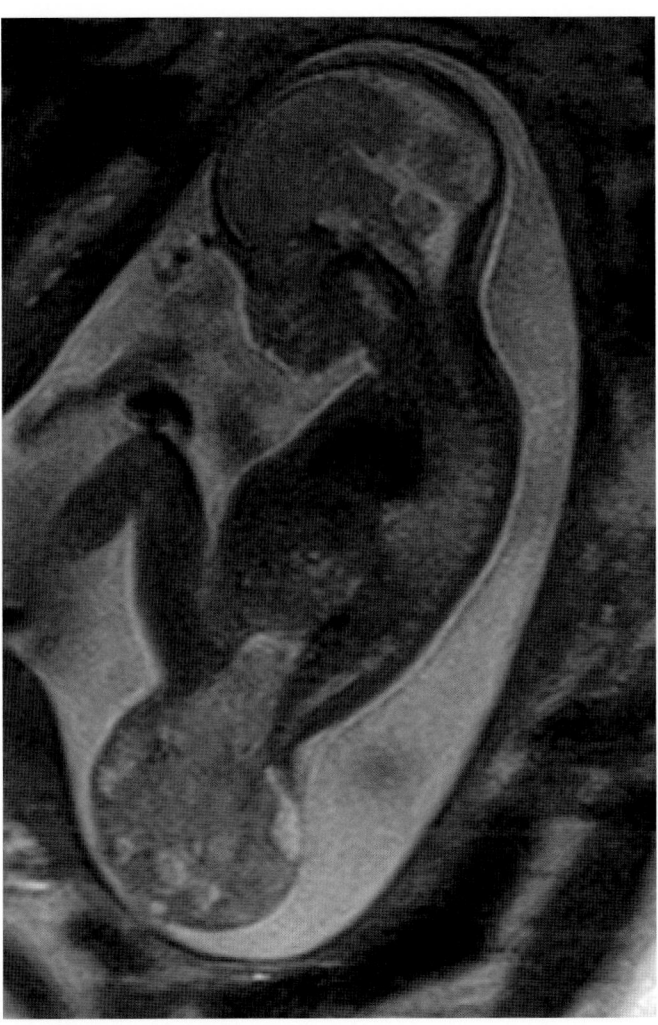

Figure 5.32 Parasagittal section through the fetal spine of a fetus with a sacral teratoma. MR is useful to assess the internal component in these cases.

associated with spinal myelomeningoceles and can demonstrate the presence, amount and location of any neural tissue in the myelomeningocele. It is still uncertain whether the size and location of the spinal defect affect the severity of the Chiari malformation. In utero spinal surgery is also still under evaluation but fetal MR is important in the selection criteria and post-surgery assessment in this prospective trial (Adzick & Walsh 2003, Bruner et al 2004, Sutton et al 2003, Walsh & Adzick 2003). Fetal MR is useful in cases with diastematomyelia, sacral agenesis, segmental spinal dysgenesis and sacral teratomas (Fig. 5.32).

CONCLUSION

Fetal MR provides an important and accurate imaging modality for malformations of the CNS. It remains a selective investigation once an abnormality has been questioned and will never replace ultrasound as a screening modality. Further technological advances in ultrafast MR imaging will increase the clinical usefulness of the technique. Advances in understanding normal and pathological development at the histological level will increase our diagnostic capabilities further. The expansion will only continue and provide clinically useful information if a multidisciplinary team approach is used.

REFERENCES

Adamsbaum C, Moutard M L, Andre C et al 2005 MRI of the fetal posterior fossa. Pediatr Radiol 35:124–140.

Adzick N S, Walsh D S 2003 Myelomeningocele: prenatal diagnosis, pathophysiology and management. Semin Pediatr Surg 12:168–174.

Agid R, Lieberman S, Nadjari M, Gomori J M 2006 Prenatal MR diffusion-weighted imaging in a fetus with hemimegalencephaly. Pediatr Radiol 36:138–140.

Appasamy M, Roberts D, Pilling D, Buxton N 2006 Antenatal ultrasound and magnetic resonance imaging in localizing the level of lesion in spina bifida and correlation with postnatal outcome. Ultrasound Obstet Gynecol 27:530–536.

Baker P N, Johnson I R, Harvey P R et al 1994 A three-year follow-up of children imaged in utero with echo-planar magnetic resonance. Am J Obstet Gynecol 170:32–33.

Barkovich A J, Norman D 1989 Absence of the septum pellucidum: a useful sign in the diagnosis of congenital brain malformations. AJR Am J Roentgenol 152:353–360.

Blaicher W, Prayer D, Mittermayer C et al 2003 Magnetic resonance imaging in foetuses with bilateral moderate ventriculomegaly and suspected anomaly of the corpus callosum on ultrasound scan. Ultraschall Medizin 24:255–260.

Breysem L, Bosmans H, Dymarkowski S et al 2003 The value of fast MR imaging as an adjunct to ultrasound in prenatal diagnosis. Eur Radiol 13:1538–1548.

Breysem L, Cossey V, Mussen E et al 2004 Fetal trauma: brain imaging in four neonates. Eur Radiol 14:1609–1614.

Brisse H, Fallet C, Sebag G et al 1997 Supratentorial parenchyma in the developing fetal brain: in vitro MR study with histologic comparison. AJNR Am J Neuroradiol 18:1491–1497.

Brunel H, Girard N, Confort-Gouny S 2004 Fetal brain injury. J Neuroradiol 31:123–137.

Bruner J P, Tulipan N, Reed G et al 2004 Intrauterine repair of spina bifida: preoperative predictors of shunt-dependent hydrocephalus. Am J Obstet Gynecol 190:1305–1312.

Clements H, Duncan K R, Fielding K et al 2000 Infants exposed to MRI in utero have a normal paediatric assessment at 9 months of age. Br J Radiol 73:190–194.

Coakley F V, Hricak H, Filly R A et al 1999 Complex fetal disorders: effect of MR imaging on management – preliminary clinical experience. Radiology 213:691–696.

Cohen M M, Jr, Lemire R J 1982 Syndromes with cephaloceles. Teratology 25:161–72.

d'Ercole C, Girard N, Cravello L et al 1998 Prenatal diagnosis of fetal corpus callosum agenesis by ultrasonography and magnetic resonance imaging. Prenat Diagn 18:247–253.

de Laveaucoupet J, Audibert F, Guis F et al 2001 Fetal magnetic resonance imaging (MRI) of ischemic brain injury. Prenat Diagn 21:729–736.

Delle Urban L A, Righini A, Rustico M et al 2004 Prenatal ultrasound detection of bilateral focal polymicrogyria. Prenat Diagn 24:808–811.

DeMyer W 1975 Median facial malformations and their implications for brain malformations. Birth Defects Orig Artic Ser 11:155–181.

Fogliarini C, Chaumoitre K, Chapon F et al 2005a Assessment of cortical maturation with prenatal MRI. Part I: Normal cortical maturation. Eur Radiol 15:1671–1685.

Fogliarini C, Chaumoitre K, Chapon F et al 2005b Assessment of cortical maturation with prenatal MRI. Part II: Abnormalities of cortical maturation. Eur Radiol 15:1781–1789.

Fukui K, Morioka T, Nishio S et al 2001 Fetal germinal matrix and intraventricular haemorrhage diagnosed by MRI. Neuroradiology 43:68–72.

Garel C 2004a MRI of the fetal brain. Springer-Verlag, Berlin.

Garel C 2004b The role of MRI in the evaluation of the fetal brain with an emphasis on biometry, gyration and parenchyma. Pediatr Radiol 34(9):694–699.

Garel C, Alberti C 2006 Coronal measurement of the fetal lateral ventricles: comparison between ultrasonography and magnetic resonance imaging. Ultrasound Obstet Gynecol 27:23–27.

Garel C, Chantrel E, Brisse H et al 2001 Fetal cerebral cortex: normal gestational landmarks identified using prenatal MR imaging. AJNR Am J Neuroradiol 22:184–189.

Garel C, Chantrel E, Elmaleh M et al 2003 Fetal MRI: normal gestational landmarks for cerebral biometry, gyration and myelination. Childs Nerv Syst 19:422–425.

Girard N J, Raybaud C A 1992 In vivo MRI of fetal brain cellular migration. J Comput Assist Tomogr 16:265–267.

Girard N, Fogliarini C, Viola A et al 2006a MRS of normal and impaired fetal brain development. Eur J Radiol 57:217–225.

Girard N, Gouny S C, Viola A et al 2006b Assessment of normal fetal brain maturation in utero by proton magnetic resonance spectroscopy. Magn Reson Med 56:768–775.

Girard N, Ozanne A, Chaumoitre K et al 2003 MRI and in utero ventriculomegaly. J Radiologie 84:1933–1944.

Glenn O A, Barkovich A J 2006a Magnetic resonance imaging of the fetal brain and spine: an increasingly important tool in prenatal diagnosis, part 1. AJNR Am J Neuroradiol 27:1604–1611.

Glenn O A, Barkovich J 2006b Magnetic resonance imaging of the fetal brain and spine: an increasingly important tool in prenatal diagnosis: part 2. AJNR Am J Neuroradiol 27:1807–1814.

Glenn O A, Goldstein R B, Li K C et al 2005a Fetal magnetic resonance imaging in the evaluation of fetuses referred for sonographically suspected abnormalities of the corpus callosum. J Ultrasound Med 24:791–804.

Glenn O A, Norton M E, Goldstein R B, Barkovich A J 2005b Prenatal diagnosis of polymicrogyria by fetal magnetic resonance imaging in monochorionic cotwin death. J Ultrasound Med 24:711–716.

Glover P, Hykin J, Gowland P et al 1995 An assessment of the intrauterine sound intensity level during obstetric echo-planar magnetic resonance imaging. Br J Radiol 68:1090–1094.

Gorincour G, Rypens F, Lapierre C et al 2006 Fetal magnetic resonance imaging in the prenatal diagnosis of cerebellar hemorrhage. Ultrasound Obstet Gynecol 27:78–80.

Grossman R, Hoffman C, Mardor Y, Biegon A 2006 Quantitative MRI measurements of human fetal brain development in utero. Neuroimage 33:463–470.

Guibaud L 2004 Practical approach to prenatal posterior fossa abnormalities using MRI. Pediatr Radiol 34:700–711.

Guibaud L, Garel C, Annie B et al 2003 Prenatal diagnosis of capillary telangiectasia of the cerebellum — ultrasound and MRI features. Prenat Diagn 23:791–796.

Gupta J K, Lilford R J 1995 Assessment and management of fetal agenesis of the corpus callosum. Prenat Diagn 15:301–312.

Hennig J, Nauerth A, Friedburg H 1986 RARE imaging: a fast imaging method for clinical MR. Magn Reson Med 3:823–833.

Hu L S, Caire J, Twickler D M 2006 MR findings of complicated multifetal gestations. Pediatr Radiol 36:76–81.

Huang W M, Monteagudo A, Bennett G L et al 2006 Schizencephaly in a dysgenetic fetal brain: prenatal sonographic, magnetic resonance imaging, and postmortem correlation. J Ultrasound Med 25:551–554.

Huisman T A, Lewi L, Zimmermann R et al 2005 Magnetic resonance imaging of the feto-placentar unit after fetoscopic laser coagulation for twin-to-twin transfusion syndrome. Acta Radiol 46:328–330.

Jung E, Won H S, Kim S K et al 2006 Spontaneous resolution of prenatally diagnosed dural sinus thrombosis: a case report. Ultrasound Obstet Gynecol 27:562–565.

Kok R D, de Vries M M, Heerschap A, van den Berg P P 2004 Absence of harmful effects of magnetic resonance exposure at 1.5 T in utero during the third trimester of pregnancy: a follow-up study. Magn Reson Imaging 22:51–54.

Kostovic I, Jovanov-Milosevic N 2006 The development of cerebral connections during the first 20–45 weeks' gestation. Semin Fetal Neonatal Med 11:415–422.

Kuzniecky R I 1994 Magnetic resonance imaging in developmental disorders of the cerebral cortex. Epilepsia 35 Suppl 6:S44–S56.

Levine D, Barnes P D 1999 Cortical maturation in normal and abnormal fetuses as assessed with prenatal MR imaging. Radiology 210:751–758.

Levine D, Barnes P D, Madsen J R et al 1997 Fetal central nervous system anomalies: MR imaging augments sonographic diagnosis. Radiology 204:635–642.

Levine D, Barnes P D, Madsen J R et al 1999a Central nervous system abnormalities assessed with prenatal magnetic resonance imaging. Obstet Gynecol 94:1011–1019.

Levine D, Barnes P D, Madsen J R et al 1999b Fetal CNS anomalies revealed on ultrafast MR imaging. AJR Am J Roentgenol 172:813–818.

Levine D, Trop I, Mehta T S, Barnes P D 2002 MR imaging appearance of fetal cerebral ventricular morphology. Radiology 223:652–660.

Lituania M, Passamonti U, Cordone M S et al 1989 Schizencephaly: prenatal diagnosis by computed sonography and magnetic resonance imaging. Prenat Diagn 9:649–655.

Martin H P 1970 Microcephaly and mental retardation. Am J Dis Child 119:128–131.

Miller E, Ben-Sira L, Constantini S, Beni-Adani L 2006 Impact of prenatal magnetic resonance imaging on postnatal neurosurgical treatment. J Neurosurg 105:203–209.

Monteagudo A, Timor-Tritsch I E 1997 Development of fetal gyri, sulci and fissures: a transvaginal sonographic study. Ultrasound Obstet Gynecol 9:222–228.

Morris J E, Rickard S, Paley M N et al 2007 The value of in-utero magnetic resonance imaging in ultrasound diagnosed foetal isolated cerebral ventriculomegaly. Clin Radiol 62:140–144.

Myers C, Duncan K R, Gowland P A et al 1998 Failure to detect intrauterine growth restriction following in utero exposure to MRI. Br J Radiol 71:549–551.

Nakahara T, Uozumi T, Monden S et al 1993 Prenatal diagnosis of open spina bifida by MRI and ultrasonography. Brain Dev 15:75–8.

Osborn R E, Byrd S E, Naidich T P et al 1988 MR imaging of neuronal migrational disorders. AJNR Am J Neuroradiol 9:1101–1106.

Ouahba J, Luton D, Vuillard E et al 2006 Prenatal isolated mild ventriculomegaly: outcome in 167 cases. Br J Obstet Gynaecol 113:1072–1079.

Peebles D M 1998 Holoprosencephaly. Prenat Diagn 18:477–480.

Pilu G, Sandri F, Perolo A et al 1993 Sonography of fetal agenesis of the corpus callosum: a survey of 35 cases. Ultrasound Obstet Gynecol 3:318–329.

Pilu G, Tani G, Carletti A et al 2005 Difficult early sonographic diagnosis of absence of the fetal septum pellucidum. Ultrasound Obstet Gynecol 25:70–72.

Prayer D, Prayer L 2003 Diffusion-weighted magnetic resonance imaging of cerebral white matter development. Eur J Radiol 45:235–243.

Rados M, Judas M, Kostovic I 2006 In vitro MRI of brain development. Eur J Radiol 57:187–198.

Raybaud C, Levrier O, Brunel H et al 2003 MR imaging of fetal brain malformations. Childs Nerv Syst 19:455–470.

Raymond A A, Fish D R, Sisodiya S M et al 1995 Abnormalities of gyration, heterotopias, tuberous sclerosis, focal cortical dysplasia, microdysgenesis, dysembryoplastic neuroepithelial tumour and dysgenesis of the archicortex in epilepsy. Clinical, EEG and neuroimaging features in 100 adult patients. Brain 118 (Pt 3):629–660.

Rickard S, Morris J, Paley M et al 2006 In utero magnetic resonance of non-isolated ventriculomegaly: Does ventricular size or morphology reflect pathology? Clin Radiol 61:844–853.

Robson C D, Barnewolt C E 2004 MR imaging of fetal head and neck anomalies. Neuroimaging Clin North Am 14:273–291, viii.

Rofsky N M, Pizzarello D J, Weinreb J C et al 1994 Effect on fetal mouse development of exposure to MR imaging and gadopentetate dimeglumine. J Magn Reson Imaging 4:805–807.

Salomon L J, Ouahba J, Delezoide, A L et al 2006 Third-trimester fetal MRI in isolated 10- to 12-mm ventriculomegaly: is it worth it? Br J Obstet Gynaecol 113:942–947.

Simon E M 2004 MRI of the fetal spine. Pediatr Radiol 34:712–719.

Simon E M, Goldstein R B, Coakley F V et al 2000 Fast MR imaging of fetal CNS anomalies in utero. AJNR Am J Neuroradiol 21:1688–1698.

Smith A S, Levine D, Barnes P D, Robertson R L 2005 Magnetic resonance imaging of the kinked fetal brain stem: a sign of severe dysgenesis. J Ultrasound Med 24:1697–1709.

Sonigo P C, Rypens F F, Carteret M et al 1998 MR imaging of fetal cerebral anomalies. Pediatr Radiol 28: 212–222.

Stehling M K, Mansfield P, Ordidge R J et al 1990 Echo-planar imaging of the human fetus in utero. Magn Reson Med 13:314–318.

Supprian T, Sian J, Heils A et al 1999 Isolated absence of the septum pellucidum. Neuroradiology 41:563–566.

Sutton L N, Adzick N S, Johnson M P 2003 Fetal surgery for myelomeningocele. Childs Nerv Syst 19:587–591.

Timor-Tritsch I 2006 Fetal magnetic resonance imaging: luxury or necessity? Ultrasound Obstet Gynecol 28:859–860; author reply 860–861.

Timor-Tritsch I E, Monteagudo A 2003 Magnetic resonance imaging versus ultrasound for fetal central nervous system abnormalities. Am J Obstet Gynecol 189:1210–1211; author reply 1211–1212.

Walsh D S, Adzick N S 2003 Foetal surgery for spina bifida. Semin Neonatol 8:197–205.

Valsky D V, Ben-Sira L, Porat S et al 2004 The role of magnetic resonance imaging in the evaluation of isolated mild ventriculomegaly. J Ultrasound Med 23:519–523; quiz 525–526.

Weinreb J C, Lowe T W, Santos-Ramos R et al 1985 Magnetic resonance imaging in obstetric diagnosis. Radiology 154:157–161.

Whitby E H, Paley M N, Sprigg A et al 2004 Comparison of ultrasound and magnetic resonance imaging in 100 singleton pregnancies with suspected brain abnormalities. Comparison of ultrasound and magnetic resonance imaging in 100 singleton pregnancies with suspected brain abnormalities. Br J Obstet Gynaecol 111:784–792.

Whitby E, Paley M N, Davies N et al 2001 Ultrafast magnetic resonance imaging of central nervous system abnormalities in utero in the second and third trimester of pregnancy: comparison with ultrasound. Br J Obstet Gynaecol 108:519–526.

Williamson R A, Weiner C P, Yuh W T, Abu-Yousef M M 1989 Magnetic resonance imaging of anomalous fetuses. Obstet Gynecol 73:952–956.

Wininger S J, Donnenfeld A E 1994 Syndromes identified in fetuses with prenatally diagnosed cephaloceles. Prenat Diagn 14:839–843.

von Koch C S, Glenn O A, Goldstein R B, Barkovich A J 2005 Fetal magnetic resonance imaging enhances detection of spinal cord anomalies in patients with sonographically detected bony anomalies of the spine. J Ultrasound Med 24:781–789.

CHAPTER

6

Imaging of the neonatal brain

Luca A. Ramenghi and Petra Hüppi

INTRODUCTION

Understanding early human brain development is of great clinical importance, as many neurological and neurobehavioral disorders have their origin in early structural and functional cerebral organization and maturation. Technological advances in neonatal brain imaging have made a major contribution to the understanding of disorders of the neonatal brain. The combination of different imaging modalities and quantitative imaging has resulted in more accurate diagnoses and helped to characterize the nature and pathogenesis of perinatal brain injury and to predict the long-term outcome. Imaging also plays an important role in screening for congenital malformations and other significant intracranial abnormalities in infants with clinical suspicion of an underlying neurologic disorder.

Magnetic resonance imaging is still a relatively new technique for imaging the very preterm infant. Any new developments in imaging the preterm infant have to be safe and quick as time is of the essence when imaging a sick preterm infant. Fast diffusion-weighted imaging has provided understanding on the formation of white matter tracts in health and disease. Quantification of the brain and its structures is providing an accurate comparison of the structural development of the brain with the functional development of the child. This may produce more accurate neuroimaging correlates for later neurocognitive disorders. Spectroscopy is providing new insights into metabolic processes in response to injury. Functional imaging is limited in the newborn, but may also throw light on the mechanisms involved in normal and abnormal neurological functioning. The interpretation of images is greatly aided by accurate histological comparisons, although it is becoming increasingly difficult to obtain consent for postmortem with retention of the brain.

IMAGING MODALITIES

Care of the infant

Consideration of the wellbeing of the neonate should be paramount in any discussions concerning the choice of imaging modality. In many situations a compromise will be needed, taking into consideration the clinical status of the infant, suspected pathology and imaging modalities available. Although ultrasound examinations can be performed at the bedside, even minimal disturbance of the very sick neonate may provoke apneic episodes and bradycardia during ultrasound examinations (Boyer 1994). The baby may be receiving respiratory support, i.e. mechanical ventilation or supplemental inspired oxygen requiring close monitoring of heart rate, blood pressure, oxygen saturation and fluid balance. The potential benefit from non-bedside imaging modalities such as magnetic resonance imaging (MRI) will always have to outweigh the additional risks of transferring the infant receiving intensive care to the radiology department. Great care must be taken not to dislodge in-dwelling catheters, endotracheal tubes and chest drains when moving a baby and for the very immature preterm baby new MR-compatible incubators are needed for secure monitoring and maintenance of temperature during the examination (Bluml et al 2004, Erberich et al 2003).

Most MRI examinations can be performed in the newborn infant without sedation, particularly if the baby is well enough to have a feed beforehand. The longer examination times for MRI increase the requirement for sedation in the older child and it is essential that MRI units have the facilities for monitoring pulse and blood oxygen saturation during the examination.

ULTRASOUND

The potential value of real-time ultrasound of the neonatal head was realized early, following its introduction in the late 1970s. For the first time the intracranial anatomy could be clearly visualized and intraventricular hemorrhage, cerebral infarction and ventricular dilatation diagnosed. Not only do further technological improvements allow us to image gross structural anatomy, but also the development of spectral, color and power Doppler imaging permits detailed assessment of the vascular anatomy of the brain.

Cranial ultrasound is usually performed through the anterior fontanelle which acts as an acoustic window. Directly following birth the fontanelle may be very small, on account of molding of the sutures, and this may limit the visualization of the intracranial anatomy. The anterior fontanelle remains open for much of the first year of life and begins to close at about 9 months, although as the infant grows the scalp tissues thicken and detailed imaging of the infant brain gradually becomes more difficult. The posterior fontanelle can also be used as an acoustic window, particularly to examine the posterior periventricular white matter and the occipital horns of the lateral ventricles. Taylor has described the advantages of scanning through the mastoid fontanelle for evaluation of the cerebellum and brain stem and has suggested that these views should be routinely incorporated into the standard imaging protocol (Di Salvo 2001, Taylor 1998). Scanning through the thin squamous temporal bone may be useful in certain clinical situations, particularly for Doppler assessment of the middle cerebral artery and branches of the circle of Willis. The transtemporal and the mastoid approaches also provide an axial view of the brain comparable with CT images and permit better visualization of the peripheral regions of the parietal lobes which are often not well visualized through the anterior fontanelle.

An ultrasound scanner for use in the neonatal unit should be easily maneuverable, have a good range of transducers to image both the extremely premature and term infant, and have facilities for image documentation, including video recording and hardcopy images. Both gray scale and color Doppler imaging should be available; in the future, power

Doppler imaging may become an important asset. The choice of transducer frequency is a compromise between resolution and penetration; high frequency transducers give better resolution but may have relatively poor penetration. In general 7–10 MHz sector transducers are appropriate for scanning the brain of the very preterm infant, whereas a 5 MHz transducer will be more appropriate for the term infant. Even lower frequency, e.g. a 3.5 MHz transducer, may be necessary to adequately visualize the posterior fossa in an older infant. High frequency, e.g. 10 MHz, linear or curved linear transducers are particularly valuable to examine the posterior fossa through posterior access (Fig. 6.1) or extra-axial space and the peripheral cerebral cortex immediately below the fontanelle, which can be useful for evaluation of the superior sagittal sinus in conjunction with color Doppler imaging.

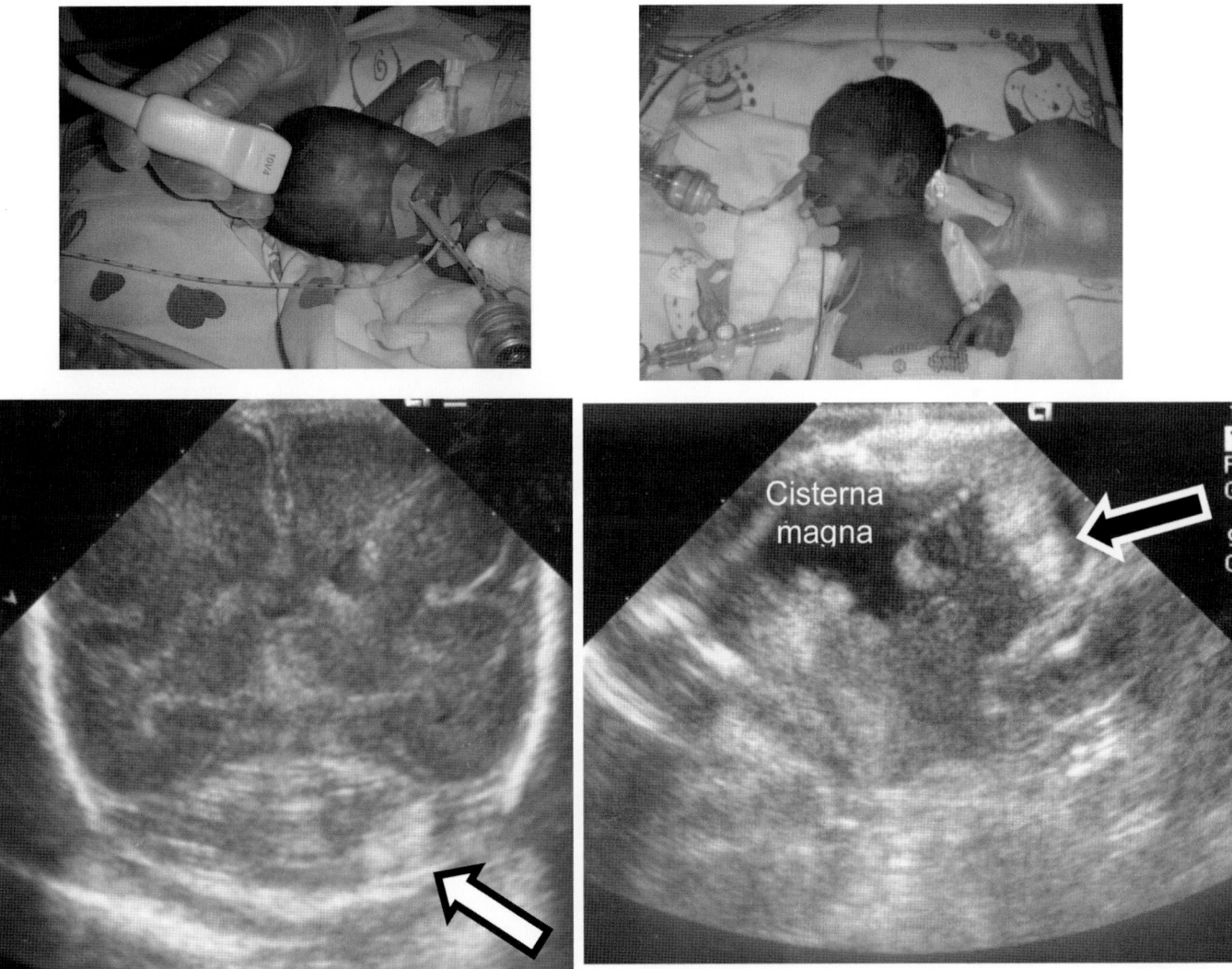

Figure 6.1 Ultrasound coronal scan obtained from conventional anterior fontanelle showing a hemorrhage in the left cerebellar hemorrhage (white arrow) of a 25 week old baby at day 3 of life. Ultrasound axial scan of cerebellum showing the same hemorrhage (black arrow); the ultrasound scan is obtained via posterior approach.

A full description of the examination technique and normal anatomy is outside the scope of this chapter but is well described elsewhere (Govaert 1997, Ramenghi et al 2005, Siegel 1995, Taylor 1998, Teele & Share 1991). Generally, scans are performed in both the coronal and sagittal plane angling as far forward, backward and as laterally as possible to interrogate the intracranial contents. It may be necessary to change transducers or scan through other acoustic windows to clarify the nature of any pathology detected. The images and reports for all ultrasound examinations should be recorded in the clinical records as these may be valuable at a later date to help time any intracranial injury, and possibly provide crucial evidence with regard to the timing of brain injury in any subsequent litigation.

Recognition of the limitations of neurosonography should indicate where additional imaging using other modalities is necessary to answer specific clinical problems. Although imaging in the near field has improved in recent years with the advent of high-frequency linear transducers, small convexity subdural collections may not be well demonstrated. In addition ultrasound is generally considered to be relatively insensitive in the detection of abnormalities in the peripheral regions of the brain and posterior fossa, and further imaging with MRI will be required to exclude a significant abnormality in these regions. It is difficult to evaluate the echogenicity of the white matter objectively other than by comparison with that of the choroid plexus. It is important to recognize the normal peritrigonal blush in the white matter (Fig. 6.2) and not confuse this with increased echodensity due to brain injury in the preterm infant (p. 443). This area of mildly increased echogenicity may be related to the white matter fibers that course radially from the cortex to the subependymal layer of the lateral ventricle, or possibly may be a reflection of the high water content of the white matter in this region (Di Pietro et al 1986). The problem is further compounded by the possibility that some specific linear-ellipsoid hyperechoic areas, appearing bilaterally adjacent to the lateral ventricle on coronal ultrasound images, can represent a normal finding as it is almost invariably seen in normal preterm infants below 32 weeks of gestation. The symmetrical and unchanged character between 26 and 31 weeks of gestational age of these linear-ellipsoid hyperechoic areas suggests that they represent part of the optic radiation and that the hyperechoic changes are due to a perpendicular insonation (Fig. 6.3) (Boxma et al 2005). A

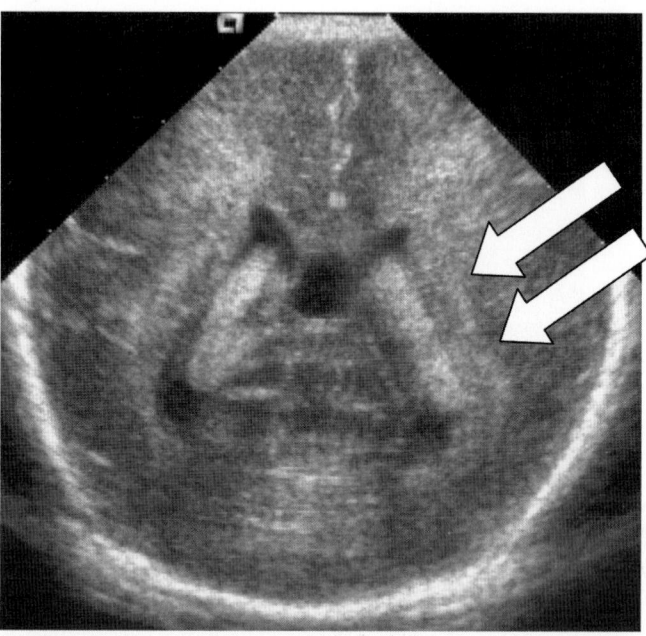

(a)

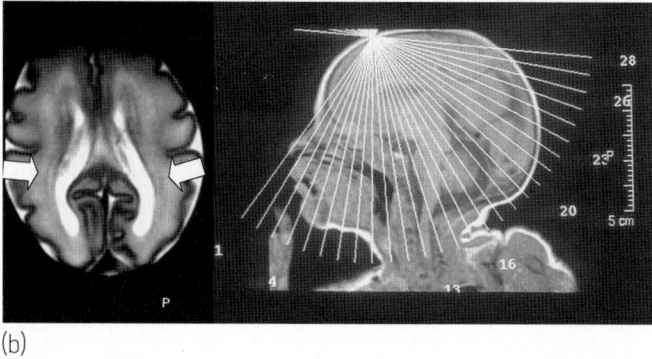

(b)

Figure 6.3 (a) Coronal ultrasound scan showing normal echogenicity with a linear appearance (arrows) consistent with the signal of optic radiation (Boxma et al 2005). (b) T2 MRI 'coronal' scan corresponding to the ultrasound cut (a) in the same baby. Optic radiations are easily seen with a linear appearance (arrows). The MRI T2 scan was obtained to mimic the ultrasound coronal scan.

Figure 6.2 Sagittal ultrasound examination demonstrating the normal peritrigonal blush (arrowheads).

wide range of definitions of hyperechoic areas is a sign of the efforts to differentiate pathological from benign ultrasound findings.

Leviton and Paneth postulated in 1990 that ultrasonographic white matter echodensities and echolucencies in low birth weight infants predicted later handicap more accurately than any other antecedent (Leviton and Paneth 1990). In the meantime though, it has become evident that up to 70% of cerebral white matter injury, particularly small focal lesions and diffuse changes as described in neuropathology, are missed by ultrasonography (Fig. 6.4) (Childs et al 2001, Inder et al 2003, Rijn et al 2001).

Image acquisition and interpretation in ultrasound are operator dependent and subject to inter-observer error. It is crucial when performing any ultrasound examination to be meticulous with the gain settings to ensure that areas of altered echogenicity are not simply due to artifact. Scanning off-center through the anterior fontanelle may give rise erroneously to the impression of unilateral increased echodensity in the parenchyma. Similarly, misdiagnosis of transient echodensity/flare may be made if the gain settings are too high or the slope of the time gain compensation (TGC) is inappropriate. Conversely, abnormality may be overlooked when the gain is too low. It is important to ensure that the focus is set at an appropriate level which may need to be altered during the scanning sequence, to examine both the periventricular regions and the structures of the posterior fossa. Subtle findings, such as mild echodensity, may not be easily reproduced on hard copy images and this may be a particular problem when the images are reported by radiologists and clinicians who have not performed the examination.

DOPPLER APPLICATIONS

The anterior fontanelle provides the best window for evaluation of the anterior cerebral, pericallosal and basilar

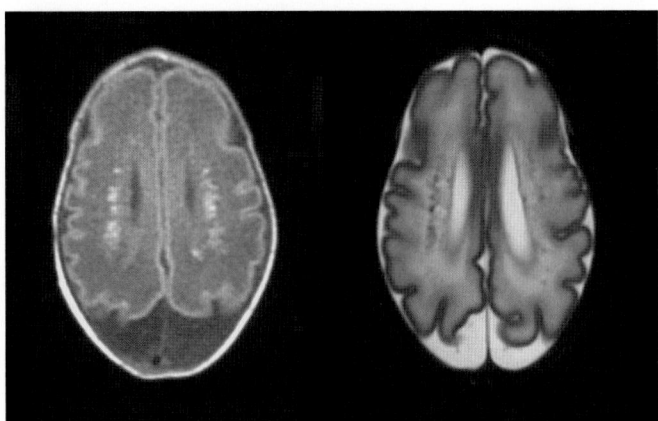

Figure 6.4 T1 and T2 MRI axial scan of a premature baby born at 27 weeks of gestation. T1 shortening with high signal intensity on T1-weighted images and low signal on T2-weighted sequences of these minor abnormalities of white matter, often showing a linear periventricular distribution.

arteries, whereas the transtemporal approach is more suited to insonation of the middle and posterior cerebral circulation. The availability of color Doppler imaging in addition to spectral Doppler imaging helps with vessel identification and choice of optimal angle for insonation. The major veins and venous sinuses can be assessed by Doppler imaging through the mastoid fontanelle (Taylor 1998). Color Doppler imaging is particularly valuable in identifying arteriovenous malformations, e.g. vein of Galen aneurysm and dural fistulae, although further imaging will be necessary for full evaluation. A number of clinical applications have been developed for spectral and color flow Doppler imaging (Archer et al 1986, Blankenberg et al 1997, McMenamin & Volpe 1983) and these are discussed in detail in Chapter 9.

Power Doppler imaging is a more recent development whereby a significant proportion of the electronic noise associated with color and spectral Doppler imaging is eliminated and the dynamic range and sensitivity of the system are increased three to five times. Power Doppler imaging is sensitive to body motion which may be a problem when scanning neonates. Power Doppler is superior to standard color and spectral Doppler imaging and is able to detect low velocity flow. Taylor has shown the feasibility of developing regional perfusion cerebral flow maps in animal studies, and future developments may see ultrasound techniques capable of assessing cerebral perfusion at the cotside (Taylor 1998).

A further development in ultrasound technology has seen the emergence of 3-D imaging. This has been shown to be useful particularly in evaluating fetal craniofacial anomalies, but a definite role in neonatal imaging has not yet been established.

COMPUTERIZED TOMOGRAPHY

The indications for CT have decreased over the last 10 years following the more widespread use of MRI, and apart from easier detection of intracranial calcification, CT has no advantage over the non-irradiating MRI and therefore little role in the evaluation of neurologic disorders in the neonate. CT can be used in the absence of MRI facilities when a very severe lesion is suspected (Fig. 6.5). Three-dimensional reconstruction from CT scans has been shown to be superior to conventional plain radiograph and CT scans in diagnosing craniosynostosis (Vannier et al 1989).

MAGNETIC RESONANCE IMAGING

The potential clinical value of magnetic resonance imaging (MRI) in the neonate was soon realized in the early 1980s. The greater soft tissue contrast inherent in MRI compared with CT permitted much better differentiation between gray and white matter and for the first time allowed us to assess the impact of pathological processes on the developing brain. Although the difficulties of performing an MRI scan are greater than for CT scanning, it is superior for most clinical indications at this age and has now become the definitive modality for imaging the neonatal brain. A full description of the basic principles of MRI scanning, choice

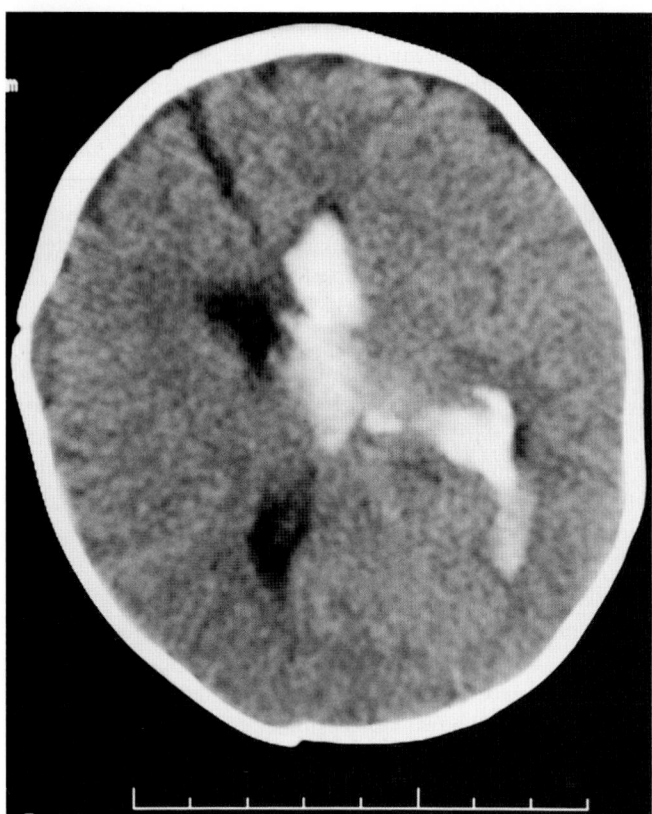

Figure 6.5 A 3-month-old infant with hemorrhagic disease of the newborn. Unenhanced axial CT scan demonstrating acute left-sided intraventricular hemorrhage.

of sequences and recognition of artifacts is available (Barkovich 1995, Boyer 1994, Flodmark 1995, Hüppi & Barnes 1997, Ramenghi et al 2005, Rutherford 2002).

High field-strength units are preferable for neonatal scanning on account of the faster scan times, ability to obtain thinner sections using a smaller field of view, better signal-to-noise ratio and improved soft tissue contrast with better differentiation of gray from white matter (Lin et al 2003, Rutherford 2004). The precise choice of sequences will depend on the model and field strength of the scanner, the age of the baby and suspected pathology (Rutherford 2002). Scanning protocols will generally be based on conventional T1- and T2-weighted spin echo, fast spin echo, inversion recovery or 3-D gradient echo sequences. Slice thickness between 1.5–4 mm is usually appropriate in the neonatal period. Although routine imaging of the brain in the adult and older child may require a single axial T2-weighted sequence, the complex changes and signal alterations associated with the developing brain require that both T1- and T2-weighted axial or coronal images are performed in most cases. A T1-weighted sagittal sequence is also useful as malformations of the brain may be associated with midline abnormalities which are well demonstrated in this plane.

Some abnormalities may be difficult to detect on standard T2-weighted images as the high water content of the premature brain may mask edema or cystic lesions at this age;

T1- and T2-weighted sequences should be heavily weighted to account for this (Boyer 1994) very long repetition time (TR) and relatively long echo-time. Other sequences may be worth considering in specific clinical situations. Fluid attenuated inversion recovery (FLAIR) sequences null the signal from cerebrospinal fluid and give heavily weighted T2 images. This is of potential value in the neonate to help differentiate the high signal seen on standard T2-weighted images due to cystic periventricular leukomalacia (PVL) from the more chronic changes of PVL, i.e. gliosis (Okuda et al 1998). T2* gradient echo sequences are particularly sensitive towards the detection of subtle areas of old hemorrhage as may be found in association with arterio-venous malformations, and may also be helpful in confirming the presence of previous hemorrhage which may not be evident on standard imaging.

Higher quality images are obtained when scanning the neonatal head using a dedicated smaller diameter quadrature head coil or specially designed phased-array coils. Currently there are commercially available head coils specifically designed for neonatal use (Erberich et al 2003).

There are few clinical indications for the administration of intravenous MRI contrast agents in the neonate. Gadopentetate dimeglumine is safe in the neonate and can be useful for the evaluation of inflammatory and neoplastic diseases, suspected phakomatoses and MR angiography, particularly venography.

The further development of gradient echo techniques and echo planar imaging has led to the development of fast and ultrafast sequences for imaging the brain which have resulted in the emergence of new MR applications of diffusion-weighted and diffusion tensor imaging (Hüppi et al 2006) and perfusion imaging (Rutherford et al 2005a, 2005b).

NORMAL ANATOMY AND BRAIN DEVELOPMENT

Development of the human brain is incomplete at birth in both the preterm and term newborn infant and continues for many months and years following birth. Although the appearance of sulci and gyri has been well documented on fetal and neonatal ultrasound, there is no doubt that MRI is superior in the comprehensive assessment of brain maturation, because gray–white matter differentiation, the progressive stages of myelination, regression of the germinal matrix and extent of glial cell migration can all be visualized and followed on conventional MRI (Fig. 6.6). The process of myelination has been studied most extensively. Early changes due to myelination tend to be better seen on T1-weighted images as evidenced by an increase in signal intensity due to the primary process of myelination. It is known that the T1 shortening correlates temporally with the increase in cholesterol and glycolipids that accompanies the formation of myelin from oligodendrocytes (Poduslo 1984). Furthermore, the T2 shortening correlates temporally with the tightening of the spiral of myelin around the axon and the conformational changes in the myelin proteins and the saturation of polyunsaturated fatty acids within the myelin membranes. Portions of the proteins, cholesterol and glycolipids that compose myelin are hydrophilic and will hydrogen bond more strongly with water molecules. With an increase in bound water to the myelin building blocks there will be a consequent decrease in free water and an increase in T1 shortening. This reduction in free water accompanying the preparation for myelination may explain the pattern of

T1-weighted MR changes preceding anatomical myelination by histological analysis (Kinney 1988). Sensory pathways are the first to myelinate: vestibular, acoustic, tactile and proprioceptive senses are myelinated by term birth. Shortening T2 relaxation and therefore T2 hypointense signal is observed in the ventrum-posterolateral nuclei of the thalamus as early as 28 weeks gestation, the posterior limb of the internal capsule as early as 36 weeks gestation, corona radiatae and the sensorimotor cortex at term.

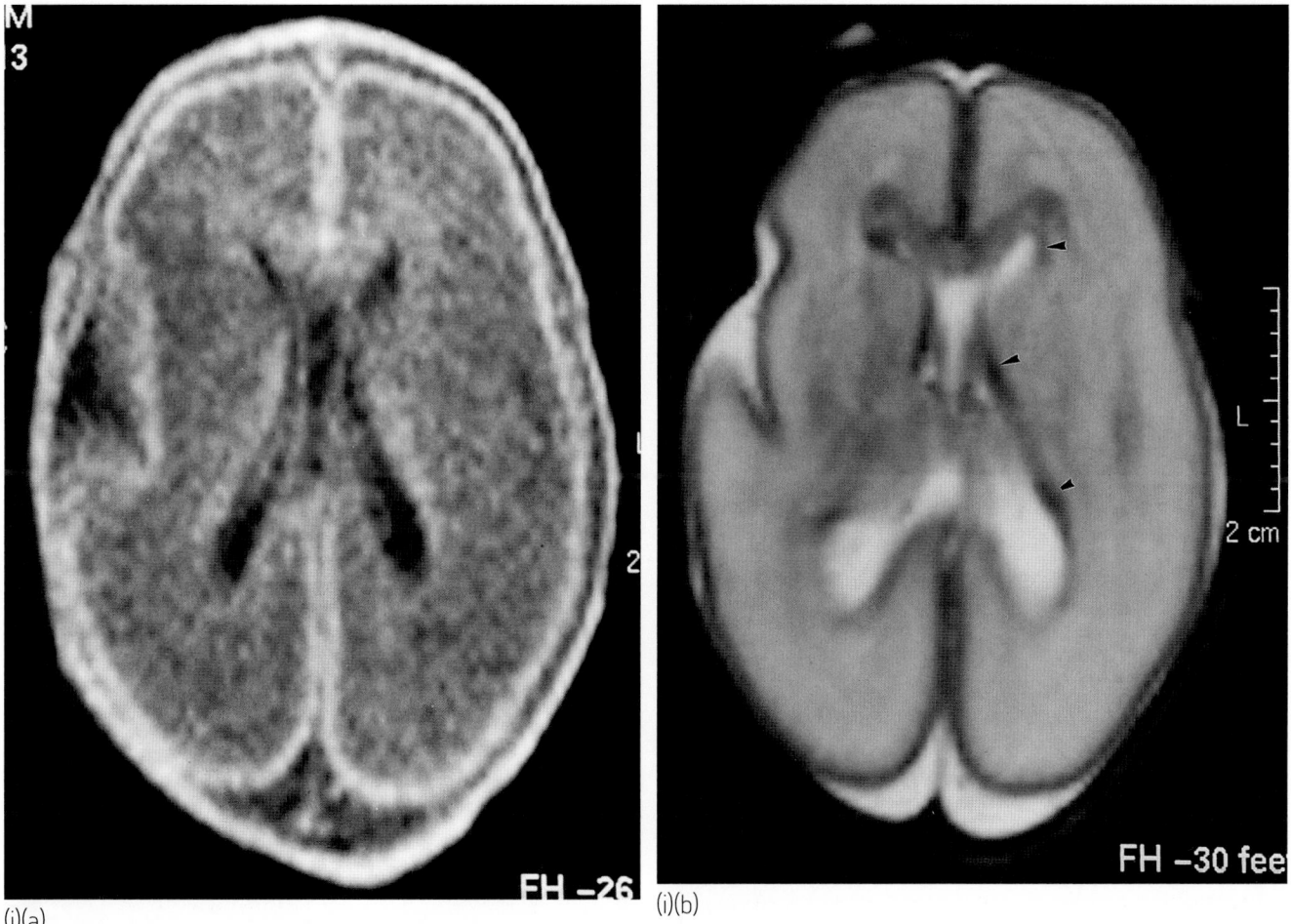

(i)(a) (i)(b)

Figure 6.6 Progression of maturation as seen at the level of the basal ganglia and lateral ventricles at the level of the foramen of Monroe. Series showing changes at increasing postmenstrual ages. (i) At 24 weeks gestation. (a) T1- and (b) T2-weighted images showing the smooth cortex and wide open insula. No myelination of the basal ganglia is visible. The germinal matrix is evident on the T2-weighted image as a low-intensity strip adjacent to the lateral ventricle around the frontal horns, caudo-thalamic notch and posterior horn (arrowheads). (ii) At 32 weeks gestation. (a) T1- and (b) T2-weighted images showing the developing sulcation. Myelination is now seen as increased signal on T1-weighted image and decreased signal on T2-weighted image in the globus pallidus and ventrolateral thalamus (arrows). Germinal matrix is less evident, being mainly visible around the frontal horn and at the caudo-thalamic notch. Discrete bands of low signal noted in the frontal white matter on T2-weighted images are thought to represent bands of migrating glial cells (arrowheads). A small GMH-IVH is present on the left. (iii) At 37 weeks gestation. (a) T1- and (b) T2-weighted images showing further development of sulcation and some infolding of the insula. Myelination is visible in the posterior limb of the internal capsule (arrow). Germinal matrix is faintly visible around the frontal horns. The bands of migrating glial cells are becoming less prominent. (iv) At 44 weeks gestation. (a) T1- and (b) T2-weighted images showing mature sulcal pattern, with gray/white matter of isointensity on T1-weighted images. Myelination is visible in the anterior (arrow) and posterior limbs (arrowhead) of the internal capsule and optic radiation (long arrow). Germinal matrix and bands of migrating glial cells are no longer visible.

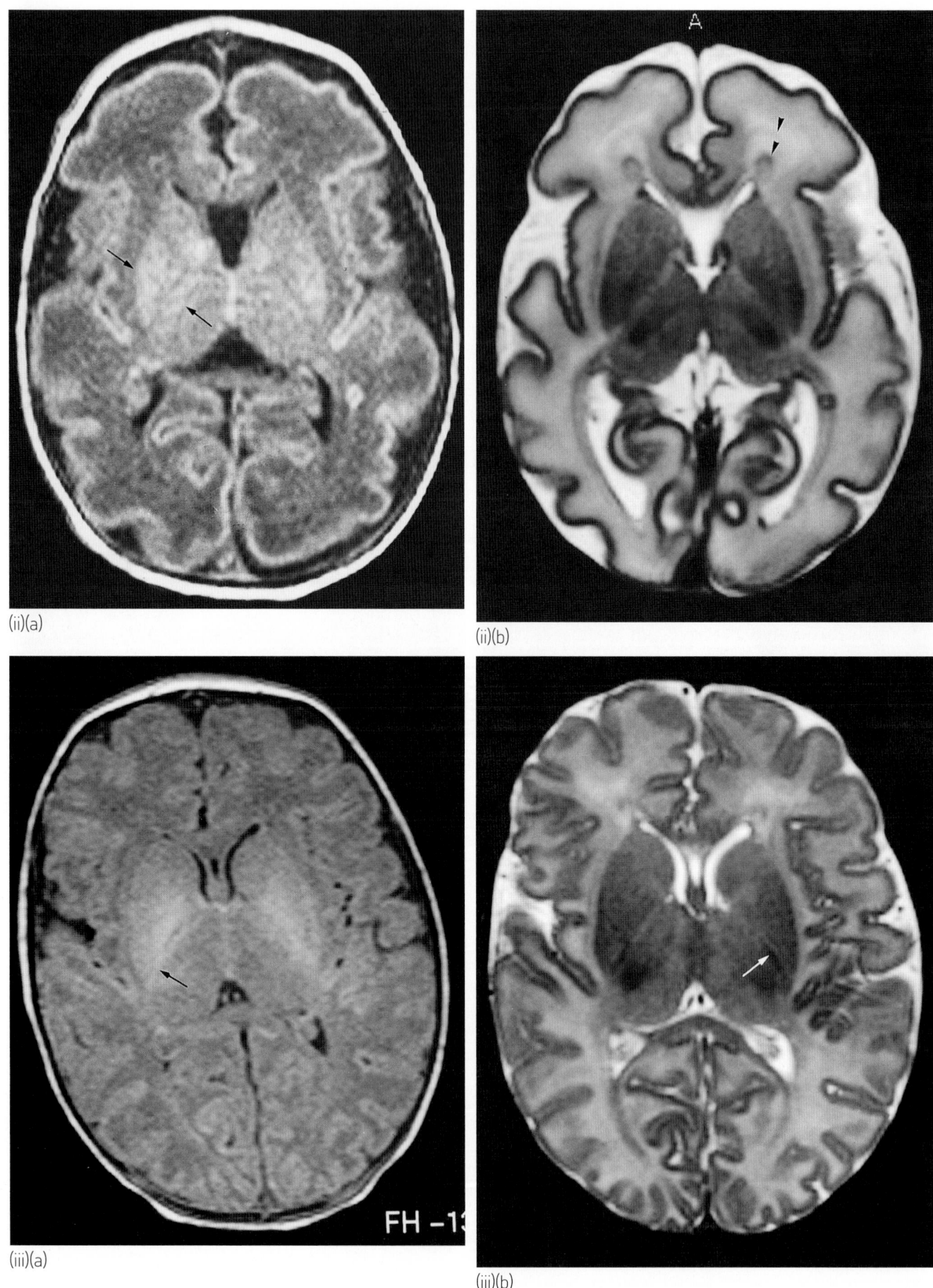

(ii)(a)

(ii)(b)

(iii)(a)

(iii)(b)

Figure 6.6 Continued

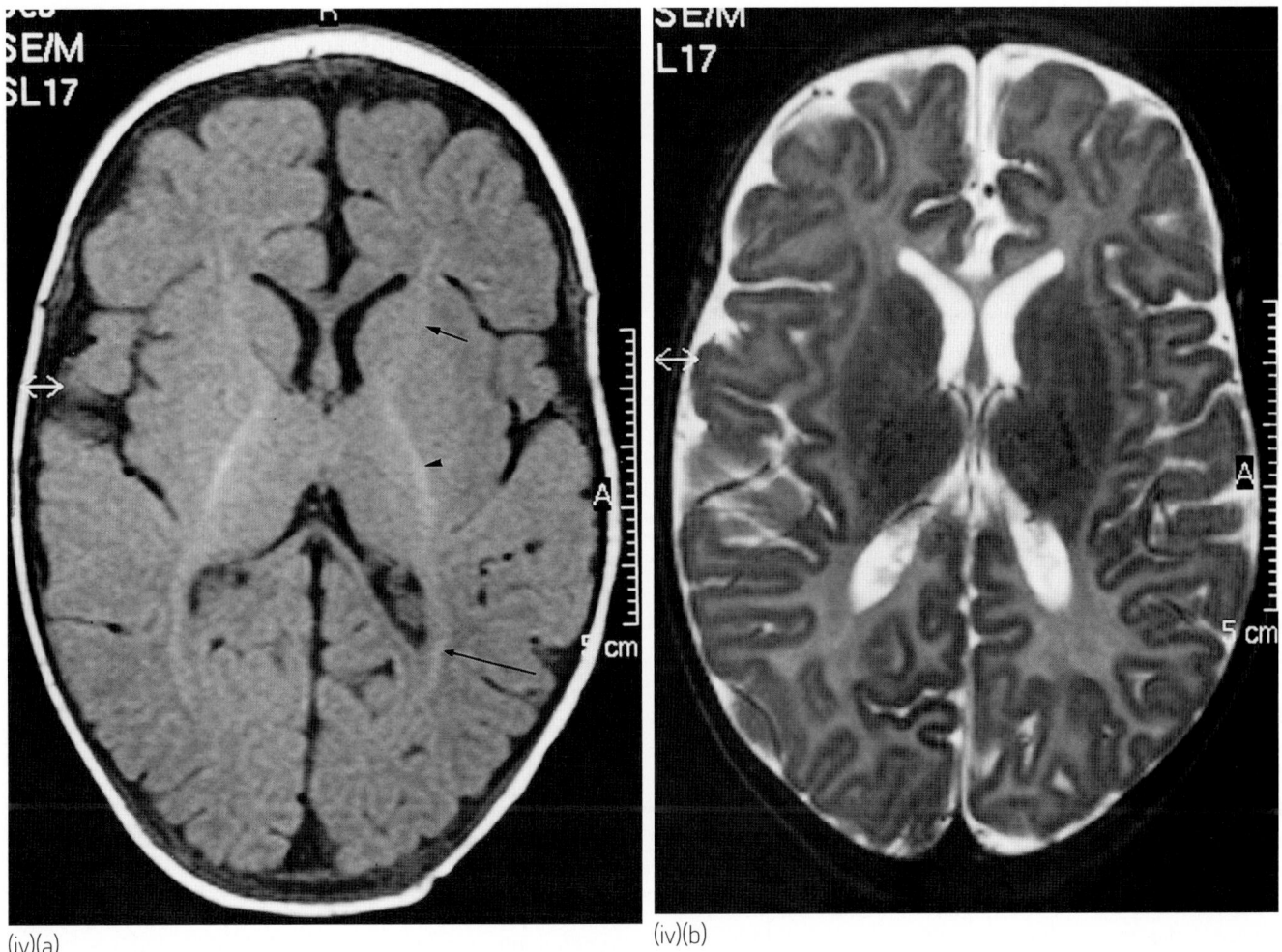

(iv)(a)   (iv)(b)

Figure 6.6 Continued

The T2-weighted images are superior to T1-weighted images to assess early maturation in the basal ganglia, cerebellum and brainstem (Barkovich 1998, 2000a, Martin et al 1991, Van der Knapp et al 1991). The T2 shortening seen in these mature nuclei is postulated to relate to the maturational changes of the neurons and, in particular, increasing synaptic density reducing the amount of free water. In a group of neurologically normal preterm and term neonates' myelin appeared on MRI in the lateral part of the posterior limb of the internal capsule and in the central part of the corona radiata between 34 and 46 weeks of postconceptional age.

The rapid process of cortical folding between 24 and 40 weeks can be readily followed on MRI. Before 24 weeks of gestation the brain is essentially lissencephalic with the exception of the sylvian fissure, which is initially very wide and appears vertically orientated. From 24 to 28 weeks the cortex shows the developing central rolandic, pericallosal and intra-parietal sulci; by 32–33 weeks an increased number of gyri and shallow sulci appear; from 34 weeks further thickening of the cerebral cortex is accompanied by the development of a nearly normal adult sulcal pattern by term (Barkovich 2000a). One can recognize almost all the gyri

seen in adult brains in the cerebral hemispheres of full-term infants at birth on MR. The marked increase in gyration is easily appreciated in Figure 6.6.

After this time brain maturation is characterized by more complexity of the sulci and gyri, which can be attributed to changes in cortical cell-packing density and the growth of cortical-subcortical fiber systems. A staging system has been devised for four major transition points in gyral development on MR imaging at postconceptional ages of 32, 34, 37 and 41 weeks gestation (Childs et al 2001, Ramenghi et al 2007).

In the very premature infant the distribution of the germinal matrix and migrating bands of glial cells can be followed on high quality MRI images (Battin et al 1998, Childs et al 1998) (Fig. 6.6). The germinal matrix appears as a strip of low signal intensity on T2-weighted images lateral to the ventricles. Its anatomical representation is inversely related to gestational age and it can be visualized throughout the subependymal areas around 24–25 weeks postconceptual age. The germinal matrix gradually regresses with the last remnants being seen around the frontal areas of the lateral ventricles, often as late as nearly 40 weeks of postconceptual age (Evans et al 1997). Discrete bands of altered signal intensity (high signal on T1-weighted images, low signal on T2-weighted images) have been described in the frontal white matter and are thought to represent bands of migrating glial cells (Childs et al 1998). These bands become more diffuse and eventually disappear towards term and may also be used as a marker of increasing maturation.

Preterm brain at term

In some ex-preterm infants there is ventricular dilation and widening of the extracerebral space at term, findings that suggest an incomplete maturation or a degree of cerebral atrophy. However these findings may not be so clear at later follow-up imaging.

In some infants approaching term the white matter develops a long T1, long T2 component, the so-called diffuse excessive high signal intensity (DEHSI) on T2-weighted images. This is probably normal if restricted to the arrowheads and caps, but in some infants is more diffuse and extends beyond these areas towards the subcortical white matter (see later in section on diffuse white matter injury). Infants with DEHSI show higher apparent diffusion coefficient (ADC) values on diffusion-weighted imaging (DWI) associated with the development of abnormal long T2, consistent with glial tissue, in the periventricular white matter at two years of age. These later changes could be described as a mild form of periventricular leukomalacia, but while they may be associated with ventricular dilation, the ventricular outline is usually abnormal. The corpus callosum may be thin. These periventricular and corpus callosal changes are a common finding when ex-preterm children and adolescents are imaged, but the exact relationship to later neurodevelopmental and neurocognitive deficits remains unclear. It is possible that these relatively focal changes are the visible side of a process that may have affected a much larger amount of developing brain, so-called perinatal teloleucoencehalopathy or white matter disease of prematurity (Counsell et al 2003, 2006).

QUANTITATIVE ASSESSMENT OF BRAIN DEVELOPMENT BY IMAGE POST-PROCESSING TOOLS

For the objective assessment of brain development measurement of accurate specific cerebral tissue volumes and morphology is required. More recently, volumetric analysis of MR imaging data sets was achieved by segmentation of the imaged volume into tissue types followed by 3-dimensional renderings. Segmentation is the process whereby contours are constructed that partition the brain into representative structures of interest depending on their signal intensity (e.g. gray matter, myelinated white matter, CSF) using mathematical algorithms (Cline et al 1990, Hüppi et al 1998, Kapur et al 1996). Several groups have been further developing the segmentation techniques working on model-driven segmentation using atlas information to guide segmentation algorithms (Prastawa et al 2005, Warfield et al 2002). These techniques have been applied in the neonatal brain, infants and adults to provide absolute quantification (Caviness et al 1996, Giedd et al 1996, Hüppi et al 1998, Inder et al 2005, Pfefferbaum et al 1994).

DIFFUSION-WEIGHTED AND DIFFUSION-TENSOR IMAGING

Diffusion-weighted imaging (DWI) or diffusion-tensor imaging (DTI) is a relatively new MR modality that assesses water diffusion in biological tissues at a microstructural level (LeBihan et al 1986). Tissue organization can be probed non-invasively, and the age-related changes of diffusion parameters (mean diffusivity, anisotropy) reveal crucial maturational processes, such as white matter connectivity and myelination. DWI/DTI may further be used to detect brain injury well before conventional MRI, as water diffusion changes are an early indicator of cellular injury. This is particularly critical in infants in the context of administration of neuroprotective therapies. Finally, with the development of 3D fiber tractography, the maturation of white matter connectivity can be followed throughout infant development into adulthood with the potential to study correlations between abnormalities on DTI and ultimate neurologic/cognitive outcome (Hüppi & Dubois 2006).

The general principle underlying the measurement of diffusion with MRI is to add a pair of strong gradient pulses along a single axis to the otherwise standard pulse sequence. The first diffusion pulse gradient dephases the spins and the second gradient completely rephases the spins that have not moved along that axis. As a result, the signal intensities of these protons are maintained. Where there is a net movement, or translation, of protons between the applications of the diffusion-sensitizing gradients, these spins are not perfectly rephased and their signal is attenuated. The normal mature brain parenchyma therefore appears high intensity relative to the cerebrospinal fluid. The self-diffusion of water in tissue is referred to as 'apparent diffusion' and its calculated rate as the apparent diffusion coefficient (ADC), a scalar representation of the total net water diffusion present in each voxel. On the calculated images, or ADC images, the gray scale intensities are inverted (Fig. 6.7). DWI and ADC

Figure 6.7 Diffusion-weighted imaging (DWI). Term baby with (a) T2-weighted image on day 4 demonstrating diffuse hyperintensity of the white matter, with subtle loss of differentiation between the cortex and subcortical white matter in both frontal and right parieto-occipital regions (arrows). (b) DWI performed the same day demonstrating corresponding areas of markedly increased signal intensity due to low diffusivity. (c) At 14 days later, T2-weighted image shows diffuse increased signal intensity of the white matter, most marked in the right parieto-occipital region. (d) DWI demonstrates regions of decreased signal intensity, due to increased diffusivity, in both frontal as well as the right posterior-parietal area.

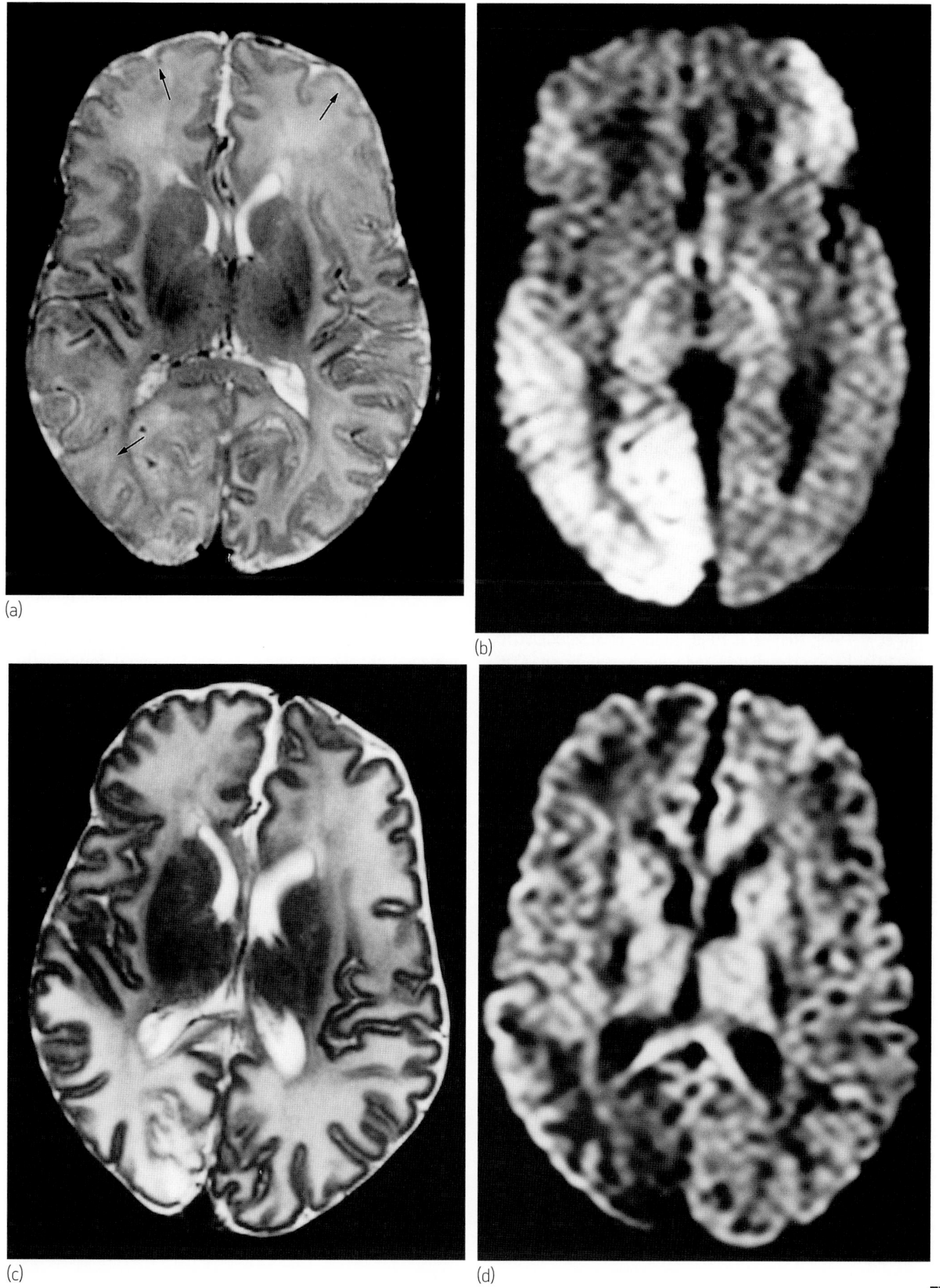

(a)

(b)

(c)

(d)

maps may also depend on the direction along which the diffusion gradient is applied. The variations in the diffusion of water molecules in different spatial directions (e.g. parallel vs. perpendicular to white matter tracts) are known as diffusion anisotropy. Anisotropy is zero for isotropic diffusion (diffusion that is equal in all directions), and increases with anisotropy up to 1. Vector maps, or RGB color-coded directionality maps, indicate the orientation of the major diffusivity, and are typically overlaid on structural images. They provide an indication of the direction in which water diffusion is highest, which typically is parallel to white matter fiber fascicles.

The main interests in the clinical use of DWI are in the evaluation of brain maturation and the early detection of cerebral ischemia. On DWI, regions of low diffusivity appear hyperintense and thus areas of acute ischemia which demonstrate decreased water diffusion, possibly as a result of the development of cytotoxic edema, will appear as areas of increased intensity compared with the surrounding brain parenchyma. These changes may be apparent on DWI prior to any abnormality being detected on conventional sequences (Beaulieu et al 1999, Cowan et al 1994, Hüppi & Barnes 1997, Inder et al 1999a). Following the acute insult, the ADC values begin to rise due to increased diffusion of water possibly related to cell lysis (Fig. 6.7). ADC maps may change with age due to the decreasing water content of the developing brain and to increasing myelination and these changes must be taken into account when interpreting DWI (Hüppi et al 1998, Neil et al 1998, Tanner et al 2000). ADC values differ between pediatric and adult human brain. ADC values are higher for neonatal brain than adult. For example, ADC values for the white matter of the centrum semiovale in premature infants approach 2.0×10^{-3} mm^2/s, while values for adult brain are typically 0.7×10^{-3} mm^2/s (for reference, ADC in free water at body temperature is approximately 3.0×10^{-3} mm^2/s). Thus, there is some restriction to water motion even for the highest ADC values measured in premature infants. ADC values decrease with increasing age during development until they reach adult values (Hüppi et al 1998, Mukherjee et al 2001, Pierpaoli et al 1996). ADC maps of pediatric brain show contrast between white and gray matter, with the ADC values for white matter being higher than those for gray matter (see Fig. 6.7). Regional differences in ADC values are observed with hemispheric white matter showing the highest values in the newborn, and internal capsule and thalami/basal ganglia already low ADC levels.

The geometric nature of the diffusion-tensor can be used to display the architecture of the brain white matter. Studies in the adult human brain have elegantly demonstrated the use of diffusion anisotropy measurements to depict human white matter pathways and characterize cortical connectivity. The increase in white matter anisotropy values during development appears to take place in two steps. The first increase takes place *before* the histologic appearance of myelin (Hüppi et al 1998, Wimberger et al 1995). This increase has been attributed to changes in white matter structure which accompany the 'premyelinating state'. This state is characterized by a number of histologic changes, including an increase in the number of microtubule-associated proteins in axons, a change in axon caliber, and a significant increase in the number of oligodendrocytes. The second, more sustained increase in anisotropy is associated with the histologic appearance of myelin and its maturation. The earliest signs of this second stage change in anisotropy are observed in the projection fibers of the posterior limb of the internal capsule in the newborn period.

Another brain area in which anisotropy values differ between immature and mature brain is the cerebral cortex. As has been shown in several human studies, values for cortical gray matter in immature brain are transiently non-zero during development (Deipolyi et al 2005, McKinstry et al 2002a, 2002b). The tensor principal eigenvectors are then oriented radially to the cortical surface. A recent study on the human fetal brain has shown that cortical anisotropy increases from 15 weeks gestation to approximately 27 weeks gestation and then shows a gradual decline to 32 weeks gestation (Gupta et al 2005). The increase of aniso-tropy in this time period coincides with active neuronal migration along the radial glial scaffolding, whereas the decrease coincides with the phase of neocortical maturation with transformation of the radial glia into the more complex astrocytic neuropil. Thus developmental changes in aniso-tropy of cerebral cortex reflect changes in its microstructure, such as the arborization of basal dendrites of cortical neurons, the innervation of the cortical plate by thalamocortical and cortico-cortical fibers, transformation of radial glia into mature astrocytes, all processes which are an important basis of later functional connectivity.

Fiber tracking is another recent technique applied to the developing brain to study quantitative assessment of specific pathway maturation in white matter (Fig. 6.8) (Hüppi et al 2006, Mori et al 2002, Watts et al 2003). Berman et al (2005) were able to show significant differences in the maturational changes in fractional anisotropy and transverse diffusion between the motor and the somatosensory pathway in premature infants between 30 and 40 weeks gestational age. This approach further allowed the measurement of diffusion changes across multiple levels of the functional tract.

MAGNETIC RESONANCE ANGIOGRAPHY AND VENOGRAPHY

MR angiography (MRA) and MR venography (MRV) are now established non-invasive techniques for the evaluation of both intracranial and extracranial vascular disorders in adults. Experience with children is more limited and there are only occasional reports of its use in the neonate (Boyer 1994, Hüppi & Barnes 1997, Lee et al 1995). 3-D time of flight techniques are generally used to examine the arterial anatomy and 2-D time of flight for the venous anatomy, although other techniques using phase contrast methods have been used. Arterial and venous 'maps' are subsequently reconstructed from the raw data using maximal intensity projections at a workstation. Image quality is generally considered to be good, but the resolution is inferior to that of conventional angiography. MRA is generally good at detecting major stenoses or displacement of vessels, but currently cannot replace angiography for the evaluation of small vessel disease. Lee et al (1995) have shown that these techniques are particularly useful in demonstrating the arterial and venous anatomy related to congenital malformations, in particular with regard to the patency and course of the superior sagittal sinus in relation to an occipital encephalocele. MR venography is increasingly used in neonates in order to assess the patency of venous vessels when venous thrombosis is clinically suspected (p. 456). The most common type of MRV used, 2-D time-of-flight (TOF), often shows flow gaps in venous sinuses, particularly in the superior sagittal sinus, transverse sinus and sigmoid sinuses with normal filling of contrast on CT venography. This high proportion of flow gap during neonatal age can be due to different factors such as a slower venous flow, the smaller caliber and the skull molding (Widjaja E et al 2006). MRV was considered superior to conventional angiography in the assessment of thrombosis and compression of the dural venous sinuses.

Other MRI techniques have also been developed including perfusion imaging and functional imaging. Perfusion imaging and functional MRI imaging are still mainly research tools in the neonate. As yet there are no established clinical applications for these techniques.

FUNCTIONAL MRI (fMRI)

Functional neuroimaging techniques permit the investigation of the functional organization of infants' and children's brains. Although functional neuroimaging has produced a wealth of new information in adults, it has been less frequently applied to the developing brain. As a relatively young field, there are many aspects of human brain development that still need to be explored, such as neurosensory and neuromotor development, development of cognition with learning processes, memory and language acquisition, as well as brain repair and plasticity after perinatal injury. In this context, functional neuroimaging techniques can bring valuable data in both healthy and diseased newborns. fMRI technically refers to the use of the non-invasive MR technology to detect regional changes in signals that are correlated with brain functional activity. This method is widely available and can be performed with any clinical or research MRI scanner with a magnetic field strength of 1.5T or higher. Principally, fMRI uses deoxygenated hemoglobin (dHb) as an endogenous contrast agent to indirectly depict cortical activated regions. The paramagnetic properties of

dHb disrupt the homogeneity of the magnetic fields generated by the powerful permanent magnetic field within the scanner. Generally, neuronal activation within a given cortical region leads to a local increase of the cerebral blood flow (CBF) accompanied by a weak oxygen consumption, and therefore to a decrease of dHb concentration in this region. This local dHb concentration drop provokes an alteration of the local magnetic field in the cortical region that fMRI can detect with appropriate sequences. This effect, known as the BOLD contrast (blood oxygenation level dependent), exploits these hemodynamic modifications that accompany neuronal activity. In 1996 Born et al (Born et al 1996) first showed brain activation in healthy newborns using visual stimulation. To date, more than twenty studies of the development and organization of different brain functions have been successfully performed in the newborn with fMRI. These studies have principally explored the visual system of healthy newborns, but others have attempted to monitor brain activity during auditory, sensory-motor, and language stimulations (Seghier et al 2006). Several interesting studies that support the utility of fMRI as a valid diagnostic tool have investigated functional responses after brain insult, in particular in infants with an abnormal visual system.

A combination of DTI and fMRI was used in a newborn showing a large lesion involving the left temporo–parieto–occipital region, compatible with acute stage of infarction. During early childhood, clinical assessment of the visual field is difficult and unilateral central blindness is therefore impossible to diagnose. fMRI was performed to assess functional outcome of this unilateral perinatal lesion. With visual stimuli presented in both block and event-related paradigms, fMRI showed a response in the visual cortex of the intact right hemisphere, principally in the anterior part, but no activation in the injured left hemisphere (Seghier et al 2004). A second fMRI experiment was performed in the same infant at 20 months of age, showing significant activation also in the visual cortex of the injured left hemisphere (Seghier et al 2005). This functional recovery occurred in parallel with new structural development that was monitored by DTI techniques (Fig. 6.8). These neuroimaging techniques might contribute to the comprehension of mechanisms of plasticity and to the elaboration of a pertinent strategy in terms of diagnosis and rehabilitation in very young infants.

Advanced quantitative MRI with image analysis tools

These techniques allow exact definition of brain volume and can therefore accurately monitor brain growth, measure cerebrospinal fluid volume and volume changes in white matter and cortical gray matter and myelination potentially affected by early injury to the developing brain. 3-D MRI volumetric techniques were used to evaluate the effect on subsequent brain development of prematurity and early

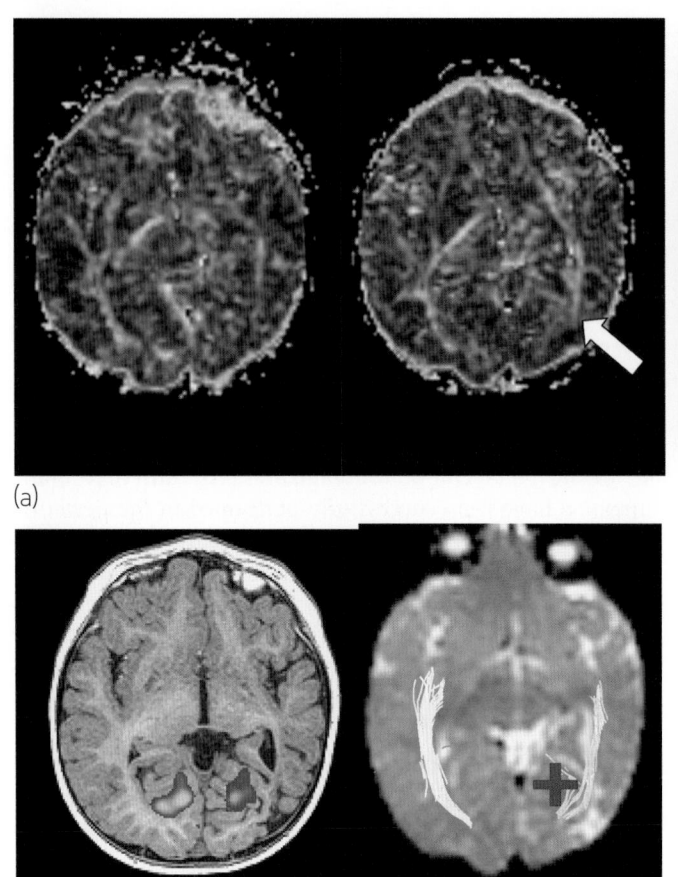

(a)

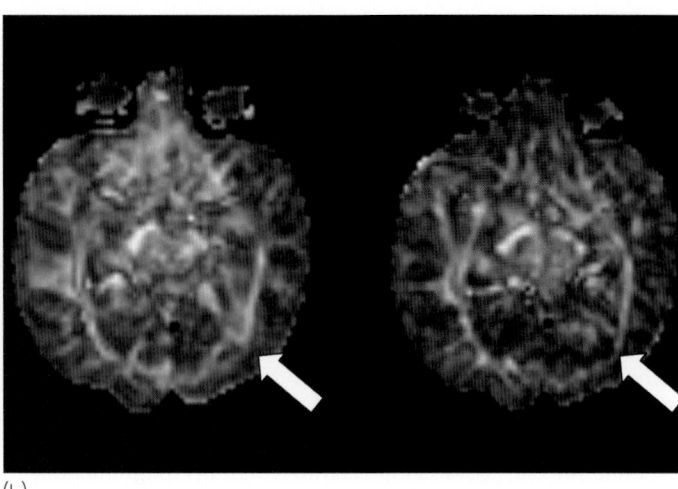

(b)

(c)

Figure 6.8 Diffusion tensor imaging with anisotropy maps at 12 months (a) and 20 months (b). Arrows indicate recovery of optic radiation fibers visualized by DTI. (c) fMRI response to visual stimulation at 20 months of age shows recovery of cortical vision in the area of tract recovery. (Reproduced from Hüppi et al in Questions and Controversies in Neonatology Series Perlman: Neurology Volume Elsevier 2007 in press).

white matter injury in premature infants in several studies (Inder et al 1999, 2005, Kesler et al 2004, Peterson et al 2000, 2003). In the premature infants with preceding white matter injury, the volume of myelinated white matter at term was significantly lower than in the premature infants without prior white matter injury and the infants born at term when measuring the degree of delay of myelination. Furthermore, this study showed a marked decrease in cortical gray matter volume in the preterm infants with prior periventricular white matter injury indicating impaired cerebral cortical development after early white matter injury (Inder et al 1999). In a recent population study similar volumetric changes of overall brain development in preterm infants were confirmed with significant reduction of myelinated white matter and cortical gray matter in preterm infants compared to full-term infants, with a reduction also of deep nuclear gray matter (basal ganglia) most pronounced in the lowest gestational ages (Inder et al 2005). Assessing moderately preterm infants without signs of white matter injury cortical development was similar to full-term infants (Zacharia et al 2006). Regional assessment of white matter myelination in preterm infants further revealed particular delay in myelination in the central and posterior part of the brain (Mewes et al 2006). When assessing cerebellar volume at term there was a significant reduction of cerebellar volume

of preterm infants when compared to term infants (Limperopoulos et al 2005). Unilateral cerebral white matter lesions resulted in contralateral reduction of cerebellar volume indicating the trophic interplay due to loss of cerebro-cerebellar connectivity (Limperopoulos et al 2005).

Long-term follow-up studies of preterm infants have confirmed the permanent character of these disruptive/adaptive changes in brain development. Recent evaluations of 8-year-old preterm infants with volumetric brain assessment showed persistence of cortical gray matter reduction in preterm infants accompanied with a reduction in the volume of hippocampus, which correlated with cognitive scores indicating long-term functional consequences (Lodygensky et al 2005). Both cortical volume and cortical thickness were shown to be reduced in 15-year-old adolescents born prematurely (Martinussen et al 2005).

MR spectroscopy (see also Ch. 11)

Commercial MRI systems nowadays provide automated reconstruction of acquired imaging and spectroscopy. Although the principle of spectroscopic quantification is rather simple because the peak area is proportional to the molecular proton concentration, this task is not straightforward in practice. Accurate estimation of peak intensities by traditional spectral peak integration is often not possible and more sophisticated approaches using a priori information are necessary. This technique is discussed in detail on page 174.

RADIONUCLIDE IMAGING

Modern radionuclide imaging techniques are becoming increasingly important in the investigation of neurologic disorders in both adults and children, although currently their role in imaging the neonatal brain is mainly confined to research applications. Cerebral single photon emission computerized tomography (SPECT) imaging assesses brain perfusion following the intravenous injection of ^{99m}Tc-labeled hexamethyl-propylene amine oxime and is particularly valuable in the evaluation of suspected cerebrovascular disease (Bloom et al 1996, Peter 1996). Positron emission tomography (PET) scanning is a relatively non-invasive method for studying brain activity which involves the intravenous injection of a tracer labeled with an unstable positron-emitting isotope which can be subsequently mapped by the sensors in the PET scanner. In the neonatal age group, PET scanning is largely used as a research tool. To give further insight into the cerebral metabolism after some common neonatal conditions such as asphyxia, Thorngren-Jerneck et al demonstrated that after perinatal asphyxia in neonates deep subcortical parts, thalamus and basal ganglia and the sensorimotor cortex, were the most metabolically active in newborn infants and therefore the most vulnerable to a hypoxic–ischemic insult.

In older children perhaps a more clinical application for PET can be observed for identification of focal cortical abnormalities and epileptogenic foci in the investigation of intractable epilepsy, particularly when the MRI is normal (Kuzniecky 1996, Mohan et al 1999, Shulkin 1997).

RADIOGRAPHIC PATHOLOGY

INTRACRANIAL HEMORRHAGE (see also Ch. 20)

Although the majority of intracranial hemorrhages seen in the neonate affect the low birth weight premature infants, intracranial hemorrhage may also occur in the term infants, particularly in response to birth trauma or as an effect of coagulation disorders (venous thrombosis often associated with prothrombotic mutations or platelet abnormalities) although the cause can remain a mystery in many full-term newborns (Perlman 2004, Ramenghi et al 2005).

Hemorrhage into the germinal matrix and ventricular system is a particular feature of the neonate with a gestational age of less than 32 weeks. Term infants are more likely to suffer extra-axial hemorrhage in the subdural and subarachnoid compartments, but bleeding into the choroid plexus and subsequently the ventricles may occur.

Ultrasound

Acute intracranial hemorrhage is very echogenic on ultrasound and will generally appear much more echogenic than the choroid plexus in the first week following the bleed

(Fig. 6.9). Acute hemorrhage into the ventricular system may be difficult to see if the scan is performed immediately before the blood consolidates to form a clot. Between 1 and 2 weeks the degree of echogenicity begins to reduce with the center of the hematoma becoming more sonolucent than the rim, after which time the clot gradually becomes smaller and retracts from the margins of the brain or ventricular wall; the clot will usually have completely resorbed by 2–3 months (Siegel 1995).

Magnetic resonance imaging

The appearances of intracranial hemorrhage are quite complex and have been extensively discussed in the literature, particularly in the mature brain (Barkovich 1995, Hüppi & Barnes 1997, Zuerrer et al 1991). A number of factors affect the appearance of hemorrhage on MRI scanning including the site of bleeding, i.e. whether the bleeding is intracerebral or into cerebrospinal fluid (CSF), the magnetic field strength and the level of T1- and T2-weighting of the scans and the age of the patient (Hüppi & Barnes 1997, Zuerrer et al 1991). The changes of the MRI appearances of hemorrhage as imaged on lower field strength MRI scanners (<1.5T) are summarized in Table 6.1. In the hyperacute stage, intracerebral hemorrhage appears indistinguishable from water or edema at most field strengths. At higher field strength acute hemorrhage may appear iso- to hypointense on T1-weighted images and iso- to hypointense on T2-weighted images due to the enhanced susceptibility of deoxyhemoglobin, which is proportional to the strength of the magnet. Over the next few days, as intracellular oxyhemoglobin is deoxygenated to deoxyhemoglobin, the hemorrhage becomes very hypointense on T2-weighted images caused by selective shortening of T2. After approximately 7

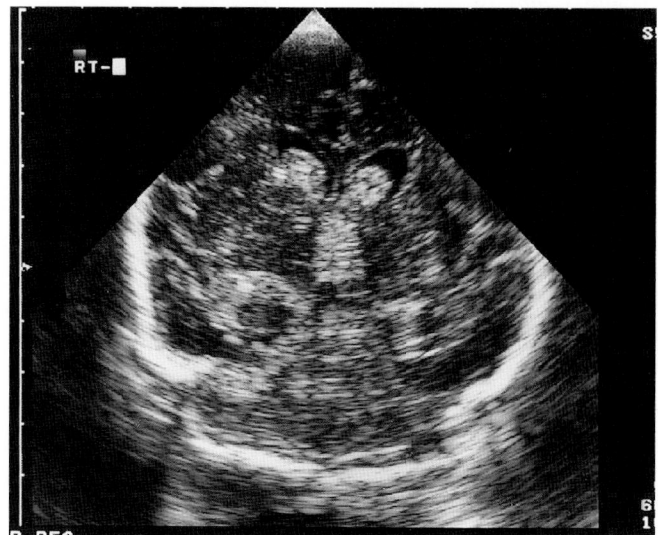

Figure 6.9 Coronal ultrasound image showing increased echogenicity due to bilateral intraventricular hemorrhages, with further hemorrhage evident in the third ventricle.

Table 6.1 Outline of MRI signal changes following intracranial hemorrhage

	Time from hemorrhage	T1	T2
Hyperacute	<24 hours	Iso- or hypointense	Iso-hyperintense[a]
Acute	24–72 hours	Iso- or hypointense	Hypointense
Subacute	4 days–2 weeks	Hyperintense	Hypointense
Early chronic	2–8 weeks	Hyperintense	Hyperintense
Late chronic	>8 weeks (hemosiderin)	Iso- or hypointense	Hypointense

[a]T2 shortening may occur after a few hours with higher field strength magnets and acute hemorrhage may appear hypointense even in the early acute phase on T2-weighted images (Fig. 6.7).
Source: Adapted from Hüppi and Barnes 1997.

days intracellular deoxyhemoglobin metabolizes to para-magnetic methemoglobin, which causes T1 shortening, i.e. high signal intensity on T1-weighted images. Lysis of erythrocytes then begins and hemorrhage becomes hyperintense on both T1- and T2-weighted images. In the chronic stages methemoglobin is metabolized to ferritin and hemosiderin, which appear as iso- or hypointense on T1-weighted images and hypointense on T2-weighted images.

The pattern of signal intensity change differs for hemorrhage into CSF, e.g. ventricular fluid compared to intra-cerebral bleeding. The deoxygenation of oxyhemoglobin is slower on account of the higher PO_2 in the CSF compared with the white matter, and the pattern of signal changes appears more slowly (Zuerrer et al 1991).

Thus with lower field strengths MRI is less sensitive than CT scanning in the detection of hyperacute and acute hemorrhage, as hemorrhage is indistinguishable from water or edema (Boyer 1994). However, MRI is very sensitive in the detection of subacute and chronic hemorrhage and is a valuable tool in helping to determine the age of a hemorrhage. Hemosiderin staining occurs after about one month and may remain visible for many months (Boyer 1994).

GERMINAL MATRIX HEMORRHAGE-INTRAVENTRICULAR HEMORRHAGE (GMH-IVH)

This is the most frequent and important cause of intracranial hemorrhage in the neonate (Ch. 20). Ultrasound is now accepted as the primary modality for the diagnosis of GMH-IVH and full descriptions of the ultrasonic findings are well reported (Hay et al 1989, Siegel 1995, Teele & Share 1991). GMH can be recognized as a globular area of intense increased echogenicity beneath the floor of the lateral ventricle, just anterior to the caudothalamic notch. The abnormality should be demonstrated in two planes and should be distinguished from other normal echogenic structures such as the normal choroid plexus. Larger hemorrhages may rupture into the lateral ventricle and when acute appear as an echogenic clot within the ventricle which may distend the ventricular lumen.

The appearance of GMH-IVH and venous infarction changes with time. GMHs resolve leaving a small subependymal cyst or a linear echodense line. The margins of a clot

Table 6.2 Grading system for the classification of GMH–IVH

Grade I	Small germinal matrix hemorrhage (GMH)
Grade IIa	GMH plus intraventricular hemorrhage (IVH) filling the ventricle <50%
Grade IIb	Large IVH distending lateral ventricle in the acute phase >50%
Grade III	IVH associated with unilateral parenchymal involvement

Source: de Vries et al 1998.

within the lateral ventricles remain echogenic whilst the more central region gradually becomes increasingly echo-poor and smaller until the hemorrhage finally resolves by approximately 12 weeks of age. Several grading systems have been proposed to classify GMH-IVH, the majority of which are based on the extent of bleeding into the germinal matrix and lateral ventricle, the development of venous infarction and the presence of ventricular dilatation (de Vries et al 1985, 1998, Papile et al 1978). The classification proposed by de Vries is given in Table 6.2.

The accuracy of ultrasound imaging in the diagnosis of GMH-IVH is reported to be approximately 90% which is comparable to diagnosis by CT (Babcock et al 1982, Dewbury & Bates 1981, Pape et al 1983, Trounce et al 1986b). Thus ultrasound imaging has now become the imaging modality of choice for the detection of GMH-IVH, as it can be performed on a daily basis if necessary, with no risk of exposure to ionizing radiation or the need to move the infant to the imaging department.

A wider use of MRI on premature babies has shown excellent visualization of the germinal matrix (GM) with high signal on T1 and low signal on T2-weighted images, especially up to the 30th week of gestation. After this time, T2-weighted images remain the best sequence to follow the physiological GM involution occurring with increasing gestational age. Germinal matrix hemorrhage has similar characteristics to normal germinal matrix, but is detectable due to its irregular shape and asymmetry. Very preterm babies may show small lesions consistent with subependymal hemorrhage in different areas than the classic sites of caudo-thalamic notch, more often in the posterior horns (Fig. 6.10). These hemorrhages seem not to be visible on ultrasound (Blankenberg et al 1996). Intraventricular hemorrhage, more often identified in the posterior horns of the lateral ventricle, is an obvious diagnosis with MRI, making this technique the most accurate for GMH-IVH investigation, although MRI scanning is not very practical for sick unstable neonates during the first days of life.

MRI has improved the detection of venous infarction associated with GMH-IVH, although caution is needed as subependymal hemorrhages may appear to have white matter involvement due to partial volume effects. Nevertheless, Keeney demonstrated that an MRI performed between 29 and 44 weeks postconceptual age was superior to both US and CT in assessing the extent of any parenchymal injury associated with GMH-IVH (Keeney et al 1991).

MRI signal shows changes following any form of intracranial hemorrhage, including IVH, according to the timing of hemorrhage. The typical hyperintense intraventricular hemorrhagic signal on T1 usually appears in the so-called subacute phase, usually between 4 days and 2 weeks after the initial bleed, while the long-lasting hemosiderin deposition seems to be visible only after 3–4 weeks (Arthur & Ramenghi 2001, Levene & deVries 2001).

Parenchymal hemorrhage/venous infarction

In general, ultrasound scanning should be chosen as the first imaging modality, but if the ultrasound scan is normal and there is a strong clinical suspicion of acute hemorrhage, an MRI should be considered. Hemorrhage occurring peripherally in the brain or in the cerebellum may not be easy to visualize by ultrasound, particularly if the anterior fontanelle is relatively small (Boyer 1994, Hay et al 1989). MRI scanning is the most sensitive technique and should be substituted for CT at all times.

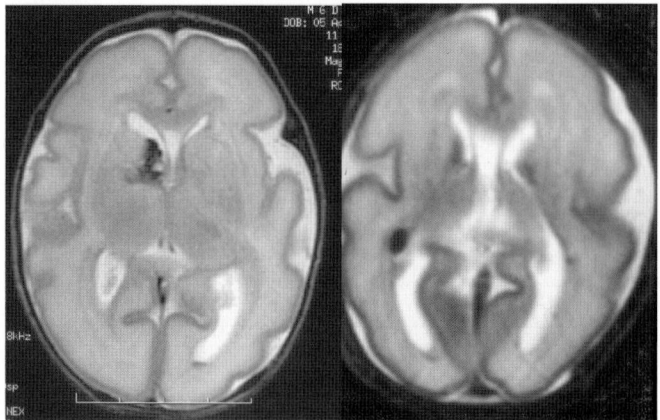

Figure 6.10 T2 axial scan showing a classic GMH originating at the caudo-thalamic notch in 26-week-old preterm baby scanned at 3 days of life; on the left an atypical origin of GMH at the posterior horn of the lateral ventricle in a 25-week-old baby at 5 days of life.

GMH-IVH can present with unilateral parenchymal hemorrhage, better known as venous infarction at the first scan, or more commonly within a few hours in a later scan. The region involved can be quite large, just dorsal and lateral to the external angle of the lateral ventricle, usually saving the cortical mantle, but location and size can vary (Ramenghi et al 2005, Volpe 2001). Less often, the lesion develops in more posterior parts of the brain, in the temporal lobe or around the atrium. In these cases, the inferior ventricular veins or lateral atrial veins are involved. It is still possible to have bilateral venous infarction, but this condition is extremely rare and well differentiated from PVL.

At the beginning the lesion appears as a triangular density often not touching the ventricle, but later the lesion grows and extends to the ventricle merging the area of increased density due to matrix hemorrhage (Govaert & deVries 1997). Sometimes there is no progression to this stage and the lesion remains as a triangular density. The hyperdensity area tends to decrease in size during the second week and the real infarcted area can as a result be smaller than expected. Cystic degeneration is the most common evolution of severe cases with a smooth-walled cavity in the parenchyma communicating with the ventricle (unlike in periventricular leukomalacia) (Govaert & deVries 1997, Ramenghi et al 2005).

Hydrocephalus

Ultrasound imaging is the most appropriate modality for the initial assessment of ventricular size. The slightly rounded shape of the frontal horns can represent the initial appearance of dilatation while balloon-shaped frontal horns are a sign of severe dilatation. Latero-lateral and diagonal measurements of the diameter are a well established modality to monitor ventricular dilatation. Absence of widening of the frontal horns may be falsely reassuring as neonates tend towards overdilatation of the occipital horns ('colpocephaly'). Many units have their own guidelines for measuring frontal horns, but very often not for the posterior horns (Govaert & deVries 1997).

MRI can be useful as detailed imaging is often required prior to shunting surgery and also after surgery to verify the functioning of the shunt, provided the proven MRI compatibility of the intraventricular device.

Pseudocysts

Cavitation within the germinal matrix represents a phenomenon called germinolysis and it results, typically at the caudo-thalamic notch, in a 'pseudocyst' due to the lack of a proper epithelium (Larroche 1972a, 1972b). During the postnatal period, pseudocysts occur mainly following small to moderate GMH-IVH, although a mechanism based on 'pure infarction' of the germinal matrix has been hypothesized. Accordingly, we have sometimes detected pseudocysts at the caudo-thalamic notch a few weeks after birth in 'normal' preterm babies with no obvious reason for this (Ramenghi et al 2005).

Pseudocysts can also be present at birth. In these cases many different prenatal conditions such as rubella, *Toxoplasma gondii* or cytomegalovirus infections (in these circumstances the cysts are often multilocated) have to be excluded. Less often, prenatal asphyxia, feto-fetal transfusion, metabolic diseases, intrauterine growth retardation and karyotype anomaly should be investigated (Paneth et al 1994). Prenatal pseudocysts are thought to incidentally arise when the developing germinal matrix outgrows its blood supply (Larroche 1972).

Pseudocysts can also be located around the frontal horns of the lateral ventricles. In this case, they are always prenatal and do not seem to correlate with GMH (see Congenital Periventricular Cavitations) (Rademaker et al 1993, Ramenghi et al 1993, 1997). Although the germinal matrix may persist around the frontal horns even in late gestation we have never observed a hemorrhage in this area with MRI studies (Ramenghi et al 2005).

CHOROID PLEXUS HEMORRHAGE (p. 418)

In vivo, this diagnosis is very complex and intricate. Ultrasound diagnosis should be based on sequential scans showing cavitation in the hematoma adjacent to the choroid plexus, while a simple intraventricular clot adjacent to the choroid plexus is not sufficient to diagnose a primitive choroid plexus hemorrhage (Govaert & deVries 1997).

In our experience MRI diagnosis of choroid plexus hemorrhage has proved to be quite difficult. We have imaged a number of scans of premature babies in their first days of life and at term corrected age but it was rarely possible to be sure of the choroid plexus origin in case of intraventricular bleeding (Fig. 6.11). In minor intraventricular bleeding of premature babies a hemorrhagic germinal matrix was almost always detectable.

CEREBELLAR HEMORRHAGE (p. 419)

Data based on MRI studies show that 8% of preterm infants less than 32 weeks gestation present cerebellar hemorrhages, although the incidence is increasing with

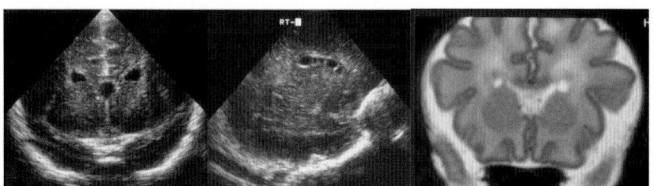

Figure 6.11 Coronal T2 scan and sagittal T1 scan of an ex preterm baby born at 24 weeks of gestation and scanned at term. In the coronal scan the hemorrhagic disruptive lesions of the cerebellar hemispheres are noted. In the sagittal scan a severe flattening of the pons is visible.

decreasing GA. Ultrasound studies performed via posterior fontanelle, more sensible than the conventional anterior fontanelle, show a lower incidence of about 3% but, especially in extremely low birth weight, ultrasound using the occipital window appears to be the best approach and the supposed incidence is probably higher (Ramenghi et al 2005) (Fig. 6.1). In some cases, cerebellar hemorrhages can be severe and associated with flattening of the pons (Fig. 6.12).

SUBDURAL AND SUBARACHNOID HEMORRHAGE

MRI scanning is particularly valuable at detecting hemorrhage in the extra-axial space although CT scanning might still play a role, especially during the very acute phase (Fig. 6.13). The multiplanar capability of MRI scanning also increases its sensitivity, since scanning in the sagittal and coronal planes may be helpful in demonstrating hemorrhage around the tentorium. If MRI is not available, an acute subdural hemorrhage may be detected as an echogenic fluid collection in the extra-axial space on an ultrasound scan. The fluid collections result in easier visualization of the cortical surface of the brain and separation of the interhemispheric fissure. The gyri may become flattened and the ventricles compressed. An increased echogenicity of the extra-axial fluid should be considered suspicious for hemorrhage. Subarachnoid hemorrhage is poorly demonstrated by ultrasound although large acute presentations may be visualized as echogenic fluid collections over the convexities.

CONGENITAL GERMINOLYSIS

Preterm newborn babies do infrequently present small cavitations around the frontal horns of the lateral ventricles, more often in twin pregnancies. This abnormality can be easily missed on routine ultrasound scan or misdiagnosed for congenital leukomalacia, but it should be referred to as congenital germinolysis and it generally carries a good prognosis, especially when it represents an isolated finding (Ramenghi et al 1997) (Fig. 6.14).

On ultrasound, these cavitations are visible on coronal and parasagittal lateral scans. They are echo-free areas and do not often divide into two or three smaller (pseudo)cysts separated by very thin septa. On coronal scans, they often appear isolated from the ventricles in more frontal sections or adjacent to the frontal horns in the slightly posterior cuts, but they can be differentiated without difficulty from PVL lesions which are located at the superior and external angle of the frontal horns of the lateral ventricle (Govaert & de Vries 1997). On parasagittal scans they appear in the more external cuts, often when the lateral ventricle is no longer visible. In more rare cases, these pseudocysts are detectable also in the temporal horns and attention should be paid to congenital rubella and cytomegalovirus (CMV), although we have also observed these abnormalities in the absence of obvious congenital infections (Ramenghi et al 2005).

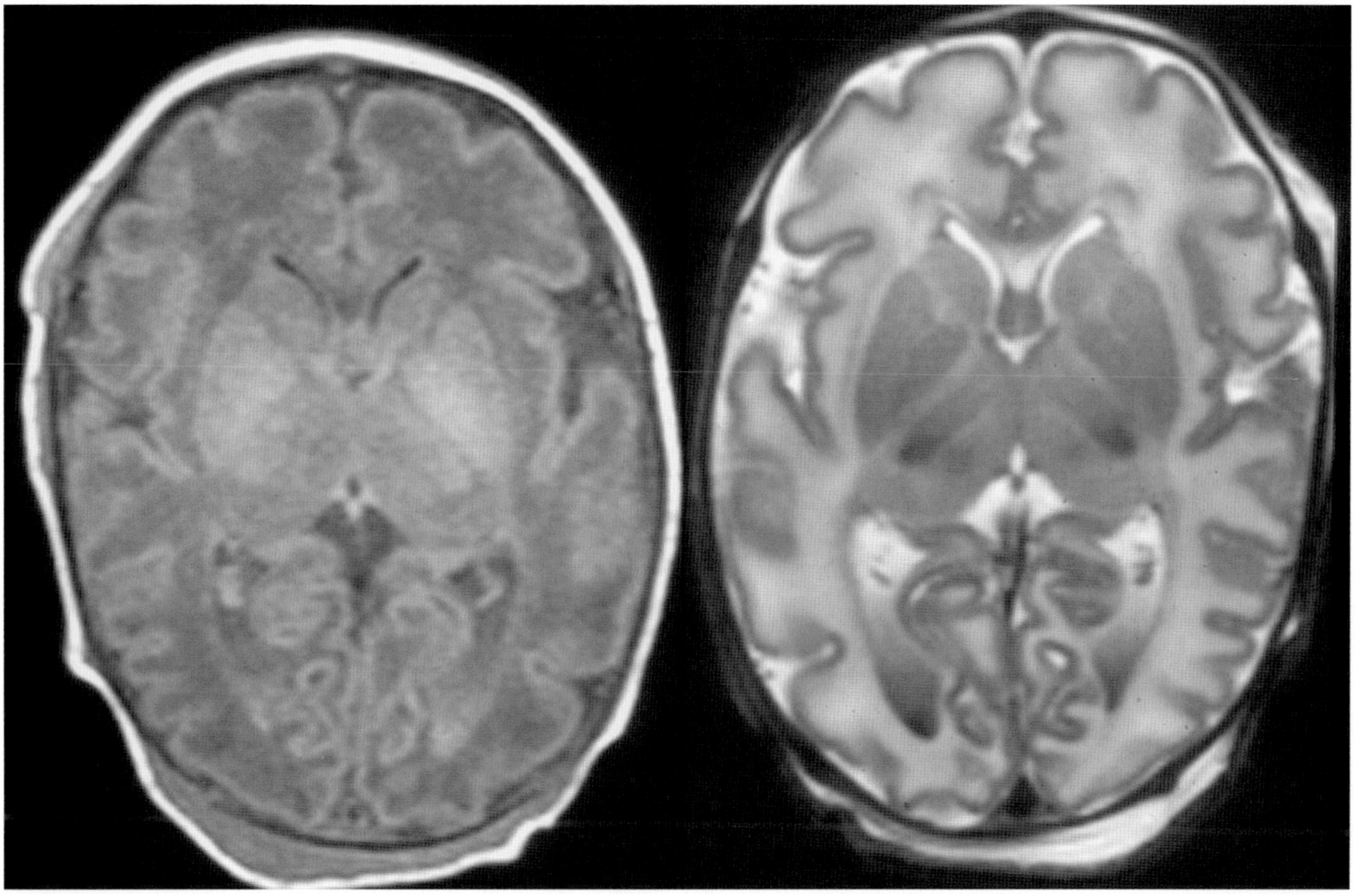

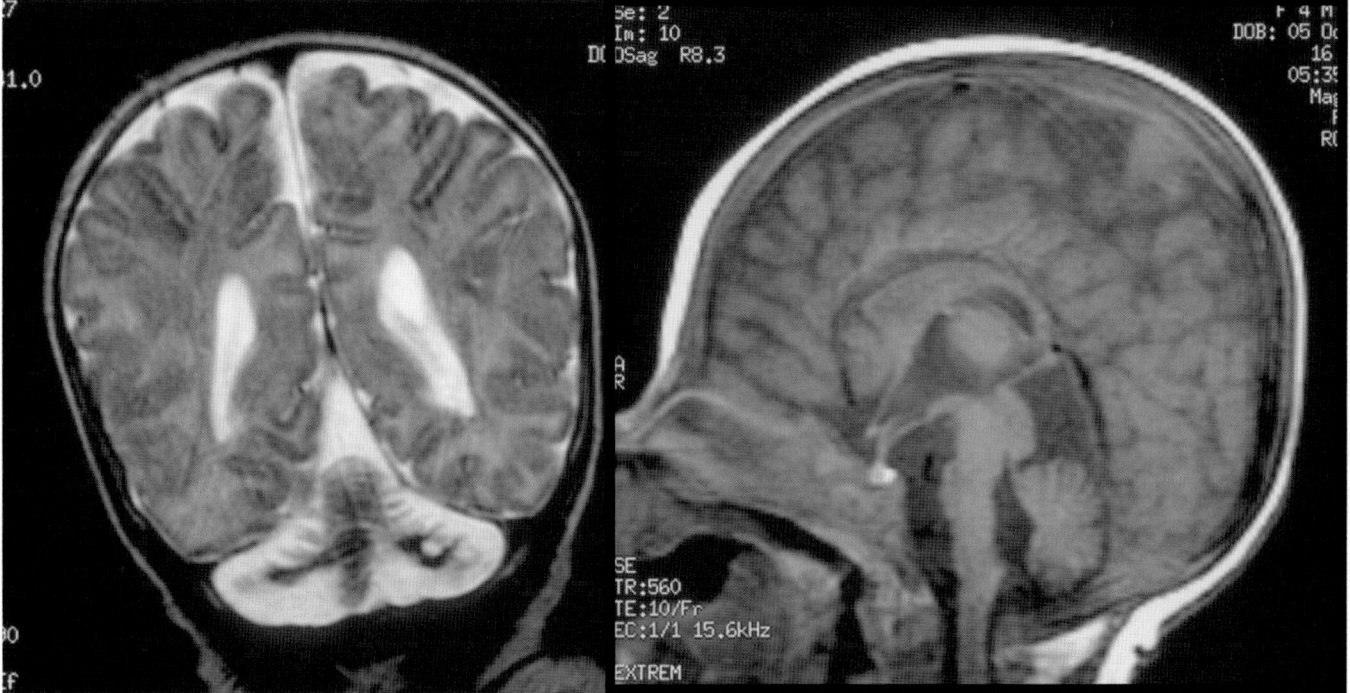

Figure 6.12 T1 and T2 MRI axial scans of a 35-week-old baby with mild intraventricular bleeding with no obvious hemorrhage from the germinal matrix, but possible origin from the choroid plexuses.

Figure 6.13 Frontal congenital cavitations as they appear in ultrasound scans (coronal and parasagittal) and T2 coronal scan. These cysts have to be considered 'benign' and are very likely to represent idiopathic germinolytic lesions.

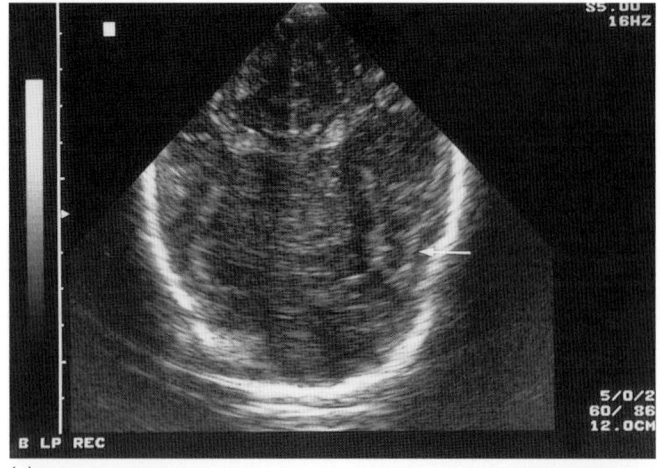

(a)

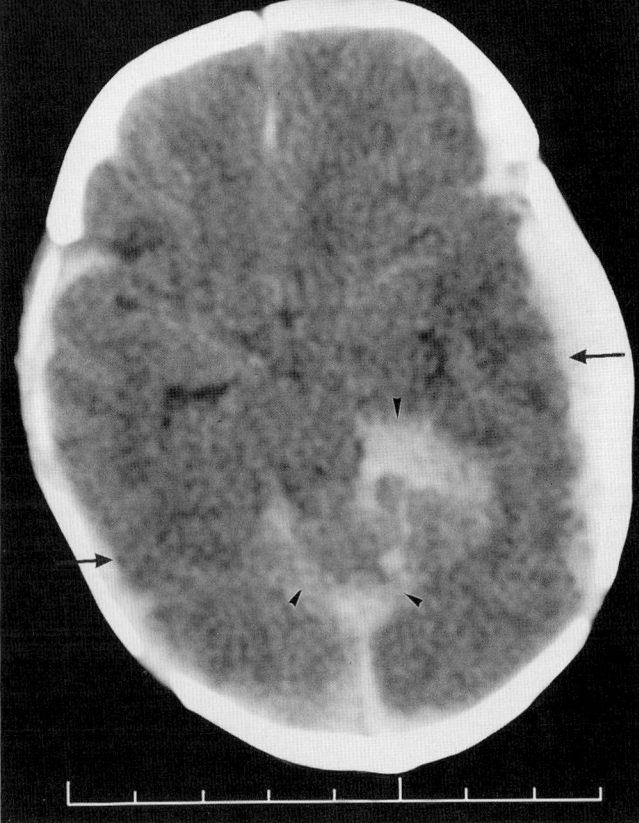

(b)

Figure 6.14 Acute extra-axial (subdural and subarachnoid) hemorrhages. (a) Coronal ultrasound scan from the posterior fontanelle showing subtle widening of the extra-axial space along the left parieto-occipital bone (white arrow) compared to the right. (b) Unenhanced CT scan at 1 day of age demonstrating bilateral extra-axial hemorrhages (arrows) and further hemorrhage in the region of the tentorium (arrowheads). Shift of the midline to the right is also noted.

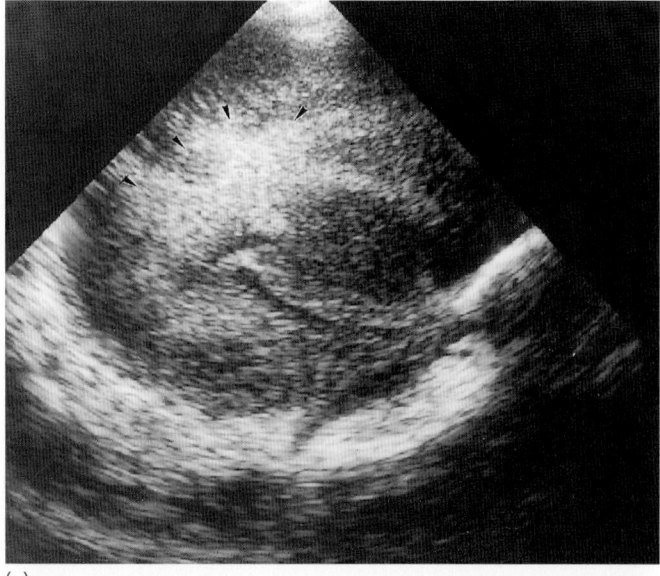

(a)

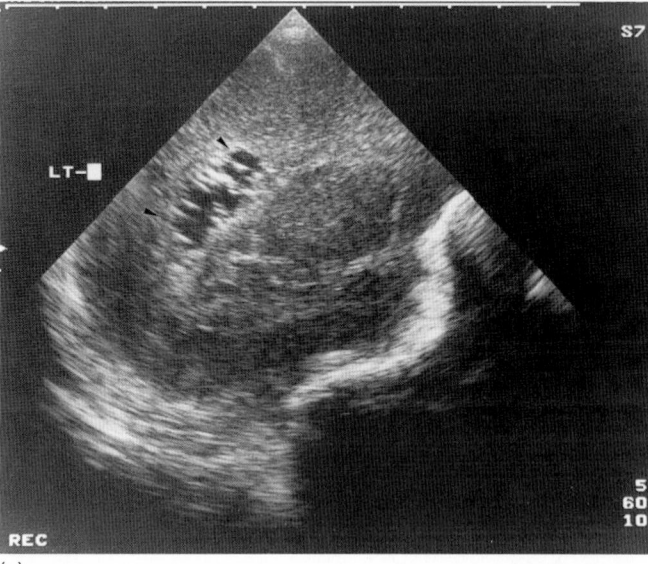

(b)

Figure 6.15 Hypoxic–ischemic injury in a premature infant. Sagittal ultrasound scans showing (a) pathological increased echodensity in the posterior parietal region (arrowheads) and (b) cavitational PVL (arrowheads).

In general, we believe these pseudocysts have a very good prognosis when they are isolated findings, but caution is needed when in association with other findings as they can derive from congenital infections or even chromosomal abnormalities.

WHITE MATTER DISEASE

Increased periventricular echodensity in the frontal or peritrigonal white matter may be the first indication on cranial sonography of injury to the white matter in a preterm infant. These echodensities may be transient and disappear

Table 6.3 Grading system for PVL lesions detected on ultrasound imaging

Grade	Description
Grade I	Periventricular echodense area, present for >7 days or more
Grade II	Periventricular echodense areas evolving into localized frontoparietal cysts
Grade III	Periventricular echodense areas evolving into multiple cysts in the parieto-occipital white matter
Grade IV	Echodense areas in the deep white matter, with evolution into multiple subcortical cysts

Source: de Vries et al 1992.

over the course of the next few days or weeks, persist unchanged, or undergo cystic degeneration to give rise to the classic ultrasonic appearances of cystic periventricular leukomalacia (PVL) (de Vries et al 1988a, 1988b, Ringelberg & van der Bor 1993, Trounce et al 1986a) (Fig. 6.15). deVries et al postulated an ultrasound-based classification for PVL of four grades (see Table 6.3), increasing grades being associated with increasing neurodevelopmental handicap, Grade I being the transient (>7days) periventricular densities without cyst formation. If cysts develop and are few in number, localized primarily in frontal and frontoparietal white matter, this is classified as Grade II. When they are widespread and extend into the parieto-occipital region, they are referred to as Grade III, and may grow and gradually disappear leaving an irregularly dilated lateral ventricle. If cysts are present all the way into the subcortical area resembling porencephaly, this is referred to as Grade IV in Table 6.3.

Cystic changes usually occur 2–4 weeks after the initial insult but may take much longer to appear (Goetz et al 1995). Cysts may be of varying sizes which may change over time, with some coalescing to become larger and others disappearing. In time, the cysts become less apparent and may not be seen on ultrasound scans, particularly three months after the initial insult. As the cysts disappear, evidence of white matter injury may become apparent on subsequent ultrasound scans, as indicated by ventricular dilatation, the development of an irregular wavy outline to the ventricular margins, and widening of the interhemispheric fissure and cortical sulci (Bozynski et al 1985, Dubowitz et al 1985, Volpe 1997).

Pathological echodensity can usually be differentiated from the normal physiological peritrigonal blush as the margins of an echodensity are usually more discrete and the echodensity more intense and inhomogeneous than the diffuse area of relatively mild echodensity that characterizes the normal peritrigonal blush (Fig. 6.2). In coronal section pathological echodensity is generally triangular in shape, with the apex pointing towards the angle of the lateral ventricle (Di Pietro et al 1986, Grant et al 1983).

Although some authors have reported a high sensitivity and specificity for the detection of PVL, this has been ques-

tioned by others. Hope et al demonstrated a sensitivity of 28% and specificity of 86% compared with Trounce who reported an accuracy of 90%, sensitivity 91%, and specificity 93% (Hope et al 1988, Trounce et al 1986a). The presence of cystic change and hemorrhage within the area of infarction is said to increase the detection of PVL on ultrasound examination (Baarsma et al 1987, de Vries et al 1988b, Nwaesei et al 1984, Paneth et al 1990). False negative ultrasound examinations can be associated with failure to detect small areas of PVL and areas of gliosis in the periventricular white matter (Baarsma et al 1987, Di Pietro et al 1986, Goetz et al 1995, Skranes et al 1993).

Ultrasound can be viewed as the ideal mode of imaging to detect cystic PVL, but has very limited value for detecting diffuse white matter injury as shown in studies comparing neonatal sonography with MRI (Childs et al 2001, de Vries et al 1993, Maalouf et al 2001, Rijn et al 2001).

The high soft tissue contrast inherent in MRI scanning is an excellent modality for detecting all stages of PVL (Barkovich 1997, Boyer 1994, de Vries et al 1993). Signal abnormality due to brain injury may be shown within 2–3 days of the insult as areas either punctate or more extensive areas of T1 shortening (high signal intensity on T1-weighted images and low signal on T2-weighted sequences) (Barkovich 1997) (Figs 6.4, 6.16).

Punctate (or petechial) lesions are predominantly seen in preterm neonates; most commonly they are linearly organized and border the lateral ventricles. Their origin is most probably hemorrhagic, and they may represent a mild form of PVL. Caution is needed when interpreting isolated punctate lesions seen on MRI as their clinical significance with regard to long-term outlook is uncertain (Childs et al 2001, Cornette et al 2000). Early reports suggest that diffusion-weighted imaging may have the potential to demonstrate abnormality in the diffusion of water in the cerebral white matter before abnormality can be detected by conventional MRI (Inder et al 1999). A reduced ADC in an otherwise normal preterm brain is considered an early indicator of white matter damage (just as a reduced ADC is seen shortly after the onset of an acute cerebral ischemic lesion in the full-term newborn). The typical histologic changes in the acute phase of PVL such as cellular and axonal swelling and astrocytic hyperplasia are characterized by some of the same mechanisms leading to restriction of water diffusivity. They considerably change the microstructure of white matter and therefore change water diffusivity.

Thus MRI has the potential to confirm the presence of brain injury prior to the detection of cystic PVL on ultrasound examination, although its potential clinical value in the management of the critically ill neonate has not yet been fully evaluated.

The longer-term sequelae of cystic PVL are well demonstrated both on ultrasound as well as on MRI scans. The more common diffuse injury to the white matter is characterized by diffuse T2 hyperintensities or DEHSI associated with higher ADC values which confirm the locally higher

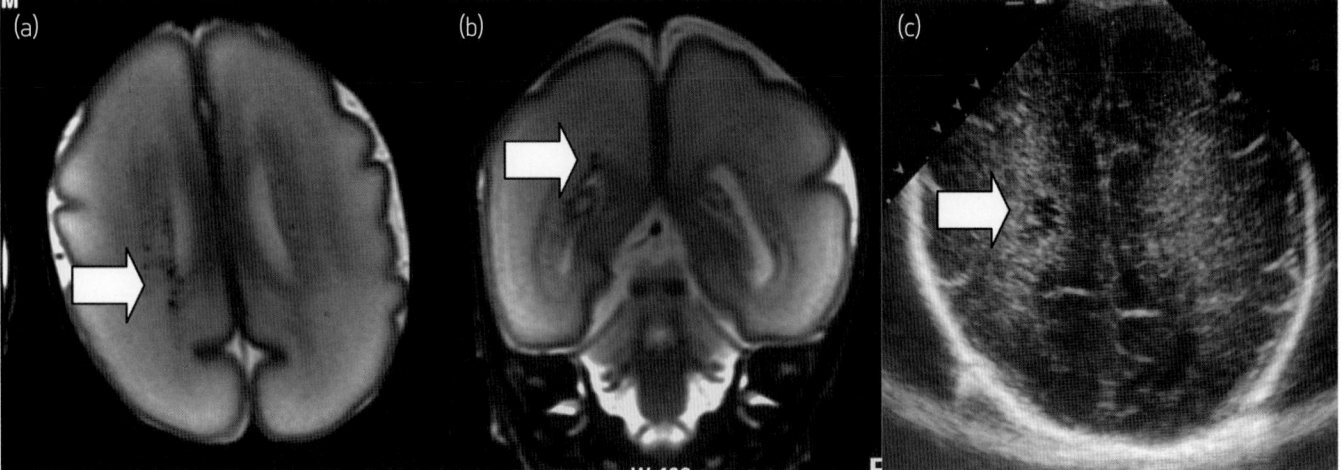

Figure 6.16 'Punctate' lesions in the white matter as they appear on T2-weighted MRI images in a 26-week-old baby at 5 days of life. On the left the ultrasound shows cavitation 2 weeks after the MRI scan was performed; ultrasound was performed with a 9 MHz high-resolution probe.

tissue water content and loss of microstructure impeding water diffusion in those areas (Counsell et al 2003, 2006, Hüppi et al, Maalouf et al 2001). These high ADC values are similar to those seen in the very immature healthy white matter, therefore a potential explanation for the failure of ADC to decline from high levels in the extremely premature infant to lower levels in the term infant in the presence of DEHSI might be related to prior injury with destruction of normal cellular elements (e.g. pre-oligodendrocytes). Further quantitative measures of diffusion at term among premature infants with perinatal white matter lesions, when compared to preterm infants without white matter injury, showed lower anisotropy values in the area of the previous injury, i.e. central periventricular white matter, but also in the underlying posterior limb of internal capsule (Hüppi et al 2001). The lower anisotropy in the injured cerebral white matter suggests that white matter fiber tracts were destroyed or their subsequent development was impaired. The lower anisotropy in the internal capsule further suggests a disturbance in the development of the descending corticospinal tracts (Mazumdar et al 2003). Diffusion-weighted imaging with diffusion-tensor analysis (DTI) has provided new insights into the microstructural white matter development and seems to be an ideal tool to assess alteration of white matter pathways in neurologic disease.

ASPHYXIA IN TERM INFANT (see also Ch. 26)

Brain injury in term babies with clinical evidence of hypoxic–ischemic encephalopathy (HIE) arising from perinatal asphyxia tends to affect the basal ganglia, particularly the ventro-lateral thalami and posterior putamen. Less frequently, injury may occur to the hippocampi, the cerebral cortex and subcortical white matter, particularly the perirolandic region (Babcock & Ball 1983, Banker & Laroche

1962, Barkovich 1992, 2000b, Connolly et al 1994, Cowan et al 1994, Grant & Barkovich 1998/1999, Leech & Ellsworth 1977, Pasternak et al 1991, Pasternak & Gorey 1998, Roland et al 1998, Rutherford et al 1994, Takashima & Tanaka 1978). Injury to the brainstem nuclei is most commonly associated with severe hypoxic–ischemic encephalopathy although these lesions have also been described in association with less severe injury to the basal ganglia (Barkovich 2000b, Leech & Ellsworth 1977). While changes due to HIE are poorly identified both on ultrasound and CT, MRI is now considered the imaging of choice for the evaluation of extent and distribution of injury in the term newborn (Barkovich et al 1998, 2006).

Ultrasound

In the very acute phase the brain may appear normal on ultrasound imaging even following a significant episode of HIE. Cerebral edema and raised intracranial pressure may be suspected by demonstrating a subtle generalized increase in echogenicity of the white matter, in association with slit-like ventricles. Areas of infarction, particularly when associated with hemorrhage in the cerebral cortex, deeper white matter and basal ganglia, may be detected as areas of abnormal increase in echogenicity. In the chronic phase, ultrasound scanning may demonstrate the development of periventricular or multicystic encephalomalacia.

Computed tomography

Hemorrhagic infarction and extra-axial hemorrhage are well demonstrated on CT, but non-hemorrhagic lesions, particularly in the cerebral cortex and deep white matter, are less well seen especially in the acute phase, as edema may be difficult to differentiate from the physiologically normal low attenuation seen in the frontal and occipital regions in the newborn infant (Cowan et al 1994). CT is also relatively insensitive for the detection of injury involving the brain stem nuclei which are known to be associated with an adverse outcome.

Conventional magnetic resonance imaging

MRI is thought to be the most appropriate technique to image brain injury following perinatal asphyxia in the term newborn infant (Barkovich et al 2006, Hüppi et al 2002, Rutherford et al 2005). Although a number of pathological features of HIE may be demonstrated on MRI, abnormal signal in the basal ganglia is the most characteristic lesion (Fig. 6.17). These lesions have a variable appearance relating to the time following the insult as summarized in Table 6.4.

Characteristic changes representing selective neuronal necrosis in these areas on T1-weighted images are T1-hyper-intensities, which become apparent 3–7 days after the insult.

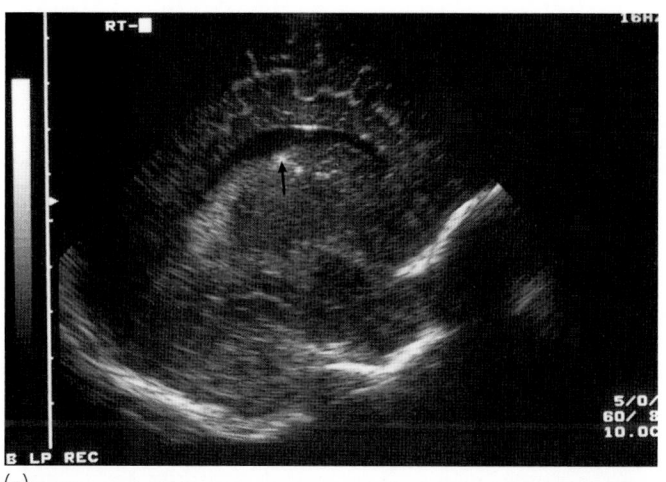

(a)

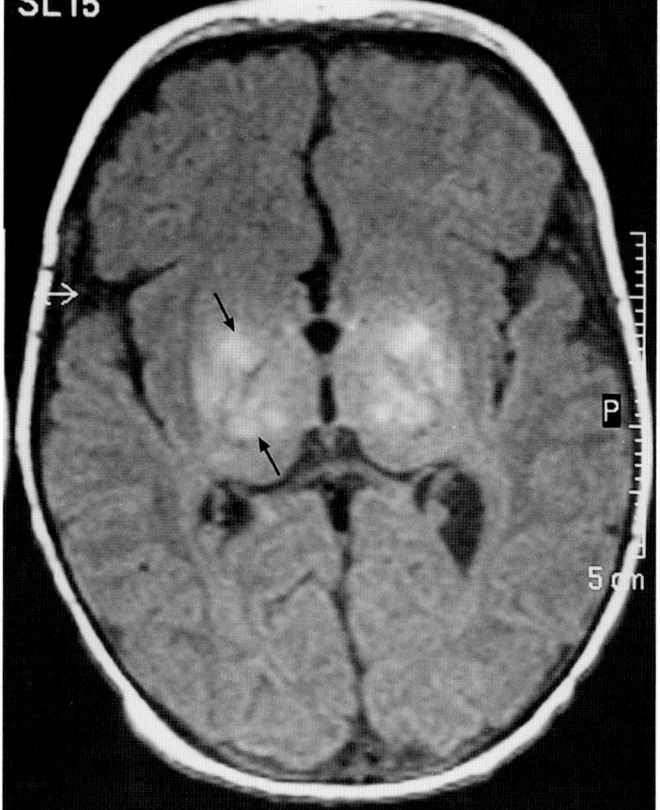

(b)

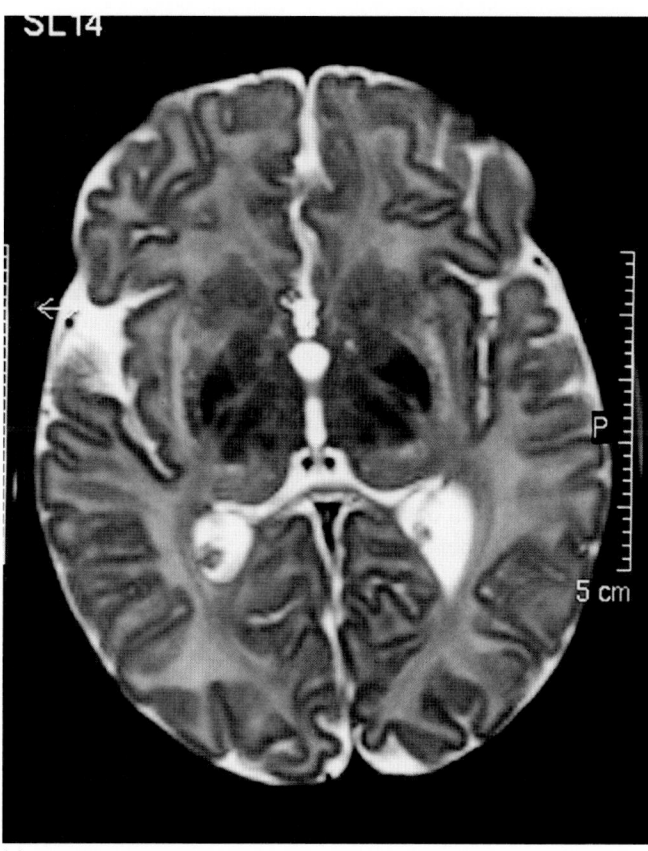

(c)

Figure 6.17 Hypoxic–ischemic encephalopathy. (a) Sagittal ultrasound examination at 26 days of age, demonstrating punctate echogenic lesions in the head of the caudate nucleus (arrow). (b) T1-weighted axial MRI (on the same day) showing patchy high signal and (c) T2-weighted axial MRI showing patchy low signal in the basal ganglia (arrows).

Table 6.4 Summary of changes seen on MRI in the basal ganglia in infants with hypoxic–ischemic encephalopathy

Timing	MRI T1	MRI T2	Diffusion-weighted MRI	CT	Ultrasound
0–24 hours	Normal	Normal	Not known, likely to be abnormal	Normal	Diffuse hyperechogenicity or normal
2–3 days	Subtle, diffuse high signal	Subtle, isointense with white matter	Abnormal, areas of increased signal	Low attenuation or normal	Diffuse hyperechogenicity
7–10 days	More globular, patchy high signal	Patchy high and low signal	Abnormal or normal	Increased attenuation or normal	Better definition of echodensities

These T1-hyperintensities might represent cellular reaction of glial cells and macrophages containing lipid droplets and/or some mineralization of necrotic cells. Some difficulties identifying these lesions arise from the fact that early myelination shows the same image characteristics. T1-hyperintensities in the internal capsule due to myelination need to be differentiated from lateral thalamic and putamenal lesions. Often the posterior limb appears swollen and has lost its normal T1-hyperintensity/T2-hypointensity, which has a bad prognostic value (Rutherford et al 1998). On T2-weighted images thalami might appear slightly hyperintense in the acute phase, but these signal changes tend to be very difficult to detect. T2-hyperintensities become more apparent at a later stage, illustrated also by well-defined lesions on proton-density images. Evolution of these lesions is marked by progressive atrophy of the involved area (i.e. putamen, thalami, rolandic cortex) with persistent T2-hyperintensity and possible cavitation (Rutherford et al 2005).

Of note, similar lesions in the bilateral thalami, lenticular nucleus and globus pallidum can also be detected in premature infants with documented severe anoxic insults.

Isolated parasagittal injury refers to a lesion of the cerebral cortex and the subcortical white matter with a defined distribution, i.e. parasagittal, superomedial aspects of the cortical convexities, usually bilateral but often asymmetric in its extension (Pasternak 1987, Pasternak et al 1991). In conventional MR imaging illustrated by cortical highlighting and evidence of subdural and subarachnoid hemorrhage, single or multiple punctate lesions of high signal on T1-weighted images and low signal on T2-weighted images may be demonstrated in the deep white matter in addition to more generalized alteration in signal intensity due to cerebral edema.

Multicystic encephalomalacia is characterized by a diffuse T1-hypointensity and T2-hyperintensity involving both the cortex and the subcortical white matter, but sparing the cerebellum and the more basal structures of the medulla. Late intrauterine generalized prolonged systemic circulatory insufficiency is probably at the origin of these lesions, which evolve into severe cortical atrophy with cavitation and are invariably associated with a severe neurological syndrome.

Diffusion-weighted imaging

There is still debate on the precise mechanism for the decrease in the apparent diffusion coefficient (ADC) associated with acute brain injury. Changes in ADC following injury are dynamic. ADC values are initially decreased, but subsequently increase so that they are greater than normal and remain so in the chronic phase of injury. During the transition between decreased and increased values, there is a brief period during which values are normal, a process referred to as 'pseudonormalization' (Fig. 6.18). Preliminary data indicate that the timing of pseudonormalization in human newborns follows more closely that of adult humans than that of rodents, taking place at roughly seven days following the injury (McKinstry et al 2002). Interpretation of ADC values to detect acute brain injury in the developing brain needs to be further adjusted for the regional differences in ADC values according to age (Rutherford et al 2004). DWI obtained less than 24 hours after injury may only partly demonstrate focal abnormalities when measuring ADC values and comparing them to regional age-corresponding values, however the full extent of lesions might not be detected yet (Soul et al 2001). MR spectroscopy in this situation can be helpful to detect early metabolic breakdown (McKinstry et al 2002).

MR-spectroscopy

Proton magnetic resonance spectroscopy (^{1}H-MRS) has also entered the clinical arena of MR techniques routinely used for the evaluation of the brain and permits the non-invasive study of metabolic alterations in the brain tissue. When oxidative phosphorylation is impaired, energy metabolism follows the alternative route of anaerobic glycolysis and produces lactic acid. Lactate has a chemical shift of 1.3 ppm and presents as a doublet peak in the in vivo ^{1}H-MRS due to coupling effects. Groenendaal et al (1994) first described markedly elevated lactate levels in five infants with severe

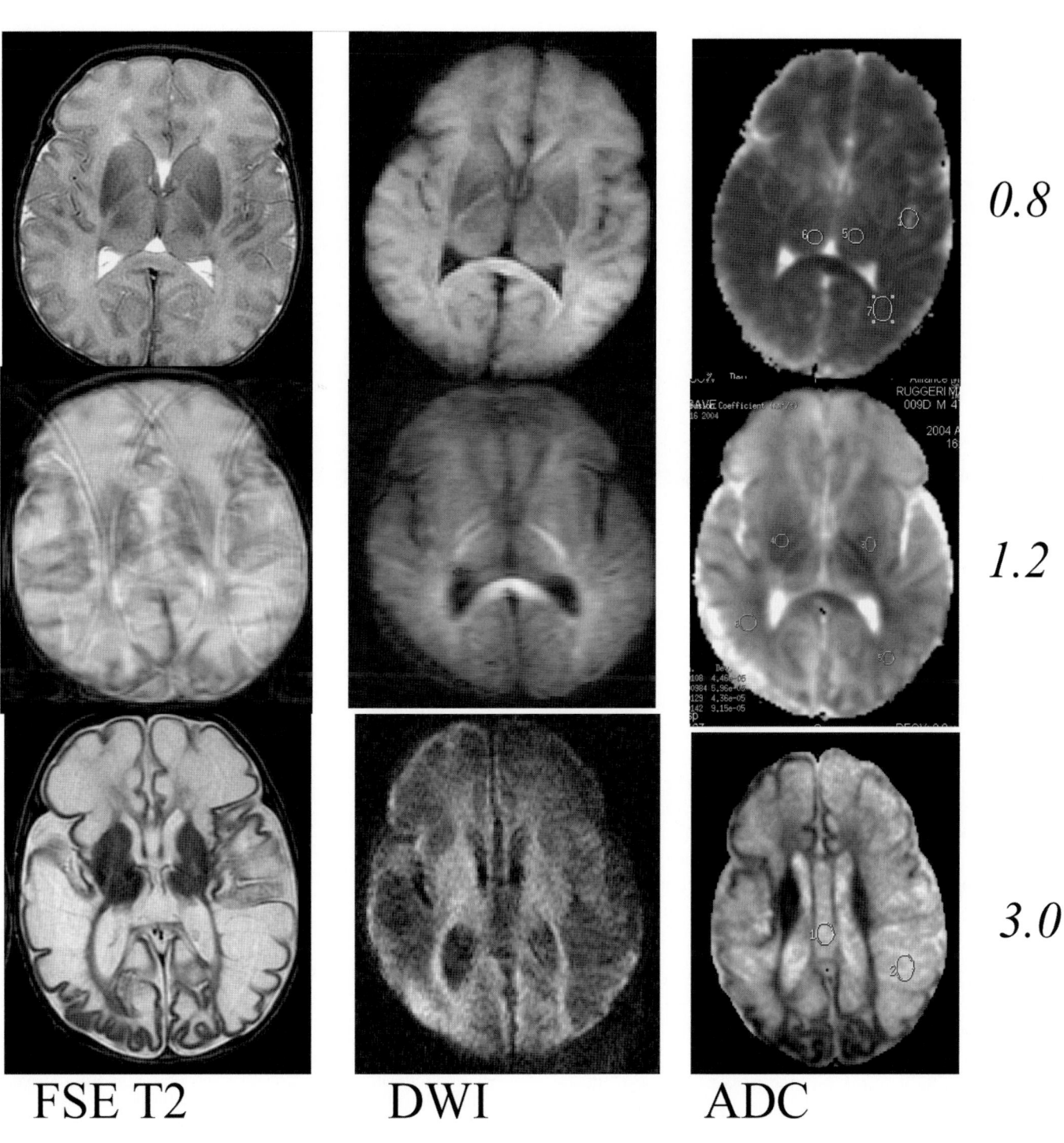

FSE T2   DWI   ADC

0.8

1.2

3.0

μm2/ms

Figure 6.18 T2, DWI and ADC maps scan at 2, 9 and 23 days of life of a severely asphyxiated baby. First line represents scans at 2 days of life, second line at 9 days and third line at 23 days. The phenomenon of ADC pseudonormalization is observed at day 9. At day 23 of life multicystic encephalomalacia is seen on T2, corresponding to high values of ADC.

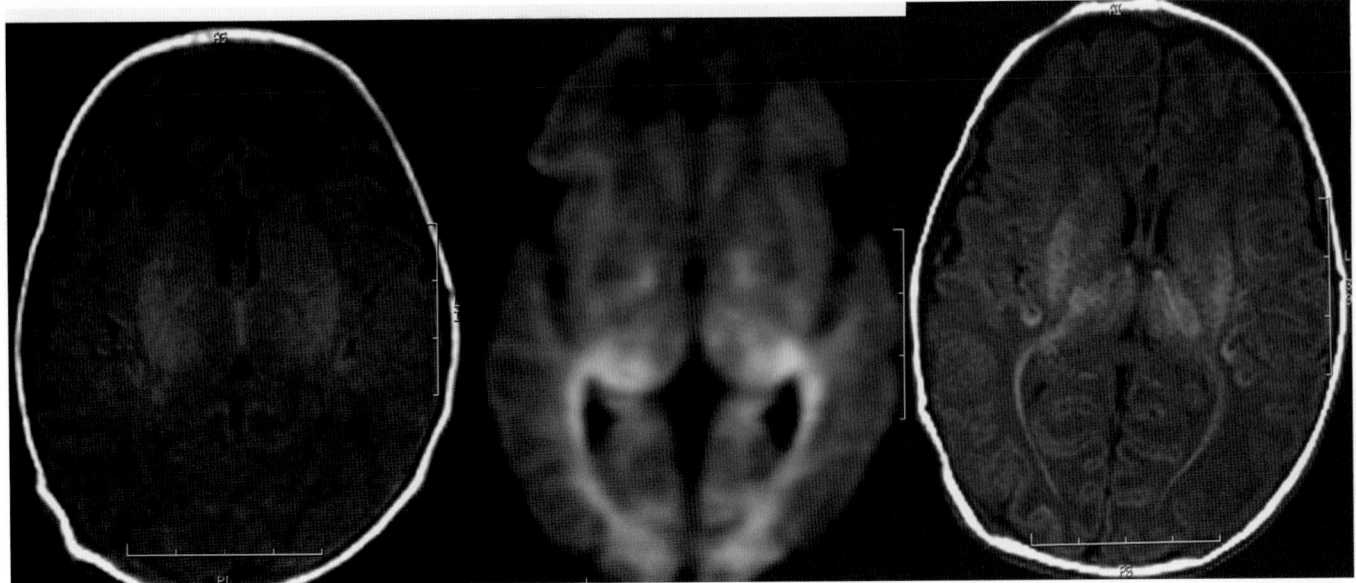

Figure 6.19 T1 MRI axial scan of a term baby with moderate 'asphyxia' at day 4 of life showing a swollen brain but no obvious focal abnormality (left). Areas of pathological 'restriction' of DWI in the optic radiations and thalami are visible at that time (middle). T1 MRI axial scan at day 10 of life showing putaminal-thalamic hyperintensity and other hyperintensities at the level of primary auditory cortex as well as in the optic radiation (right). The extent of the neuronal injury was predicted by the previous DWI with a degree of underestimation.

perinatal asphyxia. Single volume ^{1}H-MRS in acute HIE showed greater increase of the Lac/NAA ratio in the basal ganglia than in the occipitoparietal cerebrum (Penrice et al 1996). Early spectroscopy (<18 hours after event) and measurement of high Lac/Cr ratio in ^{1}H-MRS correlated well with neurodevelopmental outcome at 1 year (Hanrahan et al 1999). Studies using ^{1}H-MRS at a distance (>1–2 weeks) to the hypoxic–ischemic event showed good correlation between reduced NAA ratios with adverse neurodevelopmental outcome (Barkovich et al 2001, Groenendaal et al 1994, Hüppi et al 2001, Miller et al 2002, Robertson et al 2001) whereas in early (acute stage) ^{1}H-MRS NAA ratios are not correlated with outcome (Roelants-Van Rijn et al 2001). ^{1}H-MRS performed in the first 24 hours after the insult is sensitive to the presence of hypoxic–ischemic brain injury, and seems to be suitable for the detection of brain injury on the first day when conventional MR imaging and DWI might not yet detect the injury (Barkovich et al 2006). Early MR spectroscopy has recently been shown to predict outcome more accurately than very early DWI alone (Zarifi et al 2002).

The prognostic value of MR in asphyxia

MR has become the technique of choice to evaluate the ischemic brain both in adults and in the newborn. Advanced MR imaging techniques, such as the use of diffusion-weighted imaging and MR spectroscopy, have further improved the MR capability to investigate the neonatal brain.

The current role of DWI in the evaluation of the term newborn with perinatal asphyxia is:

(1) DWI obtained less than 24 hours after injury may demonstrate focal abnormalities when measuring ADC values and comparing them to regional age-corresponding values; however the full extent of lesions might not be detected.
(2) DWI with ADC measurement obtained between day 2 and 4 may detect lesions not detected by conventional MRI (Fig. 6.19).
(3) DWI at 7–10 days is less sensitive then conventional MRI due to the 'pseudonormalization'.

The current role of ^{1}H-MRS in the evaluation of the term newborn with perinatal asphyxia:

(1) MRS can play an important role in the assessment of encephalopathic term infants. Elevated lactate/NAA, lactate/creatine and lactate/choline ratios or elevated absolute concentrations of lactate at less than 24 hours reliably indicate cellular injury.
(2) MRS might therefore be more useful than DWI techniques in identifying infants who would benefit from early therapeutic interventions.

FOCAL ISCHEMIC LESIONS (see also p. 457)

During the neonatal age, infarction of the major or minor branches of the cerebral arteries can be revealed by ultrasound, CT and MRI. MRI and diffusion-weighted imaging seem to be the most appropriate especially in the earliest stages of the disease. Areas of asymmetrical echogenicity will be detected on ultrasound in the first 12–36 hours following the onset of seizures. The areas of abnormality often only show a subtle increase in echogenicity at first and may be overlooked on account of their more peripheral position. On conventional MRI, areas involved by the infarction will show low signal on T2-weighted images and sometimes an increase on T1-weighted images secondary to hemorrhagic reperfusion. However, the MRI scan may be normal in the first few hours following the infarction. Diffusion-weighted imaging is particularly valuable as it may demonstrate the area of signal alteration secondary to infarction when conventional MRI imaging is still normal (Baird et al 1997, Cowan et al 1994, D'Arceuil et al 1998, Tuor et al 1998). In our experience, ultrasound is often adequate to suggest the diagnosis of a middle cerebral artery infarction. The cavitational phase of the infarcted area is equally recognizable with all techniques and it occurs at a variable time after the initial insult. The majority of these focal lesions tend to affect term babies, although they can affect premature infants, especially those above 30 weeks of gestation. Lesions in the subcortical regions are often difficult to demonstrate by ultrasound scanning, and are most appropriately imaged by MRI (Figs 6.20 and 6.21).

HYPOGLYCEMIA (see also Ch. 35)

Although hypoglycemia may be common among neonates, brain damage resulting from isolated neonatal hypoglycemia is rare. A diffuse brain damage, with the most severe injury localized primarily to the parietal and particularly the occipital cortex of the brain, seems to characterize the pattern of this lesion (Fig. 6.22).

The differential diagnosis of this pattern of damage in the neonatal brain is not very extensive and includes severe sagittal sinus thrombosis, bilateral posterior cerebral artery compression and neonatal hypoxic–ischemic injury (Barkovich et al 1998).

CEREBRAL VEIN THROMBOSIS (p. 456)

Cerebral vein thrombosis is an uncommon disease affecting major sinovenous vessels (CVST) of the neonatal brain. CVST is a vaso-occlusive event with a likely gradual evolution quite unique in neonates due to their coagulation system which favors thrombosis, the presence of smaller blood vessels and a not always so straightforward neuroimaging confirmation. The two major goals of radiological diagnosis are imaging the thrombus and the associated cerebral lesions like hemorrhages and venous infarcts. An unexplained intraventricular hemorrhage in a term baby or a late-onset intraventricular hemorrhage in a 'late' preterm baby should raise the suspicion of a CVST. MRI is an excellent tool for imaging parenchyma, but it is difficult to interpret signals in sinovenous channels (Ramenghi et al 2001). On conventional MRI, the abnormality appears as an increased signal on T1-weighted images and decreased signal on T2-weighted images along the vessels involved due to the thrombotic lesion (Fig. 6.23), usually in major venous sinuses of the brain, but also in the inner small veins of the deep venous system draining the blood from the germinal matrix and periventricular white matter. MR venogram is an excellent aid although caution is needed as the slow-flow signal can be misdiagnosed as a no-flow signal.

The diagnosis with CT scanning is possible but difficult and requires administration of intravenous contrast medium (Fig. 6.24). Although color flow Doppler can be useful in

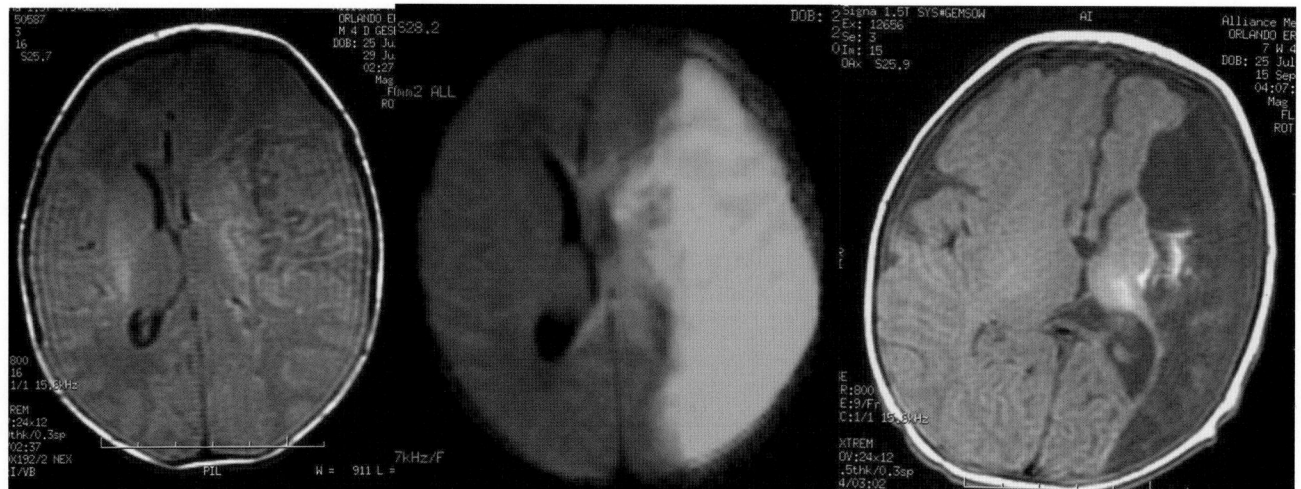

Figure 6.20 T1 axial scan and DWI of a term baby presenting with seizure and scanned at day 2 of life (left). The severe involvement of the left hemisphere is visible on T1, with a large area of restriction on DWI (middle). At 3 weeks of life the severe necrosis of the left hemisphere is noted (right).

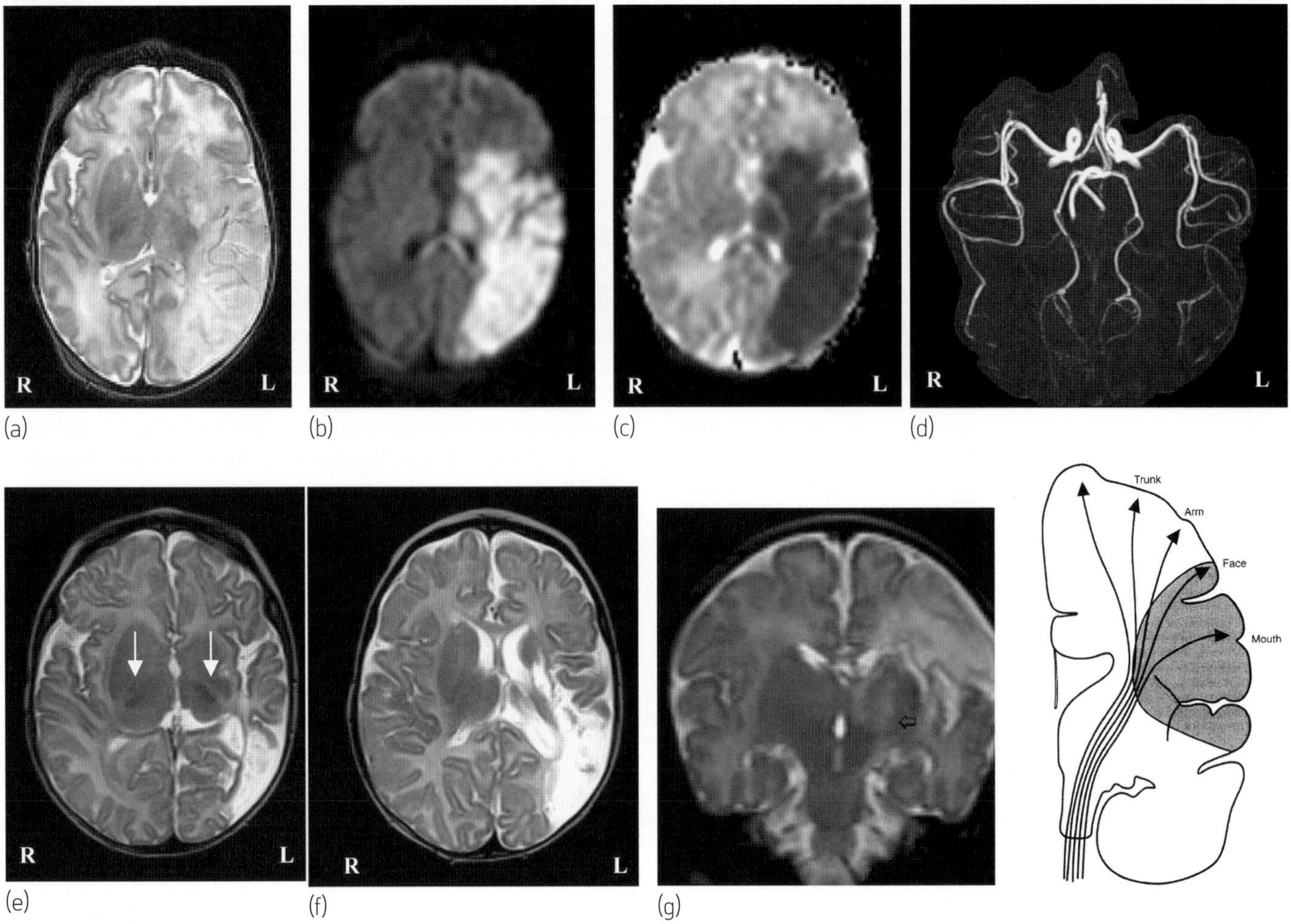

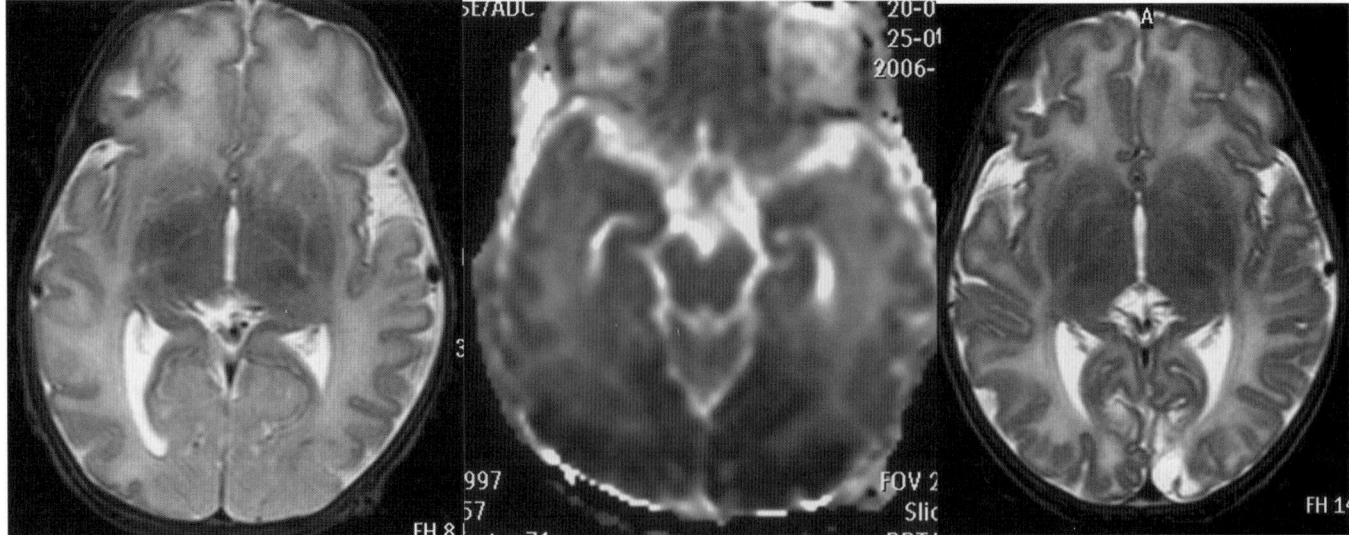

Figure 6.21 Acute left middle cerebral artery infarction in the newborn. (A) Axial T2-weighted image where infarction appears as 'missing cortex' with absence of cortical-subcortical differentiation due to acute edema. (B) Diffusion-weighted image and (C) ADC map with clear demarcation of ischemic zone. (D) Shows reperfused middle cerebral artery on the left with MR angiography. (E) and (F) Axial T2-weighted images in the chronic phase of infarction with cystic transformation of the initial ischemic zone and absence of left-sided myelination in the posterior limb of interna capsule (arrows). (G) Coronal T2-weighted image corresponding to figure representing corticospinal tracts and innervation. Lesion predicts hemiplegia with predominant involvement of arm and face. (Reproduced from Hüppi et al in Questions and Controversies in Neonatology Series Perlman: Neurology Volume Elsevier 2007 in press.)

Figure 6.22 Neonatal hypoglycemia. T2 MRI axial scan (left) and ADC map (middle) of a term baby at 4 days of life who suffered severe hypoglycemia. Both scans show an abnormality in the occipital areas. On the right panel, T2 axial scan at 21 days showing a less severe outcome affecting mainly the left part of the hemisphere.

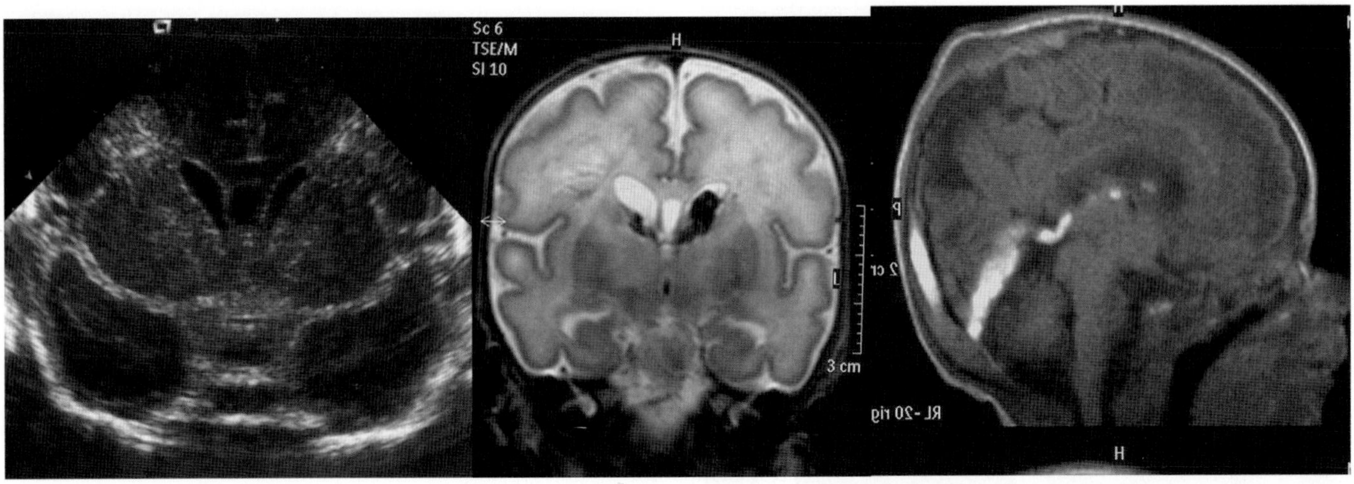

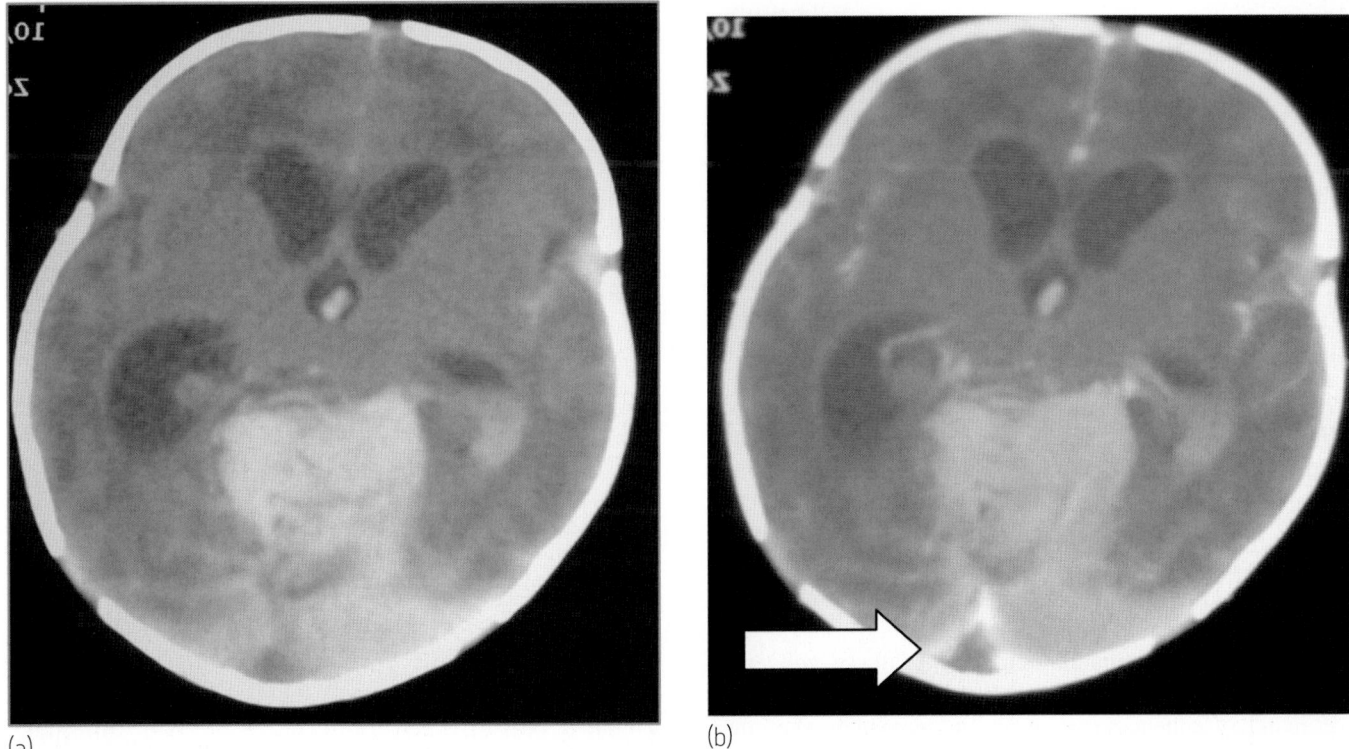

Figure 6.23 US scan (left) of a 31-week-old preterm baby with periventricular echogenicity not present on previous routine US scans. An MRI (middle) was performed which disclosed bilateral white matter lesions, IVH and diffuse sinovenous thrombosis (right).

(a)   (b)

Figure 6.24 (a) CT scan of a term baby presenting with seizure at 36 hours of life. The severe hemorrhage in the posterior fossa and the associated ventricular enlargement are noticeable. (b) CT scan after contrast shows an 'empty signal' at the torcular herophili (arrow) suggesting the presence of venous thrombosis.

identifying thrombosis in the sagittal sinus, it is difficult to visualize the other major venous sinuses and any associated infarction using this modality (Becker et al 1998, Bakac & Wardlaw 1997, De Veber et al 1998, Debus et al 1998, Grossman et al 1993, Nowak-Gottl et al 1997, Pohl et al 1998, Rivkin et al 1992).

CONGENITAL MALFORMATIONS (see also Ch. 13)

A wide range of developmental and congenital abnormalities of the brain may occur. While an ultrasound examination of the brain can identify many of the major congenital abnormalities such as agenesis of the corpus callosum, holoprosencephaly, hydrocephalus and hydranencephaly (Siegel

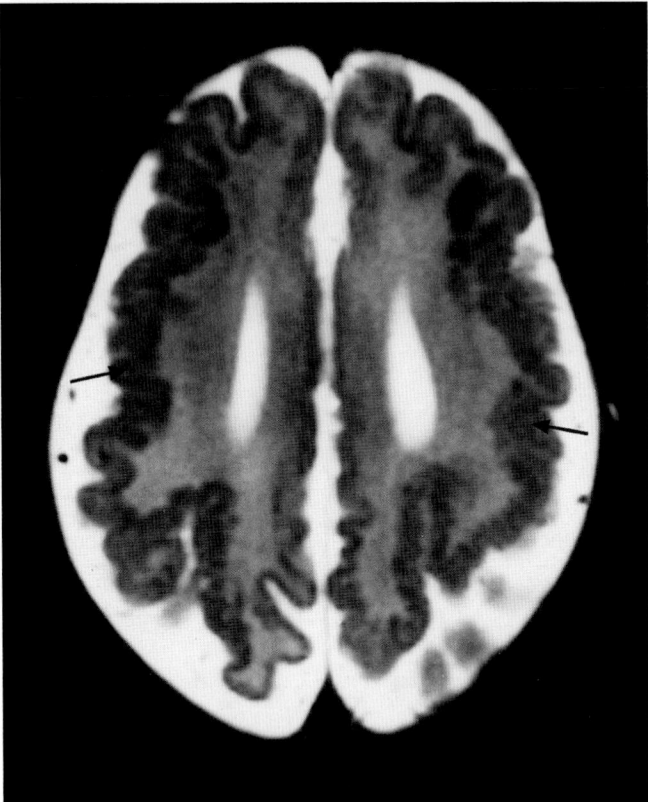

Figure 6.25 Polymicrogyria of unknown etiology despite exhaustive investigations in a term infant presenting at one day of age with seizures. T2-weighted axial MRI scan showing diffuse cortical dysplasia (long arrows).

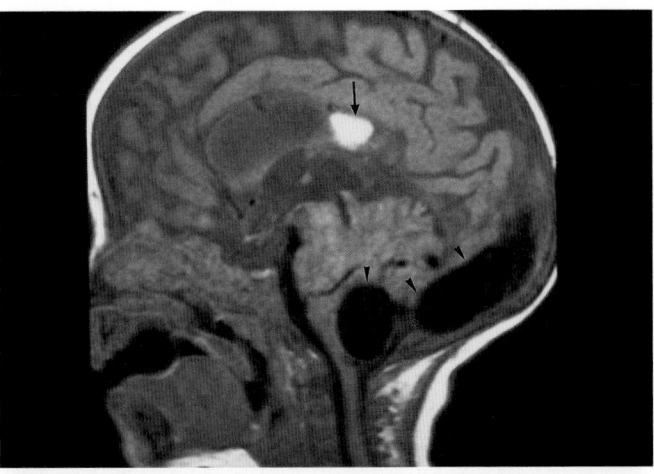

(a)

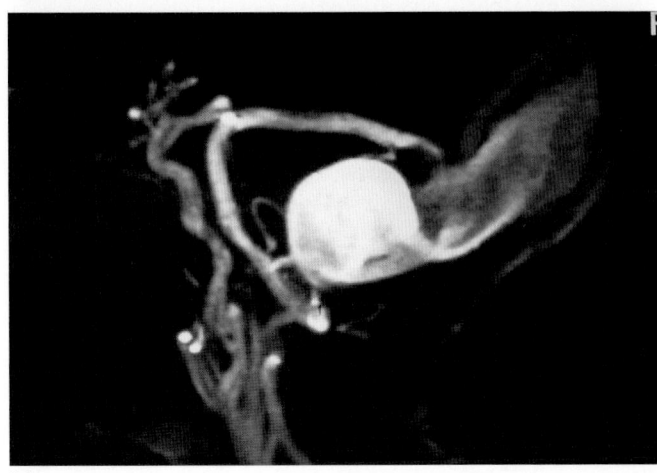

(b)

Figure 6.26 Cerebral arterio-venous malformation. (a) MRI; sagittal T1-weighted scan showing hyperintense lesion (arrow) at the level of the internal cerebral vein and large veins in the posterior fossa (arrows) displacing the cerebellum, due to an extensive arterio-venous malformation. (b) Magnified angiography of the posterior fossa showing basilar artery and its branches directly feeding into the large draining veins of the arterio-venous malformation.

1995), MRI is necessary for full evaluation and has a considerably higher exclusion value than either ultrasound examination or CT scanning (Barkovich 1995). Congenital brain disorders are often complex and may be associated with a number of other abnormalities that will be better demonstrated by MRI, e.g. disordered neuronal migration (Fig. 6.25), gray matter heterotopias, intracerebral lipomas and posterior fossa abnormalities.

Early, ideally antenatal, diagnosis of these congenital malformations is required. Recently, the use of new ultrafast MR imaging sequences such as multiplanar single-shot, fast-spin echo (SSFSE) T2-weighted images provided high resolution images of the fetus in utero with fast imaging times of less than one minute. (This is discussed further in Ch. 5.)

VASCULAR MALFORMATIONS

A number of congenital vascular anomalies in the brain may present in the neonatal period, either following prenatal diagnosis on routine ultrasound scanning or as the result of clinical abnormality, including hydrocephalus and the development of congestive cardiac failure. The vein of Galen aneurysm is the best known and includes a wide spectrum of vascular anomalies which have the common feature of

a dilated vein of Galen (Horowitz et al 1994). Ultrasound imaging with color Doppler analysis is an invaluable tool for screening for intracranial arterio-venous malformations and for monitoring the effect of therapy (Ciricillo et al 1990, Siegel 1995). While contrast-enhanced CT scanning can be used for further evaluation, MRI is superior. Multiplanar scanning and the facility for MR angiography allow the radiologist to assess not only the site and size of the malformation, the presence of any hypoxic–ischemic injury and the degree of hydrocephalus, but also helps to identify vascular access routes suitable for subsequent angiography (Fig. 6.26). Angiography remains essential for full evaluation of the arterial and venous components of the malformations

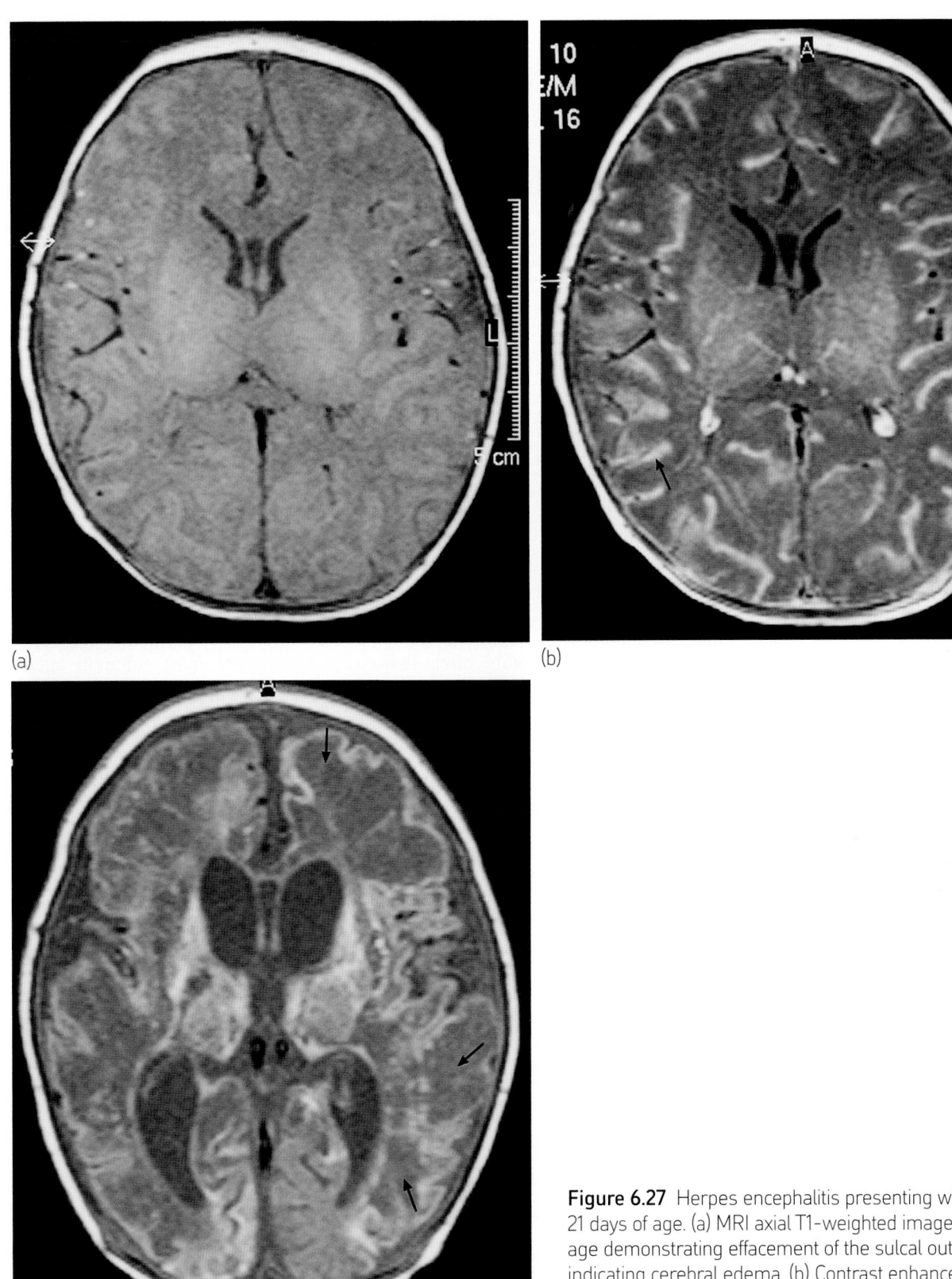

(a)

(b)

(c)

Figure 6.27 Herpes encephalitis presenting with seizures at 21 days of age. (a) MRI axial T1-weighted image at 22 days of age demonstrating effacement of the sulcal outline, possibly indicating cerebral edema. (b) Contrast enhanced T1-weighted image demonstrating abnormal meningeal enhancement (arrows). (c) T1-weighted image at 5 weeks of age demonstrating multicystic encephalomalacia (arrows).

prior to treatment, which is generally by endovascular embolization (Barkovich 1995, Brunelle 1997, Lasjaunias et al 1991).

CEREBRAL INFECTION (see also Chs 30–32)

The clinical and radiological manifestations of intracranial infection are quite different in those infants who acquire the infection prenatally from those in whom the infection occurs in the neonatal period, and the extent of subsequent injury is related to the age of the fetus at the time of infection.

Ultrasound imaging is useful in the initial assessment of an infant with possible prenatally acquired infection (Fig. 6.27). Intracerebral calcifications are seen as dense echogenic foci, which may or may not demonstrate acoustic shadowing in the periventricular white matter, basal ganglia, or in the gyri due to cortical involvement. The extent, nature and distribution of intracranial calcification vary according to the infecting organism (Flodmark 1995). Abnormal linear densities may be demonstrated in the basal ganglia in the line of normal vascular channels and are thought to represent a thalamo-striate vasculopathy (Teele et al 1988). This finding is not specific for prenatal infection and has also been demonstrated following hypoxic–ischemic injury and in association with a number of chromosomal abnormalities. In addition to ventricular dilatation, ultrasound imaging may also show evidence of a ventriculitis by demonstrating evidence of echogenic debris and septa within the lateral ventricles (Carey et al 1987). While ultrasound imaging is an important screening tool, MRI offers the potential for a comprehensive assessment of the extent of injury. Although small foci of calcification may not be as evident as on CT or ultrasound scanning, MRI has the advantage of better demonstration of the extent of white matter injury and its effect on myelination, gyration and neuronal migration.

Herpes simplex infection acquired during delivery may result in very severe necrotizing encephalitis in the first few weeks of life with devastating consequences. Ultrasound imaging may demonstrate massive foci of calcification. Both CT and MRI demonstrate widespread white matter edema in the acute phase. There is prominent meningeal enhancement following the injection of intravenous contrast agents which, together with the white matter abnormalities, are suggestive of herpes simplex infection (Fig. 6.28).

Cerebral infection may be acquired postnatally, most commonly from infection by gram-negative organisms, which may give rise to meningitis, ventriculitis, cerebritis and abscess formation. Ultrasound imaging is useful for monitoring the development of ventricular dilatation and subdural effusions. Ultrasound may also demonstrate the development of ventriculitis by the demonstration of echogenic CSF and the development of ventricular septa. While the development of subdural collections and abscess formation may be suspected on an ultrasound examination, contrast-enhanced CT or MRI is usually necessary where a cerebral abscess is suspected (Barkovich 1995).

There is no specific infection affecting premature babies more often than term babies. The most common agents causing congenital infections in term babies can also affect the developing brain of preterm babies, with special regard to CMV which produces a different pattern of lesions depending on the gestational age at which the infection begins. The importance of this concept can be generalized to other infections and be considered more important than the nature of the infection as suggested by Barkovich (1995).

REFERENCES

Appleton R E, Lee R E J, Hey E N 1990 Neurodevelopmental outcome of transient neonatal intracerebral echodensities. Arch Dis Child 65:27–29.

Archer L N J, Levene M I, Evans D H 1986 Cerebral artery Doppler ultrasonography for prediction of outcome after perinatal asphyxia. Lancet 2(8516):1116–1117.

Arthur R, Ramenghi L 2001 Imaging of the neonatal brain. In: Levene M I, Chevernack F A, Whittle M (eds) Fetal and neonatal neurology and neurosurgery, 2nd edn. Churchill Livingstone, Edinburgh, pp. 105–128.

Baarsma R, Laurini R N, Baerts W, Okken A 1987 Reliability of sonography in non-hemorrhagic periventricular leukomalacia. Pediatr Radiol 17:189–191.

Babcock D S, Ball W S 1983 Postasphyxial encephalopathy in fullterm infants: ultrasound diagnosis. Radiology 148:417–423.

Babcock D S, Bove K E, Han B K 1982 Intracranial haemorrhage in premature infants: sonographic pathologic correlation. Am J Neuroradiol 3:309–317.

Babcock D S, Han B K, Dine M S 1988 Sonographic findings in infants with macrocrania. Am J Radiol 150:1359–1365.

Baird A E, Benfield A, Schlaug S et al 1997 Enlargement of human cerebral ischemic lesion volumes measured by diffusion-weighted magnetic resonance imaging. Ann Neurol 41:581–589.

Bakac G, Wardlaw J M 1997 Problems in the diagnosis of intracranial venous infarction. Neuroradiology 39:566–570.

Banker B Q, Larroche J C 1962 Periventricular leukomalacia of infancy. Arch Neurol 7:386–410.

Barkovich A J 1992 MR and CT evaluation of profound neonatal and infantile asphyxia. Am J Neuroradiol 13:959–972.

Barkovich A J 1995 Pediatric neuroimaging. Raven, New York, NY.

Barkovich A J 1997 The encephalopathic neonate: choosing the proper imaging technique. Am J Neuroradiol 18:1816–1820.

Barkovich A J 1998 MR of the normal neonatal brain, assessment of deep structures. Am J Neuroradiol 19:971–976.

Barkovich A J 2000a Normal development of the neonatal and infant brain, skull, and spine. In: Pediatric neuroimaging, 3rd edn. Lippincott Williams & Wilkins, Philadelphia, PA, pp. 13–69.

Barkovich A J 2000b Brain and spine injuries in infancy and childhood In: Pediatric neuroimaging, 3rd edn. Lippincott Williams & Wilkins, Philadelphia, PA, pp. 157–250.

Barkovich A J, Edwards M S B 1992 Applications of neuroimaging in hydrocephalus. Pediatr Neurosurg 18:65–83.

Barkovich A J, Firas A A, Howard et al 1998b Imaging patterns of neonatal hypoglycemia. AJNR Am J Neuroradiol 19:523–528.

Barkovich A J, Hajnal B L, Vigneron D et al 1998a Prediction of neuromotor outcome in perinatal asphyxia: evaluation of MR scoring systems. Am J Neuroradiol 19:143–149.

Barkovich A J, Miller S P, Bartha A et al 2006 MR imaging, MR spectroscopy, and diffusion tensor imaging of sequential studies in neonates with encephalopathy. Am J Neuroradiol 27:533–547.

Barkovich A J, Westmark K D, Bedi H S et al 2001 Proton spectroscopy and diffusion imaging on the first day of life after perinatal asphyxia: preliminary report. Am J Neuroradiol. 22:1786–1794.

Battin M R, Maalouf E F, Counsell S J et al 1998 Magnetic resonance imaging of the brain in very preterm infants: visualization of the germinal matrix, early myelination and cortical folding. Pediatrics 101:957–962.

Beaulieu C, D'Arceuil H, Hedahus M et al 1999 Diffusion-weighted magnetic resonance imaging: theory and potential applications to child neurology. Semin Pediatr Neurol 6:87–100.

Becker S, Heller C, Gropp F et al 1998 Thrombophilic disorders in children with cerebral infarction. Lancet 352:1756–1757.

Berman J I, Mukherjee P, Partridge S C et al 2005 Quantitative diffusion tensor MRI fiber tractography of sensorimotor white matter development in premature infants. Neuroimage 27:862–871.

Blankenberg F G, Loh N N, Norbash A M et al 1997 Impaired cerebrovascular autoregulation after hypoxic-ischemic injury in extremely low birth weight neonates: detection with power and pulsed wave Doppler US. Radiology 205:563–568.

Blankenberg F G, Norbash A M, Lane B et al 1996 Neonatal intracranial ischemia and hemorrhage: diagnosis with US, CT, and MR imaging. Radiology 199:253–259.

Bloom M, Jacobs S, Pile-Spellman J et al 1996 Cerebral SPECT Imaging: effect on clinical management. J Nuclear Med 37:1070–1073.

Bluml S, Friedlich P, Erberich S et al 2004 MR imaging of newborns by using an MR-compatible incubator with integrated radiofrequency coils: initial experience Radiology 231:594–601.

Boxma A, Lequin M, Ramenghi L A et al 2005 Sonographic detection of the optic radiation. Acta Paediatr 94:1455–1461.

Boyer R S 1994 Neuroimaging of premature infants. Neuroimag Clin N Am 4:241–259.

Bozynski M E, Nelson M N, Matalon T A S 1985 Cavitatory periventricular leukomalacia: incidence and short term outcome in infants weighing <1200 g at birth. Dev Med Child Neurol 27:572–577.

Braffman B H, Bilaniuk L T, Naidich T P 1992 MR imaging of tuberous sclerosis: pathogenesis of this phakomatosis. Use of gadopentetate dimeglumine and literature review. Radiology 183:227–238.

Brunelle F 1997 Arterio-venous malformation of the vein of Galen in children. Pediatr Radiol 27:501–513.

Cady E B 1992 MRS of the newborn human infant. In: deCertaines J D, Bovee W M M J, Podo F (eds) Magnetic resonance spectroscopy in biology and medicine. Pergamon, Oxford, pp. 437–477.

Carey B, Arthur R J, Houlsby W T 1987 Ventriculitis in congenital rubella: ultrasound demonstration. Pediatr Radiol 17:415–416.

Casselden P A 1988 Ocular lens dose in cerebral vascular imaging. Br J Radiol 61:202–204.

Caviness V S, Kennedy D N, Richelme C et al 1996 The human brain age 7–11 years: A volumetric analysis based upon magnetic resonance images. Cereb Cortex 6:726–637.

Chan C, Wong Y, Chau L et al 1999 Radiation dose reduction in pediatric CT. Pediatr Radiol 29:770–775.

Childs A M, Cornette L, Ramenghi L A et al 2001a Magnetic resonance and cranial ultrasound characteristics of periventricular white matter abnormalities in newborn infants. Clin Radiol 56:647–655.

Childs A M, Ramenghi L A, Cornette L et al 2001b Cerebral maturation in premature infants: quantitative assessment using MR imaging. Am J Neuroradiol 22:1577–1582.

Childs A M, Ramenghi L A, Evans D J et al 1998 MR features of developing periventricular white matter in preterm infants: evidence of glial cell migration. Am J Neuroradiol 19:971–976.

Ciricillo S F, Schmidt K G, Silverman N H et al 1990 Serial ultrasonographic evaluation of neonatal vein of Galen malformations to assess the efficacy of interventional neuroradiological procedures. Neurosurgery 27:544–548.

Cline H E, Lorenson R, Kikinis R et al 1990 Three-dimensional segmentation of MR images of the head using probability and connectivity. J Comput Ass Tom 14:1037–1045.

Connolly B, Kelehan P, O'Brien N et al 1994 The echogenic thalamus in hypoxic-ischemic encephalopathy. Pediatr Radiol 24:268–271.

Counsell S J, Alleop J M, Harrison M C et al 2003 Diffusion-weighted imaging of the brain in preterm infants with focal and diffuse white matter abnormality. Pediatrics 112:1–7.

Counsell S J, Shen Y, Boardman J P et al 2006 Axial and radial diffusivity in preterm infants who have diffuse white matter changes on magnetic resonance imaging at term-equivalent age. Pediatrics 117:376–386.

Cowan F M, Pennock J M, Hanrahan J D et al 1994 Early detection of cerebral infarction and hypoxic ischemic encephalopathy in neonates using diffusion weighted magnetic resonance imaging. Neuropediatrics 25:172–175.

D'Arceuil H E, de Crespigny A J, Rother J et al 1998 Diffusion and perfusion magnetic resonance imaging of the evolution of hypoxic ischemic encephalopathy in the neonatal rabbit. J Magn Reson Imag 8:820–828.

De Veber G, Monagle P, Chan A et al 1998 Prothrombotic disorders in infants and children with cerebral thromboembolism. Arch Neurol 55:1539–1543.

de Vries L S, Dubowitz L M S, Dubovitz V et al 1985 Predictive value of cranial ultrasound in the newborn baby: a reappraisal. Lancet 2(8447):137–140.

de Vries L S, Eken P, Dubowitz L M S 1992 The spectrum of leukomalacia using cranial ultrasound. Behav Brain Res 49:1–6.

de Vries L S, Eken P, Groenendaal F et al 1993 Correlation between the degree of periventricular leukomalacia diagnosed using cranial ultrasound and MRI later in infancy in children with cerebral palsy. Neuropediatrics 24:263–268.

de Vries L S, Levene M I 1995 Cerebral ischaemic lesions. In: Levene M I L, Lilford R J (eds) Fetal and neonatal neurology and neurosurgery, 2nd edn. Churchill Livingstone, Edinburgh, pp. 367–386.

de Vries L S, Rademaker K J, Groenedaal F et al 1998 Correlation between neonatal cranial ultrasound, MRI in infancy and neurodevelopmental outcome in infants with a large intraventricular haemorrhage with or without unilateral parenchymal involvement. Neuropediatrics 29:180–188.

de Vries L S, Regev R, Pennock J M et al 1988a Ultrasound evolution and later outcome of infants with periventricular densities. Early Hum Dev 16:225–233.

de Vries L S, Smet M, Ceulemans B et al 1990 The role of high resolution ultrasound and MRI in the investigation of infants with macrocephaly. Neuropediatrics 21:72–75.

de Vries L S, Wigglesworth J S, Regev R, Dubowitz L M S 1988b Evolution of periventricular leukomalacia during the neonatal period and infancy: correlation of imaging and postmortem findings. Early Hum Dev 17:205–219.

Debus O, Koch H G, Kurlemann et al 1998 Factor V Leiden and genetic defects of thrombophilia in childhood porencephaly. Arch Dis Child 78:F121–F124.

Deguchi K, Mizuguchi M, Takashima S et al 1996 Immunohistochemical expression of tumor necrosis factor alpha in neonatal leukomalacia. Pediatr Neurol 14:13–16.

Deguchi K, Oguchi K, Takashima S et al 1997 Characteristic neuropathology of leukomalacia in extremely low birth weight infants Pediatr Neurol 16:296–300.

Deipolyi A R, Mukherjee P, Gill K et al 2005 Comparing microstructural and macrostructural development of the cerebral cortex in premature newborns: diffusion tensor imaging versus cortical gyration. Neuroimag 27:579–586.

Dewbury K C, Bates R I 1981 The value of transfontanellar ultrasound in infants. Br J Radiol 54:1044–1052.

Di Pietro M A, Brody B A, Teele R L 1986 Peritrigonal echogenic 'blush' on cranial sonography: pathologic correlates. Am J Roentgenol 146:1067–1072.

Di Salvo D N 2001 A new view of the neonatal brain: clinical utility of supplemental neurologic US imaging windows. RadioGraphics 21:943–955.

Dubowitz L M S, Bydder G M, Mushin J 1985 Development sequence of periventricular leukomalacia. Arch Dis Child 60:349–355.

Enzmann D, Pelc N 1991 Normal flow patterns of intracranial and spinal cerebrospinal fluid defined with phase-contrast cine MR imaging. Radiology 178:467–474.

Erberich S G, Friedlich P, Seri I et al 2003 Functional MRI in neonates using neonatal head coil and MR compatible incubator. Neuroimage 20: 683–692.

Evans D J, Childs A M, Ramenghi L A et al 1997 Magnetic resonance imaging of the brain of premature infants. Lancet 2(9076):350.

Flodmark O 1995 Imaging of the neonatal brain. In: Levene M I L, Lilford R J (eds) Fetal and neonatal neurology and neurosurgery, 2nd edn. Churchill Livingstone, Edinburgh, pp. 105–128.

Flodmark O, Becker L E, Harwood Nash D C et al 1980a Correlation between computed tomography and autopsy in premature and full-term neonates that have suffered perinatal asphyxia. Radiology 137:93–103.

Flodmark O, Fitz C R, Harwood-Nash D C 1980b CT diagnosis and short term prognosis of intracranial hemorrhage and hypoxic/ischemic brain damage in neonate. J Comput Assist Tomog 4:775–787.

Frigieri G, Guidi B, Costa Zacarelli S et al 1996 Multicystic encephalomalacia in term infants. Child Nerv Syst 12:759–764.

Giedd J, Snell J, Lange N et al 1996 Quantitative magnetic resonance imaging of human brain development: Ages 4–18. Cereb Cortex 6:551–560.

Goetz M C, Gretebeck R J, Sang Oh S et al 1995 Incidence, timing, and follow-up of periventricular leukomalacia. Am J Perinatol 12:325–327.

Gould S J, Howard S, Hope P L, Reynolds E O 1987 Periventricular intraparenchymal cerebral haemorrhage in preterm infants: the role of venous infarction. J Pathol 151:197–202.

Govaert P, de Vries L S 1997 An atlas of neonatal brain sonography. Cambridge University Press, pp. 1–363.

Grant E G, Schellinger D 1985 Sonography of neonatal periventricular leukomalacia: recent experience with a 7.5 MHz scanner. Am J Neuroradiol 6:781–785.

Grant E G, Schellinger D, Richardson J D et al 1983 Echogenic periventricular halo: normal sonographic finding or neonatal cerebral hemorrhage. Am J Roentgenol 140:793–796.

Grant P E, Barkovich A J 1998/1999 MRI in cerebral palsy. Clin MRI/Dev MR 8:105–114.

Groenendaal F, Veehoven RH, van der Grond J et al 1994 Cerebral lactate and N-acetylaspartate/choline ratios in asphyxiated full-term neonates demonstrated in vivo using proton magnetic resonance spectroscopy. Pediatr Res 35:148–151.

Grossman R, Novak G, Patel M et al 1993 MRI in neonatal dural sinus thrombosis. Pediatr Neurol 9:235–338.

Gupta R K, Hasan K M, Trivedi R et al 2005 Diffusion tensor imaging of the developing human cerebrum. J Neurosci Res 81:172–178.

Hanrahan J D, Cox I J, Azzopardi D et al 1999 Relation between proton magnetic resonance spectroscopy within 18 hours of birth asphyxia and neurodevelopment at 1 year of age. Dev Med Child Neurol 41:76–82.

Hay T C, Rumack C M, Horgan J G 1989 Cranial sonography: intracranial hemorrhage, periventricular leukomalacia and asphyxia. Clin Diagn Ultrasound 24:25–42.

Hirayama A, Okoshi Y, Hachiya Y et al 2001 Early immunohistochemical detection of axonal damage and glial activation in extremely immature brains with periventricular leukomalacia. Clin Neuropathol 20:87–91.

Hope P J, Gould S J, Howard S et al 1988 Ultrasound diagnosis of pathologically verified lesions in the brains of very preterm infants. Dev Med Child Neurol 30:457–471.

Horowitz M B, Jungreis C A, Quisling R G, Pollack I 1994 Vein of Galen aneurysms: a review and current perspective. Am J Neuroradiol 15:1486–1496.

Hüppi P S, Barnes P D 1997 Magnetic resonance techniques in the evaluation of the newborn brain. Clin Perinatol 24:693–723.

Hüppi P S, Dubois J 2006 Diffusion tensor imaging of brain development. Semin.Fetal Neonatal Med. 11:489–497.

Hüppi P S, Fusch Ch, Boesch Ch et al 1995 Regional metabolic assessment of human brain during development by proton magnetic resonance spectroscopy in vivo and by high preformance liquid chromatography/gas chromatography in autopsy tissue. Pediatr Res 37:145–150.

Hüppi P S, Lazeyras F 2001 Proton magnetic resonance spectroscopy ((1)H-MRS) in neonatal brain injury. Pediatr Res 49:317–320.

Hüppi P S, Lazeyras F 2005 MR spectroscopy. In: Tortori-Donati P (ed) Pediatric neuroradiology brain. Springer, Berlin, pp. 1049–1072.

Hüppi P S, Maier S E, Peled S et al 1998b Microstructural development of human newborns cerebral white matter assessed in vivo by diffusion tensor MRI. Pediatr Res 44:584–590.

Hüppi P S, Posse S, Lazeyras F et al 1991 Magnetic resonance in preterm and term newborns: 1H-spectroscopy in developing human brain. Pediatr Res 30:574–578.

Hüppi P S, Warfield S, Kikinis R et al 1998a Quantitative magnetic resonance imaging of brain development in premature and mature newborns. Ann Neurol 43:224–235.

Inder T E, Anderson N J, Spencer C et al 2003 White matter injury in the premature infant: a comparison between serial cranial sonographic and MR findings at term. AJNR Am J Neuroradiol 24:805–809.

Inder T E, Hüppi P S, Warfield S et al 1999b Periventricular white matter injury in the premature infant is associated with a reduction in cerebral cortical gray matter volume at term. Ann Neurol 46:755–760.

Inder T E, Warfield S K, Wang H et al 2005 Abnormal cerebral structure is present at term in premature infants. Pediatrics 115:286–289.

Inder T, Hüppi P S, Zientara G P 1999a Early detection of periventricular leukomalacia by diffusion-weighted magnetic resonance imaging techniques. J Pediatr 134:631–634.

Kapur T, Grimnson W E, Wells W M et al 1996 Segmentation of brain tissue from magnetic resonance images. Med Image Anal 1:109–127.

Keeney S E, Adcock E W, McArdle C B 1991 Prospective observations of 100 high-risk neonates by high field (1.5 Tesla) magnetic resonance imaging of the central nervous system: 1. Intraventricular and extracerebral lesions. Pediatrics 87:421–430.

Kesler S R, Ment L R, Vohr B et al 2004 Volumetric analysis of regional cerebral development in preterm children. Pediatr Neurol 31:318–325.

Kinney H C, Brody B A, Kloman A S et al 1988 Sequence of central nervous system myelination in human infancy. II Patterns of myelination in autopsied infants. J Neuropathol Exp Neurol 47:217–234.

Kreis R, Hofmann L, Kuhlmann B et al 2002 Brain metabolite composition during early human brain development as measured by quantitative in vivo 1H magnetic resonance spectroscopy. Magn Reson Med 48:949–958.

Kuzniecky R I 1996 Neuroimaging in pediatric epilepsy. Epilepsia 37 Suppl 1:S10–S21.

Laitt R D, Mallucci C L, McConachie N S et al 1999 Constructive interference in steady-state 3-D Fourier-transform MRI in the management of hydrocephalus and third ventriculostomy. Neuroradiology 41:117–123.

Larroche J C 1972 Post-haemorrhagic hydrocephalus in infancy. Anatomical study. Biol Neonate 20:287–299.

Lasjaunias P, Garcia-Monaco R, Rodesch G et al 1991 Vein of Galen malformation: endovascular treatment of 43 cases. Child Nerv Syst 7:360–367.

LeBihan D, Breton E, Lallemand D et al 1986 MR imaging of intravoxel incoherent motions: application to diffusion and perfusion in neurologic disorders. Radiology 161:401–407.

Lee B C P, Park T S, Kaufmann B A 1995 MR angiography in pediatric neurologic disorders. Pediatr Radiol 25:409–419.

Leech R W, Ellsworth C A 1977 Anoxic-ischemic encephalopathy in the human neonatal period. The significance of brain stem involvement. Arch Neurol 34:109–113.

Levene M I, de Vries L 2001 Neonatal intracranial hemorrhage. In: Levene M I, Chevernak F A, Whittle M (eds) Fetal and neonatal neurology and neurosurgery. Churchill Livingstone Edinburgh.

Levene M I, de Vries L S 1984 Extension of neonatal intraventricular haemorrhage. Arch Dis Child 59:631–636.

Leviton A, Gilles F 1996 Ventriculomegaly, delayed myelination, white matter hypoplasia, and 'periventricular' leukomalacia: how are they related? Pediatr Neurol 15:127–136.

Leviton A, Paneth N 1990 White damage in preterm newborns, an epidemilogic perspectives. Early Hum Dev 24:1–22.

Limperopoulos C, Soul J S, Gauvreau K et al 2005a Late gestation cerebellar growth is rapid and impeded by premature birth. Pediatrics 115 (3):688–695.

Limperopoulos C, Soul J S, Haidar H et al 2005b Impaired trophic interactions between the cerebellum and the cerebrum among preterm infants. Pediatrics 116:844–850.

Lin W, An H, Chen Y, Nicholas P et al 2003 Practical consideration for 3T imaging Magn Reson Imaging Clin N Am 11:615–639.

Lodygensky G A, Rademaker K, Zimine S et al 2005 Structural and functional brain development after hydrocortisone treatment for neonatal chronic lung disease. Pediatrics 116:1–7.

Logan W J 1999 Functional magnetic resonance imaging in children. Semin Pediatr Neurol 6:78–86.

Maalouf E F, Duggan P J, Counsell S J et al 2001 Comparison of findings on cranial ultrasound and magnetic resonance imaging in preterm infants. Pediatrics 107:719–727.

McKinstry R C, Mathur A, Miller J H et al 2002b Radial organization of developing preterm human cerebral cortex revealed by non-invasive water diffusion anisotropy MRI. Cereb Cortex 12:1237–1243.

McKinstry R C, Miller J H, Snyder A Z et al 2002a A prospective, longitudinal diffusion tensor imaging study of brain injury in newborns. Neurology 59:824–833.

McMenamin J B, Shackleford G D, Volpe J J 1984 Outcome of neonatal intraventricular haemorrhage with periventricular echodense lesions. Ann Neurol 15:285–290.

McMenamin J B, Volpe J J 1983 Doppler ultrasonography in the determination of neonatal brain death. Ann Neurol 14(3):302–307.

Martin E, Krassnitzer S, Kaelin P, Boesch C 1991 MR imaging of the brainstem: normal postnatal development. Neuroradiology 33:391–395.

Martinussen M, Fischl B, Larsson H B et al 2005 Cerebral cortex thickness in 15-year-old adolescents with low birth weight measured by an automated MRI-based method. Brain 128:2588–2596.

Mazumdar A, Mukherjee P, Miller J H et al 2003 Diffusion-weighted imaging of acute corticospinal tract injury preceding Wallerian degeneration in the maturing human brain. Am J Neuroradiol 24:1057–1066.

Mewes A U, Hüppi P S, Als H et al 2006 Regional brain development in serial magnetic resonance imaging of low-risk preterm infants. Pediatrics 118:23–33.

Miller S P, Newton N, Ferriero D M et al 2002 Predictors of 30-month outcome after perinatal depression: role of proton MRS and socioeconomic factors. Pediatr Res 52:71–77.

Miller S P, Tasch T, Sylvain M et al 1998 Tuberous sclerosis complex and neonatal seizures. J Child Neurol 13:619–623.

Mohan K K, Chugani D C, Chugani H T 1999 Positron emission tomography in pediatric neurology. Semin Pediatr Neurol 6:111–119.

Mori S, Kaufmann W E, Davatzikos C et al 2002 Imaging cortical association tracts in the human brain using diffusion-tensor-based axonal tracking. Magn Reson Med 47:215–223.

Mukherjee P, Miller J H, Shimony J S et al 2001 Normal brain maturation during childhood: developmental trends characterized with diffusion-tensor MR imaging. Radiology 221:349–358.

Naressi A, Couturier C, Castang I et al 2001 Java-based graphical user interface for MRUI, a software package for quantitation of in vivo/medical magnetic resonance spectroscopy signals. Comput Biol Med 31:269–286.

Neil J L, Shiran S I, McKinstry R C et al 1998 Normal brain in human newborns: Apparent diffusion coefficient and diffusion anisotropy measured by using diffusion tensor MR imaging. Radiology 209:57–66.

Nowak-Gottl U, von Kries R, Gobel U 1997 Neonatal symptomatic thromboembolism in Germany: two year survey. Arch Dis Child 76:F163–F167.

Nwaesei C G, Pape K E, Martin D J et al 1984 Periventricular infarction diagnosed by ultrasound: a postmortem correlation. J Pediatr 105:106–110.

Okuda T, Korogi Y, Ikushima I 1998 Use of fluid-attenuation recovery (FLAIR) sequences in perinatal hypoxic-ischaemic encephalopathy. Br J Radiol 71(843):282–290.

Paakko E, Lopponen T L, Saukkonen A-L et al 1994 Information value of magnetic resonance imaging in shunted hydrocephalus. Arch Dis Child 70:530–535.

Paneth N, Rudelli R, Kazam E, Monte W 1994 White matter damage, terminology, typology, pathogenesis in brain damage in the preterm infant. Mac Keith — Cambridge University Press,.

Paneth N, Rudelli R, Monte W et al 1990 White matter necrosis in very low birth weight infants: neuropathologic and ultrasonographic findings in infants surviving six days or longer. J Pediatr 116:975–984.

Pape K E, Bennett-Britton S, Szymonowicz W 1983 Diagnostic accuracy of neonatal brain imaging: a postmortem correlation of computed tomography and ultrasound scans. J Pediatr 102:275–280.

Papile L A, Burstein J, Burstein R, Koffler H 1978 Incidence and evolution of subependymal and intraventricular hemorrhage: a study of infants with birth weights less than 1500 gm. J Pediatr 92:529–534.

Pasternak J F 1987 Parasagittal infarction in neonatal asphyxia. Ann Neurol 21:202–204.

Pasternak J F, Gorey M T 1998 The syndrome of acute near total intrauterine asphyxia in the term neonate. Pediatr Neurol 18:391–398.

Pasternak J F, Predley T A, Mikhael M A 1991 Neonatal asphyxia: vulnerability of basal ganglia, thalamus and brainstem. Pediatr Neurol 7:147–149.

Penrice J, Cady E B, Lorek A et al 1996 Proton magnetic resonance spectroscopy of the brain in normal preterm and term infants, and early changes after perinatal hypoxia-ischemia. Pediatr Res 40:6–14.

Peter B M 1996 Brain SPECT gets favourable review from neuroradiology panel. J Nuclear Med 37:14N.

Peterson B S, Anderson A W, Ehrenkranz R et al 2003 Regional brain volumes and their later neurodevelopmental correlates in term and preterm infants. Pediatrics 111:939–948.

Peterson B S, Vohr B, Staib L H et al 2000 Regional brain volume abnormalities and long-term cognitive outcome in preterm infants. JAMA 284 (15):1939–1947.

Pfefferbaum A, Mathalon D H, Sullivan E V et al 1994 A quantitative magnetic resonance imaging study of changes in brain morphology from infancy to late adulthood. Arch Neurol 51:874–887.

Pierpaoli C, Jezzard P, Basser P J et al 1996 Diffusion tensor MR imaging of the human brain. Radiology 201:637–648.

Poduslo S E, Jang Y 1984 Myelin development in infant brain. Neurochem Res 9:1615–162.

Pohl M, Zimmerhackl L B, Heinen F et al 1998 Bilateral renal vein thrombosis and venous sinus thrombosis in a neonate with factor V mutation (FV Leiden). J Pediatr 132:159–161.

Prastawa M, Gilmore J H, Lin W et al 2005 Automatic segmentation of MR images of the developing newborn brain. Med Image Anal 9:457–466.

Provencher S W 2001 Automatic quantitation of localized in vivo 1H spectra with LCModel. NMR Biomed 14(4):260–264.

Quencer R M 1992 Intracranial CSF flow in pediatric hydrocephalus: evaluation with cine-MR imaging. Am J Neuroradiol 13:601–608.

Rademaker K J, de Vries L, Barth P G 1993 Subependymal pseudocysts: ultrasound diagnosis and findings at follow-up. Acta Paediatr Scand 82:394–399.

Ramenghi L A, Domizio S, Quartulli et al 1993 Atypical site of congenital pseudocysts of germinal matrix. ESPR Annual Meeting, Edinburgh.

Ramenghi L A, Gill B J, Tanner S F et al 2002 Cerebral venous thrombosis, intraventricular haemorrhage and white matter lesions in a preterm newborn with factor V (Leiden) mutation. Neuropediatrics 33:97–99.

Ramenghi L A, Mosca F, Counsell S, Rutherford M 2005 Magnetic resonance imaging of the brain in preterm infants. In: Paolo Tortori Donati (eds) Pediatric neuroradiology. Springer, Berlin, pp. 199–234.

Ramenghi LA, Domizio S, Quartulli et al 1997 Prenatal pseudocysts of the germinal matrix in preterm infants. J Clin Ultrasound 25:169–173.

Rijn A M, Groenendaal F, Beek F J et al 2001 Parenchymal brain injury in the preterm infant: comparison of cranial ultrasound, MRI and neurodevelopmental outcome. Neuropediatrics 32:80–89.

Ringelberg J, van de Bor M 1993 Outcome of transient echodensities in preterm infants. Neuropediatrics 24:269–273.

Rivkin M J, Anderson M L, Kaye E M 1992 Neonatal idiopathic cerebral venous thrombosis: an unrecognised cause of transient seizures or lethargy. Annals Neurol 32:51–56.

Robertson N J, Cowan F M, Cox I J et al 2002 Brain alkaline intracellular pH after neonatal encephalopathy. Ann Neurol 52:732–742.

Robertson N J, Lewis R H, Cowan F M et al 2001 Early increases in brain myo-inositol measured by proton magnetic resonance spectroscopy in term infants with neonatal encephalopathy. Pediatr Res 50 (6):692–700.

Roelants-Van Rijn A M, van Der Grond J, de Vries L S et al 2001 Value of (1)H-MRS using different echo times in neonates with cerebral hypoxia-ischemia. Pediatr Res 49:356–362.

Roland E H, Hill A 1997 Intraventricular haemorrhage and posthaemorrhagic hydrocephalus. Current and potential interventions. Clin Perinat 24:589–605.

Roland E H, Poskitt K, Rodriguez E et al 1998 Perinatal hypoxic-ischemic thalamic injury: clinical features and neuroimaging. Ann Neurol 44:161–166.

Rumack C, Johnson M 1984 Perinatal and infant brain imaging. Year Book Medical, Chicago.

Rutherford M 2002 MRI of the Neonatal Brain. WB Saunders,

Rutherford M A, Malamateniou C, Zeka J et al 2004 MR imaging of the neonatal brain at 3 Tesla. Eur J Paediatr Neurol 8:281–289.

Rutherford M A, Pennock J M, Dubowitz L M S 1994 Cranial ultrasound and magnetic resonance imaging in hypoxic-ischaemic encephalopathy: a comparison with outcome. Dev Med Child Neurol 36:813–825.

Rutherford M A, Ward P, Allsop J et al 2005a Magnetic resonance imaging in neonatal encephalopathy. Early Hum Dev 81:13–25.

Rutherford M A, Ward P, Malamateniou C 2005b Magnetic resonance imaging in neonatal encephalopathy. Semin Fetal Neonatal Med 10:445–460.

Seghier M L, Lazeyras F, P S Hüppi 2006 Functional MRI of the newborn. Semin Fetal Neonatal Med 11:479–488.

Seghier M L, Lazeyras F, Zimine S et al 2004 Combination of event-related fMRI and diffusion tensor imaging in an infant with perinatal stroke. Neuroimage 21:463–472.

Seghier M L, Lazeyras F, Zimine S et al 2005 Visual recovery after perinatal stroke evidenced by functional and diffusion MRI: case report. BMC Neurol 5:17.

Shankaran S, Slovis T L, Bedard M P, Poland R L 1982 Sonographic classification of intracranial hemorrhage: a prognostic indicator of mortality, morbidity and short-term neurologic outcome. J Pediatr 100:469–475.

Shevell M I, Ashwal S, Novonty E 1999 Proton magnetic resonance spectroscopy: clinical applications in children with nervous system diseases. Semin Pediatr Neurol 6:68–77.

Shrimpton P C, Wall B F 1995 The increasing importance of X-ray computed tomography as a source of medical exposure. Rad Protect Dosim 57:413–415.

Shulkin B L 1997 PET applications in pediatrics. Q J Nuc Med 41:281–291.

Siegel M J 1995 In: Siegel C M J (ed) Pediatric sonography brain, 2nd edn. Raven, New York, pp. 29–101.

Skranes J S, Vik T, Nilsen G et al 1993 Cerebral magnetic resonance imaging (MRI) and mental and motor function of very low birth weight infants at one year of corrected age. Neuropediatrics 24:256–262.

Soul J S, Robertson R L, Tzika A A et al 2001 Time course of changes in diffusion-weighted magnetic resonance imaging in a case of neonatal encephalopathy with defined onset and duration of hypoxic-ischemic insult. Pediatrics 108:1211–1214.

Strange K, Emma F, Paredes A et al 1994 Osmoregulatory changes in myo-inositol content and Na+/myo-inositol cotransport in rat cortical astrocytes. Glia 12:35–43.

Takashima S, Mito T, Ando Y 1986 Pathogenesis of periventricular white matter hemorrhages in preterm infants. Brain Dev 8:25–30.

Takashima S, Tanaka K 1978 Subcortical leukomalacia, relationship to development of the central sulcus, and its vascular supply. Arch Neurol 35:470–476.

Tanner S F, Ramenghi L A, Ridgeway J P et al 2000 Quantitative comparison of the intra-brain diffusion in adults versus pre-term and term neonates and infants. Am J Radiol 174(6):16643–16649.

Taylor G A 1998 Recent advances in neonatal cranial ultrasound and Doppler techniques. Clin Perinatol 24:677–689.

Taylor G A, Soul J S, Dunning P S 1998 Sonographic ventriculography: a new potential use for sonographic contrast agents in neonatal hydrocephalus. Am J Neuroradiol 19:1931–1934.

Taylor H G, Minich N, Bangert B et al 2004 Long-term neuropsychological outcomes of very low birth weight: associations with early risks for periventricular brain insults. J Int Neuropsychol Soc 10(7):987–1004.

Teele R, Hernanz-Schulman M, Sotrel A 1988 Echogenic vasculature in the basal ganglia of neonates: a sonographic sign of vasculopathy. Radiology 169:423–427.

Teele R, Share J 1991 Ultrasonography of infants and children. WB Saunders, Philadelphia, PA.

Trounce J Q, Fagan D, Levene M I 1986b Intraventricular haemorrhage and periventricular leukomalacia: ultrasound and autopsy correlation. Arch Dis Child 61:1203–1207.

Trounce J Q, Rutter N, Levene M I 1986a Periventricular leukomalacia and intraventricular haemorrhage in the preterm neonate. Arch Dis Child 61:1196–1202.

Tuor U I, Kozlowski P, Del Bigio M R et al 1998 Diffusion and T2-weighted increases in magnetic resonance images of immature brain during hypoxia-ischemia: transient reversal posthypoxia. Exp Neurol 150:321–328.

Van der Knapp M S, Valk J, de Neeling N, Nauta J J P 1991 Pattern recognition in MRI of white matter disorders in children and young adults. Neuroradiology 33:478–493.

Vannier M W, Hildebolt C F, Marsh et al 1989. Craniosynostosis: diagnostic value of three-dimensional CT reconstruction. Radiology 173:669–673.

Volpe J J 1997 Brain injury in the premature infant. Neuropathology, clinical aspects, pathogenesis, and prevention. Clin Perinatol 24:567–587.

Volpe J J 2001 Neurology of the newborn, 2nd edn. Saunders, Philadelphia.

Warfield S K, Kaus M, Jolesz F A et al 2002 Adaptive, template moderated spatially varying statistical classification. Med Image Anal 4:43–55.

Watts R, Liston C, Niogi S et al 2003 Fiber tracking using magnetic resonance diffusion tensor imaging and its applications to human brain development. Ment Retard Dev Disabil Res Rev 9:168–177.

Widjaja E, Shroff M Blaser S et al 2006 2D time-of-flight MR venography in neonates: anatomy and pitfalls. AJNR Am J Neuroradiol 27:1913–1918.

Wimberger D M, Roberts T P, Barkovich A J et al 1995 Identification of 'premyelination' by diffusion-weighted MRI. J Comput Assist Tomogr 19:28–33.

Wu YW, March M, Croen LA et al 2004 Perinatal stroke in children with motor impairment: a population based study. Pediatrics 114:612–619.

Zacharia A, Zimine S, Lovbladv K O et al 2006 Early assessment of brain maturation by MR imaging segmentation in neonates and premature infants. Am J Neuroradiol 27:972–977.

Zarifi M K, Astrakas L G, Poussaint T Y et al 2002 Prediction of adverse outcome with cerebral lactate level and apparent diffusion coefficient in infants with perinatal asphyxia. Radiology 225:859–870.

Zinnermann R A, Wang Z J 1997 The value of proton MR spectroscopy in pediatric metabolic brain disease. Am J Neuroradiol 18:1872–1879.

Zuerrer M, Martin E, Boltshauser E 1991 MR imaging of intracranial haemorrhage in neonates and infants at 2.35 Tesla. Neuroradiology 33:223–229.

Functional assessment of the fetal CNS

Jan G. Nijhuis

Key Points

- Fetal behavior is an expression of the activity of the fetal CNS
- The development of fetal behavior is a continuum from conception into neonatal life
- Quality of behavioral variables is more important than quantity
- For fetal assessment near term, fetal behavioral states should be taken into account
- Only a beginning is made with the functional assessment of the fetal CNS

INTRODUCTION

Both in obstetrics and pediatrics there is growing interest in the assessment of the integrity and activity of the fetal central nervous system. As it is not yet possible to test the fetal nervous system directly, a lot of attention has been focused on fetal behavior as a measure for the neurological maturation. Fetal behavior can be studied by investigating fetal heart rate (patterns) and ultrasonic observations of fetal gross body movements and eye movements, or combinations of the above variables.

Recent studies have shown that the use of valid reference ranges appropriate for the gestation duration (Nijhuis et al 1998b, ten Hof et al 2002) and an objective analysis with strict application of techniques (Nijhuis et al 1999b, ten Hof et al 1999) are prerequisites for studying fetal behavior. Without them, comparisons with former or future measurements or between groups of patients and studies cannot be made.

In this chapter we will review the most important data on fetal behavioral states and on isolated fetal behavioral variables such as fetal body, eye, breathing and mouth movements and fetal heart rate (patterns). This will be followed by a description of fetal behavior in twins and a summary indicating the consequences of the concept of fetal behavior in clinical practice.

FETAL BODY MOVEMENTS

Fetal body movements yield important information on the condition of the fetus. Ever since the introduction of ultrasound, researchers have focused on both the quantitative and qualitative aspects of fetal movements. Most types of movement patterns emerge between 7 and 15 weeks gestation. From then onwards 15 distinct patterns can be distinguished (Table 7.1). These movements, once observed, remain present during the course of pregnancy and their appearance hardly changes (de Vries et al 1982).

Comparison of the quantitative parameters of movement between different studies is hampered by the various fetal movement definitions used and by methodological differences. One aspect which makes it difficult to compare results of different studies is the use of different procedures to smooth the data by inclusion of a certain time interval between single movements that compose a burst of movement. This effect is enhanced early in gestation due to the larger number of movements separated by short intervals while episodes of fetal quiescence develop gradually, especially after 30 weeks gestation. These different smoothing procedures explain a large part of the discrepancy in results between different studies (ten Hof et al 1999). The percentage incidence and the number of movements decrease curvilinearly from 24 weeks of gestation. This overall decline in movement incidence appears to be a developmental phenomenon, rather than just the result of the emergence of rest–activity cycles with progressively increasing episodes of fetal quiescence. During episodes of quiescence the fetus moves less than during active periods. But towards term, movements gradually disappear almost completely during these quiet episodes.

Up till now, the quality of movements might be a better indicator of the integrity of the fetal nervous system. Normal quality of general movements is defined, for both the pre- and postnatal periods, as spontaneous, gross movements involving the whole body, lasting from a few seconds to a few minutes, with a variable sequence of arm, trunk, head and leg movements, a waxing and waning in intensity, force and speed, and a gradual onset and end (Prechtl & Einspieler 1997).

ABNORMAL FETAL BODY MOVEMENTS

A delay of the appearance of fetal movement patterns with 1 to 2 weeks has been found in generally well-controlled women with type-1 diabetes mellitus (Mulder et al 1991). Abnormal movement patterns, however, have been found in fetuses with several abnormalities, e.g. chromosomal anomalies, anencephaly and growth retardation (Bekedam et al 1985). The abnormal movement patterns are indicative of altered brain and/or muscular development and are most commonly due to changes in the quality of the movements (e.g. abrupt, forceful movements or slow, monotonous movements). In some fetuses this coincides with a change in the quantity of the movements, mostly a decrease (Visser et al

Table 7.1 First appearance of several fetal movement patterns in postmenstrual weeks in both singleton and twin gestations

Fetal movement pattern	Singletons	Twins[‡]
Fetal heart activity*	5.5–6.5	
Just-discernible movement	7.5–8.5	
Startle	8.0–9.5	8.0–10.5
General movement	8.5–9.5	
Hiccup	8.5–10.5	8.0–11.0
Breathing movement	10.5–11.5	9.0–14.5
Hand/face contact	10.0–12.5	8.5–11.0
Jaw opening	10.5–12.5	8.0–12.0
Stretch	10.5–15.5	11.5–15.5
Yawn	11.5–15.5	11.5–15.5
Sucking and swallowing	12.5–14.5	10.0–13.5
Eye movements**	– slow	16.0
	– rapid	23.0
Movements patterns only in twins[‡]		
Touch without reaction		9.5–13.0
First reaction		10.0–13.5
Slow body contact		9.0–16.0
Fast body contact		11.0–15.0
Complex contact: 'embrace'		12.0–16.0
Complex mouth contact: 'kiss'		

Adapted from De Vries et al 1982, *Van Heeswijk et al 1990, **Birnholz 1981, and [‡]Arabin et al 1998).

1992). Absent fetal movements have been found in fetuses with the fetal akinesia deformation sequence. Unfortunately, it is still not feasible to use quality of movements in a single case as an instrument for clinical decision-making.

INTRAFETAL CONSISTENCY IN FETAL BODY MOVEMENTS

The intrafetal consistency for body movements is low and is probably a feature of the normal development of movements. This high inter- and intrafetal variation makes the sole measurement of fetal movements therefore an inappropriate tool to assess fetal condition. Nevertheless, a percentage incidence of movements below the lower range of normality (2.5–4.0% after 30 weeks) would warrant further investigations (ten Hof et al 2002).

FETAL HEART RATE

Antenatal fetal heart rate (FHR) monitoring is widely used to assess the fetal condition. Normal basal FHR is around 70–80 beats per minute (bpm) at 7–8 weeks gestation, has a peak of around 180 bpm at 10 weeks gestation and decreases thereafter (van Heeswijk et al 1990). Before 20 weeks gestation the normal FHR pattern sometimes resembles the 'terminal' patterns as found during late gestation before fetal uterine death. In general, good bandwidth or beat-to-beat variability and accelerations are indicative for a good fetal condition and a silent pattern (small bandwidth, no accelerations) is indicative for fetal distress, certainly in the presence of severe variable or late decelerations. During gestation, FHR-variability and the amount of accelerations increase. FHR decelerations regularly occur before 28 weeks gestation, but rapidly decrease thereafter.

An objective analysis of FHR and FHR-variability can be obtained by using a computer (e.g. Sonicaid System) (Dawes et al 1994). The numerical FHR analysis is preferred over visual analysis which is associated with considerable inter- and intraobserver variation.

Nomograms for basal FHR and its long-term (LTV) and short-term (STV) variation show that, with increasing gestational age, basal FHR decreases linearly and FHR-variability increases curvilinearly (Nijhuis et al 1998b, Ribbert et al 1991) (Fig. 7.1). The lower limit (P2.5) of the normal range of FHR-variability increases till 30 weeks of gestation and stabilizes thereafter, despite an overall increase in FHR-variability and a widening of the normal range (Nijhuis et al 1998b).

Besides gestation, many other conditions influence FHR and FHR-variability, such as fetal and maternal diseases, medication, fetal diurnal rhythm, cardiac abnormalities and fetal hypoxia (for an overview see Martin, 1978, van Geijn, 1996). Also fetal behavioral states and fetal movements like regular mouth movements and sucking can influence FHR and FHR-variation considerably, as explained below (van Woerden & van Geijn 1992). Moreover, differences in FHR-variation can be explained by about 50% by differences in heart rate (Nijhuis et al 1999a), with FHR and FHR-variation having a negative relationship.

FHR-variation has a diurnal rhythm with lowest values in the early morning and highest values around midnight (Visser et al 1982). So, the time of recording also influences the heart rate parameters. During the day, FHR decreases by 0.45 bpm every hour and LTV and STV increase by about 0.8 and 0.1 millisecond/hour, respectively (Nijhuis et al 1998a). The diurnal variation might – to a great extent – be explained by differences in the occurrence of the distinct FHR patterns and fetal behavioral states during the day (Nijhuis et al 1998a).

Reference ranges based on 1 hour recordings and those based on shorter recordings show considerable differences, with the reference ranges being lower when based on recordings of a shorter duration. The validity of normal ranges based on recordings of varying or shorter durations should therefore be reviewed (Dawes et al 1994, Nijhuis et al 1998b). Furthermore, investigation has shown that, near term, normal baseline FHR varies between 110 and 150 bpm (Nijhuis et al 1998b, Rooth et al 1987), and not between 120 and 160 bpm, as reported by others.

INTRAFETAL CONSISTENCY IN FHR

Intrafetal differences in FHR are less than interfetal differences. The FHR of the individual fetus is on average 19–55% of the total variability between fetuses (Nijhuis et al 1998b)

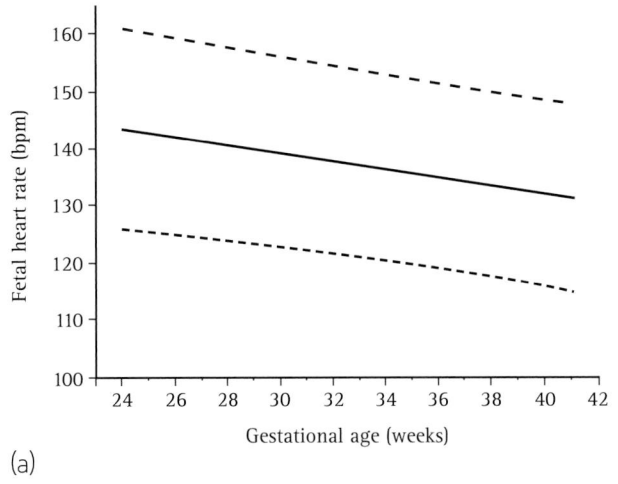

(a)

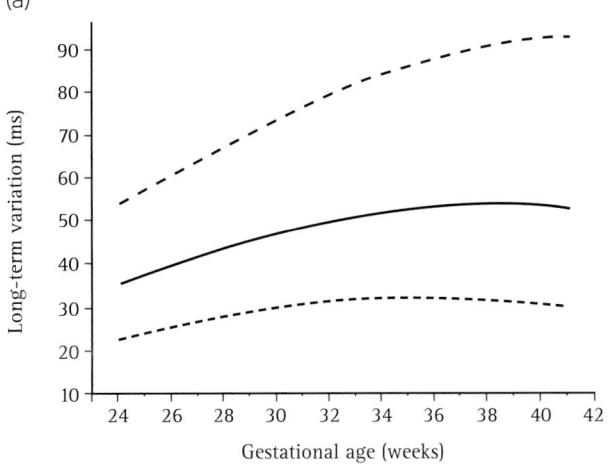

(b)

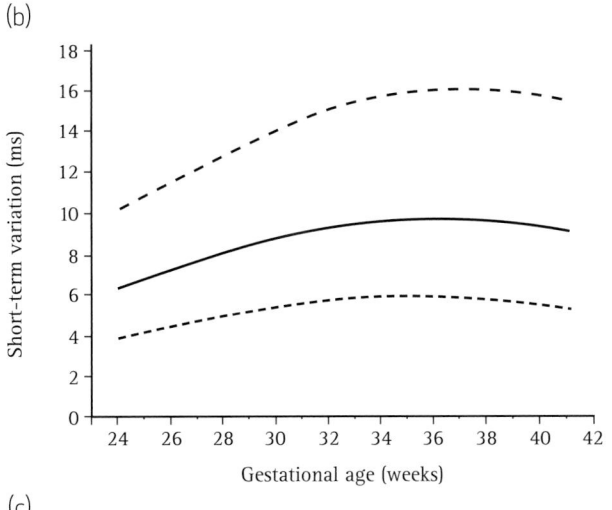

(c)

Figure 7.1 Normal ranges of (a) fetal heart rate (FHR), (b) long-term FHR variation and (c) short-term FHR variation with gestational age. Given are the p50 (solid line), the p2.5 and p97.5 (dashed lines). (From Nijhuis et al 1998.)

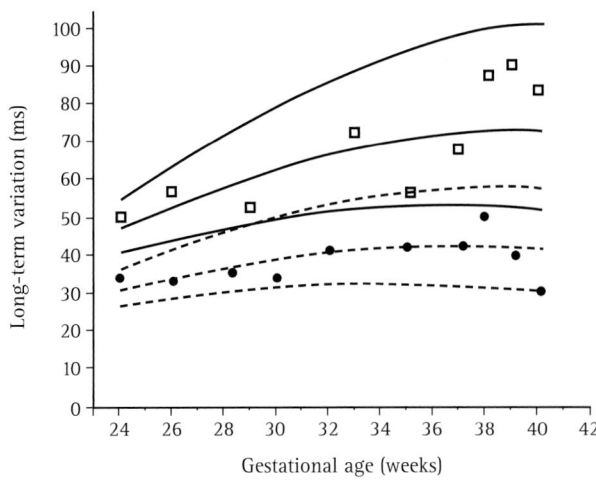

Figure 7.2 Intrafetal consistency in long-term FHR variation (LTV) as shown for two fetuses by their regression lines and 90% confidence intervals, together with the original data points. In one fetus LTV was consistently high (solid lines, squares), while the other fetus showed a consistently low variation (dashed lines, filled circles). (Reproduced from Nijhuis et al 1998, with permission from Partenon Publishing Ltd.)

using recordings of standardized duration and appropriate reference ranges (Nijhuis et al 1998b). A recording duration of 1 hour is preferred to avoid too much intrafetal variation induced by the developing sleep states. In addition, standardization for the time of the day may prevent variation induced by fetal diurnal rhythms (Nijhuis et al 1998b, Visser et al 1982).

FETAL HEART RATE IN GROWTH-RETARDED FETUSES

In intrauterine growth-restricted fetuses, LTV is about 25% less than in age-matched appropriately grown fetuses and gradually decreases with progressive compromise of the fetal condition. Correction for basal heart rate in growth-retarded fetuses does not result in a significant change in the number of recordings which are identified as having a FHR-variation below the normal range and will therefore not result in significant changes in the population identified as being at the highest risk. This correction is therefore not necessary (Nijhuis et al 1999a).

FETAL HEART RATE PATTERNS

In the course of pregnancy there is a progressive patterning of FHR into low and high variation during fetal rest and activity periods, respectively. When pregnancy progresses the amount of time spent in low variation gradually increases (Nijhuis et al 1984a). As a consequence, the existence of these rest–activity cycles has to be taken into account when interpreting the FHR tracing.

Using predefined criteria, FHR patterns (FHRP) can be classified as A, B, C or D, corresponding to different fetal

(Fig. 7.2). This intrafetal consistency is also present in growth-retarded fetuses with a low FHR-variation (Nijhuis et al 1999a).

For monitoring of trends and/or the detection of small changes, each fetus should therefore be its own control

Gedragstoestand criteria	Gedragstoestand 1F	Gedragstoestand 2F	Gedragstoestand 3F	Gedragstoestand 4F
Lichaamsbewegingen	incidenteel	regelmatig	afwezig	voortdurend
Oogbewegingen	afwezig	aanwezig	aanwezig	aanwezig
Hartfrequentiepatroon	A	B	C	D

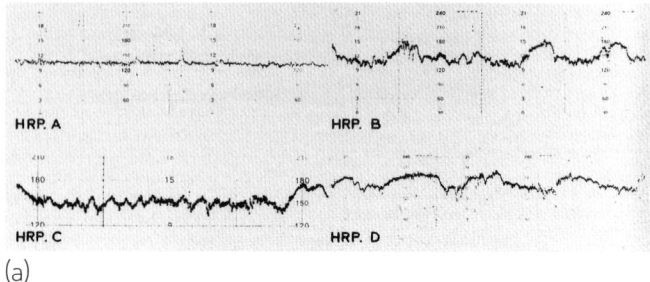

(a)

State criteria	State 1F	State 2F	State 3F	State 4F
Body movements	Incidental	Periodic	Absent	Continuous
Eye movements	Absent	Present	Present	Present
Heart rate pattern	A	B	C	D

(b)

Figure 7.3 Criteria for fetal behavioral states, with examples of the four distinct fetal heart rate patterns (HRP A–D). (Reproduced from van Vliet et al 1985b, with permission from Elsevier Science.)

Table 7.2 Differential diagnosis and proposed management in case of a silent fetal heart rate pattern (A) or a sinusoidal fetal heart rate pattern (B)

A. The silent fetal heart rate pattern

Differential diagnosis	Management
State 1F/FHRP A	Extension of the recording time
Effect of medication	Exclusion of use of medication
Tachycardia	Inspection of the baseline
Anomalies	Ultrasonographic examination
	Behavioral study
Hypoxia	Contraction stress test (CST)
Brain death	Cordocentesis
Very premature fetus	Verification of gestational age

B. The sinusoidal fetal heart rate pattern

Differential diagnosis	Management
Fetal mouth movements:	
— sucking ('major' or 'marked')	Behavioral study
— regular mouthing ('minor')	Behavioral study
Effect of medication	Exclusion of use of medication
Congenital anomalies	Ultrasonographic examination
Fetal asphyxia	Biophysical profile testing
Fetal anemia	Cordocentesis

rest–activity states, the fetal behavioral states 1F to 4F (Fig. 7.3) (Nijhuis et al 1982). These behavioral states develop during pregnancy and are generally well developed at about 36 weeks postmenstrual age. FHRP A–D are defined as follows: FHRP A is a stable heart rate, with a narrow oscillation bandwidth. Isolated accelerations occur which are strictly related to body movements. FHRP B has a wider oscillation bandwidth with frequent accelerations during movements. FHRP C is stable with a wider oscillation bandwidth than pattern A and there are no accelerations. FHRP D is unstable, with large and long-lasting accelerations, which are frequently fused into a sustained tachycardia: 'the jogging fetus'. This pattern D might easily be misinterpreted as a 'tachycardia with decelerations' if the observer is not alert to the presence of the motor activity and its effect on the FHR (Tas & Nijhuis 1992).

During gestation, normal basal FHR decreases both in FHRP A and B. FHR-variation increases during FHRP B and decreases slightly during FHRP A near term. FHRP A is therefore 'flatter' near term than at earlier gestation, with FHR-variability being below the normal range of overall FHR-variation in 50% of cases (Nijhuis et al 1998a). This may falsely suggest the presence of hypoxemia or acidemia, but in fact reflects a mature fetus with fully developed behavioral states in which state 1F (and FHRP A) is seldom interrupted by fetal movements and FHR accelerations (Table 7.2A). For an adequate assessment of the fetal condition it is therefore important to include B patterns in the analysis.

FETAL BREATHING MOVEMENTS AND HICCUPS

Both fetal breathing movements and fetal hiccups can be observed from 8–10 weeks gestation onwards (Table 7.1) (de Vries et al 1982). Breathing movements, defined as a paradoxical inward movement of the chest wall with outward movement of the abdominal wall, are considered a normal feature of fetal life and are necessary for the development of the fetal lungs. However, breathing movements are episodic in nature, subjected to diurnal and ultradian rhythms and influenced by a number of internal and external factors. They are therefore highly variable within and between individual fetuses, even under normal physiological conditions (Kisilevsky & Low 1998). For example, the postprandial increase in breathing movements, which can be found from 20–22 weeks onward, causes much variance. This high inter- and intra-individual variability makes the use of fetal breathing, as an indicator of fetal health or compromise, of little clinical value. Due to their episodic character, breathing movements can also not be used as a state variable in the fetus.

Fetal hiccups are short and powerful contractions of the diaphragm which can easily be differentiated from breathing movements. In the first trimester, periods with hiccups can be observed very regularly, while in the third trimester only 2–4 episodes with hiccups per 24 hour will be noticed.

FETAL EYE MOVEMENTS

Fetal eye movements (EM) can be observed from 16–18 weeks gestation onwards (Birnholz 1981, Bots et al 1981). Overall frequency of EM increases up to 30–33 weeks, after which frequency remains constant up to term. From about 30 weeks onwards, consolidation into long-term clusters of EM occurs. Episodes with and without (mainly rapid) EM become closely linked with the other two state variables at about 36 weeks gestation and then represent behavioral states (Nijhuis et al 1982).

ABNORMAL FETAL EYE MOVEMENTS

The frequency of EM is significantly lower in hydrocephalic fetuses than in normal fetuses, while growth-retarded fetuses show less rapid EM (Arduini et al 1988). In fetuses with dysmorphic brain structure no EM or EM of a different nature can be found (Birnholz 1981). Fetuses in breech and cephalic presentations show no difference in the EM incidence, although differences in EM directions are found (Takashima et al 1995).

FETAL MOUTH MOVEMENTS

The fetal mouth is easy to visualize using ultrasound; sucking and swallowing can be observed from 12 weeks gestation onward (Table 7.1). Recurrent clusters of 'regular mouthing movements' can be observed during the quiet state 1F, while during state 3F 'sucking movements' can be observed (for an overview, see van Woerden & van Geijn 1992). Both regular mouthing and sucking may result in 'sinusoidal-like' FHRP which may be confused with underlying pathology like severe fetal anemia (Table 7.2B) (Nijhuis et al 1984b, van Woerden et al 1988).

The fetus also swallows the amniotic fluid, and a normal amount of amniotic fluid is the resultant between fetal swallowing and fetal micturition.

FETAL BEHAVIORAL STATES

Fetal behavioral states are identified by the coincidence of specific combinations of FHRP A through D with presence or absence of body and eye movements (Fig. 7.4) (Nijhuis et al 1982). Simultaneous occurrence of specific combinations of the three parameters is classified as 'periods of coincidence 1F–4F'. If none of the specified combinations can be applied this is defined as 'no coincidence'. Fetal behavioral states are fully developed when the parameters of the three state variables show close linkage or association for prolonged periods of time and change in concert (i.e. within 3 minutes) during transitions between behavioral states. Fetal behavioral state profiles can be drawn up for each recording, indicating the on and off time of each variable and the (no-)coincidence of the three variables (Fig. 7.4). Fetal states develop during pregnancy and are almost always present from around 36 weeks gestation onwards

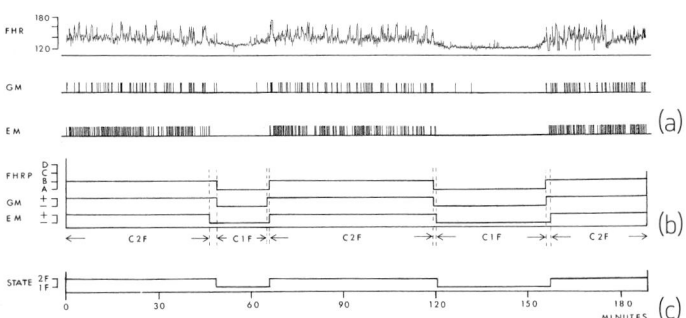

Figure 7.4 Fetal behavioral state profile of a 3-hour recording of a healthy fetus at 38 weeks gestation. It shows from above downwards: (a) the fetal heart rate (FHR) tracing, and the presence or absence of body (GM) and eye (EM) movements, (b) the on and off time of the three variables and the periods of (no-)coincidence and (c) the presence of behavioral states 1F and 2F. (Reproduced with permission form Mulder et al 1993, from S. Karger AG, Basel.)

(Nijhuis et al 1982). The development of states is generally similar in fetuses of nulli- and multiparous women, although states appear at a somewhat later gestational age in the fetuses of nulliparae (van Vliet et al 1985b). The frequency of the occurrence of state 3F and 4F has been found to be relatively low, with the incidence of 3F being so low that Pillai and James argued its very existence (Pillai & James 1990). The duration of state 1F and absence of fetal movements can be as long as 45 minutes in the near-term fetus. This emphasizes again that the fetal age should be taken into account: what is abnormal in a fetus at 20 weeks may be normal in the same fetus at 38 weeks!

Variables like fetal breathing movements, fetal micturition, and mouthing movements are called state concomitants, because they have been found to occur more frequently and/or more regularly during one specific state (Nijhuis, 1986). In the fetus, breathing episodes during fetal behavioral state 1F tend to have a much more regular rhythm than during 2F, while the breathing activity is generally higher during 2F than during 1F. This is in contrast to the continuously breathing neonate, where regular breathing is a state criterion for state 1 and irregular breathing for state 2.

Also fetal blood flow in various vessels is influenced by the different behavioral states and (Doppler) measurements in these vessels should therefore be 'standardized for states' (van Eyck & Wladimiroff 1992).

The specific sequence of change of state variables during transitions is also used to define the neurological maturation of the fetus (Groome et al 1996, Nijhuis et al 1998a). In normal-term fetuses, FHRP is the first variable to change during 1F to 2F transitions and the last variable during 2F to 1F transitions.

Periods of no-coincidence bounded on both sides by the same behavioral state or by different behavioral states have been called insertions and transitions, respectively (Groome et al 1996, Nijhuis et al 1982).

In normal post-term fetuses (>41 weeks gestation), the development of the fetal central nervous system continues, resulting in an increasing percentage of 'fetal wakefulness,' i.e. an increasing percentage of states 3F and 4F (van de Pas et al 1994). The sequence of change of state variables during transitions in these post-term fetuses differs among the various studies. These equivocal results may be due to the generally small numbers of transitions analyzed among the studies and to methodological differences (Nijhuis et al 1999b).

Linkage of pairs of state variables and coincidence of the three parameters, higher than expected by chance, can already be found from around 28–30 weeks gestation before true states can be identified (Nijhuis et al 1982, 1999b, Nijhuis & van de Pas 1992, Pillai et al 1992).

ABNORMAL FETAL BEHAVIOR

Delayed behavioral state development has been found both in growth-retarded fetuses (e.g. Van Vliet et al 1985a) and in fetuses of insulin-dependent diabetic women (Mulder et al 1987). Abnormal state development has been found in a fetus with multiple congenital anomalies with normal FHR and in a case of prolonged rupture of membranes from 26–35 weeks gestation. Abnormal behavioral patterns of three fetuses did correlate with lesion sites in the central nervous system as found after birth (Koyanagi et al 1993).

Growth-retarded fetuses show longer transitional periods than healthy fetuses and a random order in which state variables change during transitions (Nijhuis et al 1999b).

Many drugs administered to the mother have effects on fetal behavior (for reviews see Groome & Watson 1992, Kisilevsky & Low 1998). But also other influences are of importance. Abnormal fetal state cycling has been found in fetuses of cocaine-addicted mothers, a fetus exposed to maternal alcohol abuse and, temporarily, in fetuses whose mothers drank two glasses of white wine (Mulder et al 1998). The fetus has been described to respond to touch, temperature, (maternal) sound, vibration, chemical stimuli and perhaps light from 24 weeks of gestation onwards or even earlier (Hepper & Shahidullah 1992).

Another important issue is the effect of corticosteroids. Mulder et al (2004) showed a clear effect of betamethasone on fetal behavior. This drug, which is used for the enhancement of fetal lung maturation, decreases heart rate variability and the number of movements. Dexamethasone, which is used for the same purpose, seems to increase especially short-term FHR variability (Mulder et al 1997). In fact, now it was behavioral studies who showed a drug-related effect, and more recently, lung maturation with repeated doses of betamethasone becomes clearly controversial (Visser et al 2001). Therefore stricter guidelines have been proposed (Visser & Anceschi 2001), and a randomized study is in progress. Recently, Koenen et al (2005) showed that fetal heart rate tracings, which were made in the mornings, are similar with and without corticosteroid treatment, because

the effect is more a disturbance of the daily rhythm than an overall reduction of fetal movements.

Also the influence of maternal emotions or stress on the fetus has gained interest in fetal behavioral research. Evidence has been supplied that maternal emotions do affect brain development and fetal behavior in utero (Ianniruberto & Tajani 1981, Lou et al 1994) and that they might form a risk factor for the development of psychological problems in childhood (Ward 1991). The mechanisms by which maternal emotions cause behavioral changes are still speculative and largely unexplained but might also be mediated by hormonal changes in cortisol or catecholamine levels (van den Bergh 1992).

TWINS

Multiple pregnancies allow us to analyze specific twin behavior, with passive and active interactions between the two fetuses. When studying twins it must always be noted that the two fetuses are reliably distinguished.

From early gestation onward several distinct movement patterns are demonstrated (Table 7.1). Complex movements, lasting more than 5 seconds, emerge somewhat later in pregnancy (Arabin et al 1998). Investigations whether these contacts are preferably initiated by one of the multiplets or whether there are differences in the frequency and sensitivity in reaction towards touch have, up to now, not revealed a 'dominant' twin (Sherer et al 1990). Furthermore, studies could not show differences in the frequency and sensitivity in reaction towards touch between the two twin fetuses and thus no 'dominant' position was found. Monochorionic twins are described to have earlier and more numerous contacts and greater coincidence of behavior. Yet it seems impossible to define zygoticity by studying fetal heart rate and fetal behavior in twin pregnancies.

The inter-twin contacts have been supposed to cause increased simultaneous activities. So far, conflicting results have been described. In one study, FHR-accelerations are more often associated within the members of a twin pair (57%) than statistically expected (Sherer et al 1990), while in another study FHR-accelerations are simultaneous in just 36%. However, in this last study, synchronous behavioral patterns are exhibited 94.7% of time (Gallagher et al 1992). A third study, assessing fetal movements by ultrasound, demonstrates simultaneous fetal movements in only 26% of time (Zimmer et al 1988).

At advanced gestation, most investigators use the fetal actocardiograph to simultaneously monitor FHR and fetal movements in twins. Without, it is quite difficult to investigate these two parameters simultaneously in two fetuses, needing two separate cardiotocographs and two ultrasound transducers. Yet, the use of the actocardiograph might give less reliable results (De Wit & Nijhuis 2003).

Inter-twin differences are also of importance when studying (early) growth differences and twins discordant for fetal anomalies (e.g. Arabin et al 1996, Kurauchi et al 1995).

FETAL NEUROLOGY

In this chapter we have focused on fetal behavior, because fetal behavior reflects the activity of the fetal CNS. More direct insight in the fetal CNS and the development of an intra-uterine neurological investigation is an important goal in clinical perinatology (see also Nijhuis 2003).

A global assessment of the fetal condition might be made by using the biophysical profile, where 0 or 2 points are given to each of the five aspects: FHR accelerations, amount of amniotic fluid, fetal body, breathing movements and fetal tone (Manning et al 1980). However, the correlation of the biophysical profile with academia is much better than with hypoxemia, most likely because the latest three aspects only deteriorate late with worsening condition. Furthermore, a state 1F period in a perfectly healthy fetus would get a score of 2 (normal fluid), because the other criteria would be judged as 'abnormal'.

So far, direct assessment of the nervous system has been difficult. Fetuses with congenital anomalies may show bizarre behavior or dissociation of heart rate and movements (Tas & Nijhuis 1992). Other fetuses may show disrupted behavioral states or state transitions, or a delayed development of states (e.g. Mulder et al 1993, Nijhuis et al 1999b). Nevertheless, it is still difficult to draw conclusions from a single behavioral recording in a single fetus. Tas et al (1993) were able to evoke an intercostal-to-phrenic-inhibitory reflex (IPIR): compression of the ribcage results in an apnea. This seemed an interesting approach, but they were not able to find a different result in a group of growth-retarded fetuses.

Fetal habituation, i.e. the cessation of response to a repeated stimulus, is another test. Van Heteren et al showed that fetuses fail to respond after a number of vibrio-acoustic stimuli. And if such a test is repeated within 10 minutes, this number of stimuli is significantly lower. The fetus therefore seems to recognize the stimulus. This effect is also present if the test is performed after 24 hours, indicating that the fetus has a memory and is perhaps, capable of learning and memorizing (Heteren et al 2000a). This observation appeared to be state-independent (Heteren et al 2001) and in a fetus with an encephalocele, a response could not be evoked (Heteren et al 2000b). Others demonstrated (Hepper & Shahidulla 1992) that fetuses with Down syndrome take longer to habituate than normal fetuses.

It still remains difficult to perform a prenatal neurologic examination. It is quite likely that no single, isolated aspect of behavior alone will evolve to conduct a fetal neurologic investigation, but rather a combination of behavioral tests.

SUMMARY: CLINICAL RELEVANCE OF FETAL BEHAVIOR

It must be clear that insight into fetal behavior is crucial for the understanding of normal fetal wellbeing and in the evaluation of the possibly compromised fetus. It has introduced a completely different way of looking at the developing human being. However, it is very time-consuming to study fetal behavior as a routine screening method. Furthermore, although the patterns of development of fetal behavior exist for most healthy fetuses, there is a wide normal range which makes the identification of the compromised fetus very complex (Nijhuis et al 1999b). Therefore, it is difficult to differentiate between normal and impaired neurological maturation. These large normal ranges are mainly caused by considerable inter-individual differences, but the influence of factor(s) complicating pregnancy (maternal and fetal) and drug-induced effects also play a role in this. Much more investigation is therefore needed to unravel the (possible) effects of specific drugs on human fetal behavior.

When assessing the fetus it is essential to use appropriate reference ranges, to analyze objectively with strict application of techniques and, even more important, to be aware of the influence of fetal behavior (e.g. Table 7.2) and fetal behavioral patterns.

REFERENCES

Arabin B, Bos R, Rijlaarsdam R, Mohnhaupt A, Van Eyck J 1996 The onset of inter-human contacts: longitudinal ultrasound observations in early twin pregnancies. Ultrasound Obstet Gynecol 8:166–173.

Arabin B, Mohnhaupt A, Van Eyck J 1998 Intrauterine behavior of multiplets. In: Kurjak A, ed. Textbook of perinatal medicine, New York: Parthenon, pp. 1506–1531.

Arduini D, Rizzo G, Romanini C, Mancuso S 1988. Computerized analysis of behavioural states in asymmetrical growth retardedfetuses. J Perinat Med 16:357–363.

Bekedam D J, Visser G H A, de Vries J J, Prechtl H F R 1985 Motor behaviour in the growth retarded fetus. Early Hum Dev 12:155–165.

Birnholz J C 1981 The development of human fetal eye movement patterns. Science 213:679–681.

Bots R S G M, Nijhuis J G, Martin C B, Jr, Prechtl H F R 1981 Human fetal eye movements: detection in utero by ultrasonography. Early Hum Dev 5:87–94.

Dawes G S, Meir Y J, Mandruzzato G P 1994 Computerized evaluation of fetal heart-rate patterns. J Perinat Med 22:491–499.

de Vries J I P, Visser G H A, Prechtl H F R 1982 The emergence of fetal behaviour. I. Qualitative aspects. Early Hum Dev 7:301–322.

de Wit AC, Nijhuis JG 2003 Validity of the Hewlett-Packard actograph in detecting fetal movements. Ultrasound Obstet Gynecol 22(2):152–156.

Gallagher M W, Costigan K, Johnson T R 1992 Fetal heart rate accelerations, fetal movement, and fetal behavior patterns in twin gestations. Am J Obstet Gynecol 167:1140–1144.

Groome L J, Benanti J M, Bentz L S, Singh K P 1996 Morphology of active sleep–quiet sleep transitions in normal human term fetuses. J Perinat Med 24:171–176.

Groome L J, Watson J E 1992 Assessment of in utero neurobehavioral development. 1. Fetal behavioral states. J Matern-Fetal Invest 2: 183–194.

Hepper P G, Shahidullah S 1992 Habituation in normal and Down's syndrome fetuses. Q J Exp Psychol B 44:305–317.

Heteren C F van, Boekkooi P C, Jongsma H W, Nijhuis J G 2000a Fetal learning and memory. Lancet 356:1169–1170.

Heteren C F van, Boekkooi P C, Jongsma H W, Nijhuis J G 2000b Responses to vibroacoustic stimulation in a fetus with an encephalocele compared to responses of normal fetuses. J Perinat Med 28:306–308.

Heteren C F van, Boekkooi P F, Jongsma H W, Nijhuis J G 2001 Fetal habituation to vibroacoustic stimulation in relation to fetal states and fetal heart rate parameters. Early Hum Dev 61:135–145.

Ianniruberto A, Tajani E 1981 Ultrasonographic study of fetal movements. Semin Perinatol 5:175–181.

Kisilevsky B S, Low J A 1998 Human fetal behavior: 100 years of study. Dev Review 18:1–29

Koenen S V, Blom I, Visser G H A 2004 The effects of antenatal betamethasone administration on fetal heart rate and behaviour depend on gestational age. Early Hum Dev 76:65–77.

Koenen S V, Mulder E J H, Wijnberger L D, Visser G H A 2005 Transient loss of the diurnal rhythms of fetal movements, heart rate, and its variation after maternal betamethasone administration. Pediatr Res 57:662–666.

Koyanagi T, Horimoto N, Maeda H et al 1993 Abnormal behavioral patterns in the human fetus at term: correlation with lesion sites in the central nervous system after birth. J Child Neurol 8:19–26.

Kurauchi O, Ohno Y, Mizutani S, Tomoda Y 1995 Longitudinal monitoring of fetal behavior when one is anencephalic. Obstet Gynecol 86:672–674.

Lou H C, Hansen D, Nordentoft M et al 1994 Prenatal stressors of human life affect fetal brain development. Dev Med Child Neurol 36:826–832.

Manning F A, Platt L D, Sipos L 1980 Antepartum fetal evaluation: development of a fetal biophysical profile. Am J Obstet Gynecol 136:787–795.

Martin C B Jr 1978 Regulations of the fetal heart rate and genesis of FHR patterns. Semin Perinatol 2:131–146.

Mulder E J H 1993 Diabetes in pregnancy as a model for testing behavioural teratogenicity. Dev Brain Dysfunct 6:210–228.

Mulder E J H, Derks J B, Visser G H A 1997 Antenatal corticosteroid therapy and fetal behaviour: a randomised study of the effects of betamethasone and dexamethasone. Br J Obstet Gynecol 104:1239–1247.

Mulder E J H, Derks J B, Visser G H A 2004 Effects of antenatal betamethasone administration on fetal heart rate and behavior in twin pregnancy. Pediatr Res 56: 35–39.

Mulder E J H, Morssink L P, van der Schee T, Visser G H A 1998 Acute maternal alcohol consumption disrupts behavioral state organisation in the near-term fetus. Ped Resiatr 44:774–779.

Mulder E J H, Visser G H A, Bekedam D J, Prechtl H F R 1987 Emergence of behavioural states in fetuses of type-1 diabetic women. Early Hum Dev 15: 231–252.

Mulder E J H, Visser G H A, Morssink L P, de Vries J I P 1991 Growth and motor development in fetuses of women with type-1 diabetes. III. First trimester quantity of fetal movement patterns. Early Hum Dev 25:117–133.

Nijhuis I J M, ten Hof J, Mulder E J H et al 1998a Fetal heart rate (FHR) parameters during FHR patterns A and B: a longitudinal study from 24 weeks' gestation. Prenat Neonat Med 3:383–393.

Nijhuis I J M, ten Hof J, Mulder E J H et al 1998b Numerical fetal heart rate analysis: nomograms, minimal duration of recording and intrafetal consistency. Prenat Neonat Med 3:314–322.

Nijhuis I J M, ten Hof J, Mulder E J H et al 2000 Fetal heart rate in relation to its variation in normal and growth retarded fetuses. Eur J Obstet Gynecol Reprod Biol 89:27–33.

Nijhuis I J M, ten Hof J, Nijhuis J G et al 1999b Temporal organization of fetal behavior from 24 weeks gestation onwards in normal and complicated pregnancies. Dev Psychobiol 34:257–268.

Nijhuis J G 1986 Behavioral states: concomitants, clinical implications and the assessment of the condition of the nervous system. Eur J Obstet Gynecol Reprod Biol 21:301–308.

Nijhuis J G 2003 Fetal behavior. Neurobiol Aging 24: S41–S46.

Nijhuis J G, Martin C B, Jr, Prechtl H F R 1984a Behavioural states of the human fetus. In: Prechtl H F R (ed) Continuity of neural functions from prenatal to postnatal life, Vol 94. Clinics in Developmental Medicine. Spastics International Medical, London, pp. 65–79.

Nijhuis J G, Prechtl H F R, Martin C B Jr, Bots R S G M 1982 Are there behavioural states in the human fetus? Early Hum Dev 6:177–195.

Nijhuis J G, Staisch K J, Martin C B, Jr, Prechtl H F R 1984b A sinusoidal-like fetal heart-rate pattern in association with fetal sucking — report of 2 cases. Eur J Obstet Gynecol Reprod Biol 16:353–358.

Nijhuis J G, van de Pas M 1992 Behavioral states and their ontogeny: human studies. Semin Perinatol 16:206–210.

Pillai M, James D 1990 Behavioural states in normal mature human fetuses. Arch Dis Child 65:39–43.

Pillai M, James D K, Parker M 1992 The development of ultradian rhythms in the human fetus. Am J Obstet Gynecol 167:172–177.

Prechtl H F R, Einspieler C 1997 Is neurological assessment of the fetus possible? Eur J Obstet Gynecol Reprod Biol 75:81–84.

Ribbert L S M, Fidler V, Visser G H A 1991 Computer-assisted analysis of normal second trimester fetal heart rate patterns. J Perinat Med 19:53–59.

Rooth G, Huch A, Huch R 1987 Guidelines for the use of fetal monitoring. Int J Gynecol Obstet 25:159–167.

Sherer D M, Nawrocki M N, Peco N E et al 1990 The occurrence of simultaneous fetal heart rate accelerations in twins during nonstress testing [see comments]. Obstet Gynecol 76:817–821.

Takashima T, Koyanagi T, Horimoto N et al 1995 Breech presentation: is there a difference in eye movement patterns compared with cephalic presentation in the human fetus at term? Am J Obstet Gynecol 172:851–855.

Tas B A P J, Nijhuis J G 1992 Consequences for fetal monitoring. In: Nijhuis J G (ed) Fetal behaviour, developmental and perinatal aspects. Oxford University Press, Oxford, pp. 258–269.

Tas B A P J, Nijhuis J G, Nelen W, Willems E 1993 The intercostal-to-phrenic inhibitory reflex in normal and intra-uterine growth-retarded (IUGR) human fetuses from 26 to 40 weeks of gestation. Early Hum Dev 32:177–182.

ten Hof J, Nijhuis I J M, Mulder E J H et al 1999 Quantitative analysis of fetal generalised movements: methodological considerations. Early Hum Dev 56:57–73.

ten Hof J, Nijhuis I J M, Mulder E J H et al 2002 A longitudinal study of fetal body movements: nomograms, intrafetal consistency and relationship with the rest–activity cycle. Pediatr Res 52:568–575.

van de Pas M, Nijhuis J G, Jongsma H W 1994 Fetal behaviour in uncomplicated pregnancies after 41 weeks of gestation. Early Hum Dev 40:29–38.

van den Bergh B R H 1992 Maternal emotions during pregnancy and fetal and neonatal behaviour. In: Nijhuis J G (ed) Fetal behaviour. Developmental and perinatal aspects. Oxford University Press, Oxford, pp. 157–178.

van Eyck J, Wladimiroff J W 1992 Doppler flow measurements. In: Nijhuis J G (ed) Fetal behaviour. Developmental and perinatal aspects. Oxford University Press, Oxford, pp. 227–240.

van Geijn H P 1996 Developments in CTG analysis. Bailliere's Clin Obstet Gynaecol 10:185–209.

van Heeswijk M, Nijhuis J G, Hollanders H M 1990 Fetal heart rate in early pregnancy. Early Hum Dev 22:151–156.

van Vliet M A T, Martin C B Jr, Nijhuis J G, Prechtl H F R 1985a Behavioural states in growth-retarded human fetuses. Early Hum Dev 12:183–197.

van Vliet M A T, Martin C B, Jr, Nijhuis J G, Prechtl H F R 1985b Behavioural states in the fetuses of nulliparous women. Early Hum Dev 12:121–135.

van Woerden E E, van Geijn H P 1992 Heart-rate patterns and fetal movements. In: Nijhuis J G (ed) Fetal behaviour. Developmental and perinatal aspects. Oxford University Press, Oxford, pp. 41–56.

van Woerden E E, van Geijn H P, Caron F J, van der Valk A W, Swartjes J M 1988 Fetal mouth movements during behavioural states 1F and 2F. Eur J Obstet Gynecol Reprod Biol 29:97–105.

Visser G H A, Anceschi M M 2001 Guidelines on antepartum corticosteroids. Prenatal Neonatal Med 6(suppl 2):78–81.

Visser G H A, Csermely T, Cosmi E V 2001 Side-effects of prenatal corticosteroids. Prenatal Neonatal Med 6(suppl 2):42–49.

Visser G H A, Goodman J D S, Levine D H, Dawes G S 1982 Diurnal and other cyclic variations in human fetal heart rate near term. Am J Obstet Gynecol 142:535–544.

Visser G H A, Mulder E J H, Prechtl H F R 1992 Studies on developmental neurology in the human fetus. Dev Pharmacol Ther 18:175–183.

Ward A J 1991 Prenatal stress and childhood psychopathology. Child Psych Hum Dev 22:97–110.

Zimmer E Z, Goldstein I, Alglay S 1988 Simultaneous recording of fetal breathing movements and body movements in twin pregnancy. J Perinat Med 16:109–112.

CHAPTER

8

The development of senses

Birgit Arabin

Key Points

- Fetal sensitivity
- Fetal hearing
- Fetal olfaction and taste
- Fetal vision

INTRODUCTION

The development of senses is a multidimensional process incorporating sensory, affective and cognitive abilities. For a long time it was rather a philosophical than a scientific question how early such abilities are acquired. Aristotle anticipated the phenomenon, that the sensory development is a quiet process of the prenate gradually responding to the extrauterine world. In contrast to Hippocrates, who thought that the human soul starts to exist at conception, he combined the origin of the human soul with the completion of the development of fetal senses. However, negative thinking about prenatal sensory capabilities was more common: Rousseau referred to the fetus as a 'witless tadpole isolated from the agitation of the world'. Even the first scientific approaches by Preyer in 1885 led to doubtful conclusions about fetal sensory capacities (Preyer 1885).

The advent of ultrasound and fetal heart rate (FHR) monitoring has allowed non-invasive access to the unborn in the womb and to study the anatomical details of the organs involved in sensory functions and the fetal behavioral responses to internal or external stimuli.

In twin pregnancies, first reactions towards the co-twin were observed from around 10 weeks onward, reflecting sensory capacities of the skin (Arabin et al 1996). The forehead, nasal bridge, orbits, nose, ears, upper lips and anterior palate, the tongue with the oral cavity, the lower lip and mandible can be consistently identified from 12 weeks of gestation onwards by a series of transverse scans of the head. The more recent 3D-techniques help to prenatally visualize ears, nose and mouth at described locations in a sagittal, transverse and coronal plane and possibly to interpret facial expressions towards sensual experiences in the render mode (Kurjak et al 2005) (Fig. 8.1).

The unborn is involved in a perceptual world with increasing specification and differentiation. During the first trimester, self-generated movements are combined with somatosensory awareness resulting in co-ordination of early fetal movement (FM) patterns. Prechtl can be regarded as

the pioneer, integrating observations of endogenously evoked behavior into neonatal and prenatal surveillance, stressing the clinical importance and providing us with a tool appropriate to investigate developmental responses towards internal and external stimuli (Prechtl 1974). Sensory challenges may derive from two environments. The 'intrauterine world' includes the emotional state and daily rhythms of the mother, touch with the umbilical cord, the uterine wall and acoustic stimuli caused by maternal circulation, digestion, movements, breathing and, finally, her diet and her voice. As birth approaches, stimuli from the 'extrauterine world' are increasingly responded to. Neurological development allowing preparatory interaction involves a considerable number of genetic actions, which might be autoregulatory as well as activated or inhibited by positive or negative feedback mechanisms.

Reactive behavioral patterns towards touch, sound including maternal noise, vibration, light, taste and odor have been observed and may be integrated into a cohesive entity to describe developmental sensitivity. Behavioral responses may be mediated by physiological, pathologic, hormonal or metabolic processes. Although the fetal brain can organize and process stimulus information and encode in memory the activation of reflex responses, it is still difficult to define to what extent the 'memories' are conscious sensations that contribute to later sensory development.

It was postulated that from the second trimester onwards there is a trend towards more individualized behavior (Lecaneaut et al 1995). Early ultrasound studies have proven that the fetus reacts towards maternal negative and positive feelings such as stress and anxiety (Van den Bergh et al 1989, 2005) or even sexual intercourse (Chayen et al 1986).

Different disciplines have therefore become interested in the field of prenatal maturation of the sensual system such as embryology, genetics, neurophysiology, psychoanalysis and developmental psychology. Since pregnant mothers and most of the current methods used to detect immediate responses are in the hands of obstetricians, research and clinical investigations in perinatal medicine have been directed towards this field.

There are a large number of animal experiments evaluating the links between maternal and fetal sensory experience and the origin of fetal and neonatal senses and preferences, thus offering a source for hypotheses that can be applied to humans. The 'developmental origins of fetal senses' may have biological, medical and socioeconomic implications which we here like to summarize.

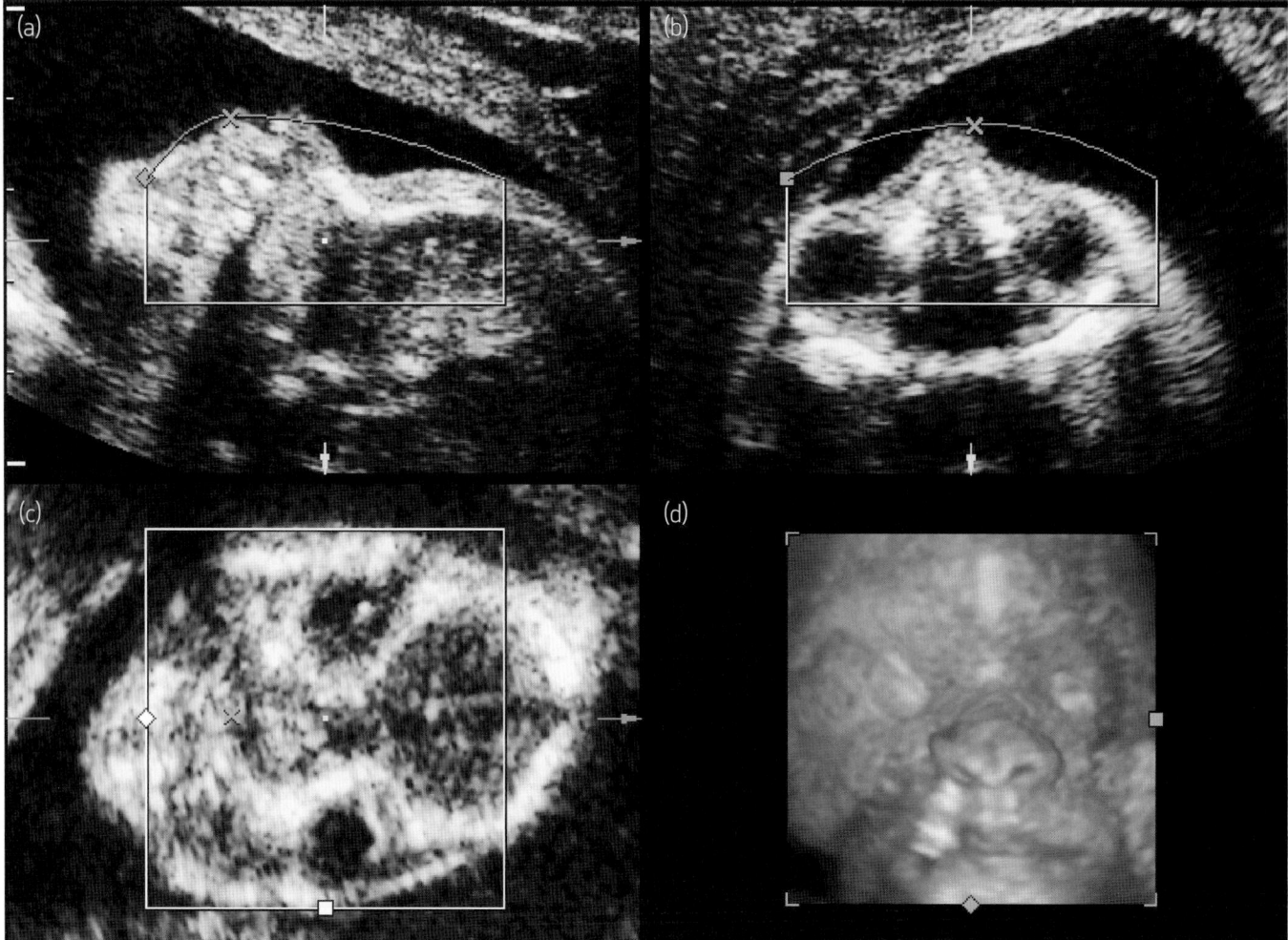

Figure 8.1 3D static planes through the fetal face with eyes, nose and lips in the sagittal view (a), axial view (b) and coronal view (c) and a rendered picture of the fetal face (d) (GE Expert 750).

SENSITIVITY AND EXPERIENCE OF PAIN

Sensitivity to touch is the cornerstone of human experience and communication. The first sensitivity to touch is based on the anatomic development and may manifest in a set of movements to protect the fetus and support neuromuscular development.

ANATOMY OF SENSITIVE RECEPTION

Cutaneous sensory receptors appear in the perioral area of the human fetus in the 7th week, spread to the face, hands and feet at around 11 weeks, to the trunk, arms and legs at around 15 weeks and to all cutaneous and mucous surfaces at around 20 weeks. The spread of cutaneous receptors is accompanied by the development of synapses between sensory fibers in the dorsal horn of the spinal cord, which first appear at around 6 weeks. Sensory nerves first grow into the spinal cord at 14 weeks' gestation. Development of the fetal neocortex begins at 8 weeks. Most sensory pathways to the neocortex have synapses in the thalamus.

Between 20 and 24 weeks, thalamocortical fibers establish synaptic connections with dendritic processes of neocortical neurons. After that time it is more likely that the fetus might not only react towards but also 'experience' touch and pain (Prechtl 1984).

In vivo measurements of glucose utilization have shown that maximal metabolic activity is located in sensory areas of the neonatal brain suggesting the functional maturity. The existence of neurotransmitters, endogenous opioids released pre- and perinatally in response to fetal stress and of stereospecific opiate receptors at spinal and supraspinal levels as well as the concomitant behavioral reactions have further increased our knowledge of sensory or painful sensation and offered implications for treatment (summary in Anand & Hickey 1987).

IMMEDIATE RESPONSIVENESS TO TOUCH

As supposed for motor activities, sensitivity to touch may develop before responding to biological or psychological relevant sensory input (Prechtl 1984). Hooker was the first to describe reactions towards cutaneous stimulation of embryos after therapeutic terminations of pregnancy by hysterotomy, maintaining them in an isotonic fluid bath (Hooker 1952).

With the introduction of real-time ultrasound, it became possible to observe early prenatal movements. The uterus and the amniotic fluid (AF) are the first environment that the human being confronts and interacts with. To study reactions of single fetuses towards touch in utero would pose ethical and practical restraints. However, during accidentally performed invasive procedures fetal reactions have been observed: Fetal blood sampling (cord needling) induced a significant decrease of pulsactility index (PI) values in all investigated vessels (umbilical artery, thoracic descending aorta, renal artery, middle cerebral artery) which was higher in the presence of a transplacental procedure than in a transamniotic procedure (Capponi et al 1996).

Similarly, a significant drop in both umbilical and MCA resistance index (RI) was found after cordocentesis with a greater drop in RI when the blood was sampled in early gestational age and transplacentally. The discussed mechanisms are probably due to changes in fetal endorphin due to 'a pain reaction' if the fetus was touched at all or to a central vasodilatator response or peripheral arterial vasoconstriction (Chitrit et al 1995, Hecher et al 1993, Teixeira et al 1996).

Furthermore, multiple pregnancies can serve as a natural research group where the members, usually twins or triplets, are exposed to cutaneous stimulations of the co-twin, enabling us to study the onset of reactions towards touch 'in vivo'.

The onset of reactions towards touch can ideally be investigated in monoamniotic multiples since first reactions towards touch are observed earlier than in monochorionic diamniotic multiples and again earlier than in dichorionic multiples (Fig. 8.2). As reported 'in vitro' for singleton aborted fetuses (Hooker 1952) we found 'in vivo' that monoamniotic multiples respond to tactile stimulation between 8 and 9 weeks (Arabin et al 1996). Early reactions towards touch in monoamniotic and monochorionic twin pregnan-

cies are more numerous compared to dichorionic pregnancies, probably because the membranes may prevent early reach and touch in utero (Arabin et al 1996). *The development of reactions towards cutaneous stimulations* of a co-twin in utero reveals different qualities. Up to 16 weeks we have analyzed several contact patterns, according to the speed of initiatives and reactions or part of the body involved (Arabin et al 1996). In advanced pregnancy, it is more difficult to differentiate fetal reactions to touch by conventional ultrasound methods. 4-D real-time ultrasound may facilitate observations in the future, but the technique is still limited in determining the speed of FM, including reactive movements. From early FHR/FM analysis of singletons and twins one can conclude that inter-twin reactions contribute to an increased number of simultaneous FHR accelerations produced by touch.

Gender differences have been reported for cognition, aggression and sociability in humans. Explanations have focused on neuroanatomic differences and exposure to steroid hormones. We have analyzed twin pairs with different gender combinations between 8 and 16 weeks: In the group of only male twins fast initiatives combined with fast reactions were significantly increased compared to only female or mixed twin pairs (Arabin et al 1996). It is suggested that differences of testosterone levels might have an impact on early prompt reactive behavior in utero as it was described postnatally.

Limitations in the interpretation of twin studies include difficulties in differentiating either reactions to touch from a parallel onset of endogenously evoked movements or passive from active reactions.

LONG-TIME RESPONSIVENESS AND FETAL PAIN

It was speculated that the tactile stimuli of multiples might *accelerate their development and improve their quality* during early follow-up examinations up to the age of 6 years where multiples scored better than singletons and that not only activity promotes growth and dendritic branching of individual neurons, but similarly, sensation from receptor cells might promote the development of the neural system.

Pain includes feeling, suffering and learning (memory). The increasing number of prenatal techniques and procedures in premature neonates has given rise to controversial discussions on how early and to what extent fetuses and neonates feel pain. This has even implications for professionals who provide abortions. At present, it has become appreciated that the fetus and newborn perceive and respond to pain (Anand & Hickey 1987).

Recently Anand has summarized his work and the different types of neonatal pain as follows (Anand et al 2006):

Pain in the newborn is a complex, multilayered phenomenon involving different sources of pain and different types of pain, which can involve various combinations of receptors and mechanisms within the

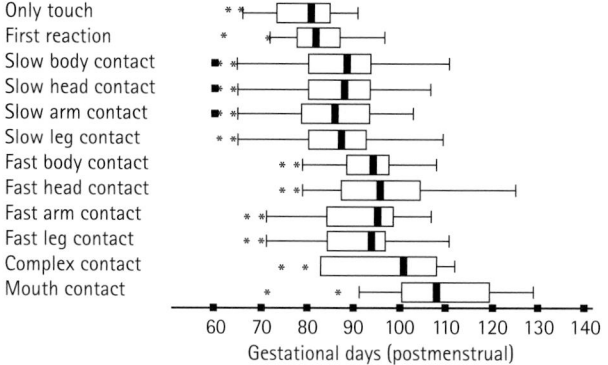

Figure 8.2 Onset of prenatal contacts in 20 dichorionic and 5 monochorionic diamniotic twin pairs (Box–Whisker plots) compared to two cases of monoamniotic twins (∗), ultrasound observations at 1-week intervals.

developing nervous system. Pain can be acute, established, or chronic. Pain can be classified as physiologic, inflammatory, neuropathic, or visceral, with each of these categories further divided according to the degree of severity.

Similar definitions might be true for the potentially viable fetus. Anand further explains the definition of pain as an unpleasant sensory and emotional experience associated with actual or potential tissue damage, whereby the inability to communicate verbally or non-verbally does not negate the possibility that an individual is experiencing pain and is in need of appropriate pain-relieving treatment (Anand et al 2006). The stress response is usually based on the individual's perception of control and predictability of its environment, generally characterized by changes in four primary domains: endocrine, autonomic, immunological and behavioral (Plotsky et al 2000). There are few publications related to immunological or endocrine responses in utero but an increasing number describing behavioral responses to acute pain and some to chronic pain.

Endocrine and behavioral fetal responses to invasive techniques were observed as blood flow redistribution from 18 weeks (Teixeira et al 1996) and as an increase of cortisol and endorphin from at least 23 weeks of gestation onwards (Giannakoulopoulos et al 1999). Within 10 minutes of needling a fetal intrahepatic vein for a transfusion, a fetus showed a 590% rise in beta-endorphin and a 183% rise in cortisol, which is interpreted as a chemical evidence of pain experience (Giannakoulopoulos et al 1999). The fetal plasma levels obtained from the intrahepatic vein were compared with those from the placental cord insertion during diagnostic procedures. Plasma levels in samples taken before transfusion from the intrahepatic vein were significantly higher than those from the placental cord insertion. After transfusion, there was a significant rise in fetal plasma noradrenaline (NA) norepinephrine levels at both sites; however, after transfusion through the intrahepatic vein, the rise was substantially greater than after transfusion through the placental cord insertion. The delta NA was significantly associated with the duration of the stimulus (the time the needle remained in situ) and with gestational age. The results indicate that the fetus is capable of mounting an independent stress response to a needle transgressing its trunk from 18 weeks gestation onwards. The effect was seen in samples taken at a mean of 5.6 minutes after needling (Giannakoulopoulos et al 1999).

Chronic fetal pain may arise in fetuses with bowel obstruction or perforation, cystic lesions such as large ovarian cysts that may lead to torsion or increased intra-abdominal pressure. Up to now, we have observed single patients where bowel obstruction and perforation were combined with a sudden decrease in variability, absence of FHR accelerations and/or tachycardia without fetal blood gas changes. In one patient we even observed normalization of the baseline after puncture of the ovarian cyst. However, these are isolated observations and not yet proven by larger series.

A new field of research deals with the role of non-specific and non-cytopathic blocking antibodies produced during pregnancy. It is hypothesized that the hypo-antigenicity of the developing human fetal system may possibly contribute to the production of this blocking antibody and thus may play a role in the lack of recognition by the host's HLA system and a reduced recognition of fetal pain. Transplantation of adrenal graft has even been used for relief of pain, inflammation and restoration of mobility in adult rheumatic patients with the medullary component contributing to endorphin-like substance liberation and the cortical component contributing to glucocorticoid synthesis (Bhattacharya et al 2002).

The most rational approach to estimating pain in the growing fetus is to make an informed guess based on knowledge of the developmental nervous system or based on measurements and observations in preterm infants. Some authors argue for placing the onset of pain sensation at somewhere between 6 and 12 weeks after conception (McCullagh 1997); others define recorded responses before 26 weeks as reflexes without conscious appreciation, suggesting that only after 26 weeks is the fetus likely to first experience pain (Lloyd-Thomas & Fitzgerald 1996). Although it seems accepted that the thalamus may assume some functions to contribute to fetal awareness of pain, no one is sure yet when the brain is mature enough to register pain. Graded cortical responses to tactile and noxious stimuli occur, implying that preterm infants are experiencing pain, not only nociception (Bartocci et al 2006). The essential physiological substrate for this study was defined by the earlier studies showing that somatosensory evoked potentials with distinct, constant components are fully developed by 29 weeks of gestation (Hrbek et al 1973, Klimach & Cooke 1988). Multiple observations, such as the cortical lateralization, the latency and duration of these responses, and their localization to the somatosensory cortex, support the idea that preterm infants are consciously processing acute pain (Bartocci et al 2006). Slater et al (2006) also reported somatosensory cortical activation, significantly greater in awake than in asleep infants, but no responses were detected after non-noxious stimulation of the heel, even when accompanied by reflex withdrawal of a foot. For the conscious processing of pain – in its widest meaning – the supraspinal processing of noxious stimuli implying activation of cortical neuronal circuits is the first step towards the formation of the primary consciousness (Edelman 2004, Seth et al 2005). Probably before the third trimester of gestation, brain cortical structures start to build re-entrant loops connecting value-category memory to current perceptual categorization. The re-entrant linkage (to frontal, temporal and parietal areas and in turn to amygdala and hippocampus) is the crucial evolutionary development that results in primary consciousness (Edelman 2004).

To avoid suffering and long-term effects it is considered to provide the fetus with analgesia during painful procedures. In addition, suffering during termination of pregnancy is a question of concern. The Royal College of

Obstetricians and Gynaecologists recommends that practitioners who undertake diagnostic or therapeutic surgical procedures upon the fetus at or after 24 weeks consider the requirements of fetal analgesia and sedation either by agents given to the mother or directly to the fetus (Gynaecologists 1997). Similarly, it is suggested to consider fetocide before performing late terminations of pregnancy (Gynaecologists 1997). Maternal analgesia which passes the placenta would be sufficient in cases of early termination of pregnancy. Research is needed to determine how the detection and treatment of pain can be extended to the fetal patient in a direct way (Anand et al 2006).

The preterm infant of 23 weeks' gestation shows reflex responses to noxious stimuli. A variety of physiological, hormonal, metabolic and behavioral changes have been observed after painful procedures such as cardiovascular variables, palmar sweating, increase of renin, epinephrine (adrenaline), norepinephrine, catecholamines and glucocorticoids. The magnitude of these changes is related to the intensity of the stimulus.

Cutaneous flexor reflex thresholds have been used as a measure of somatosensory function in preterm infants and newborn rat pups. Preterm infants of less than 30 weeks postconceptional age had very low thresholds, but by 37.5 weeks thresholds were equivalent to those in normal term babies. Newborn rat pups also have very low flexor reflex thresholds, which do not approach adult levels until 4 postnatal weeks. Repeated stimulation of the foot in preterm babies resulted in sensitization of the flexion reflex up to about 32 postconceptional weeks. After that age repeated stimulation resulted in habituation, as observed in the adult. Sensitization also occurred in newborn rat pups, which changed at 4 postnatal weeks to habituation (Fitzgerald et al 1988). The results demonstrate the sensitivity of spinal reflexes to cutaneous inputs in the neonate and it is argued that this results from lack of inhibitory control in the immature spinal cord. Therefore infants under 32 weeks might need even more analgesia to avoid stress responses and pain experience.

In our neonatal intensive care unit we score neonates from 24 weeks onwards according to the neonatal infant pain score (NIPS) looking at cry patterns, breathing, body language and facial expressions (Lawrence et al 1993). If we suspect that infants experience pain from ventilation or invasive procedures we start treatment with morphine or acetaminophen. We take advantage of the increased half-life due to a decreased clearance of the drug in preterm infants to reach higher concentrations according to the supposed lower pain threshold (van Lingen et al 2001).

Although our knowledge of pain and its management in the perinatal period has increased, little is still known about the first hours and days of life when major physiologic transition events occur. Prematurity and critical illnesses further complicate analgesic use. Increased morbidity and mortality have been shown in infants receiving placebo infusions after surgery compared with infants with analgesia, highlighting the negative consequences of pain in infants (Lawrence et al 1993, van Lingen et al 2001). Opioids can help to promote hemodynamic stability, promote respirator synchrony, and to decrease the incidence of intraventricular hemorrhages in ventilated preterm neonates (van Lingen et al 2001). Long-term follow-up studies suggest improved behavioral and cognitive outcomes in children given morphine infusions during NICU confinement. The necessity of fetal analgesia is dictated by the ability to feel pain and by the adverse effects of noxious stimuli on future sensory development. Effects of drugs given to the pregnant woman or the (preterm) infant are still not sufficiently evaluated. Consequently, dose and dose interval may vary between neonates and within individuals during the first days of life. Polymorphisms of the genes encoding for the enzymes involved in the metabolism of analgesics or in genes involved in receptor expression may contribute to the large interindividual pharmacokinetic parameter variability (van Lingen et al 2002).

Pain sensitivity may be altered after 32 weeks of gestation. Little attention has up to now been given to the experience of pain during vacuum or forceps delivery and the perinatal period. Newborns born by either of those procedures in our unit receive pain treatment directly after birth.

HEARING

Hearing is a prerequisite for the development of language and communication. Onset and development of fetal hearing are dated by extrapolation from animal studies, from premature babies and by studying prenatal reactions to acoustic stimuli. Efforts to explore prenatal recognition began in the 1920s. Peiper performed fetal sonic stimulation with the aid of a car horn and studied movement responses (Peiper 1925). Forbes and Forbes were able to acknowledge the amodal link between FM and sound by stimulating a pregnant mother lying in a water bath which was struck with a metal object (Forbes & Forbes 1927). Ray attempted to measure fetal reactions to the smacking of two boards. All authors reported habituation responses following repeated presentation of stimuli (Ray 1932).

Habituation and conditioning became more focal as researchers attempted to tighten scientific controls and FM responses to sound were observed as a major focus for fetal conditioning (Bench 1968, Sakabe et al 1969, Salk 1961).

A more detailed summary of fetal hearing can be obtained in previous publications (Arabin 2002, Arabin & Straaten 2006).

ANATOMY AND PHYSIOLOGY OF EARLY HEARING

The *external ear* is visualized by ultrasound from 10 weeks onwards (Fig. 8.3a). The outer ear collects sound energy and directs it towards the tympanic membrane (TM). The TM develops from structures associated with both the external and the middle ear. It has three layers: an outer epithelial

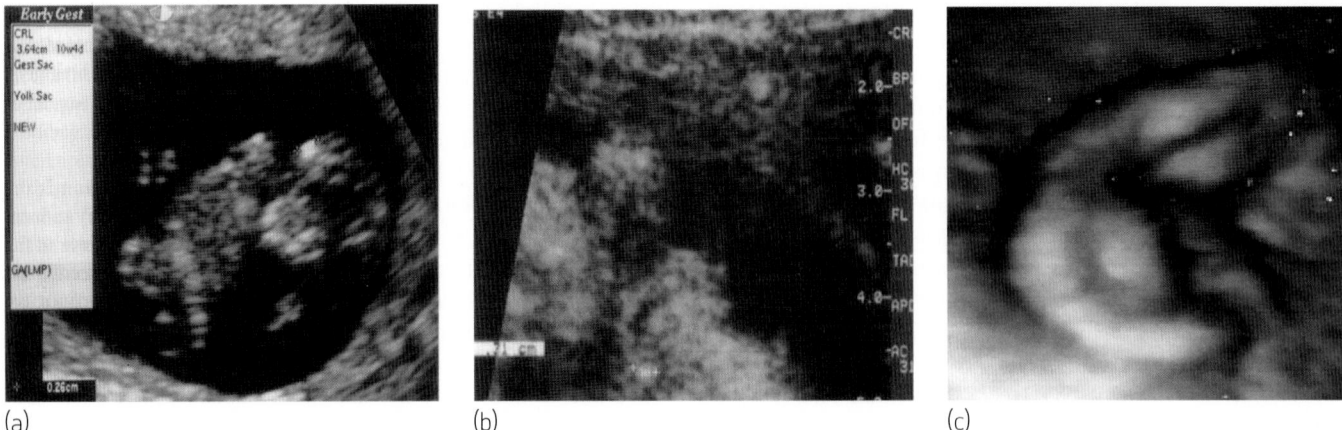

(a)   (b)   (c)

Figure 8.3 First appearance of the outer ear at 10 gestational weeks (a), the outer ear with the tympanic membrane at 28 weeks (b) (2D, ATL 5000) and the outer ear revealing more details of the individual shape obtained by 3D ultrasound at 28 weeks (c) (GE Expert 750).

layer, a middle fibrous layer and an inner mucosal layer, continuous with the lining of the tympanic cavity. The TM inserts into the tympanic ring which is complete at 16 weeks, and can be visualized by ultrasound at the end of the external auditory canal (Fig. 8.3b). The maximal diameter is of adult size in the term fetus. It develops from structures associated with both the external and the middle ear.

The size and shape of the outer ear have been proposed as a marker of a variety of syndromes in the second trimester (Birnholz 1983, Johnson et al 2005) and in aneuploid fetuses (Chitkara et al 2002, Lettieri et al 1993). The 3D/4D render mode allows a more detailed visualization of the external ear and may thus help for diagnosis in rare syndromes (Fig. 8.3c).

The *middle ear* transduces acoustic into mechanical energy. The ossicles of the middle ear develop between 4 and 6 gestational weeks. Ossicles in the middle ear are of adult size by 8 months of gestation and thus the only bones to attain their final form in the prenatal period (Anson & Winch 1974). At week 7, constriction of the midportion leads to the formation of the eustachian tube and the tympanic cavity which is subsequently filled with mucoid mesenchymal tissue becoming vacuolated. By 30–34 weeks the tympanic cavity is pneumatized.

The temporal bone derives from four separate elements: the tympanic bone, the squamous portion, the styloid process and the petromastoid. Only the first three parts have formed and ossified at birth. Postnatally, there is still no complete bony ear canal and no mastoid process. The facial nerve derives from the second branchial arch. At the end of the third gestational week the acousticofacial ganglion can be identified; by the end of the embryonic period its neuroblasts form the main trunk of the facial nerve and the chorda tympani nerve. The fully developed facial nerve transverses the internal acoustic meatus, the middle ear and, finally, exits superficially from the stylomastoid behind the TM where it can be injured by obstetric manipulations.

The *inner ear* lies in the petrous portion of the temporal bone and consists of a membranous labyrinth inside a bony labyrinth. The bony labyrinth includes the cochlea, three semicircular canals, the vestibule enclosing the utricle, the saccule and part of the cochlear duct, as well as the perilymphatic spaces. By 24 weeks, all centers have fused to form a complete bony capsule. Ossification of the inner ear does not occur until each portion has attained adult size. The configuration of the membranous labyrinth is recognizable by 10 weeks and completed at around 24 weeks. Its neurosensory elements develop from the ectodermal optic placode in the 23-day-old human embryo giving rise to the otocyst. The differentiation of the vestibular and cochlear end organs takes place during the second month of pregnancy.

Light microscopy demonstrates that the first sign of differentiation of the organ of Corti in the wall of the cochlear duct starts at 10 gestational weeks. At 14 weeks, rows of inner and outer hair cells can be observed. At around 20 weeks, the human cochlear morphology resembles the stage corresponding to the onset of cochlear function. The organ of Corti contains sensory and supporting cells. Ultrastructural development includes hair cell differentiation of inner and outer hair cells, synaptogenesis and ciliogenesis.

The role of the cochlea and structures of the inner ear is to couple the vibratory energy delivered to the oval window by the stapes footplate to the hair cells. It was postulated in 1965 by Davis that the binding of the sensory hairs of the organ of Corti depolarizes the hair-cell membrane by altering its resistance (Davis 1965). The basis of the frequency-related regional displacement of the cochlea was revealed by the Nobel laureate von Bekesy, describing it as 'traveling waves' (Bekesy 1960). Bekesy studied the inner ear by building mechanical models of the cochlea, e.g. a metal tube filled with water. Along the length of the tube ran a narrow slot covered by a stretched membrane, which served as the basilar membrane of the model. When the fluid was set in motion, the undulation traveled down the length of the membrane, but its amplitude varied with position. He also detected the same wave movement in the cochlea itself. Using first animal ears and then the ears of human cadavers, he carefully cut out the cochlea. Under the microscope he saw a bulging undulation sweep over the basilar membrane when a sound was introduced into the cochlea. It was the same traveling wave he had seen coursing along the artificial membrane of his model.

The eighth nerve ganglion also derives from the otocyst. After 4 weeks, the cells from the auditory ganglion divide into superior and inferior branches of the vestibular nerve and the cochlear nerve. The nerve cells remain bipolar throughout life, terminating in the sensory areas of the inner ear and the central processes in the brainstem. With the entry of the acoustic nerve into the brainstem auditory neurons multiply and project the information to the auditory cortex. Many auditory abilities are attributable to *sub*cortical processing. Therefore, decorticated animals are capable of detecting intensity and frequency of sounds and anencephalic fetuses demonstrate behavioral reactions to external stimuli.

Infants develop an information-processing capacity, the development of which has not yet been sufficiently studied but is essential for understanding how speech and language develop, and may have implications concerning auditory behavior, reaction to sound and diagnostic testing.

ACOUSTIC PHYSIOLOGY

Some basics about acoustics are prerequisite to understand the specific fetal situation: Sound is created by a vibratory source, causing molecules to be displaced. The amplitude is measured in Pascals (Pa). Sound pressure levels (SPL) and frequencies are given in decibel (dB) and Hertz (Hz). The SPL required to evoke a fetal response is 20–30 dB less at 35 than at 23 weeks, indicating that the fetal auditory system becomes more sensitive with age (Hepper & Shahidullah 1994). However, changes in attenuation, behavior and sensori-motor neural connections might also have an impact. The range of 20 to 20000 Hz is the bandwidth of human hearing.

Information about prenatal hearing is mainly obtained from sheep experiments since prenatal auditory sensitivity and sound attenuation are similar in sheep and humans (Armitage et al 1980). The bone conduction route implies that sound energy is diminished by 10–20 dB for frequencies <250 Hz and by 40–50 dB >500 Hz.

A reason for fetal 'sound isolation' is the sound pressure attenuation. Thereby, transmission losses range from 39 dB at 500 Hz to 85 dB at 5000 Hz. Sound attenuation decreases during late gestation. In humans, sound of at least 65–70 dB is transmitted with attenuation of 30 dB reduction in SPL for tones up to 12 kHz. Frequencies of 200 Hz are even enhanced. Sound environment in utero is dominated by frequencies <500 Hz and mean SPLs of 90 dB caused by vessel pulsations, intervillous injections, maternal digestion or breathing. This might have an 'imprinting' effect. Intelligibility is the ability to distinguish complex sounds. Music

and voices are distinguishable from the basal noise by 8–12 dB. The male voice or music with a mean frequency of 125 Hz is better transmitted, but emerges in the range with high internal noise. Female voices or music with an average of 220 Hz receive greater attenuation, but emerge in a range with low internal noise. Even intelligibility has developmental aspects (Shahidullah & Hepper 1994). Using a habituation–dishabituation technique fetuses aged 35 weeks were shown to discriminate between frequencies of 250 and 500 Hz and between speech sounds, whereas fetuses of 27 weeks were unable to make this differentiation, although they were able to differentiate between a 250 Hz pure tone and 80–2000 Hz broadband sounds.

IMMEDIATE PRENATAL AND POSTNATAL AUDITORY RESPONSIVENESS

Studies of fetal response to sound have used a variety of stimuli, not always with rationale. Studies with airborne and vibroacoustic stimuli (VAS) providing vibration *and* airborne sound should be differentiated. The electronic artificial larynx used for VAS has a spectrum between 0.5 and 1 kHz and an SPL averaging 135 dB.

To demonstrate the existence of prenatal acoustic perception, one can empirically study immediate electrophysiological and behavioral (motor and cardiovascular) responsiveness.

Prenatal electrophysiological responsiveness is obtained by recordings of electric potentials from levels of the auditory system by means of non-invasive techniques based on compound potentials (Fig. 8.4). They represent the activity of many cells by stimulus-related electroencephalographic (EEG) and magneto-encephalographic (MEG) methods. Fetal EEG responses towards acoustic signals have been performed after ruptured membranes using scalp electrodes (Barden et al 1968, Scibetta et al 1971). In MEG recordings, sensitive magnetic field detectors are used to measure prenatal neuromagnetic auditory responses to clicks of 1 kHz up to 100 dB with intact membranes. Stimulus-related auditory evoked neuromagnetic fields were recorded at 34 weeks (Blum et al 1985, 1987), comparable with postnatal recordings. In a more recent study, the earliest recordings of evoked neuromagnetic fields were detected at 29 gestational weeks. The latencies of the auditory evoked responses declined during the third trimester from 300 ms to nearly 150 ms at term (Schleussner et al 2001).

Prenatal behavioral responsiveness has been used because an association of neonatal evoked potentials with heartbeat and motor responses implies the reception of the auditory signals up to subcortical levels (Tuber et al 1980). Due to the present lack of routine technology to record neural activity in the womb, fetal sensory abilities are examined by observing behavioral reactions. Appropriate methodology has to be used to ensure that stimulus and response are correlated. Problems arise when the fetus does *not* react, since we cannot determine whether the stimulus is actually perceived or not. Ultrasound observations allow defining

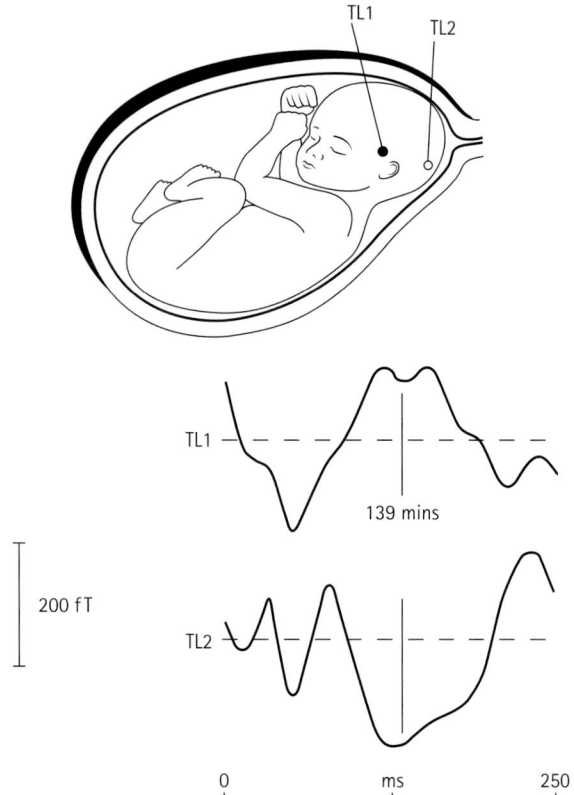

Figure 8.4 Waveforms obtained from brainstem recordings after click stimulation at 34 weeks using one-channel magnetoencephalography (54). TL = temporal lateral, ft = fentotesla.

motor responses such as twinkling or body, head, arm and leg movements (Arabin & Riedewald 1992). The methodology can be simplified by using Doppler devices for detection of FM, quantifying FM responses with a high sensitivity and specificity (Arabin et al 1988). Using this method we observed first fetal reactions towards acoustic stimulation at 25 weeks. With increasing gestational age, an increasing number of FM combined with FHR-accelerations and reactions with a prolonged change of baseline FHR lasting up to several minutes is observed.

Some factors influence fetal responsiveness, such as the behavioral state before or during the stimulus (Devoe et al 1990) or gender (Leader et al 1982). Fetal responses to speech stimuli were studied between 26–34 weeks gestation. During periods of low FHR variability, a decrease in baseline and an increase in the deviation of FHR were found (Zimmer et al 1993). This is a demonstration of prenatal responses to speech stimuli, whereby the response depends on fetal behavioral state. Female fetuses seem to respond to acoustic stimuli earlier than males (Leader et al 1982).

ENDURING EFFECTS OF PRENATAL HEARING

Considerable attention is given to the possibility that the fetus forms memories of speech and music that may influence postnatal development. In the past, most studies have used behavioral responsiveness to evaluate the reactions to sound of the fetus and the newborn. While habituation reflects short-term memory, there is also proof of long-term memory from pre- to postnatal life, as observed by studies of behavioral modifications of neonates presented with stimuli they have been confronted with prenatally.

Habituation had been described by Peiper in 1885, reporting a decrease in FM after repeated stimulation (Peiper 1925). Since then a number of studies have demonstrated a decrement in response to repeated stimulation using FHR/FM or ultrasound documentation. Habituation may be distinguished from fatigue by the recovery of response on presentation of a new stimulus ('dishabituation') and faster habituation upon re-presentation of the stimulus (Jeffrey & Cohen 1971). The intensity influences habituation time (faster habituation to more intense stimuli). Refractory times of habituation processes were studied and responses to sound were observed as one major focus for fetal conditioning (Bench 1968, Salk 1961). Habituation experiments in the fetus or newborn typically take place over a period of minutes and demonstrate that the infant retains sound characteristics long enough (up to 24 hours) (van Heteren et al 2001) to compare them with a new signal.

There is also proof of *long-term memory* from pre- to postnatal life (Querleu et al 1989), whereby the term 'fetal learning' or 'fetal enrichment' should be used with caution. Prenatal sound experience might influence postnatal sound preference and fine-tune the developing auditory system (DeCasper & Fifer 1980). In an experimental setting, newborns were taught that they could hear their mother's voice via headphones when they produced a specific sucking pattern with sucking bursts of a specific frequency and duration. Using this non-nutritive 'high-amplitude sucking procedure,' newborns were shown to prefer the voice of their mother to other voices and even to a lullaby, which had been presented by the mother during the last weeks of pregnancy, further suggesting elementary prenatal sound acquisition and discrimination.

Prenatal exposure to sound may also have an *impact on neonatal performance*. Sound stimulations resembling intrauterine noise serve as a reinforcer during sucking and can lull the newborn to sleep (Caspar & Sigafoos 1983). Similarly, postnatal feeding may be enhanced by background music (Woodward & Guidozzi 1992). Settings of talking and music were performed during pregnancy (Sallenbach 1991): within the talking group, only 58% of newborn behavioral variables were identified as positive (e.g. the child being easily comforted), 16% as ambiguous and 26% as negative (e.g. crying for obscure reasons, needing constant supervision). However, within the group exposed to music, 90% of the newborns presented with positive attitudes. It is speculated whether variations of timbre expressing care, anger or anxiety or maternal hormonal changes associated with speech and music evoke associations in the infant. Pilot studies have demonstrated a simultaneous reduction of fetal breathing and an increase of FM when mothers listened to a preferred type of music via earphones (Zimmer et al 1982) proving some kind of conditioning ('music, mother relaxed'). To have time to listen may by itself be an important intervention. Whether the unborn is more affected by the mother's emotions during listening or singing than by the sound itself is still uncertain.

In China, children who had been exposed to music stimulation during pregnancy in the neonatal period were followed by the Gesell Infant Scale. After 5 and 12 months postpartum, some abilities such as sitting, staying and walking were observed earlier in the study compared to a control group (Chen et al 1994). In Venezuela, weekly lectures to pregnant mothers about nutrition were combined with music stimulation. Significant improvement was found postnatally in orientation and autonomic stability of the infants in the experimental compared to a control group (Lamont & Dibben 2001).

In England, Lamont has demonstrated that prenatal stimuli with music induce memory tracings which can still be detected after 1 year independent of the intelligence of the test person or the kind of music (BBC program 'Child of our Time', 2000). Preferred types of music were characterized by fast rhythmic patterns (Manrique et al 1993).

Studies investigating an influence of music and sound on later development have used developmental tests such as the Early Language Milestones (ELM) test, the Brazelton, the Denver Developmental screening test, the Gesell Infant and the Bayley Scale of Infant Development. However, these tests are sensitive to subjective interpretations.

Presuming that behavioral research cannot produce standardized evidence on sound feature discrimination, some groups have used electrophysiological methods in newborns. Sensory processes underlying sound perception have been studied using the mismatch negativity (MMN) component of auditory event-related potentials (ERPs), which is not contingent on conscious perception. Thus, MMN may be suitable for studying newborns, from whom it is difficult to obtain behavioral responses. Recent studies have investigated newborns' pre-attentive analysis of sound duration and frequency changes. The majority of neonates appear to possess effective discrimination mechanisms, which is facilitated by rich sound content (Ceponiene et al 2002). The temporal dynamics of auditory sensory memory has been studied in newborns that were either awake or asleep with stimuli of 1 000 Hz tones that were occasionally replaced by 1 100 Hz tones. The results imply that the time span of auditory memory is considerably shorter in neonates than in adults (Cheour et al 2002).

ERPs elicited by music have not yet been investigated in newborns or children. In adults, the influence of a preceding musical context on music processing was examined. The amplitudes of both early and late negativities were found to be sensitive to the degree of musical expectancy and to the probability for deviant acoustic events. The results strengthen the hypothesis of an implicit musical ability of the human brain (Koelsch et al 2000). Impure chords, presented among perfect major chords, elicited a distinct MMN in professional musicians, but not in non-musicians (Koelsch et al 1999). The results demonstrate that musicians are superior in extracting information out of musical stimuli and that training might modulate sensory memory. Whether this holds true for the fetus or newborn is not yet known.

Repeated experience over longer periods of time than those afforded by the usual laboratory habituation setting is a prerequisite for 'learning' (James et al 2002). It is recognized that it is unlikely that birth marks an abrupt change in the prenate's ability to learn. In most experiments dealing with the prominence of the maternal voice to other voices it is difficult to rule out some effect of postnatal experience (Spence & Caspar 1987). However, there are some studies in which postnatal experience was excluded. Hepper et al studied the effect of prenatal music exposure of a television soap opera on infants of 2–4 days, which their mothers had watched during pregnancy (Devoe et al 1990). The 'TV learning group' experienced a decrease in heart rate and movements and a change to a more alert state whilst listening to the same melody 2–4 days after birth. No reaction was observed in the control group of mothers who had not observed the program or in newborns of the study group exposed to other melodies. Since none of the infants had heard the melody after birth, it was suggested that the fetus can learn not only from the maternal voice but also from deliberate ex utero environmental sounds throughout the perinatal period. However, neonates seem also to have the ability to forget in the absence of repetitive exposure: at day 21, recognition of the melody seemed to be lost (Hepper 1991). The response to the TV theme had prenatally been investigated using real-time ultrasound. It was concluded that the ability to recognize familiar stimuli starts between 30 and 37 weeks.

Fetal–maternal heart rate coordination has been investigated by magnetocardiograms showing that the coordination of a maternal–child pair is higher than between incidentally chosen pairs (Van Leeuwen et al 2003). It would be interesting to know whether this has a genetic, a reactive sensory, or an acoustic cause.

ACOUSTICAL RESPONSIVENESS AS A TEST FOR FETAL WELLBEING AND ENVIRONMENTAL HAZARDS

The ability of VAS to elicit FHR-accelerations has been well established. In this context, VAS was proposed to assess fetal wellbeing and to discriminate between 'non-reactive' non-stress tests (NST) due to hypoxia or just to quiet state (Pietrantoni et al 1991). FHR-reactions are reduced after VAS in intrauterine growth retardation (IUGR) fetuses. The conclusion, that nutritional deprivation is associated with delayed sensory maturation is not necessarily true, since even when there is no reaction the stimulus might well be received.

We compared the clinical value of an NST, a ratio of cerebral versus umbilical blood flow, VAS and contraction stress test (CST) to predict poor outcome for IUGR and post-term pregnancies: Doppler velocimetry and the NSTs were superior to VAS and CST in both groups (Arabin et al 1993, 1994).

In the only controlled clinical trial where VAS was compared to NST, false-positive tests were slightly lower and performance reduced from a mean of 27 to 23 minutes (Smith et al 1986). Although it has been proven that VAS does not increase catecholamine release (Fisk et al 1991) or meconium passage in healthy fetuses (Zimmer et al 1996), the question remains whether a 4-minute test of frightening or awakening an innocently sleeping fetus is justified (it is recommended that VAS is performed during quiet sleep!). What parents would appreciate this postnatally? Nevertheless, children who have been exposed in utero to VAS have been evaluated at 4 years of age by auditory tests (Arulkumaran et al 1991, Nyman et al 1992). No hearing damage or neurodevelopmental abnormalities connected to VAS were found.

Given the fact that the fetus is exposed to ongoing sound in utero, to the voice of the mother whenever she speaks or sings and to the ambient sound level of the maternal environment it seems that exaggerated acoustic stimulation with unphysiologic frequencies and intensities by audio speakers or megaphones – just in order to get any reaction – might even be risky for hearing development and behavioral state regulation in the unborn child. And this is exactly what the uncritical use of VAS to evoke some FHR changes does (Romero et al 1988). Promoting various instruments that aim to enhance neuronal ripening except within a well-defined research setting seems illogical. Conversely, several commercial products are recommended throughout pregnancy, which have been proven to be without any effect since the sound cannot even reach intrauterine hearing thresholds.

Fetal noise-induced hearing loss has been a matter of concern with regard to working or living conditions of pregnant women (Moss & Carver 1992, Pierson 1996). Epidemiological and animal research suggests that noise can adversely influence fetal hearing; however, studies in humans still lack control groups. Auditory brainstem response changes were examined in sheep suggesting that noise sources with low-frequency components and high-intensity impulses have temporary effects on auditory brainstem response waves, whereas long-term effects are still unknown (Griffiths et al 1994). In summary, the Committee on Hearing, Bioacoustics and Biomechanics, attempting to protect fetal hearing, suggested that pregnant women should avoid exposure to noise with an intensity greater than 90 dB (Statement 1982).

OLFACTION AND TASTE

Olfaction and taste have traditionally been considered to be non-functional before birth. The growing appreciation of fetal and neonatal capabilities to smell and to taste has benefited from anatomical and functional research in animal models and more recently in fetuses and newborns.

The most recent summary of Schaal et al (2004) has helped us to look for further literature and to interpret the presently existing research.

ANATOMY AND BASIC PHYSIOLOGY OF NASAL AND ORAL FLAVOR RECEPTION

About 1–2% of the human genome is allocated to receptors for the olfactory epithelium (Winberg & Porter 1998).

The *external fetal nose* and the nasal bone are well shaped between 11 and 14 weeks. The examination of the nasal bone by ultrasound has become a new topic of interest since it is proposed as an additional tool in the detection of trisomy 21, thus improving the detection rate of the combined screening by fetal nuchal translucency and maternal serum biochemistry up to 90% with a false positive rate of 2.5% during the first trimester (Cicero et al 2006).

Four anatomically distinct structures have been described to establish the intranasal chemical senses: the olfactory system, the trigeminal nerve, the vomeronasal organ and the terminal nerve (Schaal et al 2004). All systems differentiate during early pregnancy. From the end of the first trimester the receptor neurons of the main olfactory system look morphologically mature by electron microscopy (Pyatkina 1982). Olfactory receptors mediate the sense of flavor arising from low-concentration volatile substances pumped into the nasal cavity during inhalation, swallowing or chewing, mediating neuro-endocrine responses (Beauchamp & Mennella 1998, Winberg & Porter 1998).

The primary neuronal cells of the *main olfactory system* are embedded in the upper part of the nasal cavity connecting to the main olfactory bulbs through the olfactory nerves. Their dendrites merge into the mucus and bear receptor binding compounds. Receptor binding elicits an electrical signal in the neuron, which is transmitted along the axon that penetrates the lamina cribrosa to meet in one of the paired olfactory bulbs and finally arrives at the paleocortex including the hippocampus via a neuronal network (Winberg & Porter 1998).

Branches of the trigeminal system innervate the entire respiratory epithelium. Trigeminal nerve terminals are reactive to tactile stimulation from between 8 and 10 weeks prenatally (Golubeva et al 1959, Humphrey 1978) and to intranasal injection of air postnatally from 26 weeks onwards (Ramet et al 1990). This means that the fetus may respond to chemicals from this period onwards. Impulses reaching the thalamic nuclei project to the frontal cortex where the conscious perception of smell takes place, pathways to the limbic system mediate affective and neuro-endocrine responses.

The *vomero-nasal organ* is reported to degenerate or reorganize during the second trimester.

Its sensory cells on the nasal septum mediate endocrine responses activated by pheromones. More studies are required to determine the specific function in humans. By the third trimester all chemosensory receptors seem ready to be functional. The nostrils have become patent and AF is swallowed and inhaled.

Taste buds are found at as early as 12 weeks and displayed over the oral cavity concentrating at birth on the tongue and on the anterior palate (Lecanuet & Schaal 1996).

Breathing movements have been described by 2D ultrasound to emerge as early as 10 weeks at regular intervals (de Vries et al 1982, 1985). Until now 3D echography has not enabled better visualization (Andonotopo et al 2005). They are usually associated with increased AF flow through the nasal cavity and/or the fetal mouth and thus bring the AF in contact with the nasal receptors or taste buds. The chemical ecology of AF consists of a large variety of odors originating from fetal and maternal sources (Antoshechkin et al 1989, Schaal & Orgeur 1992) whereby fetal pulmonary and urinary fluids increasingly affect the composition. Furthermore, aromas of the maternal diet or habits influence the chemosensory stimulation with increasing gestational age and permeability of the placenta. Maternal oral intake of 110 g of carbohydrate significantly increases fetal breathing movements at 14 to 16 weeks of gestation, thus allowing better ultrasonographic viewing of the fetus (Goldstein et al 2003). The reason for this mechanism is still unknown. Fetal swallowing may lead to increased passage of AF as well, with a chance of eliciting local reactions by physiological or pathological chemoactive substances. Breathing movements cause a displacement of fluid in the nasal airways and mouth so that chemoreceptors are in contact with continually renewed fluid. Nasal flow of AF has been measured by color Doppler and spectrum analysis (Badalian et al 1993). Breath-to-breath interval, duration of the inspiratory phase of the fetal breathing-related nasal flow increased from 22 to 35 weeks and decreased thereafter. A positive correlation existed between the mean breathing-related nasal peak inspiratory flow velocity and between the inspiratory flow velocity acceleration with advancing gestational age (Badalian et al 1993).

IMMEDIATE PRENATAL AND PERINATAL OLFACTORY OR TASTE RESPONSIVENESS

A substantial body of data is reviewed for the rat, in which fetal chemosensation is now firmly established (Schaal & Orgeur 1992). Rat fetuses stimulated with solutions of different odorants react even more intensively than rats exposed to the same odorants in air (Smotherman & Robinson 1990). This may be interpreted as if the AF may enhance the chemosensory reaction. It may, however, also be caused by the relatively elevated concentrations of these substances in the aqueous phase. At the cellular level, the neurochemical stimulation of the olfactory tract has been traced with the olfactory marker protein (OMP) in rats (Gesteland et al 1982). In sheep, prenatal intranasal injections of odorant components induce FHR-changes (Beauchamp & Mennella 1998).

In humans OMP has been proven to be expressed from 29 weeks onwards. This was interpreted as a demonstration of a more mature function of the olfactory bulb (Chuah & Zheng 1987). It is still not possible to test in utero how fetuses differentiate different odorants since they may simultaneously swallow and taste the substances. Intra-amniotic injection of a saccharine solution leads to increased injection of bitter or acid solutions to reduced fetal swallowing signifying 'awareness' of different tastes during pregnancy (Lecanuet & Schaal 1996).

ENDURING EFFECTS OF PRENATAL ODOR AND TASTE

Several studies have tried to demonstrate fetal 'awareness' of different chemical substances and the transnatal chemosensory learning. This requires some kind of maturity of nasal chemoreceptor systems, efficient active compounds in the fetal environment, an ability to memorize chemosensory information across birth, perinatal continuity in chemical signals and the neonatal ability to detect air-borne odorants previously experienced in an aquatic environment (Schaal & Orgeur 1992, Schaal et al 2004).

The fact that specific memories of chemosensory stimuli present in the AF arise during prenatal life has been tested in infants who were exposed to consumption of alcohol by their mothers (Faas et al 2000). Babies born to frequent drinkers exhibited heightened reactivity toward ethanol odor 24–48 hours after birth when compared to newborns delivered by infrequent drinkers. No differences were observed when comparing the responses of both groups to a non-ethanol stimulus (lemon) (Faas et al 2000).

Newborns may retain olfactory memory trace: During the initial attempt to locate the mother's nipple, newborns preferred a breast with the areola moistened with AF over an untreated breast (Winberg & Porter 1998). The chemical origin of this individual AF image has not been clarified so far, but aromas might derive from the mothers' diet (Faas et al 2000, Mennella et al 2001, Schaal et al 2000). Three groups of breast-fed infants and three groups of bottle-fed infants were examined 3 days after birth for their head-turning response when exposed to paired-choice tests contrasting the odors of either familiar or unfamiliar AF or either of these AF odors and a control stimulus. In familiar versus unfamiliar AF tests, newborns oriented preferentially to the odor of familiar AF, regardless of their feeding regimen. Both groups versus controls showed that this response pattern was caused by a true positive orientation toward familiar AF and not by avoidance from unfamiliar AF odor. This highly selective neonatal response is consistent with the hypothesis that the human fetus can detect and store the unique chemosensory information available in utero and that this information becomes coupled with positive control of behavior (Schaal et al 1998).

The scent of AF has a calming effect shortly after birth as measured by infants' rate of crying (Garcia & White-Traut 1993). Finally, there is evidence that babies recognize their mothers by her scent because 6-day-old infants turn preferentially in the direction of their own mother's odor pad rather than towards an alien breast odor. Neonates respond to scents by changes in respiration, facial expression and orientation: even less than 2 days old they develop preferences (based on formation of new synapses) and orient towards an odor that had been present in their nursery for the preceding 24 hours. This phenomenon was still evident 2 weeks after the exposure was discontinued (Kenna 1996).

POSTNATAL OLFACTORY OR TASTE RESPONSIVENESS

Early olfaction was initially investigated in premature infants long before the ultrasound era. High-intensity odorants were used and the responses were interpreted to be attributable to the trigeminal effects of the stimuli. Studies using lower concentrations indicated well-developed functions of discriminization and memorization of odors in preterm infants. In general, premature infants reacted in a similar fashion but to sharp or foul odorants (aniseed oil, asa foetida) as term babies — with oral movements, head turning, gagging or crying — but needed higher concentrations. This suggests the presence of functional olfaction with higher thresholds (Kulakowskaia 1929, Stirnimann 1936) at early gestation. Another study testing that the impact of mint odor concluded that reactions before 32 weeks were less pronounced than after 32 weeks up to term (Sarnat 1978). All cited odor stimuli may stimulate both the olfactory and trigeminal system.

Low-intensity mild odorants such as diluted vanillin or butyric acid probably only stimulate the olfactory system. Two studies could demonstrate that this triggered respiratory changes or facial movements in infants of 28–34 weeks (Goubet et al 2002, Marlier et al 2001).

Taste responses have also been demonstrated in premature babies of 26 weeks. Bitter-tasting substances were reported to lead to shutting the mouth (Mennella et al 2001). In contrast, preterm infants show appetitive responses to the odor of human milk (Bingham et al 2003).

Preterm infants were not only proven to react to an odorant stimulus but also to discriminate between various odorants such as mineral oil, diluted eucalyptol or undiluted non-ionic acid when exposed to these substances between 30 and 37 weeks (Pihet et al 1996, 1997). Further, the response was influenced by gender, gestational age and no optimal adoption at birth (greater responses in males compared to females, with increasing gestational age and in infants with low Apgar scores).

Habituation, which has been extensively investigated for acoustic stimulations, may also occur to certain odors. As in acoustic stimuli, habituation to certain odors may occur. When a specific odor was presented for 10 periods of 10 seconds, the introduction of a new odorant resulted in an increase of facial responses in preterm and term infants. This again supports the concept of odor discrimination and memory in these infants (Goubet et al 2002). In addition, preterm babies were proven to demonstrate facial indicators of disgust (nose wrinkling, upper lip raising, head turning away) after unpleasant odor (butyric acid), whereas pleasant odors (vanilla) provoked appetitive reactions (licking, sucking) (Gaugler et al 2003). Some primary odor preferences such as the response to non-specific milk may result from prenatal experiences or unconditional perceptual predisposition (Marlier et al 1998). Knowledge about olfaction and taste may have not only scientific but also diagnostic and therapeutic implications, such as the initiation and stabilization of breastfeeding, newborn adaptation, attachment and the reduction of anomic episodes (Garcia & White-Traut 1993).

We therefore provide newborns admitted to our NICU with accessories of their mothers.

VISION

The ability to see — probably our most predominant sense in infant and adult life — evolves steadily during gestation but in ways difficult to study. However, at the time of birth vision is developed mainly at the distance to the mother's face when breastfeeding.

ANATOMY AND PHYSIOLOGY OF EARLY VISION

Different parts of the eye develop from different origins: The retina, iris and the optic nerve are of neuro-ectodermal origin, the lens and cornea are of ectodermal, the choroid, sclera, the ciliary body and ocular blood vessels are of mesodermal origin.

Maturation of the retina takes place from the optic disk area towards the periphery. This process is closely followed by a similar maturation of the retinal vasculature and normally completed at about 42 weeks. The maturation consists of proliferation, differentiation and migration of retinal neuronal cells and outgrowth of axons and dendrites. Neuroblastic cells differentiate into photoreceptor cells which later secrete interstitial retinol binding protein which plays a role in the defense of free radicals by binding vitamin E (Baerts & Fetter 1998). After 18 weeks, synapses appear on the eye rods. The axonal connections to the brain lay superficially in the nerve fiber layer, on the vitreous side of the retina, while the photoreceptors (rods and cones) lay on the outside, close to the choroid. Retinal surface area doubles between 26 weeks and term (Fielder & Moseley 1998).

The axons leave the eye at the optic disk and travel through the optic nerve and optic chiasma, which meanwhile can even be visualized by 3D ultrasound (Fig. 8.5) to synaptic stations in the lateral geniculate nuclei to the optic radiation and the posterior pole of the optic cortex.

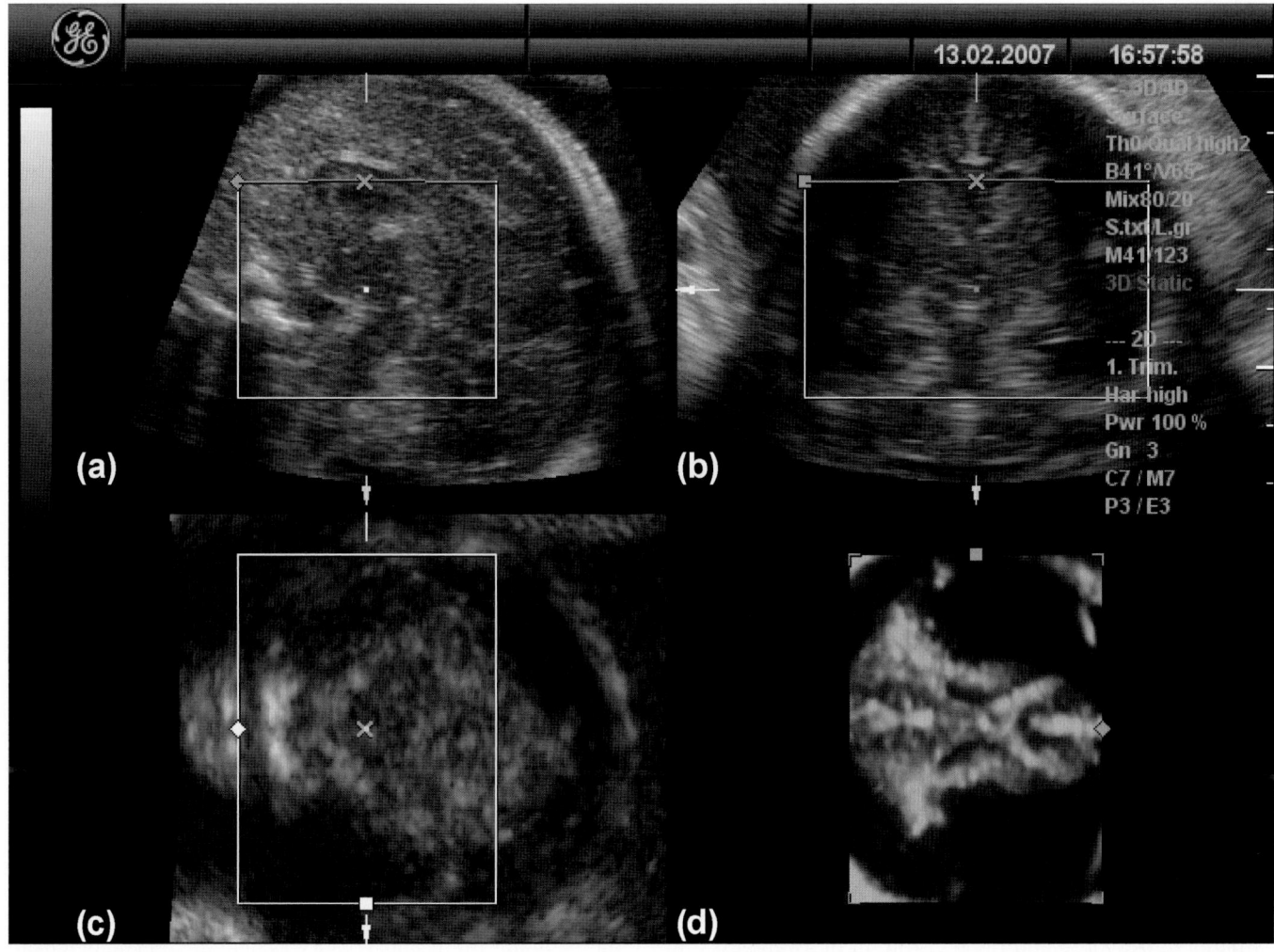

Figure 8.5 Different planes (a–c) to visualize the chiasma opticum as a rendered picture (d) by at 28 gestational weeks 3D static ultrasound (GE Expert 750).

Myelination of the optic nerve starts between 6 and 8 months, myelination of the posterior visual pathway and superior colliculus just before term (Fielder & Moseley 1998). The last part of the eye to fully develop is the fovea. This is the central area that will eventually be densely populated with cones only, to enable optimal fixation and color vision in the optical axis. This process may continue until age 4 (Lecanuet & Schaal 1996). Visual acuity at term birth has been estimated to be 20/400.

From 20 to 24 weeks fetal eyelids may open. The eye becomes fully reactive to light at about 7 months gestation, showing pupillary constriction and a blink response to exposure to light.

At term, the eye is well developed, growing only three times to reach adult size, compared to 20 times for the rest of the body.

Macula and photoreceptors start to develop: development is not completed before birth and lasts for several postnatal months (Lecanuet & Schaal 1996). In early development the eyes are placed laterally in the face like in animals with panoramic vision. With advancing gestational age they migrate towards the midline, creating favorable conditions for the development of stereoscopic vision. Birnholz first reported prenatal ocular structures during the second and third trimester as seen by ultrasound already in the 1980s (Birnholz 1985). Even at that time, the globe, lens, iris, pupil and cornea could be distinguished separately, and extraocular structures including muscles, retro-orbital fat and optic nerve were visualized as well. The hyaloid artery was seen before 20 weeks regressing by 25 weeks gestational age. Average vitreous diameter in 157 normal cases exhibited accelerated growth between 12 and 20 weeks, between 28 and 32 weeks, and near term. Associations between limited ocular growth and delayed cerebral development were reaffirmed (Birnholz 1985).

At present, 3D techniques help us not only to visualize the ocular structures by using different sections and planes (Fig. 8.1) but even to visualize internal pathways such as the chiasma opticum, as described previously (Bault 2006) (Fig. 8.5).

IMMEDIATE PRENATAL AND POSTNATAL VISUAL RESPONSIVENESS

More than sound, light is attenuated by the maternal abdomen. Transmission of external light was detected to be around only 2% at 550 nm and to reach 10% at around 650 nm (Lecanuet & Schaal 1996). In addition, the fetal position might allow not even a limited portion of light to reach the fetal retina. The restricted and irregular visual input impairs studies about behavioral responses to light in utero. Nevertheless, prenatal responses have been reported from 25 weeks onwards (Birnholz 1985).

We have observed movements of the eyeballs ('twinkling') by ultrasound as well as reactions of FHR and FM towards stimulation with flash light from 28 weeks onwards. These reactions were comparable to behavioral patterns seen during VAS. However, probably due to the described problems, reactions of FHR-FM patterns were registered in only about 10% of the tested fetuses. Stimulations with light which was introduced directly into the uterine cavity during amnioscopy were more successful (Lecanuet & Schaal 1996).

After delivery, the newborn is suddenly exposed to light but we do not know how this sudden impression is experienced. Recordings of visual responses based on compound potentials can be applied in preterm newborns such as the *electroretinogram* (ERG) or the *visual evoked potential* (VEP). The latter can be elicited even at 23 weeks. With increasing age, the latency of the response signal decreases and its morphology gets more complex, indicating visual pathway maturation (Fielder & Moseley 1998). *Behavioral tests* such as the blink response and the registration of awareness and fixation have been introduced. Dubowitz and Dubowitz used the ability of the preterm infant to focus, to follow and to track in order to draw conclusions about the integrity of the nervous system and about the developing visual system. They also observed that newborns frequently do not open their eyes in the presence of strong lighting (Dubowitz & Dubowitz 1981).

Further studies have all used *preferential looking* (PL)-based tests of visual. Although the visual development of preterm infants at different gestational ages lags behind that of term infant, both groups behave similarly when corrected for the degree acuity measurement of prematurity. Preterms sometimes even exhibit a slightly more rapid development than term infants (Fielder & Moseley 1998). However, overall around 50% of very low birth weight infants show visual impairments across a range of functions later in life (Groenendaal et al 1989). The highest incidence was found at 6 months. Beyond this age less deficit is observed, suggesting a delayed rather than a permanently impaired visual development. Visual abnormality is frequently related to neurologic impairment suggesting that the abnormality is of cerebral rather than of ophthalmological origin. Still, given time these infants may show improvement of visual functions thanks to neural plasticity.

POSSIBLE DAMAGE DURING AND AFTER PREGNANCY

The very small premature infant spends the first weeks in an excessively illuminated environment. Exposure to light has been demonstrated to cause retinal damage in animals at intensities encountered at neonatal intensive care units. It is an intriguing question whether this can be extrapolated to humans. Light is transmitted through the human eyelid at a rate of 1–10%, particularly at the red end of the spectrum (Fielder & Moseley 1998). The pupils are relatively large and react poorly to light in premature infants. Finally, retinal anti-oxidant defenses are relatively immature and may be overcome by increased oxygen concentrations during unfavorable lighting conditions. There is a trend towards lowering NICU lighting, both to prevent excessive exposure to light and to enhance sleep–wake cycling in the neonates who are being cared for.

At present, retinopathy is the most common ocular disease being characterized by abnormal proliferation of the immature retina which can progress to retinal scarring and visual handicap up to blindness (summary in: Baerts & Fetter 1998, Fielder & Moseley 1998).

CONCLUSIONS

The long history of denial and the short history of research relating to prenatal perception and the implications for future life highlight our ignorance towards early sensory development. An increasing number of data demonstrates that learning abilities of the newborn organism reflect continuity from pre- to postnatal life. It can be estimated that the neonatal brain and sensory system are as competent to extract and memorize features of external stimuli as those of the fetus of the corresponding gestational age. The fetus transits from the womb to the parent's arms or the neonatal care unit. It has been shown that the newborn remains retrospectively attentive to in utero stimuli such as rhythmic noise or odor of the AF, while the prenate is prospectively responsive to stimuli of the postnatal environment, such as the maternal voice or milk. Encoded qualities of the intrauterine environment are memorized and do have an impact on postnatal behavior. Nevertheless, premature infants are not only characterized by adaptive problems of their essential organ systems, they also face disrupted perceptional and cognitive processes.

Research about programming, in the sense of pre-adapting the fetus to features of the postnatal environment through specific maternal diets or lifestyles, has until now mainly concentrated on the fetal vegetative, cardiovascular and endocrine systems and not so much on the fetal sensory system.

During the preparation of this chapter it became evident that the first steps on the road to evaluating prenatal sensory development in humans were based on small studies with incidental character, if not a certain kind of pioneer initiative. The stimuli chosen for eliciting some kind of behavioral reactions were frequently unnatural (e.g. needles in aborted fetuses for sensory stimulation, car horns, vibroacoustic stimuli or bicycle bells at the maternal abdomen for acoustic stimulation, or mineral and aniseed oil or non-ionic acid for olfactory stimulation) and far above the normal thresholds. The aim of these stimulations was more or less to observe at least some kind of fetal or neonatal reaction, not to create a sensory environment for fetal wellbeing. In time, the studies became more subtle including more gentle and natural stimuli.

Nowadays, 'instruction programs' for parents have emerged even before basic research has proven that the stimuli might enhance postnatal cognitive functioning and neuromotor development. Since it has been established that most functions of the central nervous system follow their own maturational track (Miller 1994, Prechtl 1984), it can be doubted that sensory stimulation may enhance physiological ripening at such an early stage. From all studies cited in this article it seems that the influence of sensory stimulation on postnatal behavior and health, such as showing more stable rhythms or being more easily comforted, is mainly based on creating an environment for the start of a caring interactive relationship (Lind 1980).

Better documentation is needed of the ability of the fetus and premature baby to recognize stimuli as a function of age and functional status of the sensory system and how we might provide a rationale to use touch, sounds, or odors in the environmental or psychobiological therapy. Not just the use of modern technology to gain an understanding of pathophysiological processes and to create stimulative interventions, but even more importantly, our own respect and awareness towards the unborn and newborn infant are prerequisites to discover that this topic represents a wealth for ongoing and future research. Early capability reflects the complex neurological development and thus one of the most important objectives of perinatal care.

It is our responsibility to avoid unnecessary stress for the fetus and newborn from overstimulation by unnatural exposure to skin stimulation, light, sound, odor or taste and to treat pain as effectively as we do in adult patients.

However, health is understood as the physical, mental and social wellbeing that goes much further than just the absence of suffering or illness. As important as it is to teach children abilities at certain times, it might also be useful to create integrated stimulations for the unborn or newborn in order to enhance development or prevent sensory retardation. This should be a matter of concern of public health projects. Encouragement and avoidance of abnormal stimuli have to be considered and balanced in observational or interventional projects that are tailored to critical phases of development. Whether we go so far as to establish prenatal universities is of secondary importance, as long as we strive to understand the physiology and pathophysiology of early sensory development and to create designs suitable to induce a comprehensive expression of all our genetic potential.

ACKNOWLEDGEMENTS

The author thanks the neonatologist Dr. Wim Baerts for revising the manuscript.

REFERENCES

Anand K J, Aranda J V, Berde C B et al 2006 Summary proceedings from the neonatal pain-control group. Pediatr 117(3 Pt 2):S9–S22.

Anand K J, Hickey P R 1987 Pain and its effects in the human neonate and fetus. N Engl J Med 317(21):1321–1329.

Andonotopo W, Medic M, Salihagic-Kadic A et al 2005 The assessment of fetal behavior in early pregnancy: comparison between 2D and 4D sonographic scanning. J Perinat Med 33(5):406–414.

Anson B J, Winch T R 1974 Vascular channels in the auditory ossicles in man. Ann Otol Rhinol Laryngol 83(2):142–158.

Antoshechkin A G, Golovkin A B, Maximova L A et al 1989 Screening of amniotic fluid metabolites by gas chromatography-mass spectrometry. J Chromatogr 489(2):353–358.

Arabin B 2002 Music during pregnancy. Ultrasound Obstet Gynecol 20(5):425–430.

Arabin B, Riedewald S, Zacharias C et al 1988 Quantitative analysis of fetal behavioural patterns with real-time sonography and the actocardiograph. Gynecol Obstet Invest 26(3):211–218.

Arabin B, Becker B, Becker R et al 1993 Prediction of fetal distress and poor outcome in intrauterine growth retardation — a comparison of fetal heart rate monitoring combined with stress tests and Doppler ultrasound. Fetal Diagn Ther 8(4):234–240.

Arabin B, Becker R, Mohnhaupt A et al 1994 Prediction of fetal distress and poor outcome in prolonged pregnancy using Doppler ultrasound and fetal heart rate monitoring combined with stress tests (II) Fetal Diagn Ther 9(1):1–6.

Arabin B, Bos R, Rijlaarsdam R et al 1996 The onset of inter-human contacts: longitudinal ultrasound observations in early twin pregnancies. Ultrasound Obstet Gynecol 8(3):166–173.

Arabin B, v Straaten I 2006 Fetal and neonatal hearing. In: Karijak A, Chervenak T A (eds) Textbook of Perinatal Medicine. Wiley London, pp. 953–970.

Arabin B, Riedewald S 1992 An attempt to quantify characteristics of behavioral states. Am J Perinatol 9(2):115–119.

Armitage S E, Baldwin B A, Vince M A 1980 The fetal sound environment of sheep. Science 208(4448):1173–1174.

Arulkumaran S, Skurr B, Tong H et al 1991 No evidence of hearing loss due to fetal acoustic stimulation test. Obstet Gynecol 78(2):283–285.

Badalian S S, Chao C R, Fox H E et al 1993 Fetal breathing-related nasal fluid flow velocity in uncomplicated pregnancies. Am J Obstet Gynecol 169(3):563–567.

Baerts W, Fetter W 1998 Retinopathy of prematurity. In: Kurjak A (ed.) Textbook of perinatal medicine. Parthenon: London, pp. 129–140.

Barden T P, Peltzman P, Graham J T 1968 Human fetal electroencephalographic response to intrauterine acoustic signals. Am J Obstet Gynecol 100(8):1128–1134.

Bartocci M, Bergqvist L L, Lagercrantz H et al 2006 Pain activates cortical areas in the preterm newborn brain. Pain 122(1–2):109–117.

Bault J P 2006 Visualization of the fetal optic chiasma using three-dimensional ultrasound imaging. Ultrasound Obstet Gynecol 28(6):862–864.

Beauchamp G, Mennella J 1998 Sensitive periods in the development of human flavor perception and preference. Annales Nestle 56:19–31.

Bekesy G v 1960 Experiments in hearing. In: Ward EG (eds) McGraw Hill Series in Psychology. McGraw Hill, New York, pp. 745–755.

Bench J 1968 Sound transmission to the human foetus through the maternal abdominal wall. J Genet Psychol 113(1st Half):85–87.

Bhattacharya N, Chhetri M K, Mukherjee K L et al 2002 Human fetal adrenal transplant: a possible role in relieving intractable pain in advanced rheumatoid arthritis. Clin Exp Obstet Gynecol 29(3):197–206.

Bingham P M, Abassi S, Sivieri E 2003 A pilot study of milk odor effect on nonnutritive sucking by premature newborns. Arch Pediatr Adolesc Med 157(1):72–75.

Birnholz J C 1983 The fetal external ear. Radiology 147(3):819–821.

Birnholz J C 1985 Ultrasonic fetal ophthalmology. Early Hum Dev 12(2):199–209.

Blum T, Bauer R, Arabin B et al 1987 Prenatally recorded auditory evoked neuro-magnetic fields of the human fetus. I. In: Barber C, Blum T (eds) Evoked potentials III. Butterworth: Boston, pp. 136–142.

Blum T, Saling E, Bauer R 1985 First magnetoencephalographic recordings of the brain activity of a human fetus. Br J Obstet Gynaecol 92(12):1224–1229.

Brazelton T, Nugent K 1995 Neonatal behavioral assessment scale. 3rd ed. Cambridge University Press, Cambridge.

Capponi A, Rizzo G, Rinaldo D et al 1996 The effects of fetal blood sampling and placental puncture on umbilical artery and fetal arterial vessels blood flow velocity waveforms. Am J Perinatol 13(3):185–190.

Caspar A D, Sigafoos A 1983 The intrauterine heartbeat: A potent reinforcer. Inf Beh Dev 6:19–23.

Ceponiene R, Kushnerenko E, Fellman V et al 2002 Event-related potential features indexing central auditory discrimination by newborns. Brain Res Cogn Brain Res 13(1):101–113.

Chayen B, Tejani N, Verma U L et al 1986 Fetal heart rate changes and uterine activity during coitus. Acta Obstet Gynecol Scand 65(8):853–855.

Chen D, Huang Y, Zhang J et al 1994 Influence of prenatal music- and touch-enrichment on the IQ, motor development and behavior of infants. Chin J Psychol 8:148–151.

Cheour M, Ceponiene R, Leppanen P et al 2002 The auditory sensory memory trace decays rapidly in newborns. Scand J Psychol 43(1):33–39.

Chitkara U, Lee L, Oehlert L W et al 2002 Fetal ear length measurement: a useful predictor of aneuploidy? Ultrasound Obstet Gynecol 19(2):131–135.

Chitrit Y, Caubel P, Boulanger M C et al 1995 [Doppler velocimetry in the umbilical, middle cerebral and aortic arteries, before and after cordocentesis.] J Gynecol Obstet Biol Reprod (Paris) 24(5):516–521.

Chuah M I, Zheng D R 1987 Olfactory marker protein is present in olfactory receptor cells of human fetuses. Neuroscience 23(1):363–370.

Cicero S, Avgidou K, Rembouskos G et al 2006 Nasal bone in first-trimester screening for trisomy 21. Am J Obstet Gynecol 195(1):109–114.

Davis H 1965 A model for transducer action in the human cochlea. Cold Spring Harb Symp Quant Biol 181–193.

de Vries J I, Visser G H, Prechtl H F 1982 The emergence of fetal behaviour. I. Qualitative aspects. Early Hum Dev 7(4):301–322.

de Vries J I, Visser G H, Prechtl H F 1985 The emergence of fetal behaviour. II. Quantitative aspects. Early Hum Dev 12(2):99–120.

DeCasper A J, Fifer W P 1980 Of human bonding: newborns prefer their mothers' voices. Science 208(4448):1174–1176.

Devoe L D, Murray C, Faircloth D et al 1990 Vibroacoustic stimulation and fetal behavioral state in normal term human pregnancy. Am J Obstet Gynecol 163(4 Pt 1):1156–1161.

Dubowitz L, Dubowitz V, S 1981 The newborn assessment of the preterm and full-term newborn infant. In: Suffolk (ed) Clinics in developmental medicine. The Lavenham Press, London, pp. 48–50.

Edelman G M 2004 Biochemistry and the sciences of recognition. J Biol Chem 279(9):7361–7369.

Faas A E, Sponton E D, Moya P R et al 2000 Differential responsiveness to alcohol odor in human neonates: effects of maternal consumption during gestation. Alcohol 22(1):7–17.

Fielder A, Moseley M 1998 The immature visual syste and premature birth. In: Whitelaw A, Cooke R (eds)

The very immature infant less than 28 weeks gestation. Churchill Livingstone, London, pp. 1094–1118.

Fisk N M, Nicolaidis P K, Arulkumaran S et al 1991 Vibroacoustic stimulation is not associated with sudden fetal catecholamine release. Early Hum Dev 25(1):11–17.

Fitzgerald M, Shaw A, MacIntosh N 1988 Postnatal development of the cutaneous flexor reflex: comparative study of preterm infants and newborn rat pups. Dev Med Child Neurol 30(4):520–526.

Forbes H 1927 Fetal sense reaction: Hearing. Psychol 7:353–355.

Garcia A P, White-Traut R 1993 Preterm infants' responses to taste/smell and tactile stimulation during an apneic episode. J Pediatr Nurs 8(4):245–252.

Gaugler C, Messer J, Marlier L et al 2003 Olfaction in premature newborns: detection, discrimination and hedonic categorization. Biol Neonate 84:268.

Gesteland R C, Yancey R A, Farbman A I 1982 Development of olfactory receptor neuron selectivity in the rat fetus. Neuroscience 7(12):3127–3136.

Giannakoulopoulos X, Teixeira J, Fisk N et al 1999 Human fetal and maternal noradrenaline responses to invasive procedures. Pediatr Res 45(4 Pt 1):494–499.

Goldstein I, Makhoul I R, Nisman D et al 2003 Influence of maternal carbohydrate intake on fetal movements at 14 to 16 weeks of gestation. Prenat Diagn 23(2): 95–97.

Golubeva E L, Shuleikina K V, Vanshtein II 1959 [Development of reflex and spontaneous activity of the human fetus in the process of embryogenesis.]. Akush Ginekol (Mosk) 35(3):59–62.

Goubet N, Rattat C, Pierrat V et al 2002 Olfactory familiarization and discrimination in preterm and full-term newborns. Infancy 53–75.

Griffiths S K, Pierson L L, Gerharat K J et al 1994 Noise induced hearing loss in fetal sheep. Hear Res 74(1–2):221–230.

Groenendaal F, van Hofvan Duin J, Baerts W et al 1989 Effects of perinatal hypoxia on visual development during the first year of (corrected) age. Early Hum Dev 20(3–4):267–279.

Gynaecologists, Royal College of Obstetricians and 1997 Fetal awareness — report of a working party. RCOG, London.

Hecher K, Stettner H, Spernol R et al 1993 The effect of cordocentesis on umbilical and middle cerebral artery blood flow velocity waveforms. Br J Obstet Gynaecol 100(9):828–831.

Hepper P 1991 An examination of fetal learning before and after birth. Ir J Psychol 12:95–107.

Hepper P G, Shahidullah B S 1994 Development of fetal hearing. Arch Dis Child 71(2): F81–F87.

Hooker D 1952 The prenatal origin of behavior. Thesis. University of Kansas, Kansas.

Hrbek A, Karlberg P, Olsson T 1973 Development of visual and somatosensory evoked responses in pre-term newborn infants. Electroencephalogr Clin Neurophysiol 34(3):225–232.

Humphrey T 1978 Functions of the nervous system during prenatal life. In: Stave U (ed) Perinatal physiology. Plenum, New York, pp. 651–683.

James D K, Spencer C J, Stepsis B W 2002 Fetal learning: a prospective randomized controlled study. Ultrasound Obstet Gynecol 20(5):431–438.

Jeffrey W E, Cohen L S 1971 Habituation in the human infant. Adv Child Dev Behav 6:63–97.

Johnson J M, Benoit B, Pierre-Louis J et al 2005 Early prenatal diagnosis of oculoauriculofrontonasal syndrome by three-dimensional ultrasound. Ultrasound Obstet Gynecol 25(2):184–186.

Kenna M 1996 Embryology and developmental anatomy of the ear. In: Bluestone S S, Kenna CD (eds) Pediatric otolaryngology. Saunders, Philadelphia, pp. 113–126.

Klimach V J, Cooke R W 1988 Maturation of the neonatal somatosensory evoked response in preterm infants. Dev Med Child Neurol 30(2):208–214.

Koelsch S, Schroger E, Tervaniemi M et al 2000 Brain indices of music processing: 'nonmusicians' are musical. J Cogn Neurosci 12(3):520–541.

Koelsch S, Schroger E, Tervaniemi M 1999 Superior pre-attentive auditory processing in musicians. Neuroreport 10(6):1309–1313.

Kulakowskaia E 1929 Observations on the sense of taste and smell in newborns. Zh Izuch Rann Detsk Vospr Vorasta (Moskow) 9:15–20.

Kurjak A, Stanojevic M, Azumendi G et al 2005 The potential of four-dimensional (4D) ultrasonography in the assessment of fetal awareness. J Perinat Med 33(1):46–53.

Lamont A, Dibben N 2001 Motivic structure and the perception of similarity. Music Perception 18:145–174.

Lawrence J, Kay J, Murry S M 1993 The development of a tool to assess neonatal pain. Neonatal Network 12:59–66.

Leader R, Baillie P, Martin B et al 1982 The assessment and significance of habituation to a repeated stimulus by the human fetus. Early Hum Dev 7(3):211–219.

Lecaneaut J, Fifer W, Krasnegor N et al 1995 Fetal development: A psychobiological persepctive. Hillsdale, NJ: L.E. Ass.

Lecanuet J P, Schaal B 1996 Fetal sensory competencies Eur J Obstet Gynecol Reprod Biol 68(1–2):1–23.

Lettieri L, Rodis J F, Vintzileos A M et al 1993 Ear length in second-trimester aneuploid fetuses. Obstet Gynecol 81(1):57–60.

Lind J 1980 Music and the small human being. Acta Paediatr Scand 69(2):131–136.

Lloyd-Thomas, A R, Fitzgerald M 1996 Do fetuses feel pain? Reflex responses do not necessarily signify pain. BMJ 313(7060):797–798.

McCullagh P 1997 Do fetuses feel pain? Can fetal suffering be excluded beyond reasonable doubt? BMJ 314(7076):302–303.

Manrique B, Avarado M, Lerrobino M et al 1993 Nurturing parents to stimulate their children from prenatal stage to three years of age. In: Prenatal perception, learning and bonding. pp. 153–186.

Marlier L, Schaal B, Gaugler C et al 2001 Olfaction in premature human newborns; detection and discrimination abilities two months before birth. In: Marchelwska-Koj A, Lepri J, Schwarze D M (eds) Chemical signals in vertebrates. Klüwer Plenum, New York, pp. 205–209.

Marlier L, Schaal B, Soussignan R 1998 Bottle-fed neonates prefer an odor experienced in utero to an odor experienced postnatally in the feeding context. Dev Psychobiol 33(2):133–145.

Mennella J A, Jagnow C P, Beauchamp G K 2001 Prenatal and postnatal flavor learning by human infants. Pediatrics 107(6):E88.

Miller K D 1994 Models of activity-dependent neural development. Prog Brain Res 102:303–318.

Moss N, Carver D 1992 Pregnant women at work. Am J Indust Med 23:1–7.

Nyman M, Barr M, Westgren M 1992 A four-year follow-up of hearing and development in children exposed in utero to vibro-acoustic stimulation. Br J Obstet Gynaecol 99(8):685–688.

Peiper A 1925 Sinnesempfindungen der Kinder vor seiner Geburt. Monat Kinderheilk 29: 237–241.

Pierson L L 1996 Hazards of noise exposure on fetal hearing. Semin Perinatol 20(1):21–29.

Pietrantoni M, Angel J L, Parsons M T et al 1991 Human fetal response to vibroacoustic stimulation as a function of stimulus duration. Obstet Gynecol 78(5 Pt 1):807–811.

Pihet S, Schaal B, Bullinger A et al 1996 An investigation of olfactory responsiveness in premature newborns. Infant Behav Dev (676).

Pihet S, Mellier D, Bullinger A et al 1997 Responses comportementales aux odeurs chez le nouveau-né prémature; étude préliminaire. In: Schaal B (ed.) L 'odorat chez l' enfant: perspectives croisées. Presses Universitaire de France (Enfance), Paris, pp. 33–46.

Plotsky P, Bradley C, Anand K 2000 Behavioral and neuroendocrine consequences of neonatal stress. In: Anand K J S, S B, McGrath P J (eds) Pain in neonates. Elsevier Science, Amsterdam, pp. 77–100.

Prechtl H 1984 Continuity and change in early neural development. In: Prechtl H F R (ed.) Continuity of neural functions from prenatal to postnatal life. Clinics in developmental medicine. Blackwell, Oxford, pp. 1–15.

Prechtl H F 1974 The behavioural states of the newborn infant (a review). Brain Res 76(2):185–212.

Preyer W, Spezielle 1885 Physiologie des embryo. Grieben, Leipzig.

Pyatkina G A 1982 Development of the olfactory epithelium in man. Z Mikrosk Anat Forsch 96(2):361–372.

Querleu D, Renard X, Versyp F et al 1988 [Intra-amniotic transmission of the human voice]. Rev Fr Gynecol Obstet 83(1):43–50.

Querleu D, Renard X, Boutteville C et al 1989 Hearing by the human fetus? Semin Perinatol 13(5):409–420.

Ramet J, Praud J P, D'Allest A M et al 1990 Trigeminal airstream stimulation. Maturation-related cardiac and respiratory responses during REM sleep in human infants. Chest 98(1):92–96.

Ray W 1932 A preliminary report on a study of fetal conditioning. Child Dev 3:175–177.

Richards D S, Frentzen B, Gerhardt F J et al 1992 Sound levels in the human uterus. Obstet Gynecol 80(2):186–190.

Romero R, Mazor M, Hobbins J C 1988 A critical appraisal of fetal acoustic stimulation as an antenatal test for fetal well-being. Obstet Gynecol 71(5):781–786.

Sakabe N, Arayama T, Suzuki T 1969 Human fetal evoked response to acoustic stimulation. Acta Otolaryngol Suppl 252:29–36.

Salk L 1961 Mothers' heartbeat as an imprinting stimulus. Trans New Acad Sci 24:753–763.

Sallenbach W 1991 A theoretical framework on prenatal cognition and bonding. Int J Prenat and Perinat Studies 3:173–181.

Sarnat H B 1978 Olfactory reflexes in the newborn infant. J Pediatr 92(4):624–626.

Schaal B, Hummel T, Soussignan R 2004 Olfaction in the fetal and premature infant: Functional status and clinical implications Clin Perinatol 31:261–285.

Schaal B, Marlier L, Soussignan R 1998 Olfactory function in the human fetus: evidence from selective neonatal responsiveness to the odor of amniotic fluid. Behav Neurosci 112(6):1438–1449.

Schaal B, Marlier L, Soussignan R 2000 Human foetuses learn odours from their pregnant mother's diet. Chem Senses 25(6):729–737.

Schaal B, Orgeur P 1992 Olfaction in utero: can the rodent model be generalized? Q J Exp Psychol B 44(3–4):245–278.

Schleussner E, Schneider U, Kausch S et al 2001 Fetal magnetoencephalography: a non-invasive method for the assessment of fetal neuronal maturation. BJOG 108(12):1291–1294.

Scibetta J J, Rosen M G, Hochberg C J et al 1971 Human fetal brain response to sound during labor. Am J Obstet Gynecol 109(1):82–85.

Seth A K, Baars B J, Edelman D B 2005 Criteria for consciousness in humans and other mammals. Conscious Cogn 14(1):119–139.

Shahidullah S, Hepper P G 1994 Frequency discrimination by the fetus. Early Hum Dev 36(1):13–26.

Slater R, Boyd S, Meek J et al 2006 Cortical pain responses in human infants. J Neurosci 26(14):3662–3666.

Smith C V, Phelan J P, Platt L D et al 1986 Fetal acoustic stimulation testing. II. A randomized clinical comparison with the nonstress test. Am J Obstet Gynecol 155(1):131–134.

Smotherman W P, Robinson S R 1990 Rat fetuses respond to chemical stimuli in gas phase. Physiol Behav 47(5):863–868.

Spence M, Caspar A d 1987 Prenatal experience with low-frequency maternal voice sounds influence neonatal perception of maternal voice samples. Infant Behav Dev 10:133–142.

Statement Joint Committee on Infant Hearing Position 1982 ASHA 24:1017.

Stirnimann F 1936 Versuche über Geschmack und Geruch am ersten Lebenstag. Jahrb Kinderhk 146:211–227.

Teixeira J, Fogliani R, Giannakoulopoulos X et al 1996 Fetal haemodynamic stress response to invasive procedures. Lancet 347(9001):624.

Tuber D S, Berntson G G, Bachman D S et al 1980 Associative learning in premature hydranencephalic and normal twins. Science 210(4473):1035–1037.

Van den Bergh B R, Mulder E J, Visser G H et al 1989 The effect of (induced) maternal emotions on fetal behaviour: a controlled study. Early Hum Dev 19(1):9–19.

Van den Bergh B R, Mulder E J, Mennes M et al 2005 Antenatal maternal anxiety and stress and the neurobehavioural development of the fetus and child: links and possible mechanisms. A review. Neurosci Biobehav Rev 29(2):237–258.

van Heteren C F, Boekkooi P F, Jongsma H W et al 2001 Fetal habituation to vibroacoustic stimulation in relation to fetal states and fetal heart rate parameters. Early Hum Dev 61(2):135–145.

Van Leeuwen P, Geue D, Lange S et al 2003 Is there evidence of fetal-maternal heart rate synchronization? BMC Physiol. 3:2.

van Lingen R A, Quak C M, Deinum H T et al 2001 Effects of rectally administered paracetamol on infants delivered by vacuum extraction. Eur J Obstet Gynecol Reprod Biol 94(1):73–78.

van Lingen R A, Simons S H, Anderson B J et al 2002 The effects of analgesia in the vulnerable infant during the perinatal period. Clin Perinatol 29(3):511–534.

Winberg J, Porter R H 1998 Olfaction and human neonatal behaviour: Clinical implications. Acta Paediatr 87(1):6–10.

Woodward S C, Guidozzi F 1992 Intrauterine rhythm and blues? Br J Obstet Gynaecol 99(10):787–789.

Zimmer E Z, Divon M Y, Vilensky A et al 1982 Maternal exposure to music and fetal activity. Eur J Obstet Gynecol Reprod Biol 13(4):209–213.

Zimmer E Z, Fifer W P, Kim Y I et al 1993 Response of the premature fetus to stimulation by speech sounds. Early Hum Dev 33(3):207–215.

Zimmer E Z, Talmon R, Makler-Shiran E et al 1996 Effect of vibroacoustic stimulation on fetal meconium passage in labor. Am J Perinatol 13(2):81–83.

CHAPTER

9

Clinical assessment of the infant nervous system

Claudine Amiel-Tison and Julie Gosselin

Key Points

- A basic understanding of the chronology and direction of maturation in brainstem versus cerebral hemispheres provides helpful clinical markers when assessing the infant nervous system
- Palpation of each cranial suture is an integral part of neurological assessment, overlapping or distention often being more contributory than head circumference (HC) values alone
- Repeated assessments within the first week of life in a full-term neonate may provide the best diagnostic clues: a changing profile in the case of intrapartum insult, an unchanging profile in the case of antenatal insult
- Choice of one type of assessment over another will depend on clinical or research goals; the selected instrument should then be used as described in the literature. Temptation for short versions should be resisted
- The clinician will process in two phases: the analytic part and the synthesis, according to clinical context or circumstances. Computerization of individual items may be grossly misleading
- Preventive postural management is essential in the neonatal intensive care unit (NICU): if neglected, muscle shortening and osteocartilaginous deformities will soon occur and can be misleading in the interpretation of findings

---

INTRODUCTION

Many new technologies are aimed at documenting early central nervous system (CNS) functions. However, clinical assessment remains central to all investigations for the day-to-day medical care of the premature or sick newborn infant. Different clinical assessments are available to the pediatrician, meeting the needs for routine or research. Most have been updated in recent years and reviewed in a special issue of Mental Retardation and Developmental Disabilities Research Reviews (Allen & Lipkin 2005). We provide here a thorough description of an approach that has revealed itself to be useful not only in the neonatal period but also in the follow-up of high-risk populations.

VARIOUS ORIGINS, VARIOUS INSTRUMENTS

HISTORY OF VARIOUS TRENDS

For decades, advances in perinatology were measured by infant survival rates. By the 1950s and early 1960s, clinicians were focusing their attention on the function of the CNS in the neonatal period. These pioneers included André-Thomas and Saint-Anne Dargassies in Paris (André-Thomas & Saint-Anne-Dargassies 1952, André-Thomas et al 1960), Peiper (1963) in Leipzig, Prechtl and Beintema (1964) in Groningen. Each developed a type of assessment based on their own scientific expertise: neurology for André-Thomas, pediatrics for Peiper, ethology for Prechtl. Neonatologists, however, were unable to fully incorporate these clinical methods of assessment into their routine practice because of certain practice limitations. There was already too much physical handling of sick neonates while physicians were busy with new priorities and had less time for clinical assessment. Moreover, most pediatricians lacked the self-confidence to apply methods that they considered exceedingly complex.

Later, in the 1970s and 1980s, progressive sophistication of perinatal care restricted the clinician's access to the neonate even more. Concurrently, remarkable advances occurred in bedside brain imaging and electrophysiological techniques whose availability drove physicians to rely only on brain imaging and other investigations rather than clinical assessment. This tendency is still apparent in recent literature in which radiologists and neurophysiologists compete in the early prediction of adverse late outcome. Clinicians, however, became aware of the importance of behavioral organization of the neonate as well as interactions between neonates and their caregivers. Their behavioral studies have enriched the field of neonatal neurology.

In the 1980s, clinical evaluation in the neonatal intensive care unit (NICU) improved due to (1) a better understanding of the anatomical and physiological correlates of early neurological development, as reviewed by Sarnat (1984); (2) increased precision in research design when perinatal epidemiologists became more effective partners in the NICU. By the 1990s, with the extension of intensive care to extremely low-birth-weight (ELBW) infants, handling was replaced by observation in the NCIU.

VARIOUS INSTRUMENTS

Along with the remarkable improvement of survival of very low-birth-weight (VLBW) group of infants, three main streams for assessing the wellbeing of survivors flourished: (1) the French school, with an emphasis on tone assessment by the followers of André-Thomas; (2) the Boston school, with an emphasis on behavior and interaction by Brazelton and his followers; and (3) the Groningen school, with its emphasis on observation of spontaneous movements by Prechtl and his followers. The main characteristics and recent references are presented in Table 9.1.

The choice of assessment tool varies according to the targeted population of neonates, the clinical or research goals

Table 9.1 Major neurodevelopmental assessments for the young infant

Characteristics and domains	Als assessment of preterm infants' behavior (APIB)[a]	Amiel-Tison neurological assessment at term (ATNAT)[b]	Brazelton neonatal behavioral assessment scale (NBAS)[c]	Dubowitz neurological examination of the full-term newborn[d]	Prechtl assessment of general movements (AGM)[e]
Age range	Birth to 4 PTWs	38–42 GW	Full-term: birth to 8 PTWs; Preterm at 40 GW		From birth to 16–20 PTWs
Time to administer/ Time to score (min)	60/30–45	5/5	20–30/15	10/15	30–60 in preterm and 5–10 m in full-term/3–10 m
Number of primary reflexes tested	16	5	16	5	—
Muscle tone Limbs Axis	General/predominant tone, recoil Pull-to-sit	Popliteal, scarf, recoil Flexors and extensors	General/predominant tone, recoil Pull-to-sit	Posture, leg-arm traction/ recoil, popliteal angles Head control and lag, ventral suspension	—
Motor activity (motility)	Motor maturation. Qualitative and quantitative aspects; cuddliness, startles	Righting reaction, raise to sit, spontaneous motor activity. spontaneous thumb abduction	Motor maturation. Qualitative and quantitative aspects; cuddliness. startles	Quantity and quality of mvts, hand/toe postures, tremors, startle	Preterm general mvts, writhing mvts and fidgety (continual, intermittent and sporadic) mvts
Behavioral states/alertness	Alertness, lability of states, supplementary items*	Social interactions. crying	Alertness, lability of states, supplementary items*	Eye mvts and cry	—
Regulation	Consolability, peak of excitement, rapidity of build-up. irritability. activity. skin color. lability, self-quieting. hand-to-mouth. defensive mvts. tremulousness. startle. smiles	Excitability, adaptability	Consolability, peak of excitement, rapidity of build-up. irritability. activity. skin color. lability, self-quieting. hand-to-mouth. defensive mvts. tremulousness. startle. smiles	Irritability, consolability	—
Habituation/orientation	Habituation/orientation: visual, auditory and mixt (inanimate–animate)	Fix and track, response to voice	Habituation/orientation: visual, auditory and mixt (inanimate–animate)	Auditory and visual orientation	—
Cranial examination	—	Head circumference, sutures and fontanels	—	—	—
Required training	Certification	No formal training	Certification	No formal training	Certification

*supplementary items: these items overlap both behavioral states/alertness and regulation domain
[a]Als et al 1982
[b]Amiel-Tison 2001
[c]Brazelton 1972
[d]Dubowitz et al 1999
[e]Einspieler et al 1964

as well as national tendencies. Whatever the selected method, the clinician needs to:

1. *learn the clinical method of conducting a basic neurological assessment,* by practicing according to a precise description of each observation and manipulation with didactic support;
2. *interpret the findings,* according to the conceptual framework of the assessment;
3. *reach a clinical judgment,* based on repeated assessments and integration of step-by-step interpretation of the findings as well as results from complementary investigations.

Instead of attempting to briefly review each assessment tool, we chose to fully describe the conceptual framework and the method based on the French school legacy. In addition to its multi-domain character, this method has the advantage of not being restricted to the term period (Amiel-Tison 2002, Gosselin et al 2005). As part of a series of three instruments, it allows assessment from 32 weeks gestation (Amiel-Tison 1968, 2001) to 6 years of age (Amiel-Tison & Gosselin 2001, Gosselin & Amiel-Tison 2007).

EARLY CNS FUNCTIONS: CONCEPTUAL FRAMEWORK

FOCUS ON MOTOR CONTROL

Two systems of motor control

In order to recognize normal or abnormal neurological function, the clinician needs a basic understanding of the motor pathways, the timing and direction of their myelination as well as their role in determining motor patterns (Sarnat 1984, 1989, 2003). There are two major motor pathways: (1) the earlier (subcorticospinal) pathways (Fig. 9.1) derive from the reticular formation, vestibular nuclei and tectum; (2) the later (corticospinal) pathways originate in the motor and premotor cortex. The major component of the corticospinal pathways is the pyramidal tract, which crosses to the opposite side of the brain in the medulla. Basal ganglia are also functionally linked to this corticospinal system. The subcorticospinal pathways (brainstem) will be referred to as the 'lower motor system' and the corticospinal pathways (cerebral hemispheres) as the 'upper motor system'.

Distinct timing and direction of myelination

Myelin is easily visible and therefore used as an approximate indicator of maturation of these neuromotor pathways. In the lower motor system, myelination takes place and is completed during fetal life (between 24 and 34 weeks) and proceeds in an upward direction, from the spinal cord (Fig. 9.1). In the upper system, myelination starts later, at 32 weeks of gestation, and proceeds downward to the spinal cord, rapidly in the first 2 years of life and more slowly up to the age of 12.

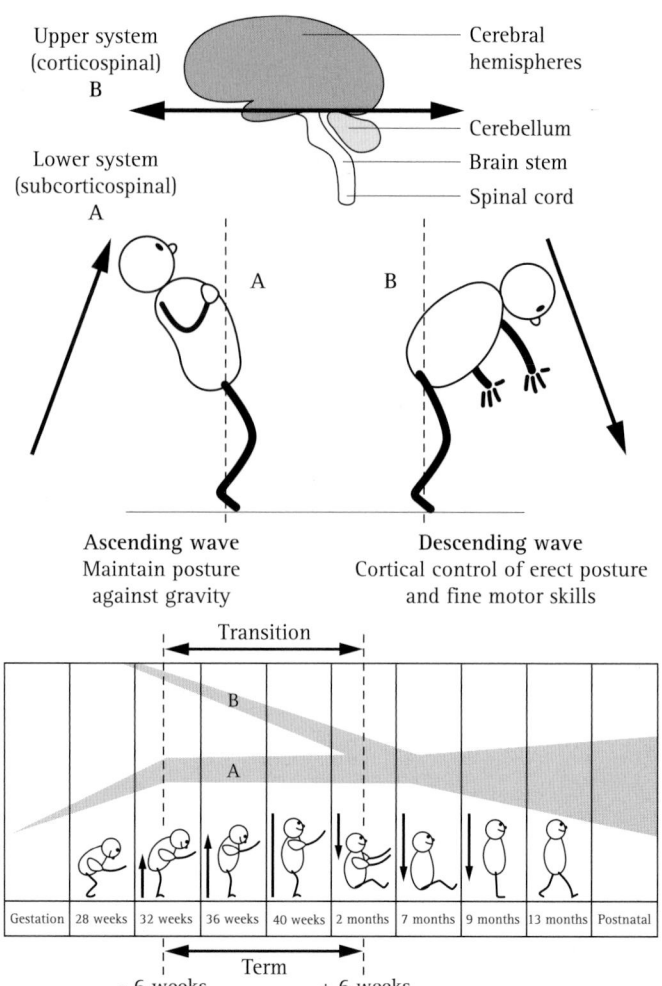

Figure 9.1 Maturation in motor control from fetal life through infancy. The subcortical pathways (lower system or extrapyramidal) derive from the brain stem with myelination taking place between 24 and 32 weeks of gestation and proceeding upward, starting in the spinal cord. Their essential role is to maintain posture against gravity. The corticospinal pathways (upper system or pyramidal) originate in cerebral hemispheres. Their myelination starts around 32 weeks of gestation, proceeds downward from the pons to the spinal cord, reaching completion at about 2 years of age. They are responsible for control of erect posture and for movements of the extremities including fine motor skills. From term onward, corticospinal control takes over, allowing development of mature head control, sitting and walking.

Distinct functions of the two motor systems

The lower (subcortical) system, which originates in the phylogenetically oldest cerebral structures, is mainly homolateral and has important connections with the cerebellum. Primary reflexes, righting reactions against gravity and flexor tone in the limbs are typically under the control of this lower motor system (Fig. 9.1). Phylogenetically speaking, the upper (corticospinal) system is a more recently developed structure. Erect posture, relaxation of flexor tone in limbs allowing fine motor skills, and integration of primary reflexes are typically under the control of this upper motor system. Intactness of both motor systems is essential for optimal neurological maturation. As an example, during fetal life, primary reflexes are mediated at the spinal cord and brain stem level; however, in the first months postnatally, they are progressively inhibited with the maturation of the upper motor system. They will persist in cases of severe damage to the latter.

CLINICAL RELEVANCY

The distinction between upper and lower motor systems became even more relevant after pathological and imaging data showed that brain damage in the neonate is located mainly in the cerebral hemispheres in the full-term with hypoxic–ischemic encephalopathy (HIE) or in the preterm with periventricular leukomalacia (PVL). Consequently, the best predictors of injury should be found in responses that depend on the upper motor system and not in responses that depend mainly on brain stem activity. These considerations have been the driving force for successive modifications of the clinical assessment at term. More emphasis has been placed on signs that depend on the integrity of the upper structures, such as axial tone and alertness, as well as cranial signs reflecting cerebral hemispheric atrophy. The signs depending on brain stem function, such as primary reflexes and passive tone in limb flexor muscles, have been de-emphasized at the neonatal period as they do not provide information about the cerebral hemispheres and basal ganglia.

METHODOLOGICAL REPERTOIRE FOR A BASIC NEUROLOGICAL ASSESSMENT

TEST PROCEDURE

In the following description of each observation and maneuver, the convention adopted is that 'typical' refers to the response expected at full-term (40 weeks). The examination usually evolves from observation to manipulation, more and more activity being demanded from the infant as the examination progresses. In individual cases, this sequence may need to be changed, depending on the infant's state of arousal. When a poor response to some procedure is obtained, it should be repeated and the best response selected. The assessment takes about 5 minutes to complete; no specific order is required. The transmission of manual skills has been facilitated by videotape (Amiel-Tison & Lafaurie-Levêque 2000).

ALERTNESS AND SLEEP

Observation of state

The most favorable time for a neurological examination is when the infant is quiet but alert, having wakened spontaneously from a 2-hour sleep after a feed. However, it is often difficult to choose such a favorable moment and the clinician is faced with waking a sleeping baby or quieting a disturbed one in the hope of obtaining a few minutes of quiet alertness. It is important that the alertness level be specified, because this information is required both for interpretation of the neurological examination and for assessment of the infant's clinical status. For these purposes, it is customary to use the following scale (Prechtl & Beintema 1964).

State 1: eyes closed, regular respiration, no movements.
State 2: eyes closed, irregular respiration, no gross movements.
State 3: eyes open, no gross movements.
State 4: eyes open, gross movements, no crying.
State 5: eyes open or closed, crying.

It is only when a few minutes of state 3 can be obtained that the neurological examination can be completed and the infant shown to be normal. The pattern of sleep and wakefulness should be noted. In term infants, it starts with periods of sleep lasting about 50 minutes and of wakefulness lasting about 10 minutes. These periods gradually lengthen during the neonatal period to 2 hours of sleep and 20–30 minutes of wakefulness.

Hyperexcitability and lethargy

If states 4 and 5 predominate with no period of quiet alertness, it may be because the infant is abnormally hyperexcitable. This conclusion is supported by the presence of tremulous movements, a high-pitched cry and a record of inadequate sleep. In contrast, if state 2 predominates and no contact can be established with the infant despite several attempts, the infant can be considered to be abnormally lethargic. When state 1 is persistent, the level is further specified by noting the presence or absence of response to vigorous stimuli.

Crying pattern

The infant's crying pattern may provide diagnostic clues. Short bursts of a high-pitched cry are characteristic of meningitis or birth asphyxia. An incessant high-pitched cry is heard in the infant of the addicted mother. A cry that the infant cannot sustain, and that may be associated with tachypnea and cyanosis or pallor, may draw attention to an underlying cardiac or pulmonary disorder. The acoustic features of crying have been shown to vary with neuromaturational development.

VISUAL AND AUDITORY COMMUNICATION; CONSOLABILITY

Vision and hearing are dealt with elsewhere in this book (Chs 37 and 38). Here we are only concerned with communication involving these modalities.

Fix and track

It is easy to test 'fix and track' in a healthy full-term infant. When the baby is held at a distance of about 30 cm, an intense gaze appears to be fixed on the observer. This eye-to-eye contact is usually present soon after birth. However, when the infant is in an incubator, the best way to obtain a visual response is to use the 'bull's eye' (Daum et al 1980). This uses a round piece of cardboard printed with glossy black and white concentric circles (Fig. 9.2) which is held some 20–30 cm from the infant's face. When the infant has fixed his or her gaze on this target, it is moved to one side and then to the other. When the response is normal, eyes and then head follow movements of the card. The test is easy to perform and it is reproducible by different observers. Indeed, with this technique, visual fixation and following (track) can be detected from 34 weeks' gestation. It constitutes one of the best neurological tests at this early gestational age (GA), as it implies a state of quiet alertness.

Response to sound

Response to sound has been shown to be present from early in fetal life by observing a change in fetal heart rate in response to sound. After birth, a response to sound in the form of a facial grimace or turning of the head can be evoked by a voice, a bell or, with greater precision, an acoustic stimulator producing 'white' noise. It may be impossible to use the simple clinical form of testing responses to sound in the noisy conditions of a NICU.

Consolability

Consolability, which is defined by the response of the crying infant to voice or soothing, has been widely used as a test of communication (Brazelton 1973, Brazelton & Nugent 1995). With the infant supine and crying, soothing tactile stimuli are applied to the arms and chest. If this is not enough to quiet the infant, he or she is gently rocked to and

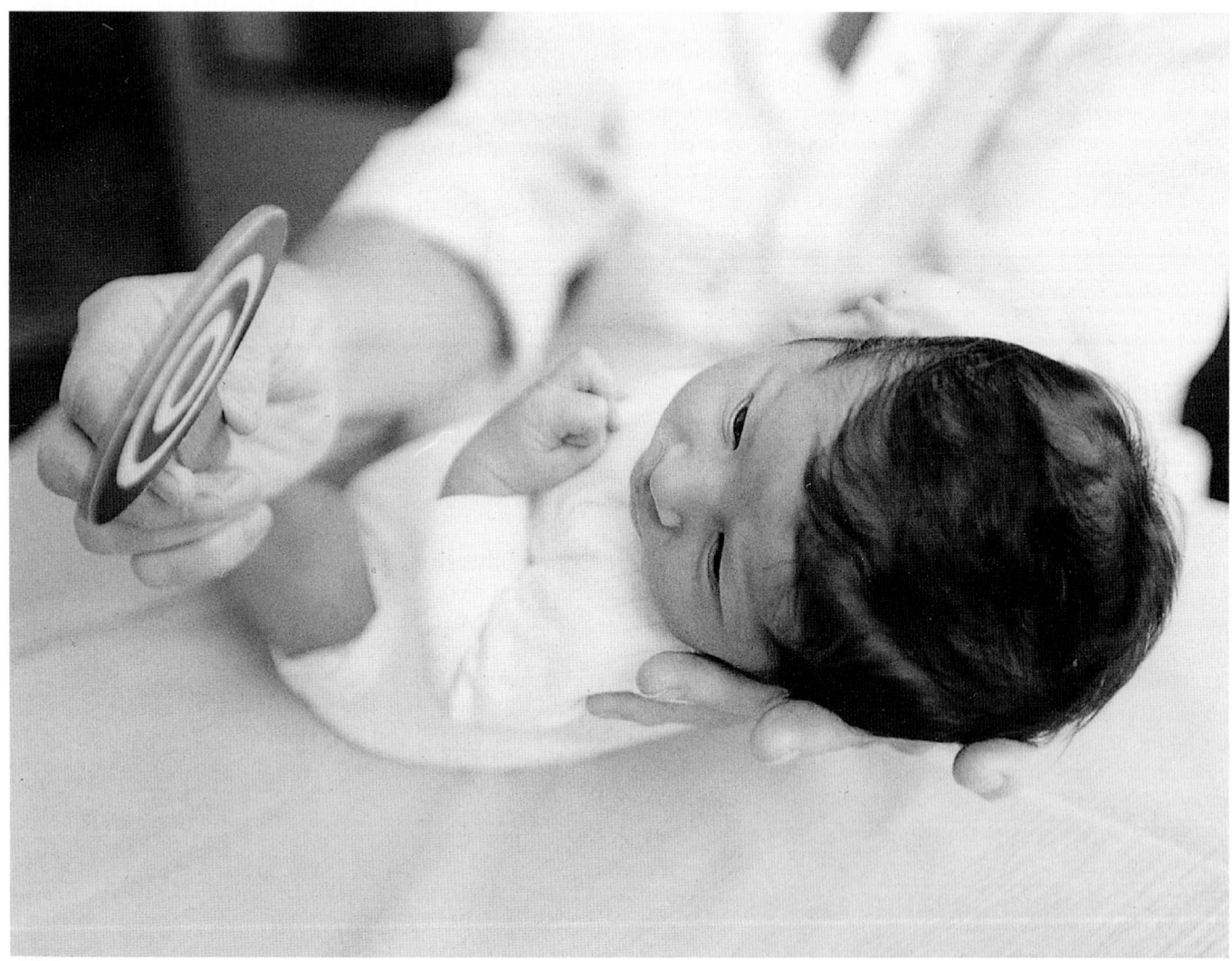

Figure 9.2 Testing for fixing and tracking with the 'bull's eye'. Note the testing position, head able to rotate on the examiner's hand.

fro, either in the supine or, preferably, the prone position. Consolability can be classified in three grades: (1) easily obtainable, (2) obtainable with difficulty within 1 min, or (3) unobtainable.

HEAD, FACE, CRANIAL NERVES

Head circumference

As the skull follows the volumetric increase of the cerebral hemispheres mostly by passive adaptation, the classic neurological assessment in infancy universally includes measurement of HC to qualify brain growth. Measurement of the maximum occipito-frontal circumference of the head provides a simple, reproducible measurement of head size. The use of paper tape measures has proven to be more reliable than cloth tape measures. In case of an extensive *caput succedaneum* at birth, a more valid measurement can be obtained after 3 days, when edema has subsided.

The numerical value of HC is reported on a normative curve, the most commonly used being Nelhaus's curve (Nelhaus 1968) (composite international and interracial graphs, with separate head growth curves for each sex). Various definitions of normal limits are found in the literature, as we reviewed elsewhere (Amiel-Tison et al 2002). Moreover an adjustment of the child head size value by the average parental value should be made in order to take into account the genetic programming of head growth (do not forget to measure maternal and paternal HC in maternity wards). There is no consensus concerning the use and value of head proportionality at birth (Amiel-Tison et al 2002). A symmetrical rate of head and body growth is often called proportionate, whereas an asymmetrical one is often called disproportionate. When disproportion is found, the pattern observed may provide etiological clues: for example, the *fetus araignée* (spider-like), characterized by a very large head in comparison to a slim, dehydrated body, may be encountered in the case of placental insufficiency. Such disproportionality (asymmetry) is believed to be the result of the brain-sparing effect. An asymmetry detrimental to HC is usually the result of fetal brain damage: hypoxic–ischemic, toxic, or resulting from viral infection. Despite the well-recognized interest in this identification of proportionate and disproportionate growth, a global appraisal (gestalt) approach is still commonly used in daily pediatric practice to relate head and body proportionality. Since the 1980s, different attempts have been made to replace the gestalt approach with a more rigorous one using different statistical models (Amiel-Tison et al 2002).

Cranial shape and sutures

Observation of cranial shape is also part of the neurological assessment. Primary craniosynostosis is due to impaired genetic programming of skull development; the abnormal shape depends on the suture or sutures involved, isolated or syndromic; this difficult topic is usually described in textbooks of genetics (Toriello 1993). Moreover, intrauterine compression is often responsible for cranial deformations (Graham 1988). The two most common examples are: (1) plagiocephaly (oblique shape), linked to an abnormal posture in utero and associated with congenital torticollis; (2) a flattened head, typical of breech pregnancies, due to molding of the cranial vault by uterus *fundus*, in the last months of fetal life.

The extreme variability of the anterior fontanel size limits its practical significance; clinical appreciation of the tension of the *dura* at this level is rarely contributory either. In our experience (Amiel-Tison et al 2002), clinical evaluation of cranial sutures provides more helpful complementary information about brain growth. The anatomy of skull bones and sutures is summarized in Figure 9.3. At an immature stage (fetal and neonatal), every suture is a 1–2 mm wide membranous zone, easily followed by palpation with the fingertip. Overlapping of sutures is felt as ridges and reinforces the suspicion of an insufficient brain growth based on a small HC. Contrarily, distension of sutures is felt as an excessive space between skull bones (5 mm or more) and reinforces the suspicion of increased intracranial pressure, even if the HC still is within normal range.

Several warning signs are worth mentioning to avoid pitfalls in the interpretation.

(1) Modifications in suture status are physiological after most cephalic deliveries; in the first hours of life, overlapping of every suture is observed, depending on the degree of intra-partum moulding. After 12 hours or so, some degree of distension, especially of the sagittal suture, is physiological, due to a mild degree of brain edema following any cephalic delivery. After 3 or 4 days, every suture is normally 'edge to edge'.

(2) Variations such as distension or overlapping can be induced by nutritional or hydration status; it is therefore mandatory to check the weight curve and to look for edema or signs of dehydration.

Systematic palpation of the temporo-parietal suture (or squamous) is particularly informative, due to its location between the cranial vault and cranial base; it resembles a bracket supporting the convex parietal bone (Fig. 9.4 part 1). When the parietal bone shifts upward, due to an increase in intracranial pressure, separation between the two edges will be felt (Fig. 9.4 part 2); when it shifts downward, due to insufficient hemispheric growth, the overlapping of the temporal bone forms a ridge (Fig. 9.4 part 3), the squamous ridge.

In conclusion, the crude information provided by HC measurement is essential but not sufficient to qualify brain growth. Significant information with respect to the integrity of the underlying cerebral hemispheres can be provided by systematic palpation of the main cranial sutures.

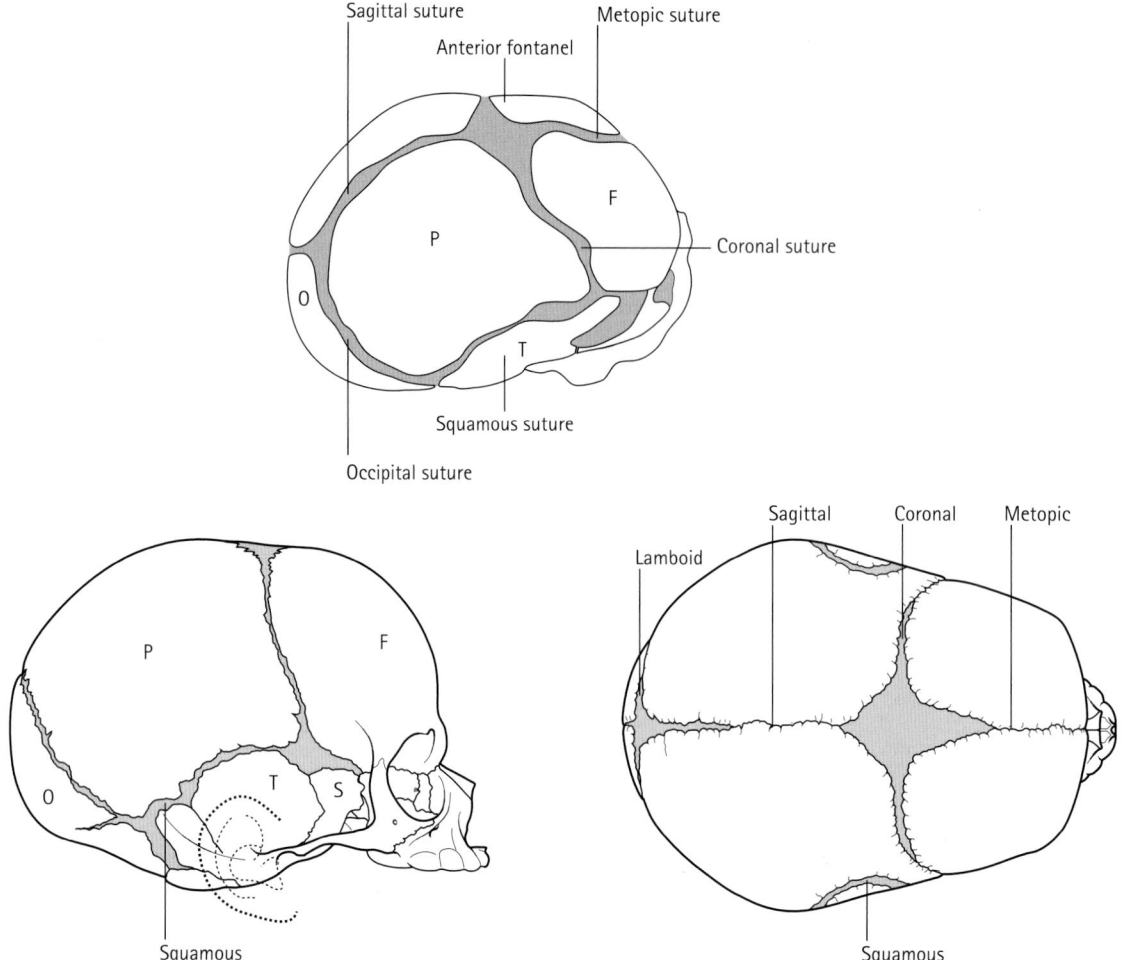

Figure 9.3 Skull bones, sutures and fontanels in fetus and neonate. Every suture is made of a 1 to 2 mm wide membranous zone. F: frontal bone, P: parietal bone, O: occipital bone, T: temporal bone. (With permission.)

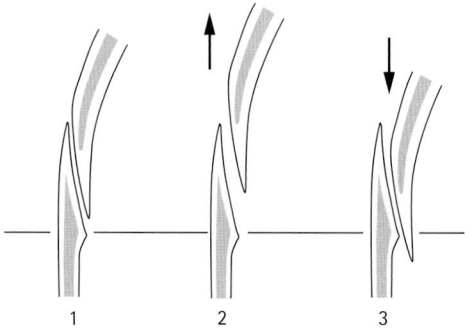

Figure 9.4 Junction between cranial vault and cranial base on a vertical section of squamous suture. (a) In normal situation, oblique edge of the temporal bone acts as a console, to sustain the parietal bone. (b) With increasing intracranial pressure, parietal edge slips upward and distension occurs between 2 edges. (c) With decreasing intracranial pressure, parietal bone slips downward and temporal edge becomes ridge-like.

Cephalhematoma and caput succedaneum

The presence of one or more cephalhematomas, which cause a fluctuant swelling due to subperiosteal bleeding limited at the suture lines, is certainly to be noted, but these lesions are quite common and are not an indication of significant trauma. A large caput succedaneum is of more significance. It consists of subcutaneous edema created by pressure at the circumference of the presenting part and is a sign of prolonged, mechanically difficult labor. Detection of its presence early in labor can be a warning sign to the obstetrician, and its localization after birth can provide a retrospective clue to the nature of a mechanical difficulty in labor. Unlike cephalhematoma, the presence of a large caput is linked statistically to abnormal neurological signs in the newborn infant (Amiel-Tison & Stewart 1994). Subgaleal hemorrhage is discussed on page 423.

Examination of the mouth and tongue

Examination of the mouth and tongue should be included in the neurological examination. A narrow, high-arched palate is a sign of abnormal motor function of the fetal tongue during a period of several weeks at least (it is the movements of tongue and oropharynx in swallowing that determine the growth and form of the fetal palate). Fasciculations of the tongue may be seen in spinal muscular atrophy (such as Werdnig–Hoffmann disease), which occasionally presents in the neonatal period. It also occurs in cases of 12th nerve damage and in some cases of hypoxic–ischemic brain injury. However, fasciculation, which is relatively rare, must be distinguished from tremulous tongue movements during crying. The latter movements are common and not abnormal. To be meaningful, fascicular movements have to be observed at rest and at the periphery of the tongue (Volpe 1995). If sucking is absent, it is important to test the gag reflex, which is done by stimulating the soft palate gently with a small spatula.

Cranial nerve examination

The infant of 28 weeks' gestation blinks when a bright light is shone into the eyes (cranial nerves II and VII). The term infant retains this reflex and, in addition, when alert may fixate on a face or large object and track it (cranial nerves II, III, IV and VI, see above). The pupillary reaction to light appears between 28 and 32 weeks of gestation (cranial nerves II and III). Funduscopic examination may reveal atrophy or hypoplasia of the optic disc or defects of the retina, indicating congenital malformations involving the optic nerve or retina. Retinitis may identify an intrauterine infection. Retinal hemorrhages are not uncommon in the neonate and do not necessarily indicate clinically significant intracranial hemorrhage. Disconjugate gaze is common in normal newborn infants when they are not fixating. The corneal reflex and withdrawal to pinprick on the face (cranial nerve V) are present in the term infant. The symmetry and amplitude of facial movements (cranial nerve VII) are observed during spontaneous and evoked facial movements, including crying (see below). Hearing (cranial nerve VIII) is assessed by eliciting a blink to a loud sound such as a hand clap. The sucking reflex is used to evaluate the function of cranial nerves V, VII and XII. The swallowing reflex is used to evaluate cranial nerves IX and X (see below). The strength of the suck and coordination of sucking and swallowing change with increasing GA (Hack et al 1985). Abnormalities of sucking and swallowing are manifested by the inability to feed adequately or even to handle saliva. Severe gastroesophageal reflux leading to aspiration may accompany disorders of swallowing. The tongue (cranial nerve XII) is observed for atrophy or fasciculations (see above) and sternocleidomastoid muscle (cranial nerve XI) for atrophy or contracture.

POSTURE AND SPONTANEOUS MOTOR ACTIVITY

Posture

The spontaneous posture of a full-term infant delivered with a cephalic presentation is one of full flexion of all four limbs and of moderate axial flexion in lateral decubitus. However,

this posture is usually modified in VLBW and sick infants by the various constraints in the NICU. At any age, arching of the trunk is abnormal and, if the neck extensor muscles are hypertonic, the infant cannot lie flat. Lying with the neck extended and the head turned to one side is described as 'retrocollis'. When the arching involves the whole body axis, the posture is described as 'opisthotonos'.

Spontaneous movements

Characteristically, the spontaneous movements of the infant are smooth, symmetrical, and varied. They stop briefly when the infant's attention is caught by a noise or other external stimulus. In contrast to the normal pattern of varied movement referred to above, slow stereotyped movements are abnormal. Persistent tremors (high frequency, low amplitude) and bursts of clonic movements (low frequency, high amplitude) with the infant at rest are also abnormal when observed after the first 2–3 days of life. Chewing movements and repetitive in-and-out movements of the tongue are also abnormal.

A growing interest has arisen in the analysis of qualitative aspects of spontaneous movements as it allows assessing optimality or non-optimality of the CNS function in the newborn. The identification of normal and abnormal general movements (GMs) is the basis of a new diagnostic tool, the Prechtl Assessment of GMs, as recently reviewed (Einspieler & Prechtl 2005). As specific training is necessary, this technique will not be detailed here.

Facial motility

Facial movements are of special interest as the facial nerve may be compressed during cephalic delivery or during late fetal life. The resulting facial palsy is usually unilateral and of the peripheral type, involving both the upper and lower parts of the face. Hence the palpebral fissure is wider and the nasolabial fold flattened on the affected side. There is often some asymmetry of the mouth, sometimes associated with dribbling, but sucking is usually normal. These signs are most obvious on crying, when the eye may not close completely on the affected side. It is important, however, to distinguish facial palsy from congenital hypoplasia of one of the minor muscles of facial expression – the depressor anguli oris. Absence of this muscle produces virtually no abnormality at rest but there is an asymmetry on crying, the affected side of the mouth not being pulled down as on the normal side. However, in these cases the upper part of the face is not involved as it is in seventh nerve paralysis. The diagnosis of facial paralysis is more difficult in bilateral than in unilateral involvement (as in the Moebius sequence p. 778) which presents with an immobile, expressionless, but symmetrical facial appearance.

Movements of the fingers

Movements of the fingers, which should be observed throughout the examination, become independent, more elegant and more controlled as term is approached. The ability to abduct the thumbs is particularly important as persistent adduction indicates a lesion involving the corticospinal tract.

PASSIVE TONE IN LIMBS AND AXIS

Definition

The extensibility of muscles, which reflects their passive tone, is examined by evaluating the amplitude of slow passive movement carried out by the observer when the infant is at rest (Amiel-Tison & Grenier 1986, André-Thomas et al 1960). Passive movement is performed slowly and gently while the observer notes the degree of resistance. The angle through which the articulation can be moved provides an objective measurement of extensibility and hence of passive tone. Alternatively, extensibility can be evaluated by reference to certain anatomical landmarks as in the 'scarf' sign, or by an estimation of gross curvature in the case of the whole trunk. In carrying out all these examinations, the examiner must carefully control the force applied to find the limit of passive movement without causing discomfort. It is also important to keep the infant's head in the midline during these maneuvers in order to avoid eliciting the asymmetric tonic neck reflex.

Passive tone in the limbs evolves from global hypotonia at 28 weeks' gestation to strong flexor tone in all four limbs at 40 weeks' gestation. This development takes place in an upward direction, starting in the lower limbs and proceeding subsequently to the upper limbs. This changing pattern of passive tone in late gestation means that abnormal hypotonia or hypertonia has to be defined with strict reference to the normal finding at a given GA. Abnormalities may be of various kinds – global hypotonia, global hypertonia, or abnormal distribution of tone. The last of these may be of various kinds; for example, an excess of extensor as compared to flexor tone in the axis, or relative hypotonicity of the upper limbs only, or lateral asymmetry of tone.

Six specific maneuvers allow relatively precise estimation of passive tone by measurement of the degree to which it limits movement or restores a spontaneously adopted posture. These maneuvers include measurement of the popliteal and foot dorsiflexion angles, the scarf sign, forearm recoil, the ventral flexion and dorsal extension of the body axis. These are specified below.

Popliteal angle

The examiner flexes the infant's thighs laterally beside the abdomen and then extends the knee to its limit. The angle formed between the leg and the thigh, which is the popliteal angle, is then measured (Fig. 9.5).

Foot dorsiflexion angle

With the infant's knee extended, the examiner dorsiflexes the ankle by applying pressure with a thumb on the sole of the foot. The angle measured is between the dorsum of the foot and the anterior aspect of the leg. In fact this angle depends on the progressive restriction of space in utero up to term and therefore has to be interpreted as a physical criterion of GA.

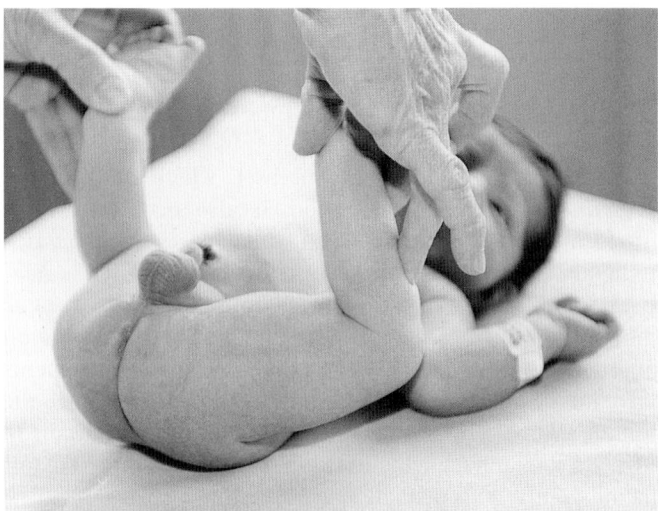

Figure 9.5 Popliteal angle. Very tight in the full-term infant (90° or less). Note the testing position, pelvis flat on the table.

Scarf sign

With one hand the examiner supports the infant in a semi-reclining supine position, keeping the head straight. One of the infant's hands is then pulled across the chest towards the opposite shoulder and the position of the elbow noted (Fig. 9.6). Three positions corresponding to states of decreasing muscle tone are described: the elbow does not reach the midline; it passes the midline; the arm encircles the neck.

Forearm recoil

This can be elicited only when the infant is in a spontaneously flexed position. It is tested by extending the arm passively at the elbow by pulling on the hand. The hand is then immediately released and the speed of recoil of the forearm to its former position is observed. If the forearm recoils normally, the test can be repeated after holding the forearm in extension for 20–30 seconds (usually not inhibited in the full-term).

Ventral flexion in the axis

With the child supine, the lower limbs are grasped and both legs and pelvis are pushed towards the head in order to achieve the maximum curvature of the spine. Some passive flexion of the trunk is normally present (Fig. 9.7a).

Dorsal extension in the axis

With the infant lying on his or her side, the flat of the palm of one hand is placed on the lumbar region and both legs pulled backwards with the other hand. Extension is normally minimal or absent (Fig. 9.7a).

Comparison of axial flexion and extension

There is a lot of individual variation in the extent of flexion and extension at all ages but in the normal individual, flexion always exceeds extension (Fig. 9.7a). Abnormal balance is observed when there is no ventral flexion and moderate or

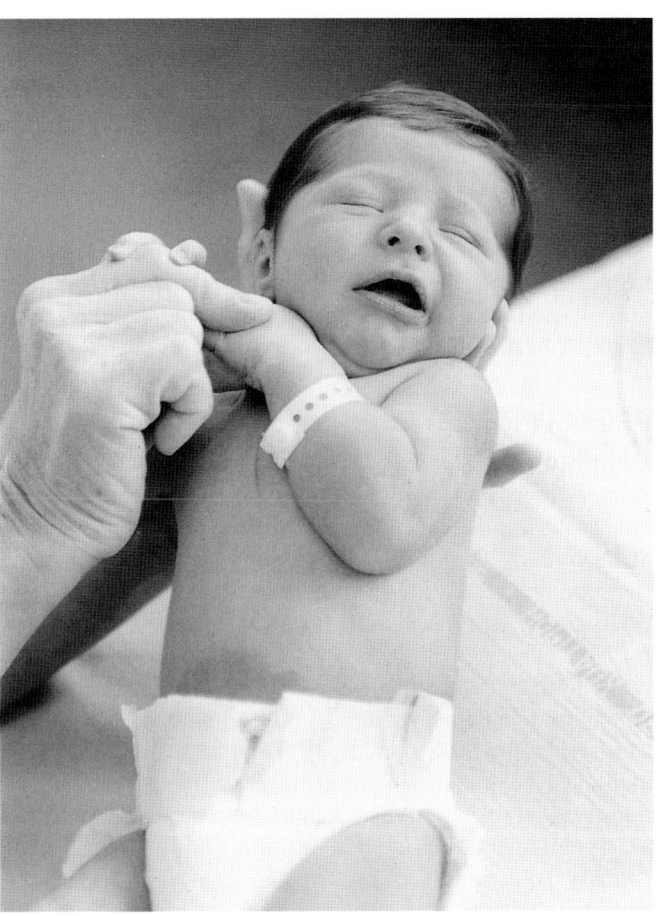

Figure 9.6 Scarf sign. The elbow does not reach the midline in the full-term infant. Note the testing position, head maintained in the axis.

FLEXION   EXTENSION

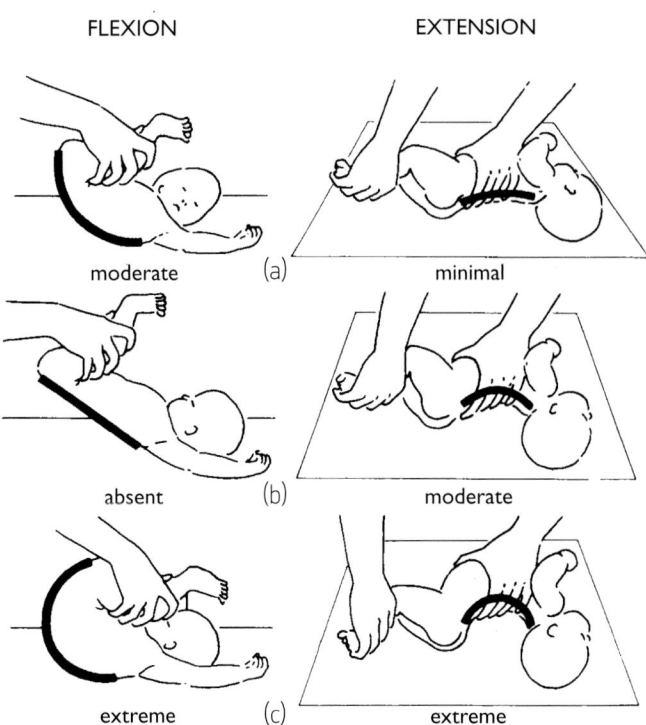

Figure 9.7 Passive tone in the body axis. (a) Ventral flexion normally exceeds dorsal extension. (b) Dorsal extension exceeding ventral flexion and (c) global hypotonia are both abnormal findings.

excessive extension (Fig. 9.7b). A global hypotonia is defined by unlimited flexion and extension (Fig. 9.7c).

ACTIVE TONE

Definition

Active tone refers to active movements of the infant in reaction to certain situations imposed by the examiner (André-Thomas & Saint-Anne-Dargassies 1952). Three responses are elicited by the following items: (1) the active global righting reaction in the upright position; (2) active passage of the head forward during the raise-to-sit maneuver; and (3) active passage of the head backward during the reverse maneuver, back to lying. These three responses permit analysis of the antigravity forces (lower system) and the control exerted on these antigravity forces by the upper system.

Righting reaction (or straightening)

To elicit this reaction, the examiner places the infant in the standing position, with the feet on a horizontal surface while supporting the trunk with one hand. A normal mature response consists of contraction of the extensor muscles of the legs and trunk so that the infant supports his or her own weight (Fig. 9.8).

Neck flexor tone tested by the 'raise-to-sit' maneuver

The examiner holds the infant's shoulders and pulls him or her from the lying to the sitting position, the relationship between the head and the trunk being noted. The forward movement elicits active contraction of the neck flexor muscles in an attempt to raise the head to a vertical position (Fig. 9.9).

Neck extensor tone tested by the reverse maneuver, 'back-to-lying'

With the infant held in the sitting position and the head hanging forwards on the chest, the examiner moves the trunk gently backwards (Fig. 9.9) while observing the reaction of the head extensor muscles. A normal reaction consists of a contraction of the neck extensor muscles in an attempt to raise the head to a vertical position. In the term infant, gentle movements of the trunk around the vertical position evoke active and symmetrical movements, which show a perfect balance between the two sets of muscles and only minimal lag. With maturation, the progressive equalization of flexor and extensor muscle activity is measurable by comparison of the responses obtained by these two maneuvers, 'raise-to-sit' and 'back-to-lying' (see Table 9.2).

In testing the neck muscles, three distinct abnormalities can be detected: (1) abnormal tone may be detectable by the weakness or absence of both flexor and extensor responses

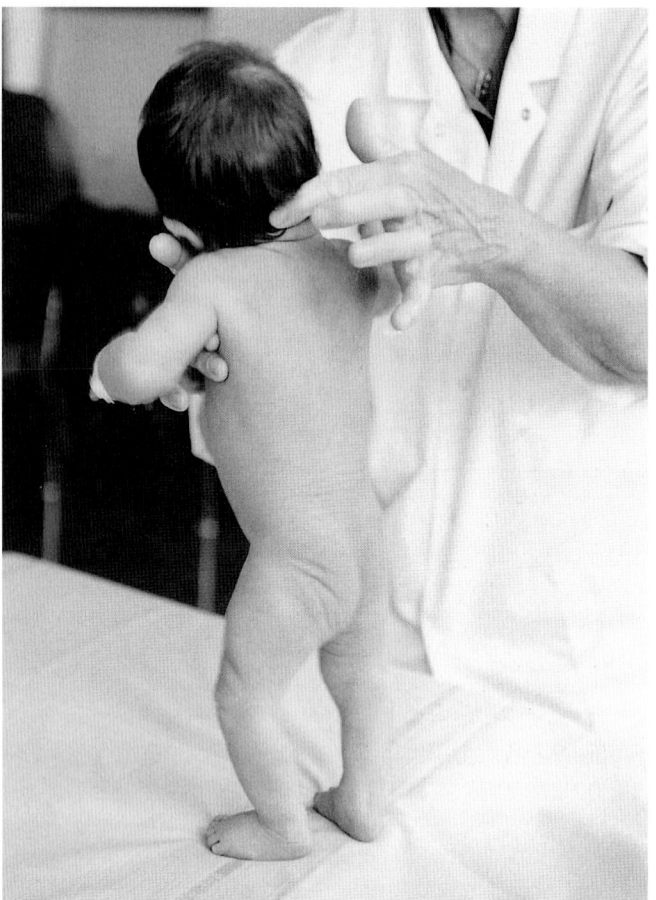

Figure 9.8 Righting reaction. When placed in the standing position, a strong contraction of the antigravity muscles is observed; the infant is able to support himself/herself for a few seconds.

(Fig. 9.10a); (2) there may be weakness or absence of flexor muscle activity, insufficient to lift the head forward (Fig. 9.10b); (3) there may be excessive action of the extensor muscles, which pull the head back too soon and too far when the trunk is moved backward from the sitting position (Fig. 9.10c). The position of the chin poking forward at the end of the raise-to-sit maneuver is easy to identify.

Interpretation of the last two maneuvers

It is essential to emphasize that the goal of these combined maneuvers is to test the active engagement of agonist muscles in reaction to passive mobilization of the trunk forward and backward. (1) Methodological deviations from the initial description have led to various misinterpretations. The most important and very frequent error is to assess the passive drop of the head backward and forward while maintaining the neonate in a sitting upright position. It must be stressed again that flexion forward (early in the raise-to-sit maneuver, i.e. before verticality is reached) and extension backward (early in the back-to-lying maneuver) are both unequivocally active movements. (2) Understanding this allows the examiner to fully appreciate the underlying neu-

rophysiological basis of this activity. Another methodological error is to hold the neonate with the arms extended: since the trapezius muscle (the main neck extensor muscle) is a multiple-joint muscle, it is essential to hold the infant at the shoulders to isolate the effect of its axial insertion.

Maturation is so fast that 2 months after term, the active responses to the raise-to-sit maneuver and reverse can no longer be analyzed separately. In other words, after the neonatal period the examiner will no longer be able to decompose the child's reactivity but will identify the acquisition of head control as the first 'gross motor milestone'.

PRIMARY REFLEXES

Definition

Primary (or primitive) reflexes are automatic responses that appear during the second half of pregnancy and are present at birth; controlled by the lower motor system (brainstem), they are later integrated by higher cortical function before 6 months of age. These reflexes are a source of fascination for most observers of the newborn infant. The walking reflex is the best known to parents and it is also the reflex about which has been most written (André-Thomas & Saint-Anne-Dargassies 1952, Peiper 1963). This fascination is easily explained by the clear demonstration of CNS preprogramming: this transient archaic behavior seems to be there just as a reminder of human evolution (Amiel-Tison 1990). Primary reflexes are a useful screening tool: when they cannot be elicited in the newborn infant, this indicates CNS depression; when persisting beyond the normal limits this indicates damage of the upper motor control. Only a few are used in routine evaluation and therefore described here.

Moro reflex

Holding both hands of the infant in abduction, the examiner lifts the infant's shoulders a few centimeters off the bed and then releases the hands briskly. The normal response is a rapid abduction and extension of the arms, followed by complete opening of the hands.

Finger grasp and response to traction

The examiner inserts his or her index fingers into the hands of the infant to obtain flexion of the infant's fingers amounting to a palmar grasp. When the examiner briskly lifts his/her index fingers, a sufficiently strong stretch reflex in the shoulder girdle is evoked to sustain the infant's weight for a few seconds. This 'response to traction' provides a very good estimate of the muscular strength (Fig. 9.11).

Automatic walking

The examiner holds the infant upright with his or her feet on the table in a standing position to obtain a supporting reaction by the infant. When the infant is tilted forward slightly, he or she should make a few steps.

Crossed extension

With one leg held in extension, the plantar surface of the foot is stroked gently, which produces a sequence of three

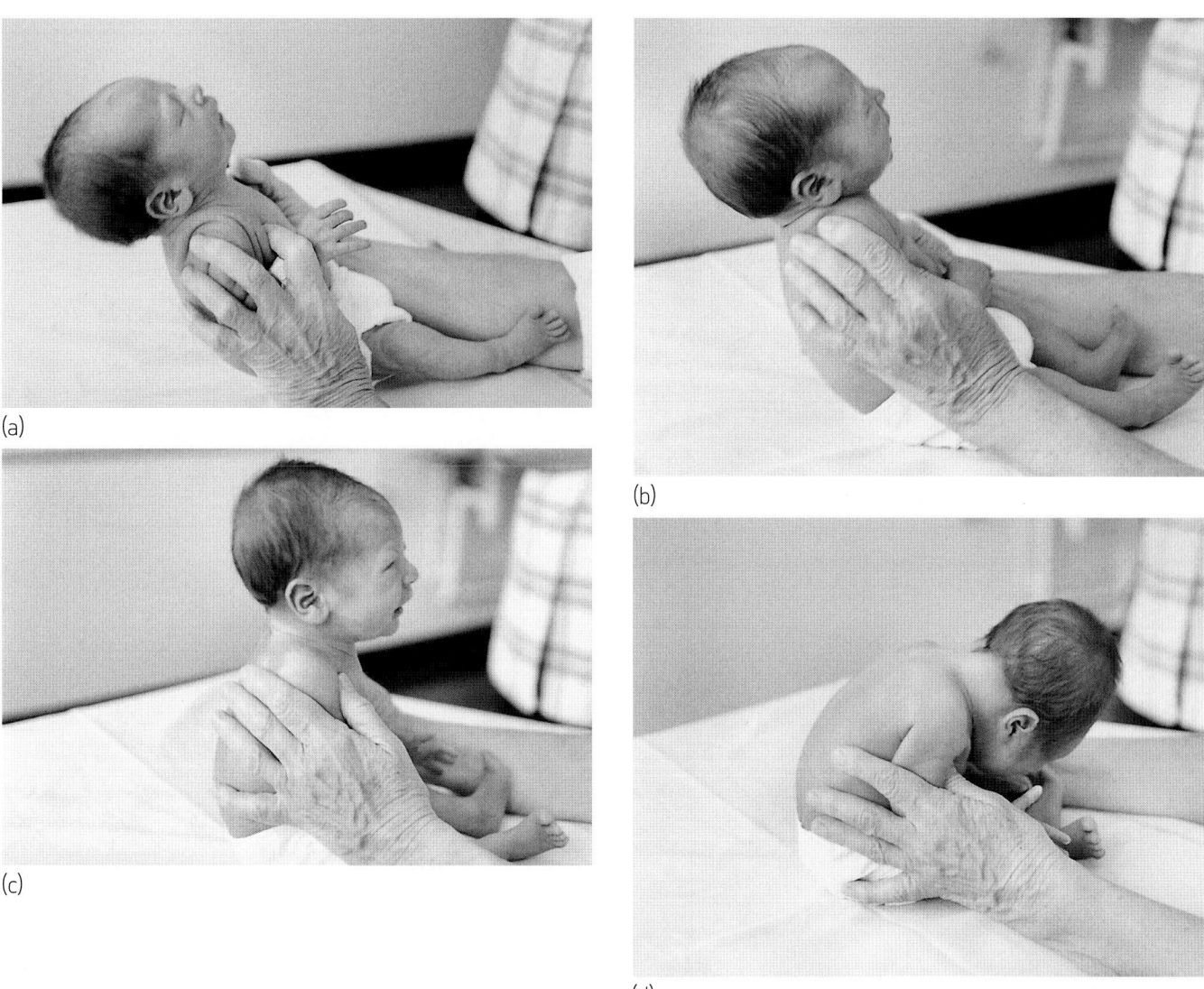

Figure 9.9 Active tone in flexor and extensor muscles of the neck. The 'raise-to-sit' response is shown in reading the pictures a to d (note the head in the axis before the trunk is vertical). The 'back-to-lying' response is shown in reading the pictures d to a. Both responses are identical in the term infant.

movements of the opposite leg (Fig. 9.12): (1) a rapid movement of withdrawal followed by extension of the leg; (2) fanning of the toes; (3) adduction of the leg towards the stimulated side. The first two parts of this response are present very early in fetal life, whereas the third component shows a distinct maturational change, first appearing at 36 weeks and becoming fully developed at 40 weeks.

Sucking reflex
The examiner places a clean finger in the infant's mouth and notes the strength and rhythm of sucking and its synchrony with swallowing. One can roughly estimate the number of movements in a burst (eight or more in the full-term infant) and the negative pressure perceived.

Asymmetric tonic neck reflex
The asymmetric tonic neck reflex (ATNR) is often observed spontaneously or elicited by turning the infant's head to one side (Fig. 9.13). The limbs on the facial side should extend and the limbs on the occipital side should flex. ATNR is normally present (but not necessarily) in the neonate and will disappear later. To avoid the consequences of the ATNR when testing passive tone in limbs, the child's head has to be maintained in the midline, particularly for comparing extensibility in the upper limbs.

DEEP TENDON REFLEXES
The deep tendon reflexes are not very helpful in the neonatal period except to confirm the presence of asymmetry. The

Table 9.2 Neurologic criteria described at 2-week intervals from 32 to 40 weeks of gestation, without scoring. Periods of rapid modification are highlighted, indicating the most discriminative period for each observation. Asterisk indicates that the items are not appropriate for maturational assessment performed after several weeks of postnatal life: sucking is modified as a result of practice; the foot dorsiflexion angle remains as it was at the time of premature birth.

Weeks gestation	Below 32	32–33	34–35	36–37	38–39	40–41
POPLITEAL ANGLE	130° or more	120°-110°	110°-100°	100°-90°	90°	90° or less
SCARF-SIGN	no resistance	very weak resistance	largely passes midline	slightly passes midline	does not reach midline	very tight
RETURN TO FLEXION OF FOREARMS	posture in extension most of the time		weak or absent	present, less than 4 times	4 times or more brisk but inhibited	4 times or more very strong & not inhibited
FINGER GRASP	present		present	present	present	present
RESPONSE TO TRACTION	absent		very weak or absent	able to lift part of the body weight	able to lift all body weight for 1 sec	maintains 2 to 3 sec with head passing forwards
RIGHTING REACTION lower limbs and trunk	no support	brief support lower limbs only	begins to maintain trunk	trunk more firm	begins to raise head	complete righting for a few secs.
RAISE-to-SIT (neck flexor muscles)	no movement of the head forwards		face view / head rolls on the shoulder	passes briskly in the axis	more powerful	perfect, minimal lag
BACK- to-LYING (neck extensor muscles)	no movement of the head backwards	head begins to lift but cannot pass backwards	BETTER BACKWARDS / passes briskly in the axis	PROGRESSIVE EQUALISATION / powerful movement backwards		SYMMETRICAL / perfect, minimal lag
CROSSED EXTENSION	good extension but no adduction			tendency to adduction	reaches the stimulated foot	crosses immediately
*SUCKING	n° mvts in a burst rate of mvts negative pressure Interburst time	3 or less 1/sec. weak or none 15–20 sec.	4 to 7 1, 5/sec. intermediate 5 to 10 sec.	8 or more 2/sec. high 5 to 10 sec.	idem	idem
*FOOT-DORSIFLEXION ANGLE	≥ 50°	40°-30°		20°-1 0°		nul

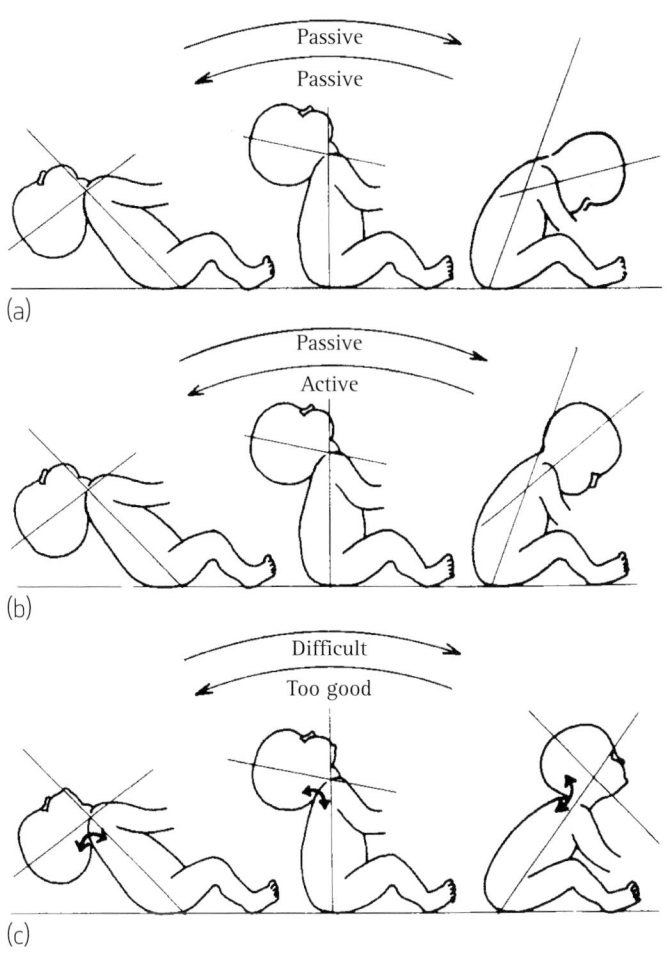

(a)

(b)

(c)

Figure 9.10 Three patterns of abnormal responses in neck muscles. (a) Weakness or absence of both flexor and extensor responses. (b) Weakness or absence of response of the flexor muscles. (c) Excessive action of the extensor muscles. Note the position of the chin poking forwards at the end of the 'raise-to-sit' maneuver.

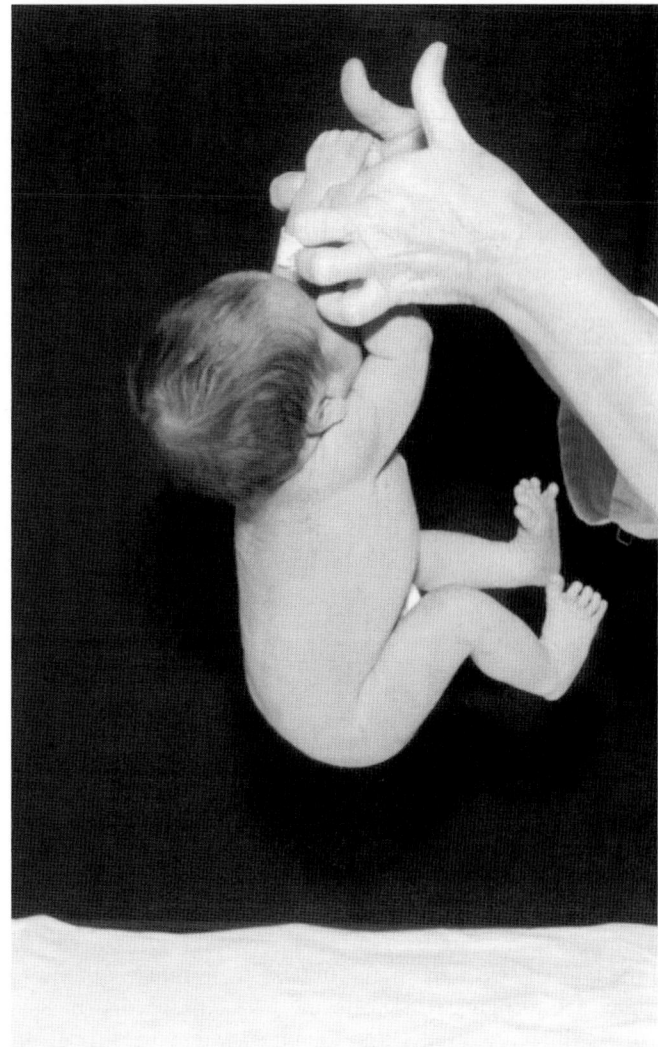

Figure 9.11 Finger grasp and response to traction. The full-term newborn infant lifts his or her whole body weight for a few seconds, the head moving forwards at the same time.

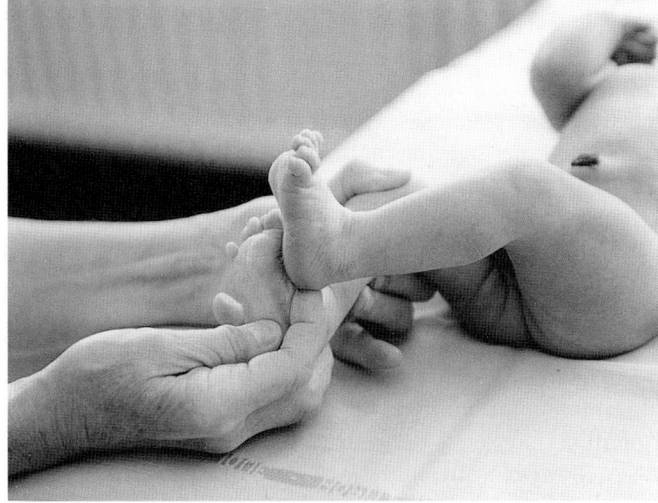

Figure 9.12 Crossed extension reflex. The three components are shown here: extension, fanning of the toes and adduction. In the full-term infant the free foot immediately crosses to the stimulated foot.

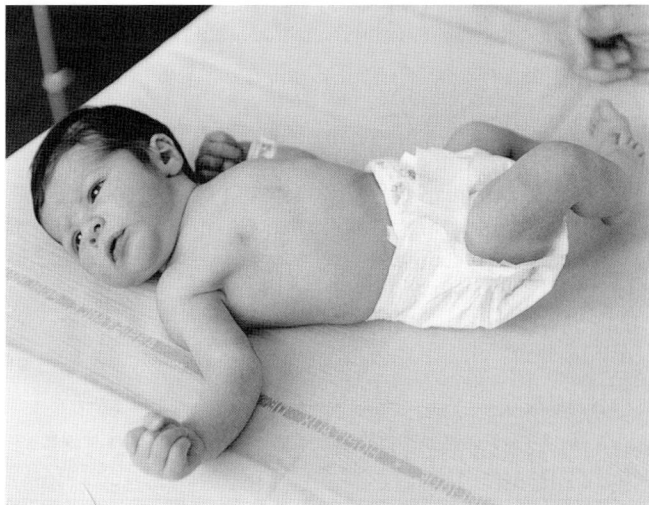

Figure 9.13 Asymmetric tonic neck reflex. Limbs extended on the facial side and flexed on the occipital side are often observed at rest in the neonatal period (fencing position).

biceps and patellar tendon jerks are easily elicited. Ankle clonus is frequently detectable and has no pathological significance at this age.

ADAPTABILITY TO MANIPULATION

Handling may have positive effects on the infant's active participation in the testing situation. For example, when assessing passive and active tone, permanent contact between the infant's body and the examiner's hands reinforces the communication already established between the two actors by voice, gaze and mimics. Handling the neonate gently and continuously helps to maintain the dialogue without rupture and obtain the best responses. However, handling may have negative effects. Destabilization can occur of any stage of the assessment, with various signs, including cardio-respiratory changes, color changes, visceral responses (e.g. gagging, hiccupping). Stability of the autonomic nervous system can be defined in three categories: excellent, transient changes and severe destabilization. According to the degree of destabilization, it is necessary either to wait a few minutes or to stop the procedure. Along with the infant's behavioral reactions to internal and external sensory stimuli, these observations are used to measure the infant's ability to tolerate his or her environment and the caregiving activities.

NURSING REPORTS ON ACUTE EVENTS

Training the nursing staff in the observation of the newborn infant in the NICU is of the utmost importance; otherwise many acute events relating to the CNS can be missed. Seizures, which are discussed in Chapter 34, may be difficult to recognize in the full-term infant and even more difficult in the VLBW infant. Rhythmic movements restricted to the hands or to the face may be the only expression of a fit. The associated signs, apnea and color change, may be masked when the infant is on a ventilator. An exact description of the event, including whether it was spontaneous or provoked, is of great diagnostic value. The report of an apneic spell may relate in fact to a seizure, often not recognized as such. In contrast, intense clonic movements of all four limbs may be wrongly interpreted as a seizure; a normal EEG may be particularly useful for excluding such an interpretation.

Similarly, observation of the states of sleep and wakefulness and any deviation according to GA should be recorded. Behavior during feeding is also relevant, as fatigue, choking and color changes may be signs of neurological abnormality. Frequent yawning is observed in cases of intracranial hypertension, although occasional yawning is normally a sign of health.

ADAPTATION OF THE ASSESSMENT TO THE PRETERM PERIOD

GENERAL CONSIDERATIONS

At a time when the duration of pregnancy is known with accuracy for most infants born in developed countries, clinical assessment of neurological maturation (Amiel-Tison 1968, Ballard et al 1991, Dubowitz et al 1970, Dubowitz & Dubowitz 1977) may appear obsolete. Moreover, with today's intensive-care apparatus, an assessment based on physical criteria (Farr et al 1966a, 1966b) is more feasible than one based on neurological criteria. As a consequence, one could deliberately ignore the assessment of neurological maturation. However, we consider this omission a real deprivation from several points of view, particularly concerning: (1) the apparent inability to demonstrate neurological signs associated with white-matter lesions and (2) the probable underestimation of accelerated maturation as a response to some stressed pregnancies (see below).

NEUROLOGICAL MATURATION MEASURED AT 2-WEEK INTERVALS

The simplified table presented (Table 9.2) derives from three tables previously published (Amiel-Tison 1968) and based on Saint-Anne Dargassies (1977). This table is based on 10 items selected from the assessment above. The progression of these 10 items is divided into 2-week stages between 32 and 40 weeks of gestation. The selected items are: four passive-tone items (popliteal angle, scarf sign, forearm recoil, dorsiflexion of the foot), three active-tone items (righting reaction, neck flexor tone, neck extensor tone), and three primary reflexes (finger grasp and response to traction, crossed extension, sucking). The passive-tone items and righting reactions allow identification of the upward wave of maturation of the subcortical system described earlier. The development of active tone in the neck flexor muscles allows the assessment of the upper system control beginning at the neck level (see Fig. 9.1). The presence of primary reflexes is linked with the function of the lower system, although some of them, including crossed extension reflex and sucking, clearly change between 35 and 40 weeks of gestation as the upper system control develops.

According to this system, between 32 and 40 weeks, a definition of the 'neurological age' can be reached when most of the responses correspond to the same 2-week gestational period; the pattern is designed as 'uniform' when seven or more results are in the same age interval. When more than three responses are off the vertical line, the pattern is designated as 'scattered' and no firm conclusion on a neurological age can be obtained. From our experience with this method, several situations can be described in the neonatal period. In some cases, the scattered pattern observed in the first few days becomes uniform by the end of the first week, when the general condition improves with adequate postnatal care. In rare cases, however, the initial scattered pattern persists into the following weeks. This is often due to poor suck and poor active-tone performances, contrasting with the other criteria. Such a situation may be indicating brain dysfunction.

APPLICATION TO THE TERM PERIOD (FULL-TERM OR 40 WEEKS CORRECTED)

SCORING SYSTEM

As maturation proceeds at about the same rate ex utero, responses in the preterm infant reaching 40 weeks are expected to be similar to those of a full-term newborn. Then, the preterm infant should be assessed following the same criteria as those applied to the full-term newborn. A single chart, presented in Appendix 1, has therefore been designed for both preterm infants reaching term (between 38 and 42 weeks corrected) and full-term neonates (Amiel-Tison 2002, Gosselin et al 2005). This chart, presented in Appendix 1, provides specific instructions for scoring each item. This scoring system has been developed to gain a more precise definition of the infant's responses but is simple enough for clinical use. A 3-point scale has been devised for each item: 0, typical; 1, moderately abnormal; 2, abnormal.

NEUROLOGICAL OPTIMALITY AT TERM

When every response is optimal (score 0), the probability of a favorable outcome is high, although the predictive value of an optimal assessment has not yet been demonstrated on a large cohort; research is under way to demonstrate this predictive value. Neurological optimality in the preterm infant is easily confirmed just as for the full-term neonate. For clinical use in maternity wards, a synthetic summary of the assessment (Amiel-Tison 1996) can be used based on the main areas of the CNS function at term: hemispheric growth, alertness and communication, motor control and adaptability. In cases of later litigation, it may be very helpful to trace such documented optimality within the first days of life in the full-term newborn.

CLUSTERS OF SIGNS AND SYMPTOMS

The following clusters of signs and symptoms can be recognized.

Seizures and hyperexcitability

Seizures may be isolated (one or two episodes) or repeated for more than 30 minutes. Hyperexcitability includes a restless sleep pattern, abnormal movements, a lowered threshold for the primary reflexes, excessive hypertonia, persistent 'fisting' and excessive crying.

CNS depression of various degrees

CNS depression may range from lethargy to coma. Lethargy means that the infant is permanently sleepy and difficult to wake and has reduced spontaneous movements, infrequent crying and poor or absent primary reflexes. Coma means that the infant does not respond to any kind of vigorous stimulation. Hypotonia is often seen in CNS depression; it may be global or confined to the upper part of the body.

Severe global hypotonia

This is defined as the absence of passive tone in the axis, limbs and face, a condition sometimes referred to as 'rag doll'. It is a common, non-specific finding in the early stages of severe types of perinatal brain damage such as HIE or intracranial hemorrhage. Global hypotonia is also seen after sedative drugs are given to the mother or infant and in systemic infections. Occasionally, a full clinical examination can provide clues to specific etiologies (extensively discussed elsewhere in this book). A few examples illustrate the value of associated findings: (1) tongue fasciculation and areflexia towards spinal muscular atrophy (Werdnig–Hoffmann disease); (2) body length more than 54 cm at birth and facial dysmorphy towards cerebral gigantism (Sotos syndrome); (3) facial diplegia and arthrogryposis towards myotonic dystrophy (Steinert disease); (4) absence of suck and swallow for several weeks towards Prader–Willi syndrome; (5) facial weakness and acute respiratory failure towards transient myasthenia gravis. Apart from these clues, the etiology of floppy-infant syndrome requires multidisciplinary assessment to identify genetic and metabolic disorders (Prasad & Prasad 2003).

Asymmetric tone

When asymmetry of muscular tone can be unequivocally demonstrated, the quandary remains, curiously enough, as to which is the abnormal side, the hypotonic or hypertonic. In recent years, repeated comparison with the results of new imaging methods has shown that (1) when the primary reflexes are depressed on the hypotonic side, this is the abnormal side, the abnormality being due to a recent lesion in the opposite hemisphere and (2) 'fisting' and an adducted thumb on the hypertonic side indicate that this is the abnormal side. In such cases the lesion may be several weeks old or more and easily confirmed by imaging.

Indeed, the association of flaccidity with a recent lesion, and of spasticity with an older one, appears to follow the well-known sequence observed in adult hemiplegia. Early asymmetry is also sometimes seen in cases of periventricular leukomalacia (PVL), reflecting inequality in the two sides of this essentially bilateral lesion.

EVOLVING PATTERNS AND GRADATION OF SEVERITY

In the early stages of extrauterine adaptation, it is difficult to separate transient effects of cardiorespiratory and metabolic problems from specific expression of brain damage. Repeated assessment provides the only good way of resolving the difficulty posed by the lability of clinical signs. When the acute phase of adaptation is complete, the clinical assessment really becomes contributory. For instance, if a lack of alertness, poor reactivity and hypotonia are found repeatedly, they are likely to be due to CNS damage, whereas the same signs, if transient or variable, may be due to disturbances in the infant's general condition from almost

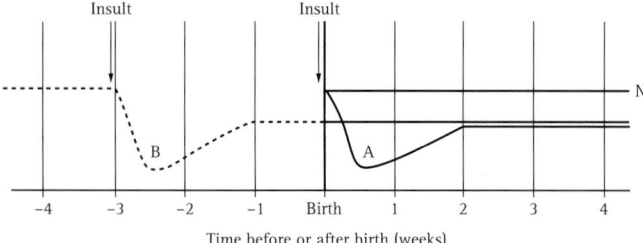

Figure 9.14 Profiles of CNS depression in the first postnatal weeks. N = normal CNS function (based on alertness, tone, primary reflexes and spontaneous motor activity). A = changing profile following an intrapartum insult. B = unchanging profile indicating a prenatal insult going back 2–3 weeks before birth, after acute changes and stabilization in utero. (From Amiel-Tison 1999.)

any cause. Repeated assessments allow distinction to be made between two different types of profile: when signs of CNS depression and tone abnormalities are found unchanged in repeated assessments, the clinical profile is defined as unchanging; this particular clinical profile constitutes an argument for a prenatal insult. *A contrario*, when signs of CNS depression increase until day 3 then tend to improve by day 5, with alertness, motor activity and sucking progressively getting better (Fig. 9.14), the clinical profile is defined as changing. This changing profile is typical of a very recent insult, most often intrapartum.

In the full-term neonate, clinical estimation of severity at the end of the first week is useful. For this purpose, it is helpful to define the following three grades of severity:

- Mild: abnormalities of tone hyperexcitability, no CNS depression, no seizures.
- Moderate: abnormalities of tone, signs of CNS depression, rarely isolated seizures (up to two).
- Severe: repeated seizures and overt CNS depression.

In the preterm infant, when neurological and/or cranial signs are found, the synthesis has to be cautious due to extra-neurological problems not yet completely resolved.

CONTRIBUTION OF CLINICAL FINDINGS TO IDENTIFICATION OF THE MOST COMMON DISORDERS

ACCELERATION OF MATURATION REFLECTING FETAL ADAPTATION TO STRESS

In most neonates, neurological and GAs are concordant, i.e. the neurological stage is what is expected from GA. Sometimes, however, they are discordant, implying that the maturational clock is not independent of adverse gestational circumstances. Advanced neurological maturation by 4 weeks or more was reported in a small series of publications (Amiel-Tison 1980, Gould et al 1977) in the late 1970s and early 1980s. The concept of advanced maturation in cases of multiple pregnancies and of intra-uterine

growth restriction was not well accepted until electrophysiological data (brain auditory evoked potentials) were presented in 1985 to support these clinical observations (Pettigrew et al 1985). Adaptive phenomena in these at-risk pregnancies have been reviewed recently (Amiel-Tison 2004, Amiel-Tison & Pettigrew 1991). As demonstrated in amphibians, humans share their adaptive capacities to stress with other species (Crespi & Denver 2005): the physiological response to experimental water volume and food deprivation results in activation of the endocrine axes that drive metamorphosis, in particular the neuroendocrine stress system. Unfavorable effects may occur however, probably due to inappropriate timing and/or duration of stress: recent experiments are converging to show a profound impairment of hippocampal functioning in the offspring of mothers exposed to prenatal stress. Moreover, fetal changes are likely one of the risk factors for a number of diseases in adulthood.

IDENTIFICATION OF FETAL BRAIN DAMAGE

Clinical clues at birth

Much litigation could be avoided by a careful neurological assessment within the first days of life as it may provide specific clues to dating brain damage as prenatal: the presence of a high-arched palate, non-reducible adduction of thumbs in a tightly clenched fist and suture ridges indicate an insult that took place some weeks (or more) earlier (Fig. 9.15). These signs are not specific; their diagnostic value is linked with their presence at birth. If not identified soon after birth, they will be of no value later in dating the insult, because an intrapartum insult will produce identical signs after a few weeks. In these cases of prenatal damage, early imaging (within the first days of life) would confirm the clinical dating by showing that a cerebral atrophy is already organized.

Subnormal head size, suspected prenatally or discovered at birth, is also significant. Head growth is so rapid during fetal life that a subnormal head size (compared to weight and height on normative curves) may indicate fetal brain damage. This finding is rarely an isolated one and a careful clinical assessment will often reveal subtle neurological abnormalities. Investigations of toxic (i.e. fetal alcohol syndrome) and viral exposures should be undertaken in the presence of subnormal head size at birth.

An unchanging profile during the first weeks of life is typical of a prenatal insult. In case of hypoxic–ischemic insult, this type of profile implies that the acute stage has ended before birth; the signs at birth are what remain after stabilization in utero (Fig. 9.14). In the case of a toxic or viral process, an unchanging profile is also observed.

Suspicion before birth

In the 1980s, fetal neurology emerged with fetal echography as a new field. More recently, the advent of 3- and 4-

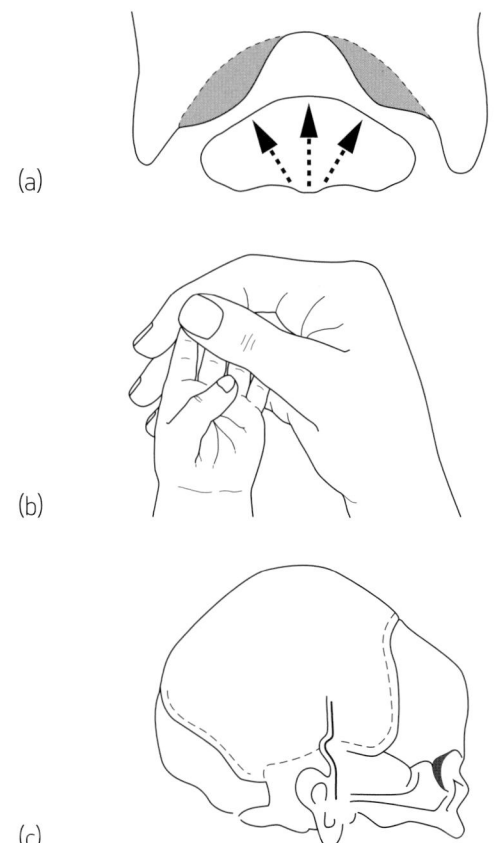

(a)

(b)

(c)

Figure 9.15 Early signs of fetal brain damage. (a) Persistence of prominent lateral ridges results in a high-arched palate, due to insufficient molding forces of the tongue (dotted lines indicate normal palate shaped by normal tongue movements. (b) Non-reducible adduction of the thumb in a clenched fist due to absence of spontaneous motor activity. (c) Cranial ridges on every suture, or restricted to the squamous suture, due to severe or moderate impairment of hemispheric growth. (From Amiel-Tison 1999, with permission.)

dimensional ultrasounds has allowed exploration of new domains of fetal motor activity, as well as more accurate evaluation of cephalic growth and cranial sutures. The conceptual framework underlying the basic neurological assessment described here now serves as a guide to complement and interpret fetal observation. Speculations on the predictive value of fetal motor behaviors are reviewed elsewhere (Amiel-Tison et al 2006).

DIAGNOSTIC ORIENTATION IN THE FULL-TERM NEONATE

The diversity of risk factors and presentations at this age often leaves the clinician considerable leeway for personal interpretation; accumulated clinical experience allows the following general empirical conclusions to be reached.

Recent years have seen a change in the pattern of perinatal brain damage. On the one hand, in well-staffed, well-equipped maternity units, cases of damage due to obstetrical factors have become uncommon. On the other hand, various possible causes of antenatal brain damage are better identified nowadays, with the expanding skills of many disciplines. This is a hot topic, due to the increasing incidence of litigation (MacLennan, for the International Cerebral Palsy Task Force 1999), and it is discussed in detail elsewhere in this book. To replace the loose terminology of 'fetal distress' and 'birth asphyxia,' more precise definitions related to the fetal status before birth and during labor will hopefully be a first step toward achieving an international consensus. The term 'neonatal encephalopathy' must be used when neurological signs are present in the neonatal period, whatever the cause may be.

The full-term neonate possesses the means to produce symptoms related to perinatal neurological damage. It is therefore unreasonable to attribute damage discovered later in life to obstetric factors if no neurological signs could be identified during the first week of life. In about one-third of cases, the cause of the symptoms remains unknown despite evaluation of all obstetrical and pediatric factors. HIE can no longer be proposed as the cause after elimination of other causes; this attitude is inappropriate and grossly misleading.

APPLICATION TO THE RECOVERY PERIOD

PARENTS' QUESTIONS ON OUTCOME

In the acute stage of a neonatal neurological disorder, the parents are usually too preoccupied with their child's survival to ask questions about long-term disability before the convalescent stage. On the medical side, there is usually a great deal of uncertainty about the outcome except at the two extremes of the spectrum. For the intermediate cases, the probabilistic approach for any given outcome is not acceptable to the vast majority of parents. There are evidently quite large cultural differences in the types of question asked and in the answers provided. In some countries, the pediatrician tries to provide comprehensive information on the evidence of damage and potential risks whereas, in others, the pediatrician tends to remain vague but optimistic. Parents often complain if they are told too early, when they are unprepared to receive this information. They may also complain if they are told too late because they may develop a retrospective feeling of mistrust linked to the fear that early intervention might also have been delayed. In either case, the messenger of ill-tidings must expect to be blamed, which is less than satisfactory for the child and for the parents, who still need medical support.

However, parental dissatisfaction with the way they are given bad news does not seem inevitable. It is possible to help the parents and the infant to both convalesce by allowing them the time for interaction and for bonding to proceed. During this convalescent period, it is advisable not to push parents into asking questions. When asked about intellectual outcome, it is possible to remain vague, emphasizing the extent of our ignorance and also the extent of individual variations. One can emphasize that assessments during the convalescent period are carried out to measure progress and not, at this stage, to reach a definitive prognosis. As often as possible, assessments are made in the presence of the parents; emphasis is placed on demonstrating newly acquired abilities. For every child suspected of neurological damage, early intervention is initiated. This helps the parents to accept that something useful has been done even when they realize how poor the outcome will be.

THE FIRST 3 MONTHS IN THE FOLLOW-UP CLINIC

The abnormalities observed within the first 2–3 months are of the same nature as those observed in the early neonatal period. After this fairly stable period, moderate neurological dysfunction may improve abruptly during the third month. Head control acquired on time is the most spectacular event, the infant becoming able to actively sustain the head in the axis for 30 seconds or longer. At the same time, passive tone in flexion begins to relax in the upper limbs, the grasp and Moro reflexes disappear and the infant begins to develop the capacity for cheerful interaction. Mothers often relate how all these changes take place quite rapidly within a few days. Insufficient head growth is another concern. (During the first 3 months of life, the head circumference normally increases at about 3 cm per month – not far short of 1 cm per week.) When transferred to a growth chart, a fall-down of the curve over a 2–3-month period clearly reveals a cerebral atrophy following HIE, even if it tends to stabilize later. In these severe cases, overlapping of all cranial sutures appears concomitantly, mimicking the findings in craniosynostosis. In moderate cases, head growth is sometimes, but not always, affected and a ridge may become evident at the site of the squamous sutures but not elsewhere. Indeed, this ridge may remain as a marker of moderate perinatal brain damage (Amiel-Tison & Stewart 1994, Gosselin et al 2002). A commonly observed but worrying pattern at 3 months is the combination of poor head growth and neurological signs (particularly imbalance between axial extensor and flexor tone and persisting primary reflexes), together with delayed developmental acquisitions such as the social smile, cooing and head control. When all these signs are present, a full recovery will rarely take place.

PITFALLS IN INTERPRETING FINDINGS

Various non-CNS factors may interfere with cranial and neurological findings, especially in ELBW infants. A few of the most common pitfalls are described briefly below, with the same question asked for each: is the abnormal response identified due to neurological or extra-neurological mechanisms?

Muscle shortenings or deformations?

Three examples of such a dilemma are common: (1) Very sick neonates and tiny premies (because they are very immature) tend to lie frog-legged in either prone or supine position. This abnormal posture within the first weeks of life will soon result in muscle shortening (mainly the adductor muscles) and osteocartilaginous deformities (Grenier 1994), abnormal posture mimicking tone abnormalities in lower limbs. (2) When adapted positioning has been neglected in sick and preterm infants, postural arching will often become permanent due to shortening of the trapezius muscle (Grenier 1994); this acquired posture will not allow the passage forward of the head in the raise-to-sit maneuver. Such findings are often wrongly interpreted as a severe neurological cluster. (3) Asymmetries may also develop when positioning is not carefully controlled; these asymmetries can be wrongly interpreted as resulting from unilateral brain damage.

It is easy to understand from these few examples that such findings are a frequent source of misinterpretation in the follow-up clinic and, also, that they negatively influence the motor function. Physical therapists will reach the right interpretation after several weeks of therapy: if posture and active responses are back to normal, the condition was environmentally induced whereas if abnormalities persist, brain damage is very likely present. Early postnatal correction of abnormal fetal postures and prevention of acquired muscle shortening therefore constitute important issues to insure valid assessment of CNS function. Interestingly, adequate positioning and handling recently became major ingredients of developmental care (Aucott et al 2002).

Extraneurological feeding problems

Bronchopulmonary dysplasia (BPD) is a frequent complication in the first months of life. Infants with BPD have difficulty achieving coordinated sucking and swallowing; less rhythmic coordination of swallowing and respiration during feeding and more apneic swallows are found in BPD compared with non-BPD infants (Gewold & Vice 2006). When BPD is well documented, it can significantly contribute to the feeding problems. However in some cases, the question is raised about a central origin explaining the abnormal sucking behavior.

Reduced rates of growth

A poor body growth curve, often multifactorial in origin, is frequent in tiny premies. The consequence will be insufficient cephalic growth, often associated with cranial ridges. As mentioned above, those cranial findings are precious clues to cerebral atrophy when associated with neurological findings but need to be interpreted with caution when body growth is likewise impaired.

In conclusion, the neurological assessment must be interpreted in the clinical context: after recording the findings analytically, the clinical synthesis will take into account persisting extra-neurological conditions as well as any unfavorable circumstances on the day of the examination.

CONCLUDING COMMENTS

Neonatologists faced with these various approaches and instruments may deplore that there is not just one tool for assessing CNS functions in the neonatal period. Each of the existing instruments provides an incomplete view, none of them being able to meet all expectations of both clinicians and researchers. Furthermore, this situation will very likely pervade, as the probability of a single instrument seems very low indeed. In fact, apart from reflecting the wide diversity of goals ranging from clinical routine to sophisticated research, this very diversity of approaches has been more stimulating than frustrating as each approach has been seen to influence the others in a positive way.

Nevertheless, the absence of a single ideal method must not be an excuse for either the clinician or the researcher not to select and rigorously apply one of the instruments available. In routine and publications, it is common not to specify which type of assessment has been chosen, an attitude which often masks the feeling of insecurity among many pediatricians as to how to perform each maneuver or how to observe and score each response. Although the transmission of manual skills has been facilitated by didactic support, a master–apprentice situation is the most efficient method of training, although not the easiest to provide.

The predictive value for the neurological outcome of any type of neonatal assessment clearly depends on the expertise of the performer. This chapter has deliberately omitted this aspect for each of the instruments mentioned because the studies published are not always totally convincing. In fact, small series in which infants are assessed by one or two very well-trained performers have a good predictive value with most of the instruments but such expectations are not fulfilled in large epidemiological studies, for instance, in which the examiners' competency varies substantially. Consequently, correlations between neonatal assessment and outcome appear loose in large epidemiological studies and the blame goes to the assessment used. Moreover, the temptation to shorten the assessment and ultimately select the items easiest to perform, albeit usually not the most meaningful, is rarely resisted. As a consequence of such methodological deviance, the results appear disappointing, except at the two extremes of the spectrum of casualties, the very abnormal or the clearly optimal.

At the present time, clinical assessment of CNS function is considered mandatory for preterm and sick neonates, as part of the standard care of high-risk infants. This is not the case for near-term and full-term neonates. The practice should be extended to this population at lower risk of brain damage, however, as it would enable pediatricians to: (1) reassure parents after a high-risk pregnancy by eliciting optimal responses in the neonate and, in addition, (2) identify unsuspected neurological abnormalities in quite a few near-term or full-term neonates (Amiel-Tison et al 2002, Raju et al 2006). Is it too much to spend a few minutes to assess the brain function of any full-term neonate in the presence of the infant's mother? It is very rewarding indeed to have the privilege of observing the self-regulatory abilities of the newborn during the assessment and, finally, the peaceful facial expression, the hands near the face, a few sucking movements: the first opportunity for a neonate to please its mother on objective grounds!

REFERENCES

Allen M C, Lipkin P H (Guest editors) 2005 Neuro developmental assessment of the fetus and young infant. MRDD Research Reviews 11:1–106.

Als H, Lester B, Tronick E et al 1982 Manual for the assessment of preterm infants' behavior (APIB). In: Fitzgerald H, Lester B, Yogman M (eds) Theory and research in behavioral pediatrics. Plenum, New York, pp. 65–132.

Amiel-Tison C 1968 Neurologic evaluation of the maturity of newborn infants. Arch Dis Child 43: 89–93.

Amiel-Tison C 1980. Possible acceleration of neurologic maturity following high risk pregnancy. Am J Obstet Gynecol 138:303–306.

Amiel-Tison C 1990 Neurological assessment of the neonate revisited: a personal view. Dev Med Child Neurol 32:1109–1113.

Amiel-Tison C 1996 Does neurological assessment still have a place in the NICU? Acta Paediatr Suppl 416:31–38.

Amiel-Tison C 2001 Clinical assessment of the infant nervous system. In: Levene M I et al (eds). Fetal and neonatal neurology and neurosurgery, 3rd edn. Churchill Livingstone, London, pp. 99–120.

Amiel-Tison C 2002 Update of the Amiel-Tison neurologic assessment for the term neonate or at 40 weeks corrected age. Pediatr Neurol 27:196–212.

Amiel-Tison C, Allen MC, Lebrun F et al 2002 Macropremies: Underprivileged newborns. MRDD Research Reviews 8:281–292.

Amiel-Tison C, Cabrol D, Denver R et al 2004 Fetal adaptation to stress. Part I: acceleration of fetal maturation and earlier birth triggered by placental insufficiency in humans. Early Hum Dev 78:15–27.

Amiel-Tison C, Gosselin J 2001 Neurologic development from birth to six years. Johns Hopkins University Press, Baltimore.

Amiel-Tison C, Gosselin J, Infante-Rivard C 2002 Head growth and cranial assessment at neurological examination in infancy. Dev Med Child Neurol 44:643–648.

Amiel-Tison C, Gosselin J, Kurjak A 2006 Neurosonography in the second half of fetal life: A neonatologist's point of view. J Perinat Med 34:437–446.

Amiel-Tison C, Grenier A 1986 Neurologic assessment during the first year of life. Oxford University Press, New York.

Amiel-Tison C, Lafaurie-Levêque M 2000 Évaluation neurologique du nouveau-né à terme. AP-HP Secteur Audiovisuel, Paris.

Amiel-Tison C, Pettigrew A G 1991 Adaptive changes in the developing brain during intrauterine stress. Brain Dev 13:67–76.

Amiel-Tison C, Stewart A 1994 The newborn infant: one brain for life. Paris: INSERM-Doin.

André-Thomas, Chesni Y, Saint-Anne Dargassies S 1960 The neurologic examination of the infant. Clin Dev Med No. 1. SIMP, London.

André-Thomas, Saint-Anne-Dargassies S 1952 Etudes neurologiques sur le nouveau-né et le jeune nourrisson. Masson, Paris.

Aucott S, Donohue P K, Atkins E et al 2002 Neurodevelopmental care in the NICU. Ment Retard Dev Disabil Res Rev 8:298–308.

Ballard J L, Khoury J C, Wedig K et al 1991 New Ballard score expanded to include extremely premature infants. J Pediatr 19:417–423.

Brazelton T B 1973 Neonatal behavioural assessment scale. Clin Dev Med No. 50. SIMP with Heinemann, Philadelphia.

Brazelton T B, Nugent J K 1995 Neonatal behavioral assessment scale 3rd ed. Clin Dev Med No. 137. Mac Keith, London.

Crespi E J, Denver R J 2005 Roles of stress hormones in food intake regulation in anuran amphibians throughout the life cycle. Comp Biochem Physiol A Mol Integr Physiol 141:381–390.

Daum C, Kurtzberg D, Ruff H et al 1980 Preterm development of visual and auditory orienting in very low birth weight infants. Pediatr Res 14:Abstr. 41.

Dubowitz L M, Dubowitz V 1977 Gestational age of the newborn. Addison-Wesley, London.

Dubowitz L M, Dubowitz V, Goldberg C 1970 Clinical assessment of gestational age in the newborn infant. J Pediatr 77:1–10.

Dubowitz L, Dubowitz V, Mercuri E 1999 The neurological assessment of the preterm and full-term newborn infant, 2nd edn. Mac Keith, London.

Einspieler C, Prechtl H F 2005 Prechtl's assessment of general movements: a diagnostic tool for the functional assessment of the young nervous system. Ment Retard Dev Disabil Res Rev 11:61–67.

Einspieler C, Prechtl H F R, Bos A F et al 2004 Prechtl's method on the qualitative assessment of general movements in preterm, term and young infants. Clin Dev Med No. 167. Mac Keith, London.

Farr V, Kerridge D F, Mitchell R G 1966b The value of some external characteristics in the assessment of gestational age at birth. Dev Med Child Neurol 8:657–660.

Farr V, Mitchell R G, Neligan G A et al 1966a The definition of some external characteristics used in the assessment of gestational age in the newborn infant. Dev Med Child Neurol 8:507–511.

Gewold I H, Vice F L 2006 Abnormalities in the coordination of respiration and swallow in preterm infants with bronchopulmonary dysplasia. Dev Med Child Neurol 48:595–599.

Gosselin J, Amiel-Tison C 2007 Évaluation neurologique de la naissance à 6 ans. Montréal: Presses de l'Hôpital Ste-Justine. Paris, Elsevier-Masson, Paris.

Gosselin J, Amiel-Tison C, Infante-Rivard C et al 2002 Minor neurological signs and developmental performance in high risk children at preschool age. Dev Med Child Neurol 44:323–328.

Gosselin J, Gahagan S, Amiel-Tison C 2005. The Amiel-Tison neurological assessment at term: conceptual and methodological continuity in the course of follow-up. Ment Retard Dev Disabil Res Rev 11:34–51.

Gould J B, Gluck L, Kulovich M V 1977 The relationship between accelerated pulmonary maturity and accelerated neurological maturity in certain chronically stressed pregnancies. Am J Obstet Gynecol 127:181–186.

Graham J M 1988 Smith's recognizable patterns of human deformation, 2nd edn. W B Saunders, Philadelphia.

Grenier A 1994 Prevention of muscle shortening and osteo-cartilaginous deformities in brain damaged infants while in the neonatal intensive care unit. In: Amiel-Tison C, Stewart A L (eds) The newborn infant: One brain for life. INSERM, Paris, pp. 175–184.

Hack M, Estabrook M M, Robertson S S 1985 Development of sucking rhythm in preterm infant. Early Hum Dev 11:133–140.

MacLennan A, for the International Cerebral Palsy Task Force 1999 A template for defining a causal relation between acute intrapartum events and cerebral palsy: international consensus statement. Br Med J 319:1054–1059.

Nelhaus G 1968 Composite international and interracial graphs. Pediatrics 41:106–112.

Peiper A 1963 Cerebral function in infancy and childhood (translation of the 3rd revised German edition by Nagler B, Nagler H). Consultants Bureau, New York.

Pettigrew A G, Edwards D A, Henderson-Smart D J 1985 The influence of intrauterine growth retardation on brainstem development of preterm infants. Dev Med Child Neurol 27:467–472.

Prasad A N, Prasad C 2003 The floppy infant: Contribution of genetic and metabolic disorders. Brain Dev 27:457–476.

Prechtl H F R, Beintema D J 1964 The neurological examination of the fullterm newborn infant. Clin Dev Med No. 12. SIMP, London.

Raju T N K, Higgins R D, Stark A R et al 2006 Optimizing care and outcome for late-preterm (near-term) infants: A summary of the workshop sponsored by the National Institute of Child Health and Human Development. Pediatrics 118:1207–1214.

Saint-Anne Dargassies S 1977 Neurological development in the full-term and premature neonate. Elsevier, Amsterdam.

Sarnat H B 1984 Anatomic and physiologic correlates of neurologic development in prematurity. In: Sarnat H B (ed.) Topics in neonatal neurology. Grune, Stratton, New York, pp. 1–24.

Sarnat H B 1989 Do corticospinal and corticobulbar tracts mediate functions in the human newborn? Can J Neurol Sci 16:157–160.

Sarnat H B 2003 Functions of the corticospinal and corticobulbar tracts in the human newborn. J Pediatr Neurol 1:3–8.

Torielo H 1993 Cranium. In: Stevenson R E, Hall J G, Goodman R M (eds) Human malformations and related anomalies Vol. II. Oxford University Press, New York, pp. 589–627.

Volpe J J 1995 Neurology of the newborn, 3rd edn. WB Saunders, Philadelphia.

1

Amiel-Tison neurological assessment at term

	M	D	Y
Name _____	Birth date	☐ ☐ ☐	
Mother's name _____	Gestational age (wk)	☐	
Chart number _____	Sex	M ☐ F ☐	

Assessments

Number	1	2	3	4
Date of assessment				
Day of life				
Corrected age (wk)				
Weight (g)				
Height (cm)				
Head circumference (cm)				

How to code?

A numerical system is proposed to code the observations. Level of severity in abnormal responses is defined.

0   indicates a typical result, within normal range
1   indicates a moderately abnormal result
2   indicates a definitely abnormal result
X   indicates examination results when scoring is considered inappropriate because the normal or abnormal character of the observation cannot be defined with certainty.

This coding system is not quantitative. Thus, any computation of quotient or total score is inappropriate.

INSTRUCTIONS

For whom?

Term neonates within the first days of life and preterm neonates closest to the term period (between 37 and 42 weeks corrected).

In order to save space, the originhal chart is reduced here, focusing on the scoring system and the clinical summary. The full chart is to be found elsewhere (Amiel-Tison 2002, Gosselin et al 2005).

Cranial assessment

		1	2	3	4
Head circumference	±2SD	0	0	0	0
	>2SD	X	X	X	X
	<2SD	X	X	X	X
Anterior fontanelle	Normal	0	0	0	0
	Tense	X	X	X	X
Squamous sutures	Edge-to-edge	0	0	0	0
	Separated	X	X	X	X
	Overlapping	X	X	X	X
Other sutures	Edge-to-edge	0	0	0	0
	Separated	X	X	X	X
	Overlapping	X	X	X	X

Neurosensory function and spontaneous motor activity during the assessment

Fix and track	Easy to obtain 4 times	0		0		0		0
	Difficult to obtain	1		1		1		1
	No response	2		2		2		2
Ocular signs	Absent	0		0		0		0
	Present, describe _____	X		X		X		X
Response to voice	Easy to obtain	0		0		0		0
	Difficult to obtain	1		1		1		1
	No response	2		2		2		2
Social interaction	Easy and spontaneous	0		0		0		0
	Poor and limited	1		1		1		1
	No interaction	2		2		2		2
Crying	Normal pitch, easy to calm	0		0		0		0
	Monotonous, abnormal pitch	1		1		1		1
	Absent	2		2		2		2
Excitability	Consolable, normal sleep	0		0		0		0
	Excessive crying, insufficient sleep	1		1		1		1
	Tremors and/or clonic movements	1		1		1		1
Convulsions	Absent	0		0		0		0
	Present (1 or 2)	2		2		2		2
	Repeated for more than 30 min.	2		2		2		2
	Describe variety							
Spontaneous motor activity	Varied, harmonious	0		0		0		0
	Insufficient, stereotyped	1		1		1		1
	Absent or barely present	2		2		2		2
	Asymmetrical (pathological side)	R	L	R	L	R	L	R	L
Spontaneous thumb abduction	Active thumb	0		0		0		0
	Inactive thumb	2		2		2		2
	Fixed thumb in adduction	2		2		2		2
	Asymmetrical (pathological side)	R	L	R	L	R	L	R	L

Passive muscle tone

			1		2		3		4	
			R	L	R	L	R	L	R	L
Upper limbs	Recoil	Quick, reproducible	0	0	0	0	0	0	0	0
		Slow, not reproducible	1	1	1	1	1	1	1	1
		Absent	2	2	2	2	2	2	2	2
	Scarf	Elbow does not reach midline	0	0	0	0	0	0	0	0
		Elbow slightly passes midline	1	1	1	1	1	1	1	1
		No resistance	2	2	2	2	2	2	2	2
Lower limbs	Recoil*	Quick, reproducible	0	0	0	0	0	0	0	0
		Slow, not reproducible	1	1	1	1	1	1	1	1
		Absent	2	2	2	2	2	2	2	2
		Value of the angle								
	Popliteal angle*	70–90°	0	0	0	0	0	0	0	0
		100–120°	1	1	1	1	1	1	1	1
		130° or more	2	2	2	2	2	2	2	2

*No coding in cases of breech delivery

			1	2	3	4
Right–left comparisons	Asymmetry	Absent or not categorized	0	0	0	0
		Right side more relaxed	X	X	X	X
		Left side more relaxed	X	X	X	X
	Ventral incurvation (flexion)	Moderate, easy to obtain	0	0	0	0
		Absent or minimal	1	1	1	1
		Unlimited	2	2	2	2
Body axis	Dorsal incurvation (extension)	Absent to moderate	0	0	0	0
		Opisthotonos (excessive)	2	2	2	2
	Comparison of curvatures	Flexion ≥ extension	0	0	0	0
		Flexion < extension	1	1	1	1
		Flexion and extension unlimited	2	2	2	2

Axial motor activity (active tone)

Righting reaction (Lower limbs + trunk)	Present, complete or not	0	0	0	0
	Excessive with arching	1	1	1	1
	Absent	2	2	2	2
Raise to sit (neck flexor muscles head forward)	Easy, in the axis	0	0	0	0
	Muscle activity but no passage	1	1	1	1
	No response	2	2	2	2
Reverse maneuver (neck extensor muscles head backward)	Easy, in the axis	0	0	0	0
	Brisk, excessive response	1	1	1	1
	No response	2	2	2	2

Primitive reflexes

		1	2	3	4
Non nutritive sucking	Rhythmic movements, efficient	0	0	0	0
	Few movements, inefficient	1	1	1	1
	No movements	2	2	2	2
Palmar grasp	Strong finger flexion	0	0	0	0
	Weak, short duration	1	1	1	1
	Absent	2	2	2	2
	Asymmetrical (pathological side)	R L	R L	R L	R L
Automatic walking	A few steps, easy to obtain	0	0	0	0
	Difficult to obtain or absent (no concern if isolated finding)	X	X	X	X
Moro reflex**	Brisk, with opening of the hands	0	0	0	0
	Incomplete	1	1	1	1
	Absent	2	2	2	2
	Asymmetrical (pathological side)	R L	R L	R L	R L
Asymmetric tonic neck reflex (ATNR)	Absent	X	X	X	X
	Present	X	X	X	X

**to assess only when other primitive reflexes are asymmetrical or absent

Palate and tongue

High arched palate	Absent	0	0	0	0
	Present	2	2	2	2
Fasciculations of tongue (peripheral, at rest)	Absent	0	0	0	0
	Present	2	2	2	2

Adaptedness to manipulations during assessment

Stability	Excellent	0	0	0	0
	Transient changes	1	1	1	1
	Severe destabilization	2	2	2	2

Feeding autonomy

Term newborn	Immediate, easy	0	0	0	0
	Incomplete	1	1	1	1
	Absent until day 7	2	2	2	2
Preterm infant close to term	Present, easy	0	0	0	0
	Incomplete	1	1	1	1
	Absent	2	2	2	2

How to achieve a synthesis of the data

- For the Preterm infant around 40 weeks corrected:
  Synthesis is based on a single assessment performed as close as possible to 40 weeks.

- For the term newborn infant:
  In the absence of any abnormality at the first assessment (day 1 or 2), synthesis relies on this single assessment. *In the presence of abnormalities at the first assessment*, synthesis relies on repeated assessments within the first week of life.

Synthesis for preterm infants around 40 weeks corrected

Absence of any neurological sign	☐

Presence of neurological signs, variable degree	☐
Minor to moderate degree	☐
Score 1 obtained on some or most of the items (imperfect responses concerning alertness, spontaneous activity, active tone, sucking)	
Severe degree	☐
Score 2 obtained on some or most of the items (no fix & track, no spontaneous activity, no activity in neck flexors excessive dorsal incurvation, no sucking)	

Persisting extraneurological pathologies	
Cardiac problems	☐
Respiratory problems	☐
Digestive problems	☐
Retinopathy	☐
Muscle shortening or deformations	☐
Other (describe)	☐

Inconclusive results	
Due to unfavorable circumstances for examination	☐

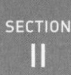

Synthesis for term newborn infants

Absence of any neurological sign ☐

Presence of neurological signs, variable degrees ☐

Minor degree, without CNS depression

Hyperexcitability ☐

Various abnormalities of passive tone ☐

	Yes		No	
Normalized by day 3	Yes	☐	No	☐
Normalized by day 7	Yes	☐	No	☐

Moderate degree, with CNS depression

Lethargy poor fix and track ☐

Hypoactivity ☐

Passive hypotonia in limbs ☐

Poor activity in neck flexors ☐

Primary reflexes poor or absent ☐

Seizures (1 or 2) ☐

	Yes		No	
Normalized by day 7	Yes	☐	No	☐

Severe degree, with deep CNS depression and repeated seizures for more than 30 minutes

Duration of status epilepticus _____ hours

Duration of assistive ventilation _____ days

Duration of absence of feeding autonomy _____ days

Evolving pattern based on repeated examinations

Dynamic (tendency to aggravation followed by improvement) ☐

Static (few or no changes) ☐

Signs in favor of a prenatal insult (present at birth)

Cortical thumb ☐

High-arched palate ☐

Overlapping sutures (with or without microcephaly) ☐

Inconclusive results

Due to unfavorable circumstances for examination ☐

CHAPTER

10

Perinatal cerebral circulation

Edgar Hernandez-Andrade, Horst Steiner and Birgit Arabin

Key Points

- Fetal cerebral blood flow
- Neonatal cerebral blood flow
- Fetal blood flow redistribution
- Fetal anemia
- IUGR
- Fetal cerebral malformation

BASIC PHYSIOLOGY AND HISTORIC STEPS IN THE DETECTION OF FETAL CEREBRAL BLOOD FLOW

The cerebral fetal and neonatal circulation has been a field of interest for many researchers and clinicians. During the 1960s and 1970s, several experimental studies were performed in the fetal lamb exploring mainly physiological changes in the fetal brain circulation (Quilligan et al 1968, Rudolph & Heymann 1968, 1970). The main limitation to study the human fetus and the neonate was the technology available at that time. We here only summarize basic features from these early investigations.

Cerebral blood flow (CBF) in man is about 50 mL/100 g of brain/minute. It has been shown that CBF, cerebral blood volume (CBV) and cerebral energy metabolism measured as the cerebral metabolic rate of oxygen ($CMRO_2$) or of glucose (CMR_{glu}) are all coupled and higher in gray than white matter. This means that the oxygen extraction fraction (OEF) remains about the same (approximately 40 percent) throughout the brain. Therefore, in normal resting human brain, CBF (i.e. flow) is a reliable reflection of $CMRO_2$ (i.e. function) (Leenders et al 1990). Cerebral circulation depends on cerebral perfusion pressure and cerebrovascular resistance. The perfusion pressure is the difference between the systemic arterial pressure and the venous pressure at the exit of the subarachnoid space, the latter being approximated by the intracranial pressure.

In the late 1950s the continuous Doppler technique was developed by Satomura to detect blood flow in human vessels (Satomura 1959). Studies on the circulation within the fetal heart were first reported by Japanese researchers as early as 1968 (Ashitaka et al 1968). However, the continuous Doppler devices did not discriminate depth and position of the targeted vessel. Since the late 1970s pulsed Doppler devices were designed.

FitsGerald and Drumm combined a continuous-wave Doppler with a 2-D static B-mode to study flow velocity waveforms in the fetal umbilical artery (FitsGerald & Drumm 1977). Later, Eik-Nes and Marsal developed the first handheld linear-array real-time apparatus coupled with rangegated Doppler (Eik-Nes et al 1982) which allowed identification of the location of the Doppler gate and dynamic blood flow changes. However, with this device only straight vessels such as the aorta or the common carotid artery (CCA) could be easily visualized (Arabin et al 1987b). The simultaneous measurement of a ratio of the fetal CCA and the umbilical artery was proposed to detect fetal blood flow redistribution (Arabin et al 1987b).

Using a sector scanner with pulsed Doppler device Wladimiroff et al (1986) were first to report Doppler studies of the fetal internal carotid arteries (ICA) and popularizing the ICA/umbilical artery Pulsatility Index (PI) ratio for the assessment of fetal compromise. They also described blood flow in the major fetal cerebral arteries, such as the middle, anterior and posterior cerebral arteries (van den Wijngaard et al 1989).

A major improvement in the localization of the fetal cerebral vessels was the development of color directional Doppler. In 1975 Brandestini's team obtained color-coded flow images superimposed on gray-scale 2-D ultrasound (US) (Eyer et al 1981). Those early systems were limited by the lack of good duplex arrays and processing, and the technique with which Doppler frequency estimation was performed.

With the introduction of the autocorrelation technique means of frequency could be estimated in real time. This approach is still in use today. Finally, analysis of the amplitude of the Doppler signals has created a new modality of color Doppler in the early 1990s (power Doppler ultrasound (PDU)) which allowed identification of vessels with low blood flow velocity (Rubin et al 1994). The application of color Doppler was reported by Kurjak et al (1987) in early pregnancy demonstrating a way to visualize the middle cerebral artery (MCA). Vyas et al (1990b) used the MCA to describe blood flow redistribution in growth-restricted fetuses and Mari et al (2005) to detect the peak systolic velocity in fetal anemia.

The prenatally detected aneurysm of the vein of Galen was described using Doppler ultrasound (Jeanty et al 1990). Later, the fetal cerebral venous circulation was described in more detail.

At present, color directional and power Doppler modes and the combined use of the inversion mode of 3D ultrasound are the favorable tools for 'state of the art' prenatal angiography. These techniques have enabled a more complex understanding of the cerebral arterial and venous circulation (Hernandez-Andrade et al 2007).

ANATOMY OF BRAIN CIRCULATION

The development of the fetal cerebral vessel system closely follows the growth and development of the brain. The basilar vertebral supplies the cerebellum and brain stem. The basic pattern of the external vessels is established by 7 weeks postgestational age and remains unchanged until term (Pape & Wigglesworth 1979). A more detailed background description of the embryology can be found in the book of Pape and Wigglesworth (1979).

THE ARTERIAL SYSTEM

Blood supply to the fetal brain or CBF is provided by the carotid and the vertebral systems joining in a remarkable anastomosis, the arterial circle of Willis (Gray 2000). In addition, branches from the external carotid artery contribute to the cerebral perfusion (Gray 2000). The fetal brain receives 5% of the total cardiac output (Cohn et al 1974) and represents approximately 2% of the total body weight under physiological conditions (Falck & Rajs 1995).

Carotid system

The CCA follow the same course with the exception of their origin. The right CCA originates in the neck from the *brachiocephalic trunk*; the left CCA arises from the *aortic arch* in the thoracic region. First descriptions of fetal blood flow in the CCA determined by Doppler velocimetry were published in 1987 (Arabin et al 1987b).

The ICA starts on both sides at the bifurcation of the CCA at the level of the fourth cervical vertebra. It passes up the neck without branching to the base of the skull where it enters the carotid canal of the petrous process and exits inside the skull just medial to the anterior clinoid process of the sphenoid bone. This vessel has a cervical, a petrous, a cavernous and a supraclinoid segment, terminal branches are the anterior cerebral and middle cerebral arteries (Fig. 10.1). First descriptions of fetal blood flow in the ICA determined by Doppler velocimetry were published in 1986 (Arabin et al 1987b, Wladimiroff 1986).

After entering the skull at the base of the brain, the ICA forms the circle of Willis by the proximal parts of the two anterior cerebral arteries connected by the anterior communicating artery, and the proximal parts of the two posterior cerebral arteries connected by the two posterior communicating arteries (Figs 10.2 and 10.3). Around 50% of circles have hypoplastic or absent segments.

Branches arising from the circle of Willis

The anterior cerebral artery (ACA) arises from the ICA at the medial extremity of the lateral cerebral fissure and passes above the optic nerve (Fig. 10.1). Both ACAs are connected

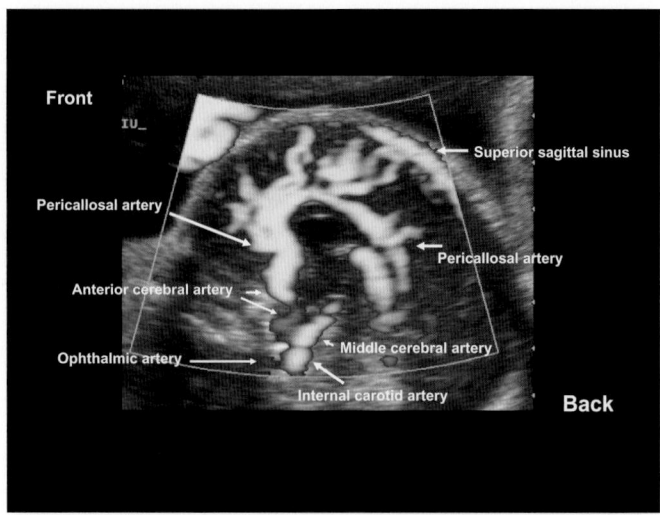

Figure 10.1 Mid sagittal view of the fetal head. The vascular network of the anterior cerebral and pericallosal arteries is observed with power Doppler ultrasound. The superior sagittal sinus runs backwards just below the skull.

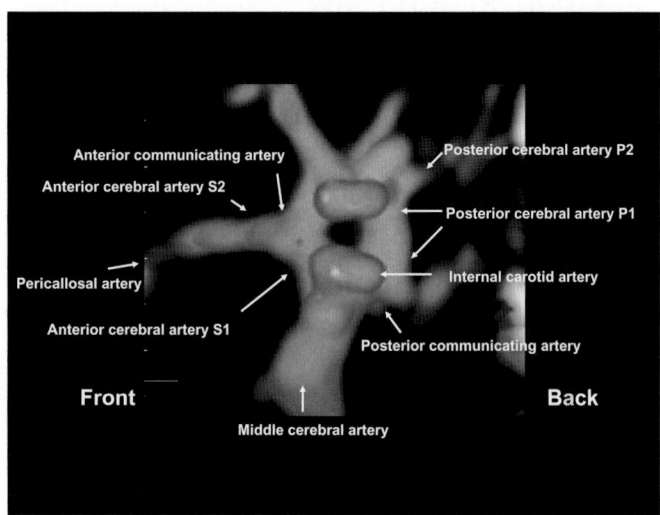

Figure 10.2 Three-dimensional power Doppler reconstruction of the circle of Willis observed from below. The two internal carotid arteries are observed in the base of the circle. S1: Segment one of the anterior cerebral artery, before the joint with the anterior communicating artery. S2: Segment two of the anterior cerebral artery, after the joint with the anterior communicating artery. P1: Part one of the posterior cerebral artery, just after the joint with the posterior communicating artery. P2: Part two of the posterior cerebral artery, after the joint with the posterior communicating artery.

by a short trunk, the anterior communicating artery (Fig. 10.2). The artery before this point is considered as segment 1 and from this point as segment 2 (Fig. 10.3). The two vessels run together following the longitudinal fissure and finish in the pericallosal arteries (PCaA) (Fig. 10.1). First

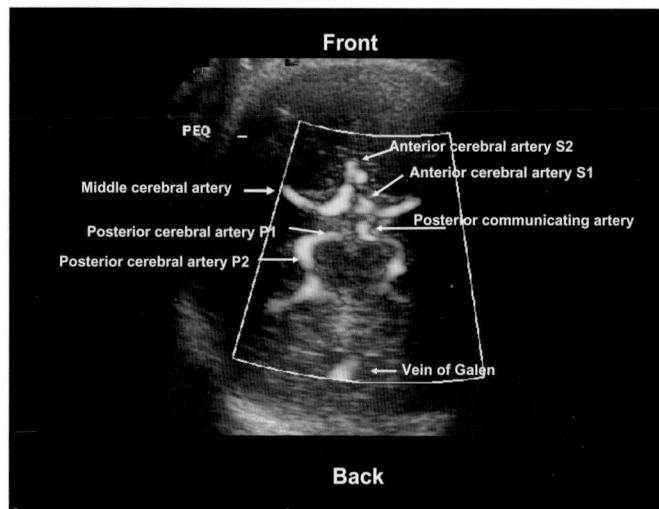

Figure 10.3 Cross sectional view of the circle of Willis and its main branches with the vein of Galen as a reference for the mid vascular structures. S1: Segment one of the anterior cerebral artery, before the joint with the anterior communicating artery. S2: Segment two of the anterior cerebral artery, after the joint with the anterior communicating artery. P1: Part one of the posterior cerebral artery before, just after the joint with the posterior communicating artery. P2: Part two of the posterior cerebral artery, after the joint with the posterior communicating artery.

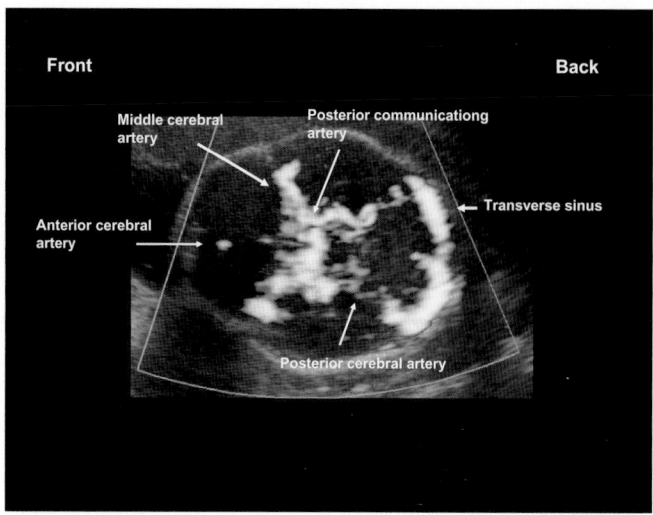

Figure 10.4 Oblique section of the fetal skull at the level of the posterior fossa. The vascular network of the posterior cerebral arteries can be observed. The posterior cerebral arteries and the transverse sinus encircle the cerebellum.

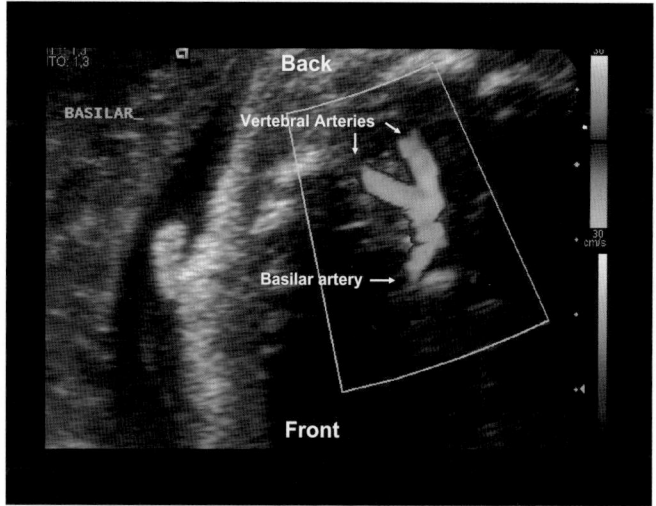

Figure 10.5 Cross sectional view of the lower part of the skull, just below the cerebellum at the level of the brain stem. The two vertebral arteries join in the middle to form the basilar artery.

blood flow velocity wave forms of this vessel were published in 1989 (van den Wijngaard et al 1989). The pericallosal artery follows the curve around the genu of the corpus callosum, turns backwards over the complete upper surface of the corpus callosum and finishes by anastomosing with the posterior cerebral artery (Figs 10.1 and 10.4). First blood flow velocity wave forms of this vessel were published in 1989 (van den Wijngaard et al 1989).

The MCA runs lateral in the sylvian fissure and then turns backward and upward on the surface of the insula, where it divides into a number of branches distributing to the lateral surface of the cerebral hemisphere (Fig. 10.4). First descriptions of fetal blood flow in the MCA determined by Doppler velocimetry were published in 1987 (Arabin et al 1987b, Woo et al 1987).

The posterior communicating arteries (PComA) are defined as a pair of *blood vessels* in the *circle of Willis* going backwards and connecting with the posterior cerebral arteries of the same side (Figs 10.2 and 10.3). Its meaning in the context of fetal cerebral circulation has been described previously (Vasovic 2004).

The anterior choroidal artery (AchoA) arises from the ICA, near the PComA passing backward and lateral between the temporal lobe and the cerebral peduncle. It enters the inferior horn of the lateral ventricle through the choroidal fissure contributing to the hippocampus, fimbria and tela choroidea of the third ventricle and ends in the choroid plexus.

Vertebral system

The vertebral artery (VA) arises from the proximal subclavian artery and ascends through the transverse foramen of the first cervical vertebra and then enters the skull through the foramen magnum. The two vertebral arteries join each other at the level of the pontomedullary junction to form the basilar artery. The vertebral artery gives rise to anterior and posterior spinal arteries, the posterior-inferior cerebellar artery and branches to the medulla.

The basilar artery (BA) is formed by the two VAs and ascends along the ventral aspect of the pons (Fig. 10.5). Main branches are the anterior inferior cerebellar artery, the superior cerebellar arteries and numerous of paramedian, short and long circumferential penetrators, the internal auditory (labyrinthine) artery, pontine and anterior-inferior cerebellar, internal auditory and superior cerebellar artery. It ends in two terminal posterior cerebral arteries. It supplies the temporal and occipital lobes, the pons, the internal ear, the cerebellum, the pineal body, the anterior medullary velum and the tela choroidea of the third ventricle.

The posterior cerebral artery (PCA) surrounds the mid-brain at the level of tentorium cerebelli; both branches anastomose with the PComAs to complete the circle of Willis (Figs 10.2 and 10.3). It supplies the occipital lobe, and the inferior part of the temporal lobe, the midbrain, thalamus, hypothalamus and geniculate bodies.

Both arterial systems also communicate through the lep-tomeningeal (cortical branches) and dural anastomoses of the ACA, MCA and PCA on the surface of the brain. In addition, the anterior choroidal artery (branch of the ICA) occasionally anastomoses with the posterior choroidal artery branch of the external carotid artery. ACA, MCA, PComA and PCAs give origin to two different systems of secondary vessels, the ganglionic and the cortical systems.

The ganglionic system supplies the thalami and corpora striata (Fig. 10.6). The vessels of this system are designated terminal arteries, meaning that they neither provide nor receive any anastomotic branch so that only a limited area of the thalamus or corpus striatum can be perfused. Gangli-onic branches from the ACA supply the rostrum of the corpus callosum, septum pellucidum, the head of the caudate nucleus, the olfactory lobe, gyrus rectus, internal orbital gyrus, part of the superior frontal gyrus, part of the superior and middle frontal gyri, the upper part of the anterior central gyrus, the cingulate gyrus, the medial surface of the superior frontal gyrus, the upper part of the anterior central gyrus, and the precuneus and adjacent lateral surface of the hemisphere.

Ganglionic branches of the MCA supply the caudate nucleus, the internal capsule; the thalamus, the anterior central gyrus, the supramarginal and angular gyri, and the posterior parts of the superior and middle temporal gyri. The temporal branches, two or three in number are distributed to the lateral surface of the temporal lobe.

Ganglionic branches of the PComA supply the medial surface of the thalami and the walls of the third ventricle, the choroid plexus. Ganglionic branches of the PCA are the postero-lateral ganglionic branches that supply a consider-able portion of the thalamus.

THE VENOUS SYSTEM

The venous system of the brain is constituted by superficial and deep cerebral veins which drain into the venous sinuses and then into the internal jugular vein. There are numerous venous connections between cerebral veins and venous sinuses. The veins of the brain possess extremely thin walls and have no valves. They also may be divided into cerebral and cerebellar veins (Gray 2000).

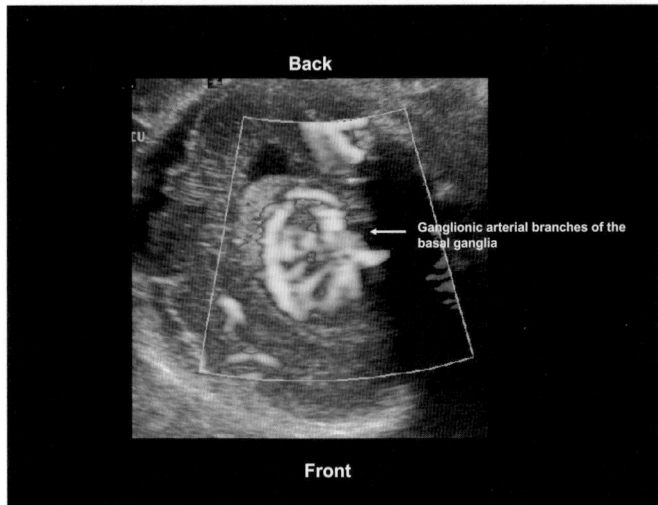

Figure 10.6 Mid parasagittal view of the fetal head, where the vascular network (ganglionic branches) of the basal ganglia is observed. The basal ganglia is delimited by the head, body and tail of the caudate nucleus which has a C-shaped structure and constitutes part of the basis of the lateral ventricle.

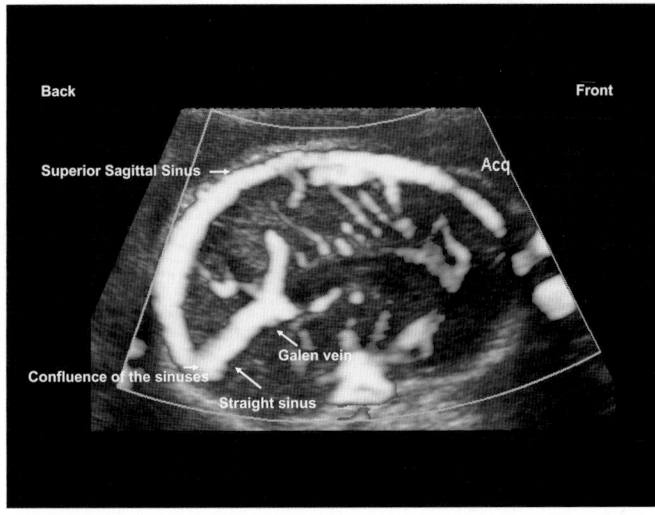

Figure 10.7 Mid sagittal view of the fetal head. The complete superior sagittal sinus is observed running backwards below the skull. The vein of Galen emerges in the central-posterior part of the brain, continuing with the straight sinus and finally draining in the confluence of the sinuses.

Cerebral veins

The superior cerebral veins drain the superior, lateral and medial surfaces of the hemispheres and open into the supe-rior sagittal sinus (Fig. 10.7).

The middle cerebral veins originate from the lateral surface of the hemisphere, and end in the sphenoparietal sinus con-necting the superior sagittal and the transverse sinuses.

The inferior cerebral veins drain the basal areas of the hemispheres and open into the superior sagittal and superior petrosal sinuses.

The basal vein is formed from the union of the anterior cerebral vein which accompanies the ACA, the deep middle (sylvian) cerebral vein and the inferior striate vein. It ends in the internal cerebral vein (vein of Galen).

The terminal vein commences between the corpus striatum and thalamus, receives numerous veins from both, and unites with the choroid vein, to form one of the internal cerebral veins.

The internal cerebral veins drain the deep parts of the hemisphere running between the layers of the third ventricle, and beneath the splenium of the corpus callosum, where they unite to form the great cerebral vein.

The great cerebral vein (great vein of Galen, GV) is formed by the union of the two internal cerebral veins. It curves backward and upward around the splenium of the corpus callosum and ends in the straight sinus.

Cerebellar veins

Cerebellar veins are placed on the surface of the cerebellum, and are disposed in two sets, superior and inferior. The superior cerebellar veins end in the straight sinus and the internal cerebellar veins in the transverse and superior petrosal sinuses. The inferior cerebellar veins end in the transverse, superior petrosal and occipital sinuses.

Diploic veins occupy channels in the diploë of the cranial bones. These veins are confined to the particular bones; when the sutures are obliterated, they unite and increase in size. They communicate with the meningeal veins and the sinuses of the dura mater and with the veins of the pericranium.

Sinuses of the dura mater

These vessels are venous channels draining the blood from the brain situated between the two layers of the dura mater. They can be divided as postero-superior at the upper and back part of the skull, and antero-inferior groups in the base of the skull. The postero-superior group comprises the superior sagittal, straight, inferior sagittal, transverse and occipital (Figs 10.7 and 10.8).

The superior sagittal sinus (SSS) runs backward from the inner surface of the frontal and between the adjacent margins of the two parietals and is continued as the corresponding transverse sinus. It increases in size as it passes backward and receives the superior cerebral veins, veins from the diploë and dura mater and veins from the pericranium (Fig. 10.8).

The inferior sagittal sinus (ISS) contains the free margin of the falx cerebri and ends in the straight sinus. It receives several veins from the falx cerebri and the medial surfaces of the hemispheres.

The straight sinus (SS) is situated at the line of junction of the falx cerebri and the tentorium cerebelli. It runs downward and backward from the end of the inferior sagittal sinus to the transverse sinus of the opposite side. Its terminal part receives the inferior sagittal sinus, the great cerebral (Galen) vein and the superior cerebellar veins (Fig. 10.8).

The occipital sinus (OS) is the smallest of the cranial sinuses. It is situated in the attached margin of the falx cerebelli and communicates with the posterior internal vertebral venous plexuses ending in the confluence of the sinuses.

The confluence of the sinuses is the term applied to the dilated extremity of the SSS (Fig. 10.7). It is of irregular form, lodged on one side (generally the right) of the internal occipital protuberance, receives blood from the OS and is connected with the transverse sinus of the opposite side.

The transverse sinuses (TS) are large and begin at the internal occipital protuberance; the right one is the direct continuation of the SSS, the left one of the SS. Each TS passes lateralward and forward, describing a slight curve, to the base of the petrous portion of the temporal bone. It reaches the jugular foramen, where it ends in the internal jugular vein. The TSs are frequently of unequal size. They receive blood from the superior petrosal sinuses at the base of the petrous portion of the temporal bone, communicate with the veins of the pericranium by means of the mastoid and condyloid emissary veins; and receive some of the inferior cerebral and cerebellar veins.

The antero-inferior group of sinuses comprises two cavernous, two superior petrosal, two intercavernous, two inferior petrosal and the basilar plexus.

TECHNICAL ASPECTS TO DETECT FETAL AND NEONATAL CEREBRAL BLOOD FLOW

The vascular anatomy within the brain can be visualized with color directional or PDU. PDU has a high sensitivity to identify low blood flow velocities in small vessels, thus allowing the visualization of the vascular architecture of several cerebral regions (Hernandez-Andrade et al 2006, Marsal & Hernandez-Andrade 2004). However, in some areas the acoustic shadow of the skull can affect the quality of the ultrasound images. Nevertheless, good-quality images can be obtained if the proper settings are used.

One of the main planes that can be obtained in the fetal brain is the mid-sagittal plane from where the blood flow to the anterior and posterior part of the brain can be visualized. In this projection, the complete anterior cerebral and pericallosal arteries and its branches can be studied. More posteriorly, the vein of Galen and the sagittal and straight sinuses are clearly observed. By using the same anatomical plane to visualize the cerebellum, the arterial circulation of the posterior fossa provided by the two PCAs and the venous flow from the TSs can be seen. Other structures, such as the basal ganglia located in the floor of the lateral ventricle, are obtained in a parasagittal view.

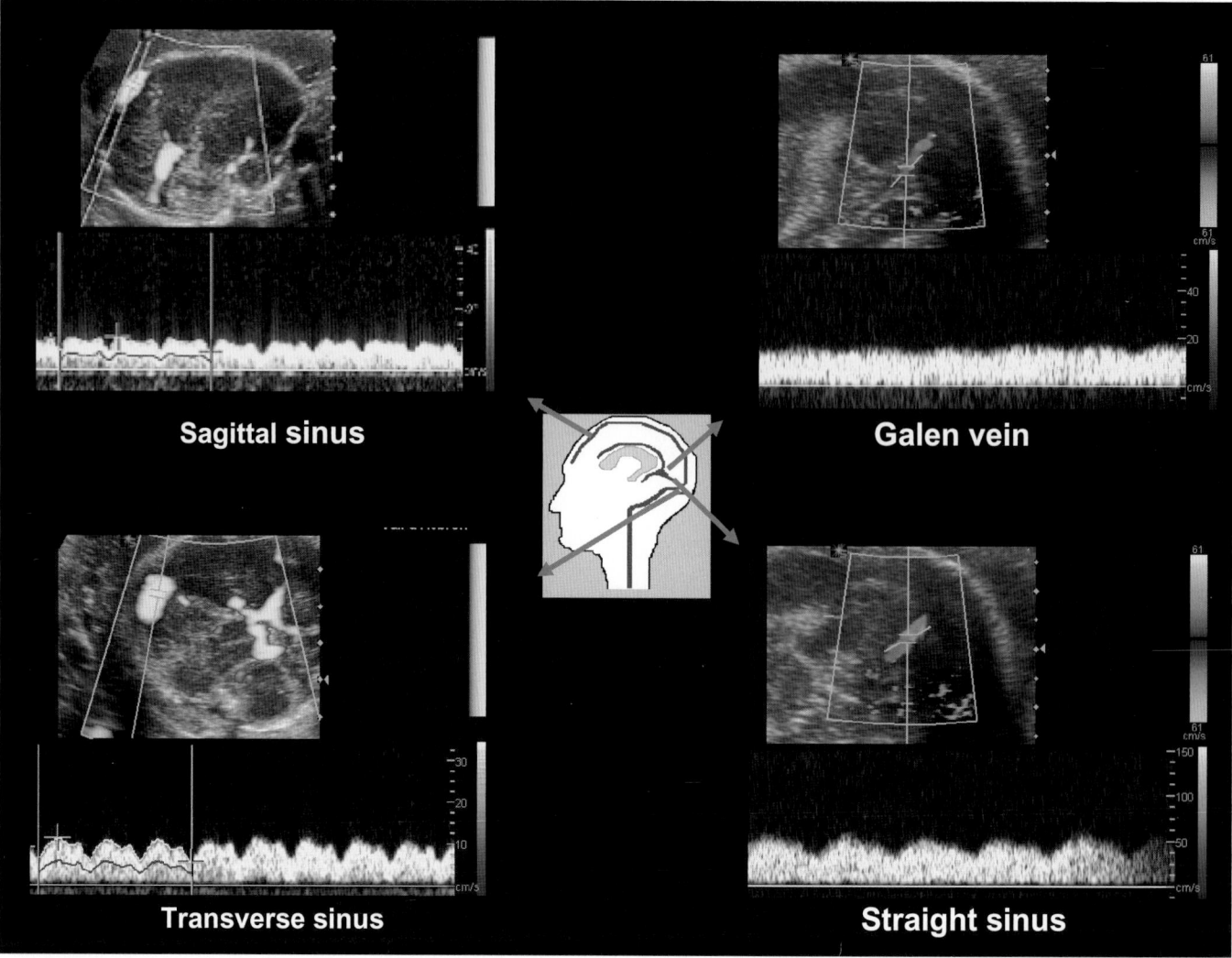

Figure 10.8 Pulsed Doppler waveforms of the three main venous sinuses and the vein of Galen in the normally grown fetus. Note that the vein of Galen is the only non-pulsatile vessel. The waveform of the transverse sinus resembles that from the ductus venosus.

Several technical recommendations should be followed to optimize the power Doppler images. The size of the color box should be maintained as small as possible to cover the studied regions and to improve the frame rate. In general, the ultrasound settings include a standard gray-scale image for obstetrics, medium persistence, high sensitivity, normal image display, medium wall filter and gain levels just above the presence of noise. The mechanical and thermal indices must always be maintained at the lowest possible level and the examination time be kept as short as possible.

Three dimensional (3-D) PDU images of the vascular anatomy provide a spatial visualization of the structures. Normal variants, abnormal patterns and increased perfusion of different vascular networks can be documented using this technique. For 3-D PDU the following settings should be used after optimizing the 2-D US and PDU settings: acquisition in Angio 3-D, or Glass Body modes, with an aperture of the US sweep between 20 and 25° and using maximum image quality (Hernandez-Andrade et al 2007).

These imaging techniques offer a new perspective in evaluating regional changes in brain perfusion, either in normal conditions or in pregnancy-associated complications.

FETAL CEREBRAL BLOOD FLOW DISTRIBUTION UNDER PHYSIOLOGIC CONDITIONS

Various factors have an impact on the blood flow distribution to the brain and within the brain, which has to be considered when interpreting the results. The authors presume a basic understanding of the principles, practice and interpretation of Doppler US which are already summarized in standard ultrasound text books.

GESTATIONAL AGE

Gestational age influences blood flow velocity waveforms of cerebral arteries. This was already shown in the first studies on fetal cerebral circulation in the CCA (Arabin et al 1987a, 1987b, Bilardo et al 1988, Malcus et al 1991) and in the ICA (Wladimiroff et al 1986).

With the introduction of color flow mapping the MCA became the gold standard to determine cerebral blood flow. Kurjak and coworkers (Kurjak et al 1992) studied early embryonic and fetal cerebral circulation from 8 weeks onwards. Diastolic frequencies (velocities) increased with advancing gestation, being constantly seen after 13 weeks. Other observational studies found a parabolic curve of the PI with gestational age between 15 and 20 weeks and a constant decrease towards term (Arduini & Rizzo 1990, Vyas et al 1990b). However, for clinical reasons and safety considerations it seems appropriate not to perform cerebral Doppler recordings during the first 20 weeks of gestation. During the late second and early third trimester all Doppler indices in the MCA such as the Resistance Index (RI), the PI and the S/D-ratio show a tendency to rise (Fig. 10.9). Later in pregnancy a decrease in these indices can be observed while diastolic velocities increase (Harrington et al 1995, Kurmanavicius et al 1997, Meerman et al 1990, Schaffer et al 1998, Vetter 1991).

A significant decrease of the RI in the MCA was observed from 38 weeks onwards, whereas there was no change of these indices in the umbilical artery, fetal aorta or renal artery (Schaffer et al 1999) (Fig. 10.10). The decrease in velocities might be due to increasing vessel diameter and to decreasing oxygen tension in the fetal blood around term. Longitudinal observations showed a continuous decrease of the RI in the MCA until spontaneous delivery allowed the prediction of the probability of spontaneous onset of labor (Schaffer et al 1999). If the RI was <0.66 between 37 and

42 weeks gestation the chance of spontaneous delivery within the next 10 days was 95% and 55% within the following 4 days respectively. However, in individual cases there might be an inverse change and an increase of the MCA-RI before a 'spontaneous' delivery.

In contrast to the RI there is no change in quantitative parameters of cerebral circulation such as the mean or peak velocities (Schaffer et al 1999).

FETAL BEHAVIORAL STATES

Fetal neurological development, expressed by the emergence of well-distinguishable fetal behavioral states, is associated with specific hemodynamic adaptations (van Eyck & Wladimiroff 1988). The asymmetrically growth-retarded human fetus is capable of modifying this relationship.

The correlation of CBF and fetal behavioral states, was examined by van Eyck et al (1987) using the fetal ICA and umbilical artery at 37–38 weeks gestation, suggesting increased fetal CBF during state 2F in normal pregnancy. In growth-retarded fetuses both vessels showed a virtual overlap of PI values originating from state 1F and 2F, reflecting behavioral state independency. It was stated that in the ICA, this state independency is associated with moderately reduced PI values (van Eyck et al 1988).

However, fetal behavioral states have been demonstrated to influence selected cerebral vascular compartments (Noordam et al 1994). Doppler recordings analyzed by the PI showed significant differences in the ACA and PCA in different states whereas the PI of the MCA did not show significant differences between fetal active and quiet (sleep) states.

In the analysis of blood flow velocity waveforms for clinical purposes, fetal behavioral states and fetal heart rate (FHR) have to be taken into account for a proper interpretation of recorded data. Nevertheless, the complete

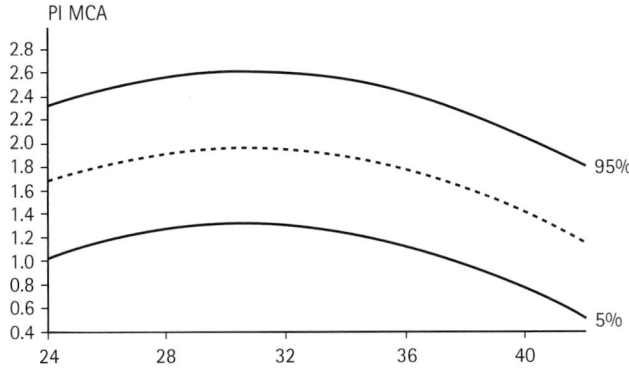

Figure 10.9 Reference values of the pulsatility index (PI) in the middle cerebral artery (MCA) between 24 and 42 gestational weeks. (Schaffer H, Steiner H, Staudach A 1998 Reference values for qualitative and quantitative analysis of uterine, fetoplacental and fetal flow velocity waveforms. J Fertil Reprod Special 2:12–13.)

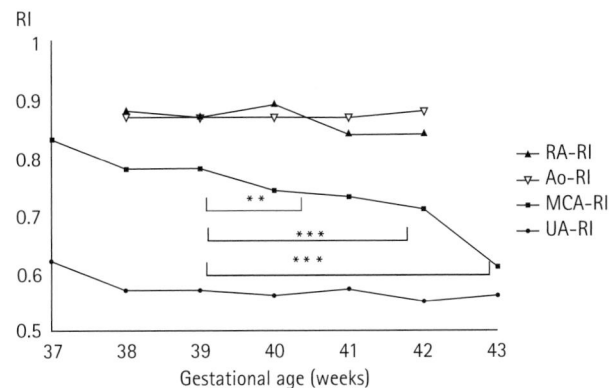

Figure 10.10 Resistance indices (RI) in the middle cerebral artery (MCA), the fetal descending aorta (Ao), the fetal renal artery (RA) and the umbilical artery (UA). ** change P < 0.01, *** change P < 0.001.

determination of behavioral states would be a time-consuming procedure. This MCA is therefore used for determination of fetal wellbeing since it seems to be most resistant to hemodynamic variance due to different fetal states (van Eyck et al 1987).

Other 'behavioral factors' influencing fetal Doppler waveforms are the FHR and respiratory movements. There is an inverse relationship between the FHR and the length of the cardiac cycle which influences the configuration of all Doppler velocity waveforms. An increase of the FHR increases end-diastolic velocities and therefore decreases the absolute values of the indices (van Eyck & Wladimiroff 1988). In fetuses with acute bradycardia, protective changes producing a 'heart-sparing' and a 'brain-sparing' effect have been observed (Gembruch & Baschat 2000).

Fetal breathing movements and hiccups have an unsystematic impact on the shape of all Doppler velocity waveforms. Therefore Doppler examinations should be conducted in the absence of both.

BLOOD VISCOSITY

Animal studies have suggested that increased blood viscosity is associated with reduced cardiac output and increased peripheral resistance. However in humans, no association was found between umbilical blood flow patterns and blood viscosity (Giles & Trudinger 1986). There are no publications with specific attention to the association between viscosity and CBF.

Special changes combined with anemia and low hematocrit are discussed below.

EXTERNAL FACTORS

Several external factors have been described to have an impact on CBF in the MCA (Vyas et al 1990a). At early gestational age, a reversal of blood flow during diastole may be an artificial finding. Increased transabdominal pressure seems to cause a decrease of mean velocities and an increase of the PI in the MCA (Vyas et al 1990a). Nevertheless, the route of Doppler application did not influence absolute values of Doppler indices when comparing values taken from the transabdominal versus the transvaginal route measured indices (Lewinsky et al 1991).

Fetal CBF has also been investigated in response to invasive techniques. No significant changes in PI values were seen after amniocentesis performed either transamniotically or transplacentally. However, fetal blood sampling (cord needling) induced a significant decrease of PI values in all investigated vessels (umbilical artery, thoracic descending aorta, renal artery, MCA) and was higher in the presence of a transplacental compared to a transamniotic procedure only in the umbilical artery, but not in the MCA (Capponi et al 1996).

Similarly, a significant drop in both umbilical and MCA RI was found after cordocentesis with a greater drop when the blood was sampled transplacentally and in early gestational age. The discussed mechanisms are hemodynamic

changes, changes in fetal endorphin and vasodilatator release or arterial vasospasm (Chitrit et al 1995, Hecher et al 1993, Teixeira et al 1996).

Vibroacoustic stimulation has been reported to increase the PI in the fetal MCA. Thereby the influence of the FHR was negligible and thus the explanation for this response remains unclear (Kofinas et al 1996).

BRAIN BLOOD FLOW DISTRIBUTION UNDER PATHOLOGIC CONDITIONS

COLOR DIRECTIONAL OR POWER DOPPLER AND CONVERSION MODE TO DIAGNOSE ABNORMAL ANATOMY OF CEREBRAL BLOOD VESSELS AND THE BRAIN

In the past, the visualization of CBF was limited due to technical reasons. The conventional pulsed Doppler transducers with linear array were limited to visualize straight vessels such as the CCA (Arabin 1990, Arabin et al 1987b). With the introduction of sector transducers, the ICA, MCA and the circle of Willis were also able to be visualized (Wladimiroff 1986).

Color directional and power Doppler modes and the combined use of the inversion mode of 3-D ultrasound have enabled us to get a more complex understanding of the cerebral arterial and venous circulations. In addition to the normal anatomy, malformations of fetal vessels can be more easily assessed (Fig. 10.11). The visualization by color mode makes Doppler recordings easy, accurate and safe, because the time of insonation to the fetal brain is minimized.

Some examples of abnormal cerebral vessel anatomy are:

Hypoechogenic lesions within the skull need vascular
   imaging to differentiate arachnoid cysts, porencephaly
   and hydrocephaly from arteriovenous fistulae such as

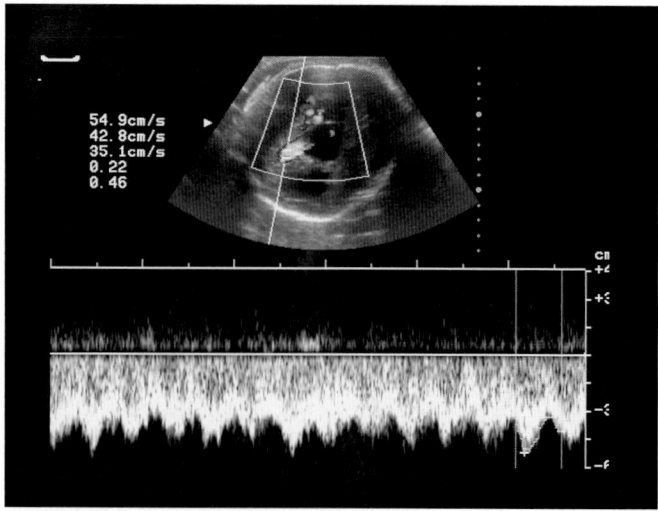

Figure 10.11 Color Doppler mapping and flow velocity waveform of the vein of Galen.

vein of Galen aneurysms, which are frequently combined with fetal hydrops and fatal outcome (Dan et al 1992, Heling et al 2000, Paladini et al 1996, Sepulveda et al 1995) (Figs 10.11 and 10.12).

Color Doppler may help in the differential diagnosis of arteriovenous fistulae which can also be found in other regions of the brain and do not always present as hypoechogenic cysts. A frequent associated finding is cardiomegaly and dilated neck veins.

Periventricular cystic lesions can be prenatally further identified by spectral Doppler analysis demonstrating pulsatile flow velocity waveforms (Fig. 10.12).

Some cerebral malformations of the fetal brain such as agenesis of the corpus callosum can either be diagnosed or excluded by visualizing the pericallosal artery (Fig. 10.1). In the case of agenesis or dysgenesis there may be an abnormal looping.

In microcephaly, holoprosencephaly or various cerebral malformations, the shape of the circle of Willis may be distorted (Guzman & Grady 1999, Pilu et al 1998).

Cerebral tumors, though rare, may be further differentiated by the vascularization within the tumor. We have observed a fetus with a tumor from the lateral skull which was post partum histologically diagnosed as infantile myofibrosis (Fig. 10.13).

CEREBRAL CIRCULATION IN FETAL HYPOXIA

Fetal hypoxia and oxygen deficiency in fetal tissue may lead to a conversion of the fetal metabolism leading to a conversion of pyruvate to lactic acid.

There are several hemodynamic mechanisms for the fetus to adapt to hypoxia favoring blood flow to the fetal brain, heart and adrenals but reducing the blood flow to kidneys, gastrointestinal tract and lower extremities. This redistribution was described in animal models as a response to acute

hypoxic stress as a brain-sparing effect (Dawes 1962, Dawes et al 1968, Rudolph 1984, Rudolph & Heymann 1968). On the basis of clinical observations from amnioscopy and microblood sampling, Saling (1996) defined these phenomena as the O_2-sparing fetal circulation. It is supposed that partial pressures of oxygen and carbon dioxide are triggering the described redistribution allowing preferential delivery of nutrients and oxygen to the vital organs. However, cerebral vascular vasodilatation is limited and no interpretable changes in resistance indices occur at least 2 weeks before the fetus is jeopardized by late FHR decelerations (Arduini et al 1992). This is why longitudinal measurements of cerebral arterial vessels are meanwhile replaced by venous Doppler measurements to determine the optimal time of early iatrogenic delivery. Animal and human studies have shown that there is also redistribution in the umbilical venous blood through the ductus venosus at the expense of hepatic blood flow allowing an increase in oxygen delivery to the fetal brain (Gudmundsson et al 1996, Kiserud et al 1998, Reuss et al 1982, 1983).

Doppler measurements in the fetal CCA (Arabin et al 1987a, 1987b, Wladimiroff et al 1986), the ICA (Arabin et al 1987a, 1987b, Arduini & Rizzo 1990, Wladimiroff et al 1986) and the MCA (Arduini & Rizzo 1990, Vyas et al 1990b) have shown that there is an increase in end diastolic velocities in fetuses with suspected fetal hypoxia, mostly in growth-retarded fetuses. By performing cordocentesis immediately before or after the Doppler investigation it became possible to directly correlate fetal blood gases with the cerebral Doppler velocity wave forms (Bilardo et al 1990, Hecher et al 1995, Rizzo et al 1995). Bilardo et al found that best predictor of asphyxia was an index comprising aortic mean velocity and the CCA artery PI. When this index was abnormal, 89% of fetuses had an 'asphyxia index' 1 SD above the mean. A normal index was always associated with normal blood gases. The indices representing the inverse relationship of impedance and velocity in the vessels that supply the brain or the abdominal viscera reflect the hemodynamic response to changes in the partial pressure of respiratory gases (Bilardo et al 1990).

Ratios from the PI or the RI of the CCA, the ICA or the MCA versus the fetal aorta or the umbilical artery were suggested as tools to diagnose and quantify fetal hemodynamic redistribution (Arabin et al 1987a, 1987b, Gramellini et al 1992, Scherjon et al 2000). Scherjon et al (2000) investigated fetuses with a raised ratio of umbilical/cerebral (MCA) blood flow. The results led to the conclusion that fetal brain-sparing, although a seemingly beneficial adaptive mechanism for intact neurologic survival is, however, later associated with a poorer cognitive outcome at 5 years of age.

Another group to investigate, in the context of impending or present hypoxia, is post-term fetuses. The prevalence of thick meconium-stained liquor in labor was inversely correlated with the MCA PI although there was no significant correlation with oligohydramnios or with the PI in the

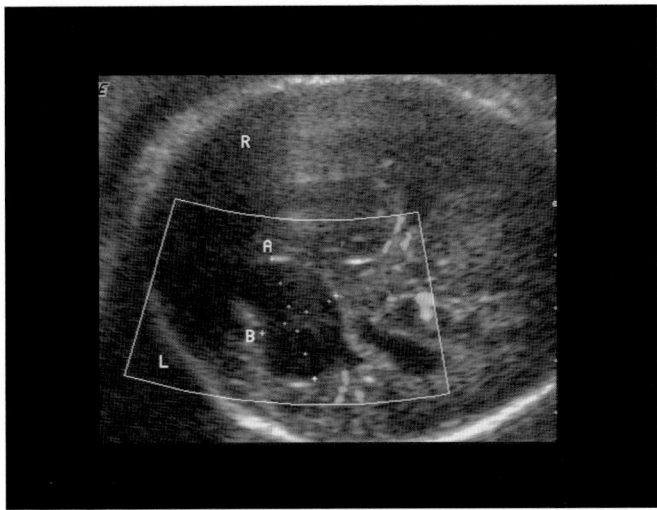

Figure 10.12 Periventricular cystic lesion in a fetus at 34 weeks gestation.

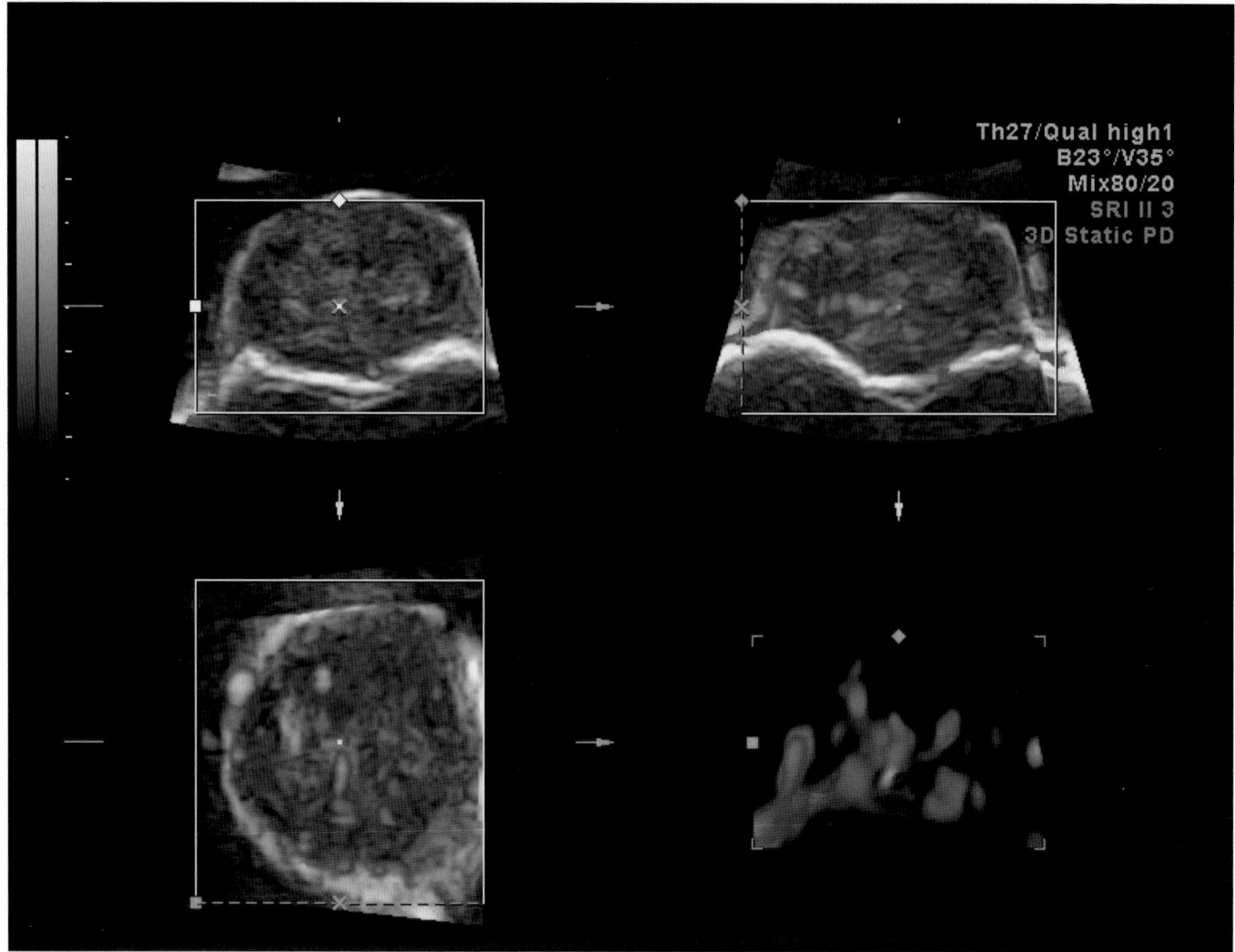

Figure 10.13 Lateral cerebral tumor (multifocal infantile myofibrosis) with vascularization, right below as three-dimensional isolated power reconstruction.

umbilical artery. Logistic regression confirmed that MCA was an independent predicting factor for a risk of thick meconium-stained liquor in uncomplicated postdated pregnancy at 41 weeks (Lam et al 2005).

FETAL ANEMIA

The hemodynamic changes due to fetal anemia are interpreted as signs of a 'hyperdynamic circulation'. Thereby the correlation of fetal CBF and anemia has been well established (Ahmed et al 2005, Chitrit et al 1995, L'Ubusky et al 2004, Mari 2005a, 2005b, Mari et al 2005, Oepkes et al 2006, Pereira et al 2003, Zimmerman et al 2002). The MCA peak systolic velocity is proven to be a highly sensitive non-invasive means for determining the degree of anemia in red blood cell alloimmunized pregnancies (RhD-, Rhc-, RhE-, or Fya-) as well as in feto-maternal hemorrhage (Sueters et al 2003) (Fig. 10.14).

The classic paper of Mari et al (2000) showed that fetal hemoglobin concentrations increase with increasing gestational age. The sensitivity of an increased peak velocity in the MCA for the prediction of moderate or severe anemia was 100% either in the presence or in the absence of hydrops with a false-positive rate of 12%. The widespread use of the Doppler method of MCA peak systolic velocity has meanwhile been used to minimize fetal complications associated with amniocentesis and fetal blood sampling to determine fetal hemoglobin. In a recent paper, Oepkes et al (2006) could prove that the peak velocity in the MCA was more sensitive and more accurate (by 12 and 9% points) than measurement of amniotic-fluid Delta OD450 in fetal hemolytic anemia. Most authors describe that determination of the Doppler velocity waveform in the MCA is only relevant in non-hydropic fetuses (Hernandez-Andrade et al 2004).

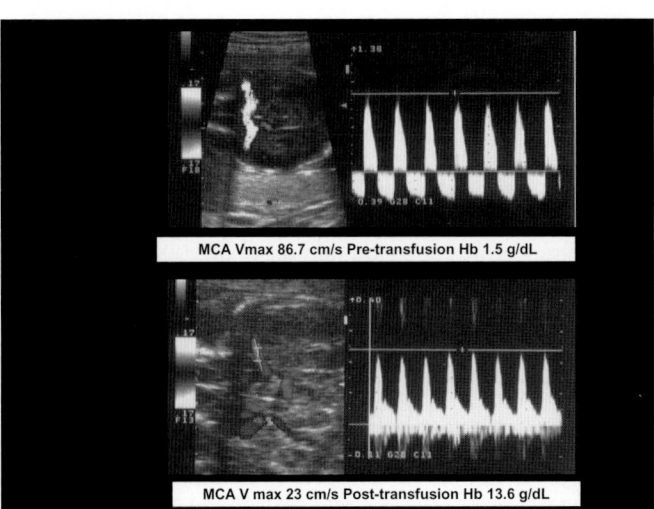

Figure 10.14 Doppler investigation of the middle cerebral artery peak systolic velocity (MCA-PSV) in a fetus affected with severe anemia due to parvovirus infection at 22 weeks of gestation (mean 28 cm/s (SD 7 cm/s)). Note the extremely high PSV and the reversed diastolic flow before the blood transfusion, a very rare sign of bad prognosis. After the blood transfusion MCA-PSV return to normal values with positive diastolic flow.

AMNIOTIC DRAINAGE AND PRETERM RUPTURE OF MEMBRANES

Amniotic fluid decompression for symptomatic polyhydramnios in discordant twin gestations has been shown to cause a significant reduction of the PI in the MCA. When considering only the larger twins in each set, the magnitude of the change in PI MCA was relatively consistent, whereas the smaller twins showed a much more variable response (Mari et al 1992). It was postulated that the acute decrease in maternal and fetal carbon dioxide tensions following relief of maternal restrictive lung dysfunction and the acute fall in amniotic fluid pressure may lead to these changes in regional vascular resistances favoring cerebrovascular perfusion (Mari et al 1992).

Preterm rupture of membranes (PROM), however, has not been proven to be associated with significant changes in cerebral circulation, not even when there were signs of amnioinfection and fetal bacteremia present (Carroll et al 1995).

This might also be explained by the fact that proinflammatory cytokines do not cross normal term placenta (Aaltonen et al 2005).

DRUGS AFFECTING EARLY CEREBRAL BLOOD FLOW

Several drugs commonly used during the transition from intrauterine to extrauterine life may affect the CBF. Prenatally, ritodrine was described as causing an increase in FHR,

the left fetal cardiac output and the PI of the MCA, a decrease in the PI of the umbilical artery (Gokay et al 2001), and oral supplementation of magnesium was reported to decrease fetal vessel resistance in the MCA (Facchinetti et al 1992). There are conflicting data when comparing antenatal magnesium sulphate and ritodrine. In one study both drugs did not induce any significant differences in CBF velocity or vascular resistance of preterm infants in the first hours of life (Pezzati et al 2001). However, another study reports on a trend of reduced CBF in the main cerebral arteries during the first hours of life in infants after treatment with magnesium sulphate but not with ritodrine (Pezzati et al 2001).

During labour, drugs used for epidural anesthesia, such as lidocaine or bupivacaine, do not alter the normal fetal–neonate heart rate. However there is a small risk of reducing the placental blood-flow and thus fetal oxygenation if the dose is prolonged leading to a reduction in CBF. According to current information there is no risk of abnormal neurodevelopment with the normal doses used for obstetric anesthesia (Hamza 1994).

In premature neonates where different therapies should be initiated, various drugs might affect CBF, some acting as protective agents and others as potentially dangerous agents. Indometacine is known to produce cerebral vasoconstriction that enables the use of this drug to prevent intraventricular hemorrhage in preterm neonates (Whitelaw 2001).

Application of steroids (dexamethasone) in the early neonatal life induces an increase of blood flow velocities in the carotid and anterior cerebral arteries, potentially causing damage to the neonatal brain or retina. Conversely, the application of hydrocortisone, combined with dopamine, did not affect CBF (Cabanas et al 1997, Noori et al 2006). In those neonates where exogenous surfactant therapy has been instilled rapidly, an increment in CBF was observed which was not seen when the surfactant was instilled gradually (Saliba et al 1994).

In severely compromised infants, some drugs used to stabilize the neonate (aminophylline) have a potentially dangerous impact on CBF (Dani et al 2000). Inotropic drugs (dopamine or epinephrine) may induce an increase in CBF mainly in infants born before 28 weeks (Pellicer et al 2005). In neonates with pulmonary hypertension, nitric oxide increases the oxygen concentration and the velocity time integral of flow velocities in the MCA (Pellicer et al 2005).

CHANGES FROM PRENATAL TO POSNATAL LIFE

CHANGES DURING CONTRACTIONS AND LABOR

Various groups have studied placental and fetal blood flow changes in the venous and arterial system and sequential changes of the cerebral and placental circulation in comparisons between basal conditions and acute hypoxic stress during uterine contractions (Li et al 2004a, 2004b, 2006, Oosterhof et al 1992).

An early study investigated CBF in the ICA during Braxton Hicks contractions. There was no change of either FHR or the PI in the ICA, suggesting that Braxton Hicks contractions have little or no effect on fetal hemodynamics and on fetal oxygenation in the healthy near-term fetus (Oosterhof et al 1992).

During active labor however, another group found a 40% reduction in MCA blood flow impedance in women in active labor compared with a control group, although the results were not significantly different in uncomplicated labor and those complicated by FHR decelerations. It was concluded that, during active labor, mechanisms that may be unrelated to low fetal blood oxygen content reduce fetal brain blood vessel impedance (Yagel et al 1992).

During labor, term fetuses with abnormal FHR and oxygen saturation values >30% and <30% were studied and peripartum outcomes were compared. MCA Doppler showed significantly lower PI and RI in the presence of reduced oxygen saturation. Differences in fetal outcomes between the two groups correlated with MCA Doppler findings. It seems that, in experienced hands, Doppler screening of fetal MCA waveforms during labor can be useful in the evaluation of intrapartum hypoxia in complicated pregnancies (Kassanos et al 2003).

More recently, placental, arterial and venous CBF during contractions and relaxations of oxytocin challenge tests (OCT) were investigated. Thereby the MCA PI decreased significantly mainly in patients with positive OCT (Li et al 2006). In growth-retarded fetuses without cardiotocograph changes after uterine contractions, de novo pulsations occurred in the GV and SS flow velocities increased during contractions. There were no significant differences in the more centrally located TS flow. It was concluded that in uncompromised intrauterine growth retardation fetuses an acute cerebral venous hyperperfusion develops in response to uterine contractions (Li et al 2004a).

CHANGES IN THE NEONATAL PERIOD

The transition from the fetal to the neonatal circulation involves the increase of arterial blood pressure after the separation of the placenta, stable gaseous lung distension, markedly increased pulmonary perfusion and effective respiratory effort. Directly after birth there is an increase in cerebral vascular resistance and a decrease in CBF in response to the increase in arterial oxygenation (Connors et al 1992). The perfusion and oxygenation of the lungs and the increase in arterial blood pressure produce a change in the direction of blood flow in the ductus venosus, ductus arteriosus and foramen ovale (Friedman & Fahey 1993).

The subsequent decrease in the cerebral RI found between 8 and 24 hours could reflect a remodeling of the circulation due to impedance matching (Connors et al 1992). The perfusion and the oxygenation of the lungs with the increase in arterial blood pressure produce a change in the direction of blood flow in the ductus venosus, ductus arteriosus and foramen ovale (Friedman & Fahey 1993).

In the first hours and days of life, CBF increases in both preterm and term infants. These changes seem to be independent of the mean arterial pressure, the PCO_2 and hematocrit (Cheung et al 1994, Kehrer et al 2005, Pellicer et al 2001, Pezzati et al 2002, Romagnoli et al 2006) and have been measured with Doppler ultrasonography in the major brain arteries such as the ACA, the MCA, the ICA and the VAs (Kehrer et al 2005, Romagnoli et al 2006).

Maesel et al (1994) reported a significant rise in vascular resistance with high systolic, diastolic and mean velocities and a low PI in term newborns following alterations in arterial oxygen content in consequence to the first breaths. The diastolic cerebral velocity may decrease by influence of the patent ductus arteriosus leading to a ductal vascular steal (Evans et al 2002). In the MCA, the mean velocity was usually higher than in the ACA and the absolute difference increased significantly over the first 48 hours of life (Evans et al 2002).

Absolute CBF and CBF velocity have been described in the first 2 days of life within the ICA, the ACA and the SAs in the absence of simultaneous changes in blood pressure and RI, representing a reliable increase in CBF (Pellicer et al 2001).

Kehrer et al (2005) performed quantitative measurements of CBF volume in ICA and VAs in preterm and term infants with gestational age between 32 and 42 weeks. They suggested that the increase in absolute CBF with fetal age might be explained by the increases in both brain weight and perfusion, indicating the demand in metabolic fuel, increasing functional brain activity and synaptic proliferation. In preterm neonates the findings were similar with a pronounced increase in CBF volume from the first to second day of life (Kehrer et al 2005).

After the third day several authors have observed a gradual increase in both the peak systolic and the end diastolic flow velocities that were related with an increase in the metabolic rate, the closure of the ductus arteriosus and an adjustment of CBF with a constant posterior CBF (Cheung et al 1994, Kojo et al 1996).

CEREBRAL CIRCULATION AND OUTCOME

The alteration in CBF is one of the most important mechanisms involved in the pathogenesis of perinatal and neonatal brain damage. Premature newborns are a particularly vulnerable population at high risk of later deficits in motor, cognitive and behavioral development (Colvin et al 2004, Msall 2006, Volpe 2001). Hemorrhagic and hypoxic-ischemic lesions are the most common injuries in the developing brain. The pathogenesis of both types of injury is likely to be associated with abnormalities of the cerebral perfusion in utero, during labor and the first days of life. In neonates with developmental disabilities, postnatal changes, such as progressive increase in CBF, seem to be absent due to a failure of the adaptive response to metabolic demands (Kehrer et al 2005, Pezzati et al 2002).

With the functional maturation of the brain the metabolic rate and consequently CBF both increase. This event is anatomically and physiologically linked with the development of cerebral vasculature which establishes different vascular responses to injuries and thus different types of brain damage in preterm and term neonates (Pearce 2006, Volpe 2001).

Different techniques have been used in the neonatal period to assess the hemodynamic changes in the developing brain including near-infrared spectroscopy imaging (Pellicer et al 2001) and positron emission tomography (Borch et al 1998). Using Doppler sonographic techniques the investigation of flow velocities in intracranial arteries allows the estimation of CBF. Doppler ultrasound has become an important tool in the study of the neonatal functional characteristics of the cerebral vasculature which allows the prediction of adverse outcomes.

PRETERM NEONATES

In preterm infants, the incomplete vascular development and the differences in regional brain perfusion imply a minimal margin of safety to supply the cerebral white matter.

Two of the most important brain lesions are intraventricular hemorrhage (IVH) and periventricular leukomalacia (PVL) (Baenziger et al 1995, Okumura et al 2002, Volpe 2001), whereby IVH seems to decline in incidence (Volpe 2001) and PVL still represents a major cause of neurodevelopmental deficits. The pathogenesis of both conditions is defined by disturbances of regional blood flow. Doppler ultrasound has been used to evaluate hemodynamic abnormalities that may predispose premature infants to these conditions and impair development, although some study results are discordant.

PVL was studied by Fukuda et al (2006) in low-birth-weight infants. The authors found a long-term reduction in CBF velocities in each of the cerebral arteries (ACA, MCA, PCA, ICA and BA) for infants with PVL with the early involvement of the PCA at 5 days of life and in the MCA, ACA, ICA and BA during the following postnatal days. The prevalence of cerebral palsy was higher within a group of infants of higher peak blood flow velocities. However, other studies comparing preterm infants with and without PVL showed no difference in the mean velocity of the ACA, but found a significantly lower RI in the same artery at the first 72 hours of life in infants developing PVL (Okumura et al 2002). The study of the ACA may not be the most adequate for the assessment of PVL since this artery contributes only in part to the vascularization of the periventricular area.

Blankenberg et al (1997) evaluated CBF in the lenticulo-striate arteries that supply the periventricular white matter in extremely low-birth-weight infants. They found an increase of higher and fluctuating velocities and a decrease in RI correlating with PVL. The authors suggest the possibility of identifying infants at risk of developing PVL by the determination of abnormal blood flow velocities.

Intraventricular hemorrhage mainly occurs in the first 72 hours of life. Its presence has been associated with cognitive and motor disabilities (Vohr et al 1992, Whitaker et al 1996).

An impaired cerebro-vascular autoregulation is one of the most important factors. The pronounced increase in CBF occurring during the first 2 days of life in healthy newborns coincides with the period of the greatest risk of IVH in preterm neonates; therefore, deviations of this adaptive response may be associated with an increased risk of brain damage (Kehrer et al 2005).

Doppler studies of preterm infants at risk of IVH may provide risk criteria of severity by means of the assessment of fluctuations of the Doppler curve (Mullaart et al 1997), abnormally low and high cerebral flow velocities (Pellicer et al 2001) and an increase of the RI (Mires et al 1994).

Mari et al (1996) studied the MCA PI in fetuses between 25 and 34 weeks of gestation complicated by intrauterine growth restriction or pre-eclampsia. They found a lower incidence of IVH in fetuses with a normal PI in the MCA. Systolic, diastolic, mean velocities and PIs in the MCA of affected and unaffected hemispheres have been investigated and it was found that the PI of the unaffected hemisphere might be a predictor of death in acute intracerebral hemorrhage (Marti-Fabregas et al 2003).

Hopefully the identification of infants at risk of PVL and IVH will allow establishing prevention strategies to diminish the long-term potential sequelae associated with this lesion.

TERM NEONATES

Term infants have a different pattern of brain lesion as a consequence of perinatal asphyxia. Although the brain is less vulnerable to white-matter damage when compared with preterm infants, the hypoxic–ischemic encephalopathy (HIE) with involvement of the cerebral cortex is an event that may result in neurodevelopment disabilities including cerebral palsy, mental retardation and learning disabilities.

The pathologic etiology of HIE includes a disturbed cerebral circulation and an impaired energy metabolism (Ilves et al 1998). At 24 to 72 hours of life infants with severe HIE show high CBF velocities and a significantly lowered RI probably related with severe vasoparalysis. Infants with CBF velocity >2SD or a RI < 2SD from the mean have a positive predictive value of 94% for death or severe impairment (Levene et al 1989). Ilves et al (1998) found that at the age of 12 ± 2 hours the mean blood flow velocity in the ACA and MCA is decreased in asphyxiated infants developing mild or moderate HIE.

In summary, cerebral Doppler studies help to identify infants who will develop hemorrhage or ischemic lesions not only in preterm, but also in term fetuses. Such information is critical for adapting current treatment strategies.

CONCLUSIONS

Intact placental function is the most important determinant of the fetal circulation and fetal CBF (Dawes 1962, Dawes et al 1968). Animal experiments with invasive detection of CBF have been the basis of our understanding of physiological and pathological mechanisms of the fetal circulation.

With the introduction of pulsed Doppler techniques it became possible to study CBF prenatally under physiologic and pathologic conditions. Venous and umbilical blood flow patterns are meanwhile preferred to detect the severity of fetal hypoxia. However, in fetal anemia the determination of the peak systolic velocity in the MCA has become the most important non-invasive tool to determine the severity of the hyperdynamic fetal circulation and fetal anemia in non-hydropic anemic fetuses.

Color Doppler and power Doppler mapping is now combined with 3-D and conversion mode techniques to visualize the cerebral vascularization in a more complete way. These tools enable future obstetricians to better dif-ferentiate local differences of CBF and may help to better understand prenatal and postnatal cerebral development and their disturbances.

In the future, new non-invasive technologies will help to detect differential CBF in specific brain regions and thus to determine the distribution of blood within the brain. The research of fetal and neonatal perfusion will remain an important parameter for clinicians and investigators to be correlated with internal and external variables and later outcome in the continuity from pre- to postnatal life.

ACKNOWLEDGMENTS

The authors thank the neonatologists Dr. Nelly Padilla and Dr. Wim Baerts for revising the manuscript.

REFERENCES

Aaltonen R et al 2005 Transfer of proinflammatory cytokines across term placenta. Obstet Gynecol 106(4):802–807.

Ahmed B et al 2005 Non-invasive diagnosis of fetal anemia due to maternal red-cell alloimmunization. Saudi Med J 26(2):256–259.

Arabin B 1990 Doppler blood flow measurement in uteroplacental and fetal vessels. Springer, Berlin.

Arabin B, Bergmann P L, Saling E 1987a Pathophysiologic and clinical aspects of measuring blood flow in utero-placental vessels, the umbilical artery, the fetal aorta and the fetal common carotid artery. Geburtshilfe Frauenheilkd 47(9):587–593.

Arabin B, Bergmann P L, Saling E 1987b Simultaneous assessment of blood flow velocity waveforms in uteroplacental vessels, the umbilical artery, the fetal aorta and the fetal common carotid artery. Fetal Ther 2(1):17–26.

Arduini D, Rizzo G 1990 Normal values of pulsatility index from fetal vessels: a cross-sectional study on 1556 healthy fetuses. J Perinat Med 18(3):165–172.

Arduini D, Rizzo G, Romanini C 1992 Changes of pulsatility index from fetal vessels preceding the onset of late decelerations in growth-retarded fetuses. Obstet Gynecol 79(4):605–610.

Ashitaka Y, Murachi K, Takemura H 1968 Analysis of the fetal heart valve with the fetal electro-cardiogram, phonocardiogram and Doppler signals. Proceedings of the 14th Scientific Meeting of the Japan Society of Ultrasonics in Medicine, pp. 29–30.

Baenziger O et al 1995 Regional differences of cerebral blood flow in the preterm infant. Eur J Pediatr 154(11):919–924.

Bilardo C M, Campbell S, Nicolaides K H 1988 Mean blood velocities and flow impedance in the fetal descending thoracic aortic and common carotid artery in normal pregnancy. Early Hum Dev 18(2–3):213–221.

Bilardo C M, Nicolaides K H, Campbell S 1990 Doppler measurements of fetal and uteroplacental circulations: relationship with umbilical venous blood gases measured at cordocentesis. Am J Obstet Gynecol 162(1):115–120.

Blankenberg F G et al 1997 Impaired cerebrovascular autoregulation after hypoxic-ischemic injury in extremely low-birth-weight neonates: detection with power and pulsed wave Doppler US. Radiology 205(2):563–568.

Borch K et al 1998 Regional cerebral blood flow during seizures in neonates. J Pediatr 132(3 Pt 1):431–435.

Cabanas F et al 1997 Effect of dexamethasone therapy on cerebral and ocular blood flow velocity in premature infants studied by colour Doppler flow imaging. Eur J Pediatr 156(1):41–46.

Capponi A et al 1996 The effects of fetal blood sampling and placental puncture on umbilical artery and fetal arterial vessels blood flow velocity waveforms. Am J Perinatol 13(3):185–190.

Carroll S G, Papaioannou S, Nicolaides K H 1995 Doppler studies of the placental and fetal circulation in pregnancies with preterm prelabor amniorrhexis. Ultrasound Obstet Gynecol 5(3):184–188.

Cheung Y F, Lam P K, Yeung C Y 1994 Early postnatal cerebral Doppler changes in relation to birth weight. Early Hum Dev 37(1):57–66.

Chitrit Y et al 1995 Doppler velocimetry in the umbilical, middle cerebral and aortic arteries, before and after cordocentesis. J Gynecol Obstet Biol Reprod (Paris) 24(5):516–521.

Cohn H et al 1974 Cardiovascular responses to hypoxemia and acidemia in fetal lambs. Am J Obstet Gynecol 120(15):817–824.

Colvin M, McGuire W, Fowlie P W 2004 Neurodevelopmental outcomes after preterm birth. Br Med J 329(7479):1390–1393.

Connors R et al 1992 Relationship of cross-brain oxygen content difference, cerebral blood flow, and metabolic rate to neurologic outcome after near-drowning. J Pediatr 121(6):839–844.

Dan U et al 1992 Prenatal diagnosis of fetal brain arteriovenous malformation: the use of color Doppler imaging. J Clin Ultrasound 20(2):149–151.

Dani C et al 2000 Brain hemodynamic changes in preterm infants after maintenance dose caffeine and aminophylline treatment. Biol Neonate 78(1):27–32.

Dawes G S 1962 The umbilical circulation. Am J Obstet Gynecol 84:1634–1648.

Dawes G S et al 1968 Vasomotor responses in the hind limbs of foetal and new-born lambs to asphyxia and aortic chemoreceptor stimulation. J Physiol 195(1):55–81.

Eik-Nes S et al 1982 Ultrasonic measurement of human fetal blood flow. Biomed Eng 4:28–36.

Evans N et al 2002 Which to measure, systemic or organ blood flow? Middle cerebral artery and superior vena cava flow in very preterm infants. Arch Dis Child Fetal Neonatal Ed 87(3):F181–F184.

Eyer M et al 1981 Color digital echo/Doppler image presentation. Ultrasound Med Biol 7:21–31.

Facchinetti F et al 1992 Oral magnesium supplementation improves fetal circulation. Magnes Res 5(3):179–181.

Falck G, Rajs J 1995 Brain weight and sudden infant death syndrome. J Child Neurol 10(2):123–126.

FitsGerald D, Drumm J 1977 Non-invasive measurement of human fetal circulation using ultrasound: a new method. Br Med J 2:1450–1451.

Friedman A, Fahey J 1993 The transition from fetal to neonatal circulation: normal responses and implications for infants with heart disease. Semin Perinatol 17(2):106–121.

Fukuda S et al 2006 Hemodynamics of the cerebral arteries of infants with periventricular leukomalacia. Pediatrics 117(1):1–8.

Gembruch U, Baschat A A 2000 Circulatory effects of acute bradycardia in the human fetus as studied by Doppler ultrasound. Ultrasound Obstet Gynecol 15(5):424–427.

Giles W B, Trudinger B J 1986 Umbilical cord whole blood viscosity and the umbilical artery flow velocity time waveforms: a correlation. Br J Obstet Gynaecol 93(5):466–470.

Gokay Z, Ozcan T, Copel J A 2001 Changes in fetal hemodynamics with ritodrine tocolysis. Ultrasound Obstet Gynecol 18(1):44–46.

Gramellini D et al 1992 Cerebral-umbilical Doppler ratio as a predictor of adverse perinatal outcome. Obstet Gynecol 79(3):416–420.

Gray H 2000 The arteries of the brain. In: Anatomy of the human body. Bartleby com, New York.

Gudmundsson S et al 1996 Venous Doppler in the fetus with absent end-diastolic flow in the umbilical artery. Ultrasound Obstet Gynecol 7(4):262–267.

Guzman R, Grady M S 1999 An intracranial aneurysm on the feeding artery of a cerebellar hemangioblastoma. Case report. J Neurosurg 91(1):136–138.

Hamza J 1994 Effect of epidural anesthesia on the fetus and the neonate. Cah Anesthesiol 42(2):265–273.

Harrington K et al 1995 Changes observed in Doppler studies of the fetal circulation in pregnancies complicated by pre-eclampsia or the delivery of a small-for-gestational-age baby. I. Cross-sectional analysis. Ultrasound Obstet Gynecol 6(1):19–28.

Hecher K et al 1993 The effect of cordocentesis on umbilical and middle cerebral artery blood flow velocity waveforms. Br J Obstet Gynaecol 100(9):828–831.

Hecher K et al 1995 Fetal venous, intracardiac, and arterial blood flow measurements in intrauterine growth retardation: relationship with fetal blood gases. Am J Obstet Gynecol 173(1):10–15.

Heling K S, Chaoui R, Bollmann R 2000 Prenatal diagnosis of an aneurysm of the vein of Galen with three-dimensional color power angiography. Ultrasound Obstet Gynecol 15(4):333–336.

Hernandez-Andrade E et al 2004 Fetal middle cerebral artery peak systolic velocity in the investigation of non-immune hydrops. Ultrasound Obstet Gynecol 23(5):442–445.

Hernandez-Andrade E et al 2007 Evaluation of fetal cerebral blood perfusion using power Doppler ultrasound and the measure of fractional moving blood volume. Ultrasound Obstet Gynecol 29:556–561.

Hernandez-Andrade E, Jansson T, Marsal K 2006 Fractional moving blood volume measurement using power Doppler ultrasound as an estimation of fetal organ blood perfusion. Curr Med Imag Rev 2:365–372.

Ilves P, Talvik R, Talvik T 1998 Changes in Doppler ultrasonography in asphyxiated term infants with hypoxic-ischaemic encephalopathy. Acta Paediatr 87(6):680–684.

Jeanty P et al 1990 In utero detection of cardiac failure from an aneurysm of the vein of Galen. Am J Obstet Gynecol 163(1 Pt 1):50–51.

Kassanos D et al 2003 The clinical significance of Doppler findings in fetal middle cerebral artery during labor. Eur J Obstet Gynecol Reprod Biol 109(1):45–50.

Kehrer M et al 2005 Development of cerebral blood flow volume in preterm neonates during the first two weeks of life. Pediatr Res 58(5):927–930.

Kiserud T, Hellevik L R, Hanson M A 1998 Blood velocity profile in the ductus venosus inlet expressed by the mean/maximum velocity ratio. Ultrasound Med Biol 24(9):1301–1306.

Kofinas A, G. MR, K. GD 1996 The effect of vibratory acoustic stimulation on fetal middle cerebral artery impedance and instantaneous fetal heart rate: a prospective cross-sectional study frtom 20–42 weeks gestational age. J Maternal Fetal Invest 6:19–22.

Kojo M, Ogawa T, Yamada K 1996 Normal developmental changes in carotid arterial blood flow measured by Doppler flowmetry in children. Pediatr Neurol 14(4):313–316.

Kurjak A et al 1987 Color flow mapping in obstetrics. J Perinat Med 15(3):271–281.

Kurjak A et al 1992 Transvaginal color Doppler study of middle cerebral artery blood flow in early normal, abnormal pregnancy. Ultrasound Obstet Gynecol 2(6):424–428.

Kurmanavicius J et al 1997 Reference resistance indices of the umbilical, fetal middle cerebral and uterine arteries at 24–42 weeks of gestation. Ultrasound Obstet Gynecol 10(2):112–120.

L'Ubusky M et al 2004 Doppler blood flow velocity in the evaluation of fetal anemia. Ceska Gynekol 69(4):316–320.

Lam H et al 2005 The use of fetal Doppler cerebroplacental blood flow and amniotic fluid volume measurement in the surveillance of postdated pregnancies. Acta Obstet Gynecol Scand 84(9):844–848.

Leenders K L et al 1990 Cerebral blood flow, blood volume and oxygen utilization. Normal values and effect of age. Brain 113 (Pt 1):27–47.

Levene M I et al 1989 Severe birth asphyxia and abnormal cerebral blood-flow velocity. Dev Med Child Neurol 31(4):427–434.

Lewinsky R M, Farine D, Ritchie J W 1991 Transvaginal Doppler assessment of the fetal cerebral circulation. Obstet Gynecol 78(4):637–640.

Li H, Gudmundsson S, Olofsson P 2004a Acute changes of cerebral venous blood flow in growth-restricted human fetuses in response to uterine contractions. Ultrasound Obstet Gynecol 24(5):516–521.

Li H, Gudmundsson S, Olofsson P 2004b Clinical significance of uterine artery blood flow velocity waveforms during provoked uterine contractions in high-risk pregnancy. Ultrasound Obstet Gynecol 24(5):429–434.

Li H, Gudmundsson S, Olofsson P 2006 Acute centralization of blood flow in compromised human fetuses evoked by uterine contractions. Early Hum Dev 82(11):747–752.

Maesel A et al 1994 Fetal cerebral blood flow velocity during labor and the early neonatal period. Ultrasound Obstet Gynecol 4(5):372–376.

Malcus P et al 1991 Diameters of the common carotid artery and aorta change in different directions during acute asphyxia in the fetal lamb. J Perinat Med 19(4):259–267.

Mari G 2005a Middle cerebral artery peak systolic velocity for the diagnosis of fetal anemia: the untold story. Ultrasound Obstet Gynecol 25(4):323–330.

Mari G 2005b Middle cerebral artery peak systolic velocity: is it the standard of care for the diagnosis of fetal anemia? J Ultrasound Med 24(5):697–702.

Mari G et al 1996 Is the fetal brain-sparing effect a risk factor for the development of intraventricular hemorrhage in the preterm infant? Ultrasound Obstet Gynecol 8(5):329–332.

Mari G et al 2000 Noninvasive diagnosis by Doppler ultrasonography of fetal anemia due to maternal red-cell alloimmunization. Collaborative Group for Doppler Assessment of the Blood Velocity in Anemic Fetuses. N Engl J Med 342(1):9–14.

Mari G et al 2005 Middle cerebral artery peak systolic velocity: technique and variability. J Ultrasound Med 24(4):425–430.

Mari G, Wasserstrum N, Kirshon B 1992 Reduction in the middle cerebral artery pulsatility index after decompression of polyhydramnios in twin gestation. Am J Perinatol 9(5–6):381–384.

Marsal K, Hernandez-Andrade E 2004 Power Doppler and fetal organ perfusion. Ultrasound Obstet Gynecol 24 Suppl:254.

Marti-Fabregas J et al 2003 Prognostic value of pulsatility index in acute intracerebral hemorrhage. Neurology 61(8):1051–1056.

Meerman R J et al 1990 Fetal and neonatal cerebral blood velocity in the normal fetus and neonate: a longitudinal Doppler ultrasound study. Early Hum Dev 24(3):209–217.

Mires G J et al 1994 Neonatal cerebral Doppler flow velocity waveforms in the uncomplicated pre-term infant: reference values. Early Hum Dev 36(3):205–212.

Msall M E 2006 Neurodevelopmental surveillance in the first 2 years after extremely preterm birth: evidence, challenges, and guidelines. Early Hum Dev 82(3):157–166.

Mullaart R A et al 1997 Cerebral blood flow velocity and pulsation in neonatal respiratory distress syndrome and periventricular hemorrhage. Pediatr Neurol 16(2):118–125.

Noordam M J et al 1994 Doppler colour flow imaging of fetal intracerebral arteries relative to fetal behavioural states in normal pregnancy. Early Hum Dev 39(1):49–56.

Noori S et al 2006 Hemodynamic changes after low-dosage hydrocortisone administration in vasopressor-treated preterm and term neonates. Pediatrics 118(4):1456–1466.

Oepkes D et al 2006 Doppler ultrasonography versus amniocentesis to predict fetal anemia. N Engl J Med 355(2):156–164.

Okumura A et al 2002 Cerebral hemodynamics during early neonatal period in preterm infants with periventricular leukomalacia. Brain Dev 24(7):693–697.

Oosterhof H, Dijkstra K, Aarnoudse J G 1992 Fetal Doppler velocimetry in the internal carotid and umbilical artery during Braxton Hicks' contractions. Early Hum Dev 30(1):33–40.

Paladini D et al 1996 Prenatal ultrasound diagnosis of cerebral arteriovenous fistula. Obstet Gynecol 88(4 Pt 2):678–681.

Pape K, Wigglesworth J 1979 Blood supply to the developing brain. In: Haemorrhage, ischemia and the perinatal brain. Spastics International Medical Publications Clinics in Developmental Medicine 69/70, London, pp. 11–38.

Pearce W 2006 Hypoxic regulation of the fetal cerebral circulation. J Appl Physiol 100(2):731–738.

Pellicer A et al 2001 Postnatal adaptation of brain circulation in preterm infants. Pediatr Neurol 24(2):103–109.

Pellicer A et al 2005 Cardiovascular support for low birth weight infants and cerebral hemodynamics: a randomized, blinded, clinical trial. Pediatrics 115(6):1501–1512.

Pereira L, Jenkins T M, Berghella V 2003 Conventional management of maternal red cell alloimmunization compared with management by Doppler assessment of middle cerebral artery peak systolic velocity. Am J Obstet Gynecol 189(4):1002–1006.

Pezzati M et al 2001 Influence of maternal magnesium sulphate and ritodrine treatment on cerebral blood flow velocity of the preterm newborn. Acta Obstet Gynecol Scand 80(9):818–823.

Pezzati M et al 2002 Early postnatal Doppler assessment of cerebral blood flow velocity in healthy preterm and term infants. Dev Med Child Neurol 44(11):745–752.

Pilu G et al 1998 Prenatal diagnosis of microcephaly assisted by vaginal sonography and power Doppler. Ultrasound Obstet Gynecol 11(5):357–360.

Quilligan E et al 1968 Fetal cephalic metabolism in sheep. Am J Obstet Gynecol 102:716–726.

Reuss M L et al 1982 Hemodynamic effects of alpha-adrenergic blockade during hypoxia in fetal sheep. Am J Obstet Gynecol 142(4):410–415.

Reuss M L, Rudolph A M, Dae M W 1983 Phasic blood flow patterns in the superior and inferior venae cavae and umbilical vein of fetal sheep. Am J Obstet Gynecol 145(1):70–78.

Rizzo G et al 1995 The value of fetal arterial, cardiac and venous flows in predicting pH and blood gases measured in umbilical blood at cordocentesis in growth retarded fetuses. Br J Obstet Gynaecol 102(12):963–969.

Romagnoli C et al 2006 Neonatal color Doppler US study: normal values of cerebral blood flow velocities in preterm infants in the first month of life. Ultrasound Med Biol 32(3):321–331.

Rubin J M et al 1994 Power Doppler US: a potentially useful alternative to mean frequency-based color Doppler US. Radiology 190(3):853–856.

Rudolph A M 1984 The fetal circulation and its response to stress. J Dev Physiol 6(1):11–19.

Rudolph A M, Heymann M A 1968 The fetal circulation. Annu Rev Med 19:195–206.

Rudolph A, Heymann M A 1970 Circulatory changes during growth in the fetal lamb. Circ Res 26:289–299.

Saliba E et al 1994 Instillation rate effects of Exosurf on cerebral and cardiovascular haemodynamics in preterm neonates. Arch Dis Child Fetal Neonatal Ed 71(3):F174–F178.

Saling E 1966 O_2 conservation by the fetal circulation. Geburtshilfe Frauenheilkd 26(4):412–419.

Satomura S 1959 Study of the flow patterns in peripheral arteries by ultrasonics. J Acoust Soc Jpn 15:151–158.

Schaffer H et al 1990 Value of the aortic/carotid ratio for predicting increased fetal acidosis. Gynakol Rundsch 30(2):123–125.

Schaffer H et al 1999 Dopplersonographie um den Geburtstermin und bei der Überschreitung. Arch Gynecol Obstet 263(2):113–116.

Schaffer H, Steiner H, Staudach A 1998 Reference values for qualitative and quantitative analysis of uterine, fetoplacental and fetal flow velocity waveforms. J Fertil Reprod Special 2:12–13.

Scherjon S et al 2000 The discrepancy between maturation of visual-evoked potentials and cognitive outcome at five years in very preterm infants with

and without hemodynamic signs of fetal brain-sparing. Pediatrics 105(2):385–391.

Sepulveda W, Platt C C, Fisk N M 1995 Prenatal diagnosis of cerebral arteriovenous malformation using color Doppler ultrasonography: case report and review of the literature. Ultrasound Obstet Gynecol 6(4):282–286.

Sueters M, Arabin B, Oepkes D 2003 Doppler sonography for predicting fetal anemia caused by massive fetomaternal hemorrhage. Ultrasound Obstet Gynecol 22(2):186–189.

Teixeira J et al 1996 Fetal haemodynamic stress response to invasive procedures. Lancet 347(9001):624.

van den Wijngaard J A et al 1989 Cerebral Doppler ultrasound of the human fetus. Br J Obstet Gynaecol 96(7):845–849.

van Eyck J et al 1987 The blood flow velocity waveform in the fetal internal carotid and umbilical artery: its relation to fetal behavioural states in normal pregnancy at 37–38 weeks. Br J Obstet Gynaecol 94(8):736–741.

van Eyck J et al 1988 The blood flow velocity waveform in the fetal internal carotid and umbilical artery: its relation to fetal behavioural states in the growth retarded fetus at 37–38 weeks gestation. Br J Obstet Gynaecol 95(5):473–477.

van Eyck J, Wladimiroff J W 1988 Human fetal behavior and blood flow in term pregnancies: a review. Fetal Ther 3(1–2):44–49.

Vasovic L P 2004 The tenth vascular component in a rare form of the cerebral arterial circle of fetuses. Cells Tissues Organs 178(4):231–238.

Vetter K. Reference values for qualitative and quantitative analysis of uterine, fetoplacental and fetal flow velocity waveforms V. Edition Medizin, Weinheim, 1991.

Vohr B et al 1992 Effects of intraventricular hemorrhage and socioeconomic status on perceptual, cognitive, and neurologic status of low birth weight infants at 5 years of age. J Pediatr 121(2):280–285.

Volpe J J 2001 Neurobiology of periventricular leukomalacia in the premature infant. Pediatr Res 50(5):553–562.

Vyas S et al 1990a Maternal abdominal pressure alters fetal cerebral blood flow. Br J Obstet Gynaecol 97(8):740–742.

Vyas S et al 1990b Middle cerebral artery flow velocity waveforms in fetal hypoxaemia. Br J Obstet Gynaecol 97(9):797–803.

Whitaker A H et al 1996 Neonatal cranial ultrasound abnormalities in low birth weight infants: relation to cognitive outcomes at six years of age. Pediatrics 98(4 Pt 1):719–729.

Whitelaw A 2001 Intraventricular haemorrhage and posthaemorrhagic hydrocephalus: pathogenesis, prevention and future interventions. Semin Neonatol 6(2):135–146.

Wladimiroff J W, Tonge H M, Stewart P A 1986 Doppler ultrasound assessment of cerebral blood flow in the human fetus. Br J Obstet Gynaecol 93(5):471–475.

Woo J S et al 1987 Middle cerebral artery Doppler flow velocity waveforms. Obstet Gynecol 70(4):613–616.

Yagel S et al 1992 Fetal middle cerebral artery blood flow during normal active labour and in labour with variable decelerations. Br J Obstet Gynaecol 99(6):483–485.

Zimmerman R et al 2002 Longitudinal measurement of peak systolic velocity in the fetal middle cerebral artery for monitoring pregnancies complicated by red cell alloimmunisation: a prospective multicentre trial with intention-to-treat. BJOG 109(7):746–752.

CHAPTER

11

Cerebral blood flow and energy metabolism in the developing brain

Gorm Greisen

Key Points

- Marginal hypoxia–ischemia takes time (30 minutes to some hours) to cause brain injury
- In a minority of ill infants pressure-flow autoregulation may be deficient and these infants may be more sensitive to moderate arterial hypotension
- It is customary to try to limit blood pressure rise in very preterm babies, e.g. by correcting hypovolemia gradually, but the effect on blood pressure must be monitored and treatment accelerated if needed
- Rapid lowering of pCO_2 can reduce CBF severely and critically at least in preterm infants; adaptation to a new level of pCO_2 takes several hours. Great care must be taken during mechanical ventilation
- There is no situation when CBF should be reduced
- The advantage of a higher blood hemoglobin for increasing oxygen-carrying capacity is nearly balanced out by greater viscosity. Optimal Hb may be 8–10 mmol/L
- Combinations of factors that are adverse to cerebral energy sufficiency, e.g. low CBF, low blood glucose, combined with seizures may add up. This in general means that ill infants are likely to be more vulnerable

---

INTRODUCTION

Cerebral perfusion may be quantified as blood flow in milliliters per 100 grams brain weight per minute (mL/100 g/min). This quantity is commonly termed cerebral blood flow (CBF) and relates to the brain as a whole or to a specified region, depending on the method of measurements.

CBF was first estimated in a few newborn infants by Garfunkel et al in 1954. However, only 20 years later did the interest in neonatal CBF appear when it was hypothesized that some important types of perinatal brain damage may be due to perturbation of CBF after observing proportionality between arterial blood pressure and CBF in eight distressed infants shortly after birth (Fig. 11.1). Lou et al (1977) proposed that the normal pressure-flow autoregulation may be abolished after asphyxia. This would allow moderate arterial hypotension to cause cerebral ischemia as well as moderate hypertension to be transmitted to the capillary bed and cause rupture and cerebral hemorrhage.

The principal role of cerebral perfusion is to provide substrates for the cerebral energy metabolism, with the final purpose of maintaining normal cellular concentrations of the high-energy phosphate metabolites adenosine triphosphate (ATP) and phosphocreatine (PCr) (Fig. 11.2). Cerebral metabolic rate (CMR) may be quantified as the consumption of oxygen and glucose as CMR_{O2} or CMR_{Glu}, respectively, in

μmol/100 g/min. In hypoglycemia, alternatives to glucose, primarily lactate and ketones, may help to support CMR and in hypoxemia or ischemia anaerobic glycolysis will speed up CMR_{Glu}. Hence, it should be noted that, although oxygen and glucose consumption is closely linked and reflects energy metabolism in the normal state, this might not be so in pathological states.

The main problem for experimental animal studies is the differences among species in cerebrovascular anatomy and physiology, in cerebral development and, to a much lesser degree, in cellular energy metabolism. The main problem in clinical research is the methodological limitations imposed by the need to limit patient risk. Risks may be associated with the measurement itself, with transport to an imaging department or a laboratory, or with the manipulation of physiological variables. Therefore, this chapter describes the clinical research methods briefly, to allow critical interpretation of the available data. Furthermore, an outline of the regulation of CBF is given along with a review of the available data concerning human perinatal CBF and cerebral energy metabolism.

CLINICAL RESEARCH METHODS

CBF as well as CMR are complex variables. CBF may change within seconds in hypoxia, seizures or with abrupt changes in blood pressure. CBF and CMR vary from one part of the brain to the other. During functional activation, or during stress, this distribution may change markedly. The methods available for use in human newborns provide only crude measures of those complexities.

THE KETY–SCHMIDT METHOD

This method is based on the Fick principle for metabolically inert tracers, stating that the change of the mean tracer concentration in a tissue equals the perfusion rate multiplied by the arterio-venous concentration difference. All CBF methods using tracers build on variations of this principle; therefore it will be presented in some detail here. Nitrous oxide, a freely diffusible inert gas, is administered by inhalation. The tracer concentration in arterial and jugular venous blood is followed by taking six to eight precisely timed blood samples over 10 minutes after the start of inhalation of 15% nitrous oxide. The tissue concentration is estimated at equilibrium as the venous concentration multiplied by the tissue–blood partition coefficient.

The assumption of equilibration may not hold if parts of the brain are perfused at low rates and therefore remain unsaturated, which often occurs in infants (Sharples et al 1991). In this situation the wash-in must be followed for 15 minutes. Completely unperfused regions of the brain will never be represented. If counter-current exchange of nitrous oxide from artery to vein takes place, the difference between venous concentration and tissue concentration will be even greater. All of these problems results in overestimation of true CBF.

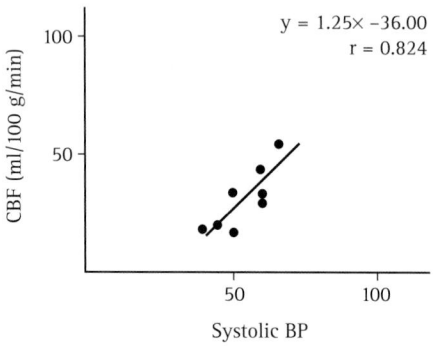

Figure 11.1 Relation of cerebral blood flow (CBF) to systolic blood pressure (BP) in eight stressed newborn infants, a few hours after birth. CBF was estimated by the intra-arterial ^{133}Xe clearance method, using an early slope index, reflecting mainly flow to gray matter. (Reproduced with permission from Lou et al 1977.)

The value of CBF obtained by the Kety–Schmidt method is a mean over the wash-in period and relates to the part of the brain drained by the jugular vein at the sampling site; even at the jugular bulb there may be a small admixture of extracerebral blood.

The Kety–Schmidt method was used in newborn infants by Garfunkel et al in 1954, and more recently by Frewen et al (1991) and Sharples et al (1991). It was made possible by the development of a micromethod for analysis of nitrous oxide (total volume of blood samples is 2–3 mL) but the application is strictly limited by the need for arterial and jugular venous blood sampling. Catheterization of the jugular bulb in infants of less than 2.5 kg is likely to be more difficult, and to carry greater risks than catheterization in larger infants and children.

The advantage is that once the jugular vein is catheterized it is possible to measure global CMR_{O_2} and CMR_{Glu} by multiplying the CBF by the cross-brain extraction of oxygen or glucose.

^{133}Xe CLEARANCE

Measurement of CBF by ^{133}Xe clearance is based on a modification of the Kety–Schmidt method. If instantaneous equilibration between brain and venous blood is assumed the venous concentrations can be derived from tissue concentrations as measured by external detection of the gamma radiation emitted by the ^{133}Xe in the brain. In this way the need for jugular vein catheterization can be circumvented.

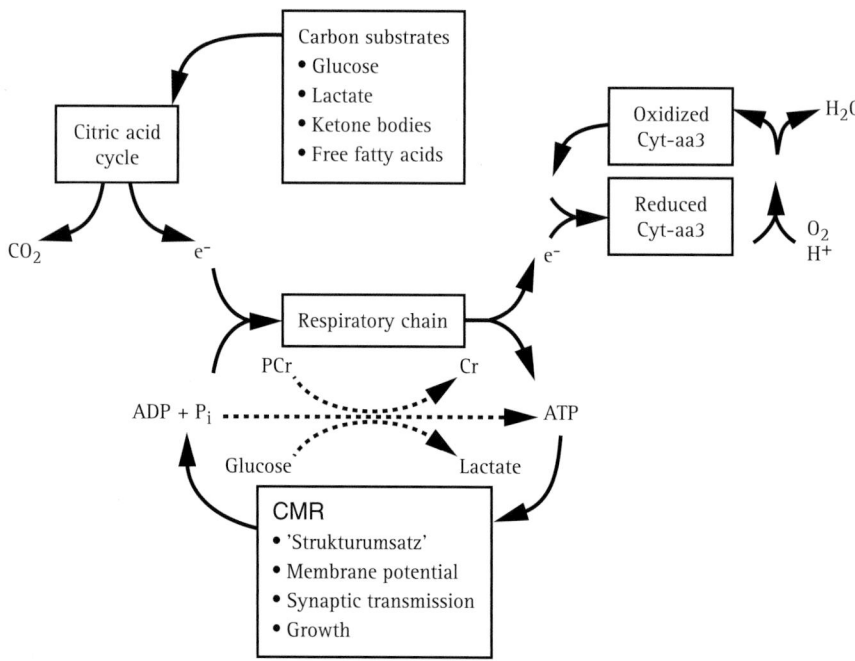

Figure 11.2 A simple, qualitative scheme of cerebral energy metabolism. Carbon passes through the citric acid cycle, yielding electrons. The passage of electrons through the respiratory chain results in phosphorylation of ADP to ATP, driving the energy consuming processes of the brain cells. The electrons are transferred to protons and oxygen by the terminal member of the respiratory chain, cytochrome-aa₃, to yield water. If this oxidative phosphorylation fails, using the phosphocreatine pool as well as anaerobic glycolysis to lactate may help to maintain ATP concentrations for some time.

In the small neonatal brain ^{133}Xe clearance provides a measure of global CBF since the detector samples from a brain volume of about 200 mL and gives an average over 5–10 minutes (Greisen & Pryds 1988).

SINGLE PHOTON EMISSION COMPUTED TOMOGRAPHY (SPECT)

Tomographic images of radiotracer localization may be obtained by methods similar to computed X-ray tomography. Gamma-emitting decays (photons) across the brain are detected and by a number of collimated detectors from a large number of angles around the circumference. The image is constructed by back-projection and usually subjected to various smoothing procedures (filters). There is no theoretical limit to the spatial resolution, but the narrow collimation required for high resolution reduces the sensitivity, and at the same time more counts are needed to fill the larger number of pixels (image elements). Furthermore, Compton scatter tends to mask 'cold' areas, whereas small high-flow structures will be underrated due to partial volume effects. Spatial resolution is 6–12 mm FWHM (full width at half-maximum). Slowly rotating gamma cameras may image the distribution of radioactively labeled substances, which is fixed in the brain tissue during the first passage, such as ^{131}I-iodoamphetamine (Rubinstein et al 1989) or ^{99m}Tc-HMPAO (hexamethylpropyleneamineoxime) (Denays et al 1992). The advantage of these compounds is that they may be injected intravenously in an acute clinical situation, e.g. a seizure, whereas the imaging may take place several hours later. The disadvantage is that only the distribution, no absolute levels, of flow is obtained. Equipment rotating in 5–10 seconds may follow the local uptake and clearance of [133]Xe (Chiron et al 1992).

STABLE XENON-ENHANCED COMPUTED TOMOGRAPHY

This method is also a variant of the Kety–Schmidt method. Detection of tracer in the brain is based on the high density of xenon to X-rays. By repeated X-ray CT scans during inhalation of 35% stable (non-radioactive) xenon, brain saturation can be followed. In principle the spatial resolution is as good as for conventional CT-scanning. Unfortunately, the low brain-blood partition coefficient of xenon in newborn brain results in a low signal-to-noise ratio. Very low levels of CBF, however, have been documented in young, brain-dead infants (Ashwal et al 1989).

POSITRON EMISSION TOMOGRAPHY

Positron emission tomography (PET) is similar to SPECT in image reconstruction, but differs in that PET utilizes the fact that positron annihilation results in two photons emitted always at an angle of 180°. Therefore, localization is done by accepting only counts occurring simultaneously at two oppositely positioned detectors and collimation is not needed. Hence the sensitivity is better than SPECT at high resolution. The resolution now approaches the theoretical minimum (3 to 5 mm) which is the average positron movement before annihilation. These improved instruments have not been used for newborn infants, and existing studies were done with instruments with much less spatial resolution, typically 10–14 mm, which for instance is insufficient for imaging of the preterm infant's cortex.

Biologically relevant positron-emitting isotopes exist, e.g. 11C, 13N and 15O, and many biochemical substances can be labeled. PET is ideally suited for receptor studies since imaging and quantification can be done with picomoles of tracer. The positron-emitting isotopes are very short-lived (2 minutes to 2 hours) and hence PET requires a nearby cyclotron facility.

CBF, CMR_{O_2}, cerebral blood volume, cerebral oxygen extraction fraction and CMR_{Glu} may all be measured by PET (Altman et al 1993, Chugani et al 1987, Powers & Raichle 1985, Volpe et al 1983).

NEAR-INFRARED SPECTROPHOTOMETRY

Near-infrared spectrophotometry (NIRS) is of great potential value since it may be used bedside and is potentially without risks, quantitative, continuous, automated and low cost. Therefore the following description is of some detail.

For in vivo NIRS, light of 3 to 6 wavelengths between 760 and 910 nm produced by laser diodes is delivered to the scalp of the infant by optical fibers. Transmitted light is picked up from another area of the scalp, at a distance of 4 to 6 cm, by another optical fiber. Optical pathlength, however, is not simply the distance between the fibers: photons are scattered several times per millimeter of tissue. The propagation of light may be likened to a diffusion process; the tissue volume interrogated by NIRS is roughly the shape of banana; the effective pathlength in human neonatal brain has been measured to 4–5 times the distance between the optodes on the average (Wyatt et al 1990a). The variant part of the optical density is assumed to be due to varying tissue concentrations of three absorbers. These are deoxyhemoglobin, oxyhemoglobin (their sum being proportional to variations in cerebral blood volume), and change in cytochrome aa3 oxidation, the terminal member of the mitochondrial respiratory chain $[CytO_2]$ (Wyatt et al 1986).

Small, induced changes in arterial oxygen saturation, SaO_2, may be used to quantify cerebral blood volume (CBV) in mL/100 g brain weight (Wyatt et al 1990b) and CBF in mL/100 g/min (Edwards et al 1988). CBF can also be determined by rapid injection of indocyanine green, an intravascular tracer, although a light guide must be inserted through an umbilical artery to trace the arterial concentration (Patel et al 1998). The values for global CBF obtained in newborn infants compare well to those obtained by the ^{133}Xe clearance (Bucher et al 1993, Skov et al 1991), although it was not possible to use the NIRS CBF technique in all the infants studied. The values obtained for CBV have not yet been compared to a reference method in babies, although the typical values (2–4 mL/100 g) are reasonable.

When infants are tilted head-down, or the jugular veins are compressed, a rapid increase in optical density over the brain is seen in most, but not all, infants. If it is assumed that the increased optical density is due exclusively to pooling of cerebrovenous blood in the brain, then the proportional increase in $[HbO_2]$ to $[HbO_2]$ + [Hb] estimates the cerebrovenous oxygen saturation (SvO_2) (Skov et al 1993, Yoxall et al 1995). The SvO_2 is a very basic physiological variable, being firmly regulated in health and a good indicator of (global) cerebral oxygen sufficiency in disease. At present the only alternative way of measuring SvO_2 is by direct blood sampling from the sagittal sinus or the internal jugular vein.

NIRS allows on-line trending of changes in O_2Hb and HHb, and hence of tHb (the sum of $[O_2Hb]$ and [HHb]), which is proportional to changes in CBV, which in its turn can be used as a surrogate measure of CBF. The appropriateness of this, however, has only been established for reactions to changes in arterial carbon dioxide tension (Pryds et al 1990). The signal has no zero-point, i.e. comparison between recording sessions or between infants is not possible. Furthermore, constant optode distance is crucial. If head circumference changes even by a fraction of a millimeter as a result of change in brain blood or brain water content, the trends are significantly biased. Minor change in optode–skin contact can induce large transients in the signal and/or a baseline shifts.

The difference between $[O_2Hb]$ and [HHb] is an indicator of the mean oxygen saturation of hemoglobin in all blood vessels in the tissue, thus the signal is dominated by venous blood. The signal is termed HbD (for difference) or OI (for oxygenation index) and is confounded by concomitant changes in tHb.

Second-generation NIRS instruments can measure regional tissue hemoglobin-oxygen saturation (rSO_2) in absolute terms without manipulation of FiO_2 or using dye (Ijichi et al 2005, Suzuki 1999, Zhao et al 2005). Values near cerebrovenous SO_2 have been found in young children in the range 40–80% (Nagdyman et al 2005), and appropriate changes have been found with changing arterial oxygen saturation, and with arterial pCO_2. The signal-to-noise ratio is not as good as that of OI, and hence rSO_2 is less useful for quantifying the response to rapid therapeutic interventions. The precision of this measurement is not better than 7–9% (Dullenkopf et al 2005, Soerensen & Greisen 2007). Presumably this is due to small differences in gyral anatomy and subarachnoidal space geometry for each placement of optodes. For comparison, the precision of pulse oximetry is better than 3%.

rSO_2 is a surrogate measure of cerebro-venous saturation. This important physiological variable is tightly regulated, normal values being 60–70%. During hypoxemia, cerebro-venous saturation will fall in parallel, whereas during cerebral ischemia, i.e. when CBF drops without

cerebral oxygen consumption dropping also, cerebrovenous saturation will fall. Hence rSO_2 is a useful measure of the sufficiency of cerebral perfusion. The problem is that a deficit in CBF by 30% will only lead to a reduction of rSO_2 from 70% to 60%, i.e. within the limits of measurement error.

Cytochrome-aa$_3$ oxidation is more difficult to measure compared to hemoglobin signals since the cytochrome signal is one order of magnitude smaller.

MAGNETIC RESONANCE SPECTROSCOPY

The nuclei of certain elements, e.g. ^{31}P and ^{1}H, are stable but magnetically asymmetric and hence behaving like magnetic dipoles. Subjected to a strong magnetic field (0.5 to 2 tesla) they will tend to align with the field, longitudinal magnetization, or rather to rotate around the axis of the field. The rotation (precession, like a spinning top) occurs at a frequency proportional to the field strength, and specific to the nucleus (about 26 MHz for ^{31}P at 1.5 T), with small differences (typically ± 1 kHz) according to its chemical environment, 'chemical shift'. Exposed to a pulse of electromagnetic energy of the proper frequencies, at 90° angle, the rotation may be synchronized, resulting in a transverse magnetization. When the pulse is discontinued the synchrony continues and, hence, emits electromagnetic energy and decay in a complex pattern due to the interference of the several slightly different resonance frequencies. Fourier analysis can transform the decay pattern into a frequency spectrum with a number of peaks representing each one the nucleus in a particular chemical constellation.

The height of each peak is proportional to the molar concentration, but due to imperfections, e.g. inhomogeneity of the magnetic field, a certain broadening of the peaks is seen, hence the area may be more informative. Due to limited signal-to-noise ratio only elements of concentrations in the millimolar range are measurable and it is necessary to use high field strengths, e.g. 1.5 tesla or above and to sum many spectra, e.g. 128 or more. If the time in between pulses are insufficient (<10 s) for complete decay (relaxation) the peak height will be underestimated.

The first use of MRS in human brain was reported by Cady et al (1983). ^{31}P spectra were obtained from a rather large hemispheric tissue volume using a 5 or 7 cm surface coil for excitation as well as resonance detection. This allowed spectra of good signal-to-noise ratio to be obtained in less than 20 minutes. The peaks which have been used subsequently are β, α and γ ATP, phosphocreatine (PCr), phosphodiesters, inorganic orthophosphate (P_i), and surprisingly prominent phosphomonoesters. The interest in the present context focuses on the PCr/P_i ratio, which is a sensitive indicator of the cellular energy charge (Fig. 11.3), as well as on intracellular pH, which may be calculated from the frequency difference (chemical shift) between Pi and PCr.

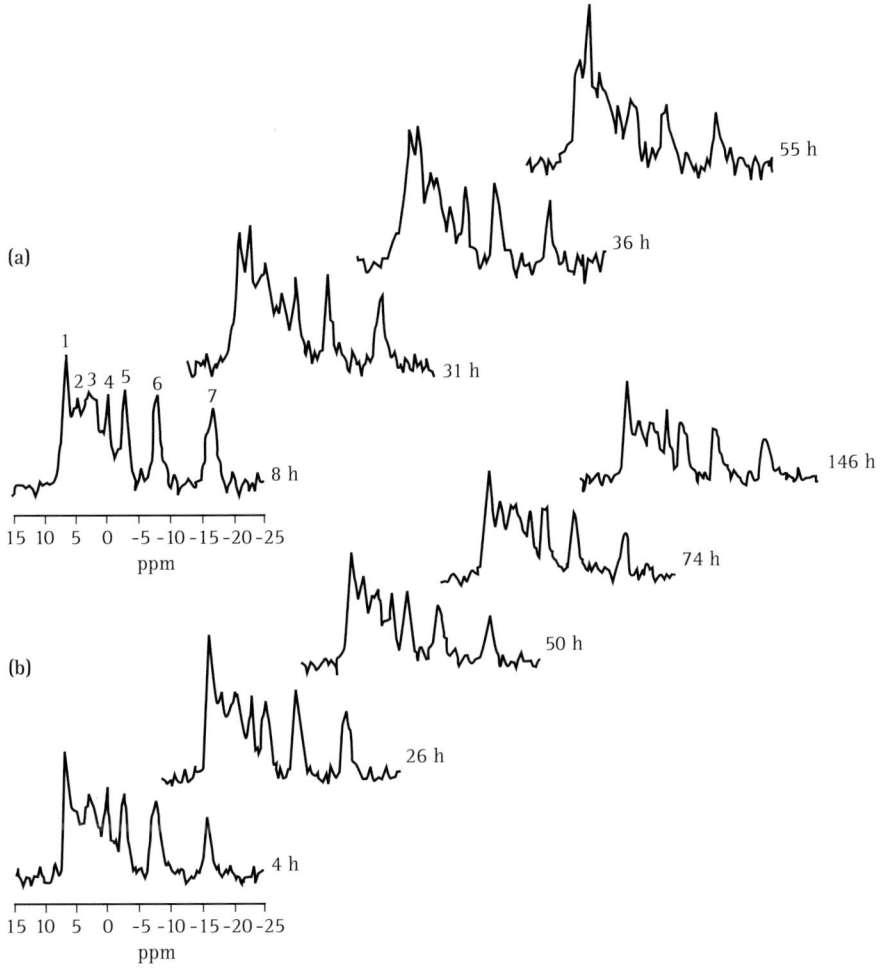

Figure 11.3 Repetitive ^{31}P MRS spectra obtained from two severely asphyxiated neonates, (a) and (b), from 4 to 146 hours after the asphyxic insult. The peaks in the spectra reflect the concentration of phosphorous atoms in various chemical environments. The 'chemical shift' indicates the resonance frequency in parts per million of the base frequency (80.5 MHz) relative to the phosphocreatine peak. The numbers in the first spectrum in (a) indicate: (1) phosphomonoesters, (2) inorganic phosphate, P_i, (3) phosphodiesters, (4) phosphocreatine, PCr and (5), (6) and (7) γ-, α- and β-ATP. The most direct information lies in the PCr/P_i peak area ratio, as well as the chemical shift of P_i relative to PCr, from which intracellular pH may be calculated. In (a) the PCr ratio is initially normal, but subsequently deteriorates. In (b) the deterioration at 50 hours recovers at 146 hours.

It is a problem that such spectra are derived from a poorly defined and large tissue volume, even including some scalp and skull. Doing magnetic resonance spectroscopy (MRS) on imaging equipment (superimposing small magnetic gradients in the X, Y and Z-plane on the main field, and hence delineating an excitable volume) may allow localization. But the relative low abundance of phosphorus and the low signal intensity from phosphorus precludes use of sample volumes smaller than several cubic centimeters and makes metabolic imaging impractical in patients. Furthermore, ^{31}P spectroscopy requires a dedicated antenna, and is therefore not routinely available.

Proton MRS, using ^{1}H, was made very useful by the invention of 'pre-saturation' pulse sequences, suppressing the large peak from water and retaining the spatial localization. Well-defined peaks became apparent: *N*-acetyl aspartate (NAA), a marker of neurons, choline (Ch) and its derivatives

and creatine + phosphocreatine associated with all types of cells (Peden et al 1990). Hence a low focal NAA/Ch ratio may prove a convenient marker of neuronal loss. Furthermore, lactate may be demonstrated by using long echo times, a strong tool in the investigation of marginal brain hypoxia-ischemia. Because of the better signal intensity from ^{1}H, smaller sample volumes may be examined, and metabolic imaging with sub-centimeter resolution is practical.

Metabolite concentrations can be expressed in mmol/L by the dividing of their peak areas with that of the unsuppressed water signal and using an estimate of the concentration of water in the brain (Toft et al 1994). Although ^{1}H spectroscopy can be done on most clinical MR machines, tuning is important and care is needed in interpretation.

Deoxyhemoglobin is paramagnetic, and hence a change in the amount of deoxyhemoglobin in tissue, e.g. as induced by a change in blood volume or in oxygen extraction, can be assessed (creating the BOLD contrast – blood oxygenation label dependence). This is termed functional magnetic resonance imaging (fMRI).

A tracer, gadolinium bound to EDTA to stay in the vascular compartment, has been used (Tanner et al 2003). Gadolinium is paramagnetic, i.e. it affects the nearby hydrogen nuclei to reduce their relaxation time, and hence strongly influence the image. When given intravenously, it will flow into brain tissue and disappear in less than 1 minute, in the same way as an intravascular dye for NIRS. In adults, it is possible to measure the gadolinium concentration in a volume near the middle cerebral arteries to obtain an arterial input function and to quantify CBF. This has not been done in newborns, so the images have been without scale. In one study (Tanner et al 2003) flow imaging was successful in 12 of 27 newborns who were examined by MRI with gadolinium contrast for clinical purposes. 'Perfusion voids' were defined as areas with tracer signal below the sensitivity threshold, and these occurred often in white matter. In one patient cortical perfusion voids did develop into cysts.

Arterial spin labeling is done by applying a radiofrequency pulse to a thick slice at the base of the skull. This labels the blood in the large arteries supplying the brain. After the arterial transit time – a little less than a second – this blood reaches the brain tissue. Regions with higher flow will contain more labeled blood (the bolus distribution principle) and hence higher signal. Flow is quantified by measuring the relative difference in signal intensity divided by the duration of the labeling pulse, and correcting for the blood–brain water partition coefficient, for any incomplete arterial labeling, and for the imaging delay compared to the relaxation time in blood (Wang et al 2003). This method was applied to 25 newborns with congenital heart disease, during normoventilation and during inhalation of added CO_2 (Licht et al 2004). All babies were mechanically ventilated and sedated and MRI was done for clinical reasons. Mean slice CBF was 19.7 ± 9.2 mL/100 g/min before and 40.1 ± 20.3 during CO_2 inhalation, an overall CBF-CO_2 reactivity of 1 mL/torr or 35%/kPa. Although all these values appear plausible, it has to be recognized that there is the potential for underestimation of CBF by overrating the arterial input since the arterial transit time at low flow is prolonged (Doppler studies show that flow velocity may go as low as 5 cm/s), and since blood near the vessel wall go even slower.

DOPPLER ULTRASOUND

Doppler ultrasound was used as soon as the interest in hemodynamic causes of damage to the newborn brain rose (Bada et al 1979) and is still a very relevant method.

According to the Doppler principle, the frequency shift of the reflected sound (the echo) is proportional to the velocity of the reflector. Since erythrocytes in blood reflect ultrasound, blood flow velocity can be measured: The frequency shift equals flow velocity multiplied by the emitted fre-

quency divided by the speed of sound in tissue. The apparent velocity has to be corrected for the angle between the blood vessel and the sound beam, and furthermore multiple frequencies are detected from a vessel, since the flow velocity decreases from the center of the stream towards the vessel wall. Even the vessel wall itself contributes to the signal. Finally velocity is pulsating, faster in systole than in diastole.

The first Doppler instruments were continuous wave (with no resolution of depth) and had no image and only a crude mean frequency shift estimator. Finding an arterial signal was done blindly, using general anatomical knowledge and using the audible signal to search for the loudest pulsating signal with the highest pitch. This left the angle and the true spatial average velocity undetermined, and therefore the scale of measurement uncertain. Indices of pulsatility (resistance index: (S-D)/S, and pulsatility index: (S-D)/mean) were often used since these are independent of scale. Indices of pulsatility reflect downstream resistance to flow. In newborn infants, however, the resistance index in the anterior cerebral artery and in the internal carotid artery was only weakly associated with cerebral blood flow as measured by ^{133}Xe clearance (Greisen et al 1984).

New instruments combined imaging and Doppler. Range-gating limits the flow measurement to a well-defined small sample volume. Signal analysis permit proper maximum and mean frequency shift estimation. Angle correction can be done accurately using the image. This all allows reliable measurement of blood flow velocity. The studies using this method have to be interpreted with care, however, since blood flow velocity in the cerebral arteries does not correlate very well with CBF (Greisen et al 1984). This is partly due to variation in arterial caliber. Blood flow in mL/min equals flow velocity (cm/s) multiplied by arterial cross-sectional area (cm²). The unknown arterial cross-sectional area precludes comparison from one infant to another, and one organ to another, but also really from one state to another, since arterial caliber varies dynamically in the immature individual (Drayton & Skidmore 1987, Malcus et al 1991).

Volumetric measurement of flow by color-coded imaging has recently been achieved in all four cerebral vessels on the neck with diameters of 1–2 mm using 10 Mz with a reproducibility of the sum of the four flows of as low as 7% (Ehehalt et al 2005) and the right common carotid artery (Sinha et al 2006) with a diameter of 2–3 mm using 15 Mz and a reproducibility of 10–15%. This method however requires training and a quiet infant and takes 10–20 minutes for a measurement.

OTHER TECHNIQUES USED IN NEWBORN INFANTS

Venous occlusion plethysmography is a standard method for measurement of limb blood flow and has been used to estimate jugular blood flow (Cross et al 1979). In spite of its virtues of technical simplicity and low risk in healthy infants, the method has fallen into disuse, mostly because of concern that low skull compliance yields falsely low values of cranial blood flow.

The transcephalic impedance, as measured by applying a small alternating electrical current, is slightly pulsatile. The pulsatility is correlated to CBF (Colditz et al 1988), although the precise basis of the impedance pulsatility is unclear. This method has theoretical risks only but gives qualitative information only and is sensitive to movement. It appears well suited for long-term monitoring, but has been used only little.

A NOTE ON RADIATION AND RISK OF CANCER

At present methods using radiation is in disuse. The topic may again become important as PET instruments with very good spatial resolution become more common. Radiation to patients from X-ray or various isotopes are compared by calculation of the 'whole-body dose,' the effective dose equivalent. This is the dose of X-ray, which if absorbed evenly in all parts of the body, will result in an identical risk of cancer or genetic damage in germ cells. In this approximation, the affinity of some tracers for certain organs is considered, and organs of high vulnerability are weighed accordingly. Recently, the International Committee of Radiation Protection reviewed the evidence, mainly from Hiroshima and Nagasaki, and increased the estimate to 5% lifetime risk of fatal cancer per sievert (1 Sv = 100 Rad = 1 joule/kg) in adults. In the last trimester and in young children the risk is estimated three times greater. This means that the added lifetime risk in an infant receiving 1 mSv as a result of an investigation is 0.00015, or 1 per 7000 compared to the average lifetime risk in western populations of 0.25 or 1 in 4. The yearly radiation from all sources averages 3 mSv. Estimated doses from the various methods described above are listed in Table 11.1.

THE PHYSIOLOGICAL REGULATION OF CBF

Blood moves as a result of a difference in pressure – from artery through capillaries to veins. This pressure gradient is called the perfusion pressure. Usually the perfusion pressure can be taken as the arterial pressure, but in some circumstances central venous pressure is significantly elevated and in some circumstances intracranial pressure is increased. When the arterial pressure is low, e.g. 25 mmHg in the extremely preterm neonate, a venous pressure of 8 cm H_2O (6 mmHg) is important.

Blood flows in proportion to perfusion pressure divided by vascular resistance. Vascular resistance is due to the limited lumen of blood vessels and due to blood viscosity. Vascular resistance is directly proportional to blood viscosity and to the length of blood vessels and inversely proportional to vessel diameter to the power of four. This means that large vessels (conduit arteries) and small vessels (intra-parenchymatous arteries and arterioles, resistance arteries) contribute about equally to vascular resistance, large arteries due to their length and small arteries and arterioles due to their small diameter. Hence the cerebrovascular resistance is partly determined by the degree of contraction of the pre-capillary arterioles, partly by the pre-arteriolar arteries (Farachi & Heistad 1990). Even a minor change in diameter induces a significant change in resistance, for instance a 10% reduction in diameter results in 35% increase in vascular resistance.

The conduit arteries of the newborn make an important contribution to the vascular resistance and are more reactive in newborns compared to adults. The diameter of the carotid artery was increased by 75% during acute asphyxia in term lambs, whereas the diameter of the descending aorta was reduced by 15% (Malcus et al 1991). Incidentally, these observations also suggest that blood flow velocity as recorded from conduit arteries by Doppler ultrasound may be potentially misleading.

Table 11.1 Typical patient radiation doses (effective dose equivalent) resulting from various techniques in use for the study of cerebral blood flow or metabolism in neonates. For comparison the mean annual dose equivalent for the population is 3 mSv

Technique	Isotope	Activity used (MBq/Kg)	Effective dose equivalent (mSv)
Xenon clearance, global CBF	^{133}Xe	40	0.2
SPECT, Xenon	^{133}Xe	60–200	0.3–1
SPECT, HMPAO	^{99m}Tc	4–50	1.5–20
SPECT, iodo-amphetamine	^{131}I	2–10	1.5–8
Xenon-enhanced tomography	X-rays	20 mSv in field	1
PET, CBF	^{15}O	30	1
PET, CMR_{O2}	^{15}O	110	5
PET, CMR_{Glu}	^{18}F	5	3

COUPLING OF CBF TO CEREBRAL ENERGY METABOLISM

Through a wide range of functional states, from deep hypothermia to electrical seizures, CBF increases in proportion to the increase in CMR. Several mechanisms operate to match local blood flow to metabolic requirements by dilating or constricting the resistance vessels. pH, adenosine, ATP, NO and local neural mechanisms all appear to play a role. It is not known when in fetal life this coupling develops. Proportionality between local CBF and local glucose metabolism is present in newborn puppies, which are rather immature at birth.

CBF, as estimated by venous occlusion plethysmography, is increased during active sleep as compared to quiet sleep (Milligan 1979, Mukhtar et al 1982, Rahilly 1980a). Using ^{133}Xe clearance after intravenous injection in preterm infants of 32 to 35 weeks post-conceptional age, Greisen et al (1985) found CBF increased in the awake state when compared to quiet or active sleep. This is evidence of flow–metabolism coupling, the action of which is also suggested by the increase in CBF seen during seizures, and the strong relation between CBF and blood hemoglobin concentration (Pryds et al 1990a, Younkin et al 1987).

The cerebrovascular response to functional activation by visual stimulation is inconsistent or non-existent in infants before term or within the first weeks of life by MRI (Born et al 1998, Martin et al 1999) or NIRS (Meek et al 1998). One possible explanation for this is that visual cortical projections are not well developed at term. Cerebral oxygenation as detected by NIRS was consistently decreased by unpleasant odors in healthy preterm newborns (Bartocci et al 2001). The neurophysiological explanation for this is uncertain.

PERFUSION PRESSURE-FLOW AUTOREGULATION

Smooth muscle cells of the arterial wall contract in response to increased intravascular pressure at the local arterial segment to a degree that more than compensates for the passive stretching of the vessel wall. The net result is that arteries constrict at higher pressures and dilate at lower pressures. This is what is called autoregulation.

Pressure induces an increase in smooth muscle cell membrane potential most likely by modification of the activity of the ATP-sensitive and Ca^{2+}-activated K^+ channels in the plasma membrane. The rate of leak of K^+ from cells to the extracellular space is regulated by plasma membrane potassium conductance and is the main determinant of resting membrane potential. The membrane potential regulates the intracellular Ca^{2+} concentration through the effect of voltage-gated Ca^{2+} channels. The intracellular Ca^{2+} concentration is the principal regulator of smooth muscle cell tone by Ca^{2+}/calmodulin myosin light chain kinase-mediated phosphorylation of the regulatory light chains of myosin with subsequent interaction of actin and myosin.

The precise mechanism of the mechano-chemical coupling is unknown, but the sequence is endothelium-independent and the arterial constriction in response to luminal pressure is an intrinsic myogenic reflex.

Pressure-flow autoregulation has been widely investigated in the immature brain since the original observation of direct proportionality of CBF to systolic blood pressure in a group of neonates during stabilization after birth (Lou et al 1977). An adequate autoregulatory plateau, shifted to the left to match the lower perinatal blood pressure, has been demonstrated in several animal species before and after birth (Hernandez et al 1980, Papile et al 1985, Pasternak et al 1985, Pryds et al 2005, Tweed et al 1983). Autoregulation was abolished by hypoxemia (arterial oxygen saturation about 50%) for 20 minutes (Tweed et al 1986), to return after 4 to 7 hours.

Unfortunately this issue is much less well investigated in the human neonate, the main reason being lack of controlled manipulation of blood pressure. All studies of global CBF in stable neonates without evidence of major brain injury suggest that autoregulation is intact (Greisen & Trojaborg 1987, Greisen 1986, Pryds et al 1989, 1990a, 1990b, Tyszczuk et al 1998, Younkin et al 1987). This means that a complete absence of relation between pressure and flow could not be statistically excluded, although typical estimates are 1–2% per mmHg corresponding to a 10–20% change in CBF per 10 mmHg change in blood pressure. The studies have included neonates with gestational age as low as 24 weeks and blood pressures as low as 25 mmHg. Overall, this suggests that the autoregulatory plateau spans the range of blood pressures commonly seen in neonatal intensive care. Three more recent studies have found absent autoregulation in preterm neonates with arterial hypotension who were treated with dopamine (Jayasinghe et al 2003, Munro et al 2004) and/or epinephrine (Pellicier et al 2005). It is likely that the discrepancy between these results and those cited above is due to the statistical uncertainty of small studies, or to methodological or clinical differences. Dopamine does not appear to have a specific (dilatory) effect on brain vessels as low-dose dopamine does not increase CBF in preterm neonates with normal blood pressure (Lundstrom et al 2000).

Based on SPECT estimates of CBF distribution during arterial hypotension in 24 preterm infants with persistently normal brain ultrasound it has been suggested that CBF to the periventricular white matter may be selectively reduced at blood pressures below 30 mmHg (Børch & Greisen 1997). Although these data support the concept of periventricular white matter being a 'watershed area' it must be realized that the statistical relation was based on differences among infants, which may have many causes.

Significantly weakened or lost autoregulation (CBF-MABP reactivity of 2-4%) has been demonstrated following severe birth asphyxia (Pryds et al 1990b) or preceding major germinal layer hemorrhage (Milligan 1980, Pryds et al 1989).

The contraction of smooth muscle cells in response to stimulation is not instantaneous. Experiments on isolated blood vessels show that typical response time to an increase in intraluminal pressure is in the order of 10 seconds. Most methods of measuring CBF take longer and hence by nature describe steady-state relations between flow and pressure, what can be called 'static' autoregulation. CBF velocity measured from second to second by Doppler, on the other hand, will vary with rapid changes in arterial blood pressure even when autoregulation operates normally (Menke et al 1997). It has been suggested that the characteristics of this 'dynamic' autoregulation may be important (Boylan et al 2000).

CARBON DIOXIDE–CBF REACTIVITY

Arteries and arterioles constrict with hypocapnia and dilate with hypercapnia. The principal part of this reaction is mediated through pH, i.e. the H^+ concentration. Perivascular pH has a direct effect on the membrane potential of arterial smooth muscle cell since the extracellular H^+ concentration is a main determinant of the potassium conductance of the plasma membrane of arterial smooth muscle cells and hence the outward K^+ current (Pearce & Harder 1996). Furthermore, increased extracellular – and to a lesser degree intracellular – H^+ concentration reduces the conductance of voltage-dependent Ca^{2+} channels, which also induces relaxation (Aalkjær & Poston 1996). Hypercapnic vasodilatation is reduced to 50% when neuronal NO synthetase is blocked in adult rat brain (Wang et al 1995). The hypercapnic response was restituted by addition of an NO donor (Ladecola & Zang 1996). This suggests that a basal level of NO level is necessary for the pH to act, at least in some species. It has more recently been suggested that it is the function of the calcium-activated K^+ and ATP-sensitive K^+ channels which are necessary for hypercapnic vasodilatation, and that the function of these receptors is dependent on a basal level of NO (Lindauer et al 2003). The role of prostanoids (Rama et al 1996, Wagerle & Mishra 1988) is less clear. The fact that indometacin abolishes the cerebral CBF-CO_2 response in preterm infants (Edwards et al 1992) may not indicate a role of prostanoids, since ibuprofen does not (Patel et al 2000). Similar differential effect is seen in other organs. This suggests that the effects of indometacin are not solely due to cyclooxygenase inhibition. Indometacin has intrinsic properties as a prostanoid receptor antagonist, but other (side) effects specific to the indometacin molecule may also be involved.

In normocapnic adults small changes in arterial carbon dioxide tension ($PaCO_2$) result in a change in CBF by 30%/kPa (4%/mmHg). Adaptation, with return of CBF to normal values, occurs within 24 hours after a chronic change of $PaCO_2$. Similar reactivity has been demonstrated in the normal human neonate by venous occlusion plethysmography (Leahy et al 1980, Rahilly 1980b) and in stable preterm ventilated infants without major germinal layer hemorrhage

by ^{133}Xe after intravenous injection (Greisen & Trojaborg 1987) (Fig. 11.4). Reactivity was less than 30%/kPa during the first 24 hours (Pryds et al 1989).

NEUROGENIC REGULATION OF CBF

Epinephrine (adrenaline) in the blood originates from the adrenals, whereas norepinephrine (noradrenaline) originates from sympathetic nerve activity and from extra-adrenal chromaffin tissue. Sympathetic nerves are present in nearly all blood vessels. The nerves are located in the adventitia and have terminals on vascular smooth muscle cells. Adrenoreceptors are widely distributed in the vascular system, located in smooth muscle cell membrane and in endothelial cell membrane as well. Several different receptors exist, alpha-1 with at least three subtypes present in arteries, alpha-2, and beta-1 and beta-2. In arteries (and veins) alpha-receptor stimulation causes vasoconstriction and beta-receptor stimulation causes vasodilatation. Often both types of receptors are present in the membrane of the same cell. The signaling pathways of the adrenoreceptors are complex, involving release of calcium from intracellular stores as a first step, cyclic AMP, but also K^+ conductance and basal level of NO. The sympathetic nerve system is activated during hypoxia, hypotension or hypovolemia from chemo- and baroreceptors via the vasomotor centers in the medulla.

From animal studies it appear that the sympathetic system may play a more marked role in the perinatal period to

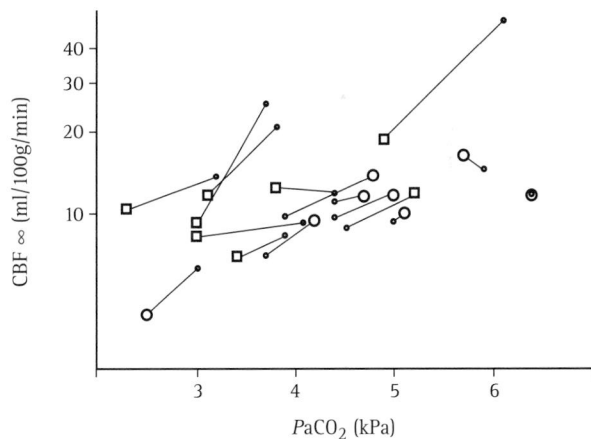

Figure 11.4 The relationship between changes in cerebral blood flow (CBF), estimated by intravenous ^{133}Xe clearance, and changes in arterial carbon dioxide tension in 16 mechanically ventilated, preterm infants. In eight infants the change occurred spontaneously (○), whereas in the other eight infants the carbon dioxide tension changed after a change in the ventilator settings (□). The intra-individual reactivity to acute changes, represented by the lines, is clearly greater than the inter-individual differences, which reflect, among other factors, more long-lasting changes in arterial carbon-dioxide tension. (Reproduced with permission from Greisen & Trojaborg 1987.)

markedly reduce blood flow to the cerebral hemispheres during circulatory stress (Goplerud et al 1991, Hayashi et al 1984, Hernandez et al 1982, Kurth et al 1988, Wagerle et al 1986). This is different from what happens in adults and is perhaps due to a relative immaturity of the nitric oxide-induced vasodilatation (Wagerle et al 1995). The mechanism is in part a constriction of conduit arteries. Human neonatal arteries in vitro (obtained post-mortem from babies with gestational age 23 to 34 weeks) show basal tone and a pressure–diameter relation quite similar to adult pial arteries (Bevan et al 1998c). Neonatal arteries, however, are significantly more sensitive to exogenous norepinephrine, to electrical field activation of adventitial sympathetic nerve fibers, and have a higher sympathetic nerve density (Bevan et al 1998b) compared to adult pial arteries (Bevan et al 1998a).

There are virtually no clinical research data on this important question. Adrenergic mechanisms may lie behind the association between low superior vena cava flow as a measure of low systemic cardiac output and cerebral injury in spite of normal blood pressure (Kluckow & Evans 2000b). The association between left ventricular output and cerebral fractional oxygen extraction in mechanically ventilated preterm infants which does not involve arterial blood pressure (Kissack et al 2004) also suggests that the vasoconstriction response to circulatory stress includes brain circulation.

The old observations of a 30–40% decrease in CBF after a feed in full-term newborn infants using venous occlusion plethysmography (Dear 1980, Rahilly 1980a) may suggest a neurogenic mechanism, although hardly mediated by increased sympathetic tone.

CBF, CEREBRAL OXYGEN DELIVERY AND CMR IN NORMAL NEONATES

The three infants studied by Garfunkel et al (1954) were all abnormal (one with myelomeningocele, one with microcephaly and one with hydrocephalus) – CBF ranged from 15 to 23 mL/100 g/min, as estimated by the Kety–Schmidt method. The CMR_{O2} ranged from 50 to 94 µmol/100 g/min (1.1–2.1 mL O_2). These values were surprisingly low compared to normal adult values of CBF of 45 mL/100 g/min and of $CMRO_2$ of 150 µmol/100 g/min.

Few entirely normal human neonates have been investigated by reliable methods. The average value of global CBF measured by ^{133}Xe clearance in 11 preterm, healthy infants during the first week of life was 20 mL/100 g/min (Greisen 1986). CBF measured by volumetric Doppler on both internal carotid arteries and both vertebral arteries was 70 mL/min, corresponding to 20 mL/100 g/min in a mixed group of normal infants born at term or born preterm and reaching term, whereas in preterm infants at 32–34 weeks of gestation CBF was 33 mL/min, corresponding to 14 mL/100 g/min (Fig. 11.5) (Kehrer et al 2003). In six term infants global CBF was 17 mL/100 g/min, as measured by MRI and arterial spin labeling, compared to 21 mL/100 g/min in 23 preterm infants

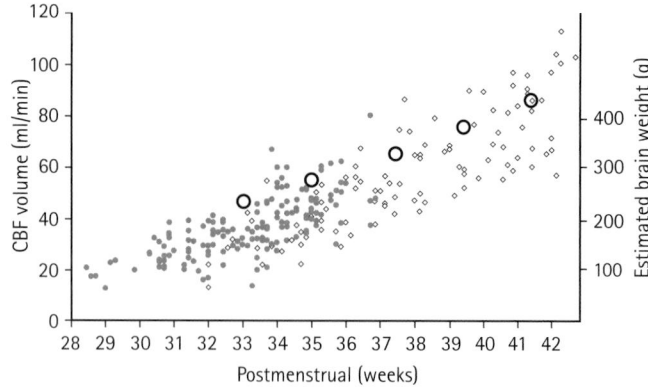

Figure 11.5 Cerebral blood flow (CBF) as measured by volumetric Doppler ultrasound as a function of age in healthy infants. The variation in age is partly due to preterm birth, partly to infants being studied at varying postnatal age. Most of the change in CBF is due to brain growth, but CBF calculated from these data and estimated brain weight (large circles) increases from about 15 to about 20 mL/100 g/min (modified from Kehrer et al 2005).

at term age (Miranda et al 2006). In a group of heterogeneous preterm infants CBF increased with postnatal age (Younkin et al 1982) and recently a 20% increase in CBF was demonstrated in the first 14 days of life in preterm infants (Kehrer et al 2005).

From EEG and behavior it is apparent that neural activity increases with increasing gestational and postnatal age. The differences in CBF, as described above, are rather small compared to that, and may not be more than what can be explained by differences in blood hemoglobin concentration, i.e. that cerebral oxygen delivery is really not increasing with increasing maturation.

Left ventricular output in the healthy term infant is approximately 500 mL/min and venous return from the upper part of the body as measured in the superior vena cava is about 250 mL/min (Kluckow & Evans 2000a). This means the CBF constitutes no more than 14% of cardiac output and less than 30% of upper body blood flow. This is only a little more than the corresponding weight, i.e. the brain is not a high-flow organ in the newborn. This is very different from the adult.

The dramatic increase from the perinatal period to 3 years of postnatal age, and later decrease to adult values (Fig. 11.6), matches maturational changes in CMR_{Glu}, as estimated from PET studies of patients (Chugani et al 1987) who later turned out to be free of neurological disease (Fig. 11.7). This pattern of development also matches the number of synapses per mm^3 of visual cortex (Huttenlocher et al 1982).

No data concerning CMR_{O2} in normal human neonates are available, although SvO_2 was entirely normal (64% ± 5) as estimated by NIRS and jugular occlusion in 11 healthy, term infants 3 days after birth (Buchvald et al 1999). Together this suggests that normal global CBF and CMRO$_2$ (expressed per 100 g of tissue) is between one-third and half of normal adult values.

The contrast between flow to white and gray matter was high compared to experimental perinatal animals in a study using HMPAO SPECT (Børch & Greisen 1998), but not in a study using MRI with arterial spin labeling (Miranda et al 2006). The reason for this discrepancy could be that the infants in the former study were very preterm in the first few days of life, whereas the infants in the latter study were term infants and preterm infants at term age. The reason could also be due to differences in the complex methodologies.

PATHOPHYSIOLOGY

ACUTE HYPOXIA–ISCHEMIA

The basic physiological quantity in hypoxic–ischemic brain injury is cerebral oxygen delivery, which is the product of CBF and arterial oxygen content. When oxygen delivery becomes insufficient to meet the cellular demands for oxygen, a sequence of events will be triggered, starting with anaerobic glycolysis and lactic acidosis, proceeding to membrane pump failure, efflux of potassium, influx of sodium and calcium. This leads to microstructural damage and cell death, possibly several days later through a process of apoptosis (see below).

During arterial hypoxemia, the normal cerebrovascular reaction leads to rising CBF and increased fractional oxygen extraction (Fig. 11.8). CBF may maximally increase two- to threefold. Oxygen extraction can increase until the critical level of venous oxygen saturation (SvO$_2$) that corresponds to a minimal oxygen tension, sufficient to provide a diffusion gradient from the venous end of the capillary to the mitochondrion. In the newborn puppy SvO$_2$ may decrease from 75% to 40% without significant lactate production ensuing (Reuter & Disney 1986). The exact minimum value will depend on the oxygen dissociation curve and hence, among other factors, be increased by alkalosis and a high fraction of fetal hemoglobin.

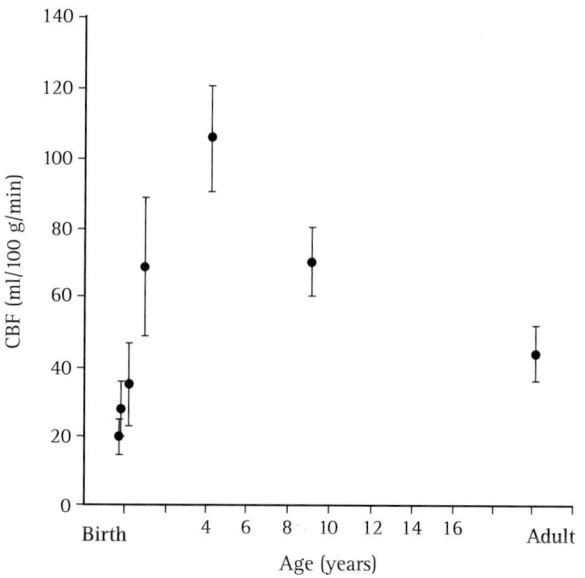

Figure 11.6 Values of cerebral blood flow (CBF) obtained in healthy, apparently normal humans from 10 weeks before term to adulthood. (From Cross et al 1979, Greisen 1986, Kennedy et al 1957, Lou et al 1984, Meyers et al 1978, Younkin et al 1982, Zettergren et al 1976.)

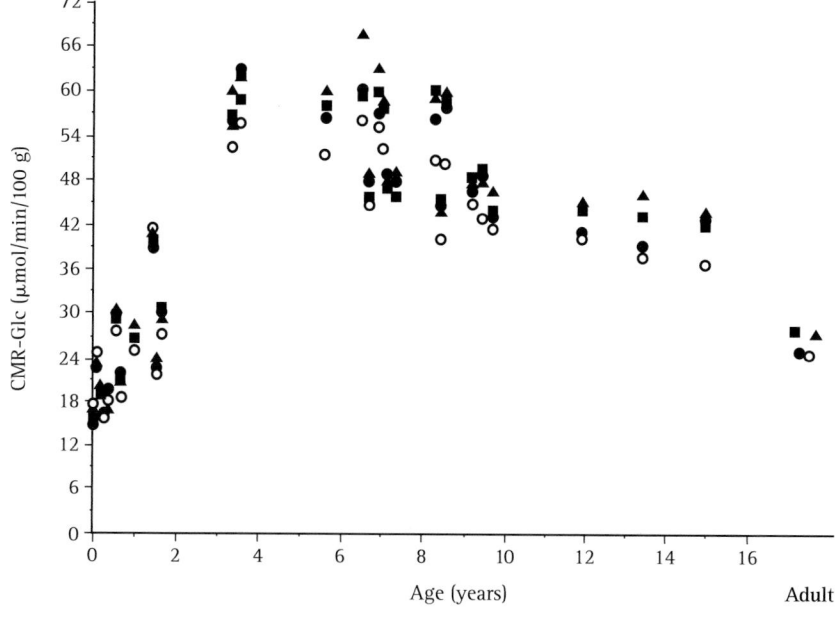

Figure 11.7 Cortical glucose uptake in patients investigated for neurological abnormality, but subsequently considered normal. There are no values for preterm neonates but the general developmental pattern is quite similar to that of CBF. (Reproduced with permission from Chugani et al 1987.)

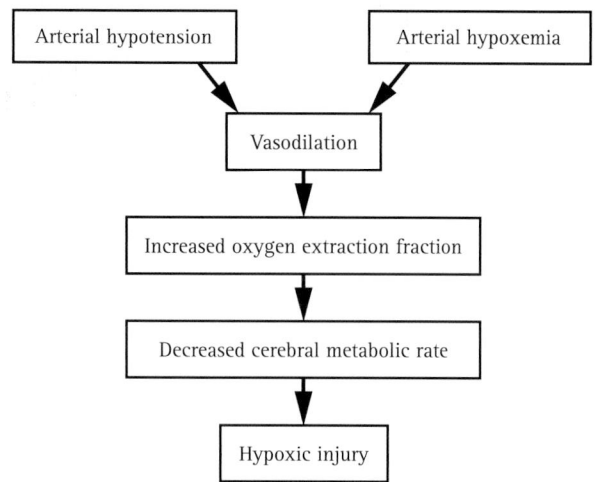

Figure 11.8 Buffering mechanisms protect the brain against hypoxic–ischemic injury. Vasodilation leads to decreased cerebrovascular resistance. Oxygen extraction fraction increases until the oxygen tension at the venous ends of the capillaries is minimized. When oxygen is no longer sufficient the metabolic rate begins to fall. Only when the metabolic rate falls markedly is injury likely to occur.

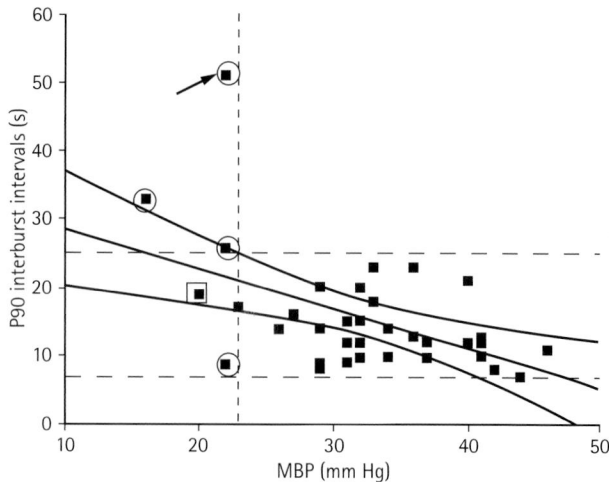

Figure 11.9 A highly statistically significant relation between the lowest recorded mean arterial blood pressure (MBP) and the incident EEG interburst interval during the first 48 hours of life in 35 infants under 30 weeks gestation. The horizontal dotted lines represent the 10–90% range for the interburst interval in stable infants of the same gestation. The dotted vertical line at 23 mmHg represents the upper limit of a blood pressure which is likely to be associated with normal EEG activity. The four circles indicate infants with qualitatively abnormal EEG. The square indicates an infant with abnormally high cerebral fractional oxygen extraction (0.44) as measured by near-infrared spectroscopy. This indicates that the low blood pressure was associated with low cerebral blood flow. The infant with the highest interburst interval (arrow), however, had normal oxygen extraction (0.31). The other three infants with blood pressure below the threshold did not have oxygen extraction measured for technical reasons. The difficulty of clinical research in extreme situations is evident (modified from Victor et al 2006).

Decrease of CBF below the threshold, when oxygen supply is no longer sufficient, is termed ischemia. In the cerebral cortex of adult baboon and adult man, the threshold of blood flow sufficient to maintain tissue integrity depends on time of exposure; for a duration of a few hours, the limit is in the range of 10 mL/100 g/min (Jones et al 1981). In acute, localized brain ischemia the concept of a border-zone or 'penumbra' has been proposed, i.e. a state in which the blood flow is sufficient to maintain the 'strukturumsatz' but fails to sustain electrical activity (Astrup 1982). The brain tissue in such a zone is electrically silent. In progressing ischemia electrical failure is a prewarning of permanent tissue injury. This concept has been used in clinical practice with EEG-monitoring during carotid surgery. In adult human brain cortex, electrical function ceases at about 20 mL/100 g/min. In subcortical gray matter and the brainstem of the adult baboon the values are 10–15 mL/100 g/min (Branston et al 1984).

The threshold values for neonates are not known but in view of the low resting levels of CBF and the comparatively much longer survival in total ischemia or anoxia, the thresholds are likely to be considerably below 10 mL/100 g/min. Thus, in ventilated preterm infants visual evoked responses were unaffected at global flow levels below 10 mL/100 g/min corresponding to a cerebral oxygen delivery of 50 μmol/100 g/min (Greisen & Trojaborg 1987, Pryds & Greisen 1990). Recently a doubling in oxygen delivery from 50 to 100 μmol/100 g/min over the first 3 days of life was demonstrated in very preterm infants on mechanical ventilation (Kissack et al 2005). Surprisingly, the low oxygen delivery on the first day of life was associated with only

modestly increased cerebral fractional oxygen extraction. Thus, either metabolic needs are much reduced during the first day of life in this situation, or oxygen consumption in the immature brain is delivery-dependent. In stable, very low-birth-weight infants on ventilatory support CBF increased by 30% from day 1 to 2 (Pellicer et al 2001), whereas in stable, spontaneously breathing very preterm infants CBF increased by only 18% from day 1 to day 2 (Kehrer et al 2005).

A weak, but statistically significant relation between discontinuity of spontaneous EEG and low CBF has been demonstrated in preterm infants (Greisen & Pryds 1989), and recently a relation between very low mean arterial blood pressure, likely to cause low CBF, and abnormally long EEG interburst intervals was demonstrated (Fig. 11.9) (Victor et al 2006). Analyzing the same data, arterial pCO_2 was inversely associated with cerebral fractional oxygen extraction to indicate a preserved CO_2-CBF reactivity and low pCO_2 was associated with slowing of the EEG, as an expected effect of hypoxia–ischemia (Victor et al 2005). High pCO₂, however, was associated with increased EEG interburst interval, usually also an indicator of hypoxia–ischemia, but here rather a direct effect of hypocapnia and/or acidosis.

THE POST ASPHYXIATED STATE

The loss of cellular energy charge during an asphyxial event can be studied by ^{31}P MRS in animals (Hope et al 1987). For logistic reasons it has not been demonstrated in human neonates; it is presumably corrected during resuscitation.

The early recovery phase lasts 4–12 hours and is not well studied in human infants. From animal studies of acute asphyxia–ischemia it is expected that CBF, CMR$_{O2}$ and CMR$_{Glu}$ is low, as witnessed by reduced EEG-activity. Clearly, in clinical practice an asphyxial event may be intermittent

or subacute during the last hours before delivery or during gradual cardio-respiratory decompensation due to severe postnatal illness. As a result, the early phase may be short or missing in some infants.

After the most severe, global injury follows a delayed phase, that lasts for several days. The PCr/P$_i$ normalizes in the early phase only to decline again (Fig. 11.3) (Hope et al 1984) when intracellular pH rises above normal, whereas the NAA/Cho ratio by ^{1}H-MRS is typically normal at this time (Fig. 11.10). This carries a poor prognosis (Fig. 11.11) (Azzopardi et al 1989), and gives more precise prediction of handicap compared to a clinical encephalopathy score (Martin et al 1996). In this delayed phase cerebral hyperperfusion has been well documented (Frewen et al 1991, Friis-Hansen 1985, Leth et al 1996, Pryds et al 1990b), i.e. high CBF with low oxygen extraction (Frewen et al 1991, Skov

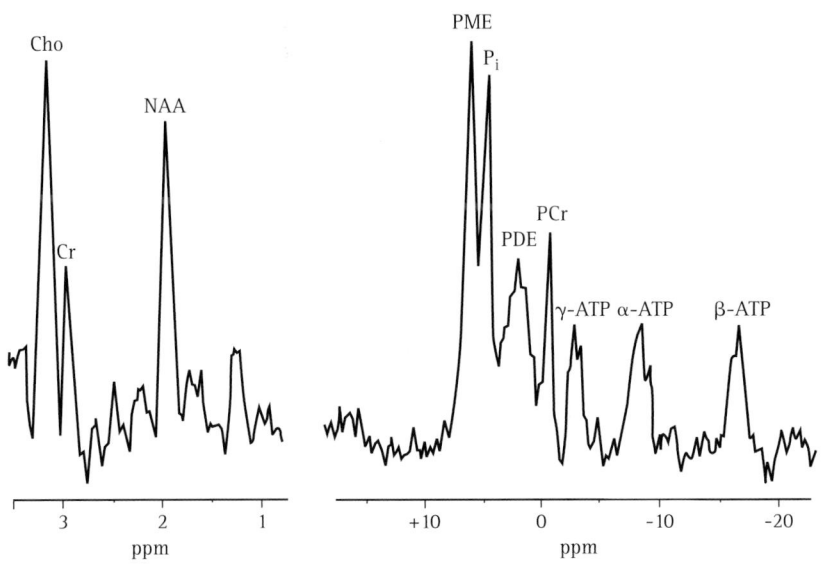

Figure 11.10 ^{1}H (left) and ^{31}P (right) spectrum from a term, asphyxiated infant 48 hours after birth. The NAA/Cho ratio is 0.8, probably within normal range. The PCr/P$_i$ ratio was 0.5, severely abnormal. The infant subsequently developed subcortical cysts. (Reproduced with permission from Peden et al 1990.)

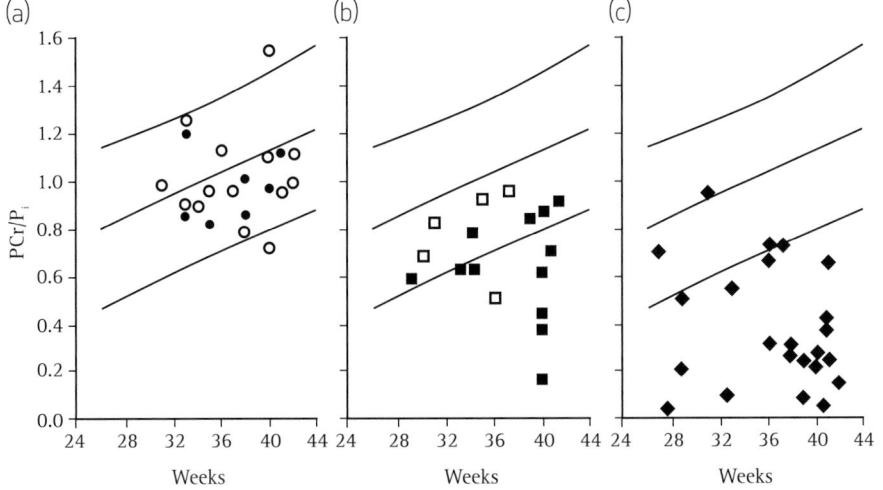

Figure 11.11 Relation between minimum values of PCr/P$_i$ ratio in 61 infants with hypoxic–ischemic brain injury and 1-year outcome. The regression line, 5 and 95 centiles for PCr/P$_i$ as a function of gestational age are indicated in each of the three panels. (a) ○ = normal progress, ● = minor impairment, (b) □ = major neuromotor impairment, ■ = multiple major impairment and (c) ◆ = death. Whereas the PCr/P$_i$ ratio is specific, since only one normal child had a low ratio, the ratio has a rather low sensitivity for neurodevelopmental impairment. (Reproduced with permission from Azzopardi 1989.)

et al 1993). A similar 'luxury perfusion' (Lassen et al 1966) has been described following head trauma, particularly in young individuals (Cohan et al 1989, Obrist et al 1984). Loss of cerebrovascular tone is suggested by the loss of reactivity to CO_2 as well as to changes in blood pressure (Fig. 11.12). In parallel, abnormally high CBV has been demonstrated by NIRS associated with a reduced reactivity of CBV to changes in $PaCO_2$ (Meek et al 1999a). The low oxygen extraction contrasts with the increased cerebral lactate concentration as shown by ^{1}H-MRS (Groenendaal et al 1994, Hanrahan et al 1996, Leth et al 1996) and increased CMR_{Glu} by PET (Blennow et al 1995). Each of these findings has been shown

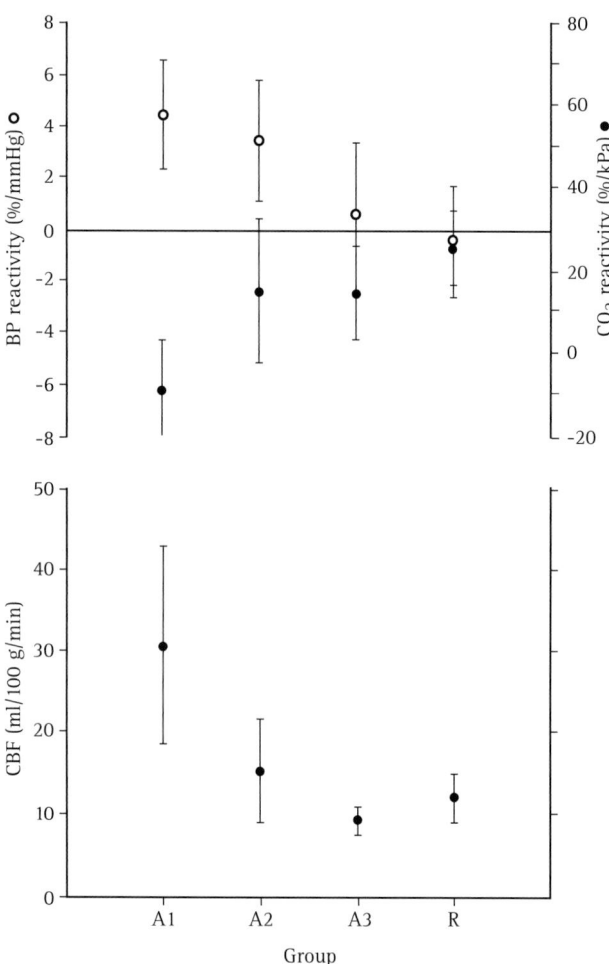

Figure 11.12 Global CBF (•, lower panel) and its reactivity to changes in $PaCO_2$ (•, upper panel) and mean arterial blood pressure (○, upper panel) in three groups of severely asphyxiated infants (A1, A2, A3) and a reference group of term infants similarly mechanically ventilated for cardio-respiratory or surgical illness (R). The asphyxiated infants were grouped according to the extent of resulting brain damage: severe and global (A1), focal (A2) and none (A3). The horizontal axis for the vascular reactivities indicates the normal value of 0%/mmHg for arterial blood pressure and 30%/kPa for $PaCO_2$. (Redrawn from Pryds et al 1990b.)

to predict later handicap and together they indicate mitochondrial failure, and support the concept of a delayed energy failure.

In infants, who develop neurological signs of focal brain damage only, slightly low levels of global CBF with abnormal pressure-flow reactivity and near-normal CBF-CO_2 reactivity have been demonstrated (Pryds et al 1990b) (Fig. 11.12).

At longer terms, Volpe et al (1985) reported local decrease in CBF, as estimated by PET, in the parasagittal regions 3 to 20 days after the insult corresponding to a decreased CMR_{Glu} in asphyxiated term neonates with poor later outcome (Suhonen-Polvi et al 1993, Thorngren-Jerneck et al 1999). The PCr/P_i ratio normalizes, whereas the N-aspartate-acetate concentration fails to develop normally (Fig. 11.13), as evidenced by ^{1}H MRS (Peden et al 1990). Since all these techniques relate to a given volume, the results do not indicate brain 'atrophy' but rather transformation of brain tissue into a 'scar' tissue of lower-energy metabolism and possibly containing fewer neurons. Interestingly, the lactate/creatine ratio appears to remain elevated for months (Hanrahan et al 1998) as well as the intracellular pH (Robertson et al 1999).

HYPOGLYCEMIA

Severe hypoglycemia lasting hours may cause brain damage by substrate insufficiency. The significance of moderate or brief hypoglycemia is less clear. Perinatal animals (Belik et al 1989) and human neonates (Kraus et al 1974) may to a large extent depend on alternative carbon sources during hypoglycemia (Fig. 11.2), but probably not fully. Furthermore, although in some situations substitutes for glucose are abundant, e.g. lactate after asphyxia or ketone bodies in fasting, in other situations they may be scarce, e.g. following a sudden discontinuation of intravenous glucose infusion.

Cerebral glucose uptake has not been studied during hypoglycemia but hypoglycemia is associated with increased CBF in preterm infants a few hours after birth (Fig. 11.14) (Pryds et al 1988b). The increase is apparent at a blood glucose slightly below 2 mM. At the lowest levels of glucose CBF increases to maximal values. The mechanism, as well as the effect on glucose uptake, is unclear. Monitoring of preterm infants with NIRS during bolus glucose administration for hypoglycemia suggests that cerebral blood volume decreases (normalizes?) in the course of the first few minutes (Skov & Pryds 1992), suggesting capillary de-recruitment. Capillary recruitment during hypoglycemia would increase the permeability-surface product and hence increase glucose flux across the blood–brain barrier. The concept of capillary recruitment, however, has been seriously questioned (Kuschinsky & Paulson 1992).

HYPERVENTILATION

Hyperventilation causes hypocapnic cerebral vasoconstriction and has been found associated with brain injury in preterm infants (Calvert et al 1987, Graziani et al 1992,

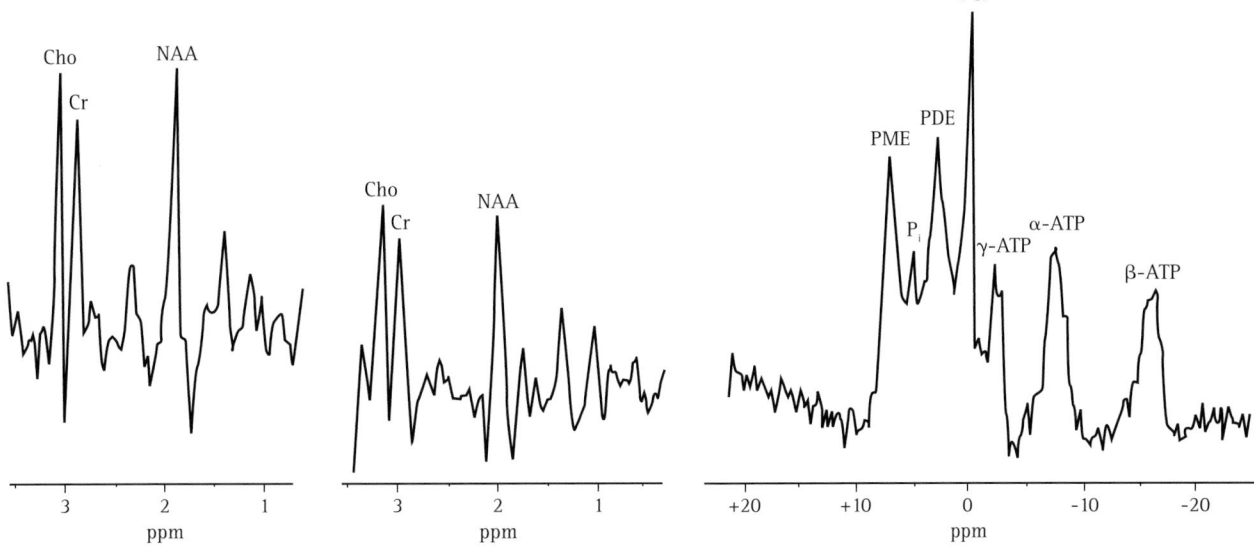

Figure 11.13 ^{1}H spectrum (left) at 5 months of age, and ^{1}H spectrum (middle) and ^{31}P spectrum (right) at 14 months of age from an infant with thalamic echo densities and subcortical cysts on cerebral ultrasound in the perinatal period. At 5 months the NAA/Cho ratio was 1.1 only, in the normal range of infants at birth. At 14 months, presenting cerebral palsy and global delay, the NAA/Cho ratio had still not developed (the normal adult range is 3.5 to 4.5), whereas in the ^{31}P spectrum the PCr/P$_i$ was quite normal, 2.5. (Reproduced with permission from Peden et al 1990.)

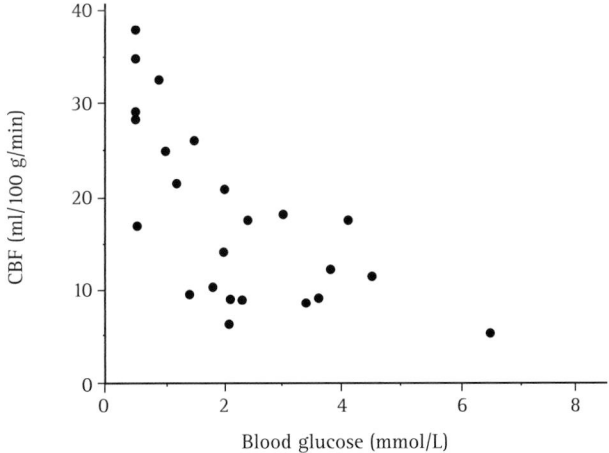

Figure 11.14 Cerebral blood flow (CBF) as a function of blood glucose concentrations a few hours after birth in 24 preterm neonates. (Reproduced with permission from Pryds et al 1988b.)

Greisen et al 1987) but not in term infants (Ferrara et al 1984) or adults. Is a question if hypocapnia alone can cause ischemia, or if it may work in combination with other factors, such as hypoxemia, hypoglycemia, sympathetic activation or seizures.

CBF adapts over time. On one side such adaptation will tend to reduce an ischemic insult, on the other side, once an infant has adapted to an abnormally high pCO$_2$, e.g. due to chronic lung disease, and then is intubated and mechani-cally ventilated, e.g. for a surgical procedure, a rapid nor-malization of pCO$_2$ may possibly cause cerebral ischemia.

SEIZURES

The clinical relevance of the flow-metabolism coupling is most clearly appreciated by considering focal electrical sei-zures. PET (Perlmann et al 1985) and SPECT (Børch et al 1998) have demonstrated increase in local CBF. The increases were less than the increase during seizures in adult experi-mental animals but the increase may be underestimated due to volume averaging of imaging with low spatial resolution. If the flow-metabolism coupling is insufficient, the highly increased local metabolic demands may not be met and neuronal injury may ensue. Ictal MRS showed a drop in PCr/P$_i$ ratio in four infants with seizures (Younkin et al 1986). Evidence of damaging effects of seizures per se is of crucial importance for the indication of aggressive anticon-vulsive therapy.

RESPIRATORY DISTRESS, OXYGEN EXPOSURE AND ARTIFICIAL VENTILATION

Respiratory distress syndrome is characterized by several circulatory features, of which decreased visceral blood flow is one. It is possible that brain blood flow is affected simi-larly. Thus, among 42 preterm infants (Fig. 11.15) artificial ventilation was associated with low levels of CBF that could not be explained by the PaCO$_2$, arterial blood pressure, or gestational age in the group of mechanically ventilated infants (Greisen 1986). This reduction of CBF may possibly increase the exposure to ischemia. Overexposure to oxygen in preterm infants in the delivery room was associated with a reduction of CBF by 23% 2 hours later (Lundstrøm et al 1995). This residual effect of hyperoxia, however, was not confirmed in newborn rats and no effect of hyper-oxygenation on CBF-CO_2 reactivity was found (Fumagalli et al 2004).

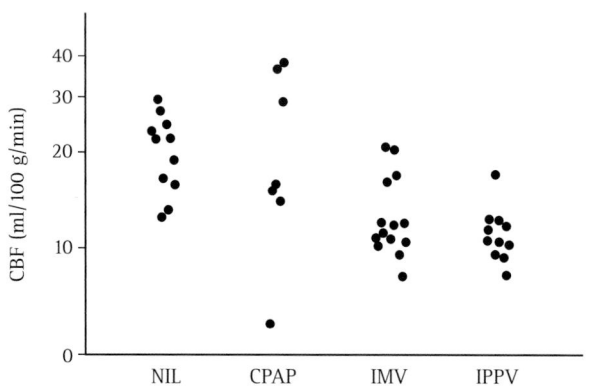

Figure 11.15 Cerebral blood flow (CBF) in 42 preterm infants less than 5 days of age, estimated by the intravenous ^{133}Xe method. Of these infants 11 required no respiratory assistance (NIL), 6 had continuous positive airway pressure (CPAP), 14 were mechanically ventilated at a rate <20/min (IMV), whereas 11 required a faster rate (IPPV). (Reproduced with permission from Greisen 1986.)

INTRACRANIAL HEMORRHAGE

Decreased levels of CBF (Meek et al 1999b, Pryds et al 1989) and impaired pressure-flow autoregulation as well as CBF-CO_2 reactivity were demonstrated in preterm infants, who went on to develop severe germinal layer hemorrhage (Pryds et al 1989). Absence of such relations, however, has also been reported (Pellicer et al 2001). Using changes in the oxygenation index (OI) of NIRS as a surrogate for changes in CBF, it was shown that ultralow-frequency coherence between OI and arterial blood pressure was higher in infants who later proved to have or who developed severe intracranial hemorrhage or cystic periventricular leukomalacia compared to those who did not (Fig. 11.16) (Tsuji et al 2000). Ultralow-frequency coherence means that OI changes in proportion with MABP when changes are slow (>30 s), i.e. impaired autoregulation. It is unknown if the CBF abnormality is part of the causation of bleeding, or whether it was just another manifestation of a primary cerebral injury. Low superior vena cava flow, as an indicator of low cardiac output and perhaps of low CBF, during the first 24 hours of life predicts subsequent severe intraventricular hemorrhage (Kluckow & Evans 2000b). This finding supports the view that a systemic circulatory compromise is behind the low CBF that precedes severe cerebral hemorrhage. It should be noted, however, that the germinal layer itself, the usual origin of hemorrhage in preterm infants, is characterized by an atypical vascularization, and

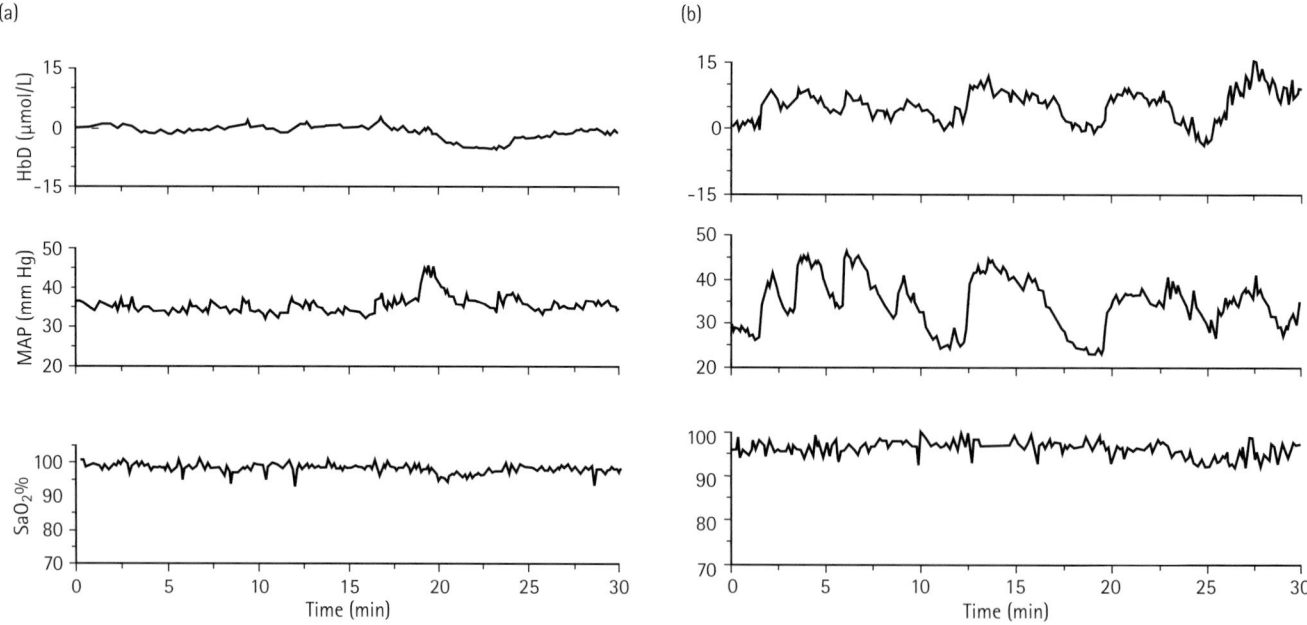

Figure 11.16 Cerebral oxygenation as monitored by near-infrared spectroscopy (here labeled HbD) over 30 minutes compared to mean arterial blood pressure (MAP) and pulse oximetry (SaO_2). In infant (a) the cerebral oxygenation does not vary in spite of some fluctuations in blood pressure lasting several minutes. In infant (b) there are wide fluctuations in cerebral oxygenation in phase with the fluctuations in blood pressure. Cerebral oxygenation fluctuates in spite of a stable arterial oxygenation and therefore can be taken as an expression of fluctuating cerebral blood flow. The high coherence of HbD and MAP in (b) is an indication of impaired pressure flow autoregulation (modified from Tsuji 2000).

that this small region will contribute little to measurements of global CBF.

Once a severe hemorrhage is established it is possible that the presence of extravascular blood induces vasospasm, leading to ischemia in the periphery (Volpe et al 1983). Alternatively, a widespread hypoperfusion may indicate a more extensive ischemic injury than evidenced by the extent of the hemorrhage or simply reflect diaschisis, i.e. far-away reduction in neuronal activity due to loss of connectivity (Børch & Greisen 1994). It is not known if the widespread perturbations of CBF that are seen in some cases of severe hemorrhage can help in identifying infants with particular risk of extensive handicap.

THE EFFECT OF DRUGS

Indometacin reduces CBF in experimental animals and in adult humans. Indometacine also reduces CBF in preterm neonates treated for persistence of the arterial duct (Pryds et al 1988a). Loss of normal CBF-CO_2 reactivity after indometacin treatment has also been demonstrated in preterm

infants (Fig. 11.17) (Edwards et al 1992). The crucial question if indometacin may actually reduce CBF to ischemic levels and cause brain injury has not yet been addressed. Interestingly ibuprofen does not have significant cerebrovascular effects (Mosca et al 1997, Patel et al 2000).

Aminophylline reduces CBF and $PaCO_2$ in experimental animals, in adults, and in preterm infants (Pryds & Schneider 1991). It is not yet clear if the reduction of CBF is a direct effect of aminophylline or rather just a result of the fall in $PaCO_2$. Studies have not addressed if aminophylline, with blockade of adenosine receptors, interferes with the CBF increase during functional activation.

Dopamine increases blood pressure and thereby may affect CBF (Jayasinghe et al 2003, Munro et al 2004, Pellicer et al 2005). It does not appear to have a specific (dilatory) effect on brain vessels (Lundstrom et al 2000, Seri et al 1998, Zhang et al 1999). Epinephrine appears not to differ from dopamine regarding the effect on cerebral oxygenation as a surrogate measure of changes in CBF (Pellicer et al 2005).

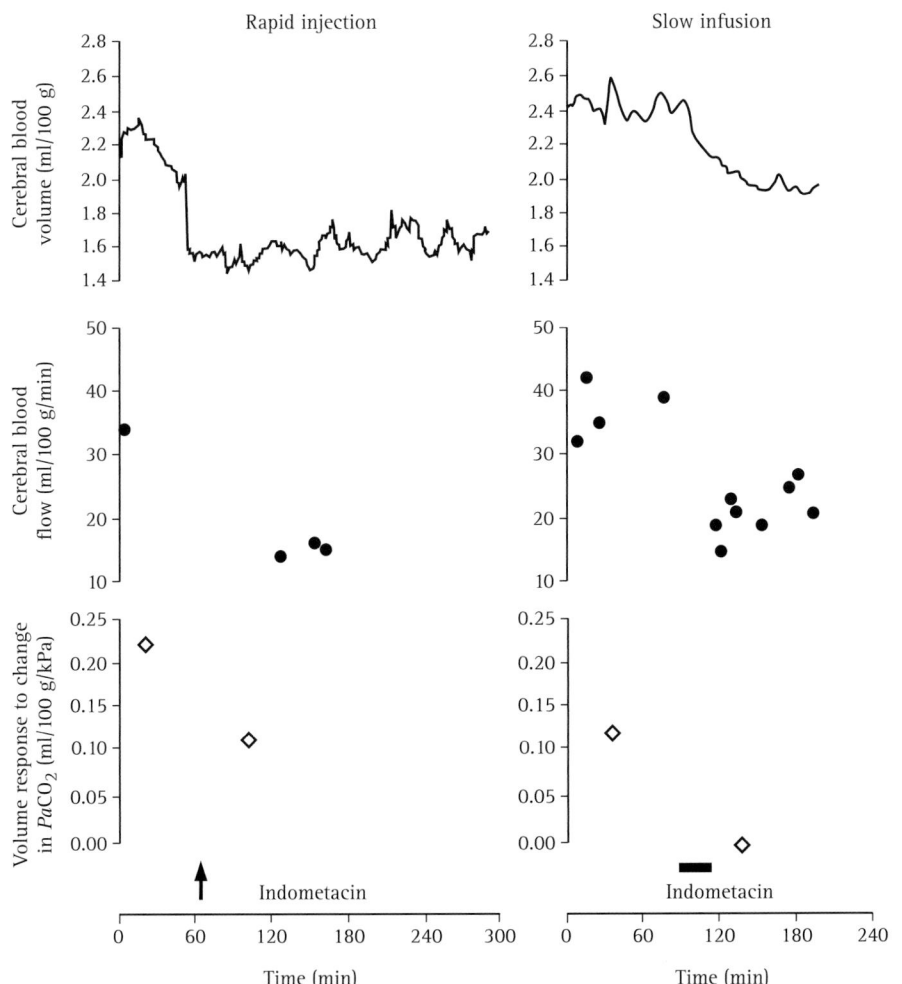

Figure 11.17 The effect of indometacin on cerebral hemodynamics as monitored and quantified by near-infrared spectrophotometry in two preterm infants treated for persistence of the arterial duct. (Reproduced with permission from Edwards et al 1990.)

MEASUREMENT OF CBF AND CMR IN CLINICAL PRACTICE

At present there is little place for measuring CBF in clinical neonatology. Low CBF or cerebral oxygen delivery carried a risk of later death, cerebral atrophy or neurodevelopmental deficit (Krageloh-Mann et al 1999, Lou & Skov 1979, Ment et al 1983, Pryds 1994). We do not know, however, with any precision the lower limit of acceptable CBF or cerebral oxygenation and furthermore it is uncertain if intervention to increase CBF can improve the outcome.

It is likely that abnormal CBF reactivity may be a forerunner of cerebral hemorrhage but it has not been demonstrated if hemorrhage may be prevented by identifying such abnormality.

The demonstration of luxury perfusion, vasoparalysis and increased cerebral lactate by ^{1}H-MRS and abnormality in the PCr/P$_i$ ratio by ^{31}P MRS provides supportive evidence of severe asphyxial vascular and neuronal injury, and demonstrating any of these abnormalities in an infant with moderate-to-severe encephalopathy may contribute to the decision to discontinue intensive care. Unfortunately these signs of delayed energy failure develop to be too late to be helpful in the selection of patients for cooling or any other anti-apoptotic therapy. They may be useful for the evaluation of its effectiveness.

MANAGING CBF

The avoidance of brain damage is a principal task for those caring for ill newborn infants. Cerebral oxygen delivery is an important variable that without monitoring methods currently has to be managed in the 'blind'. Second-generation NIRS instruments is able to monitor regional SO$_2$ — which is close to venous oxygen saturation — as pulse oximeters can monitor arterial oxygen saturation. Venous oxygen saturation is a simple measure of oxygen sufficiency. Unfortunately, at present, the precision of the measurement appears insufficient for clinical use in neonatal intensive care.

Future research will hopefully help in refining the above advice. The most directly useful monitoring equipment is a tissue oximeter. Second-generation NIRS instruments provides a measure of rSO$_2$. Unfortunately precision appears insufficient at present for clinical use.

REFERENCES

Aalkjær C, Poston L 1996 Effects of pH on vascular tension. Which are the important mechanisms? J Vasc Res 33:347–359.

Altman D I, Perlman J M, Volpe J J et al 1993 Cerebral oxygen metabolism in newborns. Pediatr 92:99–104.

Ashwal S, Schneider S, Thompson J 1989 Xenon computed tomography measuring blood flow in the determination of brain death in children. Ann Neurol 25:539–546.

Astrup J 1982 Energy-requiring cell functions in the ischaemic brain. J Neurosurg 56:482–497.

Azzopardi D, Wyatt J S, Cady E B et al 1989 Prognosis of newborn infants with hypoxic-ischaemic brain injury assessed by phosphorous magnetic resonance spectroscopy. Pediatr Res 25:445–451.

Bada H S, Hajjar W, Chua C, Sumner D S 1979 Noninvasive diagnosis of neonatal asphyxia and intraventricular hemorrhage by Doppler ultrasound. J Pediatr 95:775–779.

Bartocci M, Winberg J, Papendieck G et al 2001 Cerebral hemodynamic response to unpleasant odors in the preterm newborn measured by near-infrared spectroscopy. Pediatr Res 50:324–330.

Belik J, Wagerle L C, Stanley C A et al 1989 Cerebral metabolic response and mitochondrial activity following insulin–induced hypoglycemia in newborn lambs. Biol Neonate 55:281–289.

Bevan R D, Dodge J, Nichols P et al 1998a Weakness of sympathetic neural control of human pial compared with superficial temporal arteries reflects low innervation density and poor sympathetic responsiveness. Stroke 29:212–221.

Bevan R D, Dodge J, Nichols P et al 1998b Responsiveness of human infant cerebral arteries to sympathetic nerve stimulation and vasoactive agents. Pediatr Res 44:730–739.

Bevan R D, Vijayakumaran E, Gentry A et al 1998c Intrinsic tone of cerebral artery segments of human infants between 23 weeks of gestation and term. Pediatr Res 43:20–27.

Blennow M, Ingvar M, Lagercrantz H et al 1995 Early [^{18}F]FDG positron emission tomography in infants with hypoxic-ischaemic encephalopathy shows hypermetabolism during the postasphyctic period. Acta Paediatr Scand 84:1289–1295.

Børch K, Greisen G 1994 Widespread regional cerebral blood flow disturbances in preterm infants with intracerebral haemorrhages (abstract). Pediatr Res 36:24–24.

Børch K, Greisen G 1997 Regional cerebral blood flow during hypotension and hypoxaemia in preterm infants (abstract). Pediatr Res 42:389–389.

Børch K, Greisen G 1998 Blood flow distribution in the normal human preterm brain. Pediatr Res 43:28–33.

Børch K, Pryds O, Holm S et al 1998 Regional cerebral blood flow during seizures in neonates. J Pediatr 132:431–435.

Born P, Leth H, Miranda MJ et al 1998 Visual activation in infants and young children studied by functional magnetic resonance imaging. Pediatr Res 44:578–583.

Boylan G B, Young K, Panerai R B et al 2000 Dynamic cerebral autoregulation in sick newborn infants. Pediatr Res 48:12–17.

Branston N M, Ladds A, Symon L, Wang A D 1984 Comparison of the effects of ischaemia on early components of somatosensory evoked potentials in brainstem, thalamus, and cerebral cortex. J Cerebr Blood F Met 4:68–81.

Bucher H U, Edwards A D, Lipp A E, Duc G 1993 Comparison between near infrared spectroscopy and ^{133}Xenon clearance for estimation of cerebral blood flow in critically ill preterm infants. Pediatr Res 33:56–60.

Buchvald F F, Keshe K, Greisen G 1999 Measurement of cerebral oxyhaemoglobin saturation and jugular blood flow in term healthy newborn infants by near-infrared spectroscopy and jugular venous occlusion. Biol Neonate 75:97–103.

Cady E B, Costello A M de L, J Dawson M et al 1983 Non-invasive investigation of cerebral metabolism in newborn infants by phosphorous nuclear magnetic resonance spectroscopy. Lancet i:1059–1062.

Calvert S A, Hoskins E M, Fong K W, Forsyth S C 1987 Etiological factors associated with the development of periventricular leucomalacia. Acta Paediatr Scand 76:254–259.

Chiron C, Raynaud C, Maziere B et al 1992 Changes in regional cerebral blood flow during brain maturation in children and adolescents. J Nucl Med 33:696–703.

Chugani H T, Phelps M E, Mazziotta J C 1987 Positron emission tomography study of human brain functional development. Ann Neurol 22:487–497.

Cohan S L, Mun S K, Petite J P et al 1989 Cerebral blood flow in humans following resuscitation from cardiac arrest. Stroke 20:761–765.

Colditz P, Greisen G, Pryds O 1988 Comparison of electrical impedance and ^{133}Xe clearance for the assessment of cerebral blood flow in the newborn infant. Pediatr Res 24:461–464.

Cross K W, Dear P R F, Hathorn M K S et al 1979 An estimation of intracranial blood flow in the newborn infant. J Physiol 289:329–345.

Dear P R F 1980 Effect of feeding on jugular venous blood flow in the normal infant. Arch Dis Child 55:365–370.

Denays R, Ham H, Tondear M et al 1992 Detection of bilateral and symmetrical anomalies in technetium-99 HMPAO brain SPECT studies. J Nuclear Med 33:485–490.

Drayton M R, Skidmore R 1987 Vasoactivity of the major intracranial arteries in newborn infants. Arch Dis Child 62:236–240.

Dullenkopf A, Kolarova A, Schulz G et al. Reproducibility of cerebral oxygenation measurement in neonates and infants in the clinical setting using the NIRO 300 oximeter. Pediatr Crit Care Med 2005; 6:344–347.

Edwards A D, Wyatt J S, Ricardsson C et al 1992 Effects of indomethacin on cerebral haemodynamics in very preterm infants. Lancet i:1491–1495.

Edwards A D, Wyatt J S, Richardson C et al 1988 Cotside measurements of cerebral blood flow in ill newborn infants by near infrared spectroscopy. Lancet ii:770–771.

Ehehalt S, Kehrer M, Goelz R et al 2005 Cerebral blood flow volume measurement with ultrasound: Interobserver reproducibility in preterm and term neonates. Ultrasound Med Biol 31:191–196.

Farachi F M, Heistad D D 1990 Regulation of large cerebral arteries and cerebral microvascular pressure. Circ Res 66:8–17.

Ferrara B, Johnson D E, Chang P-N, Thompsom T R 1984 Efficacy and neurologic outcome of profound hypocapneic alkalosis for the treatment of persistent pulmonary hypertension in infancy. J Pediatr 105:457–461.

Frewen TC, Kissoon N, Kronick J et al 1991 Cerebral blood flow, cross-brain oxygen extraction, and fontanelle pressure after hypoxic-ischemic injury in newborn infants. J Pediatr 118:265–271.

Friis-Hansen B 1985 Perinatal brain injury and cerebral blood flow in newborn infants. Acta Paediatr Scand 74:323–331.

Fumagalli M, Mosca F, Knudsen G M, Greisen G 2004 Transient hyperoxia and residual cerebrovascular effects in the newborn rat. Pediatr Res 55:380–384.

Garfunkel J M, Baird H W, Siegler J 1954 The relationship of oxygen consumption to cerebral functional activity. J Pediatr 44:64–72.

Goplerud J M, Wagerle L C, Delivoria-Papadopoulos M 1991 Sympathetic nerve modulation of regional cerebral blood flow during asphyxia in newborn piglets. Am J Physiol 260:H1575–H1580.

Graziani L J, Spitzer A R, Mitchell D G et al 1992 Mechanical ventilation in preterm infants: Neurosonographic and developmental studies. Pediatr 90:515–522.

Greisen G 1986 Cerebral blood flow in preterm infants during the first week of life. Acta Paediatr Scand 75:43–51.

Greisen G, Hellstrom-Westas L, Lou H et al 1985 Sleep–waking shifts and cerebral blood flow in stable preterm infants. Pediatr Res 19:1156–1159.

Greisen G, Johansen K, Ellison P H et al 1984 Cerebral blood flow in the newborn infant: Comparison of Doppler ultrasound and 133-Xenon clearance. J Pediatr 104:411–418.

Greisen G, Munck Hm, Lou H 1987 Severe hypocarbia in preterm infants and neurodevelopmental deficit. Acta Pædiatr Scand 76:401–404.

Greisen G, Pryds O 1988 Intravenous ^{133}Xe clearance in preterm neonates with respiratory distress. Internal validation of CBF-infinity as a measure of global cerebral blood flow. Scand J Clin Lab Inv 48:673–678.

Greisen G, Pryds O 1989 Low CBF, discontinuous EEG activity, and periventricular brain injury in ill, preterm neonates. Brain Dev 11:164–168.

Greisen G, Trojaborg W 1987 Cerebral blood flow, PaCO2 changes, and visual evoked potentials in mechanically ventilated, preterm infants. Acta Paediatr Scand 76:394–400.

Groenendaal F, Veenhoven R H, van der Grond J et al 1994 Cerebral lactate and N-acetyl-aspartate/choline ratios in asphyxiated full-term neonates demonstrated in vivo using proton magnetic resonance spectroscopy. Pediatr Res 35:148–151.

Hanrahan J D, Cox I J, Edwards A D et al 1998 Persistent increases in cerebral lactate concentration after birth asphyxia. Pediatr Res 44:304–311.

Hanrahan J D, Sargentoni J, Azzopardi D et al 1996 Cerebral metabolism within 18 hours of birth asphyxia: a proton magnetic resonance spectroscopy study. Pediatr Res 39:584–590.

Hayashi S, Park M K, Kuelh T J 1984 Higher sensitivity of cerebral arteries isolated from premature and newborn baboons to adrenergic and cholinergic stimulation. Life Sci 35:253–260.

Hernandes M J, Brennan R W, Bowman G S 1980 Autoregulation of cerebral blood flow in the newborn dog. Brain Res 184:199–201.

Hernandez M J, Hawkins R A, Brennan R W 1982 Sympathetic control of regional cerebral blood flow in the asphyxiated newborn dog. In: Heistad D D, Marcus M L (eds) Cerebral blood flow, effects of nerves and neurotransmitters. Elsevier, New York, pp. 359–366.

Hope P L, Costello A M, Cady E B et al 1984 Cerebral energy metabolism studied with phosphorous NMR spectroscopy in normal and birth-asphyxiated infants. Lancet ii:366–370.

Hope PL, Cady E B, Chu A et al 1987 Brain metabolism and intracellular pH during ischaemia and hypoxia: An in vivo ^{31}P and ^{1}H nuclear magnetic resonance study in the lamb. J Neurochem 49:75–82.

Huttenlocher P R, de Courten C, Garey L J, van der Loos H 1982 Synaptogenesis in the human visual cortex — evidence for synapse elimination during normal delopment. Neurosci Lett 33:247–254.

Iadecola C, Zhang F 1996 Permissive and obligatory roles of NO in cerebrovascular responses to hypercapnia and acethylcholine. Am J Physiol 271: R990–R1001.

Ijichi S, Kusaka T, Isobe K et al 2005 Quantification of cerebral hemoglobin as a function of oxygenation using near-infrared time-resolved spectroscopy in a piglet model of hypoxia. J Biomed Optics 10:024–026.

Jayasinghe D, Gill B, Levene M I 2003 CBF reactivity in hypotensive and normotensive preterm infants. Pediatr Res 54:848–853.

Jones T H, Morawetz R B, Crowell R M et al 1981 Thresholds of focal cerebral ischaemia in awake monkeys. J Neurosurg 54:773–782.

Kehrer M, Blumenstock G, Ehehalt S et al 2005 Development of cerebral blood volume in preterm neonates during the first two weeks of life. Pediatr Res 58:927–930.

Kehrer M, Krageloh-Mann I, Goelz R, Schoning M 2003 The development of cerebral perfusion in healthy preterm and term neonates. Neuropediatrics 34:281–286.

Kennedy C, Sokoloff L 1957 An adaptation of the nitrous oxide method to the study of the cerebral circulation in children: normal values for cerebral blood flow and cerebral metabolic rate in childhood. J Clin Invest 36:1130–1137.

Kissack C M, Garr R, Wardle S, Weindling A M 2004 Cerebral fractional oxygen extraction in very low birth weight infants is high when there is low left ventricular output and hypocarbia but is unaffected by hypotension. Pediatr Res 55:400–405.

Kissack C M, Garr R, Wardle S, Weindling A M 2005 Cerebral fractional oxygen extraction is inversely correlated with oxygen delivery in the sick newborn preterm infant. J Cerebr Blood F Met 25:545–553.

Kluckow M, Evans N 2000a Superior vena cava flow in newborn infants: a novel marker of systemic blood flow. Arch Dis Child Fetal 82:F182–F187.

Kluckow M, Evans N 2000b Low superior vena cava flow and intraventricular haemorrhage in preterm infants. Arch Dis Child Fetal 82:188–194.

Krageloh-Mann I, Toft P, Lunding J et al 1999 Brain lesions in preterms: origin, consequences and compensation. Acta Paediatr 88:897–908.

Kraus H, Schlenker S, Schwedesky D 1974 Developmental changes of cerebral ketone body utilisation in human infants. Z Physiol Chemie 355:164–170.

Kurth C D, Wagerle L C, Delivoria-Papadopoulos M 1988 Sympathetic regulation of cerebral blood flow during seizures in newborn lambs. Am J Physiol 255: H563–H568.

Kuschinsky W, Paulson O B 1992 Capillary circulation in the brain. Cerebrovasc Brain Metab Rev 4:261–286.

Lassen N 1966 The luxury-perfusion syndrome and its possible relation to acute metabolic acidosis localised within the brain. Lancet ii:1113–1115.

Leahy F A N, Cates D, MacCallum M, Rigatto H 1980 Effect of CO2 and 100% O2 on cerebral blood flow in preterm infants. J Appl Physiol 48:468–472.

Leth H, Toft P B, Peitersen B et al 1996 Use of brain lactate levels to predict outcome after perinatal asphyxia. Acta Paediatr 85:859–864.

Licht D J, Wang J, Silvestre D W et al 2004 Preoperative cerebral blood flow is diminished in neonates with severe congenital heart defects. J Thorac Cardiov Sur 128:841–849.

Lindauer U, Vogt J, Schuh-Hofer S et al 2003 Cerebrovascular vasodilation to extraluminal acidosis occurs via combined activation of ATP-sensitive and Ca[2+]-activated potassium channels. J Cerebr Blood F Met 23:1227–1238.

Lou H C, Henriksen L, Bruhn P 1984 Focal cerebral hypoperfusion in children with dysphasia and/or attention deficit disorder. Arch Neurol 41:825–829.

Lou H C, Lassen N A, Friis-Hansen B 1977 Low cerebral blood flow in hypotensive perinatal distress. Acta Neurol Scand 56:343–352.

Lou H C, Skov H 1979 Low cerebral blood flow: a risk factor in the neonate. J Pediatr 95:606–609.

Lundstrøm K E, Pryds O, Greisen G 2000 The haemodynamic effect of dopamine and volume expansion in sick preterm infants. Early Hum Dev 57:157–163.

Lundstrøm K, Pryds O, Greisen G 1995 Oxygen at birth and prolonged cerebral vasoconstriction in preterm infants. Arch Dis Child 73:F81–F86.

Malcus P, Kjellmer I, Lingman G et al 1991 Diameters of the common carotid artery and aorta change in different directions during acute asphyxia in the fetal lamb. J Perinat Med 19:259–267.

Martin E, Buchli R, Ritter S et al 1996 Diagnostic and prognostic value of cerebral ^{31}P magnetic resonance spectroscopy on neonates with perinatal asphyxia. Pediatr Res 40:749–758.

Martin E, Joeri P, Loenneker T et al 1999 Visual processing in infants and children studied using functional MRI. Pediatr Res 46:135–140.

Meek J H, Elwell C E, McCormick D C et al 1999a Abnormal cerebral haemodynamics in perinatally asphyxiated neonates related to outcome. Arch Dis Child 81:F110–F115.

Meek J H, Firbank M, Elwell C E et al 1998 Regional hemodynamic responses to visual stimulation in awake infants. Pediatr Res 43:840–843.

Meek J H, Tyszczuk L, Elwell C E, Wyatt J S 1999b Low cerebral blood flow is a risk factor for severe intraventricular haemorrhage. Arch Dis Child 81: F15–F18.

Menke J, Michel E, Hillebrand S et al G 1997 Cross-spectral analysis of cerebral autoregulation dynamics in high risk preterm infants during the perinatal period. Pediatr Res 42:690–699.

Ment R L, Scott D T, Lange R C et al 1983 Postpartum perfusion of the preterm brain: relationship to neurodevelopmental outcome. Child Brain 10:266–272.

Meyer J S, Isihara N, Deshmukh V D et al 1978 Improved method for measurement of regional cerebral blood flow by [133]-xenon inhalation. I. Description of method and normal values obtained in healthy volunteers. Stroke 9:195–205.

Milligan D W A 1979 Cerebral blood flow and sleep state in the normal newborn infant. Early Hum Dev 3:321–328.

Milligan D W A 1980 Failure of autoregulation and intraventricular haemorrhage in preterm infants. Lancet i:896–899.

Miranda M J, Olofsson K, Sidaros K 2006 Noninvasive measurements of regional cerebral perfusion in preterm and term neonates by magnetic resonance arterial spin labelling. Pediatr Res 60:359–363.

Mosca F, Bray M, Lattanzio M et al 1997 Comparative evaluation of the effects of indomethacin and ibuprofen on cerebral perfusion and oxygenation in preterm infants with patent ductus arteriosus. J Pediatr 131:549–554.

Mukhtar A I, Cowan F M, Stothers J K 1982 Cranial blood flow and blood pressure changes during sleep in the human neonate. Early Hum Dev 6:59–64.

Munro M J, Walker A M, Barfield C P 2004 Hypotensive extremely low birth weight infants have reduced cerebral blood flow. Pediatr 114:1591–1596.

Nagdyman N, Fleck T, Schubert S et al 2005 Comparison between cerebral tissue oxygenation index measured by near-infrared spectroscopy and venous jugular bulb saturation in children. Intens Care Med 31:846–850.

Obrist WD. Langfitt TW, Jaggi JL et al 1984 Cerebral blood flow and metabolism in comatose patients with acute head injury. J Neurosurg 61:241–253.

Papile L A, Rudolp A M, Heyman M A 1985 Autoregulation of cerebral blood flow in the preterm fetal lamb. Pediatr Res 19:59–161.

Pasternak J F, Groothuis D R 1985 Autoregulation of cerebral blood flow in the newborn beagle puppy. Biol Neonate 48:100–109.

Patel J, Marks K, Roberts I et al 1998 Measurement of cerebral blood flow in newborn infants using near infrared spectroscopy with indocyanine green. Pediatr Res 43:34–39.

Patel J, Roberts I, Azzopardi D et al 2000 Randomized double-blind controlled trial comparing the effects of ibuprufen with indomethacin on cerebral hemodynamics in preterm infants with patent ductus arteriosus. Pediatr Res 47:36–42.

Pearce W J, Harder D R 1996 Cerebrovascular smooth muscle and endothelium. In: Mraovitch S, Sercombe R (eds) Neurophysiological basis of cerebral blood flow control: An introduction. John Libbey, London, pp. 153–158.

Peden C J, Cowan F M, Bryant D J et al 1990 Proton MR spectroscopy of the brain in infants. J Comput Assist Tomogr 14:886–894.

Pellicer A, Valverde E, Elorza M D et al 2005 Cardiovascular support for low birth weight infants and cerebral hemodynamics: a randomized, blinded, clinical trial. Pediatr 115:1501–1512.

Pellicer A, Valverde E, Gaya F et al 2001 Postnatal adaptation of brain circulation in preterm infants. Pediatr Neurol 24:103–109.

Perlman J M, Herscovitch P, Kreusser K et al 1985 Positron emission tomography in the newborn: effect of seizure on regional cerebral blood flow in an asphyxiated infant. Neurol 35:244–247.

Powers W J, Raichle M E 1985 Positron emission tomography and its application to the study of cerebrovascular disease in man. Stroke 16:361–376.

Pryds A, Pryds O, Greisen G 2005 Cerebral presure autoregulation and vasoreactivity in the newborn rat. Pediatr Res 57:294–298.

Pryds O 1994 Low neonatal cerebral oxygen delivery is associated with brain injury in preterm infants. Acta Paediatr 83:1233–1236.

Pryds O, Andersen G E, Friis-Hansen B 1990a Cerebral blood flow reactivity in spontaneously breathing, preterm infants shortly after birth. Acta Pædiatr Scand 79:391–396.

Pryds O, Greisen G 1990 Preservation of single flash visual evoked potentials at very low cerebral oxygen delivery in sick, newborn, preterm infants. Pediatr Neurol 6:151–158.

Pryds O, Greisen G, Friis-Hansen B 1988b Compensatory increase of CBF in preterm infants during hypoglycaemia. Acta Paediatr Scand 77:632–637.

Pryds O, Greisen G, Johansen K 1988a Indomethacin and cerebral blood flow in preterm infants treated for patent ductus arteriosus. Eur J Pediatr 147:315–316.

Pryds O, Greisen G, Lou H, Friis-Hansen B 1989 Heterogeneity of cerebral vasoreactivity in preterm infants supported by mechanical ventilation. J Pediatr 115:638–645.

Pryds O, Greisen G, Lou H, Friis-Hansen B 1990b Vasoparalysis is associated with brain damage in asphyxiated term infants. J Pediatr 117:119–125.

Pryds O, Schneider S 1991 Aminophylline induces cerebral vasoconstriction in stable, preterm infants without affecting the visual evoked potential. Eur J Pediatr 150:366–369.

Rahilly P M 1980a Effects of sleep state and feeding on cranial blood flow of the human neonate. Arch Dis Child 55:265–270.

Rahilly P M 1980b Effects of 2% carbon dioxide, 0.5% carbon dioxide and 100% oxygen on cranial blood flow of the human neonate. Pediatr 66:685–689.

Rama G P, Parfenova H, Leffler C W 1996 Protein kinase Cs and tyrosine kinases in permissive action of prostacyclin on cerebrovascular regulation in newborn pigs. Pediatr Res 41:83–89.

Reuter J H, Disney T A 1986 Regional cerebral blood flow and cerebral metabolic rate of oxygen during hyperventilation in the newborn dog. Pediatr Res 20:1102–1106.

Robertson N J, Cox I J, Cowan F M et al 1999 Cerebral intracellular lactic alkalosis persisting months after neonatal encephalopathy measured by magnetic resonance spectroscopy. Pediatr Res 46:287–296.

Rubinstein M, Denays R, Ham HR et al 1989 Functional imaging of brain maturation in humans using iodine [123]iodoamphetamine and SPECT. J Nuclear Med 30:1982–1985.

Seri I, Abbasi S, Wood D C, Gerdes J S 1998 Regional hemodynamic effects of dopamine in the sick preterm neonate. J Pediatr 133:728–734.

Sharples P M, Stuart A G, Aynsley-Green A et al 1991 A practical method of serial bedside measurement of cerebral blood flow and metabolism during neurointensive care. Arch Dis Child 66:1326–1332.

Sinha A K, Cane C, Kempley S T 2006 Blood flow in the common carotid artery in term and preterm infants: reproducibility and relation to cardiac output. Arch Dis Child 91:31–35.

Skov L, Pryds O 1992 Capillary recruitment for preservation of cerebral glucose influx in hypoglycemic, preterm newborns: Evidence for a glucose sensor? Pediatr 90:193–195.

Skov L, Pryds O, Greisen G 1991 Estimating cerebral blood flow in newborn infants: Comparison of near infrared spectroscopy and ^{133}Xe clerance. Pediatr Res 30:570–573.

Skov L, Pryds O, Greisen G, Lou H 1993 Cerebral mixed venous oxygen saturation and cerebral blood flow. Pediatr Res 32:52–55.

Soerensen LC, Greisen G 2007 Precision of measurement of cerebral tissue oxygenation index using near-infrared spectroscopy in preterm neonates. J Biomed Opt 11(5):054005.

Suhonen-Polvi H, Kero P, Korvenrante H et al 1993 Repeated flouroeoxyglucose positron emission tomography of the brain in infants with suspected hypoxic-ischaemic brain injury. Eur J Nucl Med 29:759–765.

Suzuki S, Takasaki S, Ozaki T, Kobayashi Y 1999 A tissue oxygenation monitor using NIR spatially resolved spectroscopy. SPIE 3597:582–592.

Tanner SF, Cornette L, Ramenghi L A et al 2003 Cerebral perfusion in infants and neonates: preliminary results obtained using dynamic susceptibility contrast enhanced magnetic resonance imaging. Arch Dis Child 88:525–530.

Thorngren-Jerneck K, Ohlsson T, Sandell A et al 1999 Cerebral glucose metabolism measured by positron emission tomography in term newborn infants with hypoxic-ischaemic encephalopathy (abstract). Pediatr Res 45:905–905.

Toft P, Christiansen P, Pryds O et al 1994 T1, T2 and concentrations of brain metabolites in neonates and adolescents estimated with H-1 MR spectroscopy. J Magn Reson Im 4:1–5.

Tsuji M, Saul P, du Plessis A J et al 2000 Cerebral intravascular oxygenation correlates with mean arterial pressure in critically ill premature infants. Pediatr 106:625–632.

Tweed W A, Cote J, Lou H et al 1986 Impairment of cerebral blood flow autoregulation in the newborn lamb by hypoxia. Pediatr Res 20:516–519.

Tweed W A, Cote J, Pash M, Lou H 1983 Arterial oxygenation determines autoregulation of cerebral blood flow in the fetal lamb. Pediatr Res 17:246–249.

Tyszczuk L, Meek J, Elwell C E, Wyatt J S 1998 Cerebral blood flow is independent of mean arterial blood pressure in preterm infants undergoing intensive care. Pediatr 102:337–341.

Victor S, Appleton R E, Beirne M et al 2005 Effect of carbon dioxide on background cerebral electrical activity and fractional oxygen extraction in very low birth weight infants just after birth. Pediatr Res 58:579–585.

Victor S, Marson A G, Appleton R E et al 2006 Relationship between blood pressure, cerebral electrical activity, cerebral fractional oxygen extraction, and peripheral blood flow in very low birth weight newborn infants. Pediatr Res 59:314–319.

Volpe J J, Herscovitch P, Perlman J M et al 1985 Positron emission tomography in the asphyxiated term newborn: parasagittal impairment of cerebral blood flow. Ann Neurol 17:287–296.

Volpe J J, Herscovitch P, Perlman J M, Raichle M E 1983 Positron emission tomography in the newborn. Extensive impairment of regional cerebral blood flow with intraventricular hemorrhage and hemorrhagic cerebral involvement. Pediatr 72:589–601.

Wagerle L C, Kumar S P, Delivoria-Papadopoulos M 1986 Effect of sympathetic nerve stimulation on cerebral blood flow in newborn piglets. Pediatr Res 20:131–135.

Wagerle L C, Mishra O P 1988 Mechanism of CO_2 response in cerebral arteries of the newborn pig: role of phospholipase, cyclooxygenase, and lipooxygenase pathways. Circ Res 62:1019–1026.

Wagerle L C, Moliken W, Russo P 1995 Nitric oxide and alpha-adrenargic mechanisms modify contractile responses to norepinephrine in ovine fetal and newborn cerebral arteries. Pediatr Res 38:237–242.

Wang J, Licht D J, Jahng G H et al 2003 Pediatric perfusion imaging using arterial spin labelling. J Magn Reson Im 18:404–413.

Wang Q, Pelligrino D A, Baughman V L et al 1995 The role of neuronal nitric oxide synthetase in regulation of cerebral blood flow in normocpania and hypercapnia in rats. J Cerebr Blood F Met 15:774–778.

Wyatt J S, Cope M, Delpy D T et al 1990a Measurement of optical pathlength for cerebral near-infrared spectrocopy in newborn infants. Dev Neurosci 12:140–144.

Wyatt J S, Cope M, Delpy D T et al 1990b Quantitation of cerebral blood volume in human infants by near-infrared spectroscopy. J Appl Physiol 68:1086–1091.

Wyatt J S, Delpy D T, Cope M et al 1986 Quantifications of cerebral oxygenation and haemodynamics in sick newborn infants by near infrared spectrophotometry. Lancet ii:1063–1066.

Younkin D P, Delivoria-Papadopoulos M, Maris J et al 1986 Cerebral metabolic effects of neonatal seizures measured with in-vivo ^{31}P NMR spectroscopy. Ann Neurol 21:513–519.

Younkin D P, Reivich M, Jaggi J et al 1982 Noninvasive method of estimating newborn regional cerebral blood flow. J Cereb Blood F Met 2:415–420.

Younkin D P, Reivich M, Jaggi J L et al 1987 The effect of haematocrit and systolic blood pressure on cerebral blood flow in newborn infants. J Cereb Blood F Met 7:295–299.

Yoxall C W, Weindling A M 1998 Measurement of cerebral oxygen consumption in the human neonate using near infrared spectroscopy: cerebral oxygen consumption increases with advancing gestational age. Pediatr Res 44:283–290.

Yoxall C W, Weindling A M, Dawani N H, Peart I 1995 Measurement of cerebral venous oxyhemoglobin saturation in children by near-infrared spectroscopy and partial jugular venous occlusion. Pediatr Res 38:319–323.

Zhang J, Penny D J, Kim N S et al 1999 Mechanisms of blood pressure increase induced by dopamine in hypotensive preterm neonates. Arch Dis Child 81: F99–F104.

Zhao J, Ding H S, Hou X L et al 2005 In vivo determination of the optical properties of infant brain using frequency-domain near-infrared spectroscopy. J Biomed Op 10:024–028.

CHAPTER

12

EEG and evoked potentials in the neonatal period

Lena Hellström-Westas and Linda S. de Vries

Key Points

- EEG is a highly sensitive indicator of brain function in newborn infants of all gestational ages
- Continuous EEG-monitoring is very useful for observing changes in brain function, such as recovery after perinatal asphyxia, diagnosis of subclinical seizures and evaluation of antiepileptic treatment
- Consistently abnormal SEP is the best predictor of poor neurologic outcome in term asphyxiated infants
- BAEP assessment at term is of clinical value in the diagnosis of hearing impairment, but has only limited positive predictive value for neurologic impairment
- Flash VEP is a good predictor of cerebral visual impairment following perinatal brain injury in term infants

INTRODUCTION

An increasing number of very preterm infants surviving the neonatal period is causing a rise in the prevalence of long-term disabilities (Fanaroff et al 2007, Himmelmann et al 2005), in spite of concurrent scientific and technological advances in perinatal care. The incidence of infants suffering from hypoxic–ischemic encephalopathy (HIE) is relatively stable, but the sequelae may be far-reaching. Therefore, it is essential to identify those infants who have sustained damage to the immature nervous system at an early stage to reduce the severity of neurologic injury as well as to instigate remedial action. For this purpose, attempts have been made to improve early prediction of neurodevelopmental outcome in at-risk infants. An objective source of evidence to see whether an infant's central nervous system (CNS) function is normal is the electroencephalogram (EEG) and evoked potentials (EPs). This chapter reviews the methodology, the maturational changes and the clinical applications for neonatal '(a)EEG' and EPs.

Hans Berger recorded the first EEG in the early 1920s. Since then thousands of studies have explored the features and dynamics of the EEG in relation to physiological states, illnesses, as well as mental and emotional processes. Initially, Berger did not believe that newborns had EEG activity. Still, and beginning in the 1950s, the EEG features of newborn infants were extensively explored especially by French investigators (Lamblin et al 1999, Monod et al 1972). The tradition of investigating and recording sequential EEGs in sick or preterm newborn infants is still very strong in France.

The EEG reflects the functional state of the brain, and can therefore be used for detection of functional abnormalities including epileptic seizure activity and for prediction of outcome. Interpretation of the neonatal EEG is an elaborate procedure and requires experience and special training. It is outside the scope of this chapter to go into details about the EEG, for this we refer to reviews or atlases of clinical neurophysiology (Lamblin et al 1999, Mizrahi et al 2004). This chapter will focus on the neonatal EEG from a neonatologists' perspective and how the EEG can be practically used in the Neonatal Intensive Care Unit (NICU) to obtain information and guide medical decisions.

EPs are averaged electrical responses to a repetitive sensory stimulus that can be either auditory, visual or sensory. EPs are providing information on both peripheral and central aspects of the sensory pathways within the CNS. The responses are recorded from the EEG, where they can be identified by their consistent temporal relationship to the stimulus event. The EEG is of higher amplitude than the EP, but it is random to the applied stimulus, whereas the EP is of small amplitude but constant relative to the stimulus. Averaging a number of responses will cause the EP to emerge from the EEG. Age-appropriate norms have to be established, as latencies of the different components of the response decrease rapidly with age in the neonatal period. Changes in latency or amplitude of the EP waveform may indicate involvement of the sensory pathway. EPs have been shown to be of great value when trying to predict neurodevelopmental outcome during the neonatal period, especially in the full-term infants, along with clinical, EEG and neuroimaging data.

METHODOLOGY AND MATURATION OF THE EEG

A standard EEG is usually derived from 9–15 electrodes applied to the scalp according to the international 10–20 system (Fig. 12.1) (Jasper 1958). The relative position of the electrodes is the 10–20% distance between four landmarks on the head (nasion-inion, and the coronal distance between the ears) and the head circumference. By applying electrodes according to the 10–20 system, it is possible to correlate electrocortical activity with anatomical landmarks, and to compare recordings from different occasions which are important especially in the neonate when the head grows. The most commonly used electrode positions include F1, F2, C3, C4, Cz, T3, T4, O1 and O2. A capital letter denotes the position, e.g. F for frontal, C for central, T for temporal, O for occipital, followed by a number with even numbers indicating the right side and odd numbers the left side. The

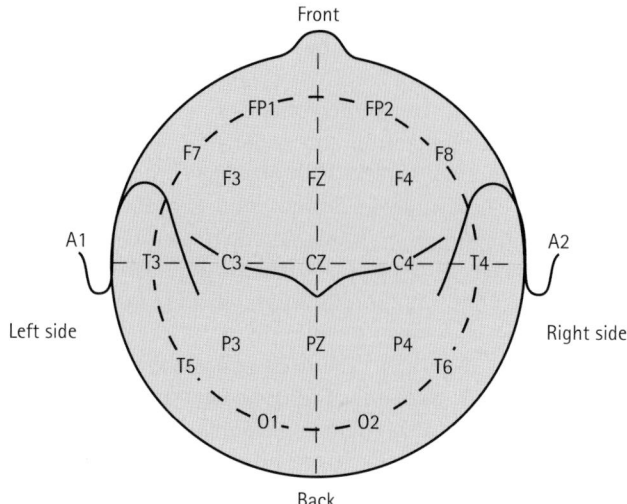

Figure 12.1 Electrode positions according to the International 10–20 system (Jasper 1958).

EEG is usually recorded with bipolar montage and shown as 'chains' of derivations over the scalp, e.g. frontal to occipital through temporal and central leads, respectively, and usually with a central coronal chain. Various types of electrodes can be used depending on the indication and the clinical setting; silver-silver chloride disc electrodes are usually used for recording EEG in the conscious patient while very thin subcutaneous needle electrodes can be used in the intensive-care setting since they are quick and easy to apply for the neonatal staff. In the extremely preterm infant, long-term EEG-monitoring has successfully been obtained through adhesive electrodes with hydrogel. Such electrodes can also be used in term infants, but the application needs training in order to get low electrode impedance and good-quality recordings. During clinical EEG-monitoring fewer electrodes are often used, although newer electrode caps also allow multiple electrode recordings with 64, 128 or more electrodes (Fifer 2006).

Initially the analog EEG was recorded on paper, often with a paper speed of 7.5, 15 or 30 mm/s and with a fixed scale, usually 70 or 100 µvolt/cm. Now digital EEG systems are increasingly being used, allowing greater flexibility. The digitally recorded EEG makes it possible to perform various ad hoc measurements of the signal, including fast Fourier transformation (FFT) and power spectral analysis. The EEG activity is categorized into four main frequency bands: delta (0.5–4 Hz), theta (4–8 Hz), alpha (8–13 Hz) and beta (13–30 Hz). It is not uncommon that artifacts from eye blinking, respiration, technical equipment including high-frequency oscillation ventilation, electrocardiogram (ECG) and muscle activity appear in the EEG recording. Such artifacts can sometimes also mimic pathologic conditions for the less experienced interpreter. Eye movements, ECG and respiration are usually recorded together with the EEG in order to facilitate the interpretation. It is common to use high-pass filters at 0.3–0.5 Hz (activity with frequencies above 0.3–0.5 Hz are selected and displayed) and low-pass filters at 70 Hz. More recently, a method called full-band EEG (FbEEG) has been developed to enable recording of all frequencies simultaneously (Vanhatalo et al 2005).

EEG DEVELOPMENT

The EEG can be recorded in newborn infants at all maturational levels, also in the extremely preterm infants (Hayakawa et al 2001). The development and normal EEG maturation in moderately preterm and term infants are well known and have been described in detail (Lamblin et al 1999, Lombroso 1985, Mizrahi et al 2004, Tharp et al 1989, Torres & Anderson 1985). However, the current knowledge about the normal EEG of the extremely low gestational age infant is more limited since only a few studies have included long-term follow-up (Vecchierini et al 2003).

The understanding and correct interpretation of neonatal EEG are based on maturational time cues that appear in the EEG. Consequently, when discussing features of the newborn EEG several terms have been used to define the maturity of the infant. Some terms that are common in the EEG literature are postconceptional/conceptional age (PCA) and postmenstrual age (PMA) which are summaries of the gestational age at which the infant was born and the postnatal age. There is a long-standing discussion whether extrauterine life and postnatal age affect EEG maturity, and whether EEGs from infants with similar PMA but different gestational ages and postnatal ages are fully comparable. This is, of course, difficult to sort out in very preterm infants in whom postnatal morbidity may significantly affect EEG maturation, although two recent studies using amplitude-integrated EEG (aEEG) indicate that postnatal age affects the maturation of the electrocortical background in preterm infants (Klebermass et al 2006, Sisman et al 2005). A few studies in preterm infants indicate that the amount of EEG activity increases during the first days of life (Greisen et al 1987, Victor et al 2005a, West et al 2006a). Whether this increase is due to initial depression and recovery related to birth, or to maturational processes is not known.

The normal EEG background in newborn infants can be described as mainly continuous or discontinuous. Discontinuous EEG activity contains periods with lower amplitudes mixed with bursts of higher voltage activity. The normal EEG background of the very preterm infant is mainly discontinuous, and is often called *tracé discontinu*. With increasing maturation the periods with low voltage activity, called interburst intervals (IBI), become shorter and the duration of the bursts increases in parallel with a decrease in burst amplitude so that the overall background becomes continuous in the awake state (Lombroso 1985). This development occurs also in the most immature infants, as shown by Hayakawa et al (2001) in a study including 16 infants with postconceptional ages 21 to 26 weeks. Vecchierini et al (2003) recorded 10 infants at 24 to 26 gestational weeks during the first days of life; nine of the infants had a normal outcome at 3 years of age. The EEGs were discontinuous and dominated by synchronous bursts of high-voltage delta activity (amplitudes >50 µV) which could last for periods up to 83 seconds. Maximum IBIs (amplitude <15 µV) did not exceed 1 minute. Crude sleep-state organization was present at 25 gestational weeks. In 17 slightly more mature infants, with conceptional ages 26–28 weeks, the EEG background was also mainly discontinuous and synchronous bursts of activity (amplitudes $\geqslant$ 30 µV) appeared with up to 3 minutes duration; no infant had IBIs exceeding 46 seconds (Selton et al 2000). There was an occipital predominance of activity, which was dominated by delta activity with superimposed theta, alpha and beta activity. Sleep-state differentiation could be seen at 26 weeks conceptional age.

The continuous EEG background can be of normal voltage (CNV) or low voltage (CLV). The CLV pattern, which denotes an undifferentiated very low amplitude EEG, is clearly abnormal and associated with poor neurological outcome in asphyxiated term infants. The discontinuous background of the preterm infant (*tracé discontinu*) and the *tracé alternant* pattern during quiet sleep in term infants are normal discontinuous background patterns. Burst-suppression (BS) is another discontinuous background pattern with more pronounced suppression during the IBIs, which are of very low voltage or entirely flat. This pattern is clearly abnormal and can be seen in association with brain injury or deep sedation. A major feature of the BS is that it is unreactive, i.e. it does not change between vigilance states, and it is also synchronous, which is not always the case with tracé discontinu. The IBI duration can be measured in both tracé discontinu and BS; in preterm infants it can be prolonged due to a response to brain injury or sedation. Table 12.1 shows average and maximum IBIs at different postmenstrual ages. The slightly modified data were obtained from several studies with varying definitions of IBIs, mainly regarding the amplitudes (Biagioni et al 2007, Connell et al 1987a, Hahn et al 1989, Hayakawa et al 2001, Selton et al 2000,

Vecchierini et al 2003). Electrocerebral silence (inactive or isoelectric EEG), represents the most abnormal EEG tracing and usually indicates a recording where no convincing electrocortical activity can be recorded.

Sleep-state organization can usually be identified in the EEG at around 28–30 weeks PCA although crude sleep–wake cycling can sometimes be found even earlier, from 25–26 weeks PCA (Selton et al 2000, Vecchierini et al 2003). With spectral analysis of the EEG, or when using a trend measure of the EEG called amplitude-integrated EEG (aEEG), sleep–wake cycling can also be identified in recordings from infants at 25–26 weeks PCA (Hellström-Westas et al 1991, Kuhle et al 2001, Scher et al 2005). Accurate evaluation of sleep–wake states also includes observation of eye movements, respiration, muscle tone and motor activity. The EEG during wakefulness and active sleep (also called rapid eye movement sleep, REM) is very similar and therefore difficult to distinguish without clinical observation of the infant. The EEG during quiet sleep, or non-REM sleep, is more discontinuous. Full-term infants consequently have continuous background when awake and during REM sleep, but during quiet sleep the EEG shows two different types of patterns, high-voltage slow activity and discontinuous EEG (also called *tracé alternant* pattern).

Other maturational aspects of the EEG

Some EEG patterns and waveforms are expected to appear, and also disappear, at specific postmenstrual ages and can be used for maturational evaluation of the EEG. Such activity includes, for example, delta brush patterns, temporal theta bursts and frontal sharp wave transients (Mizrahi et al 2004). Delta brush pattern are complexes with fast activity (alpha-beta) superimposed on delta activity; they are typical for preterm EEG. Some EEG features are normal when appearing at a certain maturational level but abnormal when present later. Temporal theta bursts ('temporal saw-tooth') are brief, rhythmic, 4–6 Hz transients that appear from 26 postconceptional weeks and reach a maximum between 30 and 32 weeks before they disappear. They are associated with normal outcome when present at 27 to 30 weeks postmenstrual age, but abnormal if present a few weeks later (Biagioni et al 1994). Temporal sharp waves may appear during the first weeks of life in infants born at 31–32 weeks gestation. However, if abundant, or persisting, they are associated with brain injury (Vecchierini-Blineau et al 1996). Frontal sharp wave transients appear from 34–35 weeks PCA and disappear around 10 weeks later. Although well defined, the underlying corresponding functional and anatomical correlates for most of these activities remain to be shown (Vanhatalo & Kaila 2006). Table 12.2 summarizes the main features of the developing EEG, as seen from a neonatologist's perspective.

FREQUENCY-BASED ANALYSIS OF THE EEG

The standard EEG interpretation is usually based on visual inspection. Power spectral analysis has been used to describe

---

Table 12.1 Mean and maximum interburst intervals (IBI) in healthy preterm and near-term infants

Postmenstrual age, wk	Mean IBI, seconds	Maximum IBI, seconds
21–22	26	
23–24	18	
25–27	12	35–45
28–30	10–12	30–35
31–33	8–10	20
34–36	6–8	10
37–40		6

Data modified from Biagioni et al 2007, Connell et al 1987a, Hahn et al 1989, Hayakawa et al 2001, Selton et al 2000, Vecchierini et al 2003.

Table 12.2 Summary of main features of the developing normal EEG

- A gradual shift in electrocortical background activity from mainly discontinuous to continuous.
- The topographical organization of the developing EEG in an occipital-frontal direction.
- Interhemispheric synchronization of activity at 24–26 weeks PCA is followed by a period of increased desynchronization between 26 and 30 weeks. Above 30 weeks PCA again increasing synchronization, more in the awake state and in active sleep.
- The emergence of sleep–wake state organization from around 25–26 weeks PCA which should become evident by 28–30 weeks PCA.

neonatal EEGs since the 1960s (Parmelee et al 1967), but for several practical reasons (as discussed also by Tolonen et al 2007) it has not yet gained widespread use for clinical interpretation of EEGs in newborns. However, an increasing number of reports indicate that power spectral analysis of the EEG can give additional information on the quality of the electrocortical background in different groups of infants. Although the utility of frequency-based analysis of the EEG for the individual infant has not been shown, it is possible that the quantitative EEG can reveal abnormalities otherwise not identified by the standard EEG, as shown by Mandelbaum et al (2000). Spectral edge frequency (SEF) is a measure that can be obtained from power spectral analysis which is calculated as the frequency below which a certain amount (often 80–95%) of the power in the power spectrum resides.

Developmental aspects of power spectral analysis

Bell et al (1991a) performed power spectral analysis on EEGs from 60 healthy infants with gestational ages 26 to 41 weeks at 3 days of age. They found a significant correlation between gestational age and absolute power within the delta band. In another study, Bell et al (1991b) investigated SEF development in 51 healthy preterm and term neonates and found that the summated SEF from four EEG channels correlated significantly with gestational age, but that the SEF also varied with behavioral state and with EEG derivation. Preterm infants had greater intra- and intervariability in SEF than term infants. Okumura et al (2003, 2006) performed serial EEGs in healthy preterm infants and found that both power within the lowest delta band (0.53–1 Hz) and within the theta band showed significant maturational trends between 29 and 34 postconceptional weeks. Victor et al (2005a) also noted that the power spectra changed during the first days of life in very preterm infants with gestational ages ≤ 30 weeks, and that a relative increase in delta power occurred. Manual measurements of IBIs also showed that these became progressively shorter during the same time

period. Similar to findings achieved with conventional EEG, Tolonen et al (2007) recorded developmental changes in FbEEG of 16 infants at 32.8 to 40 weeks conceptional ages and showed maturational increases in power within the theta-alpha frequency bands (4–9 Hz). Several reports by Scher and collaborators have shown that EEG power spectral measurements of preterm infants recorded at term differ significantly from recordings made in infants born at term, and concluded (some years before this was supported by magnetic resonance imaging studies) that 'these findings suggest a functional alteration of brain development of the preterm infant . . .' (Scher et al 1994a, 1994b, 1997).

Power spectral analysis in brain injury

Bell et al (1990) studied 16 asphyxiated term infants during the first 5 days of life. Total power, and especially delta power, was significantly reduced in infants with poor outcome. Thordstein et al (2004) performed spectral analysis within bursts during quiet sleep in asphyxiated term infants and compared this with control infants. They also found differences in spectral power mainly affecting the lower frequencies. A recent study (Wong et al 2007) did not find any differences in total power between normal infants and infants with HIE or resuscitated infants without HIE. However, the normal infants had greater variability in the total power during the analyzed epochs than the other two groups of infants. One study suggested that abnormal EEG activity in preterm infants with white matter injury can also be detected by a decrease in SEF, which was associated with severe white matter damage (Inder et al 2003).

Infraslow EEG activity

When using standard high-pass filters for EEG recordings the very-low-frequency content of the electrocortical activity is lost (Fig. 12.2) (Vanhatalo & Kaila 2006). In preterm and newly born term infants slow (0.1–0.5 Hz) high-amplitude activity called *spontaneous activity transients* (SAT) can be recorded with FbEEG, during both continuous and discontinuous EEG periods (Tolonen et al 2007, Vanhatalo et al 2002). The SAT events correspond to intermittent periods with delta activity, as recorded by the standard EEG, and thus could be present as early as 24 weeks conceptional age (Vanhatalo & Kaila 2006). Experimental data indicate that cortical events with infraslow EEG activity may be related to development of brain wiring processes (Khazipov & Luhmann 2006, Vanhatalo & Kaila 2006). Also full-term asphyxiated infants have infraslow activity and the amount of this activity may correlate to outcome (Thordstein et al 2005). Gender differences may exist at full term in healthy neonates, which has been speculated to reflect different maturational stages (Thordstein et al 2006). It is notable here that the infraslow activity should not be seen as an activity of its own kind, but it is rather a complementary aspect for demonstrating brain events (such as SATs), which take place at multiple frequencies of brain and hence can be jointly recorded with an FbEEG technique (Vanhatalo et al 2005).

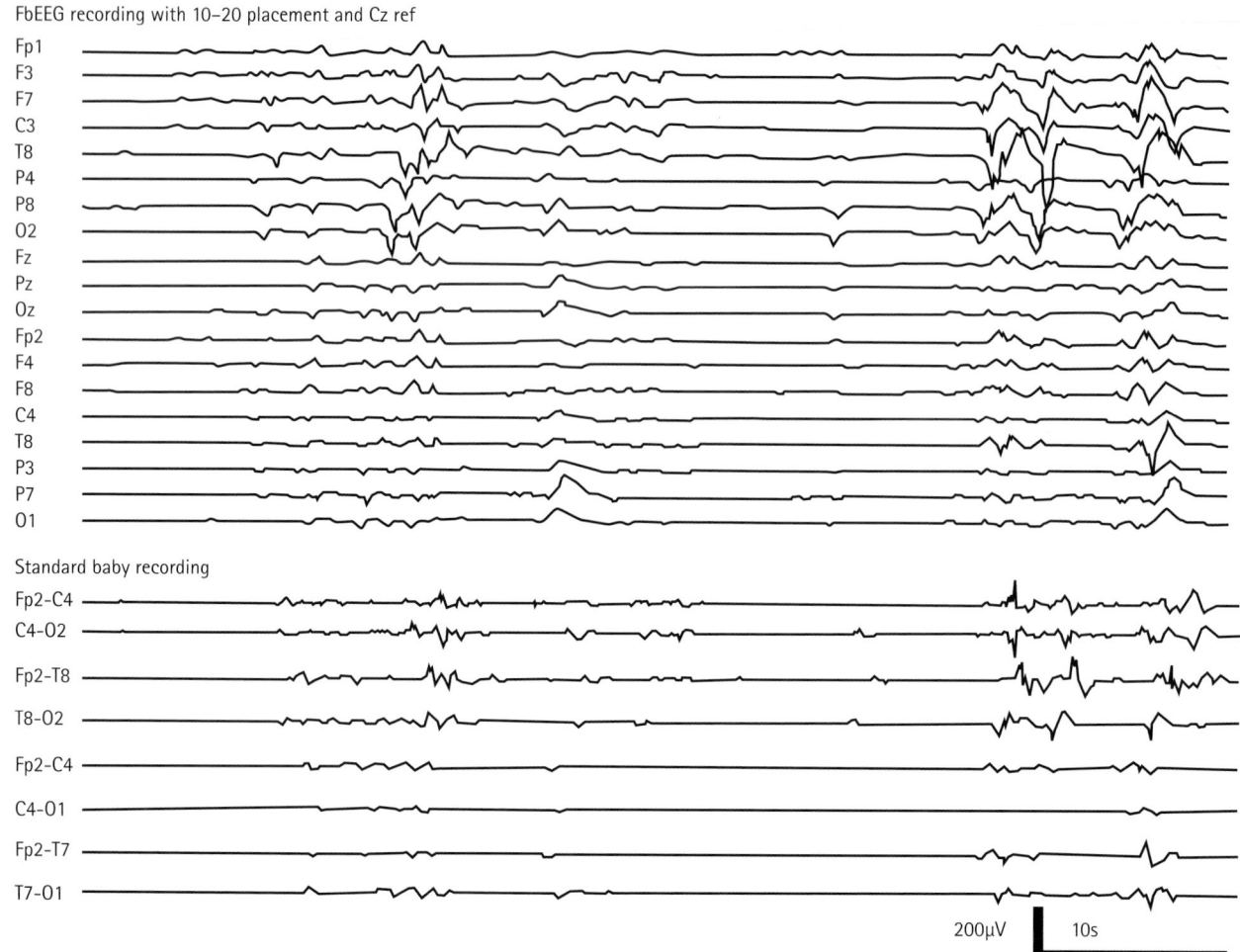

Figure 12.2 Comparison between EEGs from the same infant, recorded with standard recording method (below) and full-band EEG (upper), respectively. Note the infraslow activity which is revealed by the full-band EEG but not visible in the standard EEG. (Figure courtesy of Sampsa Vanhatalo.)

The clinical utility of this approach to show pathologies still remains to be shown.

Topographic mapping, coherence and MEG

The increasing use of digital EEG set off various new possibilities for analysis and evaluation of the EEG, including topographic mapping of electrocortical activity (Paul et al 2006, Pereda et al 2006), analysis of coherence (how electrocortical activity in different areas of the brain interact), and dipole analysis which currently is used mainly in older children and adults for identification of epileptic foci (Als et al 2004, Eiselt et al 2001, Roche-Labarbe et al 2007). Magnetoencephalography (MEG) records spontaneous and evoked magnetic fields from the brain and can also obtain intrauterine recordings of fetuses. The recordings show interesting similarities with EEG recordings in preterm infants at equivalent ages. Consequently, this method, that may have a great potential to increase our understanding of fetal physiology and changes that occur during transition from fetal to newborn life, is currently only available at a few centers worldwide. Evoked responses recorded with

MEG have been used to study fetal visual responses, auditory discrimination and short-term memory functions (Draganova et al 2007, Eswaran et al 2002, Haddad et al 2006, Huotilainen et al 2005).

EEG IN NEONATAL BRAIN INJURY

During and after an acute cerebral insult the EEG undergoes certain characteristic changes in a similar time-sequence. These changes have been characterized by Watanabe as 'acute-stage abnormalities' and 'chronic-stage abnormalities' (Table 12.3 and Fig. 12.3) (Watanabe et al 1999). The acute-stage abnormalities can be seen during and shortly (days) after an insult and are characterized by amplitude depression, increased discontinuity, seizures and loss of sleep–wake cycling. There is a recovery of the EEG background over time. However, if brain damage develops, chronic abnormalities can be detected in the EEG during the following weeks, especially in preterm infants. Chronic-stage abnormalities include, for example, presence of positive rolandic sharp waves, disorganized background patterns

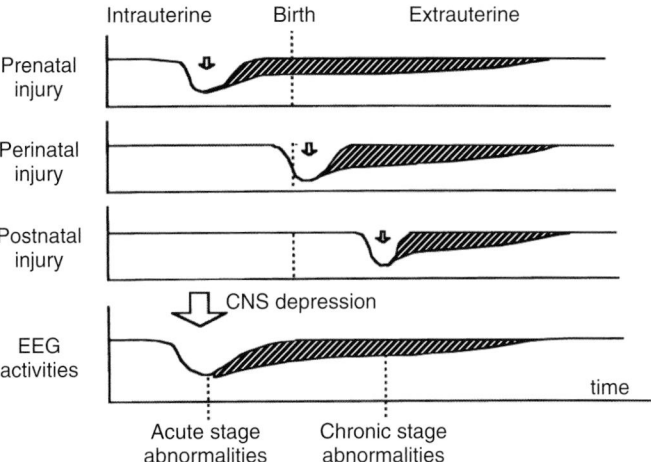

Figure 12.3 Schematic overview showing how acute and chronic EEG changes develop after an acute insult. Furthermore, how the timing of the insult, in relation to birth and when the EEG is recorded, influences the EEG findings. (Figure from Watanabe K, Hayakawa F, Okumura A 1999 Neonatal EEG: A powerful tool in the assessment of brain damage in preterm infants. Brain Dev 21:361–372, with permission.)

Table 12.3 Neonatal EEG abnormalities associated with brain injury

ACUTE-STAGE ABNORMALITIES
Increased discontinuity, amplitude depression
Decrease/loss of sleep–wake cycling
Epileptic seizure activity

CHRONIC-STAGE ABNORMALITIES
Presence of abnormal wave forms, e.g. temporal sharp waves, positive rolandic sharp waves (PRSW)
Disorganized background activity, abnormal sleep–wake cycles
Maturational delay (>2 weeks)

Watanabe et al 1999.

and delayed maturation (>2 weeks). Subtle changes of the EEG, indicating maturational delay, including various sleep measures, can also be found with power spectral analysis in preterm infants recorded at term age (Scher et al 1994a, 1994b). Most EEG abnormalities that appear in preterm infants are non-specific and not diagnostic for a certain type of brain injury. The only exception to this is positive rolandic sharp waves, which are sensitive indicators of white matter injury and associated with development of cerebral palsy (see below).

SEIZURES (see also Ch. 34)

Epileptic seizures are clearly abnormal events that may appear in the EEGs of ill newborn infants, although a majority of seizures demonstrate only subtle clinical symptoms or will remain clinically unrecognized. The most common

etiologies to seizures in the neonatal period include hypoxic–ischemic or hemorrhagic brain injury, hypoglycemia, severe infections such as sepsis and meningitis, congenital malformations and maternal drug abuse. A seizure pattern in the EEG is characterized by repetitive, stereotyped waveforms that usually wax and wane in frequency and amplitude with a definite onset, middle and end. There are no definite criteria for the duration of a seizure. In many studies a minimum duration of 10 seconds has been used but it is possible that briefer seizures, 5–10 seconds, also should be assessed since this type of activity has been associated with neurological injury (Oliveira et al 2000). Status epilepticus is often defined as continuously ongoing or repetitive seizures with a duration of at least 30 minutes, or more than 50% of the recording time. The duration of individual seizures in neonates is probably quite short, although this has been measured mainly in infants who already received antiepileptic treatment. Clancy and Legido (1987) estimated that a majority of neonatal seizures had a duration of less than 1 minute. Scher et al (1993) had an average seizure duration of 5 minutes in term infants and 2 minutes in preterms. One difference between the two studies, which may have affected the seizure durations, was that 87% of the infants in the study by Clancy and Legido (1987) received antiepileptic treatment, as compared to 50% in the study by Scher et al (1993). Epileptic seizure activity is often classified as being either electroclinical, i.e. electrographic changes with clinical symptoms, or electrographical, i.e. 'occult' or clinically silent. Newborn infants often show a mixture of these seizure types, but a majority of seizures are electrographical and thus clinically silent (Clancy et al 1988, Hellström-Westas et al 1985, Mizrahi and Kellaway 1987). It is not uncommon that electroclinical seizures continue as electrographical seizures after administration of antiepileptic treatment; a phenomenon that has been called 'uncoupling' (Boylan et al 2002, Connell et al 1989, Hellström-Westas et al 1985, Radvanyi-Bouvet et al 1985, Scher et al 2003, Toet et al 2002).

EEG AND OUTCOME IN TERM INFANTS

Several features of the EEG are associated with neurological outcome, although the electrocortical background activity seems to be the most sensitive parameter of acute brain injury. As mentioned above, a hypoxic–ischemic insult is associated with acute EEG depression which later recovers. The severity and duration of the EEG depression are predictive of outcome, especially when recorded early after an insult. The EEG usually improves and can even normalize within some days-first week after an insult also in infants developing brain damage. However, the longer the EEG remains abnormal the higher the risk for subsequent adverse outcome (Holmes & Lombroso 1993). Pezzani et al (1986) recorded EEGs during the first 24 hours of life in 80 full-term infants requiring intensive-care for different reasons. Severe background abnormalities such as BS with IBI greater than 40 seconds, inactive (isoelectric) tracings and seizures were associated with poor outcome, while minor abnormalities and preserved sleep–wake cycling were associated with normal outcome or minor sequelae. BS is still an ominous sign in the newborn term EEG and associated with high mortality and subsequent handicap. Still, some asphyxiated infants with BS do recover and have a good outcome (van Rooij et al 2005). Non-reactive BS and a predominant IBI duration of more than 30 seconds seem to identify infants with the poorest outcomes, i.e. death or severe neurologic handicap (Douglass et al 2002, Menache et al 2002).

Some metabolic diseases, e.g. non-ketotic hyperglycinemia and syndromes with neonatal encephalopathy, e.g. Ohtahara syndrome, typically demonstrate BS, and often also seizures, on the EEG. The prognosis in these infants is generally related to the underlying illness.

EEG background, and specifically the overall EEG description, is informative of outcome in newborn infants with meningitis. A moderately to markedly abnormal EEG was predictive (sensitivity 88%, specificity 90%) of death or survival with poor outcome in 37 infants with bacterial meningitis (Klinger et al 2001). Severe hyperbilirubinemia and development of kernicterus are associated with seizures and EEG abnormalities (AlOtaibi et al 2005). Also less severe hyperbilirubinemia may be associated with transient increases in delta activity, which correlates with the bilirubin level and decreases after several weeks (Gürses et al 2002).

Infants with seizures have a high risk for adverse neurodevelopmental outcome. Such infants often also demonstrate EEG background abnormalities. Several studies including infants with seizures have shown that the presence of seizure activity per se does not seem to affect overall outcome; instead there is a closer relation between the EEG background and outcome (Ortibus et al 1998, Radvanyi-Bouvet et al 1985, Rose & Lombroso 1970, Thorngren-Jerneck et al 2003). However, when investigating 'seizure burden,' i.e. total duration of seizures, as recorded with EEG-monitoring and in relation to outcome, there is a clear association between seizure burden and outcome. Infants with a large seizure burden have worse outcomes than infants with fewer seizures (McBride et al 2000, van Rooij et al 2007).

Infants with cardiac malformations constitute a high-risk group for hypoxic–ischemic brain injury and seizures. Around 10–20% of these infants develop postoperative seizures which are mainly subclinical (Clancy et al 2005, Helmers et al 1997). However, neonatal neurological compromise and abnormal EEG do not seem to be directly associated with long-term neurocognitive outcome in these infants (Gaynor et al 2006, Robertson et al 2004).

Infants with severe respiratory failure and need for extracorporeal membrane oxygenation (ECMO) are at risk for subsequent hypoxic–ischemic or hemorrhagic brain injury. The early EEG in these infants is clearly associated with outcome while the later recorded EEG is not, even if it is abnormal (Kumar et al 1999). Graziani et al (1994) recorded serial EEGs during ECMO in 119 infants. Infants with two or more EEGs showing BS or electrographic seizures had an odds ratio of 6.6 (95% confidence limits 2.2–20.2) for a poor outcome (death, low developmental assessment score or cerebral palsy) as compared to infants without EEG abnormalities on sequential EEGs.

EEG AND OUTCOME IN PRETERM INFANTS

Development of germinal matrix and intraparenchymal hemorrhages as well as ischemic cerebral lesions is associated with 'acute-stage' changes in the EEG, i.e. increased discontinuity, amplitude depression, seizures (Connell et al 1987b). There is a correlation between the severity of a hemorrhage and the degree of EEG abnormality (Clancy et al 1984, Watanabe et al 1983), although a study investigating post-mortem changes in the brains of preterm infants found a closer relation between EEG changes and the number of damaged brain structures than that between EEG and severity of the hemorrhage (Aso et al 1993). Seizures, mainly subclinical, may appear in as many as 60–70% of preterm infants developing intracranial hemorrhages but their significance for prognosis is not known (Greisen et al 1987, Hellström-Westas et al 1991). The predictive value of the early recorded EEG in very preterm infants is probably lower than that of the full-term infant, since preterm infants also may suffer from illnesses later during the neonatal course which can affect outcome, e.g. pulmonary complications and late-onset sepsis. Tharp et al (1989) recorded serial EEGs in 81 preterm infants; repeated normal EEGs were closely associated with normal outcome, while the presence of a markedly abnormal EEG was associated with poor outcome. The study also showed that abnormal EEGs were not always the first EEGs to be recorded in an infant. A later study, including 295 preterm infants between 27 and 32 gestational weeks, showed that the best correlation between EEG and severity of cerebral palsy was obtained from EEGs recorded on postnatal days 1–2. The sensitivity for prediction of outcome from EEG was significantly lower already after 3 days (Maruyama et al 2002). In another study, evaluating burst rates in relation to outcome in preterm infants surviving with large intraventricular hemorrhage (IVH) (grade 3–4), the maximum number of bursts/hour during the first 24 to 48 hours was predictive of outcome (Hellström-Westas et al 2001). Neuroprotection, aiming at limiting or reducing brain injury, may become a future option also in preterm infants. Thus, finding very early biomarkers that accurately predict outcome is of great importance.

Positive rolandic sharp waves (PRSW) and temporal sharp waves are associated with white matter injury. They appear 2–4 weeks after an insult and are associated with outcome. If a recording of a preterm infant includes more than 2 PRSW per minute, this finding is highly predictive of cerebral palsy (Baud et al 1998, Marret et al 1992, Vermeulen et al 2003). Other chronic EEG changes associated with adverse outcome include disorganized background patterns and delayed maturation. Dysmaturity or delayed maturation >2 weeks at term is associated with increased risk for handicaps in preterm infants (Biagioni et al 1996, Ferrari et al 1992). Mild prolonged depression in early EEGs and dysmaturity in later recorded EEGs also seem to be associated with impaired cognitive development in preterm infants (Hayakawa et al 1997).

EEG AND MEDICATIONS

A common clinical dilemma is that a baby treated with antiepileptic or sedative medication also needs to have the EEG recorded (Table 12.4). Sedative and antiepileptic drugs often affect and depress the electrocortical background activity, thereby obscuring the 'true' status of the brain. If the EEG background is considered normal there is usually no problem with the interpretation. However, often the EEG background is more discontinuous and depressed than what could be expected for the conceptional age, and in these cases the clinician and the neurophysiologist must try to sort out what could be real effects on the brain from, for example, previous hypoxia–ischemia or possible effects from medications. Several studies have evaluated drug effects on the neonatal EEG. However, it is not possible and ethically justified to administer medications to healthy newborns just to evaluate effects on the EEG, and therefore there are methodological problems with these studies since the medications were usually given to sick infants on clinical indications.

In general most sedative and antiepileptic drugs depress electrocortical background activity; the degree of background depression is associated with the type of medication, the dose and the time the drug was given in relation to the EEG (Bell et al 1993, Hellström-Westas et al 1988, 1992, Nguyen The Tich et al 2003, Young & da Silva 2000, van Leuven et al 2004). The EEG response to some medication also seems to be associated with illness severity; healthier babies seem to respond less than severely ill neonates and infants with severe hypoxic–ischemic brain injury, although this has not been formally evaluated in any study. Most of the current knowledge about drug effects on the EEG background is derived from studies using continuous EEG-monitoring (see below). Sleep–wake cycles may be obscured by sedatives and antiepileptic drugs in both term and preterm infants.

The effects on the EEG from small bolus doses and continuous infusion of opioids such as morphine and fentanyl seem to be only minor in term infants and moderately preterm infants. A loading dose of phenobarbital does not seem to affect the EEG background pattern to a large extent in term infants after moderate birth asphyxia; continuous EEG background may become slightly-moderately discontinuous, while the EEG background in infants with more severe birth asphyxia and discontinuous EEG may react more, e.g. change into BS or low voltage. Phenobarbital treatment with concentrations within therapeutic levels also appear to only moderately affect the EEG background and does not seem to affect EEG recovery in term asphyxiated infants (Bjerre et al 1983). Furthermore, therapeutic concentration of phenobarbital does not appear to affect the predictive sensitivity of the aEEG background in preterm infants with grade 3-4 IVHs (Hellström-Westas et al 2001). When using long-term EEG-monitoring it is clear that there is variability in the EEG background; effects from boluses of medications such as phenobarbital, phenytoin, diazepam, midazolam, morphine are mainly seen on the EEG background 1–2 hours immediately following administration of the medication. Administration of the antiepileptic medication lidocaine may change the EEG background to BS, both in term and in preterm infants. However, lidocaine is usually given when other medications such as phenobarbital and midazolam/diazepam failed to control seizures, and the effect on the EEG background may be influenced by the add-on effects of the medications (Hellström-Westas et al 2003). Endotracheal administration of surfactant for respiratory distress syndrome often results in a short, but very profound, depression of electrocortical activity which may become transiently inactive for about 10 minutes (Hellström-Westas et al 1992a). Several studies have shown changes in cerebral blood flow associated with surfactant administration but the physiological background to this EEG reaction is not known; it did coincide with a transient increase in total cerebral hemoglobin (corresponding to cerebral blood volume) as measured by near infrared spectroscopy (NIRS) but it did not correlate with blood gases or arterial blood pressure (Skov et al 1992).

Table 12.4 Practical recommendations for recording and interpretation of EEG background in infants given sedatives, opioid analgesics or antiepileptic medications

- Preferably do not record the EEG immediately after a bolus of sedatives, analgesics or antiepileptic medications. If possible, wait at least 1–2 hours.
- Loading doses of phenobarbital (up to 20 mg/kg) results in moderate additional background depression, i.e. in term and near-term infants a continuous EEG pattern may become discontinuous, a discontinuous trace may turn into burst-suppression, and the duration of IBI may increase in a burst-suppression EEG. In very preterm infants (who normally have a discontinuous background) a discontinuous EEG pattern may change to burst-suppression, sometimes with clearly increasing duration of IBI.
- Thus, moderate doses of sedatives, analgesics or antiepileptic medications usually do not result in major electrocortical background changes. If a term infant, who was given a loading dose of phenobarbital (20 mg/kg), has a burst-suppression background this is likely due to a combination of medication and affected brain function.
- Continuous EEG-monitoring makes it easier to appreciate the impact on the electrocortical background activity from various types of medications in the individual infant, and can therefore be of help when interpreting the EEG.

EXTRACEREBRAL FACTORS AFFECTING THE PRETERM EEG

Several extracerebral factors can affect the EEG of the preterm infant and should be considered when evaluating EEG or EEG-monitoring. Cardiac output and arterial blood pressure are strong determinants of cerebral blood flow and also show clear correlations with early EEG background in preterm infants (Victor et al 2006a, 2006b, West et al 2006b). West et al (2006b) showed that EEG amplitude correlated with right ventricular outflow measures and EEG continuity correlated with mean arterial blood pressure. Victor et al (2006a) also showed that the EEG became depressed (decrease in relative delta activity and prolonged IBI) when mean arterial blood pressure was below 23 mmHg in a group of very low birth weight infants. Greisen et al (1988) noted a slow increase in aEEG burst rate in five out of 12 hypotensive preterm infants receiving volume substitution to increase blood pressure. Also carbon dioxide level, which is closely associated with cerebral blood flow, and acidosis seem to elicit reversible changes in electrocortical activity as shown by two studies in preterm infants (Eaton et al 1984, Victor et al 2005b).

Pharmacological closure of the ductus arteriosus is associated with changes in cerebral blood flow, which can be quite dramatic during surgical ligation of the persistent ductus arteriosus. However, few studies have investigated effects from persistent ductus arteriosus on the neonatal EEG. In a group of preterm infants with a persistent ductus arteriosus and controls with a closed ductus, Kurtis et al (1995) did not find any differences in EEG spectral analysis before or after closure of the ductus arteriosus, and when comparing with controls.

EEG-MONITORING

Video-EEG monitoring with a full EEG is probably the 'gold standard' for clinical monitoring of seizures. However, not many hospitals have this service with on-line interpretation 24 hours per day, 7 days per week. Instead, EEG-monitors with various trend measures have been developed which enable the neonatal staff to initiate the recordings and to interpret the EEG trends around the clock. The trend measure of the EEG that has been most widely used is the aEEG, which is a method derived from the cerebral function monitor (CFM). The original CFM was created in the late 1960s by Prior and Maynard for cerebral monitoring of adult patients during intensive care or surgery (Maynard et al 1969). The CFM was created to enable long-term monitoring of trends in electrocortical background activity with a monitor that was easy to apply and to interpret for the intensive-care staff. The basic features of the aEEG include recording of the EEG from 1 or 2 channels, an asymmetric band pass filter, rectifying and smoothing, a time-compressed signal and semilogarithmic output. This method of modifying the EEG-signal is used also in the new digital monitors that have been available since the late 1990s. The original EEG could not be displayed in the CFM and in the earlier aEEG monitors, so the EEG had to be recorded intermittently. The newly developed digital EEG-monitors have introduced increased flexibility, including various trend measures of the EEG and number of recording channels that can be displayed. Consequently, some of them can be used for both recording of the EEG (during the day) and for trend-monitoring (e.g. during the night).

Similar to other monitoring equipment used in the NICU, the utility of aEEG in terms of improving outcomes or lowering costs has not been evaluated. Although the majority of neonatologists caring for critically ill infants are enthusiastic about aEEG/EEG-monitoring, since they receive continuous valuable information about the infants' brain functions, which they can use to guide medical decisions and inform parents, questions about the methods' efficiency and reliability have been raised. A key issue has been the aEEG's ability to adequately detect epileptic seizure activity with the reduced number of electrodes that are used (Freeman 2007, Rennie et al 2004). In infants with clearly identified epileptic seizure activity on the EEG it can be estimated that a single or two-channel EEG/aEEG identifies at least 80–90% of infants with seizures (Shah et al 2008, Shellhaas et al 2007, Toet et al 2002). The precision of the aEEG for detecting seizures when there is no display of the real EEG is considerably lower (25–35%). The reason for this is the short duration of neonatal seizures which makes them impossible to identify in the very time-compressed display of the aEEG. An example of this is that only 15 out of 48 EEG-verified single seizures were detectable in the aEEG (without display of the EEG); this in turn corresponded to only four clinically recognized seizures (Hellström-Westas 1992). The seizures that were not detectable by the aEEG were all of short duration, 5–30 seconds. Shellhaas et al (2007) recorded a full EEG in 125 neonates with seizures and detected a total of 851 seizures. A single-channel EEG from the C3–C4 positions identified 78% of the seizures and 94% of the EEGs with seizures. Six neonatologists, all with previous experience of the aEEG, evaluated the aEEG tracings from the same electrode positions but without simultaneous display of the EEG, and identified on average only 26% of seizures but 40% of infants with seizures. It has not been evaluated how many infants without previously known epileptic seizures are diagnosed when using aEEG, although the figure is probably significant. Two studies that included aEEG for diagnosis and treatment of epileptic seizures (including treatment of repetitive subclinical seizures) reported significantly lower risks for postnatal epilepsy (8–10%) when treating clinical as well as subclinical aEEG detected seizures, as compared to study populations where only clinical seizures or seizures diagnosed with intermittent EEGs were treated (20–50%) (Brunquell et al 2002, Clancy & Legido 1991, Hellström-Westas et al 1995b, Toet et al 2005). While clinical monitoring in the NICU always includes risks for misinterpretation due to both lack of knowledge and technical errors, it is clear that modern EEG-monitoring increases the demands on the bedside users. There are not only risks that important information may be missed, there are also risks for overinterpretation of findings, which could lead to unnecessary administration of medications, e.g. if epileptic seizure activity is suspected but later not verified. Development is currently in progress to reduce such risks and, in the near future, monitors will probably have alarms or alerts (e.g. suspected seizures, deterioration of electrocortical activity) and possibilities for on-line interpretation of the EEG trends (Lommen et al 2007, Navakatikyan et al 2006).

Recommendations for clinical aEEG/EEG-monitoring in the neonatal intensive care unit:

1. Provide adequate and regular training for all neonatal staff using aEEG-monitoring.
2. Establish close collaboration with neurologists/clinical neurophysiologists; this will improve possibilities for optimal evaluation/interpretation of recordings.
3. Record at least one standard EEG in all monitored infants, preferably as early as possible.
4. Frequent clinical notes/annotations should be made during the recording (care/procedures, etc.) since they facilitate interpretation of the recordings.

CLINICAL APPLICATIONS OF EEG-MONITORING

There are now several publications describing the normal aEEG background in term and preterm infants, including numerical values as well as pattern descriptions (Burdjalov et al 2003, Hellström-Westas et al 2006, Olischar et al 2004, Thornberg & Thiringer 1990, Verma et al 1984, Viniker et al 1984).

A main indication for long-term EEG recording is often a need for clinical monitoring of 'high-risk' infants and infants with neurological symptoms, e.g. during the first 3 days of life in infants requiring intensive care (when a majority of postasphyctic seizures, intracranial hemorrhages and hypoglycemic episodes occur); in infants with clear or suspected clinical seizures; in infants with uncharacteristic neurological symptoms (hypotonia, irritability, or apnea in term infants). A full standard EEG should be recorded in all infants early during the monitoring period and repeated as required. Close collaboration with neurologists and/or clinical neurophysiologists increases the likelihood for optimal use of EEG-monitoring.

Full-term infants with HIE (p. 557)

It was shown in the mid 1990s that the aEEG background was sensitive for prediction of outcome in asphyxiated newborns as early as 3 to 6 hours after birth (Eken et al 1995, Hellström-Westas et al 1995a, Toet et al 1999). Asphyxiated infants with normal aEEG background were likely to have a good outcome, while infants with abnormal electrocortical background had a high risk for developing handicap. It was shown in several studies that the accuracy of the early aEEG background to predict outcome in infants with neonatal

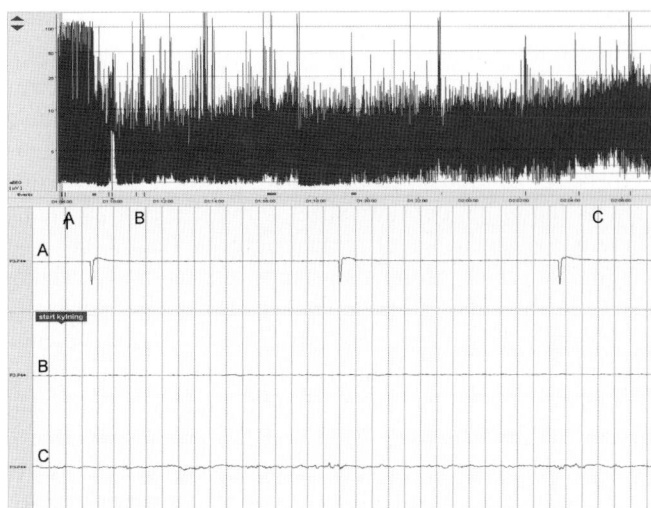

Figure 12.4 A 20-hour aEEG recording of a severely asphyxiated infant with three representative EEG samples below, each with a duration of 38 seconds. In the beginning of the recording, when the infant was 2 hours old, only occasional hiccups are seen in the upper EEG trace (A). However, there is no electrocortical activity either at 2 hours or at 5 hours (B), when cooling was started. The lower trace (C) shows the EEG 18 hours after cooling was initiated, and shows a continuous but rather low-voltage EEG. Cerebral activity continued to recover and the infant had a good recovery with normal outcome at 1 year.

encephalopathy and after perinatal asphyxia was a very stable measure and that the neurological outcome in 80–90% of infants could be correctly predicted (al Naqeeb et al 1999, Eken et al 1995, Hellström-Westas et al 1995a, Ter Horst et al 2004, Thornberg & Ekström-Jodal 1994, Toet et al 1999). The accuracy of prediction could be further increased when the aEEG was combined with a clinical examination (Shalak et al 2003). Shany et al (2006b) investigated whether aEEG background patterns or voltages were more sensitive for early prediction of outcome in near-term asphyxiated infants. Background patterns were associated with outcome both at 3 and 6 hours, while amplitudes were associated with outcome at 6 hours. Shah et al (2006b) found a correlation between the minimum amplitude of the aEEG tracing and abnormalities on magnetic resonance imaging (MRI) in a cohort of encephalopathic term infants, almost half of them with hypoxic–ischemic brain injury. The aEEG background pattern was recently used for inclusion of asphyxiated infants in a multicenter randomized controlled trial for treatment with moderate hypothermia. It was shown that infants with moderately abnormal aEEG background before 5.5 hours of life had the best effect of the hypothermia (Gluckman et al 2005). Figure 12.4 shows a 20-hour aEEG recording of a cooled infant who recovered completely.

The aEEG pattern that is recorded after the first hours of life is also strongly associated with outcome, but only if it is recorded within the first 48–72 hours, since the electro-cortical background recovers over time, even in severely asphyxiated infants (Ter Horst et al 2004, Thorngren-Jerneck et al 2003). If the early aEEG in asphyxiated infants shows BS, but normalizes within the first 24 hours, there is a 50% chance of normal outcome (van Rooij et al 2005). The timing of the appearance of sleep–wake cycling (SWC) in the aEEG is also a marker of outcome, especially in infants with moderate HIE. Osredkar et al (2005) evaluated aEEG recordings from 171 asphyxiated term infants; the median times for onset of SWC in infants with HIE grades I, II and III were 7, 33 and 62 hours, respectively. Neurodevelopmental outcome (good/poor) was correctly predicted in 82% of infants by a cut-off for onset of SWC at 36 postnatal hours. A combination of aEEG with other methods such as NIRS can also increase the predictive accuracy when recordings start around 24 hours of life (Toet et al 2006). Epileptic seizure activity is mainly present in infants with moderate HIE; this is probably the reason why the presence of seizures has not been associated with outcome after asphyxia since at least 50% of infants with moderate HIE do well and since seizures may not be as common in severe HIE, with much worse prognosis, as in moderate HIE. However, it was recently shown that both the duration of status epilepticus and the electrocortical background pattern in the aEEG were associated with long-term outcome in infants with moderate HIE (van Rooij et al 2007).

Perinatal stroke

The typical clinical presentation in an infant with perinatal stroke is unilateral clinical seizures appearing during the first 1–2 days of life in a term infant who is otherwise usually doing well. There is also an increased risk for stroke in infants who suffered from perinatal asphyxia and dehydration and in infants with cardiac malformations. Monitoring of the aEEG is often very useful in these infants, not least for evaluation of treatment with antiepileptic drugs. If bilateral EEG-traces are obtained, asymmetry can sometimes be seen with seizures and amplitude depression appearing mainly over the affected hemisphere. Abnormal EEG background (unilateral or bilateral) is associated with an increased risk for hemiplegia (Mercuri et al 1999). Figure 12.5 shows a 6-hour recording of three EEG trends (aEEG, SEF and spectrogram, which demonstrates the frequency distribution) and the original EEG in a term infant with a left-sided stroke.

EEG-monitoring during high-frequency ventilation and ECMO

High-frequency ventilation (HFV) often interferes with the EEG-monitoring, especially when there is pressure from, for example, bedding on the electrodes. In spite of the HFV, the EEG-monitor can often be used although the evaluation of the background becomes cruder. Figure 12.5 shows an example of an aEEG tracing in an infant on HFV who suf-

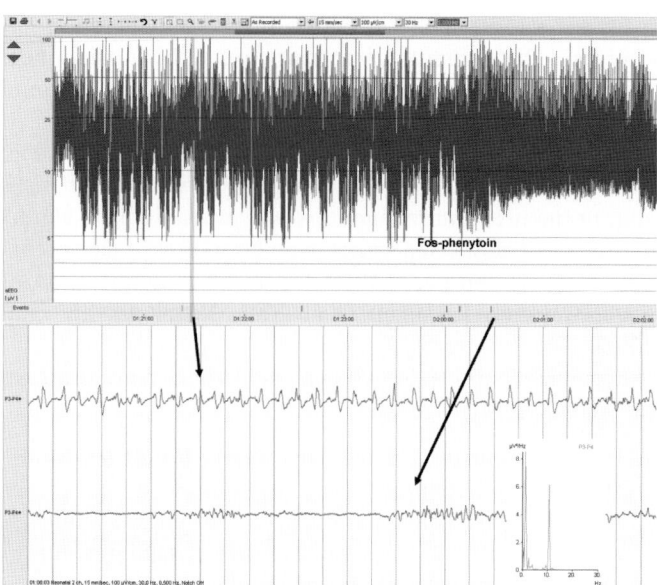

Figure 12.5 'Saw-tooth' pattern in the aEEG representing repetitive subclinical seizures in an infant with meconium aspiration syndrome and moderate hypoxic–ischemic encephalopathy. Administration of fos-phenytoin results in disappearance of seizures and the EEG background becomes discontinuous. Interference from high-frequency oscillation ventilation at 11 Hz raises the aEEG tracing.

fered from meconium aspiration syndrome and HIE with subclinical status epilepticus.

As mentioned above, the early recorded EEG in infants treated with ECMO is predictive of outcome (Graziant et al 1994). Pappas et al (2006) continuously recorded aEEG in 20 neonates treated with ECMO. There was no change in aEEG during cannulation for ECMO. An abnormal aEEG was predictive of death or moderate to severe intracranial neuropathology with 100% sensitivity and 75% specificity, PPV 86% and NPV 100%. On the other hand, Trittenwein et al (2006) compared EEG spectral power in seven infants on ECMO with 10 mechanically ventilated 'control' infants and found a significant but transient decrease in EEG power during the ECMO treatment, but not after. Recently, Horan et al (2007) investigated aEEG during ECMO and moderate hypothermia in 26 infants. One-third of the recordings were moderately to severely abnormal and 3 infants (11%) had seizures, but the aEEG was not affected by the hypothermia per se.

EEG-monitoring of seizures

Continuous EEG-monitoring is clearly superior to clinical recognition of neonatal seizures since a majority are either entirely subclinical or appear with only subtle clinical manifestations. It has been estimated that 50 to 80% of epileptic seizures are subclinical (Clancy et al 1988, Scher et al 2003), a fact that is usually evident when using EEG-monitoring (Hellström-Westas et al 1985, Shany et al 2006a). Interictal

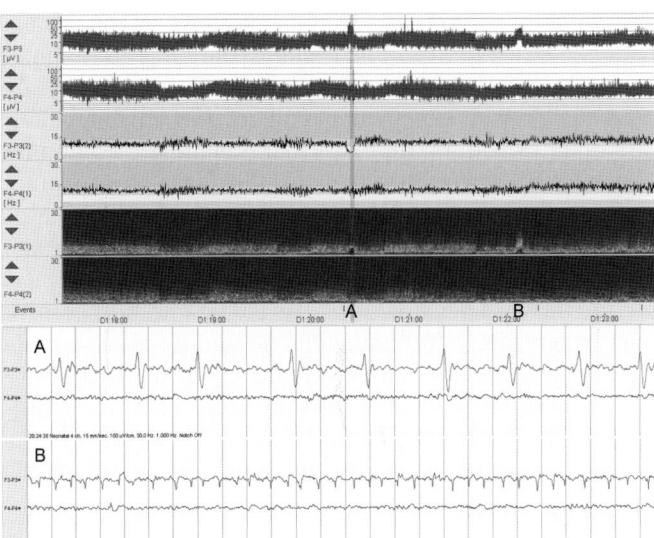

Figure 12.6 EEG-monitoring from two bilateral channels in a term infant with a left-sided stroke. The upper six panels show 6 hours of three different trends (aEEG, SEF and spectrogram) from the F3-P3 (left) and F4-P4 (right) positions. The EEG background is mainly continuous, as can be seen in the aEEG tracings, with some cyclicity indicating sleep–wake cycling. Below the trends are two 25-second displays of the EEGs during two seizures (marked A and B) that occurred on the left side during the recording. Note the corresponding changes in the trends above the EEG.

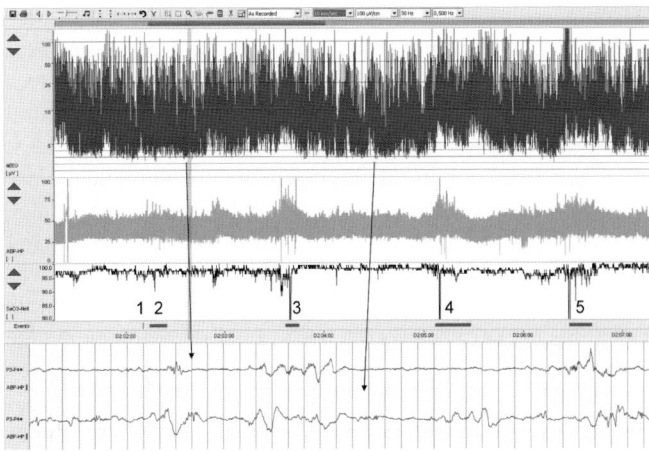

Figure 12.7 Six-hour recording of aEEG, arterial blood pressure and oxygen saturation in a newborn infant with gestational age 26 weeks who was spontaneously breathing with CPAP below the trend recording is 38 seconds of EEG from two aEEG periods. The aEEG is normal for the gestational age and shows cyclicity indicating sleep–wake cycling. Five care procedures are noted: (1) abdominal X-ray; (2) feeding; (3) turned; (4) feeding and turned, cries; (5) turned, abdominal pain? The blood pressure increases in conjunction with the care procedures, although the infant seems to tolerate these quite well, as evaluated by the stable aEEG and oxygen saturation trends.

sharp waves and other epileptiform activity can also be seen during EEG-monitoring, but for a correct estimate of amount and localization at least one standard EEG, or video-EEG-monitoring, should always be performed in infants with identified seizures.

The optimal method for EEG-monitoring is currently under debate. Some researchers advocate full video-EEG monitoring, although this is only available in some centers and also requires interpretation by trained neurologists or neurophysiologists. Trend-measures of the EEG, e.g. the aEEG, assist the clinicians to 'see the forests and the trees' of the EEG and to identify seizures more easily – not least during nights and weekends when many EEG-departments are closed (Scheuer & Wilson 2004). Figure 12.6 demonstrates how various EEG trend-measures can be used in order to enhance the identification of seizures during long-term monitoring. Continuously ongoing spiking is difficult to identify in EEG trends and may thus be missed, since there is no change in the background pattern. Repetitive and single seizures are easier to identify in the trends since they display the classic waxing and waning of rhythmic activity over at least 5–10 seconds, which shows as a change in the trend and as a transient abrupt rise in aEEG activity. A rare type of seizure is characterized by a transient EEG flattening; this has been seen in, for example, hypsarrhythmia with desynchronization of high-voltage activity (Hellström-Westas et al 2003).

The reduced number of electrodes/channels used in EEG-monitoring is an issue for the accuracy of detection of epileptic seizures during, especially, short-term recordings. The lack of recognition of seizures when using only 1–2 channels is associated with a 6–20% risk that an infant with subclinical seizures may pass unrecognized even when the EEG-monitor displays the real EEG (Shellhaas et al 2007, Toet et al 2002). Studies involving standard EEG have shown that, reducing the number of electrodes, seizures may pass undetected and infants with seizures may not be recognized (Bye & Flanagan 1995, Tekgul et al 2005).

EEG-monitoring in preterm infants

EEG-monitoring can also be used in preterm infants, and several studies have described normative values for aEEG measures in preterm infants (Burdjalov et al 2003, Olischar et al 2004, Thornberg & Thiringer 1990, Viniker et al 1984). The EEG-monitor can be used for continuous evaluation of cerebral function in high-risk preterm infants during intensive-care treatment during the first days of life or after adverse events such as hypoglycemia, pneumothorax or sepsis. Continuous EEG-monitoring of very preterm infants will probably increase our understanding of pathophysiological mechanisms leading to brain damage in the future. Simultaneous recordings of EEG and other parameters such as blood pressure and oxygen saturation monitoring will probably contribute to this development (Fig. 12.7).

Comparable to EEG findings in preterm infants with germinal matrix hemorrhages, the aEEG has also shown clear correlations between severity of the hemorrhages and electrocortical background depression. The aEEG was initiated during the first 24 hours of life and continued for at least 50 hours in a cohort of 32 mechanically ventilated very preterm infants. Absence of germinal matrix hemorrhage was associated with increasingly continuous activity during the second day of life, although this development was slightly delayed in infants with, for example, hypocalcemia. The aEEG background was depressed before the hemorrhage appeared in four infants and in six out of 10 infants, where the hemorrhage occurred during the recording, the electrocortical background decreased (Greisen et al 1987). Similar findings were found in an aEEG study on somewhat more immature infants; both studies showed that seizures, mainly subclinical, may be present in up to 60–70% of infants developing germinal matrix hemorrhages (Greisen et al 1987, Hellström-Westas et al 1991). Development of white matter injury, i.e. periventricular leukomalacia (PVL), is also associated with acute changes that can be identified on EEG-monitoring, including background depression and seizures (Connell et al 1987b).

Conclusion EEG

EEG and continuous EEG-monitoring are sensitive indicators of brain function in newborn infants. The severity and duration of acute electrocortical background changes have been shown to correlate with brain injury and later outcome. More subtle, chronic abnormalities can be seen in the EEG at later stages after an insult and are also associated with adverse outcome. aEEG-monitoring has proved to be useful for very early identification of high-risk infants who can benefit from specific interventions aiming at reducing or limiting brain injury after birth asphyxia. An increased use of EEG-monitoring in ill neonates in the NICU will probably increase our understanding of pathophysiological mechanism leading to brain injury, both in term and in preterm infants.

METHODOLOGY AND MATURATION OF EVOKED POTENTIALS

Over the last decades, there has been an increasing interest in recording EPs, both in preterm infants as well as in asphyxiated full-term babies. The brainstem auditory evoked potentials (BAEPs) and the visual evoked potentials (VEPs) are technically easier to perform than the somatosensory evoked potentials (SEPs). Initially, a high failure rate was reported in normal neonates, most likely due to the fact that the recording technique had not been adjusted from the adult settings. Only when the filter settings, stimulation rate and number of stimuli are adapted to the immature nervous system, will the success rate be sufficient.

Applying Ag/AgCl disc electrodes to the scalp should be performed without causing irritation of the vulnerable skin and without disturbing the infant. Restless infants should better be tested in the prone position. During registration of EPs it is standard procedure to repeat the test to ensure reproducibility. When in doubt about the reliability it is important to perform an extra trial, sampling the raw EEG without administering the stimulus. Following the stimulus, a series of positive and negative deflections can be measured. In some laboratories the components of the SEPs and VEPs are named according to the order of appearance, e.g. N1 for the first negative peak, or P1 for the first positive one; others use a denomination according to the mean latency of a specific age group, e.g. N19, the first scalp-derived component in adult SEPs, or P200, a positive deflection in the VEP of term neonates. In BAEPs, all laboratories use the same nomenclature (roman numerals) to indicate the different positive peaks.

BRAINSTEM AUDITORY EVOKED POTENTIALS (BAEPS)

BAEPs are responses generated within the auditory brainstem pathway following an acoustic stimulus. They are the far-field reflection of sequentially activated neurons at successively higher levels of the auditory pathway. They are used to assess both the peripheral sensitivity as well as the neurologic integrity of the auditory brainstem. The response consists of a sequence of seven positive waves of which the first two (waves I and II) represent the action potentials of the extracranial and intracranial portions of the eighth nerve; wave III is derived from the cochlear nucleus; wave IV arises from the superior olivary complex and wave V from the lateral lemniscus. Waves VI and VII are thought to arise from the inferior colliculus (Jewett & Williston 1971). The I–V peak latency is considered to be a measure of central auditory conduction time. The waves arise in the first 10 milliseconds after the acoustic stimulus.

To record the response, the active electrode is best positioned on the mastoid bone or earlobe ipsilateral to the stimulus; the reference electrode is placed on the vertex, and the forehead or the contralateral ear is grounded (Stuart et al 1996). Impedance must be below $5\,\Omega$. Most laboratories use rarefaction broadband click stimuli with a peak power of 2–4 kHz, because they produce clearer wave morphologic features than do condensation clicks (Pope-Stockard & Sharbrough 1992). The rectangular pulses have a duration of $100\,\mu s$ and usually are presented at a repetition rate of 10 per second. Increasing the repetition rate increases the latencies and decreases the amplitude of the response (Jiang et al 2001, Klein et al 1992, Lasky 1984). The pulse is calibrated in decibels above the hearing threshold of normally hearing subjects (dBnHL). The signals are presented monaurally through a special cushioned earphone (TDH-39 pediatric earphones) which may be held over the ear. Ideally, when stimulating at 80 dBnHL or higher, constant white noise should be used to mask the contralateral ear to prevent cross-hearing by bone conduction. Jiang et al (2000, 2003) have extensively studied the use of maximum length sequence (MLS) BAEPs to study functional integrity and maturation of the brainstem, using click rates as high as 91–910/s and were able to show that an increasing repetition rate of click stimuli can improve the detection of neurologic abnormalities.

BAEPs are best recorded in a quiet area of the nursery. BAEP latencies are not affected by behavioral state, but they can be obtained more reliably during a period of quiescence (McCall & Ferraro 1991). Also, the responses are not influenced by general anesthetics or drugs. Since the BAEPs are very small compared with the electrical background noise, it is necessary to average at least 1000 individual sweeps to improve the signal-to-noise amplitude ratio. Automatic artifact rejection may be used to reduce the inclusion of high-amplitude muscular activity in the averaged response (Jiang 1995). Analysis-time for the signal average is usually between 15 and 20 ms, the EEG-amplifier filter bandpass is preferably 30–3000 Hz (Sininger 1995, Spivak 1993, Stuart & Yang 1994). This relatively high-pass recording filter of 30 Hz reveals a larger amplitude and enhances the overall signal-to-noise ratio, as BAEPs from neonates comprise greater low-frequency spectral components than do adult BAEPs.

With high-intensity stimuli presented at a low rate it is possible to recognize the presence of waves I, III, and V in infants from as early as 25 weeks of gestation onwards (Cox et al 1993, Despland 1985, Fawer & Dubowitz 1982, Lary et al 1985). The peak latencies decrease progressively with increasing gestational age, and subsequently waves II and IV will appear (Vles et al 1985). The maximal change is between 29 and 36 weeks of gestational age. The maturational changes reflect the changes in myelination, axon diameter and synaptic efficacy in the brainstem auditory pathways. The latency of wave V decreases more rapidly with age than that of wave I, resulting in a wave I–V peak interval also decreasing with age. Whether preterm birth affects the maturation of the auditory system is still equivocal, but using different click rates, Jiang et al (2002) found that very preterm infants have an advanced peripheral development of the brainstem auditory pathway, probably related to early exposure to sound ex utero, but a delayed central development.

At term age, the morphology of the BAEP is similar to that of adults, but with longer latencies (Picton et al 1992). At the age of 2 years, near adult values are reached. Slight gender differences are reported, with shorter latencies and higher amplitudes in females, as well as a significant right-ear advantage in males and females attributed to cerebral laterality in auditory function (Eldredge & Salamy 1996). A high interindividual variability has been reported in several cross-sectional studies, but intraindividual maturation is consistent (Mercuri et al 1994, Vles et al 1985). To rate the maturational changes at their true value, age-specific normative data should be obtained for each laboratory. Auditory thresholds improve significantly with age (Lary et al 1985). Establishing amplitude norms in neonates is difficult, since the overall amplitudes are low and amplitude is influenced by the low frequency cut-off. Only the wave V : I amplitude ratio is being used for clinical purposes in neonates.

VISUAL EVOKED POTENTIALS (VEPS)

The VEP is a gross electrical signal generated by the occipital area of the cortex in response to a visual stimulus. The stimulus may either be a diffuse flashing light or a patterned visual stimulus. VEPs has been used widely for 40 years (Ellingson 1960) in the evaluation of maturational processes in both preterm and term infants, because of the ease with which they can be applied in longitudinal studies. VEPs show systematic changes in electrographical characteristics with advancing gestational age, which are thought to reflect the progress in myelination in the developing human brain (Minami et al 1996, Tsuneishi & Casaer 1997). In adults, the N70 and P100 peaks are the most important features, while in neonates and infants the P200 and N300 peaks are the major components. Monocular stimulation, using a combination of electroretinography and VEP measurement, will allow, by comparison of the response elicited at the two separate visual cortices, differentiation between pre- and postchiasmatic lesions.

Flash-VEPs (FVEPs) are not suitable for neurophysiological measurement of visual acuity. For this purpose the pattern-VEPs (PVEPs) are better, because they are a sensitive and quantitative measure of visual function, especially in the distinction between cortical and subcortical visual function. However, in the neonatal unit PVEPs have not been widely used, as they can only be elicited in infants who are able to fixate on a stimulus during a period of alertness.

FLASH-VEPS

In the neonatal unit, light-emitting diode (LED) goggles or small LED screens which can be placed inside the incubator are most feasible to use as a stimulus source. A stroboscopic flashlight has to be placed outside the incubator, thus producing variable stimulus intensities, and has also been shown to produce more complex waveforms (Mushin et al 1984). FVEPs are recorded from a single midline channel, the positive electrode being placed on Oz, referenced to Fz, and using the forearm as a ground. The analysis time should be 1000 ms, as the components emerge between 200 and 500 ms. The stimulus with a duration of 10 ms has to be delivered sufficiently infrequently to allow the visual system to return to its resting state between the successive stimuli, usually 0.5 Hz.

The recommended filter bandpass is 1–100 Hz, and the impedance needs to be below 5 Ω. At least two series of 40–60 trials have to be collected to ensure reproducibility, although reproducible VEPs can easily be obtained with a few trials using a long interstimulus interval (Pryds 1992). Several authors emphasized the need for looking at the behavioral state of the infant during the VEP recording, since the P200 was noted to decrease in amplitude and increase in latency in both active and quiet sleep states

(Apkarian et al 1991, Watanabe et al 1973, Whyte et al 1987).

FVEPs can be elicited as early as 23, 24 and 25 weeks of gestational age (Chin et al 1985, Hrbek et al 1973, Purpura 1975, Taylor et al 1987). At this early stage, the response consists mainly of a large negative wave occurring at approximately 300 ms (N300). The N300 shortens in latency as the infant matures by a rate of 4.6–5.5 ms a week (Pike et al 1999, Tsuneishi et al 1995). Tsuneishi and Casaer (1997) have, however, demonstrated a stepwise decrease of the latency with 'acceleration weeks,' during which the latency decreases at a rate of more than 6 ms a week. These acceleration weeks occur most prominently at 37 weeks postmenstrual age, and this was attributed to an initiation of myelination in the optic radiation. Likewise, Minami et al (1996) reported a faster decrease in latency of the N300 from 35 to 38 weeks, compared with 32 to 35 weeks. After 27 weeks a late positive component is present (P400), but this wave has a variable latency and morphology.

A smaller positive peak, preceding the N300, will emerge at around 34 weeks of gestational age (P200) and become the most consistent feature of the VEP (Ellingson 1970, Taylor et al 1987, Umezaki & Morell 1970). The latency of the P200 also decreases rapidly until term age. At term, the response consists of a negative–positive–negative complex, which will transform into the more complex adult waveform over the next few months (Benavente et al 2005).

The N300 peak is supposed to arise from the basilar dendrites of the pyramidal cells in the visual cortex, while the P200 is suggested to arise from the apical dendrites, which develop in the last trimester (Taylor et al 1987). Subcortical components may also be present, since a negative wave has also been reported in infants with severe occipital lesions (Dubowitz et al 1986).

Comparison of FVEPs recorded in preterm infants with those from term infants at equivalent postconceptional ages suggests faster maturation of particularly the P200 peak in the extrauterine versus the intrauterine environment (Leaf et al 1995, Taylor et al 1987). Tsuneishi et al (1995), however, reported that extrauterine life may accelerate the maturation of the N300 waveform, but does not affect the absolute peak latencies. Inter- and even intra-subject variability of the FVEP latencies is high, inducing a wide normal range, but Apkarian et al (1991) stressed that careful control of state during the recording reduces inter- and intra-subject variability.

The rapid maturational changes in both preterm and term born infants, the differences in recording technique among various laboratories and the differences found in intrauterine versus extrauterine development, require the establishment of normative values, ideally taking both postmenstrual and gestational age at birth into consideration.

PATTERN VEPS

Several stimulation techniques may be used, like flashed checkerboards, steady-state stimulation, and pattern-sweep,

but most studies in infants use pattern-reversal checkerboard stimulation where black and white squares exchange places with a constant luminance (McCulloch & Taylor 1994). The first reports on PVEPs in preterm infants were published by Harding's group (Grose et al 1989, Harding et al 1989) and Birch et al (1990). They obtained PVEPs in healthy preterm infants at 33 and 36 weeks of gestation, respectively. Kos-Pietro et al (1997) were able to elicit a response as early as 32 weeks of gestation, but stressed that, even in low-risk infants, they managed to obtain a PVEP to large check sizes in only 11% of their infants at 34 weeks of gestation.

PVEPs in preterm infants show a similar morphology to that of the full-term infant. The waveform morphology becomes more reproducible with larger check sizes and increasing gestational age. As in FVEPs, a gradual decrease in latency of the PVEP components is observed during development in preterm (Grose et al 1989) and in term infants (Kurtzberg & Vaughan 1985, McCulloch & Skarf 1991, Marg et al 1975).

Promising results considering the establishment of cortical visual maturation have been obtained by Mercuri et al (1998) and Braddick et al (2005), who used a combination of orientation reversal VEP, which is a pure cortical property and can be obtained from 6 weeks postnatally using slow reversal rates, and phase reversal VEP, which requires a lesser degree of cortical maturation and is already present at birth.

SOMATOSENSORY EVOKED POTENTIALS (SEPS)

SEPs are technically the most difficult to perform and more time-consuming, compared to the auditory brain stem evoked responses and VEPs and they require sophisticated electronic equipment. Following the sensory stimulus, usually to the median nerve or the posterior tibial nerve, a series of positive and negative potentials can be detected and measured. The main neuraxis of the tract from periphery to cortex contains the peripheral nerve, brachial plexus, dorsal root, posterior column, cuneate nucleus and, following decussation, medial lemniscus, thalamus and parietal cortex. After median nerve stimulation, the first negative wave, which can be recorded from an electrode placed over the Erb point (brachial plexus), is the N9. Negative waves N11 and N13 can be measured over the lower cervical vertebrae. At the scalp, contralateral to the site of stimulation and overlying the primary somatosensory cortex, wave N19 is recorded, which is considered to be cortically generated. In the newborn this component is usually referred to as the N1.

There has been a lot of discussion about the origin of the N1. According to Chiappa (1985) the component is partially derived from the thalamus. Using principal component analysis, Karniski (1992) was, however, able to show in preterm infant, that the N1 represents a tangential dipole located in the postcentral gyrus. In adults the N19 is followed by a positive component, the P22. This component is usually not yet present in the preterm infant, but can be present at term age. Following stimulation of the posterior tibial nerve, N19 and P22 can be recorded over the lumbar spine. The P35 is recorded over the somatosensory cortex.

SEPs are usually elicited following an electrical stimulus applied over the median or the posterior tibial nerve (Fig. 12.8). Stimulation of the median nerve is better tolerated than stimulation of the posterior tibial nerve. The newborn infant can be tested without the use of sedation following a feed. The cortical SEP after median nerve stimulation has been found to be dependent upon the state of alertness (Bongers-Schokking et al 1989, Desmedt & Manil 1970, Laget 1982). George and Taylor (1991) showed longer latencies and lower amplitudes of the cortical median nerve SEP with deep sleep. Klimach and Cooke (1988a), White and Cooke (1989) and Pike et al (1997) recorded all of their preterm SEPs whilst the babies were asleep.

The negative electrode is placed over the somatosensory area for the upper extremities on C3', which is 2 cm posterior to C3 in the 10–20 system, or over pCz-L/R, just lateral to pCz for the posterior tibial nerve SEP. The reference electrode is placed in the midfrontal position on Fz and the neutral electrode on the lower arm.

MEDIAN NERVE SEPS

Some of the earlier studies of SEPs in neonates were unable to identify components in a percentage of normal infants

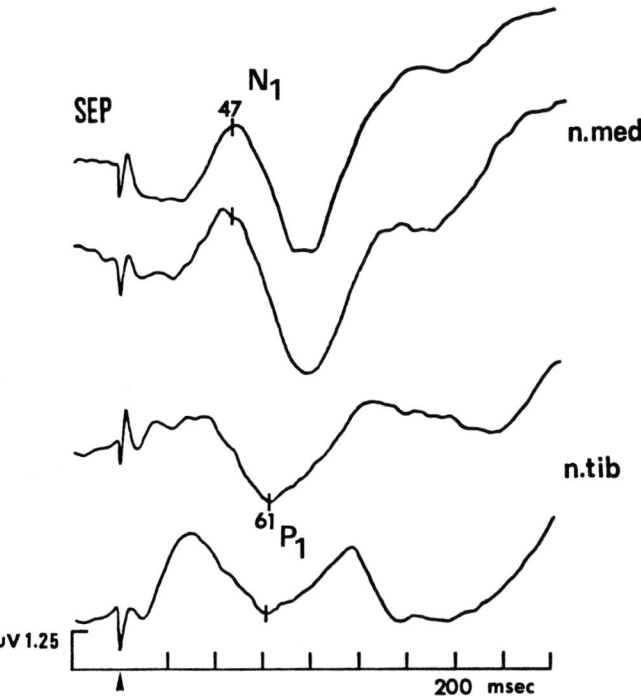

Figure 12.8 A normal response following stimulation of the median nerve (n. med) and posterior tibial nerve (n. tib) in a normal preterm infant with gestational age of 31 weeks. N1, first negative wave; P1, first positive wave; arrowhead, moment of stimulus. (Reproduced from Pierrat et al 1997.)

(15% in Laureau et al 1988, 30% in Willis et al 1984). This is mainly due to the fact that adult filter settings and stimulation rates were used. There is no agreement in the literature about stimulation rate and bandpass; however, studies using slow stimulation rates, long sweep times and lower filters appeared to be most successful in obtaining SEPs in infants (Araki et al 1999, Desmedt et al 1976, Laget et al 1976).

Bongers-Schokking et al (1989) investigated combinations of these factors and recommended a low bandpass (1–100 Hz) and few stimuli (25–50) for recording cortical SEPs. George and Taylor (1991) found two different bandpasses (5–1500 Hz, 30–3000 Hz) to be useful. Gibson et al (1992a) also recorded SEPs with a higher bandpass (10–3000 Hz). Scalais et al (1998) compared different filter settings and showed a longer latency of the N1 when a low bandpass (1–100 Hz) was used compared to a higher bandpass (30–3000 Hz). The impedance should be less than 2 K. Electrical stimuli of 0.1 ms in duration may be delivered at a rate of 0.5 Hz, using a hand-held device placed over the ventral wrist overlying the median nerve. The stimulation intensity needs to be higher than that used in children and adults in order to produce a motor response. It is now however widely accepted that, given modification in testing procedures, SEPs can be reliably recorded in all normal neonates.

It is possible to record SEPs in preterm neonates from 25 weeks gestational age onward (Karniski 1992, Klimach & Cooke 1988a, Taylor et al 1996a), using a low bandpass (1–100 Hz) and an analysis time between 100 and 500 ms. Taylor et al (1996a) were able to study very preterm infants (gestational age 27–32 weeks), with the first test being performed at an average of 5 days of age. Identifiable cortical SEPs were found in all cases studied by Taylor et al (1996a) but not in a small percentage of preterm infants (10–12%) studied by others (Karniski 1992, Klimach & Cooke 1988a).

In preterm neonates the latency of the cortical peaks decreases as the infants mature. At 27 weeks of gestational age the N1 has a latency of over 75 ms which decreased to the value observed in term neonates at 40 weeks postmenstrual age. No differences have been found between term and preterm infants tested at the same conceptional age (Karniski 1992, Klimach & Cooke 1988a, Taylor et al 1996a). Gibson et al (1992a) also reported increased waveform complexity with increasing gestational age. Karniski (1992), however, found that the late components and their scalp topography changed little over the preterm period except for the amplitude. Hrbek et al (1973) noted that the most prominent SEP response in preterm infants was a large amplitude slow wave. Recent studies by Kostovic (2006) have shed light on thalamo-cortical connections which pass through three stages. First thalamic axons form a dense synaptic network in the subplate, some weeks later thalamic fibers continue their growth from subplate to deep cortical layers. Finally these thalamic fibers reach into more superficial layers of the cortex. In a recent review by Vanhatalo and Lauronen (2006) it was suggested that the low response, first noted by Hrbek et al (1982), might provide clinically important information about the functional status of the subplate, which is believed to be crucial for thalamo-cortical connectivity. It should thus be kept in mind that SEPs in very preterm infants are responses following activation of the subplate and deep cortical layers, i.e. from transient structures during a period of rapid brain maturation.

POSTERIOR TIBIAL NERVE SEPS

Recording posterior tibial nerve SEPs was noted to be more difficult in neonates. Most of the studies reported difficulties in obtaining responses, with success rates varying between 55 and 73% (Gilmore et al 1987, Laureau & Marlot 1990). In preterm neonates, White and Cooke (1989), using a lower bandpass, as already described for median nerve SEPs, recorded SEPs following posterior tibial nerve stimulation in 93% of preterm neonates born between 26 and 41 weeks of gestational age. Good responses were also obtained by Pike et al (1997).

CLINICAL APPLICATIONS OF BAEPS AND MAXIMUM LENGTH SEQUENCE BAEPS

ASSESSMENT OF AUDIOLOGICAL DISORDERS
(see also Ch. 38)

When the diagnosis of congenital or perinatally acquired hearing loss is made before the age of 3 months, and treatment using amplification and communication therapy is started before the age of 6 months, there are better chances for language and speech development (Davis et al 1986, Markides 1986, Ramkalawan & Davis 1992, Yoshinaga-Itano 2003). As infants who have graduated from neonatal intensive care units have a higher prevalence of moderate-to-severe hearing impairment than healthy newborns, it is important to carry out screening during the neonatal period in those with risk factors associated with sensorineural and/or conductive hearing loss (Joint Committee on Infant Hearing 1994, Position Statement 1995, Uus and Bamford 2006).

BAEPs using broad-band clicks, either performed by a skilled technician using conventional equipment, or performed by a research nurse using automated equipment, is regarded as the most objective and reliable method of evaluating peripheral auditory function in neonates. A prolonged latency of wave I, associated with a normal I–V interpeak latency, is suggestive of an audiological abnormality, while a normal wave I latency, associated with a prolonged I–V interpeak latency, indicates a delay in central conduction time (Guinard et al 1988). When BAEP threshold abnormalities are found (i.e. absent responses at 30–40 dBnHL at term age), the test should be repeated 3 months later, preferably using frequency-specific and bone conduction BAEPs. Frequency-specific techniques may be used to evaluate hearing thresholds at different frequencies, whereas bone conduction

BAEPs are useful to assess the extent of a conductive loss (Picton et al 1994).

ASSESSMENT OF OTHER DISORDERS
Prediction of outcome in high-risk neonates

Given that BAEPs assess the integrity of the ascending neuraxis projecting through the brainstem, abnormalities may reflect more diffuse injury to the CNS structures along the auditory pathway (Jewett & Williston 1971). This assumption has instigated several attempts to correlate neonatal BAEP with neurologic outcome. The results of these studies are not always in agreement, possibly because of significant variations in the methodology used and the different samples tested. In high-risk infants it is recommended to perform BAEPs as close to discharge as possible. Both peripheral and central abnormalities may be transient and will have resolved at term age in a number of cases, thus increasing the positive predictive power for the development of neurologic sequelae (Stockard et al 1983).

FULL-TERM INFANTS

HYPOXIC–ISCHEMIC ENCEPHALOPATHY (see Ch. 26)

A mixture of BAEP abnormalities can be found following perinatal asphyxia (elevated response threshold, increased wave latencies and interpeak intervals, reduced wave amplitudes and decreased V/I amplitude ratios) (Hecox & Cone 1981, Jiang et al 1998). In a study by Jiang et al (1998) a reduction in amplitude of wave V was found to be the main abnormality. These are signs of increased central conduction time (for a review of 32 studies, see Murray et al 1985). A study of 56 very low birth weight infants showed that bilateral abnormalities in predischarge BAEPs were predictive of subsequent performance on measures of intelligence quotient, language and reading at the age of 8 years, whereas there was no correlation with unilateral BAEP abnormalities (Cox et al 1992). Using different repetition rates, Jiang et al (2001, 2004a) showed that a click rate of 91/sec improved detection of hypoxia–ischemic brainstem impairment mainly manifesting as an abnormal reduction of wave V amplitude. Using MLS-BAEPs, Jiang et al (2000, 2003) showed dynamic changes during the first month after birth using higher click rates (91–910/s): wave III and V latencies, as well as I–V interpeak intervals, increased over the first few days to finally normalize by day 30 (Fig. 12.9).

BAEPS IN MYELOMENINGOCELE (Ch. 44)

In infants with myelomeningocele, often associated with Arnold–Chiari malformation, the BAEPs may have predictive power as to the severity and emergency of clinical brainstem symptoms, as the brainstem is distorted and elongated due to the downward dislocation of the pons, medulla oblongata and the fourth ventricle. Many reports consider data in infants beyond the neonatal period: infants with normal BAEPs do not develop symptomatic Arnold–Chiari malformation, whereas abnormal BAEPs have been reported

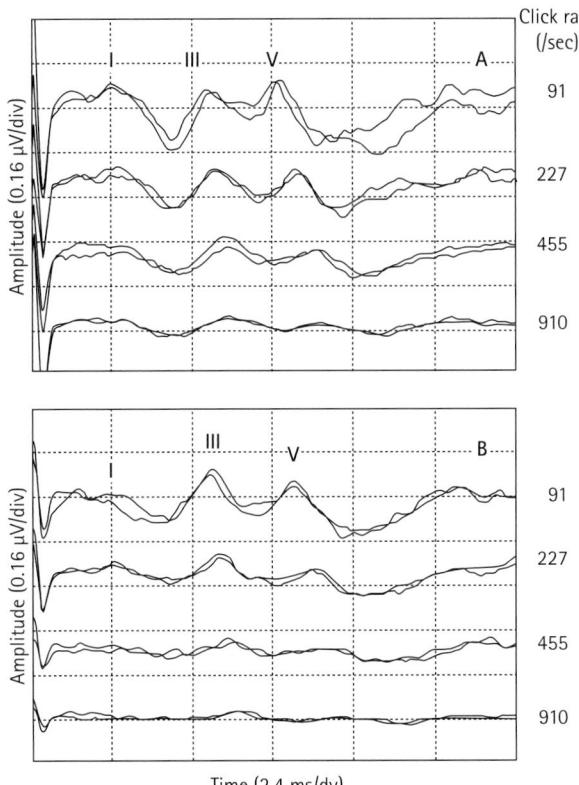

Figure 12.9 Maximum length sequence brainstem auditory evoked potential responses in term neonates who have perinatal hypoxia–ischemia. MLS-BAEP in a normal term neonate (a) and a term neonate with HIE (b). (From Jiang Z D 2000 Pediatr Res 48: 639–645 with permission).

to be associated with neurologic symptoms. These findings were confirmed in neonates (Mori et al 1988, Taylor et al 1996b, Worley et al 1994).

BAEPS IN HYPERBILIRUBINEMIA (Ch. 37)

The major reason for performing BAEPs in infants with hyperbilirubinemia is the possibility to study the correlation of BAEP abnormalities with changes in bilirubin levels and thus assess the effect of exchange transfusions, keeping in mind that careful management of hyperbilirubinemia may reduce the incidence of sensorineural deafness. De Vries et al (1987b) found sensorineural deafness to be strongly associated with the duration of hyperbilirubinemia. Most abnormalities disappear when the serum bilirubin decreases (Hung 1989), but Soares did not find significant abnormalities in neonates sustaining either mild or severe hyperbilirubinemia (Soares et al 1989). This supports the hypothesis that additional risk factors like acidosis may be operating.

BAEPS IN EXTRACORPOREAL MEMBRANE OXYGENATION (ECMO)

A relatively new hazard in neonatology is the sequelae of ECMO, a rescue therapy in severe respiratory failure in term

neonates. Since hypoxia and ischemia are related to their underlying illness and the invasive ECMO-procedure, they are at risk of neurologic impairment and sensorineural deafness. Desai et al (1997) found a sensitivity of only 42% and a specificity of 76% for elevated thresholds in neonatal BAEP to predict subsequent hearing loss in a sample of 80 neonates. However, abnormal neonatal BAEPs increased the probability of developing a receptive language delay, even when the BAEP subsequently normalized. Their high abnormality rate may be due to the threshold criteria as to what is considered to be a normal BAEP. Other studies reported abnormal BAEPs in 16–75% of infants treated with ECMO, which was associated with either sensorineural hearing loss and/or developmental delay (Hofkosh et al 1991, Kawashiro 1994, Lasky et al 1998, Schumacher et al 1991). In the latter report it was striking that 7/9 ECMO survivors with hearing loss passed their newborn BAEP screen, although high false-negative rates were found in the other reports as well. The risk of progressive hearing loss warrants a repeated test at the age of 3–4 months (Desai et al 1997, Fligor et al 2005).

BAEPS IN CYTOMEGALOVIRUS (CMV) INFECTION (Ch. 31)

CMV infection is a well-known cause of severe neurologic handicap. Sensorineural hearing loss, especially when the infection occurs in early pregnancy, is well recognized, but hearing deficits and minor neurologic handicap may occur in late infections (Steinlin et al 1996). Barbi et al (2003) found that more than 40% of deafness cases with an unknown cause, needing rehabilitation, are caused by congenital CMV. Recent reports show that among children with documented asymptomatic congenital CMV, associated with hearing loss, further deterioration occurred in 50% or more of the cases; a delayed onset of sensorineural hearing loss was observed in 18%. Infants with symptomatic congenital CMV infection show an even higher and cumulating incidence of sensorineural hearing loss (Fowler et al 1997, 1999). This progressive nature of the hearing loss emphasizes the need for continued monitoring of the hearing status in these infants (Iwasaki et al 2007).

PRETERM INFANTS

BAEPS IN HEMORRHAGES AND HYDROCEPHALUS

There is discussion in the literature as to whether BAEP latencies change in infants with periventricular and/or intraventricular hemorrhages (PVH/IVH). Beverley did not find significantly different latencies and amplitudes in preterm infants with severe PVH/IVH (Beverley et al 1990). Karmel found abnormal waveforms and prolonged latencies, but this study did not discriminate between hemorrhagic and/or ischemic lesions (Karmel et al 1988). Earlier, Fawer et al (1983) had found three of four preterm infants who were shunted for post-hemorrhagic hydrocephalus to have shortened interpeak latencies. Other groups studying infants with hydrocephalus reported a decrease of the wave V:I amplitude ratio associated with elevated thresholds (Edwards et al 1985, Lary et al 1989).

EFFECT OF INTRAUTERINE GROWTH RESTRICTION ON BAEPS

Considering the effects of intrauterine growth restriction (IUGR) on BAEPs, infants who were small for gestational age showed shorter wave V latencies and interpeak latencies relative to those appropriate for gestational age infants (Eldredge & Salamy 1996, Pettigrew et al 1985). These studies lend support to the view that infants with IUGR show accelerated neurologic maturation, but Soares posed the idea that the changes may be due to immaturity of the basal cochlea (Soares et al 1992).

Sarda et al (1992) compared the BAEPs of IUGR infants born to hypertensive and non-hypertensive mothers. IUGR infants of the hypertensive mothers showed significantly shortened interpeak latencies. These authors suggest that the reduced interpeak latencies may have been caused by a change in the development of neurotransmitters and catecholaminergic systems due to a major chronic stress. Jiang et al (2004b) used different repetition rates and found no major changes using BAEPs up to 91/sec clicks but a slight increase in III-V interval at high rate stimulation suggesting a subtle degree of central neural dysfunction or developmental delay.

CLINICAL APPLICATIONS OF VISUAL EVOKED POTENTIALS

ASSESSMENT OF OPHTHALMOLOGIC DISORDERS (see also Ch. 37)

The development of visual function is usually not the major concern for infants in the neonatal intensive care unit, although early application of rehabilitation programs may reduce the consequences of a visual handicap. However, when the infant has stabilized, there are several possibilities to obtain information about the visual system (Ricci et al 2007). Absence of fixation and following, absent blink reflex, or nystagmus may indicate disturbance of vision and these require further investigation. Although FVEPs are not suitable for measurement of visual acuity, they may be used to test the light sensitivity of the visual system, even when ophthalmologic disorders such as congenital cataract or optic nerve hypoplasia are present. PVEPs are a sensitive and quantitative indicator of lesions in the visual pathway and have the advantage that they show less intra- and inter-subject variability of latency and waveform than do FVEPs. The use of a psychophysical method like the acuity card procedure (McDonald et al 1985), which can easily be performed in stable, alert neonates, in combination with a VEP-modality may be very useful, for example, in infants with delayed visual maturation (Lambert et al 1989, Russell-Eggitt et al 1998).

FVEPS AS PREDICTOR FOR CEREBRAL VISUAL IMPAIRMENT

FVEPs are good predictors of cerebral visual impairment (CVI) following perinatal asphyxia as shown by McCulloch and Skarf (1991), Wong (1991) and McCulloch and Taylor (1992), who reported a strong association between neonatal FVEPs and visual outcome at 2.5–4.5 years. Others found a high predictive value of abnormal or absent FVEPs for the development of CVI in infants who showed extensive cystic leukomalacia on cranial ultrasound (de Vries et al 1987a), especially when this was associated with abnormal findings using the acuity card procedure (Eken et al 1996).

ASSESSMENT OF OTHER DISORDERS
Prediction of outcome in high-risk neonates

From the late 1970s onward, several authors assessed the predictive value of FVEPs for neurodevelopmental outcome in neonates. The first reports, however, did not make a distinction between term and preterm infants, but assessed heterogeneous groups of high-risk infants including those who had sustained asphyxia, respiratory distress, neurologic disorders, etc. Permanent VEP-abnormalities at repeated investigations were considered to be a serious prognostic sign in 57 term and preterm newborns with different degrees of perinatal asphyxia studied by Hrbek et al (1977). However, no correlation could be drawn between FVEPs and long-term prognosis, given that the serial examinations were conducted over a 3-week period. Hakamada et al (1981) studied BAEPs and FVEPs in 41 infants with a gestational age of 36–41 weeks who had various perinatal disorders, including 21 infants with perinatal asphyxia, during the first year of life. Absent responses or abnormal waveforms were associated with severe neurologic damage. In infants with cerebral palsy or mental retardation, initially abnormal VEPs recovered within 2–3 months of age.

PRETERM INFANTS

Several studies have shown variable associations between abnormal FVEPS in the neonatal period and abnormal neurological outcome (Beverley et al 1990, Häkkinen et al 1987, Placzek et al 1985, Pryds & Greisen 1990).

Ekert et al (1997a) were not able to predict abnormal developmental outcome in 123 preterm infants on the basis of abnormal FVEPs. Although there was a significant association between abnormal VEPs and PVL ($P < 0.04$) false positive recordings were twice as frequent as true positive recordings. In a study of 81 preterm infants, a sensitivity and specificity of 60% and 92% respectively were found for abnormal FVEPs in the subsequent development of cerebral palsy (Shepherd et al 1999). A delayed negative wave N300 before term and an absent positive wave P200 at term age were associated with adverse outcome.

Pike and Marlow (2000) studied 92 preterm infants ≤ 32 weeks gestation on day 5 and before discharge. FVEPS predicted cerebral palsy with a sensitivity of 71% and a specificity of 90%. Kato et al (2000) made very similar observations in 60 preterm infants (sensitivity 78%, specificity 94%).

Kato et al (2005) did a longitudinal study in 14 preterm infants with cystic periventricular leukomalacia. Several FVEPS were performed over a 3-week period showing loss of the response in 13/14 infants. Changes from normal to abnormal were observed during the first 10 days after birth.

EFFECT OF IUGR ON FVEPS

FVEPs have been used widely to assess the influence of IUGR on the development of the nervous system, but the results are not always in agreement. Watanabe et al (1972) and Pryds et al (1989) compared the FVEPs of appropriate for gestational age (AGA) infants and small for gestational age (SGA) infants and noted no differences in latencies and waveforms. In contrast, Hrbek et al (1982) reported a tendency towards longer latencies in SGA infants. They also noted late slow waves, which they attributed to neurologic immaturity. On the other hand, Petersen et al (1990) found shorter latencies in SGA infants, which they attributed to the smaller head circumference rather than to stress-induced maturation. Stanley et al (1991) reported normal short latency components and delayed long latency negative components and suggested that IUGR may affect the development of secondary activity in the striate cortex.

FVEPS IN INFANT RESPIRATORY DISTRESS SYNDROME

Small groups of infants who sustained severe respiratory disorders were studied (Gambi et al 1980, Graziani et al 1972, Pryds et al 1989), showing decreased amplitudes or even complete loss of VEPs during periods of severe hypoxemia with good recovery in most following resuscitation.

FVEPS AND DIETARY LONG-CHAIN POLYUNSATURATED FATTY ACIDS

Over the last few years attention has been drawn to the influence of dietary long-chain polyunsaturated fatty acids (LCP) on the rapid maturation of the nervous system and photoreceptors. Preterm infants may be LCP-deficient, and both FVEPs and PVEPs have been used to assess the effect of LCP suppletion. Faldella et al (1996) found morphological differences and significantly longer latencies in infants who were fed on traditional preterm formula, as compared to infants who were fed on breast milk or a preterm formula supplemented with LCP. Makrides et al (1995) found higher PVEP acuities in breast-fed and LCP supplemented formula-fed infants at 16 and 30 weeks of age, than in traditional formula-fed infants. However, it still has to be determined whether these changes are transient (Neuringer et al 1994). FVEPs were also assessed in the study of Auestad et al (1997) and no effect of supplementation was found at any time point over the first year. This contrasts with the study of Birch et al (1998) where VEP acuity was better in the supplemented group compared with the control group at 6 weeks,

4 and 12 months but not at 6 months. Van Wezel-Meijler et al (2002) randomized 42 formula-fed preterm infants and studied the progress of myelination, mental and motor development and latencies of visual evoked potentials. None of these measurements were positively influenced by supplementation of long-chain polyunsaturated fatty acids. At each test age, visual acuity was slightly better in the supplemented infants than in the non-supplemented infants, but the difference never reached statistical significance.

TERM INFANTS

In groups of term infants, very high correlations of FVEP and outcome was found (Scalais et al 1998, Taylor et al 1992). This was especially reported by Taylor's group, who found a high correlation of FVEPs with neurodevelopmental outcome in several groups of full-term asphyxiated infants studied from birth to 24 months of age (McCulloch et al 1991, Muttitt et al 1991, Taylor et al 1992, Whyte et al 1986). Repeated FVEPs were recorded during the first week of life. Absent FVEPs, and persistently abnormal FVEPs predicted an abnormal outcome. Normal FVEPs before the end of the first week had an accuracy rate of 87% for a normal outcome for the whole group and up to 93% for infants who sustained HIE Sarnat stage II. When comparing SEPs with VEPs, the VEPs appeared to be more resistant to an insult than SEPs, as normal VEPs were not always associated with a normal outcome. The association of SEPs and VEPs increases the prognostic reliability. Eken et al (1995) studied 34 full-term asphyxiated infants within the first six hours of life, to be able to select infants at risk of developing a major handicap who might benefit from treatment with neuro-protective agents. FVEPs were found to have a lower predictive value (PPV 77%) than did cerebral function monitoring (PPV 84.2%) and SEPs (PPV 81.8%) at this early stage.

We compared the predictive value of SEPs and VEPs for adverse neurologic outcome in all stages of HIE (Table 12.5), and separately for HIE stage II (Table 12.6), as prediction of outcome in this subgroup is more difficult than in either stages I or III. The predictive value in HIE stage II is lower than in the group as a whole. SEPs predict adverse outcome better than VEPs.

Table 12.5 Predictive value (%) of SEPs and VEPs on days 1 and 3 for adverse neurologic outcome in all stages of HIE				
Stage I-II-III	SEP		VEP	
	Day 1 (126)	Day 3 (82)	Day 1 (126)	Day 3 (82)
Sensitivity	90	87	90	78
Specificity	78	91	64	77
PPV	80	83	70	70
NPV	89	91	87	84

PPV, positive predictive value; NPV, negative predictive value.

Table 12.6 Predictive value (%) of SEP and VEP on days 1 and 3 in stage II HIE				
Stage II	SEP		VEP	
	Day 1 (43)	Day 3 (47)	Day 1 (43)	Day 3 (47)
Sensitivity	80	77	70	69
Specificity	70	85	61	73
PPV	44	67	35	50
NPV	92	91	87	86

PPV, positive predictive value; NPV, negative predictive value.

FVEPS IN HYDROCEPHALUS (Ch. 42)

Ehle and Sklar (1979) found delayed latencies, fatigability and asymmetries in 15 infants with documented hydrocephalus. The abnormalities improved in the post-shunt period, whereas VEPs worsened in cases of clinical progression of the hydrocephalus. Significant changes in the maturation curve of the P200 latency were noted by Guthkelch et al (1982, 1984), particularly when the hydrocephalus was associated with an enlarged head or with infection. However, Placzek et al (1985) found no relation between the presence of ventricular dilatation and the delay in maturation of the FVEPs. In infants who were successfully shunted, FVEP abnormalities improved rapidly, although the abnormalities did not correlate with head circumference or clinical status (George & Taylor 1987, Taylor 1992, see also Fig. 12.10). FVEP was not found to be a valuable prognostic tool for neurologic outcome in infants with myelomeningocele (Taylor et al 1996b).

FVEPS IN HYPERBILIRUBINEMIA

Usually, BAEPs are recorded in infants with hyperbilirubinemia. However, Chen and Kang (1995) studied the effect of hyperbilirubinemia on serial visual evoked potentials up to 8 weeks after birth and found prolonged latencies and lower amplitudes in the infants with moderate or severe hyperbilirubinemia. In a later study they suggested that the effects of hyperbilirubinemia on visual evoked potentials might be transient (Chen & Wong 2006).

FVEPS IN SUBSTANCE USE

The effect of prenatal substance use on FVEPs was investigated by Scher et al (1998). Maternal alcohol use during the first trimester was associated with prolonged positive wave P200 latencies at 1 month of age, while tobacco use in any trimester was associated with prolonged P200 latencies at birth and at 18 months.

CLINICAL APPLICATIONS OF SOMATOSENSORY EVOKED POTENTIALS

As there is a close proximity between the somatosensory and motor tracts, it was expected that abnormal SEPs in the

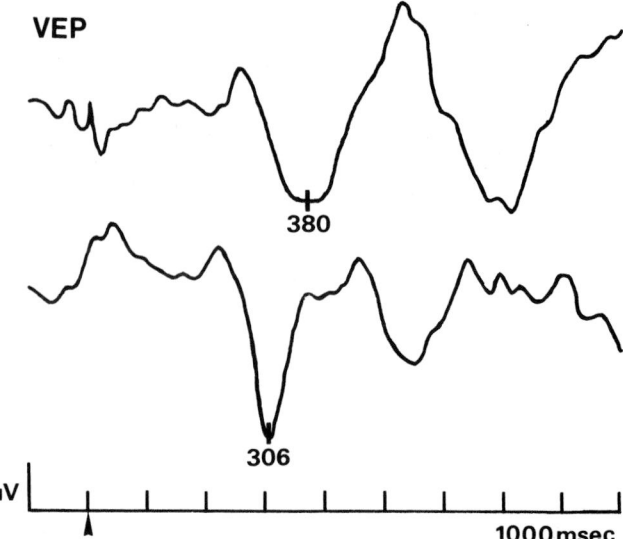

Figure 12.10 FVEPs in a preterm infant born at 28 weeks gestational age, who showed a large grade III hemorrhage with subsequent development of a large porencephalic cyst and posthemorrhagic ventricular dilatation on cranial ultrasound. At 30 weeks gestational age, a Rickham reservoir was inserted and cerebrospinal fluid was removed twice daily. FVEPs were recorded before the insertion of the reservoir, showing a broad and delayed N300 (upper trace) and 2 weeks later, showing normalization of the N300 (lower trace). Arrowhead, moment of stimulus.

neonatal period would be most predictive for an abnormal neurodevelopment.

PRETERM INFANTS
Intracranial lesions

SEPs have been used in preterm babies to identify children at risk of adverse neurologic sequelae. Klimach and Cooke (1988b) found a close relation between SEPs recorded around term and the outcome at 6–16 months. In this study the SEP findings at discharge were more predictive of outcome than those at the first test. All children with bilateral abnormalities in negative wave N1 latency had a developmental delay. Majnemer et al (1987, 1990) presented data of 34 low birth weight infants and those with an absent or persistently delayed N1 latency were found to have a major handicap. At reassessment aged 5 years of age they showed a high sensitivity (100%) and specificity (80%) for early SEP in relation to the long-term outcome (Majnemer & Rosenblatt 1995). Willis et al (1989) studied 39 very low birth weight preterm infants with periventricular hemorrhage at 2, 4 and 6 months of age corrected for prematurity. A delayed N1 latency was predictive of an abnormal outcome but a single normal SEP predicted normal motor development in only 19 of 36 infants. Scalais et al (1992) studied VEPs and SEPs in preterm neonates suffering from perinatal asphyxia and demonstrated a good correlation between VEPs and SEPs and subsequent neurologic outcome.

In a larger series, de Vries et al (1992), found SEPs recorded around term in preterm babies to be less reliable than cranial ultrasonography. A normal N1 latency was no guarantee of a normal outcome as 14 of the 25 infants who developed cerebral palsy had a normal N1 latency at, or even before, 40 weeks postmenstrual age. Pierrat et al (1993) studied 33 infants with extensive cystic leukomalacia: 27 had cysts in the periventricular white matter and 6 developed extensive cysts in the deep white matter. All but two of the 27 surviving infants had a reproducible N1 at discharge; in only 11 was it delayed and normal in 14 infants. No N1 peak could be recorded in any of the infants with cysts in the deep white matter. All surviving infants developed cerebral palsy, irrespective of the N1 latency.

Ekert et al (1997b) hypothesized that SEPs performed at a very early stage would be more predictive than SEPs performed at discharge, and therefore studied 88 preterm infants twice during their first 3 weeks of life. They were able to show a significant correlation between the early SEP appearance and subsequent development of cerebral palsy, but found a high number of false positives. In this study SEPs were less accurate than cranial ultrasound in the prediction of cerebral palsy. However, a normal early SEP, even in the presence of periventricular echogenicity on ultrasound, predicted a normal outcome in all but 1 of the 9 cases.

As preterm infants tend to develop spastic diplegia rather than quadriplegia, it was subsequently hypothesized that posterior tibial nerve SEPs would be more predictive than median nerve SEPs. White and Cooke (1994) were the first to test this hypothesis in preterm infants. They were indeed able to show a highly significant relation between bilaterally abnormal posterior tibial nerve SEPs and the presence of cerebral palsy at 3 years of age in a group of 50 neonates at risk of future neurodevelopmental impairment. Normal posterior tibial nerve SEPs were associated with a normal outcome in 24 of 25 infants. In this group of neonates posterior tibial nerve SEPs were more predictive of outcome than late cranial ultrasonography. Pierrat et al (1997) subsequently compared the predictive value of SEPs following stimulation of both the median as well as the posterior tibial nerve with that of cranial ultrasound in 39 preterm infants. A normal posterior tibial nerve response almost guaranteed a normal outcome, but the test was very time-consuming and the number of false positives was very high (sensitivity 95.6%, specificity 50%). The presence of a parenchymal lesion on ultrasound predicted cerebral palsy with a sensitivity of 95.6% and a specificity of 68.5%. The combination of an abnormal posterior tibial response and the presence of parenchymal brain lesions had the best predictive value, with a sensitivity of 91.3% and a specificity of 81.2%.

HYDROCEPHALUS

George and Taylor (1987) recorded VEPs and median nerve SEPs in hydrocephalic neonates of less than 10 weeks of age and found that 83% had abnormal VEPs while less than half had abnormal SEPs. No correlation was found in this study between EP abnormalities and head circumference or clinical status, but the abnormalities improved dramatically within days of shunting in those infants in whom the shunting procedure was successful. De Vries et al (1990) were able to show a decrease in N1 latency within 1 week following shunt insertion in 7 cases.

HYPOTHYROIDISM

Smit et al (1998) measured median nerve SEPs in 200 preterm infants (gestational age <30 weeks) who were randomized to receive thyroxine or a placebo during the first 6 weeks of life. SEPs were recorded at 2 weeks of age, at term and at 6 months corrected age. No effect of thyroxine administration was noted on the N1 latency.

SMALL FOR GESTATIONAL AGE

Only a few studies have so far looked at the influence of IUGR on SEPs. Kjellmer et al (1992) recorded SEPs and VEPs in a group of SGA infants. A high frequency of abnormal recordings was obtained in SGA babies and they had significantly longer latency periods for the primary SEPs than appropriately grown controls. Pierrat et al (1996), performing median nerve SEPs in a large cohort of SGA preterm neonates, found a persistently delayed N1 latency in 25 out of 56 infants. None of these infants had ultrasound abnormalities and none developed cerebral palsy at follow-up. There was a trend for a higher developmental quotient in the infants with a normal SEP, but this did not reach statistical significance.

FULL-TERM INFANTS

Birth asphyxia (Ch. 26)

Hrbek et al (1977) were the first to investigate the value of median nerve SEPs as a means of assessing cortical damage and predicting outcome in the asphyxiated newborn. In this study, however, neonates and infants were included. Asphyxia was defined according to Apgar score only and the duration of follow-up was variable. Lütschg et al (1983), Majnemer et al (1987) and Willis et al (1987) reported SEPs to be reliable predictors of neurologic outcome in term and preterm infants but recorded SEPs after the early neonatal period. Gibson et al (1992b) recorded SEPs during the first week of life in a population of term asphyxiated neonates. They found that the sensitivity of SEPs for adverse outcome was 100% with a specificity of 76%. De Vries (1993, De Vries 1991) demonstrated that the predictive value of median nerve SEPs was better after the first few days of life. On day 3, SEPs had a sensitivity and a specificity of 89.6% and 86% respectively, and at discharge the value of both sensitivity and specificity was 91%. Others studied the prognostic value of multimodality evoked potentials in asphyxiated babies. Taylor et al (1992) recorded SEPs and VEPs several times in the first week and found SEPs to be more variable than VEPs but stated that normal SEPs in the first week were virtually always associated with a normal neurologic outcome (Fig. 12.11a).

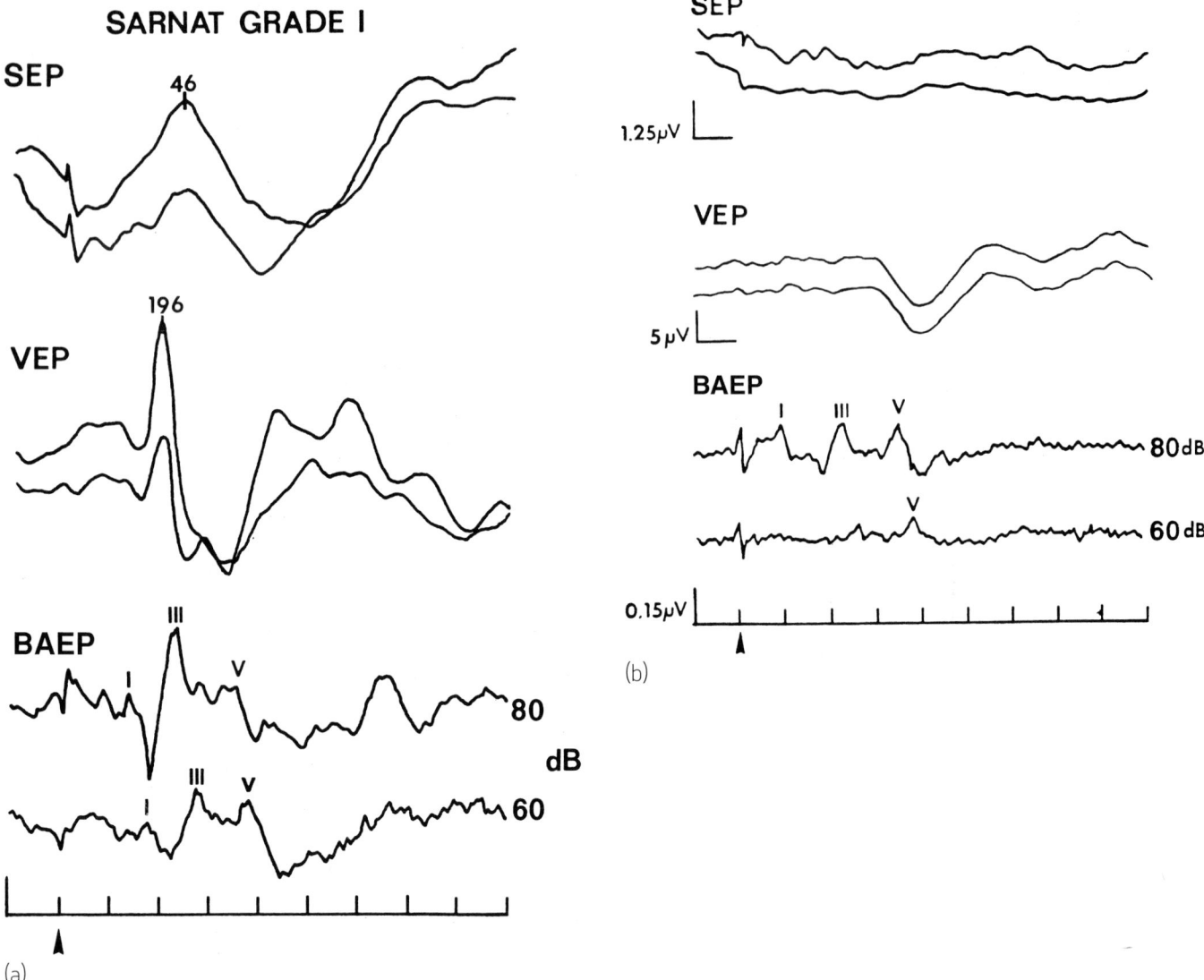

Figure 12.11 Effects of HIE on evoked potentials. (a) Normal SEP, FVEP and BAEP on day 3 in a full-term infant with HIE stage I. Subsequent neurodevelopmental outcome was normal. (b) Absent SEP, delayed latencies and abnormal waveform in the FVEP and increased threshold in the BAEP on day 3 in a full-term infant with HIE stage III. The infant subsequently died. Arrowheads, moments of stimuli.

Consistently abnormal SEPs were associated with a poor neurologic outcome in 85% of the cases (Fig. 12.11b). Scalais et al (1998) recorded SEPs and VEPs in a group of 40 term infants with perinatal asphyxia. SEPs and VEPs demonstrated a good correlation with neurodevelopmental outcome, but SEPs proved to be superior to VEPs with an accuracy of 96% for SEPs and 86% for VEPs. A combination of the two techniques gave a higher predictive power; abnormal SEPs and VEPs were also more accurate in prediction of neurologic outcome compared with the Sarnat score. Of the 24 infants with a Sarnat stage II hypoxic–ischemic encephalopathy (HIE), 5 had a normal outcome and all had a normal SEP, while none of the 18 with a mild (3), moderate (4), or severe (11) handicap had a normal SEP within the first 72 hours of life. We also calculated the predictive value of SEPs and VEPs in HIE stage II on day 1 and day 3, but found lower predictive values than Scalais et al (Table 12.6).

Most of these studies were performed beyond the first 24–48 hours (de Vries et al 1991, 1993, Gibson et al 1992b, Hrbek et al 1977, Taylor et al 1992). With the introduction of medical intervention trials, selection of infants who might benefit from early intervention should be carried out as soon as possible after delivery. Eken et al (1995) therefore decided to study 34 full-term infants with HIE within 6 hours after delivery. Besides SEPs they also performed cranial ultrasonography, the resistance index of the middle cerebral artery, obtained with Doppler ultrasonography, VEPs and amplitude integrated EEG (aEEG) (see p. 557) recordings. The SEP and the aEEG had the best predictive value, with the SEP being slightly more predictive compared with the VEP. As might

Table 12.7 Predictive values of different tests in infants with HIE and <6 h of age (n = 34) (Eken et al 1995)

	US	RI	SEP	VEP	CFM
Sensitivity	42	24	95	89	94
Specificity	60	100	73	67	79
PPV	57	100	82	77	84
NPV	45	54	92	83	92

US: ultrasound; RI: resistance index; CFM: cerebral function monitor; PPV: positive predictive value; NPV: negative predictive value.

be expected, the role of cranial ultrasound and Doppler studies was very limited at this early stage. As the aEEG is a quicker and easier tool to use, this technique is now mainly used to select infants (Table 12.7).

Hypothyroidism

Bongers-Schokking et al (1991) studied SEPs in neonates with primary congenital hypothyroidism during the first week of therapy. A maturational delay was found for all SEP parameters in neonates with congenital hypothyroidism. However, a delay of the N1 latency was not related to the initial T4 level or to the T4 level at the time of examination. The comparison of the results of the SEPs with bone age suggested that SEPs are superior to bone age as a parameter for the evaluation of neurologic maturation in infants with congenital hypothyroidism.

HYPERBILIRUBINEMIA (Ch. 36)

Neonatal hyperbilirubinemia can lead to serious neurologic sequelae and auditory impairment (Johnston et al 1967). However, the toxicity of bilirubin on the neonatal CNS depends on many factors and outcome cannot be accurately predicted. One study (Bongers-Schokking et al 1990) investigated SEPs in normal term neonates with neonatal jaundice, on the day the highest bilirubin values were reached, 2–3 days later, and at 5 weeks. In this study the central conduction time correlated positively with the bilirubin level, and both the peripheral and the central components of the SEPs were affected by neonatal jaundice. Full recovery was not yet obtained at 5 weeks. They suggested the use of SEPs to monitor daily the effect of bilirubin on the CNS.

Table 12.8 Summary of the clinical value of EPs in management of neonates

BAEPs	Reliable in screening for hearing loss in high-risk neonates Record as near to term as possible Repeat at 3 months post-term Predictive value for subsequent neurological outcome both in term and preterm infants is limited
VEPs	Most convenient of the EPs to perform Poor predictor of outcome in preterm infants (FVEPs identify infants with extensive cystic PVL likely to develop cortical visual impairment) High predictive value for adverse outcome in asphyxiated full-term infants (abnormal or absent VEPs)
SEPs	Highest predictive value for adverse outcome in asphyxiated full-term infants May predict cerebral palsy in infants with preterms with PVL (only when recorded in the second week of life) Posterior tibial nerve SEPs are difficult to record, but may be better predictor of outcome in PVL than median nerve SEP

HYPOGLYCEMIA (Ch. 35)

There is controversy over both the definition of hypoglycemia in neonates and children and its significance when there are no symptoms. Koh et al (1988) measured EPs, either SEPs or BAEPs, in relation to blood glucose concentration in 17 neonates and infants. With hypoglycemia they were able to show that the latency to the peak of N1 became prolonged and that the waveform was less well defined. They concluded that the blood glucose concentration should be maintained above 2.6 mmol/L to ensure normal EP function in children, irrespective of the presence or absence of abnormal clinical signs.

CONCLUSIONS

A summary of the clinical value of EPs is shown in Table 12.8.

REFERENCES

al Naqeeb N, Edwards A D, Cowan F, Azzopardi D 1999 Assessment of neonatal encephalopathy by amplitude integrated electroencephalography. Pediatrics 103:1263–1271.

AlOtaibi S F, Blaser S, MacGregor D L 2005 Neurological complications of kernicterus. Can J Neurol Sci 32:311–315.

Als H, Duffy F H, McAnulty G B et al 2004 Early experience alters brain function and structure. Pediatrics 113:846–857.

Apkarian P, Mirmiran M, Tijssen R 1991 Effects of behavioural state on visual processing in neonates. Neuropediatrics 22:85–91.

Araki A, Takada A, Yasuhara A, Kobayashi Y 1999 The effects of stimulus rates on the amplitude of median nerve somatosensory evoked potentials: the developmental change. Brain Dev 21:118–121.

Aso K, Abdad-Barmada M, Scher M S 1993 EEG and the neuropathology in premature neonates with

intraventricular hemorrhage. J Clin Neurophysiol 10:304–313.

Auestad N, Montalto M B, Hall R T et al 1997 Visual acuity, erythrocyte fatty acid composition, and growth in term infants fed formulas with long chain polyunsaturated fatty acids for one year. Ross Pediatric Lipid Study. Pediatr Res 41:1–10.

Barbi M, Binda S, Caroppo S et al 2003 A wider role for congenital cytomegalovirus infection in sensorineural hearing loss. Pediatr Infect Dis J 22(1):39–42.

Baud O, d'Allest A M, Lacaze-Masmonteil T et al 1998 The early diagnosis of periventricular leukomalacia in premature infants with positive rolandic sharp waves on serial electroencephalography. J Pediatr 132:813–817.

Bell A H, Greisen G, Pryds O 1993 Comparison of the effects of phenobarbitone and morphine administration on EEG activity in preterm babies. Acta Paediatr 82:35–39.

Bell A H, McClure B G, Hicks E M 1990 Power spectral analysis of the EEG of term infants following birth asphyxia. Dev Med Child Neurol 32:990–998.

Bell A H, McClure B G, McCullagh P J, McClelland R J 1991a Variation in power spectral analysis of the EEG with gestational age. J Clin Neurophysiol 8:312–319.

Bell A H, McClure B G, McCullagh P J, McClelland R J 1991b Spectral edge frequency of the EEG in healthy neonates and variation with behavioural state. Biol Neonate 60:69–74.

Benavente I, Tamargo P, Tajada N et al 2005 Flash visually evoked potentials in the newborn and their maturation during the first six months of life. Doc Ophthalmol 110(2–3):255–263.

Beverley D W, Smith I S, Beesley P et al 1990 Relationship of cranial ultrasonography, visual and auditory evoked responses with neurodevelopmental outcome. Dev Med Child Neurol 32:210–222.

Biagioni E, Bartalena L, Biver P et al 1996 Electroencephalographic dysmaturity in preterm infants: a prognostic tool in the early postnatal period. Neuropediatrics 27:311–316.

Biagioni E, Bartalena L, Boldrini A et al 1994 Background EEG activity in preterm infants: correlation of outcome with selected maturational features. Electroencephalogr Clin Neurophysiol 91:154–162.

Biagioni E, Frisone M F, Laroche S et al 2007 Maturation of cerebral electrical activity and development of cortical folding in young very preterm infants. Clin Neurophysiol 118:53–59.

Birch E E, Birch D G, Petrig B, Uauy R 1990 Retinal and cortical function of very low birthweight infants at 36 and 57 weeks postconception. Clin Vis Sci 5:363–373.

Birch E E, Hoffman D, Uauy R et al 1998 Visual acuity and the essentiality of docosahexaenoic acid in the diet of term infants. Pediatr Res 44:201–209.

Bjerre I, Hellström-Westas L, Rosén I, Svenningsen N W 1983 Monitoring of cerebral function after severe birth asphyxia in infancy. Arch Dis Child 58:997–1002.

Bongers-Schokking C J, Colon E J, Hoogland R A et al 1989 The somatosensory evoked potentials of normal infants: influence of filter bandpass, arousal state and number of stimuli. Brain Dev 11:33–39.

Bongers-Schokking C J, Colon E J, Hoogland R A et al 1990 Somatosensory evoked potentials in neonatal jaundice. Acta Paediatr Scand 79:148–155.

Bongers-Schokking C J, Colon E J, Hoogland R A et al 1991 Somatosensory evoked potentials in neonates with primary congenital hypothyrodism during the first week of therapy. Pediatr Res 30:34–39.

Boylan G B, Rennie J M, Pressler R M et al 2002 Phenobarbitone, neonatal seizures, and video-EEG. Arch Dis Child Fetal Neonatal Ed 86:F165–170.

Braddick O, Birtles D, Wattam-Bell J, Atkinson J 2005 Motion- and orientation-specific cortical responses in infancy. Vision Res 45(25–26):3169–3179.

Brunquell P J, Glennon C M, DiMario F J et al 2002 Prediction of outcome based on clinical seizure type in newborn infants. J Pediatr 140:707–712.

Burdjalov V F, Baumgart S, Spitzer A R 2003 Cerebral function monitoring: A new scoring system for the evaluation of brain maturation in neonates. Pediatrics 112:855–861.

Bye A M, Flanagan D 1995 Spatial and temporal characteristics of neonatal seizures. Epilepsia 36:1009–1016.

Chen W X, Wong V 2006 Visual evoked potentials in neonatal hyperbilirubinemia. J Child Neurol 21(1):58–62.

Chen Y J, Kang W M 1995 Effects of bilirubin on visual evoked potentials in term infants. Eur J Pediatr 154:662–666.

Chiappa K H 1985 Evoked potentials in clinical medicine: short latency somatosensory evoked potentials. In: Baker A B, Joynt R J (eds) Clinical neurology. JB Lippincott, Philadelphia, PA, pp. 26–55.

Chin K C, Taylor M J, Menzies R, Whyte H 1985 Development of visual evoked potentials in neonates. Arch Dis Child 60:1166–1168.

Clancy R R, Legido A 1987 The exact ictal and interictal duration of electroencephalographic neonatal seizures. Epilepsia 28:537–541.

Clancy R R, Legido A 1991 Postnatal epilepsy after EEG-confirmed neonatal seizures. Epilepsia 32:69–76.

Clancy R R, Legido A, Lewis D 1988 Occult neonatal seizures. Epilepsia 29:256–261.

Clancy R R, Sharif U, Ichord R et al 2005 Electrographic neonatal seizures after infant heart surgery. Epilepsia 46:84–90.

Clancy R R, Tharp B R, Enzman D 1984 EEG in premature infants with intraventricular hemorrhage. Neurology 34:583–590.

Collet L, Soares I, Morgon A, Salle B 1989 Is there a difference between extrauterine and intrauterine maturation on BAEP? Brain Dev 11:293–296.

Connell J A, Oozeer R, Dubowitz V 1987a Continuous 4-channel EEG monitoring: A guide to interpretation, with normal values, in preterm infants. Neuropediatrics 18:138–145.

Connell J, Oozeer R, de Vries L et al 1989 Clinical and EEG response to anticonvulsants in neonatal seizures. Arch Dis Child 64:459–464.

Connell J, Oozeer R, Regev R et al 1987b Continuous four-channel EEG monitoring in the evaluation of echodense ultrasound lesions and cystic leukomalacia. Arch Dis Child 62:1019–1024.

Cox C, Hack M, Aram D, Borawski E 1992 Neonatal auditory brainstem response failure of very low birth weight infants: 8-year outcome. Pediatr Res 31:68–72.

Cox L C, Martin R J, Carlo W A, Hack M 1993 Early ABRs in infants undergoing assisted ventilation. J Am Acad Audiol 4:13–17.

Davis J M, Elfenbein J, Schum R, Bentler R A 1986 Effects of mild and moderate hearing impairments on language, educational and psychosocial behavior of children. J Speech Hear Disord 51:53–62.

De Vries L S, Hellström-Westas L 2005 Role of cerebral function monitoring in the newborn. Arch Dis Child Fetal Neonatal Ed 90:F201–F207.

De Vries L S 1993 Somatosensory evoked potentials in term neonates with postasphyxial encephalopathy. Clin Perinatol 20:463–482.

De Vries L S, Connell J A, Dubowitz L M S et al 1987a Neurological, electrophysiological and MRI abnormalities in infants with extensive cystic leukomalacia. Neuropediatrics 18:61–66.

De Vries L S, Eken P, Pierrat V et al 1992 Prediction of neurodevelopmental outcome in the preterm infant: short latency cortical somatosensory evoked potentials compared with cranial ultrasound. Arch Dis Child 67:1177–1181.

De Vries L S, Lary S, Whitelaw A G, Dubowitz L M 1987b Relationship of serum bilirubin levels and hearing impairment in newborn infants. Early Hum Dev 15:269–277.

De Vries L S, Pierrat V, Eken P et al 1991 Predictive value of early somatosensory evoked potentials in full term infants with birth asphyxia. Brain Dev 13:320–325.

De Vries L S, Pierrat V, Minami T, Casaer P 1990 Short latency cortical somatosensory evoked potentials in infants with hydrocephalus. Neuropediatrics 21:136–139.

Delorme C, Collet L, Morgon A, Salle B 1986 Study of auditory evoked potentials in preterm newborns with same conceptional ages at birth. In: Gallai V (ed) Maturation of the CNS and evoked potentials. Elsevier, Amsterdam, pp. 352–355.

Desai S, Kollros P R, Graziani L J et al 1997 Sensitivity and specificity of the neonatal brain-stem auditory evoked potential for hearing and language deficits in survivors of extracorporeal membrane oxygenation. J Pediatr 131:233–239.

Desmedt J E, Brunko E, Debecker J 1976 Maturation of the somatosensory evoked potentials in normal infants and children with special reference to the early N1 component. Electroencephalogr Clin Neurophysiol 40:43–58.

Desmedt J E, Manil J 1970 Somatosensory evoked potentials of the normal human neonate in REM sleep, in slow wave sleep and waking. Electroencephalogr Clin Neurophysiol 29:113–126.

Despland P A 1985 Maturation changes in the auditory system as reflected in human brainstem evoked responses. Dev Neurosci 7:73–80.

Douglass L M, Wu J Y, Rosman N P, Stafstrom C E 2002 Burst suppression electroencephalogram pattern in the newborn: predicting the outcome. J Child Neurol 17:403–408.

Draganova R, Eswaran H, Murphy P et al 2007 Serial magnetoencephalographic study of fetal and newborn auditory discriminative evoked responses. Early Hum Dev 83:199–207.

Dubowitz L M S, Mushin J, de Vries L S, Arden G B 1986 Visual function in the newborn infant, is it cortically mediated? Lancet ii:1139–1141.

Eaton D G, Wertheim D, Oozeer R et al 1984 Reversible changes in cerebral activity associated with acidosis in preterm neonates. Acta Paediatr 83:486–492.

Edwards C G, Durieux-Smith A, Picton T W 1985 Auditory brainstem response audiometry in neonatal hydrocephalus. J Otolaryngol 14:40–46.

Eggermont J J, Salamy A 1988 Maturational time course for the ABR in preterm and fulterm infants. Hearing Res 33:35–48.

Ehle A, Sklar F 1979 Visual evoked potentials in infants with hydrocephalus. Neurology 29:1541–1544.

Eiselt M, Schindler J, Arnold M et al 2001 Functional interactions within the newborn brain investigated by adaptive coherence analysis of EEG. Neurophysiol Clin 31(2):104–113.

Eken P, de Vries L S, van Nieuwenhuizen O et al 1996 Early predictors of cerebral visual impairment in infants with cystic leukomalacia. Neuropediatrics 27:16–25.

Eken P, Toet M C, Groenendaal F, de Vries L S 1995 Predictive value of early neuroimaging, pulsed Doppler and neurophysiology in full term infants with hypoxic-ischaemic encephalopathy. Arch Dis Child 73:F75–F80.

Ekert P G, Keenan N K, Whyte H E et al 1997a Visual evoked potentials for prediction of neurodevelopmental outcome in preterm infants. Biol Neonate 71:148–155.

Ekert P G, Taylor M J, Keenan N K et al 1997b Early somatosensory evoked potentials in preterm infants: their prognostic utility. Biol Neonate 71:83–91.

Eldredge L, Salamy A 1996 Functional auditory development in preterm and fullterm infants. Early Hum Dev 45:215–228.

Ellingson R J 1960 Cortical electrical responses to visual stimulation in the human infant. Electroencephalogr Clin Neurophysiol 12:663–677.

Ellingson R J 1970 Variability of visual evoked responses in the human newborn. Electroencephalogr Clin Neurophysiol 29:10–19.

Eswaran H, Wilson J, Preissl H et al C 2002 Magnetoencephalographic recordings of visual evoked brain activity in the human fetus. Lancet 360:779–780.

Faldella G, Govoni M, Alessandroni R et al 1996 Visual evoked potentials and dietary long chain polyunsaturated fatty acids in preterm infants. Arch Dis Child 75:F108–F112.

Fanaroff A A, Stoll B J, Wright L L et al NICHD Neonatal Research Network 2007 Trends in neonatal morbidity and mortality for very low birthweight infants. Am J Obstet Gynecol 196(2):147.e1–e8.

Fawer C L, Dubowitz L M S 1982 Auditory brainstem response in neurologically normal preterm and full term infants. Neuropediatrics 13:200–206.

Fawer C L, Dubowitz L M S, Levene M I, Dubowitz V 1983 Auditory brainstem responses in neurologically abnormal infants. Neuropediatrics 14:88–92.

Ferrari F, Toricelli A, Giustardi A et al 1992 Bioelectric brain maturation in fullterm infants and in healthy and pathological preterm infans at term post-menstrual age. Early Hum Dev 28:37–63.

Fifer W P, Grieve P G, Grose-Fifer J et al 2006 High-density electroencephalogram monitoring in the neonate. Clin Perinatol 33:679–691.

Fligor B J, Neault M W, Mullen C H et al 2005 Factors associated with sensorineural hearing loss among survivors of extracorporeal membrane oxygenation therapy. Pediatrics 115(6):1519–1528.

Fowler K B, Dahle A J, Boppana S B, Pass R F 1999 Newborn hearing screening: will children with hearing loss caused by congenital cytomegalovirus infection be missed? J Pediatr 135:60–64.

Fowler K B, McCollister F P, Dahle A J et al 1997 Progressive and fluctuating sensorineural hearing loss in children with asymptomatic congenital cytomegalovirus infection. J Pediatr 130:624–630.

Fraser M, Bennet L, Gunning M et al 2005 Cortical electroencephalogram suppression is associated with post-ischemic cortical injury in 0.65 gestation fetal sheep. Brain Res Dev Brain Res 154:45–55.

Freeman J M 2007 The use of amplitude-integrated electroencephalography: beware of its unintended consequences. Pediatrics 119:615–617.

Gambi D, Rossini P M, Albertini G et al 1980 Follow-up of visual evoked potential in full-term and preterm control newborns and in subjects who suffered from perinatal respiratory distress. Electroencephalogr Clinical Neurophysiol 48:509–516.

Gaynor J W, Jarvik G P, Bernbaum J et al 2006 The relationship of postoperative electrographic seizures to neurodevelopmental outcome at 1 year of age after neonatal and infant cardiac surgery. J Thorac Cardiovasc Surg 131:181–189.

George S R, Taylor M J 1987 VEPs and SEPs in hydrocephalic infants before and after shunting. Clin Neurol Neurosurg (Suppl) 1:Abstr. 96.

George S R, Taylor M J 1991 Somatosensory evoked potentials in neonates and infants: developmental and normative data. Electroencephalogr Clin Neurophysiol 80:94–102.

Gibson N A, Brezinova V, Levene M I 1992a Somatosensory evoked potentials in the term newborn. Electroencephalogr Clin Neurophysiol 84:26–31.

Gibson N A, Graham M, Levene M I 1992b Somatosensory evoked potentials and outcome in perinatal asphyxia. Arch Dis Child 67:393–399.

Gilmore R L, Brock J, Hermansen M C, Baumann R 1987 Development of lumbar and spinal cord and cortical evoked potentials after tibial nerve stimulation in the preterm newborns: effects of gestational age and other factors. Electroencephalogr Clin Neurophysiol 68:28–39.

Gluckman P D, Wyatt J S, Azzopardi D et al 2005 Selective head cooling with mild systemic hypothermia after neonatal encephalopathy: multicentre randomised trial. Lancet 365:663–670.

Graziani L J, Streletz L J, Baumgart S et al 1994 Predictive value of neonatal electroencephalograms before and during extracorporeal membrane oxygenation. J Pediatr 125:969–975.

Graziani L J, Weitzman E D, Pineda G 1972 Visual evoked responses during neonatal respiratory disorders in low birth weight infants. Pediatr Res 6:203–210.

Greisen G, Hellström-Westas L, Lou H et al 1987 EEG depression and germinal layer haemorrhage in the newborn. Acta Paediatr Scand 76:519–525.

Greisen G, Pryds O, Rosén I, Lou H 1988 Poor reversibility of EEG abnormality in hypotensive, preterm neonates. Acta Paediatr Scand 77:785–790.

Grose J, Harding G F A, Wilton A Y, Bissenden J G 1989 The maturation of the pattern reversal VEP and flash ERG in pre-term infants. Clin Vis Sci 4:239–246.

Guinard C, Fawer C L, Despland P A, Calame A 1988 Auditory brainstem responses and ultrasound changes in a high-risk infants population. Helvet Pediatr Acta 43:377–388.

Gürses D, Kiliç I, Sahiner T 2002 Effects of hyperbilirubinemia on cerebrocortical electrical activity in newborns. Pediatr Res 52:125–130.

Guthkelch A N, Sclabassi R J, Hirsch R P, Vries J K 1984 Visual evoked potentials in hydrocephalus: relationship to head size, shunting, and mental development. Neurosurgery 14:283–286.

Guthkelch A N, Sclabassi R J, Vries J K 1982 Changes in the visual evoked potentials of hydrocephalic children. Neurosurgery 11:599–602.

Haddad N, Shihabuddin B, Preissl H et al 2006 Magnetoencephalography in healthy neonates. Clin Neurophysiol 117:289–294.

Hagberg B, Hagberg G, Zetterstrom R 1989 Decreasing perinatal mortality — increase in cerebral palsy morbidity? Acta Paediatr Scand 78:664–670.

Hahn J S, Monyer H, Tharp B R 1989 Interburst interval measurements in the EEGs of premature infants with normal neurological outcome. Electroencephalogr Clin Neurophysiol 73:410–418.

Hakamada S, Watanabe K, Hara K, Miyazaki S 1981 The evolution of visual and auditory evoked potentials in infants with perinatal disorder. Brain Dev 3:339–344.

Häkkinen V K, Ignatius J, Koskinen M 1987 Visual evoked potentials in high-risk infants. Neuropediatrics 18:70–74.

Harding G F A, Grose J, Wilton A, Bissenden J G 1989 The pattern reversal VEP in short-gestation infants. Electroencephalogr Clin Neurophysiol 74:76–80.

Hayakawa F, Okumura A, Kato T et al 1997 Dysmature EEG pattern in EEGs of preterm infants with cognitive impairment: maturation arrest caused by prolonged mild CNS depression. Brain Dev 19:122–125.

Hayakawa F, Okumura A, Kato T et al 1999 Determination of timing of brain injury in preterm infants with periventricular leukomalacia with serial neonatal electroecencephalography. Pediatrics 104:1077–1081.

Hayakawa M, Okumura A, Hayakawa F et al 2001 Background electroencephalographic (EEG) activities of very preterm infants born at less than 27 weeks gestation: a study on the degree of continuity. Arch Dis Child Fetal Neonatal Ed 84:F163–F167.

Hecox K E, Cone B 1981 Prognostic importance of brainstem auditory evoked responses after asphyxia. Neurology 31:1429–1434.

Hellström-Westas L 1992 Comparison between tape-recorded and amplitude-integrated EEG monitoring in sick newborn infants. Acta Paediatr 81:812–819.

Hellström-Westas L, Bell A H, Skov L, Greisen G, Svenningsen N W 1992 Cerebroelectrical depression following surfactant treatment in preterm neonates. Pediatrics 89:643–647.

Hellström-Westas L, Blennow G, Lindroth M et al 1995b Low risk of seizure recurrence after early withdrawal of antiepileptic treatment in the neonatal period. Arch Dis Child 72:F97–F101.

Hellström-Westas L, de Vries L S, Rosén I 2003 An atlas of amplitude-integrated EEG's in the newborn. Parthenon, London, UK, pp. 1–150.

Hellström-Westas L, Klette H, Thorngren-Jerneck K, Rosén I 2001 Early prediction of outcome with aEEG in preterm infants with large intraventricular hemorrhages. Neuropediatrics 32:319–324.

Hellström-Westas L, Rosén I, de Vries L S, Greisen G 2006 Amplitude integrated EEG: Classification and interpretation in preterm and term infants. Neoreviews 7:e76–e87.

Hellström-Westas L, Rosén I, Svenningsen N W 1985 Silent seizures in sick infants in early life. Acta Paediatr Scand 74:741–748.

Hellström-Westas L, Rosen I, Svenningsen N W 1991 Cerebral function monitoring during the first week of life in extremely small low birthweight (ESLBW) infants. Neuropediatrics 22:27–32.

Hellström-Westas L, Rosén I, Svenningsen N W 1995a Predictive value of early continuous amplitude integrated EEG recordings on outcome after severe birth asphyxia in full term infants. Arch Dis Child 72:F34–F38.

Hellström-Westas L, Westgren U, Rosén I, Svenningsen N W 1988 Lidocaine treatment of severe seizures in newborn infants. I. Clinical effects and cerebral electrical activity monitoring. Acta Paediatr Scand 77:79–84.

Helmers S L, Wypij D, Constantinou J E et al 1997 Perioperative electroencephalographic seizures in infants undergoing repair of complex congenital cardiac defects. Electroencephalogr Clin Neurophysiol 102:27–36.

Himmelmann K, Hagberg G, Beckung E et al 2005 The changing panorama of cerebral palsy in Sweden. IX. Prevalence and origin in the birth-year period 1995–1998. Acta Paediatr 94(3):287–294.

Hofkosh D, Thompson A, Nozza R et al 1991 Ten years of extracorporeal membrane oxygenation: neurodevelopmental outcome. Pediatrics 87:549–555.

Holmes G L, Lombroso C T 1993 Prognostic value of background patterns in the neonatal EEG. J Clin Neurophysiol 10:323–352.

Horan M, Azzopardi D, Edwards A D et al 2007 Lack of influence of mild hypothermia on amplitude integrated-electroencephalography in neonates receiving extracorporeal membrane oxygenation. Early Hum Dev 83:69–75.

Hrbek A, Iversen N, Olsson T 1982 Clinical applications of evoked potentials in neurology. Raven, New York, NY.

Hrbek A, Karlberg P, Kjellmer I et al 1977 Clinical application of evoked electroencephalographic responses in newborn infants. I. Perinatal asphyxia. Dev Med Child Neurol 19:34–44.

Hrbek A, Karlberg P, Olsson T 1973 Development of visual and somatosensory evoked responses in pre-term newborn infants. Electroencephalogr Clin Neurophysiol 34:225–232.

Hung K L 1989 Auditory brainstem responses in patients with neonatal hyperbilirubinaemia and bilirubin encephalopathy. Brain Dev 11:297–301.

Huotilainen M 2006 Magnetoencephalography of the newborn brain. Semin Fetal Neonatal Med 11:437–443.

Huotilainen M, Kujala A, Hotakainen M et al 2005 Short-term memory functions of the human fetus recorded with magnetoencephalography. Neuroreport 16:81–84.

Inder T E, Buckland L, Williams C E et al 2003 Lowered electroencephalographic spectral edge frequency predicts the presence of cerebral white matter injury in premature infants. Pediatrics 111:27–33.

Iwasaki S, Yamashita M, Maeda M et al 2007 Audiological outcome of infants with congenital cytomegalovirus infection in a prospective study. Audiol Neurootol 12(1):31–36.

Jasper HH 1958 The ten-twenty electrode system of the International Federation. Electroencephalogr Clin Neurophysiol 10:371–373.

Jewett D L, Williston J S 1971 Auditory-evoked far fields averaged from the scalp of humans. Brain 94:681–696.

Jiang Z D 1995 Maturation of the auditory brainstem in low risk preterm infants: a comparison with age-matched full term infants up to 6 years. Early Hum Dev 42:49–65.

Jiang Z D, Brosi D M, Shao X M, Wilkinson A R 2000 Maximum length sequence brainstem auditory evoked responses in term neonates who have perinatal hypoxia-ischemia. Pediatr Res 48(5):639–645.

Jiang Z D, Brosi D M, Wang J et al 2003 Time course of brainstem pathophysiology during first month in term infants after perinatal asphyxia, revealed by MLS BAER latencies and intervals. Pediatr Res 54(5):680–687.

Jiang Z D, Brosi D M, Wang J, Wilkinson A R 2004b Brainstem auditory-evoked responses to different rates of clicks in small-for-gestational age preterm infants at term. Acta Paediatr 93(1):76–81.

Jiang Z D, Brosi D M, Wilkinson A R 2001 Comparison of brainstem auditory evoked responses recorded at different presentation rates of clicks in term neonates after asphyxia. Acta Paediatr 90(12):1416–1420.

Jiang Z D, Brosi D M, Wilkinson A R 2002 Auditory neural responses to click stimuli of different rates in the brainstem of very preterm babies at term. Pediatr Res 51(4):454–459.

Jiang Z D, Yin R, Shao X M, Wilkinson A R 2004a Brain-stem auditory impairment during the neonatal period in term infants after asphyxia: dynamic changes in brain-stem auditory evoked response to clicks of different rates. Clin Neurophysiol 115(7):1605–1615.

Johnston W H, Angara V, Baumal R et al 1967 Erythroblastosis fetalis and hyperbilirubinemia: a five year follow-up with neurological psychological and audiologic evaluation. Pediatrics 39:88–92.

Joint Committee On Infant Hearing 1994 Position statement 1995. Pediatrics 95:152–156.

Karmel B Z, Gardner J M, Zappulla R A et al 1988 Brain-stem auditory evoked responses as indicators of early brain insult. Electroencephalogr Clin Neurophysiol 71:429–442.

Karniski W 1992 The late somatosensory evoked potential in premature and term infants. I. Principal

component topography. Electroencephalogr Clin Neurophysiol 84:32–43.

Kato T, Hayakawa F, Okumura A et al 2000 Flash visual evoked potentials in preterm infants; correlation with neurodevelopmental outcome [in Japanese]. J Jpn Soc Perinat Neonat Med 36:248.

Kato T, Okumura A, Hayakawa F et al 2005 The evolutionary change of flash visual evoked potentials in preterm infants with periventricular leukomalacia. Clin Neurophysiol 116(3):690–695.

Kawashiro N, Tsuchihashi N, Koga K et al 1994 Idiopathic deafness or hearing loss of unknown etiology following discharge from the NICU. Acta Otolaryngol Suppl 514:81–84.

Kennedy C R, Kimm L, Cafarelli Dees D et al 1991 Otoacoustic emissions and auditory brainstem responses in the newborn. Arch Dis Child 66:1124–1129.

Khazipov R, Luhmann H J 2006 Early patterns of electrical activity in the developing cerebral cortex of humans and rodents. Trends Neurosci 29:414–418.

Kjellmer I, Thordstein M, Sultan B, Wennergen M 1992 Cerebral function in the growth-retarded fetus and neonate. Biol Neonate 62:265–270.

Klebermass K, Kuhle S, Olischar M et al 2006 Intra- and extrauterine maturation of amplitude-integrated electroencephalographic acitivity in preterm infants younger than 30 weeks gestation. Biol Neonate 89:120–125.

Klein A J, Alvarez E D, Cowburn C A 1992 The effects of stimulus rate on detectability of the auditory brain stem response in infants. Ear Hear 13:401–405.

Klimach V J, Cooke R W I 1988a Maturation of the neonatal somatosensory evoked response in preterm infants. Dev Med Child Neurol 30:208–214.

Klimach V J, Cooke R W I 1988b Short latency somatosensory cortical evoked responses of preterm infants with ultrasound abnormalities. Dev Med Child Neurol 30:215–221.

Klinger G, Chin C N, Otsubo H et al 2001 Prognostic value of EEG in bacterial meningitis. Pediatr Neurol 24:28–31.

Koh T H H G, Aynsley-Green A, Tarbit M, Eyre J A 1988 Neural dysfunction during hypoglycemia. Arch Dis Child 63:1353–1358.

Kos-Pietro S, Towle V L, Cakmur R, Spire J-P 1997 Maturation of human visual evoked potentials: 27 weeks conceptional age to 2 years. Neuropediatrics 28:318–323.

Kubota T, Okumura A, Hayakawa F et al 2002 Combination of neonatal electroencephalography and ultrasonography: sensitive means of early diagnosis of periventricular leukomalacia. Brain Dev 24:698–702.

Kuhle S, Klebermass K, Olischar M et al 2001 Sleep-wake cycles in preterm infants below 30 weeks of gestational age. Preliminary results of a prospective amplitude-integrated EEG study. Wien Klin Wochenschr 113:219–223.

Kumar P, Gupta R, Shankaran S et al 1999 EEG abnormalitites in survivors of neonatal ECMO: Its role as a predictor of neurodevelopmental outcome. Am J Perinatol 16:245–250.

Kurtis P S, Rosenkrantz T S, Zalneraitis E L 1995 Cerebral blood flow and EEG changes in preterm infants with patent ductus arteriosus. Pediatr Neurol 12:114–119.

Kurtzberg D, Vaughan H G 1985 Electrophysiological assessment of auditory and visual function in the newborn. Clin Perinatol 12:277–299.

Laget P 1982 Clinical applications of cerebral evoked potentials in pediatric medicine: maturation of the somesthetic evoked potentials in normal children. In:

Chiarenza G A, Papakostopoulos D (eds) Proceedings of international conference on clinical application of cerebral evoked potentials in pediatric neurology. Excerpta Medica, Amsterdam, pp. 185–206.

Laget P, Raimbault J, D'Allest A M et al 1976 La maturation des potentiels évoqués somesthésiques (PES) chez l'homme. Electroencephalogr and Clin Neurophysiol 40:499–415.

Lambert S R, Kriss A, Taylor D 1989 Delayed visual maturation. A longitudinal clinical and electrophysiological assessment. Ophthalmology 96:524–529.

Lamblin M D, Andre M, Challamel M J et al 1999 Electroencephalography of the premature and term newborn. Maturational aspects and glossary. Neurophysiol Clin 29:123–219.

Lary S, Briassoulis G, de Vries L S et al 1985 Hearing threshold in preterm and term infants by auditory brainstem responses. J Pediatr 107:593–599.

Lary S, de Vries L S, Kaiser A et al 1989 Auditory brain stem responses in infants with posthaemorrhagic ventricular dilatation. Arch Dis Child 64:17–23.

Lasky R E 1984 A developmental study on the effect of stimulus rate on the auditory evoked brain-stem response. Electroencephalogr Clin Neurophysiol 59:411–419.

Lasky R E, Wiorek L, Becker T R 1998 Hearing loss in survivors of neonatal extracorporeal membrane oxygenation (ECMO) therapy and high-frequency oscillatory (HFO) therapy. J Am Acad Audiol 9:47–58.

Laureau E, Majnemer A, Rosenblatt B, Riley P 1988 A longitudinal study of short latency evoked responses in healthy newborns and infants. Electroencephalogr Clin Neurophysiol 71:100–108.

Laureau E, Marlot D 1990 Somatosensory evoked potentials after median and tibial nerve stimulation in healthy newborns. Electroencephalogr Clin Neurophysiol 76:453–458.

Leaf A A, Green C R, Esack A et al 1995 Maturation of electroretinograms and visual evoked potentials in preterm infants. Dev Med Child Neurol 37:814–826.

Lombroso C T 1985 Neonatal polygraphy in full-term and premature infants: a review of normal and abnormal findings. J Clin Neurophysiol 2:105–155.

Lommen C M, Pasman J W, van Kranen V H et al 2007 An algorithm for the automatic detection of seizures in neonatal amplitude-integrated EEG. Acta Paediatr 96:674–680.

Lütschg J, Hänggeli C, Huber P 1983 The evolution of cerebral hemispheric lesions due to pre- or perinatal asphyxia (clinical and neuroradiological correlation). Helvet Paediatr Acta 38:245–254.

McBride M C, Laroia N, Guillet R 2000 Electrographic seizures in neonates correlate with poor neurodevelopmental outcome. Neurology 55:506–513.

McCall S, Ferraro J A 1991 Pediatric ABR screening: pass-fail rates in awake versus asleep neonates. J Am Acad Audiol 2:18–23.

McCulloch D L, Taylor M 1994 Early maturation of the visual evoked potential (VEP): comparison of flash and pattern. Invest Ophthalmol Vis Sci Abstr. 35:2028.

McCulloch D L, Taylor M J 1992 Cortical blindness in children: utility of flash VEPs. Pediatr Neurol 8:156 [Brief commun].

McCulloch D L, Taylor M J, Whyte H E 1991 Visual evoked potentials and visual prognosis following perinatal asphyxia. Arch Ophthalmol 109:229–233.

McDonald M A, Dobson V, Sebris S L et al 1985 The acuity card procedure: a rapid test of infant acuity. Invest Ophthalmol Vis Sci 26:1158–1162.

Majnemer A, Rosenblatt B 1995 Prediction of outcome at school entry in neonatal intensive care unit survivors, with use of clinical and electrophysiologic techniques. J Pediatr 127:823–830.

Majnemer A, Rosenblatt B, Riley P 1988 Prognostic significance of the auditory brainstem evoked response in high-risk neonates. Dev Med Child Neurol 30:43–52.

Majnemer A, Rosenblatt B, Riley P et al 1987 Somatosensory evoked response abnormalities in high-risk newborns. Pediatr Neurol 3:350–355.

Majnemer A, Rosenblatt B, Riley P S 1990 Prognostic significance of multimodality evoked response testing in high-risk newborns. Pediatr Neurol 6:367–374.

Makrides M, Neumann M, Simmer K et al 1995 Are long-chain polyunsaturated fatty acids essential nutrients in infancy? Lancet 345:1463–1468.

Mandelbaum D E, Krawciw N, Assing E et al 2000 Topographic mapping of brain potentials in the newborn infant: the establishment of normal values and utility in assessing infants with neurological injury. Acta Paediatr 89:1104–1110.

Marg E, Freeman D N, Peltzman P, Goldstein P J 1975 Visual acuity development in human infants: evoked potential measurements. Invest Ophthalmol Vis Sci 15:150–153.

Markides A 1986 Age at fitting of hearing aids and speech intelligibility. Br J Audiol 20:165–167.

Marret S, Parain D, Jeannot E et al 1992 Positive rolandic sharp waves in the EEG of the premature newborn: a five year prospective study. Arch Dis Child 67:948–951.

Maruyama K, Okumura A, Hayakawa F et al 2002 Prognostic value of EEG depression in preterm infants for later development of cerebral palsy. Neuropediatrics 33:133–137.

Maynard D, Prior P F, Scott D F 1969 Device for continuous monitoring of cerebral activity in resuscitated patients. Br Med J 4:545–546.

Menache C C, Bourgeois B F, Volpe J J 2002 Prognostic value of neonatal discontinuous EEG. Pediatr Neurol 27:93–101.

Mercuri E, Braddick O, Atkinson J et al 1998 Orientation-reversal and phase-reversal visual evoked potentials in full term infants with brain lesions: a longitudinal study. Neuropediatrics 29:169–174.

Mercuri E, Rutherford M, Cowan F et al 1999 Early prognostic indicators of outcome in infants with neonatal cerebral infarction: a clinical, electroencephalogram, and magnetic resonance imaging study. Pediatrics 103:39–46.

Mercuri E, von Siebenthal K, Daniels H et al 1994 Multimodality evoked responses in the neurological assessment of the newborn. Eur J Pediatr 153:622–631.

Minami T, Kukita J, Nakayama H, Ueda K 1996 Maturational changes of VEPs in normal premature neonates: a longitudinal study. Brain Dev 18:46–49.

Mizrahi E M, Hrachovy R A, Kellaway P 2004 Atlas of neonatal encephalography, 3rd edn. Lippincott Williams & Wilkins, Philadelphia, pp. 1–250.

Mizrahi E M, Kellaway P 1987 Characterization and classification of neonatal seizures. Neurology 37:1837–1844.

Monod N, Pajot N, Guidasci S 1972 The neonatal EEG: Statistical studies and prognostic value in full-term and pre-term babies. Electroencephalogr Clin Neurophysiol 32:529–544.

Mori K, Uchida Y, Nishimura T, Eghwrudjakpor P 1988 Brainstem auditory evoked potentials in Chiari-II malformation. Child Nerv Syst 4:154–157.

Murray A D, Javel E, Watson C S 1985 Prognostic validity of auditory brainstem evoked response screening in newborn infants. Am J Otolaryngol 6:120–131.

Mushin J, Hogg C R, Dubowitz L M S et al 1984 Visual evoked responses to light emitting diode (LED) photostimulation in newborn infants. Electroencephalogr Clin Neurophysiol 58:317–320.

Muttitt S C, Taylor M J, Kobayashi J S, Whyte H E 1991 Serial visual evoked potentials and outcome in full-term birth asphyxia. Pediatr Neurol 7:86–90.

Navakatikyan M A, Colditz P B, Burke C J et al 2006 Seizure detection algorithm for neonates based on wave-sequence analysis. Clin Neurophysiol 117:1190–1203.

Neuringer M, Reisbick S, Janowsky J 1994 The role of n-3 fatty acids in visual and cognitive development: current evidence and methods of assessment. J Pediatr 125:S39–S47.

Nguyen The Tich S, Vecchierini M F, Debillon T, Pereon Y 2003 Effects of sufentanil on electroencephalogram in very and extremely preterm neonates. Pediatrics 111:123–128.

Okumura A, Kubota T, Toyota N et al 2003 Amplitude spectral analysis of maturational changes of delta waves in preterm infants. Brain Dev 25:406–410.

Okumura A, Kubota T, Tsuji T et al 2006 Amplitude spectral analysis of theta/alpha/beta waves in preterm infants. Pediatr Neurol 34:30–34.

Olischar M, Klebermass K, Kuhle S et al 2004 Reference values for amplitude-integrated electroencephalographic activity in preterm infants younger than 30 weeks' gestational age. Pediatrics 113:e61–e66.

Oliveira A J, Nunes M L, Haertel L M et al 2000 Duration of rhythmic EEG patterns in neonates: new evidence for clinical and prognostic significant of brief rhythmic discharges. Clin Neurophysiol 111:1646–1653.

Ortibus E L, Sum J M, Hahn J S 1998 Predictive value of EEG for outcome and epilepsy following neonatal seizures. Electroencephalogr Clin Neurophysiol 98:175–185.

Osredkar D, Toet M C, van Rooij L G M et al 2005 Sleep-wake cycling on amplitude-integrated EEG in full-term newborns with hypoxic-ischemic encephalopathy. Pediatrics 115:327–332.

Pappas A, Shankaran S, Stockmann P T, Bara R 2006 Changes in amplitude-integrated electroencephalography in neonates treated with extracorporeal membrane oxygenation: a pilot study. J Pediatr 148:125–127.

Parmelee A H, Akiyama Y, Schulte F J 1967 Power spectral analysis of the EEG in newborn infants during sleep. Electroencephalogr Clin Neurophysiol 23:81–82.

Pasman J W, Rotteveel J J, de Graaf R et al 1992 The effect of preterm birth on brainstem, middle latency and cortical auditory evoked potentials (BMC AERs). Early Hum Dev 31:113–129.

Paul K, Krajca V, Roth Z et al 2006 Quantitative topographic differentiation of the neonatal EEG. Clin Neurophysiol 117:2050–2058.

Pereda E, de La Cruz D M, Manas S et al 2006 Topography of EEG complexity in human neonates: effect of the postmenstrual age and the sleep state. Neurosci lett 394:152–157.

Petersen S, Pryds O, Trojaborg W 1990 Visual evoked potentials in term light-for-gestational age infants and infants of diabetic mothers. Early Hum Dev 23:85–91.

Pettigrew A G, Edwards D A, Henderson-Smart D J 1985 The influence of intrauterine growth retardation on brainstem development of preterm infants. Dev Med Child Neurol 27:467–472.

Pezzani C, Radvanyi-Bouvet M F, Relier J P et al 1986 Neonatal electroencephalography during the first twenty-four hours of life in full-term newborn infants. Neuropediatrics 17:11–18.

Picton T W, Durieux-Smith A, Moran L M 1994 Recording auditory brainstem responses from infants. Int J Pediatr Otorhinolaryngol 28:93–110.

Picton T W, Taylor M J, Durieux-Smith A 1992 Brainstem auditory evoked potentials in pediatrics. In: Aminoff M (ed) Electrodiagnosis in clinical neurology, 3rd edn. Churchill Livingstone, New York, NY, pp. 537–567.

Pierrat V, Eken P, de Vries L S 1997 The predictive value of cranial ultrasound and of somatosensory evoked potentials after nerve stimulation for adverse neurological outcome in preterm infants. Dev Med Child Neurol 39:398–403.

Pierrat V, Eken P, Duquennoy C et al 1993 Prognostic value of early somatosensory evoked potentials in neonates with cystic leukomalacia. Dev Med Child Neurol 35:683–690.

Pierrat V, Eken P, Truffert P et al 1996 Somatosensory evoked potentials in children with intrauterine growth retardation. Early Hum Dev 44:17–25.

Pike A A, Marlow N 2000 The role of cortical evoked responses in predicting neuromotor outcome in very preterm infants. Early Hum Dev 57(2):123–135.

Pike A A, Marlow N, Dawson C 1997 Posterior tibial somatosensory evoked potentials in very preterm infants. Early Hum Dev 47:71–84.

Pike A A, Marlow N, Reber C 1999 Maturation of the flash visual evoked potential in preterm infants. Early Hum Dev 54:215–222.

Placzek M, Mushin J, Dubowitz L M S 1985 Maturation of the visual evoked response and its correlation with visual acuity in preterm infants. Dev Med Child Neurol 27:448–454.

Preissl H, Lowery C L, Eswaran H 2004 Fetal magnetoencephalography: current progress and trends. Exp Neurol 190 Suppl 1:S28–S36.

Pryds O 1992 Stimulus rate-induced VEP attenuation in preterm infants. Electroencephalogr Clin Neurophysiol 84:188–191.

Pryds O, Greisen G 1990 Preservation of single-flash visual evoked potentials at very low cerebral oxygen delivery in preterm infants. Pediatr Neurol 6:151–158.

Pryds O, Trojaborg W, Carlsen J, Jensen J 1989 Determinants of visual evoked potentials in preterm infants. Early Hum Dev 19:117–125.

Purpura D P 1975 Morphogenesis of visual cortex in the preterm infant. In: Brazier M A B (ed) Growth and development of the brain. Raven Press, New York, NY.

Radvanyi-Bouvet M F, Vallecalle M H, Morel-Kahn F et al 1985 Seizures and electrical discharges in premature infants. Neuropediatrics 16:143–148.

Ramkalawan T W, Davis A C 1992 The effects of hearing loss and age of intervention on some language metrics in young hearing-impaired children. Br J Audiol 26:97–107.

Rennie J M, Chorley G, Boylan G B et al 2004 Non-expert use of the cerebral function monitor for neonatal seizure detection. Arch Dis Child Fetal Neonatal Ed 89:F37–F40.

Rennie J, Boylan G 2007 Treatment of neonatal seizures. Arch Dis Child Fetal Neonatal Ed 92: F148–F150.

Ricci D, Romeo D M, Serrao F et al 2008 Application of a neonatal assessment of visual function in a population of low risk full-term newborn. Early Hum Dev 84:277–280.

Robertson D R, Justo R N, Burke C J et al 2004 Perioperative predictors of developmental outcome following cardiac surgery in infancy. Cardiol Young 14:389–395.

Roche-Labarbe N, Aarabi A, Kongolo G et al 2007 High-resolution electroencephalography and source localization in neonates. Hum Brain Mapp. Mar 27 [Epub ahead of print]

Rose A L, Lombroso C T 1970 Neonatal seizure states. Pediatrics 45:404–425.

Russell-Eggitt I, Harris C M, Kriss A 1998 Delayed visual maturation: an update. Dev Med Child Neurol 40:130–136.

Salamy A, Eldredge L, Sweetow R 1996 Transient evoked otoacoustic emissions: feasibility in the nursery. Ear Hear 17:42–48.

Sarda P, Dupuy R P, Boulot P, Rieu D 1992 Brainstem conduction time abnormalities in small for gestational age infants. J Perinat Med 20:57–63.

Scalais E, François-Adant A, Langhendries J P et al 1992 Multimodality evoked potentials assessment in hypoxic-ischemic preterm infants. Ann Neurol Abstr 32:480.

Scalais E, Francois-Adant A, Nuttin C et al 1998 Multimodality evoked potentials as a prognostic tool in term asphyxiated newborns. Electroencephalogr Clin Neurophysiol 108:199–207.

Scher M S, Alvin J, Gaus L et al 2003 Uncoupling of EEG-clinical neonatal seizures after antiepileptic drug use. Pediatr Neurol 28:277–280.

Scher M S, Hamid M Y, Steppe D A et al 1993 Ictal and interictal electrographic seizure durations in preterm and term neonates. Epilepsia 34:284–288.

Scher M S, Johnson M W, Holditch-Davis D 2005 Cyclicity of neonatal sleep behaviors at 25 to 30 weeks' postconceptional age. Pediatr Res 57:879–882.

Scher M S, Richardson G A, Robles N et al 1998 Effects of prenatal substance exposure: altered maturation of visual evoked potentials. Pediatr Neurol 18:236–243.

Scher M S, Steppe D A, Sclabassi R J, Banks D L 1997 Regional differences in spectral EEG measures between healthy term and preterm infants. Pediatr Neurol 17:218–223.

Scher M S, Sun M, Steppe D A et al 1994a Comparisons of EEG sleep state-specific spectral values between healthy full-term and preterm infants at comparable postconceptional ages. Sleep 17:47–51.

Scher M S, Sun M, Steppe D A et al 1994b Comparisons of EEG spectral and correlation measures between healthy term and preterm infants. Pediatr Neurol 10:104–108.

Scheuer M L, Wilson S B 2004 Data analysis for continuous EEG monitoring in the ICU: seeing the forest and the trees. J Clin Neurophysiol 21: 353–378.

Schulte F J, Stennert E, Wulbrand H et al 1977 The ontogeny of sensory perception in preterm infants. Eur J Pediatr 126:211–224.

Schumacher R E, Palmer T, Roloff D et al 1991 Follow-up of infants treated with extracorporeal membrane oxygenation for newborn respiratory failure. Pediatrics 87:451–457.

Selton D, Andre M, Hascoet J M 2000 Normal EEG in very premature infants: reference criteria. Clin Neurophysiol 111:2116–2124.

Shah D K, Lavery S, Doyle L W et al 2006 Use of 2-channel bedside electroencephalogram monitoring in term-born encephalopathic infants related to cerebral injury defined by magnetic resonance imaging. Pediatrics 118:47–55.

Shah D K, Mackay M T, Lavery S et al 2008 Accuracy of bedside electroencephalographic monitoring in comparison with simultaneous continuous conventional electroencephalography for seizure detection in term infants. Pediatrics 121:1146–1154.

Shalak L F, Laptook A R, Velaphi S C, Perlman J M 2003 Amplitude-integrated electroencephalography coupled with an early neurologic examination enhances prediction of term infants at risk for persistent encephalopathy. Pediatrics 111:351–351.

Shany E, Goldstein E, Khvatskin S et al 2006b Predictive value of amplitude-integrated electroencephalography pattern and voltage in asphyxiated term infants. Pediatric Neurol 35:335–342.

Shany E, Khvatskin S, Golan A, Karplus M 2006a Amplitude-integrated electroencephalography: a tool for monitoring silent seizures in neonates. Pediatr Neurol 34:194–199.

Shellhaas R A, Saoita A I, Clancy R R 2007 The Sensitivity of amplitude-integrated EEG for neonatal seizure detection. Pediatrics, in press.

Shepherd A J, Saunders K J, McCulloch D L, Dutton G N 1999 Prognostic value of flash visual evoked potentials in preterm infants. Dev Med Child Neurol 41:9–15.

Sininger Y S 1995 Filtering and spectral characteristics of averaged auditory brain-stem response and background noise in infants. J Acoust Soc Am 98:2048–2055.

Sisman J, Campbell D E, Brion L P 2005 Amplitude-integrated EEG in preterm infants: Maturation of background pattern and amplitude voltage with postmenstrual age and gestational age. J Perinatol 25:391–396.

Skov L, Hellström-Westas L, Jacobsen T, Greisen G, Svenningsen N W 1992 Acute changes in cerebral oxygenation and cerebral blood volume in preterm infants during surfactant treatment. Neuropediatrics 23:126–130.

Smit B J, Kok J H, de Vries L S et al 1998 Somatosensory evoked potentials in very preterm infants in relation to L-thyroxine supplementation. Pediatrics 101:865–869.

Soares I, Collet L, Delorme C et al 1989 Are click-evoked BAEPs useful in case of neonate hyperbilirubinaemia? Int J Pediatr Otorhinolaryngol 17:231–237.

Soares I, Collet L, Desreux V et al 1992 Differential maturation of brainstem auditory evoked potentials in preterm infants according to birthweight. Int J Neurosci 64:259–266.

Spivak L G 1993 Spectral composition of infant auditory brainstem responses: implications for filtering. Audiology 32:185–194.

Stanley O H, Fleming P J, Morgan M H 1991 Development of visual evoked potentials following intrauterine growth retardation. Early Hum Dev 27:79–91.

Starr A, Amlie R N, Martin W H, Sanders S 1977 Development of auditory function in newborn infants revealed by auditory brainstem potentials. Pediatrics 60:831–839.

Steinlin M I, Nadal D, Eich G F et al 1996 Late intrauterine cytomegalovirus infection: clinical and neuroimaging findings. Pediatr Neurol 15:249–253.

Stockard J E, Stockard J J, Kleinberg F, Westmoreland B F 1983 Prognostic value of brainstem auditory evoked potentials in neonates. Arch Neurol 40:360–365.

Stuart A, Yang E Y 1994 Effect of high-pass filtering on the neonatal auditory brainstem response to air- and bone-conducted clicks. J Speech Hear Res 37:475–479.

Stuart A, Yang E Y, Botea M 1996 Neonatal auditory brainstem responses recorded from four electrode montages. J Commun Disord 29:125–139.

Taylor M J 1992 The neurophysiological examination of the newborn infant. MacKeith, London.

Taylor M J, Boor R, Ekert P G 1996a Preterm maturation of the somatosensory evoked potential. Electroencephalogr Clin Neurophysiol 100:448–452.

Taylor M J, Boor R, Keenan N K et al 1996b Brainstem auditory and visual evoked potentials in infants with myelomeningocele. Brain Dev 18:99–104.

Taylor M J, Menzies R, MacMillan L J, Whyte H E 1987 VEPs in normal full-term and premature neonates: longitudinal versus cross-sectional data. Electroencephalogr Clin Neurophysiol 68:20–27.

Taylor M J, Murphy W J, Whyte H E 1992 Prognostic reliability of somatosensory and visual evoked potentials of asphyxiated term infants. Dev Med Child Neurol 34:507–515.

Tekgul H, Bourgeois B F, Gauvreau K, Bergin A M 2005 Electroencephalography in neonatal seizures: comparison of a reduced and a full 10/20 montage. Pediatr Neurol 32:155–161.

Ter Horst H J, Sommer C, Bergman K A et al 2004 Prognostic significance of amplitude-integrated EEG during the first 72 hours after birth in severely asphyxiated neonates. Pediatr Res 55:1026–1033.

Tharp B R, Scher M S, Clancy R R 1989 Serial EEGs in normal and abnormal infants with birthweights less than 1200 grams — a prospective study with long term follow-up. Neuropediatrics 20:64–72.

Thordstein M, Flisberg A, Löfgren N et al 2004 Spectral analysis of burst periods in EEG from healthy and post-asphyctic full-term neonates. Clin Neurophysiol 115:2461–2466.

Thordstein M, Löfgren N, Flisberg A et al 2005 Infraslow EEG activity in burst periods from post asphyctic full term neonates. Clin Neurophysiol 116:1501–1516.

Thordstein M, Löfgren N, Flisberg A et al 2006 Sex differences in electrocortical activity in human neonates. Neuroreport 17:1165–1168.

Thornberg E, Ekström-Jodal B 1994 Cerebral function monitoring: a method of predicting outcome in term neonates after severe perinatal asphyxia. Acta Paediatr 83:596–601.

Thornberg E, Thiringer K 1990 Normal patterns of cerebral function monitor traces in term and preterm neonates. Acta Paediatr Scand 79:20–25.

Thorngren-Jerneck K, Hellström-Westas L, Ryding E, Rosen I 2003 Cerebral glucose metabolism and early EEG/aEEG in term newborn infants with hypoxic-ischemic encephalopathy. Pediatr Res 54:854–860.

Toet M C, Groenendaal F, Osredkar D et al 2005 Postneonatal epilepsy following amplitude-integrated EEG-detected neonatal seizures. Pediatr Neurol 32:241–247.

Toet M C, Hellström-Westas L, Groenendaal F et al 1999 Amplitude integrated EEG 3 and 6 hours after birth in full term neonates with hypoxic-ischaemic encephalopathy. Arch Dis Child Fetal Neonatal Ed 81: F19–F23.

Toet M C, Lemmers P M, van Schelven L J, van Bel F 2006 Cerebral oxygenation and electrical activity after birth asphyxia: their relation to outcome. Pediatrics 117:333–339.

Toet M C, van der Meij W, de Vries L S, van Huffelen A C 2002 Comparison between simultaneously recorded amplitude integrated EEG (Cerebral Function Monitor) and standard EEG in neonates. Pediatrics 109:772–779.

Tolonen M, Palva J M, Andersson S, Vanhatalo S 2007 Development of the spontaneous activity transients and ongoing cortical activity in human preterm babies. Neuroscience 145:997–1006.

Torres F, Anderson C 1985 The normal EEG of the human newborn. J Clin Neurophysiol 2:89–103.

Trittenwein G, Plenk S, Mach E et al 2006 Quantitative electroencephalography values of neonates during and after venoarterial extracorporeal membrane oxygenation and permanent ligation of right common carotid artery. Artif Organs 30:447–451.

Tsuneishi S, Casaer P 1997 Stepwise decrease in VEP latencies and the process of myelination in the human visual pathway. Brain Dev 19:547–551.

Tsuneishi S, Casaer P, Fock J M, Hirano S 1995 Establishment of normal values for flash visual evoked potentials (VEPs) in preterm infants: a longitudinal study with special reference to two components of the N1 wave. Electroencephalogr Clin Neurophysiol 96:291–299.

Umezaki H, Morrell F 1970 Developmental study of photic evoked responses in premature infants. Electroencephalogr Clin Neurophysiol 28:55–63.

Uus K, Bamford J 2006 Effectiveness of population-based newborn hearing screening in England: ages of interventions and profile of cases. Pediatrics 117(5): e887–e893.

van Leuven K, Groenendaal F, Toet M C et al 2004 Midazolam and amplitude integrated EEG in asphyxiated full-term neonates. Acta Paediatr 93:1221–1227.

van Rooij L G, Toet M C, Osredkar D et al 2005 Recovery of amplitude integrated electroencephalographic background patterns within 24 hours of perinatal asphyxia. Arch Dis Child Fetal Neonatal Ed 90:F245–F251.

van Rooij L G M, de Vries L S, Handryastuti S et al 2007 Neurodevelopmental outcome in term infants with status epilepticus detected with amplitude-integrated electroencephalography. Pediatrics, in press.

van Wezel-Meijler G, van der Knaap M S, Huisman J et al 2002 Dietary supplementation of long-chain polyunsaturated fatty acids in preterm infants: effects on cerebral maturation. Acta Paediatr 91(9):942–950.

Vanhatalo S, Kaila K 2006 Development of neonatal EEG activity: from phenomenology to physiology. Semin Fetal Neonatal Med 11:471–478.

Vanhatalo S, Lauronen L 2006 Neonatal SEP-Back to bedside with basic science. Seminars Fetal and Neonatal Med 11:464–470.

Vanhatalo S, Tallgren P, Andersson S et al 2002 DC-EEG discloses prominent, very slow wave activity patterns during sleep in preterm infants. Clin Neurophysiol. 113:1822–1825.

Vanhatalo S, Voipio J, Kaila K 2005 Full-band EEG (fbEEG): a new standard for clinical electroencephalography. Clin EEG Neurosci 36:311–317.

Vecchierini M-F, d'Allest A-M, Verpillat P 2003 EEG patterns in 10 extreme premature neonates with normal neurological outcome: qualitative and quantitative data. Brain Dev 25:330–337.

Vecchierini-Blineau M F, Nogues B, Louvet S, Desfontaines O 1996 Positive temporal sharp waves in electroencephalograms of the premature newborn. Neurophysiol Clin 26:350–362.

Verma U L, Archbald F, Tejani N, Handwerker S M 1984 Cerebral function monitor in the neonate. I. Normal patterns. Dev Med Child Neurol 26:154–161.

Vermeulen R J, Sie L T, Jonkman E J et al 2003 Predictive value of EEG in neonates with periventricular leukomalacia. Dev Med Child Neurol 45:586–590.

Vespa P M, Nenov V, Nuwer M R 1999 Continuous EEG monitoring in the intensive care unit: early findings and clinical efficacy. J Clin Neurophysiol 16:1–13.

Victor S, Appleton R E, Beirne M et al 2005a Spectral analysis of electroencephalography in premature newborn infants: normal ranges. Pediatr Res 57:336–341.

Victor S, Appleton R E, Beirne M et al 2005b Effect of carbon dioxide on background cerebral electrical activity and fractional oxygen extraction in very low birth weight infants just after birth. Pediatr Res 58:579–585.

Victor S, Appleton R E, Beirne M et al 2006b The relationship between cardiac output, cerebral electrical activity, cerebral fractional oxygen extraction and peripheral blood flow in premature newborn infants. Pediatr Res 60:454–460.

Victor S, Marson A G, Appleton R E et al 2006a Relationship between blood pressure, cerebral electrical activity, cerebral fractional oxygen extraction, and peripheral blood flow in very low birth weight newborn infants. Pediatr Res 59:314–319.

Viniker D A, Maynard D E, Scott D F 1984 Cerebral function monitor studies in neonates. Clin Electroenceph 15:185–192.

Vles J S H, Casaer P, Kingma H et al 1985 A longitudinal study of brainstem auditory evoked potentials of preterm infants. Dev Med Child Neurol 29:577–585.

Watanabe K, Hakamada S, Kuroyanagi M et al 1983 Electroencephalographic study of intraventricular hemorrhage in the preterm newborn. Neuropediatrics 14:225–230.

Watanabe K, Hayakawa F, Okumura A 1999 Neonatal EEG: A powerful tool in the assessment of brain damage in preterm infants. Brain Dev 21:361–372.

Watanabe K, Iwase K, Hara K 1972 Maturation of visual evoked responses in low-birthweight infants. Dev Med Child Neurol 14:425–435.

Watanabe K, Iwase K, Hara K 1973 Visual evoked responses during sleep and wakefulness in pre-term infants. Electroencephalogr Clin Neurophysiol 34:571–577.

Watkin P M 1996 Neonatal otoacoustic emission screening and the identification of deafness. Arch Dis Child 74:F16–F25.

West C R, Groves A M, Williams C E et al 2006b Early low cardiac output is associated with compromised electroencephalographic activity in very preterm infants. Pediatr Res 59:610–615.

West C R, Harding J E, Williams C E et al 2006a Quantitative electroencephalographic patterns in normal preterm infants over the first week after birth. Early Hum Dev 82:43–51.

White C P, Cooke R W 1989 Maturation of the cortical evoked response to posterior nerve stimulation in the preterm neonate. Dev Med Child Neurol 31:657–664.

White C P, Cooke R W I 1994 Somatosensory evoked potentials following posterior tibial nerve stimulation predict later outcome. Dev Med Child Neurol 36:34–41.

Whyte H E, Pearce J M, Taylor M J 1987 Changes in the VEP in preterm neonates with arousal states, as assessed by EEG monitoring. Electroencephalogr Clin Neurophysiol 68:223–225.

Whyte H E, Taylor M J, Menzies R et al 1986 Prognostic utility of visual evoked potentials in term asphyxiated neonates. Pediatr Neurol 2:220–223.

Willis J, Duncan C, Bell R 1987 Short-latency somatosensory evoked potentials in perinatal asphyxia. Pediatr Neurol 3:203–207.

Willis J, Duncan M C, Bell R et al 1989 Somatosensory evoked potentials predict neuromotor outcome after periventricular haemorrhage. Dev Med Child Neurol 31:435–439.

Willis J, Seales D, Frazier E 1984 Short latency somatosensory evoked potentials in infants. Electroencephalogr Clin Neurophysiol 59:366–373.

Wong F Y, Barfield C P, Walker A M 2007 Power spectral analysis of two-channel EEG in hypoxic-ischaemic encephalopathy. Early Hum Dev 83:379–383.

Wong V C N 1991 Cortical blindness in children: a study of etiology and prognosis. Pediatr Neurol 7:178–185.

Worley G, Erwin C W, Schuster J M et al 1994 BAEPs in infants with myelomeningocele and later development of Chiari II malformation-related brainstem dysfunction. Dev Med Child Neurol 36:707–715.

Yoshinaga-Itano C 2003 Early intervention after universal neonatal hearing screening: impact on outcomes. Ment Retard Dev Disabil Res Rev 9(4):252–266.

Young G B, da Silva O P 2000 Effects of morphine on the electroencephalograms of neonates: a prospective, observational study. Clin Neurophysiol 111:1955–1960.

CHAPTER

13

Congenital structural defects of the brain

Gonzalo Moscoso

Key Points

- Serious malformations occur in up to 3% of newborns. These frequently involve the nervous system and in more than 60% of infants the etiology cannot be determined. Increasingly genetic, teratogenic and infectious etiologies are identified as the cause of these disorders
- Spina bifida in conjunction with myelomeningocele and hydrocephalus remains common (about 4.6 cases/10 000 births) with the evaluation and management of such infants requiring a multidisciplinary approach
- Subtle forms of the Arnold–Chiari malformation should be considered in children who present with unexplained recurrent headaches, ataxia, neck pain or swallowing difficulties
- Holoprosencephaly, due to failure of the embryonic forebrain to separate, is associated with severe developmental delay, spastic quadriplegia, seizures and failure to thrive
- Neuronal migrational disorders, neuronal heterotopias and cortical dysplasias are increasingly recognized as the cause of epilepsy syndromes and disorders of cognition based on neuroimaging or neuropathology of tissue taken at the time of epilepsy surgery. Classification of these disorders remains elusive and will depend on correlating genetic, clinical and imaging abnormalities
- Schizencephaly is associated with the presence of clefts in the cerebral hemispheres. Children with bilateral schizencephaly are likely to have severe neurologic impairments whereas those with unilateral schizencephaly are more likely to have mild or moderate disabilities
- Lissencephaly, characterized by a brain with a smooth cerebral surface, thickened cortical mantle and incomplete neuronal migration, is usually associated with severe developmental delay and epilepsy. Several forms have been recognized. Type I lissencephaly is most frequently associated with the Miller–Dieker syndrome (17p13.3 deletion) with affected infants having a characteristic facial appearance. Type I lissencephaly may also be seen with the Norman–Roberts syndrome. These patients have a different facial appearance and do not have the same chromosomal deletion. Type II lissencephaly is associated with a cobblestone, pebbled brain surface, thickened cortex, edematous cystic white matter and often

- hydrocephalus. It has been seen with congenital muscular dystrophy and the Walker–Warburg syndrome. X-linked lissencephaly and subcortical band heterotopias are both caused by mutation of a single gene, *XLIS* that encodes a 40 kDa protein, ***Doublecortin***. Almost all patients with subcortical band heterotopias are female. Both conditions are associated with epilepsy and developmental delay
- Agenesis of the corpus callosum (1–3/1000 births) is a relatively common nervous system malformation and is seen in association with a variety of other brain malformations and syndromes. Clinical symptoms and findings cover a wide spectrum of involvement
- Cerebellar agenesis or hypoplasia frequently occurs in conjunction with other nervous system malformations as well as in association with mitochondrial disorders. Agenesis of the vermis is most commonly recognized in patients diagnosed with Joubert syndrome that presents as an autosomal recessive disorder in the neonatal period with episodic hyperpnea and apnea, disorders of ocular movement, retinal dystrophy, ataxia, hypotonia and developmental delay. The majority of patients with Joubert syndrome who survive have significant long-term neurologic impairment
- The Dandy–Walker syndrome (1/30 000 births) includes cystic dilation of the fourth ventricle with hypoplasia and superior displacement of the cerebellum. Hydrocephalus, delayed development, nystagmus and spasticity are common. The majority of patients require shunting and most patients have serious long-term cognitive and cerebellar dysfunction
- Intracranial arachnoid cysts may be benign but can cause a variety of neurologic symptoms depending on their location, size and whether they create a mass effect. Surgical decompression of symptomatic patients is indicated. Cysts occur equally in supratentorial and infratentorial compartments; sometimes the cysts are seen in conjunction with hydrocephalus
- Aqueductal stenosis is a common cause of hydrocephalus and frequently occurs in conjunction with other nervous system malformations. It may be inherited as an X-linked recessive disorder

---

INTRODUCTION

Remarkable progress in developmental and molecular neurobiology has occurred in the past decade (Anderson 1997, Lendahl 1997, Levitt et al 1997, Reid & Walsh 1996). The extraordinary and ever increasing information about the sequence of molecular and structural events controlling this development, and likewise the effects of gene dysregulation in the pathogenesis of many well-recognized malformations, is emerging at an ever-accelerating pace (see Ch. 1). Neural embryogenesis is described in detail in Chapters 2 and 3. Of particular value has been the contribution of neuroimaging, especially magnetic resonance imaging, to define new syndromes and provide more refined correlations between clinical symptoms and brain dysgenesis (see Ch. 6). This chapter

highlights selected aspects of this neuropathology (Norman et al 1995, Sarnat 1992) and neonatal neurology (Volpe 2000); developmental neuroimaging (Mize & Erzurumlu 1996) and pediatric neuroimaging (Ball 1997, Barkovich 1995) provide additional information.

PATHOGENESIS

Malformations of the brain and spinal cord form during nervous system development. In theory, malformations result form 'an intrinsically abnormal developmental process' within the CNS (Spranger et al 1982); however, malformations may also arise from extrinsic factors, such as teratogens and infections (see Table 13.1). Approximately 3% of

Table 13.1 Etiology of human nervous malformations

TERATOGENS

Physical agents in utero
Trauma
Fetal position or crowding
Hyperthermia
Radiation

Infectious agents in utero
Rubella virus
Herpes virus type 1 and 2
Cytomegalovirus
Mumps virus
Varicella virus
Treponema pallidum
Toxoplasma gondii

Maternal metabolic derangement
Phenylketonuria
Diabetes mellitus
Toxemia of pregnancy
Malnutrition
Hypoxia
Iodine deficiency

Maternal toxin and drug exposure
Carbon monoxide
Ethyl alcohol
Cocaine; other substance abuse
Antimetabolites
Antiepileptic drugs (phenytoin)
Trimethadione (valproic acid)
Isotretinoin (Accutane)
Vitamin excess or deficiency
Methyl mercury (Minamata diseases)

GENETIC CONDITIONS

Chromosomal abnormality
Single-gene inheritance
Autosomal-recessive
X-linked recessive
Autosomal-dominant

Multifactorial inheritance

Table 13.2 Congenital defects related to embryonic stages

Neural tube formation
Chiari syndrome
Cranioschisis (anterior neuropore)
   Anencephaly
   Encephalocele
   Exencephaly
   Meningocele
   Rachischisis (posterior neuropore)
   Meningocele
   Myelomeningocele
Spina bifida

Segmentation and cleavage
Basilar impression
Holoprosencephaly
Klippel–Feil syndrome
Sprengel deformity

Sulcation, proliferation, neuronal migration, organization
Callosal agenesis
Cerebellar anomalies
Heterotopias
Lissencephaly
Macrogyria
Neuronal migration defects
Schizencephaly

Myelination
White matter hypoplasia

Mesodermal development
Craniosynostosis
   Fibrous dysplasia

newborns have serious multiple or localized malformations, including those of the CNS. These malformations account for 70% of fetal deaths and 40% of deaths within the first year of life (Evrard et al 1989a, Freeman 1985).

Selective defects of morphogenesis may result in readily recognizable malformations. Some may be classified by the initial morphologic phase of development responsible for the defect (see Table 13.2) (DeMyer 1971). These abnormalities of morphogenesis include a primary mesodermal abnormality, failure of neural tube closure (neurulation), abnormal segmentation and sulci formation (sulcation), faulty prolif-

eration and migration of neurons and precursor cells, and agenesis-hypoplasia (Cohen & Lemire 1982). This classification does not designate cause, as many malformations cannot be ascribed to known abnormal patterns of development; malformation processes may also span more than one developmental stage.

The etiology of CNS malformations is unknown in more than 60% of patients. Hereditary factors that cause nervous system malformations include autosomal- and X-linked conditions (7.5%) and chromosome abnormalities (6%) (Buckton et al 1980, Carter 1976). Single mutant genes may cause localized malformations (Holmes 1974). Multifactorial inheritance originates from several gene abnormalities and environmental factors, and may explain up to 20% of malformations (Carter 1976, Holmes et al 1976).

Teratogens, such as trauma, hypoxia, hyperthermia (Layde et al 1980), chemical toxins (Marsh et al 1980) and drugs (Schardein 1985); infections; radiation (Schull 1997); maternal diabetes mellitus; phenylketonuria; and intrauterine conditions, such as constricted fetal position, account for 3.5% of nervous system malformations. Malformations associated with teratogens depend on the mechanism of action and specific time and duration of exposure during gestation. For example, isotretinoin (Accutane), a vitamin A analog used to treat acne, or high oral vitamin A intake (more than 10 000 IU per day) is a well-recognized human teratogen that acts during the first trimester (Lammer et al 1985, Rothman et al 1995). Defective neural crest migration and embryogenesis produce ear anomalies, posterior fossa cysts, microcephaly, heterotopias, Dandy–Walker syndrome, hydrocephalus, cranial nerve dysfunction and congenital heart disease.

Fetal infections may lead to morphologic alterations, dysfunction without histologic change and latent infection with subsequent abnormality (Catalans & Sever 1971, Evrard et al 1989b). *Toxoplasma gondii*, rubella, herpes simplex and cytomegalovirus infections can all cause malformations (Friede 1989), as can fetal exposure to maternal human immunodeficiency virus infection (Belman et al 1988).

NEURAL TUBE DEFECTS

SPINAL DYSRAPHISM AND ASSOCIATED MALFORMATIONS

Spinal dysraphism includes neural structural defects in which the common denominator is failed fusion, either partial or complete, of the neural tube and the vertebral canal. Furthermore, the malformation may involve multiple germ layers with variable clinical manifestations. The condition includes lesions varying from a flat dermal aberration to a gross malformation of a region of the spinal canal and cord (French 1983, Norman et al 1995).

Approximately 4000 pregnancies are affected by spina bifida and anencephaly in the United States every year. The subtlest defect, spina bifida occulta, arises when the vertebral arches fail to fuse. When this abnormality is associated with an underlying malformation of the spinal cord, the condition is known as *occult spinal dysraphism*; accompanying abnormalities of the overlying skin and soft tissue usually occur (e.g. dermal sinus or dimple, skin tag, tuft of hair, port-wine stain) (Anderson 1975). When the meninges alone protrude through the defect, the malformation is termed a meningocele. Myelomeningocele, in which a portion of the spinal cord or nerve roots are displaced through the spina bifida defect into a sac, is the most complex and usually symptomatic condition. Other classifications of neural tube defects (NTDs) categorize the lesions as being either open or closed (McComb 1997, Norman et al 1995).

Pathogenesis

Several hypotheses have been suggested to explain the evolution of myelodysplasia (George & McLone 1995, Marin-Padilla 1991, Norman et al 1995). The most plausible theory is that the neural tube fails to close during embryogenesis (Laurence 1964, Osaka et al 1978). Since the neural tube in humans has multiple sites of closure, the ultimate morphologic appearance of the defect is likely to depend on the specific site where failure of fusion occurs. Each of these sites is likely to be controlled at distinct gene loci (Van Allen et al 1993). Multiple mechanisms have been described in animal models at the gene level that affect timing, location and the process of neural formation that could account for the formation of such defects (Copp et al 1990, Sarnat 1992, Van Allen 1996). Lack of closure of the posterior neuropore, the terminal location of normal neural tube fusion, may explain the reason lumbosacral malformations frequently accompany the disorder. Primary failure of neural tube closure does not account for other dysplastic characteristics of myelodysplasia unless an associated defect of neural induction in the mesoderm is involved.

Spinal dysraphism may be caused by a teratogenic agent acting before neural tube closure, which occurs during the fourth week of gestation. Teratogens capable of inducing myelodysplasia in experimental animals or human beings include radiation, maternal hyperthermia (Shiota 1982), gestational diabetes mellitus, vitamin A deficiency, or excess D-mannose or excess glucose in embryo culture, and valproic acid, carbamazepine and folic acid deficiency (Holmes 1994, Kallen 1994, Sever 1995).

The role of folic acid is now recognized as important in the pathogenesis of spina bifida, although the specific mechanism remains unknown. This is discussed in detail in Chapter 17.

A variety of genetic models of neural tube defects (NTDs) have also been reported (George & McLone 1995). F52 is a myristoylated, alanine-rich substrate for protein kinase C, and F52-deficient mice manifest severe NTDs (Wu et al 1996). Likewise, NTDs in mice have been reported in chimeric models deficient in expression of the fibroblast growth factor receptor-1 gene (Deng et al 1997), in the splotch (Sp) mouse mutant with mutations in the *Pax-3* gene (Epstein et al 1993), in mice with allelic mutations of the breast and ovarian cancer susceptibility gene (*BRCA1*) (Gowen et al 1996), and in mice lacking the platelet-derived growth factor receptor alpha (*PDGFR-a*) gene that is associated with somite mesodermal development (Payne et al 1997). In children with NTDs, isolated cases of mutations in the *PAX1* and *PAX3* gene have been reported (Hol et al 1995, 1996).

SPINA BIFIDA OCCULTA

Spina bifida occulta occurs in at least 5% of the population but is most often asymptomatic. Accompanying associated features may include dermal hyperpigmentation, a patch of hair, a lump, or a dermal sinus. This defect is located most often in the lower lumbar area involving the lamina of L5 and S1. When associated neurologic involvement is present, the condition is occult spinal dysraphism.

OCCULT SPINAL DYSRAPHISM (see also Ch. 39)

The spectrum of occult spinal dysraphism includes distortion of the spinal cord or roots by fibrous bands and adhesions, intraspinal lipomas, dermoid or epidermoid cysts, fibrolipomas, subcutaneous lipomas (lipomyelomeningoceles), tethered cord and diastematomyelia (Anderson 1975, Byrd et al 1991). A tethered cord is the most common condition (McLone & La Marca 1997).

Symptoms of occult spinal dysraphism may be absent, minimal, or severe, depending on the degree of neural involvement. The patient may exhibit static or slowly progressive weakness or sensory loss in the legs or feet, gait difficulty and foot deformity. Bowel and bladder dysfunction, such as incontinence, repeated bladder infection and enuresis may also occur. Symptoms are caused by abnormally formed neural tissue or pressure on the spinal cord or nerve roots. Common findings include diminished Achilles tendon reflexes, contracted heel cords, high arches, equinovarus deformity of the feet, decreased rectal sphincter tone, unequal leg or foot length, scattered sensory loss, Babinski signs and trophic ulcers. Because many of these patients have associated posterior fossa or cervical cord malformation, neurologic involvement of the upper extremities may

occur (Jansen et al 1991). Ophthalmologic complications, usually observed when hydrocephalus is present, are also common and require careful evaluation and follow-up (Biglan 1990). Ultrasonography and MRI have greatly facilitated the diagnosis and management of these occult lesions (Fig. 13.1) (Gundry & Heithoff 1994). A tethered spinal cord or lipomas can be detected without invasive myelography. Ultrasonography can demonstrate a poorly pulsatile, low-lying, or thickened conus medullaris in infants (Korsvik & Keller 1992). Surgical management is described on page 849.

Recurrent meningitis from external contamination of CSF may result from occult congenital malformations along the spinal canal and neuraxis. These external connections include midline dermal sinus; temporal bone fistula to the middle ear, eustachian tube, or nasopharynx; neurenteric fistula; and basal encephalocele or meningocele involving the cribriform plate, sphenoid bone, or clivus (Hemphill et al 1982). An MRI scan should be obtained, followed by appropriate surgical treatment.

MENINGOCELE

Meningocele, a protrusion of meninges without accompanying nervous tissue, is not associated with neurologic deficit.

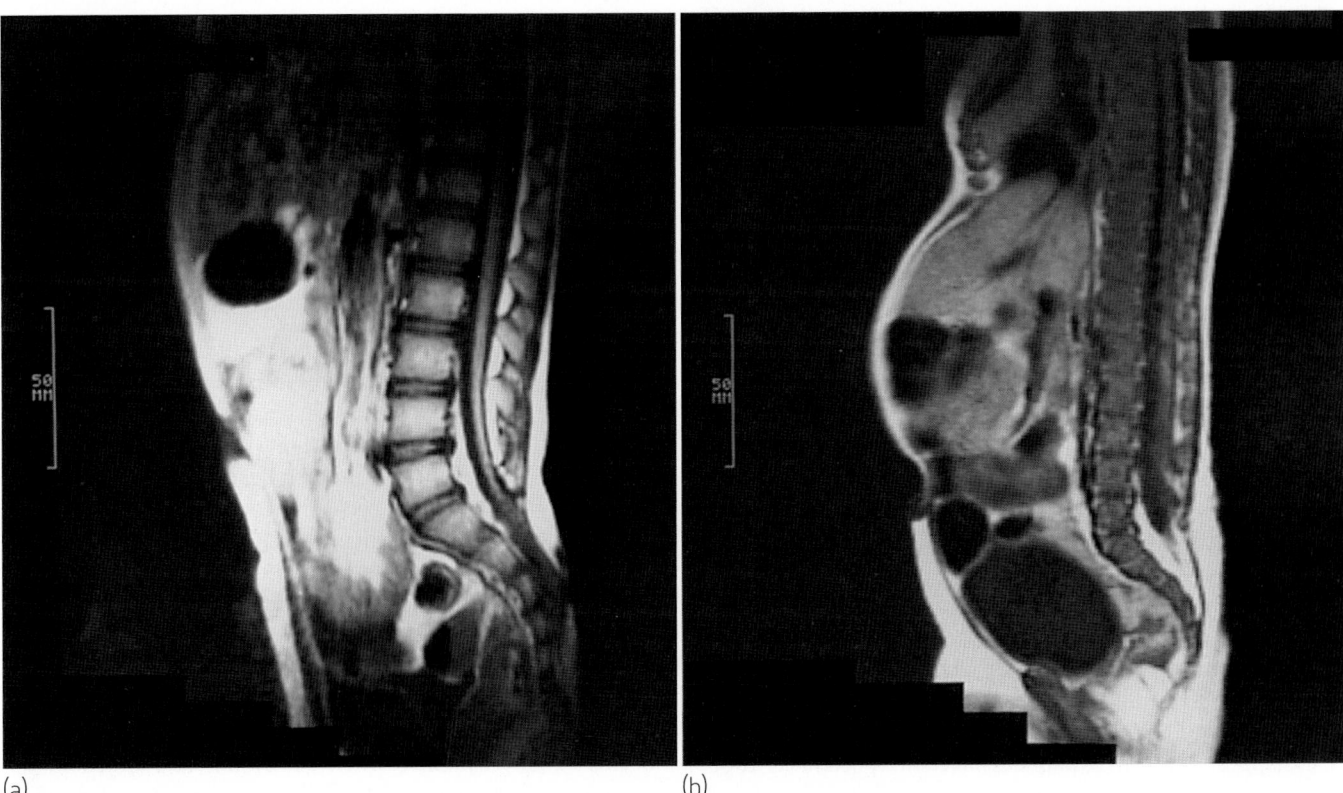

(a) (b)

Figure 13.1 (a) Tethered spinal cord. MRI scan demonstrates a low-lying spinal cord that ends at S1–S2. (A normal spinal cord terminates at L1–L2.) (b) Intraspinal lipoma: this MRI scan demonstrates a tethered spinal cord associated with lipoma. (a, Courtesy Westchester County Medical Center, Valhalla, NY; b, Courtesy Division of Neurosurgery, New York Medical College, New York.)

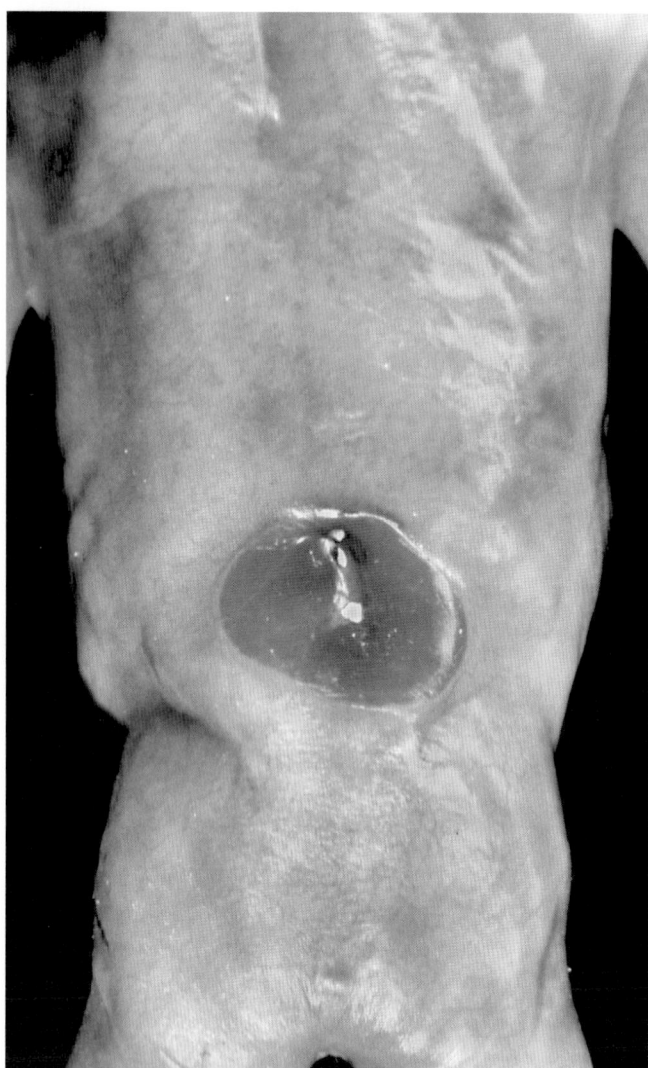

Figure 13.2 Meningocele at the level of the lumbar segment of the spine appears as fluid-filled space covered by a thin membrane in the midline. The lesion was identified during a routine second ultrasound scan (the anomaly scan) in a female fetus at 16 weeks gestation.

The mass is usually evident as a fluid-filled protrusion covered by skin or membrane in the midline (Fig. 13.2) and skin-covered lesions are more evenly distributed along the neuraxis. Very small subcutaneous lesions may remain undetected for prolonged periods.

When careful examination of patients with suspected meningocele reveals significant neurologic abnormality (e.g. equinovarus deformity, gait disturbance, abnormal bladder function) (Laurence 1964), the diagnosis of myelomeningocele is appropriate. These patients have entrapped nerve roots within the defect that can be identified during surgery.

A meningocele in the cranial or high cervical area may coexist with aqueductal stenosis, hydromyelia, or an Arnold–Chiari malformation. Membrane-covered meningoceles are more likely to be accompanied by severe abnormalities;

lesions covered with normal skin are often free of associated abnormalities (Fig. 13.3). Elective surgical treatment is recommended except for very small lesions (Steinbok & Cochrane 1991).

MYELOMENINGOCELE

Myelomeningocele, the most complex of congenital spinal deformities, involves all underlying layers, i.e. spinal cord, nerve roots, meninges, vertebral bodies, skin. The spinal cord may be exposed because of complete failure of neural closure (myeloschisis). The birth-prevalence rate for spinal bifida, which has steadily declined because of improved methods of prenatal diagnosis, has been estimated at 4.6 cases per 10 000 births (Lary & Edmonds 1996). Antenatal diagnosis is discussed in Chapters 15 and 16.

Clinical characteristics

The mortality rate of myelomeningocele is approximately 50% in the absence of therapy; surgical intervention is required because death results from hydrocephalus, meningitis and renal failure. The last complication is induced by chronic urinary tract infections, abnormal urodynamic function and genitourinary tract abnormalities, such as progressive hydronephrosis (Liptak et al 1988).

Myelomeningoceles may be situated at any longitudinal level of the neuraxis. The location and extent of the defect determine the nature and degree of neurologic impairment; rating scales have been developed in an attempt to standardize the evaluation of affected children (Oi & Matsumoto 1992). Lumbosacral involvement is most common (Fig. 13.4). Thoracic defects are the most complex and are frequently associated with serious complications. Cervical cord involvement is different from myelomeningocele of the lower spine and is characterized by two types of abnormalities: the myelocystocele herniating posteriorly into a meningocele and a meningocele with or without an underlying split cord malformation (Steinbok 1995). The protuberant and fluctuant lesion is readily observable and palpable. Varying degrees of paresis of the legs, usually profound, and sphincter dysfunction are the major clinical malformations. Congenital dislocation of the hips or deformities of the feet may also occur. Severe sensory loss and accompanying trophic ulcers may complicate the condition. Occasionally, only sphincter disturbances are present. Radiographs reveal the primary defect of a vertebral arch.

Hydrocephalus (Fig. 13.5), a frequently associated defect, is the result of the Arnold–Chiari malformation (Fig. 13.6); there may be associated aqueductal stenosis. Hydrocephalus, present in about 70% of patients with myelomeningocele, occurs most frequently when the lesion is situated in the thoracolumbar area, which is the case in 90% of patients (Lorber 1971). Although hydrocephalus was believed to be present at birth in only 25% of patients, modern imaging techniques almost always reveal the lesion to be present at birth. Lesions located more rostrally than others produce less

>

>

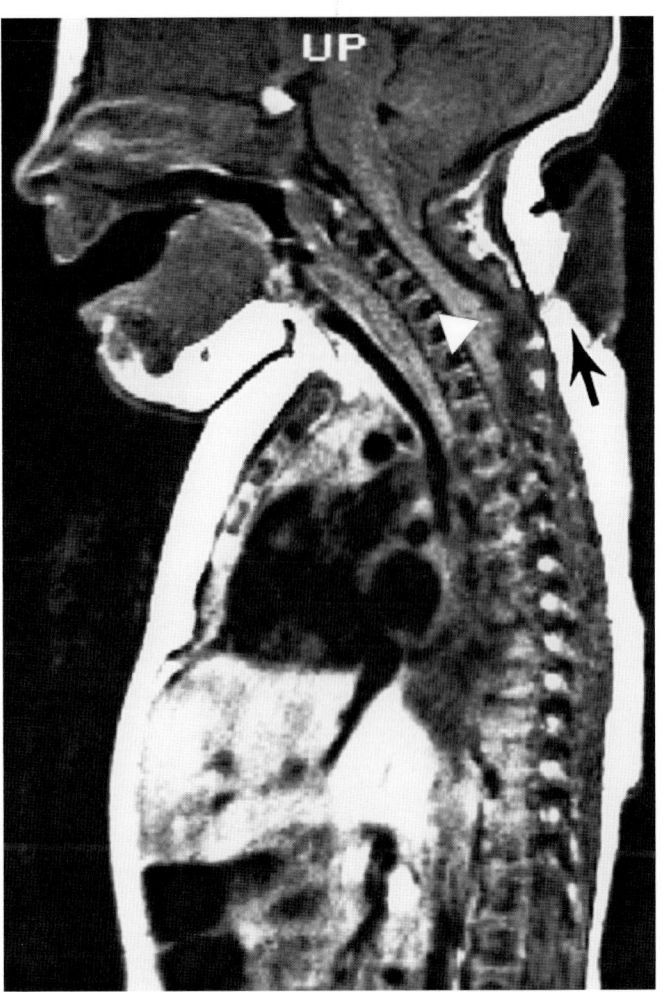

(a)

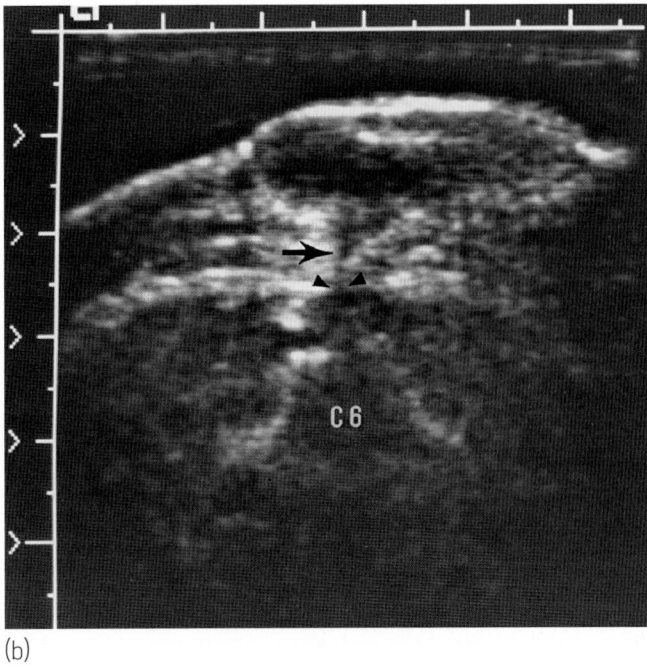

(b)

Figure 13.3 Cervical meningocele in a 3-day-old female infant. (a) C$_6$ meningocele (arrow) extending through small dorsal rachischisis, which is demonstrated on this T1-weighted sagittal MRI scan. Spinal cord is deformed (arrowhead) within focally widened thecal sac but does not extend into the dorsal cyst. (b) Small meningocele tract (arrow) and overlying meningocele are revealed well with transaxial sonogram. Note how the cord is tented toward dorsal opening (arrowheads). (Courtesy Joseph R. Thomson, Department of Radiation Sciences, Loma Linda University School of Medicine, Loma Linda, CA.)

low motor unit paralysis and sphincter involvement. Caudal lesions in the neuraxis are typically associated with bladder and sphincter involvement. The profound paralysis that accompanies caudal involvement often prevents the patient from walking.

Myelomeningocele may be transmitted as an autosomal-recessive or dominant trait, although recurrence risk statistics suggest a polygenic or environmental etiology. This is discussed in detail in Chapter 14.

MANAGEMENT

Management of a child with myelomeningocele requires the efforts of many specialists (Chambers et al 1996, Colgan 1981, Liptak et al 1988, McDonald 1995, Park 1992). Treatment includes prevention of infection, surgical reduction and covering of the myelomeningocele, control of hydro-

cephalus, management of urinary dysfunction and treatment of the paralysis and abnormalities of the hips and feet.

Neurosurgical management, antenatal and postnatal, is discussed in Chapters 42 and 45.

Seizures have been reported in up to 17% of patients with meningomyelocele and almost always occur in those with shunted hydrocephalus (Talwar et al 1995). EEG abnormalities are non-specific. Additional CNS abnormalities seen in these patients are believed to explain the cause of seizures and include encephalomalacia, previous stroke, malformations and intracranial calcifications. Seizures may be difficult to control and, frequently, exacerbation of seizures is associated with shunt malfunction or ventriculitis.

Bladder dysfunction and urinary incontinence pose major management problems and may be present at birth (Boemers et al 1996, Stone 1995). Interruption of sacral nerve roots

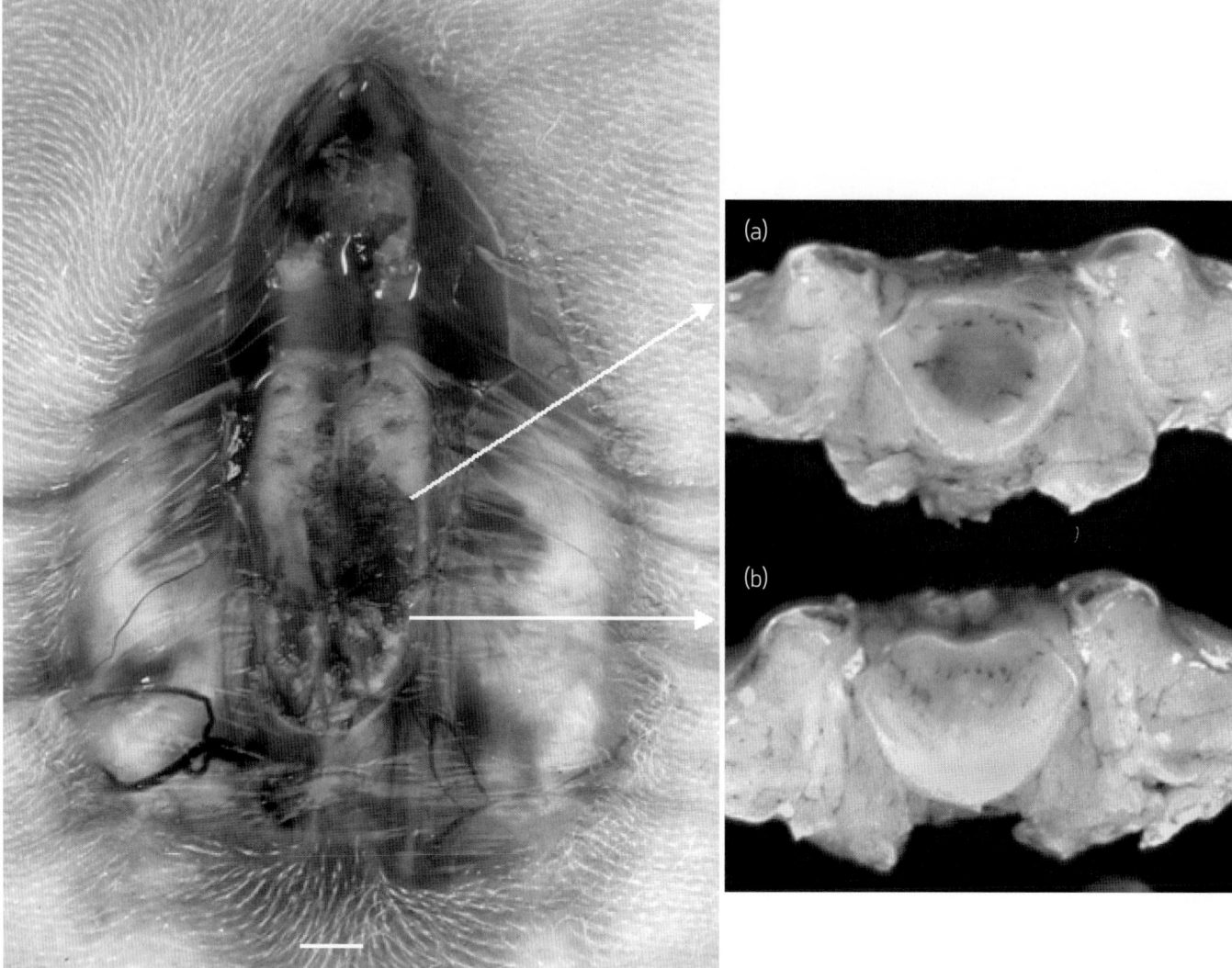

Figure 13.4 Lumbar myelomeningocele in a fetus at 24 weeks gestation. (a) and (b): transverse sections of the lumbar spine showing absent vertebral arches and some spinal cord tissue.

and fiber connections between the brainstem and sacral cord causes the dysfunction. Loss of sphincter tone, overflow incontinence, sacral and rectal loss of sensation and loss of detrusor activity on cystometry are seen. In other patients with higher lesions, dyssynergia of reflex pathways results in irregular contractions of the bladder in conjunction with outlet obstruction. Normal bladder control occurs in 10% of children with myelomeningocele. Prevention of bladder infection requires intermittent catheterization to maintain low residual urine volumes and prophylactic antibacterial drugs (Buyse et al 1995). Vesicoureteral reflux often develops during the second and third year of life and must be evaluated. Reimplantation of the ureters either directly or through an ileal conduit may be helpful. Transurethral resection of the external sphincter has been recommended when ureteral dilation occurs. The use of prosthetic devices emulating sphincters holds promise, as does selective sacral rhizotomy (Schneidau et al 1995).

Constipation and fecal incontinence are common problems in children with spinal dysraphism and usually can be managed medically (Loening Baucke 1996). Dietary manipulation, oral and rectal laxatives and manual evacuation are common treatments. Retrograde colonic enemas may also be successful (Scholler Gyure et al 1996).

Orthopedic defects associated with paralysis, muscle imbalance and spasticity may be severe and necessitate early intervention (Karol 1995, Locke & Sarwark 1996). Hip subluxation is usually treated with prosthetic splints or plaster casting (Alman et al 1996). Sensory deficits of the casted skin areas frequently enhance the likelihood of skin ulcers. Severe foot deformities are seen in up to 80% of children and are treated with splinting or casting (de Carvalho et al 1996). Physical therapy may help to preserve and extend the range of motion of the joints (McDonald 1995).

In infants and children, progressive leg or foot deformity, weakness, pain or deterioration of gait or bladder function

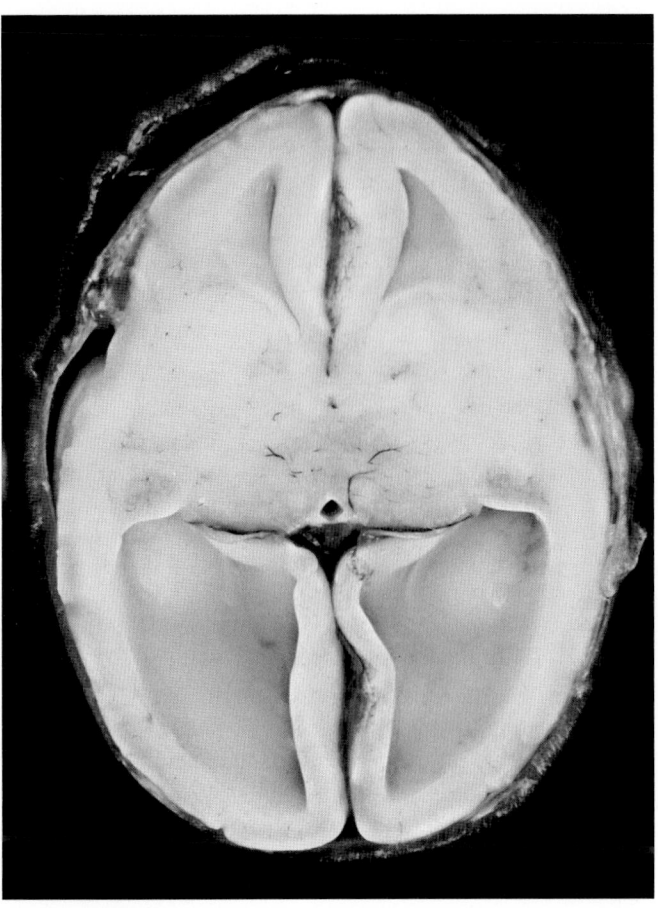

Figure 13.5 Hydrocephalus showing dilated lateral ventricles and a dilated aqueduct in a fetus at 24 weeks gestation with spina bifida.

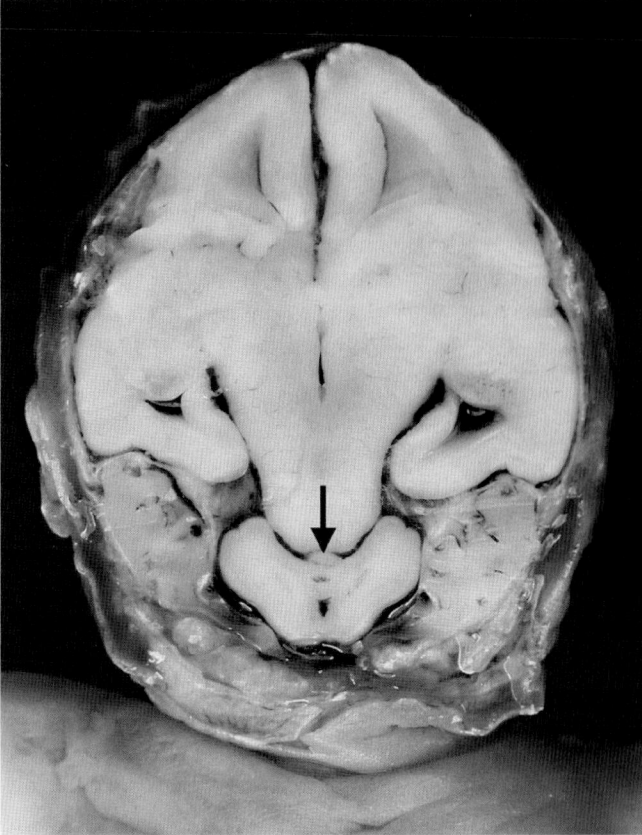

Figure 13.6 Arnold–Chiari malformation from a case shown in Figure 13.5. The cerebellum is wedged in the foramen magnum. The ventral aspect of the cerebellar vermis is pressed against the fourth ventricle (arrow).

suggests restricted growth or tethering of the spinal cord. However, cord tethering may be found in many older children with spina bifida who are neurologically stable (McEnery et al 1992). Stridor, retrocollis, weakness of the vocal cords, periodic breathing, episodes of desaturation and apnea suggest a brainstem malformation (Ward et al 1986). Evidence of brainstem dysfunction may be recorded by doing respiratory pneumograms with a carbon dioxide challenge (Petersen et al 1995) or by using brainstem auditory-evoked response testing (Docherty et al 1987, Sarnat 1992). These signs and symptoms indicate the possibility of an Arnold–Chiari malformation or a tethered spinal cord. The differential diagnosis of delayed deterioration in a child with repaired meningomyelocele includes a malfunctioning or infected shunt, seizures, scoliosis, hydrocephalus, hydromyelia, or an undetected second lesion of occult spina dysraphism, such as a dermoid, epidermoid, or arachnoid cyst. Surgical repair of a tethered spinal cord and shunting or fenestration of large hydromyelic cysts can prevent decline of function (Charney et al 1987, Iskandar et al 1994, Sakamoto et al 1991).

Outcome

Virtually all infants and children born with NTDs are provided with surgical and medical treatment. Previous studies reported that the 5-year survival rate for children with sacral lesions was 97%; for lumbar lesions, 93%; and for thoracic lesions, 75% (Welch & Winston 1987). These data suggest that selective criteria for surgical treatment offer the optimal outcome for the less severely affected child and less suffering and distress for the more handicapped patients with myelomeningocele. This is also discussed in detail in Chapter 44, p. 850.

Counseling

Counseling is essential to ensure that parents understand the nature and severity of the deformities and the necessary surgical and long-term rehabilitative efforts (Liptak et al 1988). Parents should also be aware of the patients' potential for intellectual and physical development. Also, awareness of the higher incidence of latex allergy in children with spina bifida is important to communicate to the family and others involved in their care (Konz et al 1995).

SPLIT CORD MALFORMATIONS

Recently the term *split cord malformations* (SCMs) has been applied to diastematomyelia (SCM I) and diplomyelia (SCM II) (Dias & Pan 1995). SCMs can be divided into two types, based on the composition of the dural coverings and intervening mesenchymal tissue. Type I malformations are composed of two dural sacs and a bony or fibrocartilaginous spur; type II malformations are composed of a single dural sac and intradural fibrous banks. In either case the intervening mesenchymal elements contribute to progressive neurologic, urologic and orthopedic deterioration from spinal cord tethering. The natural history of these lesions supports an early and aggressive operative approach to untether the spinal cord before clinical deterioration begins.

Diastematomyelia

In diastematomyelia a midline septum divides the spinal cord longitudinally into two usually unequal portions extending up to 10 thoracolumbar segments (Bradford et al 1991, Pang 1992). The septum may span the entire width of the spinal canal and is anchored to the ventral dura mater on the posterior aspect of the vertebral arch or dura mater. The septum is derived from mesoderm and it is composed of fibrous tissue, cartilage or bone. The etiology of diastematomyelia is currently unknown.

Clinical characteristics

Patients with diastematomyelia present with a congenital scoliosis or cutaneous lesion such as hairy patch, dimple, hemangioma, subcutaneous mass or teratoma (Kothari & Bauer 1997). They may also develop a progressive myelopathy with deformities of the feet, scoliosis, kyphosis or discrepancy in leg length. Resection of the spur frequently does not result in clinical improvement. Resection of the spur should be performed in patients who have progressive neurologic manifestations; those without worsening symptoms should be observed until progression occurs and then resection performed (Miller et al 1993). Diastematomyelia can be detected prenatally by ultrasonography (Anderson et al 1994, Sepulveda et al 1997). MRI is the preferred neuroimaging study for the evaluation of patients suspected of having this condition. Although most lesions occur in the lumbosacral region, presentations involving the cervical cord are reported. Diastematomyelia is also much more common in females (McLone & La Marca 1997). Urodynamic and electrophysiological studies are abnormal in about 80% of patients (Kothari & Bauer 1997).

Diplomyelia

Diplomyelia is a side-by-side or antero-posterior duplication or splitting of the spinal cord (Dias & Pang 1995, Norman et al 1995). Two central canals are usually present, each surrounded by gray and white matter arranged in the normal pattern. The two cords are often completely reunited caudally but may remain separated to the tip of the conus medullaris. A bony septum may partly intervene. The two cords are often unequal, may be side-by-side (the most common position), or one may be dorsal to the other. These malformations are compatible with normal function; deterioration suggests the presence of diastematomyelia or tethering. The etiology of this condition remains unknown.

HEMIVERTEBRA

This malformation can be identified as an isolated lesion or as part of a more complex sequence affecting the vertebral spine such as in caudal regression. Its etiology is unclear; it is thought to be linked to an abnormal development of the notochord. Hemivertebra is, a vertebral spine malformation. Almost invariably it affects the spinal cord (Fig. 13.7). The organs and/or segments of the body affected depend from the level at which the lesion appears and from the degree of deformity the spinal cord may suffer: the more distally placed the lesion is, the higher the chances for the patient to suffer from anal and/or uretral dysfunction as well as from varying degrees of neuromuscular pathology affecting the limbs.

SACRAL AGENESIS (see also p. 781)

Sacral agenesis, or caudal regression syndrome, is the complete or partial absence of the sacrum, hemisacrum, coccyx and lower vertebrae, and often includes genitourinary and anorectal anomalies (Davidoff et al 1991, Towfighi & Housman 1991). Although most cases are sporadic, maternal diabetes mellitus (Miller et al 1981) and an autosomal-dominant form associated with chromosome 7q36 deletion are recognized (Chatkupt et al 1994, Lynch et al 1995, Schrander-Stumpel et al 1988). The hallmark of this autosomal-dominant condition is the presence of partial sacral agenesis with an intact first sacral vertebra, a presacral mass and an anorectal malformation.

The neurologic findings are similar to those of myelomeningocele, ranging from a minimal deficit to equinovarus deformity of the feet to more extensive sensory and motor deficits of the lower extremities. The level of bone anomaly corresponds well with the level of weakness but not to sensory loss; sensation is usually preserved. The caudal spinal cord is often truncated, dysraphic and tethered (Estin & Cohen 1995). Most patients have neurogenic urinary tract and bowel impairment, visceral abnormalities, flattened buttocks and prominent iliac crests (Sarnat 1992). Constipation and perianal sepsis are common complaints. Ascending infection resulting in bacterial meningitis has also been reported.

Some patients experience progressive neurologic deficits, demonstrating that sacral agenesis is not always a static disability (O'Neill et al 1995). Slow deterioration of neurologic function may masquerade as an orthopedic or urologic problem unless the potential for progressive lesions is appreciated. Dural sac stenosis, tethered spinal cord, diastematomyelia and cauda equina lipomas and dermoids have also been associated with sacral agenesis (Brooks et al 1981). Although plain radiographs demonstrate the degree of sacral agenesis, CT or MRI is necessary to delineate the underlying

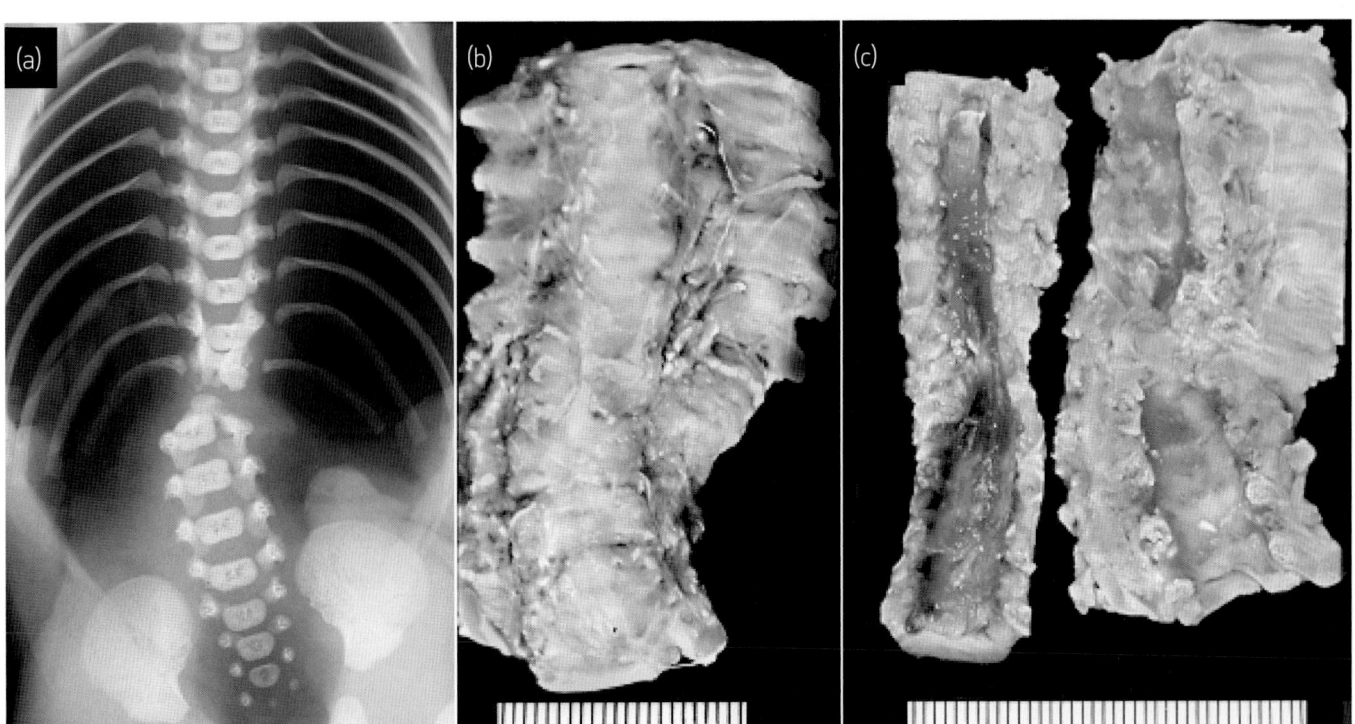

Figure 13.7 A case of hemivertebra at 23 weeks gestation observed during routine ultrasound examination at 22 weeks. (a) Post-mortem X-ray showing a 12th hemivertebral body and gross distortion of the spine best observed in (b). (c) The spinal canal is very narrow and the spinal cord shows severe constriction at this level.

spinal cord anomalies (Fig. 13.8) (Gundry & Heithoff 1994). Surgical management is discussed on page 851.

ARNOLD–CHIARI MALFORMATION

Four variations of the Arnold–Chiari malformation exist (Table 13.3) (Cai & Oakes 1997, Norman et al 1995). In type 2, the most frequently encountered, the cerebellum and medulla oblongata are shifted caudally; resultant packing into the cervical spinal canal results in deformation. Because of kinking, the thinned and elongated medulla may actually be positioned side-by-side with the upper segments of the dwarfed and deformed cervical spinal cord (Fig. 13.9). Curiously, the abnormal positioning causes the upper cervical roots to course upward before leaving the vertebral foramina. The pons is thin and narrow. By definition, type 2 Arnold–Chiari malformation is associated with myelomeningocele. Hydrocephalus occurs in most patients secondary to aqueductal stenosis or obstruction to CSF flow around the medulla.

Hydromyelia and syringomyelia of the cervical spinal cord occur in 20–50% of patients (Breningstall et al 1992, Friede 1989). Vascular lesions, including hemorrhage and infarction, are often present in the tegmentum of the medulla in children, with resultant altered respiratory control (Papasozomenos & Roessman 1981). Other CNS defects, such as small increased numbers of gyri, heterotopias, Klippel–Feil syndrome, craniolacunas and bony anomalies at the

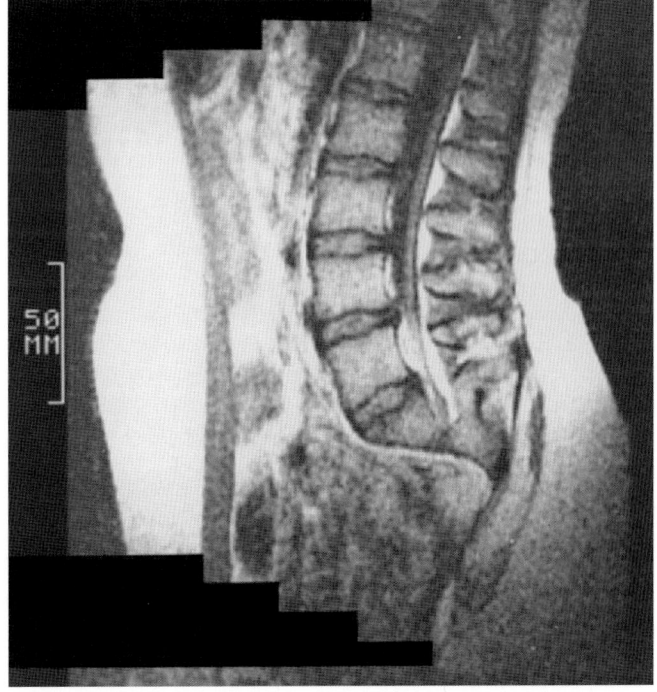

Figure 13.8 Sacral agenesis. This MRI scan demonstrates a tethered spinal cord that ends at L_5 and is associated with sacral agenesis. (Courtesy Westchester County Medical Center, Valhalla, NY.)

Table 13.3 Classification of Arnold–Chiari malformations

Type	Anatomic abnormalities	Neurologic findings
1	Downward displacement of the cerebellum and tonsils, elongated brainstem fourth ventricle	Mild and delayed onset of headache and brainstem symptoms usually beginning in adolescence. Symptoms secondary to hydrocephalus or syringomyelia
2	Downward displacement of the cerebellar vermis and cerebellar tonsils; thinned and elongated medulla may actually be positioned side-by-side with the upper segments of the atrophic cervical spinal cord	Associated with myelomeningocele in more than 95% of patients; symptoms resulting from progressive hydrocephalus and secondary brainstem dysfunction; feeding and respiratory complications are common, including apnea
3	Encephalocervical meningocele with spina bifida over the cervical area and protrusion of the cerebellum through the posterior encephalocele	Features similar to Arnold–Chiari type 2, without the same degree of association with myelomeningocele
4	Hypoplasia of the cerebellum	Variable findings from asymptomatic to classic cerebellar dysfunction

Source: From Norman et al 1995, Sarnat 1992, Friede 1989.

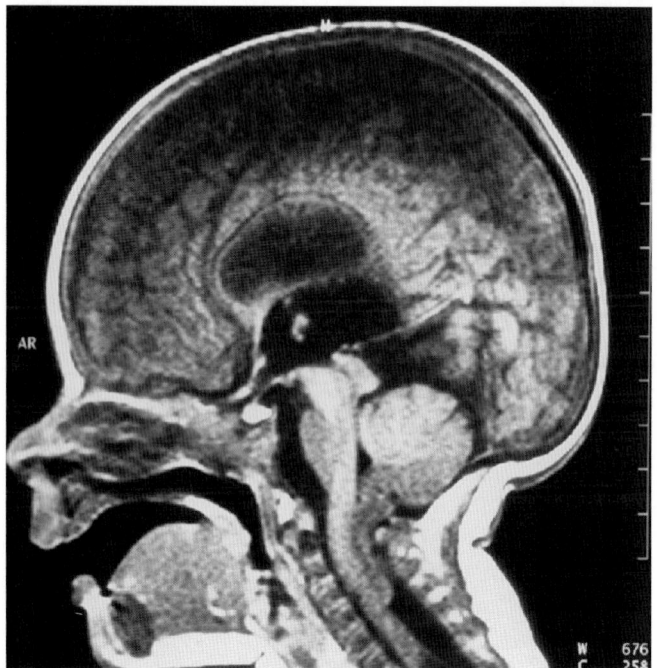

Figure 13.9 A 2-month-old male with spinal dysraphism. The mid sagittal T1-weighted MRI of the brain demonstrates a small posterior fossa, extension of the cerebellar tissue through the foramen magnum into the upper cervical spinal thecal sac, small and vertically oriented fourth ventricle and an enlarged third ventricle. The axial images, not seen, depicted enlargement of the lateral ventricles. These are classic findings of Arnold–Chiari type 2 malformation. Incidental note is made of the uppermost aspect of a cervical spinal cord syrinx, also a finding of Arnold–Chiari type 2 malformation. (Courtesy of Shahrokh Toranji, Department of Radiation Sciences, Loma Linda University School of Medicine, Loma Linda, CA.)

base of the skull, often accompany the Arnold–Chiari malformation.

Type I Arnold–Chiari malformation is similar to type 2, but the malformation is milder. The cerebellum is displaced into the cervical spinal canal. Although it is characteristically long and thin the medulla does not have a side-by-side relationship with the cervical cord. No associated myelomeningocele exists. Type 3 is essentially an encephalocervical meningocele and consists of spina bifida over the cervical area with protrusions of the cerebellum through the opening. Type 4 consists of a single abnormality, hypoplasia of the cerebellum, and may be a variation of the Dandy–Walker syndrome (Caviness 1976).

Pathophysiology

The precise mechanism causing Arnold–Chiari malformation is unknown (Cai & Oakes 1997, Gilbert et al 1986, Norman et al 1995, Sarnat 1992). At least five explanations have been proposed: (1) tethering at the brainstem-cervical cord junction; (2) altered CSF dynamics causing excessive localized brainstem pressure and distortion; (3) a primary brainstem and cerebellar malformation; (4) birth trauma; and (5) hypoplasia of the posterior cranial fossa bony structures (Nishikawa et al 1997).

Clinical characteristics

Type 1 Arnold–Chiari malformation may not be associated with clinical manifestations for many decades (Archer et al 1977). The initial symptoms are recurrent occipital and frontal headaches, neck pain, unsteady gait, progressive ataxia and difficulty in swallowing (McClone & LaMarca 1997a). The headaches are typically worsened by coughing, exertion, positional changes, or Valsalva maneuvers. Various functions of cranial nerves IX to XII are compromised. The gag reflex may be unelicitable and the soft palate paretic.

Cerebellar impairment, evidenced by ataxia and nystagmus, may be apparent. Downbeat nystagmus and periodic alternating nystagmus are characteristic of craniocervical anomalies, such as the Arnold–Chiari malformation. Extensor toe signs and deep tendon reflexes are present, and the latter are pathologically increased. The posterior columns are usually involved with compromised vibration and position sense. Increased intracranial pressure may also develop. Occasionally children with Arnold–Chiari type I malformations may present with severe spinal cord injury or death after minor injury (McClone & LaMarca 1997b).

Management

Careful monitoring of infants with known Arnold–Chiari malformations is advocated (Cai & Oakes 1997, Charney et al 1987, Venes et al 1986). Evaluation with MRI is now the procedure of choice (Gundry & Heithoff 1994). In patients with Arnold–Chiari type 1 malformations, MRI studies have demonstrated that syringomyelia was present in 70%; the remaining patients had evidence of frank herniation of the cerebellar tonsils below the foramen magnum (Amer & el-Shmam 1997). The neurosurgical management is discussed in Chapter 43.

ENCEPHALOCELE

A cephalocele is a herniation of intercranial contents through a skull defect. Cephaloceles are classified by their contents and location (Martinez-Lage et al 1996). Cranial meningoceles contain only leptomeninges and CSF, whereas encephaloceles also contain brain (Norman et al 1995). A ventriculocele is an encephalocele in which the herniated brain contents also contain portions of the ventricle. The incidence of cephaloceles is approximately 0.8 to 3.0 per 100 000 live births with encephaloceles being the most common form.

Encephaloceles are usually located in the occipital areas (75%) and frontal areas (25%). The latter condition occurs most frequently among Asians. Basal and trans-sphenoidal encephaloceles are rare; they may appear between the ethmoid and sphenoid bones and extend into the upper area of the orbit, nose, or forehead and are termed *sincipital encephaloceles* (Fig. 13.10); those in the occipital regions are termed *notencephaloceles* (Fig. 13.11). Exencephaly consists of a large out-pouching of brain tissue with surrounding thick walls. This defect may involve the spinal cord, forming an encephalomyelocele. Cranial encephalocele may contain

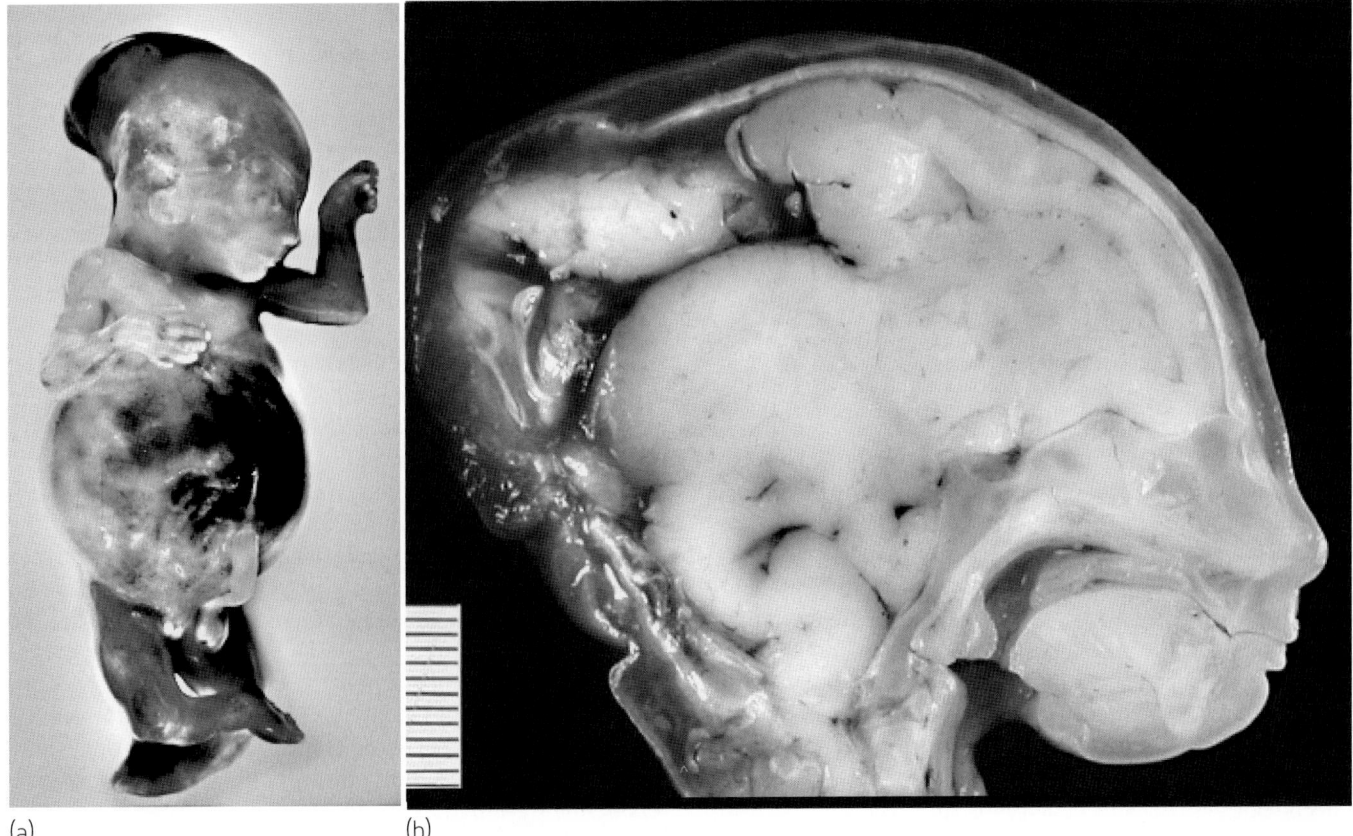

(a)   (b)

Figure 13.10 (a),(b) Sincipital encephalocele which has developed through a defect in the frontal bone in a fetus at 14 weeks gestation.

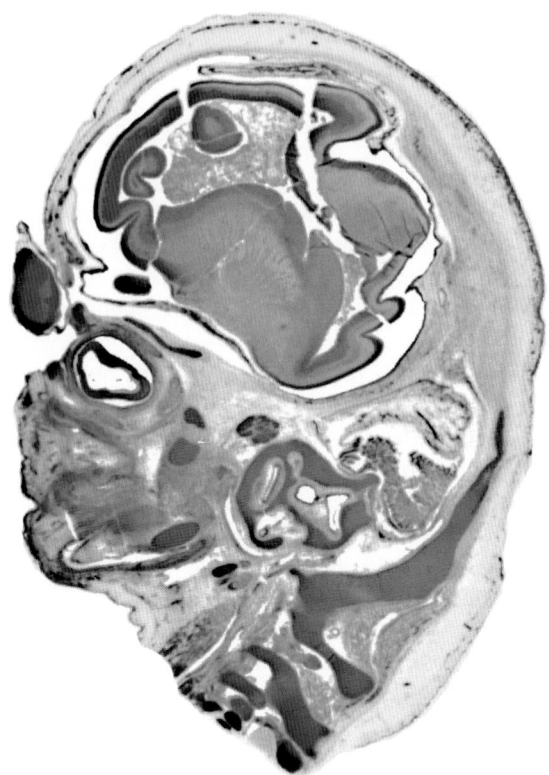

Figure 13.11 Occipital encephalocele in a case of Meckel–Gruber syndrome. Note the post axial polydactyly and the dilated abdomen due to multicystic kidneys in a fetus at 20 weeks gestation.

Table 13.4 Selected syndromes associated with encephaloceles

Syndrome	Characteristics
Walker–Warburg syndrome	Hydrocephalus, severe neurologic impairment, vermian agenesis, type 2 lissencephaly, autosomal recessive
Meckel–Gruber syndrome	Polycystic kidney, sloping forehead, polydactyly, hepatobiliary fibrosis, cleft lip and palate, autosomal recessive
Dandy–Walker syndrome	Hydrocephalus, partial or complete absence of the cerebellar vermis, posterior fossa cyst contiguous with the fourth ventricle, cranial nerve palsies, nystagmus, truncal ataxia, sporadic occurrence
Joubert syndrome	Cerebellar vermian aplasia, episodic hyperpnea, abnormal eye movements, rhythmic protrusion of the tongue, ataxia, retardation, colobomas, retinal dystrophy, renal cysts, autosomal recessive
Goldenhar–Gorlin syndrome	Orofacial abnormalities, preauricular tags, epibulbar dermoids, sporadic occurrence
Knobloch syndrome	Vitreoretinal degeneration with retinal detachment, high myopia, and occipital encephalocele, normal intelligence, chromosome 21q22.3
Roberts syndrome	Anterior encephalocele, autosomal recessive
Median cleft face syndrome	Anterior encephalocele, autosomal dominant

Source: From OMIM 2000.

a combination of meninges, ventricles and brain parenchyma (Wininger & Donnenfeld 1994).

The pathogenesis of encephalocele formation is incompletely understood but is likely related to defects in the development of the skull base (Chapman et al 1989, Marin-Padilla 1991).

Clinical characteristics

A fluctuant, round, balloon-like mass that protrudes from the cranium, usually posteriorly, is the most typical manifestation of encephaloceles. The mass may pulsate and be covered by an erythematous, translucent, or opaque membrane or by normal skin. The covering may not be uniform throughout its surface. The amount of compromised and deformed neural tissue determines the extent of cerebral dysfunction (Mealey et al 1970). Brain tissue not extending into the encephalocele may be deformed and functionally impaired.

Severe intellectual and motor delays typically occur in association with microcephaly; motor delay is accompanied by weakness and spasticity. Intellectual impairment is more prevalent in patients with posterior rather than anterior encephaloceles (Hockley et al 1990). However, some patients may have completely normal development. Occipital lobe destruction is associated with various degrees of visual impairment. When the deformity includes a ventricle, hydro-cephalus is almost inevitable. Because of increased pressure, the encephalocele may become stretched until the covering is infracted, with resultant infection and rupture.

Other malformations may accompany encephaloceles, including Dandy–Walker syndrome, Klippel–Feil syndrome, Arnold–Chiari malformation, porencephaly, agenesis of the corpus callosum, myelodysplasia, optic nerve dysplasia and cleft palate (Bindal et al 1991, Cohen & Lemire 1982, Norman et al 1995). Although ultrasonography may be helpful, the clinical diagnosis is confirmed by CT or MRI (Fig. 13.12).

Neuroendocrine disturbances occur, particularly with basal encephaloceles that involve the sella turcica or sphenoid sinus (Ellyn et al 1980). These conditions may be undetectable by gross inspection; intranasal mass or endocrine dysfunction are the cardinal features.

Encephaloceles are seen with a variety of chromosomal disorders (e.g. trisomy 13,18; 13q or 16q deletion) and syndromes (Table 13.4). They can be inherited in an

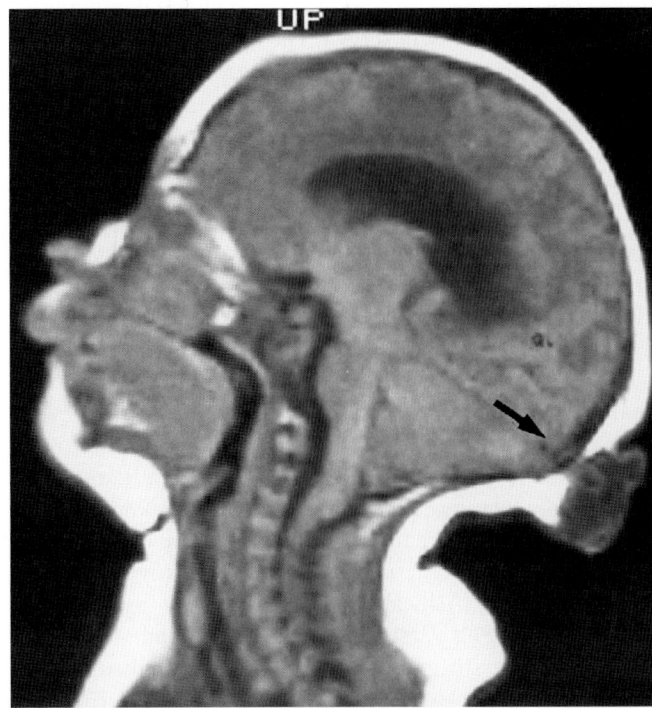

(a)

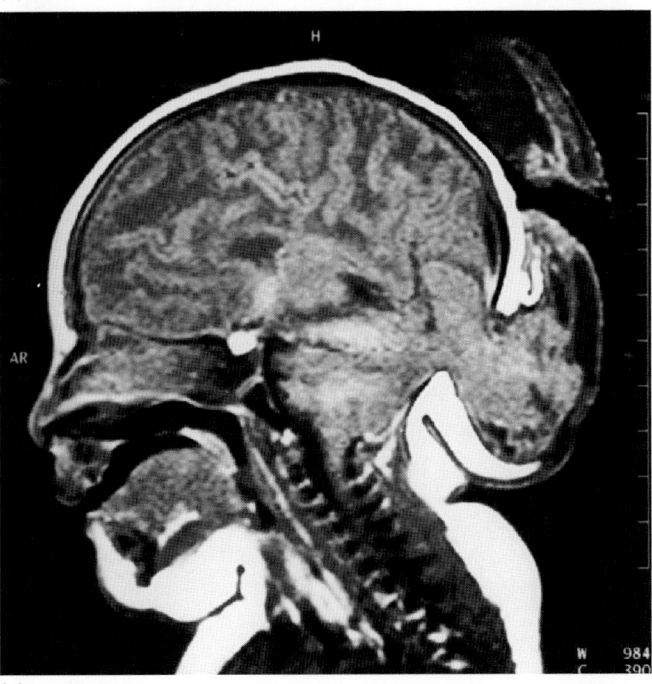

(b)

Figure 13.12 Meningoencephalocele in a 4-day-old female infant. (a) Small nubbin of brain tissue (arrow) extending into small occipital meningoencephalocele; these defects are better demonstrated with this T1-weighted sagittal MRI than with axial CT. (b) Large meningoencephalocele in a newborn infant seen on a sagittal T1-weighted image of the brain that also demonstrates a large occipital midline bony defect. (Courtesy of Shahrokh Toranji, Department of Radiation Sciences, Loma Linda University School of Medicine, Loma Linda, CA.)

autosomal-recessive mode (Cohen & Lemire 1982). Occipital encephalocele, microcephaly, cleft palate or lip, polydactyly, holoprosencephaly and polycystic kidneys constitute Meckel–Gruber syndrome (McKusick 1994). Retinal degeneration with detachment and occipital encephalocele (Knobloch syndrome) is another autosomal-recessive condition (Knobloch & Layer 1971).

Nasal glioma, a congenital tumor, appears as a fronto-nasal mass that mimics an encephalocele (Lemire et al 1975, Younus & Coode 1986). The tumor is derived from herniated brain tissue that has lost its connection to the brain; this relationship can be demonstrated by neuroimaging techniques.

Management and prognosis of encephaloceles are discussed in Chapter 44.

ANENCEPHALY

Anencephaly is a congenital malformation in which both cerebral hemispheres are absent. The cranial vault defect is an extensive cranioschisis (Medical Task Force on Anencephaly 1990). Most anencephalic infants are stillborn. Those infants born alive die shortly after birth (Botkin 1988).

Epidemiologic studies demonstrate a striking variation in prevalence rates. The highest incidence is in Great Britain and Ireland, and the lowest incidence is in Asia, Africa and South America. Other countries have intermediate rates of incidence. Anencephaly occurs six times more frequently in whites than in blacks. Females are more often affected than males.

Antenatal diagnosis is possible using assays of α-fetoprotein or acetylcholinesterase, which is increased in maternal serum and amniotic fluid (Brennand et al 1998, Brock et al 1975, Chan et al 1995, Seller et al 1974). Antenatal diagnosis is also feasible through the use of fetal ultrasonography (Goldstein & Filly 1988, Johnson et al 1997). In the past two decades, prenatal screening with ultrasound, which is near 100% accurate, and maternal α-fetoprotein determinations have resulted in earlier detection of anencephaly (Sabbagha et al 1985). Earlier detection has resulted in a dramatic decrease in the average gestational age at birth, from 35.6 weeks in the 1970s to 19.6 weeks in 1988–1990, with virtually no term live-born anencephalic infants born after 1990 in those pregnancies in which a prenatal diagnosis of anencephaly had been made (Limb & Holmes 1994).

Pathogenesis

Anencephaly follows failure of closure of the anterior neural tube (Lemire 1987). The critical period during which the neural tube closes is from approximately day 21 to day 26 of gestation; the embryonic defect probably occurs before closure of the anterior neuropore on day 26. Supportive data with anencephaly have recently been reported (Golden & Chernoff 1995). Two mechanisms leading to anterior NTDs were proposed. Anencephaly could result from failure of neural tube closure to occur at a discrete site, or if there was failure of two closure sites to meet.

The cause of anencephaly remains unknown. Various agents have been incriminated, including perinatal infections, folic acid antagonists, drinking water minerals, maternal hyperthermia, chromosomal abnormalities and an unidentified agent in blighted potato tubers (Kurent & Sever 1973, Lemire 1987, Miller et al 1978, Renwick 1972). These allegations of causal relationship remain unproven. As noted in the earlier section on spina bifida, evidence suggests a potential genetic etiology. Mutations of the *BRCA1* gene in mice embryos are associated with a 40% incidence of spina bifida and anencephaly (Gowen et al 1996). Also, mice homozygous for a deficiency in the paired class *Hox* gene, *Cart 1*, may have a form of anencephaly (meroanencephaly) at birth (Zhao et al 1996). Prenatal treatment of these mice with folic acid suppressed NTD formation. Likewise, disruption of the *MacMARCKS* gene prevents cranial neural tube closure and results in anencephaly (Chen et al 1996). The *MacMARKS* gene is a member of the MARCKS family of protein kinase C substrates that integrate calcium and kinase dependent signals to regulate actin structure at the cell membrane.

Pathology

The cranial vault is defective over the vertex, exposing a soft, angiomatous mass of neural tissue covered by a thin membrane continuous with the skin (Fig. 13.13) (Lemire et al 1978). The cranial abnormality may extend inferiorly to the cervical region with formation of a complete spina bifida. The extremely thin and flattened spinal cord (craniorachischisis) is readily observed. The optic globes are usually protuberant because of inadequate bony orbits.

Clinical characteristics

Anencephaly is a lethal condition (Lemire et al 1978, Melnick & Myrianthopoulous 1987). No specific treatment is available. Neuroendocrine defects are frequent, with failure of endocrine end-organ development secondary to a hypoplastic pituitary gland. Adrenal insufficiency may be associated with adrenocortical hypoplasia. The posterior pituitary is also hypoplastic and may cause clinical diabetes insipidus.

Recent studies have demonstrated that anencephalic infants can exhibit a wide variety of behaviors and that these can be detected prenatally (Ashwal et al 1990, Kurauchi et al 1995, Luyendijk & Treffers 1992). Term infants with anencephaly who live for several days may respond to auditory, vestibular and painful stimuli that are mediated by brainstem, diencephalic and spinal pathways without cerebral involvement (Ashwal et al 1990, Medical Task Force on Anencephaly 1990). Described behaviors include jitteriness, hyperirritability, stiffening, spontaneous or stimulus-induced myoclonus of the extremities, opisthotonic posturing and smiling (Ashwal et al 1990, Luyendijk & Treffers 1992).

By definition, anencephalic infants are permanently unconscious (Medical Task Force on Anencephaly 1990). Although some concerns have been raised that conscious-

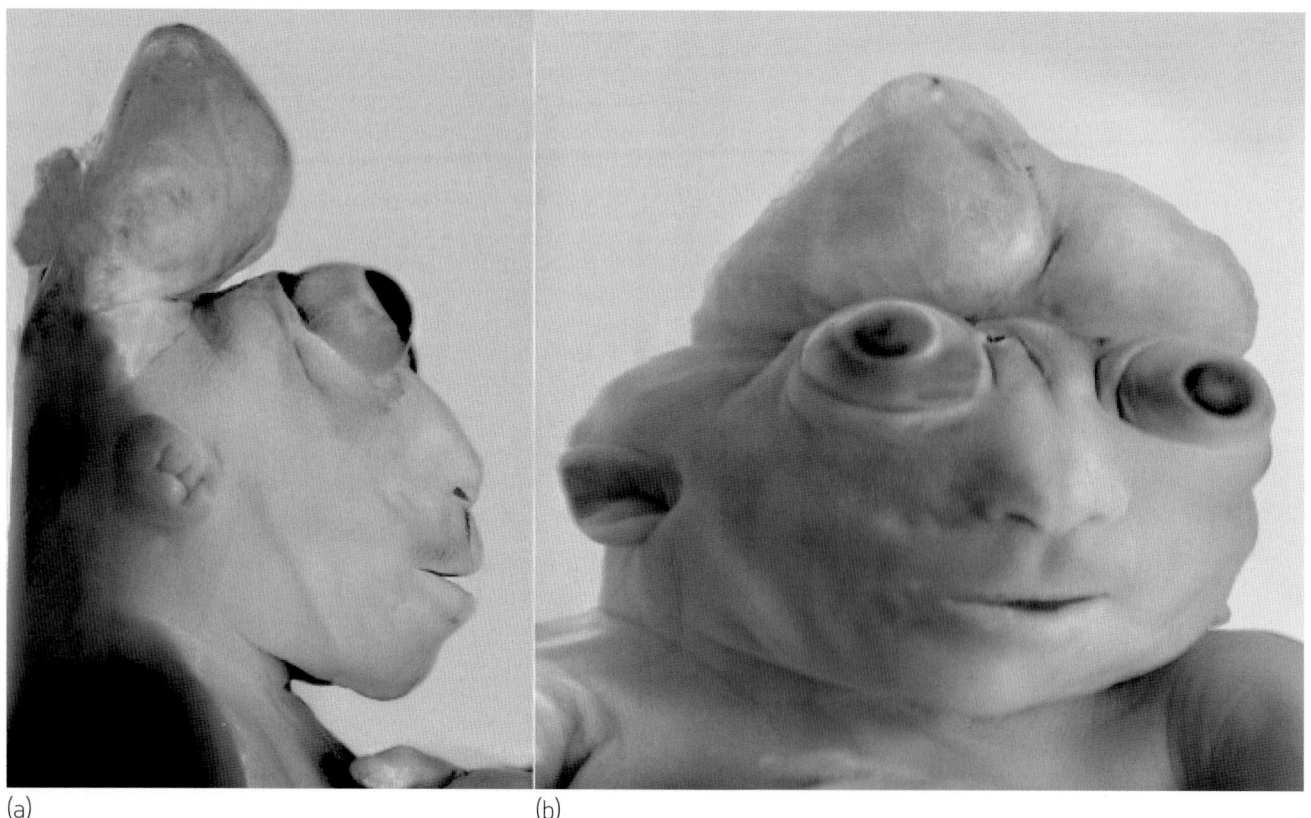

(a)   (b)

Figure 13.13 Anencephaly. (a) right lateral and (b) antero-posterior views of fetus at 24 weeks gestation. Note the absent calvarium and the vascularized membranous tissue instead.

ness may be preserved in the brainstems of such infants, because this is a developmental rather than an acquired brain lesion (Shewman et al 1989), medical evidence to support this contention has not been published (Ashwal et al 1990, Lemire et al 1978). Several studies have demonstrated that brainstem structures are rudimentary, hypoplastic and virtually devoid of neurons, fiber tracts, neural networks, or any evidence of primitive functional organization that could support conscious behaviors (Nakamura et al 1972, Vare & Bansal 1971, Walters et al 1997).

The diagnosis of brain death in anencephalic infants is problematic because of the severe CNS malformations that are present, particularly in the brainstem (Ashwal et al 1990). However, brain death can be diagnosed and depends on determining the absence of brainstem function including apnea. Difficulties in performing the examination have been previously described (Ashwal et al 1990). Serial examinations demonstrating the loss of any previously detectable cranial nerve reflexes and the performance of repeated apnea challenge studies documenting the absence of respiratory effort with PCO_2 above 60 torr over 24–48 hours are confirmatory. In anencephalic infants, in contrast to neonates with other etiologies of suspected brain death, there is no need for confirmatory laboratory studies (e.g. electroencephalography or determination of CBF), as these cannot be performed for technical reasons.

In the United States, regulations do not permit organ donation from anencephalic infants because brain death criteria are not fulfilled (Peabody et al 1989). This policy is controversial, as demonstrated by the recent action of the American Medical Association's Council on & Ethical and Judicial Affairs' withdrawal of its initial opinion calling for the direct procurement of organs from anencephalic infants (Walters et al 1997).

Iniencephaly is a rare, lethal, axial dysraphic malformation diagnosed on the basis of three cardinal features: deficiency of the occipital bone, cervicothoracic spinal retroflexion and rachischisis (Scherrer et al 1992). Iniencephaly differs from anencephaly in that the cranial cavity is present and skin covers the head and retroflexed region (Lemire et al 1972, Norman et al 1995). Severe retroflexion of the neck present on fetal ultrasound may suggest the diagnosis (Meizner et al 1992). The majority of the patients also have visceral and other severe CNS malformations. Another related condition is meroanencephaly (Isada et al 1993), a rare form of anencephaly characterized by malformed cranial bones and a median cranial defect through which protrudes the area cerebrovasculosa.

CLEAVAGE AND DIFFERENTIATION DEFECTS

HOLOPROSENCEPHALY

Holoprosencephaly (HPE) results from failure of cleavage of the embryonic forebrain, or prosencephalon, into symmetric cerebral hemispheres. The defect occurs between the 18th and the 28th day post fertilization. It affects both the brain and the face. Three types have been described following its degree of severity: (A) Lobar: where the right and left lobes are separated but with some continuity between the hemispheres at the level of the frontal cortex. (B) Semilobar: there is partial separation between the hemispheres, and (C) alobar HPE when a single lobe is present (holosphere) with a single brain. There is no interhemispheric fissure in either the anlage of the telencephalon or of the diencephalons (DeMyer 1971, Dubourg et al 2007, Christèle Norman et al 1995, Leech & Shuman 1986). Leptomeningeal glioneuronal heterotopias are commonly found in patients with HPE (Mizuguchi et al 1994). Another milder subtype of holoprosencephaly called middle interhemispheric variant or syntelencephaly has been identified (Barkovich et al 1993, Simon et al 2002).

HPE has a prevalence of 1:250 during embryogenesis and 1:16000 newborn infants (Roessler et al 1996). Children with less severe forms recently identified, i.e. syntelencephaly, will lead to a higher prevalence of the disease. The molecular basis underlying HPE is unknown. Teratogens, non-random chromosomal anomalies, and familial forms with autosomal-dominant and autosomal-recessive inheritance have been described (Balci et al 1993, Roessler et al 1996). HPE occurs more commonly in infants born to diabetic mothers (Kalter 1993). The genetics of HPE is discussed on page 272, Chapter 14.

Clinical characteristics

The majority of patients with HPE have severe delayed development, spastic quadriplegia, failure to thrive and seizures. Microphthalmia, ocular hypotelorism and colobomas, midface hypoplasia, single central upper incisor and cleft lip and palate are frequently present. Neuroendocrine dysfunction results from defects of the anterior and posterior pituitary and secondary hypoplasia of endocrine end organs (de Zegher et al 1992, Takahashi et al 1995). Cranial ultrasonography, CT and MRI demonstrate the malformation (Fitz 1994). Some patients with HPE have partial development of the posterior corpus callosum (Rubenstein et al 1996). The EEG is usually suppressed over the holoprosencephalic region, whereas in other patients asynchronous sharp waves and spikes are seen over the frontal regions with a decreasing gradient occipitally (Shah et al 1992). Children with lobar HPE usually have significant developmental delays; some children with normal or near normal development and long-term survival have been reported (Elias et al 1992, Pensler et al 1993).

Alobar holoprosencephaly arises from the rudimentary development of the prosencephalon, which includes lack of delineation of an interhemispheric fissure. The undivided telencephalon persists as a solitary lobe without olfactory bulbs or tracts (Fig. 13.14) (DeMyer 1975).

Various combinations of median facial defects are associated with the holoprosencephalic brain. The precordial mesoderm is the anlage of the median facial bones. Facial

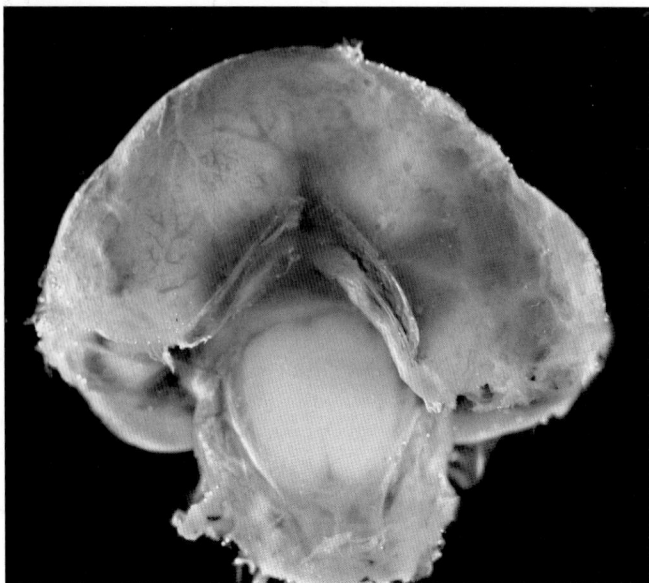

Figure 13.14 Alobar holoprosencephaly in a fetus at 14 weeks gestation. The interhemispheric fissure is absent.

anomalies accompany HPE because the induction process that eventually shapes the neural ectoderm and precordial mesoderm is flawed. When the precordial mesoderm is defective, the midline bones may be deformed. Division of the prosencephalon may be discontinued at various points during the process of formation. Conditions subsumed under alobar HPE, such as cyclopia, ethmocephaly, cebocephaly and premaxillary agenesis, are associated with identifiable facial abnormalities.

Cyclopia, a condition incompatible with life, is characterized by a single median eye and a small, grotesque shaped nose (proboscis) that arises from the supraorbital area (Liu et al 1997a). No optic chiasm exits. A single optic nerve traverses a solitary optic foramen to reach the brain; it may then separate into right and left branches.

Ethmocephaly is associated with exaggerated orbital hypotelorism; however, there are two orbits. The proboscis protrudes from the region between the eyes.

In cebocephaly, the facial features include orbital hypotelorism and a proboscis with a single midline, nasal opening. No cleft lip is present. Although the karyotype is virtually always normal, the condition has accompanied trisomies 13 and 15.

In premaxillary agenesis, facial features consist of hypotelorism, a flat nose and a midline cleft upper lip. The hard palate is normally developed. There is no nasal septum. A median angle-like protrusion of the frontal bones may occur. The calvarium may be microcephalic. Failure to thrive, delayed development, poor temperature control and seizures are common symptoms of premaxillary agenesis. Poor visual acuity, synophrys, colobomas and spastic quadriparesis are also evident. Most infants do not survive the first year of life.

In semilobar holoprosencephaly, prosencephalic cleavage is discernible, mostly posteriorly, with a hypoplastic intermaxillary segment. However, the separated cerebral lobes are grossly underdeveloped. The uncleaved cerebral neo-cortex is continuous from one side to the other (Fig. 13.15). The olfactory bulbs and tracts are present and in some cases underdeveloped. In an uncommon chromosomal abnormality 45,XX/46,XX/47,XX,+18 reported by Picone et al (2006), the corpus callosum was thickened and there were heterotopic neurons observed on microscopic examination of the vermis.

Facial abnormalities include a flattened nose, bilateral cleft lip and palate, a midline protrusion (the remnant of the premaxillary anlage) and orbital hypotelorism. Both trigonocephaly and microcephaly have been reported. Profound intellectual retardation usually occurs. Occasionally, patients live beyond infancy.

Lobar holoprosencephaly is associated with frontal lobes that are well developed and of normal weight. Normal cleavage implements formation of a normal interhemispheric fissure; however, when the frontal neocortex continues across the midline, the interhemispheric fissure is foreshortened anteriorly. Olfactory bulbs and tracts are sometimes present. Complete or partial agenesis of the corpus callosum may be present. Facial distortion may be absent or subtle. Trigonocephaly and cleft lip and palate have been described, and severe mental retardation is usually present. Neuroimaging techniques confirm the diagnosis.

NEURONAL MIGRATION DISORDERS

Neuronal migration disorders (NMDs) are perhaps the most common form of CNS malformations, yet they remain poorly understood and difficult to classify. A relatively simple division into disorders of cell proliferation and cell migration provides a framework for understanding these disorders, although substantial overlap occurs. Many other conditions are related to disturbances in neuronal organization, synaptogenesis, programmed cell death, myelination and gliogenesis. Alternatively, these disorders have been divided into two major groups: (1) abnormal cytogenesis and histogenesis in the first half of gestation, which includes disorders of neuronal proliferation and migration, and (2) abnormal growth and differentiation in the second half of gestation, which is more typically associated with destructive events to the developing nervous system (Evrard et al 1989a).

The terms *neuronal migration disorders, neuronal heterotopias* and *cortical dysplasias* are frequently and confusingly used interchangeably (Norman et al 1995). Until better correlations between clinical, neuroimaging and neuropathologic studies are obtained, clarification of the differences between these entities will remain elusive (Barkovich & Kuzniecky 1996, Battaglia et al 1996, Iannetti et al 1996, Preul et al 1997, Raymond et al 1995). As used here, the term *neuronal migrational disorders* refers to diffuse or generalized aberrant migrations of normally structured neurons, whereas the term neuronal heterotopias refers to abnormal collections of gray matter, usually lacking any type of cortical lamination that may be subependymal, subcortical or leptomeningeal. Cortical dysplasias, in contrast, consist of abnormally structured neurons that are characterized by marked neuronal and glial cytologic abnormalities with marked disruption of the normal cortical layering and architecture. Table 13.5 lists some of the CNS malformations or associated syndromes and diseases that have been associated with the presence of neuronal migration disorders, heterotopias or cortical dysplasias.

DISORDERS OF NEURONAL PROLIFERATION

Megalencephaly
Megalencephaly is a disorder of neuronal proliferation in which the brain weight and size are greater than two standard deviations above the mean. Associated with this cell and volume proliferation is the presence of neuronal

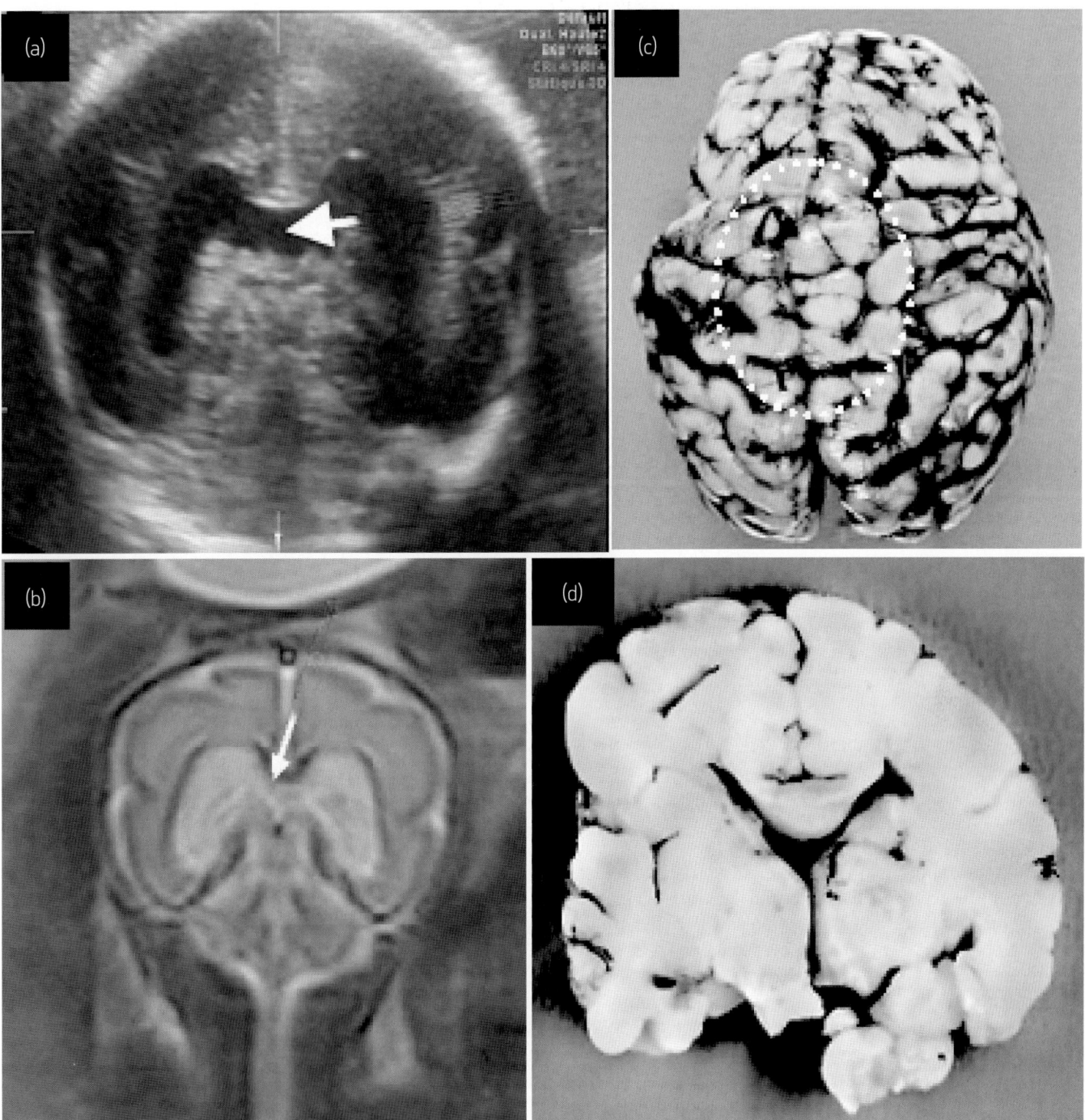

Figure 13.15 Midline interhemispheric variant of holoprosencephaly (syntelencephaly) in a 26 weeks fetus. Median coronal view of the brain showing absent septum pellucidum (arrow head): (a) Ultrasound and (b) magnetic resonance images. There is a non-cleaved segment in the interhemispheric region (dotted circle) of the brain in (c). A median coronal section of the fetal brain shows absence of the septum pellucidum (d).

Table 13.5 Diseases associated with neuronal migration disorders and heterotopias

CNS malformation syndromes	Syndromes
Cerebellar dysgenesis	Arthrogryposis multiplex congenital
Arnold–Chiari II malformation	Coffin–Siris
CRASH syndrome	Congenital muscular dystrophy
Dandy–Walker syndrome	Cornelia de Lange
Hemimegalencephaly	Duchenne muscular dystrophy
Hydrocephalus	Hypomelanosis of Ito
Lissencephaly	Incontinentia pigmenti
Pachygyria-macrogyria	Linear nevus sebaceus
Schizencephaly	Meckel–Gruber
	Myotonic dystrophy
Chromosomal/genetic disorders	Neurofibromatosis
Trisomy 9, 13, 18, 21	Orofaciodigital
Deletion 4p	Potter
	Smith–Lemli–Opitz
	Tuberous sclerosis
Metabolic disorders	
GM2 gangliosidoses	**Teratogens**
Hurler syndrome	Carbon monoxide
Menkes disease	Fetal alcohol syndrome
Mitochondrial disorders (e.g. Leigh syndrome)	
Neonatal adrenoleukodystrophy	Maternal isotretinoic acid
Non-ketotic hyperglycinemia	Mercury poisoning
Organic acidurias (glutaric aciduria type 2)	
Peroxisomal bifunctional enzyme defect	
Zellweger (peroxisomal disorder)	

Source: From OMIM 2000, Normal et al 1995, Volpe 1995.

Table 13.6 Etiology of microcephaly

Congenital
Achondroplasia
Benign familial
Cranioskeletal dysplasia
External hydrocephalus
Hydranencephaly
Hydrocephalus
Megalencephaly
Cerebral gigantism
Familial
Autosomal-dominant or autosomal-recessive
Neurocutaneous syndromes
Porencephaly

Degenerative
Alexander disease
Canavan spongy degeneration

Infectious
Abscess
Subdural empyema or effusion

Metabolic
Generalized gangliosidosis, Gm 1
Maple syrup urine disease
Metachromatic leukodystrophy
Mucopolysaccharidoses
Osteopetrosis
Rickets
Tay–Sachs disease

Toxic
Lead, vitamin A, tetracycline
Pseudotumor cerebri

Traumatic
Leptomeningeal cyst
Subdural hematoma or hygroma

heterotopias and other neuronal heterotopias and other neuronal migration abnormalities. Megalencephaly occurs in a wide variety of clinical disorders and syndromes, may be bilateral or unilateral, and is associated with an enormous spectrum of motor, cognitive (Sandler et al 1997) and behavioral symptoms including autism (Bailey et al 1993). Table 13.6 presents a list of disorders associated with a large head size (macrocephaly) and some of these conditions are related to a large brain size (megalencephaly). Of interest is a recently described syndrome with infantile onset of megalencephaly and a severe cerebral leukoencephalopathy in children who were initially normal or near normal but who developed progressive ataxia and spasticity with preserved intellect (van der Knaap et al 1995). Also of interest is the recent demonstration in patients with hemimegalencephaly of the abnormal expression of the neural cell adhesion molecule LICAM in the brains of children with hemimegalencephaly (Tsuru et al 1997).

Microcephaly

Microcephaly is present when the head circumference is greater than two standard deviations below the mean for gestational or chronologic age (whichever is approximate) and gender. The circumference and volume of the skull are abnormally decreased because of inadequate growth and development of the brain.

In general, below-average intelligence is associated with the presence of microcephaly (Dolk 1991, Nelson & Deutschberger 1970). Nevertheless, a head circumference two to three standard deviations below the mean is not inevitably linked with intellectual retardation: 7.5% of a large group of microcephalic children had normal intelligence (Martin 1970, Sells 1977).

Disruption of cellular induction, multiplication, growth or migration during the first 4 months of gestation is the presumed cause of familial microcephaly. During pregnancy, maternal, fetal and environmental factors may cause microcephaly. Many cases of microcephaly are sporadic and no underlying cause is identifiable (Cohen et al 1996). Pathologic conditions that retard brain growth after birth and during the first year or two of life also may lead to microcephaly. Microcephaly may also be associated with other brain malformations or heterotopic brain growth. Microcephaly can usually but nor uniformly be diagnosed by second trimester fetal ultrasonography (Bromley et al 1994). MRI demonstrates additional abnormalities in approximately 90% of patients (Sugimoto et al 1993).

The term *radial microbrain* (micrencephaly vera) refers to an abnormally small brain that has a normal gyral pattern, normal cortical thickness and normal cortical lamination but the number of cortical neurons is only 30% of normal (Evrard et al 1989a, 1992). A decrease in the number of radial neuronal-glial units accounts for the development of this disorder. Patients with this developmental abnormality have severe developmental retardation and profound microcephaly.

Genetic and malformation syndromes with microcephaly

Genetic counseling in individual families with microcephaly may be very difficult and is also discussed on page 272, Chapter 14.

Familial microcephaly is an autosomal-recessive, autosomal-dominant, X-linked or polygenic disorder (Gross Tsur et al 1995, McKusick 1994, Volpe 2000). The exceedingly small cerebrum contrasts with the normal cerebellum. Accompanying aberrations of cellular migration include agenesis of the corpus callosum, agyria, disrupted cortical lamination, gray matter heterotopias, macrogyria, polymicrogyria and schizencephaly. Examination reveals obvious microcephaly, a narrow forehead and a flat occiput. The face and ears may be of disproportionate normal size. Intellectual retardation is usually profound and hyperactivity may dominate the patient's behavior. Visual impairment is common and subtle-to-mild spasticity is often present. Epilepsy occurs in one-third of patients. There is a 6% risk of a family having a second microcephalic child. In families with a known pattern of inheritance, the recurrence risk may be 25–50%.

Maternal/prenatal disorders with microcephaly

The developing nervous system is highly vulnerable to infections, including toxoplasmosis, rubella, cytomegalovirus, herpes simplex and group B coxsackievirus, many of which can cause microcephaly (see Chs 30 and 31). Microcephaly has also been reported in infants of women exposed to ionizing radiation from the atomic bomb or radium implantation in the cervix during the first trimester (Dekaban 1968, Sever 1995, Wood et al 1967).

Maternal metabolic disorders that coexist with pregnancy, such as diabetes mellitus, uremia, and undiagnosed or inadequately treated phenylketonuria (Levy et al 1996, Rouse et al 1997), have been associated with neonatal microcephaly (Lenke & Levy 1982). Malnutrition, hypertension and placental insufficiency may result in microcephaly and intrauterine growth retardation. Maternal carbon monoxide poisoning results in offspring with microcephaly, polymicrogyria, mental retardation, seizures and, occasionally, hydrocephalus (Longo 1977).

Maternal alcoholism during pregnancy has also been linked with microcephaly as part of the fetal alcohol syndrome (Clarren & Smith 1978, Loebstein & Koren 1997, Ouellette et al 1977, Spohr et al 1993). Clinical features include growth and mental retardation, midfacial hypoplasia, short palpebral fissures, epicanthal folds and behavioral disturbances (Rosett & Weiner 1984). Neuropathologic findings include heterotopias, microcephaly, widespread cortical and white matter dysplasias, and defects of neuronal cortical and glial migration (Wisniewski et al 1983). Maternal cigarette smoking, as well as maternal substance abuse of cocaine and other illegal drugs, is a common cause of microcephaly (Dominguez et al 1991, Loebstein & Koren 1997).

Postnatal disorders with microcephaly

A variety of neurologic insults to the developing nervous system in neonates and infants result in microcephaly. These insults include hypoxic–ischemic encephalopathy, intracranial hemorrhage, CNS infections, malnutrition and inherited metabolic disorders. Pathologic findings include encephalomalacia, porencephaly, gliosis, abnormal myelination and atrophy.

Acquired immunodeficiency syndrome in infants causes microcephaly associated with encephalopathy, delayed development, incoordination and basal ganglia calcifications (Dickson et al 1993).

Two syndromes that have gained increasing attention and that are associated with postnatal development of microcephaly are the Rett and Angelman syndromes. Dementia, ataxia, autism and hand-wringing movements in females comprise Rett syndrome (Hagberg et al 1983). Angelman syndrome (15q11–13 deletion) is associated with seizures, hypotonia, hyperreflexia, hyperkinesis and growth failure (Fryburg et al 1991, Smith et al 1996). These children have an unusual facies and personality; the term *happy puppet* syndrome has been used to describe them.

Children with microcephaly display a wide variety of handicaps. Many infants have mental retardation, seizures, incoordination, movement disorders and spasticity (Dorman 1991).

Investigation of patients with microcephaly includes evaluation for prenatal exposure to teratogens, especially alcohol, drugs and isotretinoin (a vitamin A analog), and assessment of the family history, birth history and associated dysmorphic conditions. Laboratory studies should include: titers for toxoplasmosis, syphilis, rubella virus, cytomegalovirus and herpes simplex viruses; neuroimaging; evaluation of maternal and childhood metabolic disorders; and chromosome analysis.

DISORDERS OF NEURONAL MIGRATION

Schizencephaly

The term schizencephaly designates the presence of clefts in the cerebral hemispheres, which result from flawed development of the cortical mantle during cell migration in the first trimester of pregnancy (Yakovlev & Wadsworth 1946). The clefts are almost invariably located in the area of the sylvian fissures. The fluid-filled brain cavity is covered by normal dura or a thin pia-arachnoid membrane. The gyral pattern of the neighboring gyri is abnormal. Schizencephaly is also frequently considered to be due to an encephaloclastic process associated with fetal ischemic injury in the middle cerebral artery distribution between 31 and 35 weeks gestation (Klingensmith & Cioffi-Ragan 1986). Neuroimaging techniques may demonstrate symmetric or unilateral defects in the sylvian regions (Guillen et al 1995).

Controversy surrounds the use of the term *schizencephaly*, and abandonment of the term has been suggested by some neuropathologists (Friede 1989, Norman et al 1995), although it remains commonly used by radiologists. Recent studies, however, suggest that genetic factors may play a role in the development of this malformation (see p. 281). The recent publication of cases of intrauterine CMV infection in two children with schizencephaly also suggests another potential etiology for this malformation (Iannetti et al 1998).

The range of clinical symptoms in children with schizencephaly is currently being re-evaluated because of the availability of MRI. Children with unilateral schizencephaly are more likely to have mild or moderate impairments, whereas those with bilateral lesions usually have profound intellectual retardation, epilepsy and generalized spasticity (Granata et al 1996, Packard et al 1997). Clinical findings are usually commensurate with the size of the lesion (Aniskiewicz et al 1990). Children with closed-lip schizencephaly may present with hemiparesis or motor delay whereas those with open-lip schizencephaly are more likely to present with hydrocephalus or seizures. In one recent series, 57% of patients had seizures and 91% had associated cerebral developmental anomalies including agenesis of the septum pellucidum (45%) or focal cortical dysplasia (40%) (Packard et al 1997). In another series the severity of schizencephaly correlated with the severity of motor and cognitive disability but not with the severity of epilepsy (Granata et al 1996).

Focal transmural dysplasia

Focal transmural dysplasia is a newly described neuronal migration disorder in which cortical dysplasia extends from the cortex to the superolateral wall of the lateral ventricle (Barkovich et al 1997). MRI findings in 18 patients demonstrate this transmural malformation. Epilepsy, developmental delay and fixed neurologic deficits were observed. Neuropa-thology revealed cortical disorganization, enlarged dysplastic neurons, balloon cells, indistinct cortical gray matter–white matter junctions and variable astrogliosis. Although the etiology of this malformation is unknown, it was suggested by Barkovich et al (1997) that this malformation might be due to abnormal progenitor stem cell development.

Porencephaly

An entity that is sometimes confused with schizencephaly is porencephaly. It results from one of two abnormal processes: in one there is disruption of normal brain tissue (see p. 412) and in the other a faulty induction process and aberrant neuronal migration occur (Eller & Kuller 1995a). The terms *encephaloclastic porencephaly* and *pseudoporencephaly* indicate circumscribed defects in the cerebral mantle that rarely communicate with the ventricles and that result from destruction of cerebral tissue. Survival of the developing gray matter overlying porencephalic white matter lesions is in part due to maintenance of the independent leptomeningeal and the local anastomotic circulations (Marin-Padilla 1997). In addition, functional adaptations of local interneuronal circuitry occur. It has been suggested that the sequelae of such porencephalic lesions (e.g. cerebral palsy, epilepsy) may be, in part, due to certain of these adaptive mechanisms (Marin-Padilla 1997).

Porencephaly may also be associated with seizures. Underlying hippocampal formation atrophy may be found with postoperative pathologic changes indicative of mesial temporal sclerosis (Ho et al 1997).

Encephaloclastic porencephaly may follow severe intrauterine trauma (Viljoen 1995) and occur as a complication after amniocentesis (Eller & Kuller 1995b) or as a complication of traumatic breech and vacuum deliveries (Odita & Hebi 1996) and after periventricular intracerebral hemorrhage with ensuing encephalomalacia in preterm infants (Pasternak et al 1980). In extremely preterm infants the porencephalic lesions may involve the periphery of the brain (Cross et al 1992).

Congenital porencephaly describes familial forms of porencephaly that are primarily autosomal-dominant disorders (Berg et al 1983, Sensi et al 1990, Shastri et al 1993, Smit et al 1984). More recently, an autosomal form of bilateral porencephaly in association with absence of the septum pellucidum and pancerebellar and vermian hypoplasia has been reported (Bonnemann et al 1996).

Porencephalic cysts may be attended by an overlying encephalocele, alopecia or other cranial defects (Yokota & Matsukado 1979). Linear sebaceous nevi and developmental failure of cerebral venous sinuses may also accompany porencephaly (Chalhub et al 1975). Intracerebral cysts and porencephaly are reported in patients with the orofaciodigital syndrome type 1 (Odent et al 1998).

Clinical characteristics of porencephaly include motor dysfunction, ranging from spastic monoparesis to hemiplegia. Supranuclear bulbar palsy is associated with bilateral lesions. Basal ganglia compromise may lead to hypotonia during the neonatal period; abnormal involuntary movements, usually athetosis, may appear during the first year of life. Delayed or impaired growth and development, epilepsy and hydrocephalus are often present (Nixon et al 1974). If the cyst dilates, the ensuing increased intracranial pressure causes progressive neurologic impairment and hydrocephalus (Tardieu et al 1981).

Neuroimaging techniques, including cranial ultrasonography, reveal the cyst or cysts. In one study of 14 patients, MRI revealed porencephaly in the distribution of the middle cerebral artery in eight patients, posterior cerebral artery in three, internal carotid artery in one and multiple vessels in two (Ho et al 1997). In some patients, instilled contrast medium in conjunction with CT is necessary to determine whether the cyst communicates with the ventricular system.

A ventriculoperitoneal shunt is indicated for management of progressive enlargement of the porencephalic cyst. Furthermore, a progressive neurologic deficit may be an indication for surgical removal or shunting. In these patients, special neuroradiologic evaluation is necessary to determine the relation of the cyst to the ventricular system (Kolawole et al 1987). Most patients have static neurologic deficits that require rehabilitation.

Lissencephaly

Lissencephaly is a brain malformation manifested by a smooth cerebral surface, thickened cortical mantle and microscopic evidence of incomplete neuronal migration (Dobyns 1989, Dobyns & Truwit 1995, Dobyns et al 1992). Having established that deletion of chromosome 17p13.3 in Miller–Dieker syndrome is almost directly related to lissencephaly (Dobyns et al 1991), the understanding of neuronal migration is increasing rapidly, assisted by new imaging techniques and molecular genetics. Currently, there are five genes: *LIS1, 14-3-3e, DCX, RELN* and *ARX* which are, to a greater extent, responsible for lissencephaly in humans (Kato & Dobyns 2003). Therefore, it will be increasingly possible to determine the affected type of neuronal migration and also to evaluate and predict the degree of clinical severity in each type. Lissencephaly comprises the agyria-pachgyria spectrum of malformations, thus excluding polymicrogyria and other cortical dysplasias. The syndromes associated with lissencephaly are discussed on page 276, Chapter 14.

Type 1 lissencephaly, or classic lissencephaly, results from abnormal neuronal migration between about 10 and 14 weeks gestation (Dobyns 1987). The brain is often small and the ventricles are enlarged posteriorly. The corpus callosum may be small or absent. The structural pattern of the cerebral hemispheres and ventricles is distinctly immature and reminiscent of fetal brain. The superficial cellular layer resembles an immature cortex, with some separation into zones similar to layers III, V and VI of normal cortex, although the cell population is decreased. The heterotopic neurons are separated from the superficial layer by an acellular zone, although

this varies in thickness and may be absent. Gray matter heterotopias may be present in the white matter, which is much thinner than normal. Atypical forms of lissencephaly comprising agyria, pachygyria and other changes, such as polymicrogyria, porencephaly and intracerebral calcifications also occur. Rare variants include lissencephaly with extreme micrencephaly (head circumference at birth of 24–28 cm; brain weight less than 100 g) and lissencephaly with cerebellar hypoplasia. Seizures are common in patients with lissencephaly and the EEG shows various types of abnormalities (Gastaut et al 1987).

The *LIS-1* gene encodes a subunit of a brain platelet-activating factor acetylhydrolase. Recent studies have demonstrated that these gene products in the development human brain localize to the Cajal–Retzius cells, some subplate neurons, thalamic neurons, the ventricular neuroepithelium and, at later gestational ages, to the ependymal which suggests a potential role for these proteins in regulating neuronal migration in these structures (Clark et al 1997, Isumi et al 1997).

Type I lissencephaly occurs in several associated syndromes. Miller–Dieker syndrome (MDS) consists of severe type I lissencephaly, abnormal facial appearance and sometimes other birth defects. The facial changes include prominent forehead, bitemporal hollowing, short nose with upturned nares, protuberant upper lip with a thin vermilion border and a small jaw. Some patients have an unusual midline calcification in the region of the septum. Visible deletions of chromosome band 17p13.3 are observed in about half of all affected patients, whereas the remainder has submicroscopic deletions of the same region (Dobyns et al 1991). Isolated lissencephaly sequence consists of type I or atypical lissencephaly and minor facial changes, such as small jaw and bitemporal hollowing.

Patients with the Norman–Roberts syndrome differ from the Miller–Dieker syndrome because they have a different facies and no evidence of a 17p13.3 deletion (Iannetti et al 1993). They typically have microcephaly, bitemporal hollowing, low sloping forehead, slightly prominent occiput, widely set eyes, broad and prominent nasal bridge and severe postnatal growth deficiency. Neurologic features include generalized spasticity, seizures and profound developmental delay.

About 15–20% of patients with lissencephaly have submicroscopic deletions of 17p13.3 that are usually smaller than those observed in Miller–Dieker syndrome (Ledbetter et al 1992). Autosomal-recessive inheritance has been observed in a few families with 'pure' isolated lissencephaly, in isolated lissencephaly with neonatal death resulting from respiratory insufficiency and, in at least one family, with Norman–Roberts syndrome (Norman et al 1976).

Type II lissencephaly

Type II lissencephaly is a more complex malformation than type I and consists of agyria, pachygyria, or even polymicrogyria with a pebbled surface, thickened cortex, edematous or cystic white matter and often hydrocephalus. The cortex is severely disorganized, with no recognizable layers and widespread disruption by abnormal vascular channels and fibroglial bands. The latter often extends to the subarachnoid space, which may be partly obstructed. The white matter is poorly myelinated with large numbers of heterotopic neurons. Associated malformations include absent septum pellucidum, absent corpus callosum, vermis hypoplasia, Dandy–Walker malformation and brainstem hypoplasia. These changes reflect a protracted process beginning as early as 6 weeks gestation and continuing as late as 24 weeks gestation (Dobyns et al 1989, Evrard et al 1989a). Type II lissencephaly has been observed in several syndromes, some of which have associated congenital muscular dystrophy. Walker–Warburg syndrome includes severe eye malformations (Fig. 13.16) and either vermian hypoplasia or Dandy–Walker malformation (Rodgers et al 1994). The eye malformations may consist of microphthalmia, cataracts, Peter anomaly, congenital glaucoma and retinal malformations, although the last malformations are the most constant. Fukuyama congenital muscular dystrophy (see p. 796) is the least severe, although all patients are severely retarded. Eye and cerebellar malformations are minimal or absent (Yoshioka et al 1994). The 'cobblestone' lissencephaly that is characteristic of type II lissencephaly has recently been reported in several families who did not have eye abnormalities or muscle (Dobyns et al 1996b). Whether it is a related condition or a distinct entity remains undetermined at this time.

Type II lissencephaly is also seen in other conditions related to the Walker–Warburg syndrome. These include

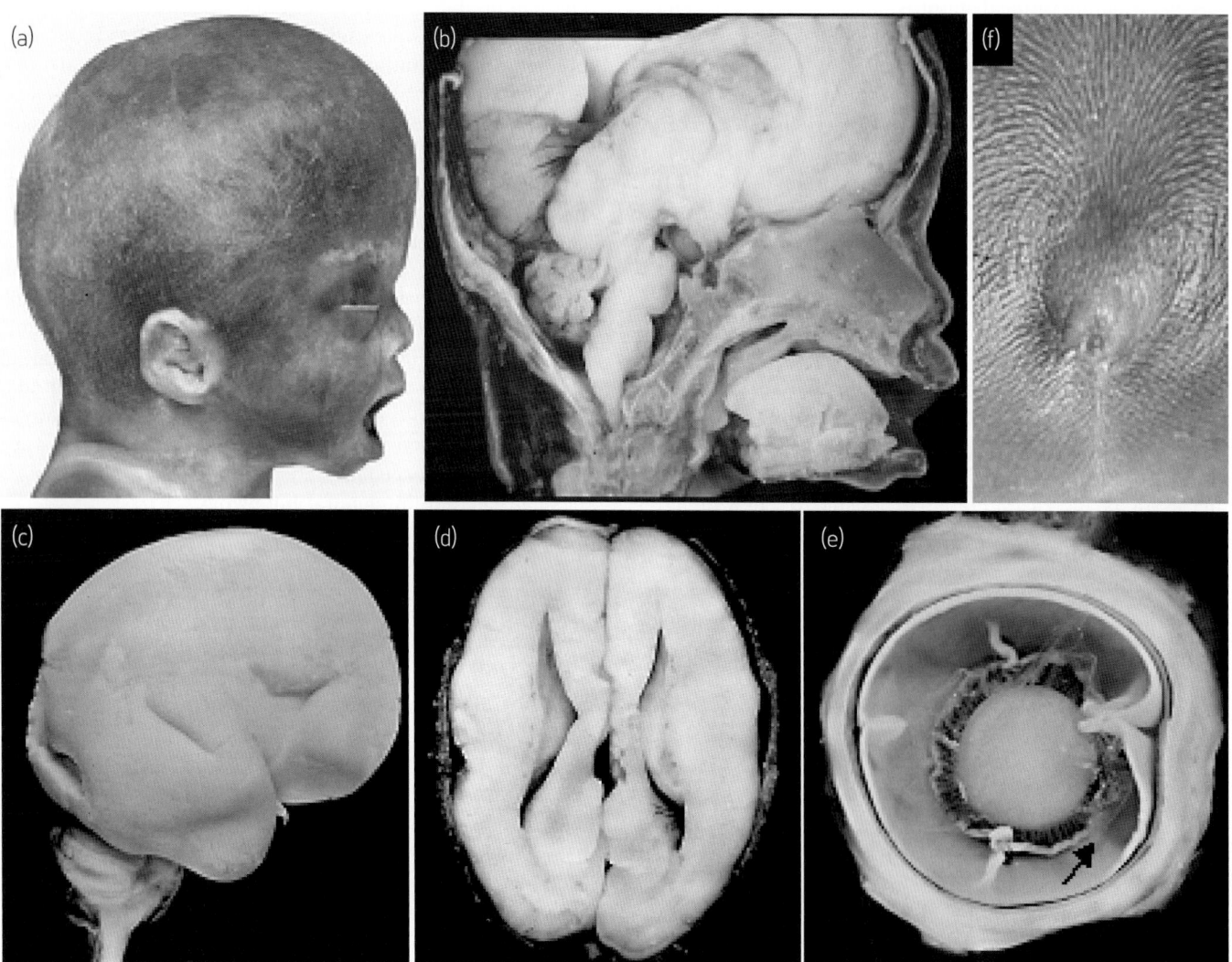

Figure 13.16 Walker–Warburg syndrome in a female fetus at 26 weeks gestation. (a) The forehead is prominent, the ears are low set, there is proptosis and a gaping mouth, the latter being the only apparent feature observed on ultrasound examination in an apparent normal pregnancy. (b) There is macroglossia forcing the mouth open. The corpus callosum is present and is normal as is the cerebellum. (c) There is classic lissencephaly and in (d) the cortical mantle is thick and the lateral ventricles are slightly dilated at the level of the posterior horns. (e) Note the marked retinal dysplasia which is bilateral. (f) There is a 'tail' and examination of the abdominal organs showed malrotation of the bowel with the cecal appendix attached near the splenic flexure.

the 'muscle, eye and brain (MEB) disease' syndrome associated with severe weakness, hypotonia with myopia, visual impairment and abnormal eye movements and the 'cerebro-oculo-muscular syndrome' (COMS) that is similar to MEB disease (Valanne et al 1994). Another rare syndrome, proliferative vasculopathy with hydranencephaly-hydrocephaly, may be related (Norman & McGillivray 1988).

Type III lissencephaly

A primary CNS disorder affecting neuronal survival in the brain and spinal cord in five fetuses with fetal akinesia sequence has been described in association with lissencephaly (Encha Razavi et al 1996). Fetal ultrasound at 23 weeks revealed polyhydramnios and severe arthrogryposis with agenesis of the corpus callosum and vermis. Postmortem examination demonstrated lissencephaly with a hypoplastic brainstem and cystic cerebellum. An autosomal-recessive pattern of inheritance was suggested in this lethal entity.

X-linked lissencephaly/subcortical band heterotopias

X-linked lissencephaly (XLIS) and subcortical band heterotopias (SBH) can be inherited alone or together in the same pedigree (Ross et al 1997). Both conditions are associated with epilepsy and several types of neurodevelopmental disorders. Available data suggests that SBH and X-linked lissencephaly are caused by mutation of a single gene, *XLIS*. The brain malformation varies from classic lissencephaly, which is observed in males, to subcortical band heterotopia, which is observed primarily in females (Dobyns et al 1996a). Almost all patients with SBH have been female, although several males with this condition have been reported (Dobyns et al 1996a, Ono et al 1997). Mutations of the gene encoding a 40 kDa protein named *doublecortin* have been reported in patients with *XLIS* (Gleeson et al 1998). X-linked lissencephaly in association with agenesis of the corpus callosum has also been observed (Berry-Kravis & Israel 1994).

Clinically, gestation is usually of normal duration, although many infants with lissencephaly (irrespective of the subtype) are small for gestational age and experience severe failure to thrive. Polyhydramnios is often present but is a non-specific feature. Appearance may be normal or abnormal, depending on the particular lissencephaly syndrome. For example, the facial appearance is always abnormal in children with Miller–Dieker syndrome and is usually abnormal in children with Walker–Warburg syndrome. Bitemporal hollowing and small jaw are common in all syndromes. Only a minority of children have microcephaly at birth, although virtually all become microcephalic within the first year of life. Many children with Walker–Warburg syndrome have congenital hydrocephalus and the head size is often large. Poor feeding and hypotonia are commonly observed in neonates and some have apnea. Seizures may occur during the first few days of life, but it is much more typical for them to begin later in the first few days of life. Seizure types in the first year include myoclonic, tonic and tonic-clonic. In over half the patients, seizures consist of or include infantile spasms. Other neurologic manifestations include severe or profound mental retardation, hypotonia that evolves to spastic quadriplegia and opisthotonus. Many patients require a gastrostomy because of poor nutrition and repeated aspiration pneumonias.

CT and especially MRI reveal the smooth surface, thickened cortex, thin white matter, lack of the normal interdigitations between cortex and white matter and enlargement of the posterior portions of the lateral ventricles (Barkovich 1995, Iannetti et al 1996). Some patients also have agenesis or thinning of the corpus callosum (Fig. 13.17a,b) (Byrd et al 1988). Cerebellar malformations, especially vermian hypoplasia or Dandy–Walker malformation, are seen in Walker–Warburg syndrome. On MRI, patients with *XLIS* show more frontal involvement in contrast to *LIS1* patients where involvement is greater in parietal and occipital regions. EEG abnormalities are common in patients with all types of lissencephalies. Hypsarrhythmia, diffuse rhythmic fast α- and β-activity and high-voltage spike discharges or 5–7 Hz slow sharp waves or δ-waves are commonly seen (Mori et al 1994).

Recurrence risks for lissencephaly

The various clinical subtypes have different risks of recurrence in siblings. Isolated lissencephaly is causally heterogeneous. The empiric recurrence risk is 5–7% (Dobyns et al 1992). The recurrence risk for Miller–Dieker syndrome depends on results of chromosome and DNA analysis; it is not inherited as an autosomal-recessive trait. The recurrence risk is 25% for isolated lissencephaly with neonatal death, Norman–Roberts syndrome, Fukuyama congenital muscular dystrophy and Walker–Warburg syndrome. The recurrence risk for unusual types of lissencephaly, such as lissencephaly with extreme micrencephaly and lissencephaly with cerebellar hypoplasia, may be as high as 25%. The recurrence risk is 50% for brothers of males having X-linked lissencephaly with microphallus. Genetic evaluation and counseling are always indicated for families with children with lissencephaly.

Pachygyria

Pachygyria indicates a simplified convolutional pattern with widened gyri and a decreased number of sulci; only one hemisphere may be involved. This disorder is caused by a defect in neuronal migration in the fourth month of gestation and children with this disorder share many of the same clinical symptoms as children with lissencephaly (Dhellemmes et al 1988). The abnormal cortical areas undergo dense gliosis and contain large, unusual neurons. Clinical findings consist of spasticity and weakness. In some patients, central rolandic and sylvian macrogyria have been associated with epilepsy, pseudobulbar palsy and mental retardation (Kuzniecky et al 1989).

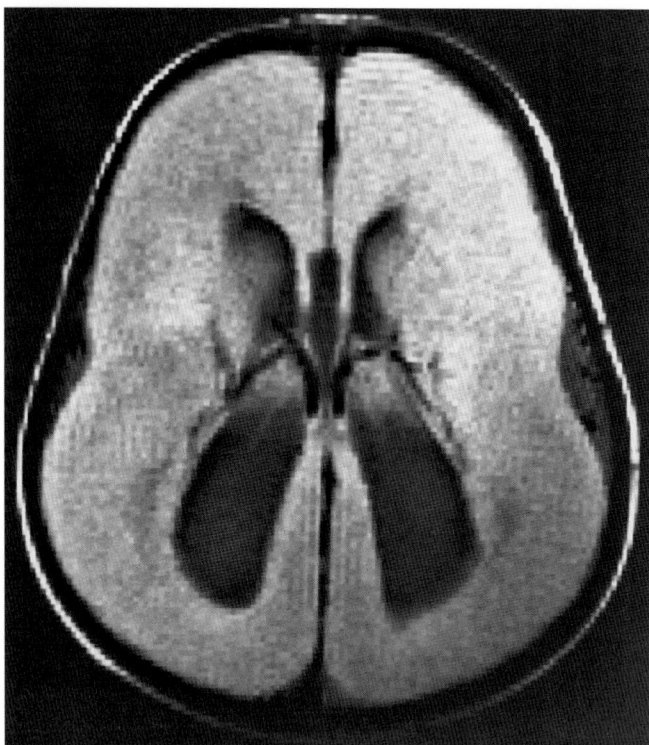

(a)

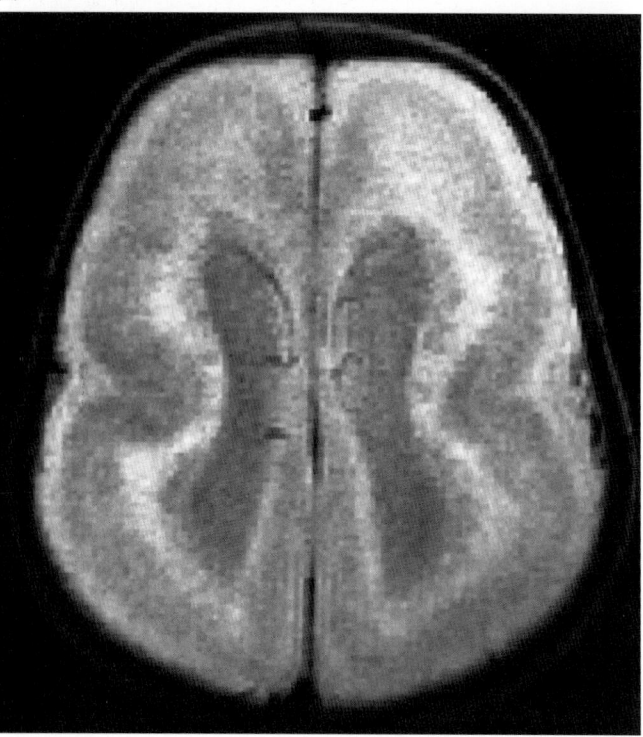

(b)

Figure 13.17 Lissencephaly in a 3-month-old female.
(a) Smooth brain surface and dilated ventricles resulting from
early arrest in neuronal migration are evident on this spin-
density axial MRI scan. (b) Note the three-layer appearance
from the primitive cortex peripherally, the darker matrix
centrally and the non-migrating neurons that have proliferated
in the periventricular region on a more T2-weighted image at
a slightly higher level. (Courtesy Joseph R. Thompson,
Department of Radiation Sciences, Loma Linda University
School of Medicine, Loma Linda, CA.)

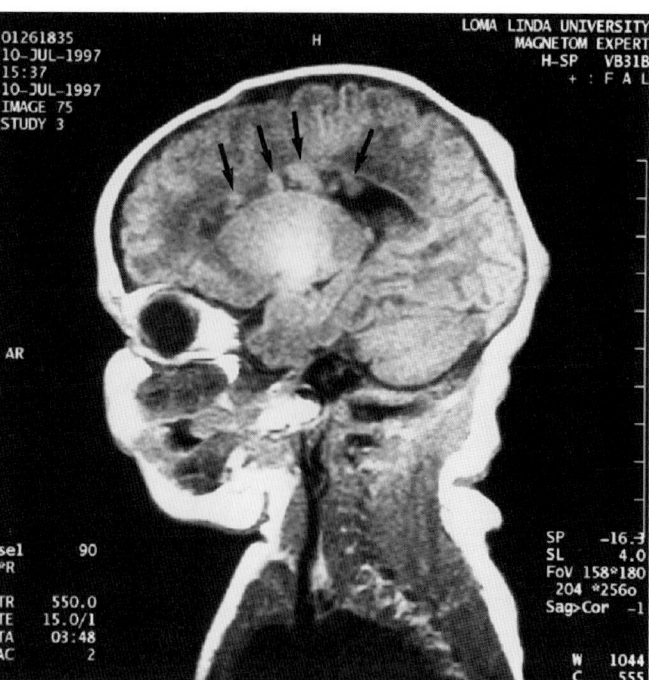

Figure 13.18 Periventricular heterotopias in a newborn infant.
This sagittal T1-weighted MRI of the brain reveals multiple
nodules of ectopic gray matter versus hamartomas in the
subependymal region protruding into the left lateral ventricle
(black arrows). (Courtesy of Shahrokh Toranji, Department of
Radiation Sciences, Loma Linda University School of
Medicine, Loma Linda, CA.)

NEURONAL HETEROTOPIAS

Neuronal heterotopias are now a commonly recognized form
of neuronal migration disorder (Friede 1989, Norman et al
1995). Resulting from the arrested migration along radial
glial elements before the fifth month of gestation, clusters
of neurons can be demonstrated pathologically and more
recently by MRI. Table 13.5 also summarizes some of the
more common disorders in which heterotopias have been
reported. Based primarily on their locations, neuronal heterotopias have been classified into three groups: (1) periventricular; (2) subcortical white matter-diffuse laminar ('band')
or focal or diffuse nodular and (3) superficial cortical or
leptomeningeal (Barkovich & Kjos 1992).

Periventricular heterotopias

Periventricular (subependymal) heterotopias (PH) are smooth
round or irregular masses of neurons that line the ventricle
(Fig. 13.18). They may extend into the ventricles and are
usually located in the corners of atria of the lateral ventricles
or the ventrolateral regions of the temporal horns (Ball
1997). A recent series of 33 patients reported unilateral PH
in 58% and bilateral lesions in 42%; 39% of patients also
have unilateral focal subcortical heterotopias (Dubeau et al
1995).

The causes of PH are multiple. Destructive lesions at the ependymal surface may affect proliferating or migrating neuroblasts or radial-glial processes, so that migration of intact neuroblasts does not occur (Sarnat 1995). The ependyma may be damaged by stretching during ventricular dilation, by ventricular wall infarction, or by intrauterine infection or inflammation. Because PH and other forms of heterotopias are seen in a wide variety of genetic and metabolic conditions, it is likely that future research will clarify the mechanisms by which early neuronal migration is perturbed by environmental and other factors that allow for the development of this form of cortical dysgenesis (Crino & Eberwine 1997, Evrard et al 1997, Kuzniecky et al 1995).

The possibility of X-linked dominant inheritance in several kindreds with epilepsy and PH has been reported and suggests that affected females are at high risk for epilepsy and that disease may be lethal in affected males (Dubeau et al 1995, Huttenlocher et al 1994). Linkage to markers in distal Xq28 in patients with PH gene may represent an important epilepsy susceptibility locus in addition to playing a key role in normal cortical development (Eksioglu et al 1996). Differentiation of this form of X-linked dominant PH from tuberous sclerosis must be considered and is based on the lack of characteristic skin lesions, more severe degrees of developmental retardation, presence of extracranial hamartomas and different chromosomal abnormalities seen in the latter condition (DiMario et al 1993, Jardine et al 1996). In one kinship involving three affected sisters with PH, developmental delay, epilepsy and dysmorphic features, including a low nasal bridge, upslanting palpebral fissures, palpebral edema, attached hypoplastic earlobes and a thickened calvarium, were reported (Musumeci et al 1996). Rectal fibrovascular polyps, urinary tract anomalies and increased foot length were also observed.

Clinically, patients with PH may have generalized or partial complex seizures; many have no or mild clinical symptoms and normal developmental function. In one series, heterotopias were associated with unilateral or bilateral independent temporal epileptic discharges in 47% of seizure patients with subependymal lesions alone and in 61% of those who had unilateral focal subcortical heterotopias (Dubeau et al 1995). Extratemporal or multifocal discharges were observed in an additional 36% of patients. Seizures may remain intractable in some patients with PH, despite temporal lobe resections suggesting a more widespread disorder with epileptogenic activity originating in or near the heterotopic tissue (Li et al 1997).

Subcortical white matter heterotopias

Heterotopias in the white matter may be classified as laminar or nodular (Barkovich 1996, Friede 1989).

Laminar or band heterotopias are diffuse symmetric single or interrupted nodular bands of gray matter that are separated from the normal-appearing cortex by a thick layer of white matter (Barkovich et al 1989, Norman et al 1995,

Palmini et al 1991a). These heterotopias form symmetric ribbons of gray matter in the centrum semiovale. Patients with laminar heterotopias usually have developmental delay, neuromotor impairment and generalized or partial complex seizures (Barkovich 1996). One form of laminar heterotopia, the double cortex, is associated with more severe neurologic involvement (Hashimoto et al 1993, Palmini et al 1991a). Affected children typically have more developmental delays and seizures that are difficult to control, including Lennox–Gastaut syndrome. Those patients, who also have overlying cortical gyral anomalies, in association with the thickened double cortex, are also more likely to be at greater risk for developmental delay (Barkovich & Kjos 1992).

Nodular heterotopias are more common and consist of single or multiple nodules of gray matter, located in the subcortical white matter that may be either focal or diffuse. They are frequently located close to the ventricular wall, lateral to the basal ganglia and thalamus or in the centrum semiovale. Microscopic examination reveals disorganized arrays of both neuronal and glial cells. These heterotopias may be seen in conjunction with other malformations such as microcephaly, agenesis of the corpus callosum, septo-optic dysplasia and chromosomal malformations. The cerebral cortex overlying subcortical heterotopia may be thin with shallow sulci and the basal ganglia dysplastic (Barkovich 1996). Seizures and developmental delays of varying degrees are the most frequent clinical manifestations (Barkovich & Kjos 1992, Gunay & Aysun 1996). EEGs depict slow-wave background activity with spike and spike-wave complexes in the affected hemisphere (Barkovich 1996, Palmini et al 1991b).

Superficial cortical or leptomeningeal heterotopias

Superficial cortical heterotopias consist of nodular collections of glial and neuronal cells derived from layers 2 and 3 of the cortex that may herniate into leptomeninges (Sarnat 1992). These glial neuronal heterotopias (brain warts) can be difficult to identify with MRI because they may be relatively as intense as the surrounding gray matter (Ball 1997). They can be seen in a variety of conditions including Walker–Warburg syndrome, congenital muscular dystrophy, Zellweger syndrome, Galloway–Mowat syndrome, 18p deletion and other chromosomal disorders (Norman et al 1995). They are commonly seen in association with many other severe forms of CNS malformations (e.g. microcephaly or lissencephaly), but can also occur as an isolated phenomenon.

Leptomeningeal glial-neuronal heterotopias involve ectopic collections of neurons and astrocytes that are principally located within the leptomeninges. They may have a nodular appearance but also may be present as sheets of cells overlying portions of the cortex (Norman et al 1995, Volpe 2000). They are frequently seen in patients with fetal alcohol syndrome.

AGENESIS OF THE CORPUS CALLOSUM

The corpus callosum, a forebrain commissure, originates from the primitive lamina terminalis (terminal plate). The first callosal fibers form at day 74 of gestation and formation is complete by 115 days; however, myelination continues after birth (Norman et al 1995, Yakovlev & LeCours 1967). The extent of the malformation varies from partial to complete agenesis.

Agenesis of the corpus callosum (ACC) occurs in about one to three infants per 1000 births, is usually sporadic, and may be transmitted as a sex-linked, autosomal-dominant, or autosomal-recessive trait (Castro-Gago et al 1993, Lynn et al 1980) (see p. 271, Ch. 14). Prenatal diagnosis of ACC can be established by 20 weeks gestation with ultrasonography (Bertino et al 1988, Vergani et al 1994). In about half of the reported fetal ultrasound studies, ACC is an isolated finding; in the remaining studies, other abnormalities or findings suggestive of specific syndromes are found. Male fetuses are more likely to have isolated agenesis that is considered benign.

The etiology of ACC has been associated with numerous syndromes (see Table 13.7) (Chevrie & Aicardi 1986) and several inborn errors of metabolism, including non-ketonic hyperglycinemia and fetal alcohol syndrome (Kolodny 1989, Norman et al 1995). The genetically determined sex-linked type of partial agenesis of the corpus callosum is associated with seizures that are evident during the first hours of life, with subsequent profound developmental retardation (Menkes et al 1964). In females, Aicardi syndrome, a sex-linked dominant condition, is associated with ACC, infantile spasms, intellectual retardation, vertebral anomalies and chorioretinal lacunae (Fig. 13.19) (Chevrie & Aicardi 1986). The condition is probably lethal in males. Gray matter heterotopias are common. Hypsarrhythmia and burst suppression are often visualized by EEG.

ACC is also seen in association with many of the major CNS malformations. An unusual association with intraventricular lipomas (Vade & Horowitz 1992) or intracranial arachnoid cysts (Pascual-Castroviejo et al 1991a) is recognized, but most commonly ACC occurs in patients with lis-

Table 13.7 Conditions associated with abnormal development of the corpus callosum

Associations with other organ development	Metabolic disorders	Hypohidrotic ectodermal dysplasia
Asplenia, anophthalmia, coloboma	Carbohydrate-deficient glycoprotein	Jeune thoracic asphyxiating dystrophy
Blepharophimosis, coloboma, hearing loss	syndrome	Kallmann
Congenital choanal atresia	Hurler syndrome	Marshall–Smith
Hirschsprung disease	Leprechaunism (insulin receptor defect)	Meckel–Gruber
Median cleft face syndrome	Mitochondrial disorders (e.g. Leigh syndrome)	Microcephalic osteodysplastic primordial dwarfism
Morning glory syndrome	Non-ketonic hyperglycinemia	Muscle, eye and brain disease
Ocular albinism	Organic acidurias (3-OH-isobutyric aciduria)	Neu-Laxova
Osseous lesions	Pyruvate decarboxylase deficiency	Neurofibromatosis
CNS malformation syndromes	Zellweger (peroxisomal disorder)	Norman–Roberts
Arachnoid cysts		Oculo-cerebro-cutaneous
Arnold–Chiari II malformation	**Syndromes**	Oral-facial-digital
Cerebellar dysgenesis	Acrocallosal	Pena–Shokeir II
CRASH syndrome	Adams–Oliver	Proteus
Dandy–Walker syndrome	Aicardi	'Reverse' Shapiro
Hydrocephalus	Andermann	Rubinstein–Taybi
Interhemispheric cyst	Apert	Seckel
Intraventricular lipomas	Baller–Gerold	Shapiro
Lissencephaly	Basal cell nevus	Shprintzen–Goldberg
	Cerebrofaciothoracic dysplasia	Smith–Lemli–Opitz
	Coffin–Siris	Thanatophoric dwarfism
Chromosomal/genetic disorders	Cranioectodermal dysplasia	Tuberous sclerosis
Aneuploidies (45, X; 47, XXY)	Di George	Walker–Warburg
Autosomal recessive	Ectodermal dysplasia	Whistling face
Pseudotrisomy 13	Edward micro-ophthalmia	
Trisomy 8, 11q-, 13, 16, 18	Frontonasal dysplasia and polydactyly	**Teratogens**
X-linked recessive	Fryns	Fetal alcohol syndrome
	Fukuyama congenital muscular dystrophy	Maternal valproate use
	Goldenhar	Maternal phenylketonuria

Source: From OMIM 1998, Norman et al 1995, Ball 1997.

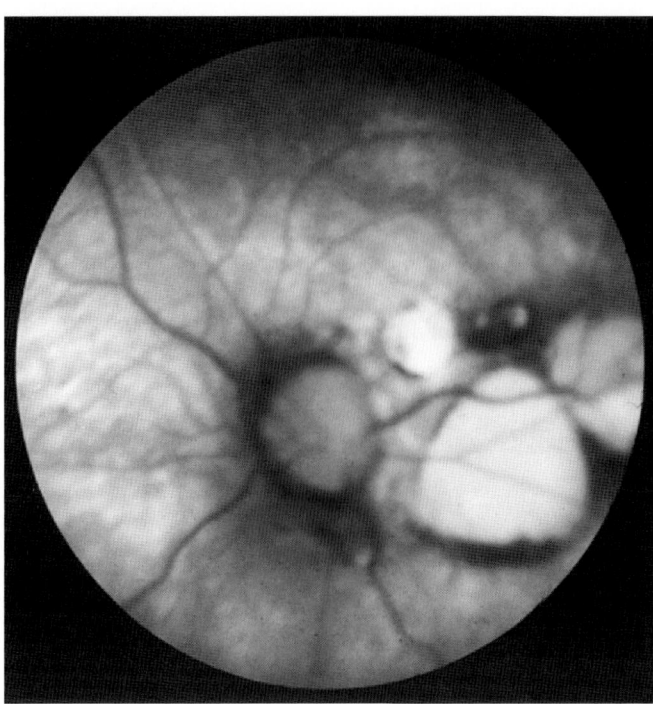

Figure 13.19 Aicardi syndrome. This fundus photograph depicts the retinal lacunae characteristic of the syndrome. (Courtesy of Pediatric Neurology, University of Minnesota Medical School, Minneapolis, MN.)

sencephaly, Dandy–Walker syndrome and Arnold–Chiari II malformations. Of interest is the recent discovery that X-linked hydrocephalus, MASA syndrome (microcephaly, adducted thumbs, spasticity, ACC), and certain forms of X-linked spastic paraplegia and agenesis of corpus callosum are now known to be due to mutations in the gene for the neural cell adhesion molecule L1CAM (Serville et al 1992, Yamasaki et al 1997). These syndromes have been reclassified as CRASH syndrome, an acronym for *corpus callosum hypoplasia, retardation, adducted thumbs, spasticity and hydrocephalus* (Fransen et al 1995). L1CAM is a transmembrane glycoprotein that is mainly expressed on neurons and Schwann cells and participates in the regulation of axon outgrowth (Fransen et al 1997). Mutations of the *L1* gene (chromosome Xq28) are responsible for a wide spectrum of neurologic abnormalities and mental retardation.

An association between certain anti-epileptic drugs, particularly valproic acid and various neural tube or midline defects including ACC, has also been suggested (Lindhout et al 1992).

Chromosomal disorders, particularly trisomies 8, 13 and 18 and pseudotrisomy 13 syndromes, are also associated with ACC (Lurie et al 1995). Rare associations with monosomy 11q and other deletions have also been reported (Hustinx et al 1993). ACC can also be seen in patients with Hirschsprung disease (Sayed & al-Alaiyan 1996), asplenia (Devriendt et al 1997) and an unusual disorder associated with mental retardation and osseous lesions (Kozlowski & Ouvrier 1993).

Other syndromes associated with ACC include the following: (1) the Meckel–Gruber syndrome, which is an autosomal-recessive disorder with principal features of renal dysplasia, polydactyly, holoprosencephaly, occipital exencephalocele and other CNS malformations (Ahdab-Barmada & Claassen 1990); (2) Andermann syndrome, which is also an autosomal-recessive disorder described primarily in individuals from certain regions of Canada and associated with a peripheral sensorimotor neuropathy, mental retardation and various dysmorphic features (Guturbay et al 1997) and (3) the acrocallosal syndrome (ACS), which is an autosomal-recessive disorder first reported by Schinzel in 1979 and characterized by the association of craniofacial anomalies, total or partial ACC, seizures, preaxial polysyndactyly, 'hallux duplex' of both feet, mental retardation and, in some patients, diabetes insipidus (Fryns et al 1997, Gelman-Kohan et al 1991). In some patients, inverted tandem duplication of chromosome band 12p11.2-p13.3 has been observed (Pfeiffer et al 1992).

Rare cases of frontonasal dysplasia (Toriello et al 1986) and Fryns syndrome may be associated with ACC (Ayme et al 1989). Patients with Fryns syndrome usually die in the neonatal period because of the presence of multiple congenital anomalies, including diaphragmatic defects, lung hypoplasia, cleft lip and plate, cardiac septal defects and aortic arch anomalies, renal cysts, urinary tract malformation, hypoplastic genitalia and distal limb hypoplasia. Various forms of the orofaciodigital syndrome may also be associated with ACC (Leao et al 1995).

An unusual condition with ACC is Shapiro syndrome, which is associated with spontaneous periodic hypothermia (Shapiro et al 1969). Variants of this syndrome have been reported with abnormalities of water metabolism (i.e. polydipsia, polyuria and hyponatremia) not associated with endocrine dysfunction (Mooradian et al 1984) or with episodic hyperhidrosis and hypothermia (LeWitt et al 1983). During attacks, patients are described as confused, withdrawn, lethargic or ataxic. More recently a 'reverse' Shapiro syndrome has been reported (Hirayama et al 1994). These patients have periodic hyperthermia rather than hypothermia. The existence of Shapiro syndrome, however, has been questioned (Norman et al 1995). Because many of the patients first present in adulthood, the relation to the congenital malformation of ACC seems unlikely.

Pathologic findings in ACC are various. The lateral ventricles are shifted laterally, with the resultant formation of a large, midline interhemispheric subarachnoid space. The foramina of Monro are malformed and elongated to reach the lateral ventricles and the third ventricle is enlarged, its roof extending dorsally (Friede 1989, Sarnat 1992). Accompanying abnormalities may include heterotopias, microgyria, abnormal cerebral fissures, porencephalic cysts and hydrocephalus. The sulci over the medial surface of the hemisphere may manifest an unusual radial pattern. Failure of decussation causes the fiber tracts to form large ipsilateral bundles of Probst. More profound pathologic deviations from normal have been typical of either the X-linked hereditary type or Aicardi syndrome (Fig. 13.19).

Clinically, the extent and nature of neurologic compromise result form the congenital absence of the corpus callosum and the associated brain abnormalities. Absence of the corpus callosum may be accompanied by mild or subtle clinical manifestations (Parrish et al 1979). Normal intelligence is not unusual. Mild compromise of skills requiring matching of visual patterns and crossed tactile localization has been described. Severe compromise may be present, including intellectual retardation, epilepsy, failure to thrive, spasticity and hydrocephalus; these findings are particularly likely to occur in children with extensive malformations (Lacey 1985).

Patients with agenesis of the corpus callosum often have asynchrony of sleep spindles, and hemispheric electrical activity may appear to be independent of the other side (Lynn et al 1980). Neuroimaging techniques document the unique pattern resulting from the abnormal space between the lateral ventricles and the upward displacement and enlargement of the third ventricle (see Fig. 6.19).

Wide or persistent cavum septum pellucidum

Persistence of the cavum septum pellucidum is believed to be a variant of normal. Recent studies suggest that children who have this finding may have subtle forms of cerebral dysgenesis and are at risk for a variety of neurodevelopmental disorders, although this has been disputed (Schaefer et al 1996).

CEREBELLAR MALFORMATIONS

Malformations of the cerebellum and vermis may be categorized as related to agenesis, hypoplasia or hyperplasia. These classifications are descriptive and are likely to undergo substantial revision as the genetic regulation of posterior fossa structures and its relation to malformations or disease processes are increasingly understood. Associated conditions that can be seen with cerebellar and vermian malformations are listed in Table 13.8.

AGENESIS

Isolated agenesis of the cerebellum is distinctly uncommon and usually associated with motor deficits (Glickstein 1994, Hamilton & Grafe 1994). The dentate nuclei, vermis and cerebellar peduncles are poorly developed (Macchi & Bentivoglio 1987). This condition and related conditions are diagnosed more frequently since the advent of modern neuroimaging techniques (Adamsbaum et al 1994). Cerebellar agenesis has been associated with chromosomal defects, such as trisomies 13 and 18. Cerebellar agenesis has been described in association with a variety of CNS malformation and syndromes. It can occur with arrhinencephaly (Leech et al 1997).

Table 13.8 Conditions associated with abnormal cerebellar development

Associations with other organ involvement		Syndromes
Congenital hepatic fibrosis	Porencephaly	CHARGE association
Congenital hip dislocation	Posterior fossa cyst	COACH
Congenital lymphedema	Rhombencephalosynapsis	Cornelia de Lange
Hirschsprung disease	Spinal dysraphism	Dekaban
Hypogonadotropic hypogonadism	Tectocerebellar dysraphia	Down syndrome
Immunodeficiency syndromes	Werdnig–Hoffmann disease	Fukuyama congenital muscular dystrophy
Optic coloboma		Fryns
Progressive pancytopenia	**Chromosomal/genetic disorders**	Hoyeraal–Hreidarsson
Tapeto-retinal degeneration	Autosomal dominant	Marinesco–Sjögren
	Autosomal recessive	Meckel–Gruber
	Down syndrome	Menkes
CNS/PNS malformation syndromes	Chromosome 5 deletion (cri-du-chat)	Neu–Laxova
Arrhinencephaly	Trisomy 9, 13, 10, 18	Neurocutaneous melanosis
Arnold–Chiari II malformation	X-linked	Oral-facial-digital (type II, type VI)
Cranial meningocele		Otopalatal-digital
CRASH syndrome	**Metabolic disorders**	Ritscher–Schinzel (3C)
Dandy–Walker	Carbohydrate-deficient glycoprotein	Walker–Warburg
Hydrocephalus	syndrome	Whistling face
Joubert	Mitochondrial disorders	
Lissencephaly/pachygyria	Muscle phosphofructokinase deficiency	
Microcephaly		**Teratogens**
Occipital meningomyelocele		Fetal alcohol syndrome
Pontocerebellar hypoplasia		Maternal isotretinoin use

Source: From OMIM 2000, Norman et al 1995, Ball 1997.

In contrast to complete agenesis of the cerebellum, hypoplasia of varying degrees occurs more commonly (de Souza et al 1994, Shevell & Majnemer 1996). Cerebellar hypoplasia can occur in the majority of the conditions listed in Table 13.8. It may also occur sporadically or be inherited as a familial (X-linked) trait (al Shahwan et al 1995). Cerebellar hypoplasia has also been detected in patients with mitochondrial respiratory chain disorders (Lincke et al 1996). Findings on examination include mild-to-moderate developmental disability, microcephaly, typical 'cerebellar' findings and impaired fine motor skills.

Unilateral cerebellar defects are more common than bilateral hemispheric agenesis of hypoplasia and are usually asymptomatic (Boltshauser et al 1996). Hemiagenesis is accompanied by poor development of the red nucleus, contralateral inferior olive and ipsilateral brachium conjunctivum. Presenting signs may include delayed motor development, contralateral torticollis, unusual head nodding and ataxia.

Recent studies have found that mice lacking the *Math 1* gene fail to form granule cells and are born with a cerebellum that is devoid of an external germinal layer (Ben Arie et al 1997). *Math 1*, the mouse homolog of the *Drosophila* gene atonal, encodes a basic helix-loop-helix transcription factor that is specifically expressed in the precursors of the external germinal layer. Since the granule cells are the predominant neurons in the cerebellum, these findings suggest one potential mechanism for the pathogenesis of malformations involving the cerebellum.

Pontocerebellar hypoplasia

Pontocerebellar hypoplasia (PCH) is distinct from disorders associated with cerebellar hypoplasia because the ventral pons is affected (Barth 1993, Malandrini et al 1997). Barth has described the following two variants: (1) PCH-1, which is associated with a form of spinal anterior horn degeneration similar to Werdnig–Hoffmann disease; and (2) PCH-2, which is associated with an early-onset choreiform and dystonic movement disorder that is often severe. PCH-1 presents in the neonatal period with respiratory insufficiency, frequent congenital contractures and a combination of central and peripheral motor signs; patients usually die before the age of 1 year. PCH-2 is likely an autosomal-recessive disorder. Patients do not have spinal anterior horn pathology but do have microcephaly and severely impaired mental and motor development and are likely to die during childhood (Barth et al 1995).

Tectocerebellar dysraphia

Tectocerebellar dysraphia (TCD) is an extremely rare condition in which both the cerebellar hemispheres and brainstem tectum are hypoplastic (Demaerel et al 1995, Hori 1994). Occipital encephaloceles are also common and some relation to rhombencephalosynapsis in which the cerebellar hemispheres are fused has been proposed.

AGENESIS OF THE VERMIS

Agenesis of the vermis is usually partial but may be complete. In partial agenesis the posterior vermis is absent, which is consistent with its embryologic development; the anterior part of the vermis is formed before the posterior area. The posterior segment of the vermis is fully formed by the 18th week of gestation. This is relevant as it would be unwise to rule out a variant of Dandy–Walker syndrome during ultrasound examination of the posterior fossa before that gestational age. In cases of complete vermian agenesis the insult occurs earlier than in partial agenesis.

Clinically, agenesis of the vermis may be asymptomatic. Neurologic findings result from abnormalities in cerebellar hemispheres, nuclei and associated brainstem pathways. Neurologic features include hypotonia in infants and incoordination, tremor and truncal ataxia in children. Delayed fine and gross motor milestones, nystagmus and decreased deep tendon reflexes also occur. Mild neurologic symptoms may improve with maturation. Agenesis of the vermis may be an associated finding with myelomeningocele, cranial meningoceles, agenesis of the corpus callosum, heterotopias, HPE and other conditions listed in Table 13.7 (Schaefer et al 1996). Vermian agenesis can also occur with fusion of the cerebellar hemispheres (rhombencephalosynapsis) and on rare occasions cerebral hemispheric fusion may also be present (Aydingoz et al 1997, Romanengo et al 1997, Sergi et al 1997). Vermian agenesis may also be inherited as an autosomal-dominant (Rivier & Echenne 1992) or X-linked disorder (Illarioshkin et al 1996).

Cerebellar hypoplasia or vermian agenesis can be detected using fetal ultrasound, usually by the end of the first trimester or early in the second trimester (van Zalen-Sprock et al 1996). Findings of isolated vermian agenesis without evidence of a Dandy–Walker malformation are usually but not universally indicative of a good prognosis (Keogan et al 1994). Diagnosis of vermian agenesis or the Dandy–Walker syndrome should not be made before 18 weeks gestation, because the development of the cerebellar vermis may be incomplete at that time (Bromley et al 1994).

Joubert syndrome

Joubert syndrome is an autosomal-recessive form of agenesis of the cerebellar vermis (Joubert et al 1969, King et al 1984, Maria et al 1997, Saraiva & Baraitser 1992). It consists of episodic hyperpnea and apnea, disorders of ocular movement, ataxia, hypotonia and mental retardation. The respiratory abnormality worsens with stimulation and improves with maturation. Abnormal respiration with episodic tachypnea and apnea can occur in several other syndromes (e.g. Rett, Mohr or Dandy–Walker), but these usually present later in childhood (Boltshauser et al 1987). Joubert syndrome has been classified into two subtypes by some investigators with the differentiating feature being the absence (type A) or presence (type B) of retinal dystrophy (Saraiva & Baraitser 1992).

The retinal dystrophy has been previously classified as a variant of Leber congenital amaurosis (Lambert et al 1989). The retinal dystrophy is always present in those patients in whom renal cysts occur. Also present are abnormalities of smooth pursuit: pendular, torsional, optokinetic, or other forms of nystagmus or oculomotor apraxia. Vestibulo-ocular reflexes are usually intact, but smooth pursuit movements are impaired. Congenital hepatic fibrosis has also been reported in some patients, usually in association with congenital medullary cystic renal disease (Lewis et al 1994). The renal cysts are multiple, small and cortical and affected kidneys also have interstitial chronic inflammation and fibrosis.

Neuroimaging techniques reveal an enlarged fourth ventricle and interpeduncular fossa, dilated cisterna magna, thickened superior cerebellar peduncles and varying degrees of vermian hypoplasia (Fig. 13.20) (Kendall et al 1990, Maria et al 1997). As a result of midbrain, vermian and superior cerebellar peduncle abnormalities, axial neuroimaging reveals a unique 'molar tooth' appearance of these structures (Maria et al 1997). Also reported with MRI are thinned optic tracts, enlarged temporal horns in the absence of hydrocephalus, high signal of the cerebral periventricular white matter, abnormal signal in the decussation of the superior cerebellar peduncles and abnormal embryonic vessels associated with the dysplastic folia of the cerebellar hemispheres (Sener 1995).

Joubert syndrome with retinal dystrophy and renal cysts may represent a variant of the carbohydrate-deficient glycoprotein syndrome (Hagberg et al 1993, Jensen et al 1995). Others have suggested that Joubert syndrome is a member of a spectrum of congenital malformation syndromes involving the CNS, eye, liver and kidneys (Lewis et al 1994, Silverstein et al 1997). Joubert syndrome should also be differentiated from the COACH syndrome, which consists of cerebellar vermis hypo/aplasia, *o*ligophrenia, *a*taxia, coloboma and *h*epatic fibrosis (Gentile et al 1996).

Several other syndromes with vermian agenesis need to be differentiated from Joubert syndrome. The Ritscher–Schnizel syndrome or 3C (craniocerebello-cardiac) syndrome is another condition with vermian agenesis or hypoplasia that is associated with cardiac and cranial defects (Kosaki et al 1997). Cardiac lesions include endocardial cushion or conotruncal defects. Speech, and to a lesser extent motor, delays are the major developmental disabilities and postnatal growth deficiencies are common. Characteristic dysmor-

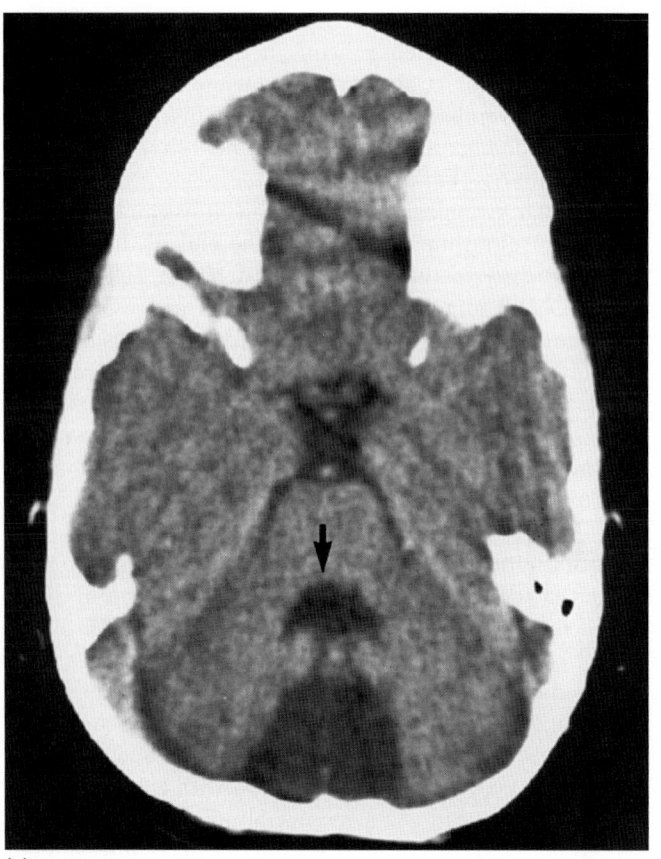

(a)

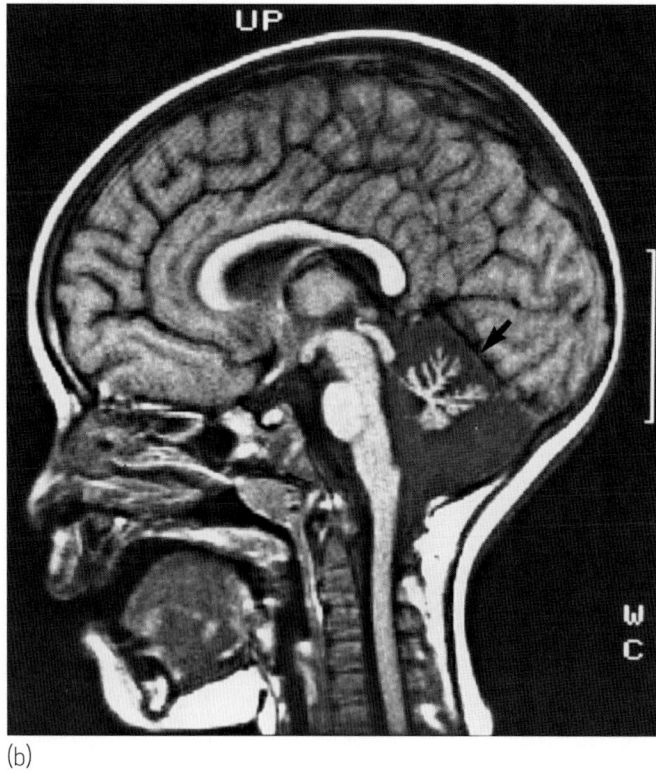

(b)

Figure 13.20 Cerebellar vermian hypoplasia in a 3-year-old male. (a) Moderate fourth ventricle dilatation (arrow) and large cisterna magna with little intervening vermian tissue seen on this axial CT scan. (b) Midsagittal T1-weighted MRI revealing leaflike small cerebellar vermis (arrow) surrounded by CSF. (Courtesy Joseph R. Thompson, Department of Radiation Sciences, Loma Linda University School of Medicine, Loma Linda, CA.)

phic features of this disorder are present, as well as coloboma, cleft palate, bifid uvula, short neck, syndactyly and hypoplasia of the nails. Also, patients with CHARGE association (coloboma of the eye, heart defect, atresia of the choana, retarded growth and development, genital hypoplasia and ear anomalies or deafness) may be intermittent hyperpnea and cerebella hypoplasia, and thus need to be distinguished from patients with Joubert syndrome (Menenzes & Coker 1990).

Recent studies suggest that Joubert syndrome and other forms of vermian agenesis may result from specific gene defect (Maria et al 1997). Several members of the *PAX* family of genes (*PAX2*, *PAX5*, *PAX8*) contribute to mid-hindbrain formation (Hatten & Heitz 1995). The *EN* family of genes also encodes for cerebellar development and targeted disruption of certain of these genes results in abnormalities of cerebellar development (Maria et al 1997). Although *EN* gene family members are regulated by the *WNT1* gene, mutations in *WNT1* in a series of Joubert syndrome patients were not detected (Pellegrino et al 1997).

Other recent investigations have identified the nephronophthisis (*NPH*) gene complex as potentially causing Joubert syndrome (type A), homozygous deletions have been described as causative in more than 80% of patients. In type B Joubert syndrome, different combinations of the extra-renal symptoms with the *NPH* gene occur. Homozygous deletions of *NPH1* region in type B Joubert syndrome patients have not been found.

A recent study reported on the follow-up of 19 children with Joubert syndrome (Steinlin et al 1997). Three children who died before 3 years of age demonstrated marked respiratory dysfunction and profound development delay. The remaining children had variable motor development; walking was typically achieved between 2 and 10 years of age. Developmental testing found that four children had profound delays, nine were mild to moderately delayed and the rest were untestable. Renal involvement was present in four children. It was also observed that ophthalmologic and renal involvement could develop over several years and required periodic monitoring. Normal intelligence despite multiple handicaps has been noted by other observers (Ziegler et al 1990). Several children with Joubert syndrome showing autistic behavior have been described (Holroyd et al 1991).

CEREBELLAR HYPERPLASIA

Unilateral cerebellar enlargement has been reported in some patients with hemimegalencephaly (Sener 1997). Ipsilateral brainstem enlargement also is present. The term total hemi-megalencephaly has been suggested to differentiate it from unilateral megalencephaly in which just the cerebral hemispheres are involved. Hemi-enlargement of the cerebellum has also been recognized in several disorders associated with somatic hemihypertrophy, including Beckwith syndrome, Russell–Silver syndrome and Klippel–Trenaunay–Weber syndrome (Bodensteiner et al 1997).

Macrocerebellum, consisting of diffusely enlarge bilateral cerebellar hemispheres, has been reported in four children with developmental delay, hypotonia, preserved reflexes, delayed or abnormal maturation of the visual system, oculomotor apraxia and delayed cerebral myelination (Bodensteiner et al 1997). The diagnosis was established by MRI volumetric determinations and differentiated from the Lhermitte–Duclos syndrome in which there is diffuse hamartomatous enlargement of the cerebellum.

MACRO CISTERNA MAGNA

The cisterna magna comprises the subarachnoid space posterior to the inferior half of the cerebellum. It may appear prominent as a normal variant. About 1% of children will have an enlarged cisterna magna as determined by neuroimaging studies. A recent review of a group of pediatric patients with macro cisterna magna has suggested that they are at greater risk for neurodevelopmental impairment including incoordination, ataxia, hypotonia, oculomotor abnormalities and seizures (Schaefer et al 1994).

DANDY–WALKER SYNDROME

The Dandy–Walker syndrome (DWS) consists of a malformation of the fourth ventricle and cerebellum and occurs in approximately 1 in 30 000 live births. The recurrence risk is low (1–5%) when DWS is not associated with a mendelian disorder (see p. 286, Ch. 14). The malformation is most likely due to a developmental cerebellar defect that originates before embryologic differentiation of the foramina of the fourth ventricle (Golden et al 1987, Normal et al 1995). The cystic transformation of the fourth ventricle and attendant hydrocephalus have been ascribed to atresia of the foramina of the fourth ventricle, the foramen of Magendie and the lateral paired foramina of Luschka (Epstein & Johanson 1987). Post-mortem studies often reveal intact foramina (Hart et al 1972). The massive cystic formation may originate from compromised absorption of ventricular fluid and subsequent increased pressure because of failure of the normal perforation of the superior coverings of the third and fourth ventricles (Gardner 1977).

Pathologic findings

The fourth ventricle is grossly misshapen and is a large, ependymal-lined cyst that extends into the spinal canal (Norman et al 1995, Pascual-Castroviejo et al 1991b). The cerebellar hemispheres are rudimentary and displaced superiorly and the posterior vermis is hypoplastic or absent (Fig. 13.21). Rostral fluid-containing spaces, including aqueduct of Sylvius, third ventricle and lateral ventricles, are grossly enlarged. The posterior fossa is enlarged with upward displacement of the lateral sinuses, tentorium and torcular.

Numerous brain abnormalities accompany the Dandy–Walker malformation, including agenesis of the corpus callosum, polymicrogyria, agyria, gray matter heterotopias,

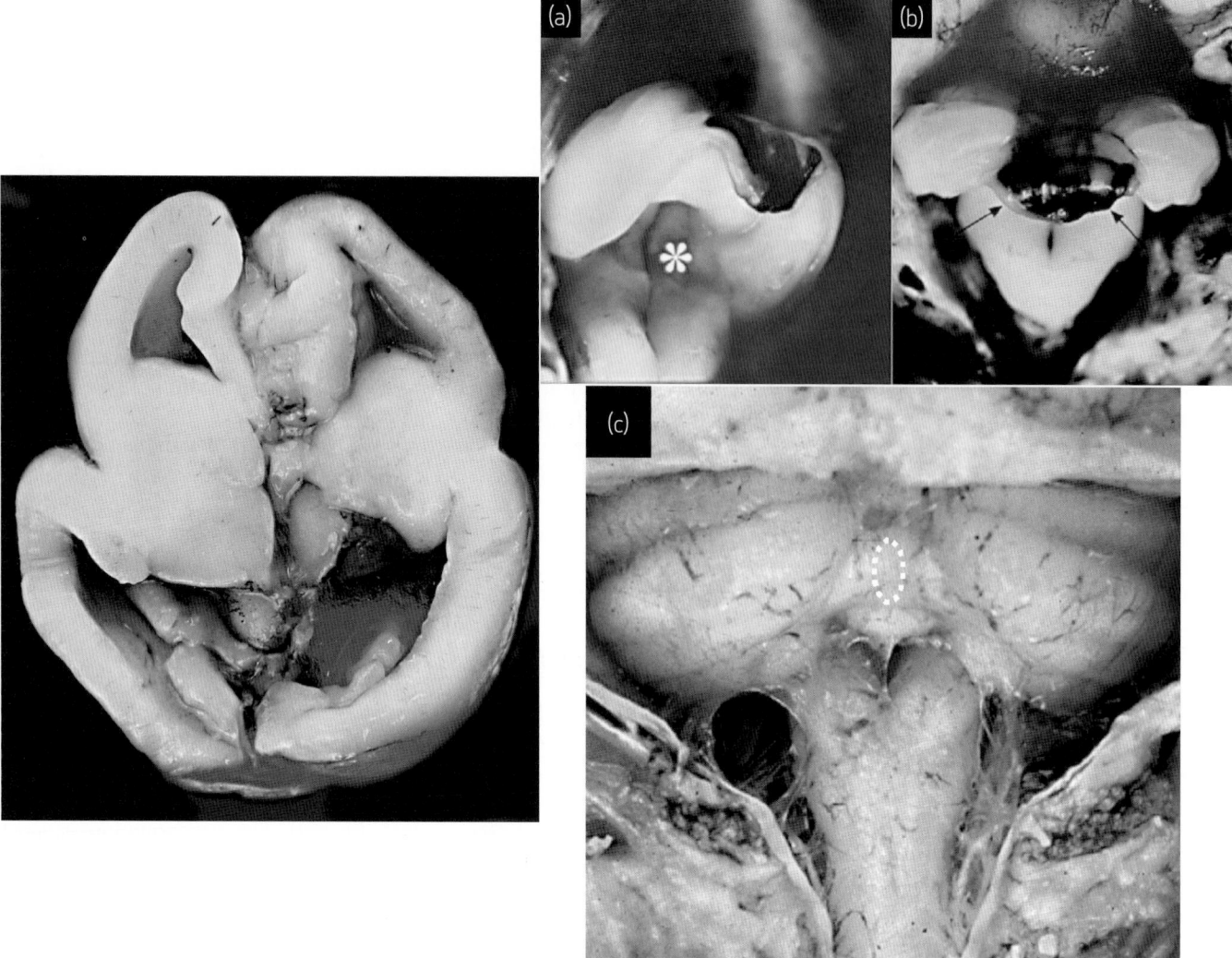

Figure 13.21 Dandy–Walker syndrome in a fetus at 23 weeks gestation. The panel on the left shows gross dilatation of the posterior horns of lateral ventricles which appear 'pushed' upwards from underneath and somehow displaced forwards (compare with Fig. 13.5). There is lissencephaly. (a) Left oblique and (b) posterior view of the cerebellum which appears displaced upwards. The vermis is abnormal and is partially covered with a richly vascularized membrane. (c) Cerebellum and posterior fossa form a normal fetus at 22 weeks gestation.

aqueductal stenosis, Klippel–Feil syndrome, microcephaly, posterior fossa lymphomas, hamartomas of the infundibulum, hemimegalencephaly and syringomyelia (Hart et al 1972, Parikh et al 1994). Other non-neural associated abnormalities include polydactyly, syndactyly, cleft palate, polycystic kidneys and abnormal lumbar vertebrae.

Chitayat et al (1994) have summarized the various single gene disorders, chromosomal aberrations, teratogen-induced conditions and other disorders that are sporadic or of undetermined inheritance associated with the Dandy–Walker malformation. Among the syndromes associated with DWS are the Marden–Walker syndrome (Ozkinay et al 1995), Fryns syndrome (Ayme et al 1989, Riela et al 1995), Neu-Laxova syndrome (Shapiro et al 1992), molybdenum cofactor deficiency (Pintos Morell et al 1995), Coffin–Siris syndrome (Norman et al 1995) and neurocutaneous melanosis (Kadonaga et al 1992).

Clinical characteristics

Clinical manifestations are often evident during infancy. Delayed motor development, hydrocephalus, nystagmus, spasticity, titubation and apnea are common features. The posterior portion of the head is enlarged and a flattened protuberance is present in the inferior occipital area (Tal et al 1980). Difficulties in older children and adults may be manifestations of increased intracranial pressure and ataxia (Maria et al 1987). In a retrospective long-term follow-up study of 20 patients with DWS surgically treated, normal cerebellar function was seen in 50% of patients and intellectual function was normal in 45% (Gerzten & Albright 1995). There was no correlation between cerebellar size and intellectual development or cerebellar function. There was also no correlation between the type of shunt and the subsequent cerebellar size.

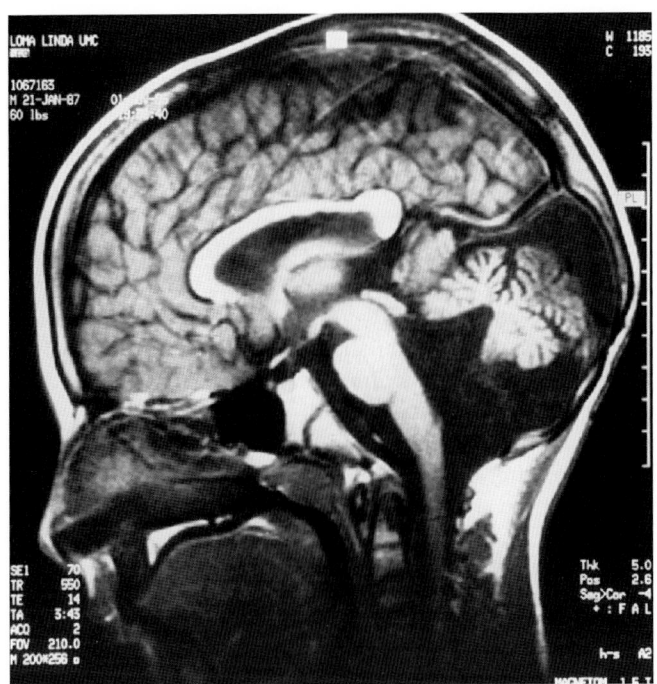

Figure 13.22 Large 2-cm posterior fossa arachnoid cyst in an 8-year-old male status after cystoperitoneal shunting is seen on a T2-weighted axial MRI image. Also present is a large fourth ventricle that interconnects with this cyst and that also distorts cerebellum. (Courtesy of Shahrokh Toranji, Department of Radiation Sciences, Loma Linda University School of Medicine, Loma Linda, CA.)

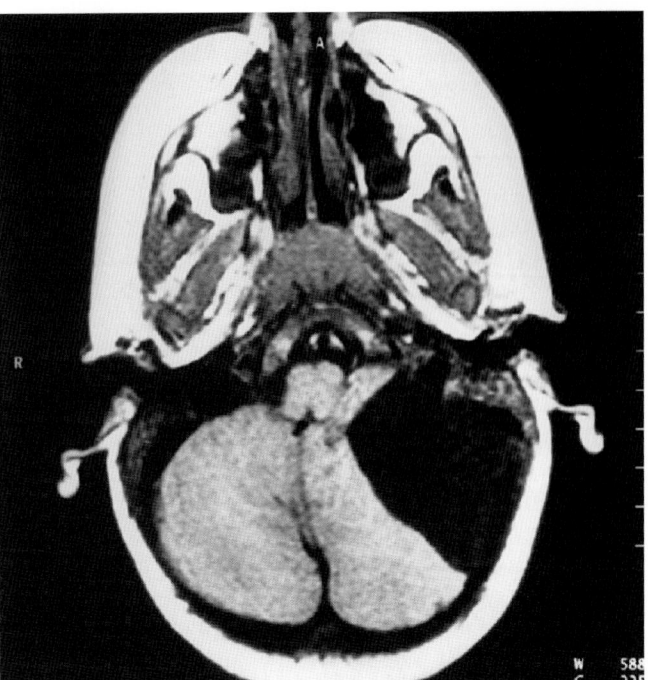

Figure 13.23 Posterior fossa arachnoid cyst in a 3-year-old male presenting with seizures. T1-weighted axial image of the posterior fossa demonstrates a sharply marginated cystic lesion of the left aspect of the posterior cranial fossa compressing and deforming the left cerebellar hemisphere and mildly compressing and displacing the fourth ventricle to the right. (Courtesy of Shahrokh Toranji, Department of Radiation Sciences, Loma Linda University School of Medicine, Loma Linda, CA.)

An uncommon but well-recognized occurrence in patients with Dandy–Walker malformation is sudden unexpected death that may occur without uncal or tonsillar herniation (Elterman et al 1995). Vascular compromise of the posterior fossa circulation secondary to local increases in intracranial pressure may be a factor.

Cranial ultrasonography accurately defines the posterior fossa cyst and hydrocephalus. Lateral plain radiographs may prove diagnostic; the posterior fossa is enlarged, with superior placement of the torcular herophili and lateral sinus grooves. CT, MRI, or cranial ultrasonography best demonstrates the characteristic pattern of hydrocephalus and cystic enlargement of the fourth ventricle (Fig. 13.22). Prenatal sonographic features include ventriculomegaly and concurrent non-CNS anomalies in about half the patients (Bromley et al 1994, Estroff et al 1992).

Familial forms of DWS have been described with autosomal-recessive or X-linked-recessive inheritance. DWS or cerebellar hypoplasia may be associated with maternal exposure to isotretinoin in the first trimester and can be detected prenatally (Nyberg et al 1988).

The presence of an arachnoid cyst may prove confounding because clinical findings may be similar (Arai & Sato 1991). This condition must be distinguished from DWS (Haller et al 1971, Menezes et al 1980). Neuroimaging techniques reveal a normal-sized fourth ventricle that is displaced anteriorly by the arachnoid cyst (Fig. 13.23) (Rock et al 1986). If necessary, metrizamide CT will demonstrate whether the cyst communicates with the ventricular system.

Management

A shunt from the ventricles, cyst, or both has replaced removal of the cyst wall as the primary treatment for Dandy–Walker or posterior fossa cysts (Kalidasan et al 1995). Surgery may be indicated when there is occipital bossing, distortion, or obliteration of CSF cisterns of the posterior fossa, compression and deformity of the brain surrounding the cyst, disturbed CSF circulation or a non-communicating cyst (Arai & Sato 1991, Domingo & Peter 1996). When the ventricles and cyst communicate, a cystoperitoneal shunt may suffice (Sawaya & McLaurin 1981).

INTRACRANIAL ARACHNOID CYSTS

Intracranial arachnoid cysts are benign, non-genetic development cysts that contain spinal fluid and occur within the arachnoid membrane (Pascual-Castroviejo et al 1991a, Rengachary & Watanabe 1981). The gross and macroscopic features were described by Scherer (1935) and by Sarkman et al (1958). The walls result from splitting of the arachnoid

Table 13.9 Distribution of arachnoid cysts

Location	Percentage
Sylvian fissure	49
Cerebellopontine angle	11
Quadrigeminal area	10
Vermian area and sellar-suprasellar area	9
Interhemispheric fissure	5
Cerebral convexity	4
Clival area	3

Source: Modified from Rengachary and Watanabe 1981.

membrane, they may contain very few blood vessels and are made up of fibrous and connective tissue slightly denser than that of the archnoid membrane. There is no epithelium lining the cystic space and the fluid it contains is translucent. The cysts occur in proximity to arachnoid cisterns, most often in the sylvian fissure (Table 13.9). The retrocerebellar and infratentorial cysts are often observed in the midline and depending on their size, they can compress the vermis and shift the cerebellum. At present the use of ultrasound allows the identification of arachnoid cysts in the first half of pregnancy (Fretelle et al 2002), and in uncomplicated cases, follow up of presumed arachnoid cysts has resolved spontaneously before birth (Elbers & Furness 1999).

Arachnoid cysts occur most often in males and in patients with Marfan syndrome and there are few reports of familial middle and posterior fossa arachnoid cysts (Handa et al 1981, Sinha & Brown 2004, Toline et al 1997). The mechanism of formation during embryogenesis is uncertain (Naidich et al 1985/86).

In a recent series of 61 children with arachnoid cysts, about 53% of cases were diagnosed before age 1 year, 42% were supratentorial and 46% infratentorial (Pascual-Castroviejo et al 1991a). Macrocephaly was the presenting symptom in 72% and associated features included the following: cranial asymmetry in 39%, aqueductal stenosis in 16% and agenesis of the corpus callosum in 13%. Developmental delay was a common finding. Skull radiographs may suggest the diagnosis. However, today CT or MRI is used as the definitive diagnostic procedure (Weiner et al 1987). Injection of contrast medium into the cyst to document communication with the ventricular system is seldom necessary.

Common neurological features are headache, seizures, hydrocephalus, focal enlargement of the skull, and signs and symptoms of elevated intracranial pressure and developmental delay, as well as specific signs or symptoms resulting from neural compression. Some arachnoid cysts remain asymptomatic (Mason et al 1997). Progressive enlargement and intracystic or subdural hemorrhage are potential complications. Suprasellar arachnoid cysts may produce neuroendocrine dysfunction, hydrocephalus and optic nerve compression. Posterior fossa cysts are now more frequently recognized with the use of MRI and CT and frequently require surgical treatment (Domingo & Peter 1996).

Management

When symptoms warrant, surgical intervention to decompress the cyst, including shunting procedures, is required (Harsh et al 1986, Pascual-Castroviejo et al 1991a, Raffel & McComb 1988). Arachnoid cysts may occur with or without hydrocephalus. The success rate of fenestration is higher in those patients without hydrocephalus (i.e. 73% required no additional treatment) compared with hydrocephalus patients (32%) (Fewel et al 1996). About 12% of patients treated with fenestration alone may require a cystoperitoneal shunt. In general, cyst fenestration should be the primary procedure in patients without hydrocephalus. If hydrocephalus is present, cyst fenestration is still recommended, but a ventriculoperitoneal shunt should be placed if hydrocephalus is marked or after fenestration if the hydrocephalus is progressive (Fewel et al 1996).

POSTNEURONAL MIGRATION DEFECTS

HYDROCEPHALUS

The diagnosis, clinical features, management and prognosis of fetal and neonatal hydrocephalus are discussed in detail in Section XI of this book.

Aqueductal stenosis

Aqueductal stenosis leads to a form of non-communicating hydrocephalus. Partial or complete obstruction of the aqueduct of Sylvius is associated with congenital structural malformations, hemorrhage, infection, neoplasms and vascular malformations. Concomitant occlusion of the subarachnoid space may occur. Specific pathologic types of aqueductal stenosis, including congenital narrowing, aqueductal forking, septum formation and aqueductal gliosis, are difficult to differentiate clinically (Drachman & Richardson 1961). The inflammatory process subsequent to neonatal meningitis and intraventricular hemorrhage can cause aqueductal gliosis. Hereditary aqueductal stenosis is transmitted as an X-linked recessive trait (Edwards 1961). Rare cases of autosomal-recessive inheritance are also reported (Castro Gago et al 1996).

Aqueductal stenosis may accompany Arnold–Chiari malformations, myelomeningocele and neurofibromatosis. Aqueductal stenosis may also be secondary to an existing communicating hydrocephalus (Nugent et al 1979).

In experimental animals, vitamin A excess, mumps encephalitis and other viruses cause aqueductal gliosis with associated aqueductal stenosis and hydrocephalus (Volpe 2000). In humans, mumps encephalitis has been associated with acquired aqueductal stenosis and hydrocephalus after a latent period of 3 months to 4 years (Spataro et al 1976). The pathogenesis in experimental animals and humans may be the propensity for selective infection of ependymal cells by the mumps virus (Volpe 2000).

Patients with congenital aqueductal stenosis are hydrocephalic at birth. Cranial ultrasonography demonstrates enlarged lateral and third ventricles with a normal or small fourth ventricle. Other neuroimaging techniques may detect tumor, vascular malformation and associated congenital anomalies.

Remarkably, some patients with congenital and even early acquired aqueductal stenosis are asymptomatic until later childhood or early adult life; some remain free of symptoms. When they become apparent, manifestations include findings consistent with chronic increased intracranial pressure, such as an enlarged head, headache, seizures, gait disturbance, decreased visual acuity, dementia and occasionally CSF rhinorrhea (Little et al 1975).

Hypothalamic-pituitary disturbance may occur, including precocious or delayed puberty, impotence, short stature, obesity, hypothyroidism, temperature instability, diabetes insipidus and amenorrhea. Abnormalities of growth hormone, antidiuretic hormone, thyroid stimulating hormone, gonadotropins and gonadotropin-releasing hormone have been documented (Fiedler & Krieger 1975, Hier & Wiehl 1977). Treatment is similar to that for progressive hydrocephalus. After shunting procedures, patients with hypothalamic-pituitary disturbance often improve.

HYDRANENCEPHALY

Hydranencephaly is a devastating CNS malformation consisting of near complete absence of the cerebral hemispheres. A variety of destructive or developmental abnormalities occurring after the fourth month of gestation may lead to hydranencephaly (Evrard et al 1989a, Halsey et al 1971). Animal models of hydranencephaly have demonstrated that different intrauterine viruses (Flanagan & Johnson 1995) or vascular occlusion (Wintour et al 1996) can cause this malformation. Intrauterine CMV and toxoplasmosis have also been reported to cause hydranencephaly (Kubo et al 1994).

Pathologic findings

The cranium is intact and therefore does not suggest anencephaly. Only small portions of the frontal, temporal and occipital cortex are identifiable. A well formed and somewhat thickened sac consists of an outer leptomeningeal layer and rudimentary representation of the cerebral cortex; no suggestion of normal ventricular configuration or ependymal lining can be delineated. The optic nerves are attenuated. The brainstem is also involved, as evidenced by underdeveloped cerebellar peduncles, pons and medulla.

Compromise of blood flow within the fetal internal carotid arteries, toxoplasmosis or CMV may be the basis of the extensive CNS malformation (Altschuler 1973, Vogel & McClenahan 1952). Hydranencephaly has also been reported as a result of maternal cocaine use (Rais-Bahrami & Naqvi 1990) and in association with a younger maternal age (Lubinsky 1997). Fetal ultrasound can be used for diagnosis (Agrawal et al 1996).

At least four cases have been reported of hydranencephaly in association with a proliferative vasculopathy that is believed to occur in the first trimester (Harding et al 1995). It has been suggested that this is an autosomal-recessive disorder that differs from encephaloclastic forms of hydranencephaly.

Hydranencephaly may develop in neonates and older infants after widespread cerebral infarction associated with extensive meningitis, intracerebral hemorrhage and ischemia (Lindberg & Swanson 1967). Hydranencephaly has been reported in association with 13q22 deletion (Gershoni-Baruch et al 1996).

Clinical characteristics

Neonates may appear normal in the perinatal period. The head circumference is usually within normal limits. After a few weeks, abnormal neurologic findings become apparent, including spasticity, myoclonic seizures and an enlarged head circumference from hydrocephalus.

Cranial ultrasonography readily demonstrates this malformation (Fig. 13.24a). Transillumination of the skull is startling because the islands of tissue, sagittal sinus and meningeal blood vessels are quite visible. Islands of preserved cortical tissue are seen as small opacities. Other neuroimaging techniques provide detailed documentation of the extent of the malformation (Fig. 13.24b) and may be required to distinguish severe hydrocephalus or severe subdural effusions from hydrocephalus or severe subdural effusions from hydranencephaly. EEG reveals suppressed or absent activity corresponding to the loss of brain tissue. Other EEG abnormalities have been described in hydranencephalic infants with Lennox–Gastaut syndrome (Velasco et al 1997). Somatosensory evoked response studies usually demonstrate an absent cortical response (Tayama et al 1992).

Although an infant may occasionally survive for one or two years, most die before one year of age. Ventriculoperitoneal shunting may be necessary in selected patients with associated progressive hydrocephalus.

POLYMICROGYRIA

Cytoarchitectonic analysis of the microgyric layers and their continuity with the layers of normal cortex allows some understanding of the mechanism that underlies microgyria formation (Evrard et al 1989a, Richman et al 1974). The superficial and deep cellular layers of microgyri appear as normal cortical layers II (the most superficial layer), III, IV and VI. The defect in microgyria is in the middle cortical layer, which has a reduced cellular population. Because the last cells to migrate form the superficial cortex, the presence of a normal superficial cortical layer documents normal neuronal migration. Microgyria, which most likely results from a postmigratory encephaloclastic injury presumably resulting from perfusion failure, produces laminar destruction of the middle layers of the cerebral cortex rather than an arrest of neuronal migration (Fig. 13.25a,b).

Polymicrogyria may be caused be intrauterine hypoxia of ischemia (Evrard et al 1989a), maternal cytomegalic

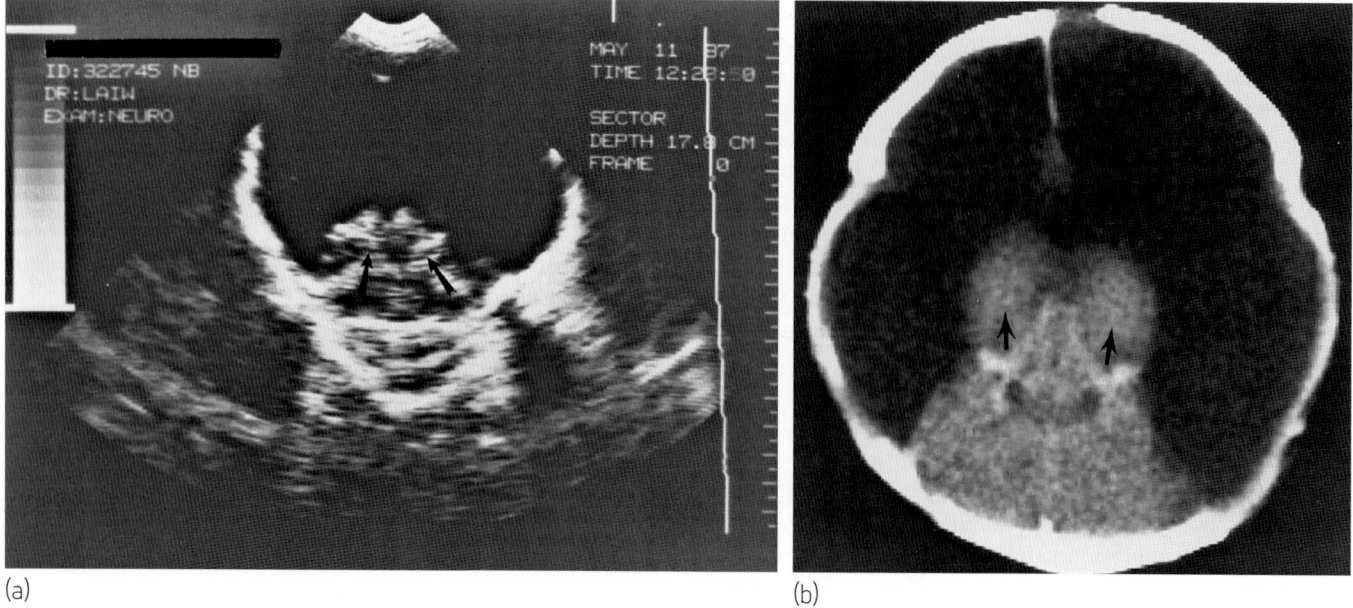

(a)

(b)

Figure 13.24 Hydranencephaly in a 1-day-old female. (a) CSF-filled cranial cavity with posterior fossa and diencephalic structures (arrows) depicted on coronal, transbregmatic cranial sonogram. (b) Axial CT scan demonstrating CSF-filled supratentorial compartment except for thalamic nuclei (arrows) and small residuum of medial right occipital lobe tissue. (Courtesy Joseph R. Thompson, Department of Radiation Sciences, Loma Linda University School of Medicine, Loma Linda, CA.)

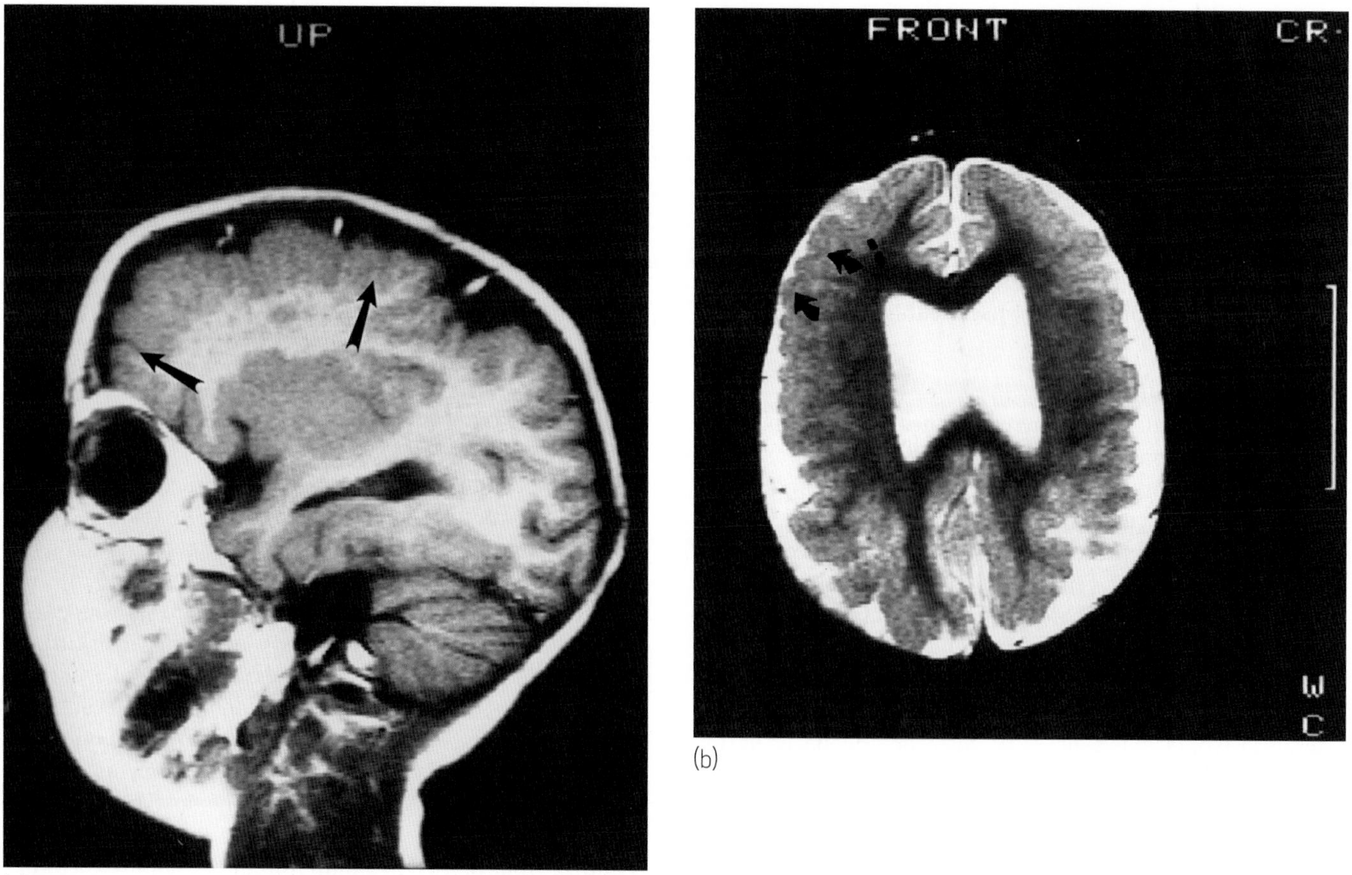

(a)

(b)

Figure 13.25 Polymicrogyria. (a) T1-weighted spin-echo sagittal view demonstrating irregular, closely spaced small frontal gyri (arrows). Note normal occipital lobe gyri for comparison. (b) T2-weighted spin-echo axial view at level of body of lateral ventricles. Note closely spaced, small gyri of right frontal lobe (arrows). Note normal occipital lobe gyri for comparison.

inclusion disease or toxoplasmosis (Crome & France 1959, Iannetti et al 1998), maternal carbon monoxide poisoning (Ginsberg & Myers 1978), or an associated finding with the type II Arnold–Chiari malformation, lissencephaly, schizencephaly and other CNS malformation. Selected groups of patients have been reported in whom polymicrogyria has been detected with MRI in bilateral perisylvian regions (Gropman et al 1997), occipital cortex (Kuzniecky et al 1997) and in the cerebellum (Sasaki et al 1997).

REFERENCES

Adamsbaum C, Moreau V, Bulteau E et al 1994 Vermian agenesis without posterior fossa cyst. Pediatr Radiol 24:543.

Agrawal P K, Agrawal U, Agrawal N K 1996 Prenatal sonographic diagnosis of hydranencephaly. J Indian Med Assoc 94:322.

Ahdab-Barmada M, Claassen D 1990 A distinctive triad of malformations of the central nervous system in the Meckel–Gruber syndrome. J Neuropathol Exp Neurol 49:610.

Al Shahwan S A, Bruyn G W, Deeb S M et al 1995 Non-progressive familial congenital cerebellar hypoplasia. J Neurol Sci 128:77.

Alman B A, Bhandari M, Wright J G 1996 Function of dislocated hips in children with lower level spina bifida. J Bone Joint Surg 78B:294.

Altschuler G 1973 Toxoplasmosis as a cause of hydrocephaly. Am J Dis Child 125:251.

Amer Ta, el-Shmam O M 1997 Chiari malformation type I: a new MRI classification. Magn Reson Imaging 15:397.

Anderson D J 1997 Cellular and molecular biology of neural crest cell lineage determination. Trends Genet 13:276.

Anderson F M 1975 Occult spinal dysraphism: a series of 73 cases. Pediatrics 55:826.

Anderson N G, Jordan S, MacFarlane M R et al 1994 Diastematomyelia: diagnosis by prenatal sonography. Am J Roentgenol 163:911.

Aniskiewicz A S, Frumkin N L, Brady D E et al 1990 Magnetic resonance imaging and neurobehavioral correlates in schizencephaly. Arch Neurol 74:911.

Arai H, Sato K 1990 Posterior fossa cysts: clinical, neuroradiological and surgical features. Childs Nerv Syst 7:156.

Archer C R, Horenstein S,, Sundaram M 1977 The Chiari malformation presenting in adult life. J Chronic Dis 30:369.

Aronyk K E 1993 The history and classification of hydrocephalus. Neurosurg Clin N Am 4:599.

Ashwal S, Peabody J L, Schneider S et al 1990 Anencephaly: clinical determination of brain death and neuropathologic studies. Pediatr Neural 6:233.

Aydingoz U, Cila A, Aktan G 1997 Rhombencephalosynapsis associated with hand anomalies. Br J Radiol 70:764.

Ayme S, Julian C, Gambarelli D et al 1989 Fryns syndrome: report on 8 new cases. Clin Genet 35:191.

Bailey A, Luthert P, Bolton P et al 1993 Autism and megalencephaly. Lancet 341:1225.

Balci S, Onol B, Ercal M D et al 1993 Autosomal recessive alobar holoprosencephaly with cyclops in three female sibs: prenatal ultrasonographic diagnosis at 18th week. Clin Dysmorphol 2:165.

Ball W S Jr 1997 Pediatric neuroradiology. Lippincott-Raven, New York, NY.

Barkovich A J 1995 Pedriatric neuroimaging, 2nd edn. Raven, New York, NY.

Barkovich A J 1996 Subcortical heterotopia: a distinct clinicoradiologic entity. AJNR Am J Neuroradiol 17:1315.

Barkovich A J, Jackson D E Jr, Boyer R S 1989 Band heterotopias: a newly recognized neuronal migration anomaly. Radiology 171:455.

Barkovich A J, Kjos B O 1992 Gray matter heterotopias: MR characteristics and correlation with developmental and neurologic manifestations. Radiology 182:493.

Barkovich A J, Kuzniecky R I 1996 Neuroimaging of focal malformations of cortical development. J Clin Neurophysiol 13:481.

Barkovich A J, Kuzniecky R I, Bollen A W et al 1997 Focal transmantle dysplasia: a specific malformation of cortical development. Neurology 49:1148.

Barkovich A J, Quint D J 1993 Middle interhemispheric fusion: an unusual variant of holoprosencephaly. AJNR Am J Neuroradiol, 14:431–440.

Barth P G 1993 Pontocerebellar hypoplasias. An overview of a group of inherited neurodegenerative disorders with fetal onset. Brain Dev 15:411.

Barth P G, Blennow G, Lenard H G et al 1995 The syndrome of autosomal recessive pontocerebellar hypoplasia, microcephaly and extrapyramidal dyskinesia (pontocerebellar hypoplasia type 2): compiled data from 10 pedigrees. Neurology 45:311.

Battaglia G, Arcelli P, Granata T et al 1996 Neuronal migration disorders and epilepsy: a morphological analysis of three surgically treated patients. Epilepsy Res 26:49.

Becker L E, Hinton D R 1995 Pathogenesis of craniosynostosis. Pedriatr Neurosurg 22:104.

Belman A L, Diamond G, Dickson D et al 1988 Pediatric acquired immunodeficiency syndrome: neurologic syndromes. Am J Dis Child 142:29.

Ben Arie N, Bellen H J, Armstrong D L et al 1997 Math 1 is essential for genesis of cerebellar granule neurons. Nature 390:169.

Berg R A, Aleck K A, Kaplan A M 1983 Familial porencephaly. Arch Neurol 40:567.

Berry-Kravis E, Israel J 1994 X-linked pachygyria and agenesis of the corpus callosum evidence for an X-chromosome lissencephaly locus. Ann Neurol 36:229–233.

Bertino R E, Nyberg D A, Cyr D R et al 1988 Prenatal diagnosis of agenesis of the corpus callosum. J Ultrasound Med 7:251.

Biglan A W 1990 Ophthalmologic complications of meningomyelocele: a longitudinal study. Trans Am Ophthalmol Soc 89:389.

Bindal A K, Storrs B B, McLone D G 1991 Occipital meningoceles in patients with Dandy-Walker syndrome. J Neurosurg 28:844.

Bodensteiner J B, Schaefer G B, Keller G M et al 1997 Macrocerebellum: neuroimaging and clinical features of a newly recognized condition. J Child Neurol 12:365.

Boemers T M, Soorani Lunsing I J, de Jong T P et al 1996 Urological problems after surgical treatment of scoliosis in children with myelomeningocele. J Urol 155:1066.

Boltshauser E, Lange B, Dumermuth G 1987 Differential diagnosis of syndromes with abnormal respiration (tachypnea-apnea). Brain Dev 9:462.

Boltshauser E, Steinlin M, Martin E et al 1996 Unilateral cerebellar aplasia. Neuropediatrics 27:50.

Bonnemann C G, Meinecke P 1996 Bilateral porencephaly, cerebellar hypoplasia, and internal malformations: two siblings representing a probably new autosomal recessive entity. Am J Med Genet 63:428.

Botkin J R 1988 Anencephalic infants as organ donors. Pediatrics 82:250.

Bradford D S, Heithoff K B, Cohen M 1991 Intraspinal abnormalities and congenital spine deformities: a radiographic and MRI study. J Pediatr Orthop 11:36.

Breningstall G N, Marker S M, Tubman D E 1992 Hydrosyringomyelia and diastematomyelia detected by MRI in myelomeningocele. Pediatr Neurol 8:267.

Brennand D M, Jehanli A M, Wood P J et al 1998 Raised levels of maternal serum secretory acetylcholinesterase may be indicative of fetal neural tube defects in early pregnancy. Acta Obstet Gynecol Scand 77:8.

Brock D J H, Scrimgeour J B, Nelson M N 1975 Amniotic fluid alpha-fetoprotein measurements in the early prenatal diagnosis of central nervous system disorders. Clin Genet 7:163.

Bromley B, Benacerraf B R 1995 Difficulties in the prenatal diagnosis of microcephaly. J Ultrasound Med 14:303.

Bromley B, Nadel A S, Pauker S et al 1994 Closure of the cerebellar vermis: evaluation with second trimester US. Radiology 193:761.

Brooks B S, El-Gammal T, Hartlage P et al 1981 Myelography of sacral agenesis. AJNR Am J Neuroradiol 2:319.

Buckton K E, O'Riordan M L, Ratcliffe S et al 1980 AG-band study of chrososomes in liveborn infants. Ann Hum Genet 43:227.

Buyse G, Verpoorten C, Vereecken R et al 1995 Treatment of neurogenic bladder dysfunction in infants and children with neurospinal dysraphism with clean intermittent (self) catheterization and optimised intravesical oxybutynin hydrochloride therapy. Eur J Pediatr Surg 1[5 Suppl]:31.

Byers P H 1993 Osteogenesis imperfecta. In: Royce P M, Steinmann B (eds.) Connective tissue and its heritable disorders: molecular, genetic, and medical aspects. Wiley-Liss, New York.

Byrd S E, Bohan T P, Osborn R E et al 1988 The CT and MR evaluation of lissencephaly. AJNR Am J Neuroradiol 9:923.

Byrd S E, Darling C F, McLone D G 1991 Developmental disorders of the pediatric spine. Radiol Clin North Am 29:711.

Cai C, Oakes W J 1997 Hindbrain herniation syndromes: the Chiari malformations (I and II). Semin Pediatr Neurol 4:156.

Carter C O 1976 Genetics of common single malformations. Br Med Bull 25:52.

Casey A T, Kimmings E J, Kleinlugtebeld A D et al 1997 The long-term outlook for hydrocephalus in childhood. A ten-year cohort study of 155 patients. Pediatr Neurosurg 27:63.

Castro-Gago M, Alonso A, Eiris Punal J 1996 Autosomal recessive hydrocephalus with aqueductal stenosis. Childs Nerv Syst 12:188.

Castro-Gago M, Rodriguez Nunez A, Eiris J et al 1993 Familial agenesis of the corpus callosum: a new form. Arch Fr Pediatr 50:327.

Catalans L W, Sever J L 1971 The role of viruses as causes of congenital defects. Ann Rev Microbiol 25:255.

Caviness V S 1976 The Chiari malformations of the posterior fossa and their relation to hydrocephalus. Dev Med Child Neural 18:103.

Chalhub E G, Volpe J J, Gado M H 1975 Linear nevus sebaceous syndrome associated with porencephaly and non-functioning major cerebral venous sinuses. Neurology 25:857.

Chambers G K, Cochrane D D, Irwin B et al 1996 Assessment of the appropriateness of services provided by a multidisciplinary meningomyelocele clinic. Pediatr Neurosurg 24:92.

Chan A, Robertson E F, Haan E A et al 1995 The sensitivity of ultrasound and serum alpha-fetoprotein in population-based antenatal screening for neural tube defects. South Australia 1986–1991. Br J Obstet Gynaecol 102:370.

Chapman P H, Swearingen B, Caviness V S 1989 Subtorcular occipital encephaloceles: anatomical considerations relevant to operative management. J Neurosurg 71:375.

Charney E G B, Rorke L B, Sutton L N et al 1987 Management of Chiari II complications in infants with myelomeningocele. J Pediatr 111:364.

Chatkupt S, Speer M C, Ding Y et al 1994 Linkage analysis of a candidate locus (HLA) in autosomal dominant sacral defect with anterior meningocele. J Med Genet 52:1.

Chen J, Chang S, Duncan S A et al 1996 Disruption of the MacMARCKS gene prevents cranial tube closure and results in anencephaly. Proc Natl Acad Sci USA 93:6275.

Chevrie J J, Aicardi J 1986 The Aicardi syndrome. In: Pedley T, Meldrum B (eds.) Recent advances in epilepsy. Churchill Livingstone, Edinburgh.

Chitayat D, Moore L, Del Bigio M R et al 1994 Familial Dandy–Walker malformation associated with microcephaly, facial anomalies, developmental delay, and brain stem dysgenesis: prenatal diagnosis and postnatal outcome in brothers. A new syndrome? Am J Med Genet 52:406.

Clark G D, Mizuguchi M, Antalffy B et al 1997 Predominant localization of the LIS family of gene products to Cajal-Retzius cells and ventricular neuroepithelium in the developing human cortex. J Neuropathol Exp Neurol 56:1044.

Clarren S K, Smith D W 1978 The fetal alcohol syndrome. N Engl J Med 298:1063.

Cohen M M, Lemire R J 1982 Syndromes with cephaloceles. Teratology 25:161.

Cohen T, Zeitune M, McGillivray B C et al 1996 Segregation analysis of microcephaly. Am J Med Genet 65:226.

Colgan M T 1981 The child with spina bifida: role of the pediatrician. Am J Dis Child 135:854.

Copp A J, Brook F A, Estibeiro J P et al 1990 The embryonic development of mammalian neural tube defects. Prog Neurobiol 35:363.

Cowan W M 1992 Development of the nervous system. In: Asbury A K, McKhann G M, McDonald W I (eds) Diseases of the nervous system, clinical neurobiology. W B Saunders, Philadelphia.

Crino P B, Eberwine J 1997 Cellular and molecular basis of cerebral dysgenesis. J Neurosci Res 50:907.

Crome L K, France N E 1959 Microgyria and cytomegalic inclusion disease in infancy. J Clin Pathol 12:427.

Cross J H, Harrison C J, Preston P R et al 1992 Postnatal encephaloclastic porencephaly-a new lesion? Arch Dis Child 67:307.

Davidoff A M, Thompson C V, Grimm J M et al 1991 Occult spinal dysraphism in patients with anal agenesis. J Pediatr Surg 26:1001.

de Carvalho Neto J, Dias L S, Gabrieli A P 1996 Congenital talipes equinovarus in spina bifida: treatment and results. J Pediatr Orthop 16:782.

De Souza N, Chaudhuri R, Bingham J et al 1994 MRI in cerebellar hypoplasia. Neuroradiology 36:148.

De Zegher F, Devlieger H, De Cock P 1992 Alternating diabetes insipidus and inappropriate antidiuresis in holoprosencephaly: relationship to intracranial pressure. J Pediatr 120:161.

Dekaban A S 1968 Abnormalities in children exposed to X-radiation during various stages of gestation: tentative time table of radiation injury to the human fetus. Part 1. J Nucl Med 9:471.

Demaerel P, Kendall B E, Wilms G et al 1995 Uncommon posterior cranial fossa anomalies: MRI with clinical correlation. Neuroradiology 37:72.

DeMyer W 1971 Classification of cerebral malformations. Birth Defects 7:78.

DeMyer W 1975 Median facial malformations and their implication for brain malformation. Birth Defects 11:155.

Deng C, Bedford M, Li C et al 1997 Fibroblast growth factor receptor-1 (FGFR-1) is essential for normal neural tube and limb development. Dev Biol 185:42.

Devrient K, Naulaers G, Matthijs G et al 1997 Agenesis of corpus callosum and anophthalmia in the asplenia syndrome. A recognizable association? Ann Genet 40:14.

Dhellemmes C, Girard S, Dulac O et al 1988 Agyria-pachygyria and Miller–Dieker syndrome: clinical, genetic and chromosome studies. Hum Genet 79:163.

Dias M S, Pang D 1995 Split cord malformations. Neurosurg Clin N Am 6:339.

Dickson D W, Llena J F, Nelson S J et al 1993 Central nervous system pathology in pediatric AIDS. Ann NY Acad Sci 693:93.

DiMario F J Jr, Cogg R J, Ramsby G R et al 1993 Familial band heretotopias simulating tuberous sclerosis. Neurology 43:1424.

Dobyns W B 1987 Developmental aspects of lissencephaly and the lissencephaly syndromes. In: Gilbert E F, Opitz J M (eds) Genetic aspects of developmental pathology. Alan R Liss, New York NY. For the March of Dimes Birth Defects Foundation, Birth Defects: Original Article Series 23: p. 225.

Dobyns W B 1989 The neurogenetics of lissencephaly. Neurol Clin 7:89.

Dobyns W B, Andermann E, Andermann F et al 1996a X-linked malformations of neuronal migration. Neurology 47:331.

Dobyns W B, Curry C J R, Hoyme H E et al 1991 Clinical and molecular diagnosis of Miller–Dieker syndrome. Am J Med Genet 48:584.

Dobyns W B, Elias E R, Newlin A C et al 1992 Causal heterogeneity in isolated lissencephaly. Neurology 42:1375.

Dobyns W B, Pagon R A, Armstrong D et al 1989 Diagnostic criteria for Walker–Warburg syndrome. Am J Med Genet 32:195.

Dobyns W B, Patton M A, Stratton R F et al 1996b Cobblestone lissencephaly with normal eyes and muscle. Neuropediatrics 27:70.

Dobyns W B, Truwit C L 1995 Lissencephaly and other malformations of cortical development: 1995 update. Neuropediatrics 26:132.

Docherty T B, Herbaut A G, Sedgwick E M 1987 Brainstem auditory evoked potential abnormalities in myelomeningocele in the older child. J Neurol Neurosurg Psychiatry 50:1318.

Dolk H 1991 The predictive value of microcephaly during the first year of life for mental retardation at seven years. Dev Med Child Neurol 33:974.

Domingo Z, Peter J 1996 Midline developmental abnormalities of the posterior fossa: correlation of classification with outcome. Pediatr Neurosurg 24:111.

Dominguez R, Vila-Coro A A, Slopis J M et al 1991 Brain and ocular abnormalities in infants with in utero exposure to cocaine and other street drugs. Am J Dis Child 145:688.

Dorman C 1991 Microcephaly and intelligence. Dev Med Child Neurol 33:267.

Drachman D A, Richardson E P 1961 Aqueductal narrowing, congenital and acquired: a critical review of the histologic criteria. Arch Neurol 5:552.

Dubeau F, Tampieri D, Lee N et al 1995 Periventricular and subcortical nodular heterotopia. A study of 33 patients. Brain 118:1273.

Dubourg Ch, Bendavid C, Pasquier L et al 2007 Holoprocencephaly (rev) http//www.OJRD.com/content/2/1/8.

Dyste G N, Menezes A H, VanGilder J C et al 1989 Symptomatic Chiari malformations. An analysis of presentation, management, and long-term outcome. J Neurosurg 71:159.

Edwards J H 1961 The syndrome of sex-linked hydrocephalus. Arch Dis Child 36:486.

Eksioglu Y Z, Scheffer I E, Cardenas P et al 1996 Periventricular heterotopia: an X-linked dominant epilepsy locus causing aberrant cerebral cortical development. Neuron 16:77.

Elbers S E L, Furness M E 1999 Resolution of presumed arachnoid cyst in utero. Ulrasound Obstet Gynecol 14:353.

Elias D L, Kawamoto H K Jr, Wilson L F 1992 Holoprosencephaly and midline facial anomalies: redefining classification and management. Plast Reconstr Surg 90:951.

Eller K M, Kuller J A 1995a Fetal porencephaly: a review of etiology, diagnosis, and prognosis. Obstet Gynecol Surv 50:684.

Eller K M, Kuller J A 1995b Porencephaly secondary to fetal trauma during amniocentesis. Obstet Gynecol 85:865.

Ellyn B, Khatir A H, Sing S P 1980 Hypothalamic — pituitary functions in patients with transsphenoidal encephalocele and midfacial anomalies. J Clin Endocrinol Metab 51:854.

Elterman R D, Bodensteiner J B, Barnard J J 1995 Sudden unexpected death in patients with Dandy-Walker malformation. J Child Neurol 10:382.

Encha Razavi F, Larroche J C, Roume J et al 1996 Lethal familial fetal akinesia sequence (FAS) with distinct neuropathological pattern: type III lissencephaly syndrome. Am J Med Genet 62:16.

Epstein D J, Vogan K J, Trasler D G et al 1993 A mutation within intron 3 of the Pax-3 gene produces aberrantly spliced mRNA transcripts in the splotch (Sp) mouse mutant. Proc Natl Acad Sci USA 90:532–6.

Epstein M H, Johanson C E 1987 The Dandy–Walker syndrome. In: Myrianthopoulos N C (ed.) Handbook of clinical neurology. Elsevier Science, Amsterdam.

Estin D, Cohen A R 1995 Caudal agenesis and associated caudal spinal cord malformations. Neurosurg Clin N Am 6:377.

Estroff J A, Scott M R, Benacerraf B R 1992 Dandy–Walker variant: prenatal sonographic features and clinical outcome. Radiology 185:755.

Evrard P, de Saint-Georges P, Kadhim H J et al 1989a
Pathology of prenatal encephalopathies. In: Evrard P,
Minkowski A (eds) Child neurology and
developmental disabilities. Paul H. Brookes,
Baltimore, MD.

Evrard P, Kadhim H J, de Saint-Georges P et al 1989b
Abnormal development and destructive processes of
the human brain during the second half of gestation.
In: Evrard P, Minkowski A, eds. Developmental
neurobiology. Nestle Nutrition Workshop Series, vol
12. Raven, New York NY.

Evrard P, Marret S, Gressens P 1997 Environmental
and genetic determinants of neural migration
and postmigratory survival. Acta Paediatr 422
[Suppl]:20.

Evrard P, Miladi N, Bonnier C et al 1992 Normal and
abnormal development of the brain. In: Rapin I,
Segalowitz S J (eds) Handbook of neuropsychology,
child psychology. Biomedical Division, Elsevier
Science, Amsterdam, Vol. 6.

Fewel M E, Levy M L, McComb J G 1996 Surgical
treatment of 95 children with 102 intracranial
arachnoid cysts. Pediatr Neurosurg 25:165.

Fiedler R, Krieger D T 1975 Endocrine disturbances in
patients with congenital aqueductal stenosis. Acta
Endocrinal 80:1.

Fitz C R 1994 Holoprosencephaly and septo-optic
dysplasia. Neuromaging Clin N Am 4:263.

Flanagan M, Johnson S J 1995 The effects of vaccination
of Merino ewes with attenuated Australian
bluetongue virus serotype 23 at different stages of
gestation. Aust Vet J 72:455.

Fransen E, Van Camp G, Vits L et al 1997 L1-associated
diseases: clinical geneticists divide, molecular
geneticists unite. Human Mol Genet 6:1625.

Freeman J M 1985 Prenatal and perinatal factors
associated with brain disorders. NIH Publication No.
85–1149. National Institute of Child Health and
Development, Washington, DC.

French B N 1983 The embryology of spinal dysraphism.
Clin Neurosurg 30:295.

Fretelle F, Senat M-V, Bernard J-P et al 2002 First
trimester diagnosis of fetal arachnoid cyst: pre-natal
implications. Ultrasound Obstet Gynecol 20:400.

Friede R L 1989 Developmental neuropathology.
Springer-Verlag, New York NY.

Fryburg J S, Breg W R, Lindgren V 1991 Diagnosis of
Angelman syndrome in infants. Am J Med Genet
38:58.

Fryns J P, Devriendt K, Legius E 1997 Polysyndactyly
and trigonocephaly with partial agenesis of corpus
callosum: an example of the variable clinical
spectrum of the acrocallosal syndrome? Clin
Dysmorphol 6:285.

Gardner W J 1977 Hemodynamic factors in Dandy–
Walker and Arnold–Chiari malformations. Childs
Brain 3:200.

Gastaut H, Pinsard N, Raybaud C et al 1987
Lissencephaly (agyriapachygyria): clinical findings
and serial EEG studies. Dev Med Child Neurol 29:167.

Gelman-Kohan Z, Antonelli J, Ankori-Cohen H et al 1991
Further delineation of the acrocallosal syndrome.
Eur J Pediatr 150:797.

Gentile M, Di Carlo A, Susca F et al 1996 COACH
syndrome: report of two brothers with congenital
hepatic fibrosis, cerebellar vermis hypoplasia,
oligophrenia, ataxia and mental retardation. Am J
Med Genet 64:514.

George T M, McLone D G 1995 Mechanisms of mutant
genes in spina bifida: a review of implications from
animal models. Pediatr Neurosurg 23:236.

Gershoni-Baruch R, Zekaria D 1996 Deletion (13)(q22)
with multiple congenital anomalies, hydranencephaly
and penoscrotal transposition. Clin Dysmorphol 5:289.

Gerzten P C, Albright A L 1995 Relationship between
cerebellar appearance and function in children with
Dandy–Walker syndrome. Pediatr Neurosurg 23:86.

Gilbert J N, Jones K L, Rorke L B et al 1986 Central
nervous system anomalies associated with
meningomyelocele, hydrocephalus, and the Arnold–
Chiari malformation: reappraisal of theories
regarding the pathogenesis of posterior neural tube
closure defects. Neurosurgery 18:559.

Ginsberg M D, Myers R E 1978 Fetal brain injury after
maternal carbon monoxide intoxication. Neurology
26:15.

Gleeson J G, Allen K M, Fox J W et al 1998 Doublecortin,
a brain-specific gene mutated in human X-linked
lissencephaly and double cortex syndrome, encodes
a putative signalling protein. Cell 92:63.

Glickstein M 1994 Cerebellar agenesis. Brain 117:1209.

Golden J A, Chernoff G F 1995 Multiple sites of anterior
neural tube closure in humans: evidence from
anterior neural tube defects (anencephaly).
Pediatrics 95:506.

Golden J A, Rorke L B, Bruce D A 1987 Dandy–Walker
syndrome and associated anomalies. Pediatr
Neurosci 13:38.

Goldstein R B, Filly R A 1988 Prenatal diagnosis of
anencephaly: spectrum of sonographic appearances
and distinction from the amniotic band syndrome.
Am J Radiol 151:547.

Gowen L C, Johnson B L, Latour A M et al 1996 Bracal
deficiency results in early embryonic lethality
characterized by neuroepithelial abnormalities. Nat
Genet 12:19.

Granata T, Battaglia G, D'Incerti L et al 1996
Schizencephaly: neuroradiologic and epileptologic
findings. Epilepsia 37:1185.

Gropman A L, Barkovich A J, Vezina L G et al 1997
Pediatric congenital bilateral perisylvian syndrome:
clinical and MRI features in 12 patients.
Neuropediatrics 28:198.

Gross Tsur V, Joseph A, Blinder G et al 1995 Familial
microcephaly with severe neurological deficits: a
description of five affected siblings. Clin Genet 47:33.

Guerrini R, Dubeau F, Dulac O et al 1997 Bilateral
parasagittal parietoccipital polymicrogyria and
epilepsy. Ann Neurol 41:65.

Guillen D, Pascual Castroviejo I, Lopez Martin V et al
1995 Neuronal migration disorders: clinical-
radiological radiological correlation. Rev Neurol
23:43.

Gunay M, Aysun S 1996 Neuronal migration disorders
presenting with mild clinical symptoms. Pediatr
Neurol 14:153.

Gundry C R, Heithoff K B 1994 Imaging evaluation of
patients with spinal deformity. Orthop Clin North Am
25:247.

Guturbay I G, Yoldi M E, Carrera B et al 1997
Andermann syndrome: presentation of a case. Rev
Neurol 25:1087.

Hagberg B A, Blennow G, Kristiansson B, Stibler H 1993
Carbohydrate-deficient glycoprotein syndromes:
peculiar group of new disorders. Pediatr Neurol
9:255.

Hagberg B, Aicardi J, Dias K et al 1983 A progressive
syndrome of autism, dementia, ataxia, and loss of
purposeful hand use in girls: Rett's syndrome: report
of 35 cases. Ann Neurol 14:471.

Haller J S, Wolpert S M, Rabe E F et al 1971 Cystic
lesions of the posterior fossa in infants: a
comparison of the clinical, radiological, and
pathological findings in Dandy–Walker syndrome in
extra-axial cysts. Neurology 21:494.

Halsey J H Jr, Allen N, Chamberlin H R 1971 The
morphogenesis of hydranencephaly. J Neurol Sci
12:187.

Hamilton R L, Grafe M R 1994 Complete absence of the
cerebellum: a report of two cases. Acta Neuropathol
Berl 88:258.

Handa j, Okamoto K, Sato M 1981 Arachnoid cyst of the
middle cranial fossa: report of bilateral cysts in
siblings. Surg Neurol 16:127.

Harding B N, Ramani P, Thurley P 1995 The familial
syndrome of proliferative vasculopathy and
hydranencephaly-hydrocephaly;
immunocytochemical and ultrastructural evidence
for endothelial proliferation. Neuropathol Appl
Neurobiol 21:61.

Harley E H 1991 Pediatric congenital nasal masses. Ear
Nose Throat J 70:28.

Harsh G R, Edwards M S B, Wilson C B 1986
Intracranial arachnoid cysts in children. J Neurosurg
64:835.

Hart M N, Malamud N, Ellis W G 1972 The Dandy–
Walker syndrome, a clinicopathological study based
on 28 cases. Neurology 22:771.

Hashimoto R, Seki T, Takuma Y et al 1993 The 'double
cortex' syndrome on MRI. Brain Dev 15:57.

Hatten M E, Heintz N 1995 Mechanisms of neural
patterning and specification in the developing
cerebellum. Ann Rev Neurosci 18:385.

Hemphill M, Freeman J M, Martinez C R et al
1982 A new, treatable source of recurrent
meningitis: basiooccipital meningocele. Pediatrics
70:941.

Hier D B, Wiehl A C 1977 Chronic hydrocephalus
associated with short stature and growth hormone
deficiency. Ann Neurol 2:246.

Hildebrandt F, Nothwang H G, Vossmerbaumer U et al
1998 Lack of large, homozygous deletions of the
nephronophthisis 1 regions in Joubert syndrome type
B. APN Study Group. Arbeitsgemeinschaft fur
Padiatrische nephrologie. Pediatr Nephrol 12:16.

Hirayama K, Hashino Y, Kumashiro H et al 1994
Reverse Shapiro's syndrome. A case of agenesis of
corpus callosum associated with periodic
hyperthermia. Arch Neurol 51:494.

Ho S S, Kuznieckky R I, Gilliam F et al 1997 Congenital
porcencephaly and hippocampal sclerosis. Clinical
features and epileptic spectrum. Neurology 49:1382.

Hockley A D, Goldin J H, Wake M J 1990 Management of
anterior encephalocele. Childs Nerv Syst 6:444.

Hol F A, Geurds M P, Chatkupt S et al 1996 PAX genes
and human neural tube defects: an amino acid
substitution in PAX1 in a patient with spina bifida.
J Med Genet 33:655.

Hol F A, Hamel B C, Geurds M P et al 1995 A frameshift
mutation in the gene for PAX3 in a girl with spina
bifida and mild signs of Waardenburg syndrome.
J Med Genet 32:52.

Holmes L B 1974 Inborn errors of morphogenesis: a
review of localized hereditary malformations. N Engl
J Med 291:763.

Holmes L B 1994 Spina bifida: anticonvulsants and other
maternal influences. Ciba Found Symp 181:232.

Holmes L B, Driscoll S G, Atkinks L 1976, Biologic
heterogenicity of neural tube defects. N Engl J Med
294:365.

Holroyd S, Reiss A L, Bryan R N 1991 Autistical features
in Joubert syndrome: a genetic disorder with
agenesis of the cerebellar vermis. Biol Psychiatry
29:287.

Hori A 1994 Tectocerebellar dysraphia with posterior
encephalocele (Friede): report of the youngest case.
Reappraisal of the condition uniting Cleland–Chiari
(Arnold–Chiari) and Dandy–Walker syndromes. Clin
Neuropathol 13:216.

Hustinx R, Verloes A, Grattagliano B et al 1993
Monosomy 11q: report of two familial cases and
review of the literature. Am J Med Genet 47:312.

Huttenlocher P R, Taravath S, Mojtahedi S 1994 Periventricular heterotopia and epilepsy. Neurology 44:51.

Iannetti P, Nigro G, Spalice A et al 1998 Cytomegalovirus infection and schizencephaly: case reports. Ann Neurol 43:123.

Iannetti P, Schwarts C E, Dietz Band J et al 1993 Norman–Roberts syndrome: clinical and molecular studies. Am J Med Genet 47:95.

Iannetti P, Spalice A, Atzei G et al 1996 Neuronal migrational disorders in children with epilepsy: MRI, interictal SPECT and EEG comparisons. Brain Dev 18:269.

Illarioshkin S N, Tanaka H, Markova E D et al 1996 X-linked nonprogressive congenital cerebellar hypoplasia: clinical description and mapping to chromosome Xq. Ann Neurol 40:75.

Isada N B, Qureshi F, Jacques S M et al 1993 Meroanencephaly: pathology and prenatal diagnosis. Fetal Diagn Ther 8:423.

Iskandar B J, Oakes W J, McLaughlin C et al 1994 Terminal syringohydromyelia and occult spinal dysraphism (see comments) J Neurosurg 81:513.

Isumi H, Takashima S, Kakita A et al 1997 Expression of the LIS-1 gene product in brain anomalies with a migration disorder. Pediatr Neurol 16:42.

Jansen J, Taudorf K, Pedersen H et al 1991 Upper extremity function in spina bifida. Childs Nerv Syst 7:67.

Jardine P E, Clarke M A, Super M 1996 Familial bilateral periventricular nodular heterotopia mimics tuberous sclerosis. Arch Dis Child 74:244.

Jensen R, Hansen F J, Skovby F 1995 Cerebellar hypoplasia in children with the carbohydrate-deficient glycoprotein syndrome. Neuroradiology 37:328.

Johnson S P, Sebire N J, Snijders R J et al 1997 Ultrasound screening for anencephaly at 10–14 weeks of gestation. Ultrasound Obstet Gynecol 9:14.

Joubert M, Eisenring J J, Robb J P et al 1998 Familial agenesis of the cerebellar vermis. Neurology 19:813.

Kadonaga J N, Barkovich A J, Edwards M S et al 1992 Neurocutaneous melanosis in association with the Dandy–Walker complex. Pediatr Dermatol 9:37.

Kalidasan V, Carroll T, Alcutt D et al 1995 The Dandy–Walker syndrome — a 10-year experience of its management and outcome. Eur J Pediatr Surg 1 [Suppl.]:16.

Kallen A J 1994 Maternal carbamazepine and infants with spina bifida. Reprod Toxicol 8:203.

Kalter H 1993 Case reports of malformations associated with maternal diabetes: history and critique. Clin Genet 43:174.

Karol L A 1995 Orthopedic management in myelomeningocele. Neurosurg Clin N Am 6:259.

Kato M, Dobyns W B 2003 Lissencephaly and the molecular basis of neuronal migration. Human Molecular Genetics, Vol 12 review issue 1 DOI:10.109.

Kendall B, Kingsley D, Lambert S R et al 1990 Joubert syndrome: a clinico-radiological study. Neuroradiology 31:502.

Keogan M T, DeAtkine A B, Hertzberg B S 1994 Cerebellar vermian defects: antenatal sonographic appearance and clinical significance. J Ultrasound Med 13:607.

King M D, Dudgeon J, Stephenson J B P 1984 Joubert's syndrome with retinal dysplasia: neonatal tachypnea as due to a genetic brain-eye malformation. Arch Dis Child 59:709.

Klingensmith W C 3rd, Cioffi-Ragan D T 1986 Schizencephaly. Diagnosis and progression in utero. Radiology 159:617.

Knobloch W H, Layer J M 1971 Retinal detachment and encephalocele. J Pediatr Ophtalmol 8:181.

Kolawole T M, Patel J J, Mahdi A H 1987 Porcencephaly: computed tomography (CT) scan findings. Comput Radiol 11:53.

Kolodny E H 1989 Agenesis of the corpus callosum: a marker for inherited metabolic disease? Neurology 39:847.

Konz K R, Chia J K, Kurup V P et al 1995 Comparison of latex hypersensitivity among patients with neurologic defects. J Allergy Clin Immunol 95:950.

Korsvik H E, Keller M S 1992 Sonography of occult dysraphism in neonates and infants with MR imaging correlation. Radiographics 12:297.

Kosaki K, Curry C J, Roeder E et al 1997 Ritscher–Schinzel (3C) syndrome: documentation of the phenotype. Am J Med Genet 68:421.

Kothari M J, Bauer S B 1997 Urodynamic and neurophysiologic evaluation of patients with diastematomyelia. J Child Neurol 12:97.

Kozlowski K, Ouvrier R A 1993 Agenesis of the corpus callosum with mental retardation and osseous lesions. Am J Med Genet 48:6.

Kubo S, Kishino T, Satake N et al 1994 A neonatal case of hydranencephaly caused by atheromatous plaque obstruction of aortic arch: possible association with a congenital cytomegalovirus infection? J Perinatal 14:483.

Kurauchi O, Ohno Y, Mizutani S et al 1995 Longitudinal monitoring of fetal behaviour in twins when one is anencephalic. Obstet Gynecol 86:672.

Kurent J E, Sever J L 1973 Perinatal infections and epidemiology and anencephaly and spina bifida. Teratology 8:359.

Kuznicky R, Andermann F, Tampieri D et al 1989 Bilateral central macrogyria: epilepsy, pseudobulbar palsy, and mental retardation — a recognizable neuronal migration disorder. Ann Neurol 25:547.

Kuznicky R, Gilliam F, Faught E 1995 Discordant occurrence of cerebral unilateral heterotopia and epilepsy in monozygotic twins. Epilepsia 36:1155.

Kuznicky R, Gilliam F, Morawetz R 1997 Occipital lobe developmental malformations and epilepsy: clinical spectrum, treatment and outcome. Epilepsia 38:175.

Lacey D J 1985 Agenesis of the corpus callosum: clinical features in 40 children. Am J Dis Child 139:653.

Lambert S R, Kriss A, Gresty M et al 1989 Joubert syndrome. Arch Ophthalmol 107:709.

Lammer E J, Chen D T, Hoar R M et al 1985 Retinoic acid embryopathy. N Engl J Med 313:837.

Lary J M, Edmonds L D 1996 Prevalence of spina bifida at birth — United States, 1983–1990: a comparison of two surveillance systems. MMWR CDC Surveill Sum 45:15.

Laurence K M 1964 The natural history of spina bifida cystica. Arch Dis Child 39:41.

Layde P M, Edmonds L D, Erickson J D 1980 Maternal fever and neural tube defects. Teratology 21:105.

Leao M J, Ribeiro Silva M L 1995 Orofaciodigital syndrome type I in a patient with severe CNS defects. Pediatr Neurol 13:247.

Ledbetter S A, Kuwano A, Dobyns W B et al 1992 Microdeletions of chromosome 17p13 as a cause of isolated lissencephaly. Am J Hum Genet 50:182.

Leech R W, Johnson S H, Brumback R A 1997 Agenesis of cerebellum associated arrhinencephaly. Clin Neuropathol 16:90.

Leech R W, Shuman R M 1986 Holoprosencephaly and related midline cerebral anomalies: a review. J Chil Neurol 1:3.

Lemire R J 1987 Anencephaly. In: Myrianthopoulos NC (ed.) Handbook of clinical neurology. Elsevier Science, Amsterdam.

Lemire R J, Beckwith J B, Shepard T H 1972 Iniencephaly and anencephaly with spinal retroflexion. A comparative study of eight human specimens. Teratology 6:27–36.

Lemire R J, Beckwith J B, Warkany J 1978 Anencephaly. Raven, New York, NY.

Lemire R J, Loeser J D, Leech R W et al 1975 Normal and abnormal development of the human nervous system. Harper & Row, New York, NY.

Lendahl U 1997 Gene regulation in the formation of the central nervous system. Acta Paediatr Suppl 422:8.

Lenke R R, Levy H L 1982 Maternal phenylketonuria: results of dietary therapy. Am J Obstet Gynecol 142:548.

Levitt P, Barbe M F, Eagleson K L 1997 Patterning and specification of the cerebral cortex. Ann Rev Neurosci 20:1.

Levy H L, Lobbregt D, Barnes P D et al 1996 Maternal phenylketonuria: magnetic resonance imaging of the brain in offspring. J Pediatr 128:770.

Lewis S M, Roberts E A, Marcon M A et al 1994 Joubert syndrome with congenital hepatic fibrosis: an entity in the spectrum of oculo-encephalo-hepato-renal disorders. Am J Med Genet 52:419.

LeWitt P A, Newman R P, Greenberg H S et al 1983 Episodic hyperhidrosis, hypothermia, and agenesis of corpus callosum. Neurology 33:1122.

Limb C J, Holmes L B 1994 Anencephaly: changes in prenatal detection and birth status, 1972 through 1990. Am J Obstet Gynecol 170:1333.

Lincke C R, van den Bogert C, Nijtmans L G et al 1996 Cerebellar hypoplasia in respiratory chain dysfunction. Neuropediatrics 27:216.

Lindenberg R, Swanson P D 1967 Infantile hydranencephaly — a report of five cases of both cerebral hemispheres in infancy. Brain 90:839.

Lindhout D, Omtzigt J G, Cornel M C 1992 Spectrum of neural-tube defects in 34 infants prenatally exposed to antiepileptic drugs. Neurology 42:111.

Liptak G S, Bloss J W, Briskin H et al 1988 The management of children with spinal dysraphism. J Child Neurol 3:3.

Little J R, Houser O W, MacCarty C S 1975 Clinical manifestations of aqueductal stenosis in adults. J Neurosurg 43:546.

Liu D P, Burrowes D M, Qureshi M N 1997a Cyclopia: craniofacial appearance on MR and three-dimensional CT. AJNR Am J Neuroradiol 18:543.

Locke M D, Sarwark J F 1996 Orthopedic aspects of myelodysplasia in children. Curr Opin Pediatr 8:65.

Loebstein R, Koren G 1997 Pregnancy outcome and neurodevelopment of children exposed in utero to psychoactive drugs: the mother's experience. J Psychiatry Neurosci 22:192.

Longo L D 1977 The biological effects of carbon monoxide on the pregnant woman, fetus and newborn infant. Am J Obstet Gynecol 129:69.

Lorber J 1971 Results of treatment of myelomeningocele: an analysis of 524 unselected cases with special reference to possible selection for treatment. Dev Med Child Neurol 13:279.

Lubinsky M S 1997 Association of prenatal vascular disruptions with decreased maternal age. Am J Med Genet 69:237.

Lurie I W, Ilyina H G, Gurevich D B et al 1995 Trisomy 2p: analysis of unusual phenotypic findings. Am J Med Genet 55:229.

Luyendijk W, Treffers P D 1992 The smile in anencephalic infants. Clin Neurol Neurosurg 94:S113.

Lynch S A, Bond P M, Copp A J et al 1995 A gene for autosomal dominant sacral agenesis maps to the holoprosencephaly region at 7q36. Nat Genet 11:93.

Lynn R B, Buchanan D C, Fenichel G M et al 1980 Agenesis of the corpus callosum. Arch Neurol 37:444.

Macchi G, Bentivoglio M 1987 Agenesis or hypoplasia of cerebellar structures. In: Myrianthopoulos NC (ed.) Handbook of clinical neurology. Elsevier Science, Amsterdam.

McComb J G 1997 Spinal and cranial neural tube defects. Semin Pediatr Neurol 4:156.

McDonald C M 1995 Rehabilitation of children with spinal dysraphism. Neurosurg Clin N Am 6:393.

McEnery G, Borzyskowski M, Cox T C et al 1992 The spinal cord in neurologically stable spina bifida: a clinical and MRI study. Dev Med Child Neurol 34:342.

McKusick V A 1994 Mendelian inheritance in man: a catalog of human genes and genetic disorders, 11th edn. John Hopkins University Press, Baltimore.

McLone D G, La Marca F 1994 The tethered spinal cord: diagnosis, significance, and not prepattern. Development 120:2271.

McLone D G, La Marca F 1997a The tethered spinal cord: diagnosis, significance, and management. Semin Pediatr Neurol 4:192.

McLone D G, La Marca F 1997b The tethered spinal cord: diagnosis, significance, and management. Semin Pediatr Neurol 473:192–208.

Malandrini A, Palmeri S, Villanova M et al 1997 A syndrome of autosomal recessive pontocerebellar hypoplasia with white matter abnormalities and protracted course in two brothers. Brain Dev 19:209.

Maria B L, Hoang K B, Tusa R J et al 1997 'Joubert syndrome' revisited: key ocular motor signs with magnetic resonance imaging correlation. J Child Neurol 12:423.

Maria B L, Zinreich S J, Carson B C et al 1987 Dandy–Walker syndrome revisited. Pediatr Neurosci 13:45.

Marin-Padilla M 1991 Embryology and pathology of axial skeletal and neural dysraphic disorders. Can J Neurol Sci 18:153.

Marin-Padilla M 1997 Developmental neuropathology and impact of perinatal brain damage. II: White matter lesions of the neocortex. J Neuropathol Exp Neurol 56:219.

Marsh D O, Myers G J, Clarkson T W et al 1980 Fetal methylmercury poisoning: clinical and toxicological data on 9 cases. Ann Neurol 7:343.

Martin H 1970 Microcephaly and mental retardation. Am J Dis Child 119:128.

Martinez Lage J F, Poza M, Sola J et al 1996 The child with a cephalocele: etiology, neuroimaging, and outcome. Childs Nerv Syst 12:540.

Mason T B 2nd, Chiriboga C A, Feldstein N A et al 1997 Intracranial arachnoid cyst in a developmentally normal infant: case report and literature report. Pediatr Neurol 16:59.

Mealey J Jr, Dzentis A J, Hockey A A 1970 The prognosis of encephaloceles. J Neurosurg 32:209.

Medical Task Force on Anencephaly 1990 The infant with anencephaly. N Engl J Med 322:669.

Meizner I, Levy A, Katz et al 1992 Iniencephaly: a case report. JReprod Med 37:885.

Melnick M, Myrianthopoulos N C 1987 Studies in neural tube defects. II. Pathologic findings in a prospectively collected series of anencephalics. Am J Med Genet 26:783.

Menenzes M, Coker S B 1990 CHARGE and Joubert syndromes: are they a single disorder? Pediatr Neurol 6:428.

Menezes A H, Bell W E, Perret G E 1980 Arachnoid cysts in children. Arch Neurol 55:457.

Menkes J H, Philippart M, Clark D B 1964 Hereditary partial agenesis of the corpus callosum. Arch Neurol 11:198.

Miller A, Guille J T, Bowen 1993 Evaluation and treatment of diastematomyelia. J Bone Joint Surg 75A:1308.

Miller E, Hare J W, Cloherty J P et al 1981 Elevated maternal hemoglobin Alc in early pregnancy and major congenital anomalies in infants of diabetic mothers. N Engl J Med 304:1331.

Miller P, Smith D W, Shepard T H 1978 Maternal hyperthermia as a possible cause of anencephaly. Lancet 1:519.

Mize R R, Erzurumlu R S 1996 Neural development and plasticity. Progress in brain research. Vol. 108. Elsevier, New York.

Mizuguchi M, Maekawa S, Kamoshita S 1994 Distribution of leptomeningeal glioneuronal heterotopia in alobar holoprosencephaly. Arch Neurol 51:951.

Mooradian A D, Morley G K, McGeachie R et al 1984 Spontaneous periodic hypothermia. Neurology 34:79.

Mori K, Hashimoto T, Tayama M et al 1994 Serial EEG and sleep polygraphic studies on lissencephaly (agyria-pachygyria). Brain Dev 16:365.

Musumeci S A, Ferri R, Elia M et al 1996 A new family with periventricular nodular heterotopia and peculiar dysmorphic features. A probable X-linked dominant trait. Arch Neurol 54:61.

Naidich T P, McLone D G, Radkowski M A 1985/86 Intracranial arachnoid cysts. Pediatr Neurosci 12:112.

Nakamura K, Hanabusa M, Okamoto N 1972 A classification of the anencephalic brain. Teratology 6:115.

Nelson K B, Deutschberger J 1970 Head size at one year as a predictor of four-year I.Q. Dev Med Child Neurol 12:487.

Nishikawa M, Sakamoto H, Hakuba A et al 1997 Pathogenesis of Chiari malformation: a morphometric study of the posterior cranial fossa. J Neurosurg 86:40.

Nixon G W, Johns R E Jr, Myers F F 1974 Congenital porencephaly. Pediatrics 54:43.

Norman M G, McGillivray B 1988 Fetal neuropathology of proliferative vasculopathy and hydranencephaly-hydrocephaly with multiple limb pterygia. Pediatr Neurosci 14:301.

Norman M G, McGillivray B C, Kalousek D K et al 1995 Congenital malformations of the brain. Oxford University Press, New York.

Norman M G, Roberts M, Sirois J et al 1976 Lissencephaly. Can J Neurol Sci 3:39.

Nugent F R, Al-Mefty O, Chou S 1979 Communicating hydrocephalus as a cause of aqueductal stenosis. J Neurosurg 51:812.

Nyberg D A, Cyr D R, Mack L A et al 1988 The Dandy–Walker malformation: prenatal sonographic diagnosis and its clinical significance. J Ultrasound Med 7:87.

O'Neill O R, Piatt J H Jr, Mitchell P et al 1995 Agenesis and dysgenesis of the sacrum: neurosurgical implications. Pediatr Neurosurg 22:20.

Odent S, Le Marec B, Toutain A et al 1998 Central nervous system malformations and early end-stage renal disease in oro-facial-digital syndrome type I: a review. Am J Med Genet 75:389.

Odita J C, Hebi S 1996 CT and MRI characteristics of intracranial hemorrhage complicating breech and vacuum delivery. Pediatr Radiol 26:782.

Ohnuma K, Imaizumi K, Masuno M et al 1997 Magnetic resonance imaging abnormalities of the brain in Goldberg–Shprintzen syndrome. Am J Genet 73:230.

Oi S, Matsumoto S 1992 A proposed grading and scoring system for spina bifida: Spina Bifida Neurological Scale (SBNS). Childs Nerv Syst 8:337.

OMIM 98 Online Mendelian Inheritance in Man. http://ncbi.nlm.gov/Omim.

Ono J, Mano T, Andermann E et al 1997 Band heterotopia or double cortex in a male: bridging structures suggest abnormality of the radial glial guide system. Neurology 48:1701.

Osaka K, Matsumoto S, Tanimura T 1978 Myeloschisis in early human embryos. Childs Brain 4:347.

Ouellette E M, Rosett H L, Rosman N P et al 1977 Adverse effects on offspring of maternal alcohol abuse during pregnancy. N Engl J Med 297:528.

Ozkinay F, Ozyurek A R, Bakiler A R et al 1995 A case of Marden–Walker syndrome with Dandy-Walker malformation. Clin Genet 47:221.

Packard A M, Miller V S, Delgado M R 1997 Schizencephaly: correlations of clinical and radiologic features. Neurology 48:1427.

Palmini A, Andermann F, Aircardi J et al 1991a Diffuse cortical dysplasia, or the double cortex syndrome: the clinical and epileptic spectrum in 10 patients. Neurology 41:1656.

Palmini A, Andermann F, Olivier A et al 1991b Focal neuronal migration disorders and intractable partial epilepsy: results of surgical treatment. Ann Neurol 30:750.

Pang D 1992 Split cord malformation. Part II. Clinical syndrome. Neurosurgery 31:481.

Papasozomenos S, Roessman U 1981 Respiratory distress and Arnold–Chiari malformation. Neurology 31:97.

Parikh J R, Mak K, Shalay K M 1994 Unilateral megalencephaly in association with Dandy–Walker complex. Can Assoc Radiol J 45:394.

Park T S 1992 Spinal dysraphism. Contemporary issues in neurological surgery. Blackwell Scientific, Boston, MA.

Parrish M L, Roessmann U, Levinsohn M W 1979 Agenesis of the corpus callosum: a study of the frequency of associated malformations. Ann Neurol 6:349.

Pascual-Castroviejo I, Roche M C, Martinez Bermejo A et al 1991a Primary intracranial arachnoidal cysts: a study of 67 childhood cases. Child Nerv Syst 7:257.

Pascual-Castroviejo I, Velez A, Pascual-Pascual S I et al 1991b Dandy–Walker malformation: analysis of 38 cases. Child Nerv Syst 7:88.

Pasternak J F, Mantovani J F, Volpe J J 1980 Porencephaly from periventricular intracerebral hemorrhage in a premature infant. Am J Child 134:673.

Payne J, Shibasaki F, Mercola M 1997 Spina bifida occulta in homozygous Patch mouse embryos. Dev Dyn 209:105.

Peabody J, Emery J, Ashwal S 1989 Experience with anencephalic infants as prospective organ donors. N Engl J Med 321:344.

Pellegrino J E, Lensch M W, Muenke M et al 1997 Clinical and molecular analysis in Joubert syndrome. Am J Med Genet 72:59.

Pensler J M, Giese S, Charrow J 1993 Surgical treatment of patients with lobar holoprosencephaly: a personal note. J Craniofac Surg 4:2.

Petersen M C, Wolraich M, Sherbondy A et al 1995 Abnormalities in control of ventilation in newborn infants with myelomeningocele. J Pediatr 126:1011.

Pfeiffer R A, Legat G, Trautmann U 1992 Acrocallosal syndrome in a child with de novo inverted tandem duplication of 12p11.2-p13.3. Ann Gent 35:41.

Picone O, Hirt R, Suarez B, Coulomb A et al 2006 Prenatal diagnosis of a possible new middle interhemispheric variant of holoprosencephaly using sonographic and magnetic resonance imaging. Ultrasound Obstet Gynecol 28:229.

Pintos Morell G, Naranjo M A, Artigas M et al 1995 Molybdenum cofactor deficiency associated with

Dandy–Walker malformation. J Inherit Metab Dis 18:86.

Preul M C, Leblanc R, Cendes F et al 1997 Function and organization in dysgenic cortex. Case report. J Neurosurg 87:113.

Raffel C, McComb J G 1988 To shunt or to fenestrate: which is the best treatment for arachnoid cysts in pediatric patients? Neurosurgery 23:338.

Rais-Bahrami K, Naqvi M 1990 Hydranencephaly and maternal cocaine use: a case report. Clin Pediatr Phila 29:729.

Raymond A A, Fish D R, Sisodiya S M et al 1995 Abnormalities of gyration, heterotopias, tuberous sclerosis, focal cortical dysplasia, microdysgenesis, dysembryoplastic neuroepithelial tumour and dysgenesis of the archicortex in epilepsy. Clinical, EEG and neuroimaging features in 100 adult patients. Brain 118:629.

Reid C B, Walsh C A 1996 Early development of the cerebral cortex. In: Mize R R, Erzurumlu R S (eds) Neural development and plasticity. Progress in brain research, Vol 108. Elsevier, New York, pp. 17–30.

Rengachary S S, Watanabe I 1981 Ultrastructure and pathogenesis of intracranial cysts. J Neuropathol Exp Neurol 40:61.

Renwick J H 1972 Hypothesis: anencephaly and spina bifida are usually preventable by avoidance of a specific but unidentified substance present in certain potato tubers. Br J Prev Soc Med 26:67.

Richman D P, Stewart R M, Caviness V S Jr 1974 Cerebral microgyria in a 27-week fetus: an architectonic and topographic analysis. J Neuropathol Exp Neurol 33:374.

Riela A R, Thomas I T, Gonzalez A R et al 1995 Fryns syndrome: neurologic findings in a survivor. J Child Neurol 10:110.

Rivier F, Echenne B 1992 Dominantly inherited hypoplasia of the vermis. Neuropediatrics 23:206.

Rock J P, Zimmerman R, Bello W O et al 1996 Arachnoid cysts of the posterior fossa. Neurosurgery 18:176.

Rodgers B L, Vanner L V, Pai G S et al 1994 Walker–Warburg syndrome: report of three affected sibs. Am J Med Genet 49:198.

Roessler E, Belloni E, Gaudenz K et al 1996 Mutations in the human Sonic Hedgehog gene cause holoprosencephaly. Nat Genet 14:357.

Romanengo M, Tortori Donati P, Di Rocco M 1997 Rhombencephalosynapsis with facial anomalies and probable autosomal recessive inheritance: a case report. Clin Genet 52:184.

Rosett H L, Weiner L 1984 Alcohol and the fetus: a clinical perspective. Oxford University Press, New York.

Ross M E, Allen K M, Srivastava A K et al 1997 Linkage and physical mapping of X-linked lissencephaly/SBH (XLIS): a gene causing neuronal migration defects in human brain. Hum Mol Genet 6:555.

Rothman K J, Moore L L, Singer M R et al 1995 Teratogenicity of high vitamin A intake. N Engl J Med 333:1369.

Rouse B, Azen C, Koch R et al 1997 Maternal Phenylketonuria Collaborative Study (MPKUCS) offspring: facial anomalies, malformations, and early neurological sequelae. Am J Med Genet 69:89.

Rubenstein D, Cajade-Law A G, Youngman V 1996 The development of the corpus callosum in semilobar and lobar holoprosencephaly. Pediatr Radiol 26:839.

Sabbagha R E, Sheikh Z, Tamura R K et al 1985 Predictive value, sensitivity and specificity of ultrasonic targeted imaging for fetal anomalies in gravid women at high risk for birth defects. Am J Obstet Gynecol 152:822.

Sakamoto H, Hukuba A, Fujitani K et al 1991 Surgical treatment of the retethered spinal cord after repair of lipomyelomeningoceles. J Neurosurg 74:709.

Sandler A D, Knudsen M W, Brown T T et al 1997 Neurodevelopmental dysfunction among non-referred children with idiopathic megalencephaly. J Pediatr 131:320.

Saraiva J M, Baraitser M 1992 Joubert syndrome: a review [see comments]. Am J Med Genet 43:726.

Sarkman S P, Brown T C, Linell E A 1958 Cerebral arachnoid cysts. J Neuropathol Exp Neurol 17:484.

Sarnat H 1992 Cerebral dysgenesis. Embryology and clinical expression. Oxford University Press, New York.

Sarnat HB 1995 Ependymal reactions to injury. A review. J Neuropathol Exp Neurol 54:1.

Sasaki M, Ehara S, Watabe T 1997 Cerebellar polymicrogyria. AJNR Am J Neuroradiol 18:394.

Sawaya R, McLaurin R L 1981 Dandy–Walker syndrome. J Neurosurg 55:89.

Sayed M, al-Alaiyan S 1996 Agenesis of corpus callosum, hypertrophic pyloric stenosis and Hirschsprung disease: coincidence of common etiology? Neuropediatrics 27:204.

Schaefer G B, Sheth R D, Bodensteiner J B 1994 Cerebral dysgenesis. An overview. Neurologic Clin 12:773–88.

Schaefer G B, Thompson J N, Bodensteiner J B et al 1996 Hypoplasia of the cerebellar vermis in neurogenetic syndromes. Ann Neurol 39:382.

Schardein J L 1985 Chemically induced birth defects. Drug and chemical toxicology series. Marcel Dekker, New York, NY, vol 2.

Scherer E 1935 Uber cystenbildung der weinchen Hirnhäute im Liquoarrum der Sylvischen Furche mit hochgradiger Deformierung des Gehirns. Srch Psychiatr Nervenkr 152:787.

Scherrer C C, Hammer F, Schinzel A et al 1992 Brain stem and cervical cord dysraphic lesions in iniencephay. Pediatr Pathol 12:469.

Schinzel A 1979 Postaxial polydactyly, hallux duplication, absence of the corpus callosum, macrencephaly and severe mental retardation: a new syndrome? Helv Paediatr Acta 34:141–6.

Schneidau T, Franco I, Zebold K, Kaplan W 1995 Selective sacral rhizotomy for the management of neurogenic bladders in spina bifida patients: long-term followup. J Urol 154:766.

Scholler Gyure M, Nesselaar C, van Wieringen H et al 1996 Treatment of defecation disorders by colonic enemas in children with spina bifida. Eur J Pediatr Surg 1 (Suppl. 6):32.

Schrander-Stumpel C, Schrander J, Fryns J P et al 1988 Caudal deficiency sequeance in 7q terminal deletion. Am J Med Genet 30:757.

Schull W J 1997 Brain damage among individuals exposed prenatally to ionising radiation: a 1993 review. Stem Cells 15 (suppl.2):129.

Seller M J, Singer J D, Coltart T M et al 1974 Maternal serum alpha-fetoprotein levels and prenatal diagnosis of neural-tube defects. Lancet 1:428.

Sells C J 1977 Microcephaly in a normal school population. Pediatrics 59:262.

Sener R N 1995 MR imaging of Joubert's syndrome. Comput Med Imaging Graph 19:481.

Sener R N 1997 MR demonstration of cerebral hemimegalencephaly associated with cerebellar involvement (total hemimegalencephaly). Comput Med Imaging Graph 21:201.

Sensi A, Cerruti S, Calzolari E et al 1990 Familial porencephaly. Clin Genet 38:396.

Sepulveda W, Kyle P M, Hassan J et al 1997 Prenatal diagnosis of diastematomyelia: case reports and review of the literature. Prenat Diagn 17:161.

Sergi C, Hentze S, Sohn C et al 1997 Telencephalosynapsis (synencephaly) and rhombencephalosynapsis with posterior fossa ventriculocele ('Dandy-Walker cyst'): an unusual aberrant syngenetic complex. Brain Dev 19:426.

Serville F, Lyonnet S, Pelet A et al 1992 X-linked hydrocephalus: clinical heterogeneity at a single gene locus. Eur J Pediatr 151:515.

Sever L E 1995 Looking for causes of neural tube defects: where does the environment fit in? Environ Health Perspect 103(Suppl.6):165.

Shah K N, Rajadhyaksha S, Shah V S et al 1992 EEG recognition of holoprosencephaly and Aicardi syndrome. Indian J Pediatr 59:103.

Shapiro I, Borochowitz Z, Degani S et al 1992 Neu-Laxova syndrome: prenatal ultrasonographic diagnosis, clinical and pathological studies, and new manifestations. Am J Med Genet 43:602.

Shapiro W R, Williams G H, Plum F 1969 Spontaneous recurrent hypothermia accompanying agenesis of the corpus callosum. Brain 92:423.

Shastri N J, Bharani S A, Modi U J et al 1997 Familial porencephaly. Indian J Pediatr 60:459.

Shevell M I, Majnemer A 1996 Clinical features of developmental disability associated with cerebellar hypoplasia. Pediatr Neurol 15:224.

Shewman D A, Capron A M, Peacock W J et al 1989 The use of anencephalic infants as organ sources. JAMA 261:1773.

Shiota K 1982 Neural tube defects and maternal hyperthermia in early pregnancy: epidemiology in a human embryo population. Am J Med Genet 12:281.

Silverstein D M, Zacharowicz L, Edelman M et al 1997 Joubert syndrome associated with multicystic kidney disease and hepatic fibrosis. Pediatr Nephrol 11:746.

Simon E M, Hevner R F, Pinter J D et al 2002 The middle interhemispheric variant of holoprosencephaly. AJNR Am J Neuroradiol 23:151–156.

Sinha S, Brown J I M 2004 Familial posterior fossa arachnoid cyst. Childs Nerv Syst 20:100.

Smit L M, Barth P G, Valk J et al 1984 Familial porencephalic white matter disease in two generations. Brain Dev 6:54.

Smith A, Wiles C, Haan E et al 1996 Clinical features in 27 patients with Angelman syndrome resulting from DNA deletion. J Med Genet (Feb):107.

Spataro R F, Lin S R, Horner F A et al 1976 Aqueductal stenosis and hydrocephalus: rare sequelae of mumps virus infection. Neuroradiology 12:11.

Spohr H L, Willms J, Steinhausen H C 1993 Prenatal alcohol exposure and long-term developmental consequences. Lancet 341:907.

Spranger J, Benirschke K, Hall J G et al 1982 Errors of morphogenesis: concepts and terms. J Pediatr 100:160.

Steinbok P 1995 Dysraphic lesions of the cervical spinal cord. Neurosurg Clin N Am 6:367.

Steinbok P, Cochrane D D 1991 The nature of congenital posterior cervical or cervicothoracic midline cutaneous mass lesions: report of eight cases. J Neurosurg 75:206.

Steinlin M, Schmid M, Landau K et al 1997 Follow-up in children with Joubert syndrome. Neuropediatrics 28:204.

Stone A R 1995 Neurologic evaluation and urologic management of spinal dysraphism. Neurosurg Clin N Am 6:269.

Sugimoto T, Yasuhara A, Nishida N et al 1993 MRI of the head in the evaluation of microcephaly. Neuropediatrics 24:4.

Takahashi S, Miyamoto A, Oki J et al 1995 Alobar holoprosencephaly with diabetes insipidus and neuronal migration disorder. Pediatr Neurol 13:175.

Tal Y, Freigang B, Dunn H G et al 1980 Dandy–Walker syndrome: analysis of 21 cases. Dev Med Child Neurol 22:189.

Talwar D, Baldwin M A, Horbatt C I 1995 Epilepsy in children with meningomyelocele. Pediatr Neurol 13:29.

Tardieu M, Evrard P, Lyon G 1981 Progressive expanding congenital porencephalies: a treatable cause of progressive encephalopathy. Pediatrics 68:198.

Tayama M, Hashimoto T, Mori K et al 1992 Electrophysiological study on hydranencephaly. Brain Dev 14:185.

Toline J L, Day R, Fredericks B et al 1997 Dominantly inherited cerebral dysplasia: arachnoid cyst associated with mild mental handicap in a mother and her son. J Med Genet 34:1018.

Toriello H V, Radecki L L, Sharda J et al 1986 Frontonasal 'dysplasia', cerebral anomalies, and polydactyly: report of a new syndrome and discussion from a developmental field perspective. Am J Med Genet Suppl 2:89.

Towfighi J, Housman C 1991 Spinal cord abnormalities in caudal regression syndrome. Acta Neuropathol Berl 81:458.

Tsuru A, Mizuguchi M, Uyemura K et al 1997 Immunohistochemical expression of cell adhesion molecule L1 in hemimegalencephaly. Pediatr Neurol 16:45.

Vade A, Horowitz S W 1992 Agenesis of corpus callosum and intraventricular lipomas. Pediatr Neurol 8:307.

Valanne L, Pihko H, Katevuo K et al 1994 MRI of the brain in muscle-eye-brain (MEB) disease. Neuroradiology 36:473.

Van Allen M I 1996 Multisite neural tube closure in humans. Birth Defects Orig Artic Ser 30: 203–25.

Van Allen M I, Kalousek D K, Chernoff G F 1993 Evidence for multi-site closure of the neural tube in humans. Am J Med Genet 47:723.

Van der Knaap M S, Barth P G, Stroink H et al 1995 Leukoencephalopathy with swelling and a discrepantly mild clinical course in eight children. Ann Neurol 37:324.

Van Zalen-Sprock R M, van Vugt J M, van Geijn H P 1996 First-trimester sonographic detention of neurodevelopmental abnormalities in some single-gene disorders. Prenat Diagn 16:199.

Vare A M, Bansal P C 1971 Anencephaly. An anatomical study of 41 anencephalic infants. Indian J Pediatr 38:301.

Velasco M, Velasco F, Gardea G et al 1997 Polygraphic characterization of the sleep-epilepsy patterns in a hydranencephalic child with severe generalization seizures of the Lennox–Gastaut syndrome. Arch Med Res 28:297.

Venes J L, Black K L, Latack J T 1986 Preoperative evaluation and surgical management of the Chiari II malformation. J Neurosurg 64:363.

Vergani P, Ghidini A, Strobelt N et al 1994 Prognostic indicators in the prenatal diagnosis of agenesis of corpus callosum. Am J Obstet Gynecol 170:753.

Viljoen D L 1995 Porencephaly and transverse limb defects following severe maternal trauma in early pregnancy. Clin Dysmorphol 4:75.

Vogel F S, McClenahan J L 1952 Anomalies of major cerebral arteries associated with malformations of the brain, with special reference to the pathogenesis of anencephaly. Am J Pathol 28:701.

Volpe J J 2000 Neurology of the newborn. 4th edn. WB Saunders, Philadelphia, PA.

Walters J, Ashwal S, Masek T 1997 Anencephaly: where do we now stand? Semin Neurol 17:249.

Weiner S N, Pearlstein A E, Eiber A 1987 MR imaging of intracranial arachnoid cysts. J Comput Assist Tomagr 11:236.

Welch K, Winston K R 1987 Spina bifida. In: Myrianthopoulos N C (ed.) Handbook of clinical neurology. Elsevier Science, Amsterdam.

Wininger S J, Donnenefled A E 1994 Syndromes identified in fetuses with prenatally diagnosed cephaloceles. Prenat Diagn 14:839.

Wintour E M, Lewitt M, McFarlane A et al 1996 Experimental hydranencephaly in the ovine fetus. Acta Neuropathol (Berl) 91:537.

Wisniewski K, Bambska M, Sher J H et al 1983 A clinical neuropathological study of the fetal alcohol syndrome. Neuropediatrics 14:197.

Wood J W, Johnson K G, Omori Y 1967 In utero exposure to the Hiroshima atomic bomb: an evaluation of head size and mental retardation twenty years later. Pediatrics 39:385.

Wu M, Chen D F, Sasaoka T et al 1996 Neural tube defects and abnormal brain development in F52-deficient mice. Proc Natl Acad Sci USA 93:2110.

Yakovlev P I, LeCours A R 1967 The myelogenetic cycles of regional maturation of the brain. In: Minkowski A (ed.) Regional development of the brain in early life. Blackwell Scientific, Oxford.

Yakovlev P I, Wandsworth R C 1946 Schizencephalies: a study of the congenital clefts in the cerebral mantle. J Neurophatol Exp Neurol 5:116.

Yamasaki M, Thompson P, Lemmon V 1997 CRASH syndrome: mutations in L1CAM correlate with severity of the disease. Neuropediatrics 28:175.

Yokota A, Matsukado Y 1979 Congenital midline porencephaly: a new brain malformation associated with scalp anomaly. Childs Brain 5:380.

Yoshioka M, Kuroki S 1994 Clinical spectrum and genetic studies of Fukuyama congenital muscular dystrophy. Am J Med Genet 53:245.

Younus M, Coode P E 1986 Nasal glioma and encephalocele: two separate entities: report of two cases. J Neurosurg 64:516.

Zhao O, Behringer R, de Crombrugghe B 1996 Prenatal folic acid treatment suppresses acrania and meroanencephaly in mice mutant for the Cart 1 homeobox gene. Nat Genet 13:275.

Ziegler A L, Deonna T, Calame A 1990 Hidden intelligence of a multiply handicapped child with Joubert syndrome. Dev Med Child Neurol 32:261.

Genetics of neurodevelopmental anomalies

Mohnish Suri

Key Points

- Genetic factors make a major etiological contribution to most CNS malformations
- Isolated 'non-syndromal' neural tube defects (NTDs) show multifactorial inheritance with the methylenetetrahydrofolate reductase gene being the most important susceptibility locus identified to date. NTDs also occur in chromosomal abnormalities, such as trisomy 18, and single-gene disorders, such as Meckel syndrome
- Isolated hydrocephalus conveys a low empiric recurrence risk for siblings of 1–4%. X-linked hydrocephalus is associated with aqueduct stenosis and is caused by mutations in the *L1CAM* gene which encodes a neuronal cell adhesion molecule
- Most cases of hydranencephaly and porencephaly are sporadic. Autosomal dominant forms of porencephaly can be caused by mutations in the *COL4A1* gene.
- Agenesis of the corpus callosum shows striking etiological heterogeneity. When present as an isolated finding the recurrence risk for siblings is low
- Microcephaly can be caused by both genetic and environmental factors. Unexplained non-syndromal microcephaly conveys a sibling recurrence risk of at least 1 in 8
- Holoprosencephaly can be chromosomal, e.g. trisomy 13, or can be a component of a large number of single-gene multiple malformation syndromes. Several genes have been identified which can cause isolated holoprosencephaly showing autosomal dominant inheritance with reduced penetrance
- Isolated classic (type I) lissencephaly is usually caused by a mutation in either the *LIS1* gene on chromosome 17 or the *DCX* gene on Xq22.3

- Cobblestone (type II) lissencephaly almost always occurs in association with other abnormalities as a feature of Walker–Warburg syndrome, muscle-eye-brain disease, Fukuyama congenital muscular dystrophy, congenital muscular dystrophy types 1C and 1D and limb-girdle muscular dystrophy type 2I
- Polymicrogyria is etiologically heterogeneous. Non-syndromal polymicrogyria has been divided into several types based on the regions of the cerebral cortex that are affected. Bilateral perisylvian polymicrogyria is the commonest form. Bilateral asymmetric perisylvian polymicrogyria can be a feature of the 22q11.2 deletion syndrome. Mutations in the *GPR56* gene at 16q13 result in autosomal recessive bilateral frontoparietal polymicrogyria (BFPP) with white matter changes and cerebellar hypoplasia
- Schizencephaly usually represents a sporadic event with only a minority of cases resulting from new dominant mutations in the homeobox gene *EMX2*. It is almost always seen in combination with polymicrogyria
- Periventricular nodular heterotopia is usually non-syndromal and inherited in an X-linked dominant manner with male lethality. It is caused by loss of function mutations in the *FLNA* gene at Xq28. Males with *FLNA* mutations usually die in utero or soon after birth. However, there have been a few reports of surviving males with *FLNA* mutations and they can have a very variable phenotype
- Cerebellar hypoplasia is a feature of several genetic dysmorphic and metabolic syndromes. In isolation the sibling recurrence risk is at least 1 in 10
- Approximately 50% of cases of Dandy–Walker malformation (DWM) diagnosed prenatally are associated with a chromosome abnormality. A non-syndromal DWM conveys a sibling recurrence risk of less than 5%

INTRODUCTION

Congenital abnormalities of the CNS are common and make a major contribution to severe disability both in childhood and in adult life. They can present before birth, in the neonatal period, or in later childhood and can occur in isolation or as one feature of a large number of complex multiple abnormality syndromes. Their recognition is important not only for the management of the child in whom the anomaly is identified, but also because of the potential genetic implications for other family members.

There is increasing evidence that genetic factors play a major role in the etiology of many CNS malformations and associated multiple malformation syndromes. This evidence stems from several sources. First, there is the burgeoning literature on syndrome recognition and delineation which has culminated in the development of computerized resources such as the London Medical Databases (Winter & Baraitser

2006). Second, there is the added evidence provided by increasingly sophisticated neuroimaging and, finally, there is the information gained from the staggering progress achieved in molecular biology over the last decade which has resulted in the isolation and characterization of many crucially important neurodevelopmental genes.

Together these developments, occurring in parallel, have provided much greater understanding of the role of genetics in malformations such as microcephaly, holoprosencephaly, lissencephaly, periventricular nodular heterotopia and polymicrogyria (Barkovich et al 2005). By utilizing this new information in conjunction with the results of traditional empiric risk family studies it is usually possible to give parents and other relevant family members a reasonable indication of risks to future children, together with details of the availability of specific DNA-based prenatal diagnostic options. Relevant developments shall be considered in this chapter in the context of specific malformations.

NEURAL TUBE DEFECTS (NTDs)

This term embraces several relatively common malformations including anencephaly, craniorachischisis, iniencephaly, encephalocele, meningocele and myelomeningocele. These arise as a consequence of impaired closure and subsequent canalization of the ectodermal neural tube. Primary neurulation, the process whereby the neural plate folds to form the neural tube, occurs between 18 and 28 days after fertilization. Secondary neurulation, involving canalization and differentiation of the closed neural tube, takes place between 4 and 8 weeks post fertilization. Most NTDs are thought to be caused by an error in primary neurulation, although there is a school of thought that reopening of a closed neural tube may be a contributory factor (Norman et al 1995).

Whatever the precise embryologic mechanism there is general agreement that most cases of isolated non-syndromal anencephaly and spina bifida are caused by a 'multifactorial' interaction of genetic susceptibility with environmental factors. The precise nature of most of these factors is unknown. However, recent studies in mice indicate that certain developmental gene families, most notably those genes containing a paired box (*PAX*) domain, play an important role (Helwig et al 1995). In humans it has been shown that specific mutations in the methylenetetrahydrofolate reductase (*MTHFR*) gene are risk factors for NTDs and in particular homozygosity for the common 677(C > T) polymorphism in both mother and child conveys a sevenfold increased risk (van der Put et al 1998). Homozygosity for the 677C > T polymorphism is associated with hyperhomocysteinemia in the presence of folate deficiency. It has been suggested that the interaction of homozygosity for the 677C > T polymorphism with folate deficiency is associated with a higher risk for NTDs than either factor acting independently (Christensen et al 1999). Known environmental contributory factors include folate deficiency, poor socioeconomic status, maternal insulin dependent diabetes mellitus and valproate teratogenicity.

Despite extensive research in this field it is not yet possible to utilize molecular analysis to determine family risks which are still based on the results of empiric family studies. Average risk figures that are suitable for counseling purposes are summarized in Table 14.1. Ideally locally derived contemporary risks should be used but these are rarely available. The importance of offering high dose (4–5 mg daily) periconceptional folic acid supplementation to prospective mothers of 'high' risk pregnancies cannot be overemphasized. This has been shown to convey a 70–80% reduction in risk (MRC Vitamin Study Research Group 1991). It is important to remember that spinal dysraphism, embracing abnormalities such as cord tethering, diastematomyelia and intradural lipoma, also convey multifactorial recurrence risks for open NTDs so that folic acid supplementation should be offered to relevant female relatives.

NTDs also occur in several single-gene disorders and syndromes, as summarized in Table 14.2. The gene or genes

Table 14.1 Multifactorial recurrence risks for NTDs

Affected relative	Recurrence risk (%)
FIRST DEGREE (50% OF GENES SHARED)	
One sibling	4
Two siblings	10
One parent	4
One parent and one sibling	10
SECOND DEGREE (25% OF GENES SHARED)	
One uncle or aunt	1–2
One nephew or niece	1–2
One half sibling	1–2
Two second degree relatives	4
THIRD DEGREE (12.5% OF GENES SHARED)	
One first cousin	0.5–1
Two first cousins	1–2
Three or more first cousins	4

Example: A woman who has a sister with spina bifida is planning a pregnancy. This baby will have an aunt with an NTD. Thus the risk that the baby will be affected, without folic acid prophylaxis, equals 1–2%.

responsible for many of these disorders have recently been identified. It is particularly important that these are recognized, as the recurrence risk will usually be much greater than for an isolated NTD. Furthermore, syndromal NTDs will almost certainly not be susceptible to periconceptional folic acid prophylaxis. There is evidence that isolated anencephaly can occasionally show autosomal recessive inheritance, particularly in the Iranian Jewish population (Zlotogora 1995), and there have been a few reports of pedigrees consistent with X-linked recessive transmission of non-syndromal NTDs (Baraitser & Burn 1984, Toriello 1984). Molecular genetic analysis in a family in which two male siblings with spina bifida and hypopituitarism had inherited an Xq26-q27 duplication that was also present in their unaffected mother and maternal grandmother suggested the involvement of a gene at Xq27.3, the distal breakpoint of the duplication (Hol et al 2000). However, the vast majority of isolated non-syndromal NTDs are thought to be multifactorial in etiology and to convey multifactorial recurrence risks as already outlined (Table 14.1).

NTDs have also been described with a wide variety of chromosomal abnormalities including trisomy 13 and 18, triploidy, tetraploidy, duplications, deletions and rings (Lynch 2005). The chances of finding a chromosomal abnormality are higher in children with NTDs and other congenital abnormalities. Hence when assessing any child with an NTD for the purpose of genetic counseling, due consideration should be given to chromosome analysis in the evaluation protocol (Table 14.3). Finally NTDs can also occur in the amniotic band syndrome when rupture of the amnion has occurred before 45 days gestation (Higginbottom et al 1979) and in the 'schisis association,' this being the term used to account for the tendency of NTDs, oral clefts, omphaloceles and diaphragmatic herniae to occur together more often

Table 14.2 Single-gene disorders in which NTDs may occur

Disorder	Inheritance	Locus	Gene	Features
Fraser (cryptophthalmos) syndrome	AR	4q21	FRAS1	Cryptophthalmos, occipital encephalocele, renal agenesis, syndactyly
		13q13	FREM2	
Frontofacionasal dysplasia	AR	NK	NK	Frontonasal dysplasia with severe ocular anomalies, facial clefting, frontal encephalocele
Knobloch–Layer syndrome	AR	21q22	COL18A1	Myopia, occipital encephalocele
Meckel–Gruber syndrome	AR	17q23	MKS1	Occipital encephalocele, polycystic kidneys, postaxial polydactyly
		11q13	NK	
		8q21-q22	MKS3	
Roberts syndrome	AR	8p21	ESCO2	Facial clefting, radial anomalies, phocomelia, hypertelorism, frontal encephalocele
Currarino syndrome	AD	7q36	HLXB9	Anal atresia or stenosis, anterior meningocele or presacral teratoma/cyst, partial sacral agenesis
Spondylocostal syndrome	AR	19q13	DLL3	Spina bifida, multiple rib and vertebral abnormalities
		15q26	MESP2	
		7p22	LFNG	
Walker–Warburg syndrome	AR	9q34	POMT1	Encephalocele, hydrocephalus, lissencephaly, retinal dysplasia
		14q24	POMT2	
		19q13	FKRP	
XK-Aprosencephaly	AR/AD	NK	NK	Anencephaly, radial ray anomalies, congenital heart disease

Key: AD, autosomal dominant; AR, autosomal recessive; NK, not known.

Table 14.3 Genetic assessment of NTDs

• Family history	Pedigree data to include all first, second and third degree relatives, relevant terminations of pregnancy, stillbirths, and neonatal deaths
• Pregnancy history	Maternal illness, e.g. IDDM Drug exposure — especially valproate
• Examination	Examine proband for other congenital malformations and/or dysmorphic features Examine spine of both parents for hemangioma, lipoma and hairy patch
• Investigations	Chromosome analysis, if other congenital abnormalities and/or dysmorphic features noted

Key: IDDM, insulin dependent diabetes mellitus.

than would be expected by chance (Czeizel 1981). The incidence of schisis-type malformations in siblings in Czeizel's original series was seven out of 190 (3.7%).

HYDROCEPHALUS (p. 256)

Congenital hydrocephalus is a relatively common anomaly with an incidence approaching 1 in 1000 births (Blackburn & Fineman 1994). The causes are numerous and include environmental factors such as trauma and infection together with the well recognized association with NTDs. Hydrocephalus also occurs in many chromosome abnormalities, such as triploidy, trisomy 13 and 6p25 deletion. It can be a feature of several single gene multiple malformation syndromes, the more common of which are listed in Table 14.4. Communicating hydrocephalus can also be seen in patients with maternal uniparental disomy of chromosome 14 (these patients have inherited both copies of their chromosome 14 from their mother).

The recurrence risk for isolated non-syndromal ('uncomplicated') hydrocephalus is relatively low, with family study

Table 14.4 Single gene multiple malformation syndromes in which hydrocephalus is a characteristic feature

Syndrome	Inheritance	Locus	Gene	Associated features
Opitz–Kaveggia (FG) syndrome	XR	Xq12-q21	NK	Agenesis of corpus callosum, Chiari I malformation, hypotonia, constipation
		Xq12-q28	NK	
		Xp22.3	NK	
		Xp11	NK	
		Xq22.3	NK	
Hydrocephalus with VATER	AD	10q22-q23	PTEN	Vertebral malformations, anal atresia, tracheo-esophageal fistula, renal and radial anomalies
	AR	NK		
	XR	NK		
Hydrolethalus syndrome	AR	11q23-q25	*HYLS1*	Hydrocephalus with absent upper midline structures, micrognathia, polydactyly
Linear sebaceous nevus syndrome	NK	NK	NK	Hyperpigmentation, nevus sebaceous, iris coloboma, mental retardation, seizures
Osteopetrosis (severe infantile form)	AR	11q13	*TCIRG1*	Optic atrophy, deafness, anemia, hepatosplenomegaly, dense bones
		16p13	*CLCN7*	
		6q21	*OSTM1*	
Thanatophoric dysplasia	AD	4p16	*FGFR3*	Craniosynostosis, short limbs, small chest
Walker–Warburg syndrome	AR	9q34	*POMT1*	Encephalocele, hydrocephalus, lissencephaly, retinal dysplasia
		14q24	*POMT2*	
		19q13	*FKRP*	

Key: AD, autosomal dominant; AR, autosomal recessive; XR, X-linked recessive; NK, not known.

derived sibling recurrence risks of between 1 and 4% (Adams et al 1982, Burton 1979, Varadi et al 1988). It has been noted that the recurrence risk for male siblings of a male proband tends to be higher (i.e. 4%) than for female siblings of a female proband (1–2%), and it is now well recognized that a small proportion of all cases of hydrocephalus show X-linked inheritance. Most, if not all, of these X-linked cases are now known to be caused by mutations in the *L1CAM* gene which is located at Xq28 (Rosenthal et al 1992).

The *L1CAM* gene encodes a neuronal cell adhesion molecule, known as L1, which is involved in neuronal migration and axonal extension. Mutations in *L1CAM* can result in several different phenotypes, i.e. X-linked hydrocephalus, the MASA syndrome (M = mental retardation, A = aphasia, S = shuffling gait, A = adducted thumbs), complicated spastic paraplegia type 1, and X-linked agenesis of the corpus callosum. These entities are collectively designated as L1-disease and they have an estimated incidence of between 1 in 25 000 to 1 in 60 000 male births (Finckh et al 2000, Halliday et al 1986). Males with X-linked hydrocephalus show severe retardation in association with flexed adducted thumbs (Fig. 14.1) and other CNS malformations, most notably aqueduct stenosis and bilateral absence of the pyramids. This latter finding is a particularly useful discriminatory diagnostic feature (Kenwrick et al 1996). Carrier females sometimes show mild learning difficulties (Halliday et al 1986).

A large number of mutations have been found in *L1CAM*. These include missense, nonsense, and splice site mutations as well as deletions and insertions (Weller & Gärtner 2001). Most mutations appear to represent 'private' mutations. There is a genotype-phenotype correlation with truncating mutations in the extracellular domain being associated with severe phenotypes and mutations in the cytoplasmic domain being associated with the mild phenotypes (Fransen et al 1998). Mutation analysis for *L1CAM* is available from several diagnostic laboratories. The chances of detecting a mutation are high in males with congenital hydrocephalus and a family history of similarly affected males. However, a mutation can also be identified in this gene in 22.4% of isolated male cases with hydrocephalus (Finckh et al 2000). When a mutation is identified genetic counseling on the basis of X-linked inheritance is relatively straightforward. At present, screening techniques can only identify approximately 80–90% of all mutations, so that failure to identify a mutation in *L1CAM* does not exclude a diagnosis of X-linked hydrocephalus. Consequently, if the clinical and pathologic features are typical it would be unwise to counsel on the basis of a low recurrence risk even if mutation analysis is negative.

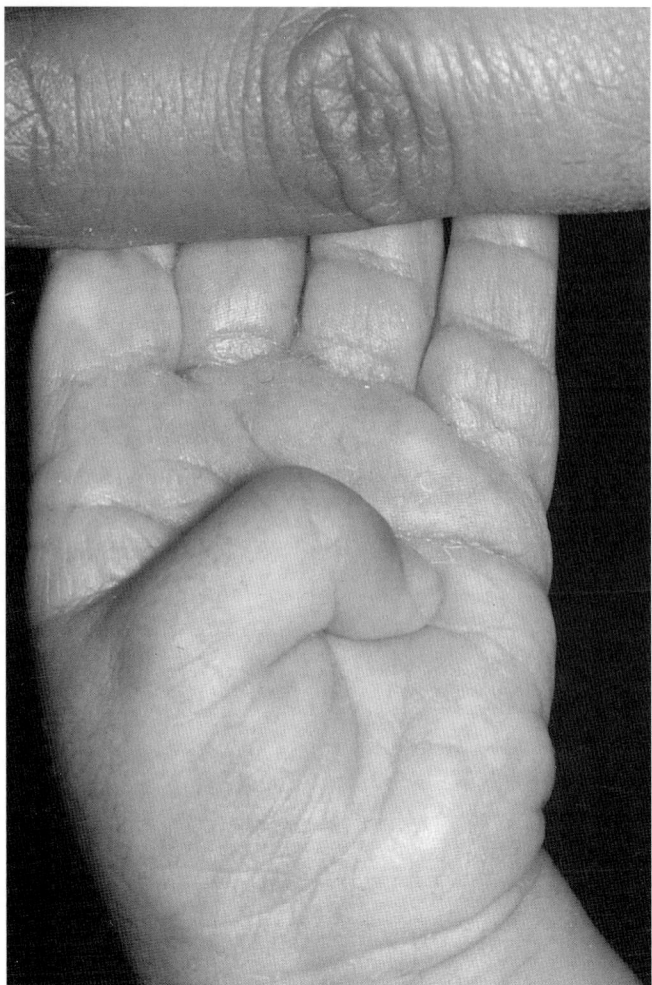

Figure 14.1 Hand of a child with X-linked hydrocephalus showing a clasped adducted thumb.

HYDRANENCEPHALY AND PORENCEPHALY

(p. 257 and p. 242)

Hydranencephaly is characterized by complete or almost complete replacement of the cerebral hemispheres by cerebrospinal fluid–filled sacs in the presence of intact meninges and a relatively normal skull. Most cases represent sporadic events within a family and are thought to be the consequence of a destructive process such as infection, trauma or a intrauterine vascular accident. Thus usually the recurrence risk for siblings is very low. However genetic counseling is complicated by several reports of a condition known as encephaloclastic proliferative vasculopathy or congenital hydranencephalic-hydrocephalic syndrome, which shows autosomal recessive inheritance (Fowler et al 1972, Harper & Hockey 1983, Moeschler & Marin Padilla 1989, Usta et al 2005, Witters et al 2002). Neuropathological features of this condition, which is now called Fowler-type hydranencephaly or Fowler syndrome, comprise hydranencephaly with a glomeruloid vasculopathy of blood vessels of the brain,

calcification of the basal ganglia and brainstem, fetal akinesia deformation sequence and muscle hypoplasia. The existence of this rare entity emphasizes the importance and value of detailed neuropathologic assessment.

Syndromic forms of hydranencephaly are rare. An X-linked form of hydranencephaly with abnormal genitalia due to mutations in the *ARX* gene has been reported recently (Kato et al 2004). Hydranencephaly has also been reported in two male siblings in association with multinucleated neurons, hypoplastic kidneys and 2/3 toe syndactyly (Bendon et al 1987), in association with hypoplastic thumbs (Norman & Donnai 1992) and in Roberts syndrome (Ekong & Rozdilsky 1978, Samson & Gardner 1996). Hydranencephaly in association with other congenital abnormalities has been described in a patient with a terminal 13q32 deletion (Gershoni-Baruch & Zekaria 1996) and in another patient with a terminal 7q32 deletion (McMorrow et al 1987).

Porencephaly refers to a fluid-filled cavity in the brain which communicates with the ventricular system. As with hydranencephaly, most cases are sporadic and are probably caused by a destructive process such as infection, hemorrhagic infarction related to venous occlusion, or trauma. Porencephaly can also be related to maternal cocaine use. Debus et al (1998) have reported that 16 out of 24 children with porencephalic cysts seen over a 10-year period had an apparent genetic risk factor for thrombophilia, such as heterozygous factor V Leiden deficiency or protein C deficiency and may be mediated through increased risk of cerebral artery infarction (p. 457). At present it is difficult to know how best to interpret the significance of these findings, as heterozygous factor V Leiden deficiency is relatively common in the general population. However, this report does raise the possibility that a proportion of cases of familial porencephaly could be caused by a hereditary tendency to thrombophilia.

As with hydranencephaly, counseling is complicated by several reports of familial porencephaly, often involving multiple generation transmission of hemiplegia with or without convulsions (Al-Shahwan & Singh 1995, Berg et al 1983, Mancini et al 2004, Sensi et al 1990, Smit et al 1984, Vilain et al 2002, Zonana et al 1986). True non-penetrance has been documented in some of these families (Vilain et al 2002). Mutations in the *COL4A1* gene at 13q34, whose protein product is a component of vascular basement membrane, have been reported in some families with an autosomal dominant form of porencephaly (Breedveld et al 2006, Gould et al 2005, van der Knaap et al 2006). It is believed that porencephaly in patients with *COL4A1* mutations may be due to an intracerebral bleed in the antenatal or perinatal period as a result of compromised structural integrity of the vascular basement membrane resulting in susceptibility to disruption during periods of increased stress.

Syndromic forms of porencephaly are rare. It has been reported as a feature of oral-facial-digital syndrome type I, which is an X-linked disorder with male lethality (Thauvin-Robinet et al 2001). There is also a single report of two siblings with bilateral porencephaly, absent septum pellucidum, cerebellar hypoplasia, situs inversus and congenital heart disease (Bonnemann & Meinecke 1996).

AGENESIS OF THE CORPUS CALLOSUM (ACC)

(p. 248)

Of all the cerebral malformations discussed in this chapter, ACC almost certainly demonstrates the greatest etiological heterogeneity with numerous reported chromosomal, single-gene, syndromal and environmental causes (Dobyns 1996). Hence counseling with regard to prognosis and recurrence risk is rarely straightforward, particularly when the abnormality is detected prenatally. The difficulty of interpreting the significance of isolated ACC is illustrated by its occasional discovery in an individual of normal intelligence, and when ACC is detected prenatally as an isolated abnormality it is associated with a probability of around 85% for normal development. However, in the presence of other abnormalities the long-term outlook for normal intellectual development is poor (Gupta & Lilford 1995).

ACC has been observed in a very large number of chromosome abnormalities (Dobyns 1996). This suggests that either many genes are involved in the development of the corpus callosum, in keeping with the 'reductionist' interpretation of the effects of chromosome imbalance, or that the corpus callosum is particularly sensitive to any disturbance in the meticulously orchestrated cascade of events which determine normal development. Chromosome abnormalities in which ACC commonly occurs include the 4p16.3 deletion (Wolf–Hirschhorn) syndrome, duplication 8p and 11q, trisomy 13 and 18, and trisomy 8 mosaicism. The long list of other rarer chromosome abnormalities in which ACC has been reported emphasizes the importance of detailed chromosome analysis in all cases.

Version 1.0.9 of the Winter–Baraitser Dysmorphology Database (2006) lists 307 syndromes that are associated with agenesis or hypoplasia of the corpus callosum. Many of these show single-gene inheritance as indicated in Table 14.5. Although some of these disorders have been mapped to particular chromosome regions, the relevant genes have been isolated in only a few instances. Notable examples include the X-linked α-thalassemia/mental retardation (ATR-X) syndrome (Gibbons et al 1995), which is caused by mutations in the *ATRX* gene at Xq13, the MASA syndrome which is caused by mutations in *L1CAM* as discussed above in the section on hydrocephalus, the X-linked form of Optiz G syndrome (Quaderi et al 1997) and Graham syndrome, a syndromic form of X-linked mental retardation (Graham et al 2003).

When present in isolation, ACC is generally stated to convey a low (<5%) recurrence risk for siblings and offspring, although the present author is not aware of any specific family studies that have been undertaken to confirm

Table 14.5 Single-gene disorders in which agenesis of the corpus callosum is a common finding

Syndrome	Inheritance	Locus	Gene	Associated features
Acrocallosal syndrome	AR	NK	NK	Mental retardation, pre- and postaxial polydactyly
	AD	7p13	GLI3	
Aicardi	XD	Xp22	NK	Chorioretinitis, infantile spasms
ATR-X	XR	Xq13	ATRX	Genital anomalies, hypotonia, mental retardation
Andermann syndrome	AR	15q13-q14	SLC12A6	Mental retardation, peripheral neuropathy
FG syndrome	XR	Xq12-q21	NK	Anal stenosis, hypotonia, macrocephaly
		Xq28	NK	
		Xp22.3	NK	
		Xp11	NK	
		Xq22.3	NK	
Graham	XR	Xq13	IGBP1	Mental retardation, iris and optic nerve colobomas, nerve deafness, micrognathia, choanal atresia, congenital heart disease, scoliosis, short stature
MASA syndrome	XR	Xq28	L1CAM	Adducted thumbs, shuffling gait, speech delay
Opitz G	XR	Xp22	MID1	Hypertelorism, hypospadias, laryngeal-tracheo-esophageal defects, anal anomalies
	AD	22q11.2	NK	
Toriello–Carey syndrome	AR	NK	NK	Cardiac and laryngeal abnormalities, Pierre-Robin anomaly, brachydactyly, hypotonia

Key: AR, autosomal recessive; XR, X-linked recessive; XD, X-linked dominant; NK, not known.

this. Counseling is complicated by several reports of multiple family members being affected with ACC, or with ACC as part of an apparently 'private' unique syndrome (e.g. da Silva 1988). Hence the genetic evaluation of every child with ACC should involve not only detailed chromosome analysis, as previously discussed, but also a full family history and thorough examination for other developmental and/or neurologic abnormalities.

MICROCEPHALY (p. 240)

This constitutes a difficult and relatively common problem in genetic counseling, particularly if microcephaly is defined as a head circumference greater than 2 standard deviations (SD) below the mean for age and sex, as this will embrace almost 2.5% of the general population. However around only 10% of such individuals will show significant mental retardation in contrast to almost 50% of the 0.15% of the population ascertained if a stricter diagnostic criterion of >3SD below the population mean is applied (Dolk 1991).

Microcephaly has numerous causes, both environmental and genetic, and in many cases it can be very difficult to establish a precise diagnosis. Known environmental causes include intrauterine infection and exposure to various agents including radiation, alcohol and high circulating levels of maternal phenylalanine. Genetic causes can be considered under the categories of chromosomal, syndromal and isolated.

Chromosomal. Almost any degree of autosomal imbalance will have severe neurodevelopmental consequences often in association with microcephaly, so that chromosome analysis is an essential step in the investigation of any microcephalic infant (Table 14.6). If a strong suspicion of a chromosome abnormality persists despite a normal chromosome result,

Table 14.6 Genetic assessment of microcephaly

• History	Family history, parental consanguinity, antenatal exposure to teratogens, including alcohol
	Possible pre, peri or postnatal asphyxia
	OFC at birth
• Examination	General for dysmorphic features
	Neurologic and ophthalmologic
• Parents	Parental OFC
	Maternal phenylketonuria
• Investigations	Chromosome analysis
	Congenital infection screen
	Metabolic screen
	Detailed eye examination
	Neuroimaging to include cranial CT and/or MRI

OFC, occipito-frontal circumference.

then consideration should be given to more detailed chromosome analysis using a technique such as fluorescent in-situ hybridization (FISH) (Flint et al 1995), multiplex amplifiable probe hybridization (MAPH) (Sismani et al 2001), multiplex ligation-dependent probe amplification (MLPA) (Rooms et al 2004), or microarray comparative genomic hybridization (array-CGH) (Veltman et al 2002) to look for subtelomeric rearrangements. The latter technique has been extensively evaluated recently for the genomewide detection of submicroscopic chromosomal abnormalities (Shaw-Smith et al 2004, Vissers et al 2003).

Syndromal. Version 1.0.9 of the Winter–Baraitser Dysmorphology Database (2006) identifies 672 syndromes in which microcephaly have been described. Some of the more commonly encountered examples are listed in Table 14.7. To this list should be added several other relatively rare disorders in which microcephaly occurs in association with ocular and/or other neurologic abnormalities (Table 14.8).

Isolated ('Simple' or 'Primary'). Non-syndromal or primary microcephaly can show both autosomal dominant and autosomal recessive inheritance. In the autosomal dominant form (or forms) intellectual impairment is usually mild and may be absent (Merlob et al 1988, Rossi et al 1987). Typical features of primary autosomal recessive microcephaly include severe microcephaly at birth that is non-progressive, a sloping forehead, relatively large ears, micrognathia, mild to severe intellectual impairment, usually normal neurology and an amiable extrovert personality. Neuroimaging in these patients shows a small brain with simplified cerebral cortex and slight reduction in the volume of the cortical white matter. This condition demonstrates remarkable allelic heterogeneity and so far six loci have been mapped for this condition and four genes identified (Cox et al 2006). These include the *MCPH1* (microcephalin) gene at 8p23 (Jackson et al 2002), the *ASPM* gene at 1q31 (Bond et al 2002), the *CDK5RAP2* gene at 9q33.3, and the *CENPJ* gene at 13q12.2 (Bond et al 2005). Mutations in *ASPM* are the most frequent cause of autosomal recessive primary microcephaly (Gul et al 2006, Kumar et al 2004, Roberts et al 2002). No loci or genes have so far been identified for autosomal dominant primary microcephaly.

Estimates of the recurrence risk for unexplained non-syndromal microcephaly vary from 1 in 8 to 1 in 5. If the parents are consanguineous then a figure of 1 in 4 should probably be quoted (Tolmie et al 1987). These empirical risks indicate that at least half of the unexplained non-syndromal cases result from autosomal recessive inheritance. The same applies when microcephaly is associated with symmetrical spastic paraplegia (Bundey 1992).

HOLOPROSENCEPHALY (HPE) (p. 237)

This is a severe malformation that is caused by a failure of cleavage of the embryonic forebrain or prosencephalon (Cohen & Sulik 1992). In normal development, the prosencephalon divides transversely into the telencephalon and the

Table 14.7 Dysmorphic syndromes in which microcephaly is a characteristic feature

Syndrome	Inheritance	Locus	Gene	Associated features
COFS	AR	NK	NK	Arthrogryposis, cataracts, microphthalmia
Cockayne	AR	10q11 5q11 2q21 19q13 13q33	*ERCC6* *ERCC8* *ERCC3* *ERCC2* *ERCC5*	Deafness, DNA repair defect, photosensitivity, premature aging
Cornelia de Lange	AD XR	5p13.1 Xp11.2	*NIPBL* *SMC1L1*	IUGR, hirsutism, limb defects, short stature, synophrys
Feingold	AD	2p24.1	*MYCN*	Esophageal and duodenal atresia, digital anomalies
Fetal alcohol	—	—	—	Congenital heart disease, short palpebral fissures, smooth philtrum
Nijmegen breakage	AR	8q21	*NBS1*	Poor growth, recurrent infections, chromosomal breakage
Rubinstein–Taybi	AD	16p13.3 22q13	*CREBBP* *EBP300*	Beaked nose, broad thumbs, downward sloping palpebral fissures
Seckel	AR	3q22-q24 18p11-q11 14q	*ATR* NK NK	IUGR, prominent nose, receding forehead, short stature

Key: AD, autosomal dominant; AR, autosomal recessive; COFS, cerebro-oculo-facio-skeletal; IUGR, intra-uterine growth retardation; NK, not known.

Table 14.8 Neurologic and ophthalmologic syndromes with microcephaly

Syndrome	Inheritance	Locus	Gene	Associated features
Aicardi–Goutieres	AR	3p21 13q14 11q13 19p13	*TREX1* *RNASEH2B* *RNASEH2C* *RNASEH2A*	Calcification of basal ganglia, leukoencephalopathy, CSF lymphocytosis, raised α-interferon in serum and CSF, seizures, severe mental retardation, chilblains
Amish microcephaly	AR	17q25	*SLC25A19*	Severe congenital microcephaly, elevated urinary α-ketoglutarate, death in infancy
Cohen	AR	8q22-q23	*COH1*	Short philtrum, myopia, progressive chorioretinal dystrophy, intermittent neutropenia, hypotonia
Jarmas	AD	NK	NK	Microphthalmia, falciform retinal folds, mild delay
Meckel–Gruber	AR	17q23 11q13 8q21-q22	*MKS1* Unknown *MKS3*	Occipital encephalocele, polycystic kidneys, postaxial polydactyly
Micro (Warburg)	AR	2q21.3	*RAB3GAP*	Microphthalmia, microcornea, congenital cataract, hypogenitalism, poor growth
Microcephaly-chorioretinopathy	AR	NK	NK	Microphthalmia, cataract, optic atrophy, chorioretinal dysplasia, mental retardation, spasticity
Microcephaly-lymphedema-chorioretinal dysplasia	AD	NK	NK	Lacunar retinal lesions, lymphedema, mild developmental delay
Microcephaly-spasticity-seizures	AR	NK	NK	Progressive severe microcephaly, spastic quadriplegia, seizures, severe mental retardation

Key: AD, Autosomal dominant; AR, autosomal recessive; NK, not known; XR, X-linked recessive.

diencephalon. The telencephalon divides in the sagittal plane to form the cerebral hemispheres and the olfactory tracts and bulbs. The paired thalamic and subthalamic nuclei, the optic chiasm and optic nerves, and the unpaired pineal gland and neurohypophysis develop from the diencephalon. In HPE there is failure of cleavage of both the telencephalon and diencephalon. The pathologic features of HPE include an undivided or partially divided cerebral hemisphere, usually with absent olfactory bulbs (arhinencephaly), absent or hypoplastic corpus callosum and fused thalami.

Pathologically, HPE is usually divided into three types. The most severe form is alobar HPE in which there is no separation of the cerebral hemispheres and there is a single cerebral ventricle (holoventricle). In semi-lobar HPE there is some division of the cerebral hemispheres with the inter-hemispheric fissure present posteriorly. In lobar HPE the cerebral hemispheres are almost completely separated with well-developed lateral ventricles. However, there is usually some degree of fusion of the frontal lobes, thalami and corpora striata. Septo-optic dysplasia and arhinencephaly (absence of olfactory tracts and bulbs) are thought to represent the mild end of the HPE spectrum.

Holoprosencephaly is seen in about 1 in 250 conceptuses (Matsunaga & Shiota 1977). However, the prevalence at birth varies from 0.48 to 1.2 per 10 000 live births (Croen et al 1996, Olsen et al 1997).

HPE is an etiologically heterogeneous disorder. Genetic causes of HPE can be discussed under the categories of chromosomal, syndromal and isolated (non-syndromal). HPE has also been described in infants of diabetic mothers, retinoic acid embryopathy and following antenatal exposure to alcohol (Cohen & Shiota 2002).

Chromosomal. About 30–40% of all affected individuals with HPE have an underlying chromosomal abnormality (Croen et al 1996, Whiteford & Tolmie 1996). This is usually a chromosome 13 abnormality such as trisomy 13, deletion or duplication of 13q, or ring 13. About 70% of patients with trisomy 13 have HPE (Taylor 1968). Other chromosomal abnormalities consistently associated with HPE include del(2p), dup(3p), del(7q), del(21q), and triploidy (Cohen & Sulik 1992). Thus chromosome analysis is strongly indicated in all children with this condition.

Syndromal. Holoprosencephaly can be a component of multiple malformation syndromes. Version 1.0.9 of the Winter–Baraitser Dysmorphology Database (2006) lists 104 syndromes in which HPE or arhinencephaly has been described. Table 14.9 lists some of the more commonly seen syndromes with HPE.

Isolated (Non-syndromal). This form of HPE can be inherited in a mendelian fashion. Familial non-syndromal HPE is usually inherited in an autosomal dominant manner. Autosomal recessive and X-linked recessive forms of non-syndromal HPE are exceedingly rare (Cohen & Gorlin 1969, Hockey et al 1988). In autosomal dominant HPE families, the transmitting parent is either clinically normal or may have subtle craniofacial malformations with normal brain imaging (Muenke et al 1994). These 'microsigns' or 'microforms' include anosmia or hyposmia, microcephaly, hypotelorism, iris coloboma, congenital nasal pyriform aperture stenosis, single central maxillary incisor, absent or abnormal midline maxillary frenulum and cleft palate.

As mentioned above, the autosomal dominant form of non-syndromal HPE can show marked intrafamilial variability as well as non-penetrance. The penetrance of autosomal dominant non-syndromal HPE is estimated to be about 70% (Cohen 1989). Eight genes have so far been identified for autosomal dominant non-syndromal HPE. These are the Sonic hedgehog (*SHH*) gene at 7q36 (Roessler

Table 14.9 Malformation syndromes in which holoprosencephaly is a characteristic feature

Syndrome	Inheritance	Locus	Gene	Associated features
Meckel–Gruber	AR	17q23 11q13 8q21–q22	MKS1 Unknown MKS3	Occipital encephalocele, polycystic kidneys, postaxial polydactyly
Pallister–Hall	AD	7p13	GLI3	Anal atresia, hypopituitarism, hypothalamic hamartoblastoma, polydactyly, syndactyly
Pseudotrisomy 13	AR	NK	NK	Congenital heart disease, cryptorchidism, microphthalmia, polydactyly
Smith–Lemli–Opitz	AR	11q12–q13	DHCR7	Genital anomaly, microcephaly, ptosis, syndactyly
Varadi–Papp (OFD VI)	AR	NK	NK	Polydactyly with Y-shaped 3rd metacarpal, midline cleft lip/palate, lingual nodules, MR
Velo-cardio-facial	AD	22q11.2	NK	Cleft palate, congenital heart disease, short stature
XK aprosencephaly	AR	NK	NK	Craniofacial anomalies, radial anomalies, congenital heart disease, anal atresia

Key: AD, autosomal dominant; AR, autosomal recessive; MR, mental retardation; NK, not known.

et al 1996, Roessler et al 1997) *ZIC2* at 13q32 (Brown et al 1998), *SIX3* at 2p21 (Wallis et al 1999), *TGIF* at 18p11.3 (Gripp et al 2000), *PTCH* at 9q22.3 (Ming et al 2002), *FAST1* at 8q24.3 (Ouspenskaia et al 2002) and *TDGF1* at 3p21-p23 (De la Cruz et al 2002), and *GLI2* at 2q14 (Roessler et al 2003). All patients with *GLI2* mutations had abnormal pituitary gland formation or function in addition to craniofacial features of HPE (Roessler et al 2003).

In a study from France 200 patients with HPE were screened for mutation in the *SHH, ZIC2, SIX3* and *TGIF* genes (Dubourg et al 2004). Mutations were only identified in 34 (17%) patients. Mutations in *SHH* accounted for half (8.5%) of all mutations identified in this cohort, whereas mutations in *ZIC2, SIX3* and *TGIF* were seen in 3.5%, 4% and 1% of patients respectively. For reasons that are unclear, the mutation detection rate was higher in living children with HPE (20.5%) compared to fetuses with this malformation (12.5%). Patients with HPE and choanal stenosis, cerebellar hypoplasia and pituitary gland anomalies predominant had *SHH* mutation, whereas patients with HPE and ocular malformations usually had mutations in *SHH* or *SIX3*. Unlike mutations in the other three genes, patients with HPE and mutations in *ZIC2* more often had minor facial anomalies. According to Cohen (2006) mutations in *SHH* can be seen in 17% of familial cases of non-syndromal HPE cases and 3.7% of sporadic cases, mutations in *ZIC2* can be seen in 3–4% of cases, mutations in *SIX3, TGIF, GLI2* each account for 1–2% of non-syndromal HPE, *TDGF1* mutations can be seen in 0.5% of cases, and *PTCH* mutations are a rare cause of HPE.

An approach to genetic counseling of parents of a child/fetus with HPE is shown in Figure 14.2.

LISSENCEPHALY (AGYRIA-PACHYGYRIA-SUBCORTICAL BAND HETEROTOPIA SPECTRUM) (p. 243)

Lissencephaly is a severe CNS malformation in which the surface of the brain is smooth with either complete absence of gyri and sulci (agyria) or only a few broad gyri and a few shallow sulci (pachygyria) (Barkovich et al 1992). Lissencephaly results from migrational arrest of primitive neurons between 12 and 16 weeks gestation. Subcortical band heterotopia (SBH) is also a neuronal migration disorder in which there is a second band of gray matter lying just below the cerebral cortex but separated by it by a thin band of white matter. There are two main histopathologic subtypes of lissencephaly: Classic (Type I) and Cobblestone (Type II) (Dobyns & Truwit 1995). Recent studies suggest that there are probably two further histopathologic subtypes of lissencephaly and that there is good correlation between the histopathological features of lissencephaly and the underlying genetic defect (Forman et al 2005).

CLASSIC (TYPE I) LISSENCEPHALY

This is the only type of lissencephaly that is associated with SBH. In this malformation the cerebral cortex has only 4 layers instead of the usual 6 layers (Barkovich et al 1992). The surface of the brain is smooth with absent or very few

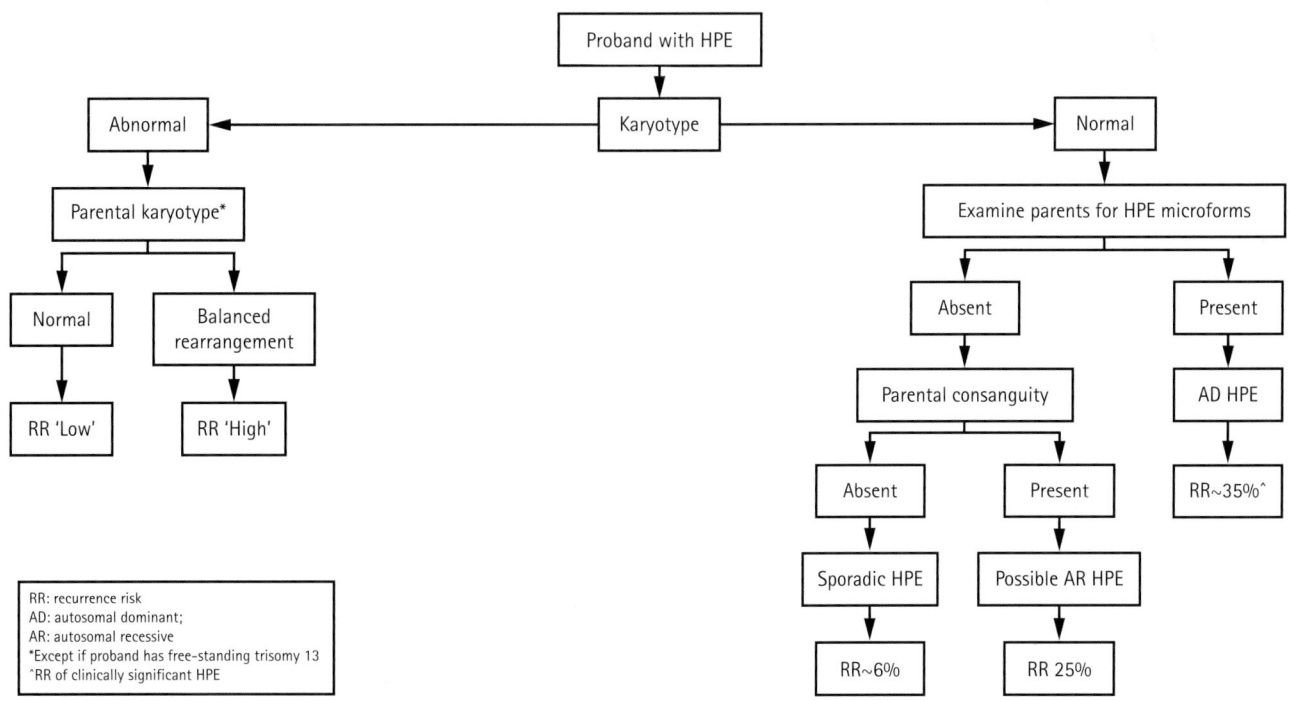

Figure 14.2 Genetic counseling for non-syndromal holoprosencephaly (HPE).

sulci. Neuroradiologic findings in classic lissencephaly include agyria or pachygyria and a thick cerebral cortex with a 'figure of eight' appearance of the cortex on axial CT/MRI cuts due to a shallow sylvian fissure. The corpus callosum and cerebellum are usually normal in classic lissencephaly, although hypoplasia/agenesis of the corpus callosum and cerebellar hypoplasia can be seen depending on the underlying genetic defect. Dobyns and Truwit (1995) have devised a grading system for classic lissencephaly based on neuroradiological findings. According to this classification, grade 1 lissencephaly is associated with diffuse agyria, grade 2 lissencephaly is associated with diffuse argyria with a few shallow sulci over the frontal, temporal or occipital poles, grade 3 lissencephaly is the combination of agyria and pachygyria, grade 4 lissencephaly comprises diffuse pachygyria, grade 5 lissencephaly the combination of pachygyria and SBH and grade 6 lissencephaly is limited to SBH.

Classic lissencephaly can be non-syndromal or syndromal. Non-syndromal classic lissencephaly is also called isolated lissencephaly sequence (ILS). Commonly seen syndromal forms of classic and other forms of lissencephaly (excluding cobblestone lissencephaly) are listed in Table 14.10. Five genes have been identified so far for non-syndromal and syndromal forms of classic lissencephaly. These include the *LIS1* gene at 17p13.3 (Lo Nigro et al 1997, Reiner et al 1993), *DCX* at Xq22.3-q23 (des Portes et al 1998, Gleeson et al 1998), *RELN* at 7q22 (Hong et al 2000), *ARX* at Xp22.13 (Kitamura et al 2002) and *14-3-3e* at 17p13.3 (Toyo-oka et al 2003).

Deletions or microdeletions of 17p13.3, which result in deletion of the *LIS1* and *14-3-3e* genes, are associated with the phenotype of Miller–Dieker syndrome (Toyo-oka et al 2003). Patients with this condition usually have grade 1 lissencephaly (diffuse agyria). Patients with partial deletions or mutations affecting the *LIS1* gene have ILS with lissencephaly of variable severity (grade 2–4) with a cortical thickness of 10–20 mm, that is more severe in the posterior regions of the cerebral cortex (i.e. the parietal and occipital regions) of the brain (Pilz et al 1998). Missense mutations in *LIS1* or somatic mosaicism for *LIS1* mutations can be associated with mild lissencephaly phenotypes or with isolated SBH affecting the posterior regions of the cortex in both males and females (Leventer et al 2001, Pilz et al 1999).

Mutations in *DCX* result in the phenotype of ILS in males with lissencephaly of variable severity (grade 1–5) with a cortical thickness of 10–20 mm that is more severe in the

Table 14.10 Syndromes with lissencephaly (excluding syndromes with cobblestone lissencephaly)

Syndrome	Inheritance	Locus	Gene	Associated features
Craniotelencephalic dysplasia	AR	NK	NK	Anterior midline encephalocele, multiple craniosynostosis, bilateral microphthalmia and severe optic nerve hypoplasia
Baraitser–Winter	AR	NK	NK	Lissencephaly, SBH, ptosis, iris coloboma, hypertelorism, MR, short stature
Barth microlissencephaly (radial microbrain)	AR	NK	NK	Extreme microcephaly (OFC < 28 cm), severe cerebellar hypoplasia, neonatal death
Miller–Dieker	AD	17p 13.3	*LIS1*, 14-3-3 ε	Prominent forehead, vertical furrowing of forehead on crying, classic lissencephaly with diffuse agyria
Norman–Roberts	AR	NK	NK	Severe microcephaly (OFC < 30 cm), prominent nasal root
Lissencephaly-congenital Lymphedema-cerebellar hypoplasia	AR	7q22	*RELN*	Severe cerebellar hypoplasia, hypotonia, congenital lymphedema, MR
Winter–Tsukahara	AR	NK	NK	Brachycephaly with large fontanelles, hypertelorism, small cystic pinnae, camptodactyly, talipes, hypoplastic lungs and kidneys, small penis with cryptorchidism in males, neonatal death
X-linked lissencephaly with ambiguous genitalia	XR	Xp22.13	*ARX*	Lissencephaly with posterior to anterior gradient, agenesis of corpus callosum, intractable neonatal seizures, ambiguous genitalia in karyotypic males, death in infancy

Key: AD, autosomal dominant; AR, autosomal recessive; MR, mental retardation; NK, not known; OFC, occipitofrontal circumference; SBH, subcortical band heterotopia; XR, X-Linked recessive.

anterior regions of the cerebral cortex (Pilz et al 1998). Somatic mosaicism for *DCX* mutations in males may be associated with mild lissencephaly phenotypes or with isolated SBH with an anterior cortical distribution (Gleeson et al 2000, Poolos et al 2002). Females with *DCX* mutations usually present with isolated diffuse SBH or SBH that is more severe in anterior regions of the cerebral cortex. This is explained by the phenomenon of random X-inactivation (lyonization) in females. The developing cortex in females with an *DCX* mutation has two populations of primitive neurons. The neurons in which the X-chromosome with the normal *DCX* gene is active migrate normally to the cortex. The neurons in which the X-chromosome with the *DCX* mutation is active do not migrate normally, and come to lie in a subcortical location, giving rise to the subcortical ribbon of gray matter seen in SBH (Fig. 14.3).

About 76% of sporadic patients with ILS have a mutation in either *LIS1* or *DCX* (Pilz et al 1998). Matsumoto et al (2001) screened 11 families with lissencephaly/SBH and 26 females with sporadic SBH for mutations in *DCX*. They showed that all lissencephaly/SBH families had mutations in *DCX* as did about 85% of females with sporadic SBH. Maternal gonadal mosaicism was found in one family suggesting that the possibility of gonadal mosaicism should be taken into account when counseling these families. Pilz et al (1999) identified mutations in the *LIS1* gene in 1 out of 11 males and mutations in *DCX* in 2 out of 11 males with SBH or mixed pachygyria-SBH. D'Agostino et al (2002) studied 24 males with SBH and showed that 7 (29%) had missense mutations in *DCX* (four patients had germline mutations and 3 had somatic mosaicism for the mutation), 1 (4%) had a germline missense mutation in *LIS1*, 1 (4%) had a possible pathogenic intronic base change in *DCX*, 1 (4%) had a possible pathogenic intronic base change in *LIS1* and 1 (4%) had partial trisomy 9p. They suggested that SBH in males could also be the result of other genetic mechanisms such as mutations in non-coding regions of the *DCX* and *LIS1* genes or mutations in other genes. A genetic approach to non-syndromal classic lissencephaly is shown in Figure 14.4.

Mutations in *RELN* and *ARX* are associated with syndromal forms of lissencephaly. Mutations in *RELN* are seen in patients with an autosomal recessive syndrome of moderate lissencephaly, severe cerebellar hypoplasia and congenital lymphedema (Hong et al 2000, Hourihane et al 1993). Neuroimaging in patients with *RELN* mutations shows lissencephaly of moderate severity (grade 4) with cortical thickness of 5–10 mm, which is more severe over the frontal and temporal regions, decreased subcortical white matter, thin corpus callosum, abnormally formed hippocampus, very small cerebellum with hypoplasia of the inferior vermis and cerebellar hemispheres and abnormal pons (Hong et al 2000). Mutations in *ARX* result in the syndrome of X-linked lissencephaly with abnormal genitalia (XLAG). This condition affects males, who present in the neonatal period with intractable seizures, ambiguous genitalia, feeding difficulties, tempera-

ture instability, poor weight gain, profound developmental delay, hypotonia leading to spasticity and death in early infancy. Neuroimaging in males with XLAG shows moderately severe lissencephaly with a cortical thickness of 5–10 mm, which is more severe in the posterior regions of the cerebral cortex, abnormal signal from the cortical white matter, agenesis of the corpus callosum and cystic or fragmented basal ganglia (Kitamura et al 2002). Female carriers of *ARX* mutations that cause XLAG in males may have agenesis of the corpus callosum (Kato et al 2004). Mutations in ARX can be associated with other phenotypes with and without developmental brain anomalies, including X-linked hydranencephaly with abnormal genitalia (XHAG), Proud syndrome (X-linked mental retardation with agenesis of the corpus callosum and abnormal genitalia), X-linked infantile spasms/West syndrome, Partington syndrome (a syndromic form of mental retardation) and non-syndromic X-linked mental retardation (Kato et al 2004, Suri et al 2005).

COBBLESTONE (TYPE II) LISSENCEPHALY

The pathologic features of this form of lissencephaly include an unlayered and severely disorganized cerebral and cerebellar cortex with neuronal and glial ectopia in the leptomeninges (Barkovich et al 1992, Dobyns & Truwit 1995). The latter give the surface of the brain a cobblestone or verrucous appearance. In addition, the surface of the brain is agyric or pachygyric. Neuroradiologic features of cobblestone lissencephaly include agyria or pachygyria, a thinner cerebral cortex than in classic lissencephaly, hydrocephalus, and hypoplastic or absent corpus callosum and septum pellucidum. Posterior fossa abnormalities seen in cobblestone lissencephaly include a small cerebellum, hypoplastic vermis, Dandy–Walker malformation and occipital encephalocele. The cerebral and cerebellar abnormalities on both CT and MRI scans help to differentiate cobblestone from classic lissencephaly. Cobblestone lissencephaly is almost always part of a wider genetic syndrome (Table 14.11). In all, six genes have so far been identified, mutations in which result in phenotypes associated with cobblestone lissencephaly. These include the *FCMD* gene at 9q31 (Kobayashi et al 1998), *FKRP* at 19q13 (Brockington et al 2001), *POMGnT1* at 1p33-p34 (Yoshida et al 2001), *POMT1* at 9q34 (Beltran-Valero de Bernabe et al 2002), *LARGE* at 22q12-q13 (Longman et al 2003) and *POMT2* at 14q24 (van Reeuwijk et al 2005). It appears that abnormal O-linked glycosylation of α-dystroglycan, a laminin-binding glycoprotein, is a key feature of all syndromes associated with cobblestone lissencephaly (van Reeuwijk et al 2004). *POMT1* and *POMGnT1* catalyze the first two steps respectively of O-linked glycosylation, a post-translational modification, of α-dystroglycan (this is the only known protein in mammals that undergoes O-linked glycosylation), and *LARGE* may play a regulatory role in this process. The precise functions of the protein products of the other genes in the O-linked glycosylation of α-dystroglycan are not known at the present time.

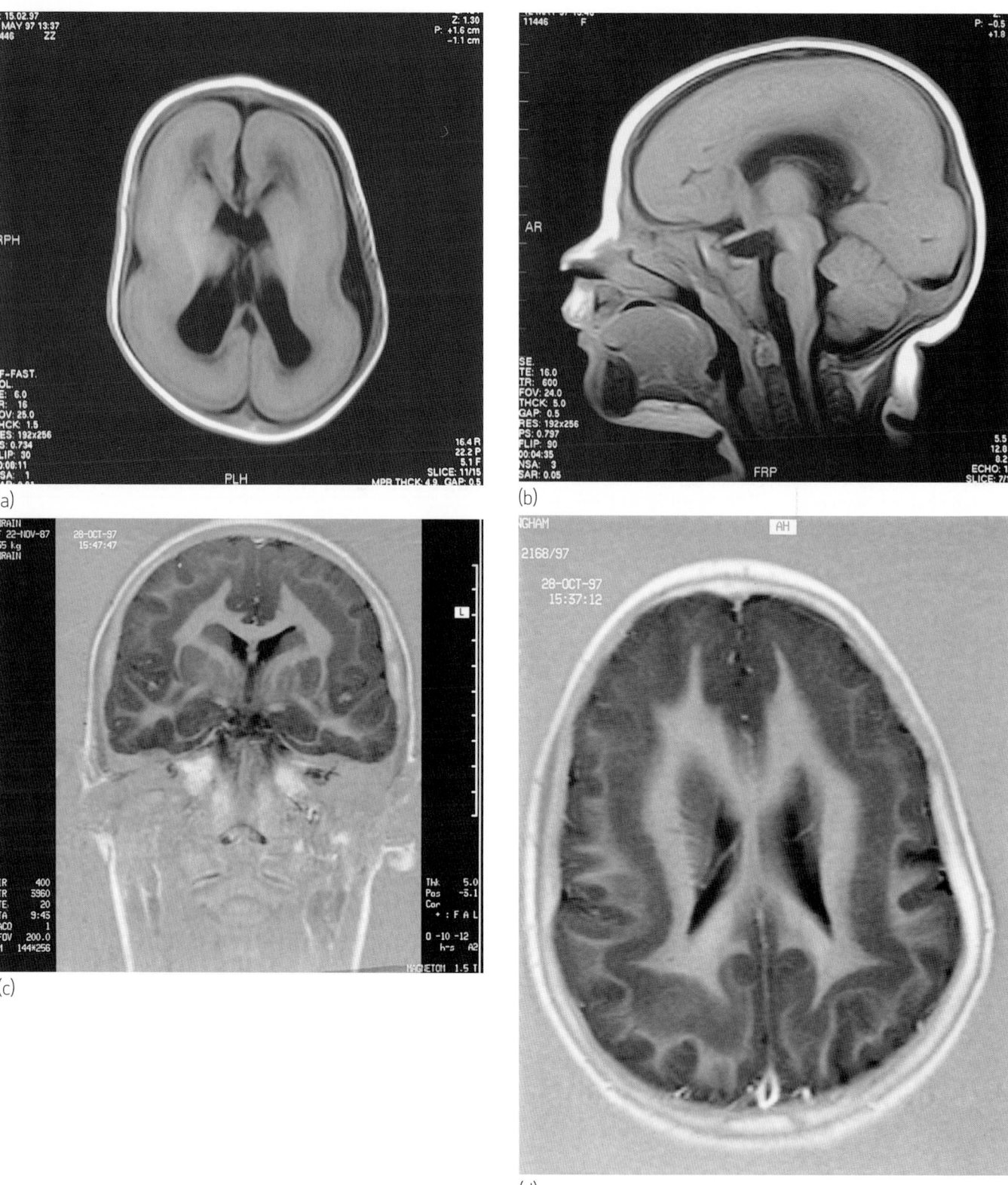

Figure 14.3 (a, b) MRI scans in a boy with X-linked lissencephaly and (c, d) his carrier sister. (Photographs kindly provided by Dr. Tim Jaspan, University Hospital, Nottingham.)

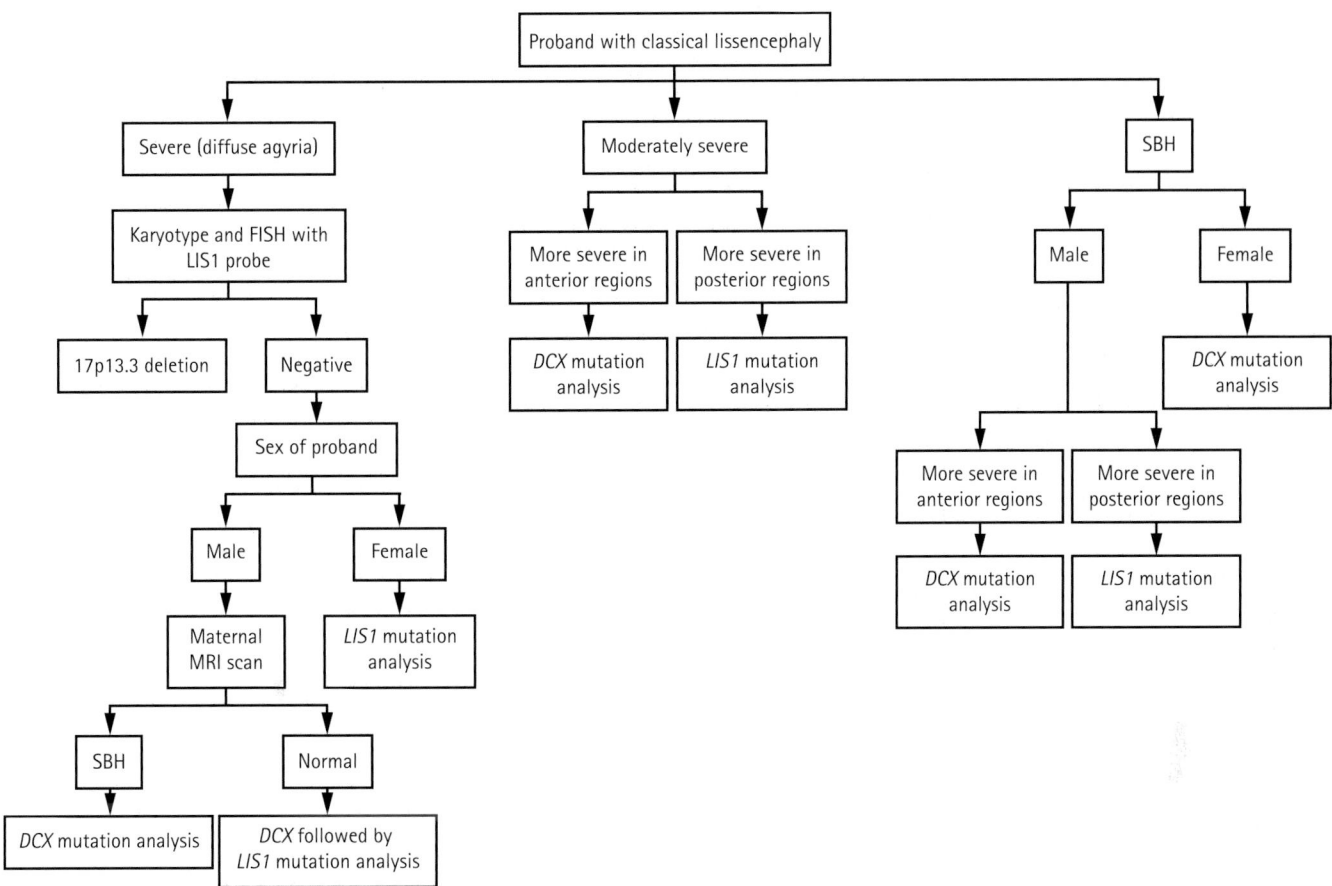

Figure 14.4 Genetic approach to non-syndromal classic lissencephaly. SBH: subcortical band heterotopia.

Table 14.11 Syndromes with cobblestone (Type II) lissencephaly				
Syndrome	Inheritance	Locus	Gene	Associated features
Congenital muscular dystrophy type 1C	AR	19q13	*FKRP*	Congenital muscular dystrophy, severe involvement of shoulder and pelvic girdles, weakness of respiratory muscles, MR, cerebellar cysts
Congenital muscular dystrophy type 1D	AR	22q12-q13	*LARGE*	Hypoplastic brainstem, congenital muscular dystrophy, severe MR
Fukuyama congenital muscular dystrophy	AR	9q31	*FCMD*	Severe progressive congenital muscular dystrophy, joint contractures, elevated CK levels, optic atrophy and retinal detachment, MR
Limb-girdle muscular dystrophy type 2I	AR	19q13	*FKRP*	Childhood or later-onset muscular dystrophy, muscle pseudohypertrophy, elevated CK levels, MR, microcephaly, white matter changes, cerebellar cysts, vermis hypoplasia
Muscle-eye-brain (MEB) disease	AR	1p33-p34 19q13	*POMGnT1* *FKRP*	Congenital muscular dystrophy, retinal hypoplasia, high myopia
Walker–Warburg	AR	9q34 14q24 19q13 9q31	*POMT1* *POMT2* *FKRP* *FCMD*	Encephalocele, hydrocephalus, anterior chamber dysgenesis, congenital cataract, retinal dysplasia, severe congenital muscular dystrophy with elevated CK levels

Key: AR, autosomal recessive; CK, creatine kinase; MR, mental retardation.

All syndromes associated with cobblestone lissencephaly are inherited in an autosomal recessive manner and families with a child with cobblestone lissencephaly should be given a 25% (1 in 4) offspring recurrence risk.

POLYMICROGYRIA (PMG)

Polymicrogyria (PMG) is a congenital abnormality of the cerebral cortex in which the cortical surface is irregular due to the replacement of the normal gyri and sulci with an excessive number of small and partly fused gyri separated by shallow sulci. Polymicrogyria and the closely related abnormality, schizencephaly, are both believed to be the result of abnormal cortical organization (Barkovich et al 2005). They may be the result of abnormal cortical development (i.e. true malformations) or a disruptive event (vascular or infective) between 16 and 24 weeks gestation. Polymicrogyria can be unilateral or bilateral. Two forms of PMG can be distinguished based on pathological findings. One form demonstrates a four-layered cortex and the other form shows an unlayered cortex. Both forms can co-exist in the same patient suggesting that they may represent a spectrum rather than distinct malformations (Robain 1996).

Polymicrogyria is probably the most commonly seen cortical malformation and it is etiologically heterogeneous. It can be associated with intrauterine hypoperfusion associated with twin-to-twin transfusion, intrauterine infections (particularly CMV infection), or antenatal exposure to alcohol. Genetic causes of PMG can be considered under the categories of chromosomal, syndromal or non-syndromal. Syn-

dromal forms of PMG are associated with congenital abnormalities affecting other systems whereas non-syndromal PMG refers to PMG that either occurs as an isolated abnormality or in association with other CNS abnormalities such as schizencephaly, white matter changes or periventricular nodular heterotopia.

A number of chromosomal abnormalities can be associated with PMG (Jansen & Andermann 2005). These include 1p36 and 22q11.2 deletions or microdeletions and several unbalanced chromosomal rearrangements. Leventer et al (2001) proposed that there are loci for PMG at 1p36, 2p13, 6q25, 21q22 and 22q11 based on the chromosomal deletions and rearrangements that have been reported in association with this abnormality. Polymicrogyria is one of the most frequently reported CNS malformation in patients with the 22q11.2 deletion. These patients usually have asymmetric perisylvian PMG of variable severity with a striking predisposition for the right hemisphere suggesting that the PMG in these patients may be the result of abnormal vascular development rather than representing a primary cortical malformation (Robin et al 2006).

Non-syndromal PMG can be unilateral or bilateral, focal or diffuse. It has been classified into several types based on the cortical regions that are primarily affected (Barkovich et al 2005, Jansen & Andermann 2005) and the associated CNS malformations (Wieck et al 2005). Table 14.12 lists the different types of non-syndromal PMG, their inheritance patterns and clinical features. Bilateral perisylvian polymicrogyria (BPP) is the most frequently seen type of PMG, accounting for about 60% of all cases of this condition (Leventer et al

Table 14.12 Classification of non-syndromal polymicrogyria based on topographical distribution

Type	Inheritance	Locus	Gene	Clinical features
Unilateral(UP)	Sporadic AD XL	NA NK NK	NA NK NK	Spastic hemiparesis, variable MR, seizures with electrical status during sleep (ESES)
Bilateral generalized (BGP)	AR	NK	NK	Variable MR, seizures, spastic hemiparesis or quadriparesis, seizures, reduced white matter, ventriculomegaly
Bilateral frontal (BFP)	AR	NK	NK	Spastic hemiparesis or quadriparesis, mild-moderate MR, seizures
Bilateral frontoparietal (BFPP)	AR	16q13	GPR56	Global developmental delay, squint, spasticity, seizures, white matter abnormalities, atrophy of brainstem and cerebellum
Bilateral perisylvian (BPP)	XL AR AD	Xq28 Xq22 NK NK	NK SRPX2 NK NK	Worster–Drought syndrome (pseudobulbar palsy with restricted tongue movements, excessive drooling, swallowing difficulties, dysarthria, seizures, variable spasticity)
Bilateral parasagittal parieto-occipital (BPOP)	Sporadic	NA	NA	Complex partial seizures with onset between 20 months – 15 years associated with cognitive slowing, average intelligence or mild MR

Key: AD, autosomal dominant; AR, autosomal recessive; MR, mental retardation; NA, not applicable; NK, not known.

2001). As mentioned previously, it can be a feature of the 22q11.2 deletion syndrome. Familial forms of BPP can demonstrate X-linked, autosomal dominant or autosomal recessive inheritance. Villard et al (2002) mapped a locus for BPP at Xq28 in five families with an X-linked form of this condition. However, the gene at this locus has not yet been identified. Roll et al (2006) identified a missense mutation in the *SRPX2* gene at Xq22 in 1 of 12 patients with BPP. This male patient presented with rolandic seizures and mild intellectual impairment and the mutation was also identified in his unaffected mother and maternal aunt as well as two other maternal aunts with mild intellectual impairment. None of the female relatives with the mutation had a cortical malformation on MRI scan. Mutations in the *GPR56* gene at 16q13 are associated with bilateral frontoparietal polymicrogyria (BFPP) with white matter changes and cerebellar hypoplasia (Piao et al 2004). No other genes have as yet been identified for the non-syndromal forms of PMG.

Multiple congenital malformation syndromes in which PMG has been reported consistently are listed in Table 14.13. Although Joubert syndrome can be caused by mutations in several different genes, cortical PMG is a consistent feature of Joubert syndrome that is caused by mutations in the *AHI1* gene at 6q23 (Dixon-Salazar et al 2004). Wieck et al (2005) recently reported several patients with the combination of periventricular nodular heterotopia (PNH) and overlying PMG. They classified these patients into three distinct groups: those with frontal-perisylvian PNH and PMG, those with posterior predominant PNH and PMG and a small group with severe congenital microcephaly with PNH and PMG. Most patients had developmental delay, mental retardation and epilepsy. Several patients also had dysmorphic features and a few had other congenital malformations such as cleft palate, malrotation of the small bowel and micropenis. These patient should therefore be classified as having a syndromic form of both PNH and PMG. Skewing of the sex ratio (many more affected males than females) in the first two groups raised the possibility of X-linked inheritance.

Metabolic disorders associated with PMG include Zellweger syndrome, peroxisomal bifunctional enzyme deficiency, non-ketotic hyperglycinemia, glutaric aciduria type II, fumarase deficiency, MELAS, respiratory complex I and IV deficiency and pyruvate dehydrogenase deficiency.

All children with PMG should have a detailed workup as shown in Table 14.14. Detailed chromosome analysis with FISH analysis for 1p36 and 22q11.2 deletions is recommended in all cases with developmental delay or congenital heart disease. Parents of a male child with bilateral perisylvian polymicrogyria (BPP) should be given a 10% (1 in 10) recurrence risk and parents of a female child with BPP should be counseled a 5% (1 in 20) recurrence risk.

SCHIZENCEPHALY (p. 242)

Schizencephaly is a rare congenital abnormality of the cerebral cortex that is characterized by a full thickness cleft of one or both cerebral hemispheres. The full thickness cortical

Table 14.13 Multiple malformation syndromes associated with polymicrogyria (PMG)

Syndrome	Inheritance	Locus	Gene	Associated features
Adams–Oliver	AD	NK	NK	Scalp defects, terminal transverse limb defects, congenital heart disease, lethal in males
Aicardi	XD	Xp22	NK	Chorioretinitis, infantile spasms, hypsarrhythmia, vertebral anomalies, MR, lethal in males
Delleman (oculo-cerebro-cutaneous)	Uncertain	NK	NK	Frontal PMG and periventricular nodular heterotopia, midbrain-hindbrain malformation, microphthalmia, orbital cysts, periorbital skin tags
Galloway–Mowat	AR	NK	NK	Microcephaly, neuronal migration defects, MR, hiatus hernia, nephrotic syndrome
Goldberg–Shprintzen	AR	10q22.1	*KIAA1279*	Microcephaly, MR, hypertelorism, cleft palate, short stature, Hirschsprung disease
Joubert	AR	6q23	*AHI1*	Cerebellar vermis hypoplasia with molar tooth sign, episodic apnea/tachypnea, oculomotor apraxia, chorio-retinal colobomas, retinopathy, renal cysts, MR
Micro (Warburg)	AR	2q21.3	*RAB3GAP*	Microphthalmia, microcornea, congenital cataract, MR, hypogenitalism, poor growth
MPPH	Uncertain	NK	NK	Megalencephaly, perisylvian PMG, tetramelic postaxial polydactyly, hydrocephalus, severe MR, seizures

Key: AD, autosomal dominant; AR, autosomal recessive; MR, mental retardation; NK, not known; XD, X-linked dominant

Table 14.14 Genetic assessment of polymicrogyria

• History	Family history of epilepsy, developmental delay, learning difficulties, hemiparesis, speech problems
	Parental consanguinity
	Pregnancy history of blood loss, viral infections, twinning with twin to twin transfusion syndrome
	Speech articulation problems
	Drooling or swallowing difficulties
	Seizures (age at onset, type, frequency, and response to treatment)
• Examination	Head circumference, facial dysmorphism, tongue movements, ability to purse lips, spastic monoparesis/hemiparesis/quadriparesis
• Investigations	Chromosome analysis
	FISH for 22q11 and 1p36 deletions if developmental delay and/or congenital heart disease
	Congenital infection screen
	Cranial MRI scan
	Metabolic investigations: urine amino acids and organic acids, plasma very long chain fatty acids (VLCFAs), CK and lactate
	Consider testing for common MELAS mutation (A3243G)

clefts are characterized by a pial-ependymal seam, which is an infolding of cortical gray matter into the ventricle. This results in the fusion of the cortical pia and ventricular ependyma within the cleft. Schizencephaly and polymicrogyria are related disorders that are believed to result from abnormal cortical organization (Barkovich et al 2005). The cortical clefts in schizencephaly are lined with gray matter and the clefts or the adjacent cortex or more distant or contralateral cortex often shows polymicrogyria (Hayashi et al 2002, Norman et al 1995). The most frequent sites of schizencephaly are along the primary cerebral fissures, usually the sylvian fissure. Barkovich et al (2005) have classified schizencephaly as a malformation of cortical development that results from abnormal cortical organization. However, schizencephaly can also result from a disruptive process before neuronal migration is complete, i.e. about 20 weeks gestation (Norman et al 1995). Neuroradiologically, schizencephaly can be of two types: 'closed-lip' (Type I) and 'open-lip' (Type II) (Barkovich et al 1992). In closed-lip schizencephaly the edges of the cortical cleft appear fused. In open-lip schizencephaly the edges of the cortical cleft are well separated. This results in a large full thickness fluid-filled cortical cleft that is lined with polymicrogyric gray matter.

Although schizencephaly is usually a sporadic abnormality, siblings with schizencephaly have been reported (Hilburger et al 1993, Hosley et al 1992, Robinson 1991). Brunelli et al (1996) found de novo dominant mutations in the homeobox gene *EMX2* on 10q26.1 in 7 out of 8 sporadic patients with open-lip schizencephaly. Faiella et al (1997) reported 10 additional patients with schizencephaly, 6 of whom were found to be heterozygous for new dominant mutations in the *EMX2* gene. These included two brothers with bilateral open-lip schizencephaly who were found to have the same 3′ splice site mutation in position 1 of exon 2. Neither parent carried this mutation suggesting that one of the parents was a gonadal mosaic for this mutation. However, other groups have not been able to replicate these results (Barkovich et al 2005) and there have been no further reports of *EMX2* mutations in schizencephaly. Tietjen et al (2005) reported a large Turkish family with three affected individuals with schizencephaly. Genome-wide linkage studies ruled out linkage to the *EMX2* locus and instead suggested additional candidate loci for the schizencephaly in this family (5q21.3-q23.2 assuming an autosomal dominant maternal mode of inheritance and 8q24.22-q24.3 assuming an autosomal recessive mode of inheritance). Therefore, schizencephaly is likely to be a genetically heterogeneous disorder with mutations in the *EMX2* gene probably accounting for only a minority of cases (Granata et al 2005).

Schizencephaly and other brain malformations such as porencephaly, hydranencephaly, agenesis of the corpus callosum, congenital hydrocephalus, septo-optic dysplasia and cerebral infarctions have all been reported in the children of mothers who abused cocaine in the antenatal period (Dominguez et al 1991). These anomalies presumably arise as a result of vascular disruption. Syndromic forms of schizencephaly are rare. It is a recognized feature of septo-optic dysplasia, and it has been described as a component of an autosomal recessive syndrome comprising hypoplasia/agenesis of the corpus callosum, enlarged cisterna magna, Moebius sequence with involvement of cranial nerves V, VI, VII, IX and XII, dysmorphic facial features, severe developmental delay, spastic tetraparesis, flexion contractures of the hips, knees and elbows and hypogenitalism (Rodríguez Cradio & Pérez Aytés 1999).

Until further advances are made in understanding the genetic basis of schizencephaly, parents with a single affected child with unilateral schizencephaly should be given a 1% (1 in 100) recurrence risk for this condition. Parents with a single affected child with bilateral schizencephaly should be given a 10% (1 in 10) recurrence risk (Baraitser 1997).

PERIVENTRICULAR NODULAR HETEROTOPIA (PNH)

Periventricular or subependymal nodular heterotopia is a developmental abnormality of the cerebral cortex, which is classified as a disorder of abnormal neuronal migration

(Barkovich et al 2005). It is characterized by the presence of groups of neurons along the walls of the lateral ventricles due to their failure to migrate to the cortex.

Periventricular nodular heterotopia can be an isolated (non-syndromal) abnormality or a component of a multiple congenital abnormality syndrome (syndromal). It has rarely been described in association with the 1p36 deletion (Neal et al 2006), Williams syndrome (7q11.23 deletion) (Ferland et al 2006), duplications of 5p15 (Sheen et al 2003a) and Xq28 (Fink et al 1997).

Isolated (non-syndromal) PNH is a rare disorder that is inherited in an X-linked dominant manner, usually with male lethality. The condition usually affects females who present with normal intelligence or mild learning difficulties and epilepsy. Less frequently seen problems in these patients include congenital heart disease (patent ductus arteriosus, aortic insufficiency), thrombocytopenia, stroke, squint, short digits and gastric immotility (Fox et al 1998, Parrini et al 2006). Fox et al (1998) identified loss of function mutations in the *filamin 1* gene (now called *filamin A* or *FLNA*) in patients with X-linked dominant PNH. Sheen et al (2001) screened affected females from 6 families with X-linked PNH, 31 sporadic female patients and 24 sporadic male patients with PNH for mutations in the *FLNA* gene. Mutations were identified in five families (83%) with X-linked PNH, six (19%) sporadic female patients, and two (9%) sporadic male patients with PNH. All mutations identified in the familial cases were predicted to result in loss of function of the *FLNA* protein, whereas mutations identified in spo-

radic female cases were thought to cause severe or partial loss of function. Mutations identified in the 2 sporadic males were not present in mosaic form but were thought to result in only partial loss of function of the *FLNA* protein. Somatic mosaicism for *FLNA* mutations has been reported in both males and females with PNH (Guerrini et al 2004, Parrini et al 2004). MRI/CT scan findings in patients with PNH due to *FLNA* mutations include bilateral near-continuous periventricular heterotopia with or without thinning of the corpus callosum, cerebellar hypoplasia and enlarged cisterna magna (Poussaint et al 2000).

Males with *FLNA* mutations usually die in the prenatal period with excessive bleeding (Moro et al 2002). However, there are a few reports of surviving males with both mosaic and non-mosaic *FLNA* mutations and these cases have a variable phenotype. Some males with *FLNA* mutations have a mild phenotype that is similar to females with *FLNA* mutation, i.e. normal intellect or mild learning difficulties with seizures (Sheen et al 2001), whereas other surviving males with *FLNA* mutations have a more severe phenotype with developmental delay, severe learning difficulties, seizures and multiple congenital malformations (Guerrini et al 2004, Parrini et al 2004). A male with PNH and an intermediate phenotype (normal development, no seizures, severe constipation, facial dysmorphism and gut malrotation) has also been reported (Hehr et al 2006).

Syndromal forms of PNH are relatively rare. Table 14.15 lists most of the syndromal forms of PNH, i.e. syndromes associated with PNH and other CNS malformations and

Table 14.15 Syndromes associated with bilateral periventricular nodular heterotopia (PNH)

Syndrome	Inheritance	Locus	Gene	Associated features
Cerebro-fronto-facial type I	Uncertain	NK	NK	Both sexes affected, coarse facies, hypertelorism, short limbs, mild MR
PNH with Ehlers–Danlos syndrome	XLD	Xq28	*FLNA*	Females affected, joint hypermobility, skin fragility, aortic dilatation, lethal in males
Frontal-perisylvian PNH with PMG	Uncertain	NK	NK	Both sexes affected, severe DD, epilepsy, dysmorphic features
PNH with frontonasal dysplasia	Uncertain	NK	NK	Both sexes affected, severe hypertelorism, widow's peak, broad nasal tip, mild MR, epilepsy, partial ACC
PNH-hippocampal malformation-CH	Uncertain	NK	NK	Both sexes affected, posterior PNH, cerebellar signs, seizures, normal intelligence or mild MR
PNH with hydrocephalus	Uncertain	NK	NK	Both sexes affected, hydrocephalus, severe DD, epilepsy
PNH with limb defects	Uncertain	NK	NK	Both sexes affected, distal limb reduction defects, mild MR
PNH with microcephaly	AR	20q13	*ARFGEF2*	Microcephaly, severe DD, seizures, recurrent infections
PNH-MR-syndactyly	XL	Xq28	NK	Males affected, cerebellar hypoplasia, severe MR, seizures facial dysmorphism, syndactyly of fingers and toes
Posterior PNH-PMG	Uncertain	NK	NK	Both sexes affected, DD/MR, epilepsy, dysmorphic features

Key: AR, autosomal recessive; CH, cerebellar hypoplasia; DD, developmental delay; MR, mental retardation; NK, not known; PMG, polymicrogyria; XL, X-linked; XLD, X-linked dominant.

syndromes associated with PNH and facial dysmorphism or other congenital abnormalities. It is interesting to note that *FLNA* mutations have been identified in patients with the syndrome of PNH with Ehlers–Danlos syndrome as patients with the classic X-linked dominant PNH can also have vascular anomalies (Parrini et al 2006, Sheen et al 2005). Parrini et al (2006) identified a frameshift mutation in *FLNA* in a proband with PNH and Ehlers–Danlos syndrome and her mother with classic PNH. They suggest that Ehlers–Danlos syndrome in the daughter could be the result of variable expressivity due to genetic modifying factors or skewed X-inactivation and PNH without Ehlers–Danlos syndrome in the mother could be the result of somatic mosaicism for the *FLNA* mutation.

Gain of function mutations in *FLNA* can result in four overlapping multiple malformation syndromes called otopalatodigital syndromes types I and II, frontometaphyseal dysplasia and Melnick–Needles syndrome (Robertson et al 2003). These syndromes are not associated with PNH. However, Zenker et al (2004) reported a female with the dual phenotype of classic PNH and frontometaphyseal dysplasia (FMD) and a point mutation in the *FLNA* gene. They proposed that the mutation created an ectopic splice donor site in exon 45 that resulted in the production of two functionally different *FLNA* proteins, one with a gain of function resulting in the FMD phenotype and the other with a loss of function giving rise to the PNH phenotype.

Mothers of children of both sexes with isolated PNH or PNH with Ehlers–Danlos syndrome should be offered an MRI scan to look for PNH. If an *FLNA* mutation has been identified in the index case then the mother should be offered testing for the mutation. If the mother's scan shows PNH or she has the *FLNA* mutation that has been identified in the proband then she should be counseled on the basis of X-linked dominant inheritance and told that her daughters will be at 50% (1 in 2) risk of being affected with PNH. Her sons would also be at 50% (1in 2 risk) of being affected but affected males are likely to die before or soon after birth. Although there have been rare instances of affected males surviving beyond the neonatal period it is difficult to predict the phenotype and prognosis in these children. If the mother's MRI scan is normal or if she does not have the *FLNA* mutation that has been identified in the proband then the recurrence risk of PNH in her next pregnancy is likely to be low.

CEREBELLAR HYPOPLASIA (p. 250)

The cerebellum develops from the alar plate of the rhombencephalon at about 28–44 days postconception (Altman et al 1992). The first part of the cerebellum to form is the flocculonodular lobe. The next part of the cerebellum to develop is the vermis followed by the anterior and posterior cerebellar hemispheres. Cerebellar hypoplasia may affect only the vermis, only the hemispheres or both. Hypoplasia of the cerebellar vermis is more frequently seen than hypoplasia of the cerebellar hemispheres or hypoplasia of the entire cerebellum. At birth, the cerebellum is normally relatively small compared with the cerebral hemispheres, and this can give the impression of cerebellar hypoplasia (Norman et al 1995).

Cerebellar hypoplasia is an etiologically heterogeneous condition (Boltshauser 2004). It can be the result of antenatal exposure to infections (e.g. cytomegalovirus) and teratogens, an underlying chromosomal abnormality or a metabolic disorder. Cerebellar hypoplasia can also be a characteristic feature of several different multiple malformation syndromes. Chromosomal abnormalities associated with cerebellar hypoplasia include trisomy 18, terminal 5p deletion, 6p25 deletion, and inversion duplication of 8p. Metabolic disorders in which cerebellar hypoplasia is a key diagnostic feature include Tay–Sachs disease, adenylosuccinase deficiency and congenital disorders of glycosylation (Friede 1964, Steinlin et al 1998). Multiple congenital malformation syndromes associated with cerebellar hypoplasia are listed in Table 14.16 and genetic syndromes associated with cerebellar hypoplasia and other CNS malformations are listed in Table 14.17.

Cerebellar hypoplasia can also occur as an isolated (non-syndromal) anomaly. Affected individuals usually present with non-progressive cerebellar ataxia or ataxic cerebral palsy. A significant proportion (10–25%) of non-syndromal cerebellar hypoplasia is genetically determined (Esscher et al 1996, Steinlin et al 1998). Norman (1940) reported an autosomal recessive form of non-syndromal cerebellar hypoplasia that was associated with atrophy of the granular layer (Norman 1940). However, this condition is probably the same as congenital disorder of glycosylation type Ia (CDG Ia) (Pascual-Castroviejo et al 2006). An autosomal recessive form of cerebellar hypoplasia is prevalent in the Cayman Islands (Johnson et al 1978). This is caused by mutations in the *ATCAY* gene at 19p13.3 (Bomar et al 2003). Other forms of autosomal recessive non-syndromal cerebellar hypoplasia have also been described (McHale et al 2000, Wichman et al 1985). Autosomal dominant and X-linked forms of non-syndromal cerebellar hypoplasia have also been reported (Fenichel & Philips 1989, Illarioshkin et al 1996, Rivier & Echenne 1992). Autosomal dominant forms of cerebellar hypoplasia are associated with mild ataxia and mild cognitive impairment that may improve with age. Dudding et al (2004) mapped one form of autosomal dominant non-syndromal cerebellar hypoplasia to 3p26, which overlaps with the SCA15 locus. However, Tsao et al (2006) were unable to demonstrate linkage to the SCA15 locus in another family with autosomal dominant non-syndromal cerebellar ataxia with progressive motor and cognitive improvement with age. X-linked recessive forms of this condition can be associated with normal intelligence or mental retardation. Philip et al (2003) have shown that mutations in the *OPHN1* gene at Xq12 cause X-linked cerebellar hypoplasia and mental retardation.

Table 14.16 Multiple congenital malformation syndromes with cerebellar hypoplasia

Syndrome	Inheritance	Locus	Gene	Associated features
3C (Ritscher–Schinzel)	AR	NK	NK	Cerebellar vermis hypoplasia, iris/retinal coloboma, congenital heart disease, mental retardation
Cerebellar hypoplasia with endosteal sclerosis	AR	NK	NK	Hypoplasia of cerebellar vermis and hemispheres, MR, microcephaly, bony sclerosis, medullary canal stenosis
COACH	AR	NK	NK	Cerebellar vermis hypoplasia with molar tooth sign, oligophrenia (MR), ataxia, coloboma, hepatic fibrosis
Dekaban–Arima	AR	NK	NK	Cerebellar vermis hypoplasia with molar tooth sign, chorio-retinal colobomas, congenital retinal blindness, polycystic kidneys
Gillespie	AR	NK	NK	Hypoplasia of cerebellar hemispheres or vermis, partial aniridia with non-reactive pupils, non-progressive ataxia, MR
Joubert	AR	9q34 11p12-q13 6q23 2q13 12q21 8q21-q22	NK NK AHI1 NPHP1 NPHP6 MKS3	Cerebellar vermis hypoplasia with molar tooth sign, episodic apnea/tachypnea, oculomotor apraxia, chorio-retinal colobomas, retinopathy, renal cysts, MR
Marinesco–Sjögren	AR	5q31	SIL1	Cerebellar atrophy, ataxia, congenital cataracts, MR, myopathy with elevated CK levels and abnormalities on EM, kyphoscoliosis
Varadi–Papp (OFD VI)	AR	NK	NK	Cerebellar vermis aplasia or hypoplasia, molar tooth sign, midline cleft lip, multiple oral frenulae, synpolydactyly, MR

Key: AR, Autosomal recessive; EM, electron microscopy; MR, mental retardation; NK, not known, OFD, oral-facial-digital.

Table 14.17 Syndrome associated with cerebellar hypoplasia (CH) and other CNS malformations

Syndrome	Inheritance	Locus	Gene	Associated features
Barth microlissencephaly (radial microbrain)	AR	NK	NK	Extreme microcephaly (OFC < 28 cm), severe cerebellar hypoplasia, neonatal death
Hutterite dysequilibrium	AR	9p24	VLDLR	Inferior cerebellar hypoplasia, mild pachygyria, moderate to profound MR, truncal ataxia, strabismus, seizures, scoliosis, pes planus
Lissencephaly-congenital lymphedema-CH	AR	7q22	RELN	Severe cerebellar hypoplasia, hypotonia, congenital lymphedema, MR
PNH-hippocampal malformation-CH	Uncertain	NK	NK	Posterior PNH, cerebellar signs, seizures, normal intelligence or mild MR
Pontocerebellar hypoplasia type 1	AR	NK	NK	Hypoplasia of cerebellar hemispheres and pons, spinal anterior horn cell degeneration, early death
Pontocerebellar hypoplasia type 2	AR	NK	NK	Hypoplasia of cerebellar hemispheres and pons, microcephaly, chorea/dystonia, epilepsy, severe MR

Key: AR, Autosomal recessive; MR, mental retardation; NK, not known; PNH, periventricular nodular heterotopia.

Table 14.18 Genetic assessment of cerebellar hypoplasia

• History	Family history of congenital ataxia or ataxic cerebral palsy Parental consanguinity Exposure to teratogens (anticonvulsants, retinoic acid, methylmercury) Extreme prematurity or very low birth weight Abnormal breathing patterns as a neonate Pericardial effusion, stroke-like episodes, abnormal movements
• Examination	Head circumference, facial dysmorphism, oral frenulae, synpolydactyly, abnormal fat distribution, inversion of nipples, abnormal saccades, retinal dystrophy, neurological findings
• Investigations	Chromosome analysis Congenital infection screen Cranial MRI scan Electroretinogram and visual evoked potentials EMG and nerve conduction studies Muscle biopsy Renal ultrasound scan Metabolic investigations: urine succinyladenosine levels, plasma CK levels, serum transferrin isoforms, white cell hexosaminidase A assay

Clinical features of cerebellar hypoplasia include speech delay, ataxia, hypotonia, autistic features and ocular signs such as nystagmus, strabismus and abnormal ocular movements (Wassmer et al 2003). In these children, every effort must be made to try and identify the cause of the cerebellar hypoplasia (Table 14.18). It can be difficult to distinguish between cerebellar hypoplasia and cerebellar atrophy by neuroimaging. It is important to enquire about extreme prematurity (gestational age less that 28 weeks) and very low birth weight (under 1085 g) in a child with cerebellar hypoplasia as severe injury to the cerebellum, presumably as a result of cerebellar infarction, has been reported in these children (Bodensteiner & Johnsen 2005, Johnsen et al 2002), who present with cerebral palsy with ataxia and athetosis or dystonia, microcephaly, developmental delay, learning difficulties and absence of the inferior cerebellar vermis and variable portions of the cerebellar hemispheres.

Metabolic disorders and genetic syndromes associated with cerebellar hypoplasia are almost all inherited in an autosomal recessive manner. If no cause is identified for the cerebellar hypoplasia the parents should be counseled about a recurrence risk of at least 10% (1 in 10). Consanguineous parents should be given a 25% (1 in 4) recurrence risk.

DANDY–WALKER MALFORMATION (DWM) (p. 253)

In this developmental abnormality, partial or complete absence of the cerebellar vermis is associated with cystic dilatation of the fourth ventricle, elevation of the tentorium and transverse sinuses and the early onset of hydrocephalus. This condition shows marked etiological heterogeneity (Chitayat et al 1994). Approximately 50% of cases diagnosed prenatally are caused by a chromosome abnormality (Nyberg et al 1991), such as one of the viable autosomal trisomy syndromes (i.e. trisomy 8, 9, 13, 18, and 21), triploidy, or more subtle imbalance such as 2q, 3q, and 6p25 deletion or 8p, 8q and 17q duplication. Known environmental causal agents include prenatal exposure to infection such as cytomegalovirus and rubella and to drugs such as warfarin and valproic acid.

A DWM is a recognized finding in a large number of multiple malformation syndromes, the most commonly encountered of which are listed in Table 14.19. Two conditions in this list have characteristic posterior fossa changes that are reminiscent of DWM but are considerably more complex. These include Joubert and Delleman (oculocerebrocutaneous) syndromes. The posterior fossa abnormalities of Joubert syndrome include a deep interpeduncular fossa at the level of the isthmus and upper pons, elongated, thick and abnormally oriented superior cerebellar peduncles and cerebellar vermis hypoplasia. These anomalies result in the 'molar tooth' sign, which can be seen on an axial MRI scan of the brain. However, the molar tooth sign is not pathognomonic of Joubert syndrome as it can be seen in other conditions including Dekaban–Arima, COACH and Senior–Loken syndromes as well as oral-facial-digital syndrome type VI (Gleeson et al 2004). The posterior fossa abnormalities of Delleman syndrome have previously been classified as DWM. However a recent study has shown that the patients with Delleman syndrome have a complex mid-hindbrain malformation that is pathognomonic for this condition (Moog et al 2005). This comprises a giant, upwardly rotated tectum, forward flexed tegmentum of the midbrain resulting in a horizontal orientation of the aqueduct, hypoplasia or aplasia of the cerebellar hemispheres, absent vermis and a large posterior fossa fluid collection.

Murray et al (1985) noted that in 23 of 113 reviewed cases of DWM there was another midline abnormality such as a cleft lip or palate, congenital heart defect or neural tube defect. They proposed that in these situations the recurrence risk quoted should be that appropriate for the other malformation, i.e. usually around 2–5%. Then if a DWM occurs in isolation the recurrence risk is low. Pooling the results from two studies gives a risk of 1% for siblings (Burton 1979, Murray et al 1985). However, it was noted that 3 out of 44 of the siblings of the index cases in one of these series had another midline defect, an observation which emphasizes the importance of offering detailed prenatal ultrasound monitoring in subsequent pregnancies.

Table 14.19 Syndromes featuring a Dandy–Walker malformation

Syndrome	Inheritance	Locus	Gene	Associated features
3C (Ritschier–Schinzel)	AR	NK	NK	Congenital heart disease, iris coloboma, cleft palate
Aicardi	XD	Xp22	NK	Chorioretinitis, infantile spasms, hypsarrhythmia, vertebral anomalies, lethal in males
Delleman (oculocerebrocutaneous)	Uncertain	NK	NK	Frontal polymicrogyria and periventricular nodular heterotopia, midbrain-hindbrain malformation, microphthalmia, orbital cysts, periorbital skin tags
Fryns	AR	NK	NK	Corneal clouding, diaphragmatic hernia, small nails
Hydrolethalus	AR	11q23-q25	*HYLS1*	Hydrocephalus with absent upper midline structures, micrognathia, polydactyly
Meckel–Gruber	AR	17q23	*MKS1*	Occipital encephalocele, polycystic kidneys, postaxial polydactyly
		11q13	Unknown	
		8q21-q22	*MKS3*	
Oro-facial-digital type I	XD	Xp22	*CXORF5*	Cleft lip, oral frenulae, polydactyly, syndactyly
PHACES	AR	NK	NK	Facial hemangiomas, congenital heart disease, arterial
	AD	NK	NK	anomalies and aortic coarctation, eye anomalies, sternal clefts
Smith–Lemli–Opitz	AR	11q12-q13	*DHCR7*	Genital anomaly, microcephaly, ptosis, syndactyly
Walker–Warburg	AR	9q34	*POMT1*	Encephalocele, hydrocephalus, lissencephaly, retinal dysplasia
		14q24	*POMT2*	
		19q13	*FKRP*	

Key: AD, autosomal dominant; AR, autosomal recessive; XD, X-linked dominant; NK, not known

REFERENCES

Adams C, Johnston W P, Nevin N C 1982 Family study of congenital hydrocephalus. Dev Med Child Neurol 24:493–498.

Al-Shahwan S, Singh B 1995 Familial congenital hemiparesis. J Child Neurol 10:413–414.

Altman N R, Naidich T P, Braffman B H 1992 Posterior fossa malformations. AJNR Am J Neuroradiol 13:691–724.

Baraitser M 1997 The genetics of neurological disorders, 3rd edn. Oxford University Press, Oxford.

Baraitser M, Burn J 1984 Neural tube defects as an X-linked condition. Am J Med Genet 17:383–385.

Barkovich A J, Gressens P, Evrard P 1992 Formation, maturation and disorders of brain neocortex. AJNR Am J Neuroradiol 13:423–446.

Barkovich A J, Kuzniecky R I, Jackson G D et al 2005 A developmental and genetic classification for malformations of cortical development. Neurology 65:1873–1887.

Beltran-Valero de Bernabe D, Currier S, Steinbrecher A et al 2002 Mutations in the O-mannosyltransferase gene POMT1 give rise to the severe neuronal migration disorder Walker–Warburg syndrome. Am J Hum Genet 71:1033–1043.

Bendon R W, Siddiqi T, de Courten-Myers G, Dignan P 1987 Recurrent developmental anomalies: 1. syndrome of hydranencephaly with renal aplastic dysplasia. 2. polyvalvular development heart defect. Am J Med Genet Suppl 3:357–365.

Berg R A, Aleck K A, Kaplan A M 1983 Familial porencephaly. Arch Neurol 40:567–569.

Blackburn B L, Fineman R M 1994 Epidemiology of congenital hydrocephalus in Utah, 1940–1979: report

of an iatrogenically related 'epidemic'. Am J Med Genet 52:123–129.

Bodensteiner J B, Johnsen S D 2005 Cerebellar injury in the extremely premature infant: newly recognized but relatively common outcome. J Child Neurol 20:139–142.

Boltshauser E 2004 Cerebellum — small brain but large confusion: a review of selected cerebellar malformations and disruptions. Am J Med Genet 126A:376–385.

Bomar J M, Benke P J, Slattery E L et al 2003 Mutations in a novel gene encoding a CRAL-TRIO domain cause human Cayman ataxia and ataxia/dystonia in the jittery mouse. Nat Genet 35:264–269.

Bond J, Roberts E, Mochida G H et al 2002 ASPM is a major determinant of cerebral cortical size. Nat Genet 32:316–320.

Bond J, Robert E, Springell K et al 2005 A centrosomal mechanism involving CDK5RAP2 and CENPJ controls brain size. Nat Genet 37:353–355.

Bonnemann C G, Meinecke P 1996 Bilateral porencephaly, cerebellar hypoplasia, and internal malformations: two siblings representing a probably new autosomal recessive entity. Am J Med Genet 63:428–433.

Breedveld G, de Coo I F, Lequin M H et al 2006 Novel mutations in three families confirm a major role of COL4A1 in hereditary porencephaly. J Med Genet 43:490–495.

Brockington M, Yuva Y, Prandini P et al 2001 Mutations in the fukutin-related protein gene (FKRP) identify limb girdle muscular dystrophy 2I as a milder allelic

variant of congenital muscular dystrophy MDC1C. Hum Mol Genet 10:2851–2859.

Brown S A, Warburton D, Brown L Y et al 1998 Holoprosencephaly due to mutations in ZIC2, a homologue of *Drosophila* odd-paired. Nat Genet 20:180–183.

Brunelli S, Faiella A, Capra V et al 1996 Germline mutations in the homeobox gene EMX2 in patients with severe schizencephaly. Nat Genet 12:94–96.

Bundey S 1992 Genetics and neurology, 2nd edn. Churchill Livingstone, Edinburgh.

Burton B K 1979 Recurrence risks for congenital hydrocephalus. Clin Genet 16:47–53.

Chitayat D, Moore L, Del Bigio M R 1994 Familial Dandy–Walker malformation associated with macrocephaly, facial anomalies, developmental delay, and brain stem dysgenesis. Am J Med Genet 52:406–415.

Christensen B, Arbour L, Tran P et al 1999 Genetic polymorphisms in methylenetetrahydrofolate reductase and methionine synthase, folate levels in red blood cells, and risk of neural tube defects. Am J Med Genet 84:151–157.

Cohen M M Jr 1989 Perspectives on holoprosencephaly: Part I. Epidemiology, genetics and syndromology. Teratology 40:211–235.

Cohen M M Jr 2006 Holoprosencephaly: clinical, anatomic, and molecular dimensions. Birth Defects Res (Part A) 76:658–673.

Cohen M M Jr, Gorlin R J 1969 Genetic considerations in a sibship of cyclopia and clefts. Birth Defects Orig Artic Ser 5:113–118.

Cohen M M Jr, Shiota K 2002 Teratogenesis of holoprosencephaly. Am J Med Genet 109:1–15.

Cohen M M Jr, Sulik K K 1992 Perpectives on holoprosencephaly: Part II. Central nervous system, craniofacial anatomy, syndrome commentary, diagnostic approach and experimental studies. J Craniofacial Genet Dev Biol 12:196–244.

Cox J, Jackson A P, Bond J et al 2006 What primary microcephaly can tell us about brain growth. Trends Mol Med 12:358–366.

Croen L A, Shaw G M, Lammer E J 1996 Holoprosencephaly: epidemiologic and clinical characteristics of a California population. Am J Med Genet 64:465–472.

Czeizel A 1981 Schisis Association. Am J Med Genet 10:25–35.

D'Agostino M D, Bernasconi A, Das S et al 2002 Subcortical band heterotopia (SBH) in males: clinical, imaging and genetic findings in comparison with females. Brain 125:2507–2522.

Da Silva E 1988 Callosal defect, microcephaly, severe mental retardation and other anomalies in three sibs. Am J Med Genet 29:837–843.

De la Cruz J M, Bamford R N, Burdine R D et al 2002 A loss-of-function mutation in the CFC domain of TDGF1 is associated with human forebrain defects. Hum Genet 110:422–428.

Debus O, Koch H G, Kurlemann G et al 1998 Factor V Leiden and genetic defects of thrombophilia in childhood porencephaly. Arch Dis Child 78:F121–F124.

des Portes V, Pinard J M, Billuart P et al 1998 A novel CNS gene required for neuronal migration and involved in X-linked subcortical laminar heterotopia and lissencephaly syndrome. Cell 92:51–61.

Dixon-Salazar T, Silhavy J L, Marsh S E et al 2004 Mutations in the AHI1 gene, encoding jouberin, cause Joubert syndrome with cortical polymicrogyria. Am J Hum Genet 75:979–987.

Dobyns W B 1996 Absence makes the search grow longer. Am J Hum Genet 58:7–16.

Dobyns W B, Truwit C L 1995 Lissencephaly and other malformations of cortical development: 1995 update. Neuropediatrics 26:132–147.

Dolk H 1991 The predictive value of microcephaly during the first year of life for mental retardation at seven years. Dev Med Child Neurol 33:974–983.

Dominguez R, Aguirre Vila-Coro A, Slopis J M et al 1991 Brain and ocular abnormalities in infants with in utero exposure to cocaine and other street drugs. Am J Dis Child 145:688–695.

Dubourg C, Lazaro L, Pasquier L et al 2004 Molecular screening of SHH, ZIC2, SIX3, and TGIF genes in patients with features of holoprosencephaly spectrum: mutation review and genotype-phenotype correlations. Hum Mutat 24:43–51.

Dudding T E, Friend K, Schofield P W et al 2004 Autosomal dominant non-progressive ataxia overlaps with the SCA15 locus. Neurology 63:2288–2292.

Ekong C E, Rozdilsky B 1978 Hydranencephaly in association with Roberts syndrome. Can J Neurol Sci 5:253–255.

Esscher E, Flodmark O, Hagberg G et al 1996 Non-progressive ataxia: origins, brain pathology and impairments in 78 Swedish children. Dev Med Child Neurol 38:285–296.

Faiella A, Brunelli S, Granata T et al 1997 A number of schizencephaly patients including 2 brothers are heterozygous for germline mutations in the homeobox gene EMX2. Eur J Hum Genet 5:186–190.

Fenichel G M, Phillips J A 1989 Familial aplasia of the cerebellar vermis. Possible X-linked dominant inheritance. Ann Neurol 46:582–583.

Ferland R J, Gaitanis J N, Apse K et al 2006 Periventricular nodular heterotopia and Williams syndrome. Am J Med Genet 140A:1305–1311.

Finckh U, Schroder J, Ressler B et al 2000). Spectrum and detection rate of L1CAM mutations in isolated and familial cases with clinically suspected L1-disease. Am J Med Genet 92:40–46.

Fink J M, Dobyns W B, Guerrini R et al 1997 Identification of a duplication of Xq28 associated with bilateral periventricular nodular heterotopia. Am J Hum Genet 61:379–387.

Flint J, Wilkie A O M, Buckle V J et al 1995 The detection of subtelomeric chromosomal rearrangements in idiopathic mental retardation. Nat Genet 9:132–139.

Fox J W, Lamperti E D, Eksioglu Y Z et al 1998 Mutations in filamin 1 prevent migration of cerebral cortical neurons in human periventricular heterotopia. Neuron 21:1315–1325.

Forman M S, Squier W, Dobyns W B et al 2005 Genetically defined lissencephalies show distinct pathologies. J Neuropathol Exp Neurol 64:847–857.

Fowler M, Dow R, White T A, Green C H 1972 Congenital hydrocephalus-hydrencephaly in five siblings, with autopsy studies: a new disease. Dev Med Child Neurol 14:173–188.

Fransen E, Van Camp G, D'Hooge R et al 1998 Genotype-phenotype correlation in L1 associated diseases. J Med Genet 35:399–404.

Friede R L 1964 Arrested cerebellar development: a type of cerebellar degeneration in amaurotic idiocy. J Neurol Neurosurg Psychiatry 27:41–45.

Gershoni-Baruch R, Zekaria D 1996 Deletion (13)(q22) with multiple congenital anomalies, hydranencephaly and penoscrotal transposition. Clin Dysmorphol 5:289–294.

Gibbons R J, Picketts D J, Villard L, Higgs D R 1995 Mutations in a putative global transcriptional regulator cause X-linked mental retardation with alpha-thalassaemia (ATR-X syndrome). Cell 80:837–845.

Gleeson J G, Allen K M, Fox J W et al 1998 Doublecortin, a brain-specific gene mutated in human X-linked lissencephaly and double cortex syndrome encodes a putative signaling protein. Cell 92:63–72.

Gleeson J G, Minnerath S, Kuzhiecky R I et al 2000 Somatic and germline mosaic mutations in the doublecostin gene are associated with variable phenotypes. AM J Hum Genet 67:574–581.

Gleeson J G, Keeler L C, Parisi M A et al 2004 Molar tooth sign of the midbrain-hindbrain junction: occurrence in multiple distinct syndromes. Am J Med Genet 125A:125–134.

Gould D B, Campbell Phalan F, Breedveld G J et al 2005 Mutations in Col4a1 cause perinatal cerebral haemorrhage and porencephaly. Science 308:1167–1171.

Graham J M, Wheeler P, Tackels-Horne D et al 2003 A new X-linked syndrome with agenesis of the corpus callosum, mental retardation, coloboma, micrognathia, and a mutation in the alpha 4 gene at Xq13. Am J Med Genet 123A:37–44.

Granata T, Freri E, Caccia C et al 2005 Schizencephaly: clinical spectrum, epilepsy, and pathogenesis. J Child Neurol 20:313–318.

Gripp K W, Wotton D, Edwards M C et al 2000 Mutations in TGIF cause holoprosencephaly and link NODAL signalling to human neural axis determination. Nat Genet 25:205–208.

Guerrini R, Mei D, Sisodiya S et al 2004 Germline and mosaic mutations in FLN1 in men with periventricular heterotopia. Neurology 63:51–56.

Gul A, Hassan M J, Mahmood S et al 2006 Genetic studies of autosomal recessive primary microcephaly in 33 Pakistani families: novel sequence variants in ASPM gene. Neurogenetics 7:105–110.

Gupta J K, Lilford R J 1995 Assessment and management of fetal agenesis of the corpus callosum. Prenat Diagn 15:301–312.

Halliday J, Chow C W, Wallace D, Danks D M 1986 X-linked hydrocephalus: a survey of a 20 year period in Victoria, Australia. J Med Genet 23:23–31.

Harper C, Hockey A 1983 Proliferative vasculopathy and a hydranencephalic-hydrocephalic syndrome: a neuropathological study of two siblings. Dev Med Child Neurol 25:232–239.

Hayashi N, Tsutsumi Y, Barkovich A J 2002 Morphological features and associated anomalies of schizencephaly in the clinical population: detailed analysis of MR images. Neuroradiology 44:418–427.

Hehr U, Hehr A, Uyanik G et al 2006 A filamin A splice site mutation resulting in a syndrome of facial dysmorphism, periventricular nodular heterotopia and severe constipation reminiscent of cerebro-fronto-facial syndrome. J Med Genet 43:541–544.

Helwig U, Imai K, Schmahl W et al 1995 Interaction between undulated and Patch leads to an extreme form of spina bifida in double-mutant mice. Nat Genet 11:60–63.

Higginbottom M C, Jones K L, Hall B D, Smith D W 1979 The amniotic band disruption complex: timing of amniotic rupture and variable spectra of consequent defects. J Pediatr 95:544–549.

Hilburger A C, Willis J K, Bouldin E, Henderson-Tilton A 1993 Familial schizencephaly. Brain Dev 15:234–236.

Hockey A, Crowhurst J, Cullity G 1988 Microcephaly, holoprosencephaly, hypokinesia — second report of a new syndrome. Prenat Diagn 8:683–686.

Hol F A, Schepens M T, van Beersum S E et al 2000 Identification and characterization of an Xq26-q27 duplication in a family with spina bifida and panhypopituitarism suggests the involvement of two distinct genes. Genomics 69:174–181.

Hong S E, Shugart Y Y, Huang D T et al 2000 Autosomal recessive lissencephaly with cerebellar hypoplasia is associated with human RELN mutations. Nat Genet 26:93–96.

Hosley M A, Abroms I F, Ragland R L 1992 Schizencephaly: case report of familial incidence. Pediatr Neurol 8:148–150.

Hourihane J O, Bennett C P, Chaudhuri R et al 1993 A sibship with a neuronal migration defect, cerebellar hypoplasia and congenital lymphedema. Neuropediatrics 24:43–46.

Illarioshkin S N, Tanaka H, Markova E D et al 1996 X-linked nonprogressive congenital cerebellar hypoplasia: clinical description and mapping to chromosome Xq. Ann Neurol 40:75–83.

Jackson A P, Eastwood H, Bell S M et al 2002 Identification of microcephalin, a protein implicated in determining the size of the human brain. Am J Hum Genet 71:136–142.

Jansen A, Andermann E 2005 Genetics of the polymicrogyria syndromes. J Med Genet 42:369–378.

Johnsen S D, Tarby T J, Lewis K S et al 2002 Cerebellar infarction: an unrecognised complication of very low birthweight. J Child Neurol 17:320–324.

Johnson W G, Murphy M, Murphy W I et al 1978 Recessive congenital cerebellar disorder in a genetic isolate: CPD type VII? Neurology 28:352–353.

Kato M, Das S, Petras K et al 2004 Mutations of ARX are associated with striking pleiotropy and consistent genotype-phenotype correlation. Hum Mutat 23:147–159.

Kenwrick S, Jouet M, Donnai D 1996 X-linked hydrocephalus and MASA syndrome. J Med Genet 33:59–65.

Kitamura K, Yanazawa M, Sugiyama N et al 2002 Mutation of ARX causes abnormal development of forebrain and testes in mice and X-linked lissencephaly with abnormal genitalia in humans. Nat Genet 32:359–369.

Kobayashi K, Nakahori Y, Miyake M et al 1998 An ancient retrotransposal insertion causes Fukuyama-type congenital muscular dystrophy. Nature 394:388–392.

Kumar A, Blanton S H, Babu M et al 2004 Genetic analysis of primary microcephaly in Indian families: novel ASPM mutations. Clin Genet 66:341–348.

Leventer R J, Cardoso C, Ledbetter D H et al 2001 LIS1 missense mutations cause milder lissencephaly phenotypes including a child with normal IQ. Neurology 57:416–422.

Leventer R J, Lese C M, Cardoso C et al 2001 A study of 220 patients with polymicrogyria delineates distinct phenotypes and reveals genetic loci on chromosomes 1p, 2p, 6q, 21q and 22q. Am J Hum Genet (Suppl 4) 69:177.

Lo Nigro C, Chong S S, Smith A C M et al 1997 Point mutations and an intragenic deletion in LIS1, the causative gene in isolated lissencephaly sequence and Miller–Dieker syndrome. Hum Mol Genet 6:157–164.

Longman C, Brockington M, Torelli S et al 2003 Mutations in the human LARGE gene cause MDC1D, a novel form of congenital muscular dystrophy with severe mental retardation and abnormal glycosylation of alpha-dystroglycan. Hum Mol Genet 12:2853–2861.

Lynch S A 2005 Non-multifactorial neural tube defects. Am J Med Genet 135C:69–76.

McHale D P, Jackson A P, Campbell D A et al 2000 A gene for ataxic cerebral palsy maps to chromosome 9p12-q13. Eur J Hum Genet 8:267–272.

McMorrow L E, Toth I R, Gluckson M M et al 1987 A lethal presentation of de novo deletion 7q. J Med Genet 24:629–631.

Mancini G M S, de Coo I F M, Lequin M H et al 2004 Hereditary porencephaly: clinical and MRI findings in two Dutch families. Eur J Pediatr Neurol 8:45–54.

Matsumotu N, Leventer R J, Kuc J A et al 2001 Mutation analysis of the DCX gene and genotype/phenotype correlation in subcortical band heterotopia. Eur J Hum Genet 9:5–12.

Matsunaga E, Shiota K 1977 Holoprosencephaly in human embryos: epidemiologic study of 150 cases. Teratology 16:261–272.

Merlob P, Steier D, Reisner S H 1988 Autosomal dominant isolated ('uncomplicated') microcephaly. J Med Genet 25:750–753.

Ming J E, Kaupas M E, Roessler E et al 2002 Mutations in PATCHED-1 the receptor for Sonic Hedgehog, are associated with holoprosencephaly. Hum Genet 110:297–301.

Moeschler J B, Marin-Padilla M 1989 Autosomal recessive encephaloclastic proliferative vasculopathy (hydrocephaly/hydranencephaly). Am J Hum Genet 45:A55.

Moog U, Jones M C, Bird L M, et al 2005 Oculocerebrocutaneous syndrome: the brain malformation defines a core phenotype. J Med Genet 42:913–921.

Moro F, Carrozzo R, Veggiotti P et al 2002 Familial periventricular heterotopia: missense and distal truncating mutations of the FLN1 gene. Neurology 58:916–921.

MRC Vitamin Study Research Group 1991 Prevention of neural tube defects: results of the Medical Research Council vitamin study. Lancet 338:131–137.

Muenke M, Gurrieri F, Bay C et al 1994 Linkage of a human malformation, familial holoprosencephaly to chromosome 7 and evidence for genetic heterogeneity. Proc Natl Acad Sci USA 91: 8102–8106.

Murray J C, Johnson J A, Bird T D 1985 Dandy–Walker malformation: etiologic heterogeneity and empiric recurrence risks. Clin Genet 28:272–283.

Neal J, Apse K, Sahin M et al 2006 Deletion of chromosome 1p36 is associated with periventricular nodular heterotopia. Am J Med Genet 140A:1692–1695.

Norman R M 1940 Primary degeneration of the granular layer of the cerebellum: an unusual form of familial cerebellar atrophy occurring in early life. Brain 63:365–374.

Norman A M, Donnai D 1992 Hypoplastic thumbs and hydranencephaly: a new syndrome? Clin Dysmorphol 1:121–123.

Norman M G, McGillivray B C, Karlousek D K et al 1995 Congenital malformations of the brain. Oxford University Press, New York.

Nyberg D A, Mahony B S, Hegge F N et al 1991 Enlarged cisterna magna and Dandy–Walker malformation: factors associated with chromosome abnormalities. Obstet Gynecol 77:436–442.

Odent S, Attie-Bitach T, Blayau M et al 1999) Expression of the Sonic Hedgehog (SHH) gene during early human development and phenotypic expression of new mutations causing holoprosencephaly. Hum Mol Genet 8:1683–1689.

Olsen C L, Hughes J P, Youngblood L G, Sharpe-Stimac M 1997 Epidemiology of holoprosencephaly and phenotypic characteristics of affected children: New York State, 1984–1989. Am J Med Genet 73:217–226.

Ouspenskaia M V, Karkera J D, Roessler E et al 2002 Role of FAST1 gene in the development of holoprosencephaly (HPE) and congenital cardiac malformations in humans. Am J Hum Genet 71 (Suppl):313.

Parrini E, Mei D, Wright M et al 2004 Mosaic mutations of the FLN1 gene cause a mild phenotype in patients with periventricular nodular heterotopia. Neurogenetics 5:191–196.

Parrini E, Ramazzotti A, Dobyns W B et al 2006 Periventricular heterotopia: phenotypic heterogeneity and correlation with filamin A mutations. Brain 129:1892–1906.

Pascual-Castroviejo I, Pascual-Pascual S I, Quijano-Roy S et al 2006 Cerebellar ataxia of Norman-Jaeken. Presentation of seven Spanish patients. Rev Neurol 42:723–728.

Philip N, Chabrol B, Lossi A-M et al 2003 Mutations in the oligophrenin-1 gene (OPHN1) cause X linked congenital cerebellar hypoplasia. J Med Genet 40:441–446.

Piao X, Hill R S, Bodell A, et al 2004 G protein-coupled receptor-dependent development of human frontal cortex. Science 303:2033–2036.

Pilz D T, Kuc J, Matsumoto N et al 1999 Subcortical band heterotopia in rare affected males can be caused by missense mutations in DCX (XLIS) or LIS1. Hum Mol Genet 8:1757–1760.

Pilz D T, Matsumoto N, Minnerath S et al 1998 LIS1 and XLIS (DCX) mutations cause most lissencephaly, but different patterns of malformation. Hum Mol Genet 7:2029–2037.

Pollin T I, Dobyns W B, Crowe C A et al 1999) Risk of abnormal pregnancy outcome in carriers of balanced reciprocal translocations involving the Miller–Dieker syndrome (MDS) critical region in chromosome 17p13.3. Am J Med Genet 85:369–375.

Poolos N P, Das S, Clark G D et al 2002 Males with epilepsy, complete subcortical band heterotopia, and somatic mosaicism for DCX. Neurology 58:1559–1562.

Poussaint T Y, Fox J W, Dobyns W B et al 2000 Periventricular nodular heterotopia in patients with

filamin-1 gene mutations: neuroimaging findings. Pediatr Radiol 30:748–755.

Quaderi N A, Schweiger S, Gaudenz K et al 1997 Opitz G/BBB syndrome, a defect of midline development, is due to mutations in a new RING finger gene on Xp22. Nat Genet 17:285–291.

Reiner O, Carrozzo R, Shen Y et al 1993 Isolation of a Miller–Dieker lissencephaly gene containing G protein beta–subunit-like repeats. Nature 364:717–721.

Rivier F, Echenne B 1992 Dominantly inherited hypoplasia of the vermis. Neuropediatrics 23:206–208.

Robain O 1996 Introduction to the pathology of cerebral cortical dysplasia. In Guerrini R, Andermann F, Canapicchi R et al (eds) Dysplasias of cerebral cortex and epilepsy. Lipincott-Raven, Philadelphia, 1–9.

Roberts E, Hampshire D J, Pattison L et al 2003). Autosomal recessive primary microcephaly: an analysis of locus heterogeneity and phenotypic variation. J Med Genet 39:718–721.

Robertson S P, Twigg S R, Sutherland-Smith A J et al 2003 Localized mutations in the gene encoding the cytoskeletal protein filamin A cause diverse malformations in humans. Nat Genet 33:487–491.

Robin N H, Taylor C J, McDonald-McGinn D M et al 2006 Polymicrogyria and deletion 22q11.2 syndrome: window to the etiology of a common cortical malformation. Am J Med Genet A 140:2416–2425.

Robinson R O 1991 Familial schizencephaly. Dev Med Child Neurol 33:1010–1014.

Rodríguez Cradio G, Pérez Aytés A 1999 Moebius sequence, hypogenitalism, cerebral, and skeletal malformations in two brothers. Am J Med Genet 86:492–496.

Roessler E, Belloni E, Gaudenz K et al 1996 Mutations in the human Sonic Hedgehog gene cause holoprosencephaly. Nat Genet 14:357–360.

Roessler E, Belloni E, Gaudenz K et al 1997 Mutations in the C-terminal domain of Sonic Hedgehog cause holoprosencephaly. Hum Mol Genet 6:1847–1853.

Roessler E, Du Y Z, Mullor J L et al 2003 Loss-of-function mutations in the human GLI2 gene are associated with pituitary anomalies and holoprosencephaly-like features. Proc Natl Acad Sci U S A 100:13424–13429.

Roll P, Rudolf G, Pereira S et al 2006 SRPX2 mutation in disorders of language cortex and cognition. Hum Mol Genet 15:1195–1207.

Rooms L, Reyniers E, van Luijk R et al 2004 Subtelomeric deletions detected in patients with idiopathic mental retardation using multiplex ligation-dependent proble amplification (MLPA). Hum Mut 23:17–21.

Rosenthal A, Jouet M, Kenwrick S 1992 Aberrant splicing of neural cell adhesion molecular L1 mRNA in a family with X-linked hydrocephalus. Nat Genet 2:107–112.

Rossi L N, Candini G, Scarlatti G 1987 Autosomal dominant microcephaly without mental retardation. Am J Dis Child 141:655–659.

Samson G, Gardner J C 1996 Craniosynostosis, microcephaly, hydranencephaly, humero-radial synostosis, and thumb aplasia: a new syndrome. Am J Med Genet 61:174–177.

Sismani C, Armour J A, Flint J et al 2001 Screening for subtelomeric chromosome abnormalities in children with idiopathic mental retardation using multiprobe telomeric FISH and the new MAPH telomeric assay. Eur J Hum Genet 9:527–532.

Sensi A, Cerruti S, Calzolari E et al 1990 Familial porencephaly. Clin Genet 38:396–400.

Shaw-Smith C, Redon R, Rickman L et al 2004 Microarray based comparative genomic hybridisation (array-CGH) detects submicroscopic chromosomal deletions and duplications in patients with learning disability/mental retardation and dysmorphic features. J Med Genet 41:241–248.

Sheen V L, Dixon P H, Fox J W et al 2001 Mutations in the X-linked filamin 1 gene cause periventricular nodular heterotopia in males as well as females. Hum Mol Genet 10:1775–1783.

Sheen V L, Jansen A, Chen M H et al 2005 Filamin A mutations cause periventricular heterotopia with Ehlers–Danlos syndrome. Neurology 64:254–262.

Sheen V L, Wheless J W, Bodell A et al 2003 Periventricular heterotopra associated with chromosome Sp anomalies. Neurology 60:1033–1036.

Smit L M E, Barth P G, Valk J, Nijiokiktjien C 1984 Familial porencephalic white matter disease in two generations. Brain Dev 6:54–58.

Steinlin M 1998 Non-progressive congenital ataxia. Brain Dev 20:199–208.

Steinlin M, Blaser S, Boltshauser E 1998 Cerebellar involvement in metabolic disorders: a pattern-recognition approach. Neuroradiology 40:347–354.

Suri M 2005 The phenotypic spectrum of ARX mutations. Dev Med Child Neurol 47:133–137.

Taylor A I 1968 Autosomal trisomy syndromes: a detailed study of 27 cases of Edwards' syndrome and 27 cases of Patau's syndrome. J Med Genet 5:227–252.

Thauvin-Robinet C, Rousseau T, Durand C et al 2001). Familial orofaciodigital syndrome type I revealed by ultrasound prenatal diagnosis of porencephaly. Prenat Diagn 21:466–470.

Tietjen I, Erdogan F, Currier S et al 2005 EMX2-independent familial schizencephaly: clinical and genetic analyses. Am J Med Genet 132A:166–170.

Tolmie J L, McNay M, Stephenson J B P et al 1987 Microcephaly: genetic counseling and antenatal diagnosis after the birth of an affected child. Am J Med Genet 27:583–594.

Toriello H V 1984 Report of a third kindred with X-linked anencephaly/spina bifida. Am J Med Genet 19:411–412.

Toyo-oka K, Shionoya A, Gambello M J et al 2003 14-3-3-epsilon is important for neuronal migration by binding to NUDEL: a molecular explanation for Miller–Dieker syndrome. Nat Genet 34:274–285.

Tsao J W, Neal J, Apse K et al 2006 Cerebellar ataxia with progressive improvement. Arch Neurol 63:594–597.

Usta I M, AbuMusa A A, Khoury et al 2005 Early ultrasonographic changes in Fowler syndrome features and review of the literature. Prenat Diagn 25:1019–1023.

van der Knaap M S, Smit L M E, Barkhof F et al 2006 Neonatal porencephaly and adult stroke related to mutations in collagen IV A1. Ann Neurol 59:504–511.

Van der Put N M J, Gabreëls F, Stevens E M B et al 1998 A second common mutation in the methylenetetrahydrofolate reductase gene: an additional risk factor for neural-tube defects? Am J Hum Genet 62:1044–1051.

Van Reeuwijk J, Brunner H G, van Bokhoven H 2004 Glyc-O-genetics of Walker–Warburg syndrome. Clin Genet 67:281–289.

van Reeuwijk J, Janssen M, van den Elzen C et al 2005 POMT2 mutations cause alpha- dystroglycan hypoglycosylation and Walker–Warburg syndrome. J Med Genet 42:907–912.

Váradi V, Tóth Z, Török O, Papp Z 1988. Heterogeneity and recurrence risk for congenital hydrocephalus (ventriculomegaly): a prospective study. Am J Med Genet 30:305–310.

Veltman J A, Schoenmakers E F P M, Eussen B H et al 2002 High-throughput analysis of subtelomeric chromosome rearrangements by use of array-based comparative genomic hybridization. Am J Hum Genet 70:1269–1276.

Vilain C, van Regemorter N, Verloes A et al 2002 Neuroimaging fails to identify asymptomatic carriers of familial porencephaly. Am J Med Genet 112, 198–202.

Villard L, Nguyen K, Cardoso C et al 2002 A locus for bilateral perisylvian polymicrogyria maps to Xq28. Am J Hum Genet 70:1003–1008.

Vissers L E L M, de Vries B B A, Osoegawa K et al 2003 Array-based comparative genomic hybridization for the genomewide detection of submicroscopic chromosomal abnormalities. Am J Hum Genet 73:1261–1270.

Wallis D E, Roessler E, Hehr U et al 1999 Mutations in the homeodomain of the human SIX3 gene cause holoprosencephaly. Nat Genet 22:196–198.

Wassmer E, Davies P, Whitehouse W P et al 2003 Clinical spectrum associated with cerebellar hypoplasia. Pediatr Neurol 28:347–351.

Weller S, Gärtner J 2001 Genetic and clinical aspects of X-linked hydrocephalus (L1 disease): mutations in the L1CAM gene. Hum Mutation 18:1–12.

Whiteford M L, Tolmie J L 1996 Holoprosencephaly in the West of Scotland 1975–1994. J Med Genet 33:578–584.

Wichman A, Frank L M, Kelly T E 1985 Autosomal recessive congenital cerebellar hypoplasia. Clin Genet 27:373–382.

Wieck G, Leventer R J, Squier W M et al 2005 Periventricular nodular heterotopia with overlying polymicrogyria. Brain 128:2811–2821.

Winter R M, Baraitser M 2006 Winter-Baraitser Dysmorphology Database. Version 1.0.9. London Medical Databases.

Witters I, Moerman P, Devriendt K et al 2002 Two siblings with early onset fetal akinesia deformation sequence and hydranencephaly: further evidence for autosomal recessive inheritance of hydranencephaly, Fowler type. Am J Med Genet 108:41–44.

Yoshida A, Kobayashi K, Manya H et al 2001 Muscular dystrophy and neuronal migration disorder caused by mutations in a glycosyltransferase, POMGnT1. Dev Cell 1:717–724.

Zenker M, Rauch A, Winterpacht A et al 2004 A dual phenotype of periventricular nodular heterotopia and frontometaphyseal dysplasia in one patient caused by a single FLNA mutation leading to two functionally different aberrant transcripts. Am J Hum Genet 74:731–737.

Zlotogora J 1995 Major gene is responsible for anencephaly among Iranian Jews. Am J Med Genet 56:87–89.

Zonana J, Adornato B T, Glass S T, Webb M J 1986 Familial porencephaly and congenital hemiplegia. J Pediatr 109:671–674.

CHAPTER
15

Antenatal assessment of CNS anomalies, including neural tube defects

Ritsuko K. Pooh and KyongHon Pooh

Key Points

- Fetus
- Central nervous system
- 3D ultrasound
- MRI
- Neuroimaging
- Congenital anomaly

INTRODUCTION

During the fetal period, the embryonal premature CNS structure rapidly develops into a mature structure with gyral formation. During this rapid change of development, various developmental disorders and/or insults result in various phenotypes of fetal CNS abnormalities. To understand fetal CNS diseases, basic knowledge of the development of the nervous system is essential. The cerebral developmental stages and major disorders are described in Table 15.1.

Recent advanced technologies of high-frequency transvaginal ultrasound (Monteagudo et al 1991, 1994, 1997, Pooh et al 1996, 1998, 1999c, Timor-Tritsch et al 1996), three-dimensional (3D) ultrasound (Monteagudo et al 2000, Pooh and Pooh 2000, 2001, 2002, Timor-Tritsch et al 2000), and magnetic resonance imaging (MRI) (Garel 2006, Glenn

and Barkovich 2006, Pooh et al 2006, Raybaud et al 2003) have revealed detailed and objective structures of many CNS congenital abnormalities. The more improved the technologies, the more new findings in utero are discovered. In this chapter, we describe CNS abnormalities in utero which can be prenatally detected using transabdominal/transvaginal sonography, 3D ultrasound and MRI.

NURAL TUBE DEFECTS

CRANIUM BIFIDUM

Cranium bifidum is classified into four types of encephaloschisis (including anencephaly and exencephaly), meningocele, encephalomeningocele, encephalocystocele and cranium bifidum occultum. Encephalocele occurs in the occipital region in 70–80%. Acrania, exencephaly and anencephaly are not independent anomalies. It is considered that dysraphia (absent cranial vault, acrania) occurs at a very early stage and disintegration of the exposed brain (exencephaly) during the fetal period results in anencephaly (Monteagudo and Timor-Tritsch 2001).

Prevalence: anencephaly is 0.29/1000 births (Martinez de Villarreal et al 2002), overall neural tube defect (NTD) is 0.58–1.17/1000 births (Mathews et al 2002, Persad et al 2002, Ray et al 2002). Many authors reported remarkable

---

Table 15.1 Cerebral developmental stages and major disorders

Developmental stage	Disorders
Primary neurulation (3–4 weeks' gestation)	Spina bifida aperta, cranium bifidum
Caudal neural tube formation (secondary neurulation, from 4 weeks' gestation)	Occult dysraphic states
Prosencephalic development (2–3 months' gestation)	Holoprosencephaly Agenesis of the corpus callosum Agenesis of the septum pellucidum, septo-optic dysplasia
Neuronal proliferation (3–4 months' gestation)	Micrencephaly Macrencephaly
Neuronal migration (3–5 months' gestation)	Schizencephaly Lissencephaly, pachygyria Polymicrogyria Other migration disorder
Organization (5 months' gestation — years postnatal)	Idiopathic mental retardation
Myelination (5 months' gestation — years postnatal)	Cerebral white matter hypoplasia

reduction of prevalence of NTDs after using folic acid supplementation and fortification (Martinez de Villarreal et al 2002, Mathews et al 2002, Persad et al 2002, Ray et al 2002), although some reported no decline in the anencephaly rate (Green 2002).

Etiology: multifactorial inheritance, single mutant genes, specific teratogens (valproic acid), maternal diabetes, environmental factors, predominant in females.

Pathogenesis: failure of anterior neural tube closure or a restricted disorder of neurulation.

Associated anomalies: open spina bifida (iniencephaly), Chiari type III malformation, bilateral renal cystic dysplasia and postaxial polydactyly with occipital cephalocele (Meckel–Gruber syndrome), hydrocephalus and polyhydramnios.

Prenatal diagnosis: acrania in Figure 15.1, anencephaly in Figure 15.2, encephalocele in Figure 15.3 and early detection of iniencephaly with acrania in Figure 15.4.

Differential diagnosis: amniotic band syndrome (ABS). In cases of ABS, cranial destruction occurs secondarily to an amniotic band, similar appearance is observed (Fig. 15.5). However, ABS has completely different pathogenesis from acrania/exencephaly.

Prognosis: anencephaly is a uniformly lethal anomaly. Other types of cranium bifidum, various neurological deficits may occur, depending on types and degrees.

Recurrence risk: used to be high recurrence risk of 5–13%, however, recently declined by use of folic acid supplementation and fortification.

Obstetrical management: termination of pregnancy can be offered in cases with anencephaly.

Neurosurgical management: for other cranium bifidum, surgical operation aims at transposition of cerebral tissue into the intracranial cavity. Ventriculoperitoneal shunt for hydrocephalus.

SPINA BIFIDA

Spina bifida aperta, a manifest form of spina bifida, is classified into 4 types: meningocele, myelomeningocele, myelocystocele and myeloschisis. In myelomeningocele the spinal cord and its protective covering (the meninges) protrude from an opening in the spine. In meningocele, the spinal cord develops normally but the meninges protrude from a spinal opening. The most common locations of the malformations are the lumbar and sacral areas of the spinal cord.

Prevalence: 0.7–2/1000 births but certain populations have a significantly greater risk. Many reported remarkable reduction of prevalence of NTDs after using folic acid supplementation and fortification (Martinez de Villarreal et al 2002, Mathews et al 2002, Persad et al 2002, Ray et al 2002).

Etiology: multifactorial inheritance, single mutant genes, autosomal recessive, chromosomal abnormalities (trisomy 18, 13), specific teratogens (valproic acid), maternal diabetes, environmental factors and predominant in females.

Pathogenesis: spina bifida aperta; an impairment of neural tube closure; spina bifida occulta; caudal neural tube malformation by the processes of canalization and retrogressive differentiation.

Associated anomalies: Chiari type II malformation, hydrocephalus, scoliosis (above L2), kyphosis, polyhydramnios and additional non-CNS anomalies,

Prenatal diagnosis: early detection in the first trimester is possible (Fig. 15.6). Surface anatomy of the fetus and appearance of clubfoot, which occasionally manifests from middle gestation, are identifiable using 3D ultrasound (Fig. 15.7). 3D ultrasound, with maximum mode, can demonstrate bony structures (Figs 15.8 and 15.9) and is helpful in detecting the spinal levels of lesions and enabling neurological prognosis prediction. Figure 15.10 shows a case of meningocele. Because in more than 80% of cases with open spina bifida, ventriculomegaly is apparent during pregnancy due to Chiari type II malformation, spina bifida is detected in many cases, following demonstration of ventriculomegaly.

Differential diagnosis: sacrococcygeal teratoma.

Prognosis: disturbance of motor, sensory and sphincter function; depends on lesion levels. Below S1: able to walk unaided, above L2: wheelchair dependent, variable at intermediate level.

Recurrence risk: decreased, almost no recurrence rate by use of folic acid supplementation and fortification (Stevenson et al 2000).

Obstetrical management: Delivery mode is controversial. Cesarean delivery has been advocated as being superior to vaginal delivery in preventing further neurologic damage in fetuses with antenatally diagnosed myelomeningocele (Luthy et al 1991). However, no difference of motor function or ambulation status is shown when the data is stratified by route of delivery (Lewis et al 2004, Merrill et al 1998).

Text continued on p. 299

Figure 15.1 Acrania in the first trimester. (upper left) Coronal image at 10 weeks. Note the normal appearance of amniotic membrane, which indicates this condition is not amniotic band syndrome. (upper middle and right) Sagittal and coronal images of acrania at 12 weeks. (lower left) 3D sonographic image of acrania at 10 weeks. (lower middle) 3D sonographic image of acrania at 14 weeks. (lower right) Macroscopic picture of acrania from an aborted fetus at 12 weeks of gestation.

Figure 15.2 Anencephaly in middle gestation. (same case as Fig. 15.1 left) (upper left) US sagittal image at 23 weeks of gestation. (upper middle) US coronal image. (upper right) 3D US image. (lower) External appearances of stillborn fetus at 25 weeks of gestation. It is clear that exencephalic brain tissue, which had existed at 10 weeks, is scattered in the amniotic space.

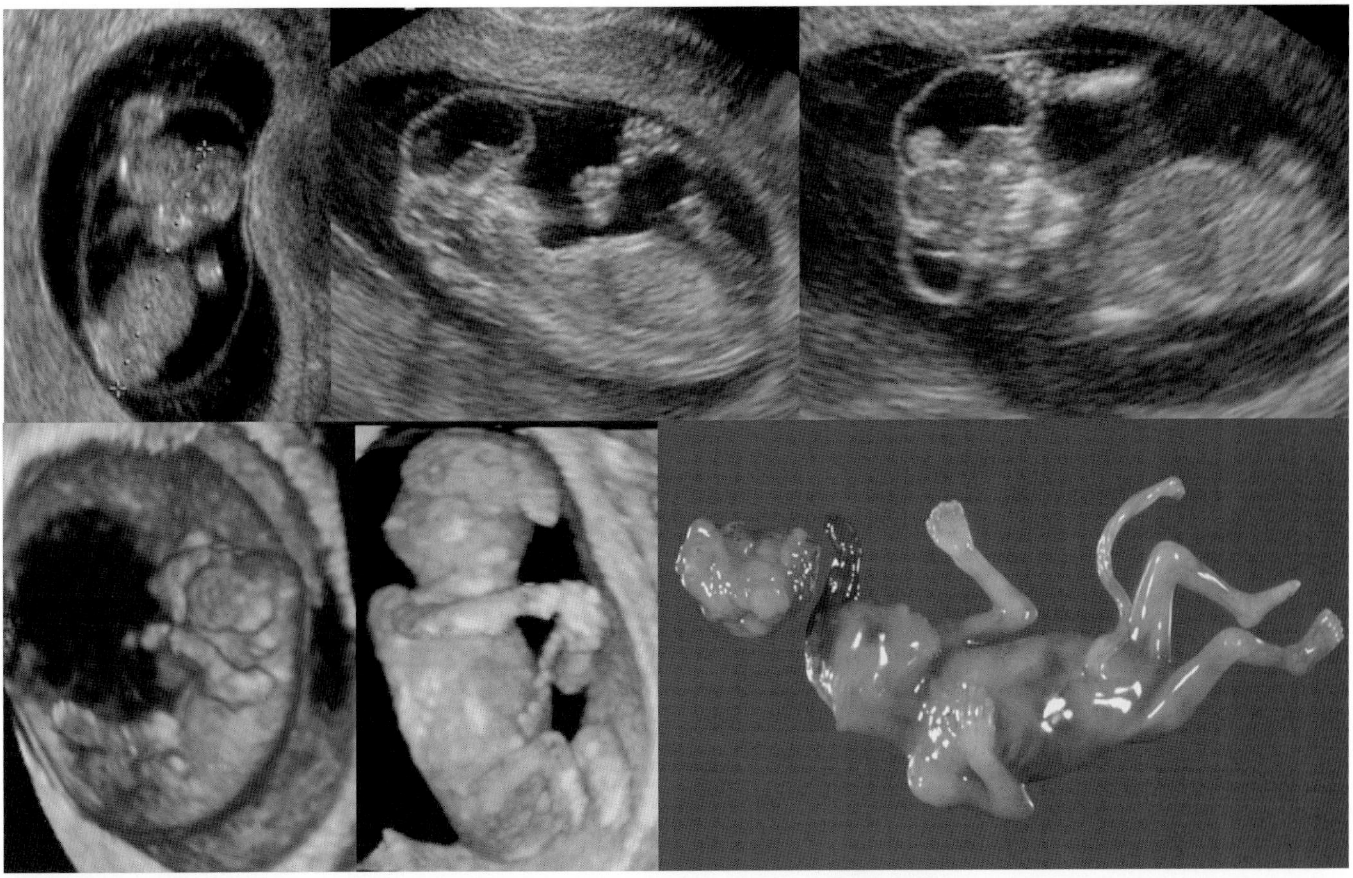

Figure 15.1

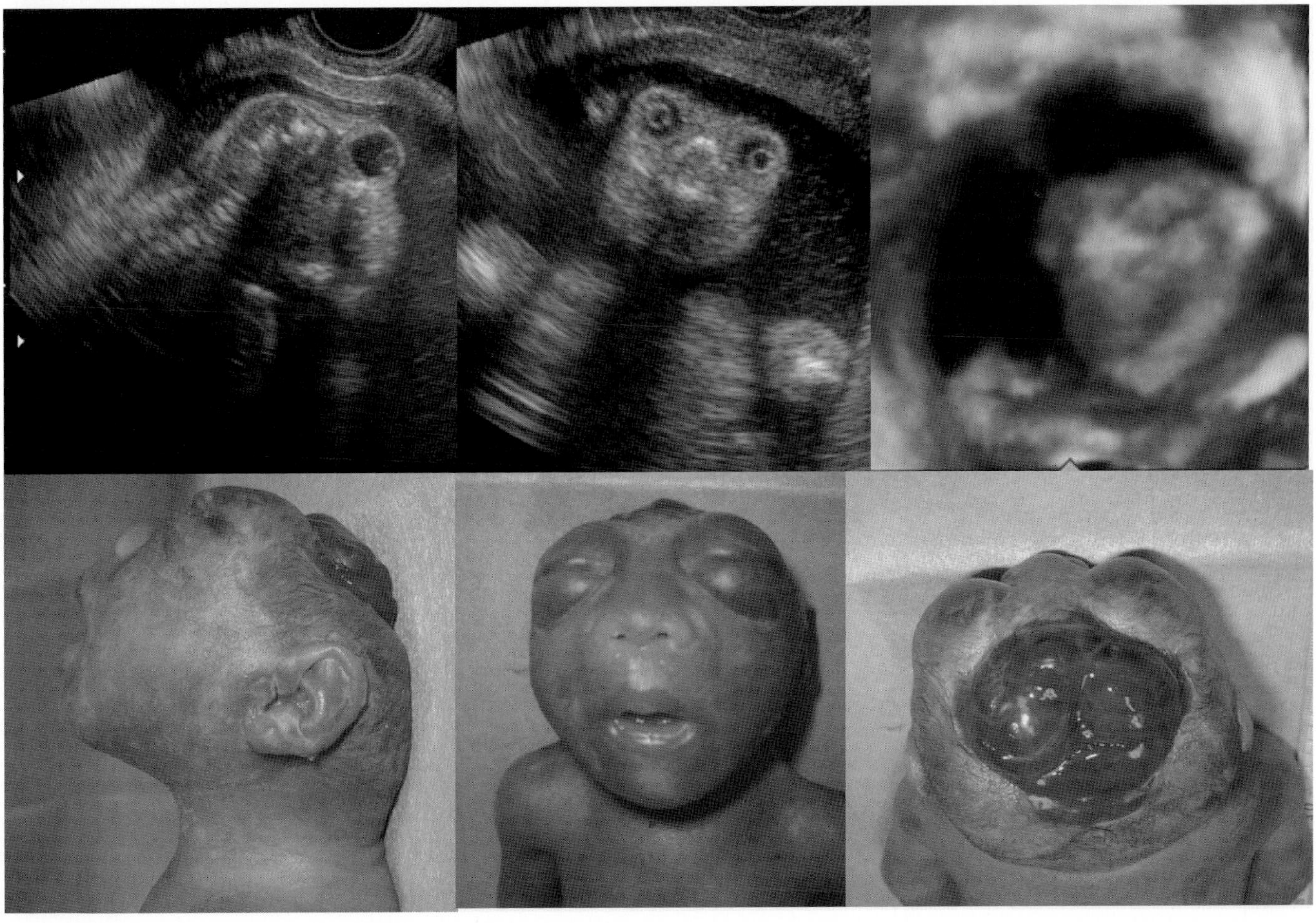

Figure 15.2

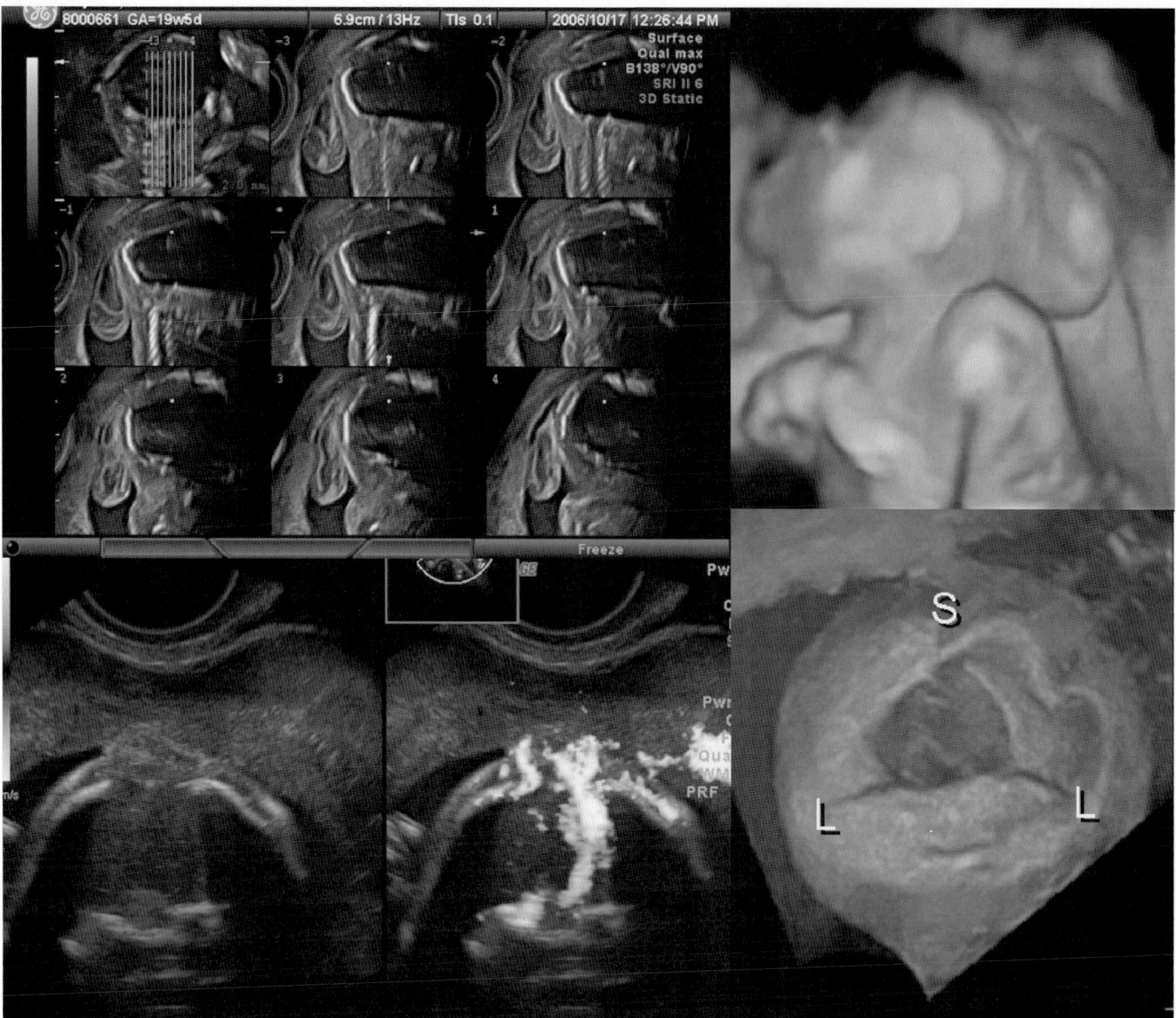

Figure 15.3 Encephalocele at 18 weeks of gestation. (upper left) Tomographic sagittal imaging of encephalocele. (upper right) 3D reconstructed image. Microcephaly and occipital encephalocele are demonstrated. (lower left) Gray scale mode and bi-directional power Doppler image of connection between intracranial brain and extracranial brain. Cerebral vessels between them are clearly visualized. (lower right) 3D maximum mode of the occipital bone defect. Ectopic cerebrum is out from this defect. S; sagittal suture, L; lambdoid suture.

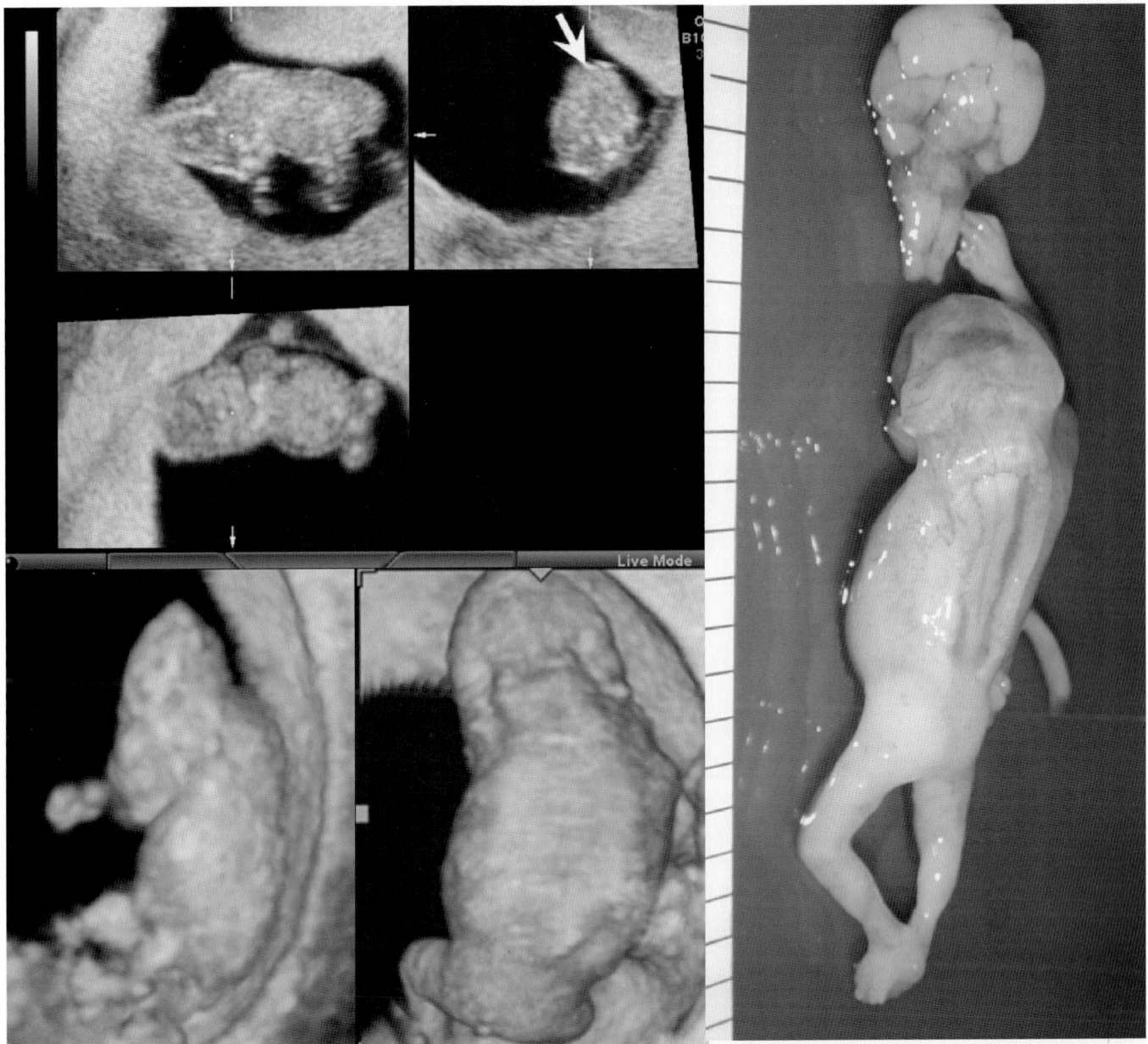

Figure 15.4 Iniencephaly and acrania at 10 weeks of gestation. (upper left) Three orthogonal view of the fetus. Spina bifida (arrow) was demonstrated in the coronal section. (lower left and middle) 3D images show the fetal lateral and dorsal views. (right) External appearance of aborted fetus. The brain and a part of spinal cord were detached at delivery.

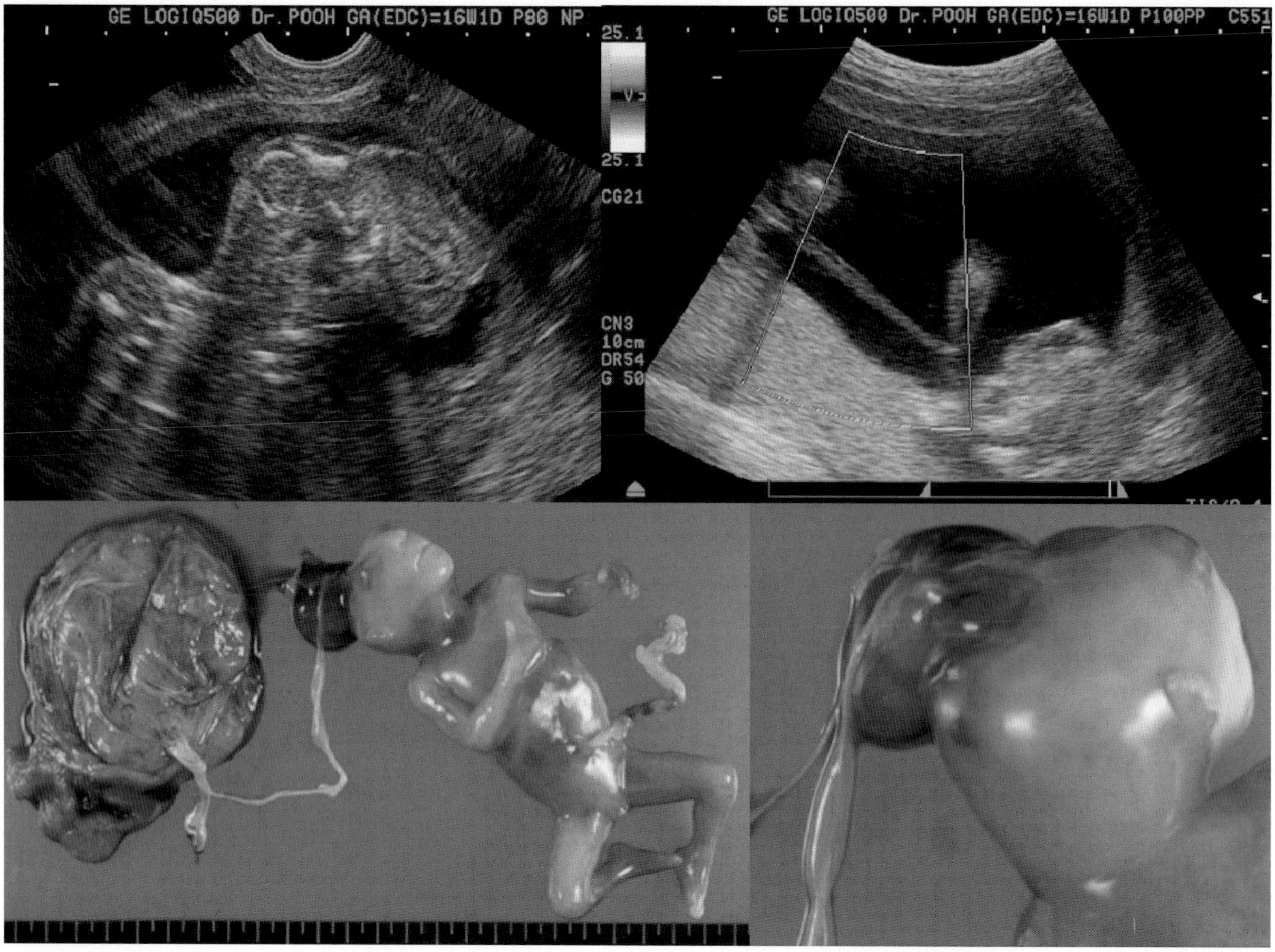

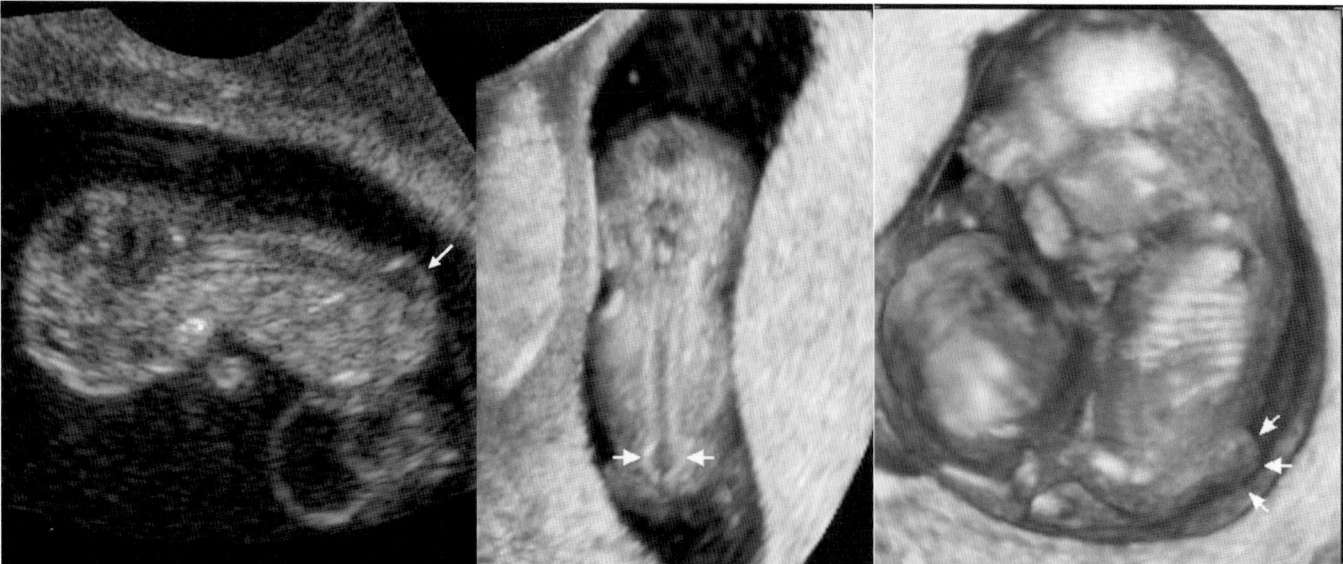

Figure 15.5 Amniotic band syndrome at 16 weeks of gestation (differentiate diagnosis from acrania). (upper left) Exencephaly with incomplete asymmetrical cranial defect. (upper right) Amniotic band between placenta and exencephalic brain. (lower left) Microscopic appearance of aborted fetus. Note the amniotic band between placenta and brain. (lower right) Magnified photograph of the head. This condition should be differentiated from neural tube defects. Amniotic band syndrome has little recurrence risk.

Figure 15.6 Myelomeningocele in the first trimester. Two dimensional US (left) and three dimensional dorsal view (middle) at 9 weeks clearly demonstrate a neural tube defect at the lower lumber level (arrows). Right figure shows the same fetus at 12 weeks of gestation. Arrows indicate the lumbar myelomeningocele.

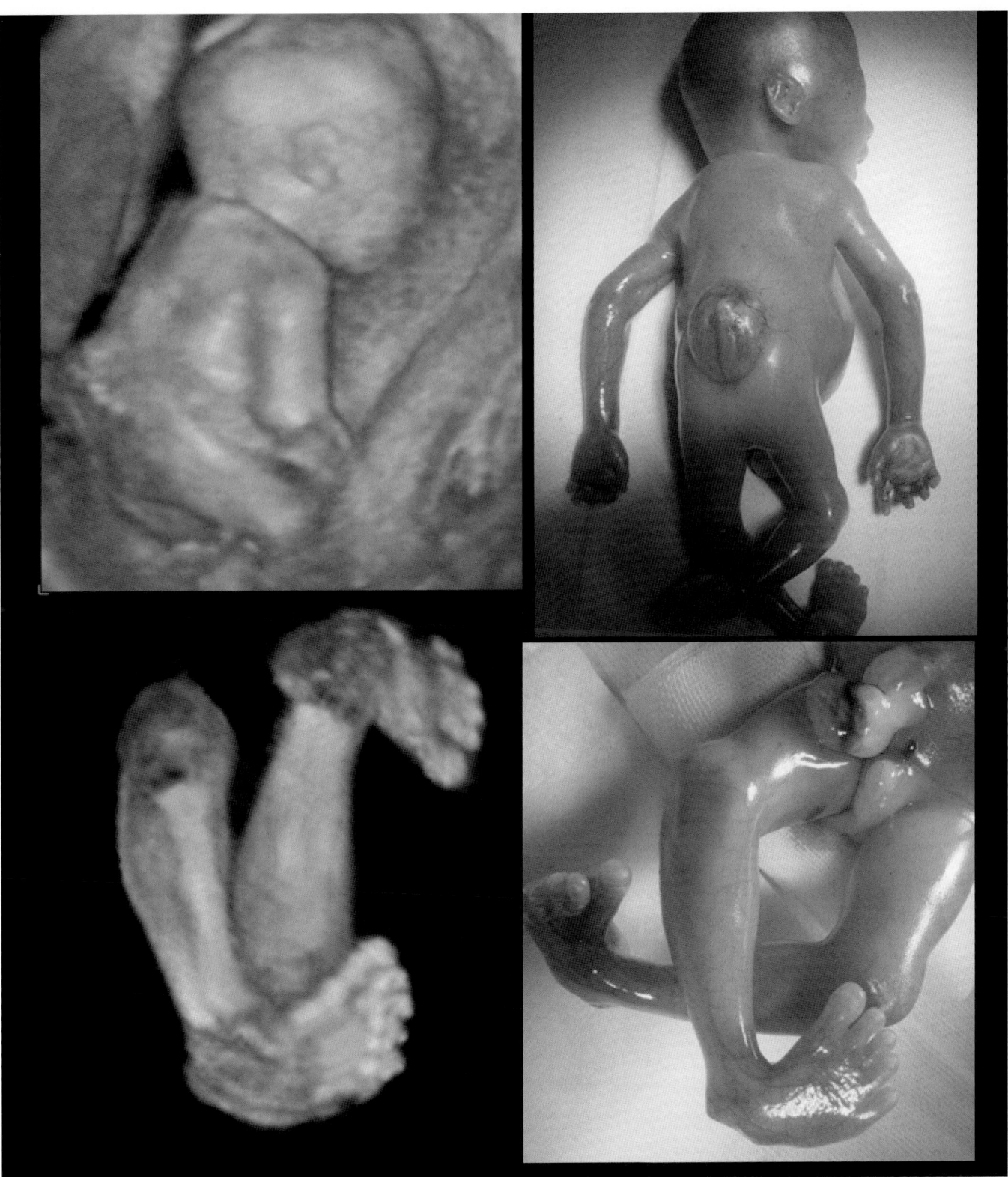

Figure 15.7 Myelomeningocele with clubfoot. (upper left) 3D image of the fetus with myelomeningocele with kyphosis at 20 weeks of gestation. (upper right) Macroscopic picture of aborted fetus at 21 weeks. Huge myelomengocele is visualized. (lower left) 3D image of the fetal legs. Severe clubfoot is demonstrated. (lower right) Appearance of lower extremities after termination of pregnancy.

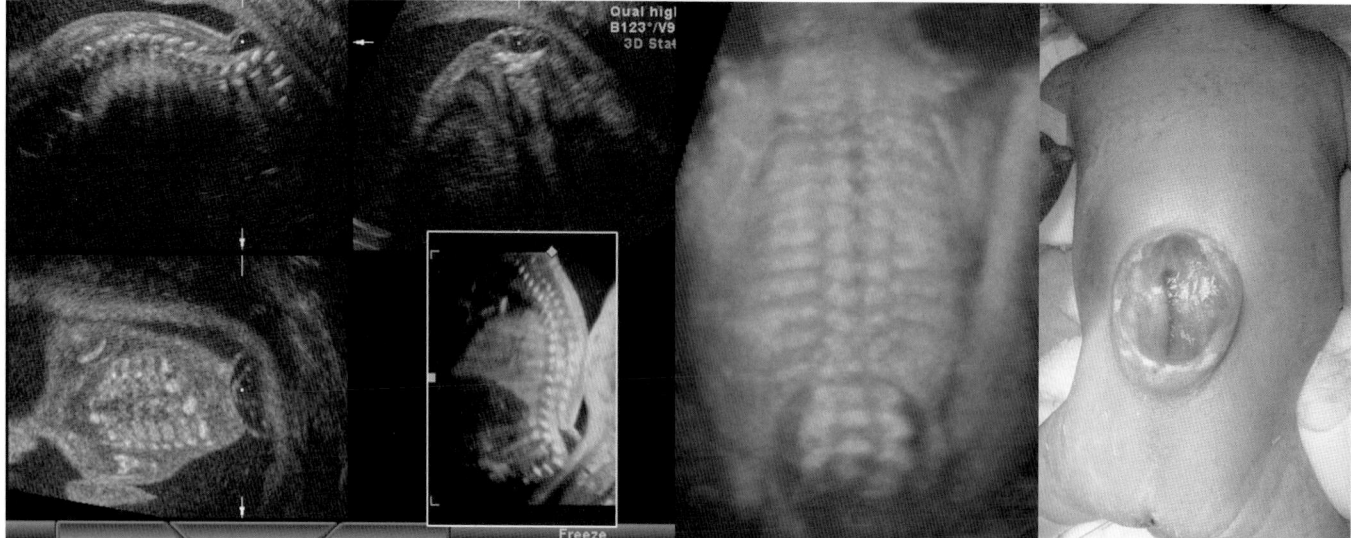

Figure 15.8 Myelomeningocele with severe kyphosis detected at 20 weeks of gestation. (left) Black-white pictures show three orthogonal view of vertebral structure and myelomeningocele with severe kyphosis. 3D reconstruction bony structure in the sagittal section clearly demonstrated the vertebral bodies. (middle) 3D surface reconstruction image of fetal back shows the large myelomeningocele from T12. (right) Macroscopic picture of the same baby born at 37 weeks.

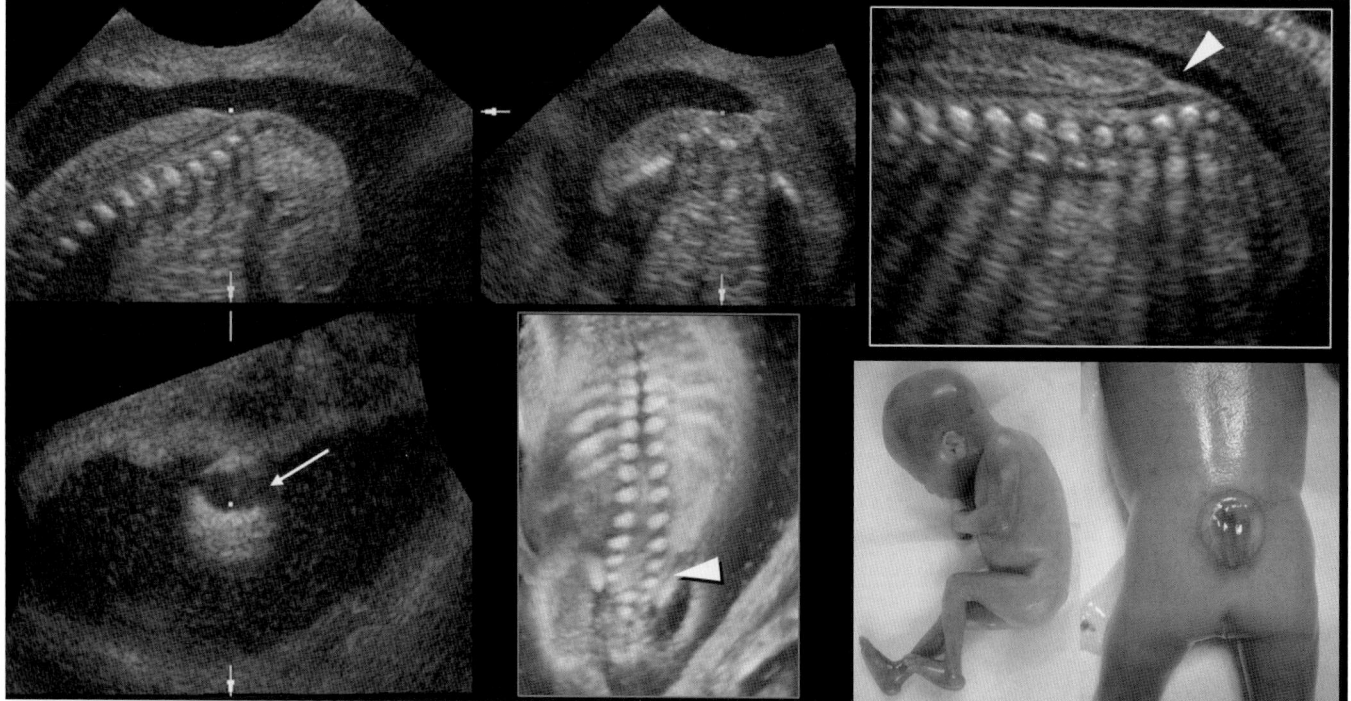

Figure 15.9 Myeloschisis detected at 18 weeks of gestation. (left) Black-white pictures show three orthogonal view of vertebral structure and myeloschisis. It is difficult to detect myeloschisis because no cyst- or meningocele is formed. Arrow indicates skin defect of lesion. 3D reconstruction bony structure shows lumbosacral spina bifida (arrowhead). (upper right) Mid sagittal section of the spine. The spinal cord runs from spinal tube directly to the surface of fetal back (arrowhead). (lower right) Macroscopic findings of aborted fetus at 21 weeks of gestation. The lesion, not demonstrated on the lateral view, is clearly visible on the posterior view.

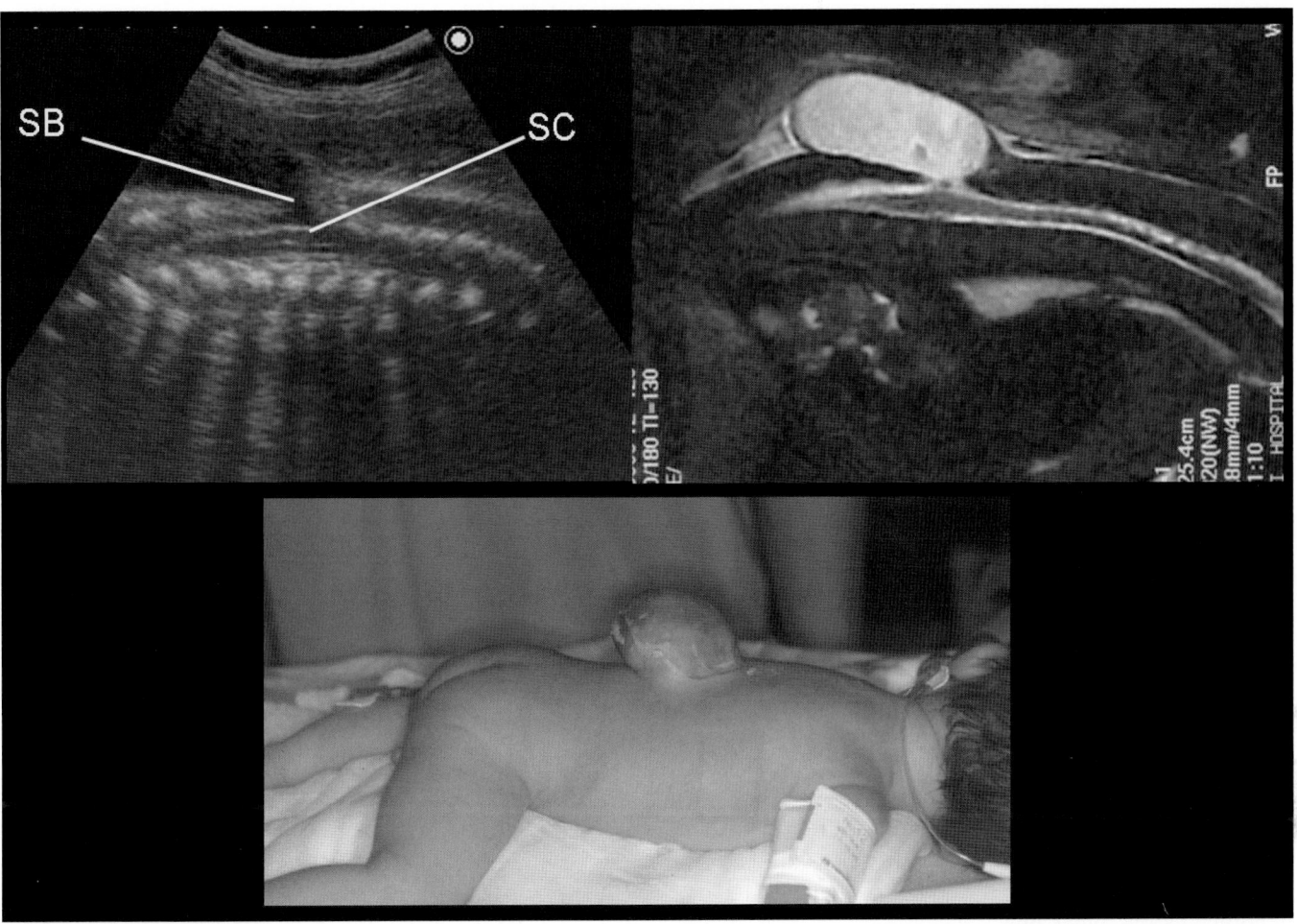

Figure 15.10 Thoracic meningocele. (upper left) Sagittal US image at 37 weeks of gestation. Spinal cord (SC) is located inside the spinal canal. Spina bifida (SB) is demonstrated. (upper right) Fetal MR sagittal image. The meninges protrude from a spinal opening and form meningocele. (lower) Postnatal appearance of meningocele, which is completely covered by skin.

Neurosurgical management: spina bifida aperta: in cases with defect of normal skin tissue, immediate closure of spina bifida after birth reduces spinal infection. Spinal cord reconstruction is the most important role of operation. Miniature Ommaya reservoir placement and subsequent ventriculoperitoneal shunt are required for hydrocephalus. For symptomatic Chiari malformation, posterior fossa decompressive craniectomy and/or tonsillectomy is performed. Spina bifida occulta: the aim of surgical treatment is decompression of the spinal cord and cutting of the tethering to the spinal cord.

HYDROCEPHALUS AND VENTRICULOMEGALY

'Hydrocephalus' and 'ventriculomegaly' are both used to describe dilatation of the lateral ventricles. However, these two conditions should be distinguished from each other. Hydrocephalus signifies dilated lateral ventricles resulting from an increased amount of CSF inside the ventricles and increased intracranial pressure, while ventriculomegaly is a dilatation of lateral ventricles without increased intracranial pressure, due to cerebral hypoplasia or CNS anomaly such

as agenesis of the corpus callosum (Pooh et al 2003, Pooh et al 1999c). Of course, ventriculomegaly can sometimes change into a hydrocephalic state. In sonographic imaging, these two intracranial conditions can be differentiated by visualization of the subarachnoid space and the appearance of the choroid plexus. Normally the condition of the subarachnoid space, visualized around both cerebral hemispheres, is well preserved during pregnancy. Choroid plexus is a soft tissue and easily affected by external pressure. Obliterated subarachnoid space and dangling choroid plexus are observed in the case of hydrocephalus. In contrast, the subarachnoid space and choroid plexus are well preserved in cases of ventriculomegaly. It is difficult to evaluate the subarachnoid space in the axial plane because the subarachnoid space is observed in the parietal side of the hemispheres. Therefore, the transabdominal approach may not differentiate accurately hydrocephalus with increased intracranial pressure from ventriculomegaly without pressure. It is suggested that the evaluation of enlarged ventricles should be done in the parasagittal and coronal views by the transvaginal approach to the fetal brain or 3D multidimensional anal-

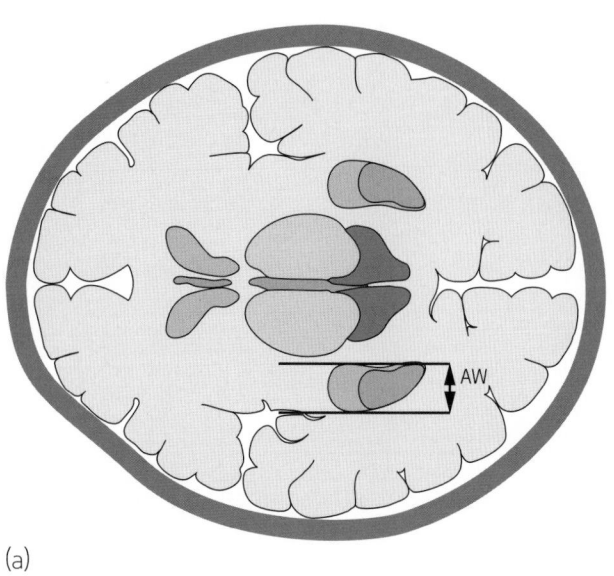

(a)

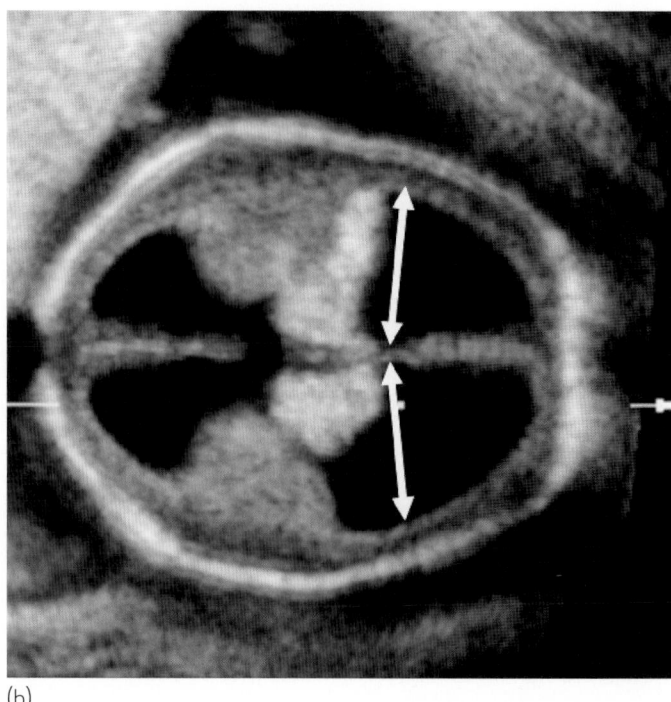

(b)

Figure 15.11 Atrial width measurement for ventriculomegaly screening.

ysis. As a screening examination of ventriculomegaly, the measurement of atrial width (AW) (Fig. 15.11) is useful with a cut-off value of 10 mm (Alagappan et al 1994, Almog et al 2003), although isolated mild ventriculomegaly with AW of 10–12 mm may be a normal variant (Signorelli et al 2004). In normal fetuses, blood flow waveforms of the dural sinuses, such as the superior sagittal sinus, vein of Galen and straight sinus, have a pulsatile pattern (Pooh et al 1999c). However, in cases with progressive hydrocephalus, normal pulsation disappears and blood flow waveforms show a flat pattern, because intracranial venous blood flow may be influenced by increased intracranial pressure (Pooh et al 1999c).

• Moderate to severe ventriculomegaly with AW >15 mm.

The term 'hydrocephalus' does not identify a specified disease, but is a generic term which designates a serial pathologic condition due to an abnormal circulation of cerebrospinal fluid (CSF). The method of treatment of hydrocephalus should be selected according to age of onset and symptoms. Congenital hydrocephalus is classified into three categories by causes which disturb the CSF circulation pathway: simple hydrocephalus, dysgenetic hydrocephalus and secondary hydrocephalus (Pooh et al 2003).

(a) Simple hydrocephalus.

Simple hydrocephalus, caused by developmental abnormality which is localized within the CSF circulation pathway, includes aqueductal stenosis, atresia of foramen Monro and maldevelopment of arachnoid granulation. Types of hydrocephalus due to various obstructive sites of CSF flow are shown in Figure 15.12.

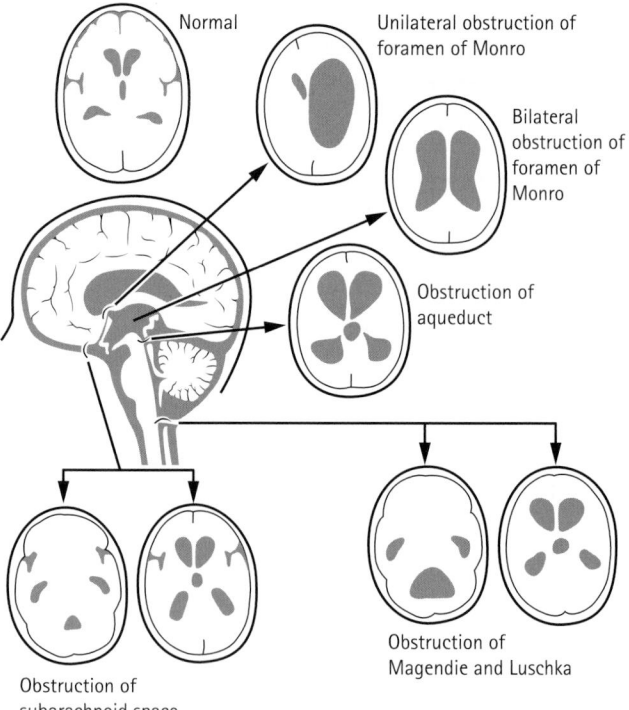

Figure 15.12 Types of hydrocephalus due to various obstructive sites of cerebrospinal fluid flow. (From Handbook on hydrocephalus for patients. Research Committee of Intractable Hydrocephalus, Japanese Ministry of Health and Welfare, ©1993, with permission: Schema by courtesy of chairman of the Committee, Professor K. Mori.)

(b) Dysgenetic hydrocephalus.

Dysgenetic hydrocephalus indicates hydrocephalus as a result of cerebral developmental disorder at an early developmental stage and includes hydranencephaly, holoprosencephaly, porencephaly, schizencephaly, Dandy–Walker malformation, dysraphism and Chiari malformation.

(c) Secondary hydrocephalus.

Secondary hydrocephalus is a generic term indicating hydrocephalus caused by an intracranial pathologic condition, such as brain tumor, intracranial infection and intracranial hemorrhage.

In cases with progressive hydrocephalus, there may be seven stages of progression: (1) increased fluid collection in the lateral ventricles, (2) increased intracranial pressure, (3) dangling choroid plexus, (4) disappearance of subarachnoid space, (5) excessive extension of the dura and superior sagittal sinus, (6) disappearance of venous pulsation and, finally, (7) enlarged skull (Pooh et al 2003). In general, both hydrocephalus and ventriculomegaly are still evaluated by the measurement of biparietal diameter (BPD) and atrial width (AW) in transabdominal axial section. As described above, however, hydrocephalus and ventriculomegaly should be differentiated from each other and the hydrocephalic state

should be assessed by the changing appearance of intracranial structure. To evaluate enlarged ventricles, examiners should carefully observe the structures below and specify the causes of hydrocephalus.

- Choroid plexus, dangling or not.
- Subarachnoid space, obliterated or not.
- Ventricles, symmetry or asymmetry.
- Visibility of third ventricle.
- Pulsation of dural sinuses.
- Ventricular size (3D volume calculation if possible).
- Other abnormalities.

Figures 15.13 to 15.15 show prenatal sonographic imaging of fetal ventriculomegaly with atrial width of over 15 mm. Although all cases have similar ventricular appearance, the causes of ventriculomegaly vary, such as Chiari type II malformation (Fig. 15.13 right), aqueductal obstruction (Fig. 15.13 left) or stenosis and cerebral hypoplasia (Fig. 15.14), or occasionally amniotic band syndrome (ABS) (Fig. 15.15). The shape of the enlarged ventricles is different in ventriculomegaly due to CSF obstruction and ventriculomegaly due to Chiari malformation. In Chari type II malformation cases, the ventricular shape is squarish and a triangle shape of enlarged ventricles is often seen in the posterior coronal section in the second trimester (Fig. 15.13). In the case of

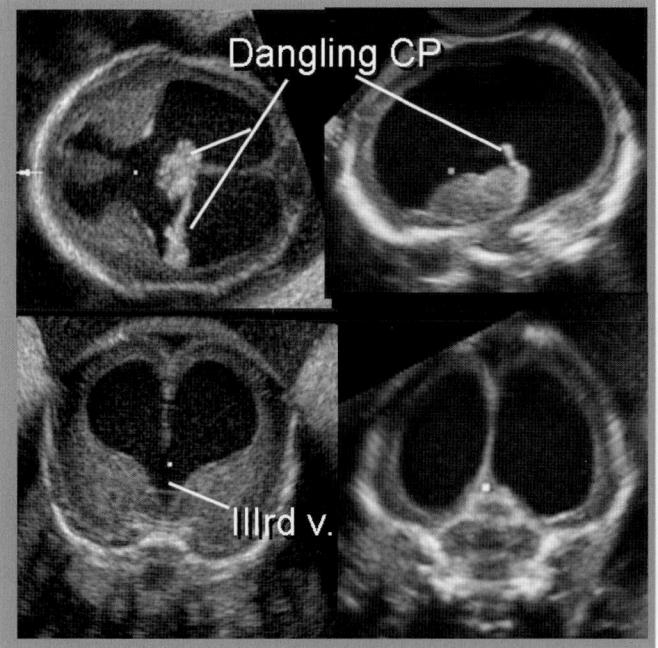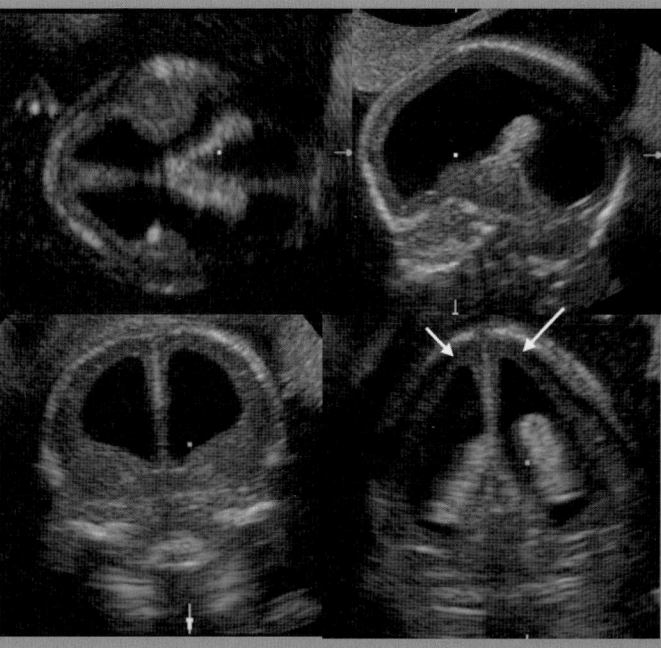

Figure 15.13 Hydrocephalus due to aqueductal obstruction (left) and Chiari type II malformation (right). (left 4 figures) Hydrocephalus due to aqueductal obstruction detected by transvaginal scan at 19 weeks of gestation. Upper left; axial section, upper right; parasagittal section, lower left; anterior coronal section, lower right; posterior coronal section. Bilateral ventriculomegaly with dilated foramen of Monro and third ventriculomegaly, with dangling choroid plexus. Note the ventricular is round shaped. (right 4 figures) Hydrocephalus due to myelomeningocele and Chiari type II malformation demonstrated by transvaginal scan at 17 weeks of gestation. Upper left; axial section, upper right; parasagittal section, lower left; anterior coronal section, lower right; posterior coronal section. Note the ventricular shape is squarish compared with ventricles in the left figures, and especially posterior coronal section; triangle shape of enlarged ventricles (arrows) is often seen in cases of Chiari II malformation in the second trimester.

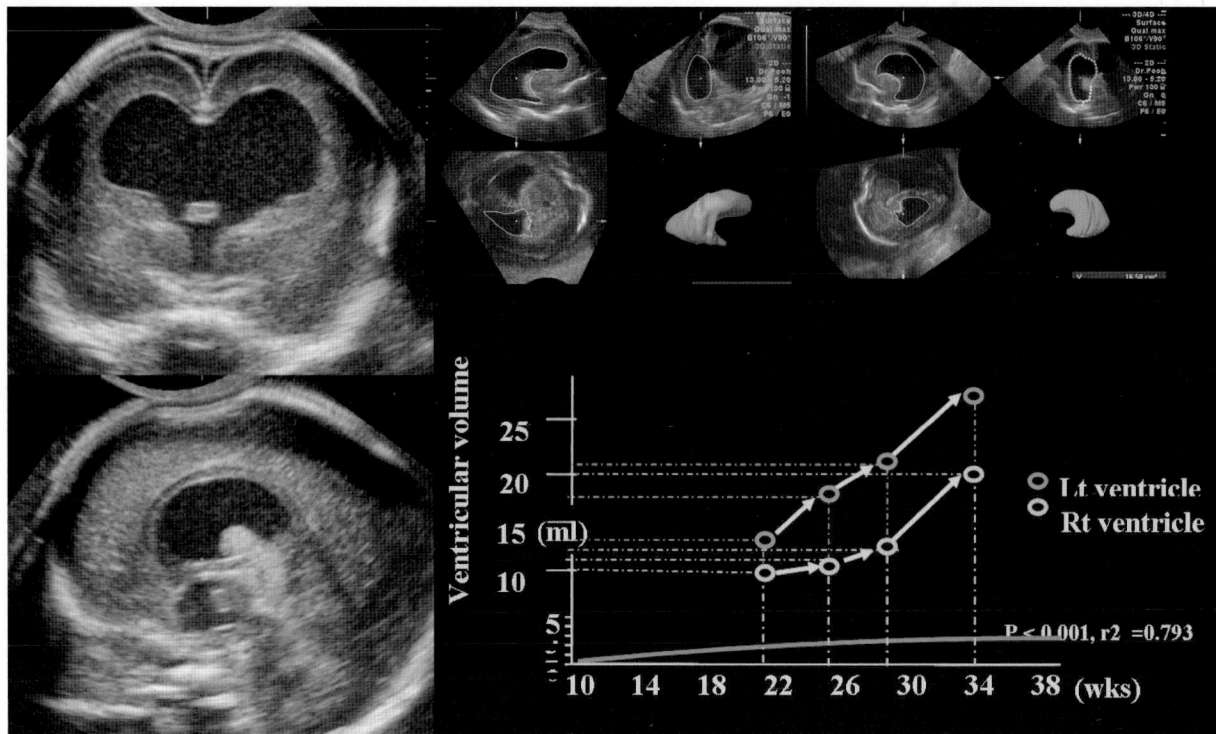

Figure 15.14 Moderate ventriculomegaly (21 weeks). (left) Ultrasound images in the coronal and sagittal sections. Fused ventriculomegaly, enlarged foramen of Monro, mild third ventriculomegaly are demonstrated in the coronal section, and no enlargement of fourth ventricle was seen in the sagittal section. Therefore, aqueductal stenosis and cerebral hypoplasia were suspected. (right upper) 3D images with volume calculation of bilateral ventricles. (right lower) Longitudinal study of ventricular size was on the graph. This case shows moderate increase of ventricular size during pregnancy.

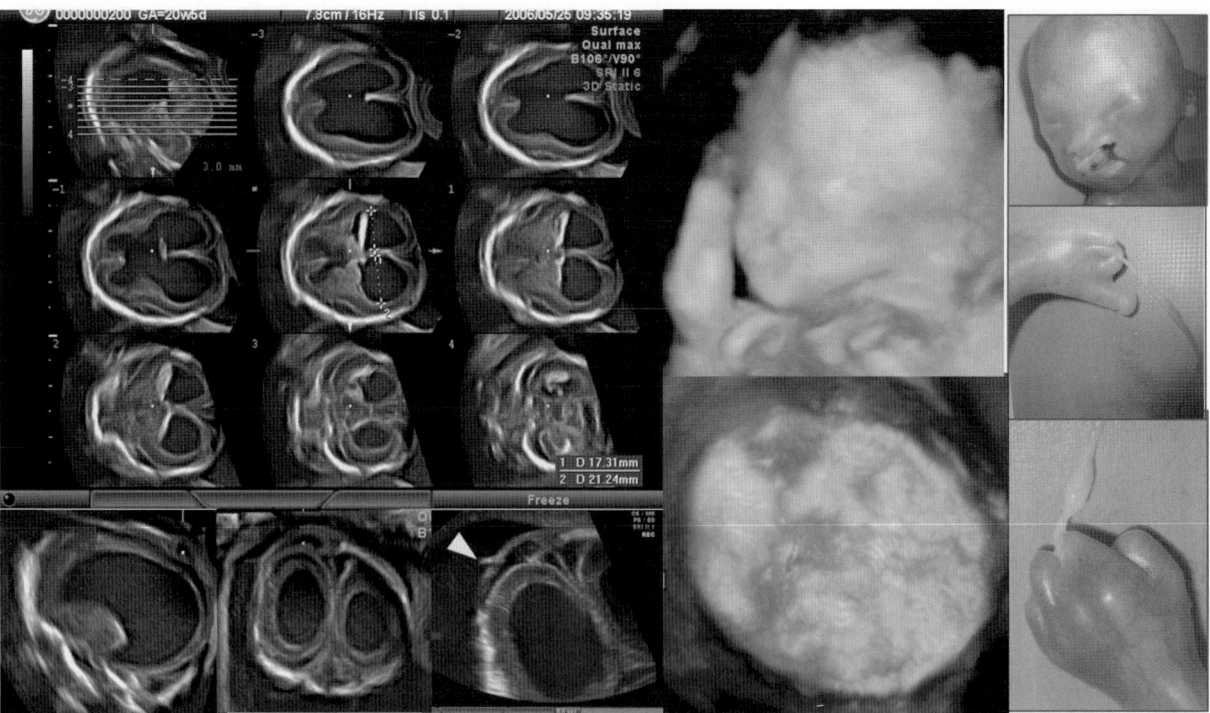

Figure 15.15 Hydrocephalus due to amniotic band syndrome (20 weeks). (left upper) Tomographic ultrasound imaging in the axial section of fetal brain at referral. Bilateral atrial width was 17 and 21 mm respectively. From the observation of enlarged ventricles, simple hydrocephalus due to Monro obstruction was suspected. However, the fetus was complicated with cleft lip, amputation of fingers and amniotic band were detected by extra CNS scan. (lower) Small cephalocele (arrows) was seen with remnant of the amniotic band (arrowhead). (middle upper) Fetal face by 3D surface mode. Cleft lip is apparent. (middle lower) Fetal cranial bone from parietal direction. Partial cranial bone defect with irregular sutural formation is visible. (right) Macroscopic view of the face and extremities after termination of pregnancy. In this case, cranial bone defect and cephalocele due to amniotic band may result in hydrocephalus.

ABS, an amniotic band attached to the skull results in a partial cranial bone defect and a small cephalocele, which may have caused Monro obstruction and enlarged ventricles.

Table 15.2 shows the summary of 23 ventriculomegaly cases with atrial width of >15 mm.

Nine cases (39.1%) had no other CNS abnormality but two out of those 9 were complicated with chromosomal aberration. Among the remaining 14 cases, holoprosencephaly was detected in 5 and myelomeningocele in 5. Four cases out of 7 without any complication had favorable postnatal prognosis after a ventricular-peritoneal shunting procedure (Pooh et al 2007).

Genetic hydrocephalus is rare but it is important in counseling couples on subsequent pregnancy. X-linked hydrocephalus, hydrocephalus due to stenosis of the aqueduct of Sylvius (HSAS), mental retardation-aphasia-shuffling gait-adducted thumbs syndrome (MASA), X-linked complicated spastic paraparesis (SP1) and X-linked corpus callosum agenesis are all due to mutations in the *L1* gene (Fransen et al 1995). The gene encoding L1 is located near the telomere of the long arm of the X chromosome in Xq28. Therefore, it was thought appropriate to refer to this clinical syndrome with the acronym CRASH, for corpus callosum hypoplasia, retardation, adducted thumbs, spastic paraplegia and hydrocephalus (Fransen et al 1995). It has been reported that mutations which produce truncations in the extracellular domain of the L1 protein are more likely to produce severe hydrocephalus, grave mental retardation or early death than point mutations in the extracellular domain or mutations affecting only the cytoplasmic domain of the protein (Yamasaki et al 1997). For the families, prenatal CNS diagnosis of male infants is important. A morphology-based approach becomes feasible between postmenstrual weeks 15 and 20. Prior to this gestational age, the diagnosis should rely on molecular biology tests (Timor-Tritsch et al 1996). Figure 15.16 shows a case of generic hydrocephalus of CRASH syndrome. Prenatal diagnosis can be done by detecting ventriculomegaly, partial or complete ACC and adducted thumbs.

• Variety of mild ventriculomegaly with AW 10–15 mm.

Mild ventriculomegaly is defined as a width of the atrium of the lateral cerebral ventricles of 10–15 mm. It has been reported that mild ventriculomegaly with atrial width 10–15 mm resolves in 29%, remains stable in 57% and progresses in 14% of the cases during pregnancy (Kelly et al 2001). Figure 15.17 shows a case with spontaneous resolution of ventriculomegaly between 17 and 25 weeks of gestation. Generally, in cases of mild fetal ventriculomegaly with a normal karyotype and an absence of malformations, the outcome appears to be favorable (Goldstein et al 2005). Pilu and his colleagues reviewed 234 cases of borderline ventriculomegaly including an abnormal outcome in 22.8% and concluded that borderline ventriculomegaly carries an increased risk of cerebral maldevelopment, delayed neuro-

Table 15.2 23 cases of ventriculomegaly of atrial width >15 mm	
Isolated ventriculomegaly	9
normal karyotype	7
abnormal karyotype	2
Holoprosencephaly	5
Myelomeningocele	5
Dandy–Walker syndrome	1
Agenesis of CC	1
ACC + IHC	1
Multiple porencephaly	1
Total	23

logical development and, possibly, chromosomal aberrations (Pilu et al 1999). Isolated mild ventriculomegaly with atrial width of 10–12 mm may be a normal variation. Signorelli and colleagues observed that their data of normal neurodevelopment between 18 months and 10 years after birth in cases of isolated mild ventriculomegaly (atrial width of 10–12 mm), should provide a basis for reassuring counseling (Signorelli et al 2004). Ouahba and colleagues recently reported the outcome of 167 cases of isolated mild ventriculomegaly and concluded that in addition to associated anomalies, three criteria are often associated with an unfavorable outcome: atrial width greater than 12 mm, progression of the enlargement, and asymmetrical and bilateral ventriculomegaly (Ouahba et al 2006).

Mild ventriculomegaly is often associated with other cranial and/or intracranial abnormalities such as cerebral hypoplasia, multiple intracerebral bleeding, brain tumor, craniosynostosis, vein of Galen aneurysmal malformation, Dandy–Walker malformation and others. Mild ventriculomegaly is also associated with extra CNS abnormalities, such as chromosomal aberration, genetic diseases, infection of cytomegalovirus, rubella, toxoplasma and others. Various outcome and prognosis followed according to complicated abnormalities. Table 15.3 summarizes 23 cases of ventriculomegaly with atrial width 10–15 mm: 13 cases with additional anomaly and 10 cases without other abnormality. More than 30% of cases with other abnormalities had chromosomal aberration or genetic disorder. However, among the cases with other complication, 30% of them have had no neurological deficit in the short-term. It is difficult to estimate postnatal prognosis simply by intra-uterine progression or resolution of ventricular enlargement during pregnancy. Normalization of ventricular enlargement during fetal period was seen in 70% of cases with no other complications. In our series, all cases with both no complications and spontaneous resolution of enlargement have had a favorable short-term prognosis (Pooh and Pooh 2007).

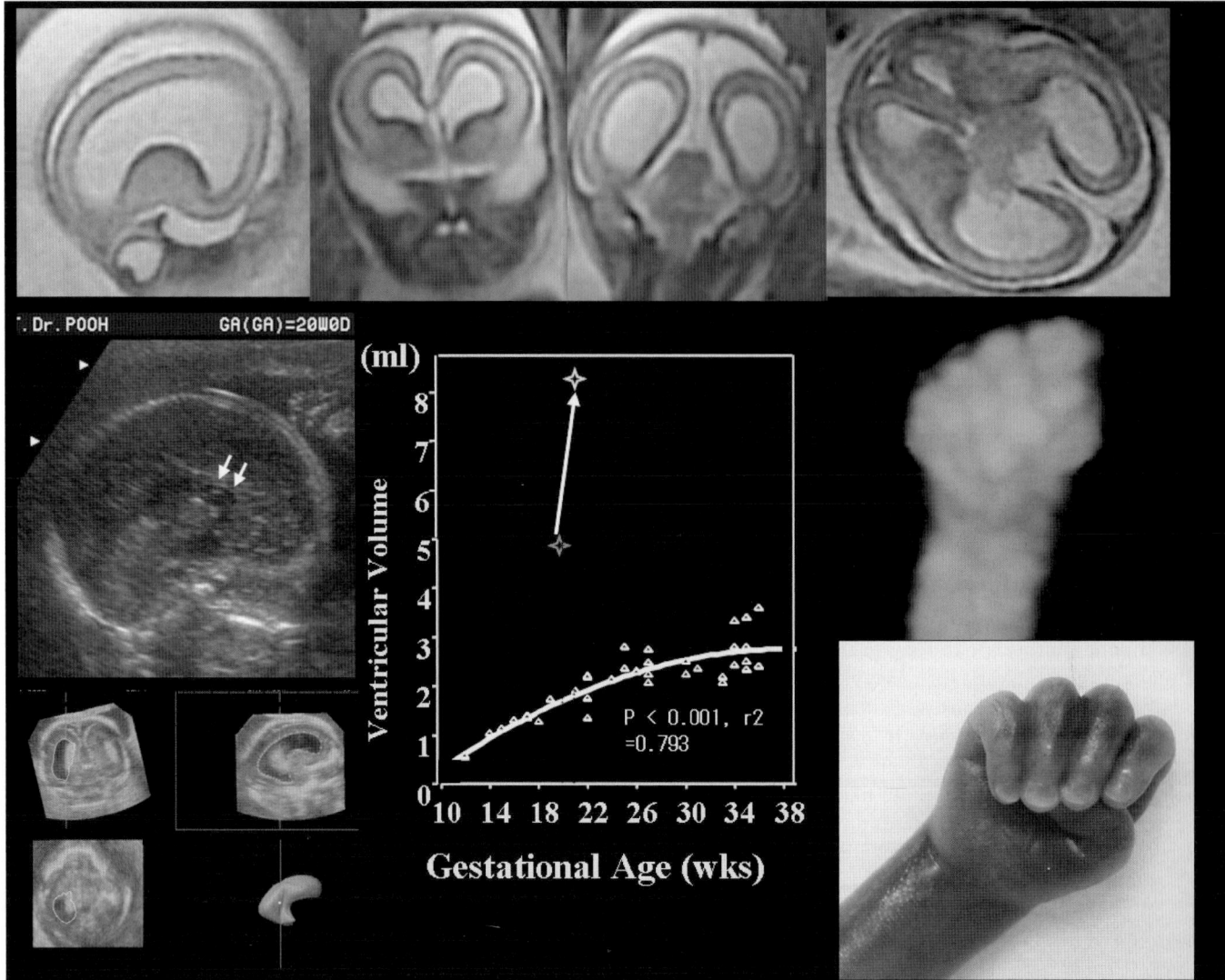

Figure 15.16 Early stage of genetic hydrocephalus at 20–21 weeks of gestation. (upper) MRI at 20 weeks of gestation. Bilateral ventriculomegaly with cerebral hypoplasia is seen, but it is difficult to diagnose as hydrocephalus because subarachnoid space is clearly visible. (middle left) Sagittal sonographic image. Partial agenesis of the corpus callosum (arrows) is demonstrated. (lower left) Three orthogonal view with extraction of enlarged ventricle. (lower middle) Graph showing ventricular volume. In this case, ventricular volume rapidly increased from 20 to 21 weeks of gestation. (middle right) 3D ultrasound image of fetal hand. Adducted thumb is demonstrated. (lower right) Macroscopic picture of fetal hand from aborted fetus at the end of 21 weeks of gestation. (Macroscopic picture is by courtesy of Dr. Tanemura, Nagoya City University.)

PROCENCEPHALIC DEVELOPMENTAL DISORDER

HOLOPROSENCEPHALY

Holoprosencephalies are classified into three varieties:

Alobar type: a single-sphered cerebral structure with a single common ventricle, posterior large cyst of third ventricle (dorsal sac), absence of olfactory bulbs and tracts and a single optic nerve.

Semilobar type: with formation of a posterior portion of the interhemispheric fissure.

Lobar type: with formation of the interhemispheric fissure anteriorly and posteriorly but not in the midhemispheric region. The fusion of the fornices is seen (Pilu et al 1994).

Incidence: 1 in 15 000–20 000 live births; however, initial incidence may be more than sixty fold greater in aborted human embryos (Matsunaga et al 1977, Cohen 1989).

Etiology: 75% of holoprosencephaly has normal karyotype, but chromosomes 2, 3, 7, 13, 18 and 21 have been implicated in holoprosencephaly (Cohen 1982). Particularly, trisomy 13 has most commonly been observed. Autosomal dominant transmission is rare.

Pathogenesis: failure of cleavage of the prosencephalon and diencephalon during early first trimester (5–6 weeks) results in holoprosencephaly.

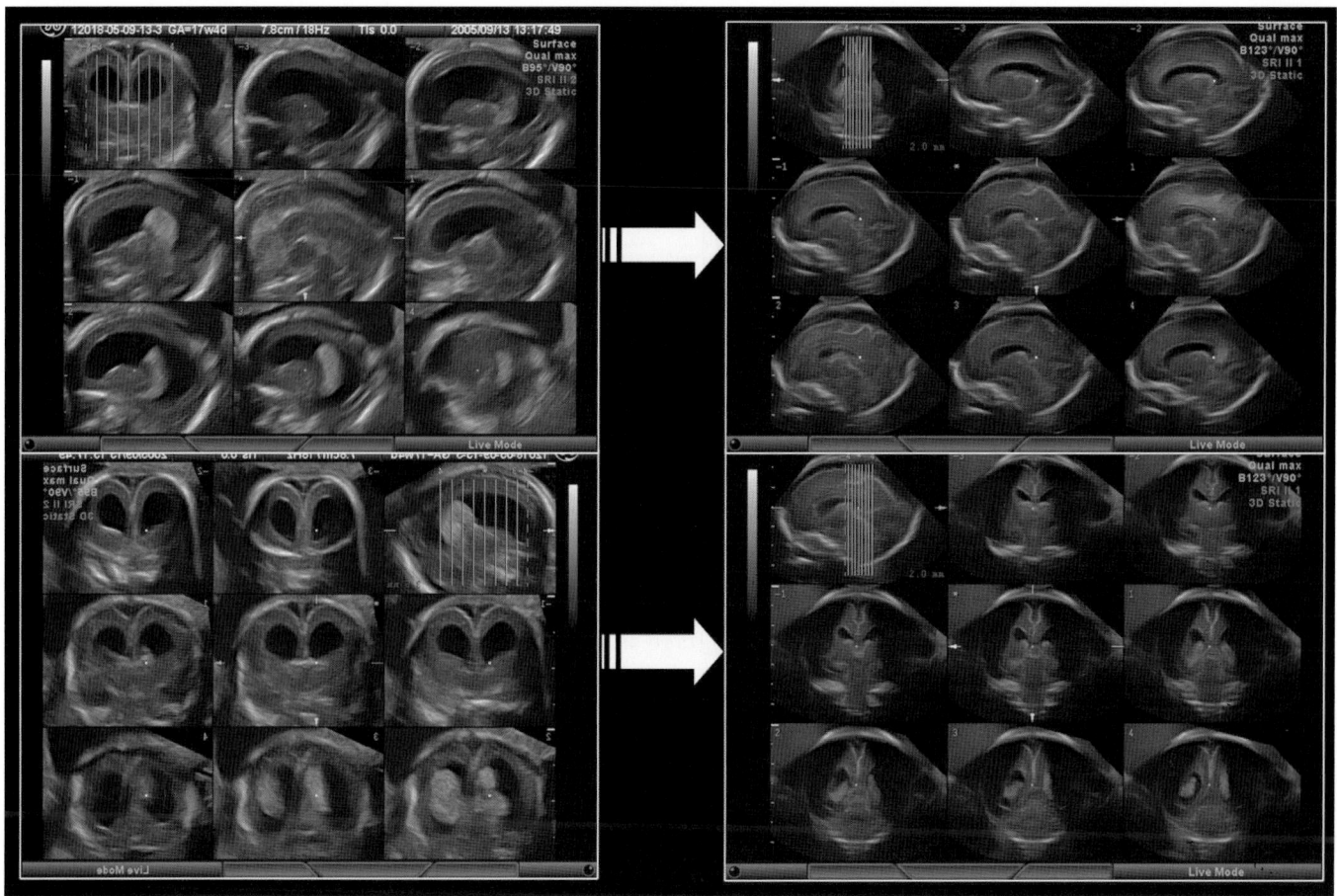

Figure 15.17 Mild ventriculomegaly with spontaneous resolution. (left) Tomographic sagittal (upper) and coronal (lower) ultrasound imaging of the brain at 17 weeks. Atrial width measurement shows 10–11 mm. (right) Tomographic sagittal (upper) and coronal (lower) brain imaging at 25 weeks. Spontaneous resolution of ventriculomegaly is seen.

Table 15.3 23 cases of ventriculomegaly of atrial width 10–15 mm	
With additional abnormality	13/23 cases (56.5%)
chromosomal/genetic abnormality	31%
other brain abnormality	69%
extra CNS abnormality	31%
MR, CP, neurological deficits	40%
no neurological deficit (<2 years)	30%
IUFD, TOP	30%
Ventriculomegaly during pregnancy	
resolved	31%
remain stable	31%
progressive	23%
uncertain	15%
With no other abnormality	10/12 cases (43.5%)
cerebral palsy	10%
epilepsy	10%
no neurological deficit (<2 years)	80%
Ventriculomegaly during pregnancy	
resolved	70%
remain stable	20%
progressive	10%

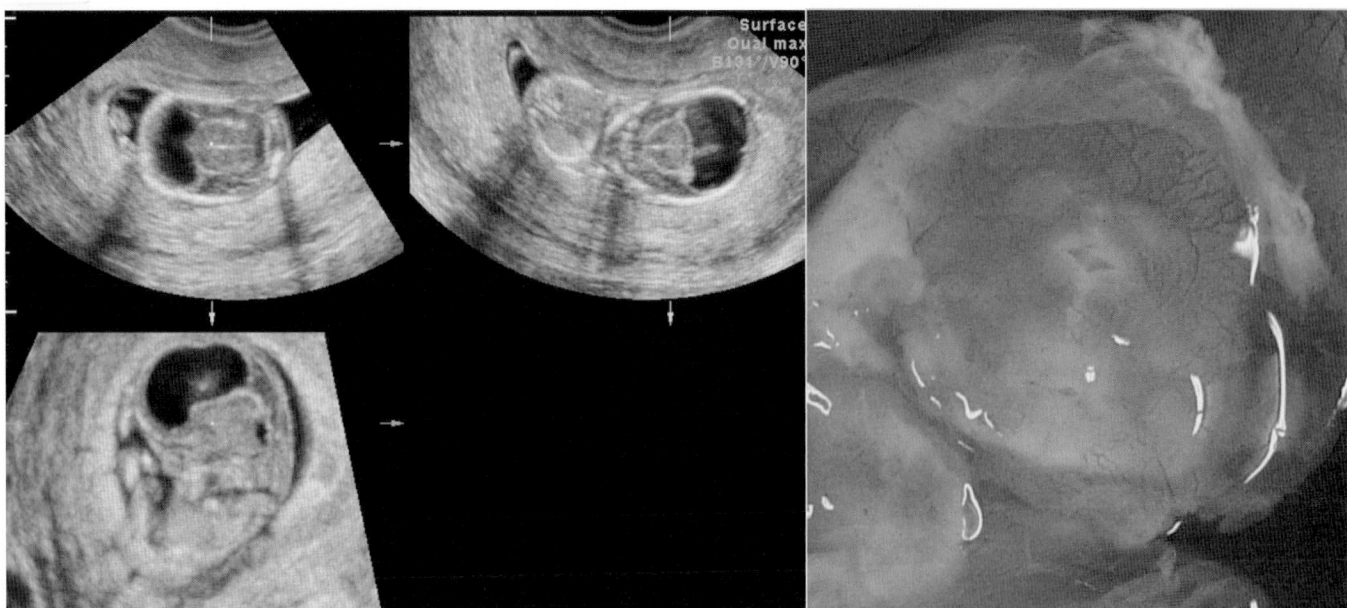

Figure 15.18 Alobar holoprosencephaly in the first trimester. Three orthogonal views demonstrate holoprosencephaly at 13 weeks. CRL was compatible to 10 weeks of gestation. Right figure shows the face of aborted fetus with cyclopia, arhinia and small mouth. Chromosome exam resulted in 69, XXX, triploidy.

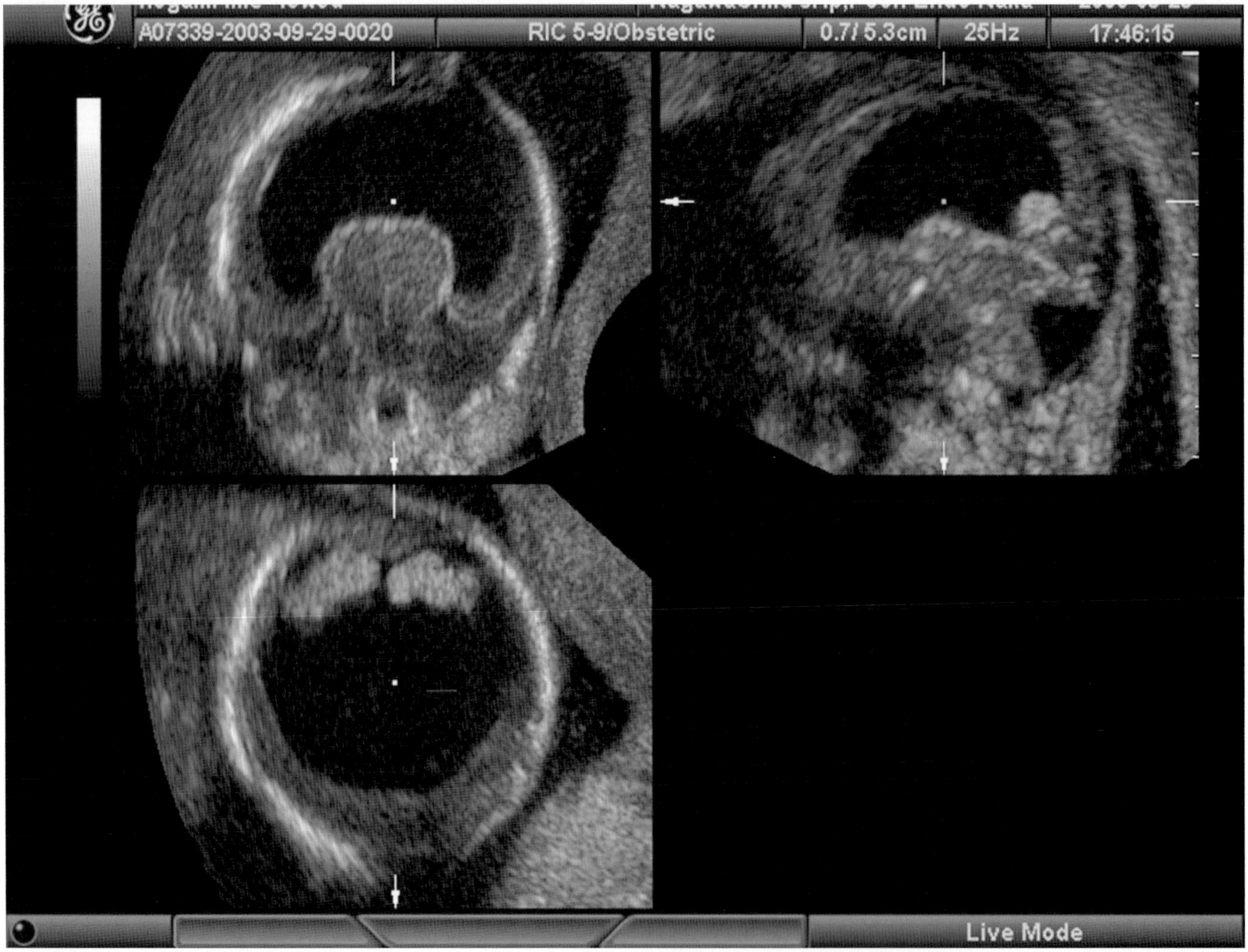

Figure 15.19 Alobar holoprosencephaly at 15 weeks of gestation. Three orthogonal images of intracranial structure show a complete single ventricle within a single-sphered cerebral structure.

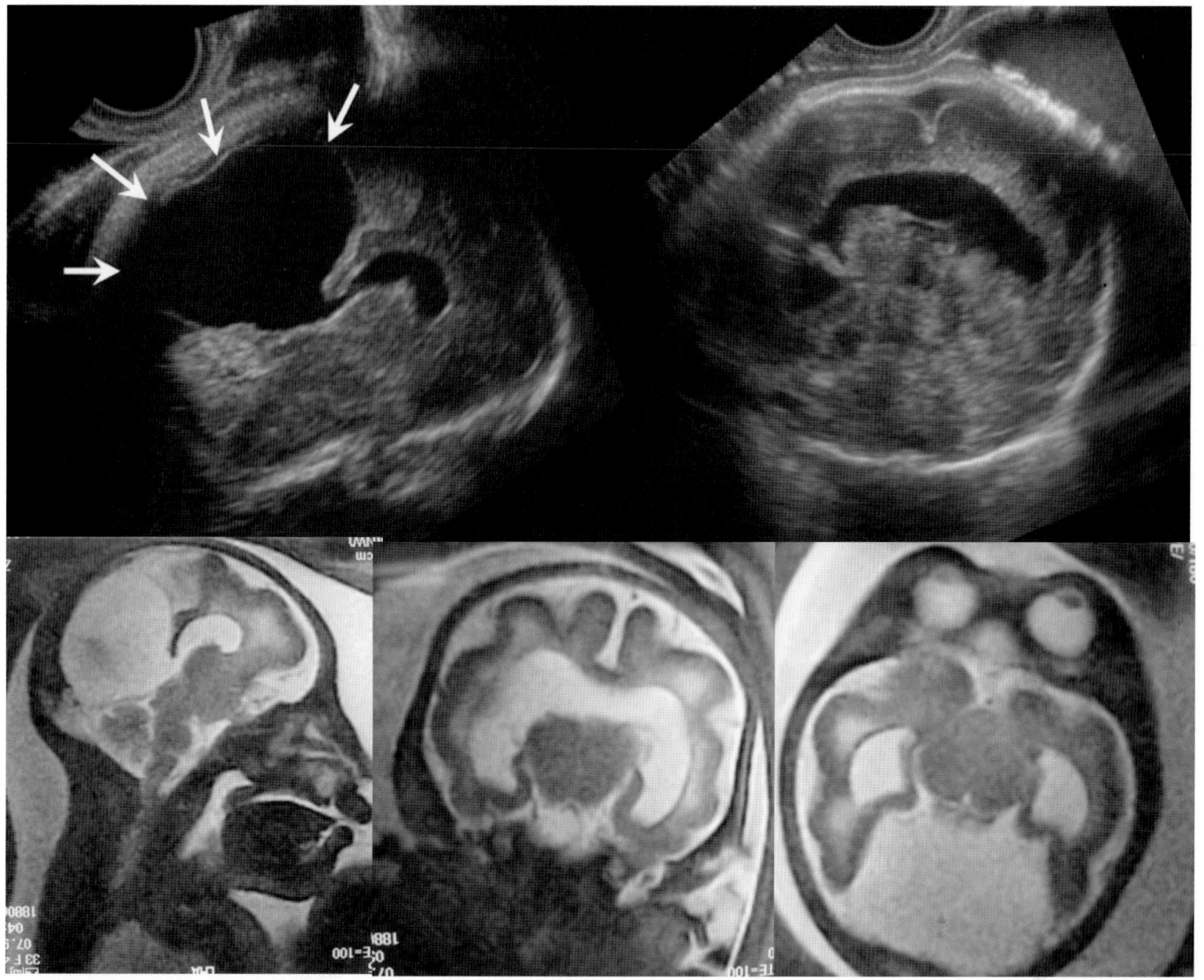

Figure 15.20 Semilobar holoprosencephaly at 33 weeks of gestation. (upper left) Sonogram in the median section. Arrows indicate a dorsal sac. (upper right) Sonogram in the coronal section. Fused ventricle is demonstrated. Lower figures are fetal MR images. Sagittal (left), coronal (middle) and axial (right) sections A blind end of nasal cavity (arrow) and hypotelorism are seen in the sagittal and axial MR images respectively.

Associated anomalies: facial abnormalities such as cyclopia, ethmocephaly, cebocephaly, flat nose, cleft lip and palate are invariably associated with holoprosencephaly. Extracerebral abnormalities are also invariably associated, such as renal cysts/dysplasia, omphalocele, cardiac disease and or myelomeningocele.

Prenatal diagnosis: alobar type in the first trimester and at 15 weeks of gestation are shown in Figures 15.18 and 15.19, and semilobar type in late pregnancy in Figure 15.20. Figure 15.21 shows facial appearance in cases of holoprosencephaly.

Differential diagnosis: hydrocephalus, hydranencephaly.

Prognosis: extremely poor in alobar holoprosencephaly; uncertain in lobar type; various but poor in semilobar type.

Recurrence risk: 6%, but much lower in sporadic or trisomy cases, much higher in genetic cases.

Management: chromosomal evaluation is offered.

AGENESIS OF THE CORPUS CALLOSUM

Agenesis of the corpus callosum is the absence of the corpus callosum, which may be divided into (complete) agenesis, partial agenesis or hypogenesis of the corpus callosum.

Complete agenesis: complete absence of the corpus callosum.

Partial agenesis (hypogenesis): absence of splenium or posterior portion in various degrees.

Prevalence: uncertain, 3–7 : 1000 in the general population is estimated.

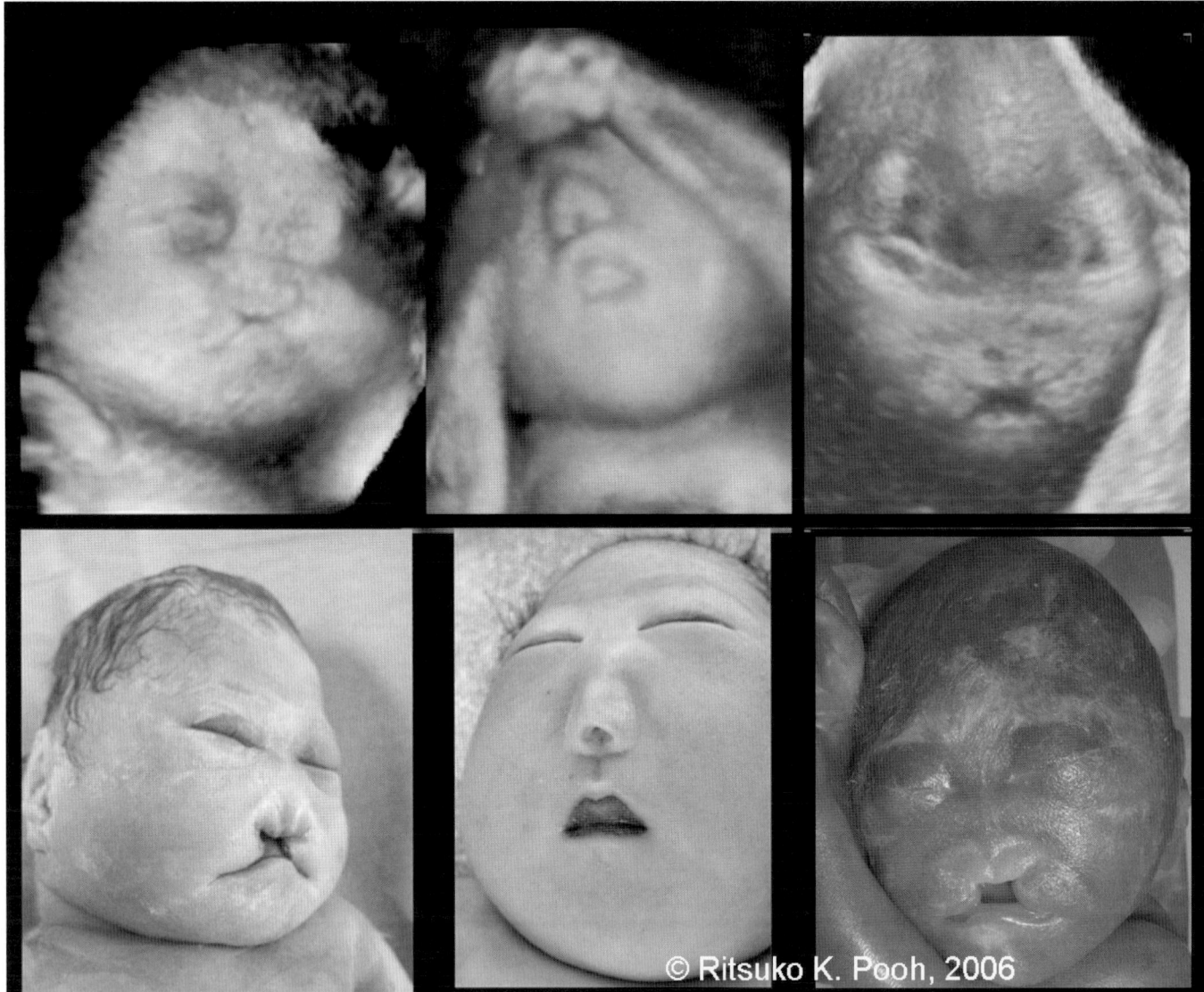

Figure 15.21 Facial abnormality in cases of holoprosencephaly. Upper figures are prenatal 3D facial images and lower figures show postpartum face appearance of each baby. Left; alobar holoprosencephaly at 20 weeks, middle and right; semilobar type in late pregnancy. Hypotelorism, exophthalmos are common. Left and middle cases had cleft lip and palate and obstruction of the nasal cavity. Right case had a single and obstructed nasal cavity.

Etiology: chromosomal aberration in 20% of affected cases, such as trisomy 18, 8 and 13; autosomal dominant, autosomal recessive, X-linked recessive, part of mendelian syndrome such as Walker–Warburg syndrome, and X-linked dominant such as Aicardi syndrome.

Pathogenesis: uncertain, but callosal formation may be associated with migration disorder.

Associated anomalies: colpocephaly (ventriculomegaly with disproportionate enlargement of trigones, occipital horns and temporal horns, not hydrocephaly), superior elongation of the third ventricle, interhemispheric cyst, lipoma of the corpus callosum.

Prenatal diagnosis: complete agenesis of the corpus callosum in the coronal and sagittal section, typical shape of enlarged ventricles detected by sonography and fetal MRI are shown in Figure 15.22. Typical radiated formation of brain vessels in the sagittal section is demonstrated in Figure 15.23.

Figure 15.23 Agenesis of the corpus callosum (AOCC). (left upper) Mid sagittal section in a case of AOCC. Typical radial sulcus formation is seen instead of normal cingulate sulcus and gyrus formed with normal development of the corpus callosum (arrows) seen in the upper right figure. (lower left) Angiostructure by 3D power Doppler. Normal callosomarginal artery (CMA, lower right) does not exist and radial formation of the branches of anterior cerebral arteries (ACA) is seen.

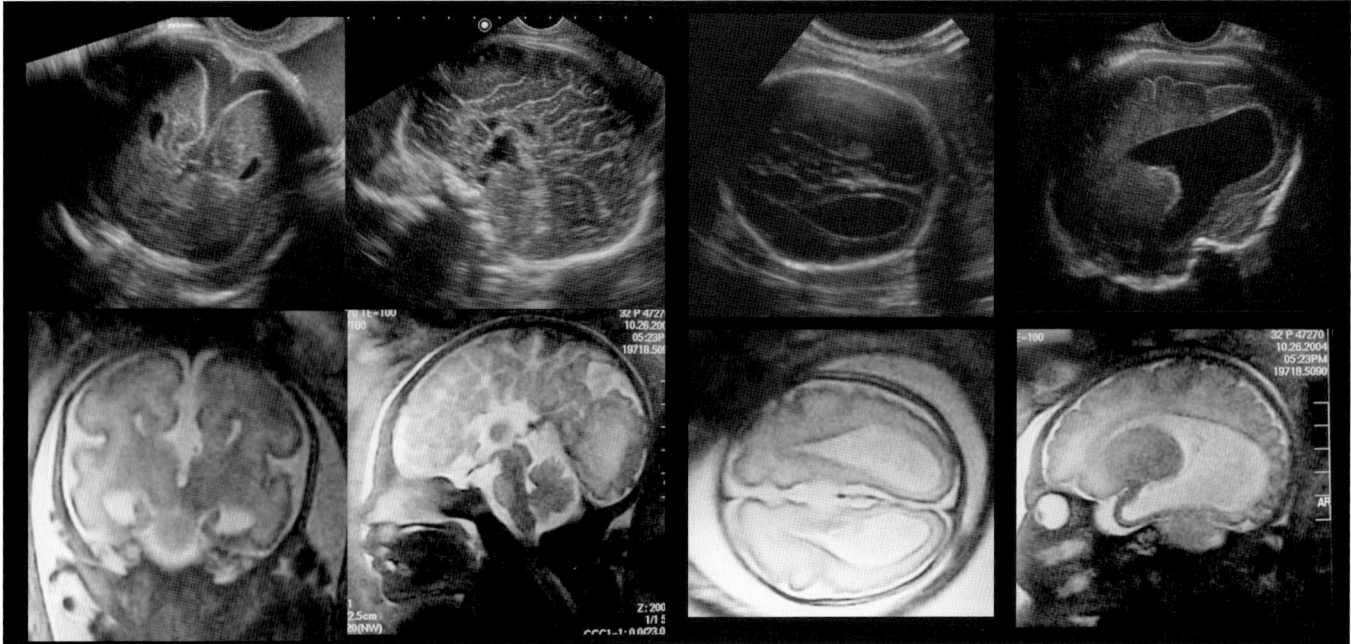

Figure 15.22 Fetal US and MR images of complete agenesis of the corpus callosum. Sonographic images (upper) and MR images (lower). Anterior coronal, mid-sagittal, axial and parasagittal sections from the left. (right) No communicated bridge is seen between bilateral hemispheres. Note the bull's horn like appearance of the anterior horns of lateral ventricle in the coronal image. Typical ventricular shape of colpocephaly is demonstrated on the axial and parasagittal sections.

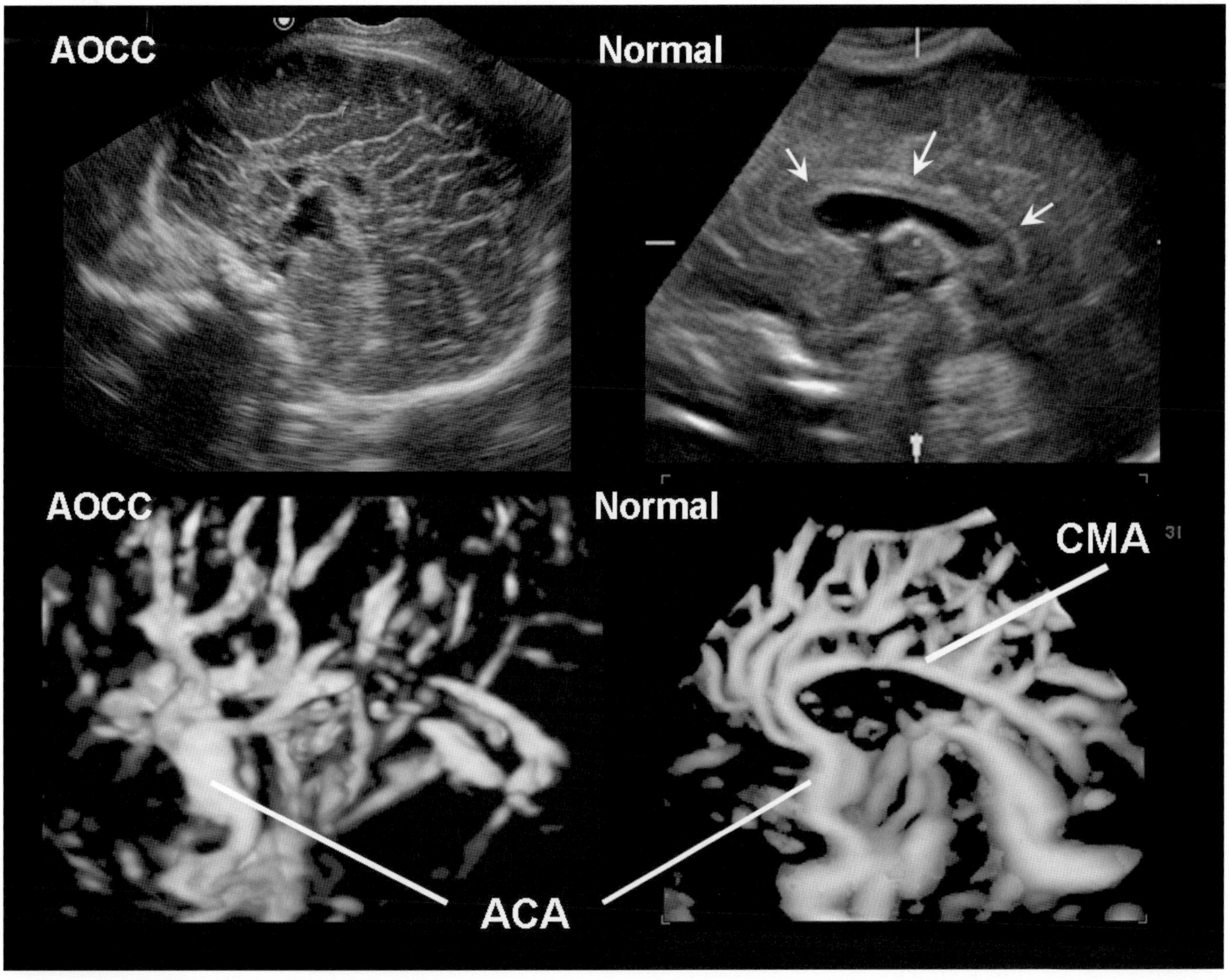

Diagnosis: as the corpus callosum is depicted after 17 or 18 weeks of gestation by ultrasound, it is impossible to diagnose agenesis of the corpus callosum prior to this age (Pilu et al 2001).

Prognosis: various; depends on associated anomalies. Most cases with isolated agenesis of the corpus callosum without other abnormalities are asymptomatic and neurological prognosis is rather good. Complete agenesis has a worse prognosis than partial agenesis (Goodyear et al 2001). Epilepsy, intellectual impairment or psychiatric disorder (Taylor and David 1998) may occur later on.

Recurrence risk: depends on etiology: chromosomal; 1%, autosomal recessive; 25%, X-linked recessive male; 50%.

Management: standard obstetrical care. Chromosomal evaluation is offered. In cases with interhemispheric cyst, postnatal fenestration or shunt procedure may be performed.

ABSENT SEPTUM PELLUCIDUM, SEPTO-OPTIC DYSPLASIA

Absent septum pellucidum: absence of the septum pellucidum with or without associated anomalies. The septum pellucidum can be destroyed by concomitant hydrocephalus or by contiguous ischemic lesions such as porencephaly. An isolated absent septum pellucidum exists (Schmidt-Riese 1994) but is rare.

Septo-optic dysplasia: absence of the septum pellucidum and unilateral or bilateral hypoplasia of the optic nerve.

Incidence: unknown, rare.

Synonyms: de Morsier syndrome (septo-optic dysplasia).

Etiology: maternal drug abuse, such as valproic acid (McMahon and Braddock 2001), cocaine (Dominguez et al 1991); autosomal recessive, HESX1 homeodomain gene mutation (Dattani et al 1998).

Pathogenesis: may occur as a vascular disruption sequence, with other prosencephalic or neuronal migration disorders.

Associated anomalies: schizencephaly, gyral abnormalities, heterotopias, hypotelorism, ventriculomegaly, communicating lateral ventricles, bilateral cleft lip and palate, hypopituitarism.

Differential diagnosis: dysgenesis of the corpus callosum, lobar holoprosencephaly.

Prenatal diagnosis: isolated absent septum pellucidum detected at 21 weeks of gestation is shown in Figure 15.24.

Prognosis: depends on associated anomalies; variable degree of mental deficit, multiple endocrine dysfunctions. In cases with isolated absent of septum pellucidum, prognosis may be good.

Recurrence risk: unknown.

Management: confirmation of diagnosis after birth is important for genetic counseling. Endocrine dysfunction should be searched for and corrected. Shunt procedure in cases with progressive ventriculomegaly.

POSTERIOR FOSSA ANOMALY

CHIARI MALFORMATION

Chiari anomalies with cerebellar herniation in the spinal canal are classified into three types by contents of herniated tissue: contents of type I is a lip of cerebellum, type II part of cerebellum, fourth ventricle and medulla oblongata, pons and type III large herniation of the posterior fossa. Thereafter, type IV with just cerebellar hypogenesis was added. However, this classification occasionally leads to confusion in neuroimaging diagnosis. Therefore, at present, the classification as below is advocated.

- Type I: herniation of only cerebellar tonsil, not associated by myelomeningocele.
- Type II: (schematic picture is shown in Figure 15.25), herniation of cerebellar tonsil and brain stem. Medullary kink, tentorial dysplasia, associated with myelomeningocele.
- Type III: associated with cephalocele or craniocervical meningocele, in which cerebellum and brainstem herniated.
- Type IV: associated with marked cerebellar hypogenesis and posterior fossa shrinking.

Prevalence: depends on prevalence of spina bifida (Chiari type II malformation). According to recent remarkable reduction of prevalence of NTDs after using folic acid supplementation and fortification, prevalence has declined. Other types are rare.

Synonyms: Arnold–Chiari malformation.

Etiology: depends on the types.

Pathogenesis: Chiari malformation occurs according to: (1) inferior displacement of the medulla and the fourth ventricle into the upper cervical canal, (2) elongation and thinning of the upper medulla and lower pons and persistence of the embryonic flexure of these structures, (3) inferior displacement of the lower cerebellum through the foramen magnum into the upper cervical region and (4) a variety of bony defects of the foramen magnum, occiput and upper cervical vertebrae (Volpe 2001c).

Associated anomalies: myelomeningocele or myeloschisis (type II), cephalocele or craniocervical meningocele (type III), cerebellar hypogenesis (type IV) and syringomyelia (type I). Hydrocephalus caused by obstruction of fourth ventricular outflow or associated aqueductal stenosis. Eighty-eight percent of fetuses with open spina bifida develop ventriculomegaly and the majority do so by 21 weeks' gestation (Biggio et al 2004).

Prenatal diagnosis: lemon and banana signs (Nicolaides et al 1986) are circumstantial evidences of Chiari malformation which are easily demonstrated in the second trimester. Lemon sign indicates deformity of the frontal bone; banana sign indicates abnormal shape of cerebellum without cisterna magna space (Fig. 15.26). Herniation of the cerebellar tonsil and medulla oblongata and medullary kink are

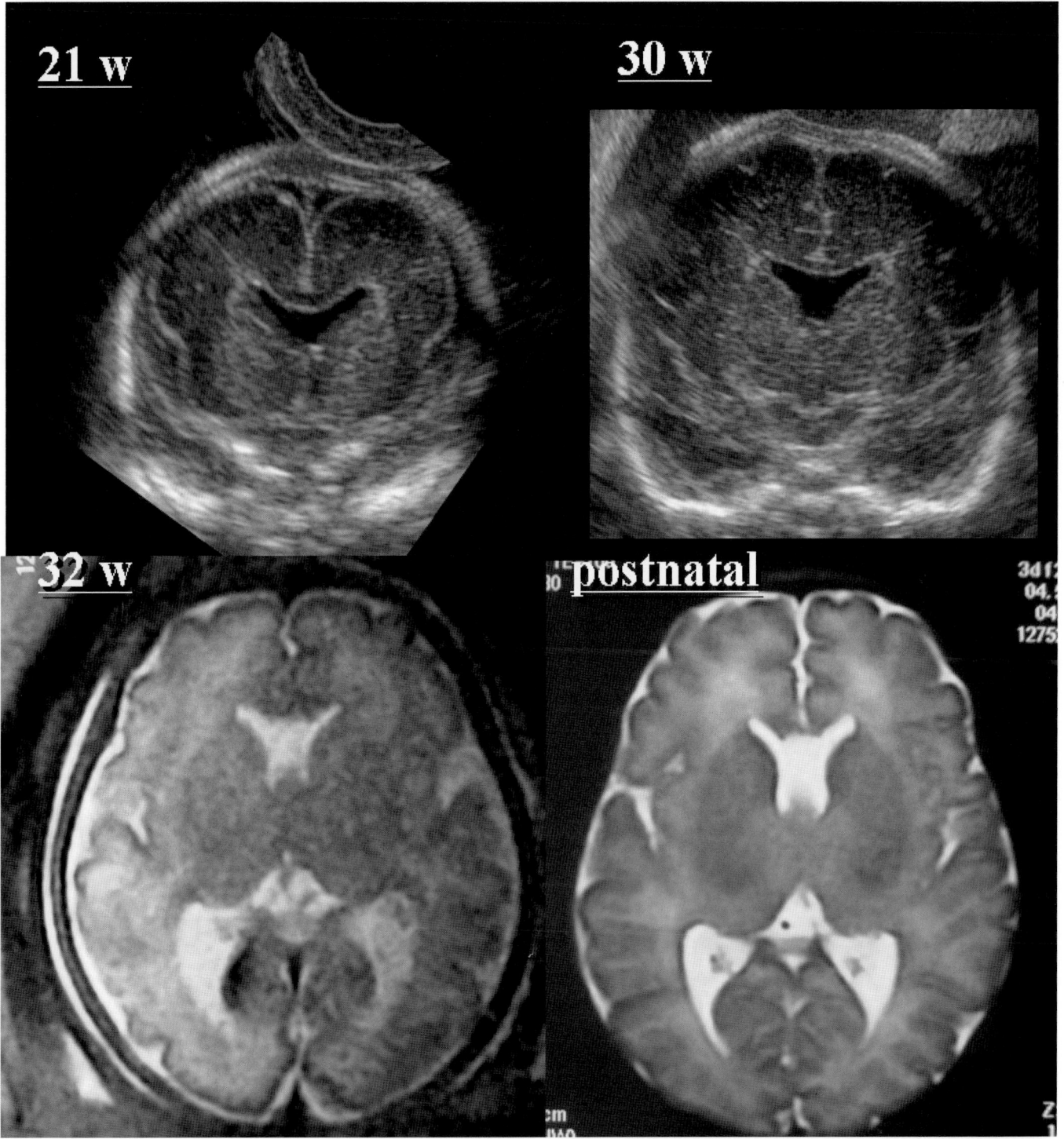

Figure 15.24 Isolated absent septum pellucidum. (upper left) 21 weeks of gestation. Absent septum pellucidum and fusion of lateral ventricles are seen. (upper right) 30 weeks. Normal development of cerebral structure is seen. (lower left) Fetal MRI at 32 weeks. (lower right) Postnatal MRI. Postnatal course has been favorable for 5 years.

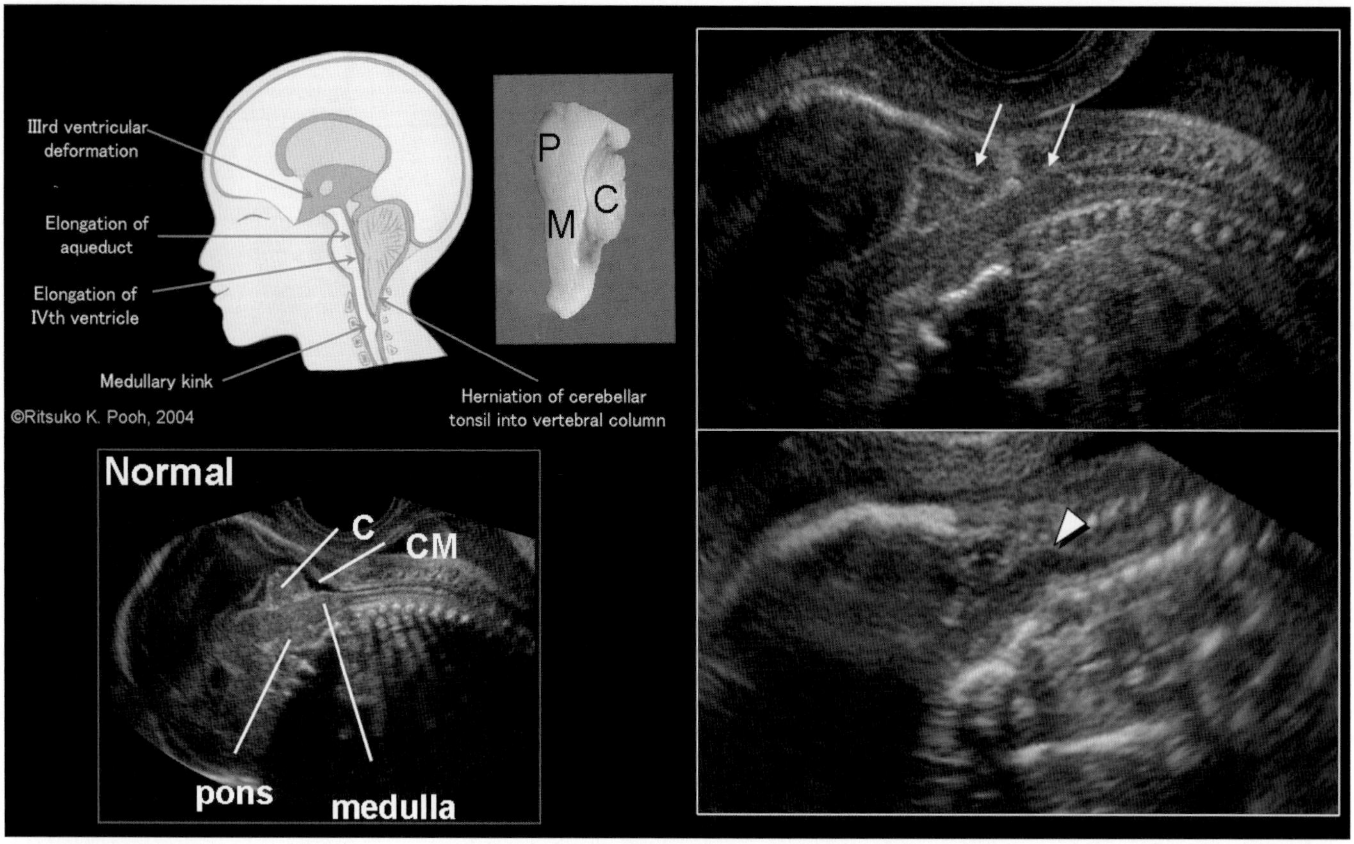

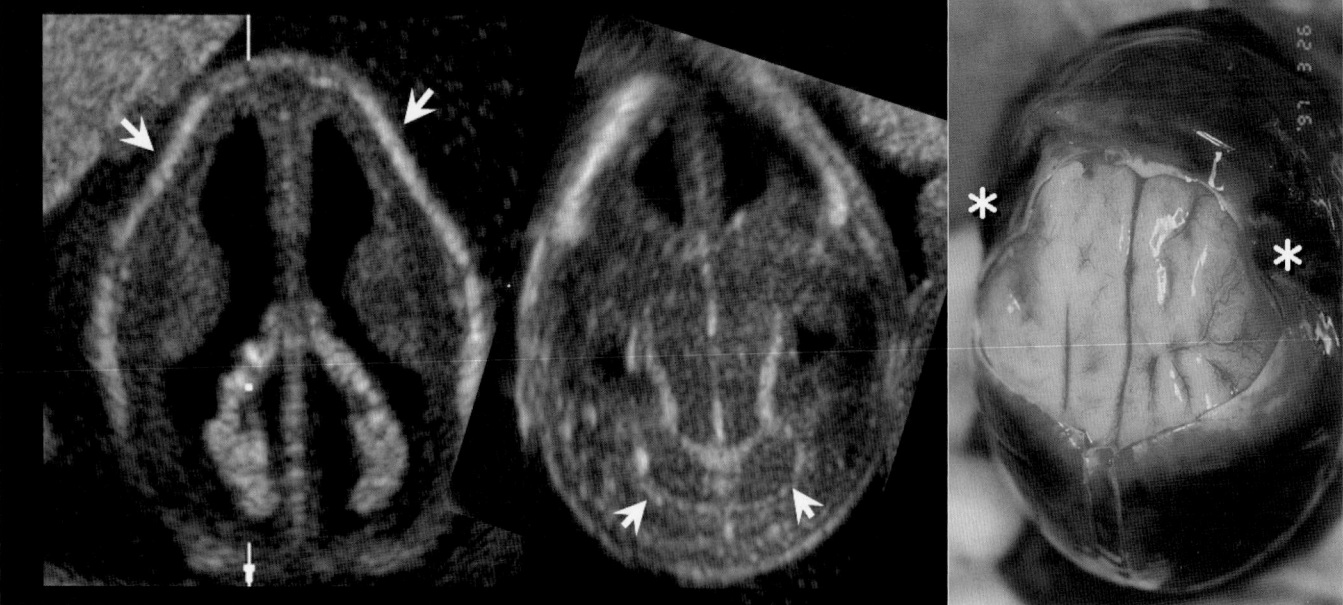

Figure 15.25 Chiari type II malformation. Schema, macroscopic picture and ultrasound. (upper left) Schema of Chiari type II malformation and macroscopic picture of specimen from aborted fetus at 21 weeks of gestation. P; pons, M; medulla oblongata, C; cerebellum. (lower left) Normal cerebrospinal region demonstrated by ultrasound in the sagittal section at 19 weeks. C; cerebellum, CM; cisterna magnum. (upper right) Sonographic picture in the sagittal section of Chiari type II malformation at 19 weeks of gestation. Herniation of the cerebellum and medulla oblongata (arrows) into spinal canal is clearly demonstrated. (lower right) Sagittal ultrasound image of medullary kink at 19 weeks (arrowhead) occasionally seen in some cases of Chiari type II malformation.

Figure 15.26 Lemon sign and banana sign of Chiari type II malformation at 16 weeks of gestation. (left) Typical lemon sign of cranial shape. Indentations of anterolateral parts (arrows) are conspicuous before 26 weeks of gestation. (middle) Typical banana sign. Disappearance of cisterna magna and cerebellar deformity (arrows) due to cerebellar tonsil herniation into spinal canal form a banana sign. (right) Macroscopic picture of lemon sign from aborted fetus at 21 weeks of gestation. Asterisks indicate anterolateral indentations.

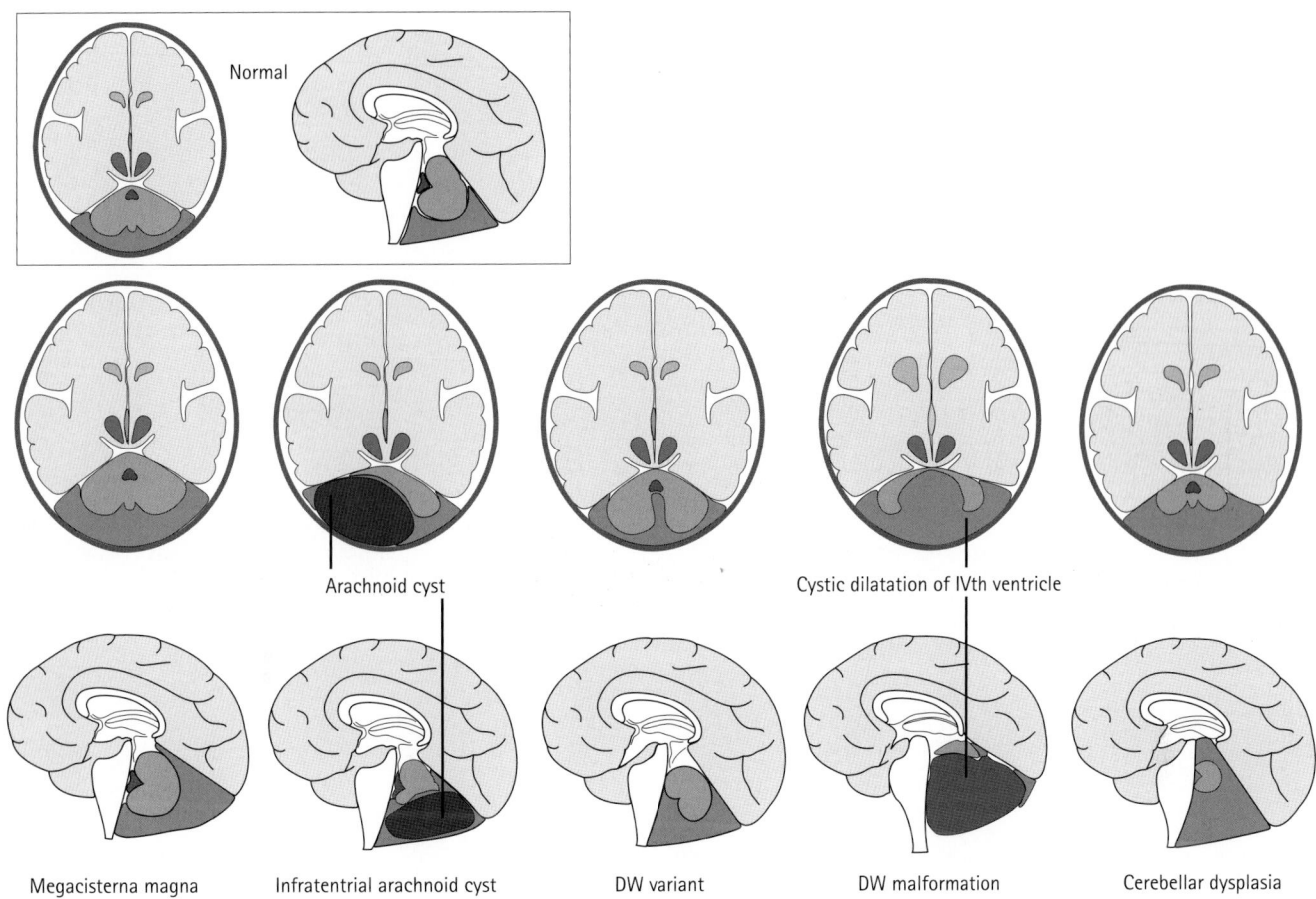

Figure 15.27 Differential diagnosis of 'hypoechoic lesion' of the posterior fossa.

demonstrable (Fig. 15.25). Small clivus-supraocciput angle is seen in cases of Chiari malformation (D'Addario et al 2001).

Prognosis: nearly every case of myelomeningocele is accompanied by morphological Chiari II malformation. Many cases with Chiari II are asymptomatic. However, clinical features due to Chiari malformation, such as feeding disturbances, laryngeal stridor or apneic episode, are found in approximately 9–30% of cases. In cases with these clinical features, vital prognosis is often poor.

Recurrence risk: depends on types of Chiari malformation; decreased according to decline of NTD recurrence rate by use of folic acid supplementation and fortification.

Neurosurgical management: neurosurgical operation of foramen magnum decompression (FMD) for any types of symptomatic Chiari malformation. Syringo-subarachnoid shunt for Chiari type I.

DANDY–WALKER MALFORMATION, DANDY–WALKER VARIANT, MEGACISTERNA MAGNA

At present, the term Dandy–Walker complex (Barkovich et al 1989) is used to indicate a spectrum of anomalies of the posterior fossa that are classified by axial CT scans.

Dandy–Walker malformation, Dandy–Walker variant and mega-cisterna magna seem to represent a continuum of developmental anomalies of the posterior fossa (Barkovich et al 1989). Figure 15.27 shows the differential diagnosis of hypoechoic lesion of the posterior fossa.

(Classic) Dandy–Walker malformation: cystic dilatation of fourth ventricle, enlarged posterior fossa, elevated tentorium and complete or partial agenesis of the cerebellar vermis.

Dandy–Walker variant: variable hypoplasia of the cerebellar vermis with or without enlargement of the posterior fossa.

Megacisterna magna: enlarged cisterna magna with integrity of both cerebellar vermis and fourth ventricle.

Incidence: Dandy–Walker malformation has an estimated prevalence of about 1:30 000 births, and is found in 4–12% of all cases of infantile hydrocephalus (Osenbach and Menezes 1991). Incidence of Dandy–Walker variant and megacisterna magna is unknown.

Etiology: mendelian disorders such as Warburg, chromosomal aberration such as 45,X, partial monosomy/trisomy, viral infections and diabetes.

Pathogenesis: during development of the fourth ventricular roof, a delay or total failure of the foramen of Magendie to open occurs, allowing a build-up of CSF and development of the cystic dilation of the fourth ventricle. Despite the subsequent opening of the foramina of Luschka (usually patent in Dandy–Walker malformation), cystic dilatation of the fourth ventricle persists and CSF flow is impaired.

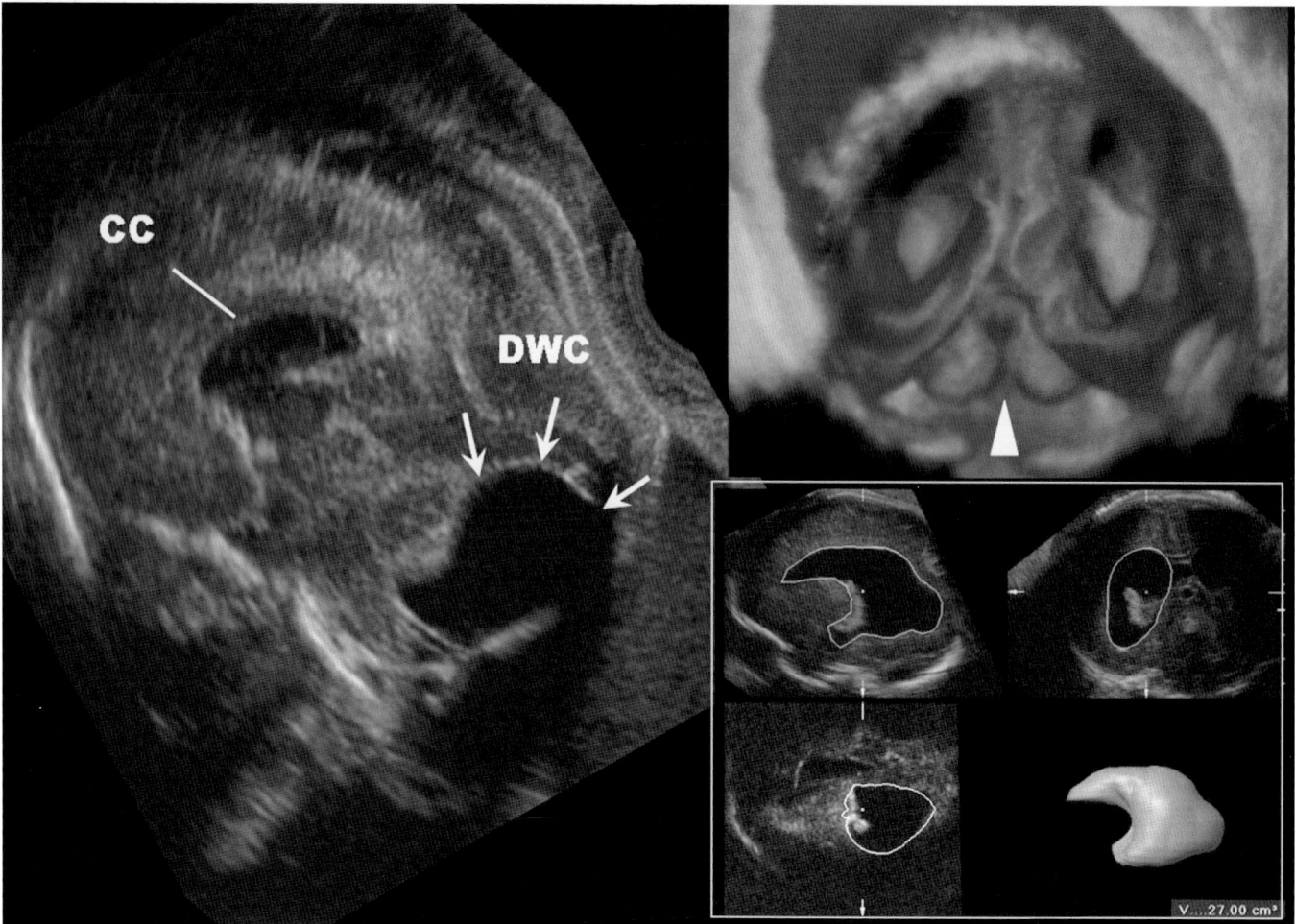

Figure 15.28 Dandy–Walker malformation at 28 weeks of gestation. Left figure shows the median section of the brain. Corpus callosum (CC) is normally demonstrated and Dandy–Walker cyst (DWC, arrows) is seen in the posterior fossa. Right upper figure is a 3D view in the posterior coronal section. Hypoplastic vermis of the cerebellum (arrowhead) is seen. Right lower figures, three orthogonal views and an extracted ventricular appearance, demonstrate moderate ventriculomegaly in this case.

Associated anomalies of Dandy–Walker malformation: hydrocephalus; other midline anomalies, such as agenesis of the corpus callosum, holoprosencephaly and occipital encephalocele; extracranial abnormalities such as congenital heart diseases, neural tube defects and cleft lip/palate. A frequency of additional anomalies ranges between 50 and 70%.

Prenatal diagnosis: DW malformation in Figure 15.28, and DW variant in Figures 15.29 and 15.30. To observe the agenesis of the cerebellar vermis, axial cutting section is preferable. To observe the elevated tentorium, sagittal section is preferable.

Differential diagnosis: infratentorial arachnoid cyst, other intracranial cystic tumor, hydrocephalus, cerebellar dysplasia.

Prognosis: progressive hydrocephalus, not observed in neonates but often progressive during the first month. Cases diagnosed in utero or the neonatal period, outcome is generally unfavorable. Nearly 40% die and 75% of survivors exhibit cognitive deficits. Prognosis of Dandy–Walker variant is good. Clinical significance of megacisterna magna is uncertain.

Recurrence risk: depends on etiology. Generally 1–5% (Dandy–Walker malformation).

Management: cystoperitoneal shunt or cyst-ventriculoperitoneal shunt.

NEURONAL PROLIFERATION DISORDER

MICROCEPHALY

Microcephaly is defined as a head circumference that is more than 2 standard deviations below the normal mean for age, sex, race and gestation.

Incidence: rare.

Etiology: infections such as with rubella, cytomegalovirus (CMV), varicella (chicken pox) virus and toxoplasmosis, radiation, medications, chromosome abnormalities and genetic diseases. It is part of many chromosomal abnormalities and other syndromes including:

• Chromosome abnormalities – trisomy 18 (Edwards syndrome), trisomy 13 (Patau syndrome), the Wolf–

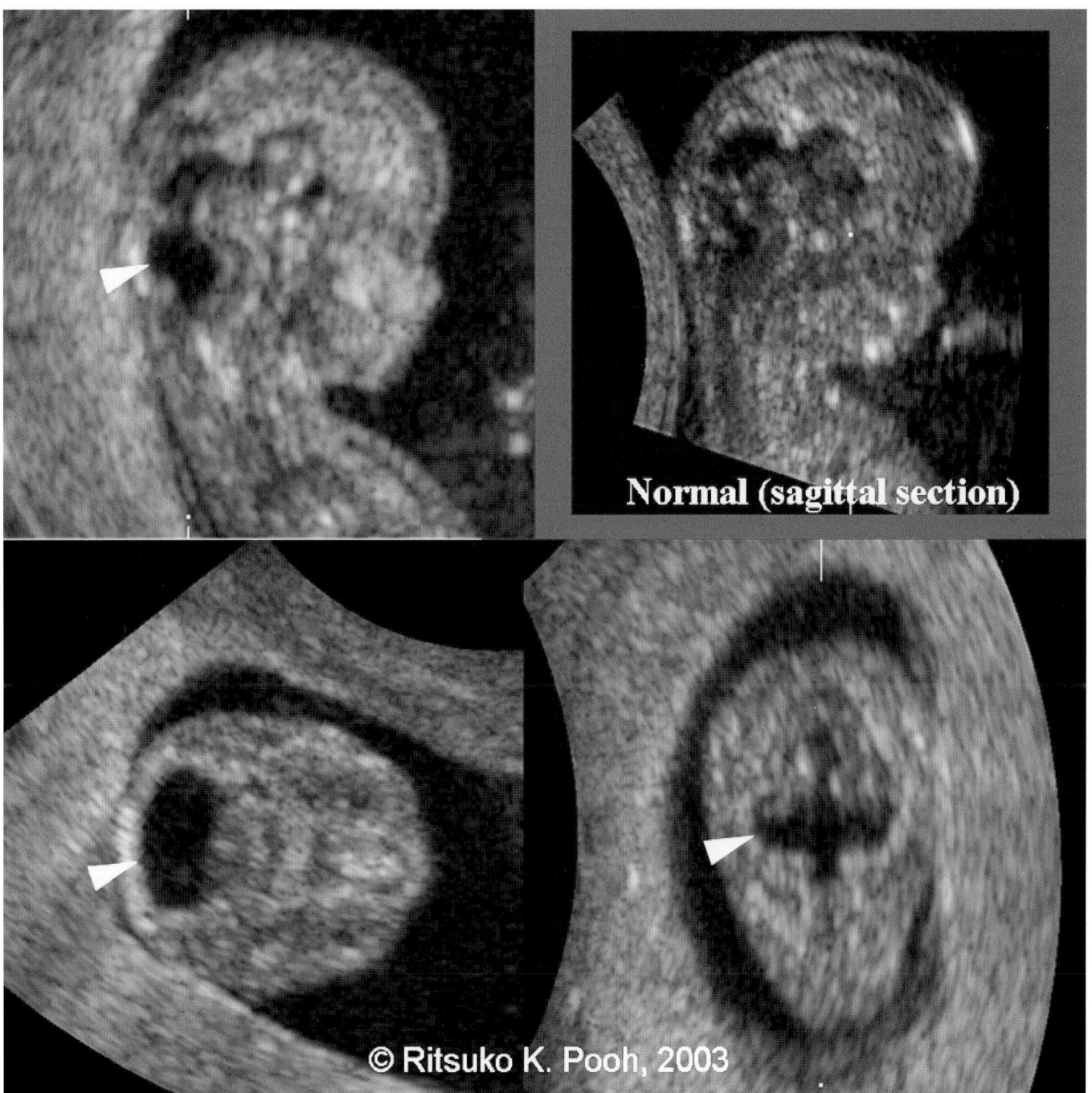

Figure 15.29 Early stage of Dandy–Walker variant at 11 weeks of gestation. Abnormal dilatation of the posterior fossa (arrowheads). Upper right figure is a sagittal image at the same gestational age in a normal case. Amniocentesis revealed trisomy 9 mosaicism and the fetus died in utero at 19 weeks.

Hirschhorn syndrome, the cat cry syndrome and partial deletion of long arm of chromosome 13.
- Contiguous gene syndromes – Miller–Dieker syndrome. Langer–Giedion syndrome, Prader–Willi syndrome and the aniridia-Wilms tumor syndrome.
- Genetic disorders – Johanson–Blizzard syndrome, Seckel syndrome and the Smith–Lemli–Opitz syndrome.

- Environmental insults – maternal PKU (mothers who have poorly controlled PKU during pregnancy) and the fetal alcohol syndrome.

Pathogenesis: may be caused by a disturbance in the proliferation of nerve cells. Abnormalities of neurocranial architecture occur in approximately two-thirds of cases (Persutte 1998).

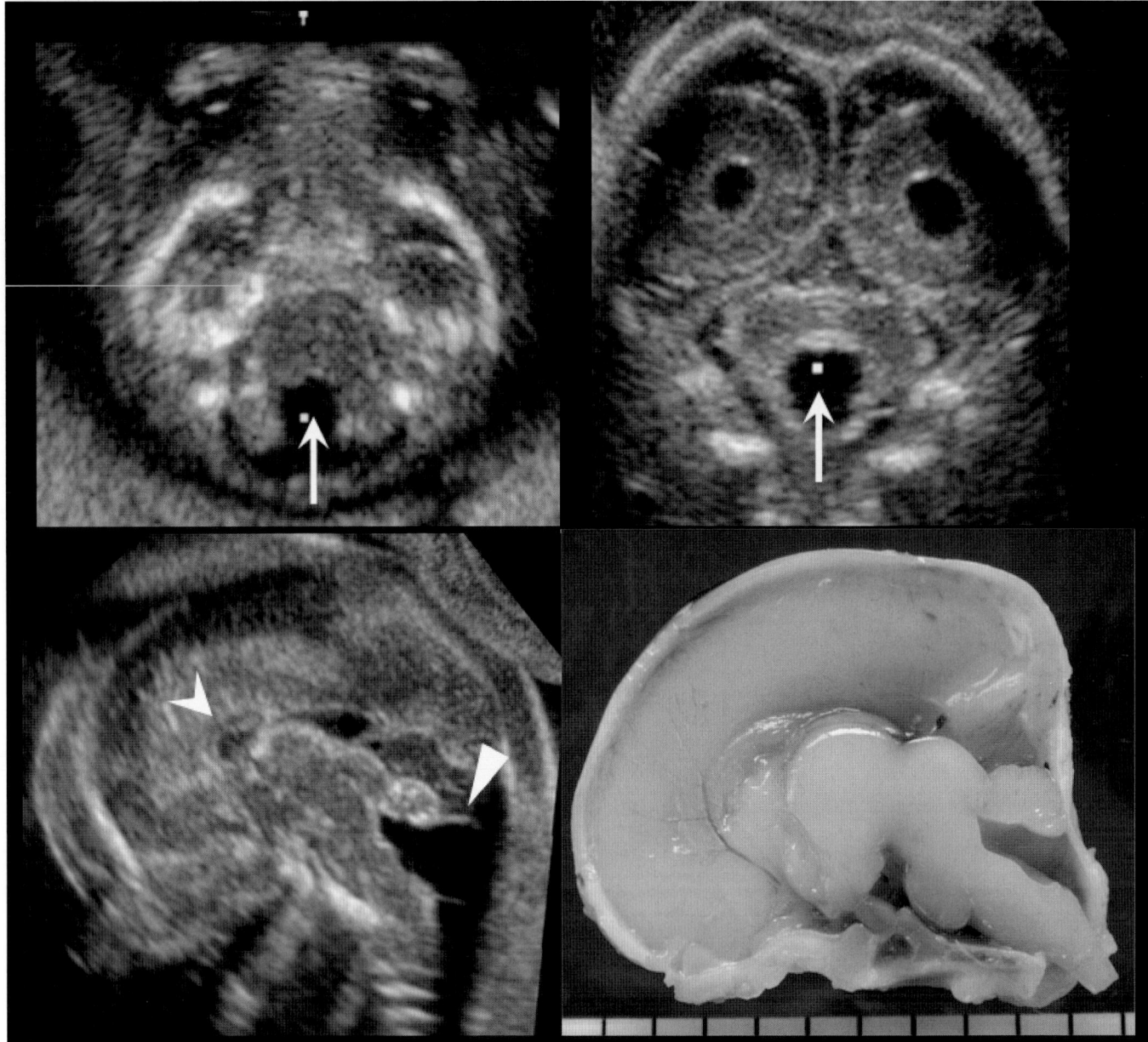

Figure 15.30 Dandy–Walker variant at 20 weeks of gestation. (upper left) Axial sonographic image. (upper right) Posterior coronal image. Hypoplasia of the vermis (arrows) is demonstrated and no marked ventriculomegaly was seen. (lower left) Median section. Partial agenesis of the corpus callosum (arrowhead), floated cerebellum and cystic formation of the posterior fossa (triangle arrowhead) are seen. (lower right) Median cutting section of the specimen from the same fetus at 21 weeks of gestation. This case had other complicated anomalies and the karyotype was partial trisomy of chromosome 10.

Differential diagnosis: craniosynostosis.

Prenatal diagnosis: ultrasonograms and MR images of typical microcephaly are shown in Figure 15.31. Occasionally, microcephaly occurs with late onset during pregnancy (Schwarzler et al 2003).

Prognosis: development of motor functions and speech may be delayed. Hyperactivity and mental retardation are common occurrences, although the degree of each varies. Convulsions may also occur. Motor ability varies, ranging from clumsiness in some to spastic quadriplegia in others.

Recurrence risk: unknown.

Treatment: no specific treatment for microcephaly. Treatment is symptomatic and supportive.

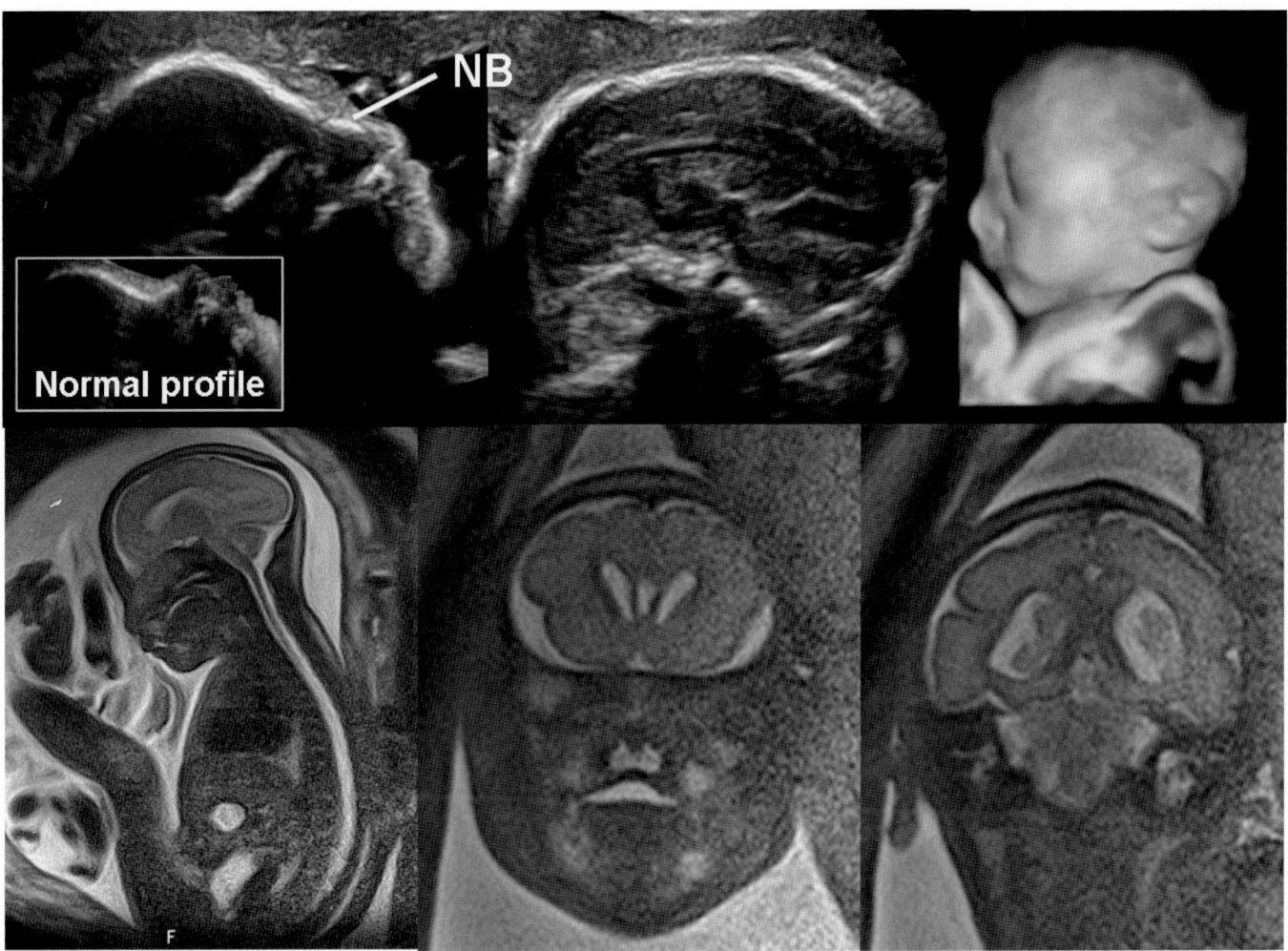

Figure 15.31 Microcephaly at 28 weeks of gestation. (upper left) Fetal face in the sagittal section. Note the flat face with the frontal bone and nasal bone (NB) on a single line, compared to the normal face in the yellow box. (upper middle) Sagittal section of the brain. Microcephaly and micro-brain are detectable. (upper right) 3D reconstruction image of fetal craniofacial expression. (lower) MR image in the sagittal, anterior-coronal and posterior-coronal sections from the left.

NEURONAL MIGRATION DISORDERS

Neuronal migration disorders are caused by the abnormal migration of neurons in the developing brain and nervous system. Neurons must migrate from the areas where they are born to the areas where they will settle into their proper neural circuits. Neuronal migration, which occurs as early as the second month of gestation, is controlled by a complex assortment of chemical guides and signals. When these signals are absent or incorrect, neurons do not end up where they belong. This can result in structurally abnormal or missing areas of the brain in the cerebral hemispheres, cerebellum, brainstem, or hippocampus, including schizencephaly, porencephaly, lissencephaly, agyria, macrogyria, pachygyria, microgyria, micropolygyria, neuronal heterotopias (including band heterotopia), agenesis of the corpus callosum and agenesis of the cranial nerves. Figure 15.32 shows unilateral maldevelopment caused by migration dis-

order detected by ultrasonography and MRI. Symptoms vary according to the specific disorder and the degree of brain abnormality and subsequent neurological losses, but often feature poor muscle tone and motor function, seizures, developmental delays, mental retardation, failure to grow and thrive, difficulties with feeding, swelling in the extremities and a smaller than normal head. Most infants with a neuronal migration disorder appear normal, but some disorders have characteristic facial or skull features.

LISSENCEPHALY

Lissencephaly is characterized by a lack of gyral development and divided into two types:

Lissencephaly type I: a smooth surface of the brain. Cerebral wall is similar to that of an approximately 12-week-old fetus (Volpe 2001d).
Isolated lissencephaly.

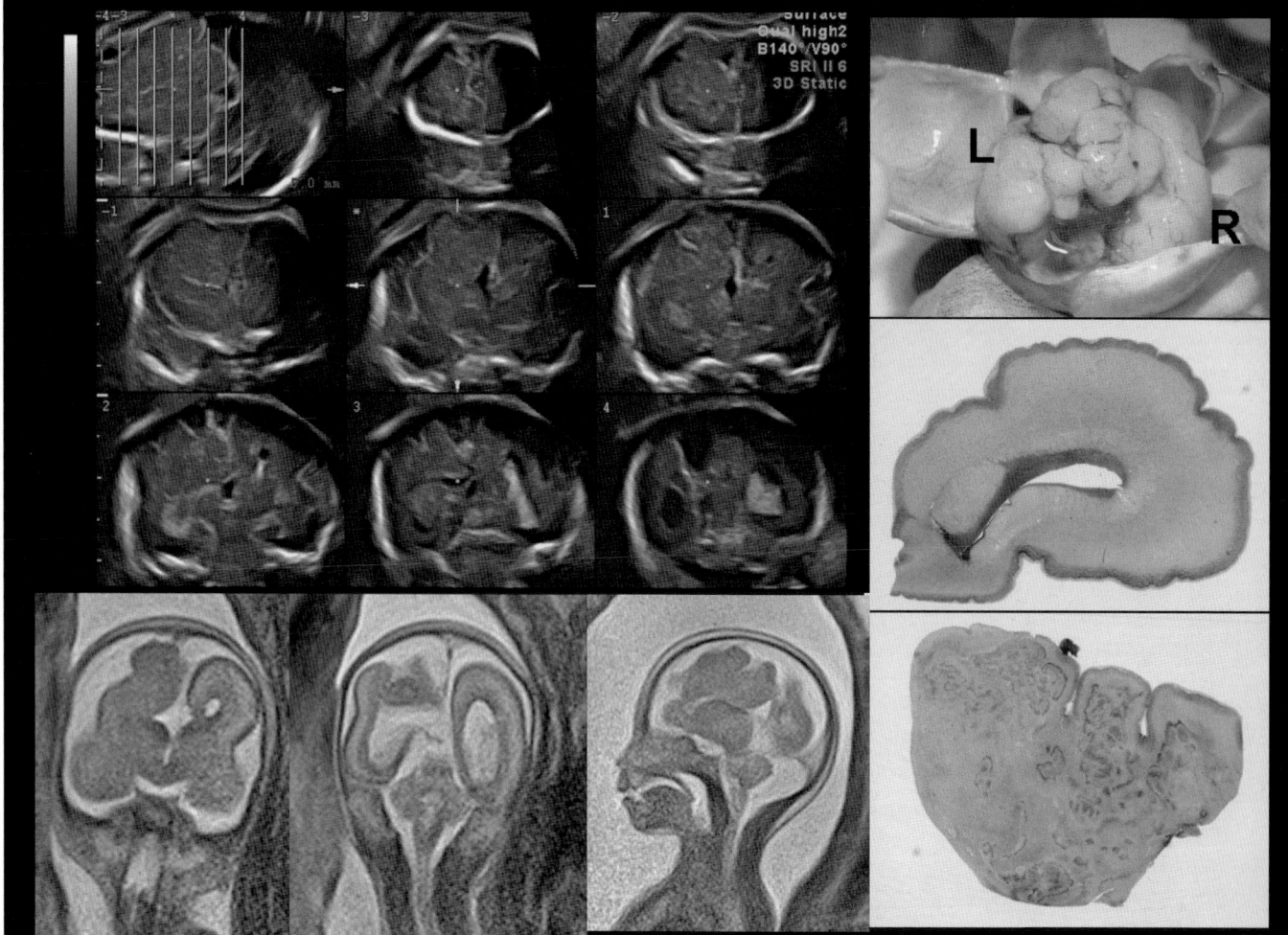

Figure 15.32 Migration disorder of unilateral hemisphere at 18 weeks of gestation. (upper left) Tomographic coronal image of the brain. Note the different development between bilateral hemispheres. (lower left) MR images at same gestational age. Anterior-coronal, posterior-coronal and sagittal sections from the left. Unilateral abnormal brain development was caused according to migration disorder. (right upper) Macroscopic intracranial finding by autopsy after termination at 21 weeks of gestation. (right middle) Normal histological findings of normal hemisphere. (right lower) Maldevelopment of the other hemisphere because of migration disorder.

Miller–Dieker syndrome with additional craniofacial abnormalities, cardiac anomalies, genital anomalies, sacral dimple, creases and/or clinodactyly.

Lissencephaly type II; cobblestone appearance.

Walker–Warburg syndrome with macrocephaly, congenital muscular dystrophy, cerebellar malformation, retinal malformation.

Fukuyama congenital muscular dystrophy with microcephaly and congenital muscular dystrophy.

Incidence: unknown, rare.

Synonyms: agyria, pachygyria, Walker–Warburg syndrome was known as HARD ± E syndrome (hydrocephalus, agyria, retinal dysplasia, with or without encephalocele).

Etiology: isolated lissencephaly is linked to chromosome 17p13.3 and chromosome Xq24-q24. Miller–Dieker syndrome is also linked to chromosome 17p13.3. Walker–

Warburg syndrome is of autosomal recessive inheritance. Fukuyama congenital muscular dystrophy is linked to chromosome 9q31, fukutin (Kobayashi et al 1998).

Pathogenesis: defective neuronal migration with four, rather than six, layers in the cortex.

Associated anomalies: polyhydramnios, less fetal movement, colpocephaly, agenesis of the corpus callosum, Dandy–Walker malformation. In Miller–Dieker syndrome, micrognathia, flat nose, high forehead, low-set ears, cardiac anomalies, genital anomalies in males are often observed.

Prenatal diagnosis: a few reports of prenatal diagnosis of lissencephaly have been published (Greco et al 1998, Kojima et al 2002, McGahan et al 1994). Without previous history of an affected child diagnosis probably cannot be reliably made until 26 to 28 weeks' gestation (Monteagudo and Timor–Tritsch 2001).

Prognosis: Type I: hypotonia, paucity of movements, feeding disturbance, seizures. The prognosis is poor and death occurs. Type II: severe seizures, mental disorders, severe muscle disease with hypotonia. Death in the first year is common.

Recurrence risk: depends on etiology.

Management: karyotyping is recommended to detect the chromosomal defect.

SCHIZENCEPHALY

Incidence: rare.

Definition: a disorder characterized by congenital clefts in the cerebral mantle, lined by pia-ependyma, with communication between the subarachnoid space laterally and the ventricular system medially. Sixty-three percent is unilateral and 37% bilateral. Frontal region in 44% and frontoparietal 30% (Volpe 2001d).

Etiology: uncertain. In certain familial case, a point mutation in the homeobox gene, EMX2 was found (Brunelli et al 1996, Granata et al 1997). Cytomegalovirus infection was also related in some cases (Iannetti et al 1998).

Pathogenesis: neuronal migration disorder.

Associated anomalies: ventriculomegaly, microcephaly, polymicrogyria, gray matter heterotopias, dysgenesis of the corpus callosum, absence of the septum pellucidum and optic nerve hypoplasia.

Prenatal diagnosis: Figure 15.33 shows sonograms and fetal MRI of bilateral schizencephaly.

Differential diagnosis: porencephaly, arachnoid cyst or other intracranial cystic masses. MR imaging is useful in diagnosis of schizencephaly (Denis et al 2001).

Prognosis: variable. Generally suffer from mental retardation, seizures, developmental delay and motor disturbances.

Recurrence risk: unknown.

Management: ventriculoperitoneal shunt for progressive hydrocephalus.

OTHER CONGENITAL ANOMALIES

ARACHNOID CYST, INTERHEMISPHERIC CYST

Congenital or acquired cyst, lined by arachnoid membranes and filled with fluid collection which is the same character as the cerebrospinal fluid. The number of cysts is mostly single, but two or more cysts can be occasionally observed. Location of arachnoid cyst is various; and it is said that approximately 50% of cysts occur from the sylvian fissure (middle fossa), 20% from the posterior fossa, and 10–20% each from the convexity, suprasellar, interhispheral and quadrigeminal cistern in the pediatric field. Interhemispheric cysts are commonly associated with agenesis or hypogenesis of the corpus callosum. Callosal agenesis with interhemispheric cyst is classified as two types (Barkovich et al 2001). Type 1 cysts appear to be an extension or diverticulation of the third or lateral ventricles, whereas Type 2 cysts are loculated and do not communicate with the ventricular system.

Prevalence: 1% of intracranial masses in newborns.

Etiology: unknown.

Pathogenesis: congenital arachnoid cyst is formed by maldevelopment of the arachnoid membrane. CSF accumulation in the subarachnoid space or intra-arachnoid layers from a choroid plexus-like tissue within the cyst wall leads to a progressive distension of the lesion.

Associated anomalies: unilateral or bilateral hydrocephalus, macrocrania.

Prenatal diagnosis: interhemispheric cyst in Figures 15.34, 15.35 and 15.36, middle fossa arachnoid cyst in Figure 15.37 and suprasellar arachnoid cyst in Figure 15.38. As intrauterine spontaneous resolution or changing cyst size is often seen during the fetal period, serial scanning is important. Detection in the first trimester was reported (Bretelle et al 2002).

Differential diagnosis: porencephaly, schizencephaly, third ventriculomegaly, intracranial cystic type tumor, vein of Galen aneurysm, Dandy–Walker malformation, large cisterna magna, external hydrocephalus.

Prognosis: generally good. Postnatally, many are asymptomatic and remain quiescent for years, although others expand and cause neurological symptoms by compressing adjacent brain, ventriculomegaly and/or expanding the overlying skull.

Recurrence risk: unknown.

Obstetrical management: arachnoid cysts may increase or decrease its size. Therefore, expectant management of antenatally diagnosed cases is suggested (Elbers and Furness 1999). In cases with accompanied hydrocephalus, mode and timing of delivery may be modified.

Postnatal management: in cases with those symptoms or with prospects of neurological symptoms, treatment should be considered. Operation methods include:

- Cyst fenestration by craniotomy.
- Cyst fenestration by neuroendoscopy.
- Cyst-peritoneal shunt.

Craniotomy, shunting or neuroendoscopic method has been controversial (Ciricillo et al 1991, Nakamura et al 2001).

BRAIN TUMORS

Incidence: extremely rare.

Histological types: brain tumors are divided into teratoma, most commonly reported, and non-teratomatous tumor. Non-teratomatous tumors include neuroepithelial tumor, such as medulloblastoma, astrocytoma, choroid plexus papilloma, choroid plexus carcinoma, ependymoma, ependymoblastoma and mesenchymal tumor such as craniopharyngioma, sarcoma, fibroma, hemangioblastoma, hemangioma and meningoma, and others of lipoma of the corpus callosum, subependymal giant-cell astrocytoma associated with tuberous sclerosis (often accompanied by cardiac rhabdomyoma) (Volpe 2001a, Wakai et al 1984).

Location of tumor: supratentorial predominance in neonatal tumor. Infratentorial predominance in medulloblastoma.

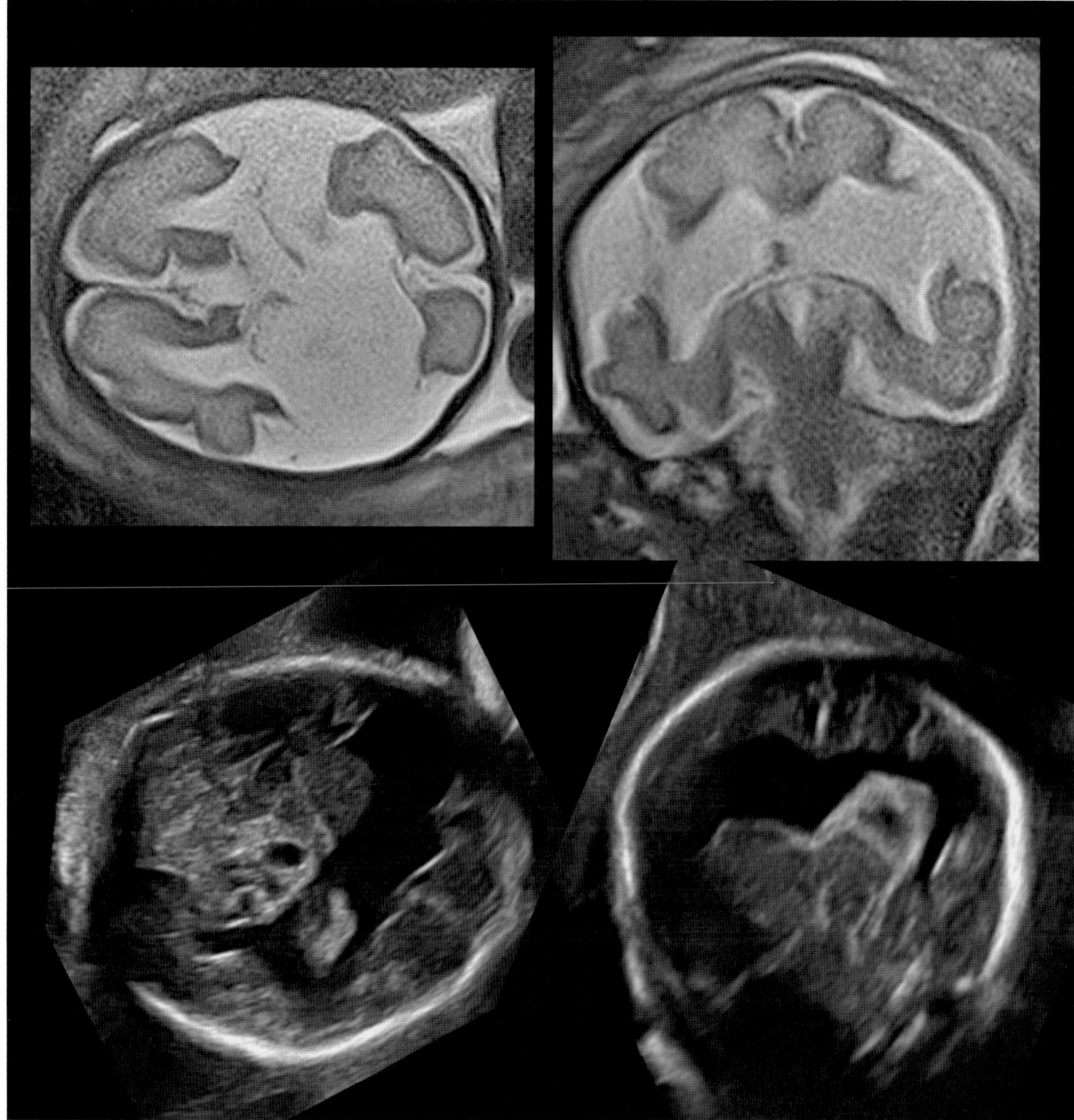

Figure 15.33 Schizencephaly at 33 weeks of gestation. (upper left) MR axial image. Bilateral schizencephaly is clearly demonstrated. (upper right) MR coronal image. (lower) Sonographic axial and coronal images.

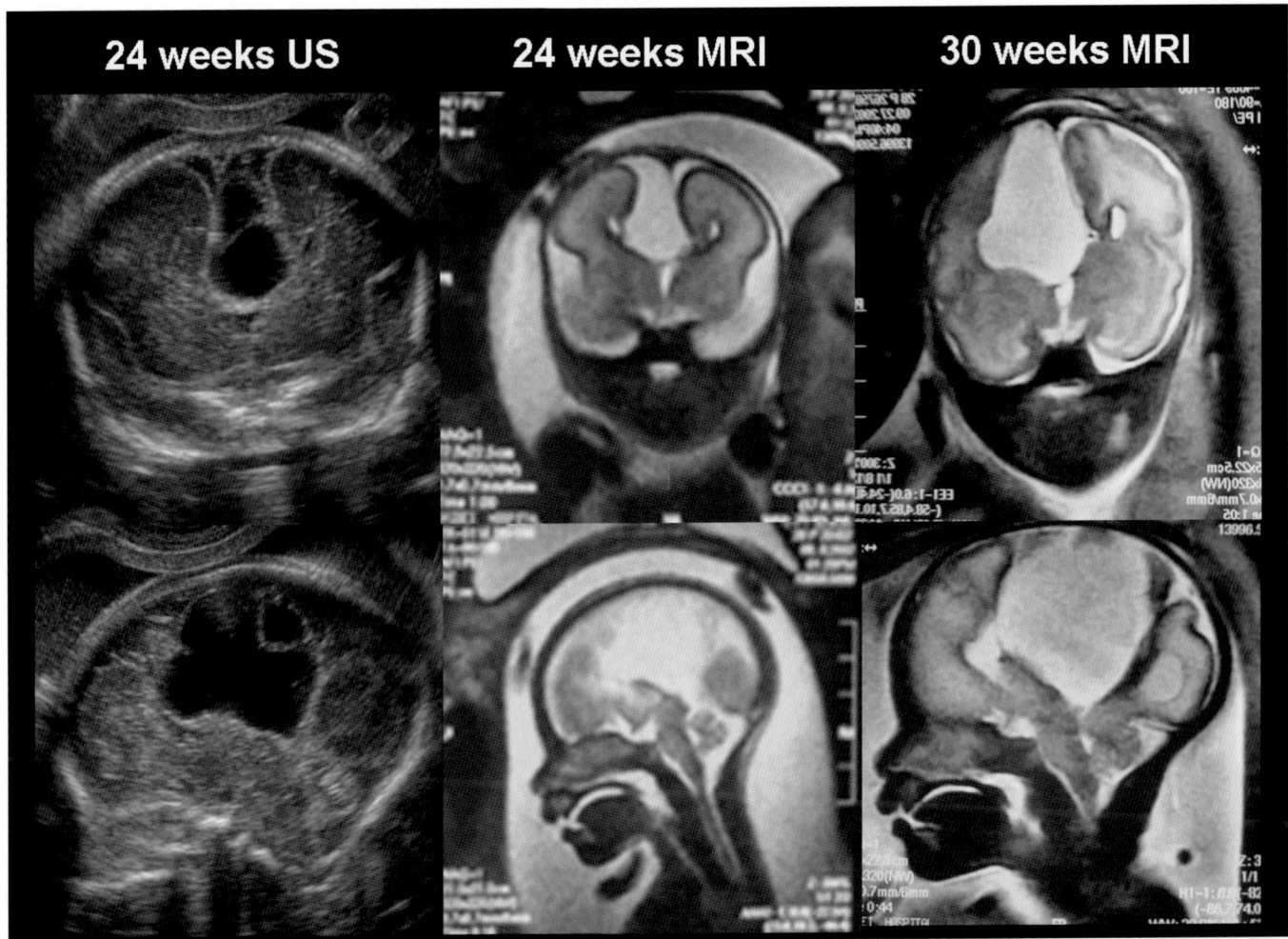

24 weeks US   **24 weeks MRI**   **30 weeks MRI**

Figure 15.34 US and MR images of interhemispheric cyst. Anterior coronal sections (upper) and mid sagittal sections (lower). At 24 weeks of gestation, interhemispheric cyst with agenesis of the corpus callosum is seen. Ultrasound shows the cysts in cyst. MR images at 30 weeks show spontaneous increased cyst-size during pregnancy.

Choroid plexus papilloma is located within the lateral ventricles.

Associated abnormalities: macrocrania or local skull swelling, epignathus, secondary hydrocephalus, intracranial hemorrhage, intraventricular hemorrhage, polyhydramnios, heart failure by high-cardiac output (Sherer et al 1993) and hydrops.

Prenatal diagnosis: intracranial masses with solid, cystic or mixture pattern with or without visualization of hypervascularity by ultrasound and fetal MRI. Brain tumor should be considered in cases with unexplained intracranial hemorrhage. Prenatal diagnosis of intracranial tumor and its vascularization by 3D power Doppler is shown in Figure 15.39, glioma at 18 weeks in Figure 15.40, immature teratoma at 14 weeks in Figure 15.41.

Differential diagnosis: arachnoid cyst, vein of Galen aneurysm, porencephaly, schizencephaly, periventricular leukomalacia, subdural hemorrhage.

Prognosis: fetal demise, stillborn may occur. Prognosis in neonates is generally poor, but depends on timing of diagnosis and the histological type of tumor. Choroid plexus papilloma has minimal mortality rate and high likelihood of neonatal outcome. Mortality rate of teratomas is over 90%, medulloblastoma over 80%. Other tumors have various prognoses.

Recurrence risk: unknown.

Management: cesarean section may be considered. Neurosurgical tumor resection including subtotal hemispherectomy by craniotomy and chemotherapy are possible treatments for neonatal tumors. Radiation therapy is usually not indicated in neonates.

CRANIOSYNOSTOSIS

Premature closure of cranial suture, which may affect one or more cranial sutures. Simple sagittal synostosis is

Text continued on p. 326

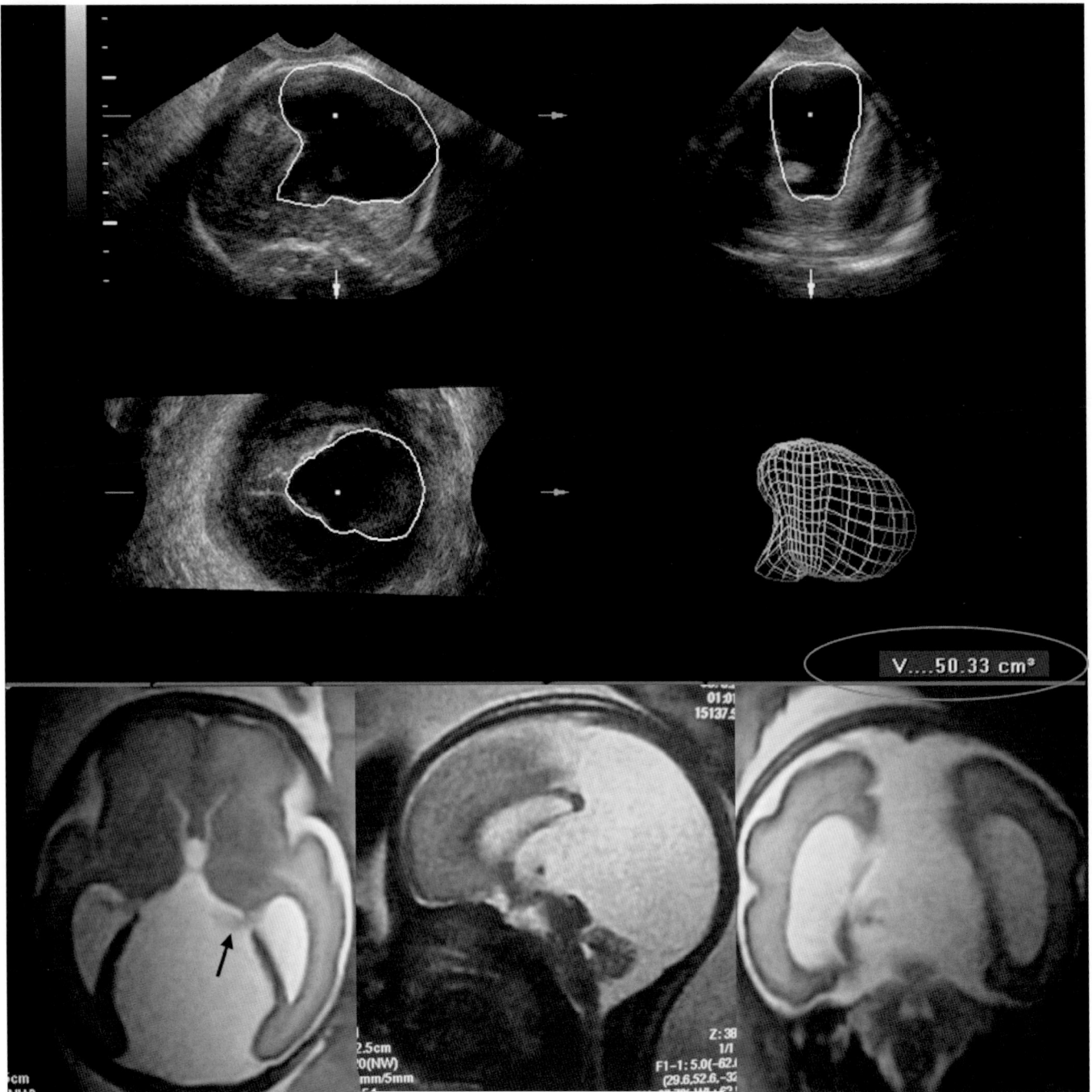

Figure 15.35 Interhemispheric cyst at 27 weeks. (upper) Three orthogonal view with tracing interhemispheric cyst. The extracted structure of the cyst is demonstrated with volume calculation of the cyst (red circle). (lower) Fetal MR images. Axial, sagittal and posterior coronal sections from the left. The choroid plexus inside the lateral ventricle comes out into the cyst (arrow). This fact indicates fusion between lateral ventricles and interhemispheric cyst.

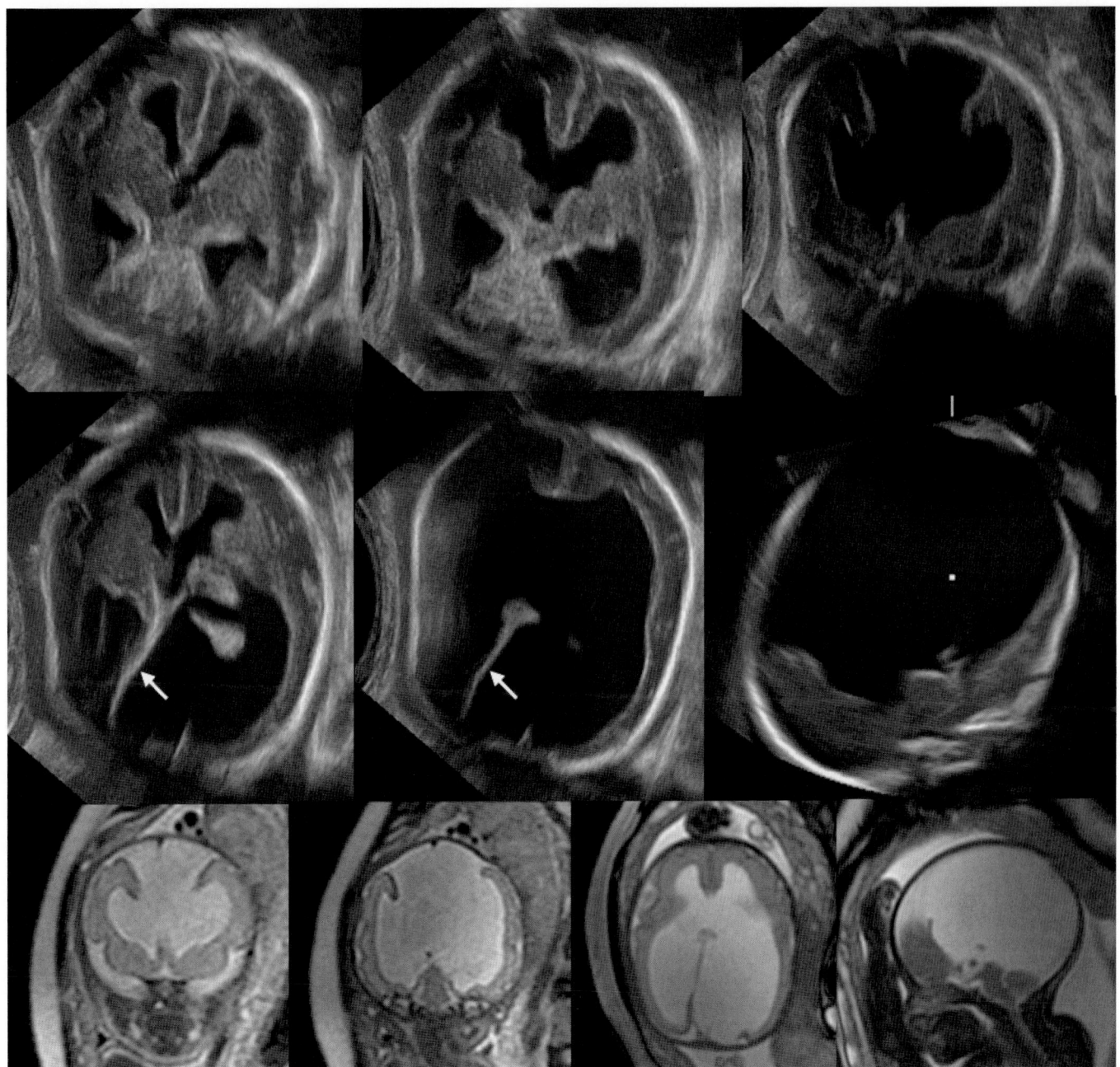

Figure 15.36 Communicating interhemispheric cyst with hydrocephalus. (upper) Oblique (coronal–axial) ultrasound images. Bilateral ventriculomegaly fused with large interhemispheric cyst. (middle) Axial images and sagittal ultrasound images. Unilateral ventricular wall is preserved (arrows). (lower) Fetal MR images. Anterior coronal, posterior coronal, axial and sagittal images from the left.

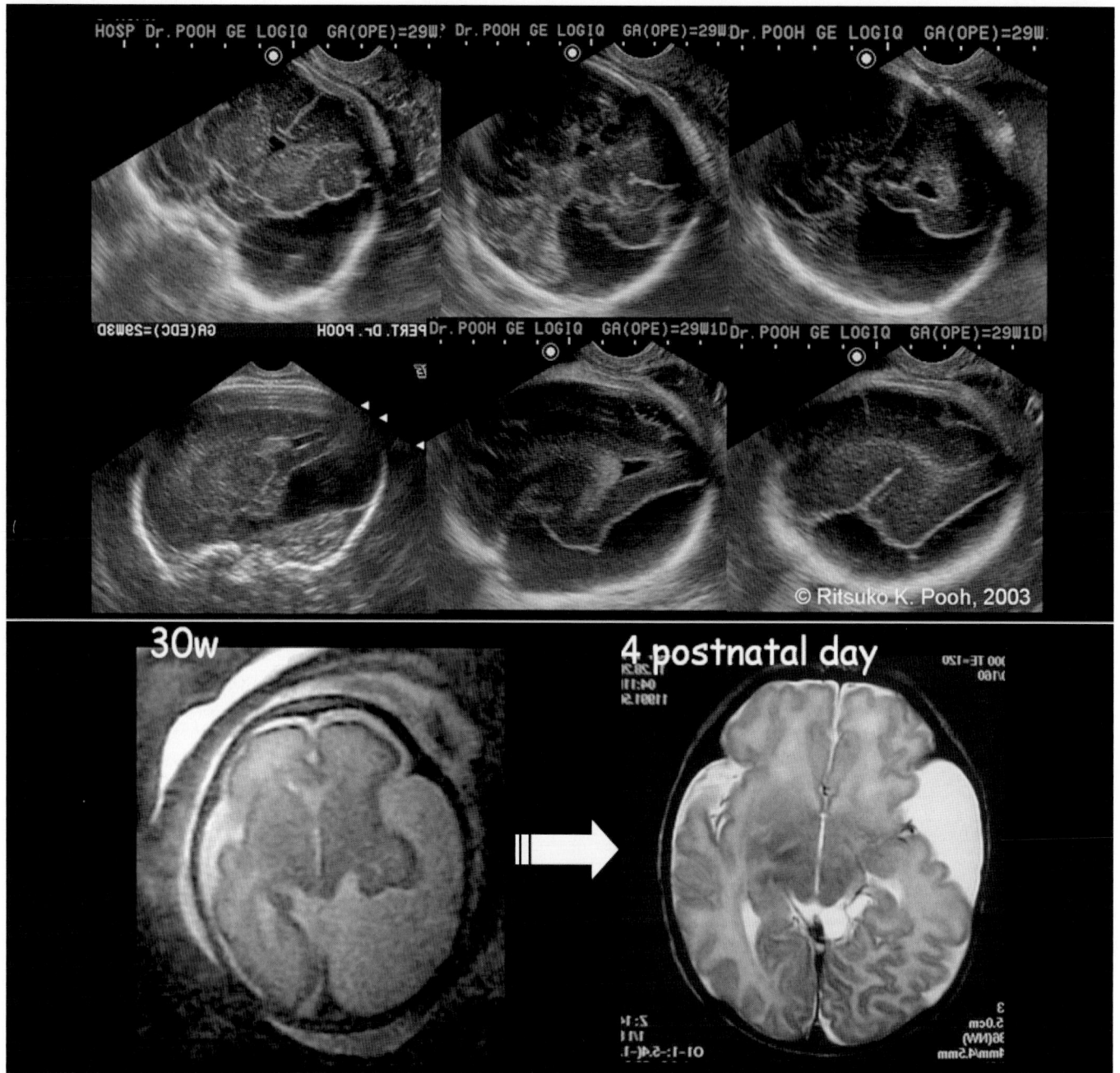

Figure 15.37 Middle fossa arachnoid cyst at 29 weeks of gestation and its spontaneous resolution. (upper) Series of coronal and sagittal sections. The arachnoid cyst arose from the middle fossa and compresses the cerebral hemisphere. (lower) MRI at 30 weeks of gestation and 4 postnatal days. Cerebral development according to spontaneous resolution of arachnoid cyst during pregnancy is seen.

Figure 15.38 Suprasellar arachnoid cyst. MR images and serial US scan images. (upper) MRI at 24 weeks of gestation. Sagittal, coronal and axial planes from the left. Suprasellar arachnoid cyst oppressing the brain stem (BS) and bilateral hemispheres. (lower) Serial scan images of the mid-sagittal section. Spontaneous size decreases from 24 to 29 weeks and increases from 29 to 33 weeks are well demonstrated. Asterisks indicate the arachnoid cyst.

Figure 15.39 Ultrasound images and tumoral vascular visualization by 3D power Doppler in a fetus of intracranial tumor with interventricular hemorrhage (35 weeks and 5 days of gestation). (upper) Sagittal, coronal and axial US images. Huge tumor (arrowheads) with hemorrhage within the tumor in the fronto-parietal lobe complicated with unilateral hydrocephalus with intraventricular hemorrhage (arrow). (left lower) Oblique sagittal view from fetal left side. (right lower) Oblique coronal view from fetal frontal side. Tumor is fed by numerous feeding arteries from anterior cerebral artery. Feeder arteries have low resistant flow waveform. One large vein which drains blood from tumor is visible. The draining vein has pulsatile flow.

BS
24w
29w
33w

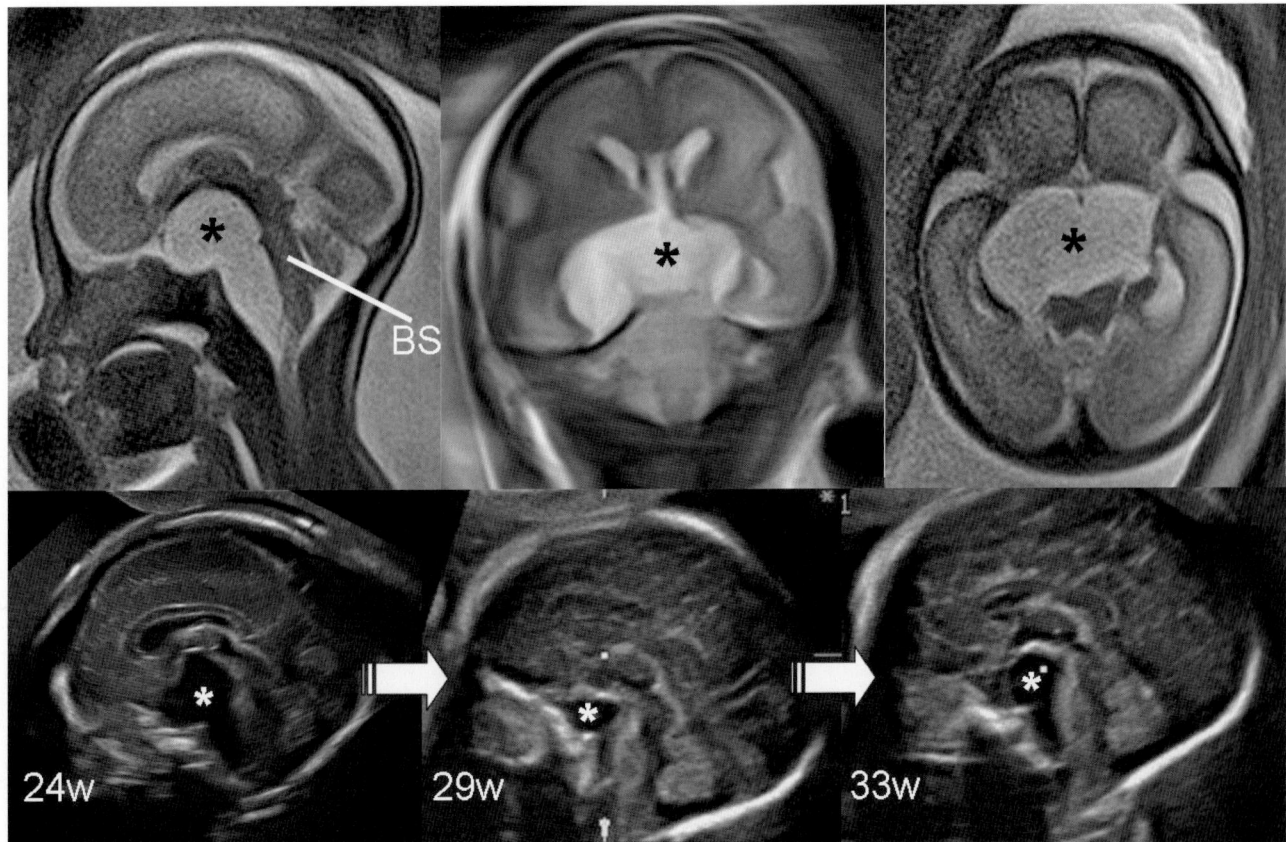

Figure 15.38

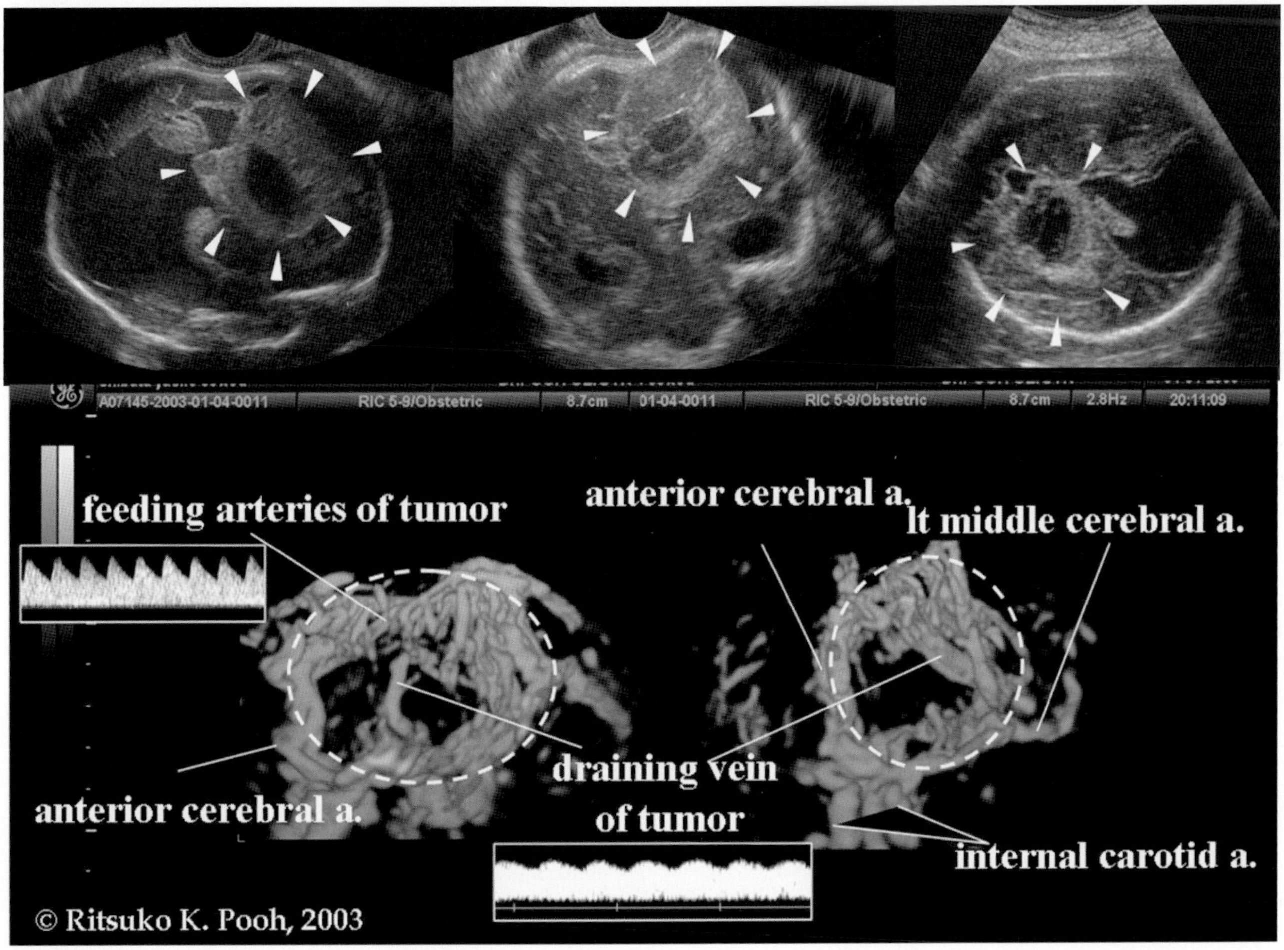

feeding arteries of tumor
anterior cerebral a.
lt middle cerebral a.
draining vein
of tumor
anterior cerebral a.
internal carotid a.
© Ritsuko K. Pooh, 2003

Figure 15.39

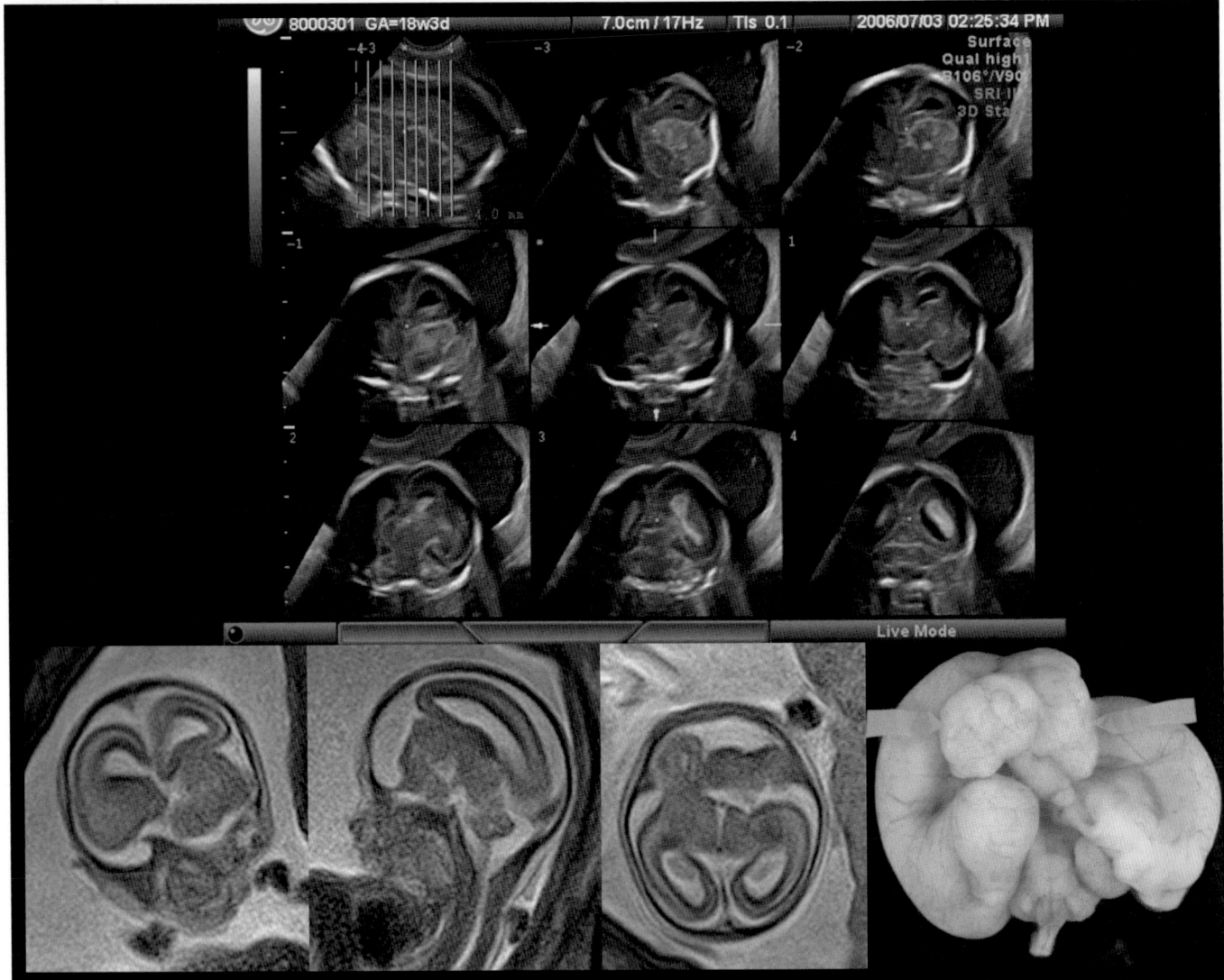

Figure 15.40 Brain tumor at 18 weeks of gestation. (upper left) Tomographic coronal image of the brain. Unilateral hemisphere is oppressed by echogenic mass. (lower left) MR images. Coronal, sagittal and axial planes from the left. (lower right) Brain specimen from aborted fetus at 21 weeks of gestation. The tumor is indicated by green arrows.

most common. Various cranial shapes depend on affected suture(s).

Sagittal suture	scaphocephaly or dolichocephaly
Bilateral coronal suture	brachycephaly
Unilateral coronal suture	anterior plagiocephaly
Metopic suture	trigonocephaly
Lambdoid suture	acrocephaly
Unilateral lambdoid suture	posterior plagiocephaly
Coronal/lambdoid/metopic or squamous/sagittal suture	cloverleaf skull
Total cranial sutures	oxycephaly

Incidence: unknown

Syndromes: Crouzon syndrome; acrocephaly, synostosis of coronal, sagittal and lambdoid sutures.

With ocular proptosis, maxillary hypoplasia

Apert syndrome; brachycephaly, irregular synostosis, especially coronal suture

With midfacial hypoplasia, syndactyly, broad distal phalanx of thumb and big toe

Pfeiffer syndrome; brachycephaly, synostosis of coronal and/or sagittal sutures

With hypertelorism, broad thumbs and toes, partial syndactyly

Antley–Bixler syndrome; brachycephaly, multiple synostoses, especially of coronal suture

With maxillary hypoplasia, radiohymeral synostosis, choanal atresia, arthrogryposis.

Etiology: Crouzon (AD, variable), Apert (AD, usually new mutation), Pfeiffer (AD), Antley–Bixler (AR).

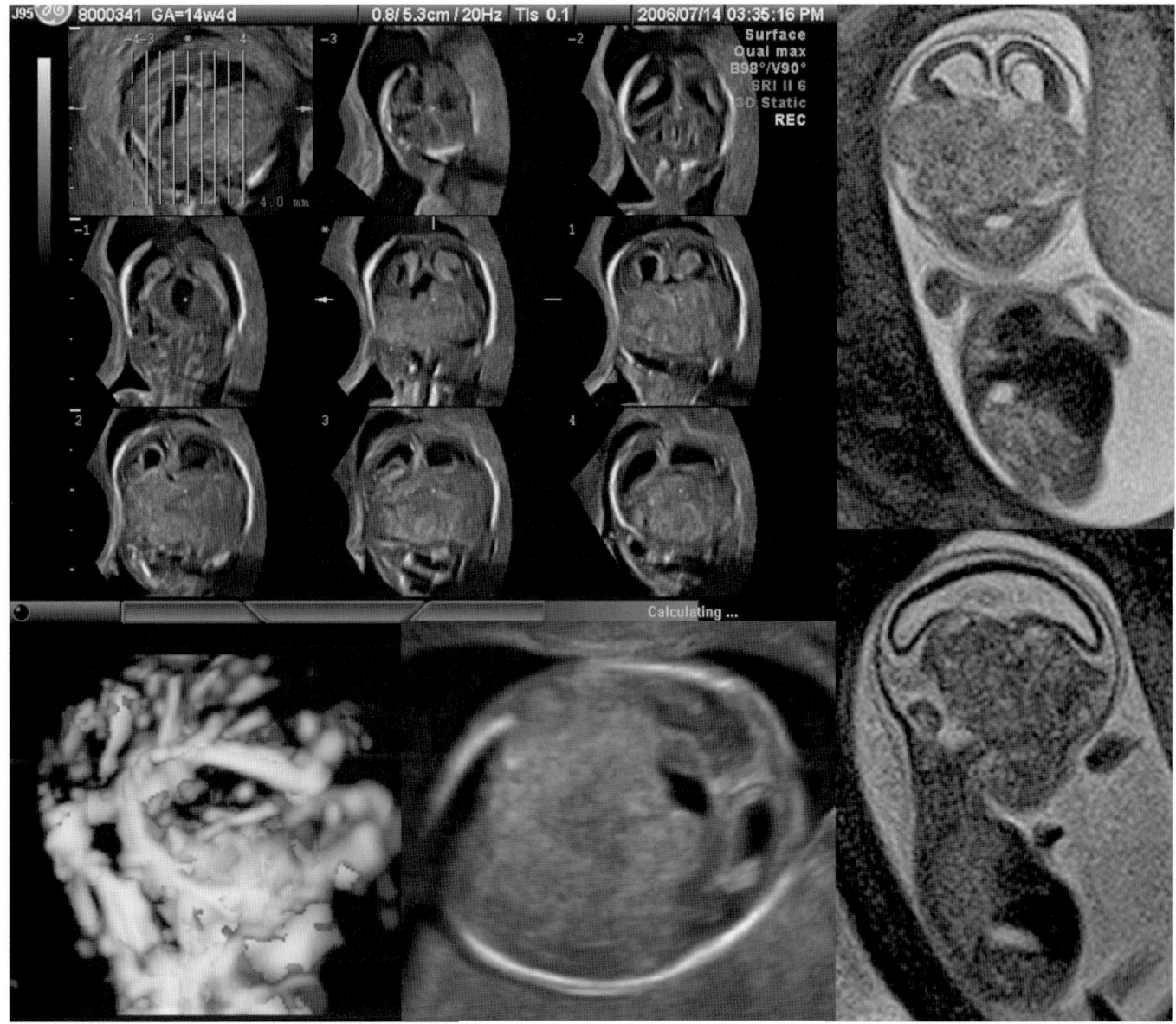

Figure 15.41 Brain tumor at 14 weeks of gestation. (upper left) Tomographic coronal image of the brain. Huge hyperechogenic mass occupies more than half of cranial cavity. (lower left) Intratumoral vascularity demonstrated by directional power Doppler. (lower middle) Axial image by ultrasound. (upper right) Fetal MR coronal image. Bilateral hemispheres are oppressed toward parietal portion. (lower right) Fetal MR sagittal image. Pregnancy was terminated and immature teratoma was confirmed.

Five autosomal dominant craniosynostosis syndromes (Apert, Crouzon, Pfeiffer, Jackson–Weiss and Crouzon syndrome with acanthosis nigricans) result from mutations in *FGFR* genes (Hollway et al 1997).

Pathogenesis (Delashaw et al 1989): (1) cranial vault bones with decreased growth potential, (2) asymmetrical bone deposition at perimeter sutures, (3) sutures adjacent to the prematurely fused suture compensate in growth more than those sutures not contiguous with the closed suture, (4) enhanced symmetrical bone deposition occurs along both sides of a non-perimeter suture continuing prematurely closed suture.

Associated anomalies: hypertelorism, syndactyly, polydactyly, exophthalmos, frontal bossing, low nasal bridge.

Prenatal diagnosis: abnormal craniofacial appearance can be detected by 2D/3D ultrasound (Benacerraf et al 2000, Faro et al 2006, Pooh et al 1999b). Longitudinal profile appearance during pregnancy, intracranial structure, postnatal findings of Apert syndrome is shown in Figure 15.42. Facial abnormality and intracranial structure

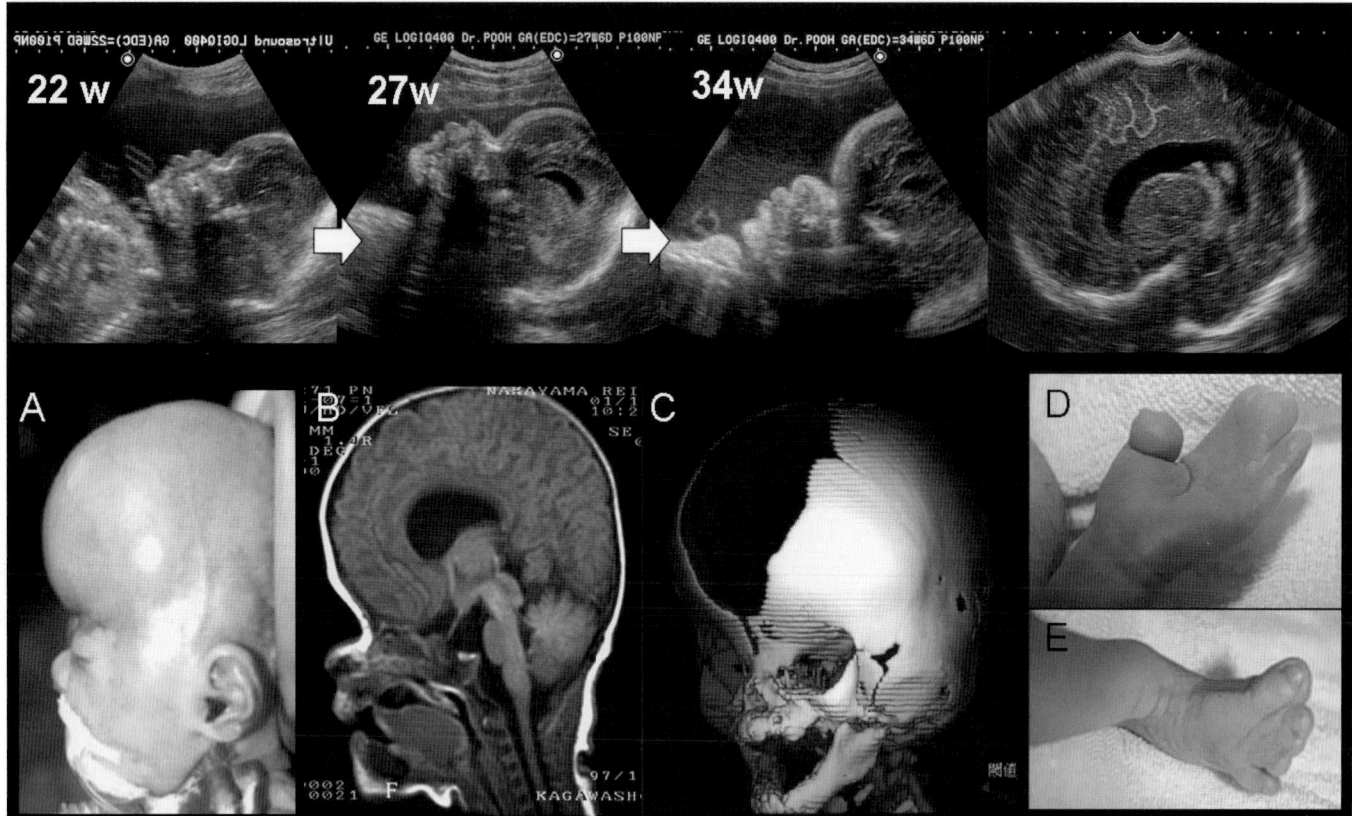

Figure 15.42 Prenatal craniofacial images and postnatal findings in Apert syndrome. (upper) Longitudinal changing appearance of profile at 22, 27 and 34 weeks of gestation. Note the gradual change of frontal bossing and low nasal bridge. (upper right) Parasagittal section of the brain at 34 weeks. Deformed mild ventriculomegaly is seen. (lower) Postnatal findings. A; postnatal profile. B; MR sagittal image. C; 3D-CT image. Fusion of coronal suture and squamous suture, defect of frontoparietal cranial bones and craniofacial bony dysplasia are recognizable. D,E; Typical appearance of syndactyly and large thumbs.

in a case of Pfeiffer syndrome are demonstrated in Figure 15.43.

Prognosis: various. In some cases of trigonocephaly and syndromic types, prognosis is poor.

Recurrence risk: depends on etiology.

Management: operative aim of cranioplasty is improvement of intracranial pressure and cosmetic change.

VEIN OF GALEN ANEURYSM

A congenital malformation of blood vessels of the brain. The main structure is direct arteriovenous fistulas in which blood shunts from choroidal and/or quadrigeminal arteries into an overlying single median venous sac. Vein of Galen aneurysm is not 'aneurysm' but 'arteriovenous malformation' (AVM).

Incidence: rare.

Synonyms: vein of Galen malformation, vein of Galen aneurysmal malformation.

Etiology: unknown.

Pathogenesis: the vein of Galen aneurysmal malformation (VGAM) is a choroidal type of arteriovenous malformation involving the vein of Galen forerunner. This is distinct from

an arteriovenous malformation with venous drainage into a dilated, but already formed, vein of Galen (Lasjaunias et al 2006).

Associated anomalies: cardiomegaly, high cardiac output, secondary hydrocephalus, macrocrania, cerebral ischemia (intracranial steal phenomenon), subarachnoid/cerebral/intraventricular hemorrhages.

Prenatal diagnosis: 2D and 3D color/power Doppler and 3D B-flow detection of VGAM and brain damage caused by cerebral ischemia or hemorrhage with mild ventriculomegaly are shown in Figure 15.44.

Differential diagnosis: arachnoid cyst, porencephalic cyst, intracranial teratoma. Color/power Doppler is helpful for differential diagnosis.

Prognosis: according to earlier review, outcome did not differ between treated and non-treated group and over 80% of cases died (Hoffman et al 1982). However, recent advances in treatment have improved outcome, such that 60–100% survive and over 60% have a good neurological outcome (Campi et al 1998, Friedman et al 1993, Lasjaunias et al 2006).

Recurrence risk: unknown.

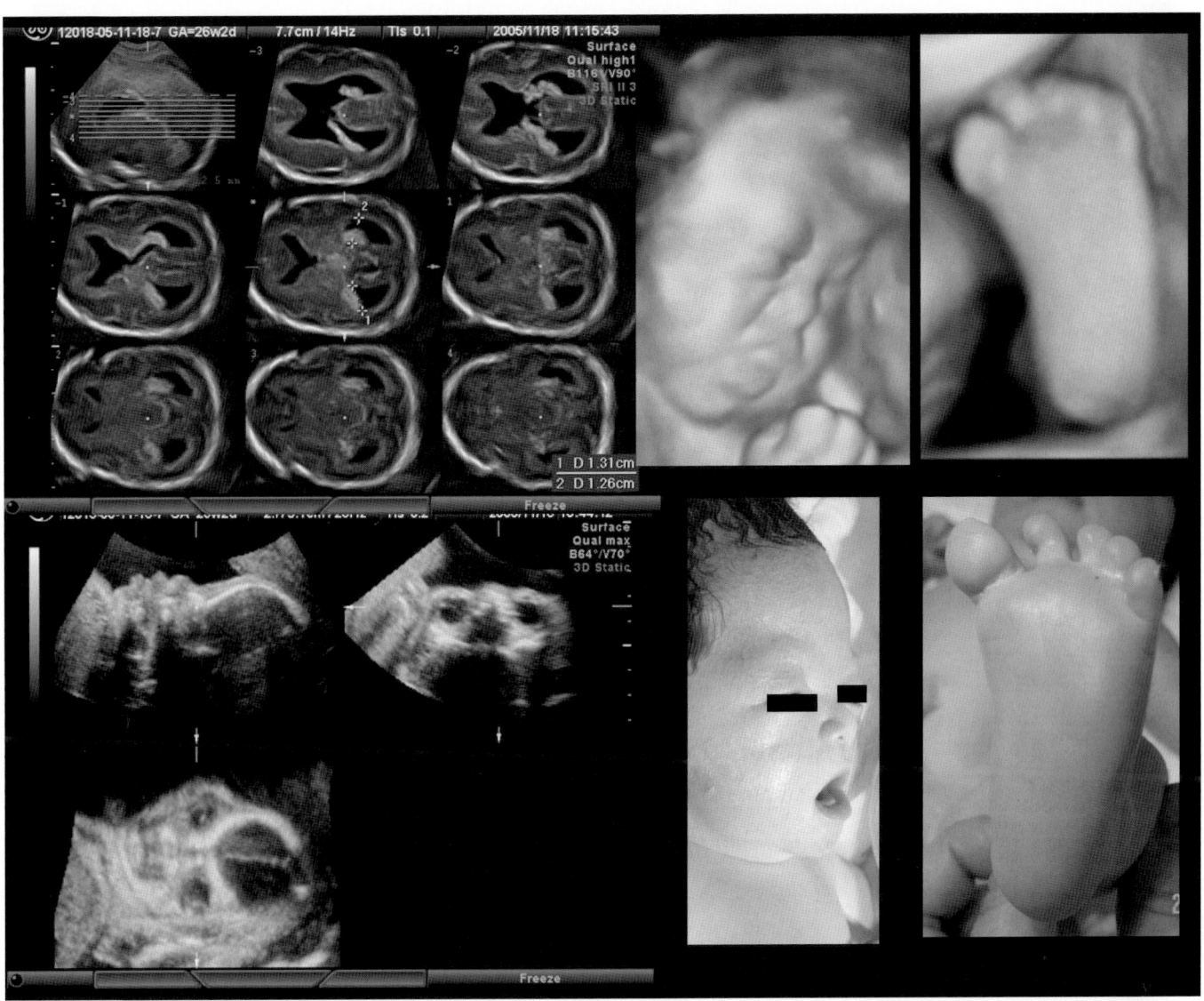

Figure 15.43 Prenatal and postnatal findings of Pfiffer syndrome. (left upper) Tomographic ultrasound imaging of the brain at 26 weeks. Fused ventricle with mild enlargement is demonstrated. Atrial width measurement shows 12 to 13 mm. (upper right) 3D surface images of fetal face and foot. Exophthalmos with flat face and large thumb are seen. (left lower) Three orthogonal view of fetal face. (right lower) Abnormal facial expression and foot appearance after birth.

Management: evaluation of the fetal high-output cardiac state for the proper obstetrical management. Percutaneous embolization by microcoils is recent main postnatal treatment and remarkably improved outcome.

PERICALLOSAL LIPOMA

Intracranial lipomas are congenital malformations composed of mature adipocytes. They are usually located in the midline, particularly in the pericallosal region, a hemispheric location accounting for only 3 to 7% of cases. Two morphologic types of pericallosal lipoma have been described (Demaerel et al 1996, Tart and Quisling 1991).

- Tubulonodular type; generally greater than 2 cm in diameter (often smaller than 2 cm in fetal period) and

have a high incidence of corpus callosum dysgenesis, frontal lobe anomalies, and frontal encephaloceles.
- Curvilinear type: comprises thin, posteriorly situated lipomas curving around the splenium, generally associated with a normal corpus callosum and otherwise have a low incidence of associated anomalies.

Incidence: rare.

Pathogenesis: considered to be the result of an abnormal resorption of the primitive meninges, which occurs between the eighth and 10th week of development. Lipomas develop much more frequently in the corpus callosal area, and interfere with its normal growth between the 11th and 20th weeks. Therefore, complete/partial agenesis or hypoplasia of the corpus callosum often coexists.

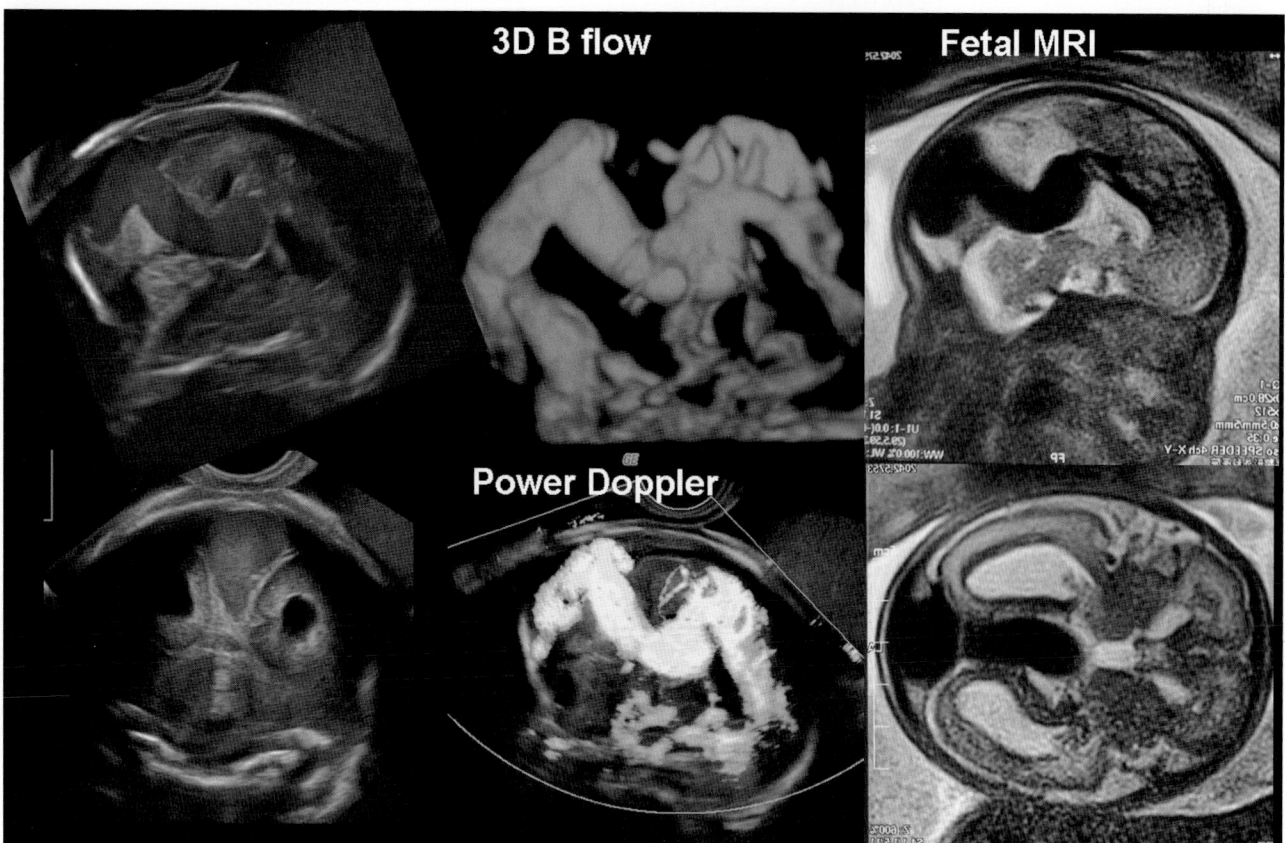

Figure 15.44 Vein of Galen aneurysm at 28 weeks of gestation. (upper left) Transvaginal sagittal image. Dilated dural sinuses are demonstrated. (lower left) Transvaginal coronal image. Interhemispheric space occupying lesion is the dilated vein. (upper middle) 3D B-flow image of intracranial vasculature. Many intracranial arteries run directly toward aneurysmal sac. (lower middle) Power Doppler image. (upper right) Fetal MR sagittal image. (lower right) Fetal MR axial image.

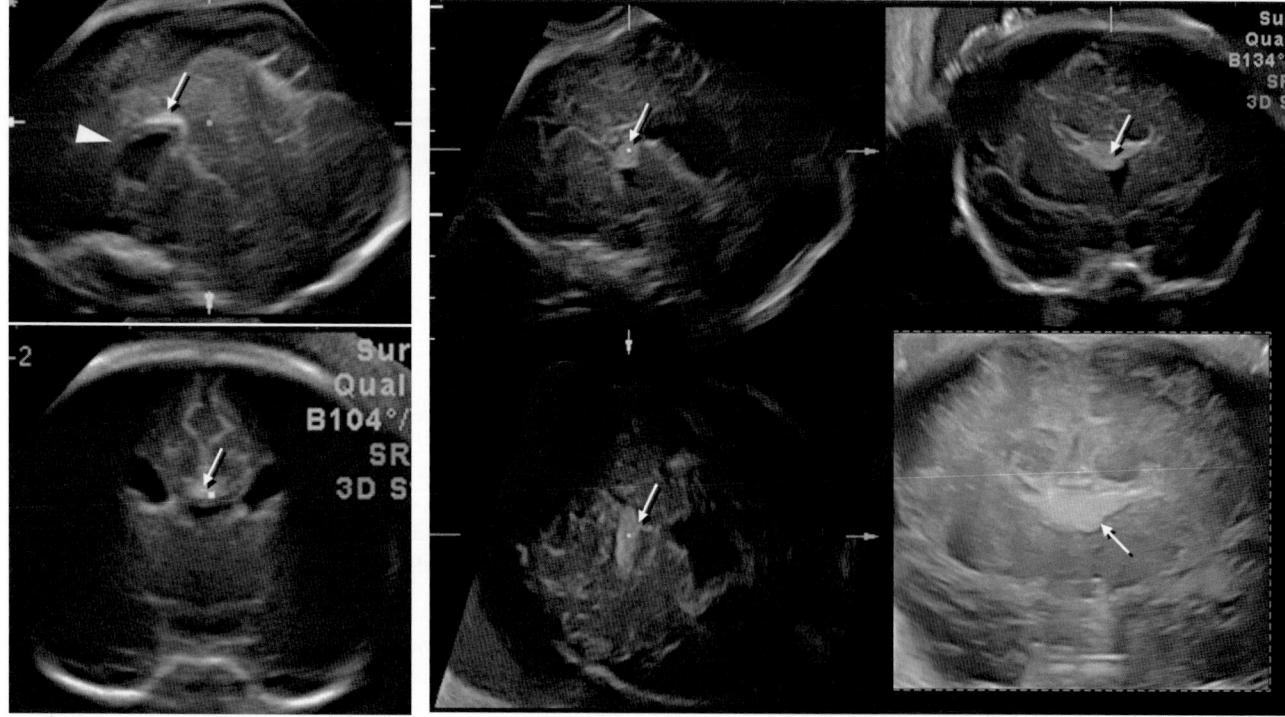

Figure 15.45 Pericallosal lipoma. curvilinear type (left) and tubulonodular type (right). (left) Curvilinear type of lipoma at 29 weeks of gestation. Partial agenesis of the corpus callosum (arrowhead) with posteriorly situated lipoma (arrows) curving around the splenium in the sagittal (upper) and coronal (lower) images. (right) Three orthogonal view and thick slice image of tubulonodular type of lipoma at 36 weeks of gestation. Complete agenesis of the corpus callosum is seen in the sagittal and coronal sections. Arrows indicate pericallosal lipoma. In this case, micrognathia, vertebral anomaly, vermis dysplasia were complicated and postnatal diagnosis was Aicardi syndrome.

Prenatal diagnosis: high echogenic mass can be easily demonstrated by ultrasound. Figure 15.45 shows prenatal detection of curvilinear type and tubulonodular type of pericallosal lipomas. Several reports on prenatal diagnosis have been published (Ickowitz et al 2001, Jeanty et al 1991, Malinger et al 2004).

Differential diagnosis: hemorrhage, teratoma and other brain tumor.

Associated anomalies: dysgenesis/agenesis of the corpus callosum. Occasionally associated with specific malformative syndromes, such as Goldenhar syndrome (Jeanty et al 1991) and chromosomal aberration.

Prognosis: very good prognosis for fetuses with isolated lipoma of the corpus callosum. Variable if other anomalies are complicated.

Management: surgical therapy is usually not indicated because symptoms are generally not related.

ACQUIRED BRAIN ABNORMALITIES IN UTERO

In terms of encephalopathy or cerebral palsy, '*timing of brain insult, antepartum, intrapartum or postpartum?*' is one of the serious controversial issues including medico-socio-legal-ethical problems (Pooh et al 2003). Although brain insults may relate to antepartum events in a substantial number of term infants with hypoxic–ischemic encephalopathy, the timing of insult cannot always be clarified. It is a hard task to give antepartum evidence of brain injury predictive of cerebral palsy. Fetal heart rate monitoring cannot reveal the presence of encephalopathy, and neuroimaging by ultrasound and MR imaging is the most reliable modality for disclosure of silent encephalopathy. In many cases with cerebral palsy with acquired brain insults, especially, term-delivered infants with reactive fetal heart rate tracing and good Apgar score at delivery are not suspected of having encephalopathy and are often overlooked for months or years. Recent imaging technology has revealed brain insult in utero.

INTRACRANIAL HEMORRHAGE

Intracranial hemorrhage includes subdural hemorrhage, primary subarachnoid hemorrhage, intracerebellar hemorrhage, intraventricular hemorrhage and intraparenchymal hemorrhage other than cerebellar hemorrhage (Sherer et al 1998).

Incidence: unknown.

Etiology: trauma, alloimmune and idiopathic thrombocytopenia, von Willebrand disease, specific medications (warfarin) or illicit drug (cocaine) abuse, seizure, fetal conditions including congenital factor-X and factor-V deficiencies, intracranial tumor, twin–twin transfusion, demise of a co-twin, vascular diseases, or fetomaternal hemorrhage, extracorporeal membrane oxygenation (ECMO) (Hardart and Fackler 1999).

Associated anomalies: hydrocephalus, hydranencephaly, porencephaly, or microcephaly.

Prenatal diagnosis: multiple intracerebral hemorrhages with unknown cause at 35 weeks and multiple hemorrhage

and ischemic change due to vein of Galen aneurysm malformation at 28 weeks are shown in Figures 15.46 and 15.47. The lesion often changes into porencephaly in a short period.

Differential diagnosis: intracranial tumor.

Prognosis: poor in premature infants. Apnea, seizures, and other neurological symptoms.

Recurrence risk: depends on etiology.

Management: ventriculoperitoneal shunt if hydrocephalus progresses.

PORENCEPHALY

Porencephaly is defined as fluid-filled spaces replacing normal brain parenchyma and may or may not communicate with the lateral ventricles or subarachnoid space.

Incidence: unknown.

Synonyms: porencephalic cyst.

Etiology: ischemic episode, trauma (Eller and Kuller 1995), demise of one twin, intercerebral hemorrhage, infection of cytomegalovirus (Moinuddin et al 2003).

Pathogenesis (Volpe 2001): easy to occur when immature cerebrum has some factors with propensity of dissolution and cavitation (high content of water, myelinated fiber bundles, and deficient astroglial response). Timing of ischemic injury (maybe as early as second trimester) is strongly related to porencephaly, hydranencephaly.

Associated anomalies: intercerebral hemorrhage, interventricular hemorrhage, hydrocephalus.

Prenatal diagnosis: Figure 15.48 shows porencephaly after intracerebral hemorrhage at 25 weeks. Some cases in utero have been reported (Meizner and Elchalal 1996, de Laveaucoupet et al 2001).

Differential diagnosis: schizencephaly, arachnoid cyst, intracranial cystic tumor, other cysts. Porencephalic cyst never causes a mass effect, which is observed in cases with arachnoid cyst or other cystic mass lesions. This condition is acquired brain insult and differentiated from schizencephaly of migration disorder.

Prognosis: various, depends on timing and size of lesion. Seizures, neurological deficits, cerebral palsy often occur (Scher et al 1991).

Recurrence risk: unknown.

Management: ventriculoperitoneal shunt if hydrocephalus progresses.

HYDRANENCEPHALY

Hydranencephaly is defined as absence of the cerebral hemispheres and a sac-like structure containing cerebral spinal fluid surrounding the brainstem and basal ganglia.

Incidence: 1–2.5 : 10 000 births.

Etiology: ischemic episode, trauma, demise of one twin, intercerebral hemorrhage, infection. There are several theories but bilateral occlusion of the supraclinoid segment of the internal carotid arteries (Stevenson et al 2001) or of the middle cerebral arteries is one of the causes of subtotal defects of cerebral hemisphere.

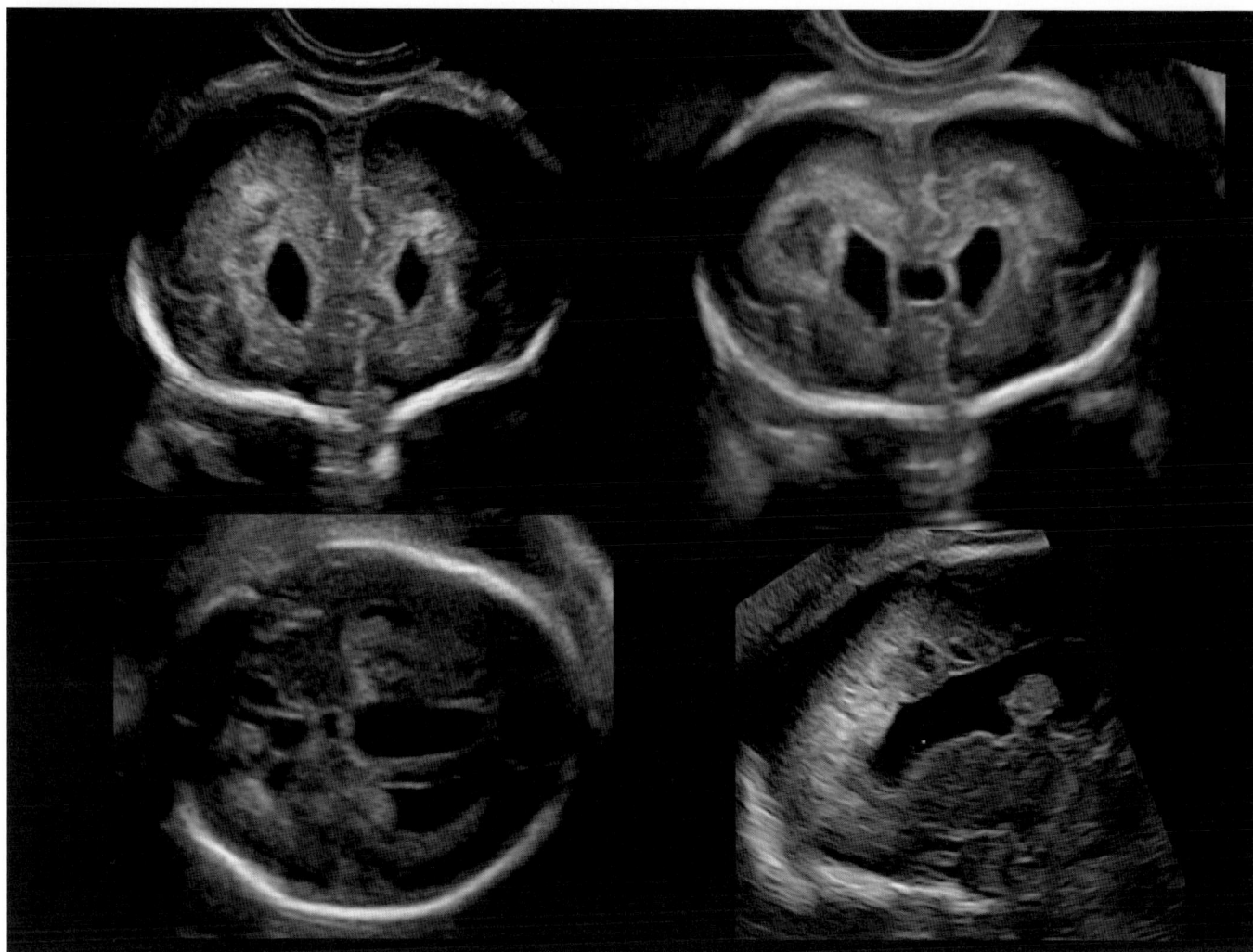

Figure 15.46 Cerebral hemorrhage and ischemic change with mild ventriculomegaly at 28 weeks of gestation. (upper) Anterior coronal sections. Multiple brain damage due to cerebral hemorrhage or ischemic–hypoxic episode. Note multiple brain damage with low and high echogenicity around mildly enlarged ventricles. The case had vein of Galen aneurysm malformation. (lower left) Axial image. Atrial width measurement was just 10 mm at this stage. (lower right) Parasagittal section. Periventricular brain damage and ventriculomegaly are seen.

Pathogenesis: easy to occur when immature cerebrum has some factors with propensity of dissolution and cavitation (high content of water, myelinated fiber bundles and deficient astroglial response). Timing of ischemic injury (maybe as early as second trimester) is strongly related to porencephaly and hydranencephaly.

Prenatal diagnosis: ultrasound and MRI (Byers 2005). Hydranencephaly from 11 weeks of gestation has been reported (Lam and Tang 2000).

Differential diagnosis: massive hydrocephalus, alobar holoprosencephaly, porencephaly.

Prognosis: extremely poor.

Recurrence risk: unknown.

Management: no active treatment. Shunt procedure for progressive increase of infant's head.

FETAL PERIVENTRICULAR LEUKOMALACIA (PVL)

Multifocal areas of necrosis found deep in the cortical white matter, which are often symmetrical and occur adjacent to the lateral ventricles. PVL represents a major precursor for neurological and intellectual impairment and cerebral palsy in later life.

Incidence: 25–75% of premature infants at autopsy are complicated with periventricular white matter injury. However, clinically, incidence may be much lower. 5 to 10% of infants less than 1500 g birth weight. In term infants, PVL is very rare.

Etiology: birth trauma, asphyxia and respiratory failure, cardiopulmonary defects, premature birth/low birthweight, associated immature cerebrovascular development and lack

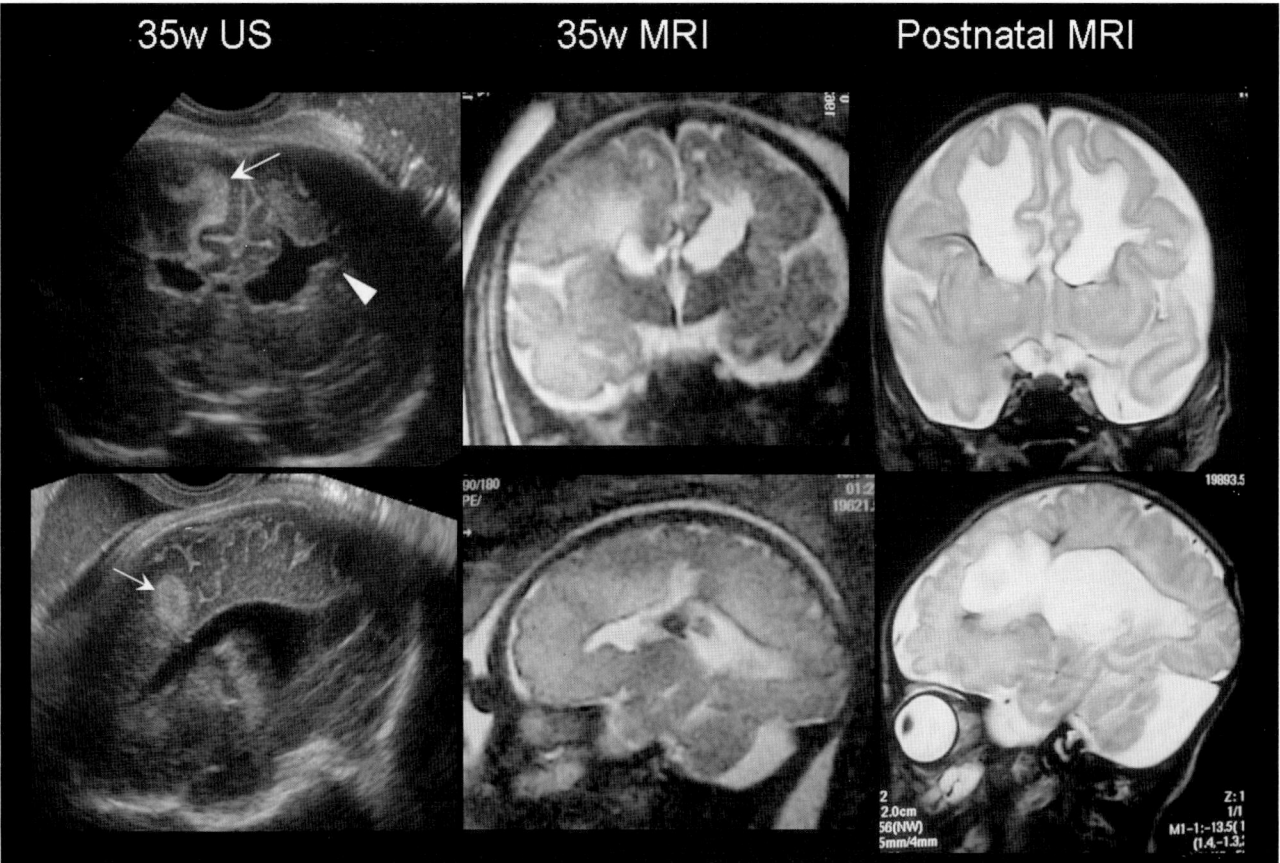

Figure 15.47 US and MR images in a fetus with cerebral hemorrhage and mild ventriculomegaly and postnatal porencephalic change. Anterior coronal sections (upper) and parasagittal sections (lower). Intracerebral hemorrhage (arrows) and porencephalic part fused with the lateral ventricle (arrowhead) are demonstrated by ultrasound. Postnatal MR images (right) show porencephalic change of bleeding lesions, fused with ventricles.

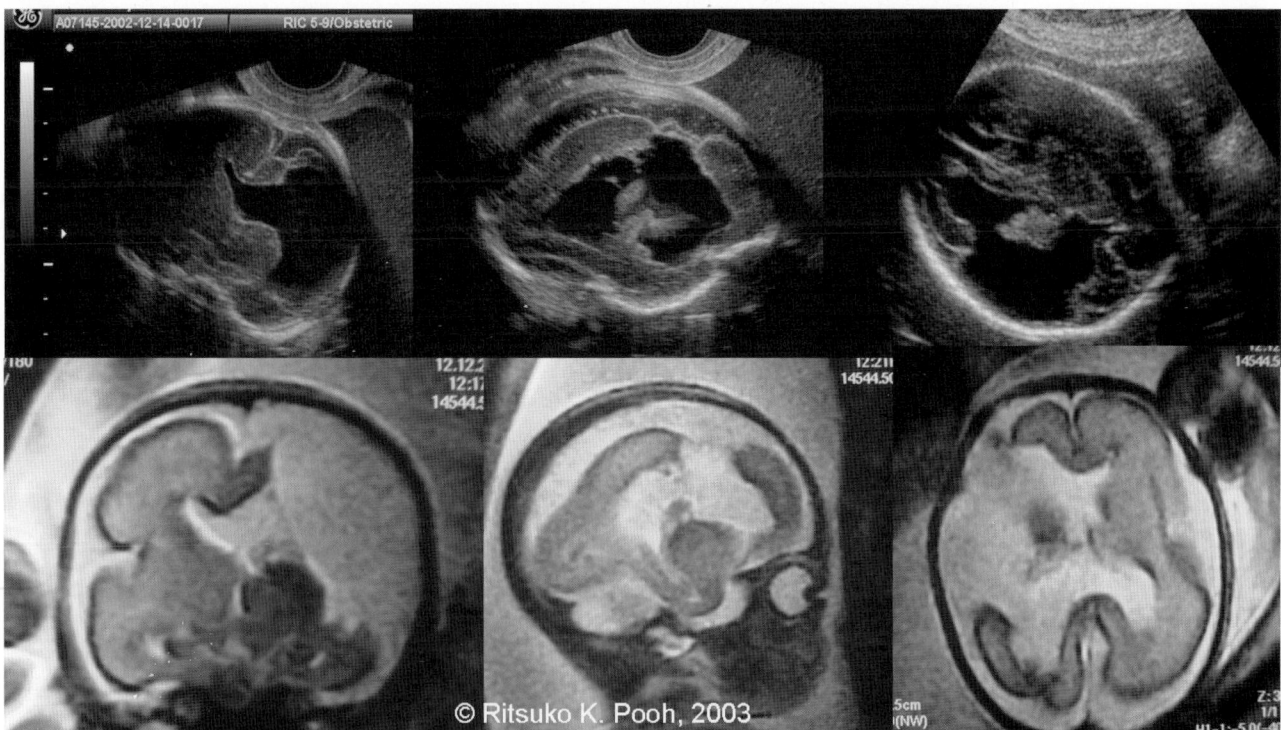

Figure 15.48 Fetal US and MR images of porencephaly at 25 weeks of gestation. (upper left) Transvaginal US coronal image. Defect of parietolateral part of the unilateral cerebrum. This case has also absent septum pellucidum. (upper middle) Parasagittal US image. Porencephalic part is fused with the unilateral ventricle. Echogenicity of inside ventricular wall indicates intraventricular hemorrhage. (upper right) Transabdominal US axial image. (lower) Fetal MR images on the same day. Coronal, parasagittal and axial sections from the left side.

of appropriate autoregulation of cerebral blood flow in response to hypoxic–ischemic insults (Rezaie and Dean 2002).

Pathogenesis: distinctive and consists primarily of both focal periventricular necrosis and more diffuse cerebral white matter injury. Two most common sites are at the level of the cerebral white matter near the trigone of the lateral ventricles and around the foramen of Monro. Volpe describes three factors, such as (1) periventricular vascular anatomical and physiological factors, (2) cerebral ischemia, (3) intrinsic vulnerability of cerebral white matter of premature newborn, are strongly related to PVL (Volpe 2001b).

Prenatal diagnosis: Figure 15.49 shows fetal PVL; its appearance changed from cystic PVL into widespread type of PVL from 27 weeks to three years after birth.

Differential diagnosis: subarachnoid (periventricular) pseudocysts, porencephaly, other intracranial cystic formation.

Prognosis: neurological features of PVL in neonatal period is probable lower limb weakness and as features of long-term sequelae, spastic diplegia, intellectual deficits and visual deficits are observed (Volpe 2001b).

Recurrence risk: unknown.

Management: early rehabilitation.

NORMAL VARIANTS

CHOROID PLEXUS CYSTS

Choroid plexus cysts are cysts with fluid collection within the choroid plexus, which may exist unilaterally or bilaterally. They are depicted in the second trimester and usually resolve by the 24th week.

Incidence: 0.61–2.89% of all fetuses scanned (Coco and Jeanty 2004, Kupferminc et al 1994, Morcos et al 1998, Nadel et al 1992, Reinsch 1997, Snijders 1994).

Pathogenesis: choroid plexus is located within the ventricular system and produces cerebrospinal fluid. Within the choroidal villi, choroid plexus cysts exists, surrounded by the loose stroma of the choroid plexus 81 (Nadel et al 1992). Choroid plexus cysts probably result from entrapment of cerebrospinal fluid within tangled villi of the fetal ventricular system (Kennedy and Carey 1993).

Associated anomalies: in cases of trisomy 18, associated anomalies include growth retardation, congenital heart diseases such as ventricular septum defect and double outlet right ventricle, overlapping finger, facial anomaly, cerebellar dysplasia and others.

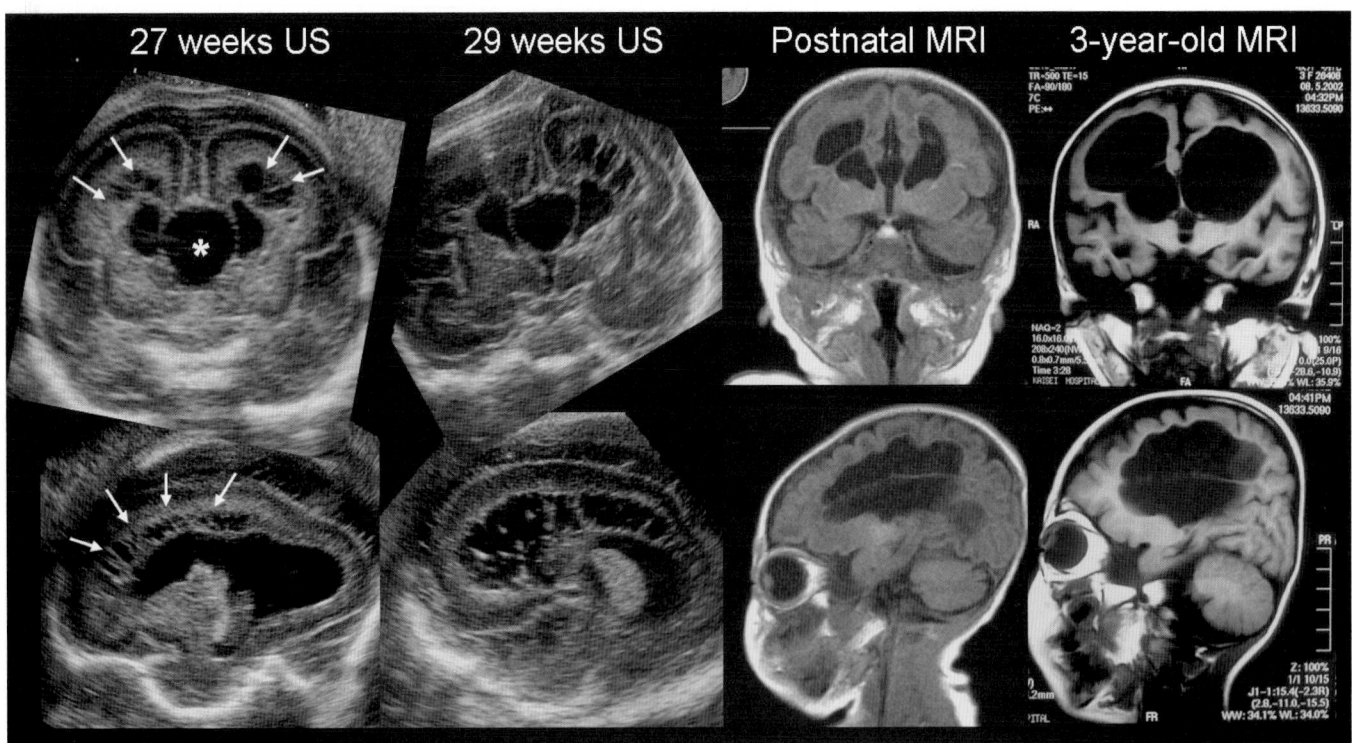

Figure 15.49 Intrauterine periventricular leukomalacia (PVL) from 27 weeks of gestation. Anterior coronal sections (upper) and parasagittal sections (lower). Cystic PVL (arrows), ventriculomegaly and enlargement of the septum pellucidi (asterisk) are clearly seen from 27 weeks of gestation. PVL rapidly exacerbated during pregnancy. At 29 weeks of gestation, cystic periventricular leukomalacia changed into widespread type. Postnatal MRI shows further exacerbation of PVL and porencephalic formation after birth.

Prenatal diagnosis: it is impossible to distinguish normal from abnormal karyotypes only by location and appearance of choroid plexus cyst (Fig. 15.50). Detection of additional anomalies is important for differential diagnosis.

Differential diagnosis: intraventricular hemorrhage.

Prognosis: choroid plexus cysts, per se, are usually asymptomatic and benign, but rarely, symptomatic and disturb CSF flow (Lam and Villanueva 1992, Parizek et al 1998). Isolated choroid plexus cysts may be a normal variation.

Recurrence risk: unknown.

Management: an isolated choroid plexus cyst is an indication to perform a detailed and accurate examination of other markers of aneuploidy. If the choroid plexus cyst is an isolated finding, there is no reason to perform amniocentesis (Coco and Jeanty 2004).

SUBEPENDYMAL PSEUDOCYSTS

Cystic formation, which is located in the caudothalamic groove or in the caudate nucleus, lateral to the wall of the anterior horns of lateral ventricles.

Prevalence: 2.6–5% of all neonates, 1% of premature newborns, unknown in fetuses.

Synonyms: periventricular pseudocysts (Lu et al 1992, Malinger et al 2002).

Etiology: infection (cytomegalovirus, rubella), subependymal hemorrhage, metabolic diseases, chromosomal deletions (del q6, delp4), cocaine exposure and others.

Pathogenesis: cystic cavity is lined by a pseudocapsule, consisting of aggregates of germinal cells and glial tissue, but no epithelium can be found. Origin of pseudocysts is uncertain. Maybe cystic matrix regression or germinolysis.

Associated anomalies: congenital infection such as cytomegalovirus, congenital heart diseases, associated CNS abnormalities.

Prenatal diagnosis: often detectable by transvaginal sonography in the sagittal and anterior-coronal sections (Fig. 15.51).

Differential diagnosis: periventricular leukomalacia.

Prognosis: good in cases with isolated subependymal pseudocysts. In cases with accompanied abnormalities, such as cardiac disease, cytomegalovirus infection, other intracranial abnormalities, or cases with atypical pseudocysts, prognosis may be poor (Bats et al 2002, Lu et al 1992, Malinger et al 2002).

Recurrence risk: unknown.

Management: in many cases, cysts regress in several months after birth. Normal obstetrical/neonatal care.

CONCLUSIONS

Recent advances of imaging technology have provided us with objective neuroimaging diagnosis as shown in this chapter. Longitudinally and carefully evaluation of neurological short-term/long-term prognosis should be required according to precise prenatal diagnosis, for proper counseling and management based on accurate evidence.

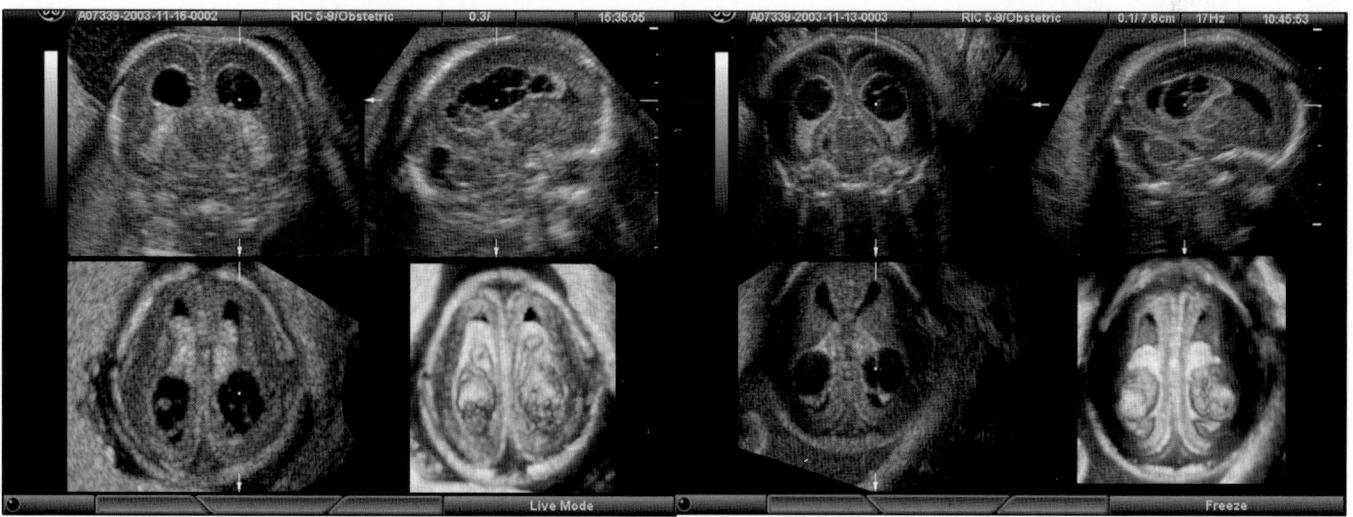

Figure 15.50 Choroid plexus cysts in trisomy 18 (left) and normal karyotype (right). (left) Three orthogonal view and inside 3D view of CPC in a case of trisomy 18 at 17 weeks of gestation. (right) Three orthogonal view and inside 3D view of CPC in a case with normal karyotype at 16 weeks. No additional abnormalities. Normal postnatal course. Impossible to distinguish normal from abnormal karyotypes only by location and appearance of choroid plexus cyst. Careful fetal screening for additional anomalies is important for differential diagnosis.

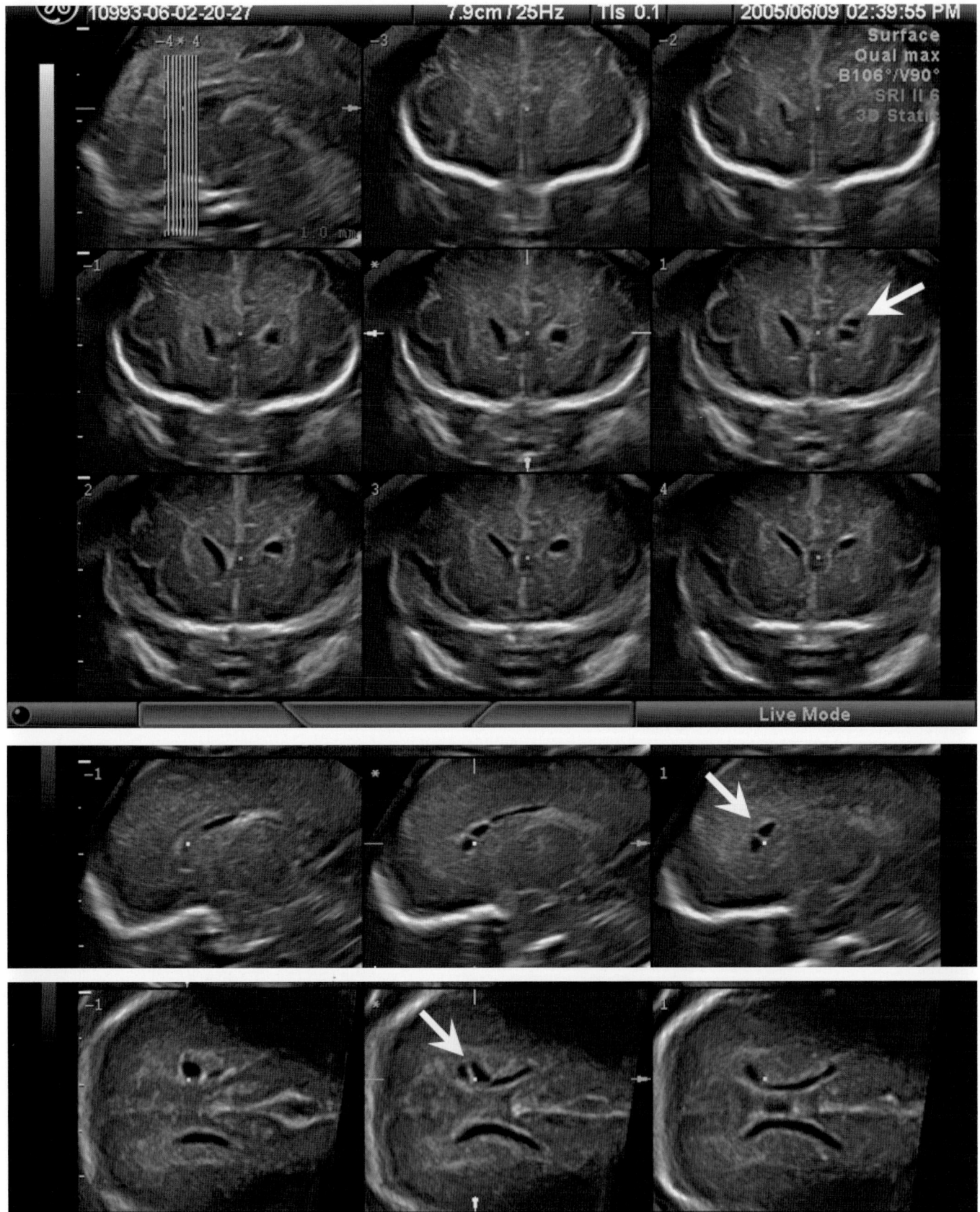

Figure 15.51 Subependymal cysts. (upper) Coronal tomographic ultrasound images of unilateral subependymal cysts. Two clear cysts are demonstrated (arrow). Middle and lower figures show sagittal and axial tomographic images.

REFERENCES

Alagappan R, Browning P D, Laorr A, McGahan J P 1994 Distal lateral ventricular atrium: reevaluation of normal range. Radiology 193:405–408.

Almog B, Gamzu R, Achiron R et al 2003 Fetal lateral ventricular width: what should be its upper limit? A prospective cohort study and reanalysis of the current and previous data. J Ultrasound Med 22:39–43.

Barkovich A J, Kjos B O, Normal D et al 1989 Revised classification of the posterior fossa cysts and cystlike malformations based on the results of multiplanar MR imaging. AJNR 10:977–988.

Barkovich A J, Simon E M, Walsh C A 2001 Callosal agenesis with cyst: a better understanding and new classification. Neurology 23,56(2):220–227.

Bats A S, Molho M, Senat M V et al 2002 Subependymal pseudocysts in the fetal brain: prenatal diagnosis of two cases and review of the literature. Ultrasound Obstet Gynecol 20(5):502–505.

Benacerraf B R, Spiro R, Mitchell A G 2000 Using three-dimensional ultrasound to detect craniosynostosis in a fetus with Pfeiffer syndrome. Ultrasound Obstet Gynecol 16:391–394.

Biggio J R Jr, Wenstrom K D, Owen J 2004 Fetal open spina bifida: a natural history of disease progression in utero. Prenat Diagn 24(4):287–289.

Bretelle F, Senat M V, Bernard J P et al 2002 First-trimester diagnosis of fetal arachnoid cyst: prenatal implication. Ultrasound Obstet Gynecol 20:400–402.

Brunelli S, Faiella A, Capra V et al 1996 Germline mutations in the homeobox gene EMX2 in patients with severe schizencephaly. Nat Genet 12:94–96.

Byers B D, Barth W H, Stewart T L, Pierce B T 2005 Ultrasound and MRI appearance and evolution of hydranencephaly in utero: a case report. J Reprod Med 50(1):53–56.

Campi A, Rodesch G, Scotti G, Lasjaunias P 1998 Aneurysmal malformation of the vein of Galen in three patients: clinical and radiological follow-up. Neuroradiology 40:816–821.

Ciricillo S F, Cogen P H, Harsh G R et al 1991 Intracranial arachnoid cysts in children. A comparison of the effects of fenestration and shunting. J Neurosurg 74:230–235.

Coco C, Jeanty P 2004 Karyotyping of fetuses with isolated choroid plexus cysts is not justified in an unselected population. J Ultrasound Med 23:899–906.

Cohen M M 1982 An update on the holoprosencephalic disorders. J Pediatr 101:865–869.

Cohen M M Jr 1989 Perspectives on holoprosencephaly. I. Epidemiology, genetics and symdromology. Teratology 40:211–235.

D'Addario V, Pinto V, Del Bianco A et al 2001 The clivus-supraocciput angle: a useful measurement to evaluate the shape and size of the fetal posterior fossa and to diagnose Chiari II malformation. Ultrasound Obstet Gynecol 18:146–149.

Dattani M T, Martinez-Barbera J P, Thomas P Q et al 1998 Mutations in the homeobox gene HESX1/Hesx1 associated with septo-optic dysplasia in human and mouse. Nat Genet 19:125–133.

de Laveaucoupet J, Audibert F, Guis F et al 2001 Fetal magnetic resonance imaging (MRI) of ischemic brain injury. Prenat Diagn 21:729–736.

Delashaw J B, Persing J A, Broaddus W C, Jane J A 1989 Cranial vault growth in craniosynostosis. J Neurosurg 70:159–165.

Demaerel P, Van de Gaer P, Wilms G, Baert A L 1996 Interhemispheric lipoma with variable callosal dysgenesis: relationship between embryology, morphology, and symptomatology. Eur Radiol 6(6):904–909.

Denis D, Maugey-Laulom B, Carles D et al 2001 Prenatal diagnosis of schizencephaly by fetal magnetic resonance imaging. Fetal Diagn Ther 16:354–359.

Dominguez R, Aguirre Vila-Coro A, Slopis J M, Bohan T P 1991 Brain and ocular abnormalities in infants with in utero exposure to cocaine and other street drugs. Am J Dis Child 145:688–695.

Elbers S E, Furness M E 1999 Resolution of presumed arachnoid cyst in utero. Ultrasound Obstet Gynecol 14:353–355.

Eller K M, Kuller J A 1995 Porencephaly secondary to fetal trauma during amniocentesis. Obstet Gynecol 85:865–867.

Faro C, Chaoui R, Wegrzyn P et al 2006 Metopic suture in fetuses with Apert syndrome at 22–27 weeks of gestation. Ultrasound Obstet Gynecol 27:28–33.

Fransen E, Lemmon V, Van Camp G et al 1995 CRASH syndrome: clinical spectrum of corpus callosum hypoplasia, retardation, adducted thumbs, spastic paraparesis and hydrocephalus due to mutations in one single gene, L1. Eur J Hum Genet 3:273–284.

Friedman D M, Verma R, Madrid M et al 1993 Recent improvement in outcome using transcatheter embolization techniques for neonatal aneurysmal malformations of the vein of Galen. Pediatrics 91:583–586.

Garel C 2006 New advances in fetal MR neuroimaging. Pediatr Radiol 36(7):621–625.

Glenn O A, Barkovich J 2006 Magnetic resonance imaging of the fetal brain and spine: an increasingly important tool in prenatal diagnosis: part 2. AJNR Am J Neuroradiol 27(9):1807–1814.

Goldstein I, Copel J A, Makhoul I R 2005 Mild cerebral ventriculomegaly in fetuses: characteristics and outcome. Fetal Diagn Ther 20:281–284.

Goodyear P W, Bannister C M, Russell S, Rimmer S 2001 Outcome in prenatally diagnosed fetal agenesis of the corpus callosum. Fetal Diagn Ther 16:139–145.

Granata T, Farina L, Faiella A et al 1997 Familial schizencephaly associated with EMX2 mutation. Neurology 48:1403–1406.

Greco P, Resta M, Vimercati A et al 1998 Antenatal diagnosis of isolated lissencephaly by ultrasound and magnetic resonance imaging. Ultrasound Obstet Gynecol 12:276–279.

Green N S 2002 Folic acid supplementation and prevention of birth defects. J Nutr 132:2356S–2360S.

Hardart G E, Fackler J C 1999 Predictors of intracranial hemorrhage during neonatal extracorporeal membrane oxygenation. J Pediatr 134:156–159.

Hoffman H J, Chuang S, Hendrick E B, Humphreys R P 1982 Aneurysms of the vein of Galen. Experience at The Hospital for Sick Children, Toronto. J Neurosurg 57:316–322.

Hollway G E, Suthers G K, Haan E A et al 1997 Mutation detection in FGFR2 craniosynostosis syndromes. Hum Genet 99:251–255.

Iannetti P, Nigro G, Spalice A et al 1998 Cytomegalovirus infection and schizencephaly: case reports. Ann Neurol 43:123–127.

Ickowitz V, Eurin D, Rypens F et al E 2001 Prenatal diagnosis and postnatal follow-up of pericallosal lipoma: report of seven new cases. AJNR 22:767–772.

Jeanty P, Zaleski W, Fleischer A C 1991 Prenatal sonographic diagnosis of lipoma of the corpus callosum in a fetus with Goldenhar syndrome. Am J Perinatol 8(2):89–90.

Kelly E N, Allen V M, Seaward G et al 2001 Mild ventriculomegaly in the fetus, natural history, associated findings and outcome of isolated mild ventriculomegaly: a literature review. Prenat Diagn 21:697–700.

Kennedy K A, Carey J C 1993 Choroid plexus cysts: significance and current management practices. Semin Ultrasound CT MR 14:23–30.

Kobayashi K, Nakahori Y, Miyake M et al 1998 An ancient retrotransposal insertion causes Fukuyama-type congenital muscular dystrophy. Nature 23,394(6691):388–392.

Kojima K, Suzuki Y, Seki K et al 2002 Prenatal diagnosis of lissencephaly (type II) by ultrasound and fast magnetic resonance imaging. Fetal Diagn Ther 17:34–36.

Kupferminc M J, Tamura R K, Sabbagha R E et al 1994 Isolated choroid plexus cyst(s): an indication for amniocentesis. Am J Obstet Gynecol 171:1068–1071.

Lam A H, Villanueva A C 1992 Symptomatic third ventricular choroid plexus cysts. Pediatr Radiol 22:413–416.

Lam Y H, Tang M H 2000). Serial sonographic features of a fetus with hydranencephaly from 11 weeks to term. Ultrasound Obstet Gynecol 16:77–79.

Lasjaunias P L, Chng S M, Sachet M et al 2006 The management of vein of Galen aneurysmal malformations. Neurosurgery 59:S184–S194.

Lewis D, Tolosa J E, Kaufmann M et al 2004 Elective Cesarean delivery and long-term motor function or ambulation status in infants with meningomyelocele. Obstet Gynecol 103:469–473.

Lu J H, Emons D, Kowalewski S 1992 Connatal periventricular pseudocysts in the neonate. Pediatr Radiol 22(1):55–58.

Luthy D A, Wardinsky T, Shurtleff D B et al 1991 Cesarean section before the onset of labor and subsequent motor function in infants with meningomyelocele diagnosed antenatally. N Engl J Med 324:662–666.

McGahan J P, Grix A, Gerscovich E O 1994 Prenatal diagnosis of lissencephaly: Miller–Dieker syndrome. J Clin Ultrasound 22:560–563.

McMahon C L, Braddock S R 2001 Septo-optic dysplasia as a manifestation of valproic acid embryopathy. Teratology 64:83–86.

Malinger G, Ben-Sira L, Lev D et al T 2004 Fetal brain imaging: a comparison between magnetic resonance imaging and dedicated neurosonography. Ultrasound Obstet Gynecol 23(4):333–340.

Malinger G, Lev D, Ben Sira L et al 2002 Congenital periventricular pseudocysts: prenatal sonographic appearance and clinical implications. Ultrasound Obstet Gynecol 20(5):447–451.

Martinez de Villarreal L, Perez J Z, Vazquez P A et al 2002 Decline of neural tube defects cases after a folic acid campaign in Nuevo Leon, Mexico. Teratology 66:249–256.

Mathews T J, Honein M A, Erickson J D 2002 Spina bifida and anencephaly prevalence — United States, 1991–2001. MMWR Recomm Rep 51:9–11.

Matsunaga E, Shiota K 1977 Holoprosencephaly in human embryos: epidemiologic studies of 150 cases. Teratology 16:261–272.

Meizner I, Elchalal U 1996 Prenatal sonographic diagnosis of anterior fossa porencephaly. J Clin Ultrasound 24:96–99.

Merrill D C, Goodwin P, Burson J M et al 1998 The optimal route of delivery for fetal meningomyelocele. Am J Obstet Gynecol 179:235–240.

Moinuddin A, McKinstry R C, Martin K A, Neil J J 2003 Intracranial hemorrhage progressing to porencephaly as a result of congenitally acquired cytomegalovirus infection — an illustrative report. Prenat Diagn 23:797–800.

Monteagudo A, Reuss M L, Timor-Tritsch I E 1991 Imaging the fetal brain in the second and third trimesters using transvaginal sonography. Obstet Gynecol 77:27–32.

Monteagudo A, Timor-Tritsch I E 1997 Development of fetal gyri, sulci and fissures: a transvaginal sonographic study. Ultrasound Obstet Gynecol 9:222–228.

Monteagudo A, Timor-Tritsch I E 2001 Fetal Neurosonography of congenital brain anomalies. In: Timor-Tritsch I E, Monteagudo A, Cohen H L (eds) Ultrasonography of the prenatal and neonatal brain, 2nd edn. McGraw-Hill, New York, NY, pp. 151–258.

Monteagudo A, Timor-Tritsch I E, Mayberry P 2000 Three-dimensional transvaginal neurosonography of the fetal brain: 'navigating' in the volume scan. Ultrasound Obstet Gynecol 16:307–313.

Monteagudo A, Timor-Tritsch I E, Moomjy M 1994 In utero detection of ventriculomegaly during the second and third trimesters by transvaginal sonography. Ultrasound Obstet Gynecol 4:193–198.

Morcos C L, Platt L D, Carlson D E et al 1998 The isolated choroid plexus cyst. Obstet Gynecol 92:232–236.

Nadel A S, Bromley B S, Frigoletto F D Jr et al 1992 Isolated choroid plexus cysts in the second-trimester fetus: is amniocentesis really indicated? Radiology 185:545–548.

Nakamura Y, Mizukawa K, Yamamoto K, Nagashima T 2001 Endoscopic treatment for a huge neonatal prepontine-suprasellar arachnoid cyst: a case report. Pediatr Neurosurg 35:220–224.

Nicolaides K H, Campbell S, Gabbe S G, Guidetti R 1986 Ultrasound screening for spina bifida: cranial and cerebellar signs. Lancet 12,2(8498):72–74.

Osenbach R K, Menezes A H 1991 Diagnosis and management of the Dandy–Walker malformation: 30 years of experience. Pediatr Neurosurg 18:179–185.

Ouahba J, Luton D, Vuillard E et al 2006 Prenatal isolated mild ventriculomegaly: outcome in 167 cases. BJOG 113:1072–1079.

Parizek J, Jakubec J, Hobza V et al 1998 Choroid plexus cyst of the left lateral ventricle with intermittent blockage of the foramen of Monro, and initial invagination into the III ventricle in a child. Childs Nerv Syst 14:700–708.

Persad V L, Van den Hof M C, Dube J M, Zimmer P 2002 Incidence of open neural tube defects in Nova Scotia after folic acid fortification. CMAJ 167:241–245.

Persutte W H 1998 Microcephaly–no small deal. Ultrasound Obstet Gynecol 11(5):317–318.

Pilu G, Ambrosetto P, Sandri F et al 1994 Intraventricular fused fornices: a specific sign of fetal lobar holoprosencephaly. Ultrasound Obstet Gynecol 34:259–262.

Pilu G, Falco P, Gabrielli S et al 1999 The clinical significance of fetal isolated cerebral borderline ventriculomegaly: report of 31 cases and review of the literature. Ultrasound Obstet Gynecol 14:320–326.

Pilu G, Porelo A, Falco P, Visentin A 2001 Median anomalies of the brain. In: Timor-Tritsch I E, Monteagudo A, Cohen H L (eds). Ultrasonography of the prenatal and neonatal brain, 2nd edn. McGraw-Hill, New York, pp. 259–276.

Pooh R K 2000 Three-dimensional ultrasound of the fetal brain. In: Kurjak A (ed.) Clinical application of 3D ultrasonography. Parthenon, Carnforth, pp. 176–180.

Pooh R K, Aono T 1996 Transvaginal power Doppler angiography of the fetal brain. Ultrasound Obstet Gynecol 8:417–421.

Pooh R K, Maeda K, Pooh K H 2003 An atlas of fetal central nervous system disease. Diagnosis and Management. Parthenon CRC, London.

Pooh R K, Maeda K, Pooh K H, Kurjak A 1999a Sonographic assessment of the fetal brain morphology. Prenat Neonat Med 4:18–38.

Pooh R K, Nakagawa Y, Nagamachi N et al 1998 Transvaginal sonography of the fetal brain: detection of abnormal morphology and circulation. Croat Med J 39:147–157.

Pooh R K, Nakagawa Y, Pooh K H et al 1999b Fetal craniofacial structure and intracranial morphology in a case of Apert syndrome. Ultrasound Obstet Gynecol 13:274–280.

Pooh R K, Pooh K H 2001 Transvaginal 3D and Doppler ultrasonography of the fetal brain. Semin Perinatol 25:38–43.

Pooh R K, Pooh K H 2002 The assessment of fetal brain morphology and circulation by transvaginal 3D sonography and power Doppler. J Perinat Med 30:48–56.

Pooh R K, Pooh K H 2007 Fetal ventriculomegaly. Donald School J Ultrasound Obstet Gynecol 2:40–46.

Pooh R K, Nagao Y, Pooh K H 2006 Fetal neuroimaging by transvaginal 3D ultrasound and MRI. Ultrasound Rev Obstet Gynecol 6:107–108.

Pooh R K, Pooh K H, Nakagawa Y et al 1999c Transvaginal Doppler assessment of fetal intracranial venous flow. Obstet Gynecol 93:697–701.

Pooh R K, Pooh K H, Nakagawa Y et al 2000 Clinical application of three-dimensional ultrasound in fetal brain assessment. Croat Med J 41:245–251.

Ray J G, Meier C, Vermeulen M J et al 2002 Association of neural tube defects and folic acid food fortification in Canada. Lancet 360:2047–2048.

Raybaud C, Levrier O, Brunel H et al 2003 MR imaging of fetal brain malformations. Childs Nerv Syst 19(7–8):455–470.

Reinsch R 1997 Choroid plexus cysts-association with trisomy: prospective review of 16,059 patients. Am J Obstet Gynecol 176:1381–1383.

Rezaie P, Dean A 2002 Periventricular leukomalacia, inflammation and white matter lesions within the developing nervous system. Neuropathology 22:106–132.

Scher M S, Belfar H, Martin J, Painter M J 1991 Destructive brain lesions of presumed fetal onset: antepartum causes of cerebral palsy. Pediatrics 88:898–906.

Schmidt-Riese U, Zieger M 1994 Ultrasound diagnosis of isolated aplasia of the septum pellucidum. Ultraschall Med 15:286–292.

Schwarzler P, Homfray T, Bernard J P et al 2003 Late onset microcephaly: failure of prenatal diagnosis. Ultrasound Obstet Gynecol 22(6):640–642.

Sherer D M, Abramowicz J S, Eggers P C et al 1993 Prenatal ultrasonographic diagnosis of intracranial teratoma and massive craniomegaly with associated high-output cardiac failure. Am J Obstet Gynecol 168:97–99.

Sherer D M, Anyaegbunam A, Onyeije C 1998 Antepartum fetal intracranial hemorrhage, predisposing factors and prenatal sonography: a review. Am J Perinatol 15:431–441.

Signorelli M, Tiberti A, Valseriati D et al 2004 Width of the fetal lateral ventricular atrium between 10 and 12 mm: a simple variation of the norm? Ultrasound Obstet Gynecol 23:14–18.

Snijders R J, Shawa L, Nicolaides K H 1994 Fetal choroid plexus cysts and trisomy 18: assessment of risk based on ultrasound findings and maternal age. Prenat Diagn 14:1119–1127.

Stevenson D A, Hart B L, Clericuzio C L 2001 Hydranencephaly in an infant with vascular malformations. Am J Med Genet 15,104:295–298.

Stevenson R E, Allen W P, Pai G S et al 2000 Decline in prevalence of neural tube defects in a high-risk region of the United States. Pediatrics 106:677–683.

Tart R P, Quisling R G 1991 Curvilinear and tubulonodular varieties of lipoma of the corpus callosum: an MR and CT study. J Comput Assist Tomogr 15:805–810.

Taylor M, David A S 1998) Agenesis of the corpus callosum: a United Kingdom series of 56 cases. J Neurol Neurosurg Psychiatry 64:131–134.

Timor-Tritsch I E, Monteagudo A 1996 Transvaginal fetal neurosonography: standardization of the planes and sections by anatomic landmarks. Ultrasound Obstet Gynecol 8:42–47.

Timor-Tritsch I E, Monteagudo A, Haratz-Rubinstein N, Levine R U 1996 Transvaginal sonographic detection of adducted thumbs, hydrocephalus, and agenesis of the corpus callosum at 22 postmenstrual weeks: the masa spectrum or L1 spectrum. A case report and review of the literature. Prenat Diagn 16:543–548.

Timor-Tritsch I E, Monteagudo A, Mayberry P 2000 Three-dimensional ultrasound evaluation of the fetal brain: the three horn view. Ultrasound Obstet Gynecol 16:302–306.

Volpe J J 2001a Brain tumors and vein of Galen malformation. Neurology of the newborn, 4th edn. WB Saunders, Philadelphia, pp. 841–856.

Volpe J J 2001b Hypoxic-ischemic encephalopathy: neuropathology and pathogenesis. Neurology of the newborn, 4th edn. WB Saunders, Philadelphia, pp. 296–330.

Volpe J J 2001c Neural tube formation and prosencephalic development. Neurology of the newborn, 4th edn. WB Saunders, Philadelphia, pp. 3–44.

Volpe J J 2001d Neuronal proliferation, migration, organization and myelination. Neurology of the newborn, 4th edn. WB Saunders, Philadelphia, pp. 45–99.

Wakai S, Arai T, Nagai M 1984 Congenital brain tumors. Surg Neurol 21:597–609.

Yamasaki M, Thompson P, Lemmon V 1997 CRASH syndrome: mutations in L1CAM correlate with severity of the disease. Neuropediatrics 28:175–178.

CHAPTER

16

Transvaginal fetal neuroscan

Nadav Schwartz, Ilan E. Timor-Tritsch and Ana Monteagudo

Key Points

- Transvaginal sonography is an vital part of the dedicated neuroscan and provides key scanning planes, particularly the median plane, that greatly contributes to the accuracy and detection rates for various CNS anomalies
- Knowledge of the developmental stages and anatomy of the fetal brain is essential to understanding and interpreting fetal neuro-imaging
- 3-D ultrasound capability provides many innovative and advanced ways to view the intricate anatomy of the developing fetal brain and promises to become an important part of routine neurosonography

---

INTRODUCTION

The fetal CNS, and more precisely the fetal brain, is in constant development from its incipient and early stages throughout the gestation and even after birth. It is therefore extremely important to understand the developmental changes of the brain that occur during the intrauterine life, since the sonographic appearance changes almost every month during gestation. All organs, other than the brain, assume their final sonographic appearance early in gestation; the only change that takes place in these organ systems is that they increase in size. As opposed to other organs and organ systems, the brain is the only fetal organ that changes its sonographic appearance throughout gestation.

In order to adequately visualize the intricate anatomic relationships in the fetal brain, our approach has always been to turn to the transvaginal imaging approach whenever possible, as the highest frequency transducers are those utilized in the transvaginal ultrasound probes. In our opinion, this approach enables us to obtain high quality and high resolution images of the fetal brain. We have previously demonstrated that trained sonographers can use the transvaginal technique to perform early anatomy scans in the late first trimester with good detection rates (Timor-Tritsch et al 2004).

In this chapter we will deal with the general technique of the fetal neuroscan and, more precisely, the transvaginal ultrasound technique, as well as the multiplanar imaging obtained by two-dimensional (2-D) and three-dimensional (3-D) scanning techniques. Several examples of the normal and abnormal fetal neuroscan obtained by 2-D and 3-D ultrasound will also be presented.

EQUIPMENT AND TECHNIQUE

Several factors serve to limit the functionality of ultrasound transducers when imaging the fetal brain. Factors to consider are the size of the fetal brain, the available surface or 'window' through which the transducer can achieve the best image, the fetal position and presentation and last, but not least, the thickness of the abdominal wall. In addition, as ultrasound resolution is dependent on the penetration of the sound wave through the tissues, progressive thickening of the fetal skull during gestation can further limit overall visualization. It should be remembered, however, that even towards the end of the pregnancy, the fetal brain can be scanned through the still-open anterior fontanelle and along the sagittal suture. Several scanning planes can be obtained through this acoustic window, including the median and paramedian, as well as (rotating the transducer) the coronal and the oblique sections. This is how neonatologists and pediatric neurologists obtain their information regarding the neonatal brain.

Due to the variable scanning conditions, several different transducers with a variety of frequencies and frequency ranges are used in order to obtain the optimal images. Both transabdominal (TA) and transvaginal (TV) ultrasound probes play important roles in fetal neuroimaging. Transvaginal ultrasound probes typically operate frequencies of 5–9 MHz, while the transabdominal probes frequencies of 3.5–7 MHz. During the first half of the pregnancy, when the fetal skull is relatively thin and hypomineralized, high-frequency (and high resolution) transvaginal probes are preferred as the deeper penetration of the low-frequency transabdominal probes is not required to adequately image the fetal brain. In addition, the relatively small size of the fetus at the earlier gestational ages allows the entire fetus to be easily scanned via the vaginal route. Furthermore, as long as the fetus remains in the cephalic presentation, we can employ the transvaginal ultrasound scanning approach anytime in pregnancy. If, however, the fetal head cannot be reached any more using the transvaginal route, transabdominal probes have to be used. Also, at later gestational ages the lower frequency probes have to be used in order to penetrate the progressively thickening skull bones.

Aside from transducer frequency and image resolution, another basic difference between the transabdominal scan and the transvaginal scan is the directional approach of the techniques. During transabdominal scanning, we usually scan through the temporal bone to obtain axial images of the fetal brain. If the circumstances are favorable we may even obtain a coronal image. The transvaginal route, however, allows us to obtain coronal and sagittal images in addition to the axial images. Taken together, 2-D transabdominal and transvaginal imaging complement each other by allowing adequate visualization of all three classic anatomic planes, i.e. axial, coronal and sagittal. Later in this chapter, we will discuss 3-D volume scanning which can capture all of the anatomic planes.

As far as the actual scanning technique is concerned, the transabdominal technique is widely used and will not be considered further here (for a review see Malinger et al 2007). More emphasis will be placed on a detailed discussion of the transvaginal sonographic examination of the fetal brain which is slowly gaining its well-deserved place among the scanning options for fetuses. The use of the transvaginal ultrasound technique for the fetal neuroscan was first introduced in the early 1990s (Achiron & Achiron 1991, Blaas et al 1994, 1995a, 1995b, Kushnir et al 1989, Malinger & Zakut 1993, Monteagudo & Timor-Tritsch 1997, Monteagudo et al 1991a, 1991b, 1993, Timor-Tritsch & Monteagudo 1991, 1996, Timor-Tritsch et al 1988, 1990, 1991a, Warren et al 1989) and relied heavily upon the experience gained from the transfontanelle examination of the neonatal brain (Babcock et al 1980, Ben-Ora et al 1980, Dewbury & Aluwihare 1980, Edwards et al 1981, Grant et al 1981, Johnson & Rumack 1980, Naidich et al 1986, Richardson & Grant 1986, Slovis & Kuhns 1981).

The TV neuroscan technique is relatively simple and the general approach is similar to neonatal transfontanelle scanning. The probe is prepared as usual for TV scanning. The tip of the probe is well covered by a plastic sheath, a clean condom, or inserted in one digit of a surgical rubber glove. The patient is instructed to empty her bladder in order to enable the transvaginal probe to come closer to the fetal head. The patient is then placed in the lithotomy position and the probe is slowly advanced into the vagina to reach the anterior cervical lip. The objective is to place the tip (the foot print) of the transvaginal probe opposite the anterior fontanelle by maneuvering the vaginal probe until the best image is obtained. The operator's second hand is placed abdominally to stabilize the fetal head in the desired position for the clearest ultrasound picture.

If a dedicated neuroscan is required to rule out brain anomaly in a fetus in breech presentation, one should strongly consider performing an external version in order to turn the fetus into vertex presentation. In most instances, this can easily be accomplished during the first and the second trimester when the small fetus is surrounded by copious amounts of amniotic fluid.

We place importance on the fact that the TV transducer should be an end-firing type that will enable symmetrical pictures on both sides of the scanning axis. The use of a non-end-firing or out-of-axis vaginal probe can cause the scanning of a perfectly symmetrical image of the brain to become extremely cumbersome, as the probe has to be continuously manipulated into the right position.

SCANNING PLANES

As mentioned before, transabdominal scanning of the fetal brain can only yield the axial and, potentially, coronal images. It is extremely difficult to obtain the sagittal planes. However, using 2-D transvaginal fetal neuroscans it is impossible to obtain all the classic orthogonal planes. By performing the transvaginal fetal neuroscan with the footprint of the probe touching the anterior fontanelle the 'coronal' and 'sagittal' planes obtained are tilted or slanted sections. Only the median and single coronal sections will conform to the classic definitions of these planes.

These angled planes are not only similar but they are also identical to those obtained by the neonatal transfontanelle imaging of the fetal brain (Ben-Ora et al 1980, Cohen & Ziprkowski 1991, Dewbury & Aluwihare 1980, Grant & Richardson 1994). This is because the neonatal 2-D scan uses the same fontanelle as the sonographic window to access the intracranial anatomy. The obvious advantage in obtaining similar planes is that it allows for easy and more direct correlation between antenatal and neonatal findings. One point that must be considered, however, is that these sonographic planes are not identical to the planes obtained with CT or MRI imaging, where the classic parallel planes are conventionally used.

CONVENTIONAL PLANES

We attempted to standardize the planes and sections by transvaginal 2-D fetal neurosonography using anatomic landmarks and adapting a new nomenclature for labeling them. The first assumption using this approach was that the planes generated are not parallel with each other, and therefore, they do not comply with the definitions of the classic planes imaging of the fetal head. First we will attempt to clarify some of the classic planes defined in the Nomina Anatomica (1989), and hope that this will allow a better understanding of the transvaginal/transfontanelle planes.

The classic planes consist of the sagittal and coronal (two vertical planes) and the axial (a horizontal plane). The coronal, or frontal sections are serial vertical sections extending from the occiput (posterior) to the forehead (anterior) and are parallel to each other. For the sagittal sections, the 'mid sagittal plane' is called the median plane. Parallel right and left sagittal planes are located to either side of the median plane. There can be multiple such right and left planes, but the term 'parasagittal' is incorrect. Axial sections, rarely obtained by 2-D transvaginal scanning, are serial horizontal sections that are also parallel to each other.

IMAGING PLANES USING THE TRANSVAGINAL APPROACH

The planes, obtained using the transvaginal probe, diverge in a fan-shaped fashion from a central point (the anterior fontanelle). Thus, it is incorrect to talk about 'sagittal' and 'coronal' planes in the classic sense. As said before, only one section is considered as the classic 'coronal' plane and only one section is considered the classic sagittal plane (the median plane) and the rest are oblique planes.

Toward a better understanding of this, we previously proposed a new nomenclature for the transvaginal neuroscan using well-defined landmarks to allow for standardization and easy description of the various planes (Timor-Tritsch & Monteagudo 1996). The landmark and ana-

tomic structures taken into consideration were: the orbit, the meninges (the falx and the tentorium), ventricles and their connections (the lateral, third and fourth ventricles), the interhemispheric foramina, the choroid plexus, and the tela-choroidea, midbrain structures such the corpus callosum, the head of the caudate nucleus, the thalamus and the cavum septi pellucidi, the cerebellum with its hemispheres and the vermis.

The different coronal and sagittal sections are illustrated in Figure 16.1). The anatomic structures visualized in each

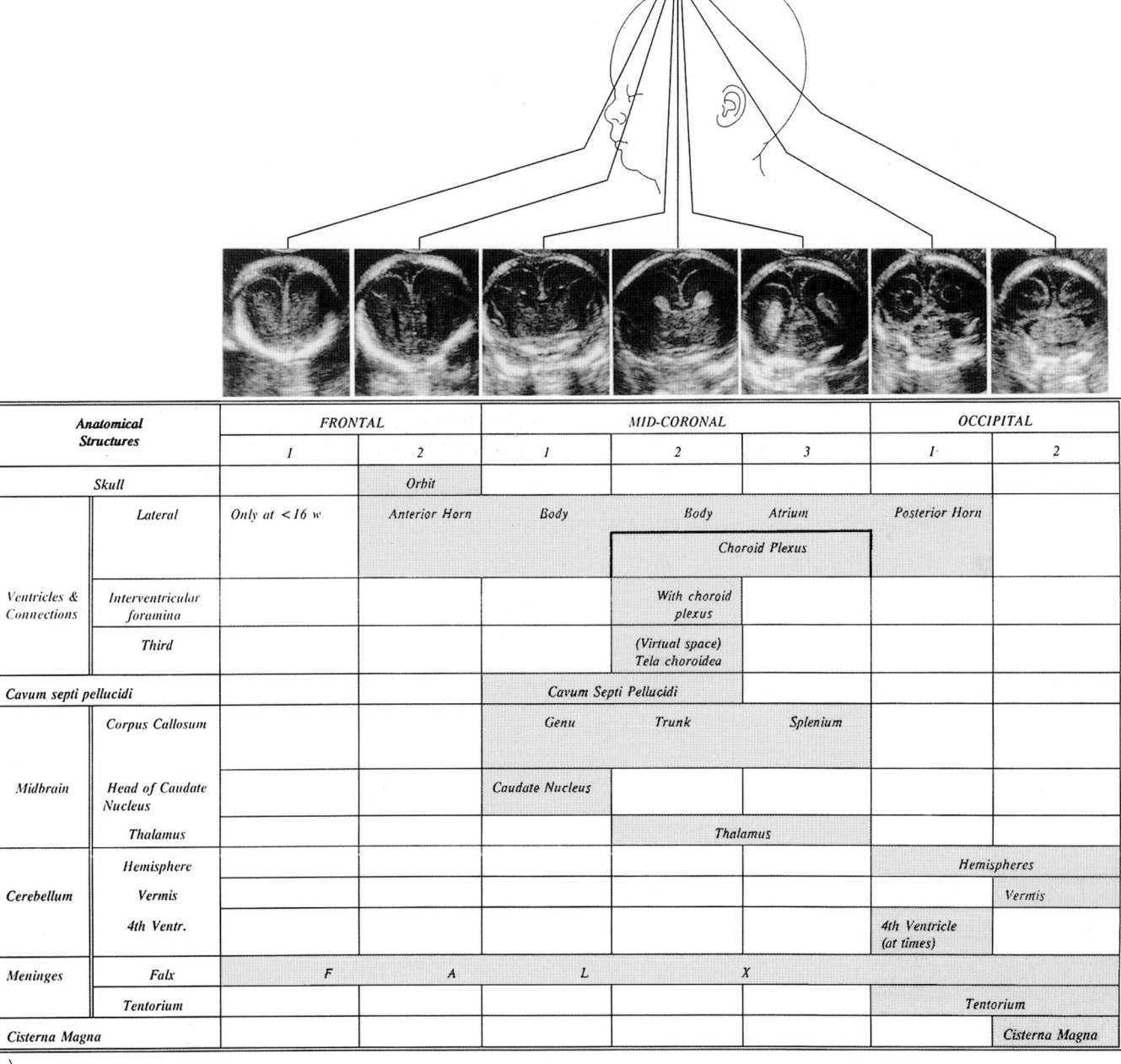

Anatomical Structures		FRONTAL		MID-CORONAL			OCCIPITAL	
		1	*2*	*1*	*2*	*3*	*1*	*2*
Skull			Orbit					
Ventricles & Connections	Lateral	Only at <16 w	Anterior Horn	Body	Body	Atrium	Posterior Horn	
					Choroid Plexus			
	Interventricular foramina				With choroid plexus			
	Third				(Virtual space) Tela choroidea			
Cavum septi pellucidi				Cavum Septi Pellucidi				
Midbrain	Corpus Callosum			Genu	Trunk	Splenium		
	Head of Caudate Nucleus			Caudate Nucleus				
	Thalamus				Thalamus			
Cerebellum	Hemisphere						Hemispheres	
	Vermis							Vermis
	4th Ventr.						4th Ventricle (at times)	
Meninges	Falx	F	A	L	X			
	Tentorium						Tentorium	
Cisterna Magna								Cisterna Magna

(a)

Figure 16.1 The newly proposed planes and sections by transvaginal sonography. (a) Pictorial table of the different structures seen on the seven 'quasi-coronal' planes seen by 2-D transvaginal sonography. The cluster of structures in any of the planes is unique only to that particular plane. (Reproduced with permission from Timor-Tritsch et al 1996).

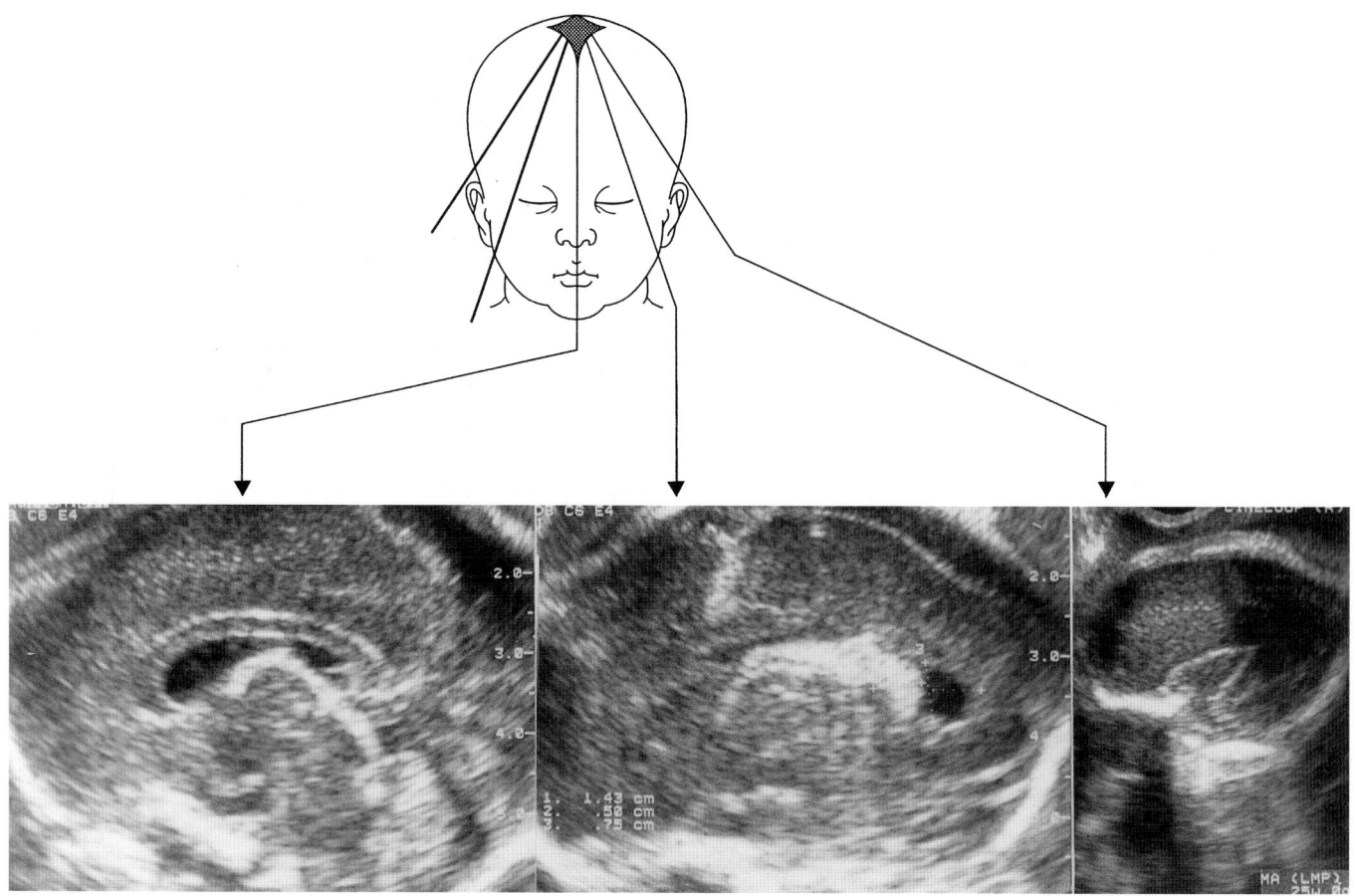

MEDIAN	OBLIQUE-1	OBLIQUE-2
Corpus callosum	Lateral ventricle	Insula
Cavum septi pellucidi	Anterior horn	Parietal operculum
Caudate nucleus	Posterior horn	Temporal operculum
Thalamus	Atrium	Lateral sulcus
Tela choroidea	Choroid plexus	
Tectum	Thalami	
Corpora quadrigemina		
Vermis		
4th ventricle		
Cisterna magna		

(b)

Figure 16.1 continued (b) The different structures seen on the 'quasi-sagittal' planes obtained by 2-D transvaginal sonography. Here too, the group of structures in each plane is unique only to the plane in question. (Reproduced with permission from Timor-Tritsch et al 1996.)

plane are listed in the accompanying table. Once again, we feel that understanding the subtleties of the transfontanalle planes is crucial to proper correlation with similar neonatal images as well as with the conventional planes seen with transabdominal 2-D scanning or with neonatal CT or MRI.

ANATOMIC EVALUATION USING 2-D TRANSVAGINAL FETAL NEUROSCAN

THE POSTERIOR FOSSA

The posterior coronal sections, such as the mid-coronal-3, occipital-1 and occipital-2, provide a sufficiently good evaluation of the posterior fossa. However, at times it is feasible to scrutinize the same area using semiaxial, or even a sagittal plane. When the tip of the transvaginal transducer is closer to the posterior fontanelle it is possible to obtain a clear scan of the posterior fossa. It is important to remember that prior to 16–18 postmenstrual weeks, the cerebellar vermis is still not completely developed and the fourth ventricle clearly communicates with the cerebellopeduncular cistern (cisterna magna) through the widely open median aperture (Fig. 16.2a). Understanding the timing of vermian development will avoid misdiagnosis of cerebellar anomalies, such as a Dandy–Walker continuum and others.

On the occipital-2 section it is possible to detect not only the cerebellar hemisphere and the vermis, but also the surrounding fluid-filled cisterns above, lateral and below the cerebellum itself (Fig. 16.2b).

In the sagittal plane it is possible to view the cerebellar vermis, cerebellomedullary cistern (cisterna magna), the medulla and even the spinal cord (Fig. 16.2c). One should be aware of the fine linear echoes of the arachnoid which are sometimes visualized in the cerebellomedullary cistern. These are normal and should not be confused with pathology. The cortex of the cerebellum is hyperechoic due to the fine invaginations of the pia mater into the cerebellar gyri and sulci, which densely cover the surface of the cerebellum. The vermis is particularly hyperechoic and easy to recognize by transvaginal sonography.

THE CORPUS CALLOSUM AND MIDBRAIN STRUCTURES

The most representative plane to study the midbrain is the median plane. The most obvious and one of the more important structures appearing on this plane is the corpus callosum (Fig. 16.3). It starts to form at around 12 weeks and completes its anterior-to-posterior development at around 20–22 weeks. The median plane is the most important scanning plane to evaluate the presence or absence of the corpus callosum. The other planes, coronal and axial, can only provide indirect sonographic clues regarding this pathology.

Three structures develop in close relation to each other: the corpus callosum, the pericallosal artery and the cavum septi pellucidi. During the second and the early third trimes-

ter of pregnancy, the cavum septi pellucidi is divided into two distinct areas. The anterior portion is the cavum septi itself, while its posterior extension is called the cavum vergae (Fig. 16.3a). The cavum vergae diminishes in size and almost disappears close to term. The cavum septi pellucidi and cavum vergae are not part of the ventricular systems, as they do not have connections with the lateral ventricle. The cavum septi pellucidi is found under the corpus callosum and the pericallosal artery runs parallel to its superior border (Fig. 16.3b). Identifying the pericallosal artery with power Doppler imaging along the entirety of the corpus callosum can aid in confirming the presence of this important structure.

The thalami, caudate nuclei, fourth ventricle and the medulla are also seen by moving the transducer slightly right or left of the median plane. The above-mentioned midbrain structures can also be studied on the consecutive mid-coronal planes, which should be used as a control of the image obtained by the median plane.

THE VENTRICULAR SYSTEM

The cerebrospinal fluid (CSF) is produced by the choroid plexuses in the atrium of the two lateral ventricles. The two symmetrically positioned, back-to-back, C-shaped lateral ventricles connect with the third ventricle in the midline through the interventricular foramina (Monroe). The fluid then drains into the fourth ventricle through the aqueduct and then through the median and lateral aperture into the cerebellomedullary cistern (cisterna magna). From there it is dispersed throughout the surface of the cerebral hemispheres.

As far as the individual components of the lateral ventricle are concerned, there are three horns that can be quite easily detected by transvaginal sonography: the anterior, posterior and inferior horns. These are sometimes referred to as the frontal, occipital and temporal horns, respectively. All three horns are relatively large at 12–14 weeks' gestation, although their relative size compared to the rest of the brain gradually diminishes as term approaches. Clinically, the size of the lateral ventricular atrium is measured as an indication of ventricular size. Traditionally, if the width of the lateral ventricle measures greater than 10 mm, four times the standard deviation of normal, it should trigger a suspicion of true ventriculomegaly (Cardoza et al 1988a). While many authors use the term 'mild ventriculomegaly' for cases where the atrial measurement is between 10 mm and 15 mm (Kelly et al 2001, Wax et al 2003), recent evidence has questioned these cutoffs as even ventricular widths between 12 mm and 15 mm are associated with an increase in morbidity and mortality (Gaglioti et al 2005).

The dilatation of the posterior horn, also called colpocephaly, is probably the most sensitive indicator of ventricular dilatation. Using the transvaginal imaging method it is easy to measure the posterior horn and compare it against published nomograms (Monteagudo et al 1993, 1994).

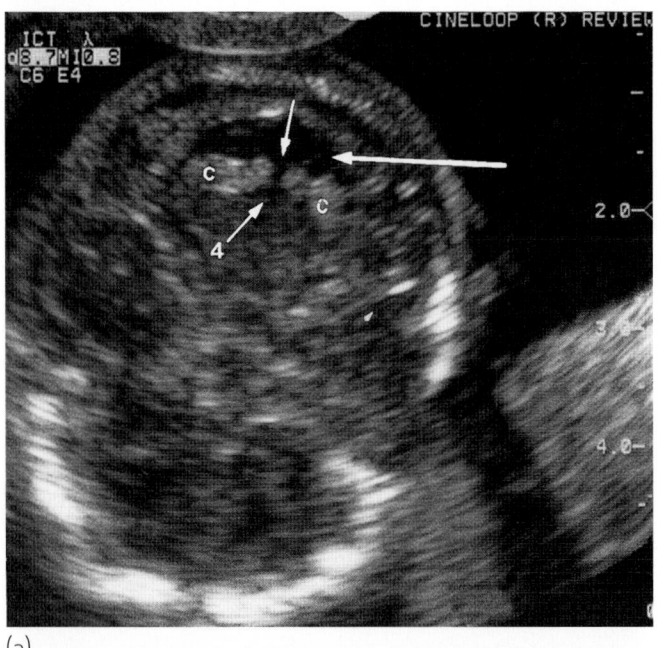

(a)

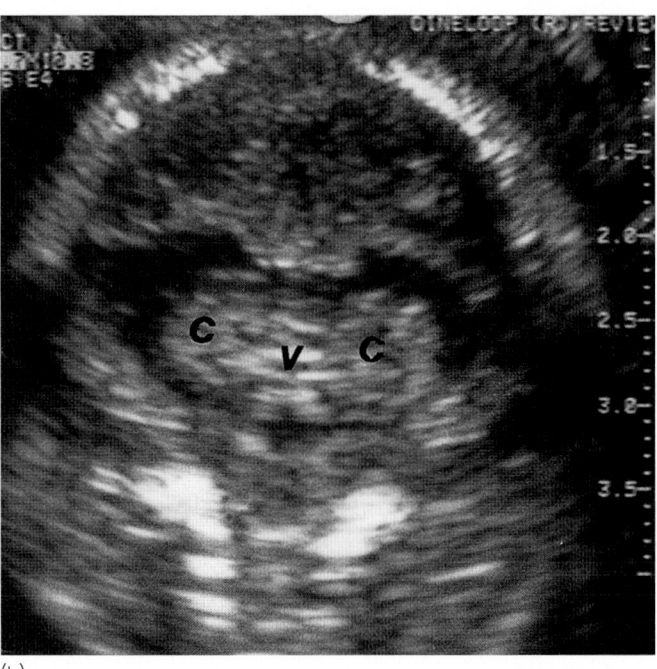

(b)

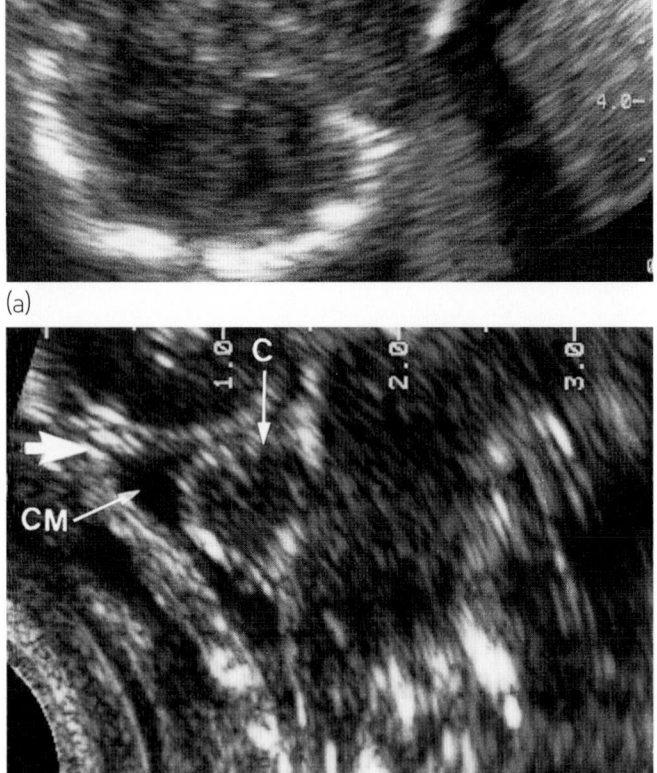

(c)

Figure 16.2 The posterior fossa at 16 postmenstrual weeks. (a) From an occipital viewpoint this low axial section demonstrates that the median aperture (Magendie) marked by two small opposing arrows is wide open and communicates with the fourth ventricle. The two hemispheres of the cerebellum, c, are also seen. The vermis, which is still not fully formed at this age, is not seen on this low axial section. (b) This posterior coronal (0–2) section of the brain demonstrates the echogenic vermis, v, connecting the two hemispheres of the cerebellum, c, as well as the surrounding cisterns. The cistern above the cerebellum is the cisterna ambiens. (c) A median section from an occipital approach depicts the tentorium (solid white arrow), the cisterna magna, CM, and the spinal canal, SpC, as well as the cerebellum, C.

The inferior horn extends laterally into the temporal lobe. After 16 weeks, the size of this horn on the oblique-1 sections remains stable while the rest of the brain is growing. After 24 weeks, however, the inferior horn should not be evident on the oblique-1 view. If, on the other hand, the inferior horns are clearly seen on the oblique-1 section (2-D TV ultrasound) or on the three horn view (3-D TV ultrasound – discussed later), ventriculomegaly should be seriously suspected. Figure 16.4 illustrates a case of ventriculomegaly in a fetus with aqueductal stenosis.

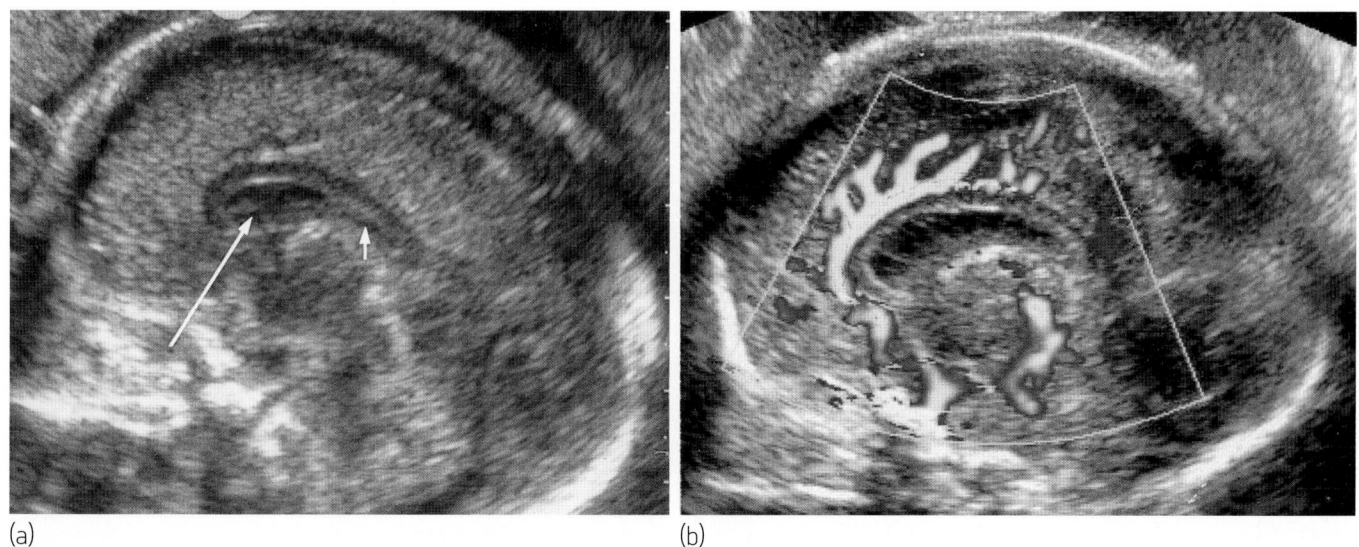

(a)   (b)

Figure 16.3 The corpus callosum at 23 postmenstrual weeks. (a) Median section demonstrating the C-shaped corpus callosum. Under it the anterior cavum septi pellucidi (long arrow) and cavum vergae (short arrow) are seen. T, thalamus. (b) Power Doppler study of the pericallosal artery above the corpus callosum.

The third ventricle is rarely imaged in the second and third trimesters. Any dilation of the 3rd ventricle above 5 mm using the mid-coronal-2 section should trigger a detailed fetal neuroscan to examine the lateral ventricular system. The fourth ventricle, seen on the median plane, usually appears as a sonolucent triangle at the level of the cerebellum.

While multiple scanning planes are necessary to fully evaluate the various components of the ventricular system, it has been shown that the etiology in the majority of cases of ventriculomegaly can be correctly identified by a simultaneous 2-D visualization of the posterior fossa, the corpus callosum and the cavum septi pellucidi in the median plane (D'Addario et al 2005).

CHOROID PLEXUSES

The choroid plexuses are found in the two lateral, the third, and fourth ventricles; however, the best place to evaluate this structure is at the atrium of the lateral ventricles using the mid-coronal-3 (Fig. 16.1a – MC-2 and MC-3) and/or the oblique-1 (Fig. 16.1b) scanning planes. Sonographically it appears as a cotton-like structure with irregular borders filling the available space of the lateral ventricles. In fetuses with ventriculomegaly, the choroids may thin out and separate from their lateral attachments. This 'dangling choroid' has been proposed as a sensitive marker for ventriculomegaly (Cardoza et al 1988b) (Fig. 16.4). Choroid plexus cysts (discussed later) can be a marker for aneuploidy, specifically trisomy 18.

THE CEREBRAL CORTEX

Aside from the medial aspect of the cerebral cortex, the other surfaces of the brain are convex, and are thus inadequately imaged using 2-D technology. The median surface, however, can be visualized with 2-D imaging if the median scanning plane is adequately obtained. As mentioned before, this median plane is most readily accessible via the transvaginal route. Therefore, it is via this approach that the sulci and gyri along the falx cerebri are best visualized.

Pathologic and developmental studies have shown that the cerebral hemispheres are still smooth at around the 22nd postmenstrual week. The cingulate sulcus is first detectable at approximately the 24th postmenstrual week (Fig. 16.5a). The biggest increase in the number and depth of the sulci takes place between 28 and 30 weeks' gestation. Using transvaginal ultrasonography we studied the development of the cingulate sulcus as well as the parieto-occipital fissure in normal fetuses from the 14th postmenstrual week to term and came to the conclusion that the developmental maturation of the normal fetal brain follows a predictable timetable which can be followed sonographically (Monteagudo & Timor-Tritsch 1997). Typically, two or three sections of the fetal brain are sufficient to study the sulci and gyri at or after the 28th postmenstrual week. In addition to the median plane, the mid-coronal-1 and -2 planes can identify the interhemispheric fissure, the falx, the budding of the cingulate sulcus, and later in gestation, its branches (Fig. 16.5b). All the above-mentioned cortical structures are detectable via TV ultrasound and may be the markers of developmental problems of the brain surface.

It is imperative to note, however, that the technologic advances afforded by 3-D ultrasound capabilities discussed below allow for visualization of the outer, convex brain surfaces in a manner that 2-D technology cannot replicate.

THE 3-D TRANSVAGINAL NEUROSCAN

Recent developments in 3-D ultrasound technology have enabled us to greatly expand our sonographic evaluation of the fetal brain. Using 3-D probes to complement our 2-D

345

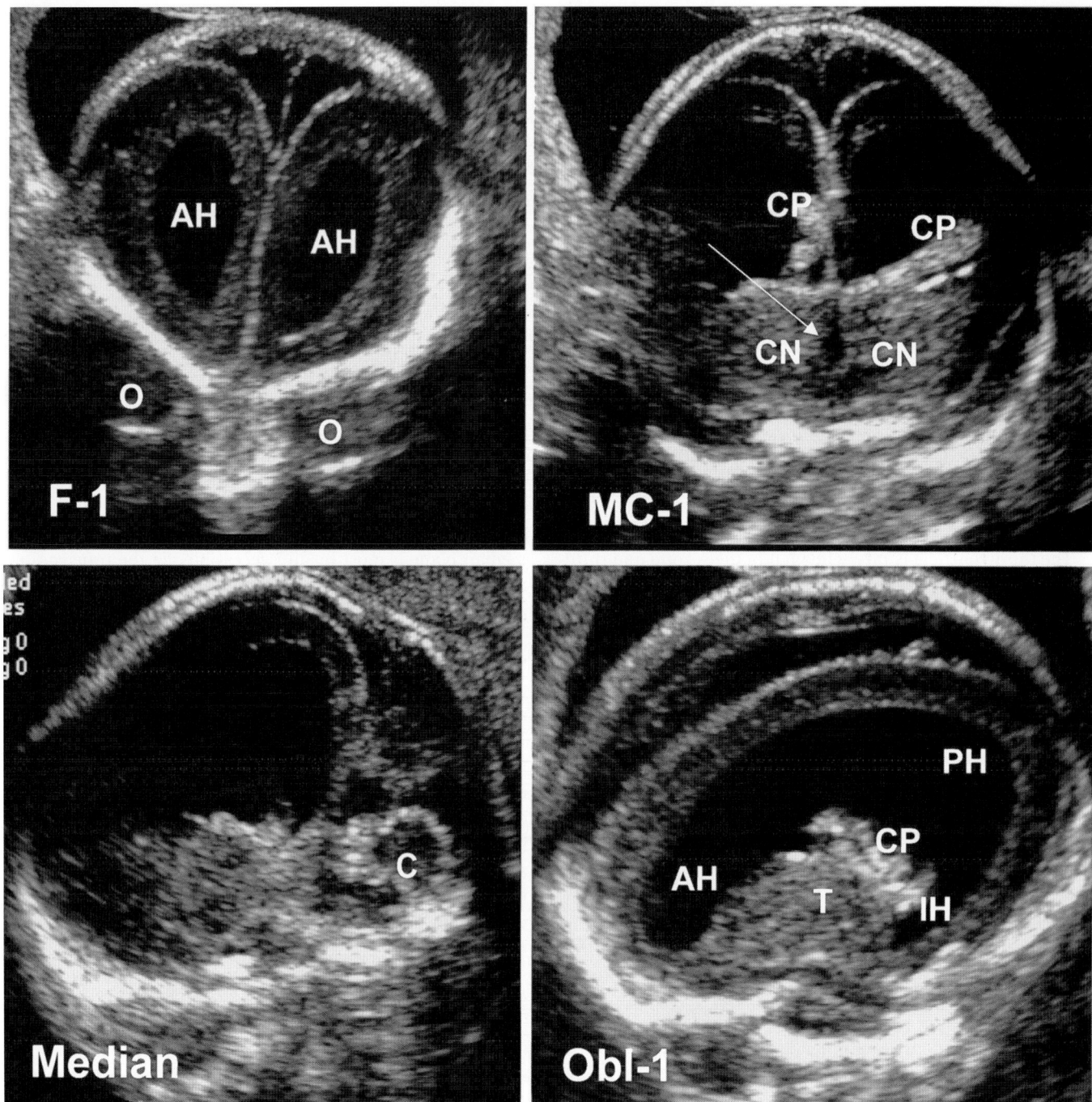

Figure 16.4 Aqueductal stenosis with hydrocephaly at 24 postmenstrual weeks. F-1, Frontal-1 section, MC-1, Midcoronal-1 section. Note the dangling choroid plexus (CP). The arrow points to the third ventricle. Obl-1, oblique-1 section (AH, anterior horn; CN, caudate nucleus; IH, inferior horn; O, orbits; T, thalamus). Median section (C, cerebellum).

transabdominal and transvaginal imagery, we can enhance the diagnostic abilities of the fetal neuroscan. While it has been suggested to include transabdominal 3-D imaging of the fetal brain into the routine imaging protocol (Correa et al 2006), we believe that as practitioners gain experience in the transvaginal route, both with 2-D and 3-D transducers, the advantages of these techniques will become self-evident.

We have gained experience over the years with several different 3-D transducers and machines, each of which has its own unique features. Below, we will describe some of the basic 3-D features that have helped bring the field of diagnostic neurosonography to the next level.

Volume acquisition – acquiring a volume adds the third dimension to the imaging capabilities. While transabdominal

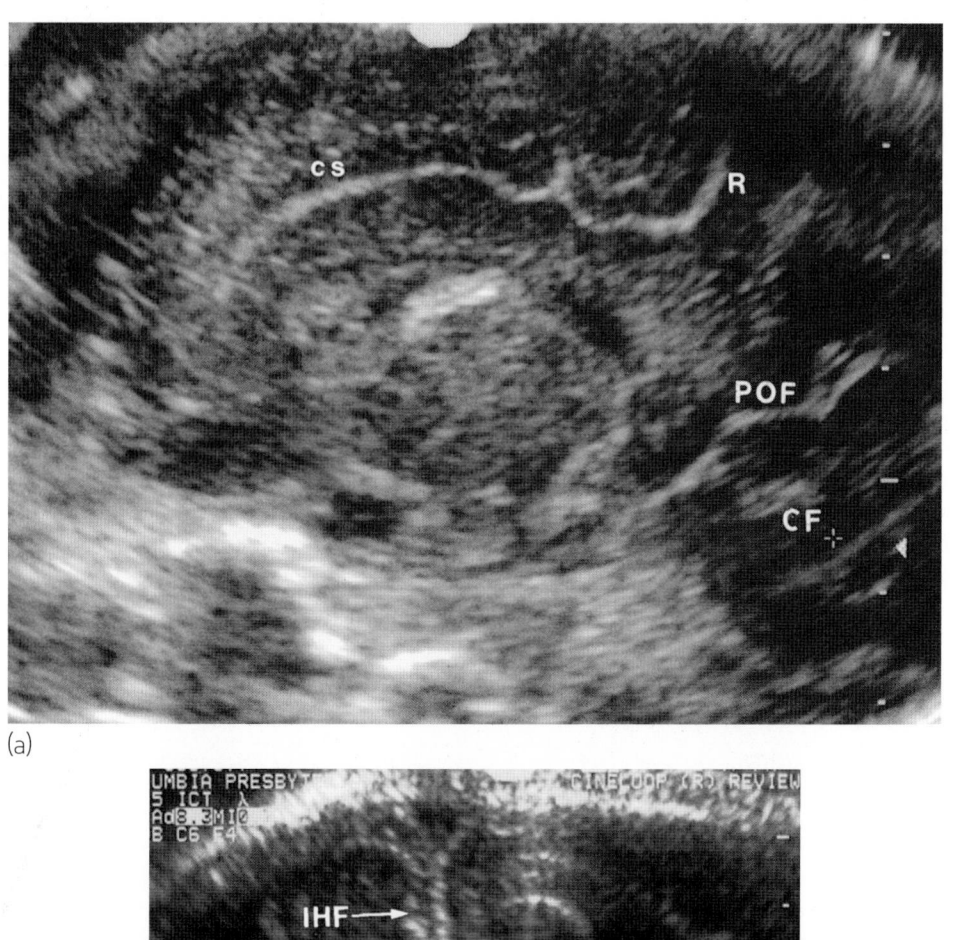

(a)

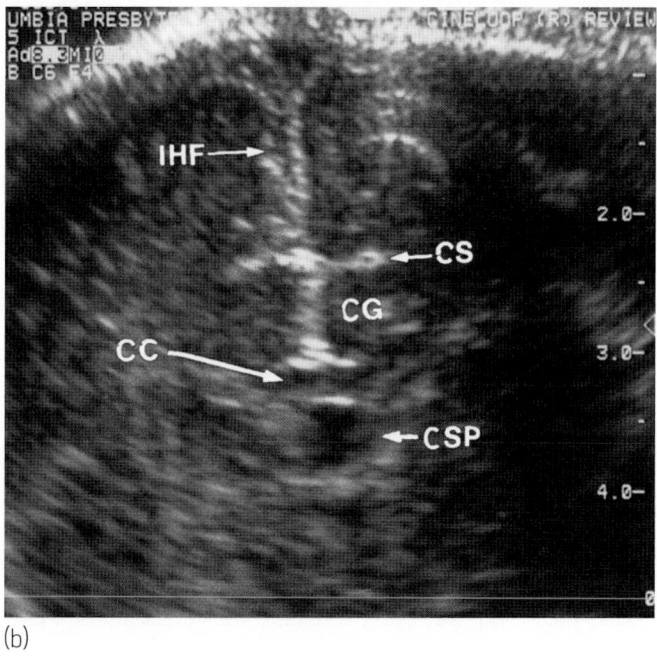

(b)

Figure 16.5 Gyri and sulci. (a) At 32 postmenstrual weeks a median section by transvaginal sonography shows the main sulci and fissures of the fetal brain on the medial aspect of the hemisphere (CS, callosal sulcus with its upward turning branch = R; POF, parieto-occipital fissure; CF, calcarine fissure). (b) A midcoronal-2 section at 32 postmenstrual weeks demonstrates the interhemispheric fissure (IHF), the callosal sulcus (CS), the callosal gyrus (CG), the corpus callosum (CC) and the cavum septi pellucidi (CSP).

2-D imaging limited us to the axial plane, and 2-D transvaginal imaging allowed us visualization of the coronal and sagittal planes, 3-D imaging, via the transabdominal ro transvaginal routes, allows us to image all three planes simultaneously. Furthermore, in most 3-D transducers the crystal array is mechanically moved, thus the successive sec-

tions within the volume are acquired at precise time intervals. This allows for accurate measurement within the volume itself, as the exact distances between the planes are known.

An additional key advantage of the volume acquisition is the ability to store the volume electronically for future manipulation and investigation. This affords for the sonologist the freedom to scrutinize the fetal anatomy well after the patient has already left the laboratory. In addition, these stored volumes can be sent to off-site providers for initial analysis or for second opinions. The technique for acquiring the 3-D volume of the brain is described elsewhere (Monteagudo et al 2000).

Multiplanar imaging – this technology allows for the simultaneous display of images in all three conventional planes (i.e. coronal, sagittal and axial planes). As the three planes are at right angles to each other this display method is also referred to as the orthogonal display. Not only are the three perpendicular images displayed, but we can scroll through the planes in all directions enabling free movement or 'navigation' within the volume. This allows for pinpoint visualization of the anatomy of interest from all three conventional planes. It is these conventional planes that are more easily correlated with neonatal CT and MRI imaging, as the planes are truly parallel to each other, and not slanted as in 2-D TV scanning.

Multi-planar technology allows for the standardization of 3-dimensional views to aid in the diagnosis of various pathologies. For example, we have previously described a 'three-horn view' (3HV) (Timor-Tritsch et al 2000) which allows for simultaneous visualization of the anterior, posterior and inferior horns of the lateral ventricle. This is possible by tilting the volume seen in Box 'A' to the right or left and then placing the scanning planes across all three horns at the same time. On the 3HV very subtle changes in size and shape during a progressively developing ventriculomegaly can be observed. (Fig. 16.6) Using 2-D transvaginal ultrasonography we published measurements of the anterior, posterior, and inferior horns in the sagittal as well as coronal planes (Monteagudo et al 1993). These measurements can be used for the 3HV. An example of obtaining the 3HV in a pathologic case with agenesis of the corpus callosum (ACC) can be seen in Figure 16.6.

Thick slice display – this added technique allows the operator to adjust the numbers of cuts that are compressed

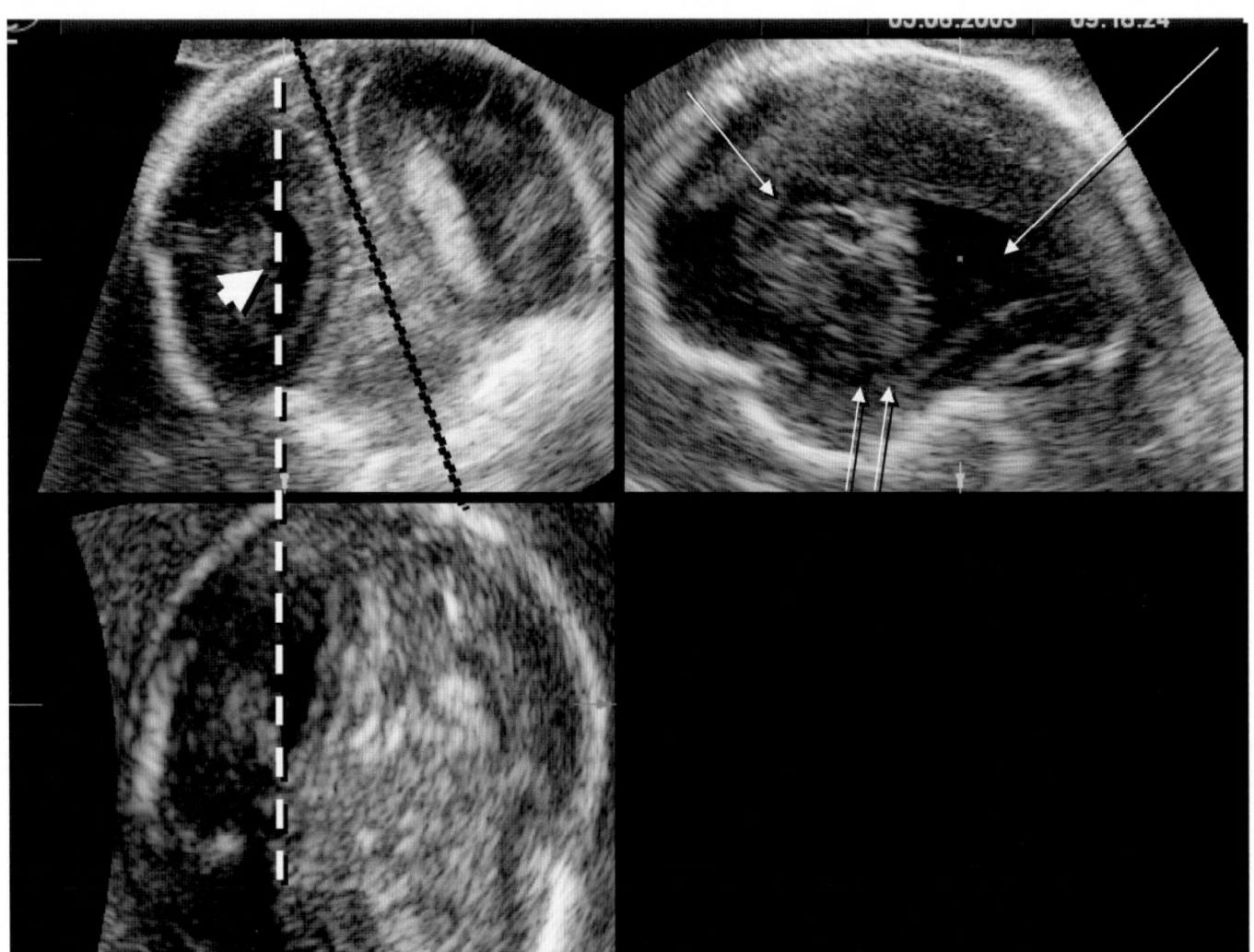

Figure 16.6 The three horn view. After the median plane (dotted black line) is tilted to the left the plane marked by the dotted white line is shifted to overlay the posterior horn (arrowhead). The result is a comprehensive view of all three horns of the lateral ventricle (anterior horn: short arrow; posterior horn: long arrow; inferior horn: double arrows).

into the final rendered image. The resulting 3-D image portrays a thicker section of the anatomy and is occasionally helpful in clarifying the anatomic relationships in the area of interest (Fig. 16.7).

Volume calculation – as mentioned previously, the precise timing of the serial sonographic cuts obtained by the mechanical 3-D probes allows accurate measurement of distances within the volume. Whereas 2-D imaging allows for the measurement of the distance between two points, the volume calculation feature available for 3-D imaging allows one to trace the structure of interest in the various 3-D planes and then calculate the volume of the structure. Several investigators have also been working to establish normal volume measurements for different fetal brain structures at various stages of development (Chang et al 2003, Endres & Cohen 2001, Roelfsema et al 2004).

3-D power angio or color Doppler mode – this feature allows us to obtain a 3-dimensional view of the vasculature of the fetal brain. This is extremely helpful when trying to characterize a vascular anomaly. In addition, we have already mentioned how visualization of certain vessels, such as the pericallosal artery, can help in evaluating the anatomy of the structure being supplied, i.e. the corpus callosum (Fig. 16.8).

Inversion – in our continuous efforts to optimally visualize the fetal brain structures, inversion allows the sonographer to invert the echogenic characteristics of the image and cancel out the background to obtain a 3-D view of the structure of interest alone. This is the technologic equivalent of the wax casting that was once done to re-create the shape and volume of an anatomic space. For example, this rendering technique can be used to reconstruct the ventricular system to help characterize the pathology present (Fig. 16.9). Also, when used in conjunction with power angio or color Doppler, inversion allows the operator to obtain an image similar to the angiography performed under fluoroscopy in adults. In this way, the vascular tree and its anastomoses can be examined for anomalies.

Tomographic imaging – this feature is the prime example of how ultrasound can now be perfectly correlated with neonatal images. This software allows the 3-D volume image

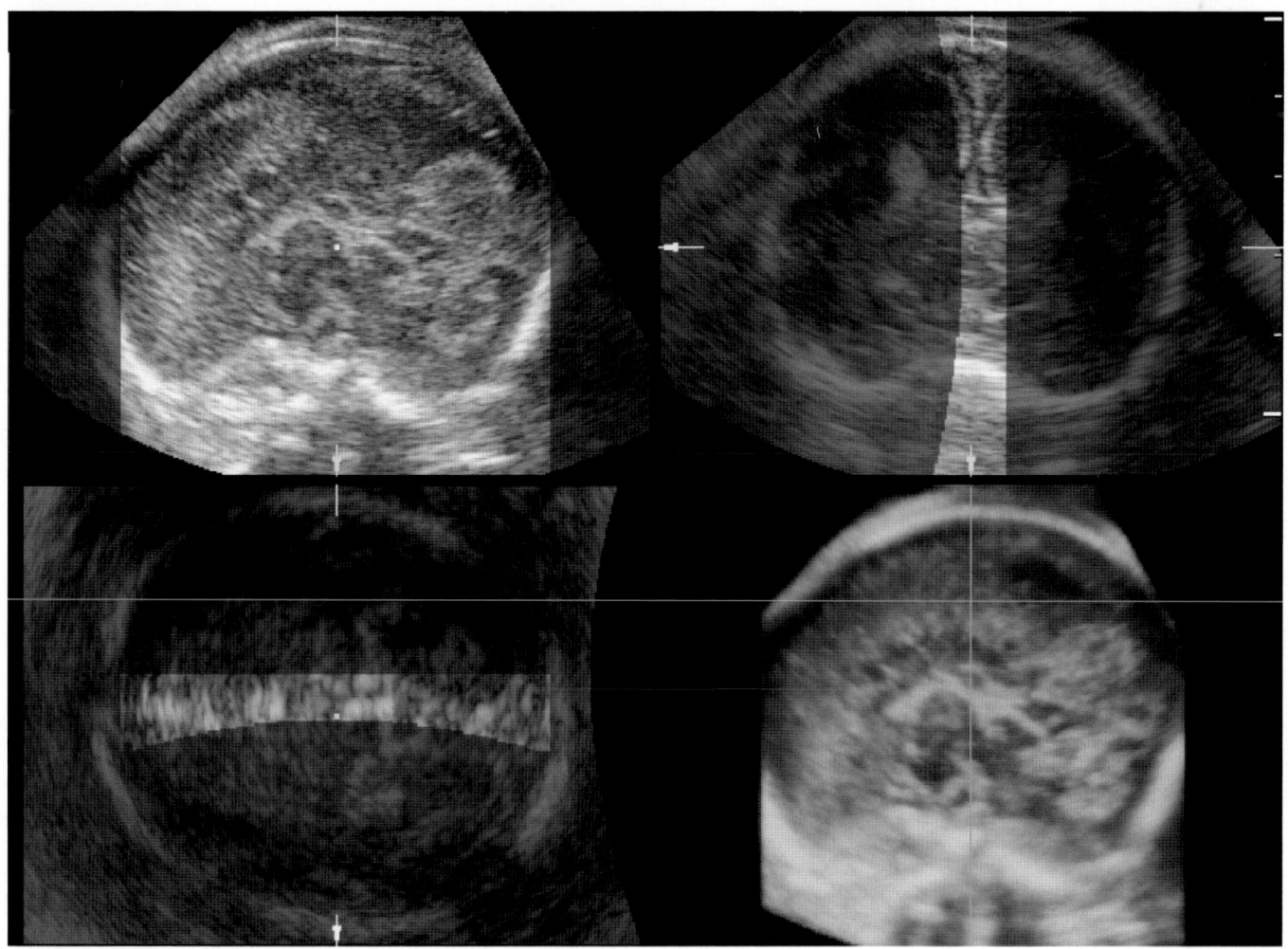

Figure 16.7 Thick slice rendering of the median plane. The diagnosis of complete agenesis of the corpus callosum is better emphasized using the thick slice display mode.

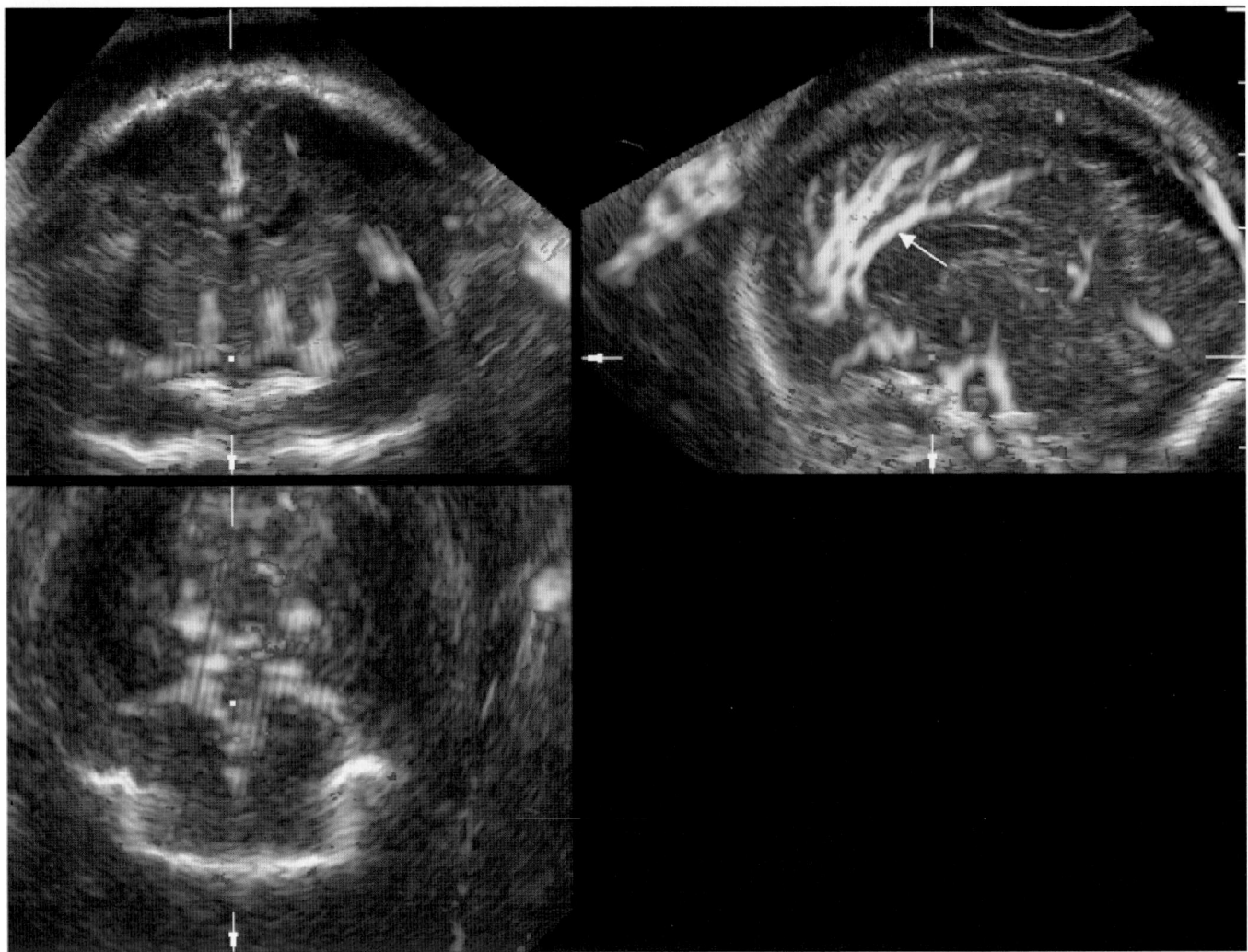

Figure 16.8 Orthogonal display of the brain vascularity using the power Doppler mode. The pericallosal artery is marked by an arrow.

to be cut into slices of a pre-determined interval and displayed just as a CT scan or MRI would be. This capability allows for pediatric neurologists and neurosurgeons to visualize the anatomy in a manner in which they are more comfortable. This facilitates patient counseling, surgical planning, and neonatal correlation. Most of all, it optimizes and standardizes the communication between the various clinicians caring for the fetus (Fig. 16.10a,b).

X-ray or transparency mode – this mode can be helpful when evaluating skeletal structures, often via the transabdominal route. In the neuroscan, this is most useful when evaluating the skull in cases of microcephaly or cephalocele. This modality can also prove useful when evaluating the vertebral column in cases of spina bifida.

Overall, there are very few limitations of 3-D ultrasound of the fetal brain; however, one important limitation is the sensitivity of this technology to fetal motion, as well as

other artifacts. Currently, it takes approximately 2 to 6 seconds to get a basic 3-D volume sweep with the TV transducer and up to 20 or more seconds to get a volume of the vasculature. Any fetal movement during that sweep can cause significant artifact. Ideally, waiting for a period of fetal quiescence can avoid this artifact. However, in a very active fetus, setting the sweep time to a shorter duration can help in acquiring a volume with minimal artifact.

To conclude, we feel that the 3-D transvaginal sonography can effectively be used to examine the fetal brain. The ability to image the brain in all scanning planes and to navigate within the volume allows the intricate anatomic relationships to be better appreciated. For instance, this technology has been used to isolate the optic chiasm and its relationship to surrounding structures in fetuses at varying gestational ages (Bault 2006). Furthermore, access to all of the conventional scanning planes allows for accurate com-

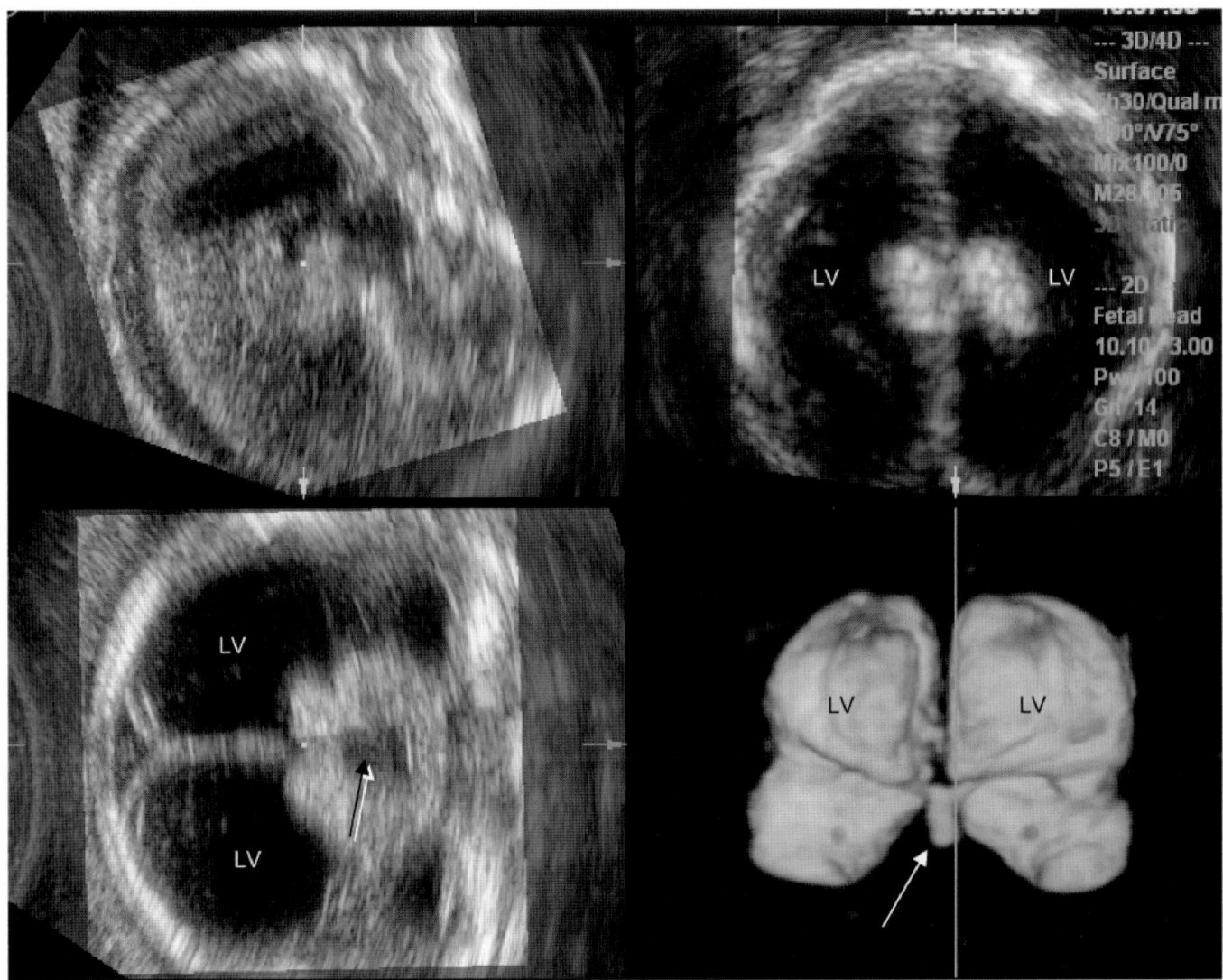

Figure 16.9 Inversion rendering of the fluid-filled lateral (LV) and third ventricle (arrow) seen in the lower right image.

parison with neonatal ultrasound, MRI, and CT studies. Lastly, the ability to save the volume for future, off-site scrutiny adds a degree of freedom to diagnostic ultrasound that will only make the entire ultrasound experience smoother for the patient as well as for the sonologist. Moreover, the ability to easily send 3-D volumes for other specialists to review allows for easy and efficient second opinions that ultimately improve patient care and counseling.

In our opinion, the largest obstacle to the widespread use of 3-D imaging of the fetal brain is lack of experience and familiarity with the scanning procedure. These can be overcome fairly easily and allow for the routine use of this amazing technology (Monteagudo et al 2000, Pooh & Pooh 2001). We are confident that 3-D fetal neuroscanning will find its way to the daily scanning routine of the imaging specialist.

SELECTED FETAL NEUROPATHOLOGY USING TRANSVAGINAL TRANSFONTANELLE SCANNING

As it is beyond the scope of this chapter to list and show all the fetal CNS anomalies, we have chosen a handful of anomalies to be presented here to enable the reader to understand the principle behind the scanning methods and their advantages.

POSTERIOR FOSSA ANOMALIES

Traditionally, posterior fossa anomalies have been diagnosed and classified based on axial views of the fetal head (Fig. 16.11). In fact, until recently, the vast majority of the fetal neuro-imaging literature was based on observations made primarily using axial views. However, many important features of the posterior fossa anatomy, such as the position

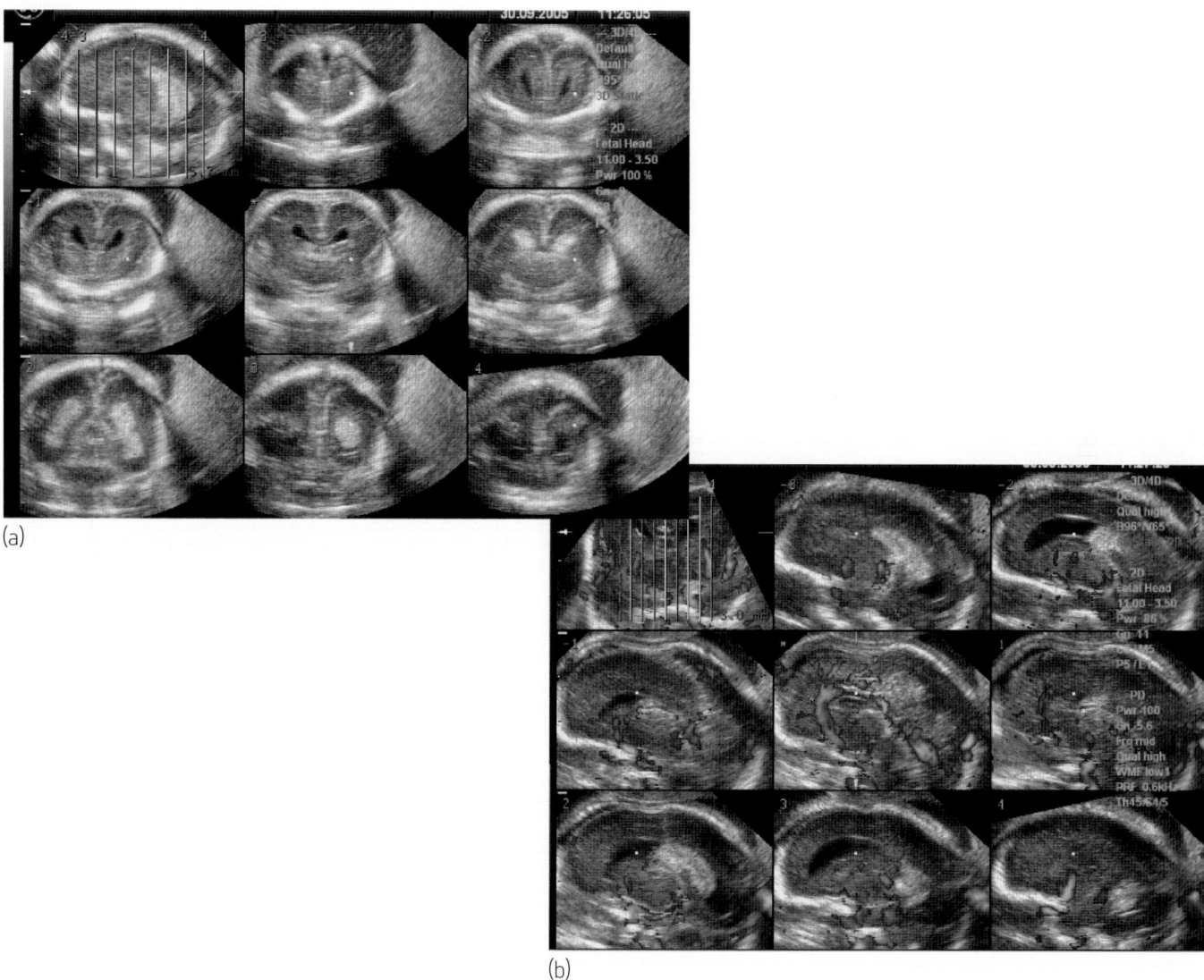

Figure 16.10 Tomographic display of the fetal brain at 20 weeks. (a) Serial coronal sections. (b) Several sagittal sections showing the brain vessels using power Doppler mode.

of the vermis, tentorium and the torcular (confluence of sinuses), cannot be adequately assessed seen on the axial views. Unfortunately, the difficulties with diagnosis and counseling have led to an increased focus on MRI instead of using the sagittal (median) plane obtainable by transvaginal sonography or 3-D scanning, which, as mentioned above, can provide important information regarding the cerebellum and its surroundings. The median view (Fig. 16.12) is especially important when establishing certain pathologies in the posterior fossa as it depicts the size and the orientation of the vermis and the position of the torcular. Table 16.1 compares the various structures seen with these two scanning planes.

Lately, several authors have emphasized the indispensable role of the sagittal plane in the neuroscan (Achiron et al 2004, Malinger et al 2001, Zalel et al 2002). In fact, one of the important contributions of 3-D imaging has been the capability to reliably and easily obtain the exact median

view (Fig. 16.13) (Pilu et al 2006). Three dimensional imaging of the posterior fossa using the various display modalities mentioned above presents a new avenue to study the cerebellum and its deviant development.

Several algorithms to evaluate the posterior fossa stand out. Guibaud and des Portes methodically outlined an anatomic approach to diagnosing posterior fossa anomalies based on the major sonographic abnormalities (Guibaud & des Portes 2006). Others base their classifications upon MRI findings (Patel et al 2002), which are difficult to apply to sonographic evaluation of the posterior fossa.

It is clear that a significant knowledge of developmental milestones of the cerebellum and its environs is needed to diagnose their malformations and pathologies. Recent advances in the transvaginal fetal neuroscan, in addition to 3-dimensional volume scanning, have particularly enhanced our diagnostic power as far as the posterior fossa is concerned.

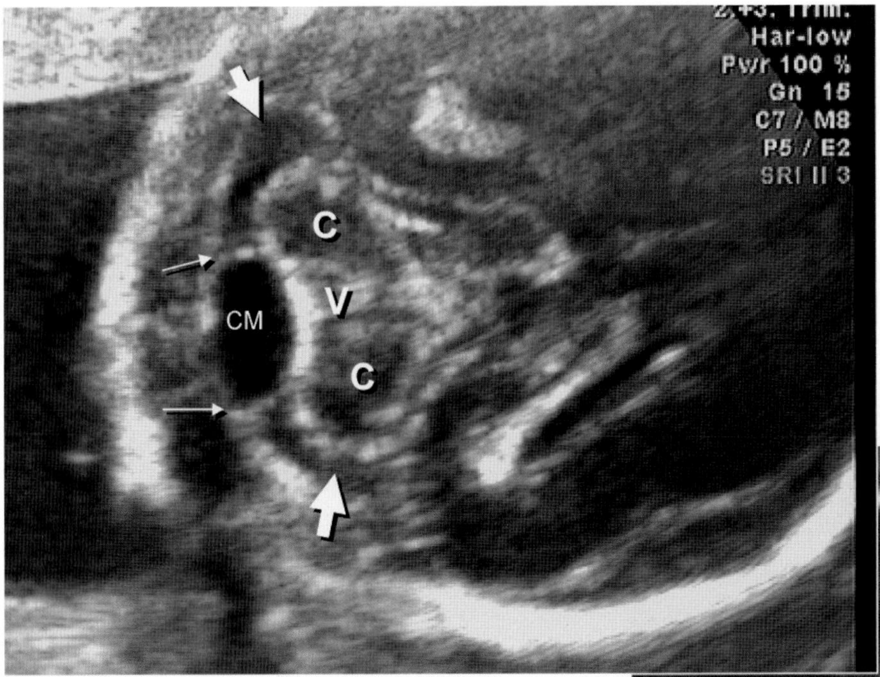

Figure 16.11 Axial scanning views of the posterior fossa. (a) A low axial section depicting the cerebellar hemispheres (c), vermis (v), cisterna magna (cm). The thin arrows point to the linear echoes representing the remnants of the lateral walls of the Blake's pouch. The space between them is anechoic, while lateral to these the subarachnoid space is somewhat more echo-filled (thick arrows). (b) A high axial view reveals the lower edge of the falx as a midline linear echo (arrow).

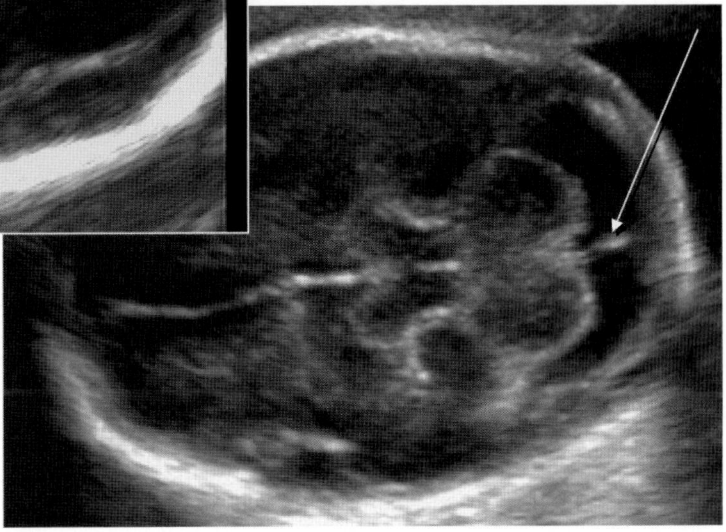

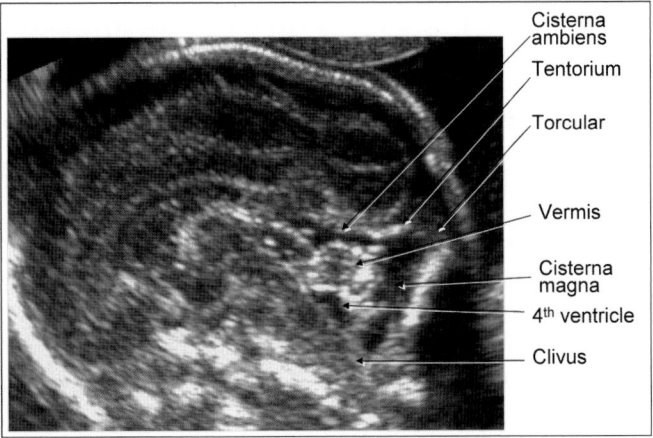

Figure 16.12 Anatomy of the posterior fossa and the vermis on a median plane.

Cisterna ambiens
Tentorium
Torcular
Vermis
Cisterna magna
4th ventricle
Clivus

Table 16.1 Imaging of anatomic structures by planes		
Structures	Axial	Median
Hemispheres, measurements	+	–
Vermis (general appearance)	+/?	+
Vermis (caudo-cranial diameter)	–	+
Vermis (foliae and sulci, ?rotation)	–	+
Torcular & tentorium (displacement)	–	+
Fourth ventricle	–/+	+
Clivus	–	+
Foramen Magendie (median aperture)	+/?	+
Cisterna magna	+	+
Pons/midbrain	–	+
Blake's cyst walls	–/+	+

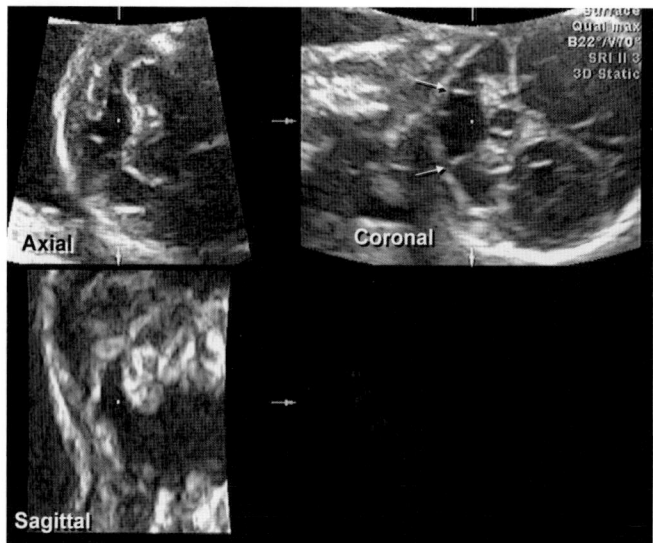

Figure 16.13 Three-dimensional imaging the posterior fossa in the three classic orthogonal planes. The arrows on the coronal plane point to the two linear echoes of the remnants of the Blake's pouch.

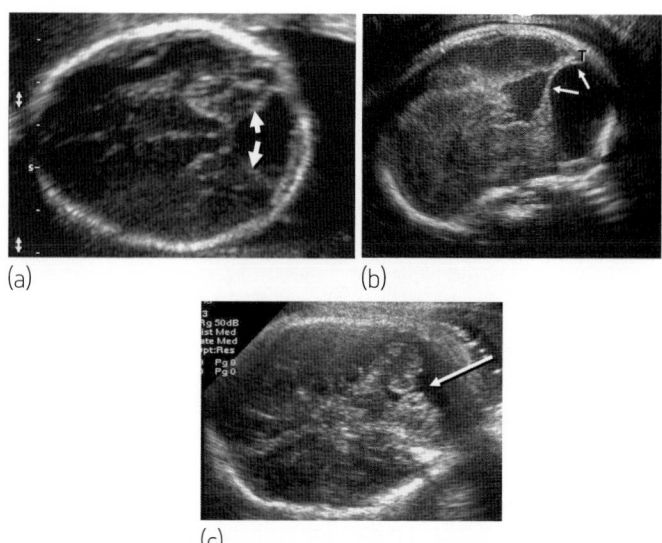

Figure 16.14 Dandy–Walker malformation. (a) Axial plane. The arrows show the pressure effect upon the cerebellar hemispheres. (b) Sagittal view. The arrows point to the elevated tentorium and the torcular (T).

The diagnostic challenges associated with posterior fossa anomalies have made prenatal counseling regarding postnatal prognosis exceedingly difficult (Klein et al 2003). In fact, accurate diagnosis and characterization of posterior fossa pathologies are considered by many to be the last frontier of fetal neurosonography (Guibaud & des Portes 2006, Guibaud 2004, Klein et al 2003, Pilu et al 2006). Thus, we have chosen to elaborate on this anatomic region and provide examples illustrating how transvaginal scanning can help elucidate the various complex pathologies associated with the posterior fossa.

The Dandy–Walker complex or continuum

This term refers to a group of posterior fossa malformations which share some basic features as far as appearance and pathologic definition. The classification and nomenclature of posterior fossa anomalies were based upon axial fetal ultrasound and neonatal or adult MRI using all three cardinal planes. This is the main reason that several pathological entities such as the Dandy–Walker malformation, Dandy–Walker variant, Blake's pouch cyst, mega-cisterna magna, posterior fossa arachnoid cyst and others are frequently mentioned as the 'Dandy–Walker continuum'. However, there is a need for more accurate definition and description of these entities since their pathogenesis, their anatomic picture, their prognosis and their treatment are different. Since the term Dandy–Walker 'complex' or 'continuum' (Barkovich et al 1989) is a confusing term, we will describe the various pathologies as individual diagnoses.

1. Dandy–Walker malformation: This diagnosis is a relatively easy one to make in utero with ultrasound

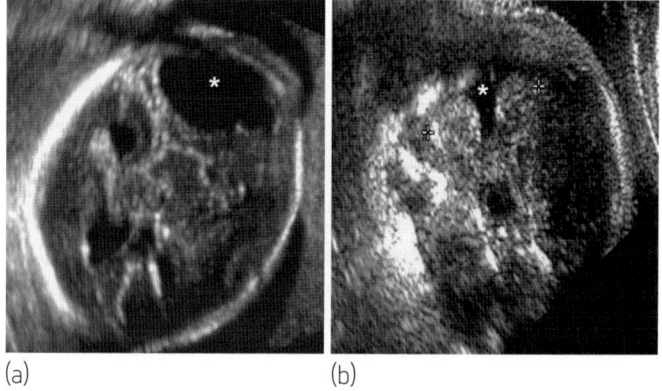

Figure 16.15 Pathologies of the cerebellum. (a) Dandy–Walker malformation. (b) Dandy–Walker variant. Note the difference between the anechoic area (asterisk) of the two cases.

(Klein et al 2003). The posterior fossa fluid content is enlarged, and there can be complete or partial agenesis of the vermis. The cerebellar hemispheres are laterally displaced and the tentorium and the torcular are elevated (Figs 16.14 and 16.15a). Despite the relative ease of diagnosis, only 60–80% is detected antenatally. However, advances in ultrasound technology have led to the ability to diagnose this condition in the first trimester using transvaginal imaging (Sherer et al 2001). The exact incidence of Dandy–Walker malformation is difficult to determine due to the confusion of definitions, but it is believed to be 1 in 30 000 births. In 50–70% of the cases it is a severe anomaly with a

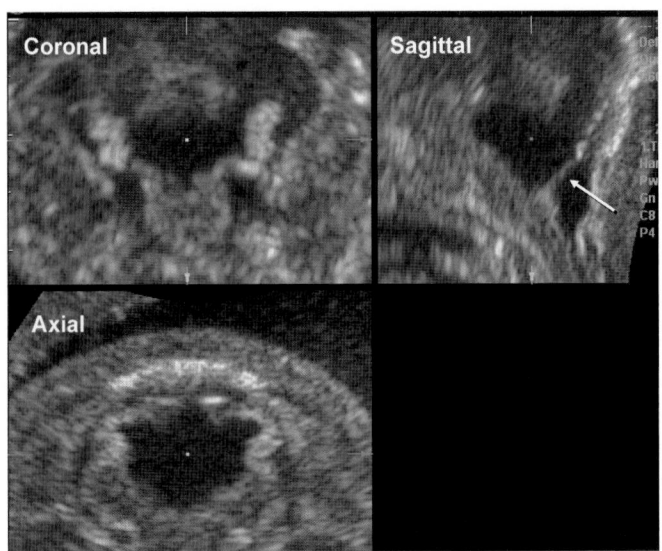

Figure 16.16 Three-dimensional orthogonal ultrasound pictures of the posterior fossa at 19 postmenstrual weeks in a case of persistent Blake's pouch cyst. The arrow points to the cyst wall on the sagittal view.

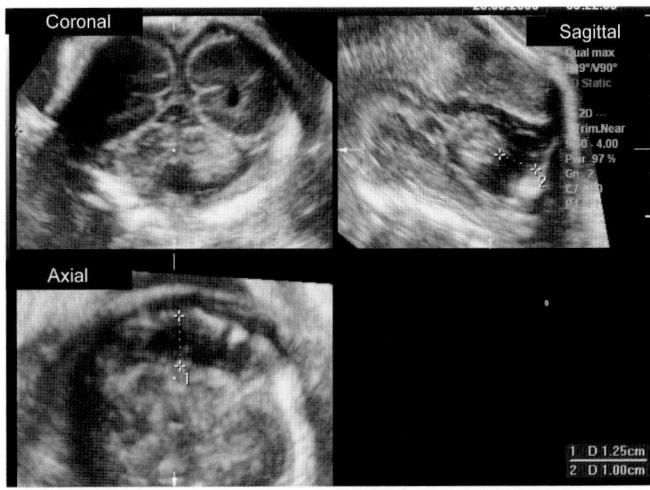

Figure 16.17 Three-dimensional orthogonal ultrasound pictures of a large cisterna magna. The measurements are also displayed.

list of associated brain anomalies. If isolated, the recurrence risk is 1–5%. In 50–70% of survivors a poor neurodevelopment is observed.

2. Dandy–Walker variant: This diagnosis consists of variable hypoplasia or agenesis of the vermis with or without enlargement of the cerebello-peduncular cistern (CM) which communicates with the fourth ventricle. It is a difficult prenatal sonographic diagnosis to make as the cerebellar hemispheres may be of normal size (Fig. 16.15b). On the other hand, it can be overdiagnosed before 18 weeks gestation, prior to complete vermian development.

Genetic factors play a major role in the etiology and agenesis of the vermis is associated with a number of anomalies such as Aicardi syndrome, chromosomal aneuploids (T8, T9, triploidy) as well as Fry, Meckel–Grubber, Nen–Laxova, Smith–Lemli–Opitz and Walker–Warburg syndromes.

3. Persistent Blake's pouch cyst: This pathology is believed to be the result of failed fenestration laterally through the lateral aperture (Luschka) and in the median plane through the median aperture (Magendie), thereby preventing connection and fluid drainage between the so created 'cyst' and the subarachnoid space (Fig. 16.16) (Calabro et al 2000, Conti et al 2003, Nelson et al 2004, Strand et al 1993, Tortori-Donati et al 1996).

This pathology can be diagnosed in utero by ultrasound since the cyst wall is evident on the axial and the sagittal planes. There is anechoic fluid inside the cyst and slightly low level echoic fluid in the surrounding subarachnoid space. As for the sonographic picture, the vermis may be displaced

upward by the mass effect which can also push the cerebellar hemispheres apart. At times ventriculomegaly can be seen if the mass effect obliterates the CSF drainage pathways.

This entity is often first diagnosed in late adulthood. The prognosis is relatively good since postnatal shunting leads to re-expansion of the displaced brain structures.

4. Megacisterna magna: An enlarged cerebello-medullary (CM) measuring >10 mm with integrity of both the cerebellar vermis and the fourth ventricle characterizes this entity (Fig. 16.17) (Barkovich et al 1989, Tortori-Donati et al 1996l). Its clinical significance is uncertain and no clear-cut prognostic data are available. It can be totally asymptomatic and has frequent association with other malformations and/or chromosomal aberrations.

5. Arachnoid cyst: Although this entity will also be discussed in greater detail below, we mention it here since 5–10% of arachnoid cysts are located in the posterior fossa (Nelson et al 2004). The anatomy of the cerebellum and the fourth ventricle remain normal although the tentorium may be slightly elevated and the vermis turned slightly upward. They have a relatively good prognosis provided they are isolated and cause no pressure effect to result in ventriculomegaly.

Walker–Warburg syndrome (Lissencephaly type II, HARD (±E) syndrome)

The descriptive acronym for this syndrome, HARD (±E), refers to the distinguishing features that this entity often displays: *h*ydrocephaly, *a*gyria (lissencephaly), *r*etinal dys-

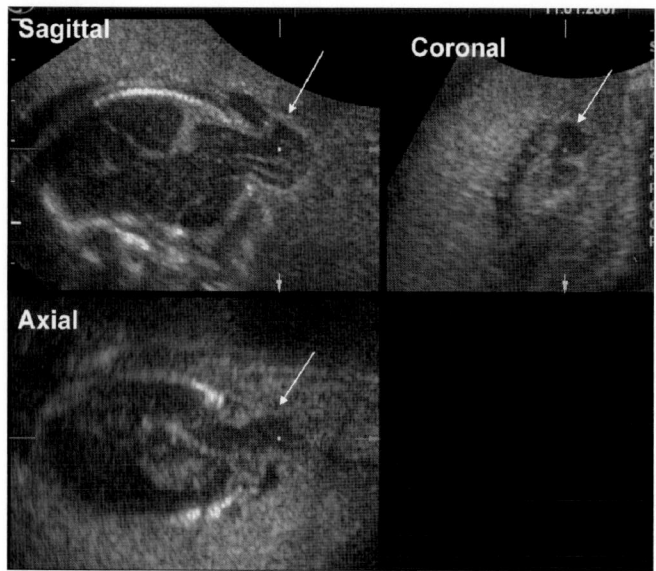

Figure 16.18 Three-dimensional orthogonal ultrasound pictures of a posterior cephalocele (arrows).

plasia, *D*andy–Walker malformation and at times encephalocele. It has an autosomal recessive inheritance with a dismal prognosis (Blin et al 2005, Low et al 2005).

Spina bifida

Although neural tube defects will be addressed in greater detail below, it is important to keep these anomalies in mind when evaluating the posterior fossa. Significant open neural tube defects will usually exhibit pathology of the posterior fossa, i.e. the impacted cerebellum in this case, as an indirect consequence of the vertebrae anomaly. The sonographic finding of an obliterated cisterna magna and an impacted cerebellum, widely known as the 'banana sign,' should alert the sonographer to the presence of a neural tube defect such as spina bifida.

Joubert syndrome

Affected infants with this clinical syndrome present with episodic apnea, abnormal eye movements, ataxia and mental retardation. There is a hypogenesis and midline clefting of the cerebellar vermis, dysplasia and heterotopia of cerebellar nuclei, absence of the pyramidal decussations and other anomalies of the nuclei and nerve tract.

This is a very difficult diagnosis as far as ultrasound is concerned. Increased nuchal translucency, agenesis of the vermis and dysmorphic facial features are the indirect signs. The MRI diagnosis is relatively easy and features the 'molar tooth' sign, which is made up of deepening of the interpeduncular fossa, thick and straight superior cerebellar peduncles and a hypoplastic vermis.

Occipital cephalocele

In the western hemisphere about 80% of cephaloceles arise from the posterior fossa (Fig. 16.18). Their sizes and content can be variable. In three quarters of the cases the extruded brain causes ventriculomegaly. In about 25% of cases the head is small (microcephaly). It is associated with several genetic syndromes, including Meckel–Gruber syndrome.

Cerebellar hypoplasia

In cerebellar hypoplasia, focal reduction in the size of the cerebellum is usually caused by abnormal development (dysplasia), ischemia or hemorrhage (Barht et al 1995, Robins et al 1998). The cerebellar measurements indicate a discrepancy between size and dates. At times unilateral hypoplasia or aplasia can be seen. Global reduction can also involve the brain stem and/or the cerebellum. Several syndromes can be associated with such cerebellar pathology, including aneuploidy, Joubert's syndrome, CHARGE sequence and CMV infection.

Rhombencephalosynapsis

This is a rare congenital developmental anomaly with fusion of the cerebellar hemispheres and the superior cerebellar peduncles with horizontal orientation of the folia (McAuliffe et al 2006). The posterior fossa appears small and other associated brain anomalies such as agenesis of the corpus callosum, hydrocephaly (aqueductal stenosis), holoprosencephaly, can be present. This syndrome is sporadic in nature with no known familial recurrence. The severity and presentation correlate with supratentorial anomalies. Most patients die in early life (<30).

Ventriculomegaly and hydrocephaly (see p. 299): These two terms are used interchangeably; however, ventriculomegaly is a denotation of the lateral ventricles when there is normal CNS fluid pressure present. As opposed to this, hydrocephaly is more than ventriculomegaly, since in this case there is an increased pressure of CFS fluid, causing increasing fetal head size and thinning of the brain tissue. Usually hydrocephaly is divided into non-communicating (Figs 16.4 and 16.9) and communicating types. The diagnosis of hydrocephaly or ventriculomegaly is relatively simple, as there are relatively large fluid-filled spaces which can be detected easily even by transabdominal fetal neuroscan.

The size of the ventricular system can be evaluated subjectively and objectively. There are several ways to assess the size of the ventricles subjectively or qualitatively using transvaginal sonography: (a) relying on indirect signs such as the thickness of the cortical mantle, detection of the inferior horn (which should normally not be seen on an oblique-1 section!), the shape and the mobility of the choroid plexus (if thin and dangling it signifies ventricular dilatation); (b) the gestalt approach, defined as relying on the observer's experience in judging the appearance of the ventricular system; (c) looking at the third ventricle on mid-coronal-1 or 2 sections. Anytime this ventricle is seen (usually it is slit-like!) attention to the entire ventricular system should be given.

As shown earlier the three-horn views are instrumental sections that provide valuable information about the extent of this pathology. The objective assessment of ventricular size is based upon the published measurements of different parts of the lateral and the third ventricles or their ratios. These measurements are based upon TAS (Cardoza et al 1988a, Pretorius et al 1986) or transvaginal sonography (Monteagudo et al 1993, 1994).

Transvaginal sonographic evaluation of the ventricular system seems to be of high specificity in detecting mild ventriculomegaly as well as asymmetric ventriculomegaly. Their implications are well documented in the literature (Achiron et al 1993, Bromley et al 1991, Mahony et al 1988). Using such an apparently sensitive and specific scanning route, one has to still remember that the most important prognostic factors in the outcome of prenatally detected hydrocephaly are: associated chromosomal anomalies, the

amount of residual brain tissue around the ventricles and the presence or absence of any other anomaly.

Agenesis of the corpus callosum (see also Ch. 13): Our aim here is to demonstrate the diagnosis of total and/or partial agenesis of the corpus callosum (ACC, PACC). Our experience in evaluating patients referred for second opinion for hydrocephaly or ventriculomegaly has led us to believe that many sonologists and sonographers often report the more obvious hydrocephaly while missing the real diagnosis.

The use of transvaginal sonography seems to us indispensable to make or rule out this diagnosis in a reliable and straightforward manner (Figs 16.7 and 16.19). The median plane provides the most direct observation of the presence

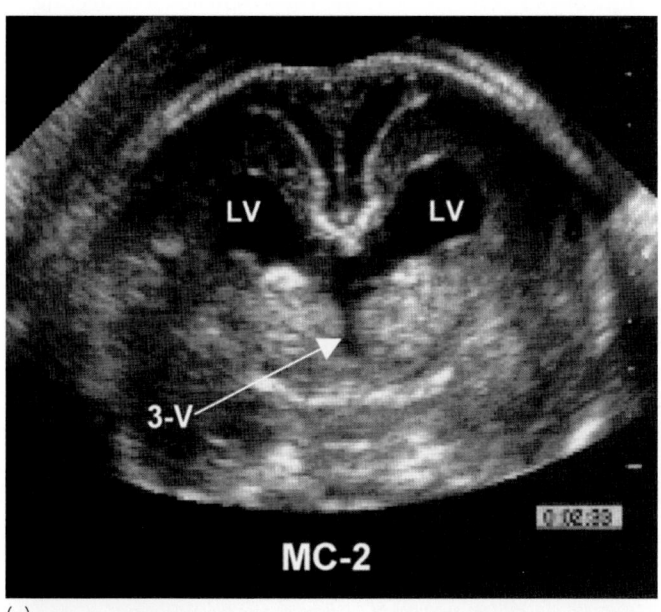

(a)

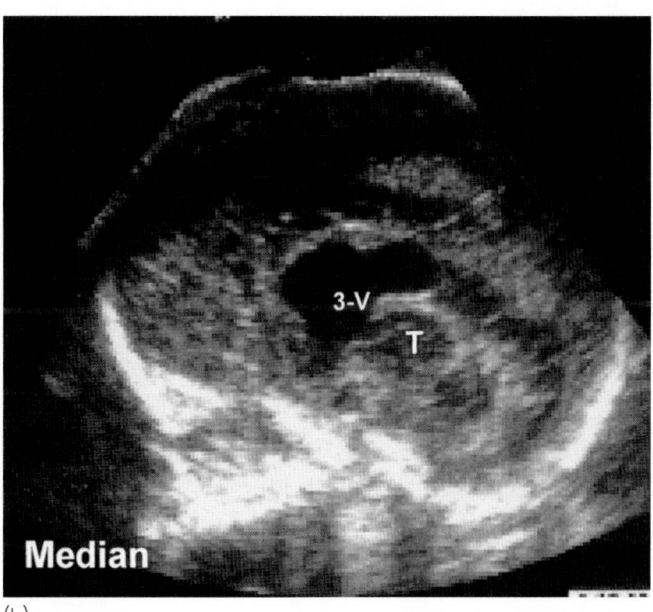

(b)

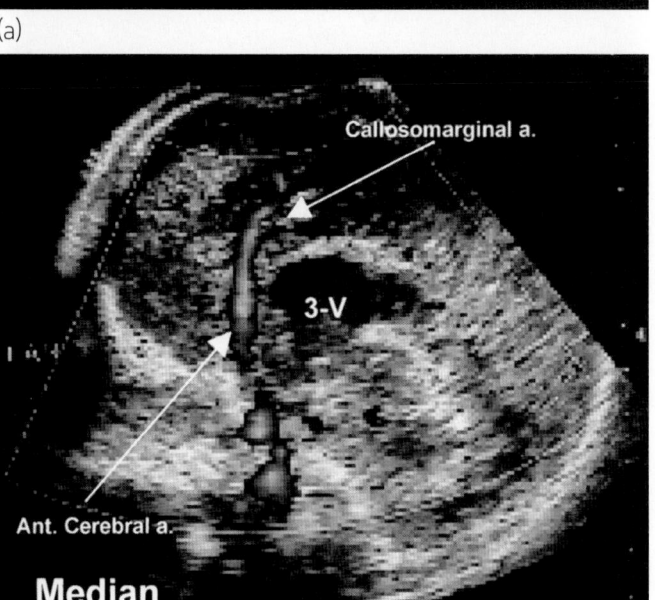

(c)

Figure 16.19 Total agenesis of the corpus callosum at 23 postmenstrual weeks. (a) MC-2, Mid-coronal-2 section with the third ventricle (3-V) communicating with the lateral ventricles (LV) without the presence of the corpus callosum or the cavum septi pellucidi. The two median sections (b, c) are practically the same showing the upward displaced third ventricle above the thalamus (T); however part (c) is a power Doppler image of the anterior cerebral and the callosomarginal arteries without the presence of the pericallosal artery.

or absence of the entire corpus callosum. As mentioned above, this plane is most reliably obtained via the transvaginal route. However, the ability to navigate and manipulate 3-D volumes has made the exact median plane more readily accessible (Pilu et al 2006). The median plane is also used to visualize the pericallosal artery via power angio or color Doppler mode. Absence of some or all of this vessel provides additional support to the diagnosis of partial or total agenesis of the corpus callosum.

Differentiating between a partial agenesis and a normal corpus callosum can be difficult when relying on subjective assessment. For this reason, Achiron and Achiron (2001) have published normative measurements of the corpus callosum to aid in standardizing this potentially subjective diagnosis. Following the course of the pericallosal artery along the length of the splenium of the corpus callosum may help as well.

While the only direct signs of this diagnosis are on the median plane, other planes can be useful in visualizing the corpus callosum. We have previously described how the mid-coronal views can demonstrate portions of the corpus

callosum in cross-section. More recently, a transfrontal approach has been advocated for cases where the fetal position or the sonographer preference requires transabdominal imaging (Visentin 2001).

The following are the indirect diagnostic features of ACC which can also be helpful in clarifying the diagnosis in cases where the direct approaches are unclear.

- Teardrop-shaped, parallel lateral ventricles on the axial section.
- Colpocephaly on sagittal or oblique views.
- 'Sunburst sign' – radial gyri and sulci on median surface (seen only after 18 weeks when gyri/sulci are normally visible) on the median section.
- 'Viking's helmet sign' – widely separated, vertically oriented lateral ventricles on anterior coronal sections.
- Upward displacement of the third ventricle connecting with the interhemispheric fissure on coronal sections.

Holoprosencephaly (see p. 237 and 272) (Fig. 16.20): At birth its incidence is 1 per 1600 births; however, at earlier

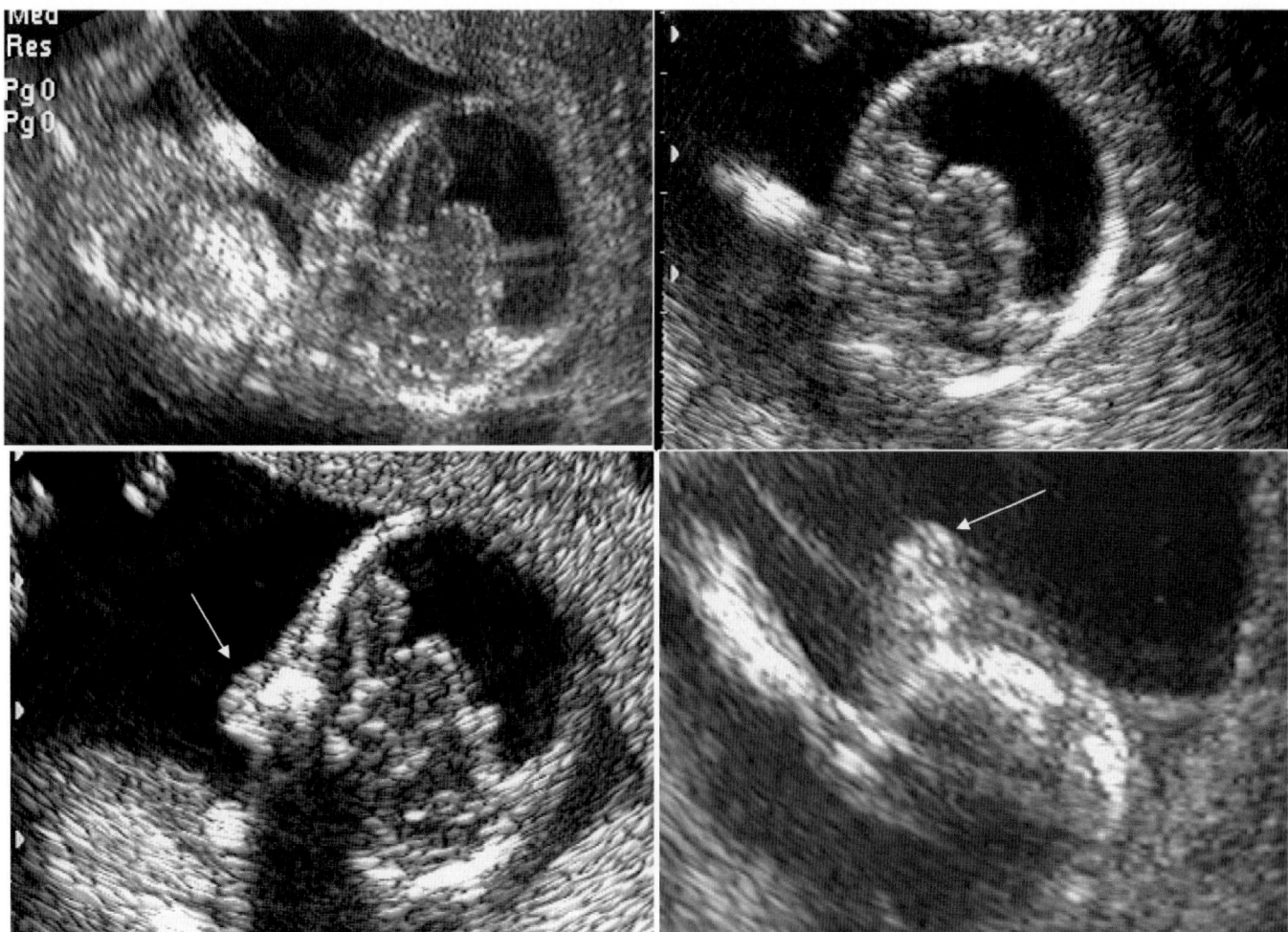

Figure 16.20 Alobar holoprosencephaly detected at 13¹/₂ postmenstrual weeks. The arrows point to the proboscis frequently seen in such cases.

scans the sonologist will encounter this anomaly more frequently (Matsunaga & Shiota 1977).

Two of the more frequent forms, alobar and semilobar types, are relatively easily diagnosed any time an exhaustive fetal neuroscan is performed. Absence of the interhemispheric fissure (total or partial), non-disjunction of the thalami, no corpus callosum and cavum septi pellucidi, and various facial anomalies (cyclops, proboscis, median clefts, etc.) are the most frequent features. 3-D capabilities have led to the accurate diagnosis of this complex syndrome in the first trimester (Hsu et al 2001, Tonni et al 2006).

The lobar type of holoprosencephaly, however, has more subtle features. At times the only signs are clustered around the corpus callosum, cavum septi pellucidi and the third ventricle. The presence of a box-shaped cavity in the midbrain below the corpus callosum without the two lateral walls of the septum pellucidum gives rise to the suggestion of lobar holoprosencephaly (Fig. 16.21) and its closest differential diagnosis: septo-optic dysplasia (Pilu et al 1996). At times the final diagnosis is only made after birth.

As mentioned above, Bault recently demonstrated the ability to image the optic chiasm using 3-D sonography (Bault 2006). This may aid in differentiating septo-optic dysplasia from lobar holoprosencephaly, since the optic nerve atrophy associated with the former diagnosis is not present in the latter.

Neural tube defects (NTDs) (see Ch. 13). Considering the incidence of NTDs in the world is 2–3 per 1000 births it is important to recognize them at the earliest possible stage. Figure 16.22 illustrates a fetus with anencephaly and rachischisis detected at 18 weeks and 5 days gestation by transvaginal sonography. Advances in sonography have allowed for first-trimester diagnosis of exencephaly-anencephaly sequence, as well as many other complex neural tube and cranial anomalies (Blaas et al 2000, Chan-

prapaph et al 2000, Cuillier et al 2003, Machado 2005, Noriega et al 2001, Roman et al 2004). The head shape in the coronal, sagittal as well as in the axial planes is part of the diagnosis at these early gestational ages. We supported the theory of Bronsthtein and Ornoy (1991), which suggests that anencephaly results from the rubbing-off of exposed brain tissue, by observing the progressively diminishing amount of brain tissue in cases of exencephaly and by detecting free-floating neural cells. It is therefore felt that the exposed brain tissue gradually disintegrates and diminishes as gestation progresses (Greenebaum et al 1997, Timor-Tritsch et al 1996).

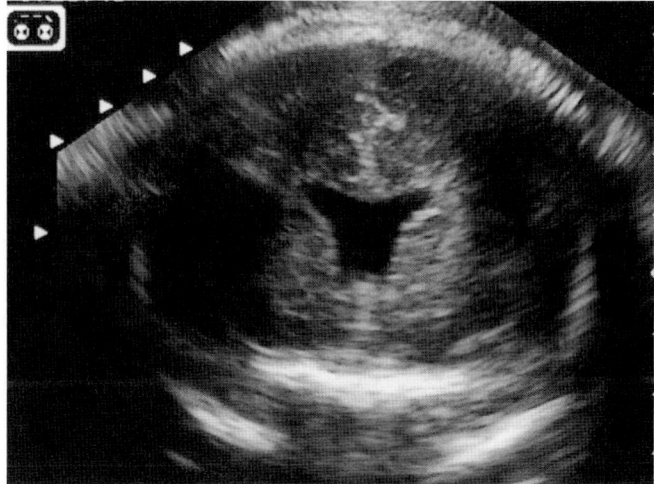

Figure 16.21 Lobar holoprosencephaly. Typical shape of the third ventricle and the cavum septi pellucid on the mid-coronal-1 section. The box-shaped sonolucent structure is created by the missing lateral walls of the cavum septi pellucidi.

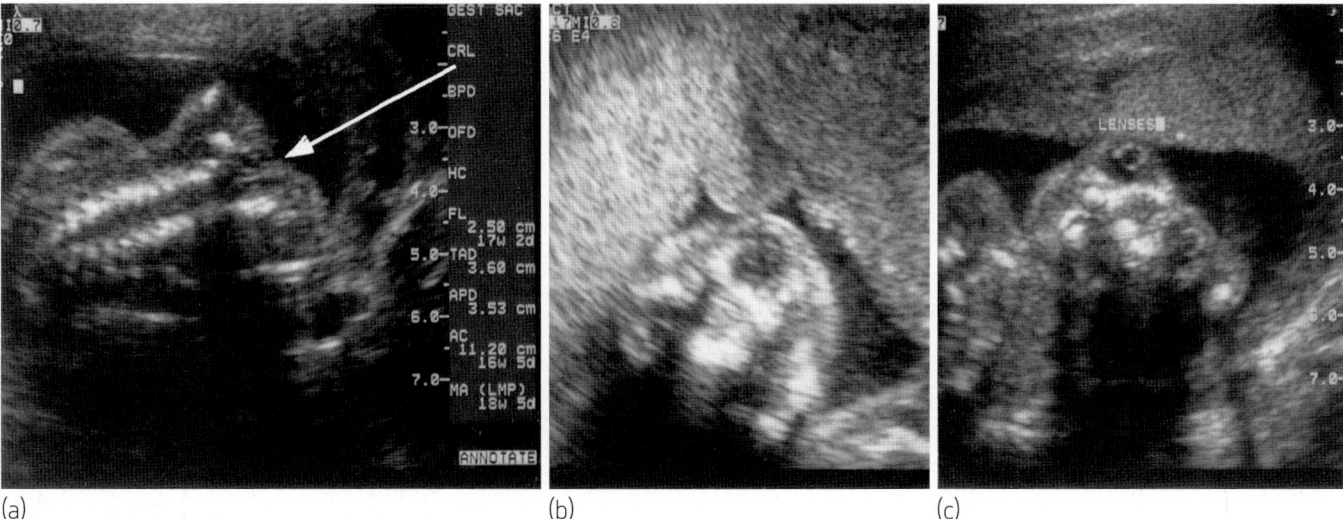

(a)   (b)   (c)

Figure 16.22 Anencephaly and upper spinal rachischisis at 18 postmenstrual weeks by transvaginal sonography. (a) The arrow points to the open upper spine; (b) sagittal section of the face and base of skull; (c) coronal section of the head.

Choroid plexus cysts (see p. 334): These fluid-filled cystic lesions in the choroid plexus are usually benign and have an approximate incidence of 1% of all pregnancies. They can be detected as early as the 11th–12th week of gestation and usually disappear by about the 24th postmenstrual week. Figure 16.23 depicts bilateral cysts on the mid-coronal-2 section. While improvements in ultrasound technology have allowed sonographers to visualize such findings with greater frequency, there remains an ongoing debate in the literature regarding their clinical significance as isolated markers of chromosomal anomalies (Doubilet et al 2004, Filly 2004, Filly et al 2004). We agree with the many authors who believe that invasive testing for karyotype is not indicated for the finding of an isolated choroid plexus cyst.

Arachnoid cysts (see p. 255): These are CSF-filled spaces which do not connect with the ventricles or the cava. They are space-occupying lesions which can compress surrounding structures; however, histologically they are benign. They appear as sonolucent, thin-walled structures. Most common are left-sided lesions and 10% are located in the quadrigeminal cistern (Fig. 16.24a). Five to ten percent are in the posterior fossa and about 10% of them are in potentially dangerous areas (e.g. the suprasellar cistern). By exerting pressure on the flow of the CSF they may cause bilateral hydrocephaly (e.g. pressure on the interventricular foramen). If they are located on the convexity of the brain, the outcome is usually good (Hudgins et al 1988).

Advances in sonogram resolution have allowed first trimester detection of these cysts (Bretelle et al 2002). Counseling patients in such situations can be difficult as many cysts remain stable in size and do not compress vital brain structures. Occasionally, very large arachnoid cysts can indent the underlying cortex and mimic a picture of lissencephaly. In our experience, reconstructing the area of the pathology with 3-D imaging helped us to differentiate between the two diagnoses (Fig. 16.24b).

Intracranial hemorrhage (see Ch. 20): This finding is relatively rare in utero. Potential causes include trauma, hypoxemia, congenital vascular anomalies, coagulation disorders, platelet dysfunction, drugs and thrombosis of the umbilical cord or its entanglement. As the blood clots, one can detect fresh clots by their hyperechoic appearance within the parenchyma (Fig. 16.25) or in the ventricles (Fig. 16.26). Sites of long standing clots may resorb and become porencephalic cysts. Periventricular leukomalacia can also result (see below).

It is important to accurately identify the anatomic location of the bleed, as the neurodevelopmental long term outcome of fetuses diagnosed with intracranial hemorrhage is related not only to the severity, but also to the location of the hemorrhage (Ghi et al 2003).

Periventricular leukomalacia (see Ch. 21): As the name implies the lesion is located in the white matter around or close to the lateral ventricles (Fig. 16.27). It is believed that the relatively poorly perfused areas between two arterial supplies ('watershed areas') are affected by changes in the blood supply, resulting in this pathology. This finding in the neonate can be a poor prognostic indicator as many of these infants end up with significant neurologic morbidity. The presence of periventricular echo-densities in the fetal brain has been shown to predict neonatal periventricular leukomalacia in high risk cases (Yamamoto et al 2000).

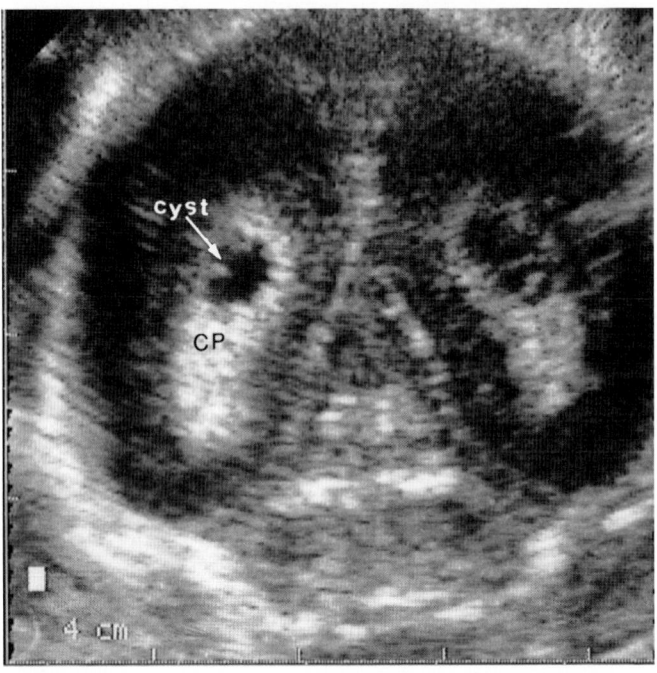

Figure 16.23 Mid-coronal-3 section obtained by transvaginal sonography at 16 postmenstrual weeks depicting the bilateral choroid plexus cysts (CP, choroid plexus) and the infratentorial cerebellar hemispheres.

Figure 16.24 Arachnoid cysts at 23 postmenstrual weeks. (a) The cyst is marked by arrows. It originates probably from the area of the quadrigeminal plate. The cyst extends anteriorly and is seen on frontal-2 (F-2) section. On the mid-coronal-1 (MC-1) section, it is clear that the cyst is predominantly on the left side of the mid-line (the falx is displaced to the right). There was already sufficient pressure on the aqueduct to cause ventriculomegaly (note the dilatation of the posterior horn on the O-1 section). The oblique-1 (Obl-1) section demonstrates the extent of the cyst anteriorly and posteriorly. (b) Three-dimensional orthogonal ultrasound pictures of an interhemispheric arachnoid cyst. The arrows point to the cyst walls.

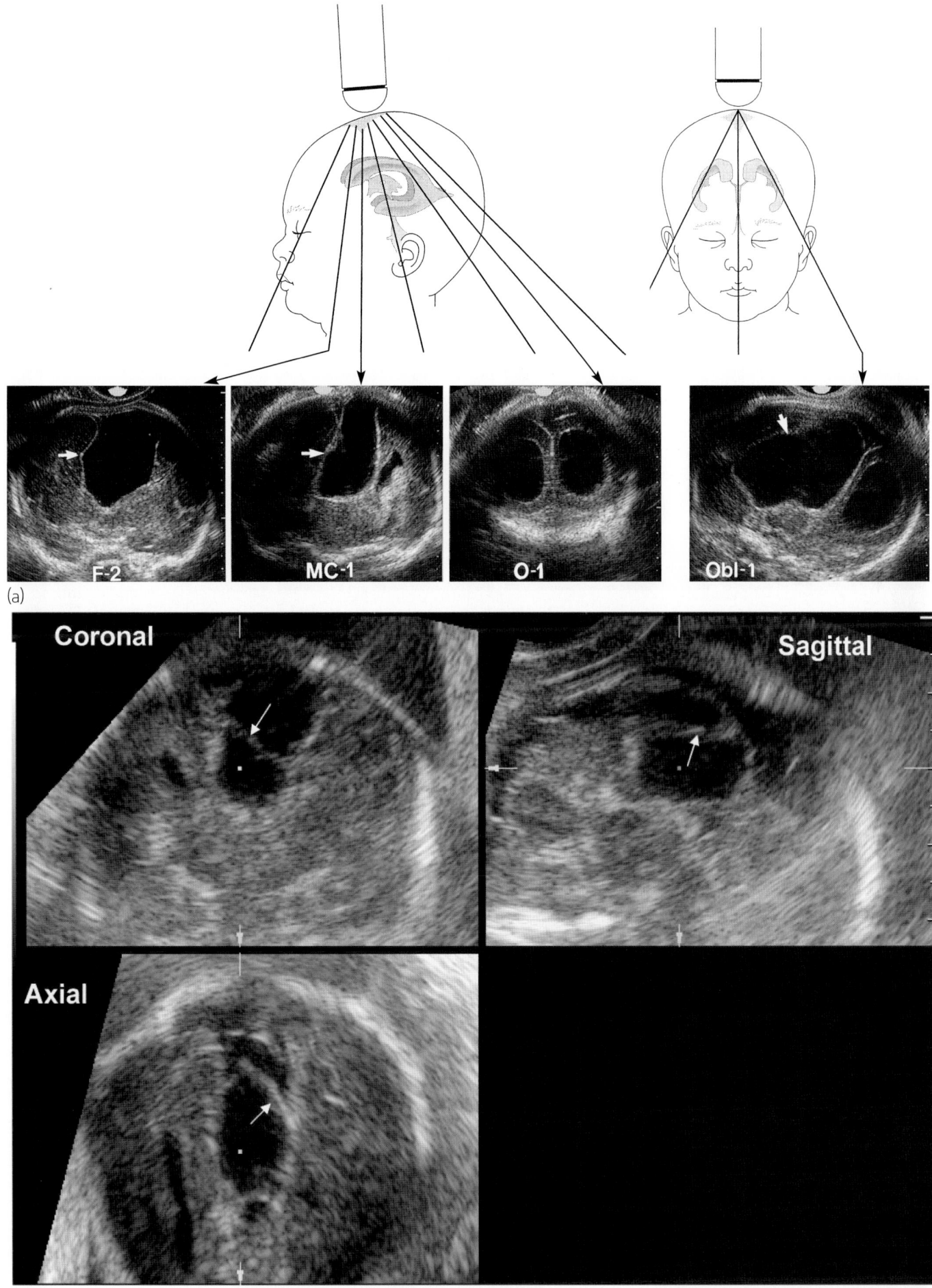

(a)

F-2

MC-1

O-1

Obl-1

(b)

Coronal

Sagittal

Axial

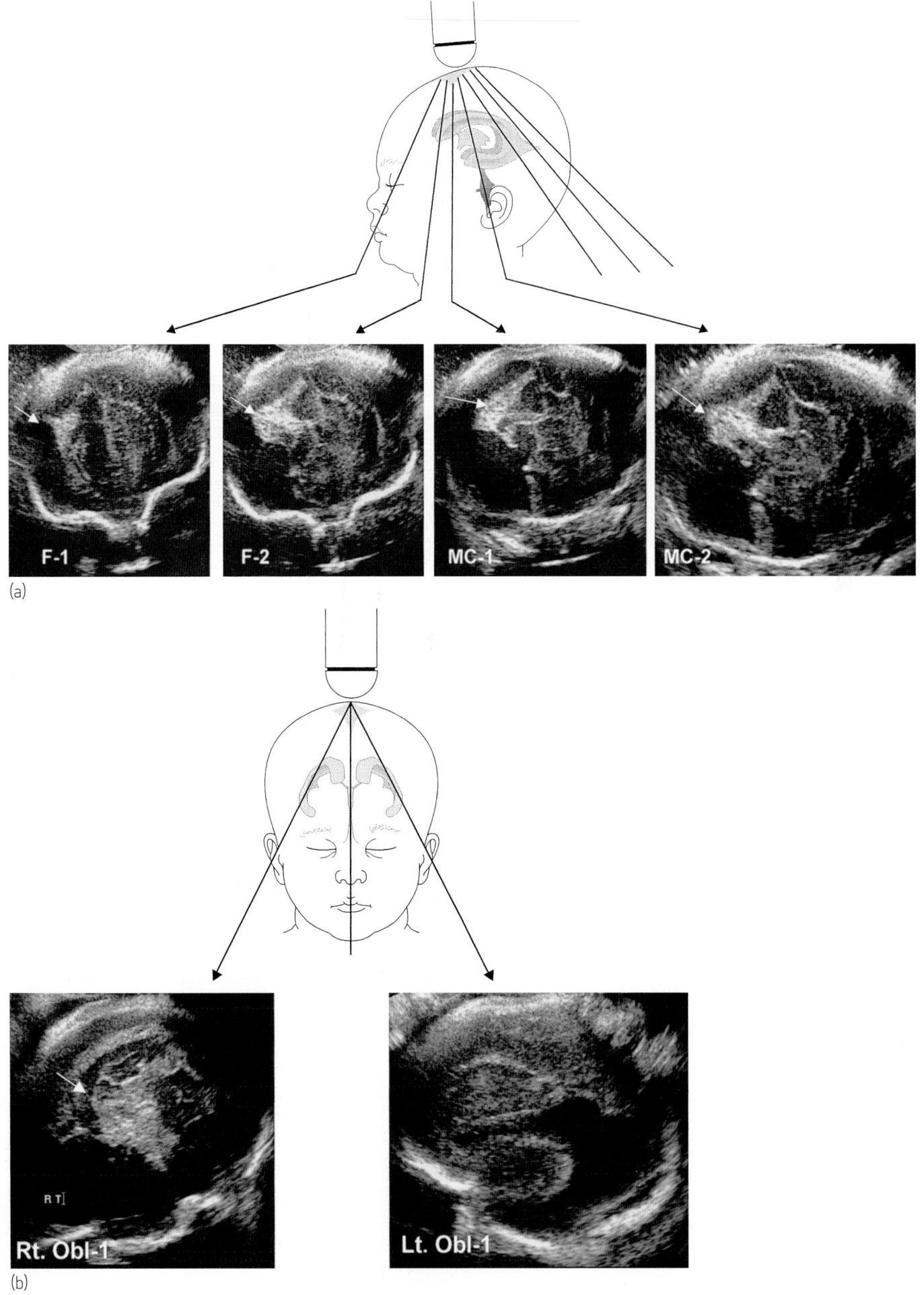

(a)

(b)

F-1

F-2

MC-1

MC-2

Rt. Obl-1

Lt. Obl-1

R T

Figure 16.25 Intraparenchymal bleeding, mostly in the right hemisphere, marked by the arrow. The right hemisphere is almost totally destroyed with excessive lateral ventriculomegaly. The left lateral ventricle is dilated however to a somewhat lesser degree. (a) Four successive coronal sections: F-1 = Frontal-1 (F-1) section, F-2 = Frontal-2 (F-2) section, MC-1 = Mid-coronal-1 (MC-1) section, MC-2 = Mid-coronal-2 (MC-2) section. (b) The right and left Oblique-1 sections.

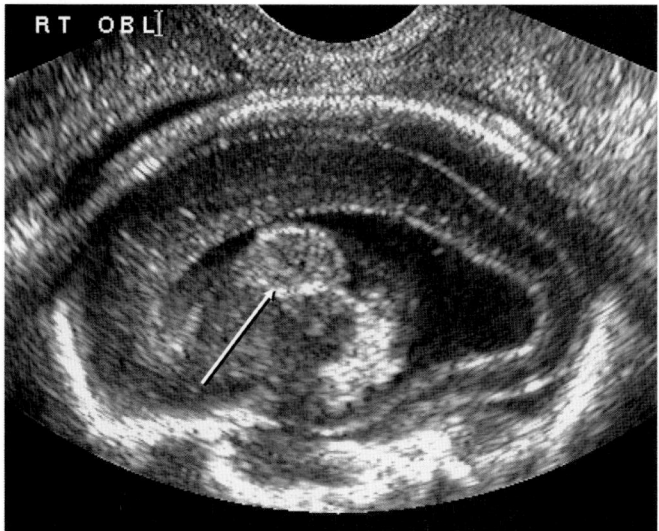

Figure 16.26 Oblique-1 section of a fetal brain with Grade 3 intraventricular hemorrhage (arrow).

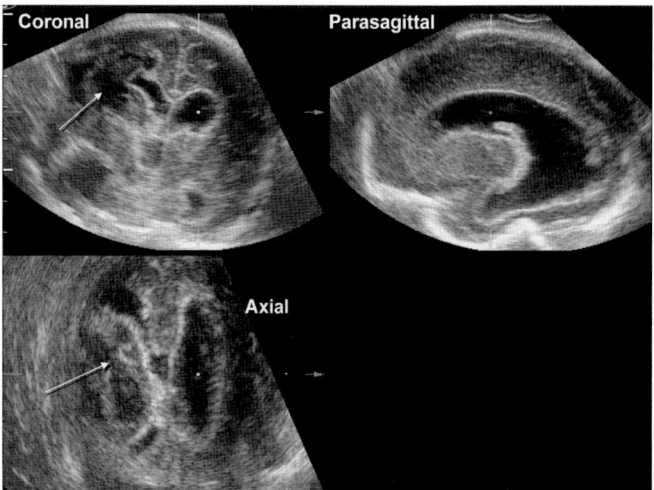

Figure 16.27 Three-dimensional orthogonal ultrasound image of periventricular leukomalacia, the result of intraparenchymal hemorrhage (arrows).

REFERENCES

Achiron R, Achiron A 1991 Transvaginal ultrasonic assessment of the early fetal brain. Ultrasound Obstet Gynecol 1:336–344.

Achiron R, Achiron A 2001 Development of the human fetal corpus callosum: a high-resolution, cross-sectional sonographic study. Ultrasound Obstet Gynecol 18(4):343–347.

Achiron R, Kivilevitch Z, Lipitz S et al 2004 Development of the human fetal pons: in utero ultrasonographic study. Ultrasound Obstet Gynecol 24(5):506–510.

Achiron R, Schimmel M, Achiron A et al 1993 Fetal mild idiopathic lateral ventriculomegaly: Is there a correlation with fetal trisomy? Ultrasound Obstet Gynecol 3:89–92.

Babcock D S, Han B K, LeQuesne G W 1980 B-mode gray scale ultrasound of the head in the newborn and young infant. AJR Am J Radiol 134:457–468.

Barht P G, Blennow G, Lenard H G et al 1995 The syndrome of autosomal recessive pontocerebellar hypoplasia, microcephaly, and extrapyramidal dyskinesia (pontocerebellar hypoplasia type 2): compiled data from 10 pedigrees. Neurology 45:311–317.

Barkovich A J, Kjos B O, Norman D et al 1989 Revised classification of posterior fossa cysts and cystlike malformations based on the results of multiplanar MR imaging. AJR Am J Roentgenol 153:1289–1300.

Bault J P 2006 Visualization of the fetal optic chiasma using three-dimensional ultrasound imaging. Ultrasound Obstet Gynecol 28(6):862–864.

Ben-Ora A, Eddy L, Hatch G et al 1980 The anterior fontanelle as an acoustic window to the neonatal ventricular system. J Clin Ultrasound 8:65–67.

Blaas H G, Eik-Nes S H, Isaksen C V 2000 The detection of spina bifida before 10 gestational weeks using two- and three-dimensional ultrasound. Ultrasound Obstet Gynecol 16(1):25–29.

Blaas H G, Eik-Nes S H, Kiserud T et al 1994 Early development of the forebrain and midbrain: a longitudinal ultrasound study from 7 to 12 postmenstrual weeks of gestation. Ultrasound Obstet Gynecol 4:183–192.

Blaas H G, Eik-Nes S H, Kiserud T et al 1995a Early development of the hindbrain: a longitudinal ultrasound study from 7 to 12 weeks of gestation. Ultrasound Obstet Gynecol 5:151–160.

Blaas H G, Eik-Nes S H, Kiserud T et al 1995b Three-dimensional imaging of the brain cavities in human embryos. Ultrasound Obstet Gynecol 5:228–232.

Blin G, Rabbe A, Ansquer Y et al 2005 First-trimester ultrasound diagnosis in a recurrent case of Walker–Warburg syndrome. Ultrasound Obstet Gynecol 26:297–299.

Bretelle F, Senat M V, Bernard J P et al 2002 First-trimester diagnosis of fetal arachnoid cyst: prenatal implication. Ultrasound Obstet Gynecol 20(4):400–402.

Bromley B, Frigoletto F D, Benacerraf B R 1991 Mild fetal lateral cerebral ventriculomegaly: clinical course and outcome. Am J Obstet Gynecol 164:863–867.

Bronshtein M, Ornoy A 1991 Acrania: anencephaly resulting from secondary degeneration of a closed neural tube: two cases in the same family. J Clin Ultrasound 19:230–234.

Calabro F, Arcuri T, Jinkins J R 2000 Blake's pouch cyst: an entity within the Dandy–Walker continuum. Neuroradiology 42:290–295.

Cardoza J D, Filly R A, Podrasky A E 1988b The dangling choroid plexus: a sonographic observation of value in excluding ventriculomegaly. AJR Am J Roentgeol 151(4):767–770.

Cardoza J D, Goldstein R B, Filly R A 1988a Exclusion of fetal ventriculomegaly with a single measurement of the width of the lateral ventricular atrium. Radiology 169:711–714.

Chang C H, Yu C H, Chang F M et al 2003 The assessment of normal fetal brain volume by 3-D ultrasound. Ultrasound Med Biol 29(9):1267–1272.

Chanprapaph P, Tongsong T, Wongtra-ngan S 2000 Sonographic diagnosis of exencephaly: omphalocele at 11 weeks of gestation. J Obstet Gynaecol Res 26(5):363–366.

Cohen H L, Ziprkowski M 1991 New diagnostic insight in pediatric neurosonography. Diagn Imag 13: 142–146.

Conti C, Lunardi P, Bozzao A et al 2003 Syringomyelia associated with hydrocephalus and Blake's pouch cyst: case report. Spine 28:E279–E283.

Correa F F, Lara C, Bellver J et al 2006 Examination of the fetal brain by transabdominal three-dimensional ultrasound: potential for routine neurosonographic studies. Ultrasound Obstet Gynecol 27:503–508.

Cuillier F, Koenig P, Lagarde L et al 2003 Transvaginal sonographic diagnosis of iniencephaly apertus and craniorachischisis at 9 weeks' gestation Ultrasound Obstet Gynecol 22(6):657–658.

D'Addario V, Pinto V, Di Cagno L, Pintucci A 2005 The midsagittal view of the fetal brain: a useful landmark in recognizing the cause of fetal cerebral ventriculomegaly. J Perinat Med 33(5):423–427.

Dewbury K C, Aluwihare A P R 1980 The anterior fontanelle as an ultrasound window for study of the brain: a preliminary report. Br J Radiol 53:81–84.

Doubilet P M, Copel J A, Benson C B et al 2004 Choroid plexus cyst and echogenic intracardiac focus in women at low risk for chromosomal anomalies: the obligation to inform the mother. J Ultrasound Med 23(7):883–885.

Edwards M K, Brown D L, Muller J et al 1981 Cribside neurosonography: real-time sonography for intracranial investigation of the neonate. AJR Am J Radiol 136:271–276.

Endres L K, Cohen L 2001 Reliability and validity of three-dimensional fetal brain volumes. J Ultrasound Med 20(12):1265–1269.

Filly R A 2004 Echogenic intracardiac foci and choroid plexus cysts. J Ultrasound Med 23(8):1135–1138, author reply 1138–1139.

Filly R A, Benacerraf B R, Nyberg D A et al 2004 Choroid plexus cyst and echogenic intracardiac focus in women at low risk for chromosomal anomalies. J Ultrasound Med 23(4):447–449.

Gaglioti P, Danelson D, Bontempo S et al 2005 Fetal cerbral ventriculomegaly: outcome in 176 cases. Ultrasound Obstet Gynecol 25:372–377.

Ghi T, Simonazzi G, Perolo A et al 2003 Outcome of antenatally diagnosed intracranial hemorrhage: case series and review of the literature. Ultrasound Obstet Gynecol 22(2):121–130.

Grant E G, Schellinger D, Borts F T et al 1981 Real-time sonography of the neonatal and infant head. AJR Am J Radiol 136:265–270.

Grant E, Richardson J 1994 Infant and neonatal neurosonography technique and normal anatomy. In: Taveras J (ed.) Radiology diagnosis-imaging-intervention, vol 3. Lippincott, Philadelphia, PA, pp. 1–7.

Greenebaum E, Mansakhani M M, Heller D S, Timor-Tritsch I E 1997 Open neural tube defects: immunocytochemical demonstration of neuroepithelial cells in amniotic fluid. Diagn Cytopathol 16(2):143–144.

Guibaud L 2004 Practical approach to prenatal posterior fossa abnormalities using MRI. Pediatr Radiol 34:700–711.

Guibaud L, des Portes V 2006 Plea for an anatomical approach to abnormalities of the posterior fossa in prenatal diagnosis. Ultrasound Obstet Gynecol May, 27(5):477–481.

Hsu T Y, Chang S Y, Ou C Y et al 2001 First trimester diagnosis of holoprosencephaly and cyclopia with triploidy by transvaginal three-dimensional ultrasonography. Eur J Obstet Gynecol Reprod Biol 96(2):235–237.

Hudgins R J, Edwards M S B, Goldstein R et al 1988 Natural history of fetal ventriculomegaly. Pediatrics 82:692–697.

Johnson M L, Rumack C M 1980 Ultrasonic evaluation of the neonatal brain. Radiol Clin North Am 18:117–131.

Kelly E N, Allen V, Seaward G et al 2001 Mild ventriculomegaly in the fetus, natural history, associated findings and outcome of isolated mild ventriculomegaly: a literature review. Prenat Diagn 21:697–700.

Klein O, Pierre-Kahn A, Boddaert N et al 2003 Dandy–Walker malformation: prenatal diagnosis and prognosis. Childs Nerv Syst 19:484–489.

Kushnir U, Shalev J, Bronshtein M et al 1989 Fetal intracranial anatomy in the first trimester of pregnancy: transvaginal ultrasonographic evaluation. Neuroradiology 31:222–225.

Low A S, Lee S L, Tan A S et al 2005 Difficulties with prenatal diagnosis of the Walker–Warburg syndrome. Acta Radiol 46:645–651.

McAuliffe FM, Chitayat D, Halliday W et al 2006 Fetal ultrasound and magnetic resonance imaging in rhombencephalosynapsis. Ultrasound Obstet Gynecol 28:412–511.

Machado R A, Brizot M L, Carvalho M H et al 2005 Sonographic markers of exencephaly below 10 weeks' gestation. Prenat Diagn 25(1):31–33.

Mahony B S, Nyberg D A, Hirsch J H et al 1988 Mild idiopathic lateral cerebral ventricular dilatation in utero: sonographic evaluation. Radiology 169:715–721.

Malinger G, Ginath S, Lerman-Sagie T et al 2001 The fetal cerebellar vermis: normal development as shown by transvaginal ultrasound. Prenat Diagn 21(8):687–692.

Malinger G, Monteagudo A, Pilu G et al 2007 Sonographic examination of the fetal central nervous system: guidelines for performing the 'basic examination' and the 'fetal neuroscan'. Ultrasound Obstet Gynecol 29:109–116.

Malinger G, Zakut H 1993 The corpus callosum: normal fetal development as shown by transvaginal sonography. AJR Am J Radiol 161:1041–1043.

Matsunaga E, Shiota Y 1977 Holoprosencephaly in human embryos: epidemiological studies of 150 cases. Teratology 16:261.

Monteagudo A, Reuss M L, Timor-Tritsch I E 1991a Imaging the fetal brain in the second and third trimesters using transvaginal sonography. Obstet Gynecol 77:27–32.

Monteagudo A, Timor-Tritsch I E 1997 Development of fetal gyri, sulci and fissures: a transvaginal sonographic study. Ultrasound Obstet Gynecol 9:222–228.

Monteagudo A, Timor-Tritsch I E, Mayberry P 2000 Three dimensional transvaginal neurosonography of the fetal brain: navigating in the volume scan. Ultrasound Obstet Gynecol 16:307–313.

Monteagudo A, Timor-Tritsch I E, Moomjy M 1993 Nomograms of the fetal lateral ventricles using transvaginal sonography. J Ultrasound Med 5:265–269.

Monteagudo A, Timor-Tritsch I E, Moomjy M 1994 In utero detection of ventriculomegaly during the second and third trimesters by transvaginal sonography. Ultrasound Obstet Gynecol 4:193–198.

Monteagudo A, Timor-Tritsch I E, Reuss M L et al 1991b Transvaginal sonography of the second and third trimester fetal brain. In: Timor-Tritsch I E, Rottem S

(eds) Transvaginal sonography, 2nd edn. Chapman & Hall, New York, NY, pp. 393–425.

Naidich T P, Yousefzadeh D K, Gusnard D A 1986 Sonography of the normal neonatal head. Supratentorial structures: state of the art imaging. Neuroradiology 28:408–427.

Nelson M D Jr, Maher K, Gilles F H 2004 A different approach to cysts of the posterior fossa. Pediatr Radiol 34:720–732.

Nomina anatomica, 6th edn 1989 Authorized by the 12th International Congress of Anatomists, London, 1985. Churchill Livingstone, Edinburgh.

Noriega C A, Fleming A D, Bonebrake R G 2001 A false-positive diagnosis of a prenatal encephalocele on transvaginal ultrasonography J Ultrasound Med 20(8):925–927.

Patel S, Barkovich A J 2002 Analysis and classification of cerebellar malformations. AJNR Am J Neuroradiol 23(7):1074–1087.

Pilu G, Perolo A, David C 1996 Midline anomalies of the brain. In: Timor-Tritsch I E, Monteagudo A, Cohen H L (eds) Ultrasonography of the prenatal and neonatal brain. Appleton, Lange, Stamford, CT, pp. 241–258.

Pilu G, Segata M, Ghi T et al 2006 Diagnosis of midline anomalies of the fetal brain with the three-dimensional median view. Ultrasound Obstet Gynecol 27(5):522–529.

Pooh R K, Pooh K 2001 Transvaginal 3D and Doppler ultrasonography of the fetal brain. Semin Perinatol 25(1):38–43.

Pretorius D H, Drose J A, Manco-Johnson M L 1986 Fetal lateral ventricular ratio determination during the second-trimester. J Ultrasound Med 5:121–124.

Richardson D J, Grant E G 1986 Scanning techniques and normal anatomy. In: Grant G E (ed.) Neurosonography of the preterm neonate. Springer-Verlarg, New York, NY, pp. 1–24.

Robins J B, Mason G C, Watters J, Martinez D 1998 Case report: cerebellar hemihypoplasia. Prenat Diagn 18:173–177.

Roelfsema N M, Hop W C, Boito S M et al 2004 Three-dimensional sonographic measurement of normal fetal brain volume during the second half of pregnancy. Am J Obstet Gynecol 190(1):275–280.

Roman A S, Monteagudo A, Timor-Tritsch I et al 2004 First-trimester diagnosis of sacrococcygeal teratoma: the role of three-dimensional ultrasound. Ultrasound Obstet Gynecol 23(6):612–614.

Sherer DM, Shane H, Anyane-Yeboa K 2001 First-trimester transvaginal ultrasonographic diagnosis of Dandy–Walker malformation. Am J Perinatol 18(7):373–377.

Slovis T L, Kuhns L R 1981 Real-time sonography of the brain through the anterior fontanelle. AJR 136:277–286.

Strand R D, Barnes P D, Poussaint T Y et al 1993 Cystic retrocerebellar malformations: unification of the Dandy–Walker complex and the Blake's pouch cyst. Pediatr Radiol 23:258–260.

Timor-Tritsch I E, Bashiri A, Monteagudo A et al 2004 Qualified and trained sonographers in the US can perform early fetal anatomy scans between 11 and 14 weeks. Am J Obstet Gynecol 191(4):1247–1252.

Timor-Tritsch I E, Blumenfeld Z, Rottem S 1991b Sonoembryology. In: Timor-Tritsch I E, Rottem S (eds) Transvaginal sonography, 2nd edn. Chapman & Hall, New York, NY, p. 241.

Timor-Tritsch I E, Farine D, Rosen M G 1988 A close look at early embryonic development with the high-frequency transvaginal transducer. Am J Obstet Gynecol 159:676–681.

Timor-Tritsch I E, Greenebaum E, Monteagudo A, Baxi L 1996 The exencephaly-anencephaly sequence: proof by ultrasound imaging and amniotic fluid cytology. Matern Fet Med 5:182–185.

Timor-Tritsch I E, Monteagudo A 1991 Transvaginal sonographic evaluation of the fetal central nervous system. Obstet Gynecol Clin North Am 18:713–748.

Timor-Tritsch I E, Monteagudo A 1996 Transvaginal fetal neurosonography: standardization of the planes and sections by anatomic landmarks. Ultrasound Obstet Gynecol 8:42–47.

Timor-Tritsch I E, Monteagudo A, Mayberry P 2000 3-D ultrasound evaluation of the fetal brain: the three horn view. Ultrasound Obstet Gynecol 16:302–306.

Timor-Tritsch I E, Monteagudo A, Warren W B 1991a Transvaginal ultrasonographic definition of the central nervous system in the first and early second trimesters. Am J Obstet Gynecol 164:747–753.

Timor-Tritsch I E, Peisner D B, Raju S 1990 Sonoembryology: an organ–oriented approach using a high-frequency vaginal probe. J Clin Ultrasound 18:286–298.

Tonni G, Centini G 2006 Three-dimensional first-trimester transvaginal diagnosis of alobar holoprosencephaly associated with omphalocele in a 46,XX fetus. Am J Perinatol 23(1):67–69.

Tortori-Donati P, Fondelli M P, Rossi A et al 1996 Cystic malformations of the posterior cranial fossa originating from a defect of the posterior membranous area. Mega cisterna magna and persisting Blake's pouch: two separate entities. Childs Nerv Syst 12:303–308.

Visentin A, Pilu G, Falco P et al 2001 The transfrontal view: a new approach to the visualization of the fetal midline cerebral structures. J Ultrasound Med 20(4):329–333.

Warren W B, Timor-Tritsch I E, Peisner D B et al 1989 Dating the early pregnancy by sequential appearance of embryonic structures. Am J Obstet Gynecol 161:747–753.

Wax J R, Bookman L, Cartin A et al 2003 Mild fetal cerebral ventriculomegaly: diagnosis, clinical associations, and outcomes. Obstet Gynecol Surv 58(6):407–414.

Yamamoto N, Utsu M, Serizawa M et al 2000 Neonatal periventricular leukomalacia preceded by fetal periventricular echodensity. Fetal Diagn Ther 15(4):198–208.

Zalel Y, Seidman D S, Brand N et al 2002 The development of the fetal vermis: an in-utero sonographic evaluation. Ultrasound Obstet Gynecol 19(2):136–139.

Epidemiology and prevention of neural tube defects

Aubrey Milunsky

Key points

- Neural tube defects (NTDs) are among the most common congenital malformations worldwide
- Etiology is largely multifactorial (polygenic and environmental factors together)
- NTDS also occur in association with chromosome abnormality and much less often with monogenic disorders
- The prevalence of NTDs has been steadily decreasing as socio-economic status improves together with better diets
- Maternal serum screening and prenatal diagnosis have clearly assisted in further decreasing the prevalence of NTDs
- Folic acid deficiency is the major environmental recognized factor in causation of NTDs
- Daily consumption of at least 0.4 mg of folic acid three months prior to and at least six weeks after conception avoids about 70% of all NTDs
- Governments worldwide need to be more active in educating the public and fortifying the food supply with folic acid

---

The occurrence of neural tube defects (NTDs) dates back to antiquity. Archeological excavations in the Andean region of Southern Peru and Northern Chile have revealed evidence of NTDs some 8000 years ago (Carod-Artal & Vasquez-Cabrera 2006). Carbon dating of skeletons found in Morocco suggested a period some 10 000 years BC (Smith 2001). An adolescent skeleton with spina bifida was uncovered at the Early Archaic Windover site in the state of Florida and dated some 7500 years ago (Dickel & Doran 1989). Skeletal remains showing spina bifida have also been reported in ancient Canadian Inuits (Merbs 2004). An Egyptian mummy was found with spina bifida (Lie 2006). Other ancient texts from the Greek and Roman period, from India and elsewhere, also recount the occurrence of NTDs (Elwood et al 1992).

DEFINITIONS

Failure or incomplete closure of the neural tube results in different types of NTDs. Failure of closure of the neural tube at the cephalic end may result in anencephaly which results in an open cranium. Other defects that may occur at the cephalic end of the neural tube include herniation of brain through a skull defect, most often occipital, termed encephalocele. Extrusion of membranes through a cranial defect or elsewhere down the vertebral column is termed meningocele. Dorsal closure failures in the midline of the vertebral column result in variable sized defects called spina bifida with extrusion of neuronal tissue and membranes (myelomeningocele) or simply membranes (meningocele). Ventral lesions occur much more rarely. Open spina bifida refers to lesions where neural tissues are exposed with an open spinal canal and no skin cover. Where skin cover exists, the lesion is usually cystic (spina bifida cystica). Craniorachischisis refers to a combination of anencephaly and extensive opening of the vertebral column and exposure of the spinal cord. Spina bifida occulta simply describes defects in the vertebrae which are covered with normal skin, are not obvious other than radiologically and are almost always clinically silent. Overlying skin, however, may be dimpled, pigmented or signaled by an abnormal tuft of hair or hemangioma.

EMBRYOLOGY

The neural crest is derived from embryonic ectoderm and through migration of its constituent cells forms numerous derivative tissues including the peripheral nervous system, dorsal root and autonomic ganglia, melanocytes, the craniofacial skeleton and multiple other tissues where they undergo terminal differentiation (Sarnat & Flores-Sarnat 2005). The development of the neural tube is dependent upon multiple interacting genes that control both the formation and migration of constituent cells. The key genes that promote neural crest differentiation and migration in the formation of the vertical axis of the neural tube include *PAX3*, *BMP4*, *ZIC2*, segmentation genes such as *WNT1*, inhibitory neural crest genes such as *EGR2* and differentiating genes *SLUG* and *SOX10* (Sarnat & Flores-Sarnat 2005). The complexity of neural tube formation is reflected in the increasing understanding of the molecular genetic control and involvement of neural crest cells in migration, proliferation and differentiation including involvement in intercellular signaling and inter-tissue reactions. Interference by environmental factors (e.g. diet) further complicates molecular control of neural tube formation.

The neural tube closure occurs between 26–29 days following conception and failure to close results in anencephaly when the cephalic region is involved and variable spinal defects eventuate when the thoracic and lumbar-sacral regions are affected.

ETIOLOGY

NTDs are recognized as having heterogeneous origins. An identifiable cause is recognized only in 6–20% of cases (Holmes et al 1976, Khoury et al 1982, Martin et al 1983).

Reported and recognizable 'environmental' causal associations with NTDs are shown in Table 17.1 and putative causal associated genetic factors in Table 17.2.

A range of chromosomal disorders are also known to have associations with NTDs (Milunsky & Canick 2004). There are many uncommon to rare syndromes that may also have NTDs as a feature (Milunsky & Canick 2004). For the most part however, genetic-environmental interactions are thought to account for the multifactorial origin of NTDs, key observations of which are reflected in Table 17.1.

For over forty years, folic acid deficiency has been postulated as a crucial factor in the pathogenesis of NTDs (Hibbard & Smithells 1965). Daly et al (1995) elegantly showed that the risk of NTD is clearly associated with low red blood cell folate levels in a continuous dose–response relationship. They demonstrated more than an 8-fold difference in risk between those patients with the lowest and those with the highest red blood cell folate levels.

Polygenic causation of NTDs has been an accepted theory for many years but only recently has evidence accrued pointing to certain susceptibility genes. Not unexpectedly, functional polymorphisms of several genes that encode enzymes involved in folate metabolism (such as MTHFR, MTR and MTRR) have been observed in some studies to increase the risk of spina bifida (Mitchell et al 2004). Homozygosity for the *C677T MTHFR* gene polymorphism is associated with a moderately increased risk for spina bifida (Botto & Yang 2000). Maternal *C677T* homozygosity is also associated with a moderate increased risk to mothers for having a child with spina bifida. An Italian study concluded that heterozygosity and homozygosity for the methylene tetrahydrofolate dehydrogenase I gene polymorphism 1958G/A increased the mother's risk 1.69-fold for having a child with an NTD (DeMarco et al 2006).

Stamm et al (2006) in a study of 44 multiplex families and using a genome-wide scan focused on one particular family demonstrating likely gene susceptibility loci for NTDs proximate to the telomeric regions of chromosomes 2q33.1-q35 and 7p21.1-pter. Given evidence that early first trimester exposure to hyperthermia is associated with an increased risk of spina bifida (Milunsky et al 1992), Jensen et al (2006), hypothesized that processes involved in inflammation and elevated body temperature, such as chemokines, could be involved in the pathogenesis of spina bifida. These authors focused on the gene encoding a potent chemokine monocyte

Table 17.1 Reported 'environmental' causal associations with neural tube defects
'Environmental' factors
Aminopterin
Carbamazepine
Clomiphene citrate
Copper in drinking water
Efavirenz (reverse transcriptase inhibitor)
Fetus interaction with residual trophoblast
First-trimester surgery
Folic acid deficiency
Hyperthermia
Industrial/agricultural exposure
Magnesium or calcium content of drinking water
Maternal alcohol ingestion
Maternal age <20 or >35 years
Maternal diabetes mellitus
Maternal health
Maternal obesity
Maternal weight reduction (early pregnancy)
Maternal zinc deficiency
Nitrates, nitrites, and magnesium salts in foods
Oral contraceptives
Parity
Paternal age
Potato blight
Previous spontaneous abortions/stillbirth
Season, epidemics
Social class/poverty/illegitimacy
Subfertility
Tea drinking
Thalidomide
Twinning
Valproic acid
Vitamin A
Vitamin B_{12} deficiency
Warfarin (Coumadin)

Modified from: Milunsky A and Canick 2004.

Table 17.2 Evidence for a putative causal association of genetic factors with neural tube defects
Observations implicating genetic factors
Polygenic nature of most disorders
Bias in sex ratio toward higher number of females
High percentage of males in low-prevalence areas
Increased susceptibility if parent has HLA-DR locus
Increased frequency in consanguineous matings
Monozygotic twin concordance
Racial/ethnic bias in incidence
Familial recurrence pattern: affected parent: affected sibling/ aunt/uncle/cousin
Increased incidence when there is a previous child with hydrocephaly
Increased incidence when there is a previous child with germ-cell tumor
Susceptibility of midline 'developmental field'
Mitochondrial uncoupling gene
Mutations in *PAX-3* gene
Abnormalities in folate and/or cobalamin metabolism

Modified from: Milunsky A and Canick J 2004.

chemoattractant protein, a product of the *CCL-2* gene. They discovered a polymorphism (A)(-2518)G in the promoter region of this gene and studied 469 families who had at least a single member with spina bifida. They identified this promoter polymorphism as a significant maternal risk factor for spina bifida. Women with this polymorphism had a 1.5-fold higher risk than women without this polymorphism of having a child with an NTD.

Certain genetic variants may protect against having spina bifida offspring or at least modify risk. One such protective gene polymorphism is that of the myo-inositol synthase gene polymorphism *ISYNA1 1029A > G* (Groenen et al 2004). A specific polymorphism (Ile120Val) of the *PCMT1* gene whose product is involved in protein repair appears to be a genetic modifier in reducing the risk of spina bifida (Zhu et al 2006).

N-acetyltransferase I (NAT1) is another gene involved in the catabolism of folates and the acetylation of aromatic and heterocyclic amines. Functional polymorphisms in this gene have also been shown to have a protective effect against having offspring with spina bifida (Jensen et al 2006).

To complicate etiological considerations further, evidence accumulating over the past three decades has pointed to an excess rate of NTDs among the relatives of mothers bearing affected offspring. More recently, another study from Ireland focused on 1033 singleton first cousin pregnancies with reference to pregnancy outcome and compared NTD risks among maternal and paternal relatives (Byrne & Carolan 2006). The authors concluded that maternal first cousin pregnancies were more likely to end with an NTD when compared to paternal first cousin pregnancies (17.4% vs. 11.7%, $P = 0.01$).

EPIDEMIOLOGY

An accurate determination of the incidence or prevalence of NTDs has always faced considerable challenges. To begin with, the phenotype of a relatively common malformation is variable, not evenly distributed across populations and in fact not always easily detected (such as some forms of dysraphism or following second trimester pregnancy termination). Typically phenotypes of anencephaly, spina bifida, craniorachischisis, meningocele and encephalocele are readily determined while dysraphism and lipomeningocele as well as spina bifida occulta may be less obvious. The concurrence with NTDs of associated malformations may end up being recorded without mention of, for example, spina bifida. There are scores of recognized syndromes in which NTDs invariably, often or occasionally, occur (Milunsky & Canick 2004, Stevenson & Hall 2006). Etiologies include chromosomal, monogenic, multifactorial and idiopathic categories. Widely varying frequencies of NTDs in different global regions include changes in the rate of occurrence with seasons. Genetic susceptibility (for example to the methylene tetrahydrofolate reductase polymorphisms),

discussed earlier, further influences occurrence and probably recurrence. The remarkable advances occasioned by the introduction of maternal serum screening for NTDs and the associated availability of prenatal diagnosis have had important effects on decreasing the birth frequency of NTDs. The value of these advances has been exceeded only by the introduction of dietary folic acid supplementation. Nevertheless, these advances over the past quarter of a century have had significant effects on the frequency of occurrence of NTDs and have also confounded efforts at comparative studies of incidence and prevalence.

Methodological approaches to the investigation of prevalence or incidence of NTDs have varied enormously (Hulley et al 2001, Kirby 2006). These authors have critically reviewed the design and analytical issues of epidemiologic studies and focused on specific methodological concerns and problems. For *cross-sectional and descriptive studies*, these authors draw attention to the limitations that include recall bias, selection bias and survival bias. They emphasize that the cross-sectional study as an initial effort is of value in determining demographic patterns, trends and prevalence patterns.

A second method involves *case-control studies* which largely rely on birth defect surveillance data linked to established databases that identify NTD cases. These studies are often retrospective. Reporting bias between parents of cases and controls may occur in these studies and recall bias may again be a problem.

Cohort and longitudinal studies prospectively focus on a study population for a specified length of time or given outcome. One key issue can be the failure to study and identify individuals prior to conception of the pregnancy at risk and failure to follow pregnancy outcome.

Randomized controlled trials and intervention studies focus on at least two or more treatment and control groups. The critical issue in this approach is to certify that it is a blinded study.

REASONS FOR EPIDEMIOLOGICAL STUDY

Key to the initiation of public health programs aimed at the prevention of congenital malformations is the determination of both prevalence and incidence. Such data provide an opportunity to assess population risk and to focus public health efforts. Such data assessment also enables economic estimates relative to predicted health care needs and the establishment of priorities in a cost-conscious society with rapidly escalating health care expenses. Epidemiologic data also has an important role in the recognition of actual or contributing causes of NTDs such as the recognition of NTD risk as a consequence of hot tub and sauna use (Milunsky et al 1992). Carefully assembled epidemiologic data also enable study of the effects of preventive regimens such as dietary improvements or actual supplementation (e.g. by folic acid).

Regardless of the study designs as noted above, an enormous portion of the published literature on NTD prevalence and incidence has failed to address major or important factors that may influence conclusions. One or more of the following items have frequently been overlooked in published studies of NTD incidence/prevalence:

- Ascertainment bias.
- Recall bias.
- Survival bias.
- Failure to include spontaneous abortion.
- Failure to include elective abortion.
- Failure to account for prenatal diagnosis.
- Failure to account for stillbirths.
- Dependence on death certificates.
- Failure to recognize a syndromic etiology.
- Failure to study a population of adequate size to power a necessary calculation.
- Failure to recognize economic class differences.
- Failure to account for pregnancy outcome among insulin-dependent diabetics.
- Failure to account for pregnancy outcome in epileptics on anticonvulsant medications.
- Failure to identify those who do and do not use folic acid supplements.

PREVALENCE OF NTDs

While prevalence is defined as the number of infants and/or fetuses with an NTD born per annum, affected fetuses aborted spontaneously or electively could also be included. The first and second trimester affected fetuses have frequently not been included in prevalence estimates. Considerable differences in prevalence rates for both anencephaly and spina bifida in published studies reflect data collected from hospitals or have been purely population-based (Lie 2006). Not unexpectedly, prevalence rates for both these defects were higher in the hospital-based studies. This was especially the case when pregnancy terminations were not included.

Confounding comparative prevalence rates for anencephaly and spina bifida over the past 40 years is the advent of certain major environmental changes and advances in medicine. Dietary supplementation or direct ingestion of supplements of folic acid (see below) ranks as the most important factor in reducing prevalence rates for these defects. The introduction and progressive improvement in the use of obstetrical ultrasound have facilitated earlier diagnosis and the option for pregnancy termination. The introduction of maternal serum alpha fetoprotein screening for NTDs was a milestone development in the avoidance of these defects (Milunsky 2004). Notwithstanding the dietary supplementation and technical advances, clear evidence has been presented showing a significant decline in prevalence rates for NTDs prior to 1975 (Wald & Leck 2000). These authors point to the dramatic decline in prevalence rates and indicate that

in 1965 in England and Wales there were 2800 NTD births, while in 1997 there were fewer than 100. Coupled economic and dietary improvements probably explain the initiation of the early decline in prevalence rates. Studies of NTD prevalence prior to 1990 were extensively reviewed by Elwood et al (1992).

Striking differences in prevalence rates for anencephaly and spina bifida (Tables 17.3 and 17.4) are reported from various geographical regions. Tables 17.2 and 17.3 reflect selected extrapolated data from Lie (2006) in which there was reported rates for 1991–1995, as well as 1996–2000. Data for *both* periods were mostly not available for some high prevalence areas such as Turkey, Russia, China, India, Thailand and Ireland. In another study that included NTDs in all live births and stillbirths at University Hospitals throughout Turkey in a single year period (1993–1994), a rate of 30.1 per 10 000 births was reported among the total 21 907 births (Tuncbilek et al 1999). In a hospital-based study in Bangkok, Thailand, among 18 000–20 000 deliveries in the period 1990–1999, an NTD incidence of 0.67 per thousand births was reported (Wasant & Sathienkijkanchai 2005). In another Thai hospital study focused on sonographic prenatal diagnosis of NTDs, the striking result reflected an overall rate of 0.66 per thousand births among which only 0.06 per thousand were due to spina bifida (Kitisomprayoonkul & Tongsong 2001). A study from Pondicherry in India revealed a higher frequency of NTDs in babies born to some consanguineous parents (Mahadevan & Bhat 2005). Prevalence rates were as high as 21.3 per 10 000 births in 1991–1995 from India's Uttar Pradesh region (Argarwal et al 1991, Kumar & Singh 2003). A remarkable rate of 38.2 per 10 000 births in the Elazig region of Turkey was reported by Guvene et al (1993). For the most severe NTD, craniorachischisis, Johnson et al (2004) reported a remarkable 0.52 per 10 000 live births among Mexican Americans living in a Texas–Mexico border population. Since congenital defects associated with NTDs were observed in 12.6% of the cases studied, autosomal recessive inheritance may have played a greater than usual role in causation.

THE IMPACT OF PRENATAL SCREENING AND DIAGNOSIS ON THE PREVALENCE OF NTDs

Maternal serum screening by assaying for alpha fetoprotein took about 20 years to be fully integrated into medical practice. Notwithstanding this tardy pace, this screening method, especially coupled with advances in sonography, has enabled the prenatal detection of 100% of fetal anencephaly and at least 90% for spina bifida (Milunsky & Canick 2004). A precise fix on the efficacy of maternal serum screening and prenatal diagnosis on the birth prevalence of NTDs has been difficult to achieve. The Eurocat Working Group (1991) evaluated the impact of prenatal diagnosis especially noting the frequency and timing of pregnancy termination. That study focused on 3113 cases

Table 17.3 Selected prevalence rates for anencephaly in the period 1991–2000 for different geographic areas (as extracted and modified from Lie 2006)

Geographical region	1991–1995		1996–2000		Source type*	Prevalence type†	Reference
	Total births	Prevalence (per 10 000)	Total births	Prevalence (per 10 000)			
Australia	1 109 159	2.6	757 724	4.4	P	LST(95-)	ICBDMS (1993–2002)
Canada, Alberta	38 784	1.8	187 359	2.8	P	LST(97-)	ICBDMS (1997–2002)
Czech Republic	577 964	1.1	453 465	3.1	P	LST	ICBDMS (1993–2002)
England/Wales	3 388 435	1.4	3 168 907	2.8	P	LST	ICBDMS (1993–2002)
Finland	326 669	0.3	292 234	3.1	P	LST(96-)	ICBDMS (1993–2002)
Hungary	595 926	0.7	497 741	1.4	P	LST	ICBDMS (1993–2002)
Japan	554 477	3.5	482 195	1.7	H	LS	ICBDMS (1993–2002)
Mexico	288 684	16.0	181 013	13.5	H	LS	ICBDMS (1993–2002)
Norway	303 092	3.2	299 153	3.4	P	LST	ICBDMS (1993–2002)
South Africa	222 614	0.8	123 879	2.2	H	L	ICBDMS (1994–97, 1999, 2001–2)
Sweden	247 271	0.4	179 308	3.1	P	LST (99-)	ICBDMS (1993–94, 2001–2)
USA	24 726 932	1.4	4 381 901	1.0	P	LS	Honein et al (2001)

*Source types: H, hospital-based; P, population-based
†Prevalence type: L, including live births; M, medical insurance data; S, including stillbirths; T, including terminations after prenatal diagnoses (period indicated).

of NTDs in 20 regions. In the centers whose data could be evaluated and in which elective abortion was recorded, at least 80% of pregnancies with anencephaly and 40% with spina bifida ended in termination. A 1995 study by Cragan et al of birth defect surveillance in six USA states found that elective pregnancy termination for anencephaly or spina bifida ranged from 9–42%. As expected, pregnancies with fetal anencephaly ended up with termination much more frequently than those with spina bifida (Forrester and Merz 2000). Reported data from the Hawaii Birth Defects Program have indicated that 74% of NTDs were detected prenatally and 48% of pregnancies were terminated (Cragan et al 1995).

FOLIC ACID SUPPLEMENTATION AND DIETARY FORTIFICATION

For over four decades, repeated publications have pointed to a probable folate deficiency as key to the pathogenesis of NTDs. In 1989, we reported our results of the first prospective, broadly based, large (22 776 women) mid-trimester study which showed a prevalence of NTDs of 3.5 per thousand among women who never use multi-vitamins before or after conception and 0.9 per thousand among those who did use the supplements during the first six weeks of pregnancy. We concluded that multi-vitamins with folic acid taken when planning pregnancy and for the first six weeks after conception provided about a 70% degree of protection against NTDs (Milunsky et al 1989). We also observed a strikingly higher prevalence of NTDs in women with a positive family history who did not take supplements (13.0 per 1000) compared with those with a family history who did (3.5 per thousand).

The results of our observational study were confirmed by the UK Medical Research Council Multi-Country, randomized, double-blind intervention trial published in 1991 (Medical Research Council Vitamin Study Research Group 1991). The UK study concluded that for women who had at least one previous affected offspring, there was a 72% protective effect. In that study, a large daily dose (4 mg) of folic acid was used. Both we and others have reported lower effective doses (0.4 mg daily). A double blind, randomized inter-

Table 17.4 Selected prevalence rates for spina bifida in the period 1991–2000 for different geographic areas (as extracted and modified from Lie 2006)

Geographical region	1991–1995		1996–2000		Source type*	Prevalence type†	Reference
	Total births	Prevalence (per 10 000)	Total births	Prevalence (per 10 000)			
Australia	1 109 159	4.7	757 724	5.2	P	LST(95-)	ICBDMS (1993–2002)
Canada, Alberta	38 784	6.5	187 359	3.7	P	LST(97-)	ICBDMS (1997–2002)
Czechoslovakia	577 964	2.2	453 465	4.2	P	LST	ICBDMS (1993–2002)
England/Wales	3 388 435	1.7	3 168 907	2.9	P	LST	ICBDMS (1993–2002)
Finland	326 669	2.4	292 234	4.7	P	LST(96-)	ICBDMS (1993–2002)
France, Central East	513 514	3.0	521 168	3.6	P	LST	ICBDMS (1993–2002)
Hungary	595 926	1.8	497 741	3.0	P	LST	ICBDMS (1993–2002)
Israel	78 764	2.4	101 249	2.6	H	LST (95-)	ICBDMS (1993–2002)
Italy, Emilia-Romagna	126 923	3.9	123 541	3.6	P	LST	ICBDMS (1993–2002)
Japan	554 477	3.6	482 195	3.8	H	LS	ICBDMS (1993–2002)
Mexico	288 684	15.8	181 013	14.4	H	LS	ICBDMS (1993–2002)
Netherlands, Northern	77 106	4.3	98 999	5.4	P	LST	ICBDMS (1993–2002)
Norway	303 092	4.9	299 153	5.5	P	LST	ICBDMS (1993–2002)
South Africa	222 614	4.4	123 879	5.8	H	L	ICBDMS (1994–97, 1999,2001–2)
South America	952 372	7.9	766 460	10.4	H	LS	ICBDMS (1993–2002)
Spain	430 098	3.1	499 650	2.1	H	LS	ICBDMS (1993–2002)
Sweden	247 271	4.9	179 308	5.1	P	LST (99-)	ICBDMS (1993–94, 2001–2)
USA	24 726 932	2.5	4 381 901	2.0	P	LS	Honein et al (2001)

*Source types: H, hospital-based; P, population-based
†Prevalence type: L, including live births; M, medical insurance data; S, including stillbirths; T, including terminations after prenatal diagnoses (period indicated).

vention trial in Hungary also demonstrated the efficacy of periconceptional folic acid supplementation (Czeizel & Dudas 1992). The dosage of multi-vitamins used in that study was 0.4–0.8 mg folic acid taken at least one month before and three months after conception. NTDs occurred in 6 of 2104 women who did not take supplements while no cases occurred among the 2052 women who did take supplements.

As a direct consequence of these studies and the weight of evidence presented, a change in public health policy

ensued. Clear recommendations were issued by the Centers for Disease Control and Prevention (CDC) in the United States on September 12, 1992, that all women of childbearing age who are capable of becoming pregnant take 0.4 mg/day of folic acid. This recommendation was echoed by an Advisory Group in the United Kingdom who included a recommendation of 4–5 mg/day of folic acid for women who had previously had an affected child. Difficulties in implementing this new public health policy were encountered and included economic, educational and personal hurdles. Consequently an alternative policy of food fortification emerged. Fortification of grain products with folic acid was approved by the US Food and Drug Administration in 1996 with a mandatory requirement for compliance by January, 1998.

Subsequently, a CDC study of live-births in the United States between 1996–2001 revealed a 23% decline in NTDs. Spina bifida cases declined 24% and anencephaly 21% during this period. The authors calculated that these figures translated to approximately 920 infants being born without NTDs (Matthews et al 2002). A study in Nova Scotia after fortification had been implemented showed that the incidence of open NTDs decreased by over 50% (Persad et al 2002). Their mean annual rate was 2.58 per thousand births during 1991–1997 and 1.17 per thousand births during 1998–2000. In the northeastern Mexico state of Nuevo Leon situated near the border with Texas, a prospective study was based on cases ascertained from hospitals, clinics, death certificates and fetal death registries. The regimen used was a 5.0 mg pill taken once per week and provided at no cost to the patient. In 1999, they recorded 95 NTD cases and in the years 2000 and 2001, there were 59 and 55 cases respectively. They concluded that after 2 years, there was a 50% decrease in the incidence of anencephaly and spina bifida (Martinez de Villarreal et al 2002).

Shanxi Province in North Central China has very high rates of NTDs (Xiao et al 1990). Li et al (2006) collected data from a population-based birth defects surveillance program in four counties that captured information on all live-births, stillbirths of at least 20 weeks gestation and all abortions resulting from prenatal diagnosis of a fetal malformation. Among 11 534 births, these authors recorded an NTD prevalence of 13.87 per thousand births. They noted that among 143 mothers with NTD offspring, only 6 (4.2%) used folic acid supplements during the periconceptional period. In continuing studies, this team (Zhang et al 2006) showed that women in rural areas of Shanxi Province had low plasma and erythrocyte folate levels.

ETIOLOGY OF NTDs

Development and closure of the neural tube are usually completed by 26–29 days following conception.

Epidemiologic studies frequently fail to take into account environmental and genetic factors that may influence prevalence of NTDs specifically in certain population groups. Milunsky and Canick (2004) reviewed genetic, environmental and syndromic causes or contributing factors that result in NTDs. NTDs in association with chromosomal abnormality or a monogenic disorder (such as Waardenburg syndrome) are uncommon and not a significant contributor to population prevalence. Multifactorial etiology remains most common with increasing research focused on predisposing genetic polymorphisms such as in the methylene tetrahydrofolate reductase gene (Van der Put et al 1997) and plate-

let-derived growth factor alpha-receptor gene (Joosten et al 2001).

Environmental factors such as maternal insulin-dependent diabetes, maternal use of anticonvulsants, first trimester heat exposure (Milunsky et al 1992) and obesity represent significant risk factors for individuals, but are not likely singly to significantly influence population prevalence rates. Similarly recurrent NTDs or those occurring as a consequence of parental consanguinity (Murshid 2000) are not likely to significantly influence population prevalence rates. Factors that dominate the causation for NTDs are likely to be low socioeconomic class almost certainly related to folate deficiency.

A study by Williams et al (2005) focused on 21 population-based birth defect surveillance systems for trends in the prevalence of NTDs with specific attention to racial/ethnic groups between 1995–2002. That study concentrated on periods prior to food fortification, a period during optional fortification and mandatory fortification of enriched serial-grain products. These authors recorded prevalence values per 10 000 births for spina bifida in 3 groups of women – Hispanic, non-Hispanic White and non-Hispanic Black. Prior to food fortification by folate enrichment, the rates were 6.49, 5.13 and 3.57 respectively, compared to post-fortification rates of 4.18, 3.37 and 2.90, respectively. This data reflected a significant decrease in the prevalence of spina bifida among non-Hispanic White and Hispanic births (34% and 36% decreases respectively). There was a 19% decline in the prevalence of spina bifida among non-Hispanic Black births, but the result was considered to be of borderline statistical significance.

Considerable debate has followed after the folate fortification policy was made mandatory. A major claim was the inadequacy of the folic acid enrichment (Brent & Oakley 2005). Two particular concerns regarding safety of food-folate enrichment is the possible masking of cobalamin deficiency which could precipitate neurologic complications of pernicious anemia. Other medications such as methotrexate, certain anticonvulsants and some sulfa drugs may prove less effective for patients taking folic acid. The claim by Brent and Oakley about inadequate folate fortification invoked a strong opposing view from the US Food and Drug Administration (Rader & Schneeman 2006).

Berry et al (1999) studied the birth prevalence of NTDs in Northern China where the rate of NTDs is high and in Southern China with a much lower NTD rate during the 1993–1995 period. Data came from 130 000 women who took folic acid (400 µg per day) supplements at any time before or during pregnancy and 118 000 who took no supplements. The prevalence rate in the high risk area declined by almost 79% (from 4.8 to 1.0 per thousand) and in the low risk region, the prevalence declined by 40% (from 1.0 to 0.6 per thousand).

Prevention and avoidance of NTDs are paramount given the high morbidity and mortality rates. Anencephalics in Western countries are mostly detected prior to delivery and most affected pregnancies are electively terminated or fetal loss/stillbirth occurs. Approximately 30–40% are live-born, but virtually all demise within one week. Rarely an anencephalic infant may survive up to 10 months, more especially when extraordinary means are used to maintain life.

The outcome for spina bifida is vastly different. Two major long term studies of survival with spina bifida have been reported (Bowman et al 2001, Hunt 1990, 1995, Hunt & Oakeshoff 2003). Studies of these two large cohorts extend to 20–25 years and up to 38 years respectively. In the first study of 117 children assessed at 16–20 years of age, only 7% had little or no disability, while 21% had died within the first year. Some 41% had died by 16 years of age. Among the 69 (59%) who survived to aged 16 years, a long series of complications were experienced and included shunting for hydrocephalus, blindness, mental retardation, seizures,

incontinence (44%) and wheel-chair dependence (30%). At 25 years, 48% had died and at 32–38 years, 54% had died.

In the second study (details in Milunsky & Canick 2004), 60% survived to 20–25 years. Being wheel-chair bound, mentally handicapped and requiring lifelong continuous care remain serious issues. However, some 49% achieved university entrance and 45% were employed. The most common causes of death were shunt malfunction and renal failure.

The personal, family and public burden engendered by the commonly occurring NTDs challenges governments worldwide to proactively provide dietary folate supplementation, public education and relief of socioeconomic privation. Sadly, few governments have taken any significant preventive steps to avoid NTDs.

REFERENCES

Argawal S S, Singh U, Singh P S et al 1991 Prevalence and spectrum of congenital malformations in a prospective study at a teaching hospital. Indian J Med Res 94:413–419.

Berry R J, Li Z, Erickson J D et al 1999 Prevention of neural-tube defects with folic acid in China. N Engl J Med 341:1487.

Botto L D, Yang Q 2000 5,10-Methylenetetrahydrofolate reductase gene variants and congenital anomalies: a HuGE review. Am J Epidemiol 151(9):862–877.

Bowman R M, McLone D G, Grant J A et al 2001 Spina bifida outcome: a 25-year prospective. Pediatr Neurosurg 34:114.

Brent R L, Oakley G P 2005 The Food and Drug Administration must require the addition of more folic acid in 'enriched' flour and other grains. Pediatrics 116:753–755.

Byrne J, Carolan S 2006 Adverse reproductive outcomes among pregnancies of aunts and (spouses of) uncles in Irish families with neural tube defects. Am J Med Genet 140A:52–61.

Carod-Artal F J, Vasquez-Cabrera C B 2006 Myelomeningocele in a Peruvian mummy from the Moche period. Neurology 66:1775–1776.

Cragan J D, Roberts H E, Edmonds L D et al 1995 Surveillance for anencephaly and spina bifida and the impact of prenatal diagnosis — United States, 1985–1994. MMWR CDC Surveill Summ 25:44(4):1–13.

Czeizel A E, Dudas I 1992 Prevention of the first occurrence of neural-tube defects by periconceptional vitamin supplementation. N Engl J Med 327:1832.

Daly L E, Kirke P N, Molloy A et al 1995 Folate levels and neural tube defects. JAMA 274:1698.

DeMarco P, Merello E, Calevo M G et al 2006 Evaluation of a methylene tetrahydrofolate-dehydrogenase 1958G > A polymorphism for neural tube defect risk. J Hum Genet 51(2):98–103.

Dickel D N, Doran G H 1989 Severe neural tube defect syndrome from the Early Archaic of Florida. Am J Phys Anthropol 80(3):325–334.

Elwood J M, Little J, Elwood J H. 1992 Epidemiology and control of neural tube defects. Oxford University Press, Oxford.

EUROCAT Working Group 1991 Prevalence of neural tube defects in 20 regions of Europe and the impact

of prenatal diagnosis, 1980–1986. J Epidemiol Commun Health 45:52–58.

Forrester M B, Merz R D 2000 Prenatal diagnosis and elective termination of neural tube defects in Hawaii, 1986–1997. Fetal Diagn Ther 15:146–151.

Groenen P M W, Klootwijk R, Schijvenaars M M V A P et al 2004 Spina bifida and genetic factors related to myo-inositol, glucose, and zinc. Mol Gen Genet 82:154–161.

Guvene H, Uslu M A, Guvene M et al 1993 Changing trend of neural tube defects in eastern Turkey. J Epidemiol Community Health 47:40–41.

Hibbard E D, Smithells R W 1965 Folic acid metabolism and human embryopathy. Lancet 1:1254.

Holmes L B, Driscoll S G, Atkins L 1976 Etiologic heterogeneity of neural-tube defects. N Engl J Med 294:365.

Honein M A, Paulozzi L J, Mathews T J et al 2001 Impact of folic acid fortification of the U.S. food supply on the occurrence of neural tube defects. JAMA 285:2981–2986.

Hulley S B, Cummings S R, Browner W S et al 2001 Designing Clinical Research, 2nd edn. Lippincott Williams & Wilkins, Philadelphia.

Hunt G M 1990 Open spina bifida: outcome for a complete cohort treated unselectively and followed into adulthood. Dev Med Child Neurol 32:108.

Hunt G M, Oakeshoff P 2003 Outcome in people with open spina bifida at age 35: prospective community based cohort study. BMJ 326:1365.

Hunt G M, Poulton A 1995 Open spina bifida: a complete cohort reviewed 25 years after closure. Dev Med Child Neurol 37:19.

ICDMS 1993 The International Centre for Birth Defects. Annual Report 1993 (with Data for 1991)– International Clearinghouse for Birth Defects Monitoring Systems. International Centre for Birth Defects, Rome.

ICDMS 1994 Annual Report 1994 (with Data for 1992)– International Clearinghouse for Birth Defects Monitoring Systems. International Centre for Birth Defects, Rome.

ICDMS 1995 Annual Report 1995 (with Data for 1993)– International Clearinghouse for Birth Defects Monitoring Systems. International Centre for Birth Defects, Rome.

ICDMS 1996 Annual Report 1996 (with Data for 1994)– International Clearinghouse for Birth Defects Monitoring Systems. International Centre for Birth Defects, Rome.

ICDMS 1997 Annual Report 1997 (with Data for 1995)– International Clearinghouse for Birth Defects Monitoring Systems. International Centre for Birth Defects, Rome.

ICDMS 1998 Annual Report 1998 (with Data for 1996)– International Clearinghouse for Birth Defects Monitoring Systems. International Centre for Birth Defects, Rome.

ICDMS 1999 Annual Report 1999 (with Data for 1997)– International Clearinghouse for Birth Defects Monitoring Systems. International Centre for Birth Defects, Rome.

ICDMS 2000 Annual Report 2000 (with Data for 1998)– International Clearinghouse for Birth Defects Monitoring Systems. International Centre for Birth Defects, Rome.

ICDMS 2001 Annual Report 2001 (with Data for 1999)– International Clearinghouse for Birth Defects Monitoring Systems. International Centre for Birth Defects, Rome.

ICDMS 2002 Annual Report 2002 (with Data for 2000)– International Clearinghouse for Birth Defects Monitoring Systems. International Centre for Birth Defects, Rome.

Jensen L E, Etheredge A J, Brown K S et al 2006 Maternal genotype for the monocyte chemoattractant protein 1 A(-2518)G promoter polymorphism is associated with the risk of spina bifida in offspring. Am J Med Genet Part A 140A:1114–1118.

Jensen L E, Hoess K, Mitchell L E et al 2006 Loss of function polymorphisms in NAT1 protect against spina bifida. Hum Genet 120:52–57.

Johnson K M, Suarez L, Felkner M M et al 2004 Prevalence of craniorachischisis in a Texas-Mexico border population. Birth Defects Res A Clin Mol Teratol Feb;70(2):92–94.

Joosten P H, Toepoel M, Mariman E C et al 2001 Promoter haplotype combinations of the platelet-derived growth factor alpha-receptor gene predispose to human neural tube defects. Nat Genet 27:215.

Khoury M F, Erickson J D, James L M et al 1982 Etiologic heterogeneity of neural tube defects. II. Clues from family studies. Am J Hum Genet 34:980.

Kirby R S 2006 Methodological issues in the study of neural tube defects. In: Wyszynski D F (ed.) Neural tube defects, from origin to treatment. Oxford University Press, New York, pp. 103–108.

Kitisomprayoonkul N, Tongsong T 2001 Neural tube defects: a different pattern in northern Thai population. J Med Assoc Thai Apr;84(4):483–488.

Kumar R, Singh S N 2003 Spinal dysraphism: Trends in northern India. Pediatr Neurosurg 38(3):133–145.

Li Z, Ren A, Zhang L, Ye R et al 2006 Extremely high prevalence of neural tube defects in a 4-county area in Shanxi Province, China. Birth Defects Research (Part A) 76(4):237–240.

Lie R T 2006 An international perspective on anencephaly and spina bifida: Prevalences by the turn of the century. In: Wyszynski D F (ed.) Neural tube defects. Oxford University Press, New York, p. 117.

Mahadevan B, Bhat B V 2005 Neural tube defects in Pondicherry. Indian J Pediatr 72(7):557–559.

Martin R A, Fineman R M, Jorde L B 1983 Phenotypic heterogeneity in neural tube defects: a clue to causal heterogeneity. Am J Med Genet 16:519.

Martinez de Villarreal L, Perez J Z, Vazquez P A et al 2002 Decline of neural tube defects cases after a folic acid campaign in Nuevo Leon, Mexico. Teratology Nov; 66(5):249–256.

Mathews T J, Honein M A, Erickson J D 2002 Spina bifida and anencephaly prevalence — United States, 1991–2001. MMWR Recomm Rep Sep 13;51 RR-13):9–11.

Medical Research Council Vitamin Study Research Group 1991 Prevention of neural tube defects: results of the Medical Research Council vitamin study. Lancet 228:131.

Merbs C F 2004 Sagittal clefting of the body and other vertebral developmental errors in Canadian Inuit skeletons. Am J Phys Anthropol 123:236–249.

Milunsky A 2004 Genetic disorders and the fetus: diagnosis, prevention and treatment, 5th edn. Johns Hopkins University Press, Baltimore.

Milunsky A, Canick J 2004 Maternal serum screening for neural tube and other defects. In: Milunsky A (ed.) Genetic disorders of the fetus: diagnosis, prevention and treatment. Johns Hopkins University Press, Baltimore, p. 719.

Milunsky A, Ulcickas M, Rothman K et al 1992 Maternal heat exposure and neural tube defects. JAMA 268:882–885.

Milunsky, A, Jick H, Jick SS et al 1989 Multivitamin/folic acid supplementation in the earliest weeks of pregnancy reduces the prevalence of neural tube defects. JAMA 262:2847.

Mitchell L F, Adzick N S, Melchionne J et al 2004 Spina bifida. Lancet 364:1885–1895.

Murshid W R 2000 Spina bifida in Saudi Arabia: is consanguinity among the parents a risk factor? Pediatr Neurosurg 32(1):10–12.

Persad V L, Van den Hof M C et al 2002 Incidence of open neural tube defects in Nova Scotia after folic acid fortification. CMAJ 167(3):241–245.

Rader J I, Schneeman B O 2006 Prevalence of neural tube defects, folate status, and folate fortification of enriched cereal–grain products in the United States. Pediatrics 117(4):1395–1399.

Sarnat H B, Flores-Sarnat F 2005 Embryology of the neural crest: its inductive role in the neurocutaneous syndromes. J Child Neurol 20:637–643.

Smith G K 2001 The history of spina bifida, hydrocephalus, paraplegia, and incontinence. Pediatre Sur Int 17:424–432.

Stamm D S, Rampersaud E, Slifer SH et al 2006 High-density single nucleotide polymorphism screen in a large multiplex neural tube defect family refines linkage to loci at 7p21.1-pter and 2q33.1-q35. Birth Defects Research (Part A) 76:499–505.

Stevenson R E, Hall J G (eds) 2006 Human malformations and related anomalies, 2nd edn. Oxford University Press, New York.

Tuncbilek E, Boduroglu K, Alikasifoglu M 1999 Neural tube defects in Turkey: prevalence, distribution and risk factors. Turk J Pediatr 41(3):299–305.

Van der Put N M J, Eskes T K A B et al 1997 Is the common 677C? T mutation in the methylenetetrahydrofolate reductase gene a risk factor for neural tube defects? A meta-analysis. Q J Med 90:111.

Wald N, Leck I 2000 Antenatal and neonatal screening. Oxford University Press, Oxford.

Wasant P, Sathienkijkanchai A 2005 Neural tube defects at Siriraj Hospital, Bangkok, Thailand — 10 years review (1990–1999). J Med Assoc Thai 88 Suppl 8:592–599.

Williams L J, Rasmussen S A, Flores A et al 2005 Decline in the prevalence of spina bifida and anencephaly by race/ethnicity: 1995–2002. Pediatrics 116(3):580–586.

Xiao K Z, Zhang Z Y, Su Y M et al 1990 Central nervous system congenital malformations, especially neural tube defects in 29 provinces, metropolitan cities and autonomous regions of China: Chinese Birth Defects Monitoring Program. Int J Epidemiol 19:978–982.

Zhang L, Ren A, Li Z et al 2006 Folate concentrations and folic acid supplementation among women in their first trimester of pregnancy in a rural area with a high prevalence of neural tube defects in Shanxi, China. Birth Defects Research (Part A) 76:461–466.

Zhu H, Yang W, Lu W et al 2006 A known functional polymorphism (Ile120Val) of the human PCMT1 gene and risk of spina bifida. Mol Genet Metab 87(1):66–70.

CHAPTER

18

Fetal brain injury and multiple pregnancies

Isaac Blickstein

Key Points

- A 6- to 8-fold increased prevalence of cerebral palsy (CP) exists in twins compared with singletons and that in triplets is more than thrice the prevalence of CP in twins. This trend in CP prevalence is similar to the trend of preterm birth and very low birth weight (VLBW) among multiples
- Assisted reproductive techniques (ART) are associated with increased frequencies of multiples, but when the effect of preterm birth is controlled, no clear-cut cause-and-effect relationship exists between the contribution of ART and brain injury in multiples
- Multiple and singleton pregnancies have similar risks for CP until near term. Although VLBW and preterm birth are apparently the most significant risk factor for CP among multiples, the disadvantage (at least for twins) becomes evident near term
- MC twins are at increased risk of CP compared to DC twins. This statement is true also when both twins are live born
- Neurological damage in the twin-twin transfusion syndrome (TTTS) is primarily gestational age-dependent, associated with syndrome-related death of one of the twins, and seems to depend on the severity of the TTTS
- There are conflicting data related to the effects of fetal growth aberrations, the vanishing twin syndrome and mode of delivery on the brain injury in multiples

INTRODUCTION

Although the association between fetal brain injury and multiple pregnancies was not included in previous editions of this book, the concern about this relationship is not new (Blickstein 2004, 2006b, Pharoah 2005a, Scher et al 2002). The importance of this association emerges from two observations. First, multiple birth rates increased in most developed countries, with a twice to thrice rate compared to the roughly 1% before the so-called 'epidemic' of multiple births (Blickstein & Keith 2005). The most recent data from United States births show, for example, that twin birth rates have increased 65% since 1980, and the rate of triplet births has increased more than 400% (Martin et al 2003). Thus, multiples are not anymore considered rare curios of Nature (Fig. 18.1). The only potential 'advantage' of the increased numbers of multiples is the replacement of many small size series by adequately powered studies that improved our understanding of the adverse impact of multiple gestations on perinatal outcomes. The importance of the association between fetal brain injury and multiple pregnancies is further highlighted by the observation that all published registries unanimously found higher rates of fetal brain injury among multiples (Scher et al 2002).

The association between fetal brain injury and multiple pregnancies is discussed under two main headings according to the presumptive etiology, namely cases resulting from preterm birth and low birth weight and those resulting from circumstances that are unique to multiple gestations and births. Admittedly, the former is definitely the principal etiology for brain injury among multiples because twins and higher-order multiples are over-represented among severe preterm births: 11.9% and 36.1% of twins and triplets are born at less than 32 completed weeks of gestation, respectively (Martin et al 2003).

The entire spectrum of brain injury in multiples is difficult to cover for several reasons. First, as in singletons, the presence and extent of cerebral palsy (CP) are usually appreciated later in infancy and the link to perinatal events is frequently unavailable. This is particularly true for a lesser extent of brain damage, or so-called minor neurological deficits. Second, population-based studies are extremely difficult to conduct and, moreover, they frequently lack essential information such as mode of conception and chorionicity. Third, available large-scale series predate the peak years of the 'epidemic' and, hence the true impact of assisted procreation (ovulation induction and assisted reproductive techniques (ART)) is unknown. Fourth, most large scale studies were conducted before a more liberal use of cesarean section had been implemented and, therefore, the association of neurological outcomes with labor and delivery events is unknown. Fifth, as the threshold of viability has been lowered over the past decades, increasingly more multiples survive the perils of preterm birth but do not escape the prematurity-related risks. Most registries, however, do not account for these changes in neonatal treatment. Finally, the diagnostic and therapeutic approach to the twin-twin transfusion syndrome (TTTS) and to other complex situations in monochorionic twins has been changed over the last few years and led to higher salvage rates of hitherto 'lost' cases and to improved long-term outcomes (Senat et al 2004). However, data concerning brain injury in monochorionicity-related circumstances are far from being comprehensive.

This chapter discusses the available data regarding the association between fetal brain injury and multiple pregnancies.

EPIDEMIOLOGY

As noted earlier, American figures for the year 2003 represent 7.4 and 9.3-fold increases for twins and 22.6 and

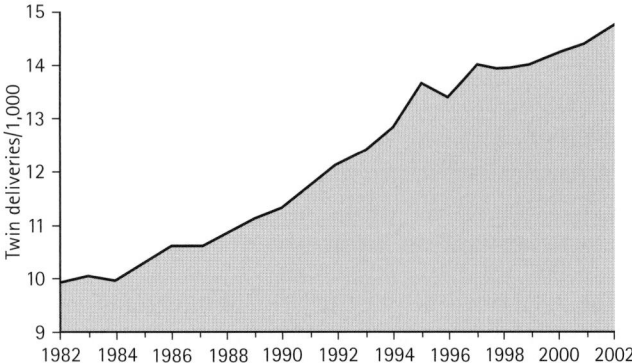

Figure 18.1 The 'epidemic' dimensions of twin births, United Kingdom and Wales. Data derived from the Twin and Multiple Birth Association (TAMBA, http://www.tamba.org.uk).

31.4-fold increases for triplets compared with figures in singletons for preterm birth (<32 weeks) and very low birth weight (VLBW, <1500 g), respectively (Martin et al 2003). Since CP rates are increased among preterm and low birth weight infants, it is not surprising that CP rates parallel the plurality-depended incidence of preterm and low birth weight infants among twins and higher-order multiples. Indeed, several epidemiological studies, from all over the world, confirmed the plurality-dependent exponentially increased risk of CP in infants from multiple births (Blickstein 2004, 2006b). Interestingly, a trend in CP similar to the trend of preterm birth was reported, indicating a 7.4% average prevalence of twins among CP cases, and a 6 to 8-fold increased prevalence of CP in twins compared with singletons (Grether et al 1993, Laplaza et al 1992, Liu et al 2000, Touyama et al 2000, Williams et al 1996). Data further indicate that the prevalence of CP in triplets exceeds that of twins and of singletons – 28 vs. 7.3 vs. 1.6 per 1000 survivors to 1 year (Petterson et al 1993) and 44.8 vs. 12.6 vs. 2.3 per 1000 survivors (Pharoah & Cooke 1996), whereas data from Japan confirmed this plurality dependent trend in quadruplets: 0.9% vs. 3.1% vs. 11.1% for twins, triplets and quadruplets, respectively (Yokoyama et al 1995).

Recent studies provided similar conclusions. Data from 12 European population-based CP registers on 6613 children born between 1975–1990 found that the rate of multiple births increased more than 25% (from 1.9% in 1980 to 2.4% in 1990), but the proportion of multiples among CP infants increased nearly 120% (from 4.6% in 1976 to 10% in 1990) (Topp et al 2004). This study also found that multiples have a 4-times higher rate of CP than singletons (7.6 vs. 1.8 per 1000 live births, RR 4.36; 95% CI 3.76–4.97). In a recent Scottish study, Bonellie et al (2005) examined data from the Scottish Register of Children with a Motor Deficit of Central Origin and the Scottish Morbidity Record series. The cohort of 646 children with CP born in Scotland between 1984 and 1990 included 57 children from twin pregnancies. The OR in twins compared to singletons for the CP prevalence per 1000 neonatal survivors was 4.83 (95% CI 3.8, 6.1) (Bonellie et al

2005). Finally, vital statistics from five populations in the United States and Australia of more than 25 000 twins suggested that twins were at an approximately 4-fold increased risk of CP compared with singletons (Scher et al 2002).

In retrospect, these data suggest a reduction in the increased risk of CP in twins in more recent compared to earlier studies (4- to 5-times vs. 6- to 8-times, respectively). At present, it is unknown whether this reduced risk is real or whether it is related to different methodologies of risk estimation. It is expected, however, that the increased proportions of multiple births as a result of assisted conceptions would result in a parallel increased prevalence of CP in the population at large. It should be noted that even the more recent series (Bonellie et al 2005, Scher et al 2002, Topp et al 2004) only cover the period until 1990, during which widespread availability of in vitro fertilization (IVF) procedures had just begun.

THE CONTRIBUTION OF ASSISTED REPRODUCTIVE TECHNOLOGY

A significant proportion of multiple pregnancies follows ovulation induction or assisted reproductive technology (ART) and is rightfully termed *iatrogenic* multiple pregnancies (Blickstein & Keith 2001). Data from the East Flanders Prospective Twin Survey indicate that 1:40 compared to 1:2 twin births followed an iatrogenic conception during the late 1970s and the late 1990s, respectively (Derom & Derom 2005). Not surprisingly, ART babies are more prevalent among the cohort of VLBW infants. Data from the Israel Neonatal Network – a population-based registry of all VLBW infants – suggest that only 10% of singletons were conceived by ART compared to 60% of the twins and 90% of the triplets (Shinwell et al 2003). As such, iatrogenic conceptions are inherently associated with increased risk of complications, including CP.

It should be remembered that the possibility to control the number of fetuses is limited with ovulation induction methods; in contrast, the possibility to reduce the proportion of iatrogenic multiples can be simply achieved by reducing the number of transferred embryos in IVF-embryo transfer (IVF-ET) methods. For example, to estimate the risk of 3 ETs in producing CP, the excess risk of multiple pregnancies was integrated with the risk of CP (Blickstein & Weissman, 1999). Estimated rates of CP were significantly higher after the transfer of 3 embryos (16.86/1000), transfer of two embryos (8.77/1000), or after the transfer of three embryos with reduction of all triplets to twins (10.31/1000) than after spontaneous conception (2.7/1000 neonates). By contrast, the estimated rates of CP are expected to be similar after the reduction of triplets to twins and after the transfer of two embryos. Using a similar extrapolation methodology, Kiely et al (2000) estimated that as much as an 8% increase in the prevalence of CP is due solely to the rise in iatrogenic multiple births in the United States. The increased risk of CP among iatrogenic multiples might be even more striking because twins from assisted conceptions seem to survive to infancy more often compared with natural conception (i.e. a lower perinatal mortality rate, OR 0.58, 95% CI 0.44 to 0.77) (Helmerhorst et al 2004).

An attempt to verify the increased risk of neurological morbidity in assisted conceptions was performed in a controlled, population based, cohort study by Pinborg et al (2004). The authors evaluated 3393 twins and 5130 singletons conceived by ART and compared the data with those of 10 239 naturally conceived twins in the Danish population. The children's age at time of follow-up was 2–7 years. In contrast to what is considered as the 'current paradigm' (Lambert RD, commenting on this paper), twins from assisted conception had a similar risk of neurological sequelae as their naturally conceived peers and singletons from assisted conception (crude prevalence rates per 1000 of neurological morbidity in the 3 groups were 8.8, 8.2 and 9.6, and of CP 3.2, 2.5 and 4.0, respectively). Moreover, children born after intracytoplasmic sperm injection (ICSI) had the same risk of neurological morbidity as children born after IVF. Lambert, in his on-line comment on the study of Pinborg et al (2004), rightfully pointed that the results, as intriguing as they are, did not compare the risk of neurological morbidity in these assisted conceptions with that of appropriately matched spontaneous singleton control pregnancies. Indeed, Hvidt-jorn et al (2006) more recently examined the incidence of CP following IVF and non-IVF pregnancies. These authors worked on data from the same Danish population but found, in contrast to Pinborg et al (2004), that children born after IVF had an increased risk of CP and that this observation was largely unchanged after adjustment for maternal age, gender, parity, small-for-gestational age status and educational level. However, after additional adjustment for plurality and preterm birth, the independent effect of IVF was no longer found. Importantly, when both plurality and preterm birth were included in the multivariate analysis, the former remained strongly associated with the risk of CP.

The success of modern treatment allowed numerous infertile women to conceive, but created at the same time the so-called epidemic of multiple pregnancies associated with significant perinatal morbidity and mortality. To amend this untoward effect of assisted conceptions, multifetal pregnancy reduction (MFPR) in the late first trimester has been introduced to unselectively (or quasi-selectively) decrease the number of embryos/fetuses. As expected, outcomes of a lower number of remaining fetuses (usually twins) is better than the non-reduced set because, as a rule, twins will always do better than triplets; singleton will do better than twins and so forth. The concern, however, is whether MFPR affects by some way the remaining fetuses. Regrettably, scant information exists about affected infants following MFPR – the iatrogenic equivalent of the 'vanishing' twin syndrome (see below). It could be argued that the lack of reported CP cases following MFPR may be reassuring on one hand, and on the other misleading because subsequent CP would probably be attributed to other factors such as preterm birth or low birth weight. In a small series, Geva et al (1998)

found, in a cohort of preterm infants who developed periventricular leukomalacia (PVL), that 28.6% were exposed to MFPR compared with 1.9% of the controls (OR 20.9, 95% CI 5.5–79.4). The results suggest that, regardless of twinning and method of conception, MFPR might be an additional risk factor for brain injury in premature infants. More recently, Dimitriou et al (2004) determined whether MFPR increases the prevalence of CP by comparing women with trichorionic triplet pregnancies who had either given birth to live triplets or, following MFPR, to live twins. The authors expected a lower CP rate among the twin pregnancies because they were delivered at a significantly later gestational age. Unexpectedly, however, the CP prevalence (13.8 per 1000) of 72 triplet children reduced to twins was similar to that of 111 triplet infants (18 per 1000).

In conclusion, when the effect of preterm birth is controlled, the data concerning the contribution of ART on brain injury in multiples do not support a clear-cut, cause-and-effect relationship.

THE EFFECT OF BIRTH WEIGHT AND GESTATIONAL AGE

In contrast to the questionable effect of ART, per se, on brain injury, there is a strong cause-and-effect association between brain injury and the preterm birth. The vulnerability of preterm infants to sustain brain injury is beyond the scope of this chapter; however, it is sufficient to note here that the risk of brain damage and gestational age and birth weight have a clear inverse correlation: the lower the gestational age/birth weight the greater the risk of brain injury. Hence, preterm infants are expected to have similar gestational age as well as birth weight related outcomes regardless of being singletons or members of a multiple set. In this context one should reiterate the fact that the main contributor to the increased prevalence of CP among multiples is related to the 7 and 23-fold increased incidence of deliveries at <32 for twins and triplets compared to singletons (Martin et al 2003), figures that are remarkably similar to the prevalence of CP among twins and triplets.

In order to show that multiples, per se, are at increased risk of brain injury, the prevalence of CP in multiples and singletons should be stratified according to birth weight and gestational age. Such data, however, exist for twins only. At present, there are compelling data to suggest that CP risk is higher in twins weighing >2499 g than of singletons of similar weight (Grether et al 1993, Pharoah & Cooke 1996, Williams et al 1996) whereas the risk was comparable among VLBW twins and singletons (Grether et al 1993, Pharoah & Cooke 1996). A similar trend was observed regarding gestational age (Williams et al 1996, Yokoyama et al 1995). Specifically, Williams et al (1996) presented a strong correlation between the risk of CP in twins and gestational duration but the relative risk of CP was greatest and, significant, only for twins delivered at >36 weeks.

One possible explanation for these findings is that the lower CP prevalence among small multiples might result from a higher mortality rate among preterm multiples compared with singletons whereas normal birth weight multiples have similar mortality rates and, therefore, more survivors, to demonstrate a higher prevalence of CP than in singletons (Liu et al 2000). This explanation was more recently supported by the observation that twins weighing <2500 g fare better than singletons in terms of mortality and CP rates (Scher et al 2002).

It follows that multiple and singleton pregnancies have similar risks for CP until near term, with a potential advantage for the former. *Although low birth weight and preterm birth are apparently the most significant risk factor for CP among multiples, the disadvantage (at least for twins) becomes evident near term.* This statement is supported by Shinwell et al (2003) who recently studied data from the Israel Neonatal VLBW infant Network and compared 3717 singletons and all *complete sets* of twins (*n* = 1394) and triplets (*n* = 483). In this study, plurality did not influence the risk of adverse neurological outcomes among infants weighing <1500 g (OR 1.29, 95% CI 0.91 to 1.85).

The excess risk for CP beyond 36 weeks may suggest that 'term' occurs earlier in twins compared with singletons, because twins experience increased morbidity compared with singletons (Luke et al 1996) and are at increased risk of mortality (Minakami & Sato 1996) and severe handicap (Luke et al 1996) after reaching 38 weeks' gestation. These findings constitute a strong argument that the optimal gestational age for twin birth is 38 weeks (Blickstein 2000), a notion supported by Luke and her coworkers (2005) who recently observed that the shortest hospitalization as well as lowest birth charges for both mother and infants were noted for this gestational age at birth.

THE EFFECT OF FETAL/INFANT DEATH AND ZYGOSITY/CHORIONICITY

Brain damage is more common in the surviving twin after single fetal death. Pahroah and Adi (2000) evaluated data from England and Wales for twin sets with one stillborn. The gestational-age-specific prevalence of CP after single fetal death was much higher than that reported for the general twin population and the survivor was at an overall 20% risk of cerebral impairment (Pahroah & Adi 2000). Scher and coworkers (2002) also found that twins whose co-twins died in utero were at increased risk of both mortality and CP. The highest rates of CP were in surviving twins whose co-twin was stillborn (4.7%), died shortly after birth (6.3%) or had CP (11.8%).

Our current understanding of neurological injury following single fetal demise suggests that it is almost exclusively seen in monchorionic (MC) twins. These twins are a subset (two thirds) of monozygotic (MZ) twins, which comprise 1/3 of the population of spontaneous and about 5% of the population of iatrogenic twins. MC placentation is thus expected in about 20% and 3% of spontaneous and iatrogenic twin gestations, respectively (Blickstein 2005). Despite the fact that all MC placentas have intertwin-transplacental vascular connections, an unbalanced inter-twin shunt occurs via the vascular connection in only 10 to 15% of MC placentas and results in different severity of the twin-twin transfusion syndrome (TTTS) (Blickstein 1990). Despite the accepted relationship between CP rates and MZ twinning, large-scale datasets are not available because of the inability of ultrasound and placental examination to differentiate like-sex dichorionic-DZ twins (half of all DZ twins) from dichorionic-MZ twins (one third of all MZ twins) (Blickstein 2005). Instead, estimations were based on the Hardy-Weinberg rule or on the proxy of like-sexed vs. unlike-sexed twins for extrapolating the risk of CP in MZ twins.

For many years it was postulated that following death of one twin, thromboplastin-like material is transfused through the vascular connection from the dead fetus into the survivor's circulation, causing end-organ damage. This 'embolic' mechanism was referred to as the 'twin embolization syndrome,' although the thromboplastin-like material was not identified, emboli were rarely seen and the neurological insults were quite often ischemic in nature. Indeed, signs of ischemic injury in meticulous post-mortem studies lead to the alternative theory, the so-called 'ischemic' theory, which postulates that blood is assumed to drain via an open anastomosis into the low-resistance vascular system of the dead fetus, resulting in acute hypovolemia, ischemia and subsequent end-organ injury in the survivor (Fig.18.2).

In addition to the effect of fetal death on brain injury in the survivor, recent data suggest that an effect can be traced to infancy whereby death during infancy of one twin also affects the risk of brain injury in the co-twin that survives beyond infancy. Pharoah (2001) compared the birth weight specific neonatal death rates and CP prevalence in the surviving twin following single infant death in like-sexed and unlike-sexed sets. The author found that the prevalence of CP in those weighing <1000 g was marginally higher in like-sexed than in unlike-sexed twin survivors, whereas it was significantly higher in those weighing 1000–1999 g. The author concluded that preterm birth, per se, predisposes to brain damage but like-sexed twins are at risk of cerebral damage in excess to that expected from prematurity. More recently, the same author (Pharoah 2005) observed that in the case of single fetal death, the prevalence of CP among like-sexed twins was 103.9/1000 survivors compared to 37.6/1000 survivors from unlike-sexed pairs. Similarly, when both twin were born alive but one twin died during infancy, the prevalence of CP was 132.0 compared with 74.1/1000 survivors, in like-sexed and unlike-sexed twins, respectively. Finally, when both twins survived infancy, the figures were still higher among like-sexed twins: 8.1 vs. 4.8/1000 survivors. When the data were stratified by birth weight below or above 1500 g, the differences seem to be clearer among the heavier twins, supporting the idea that twinning, per se, increases the risk of CP beyond the effect of premature birth.

The increased vulnerability of like-sexed twins to sustain CP is supported by data provided by Javier Laplaza et al

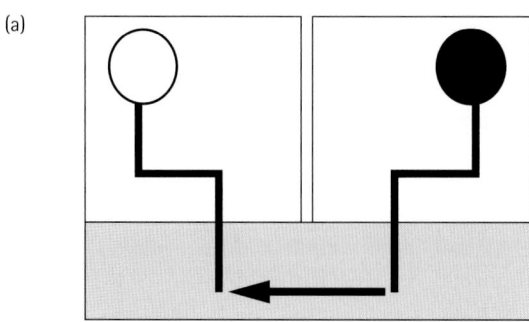

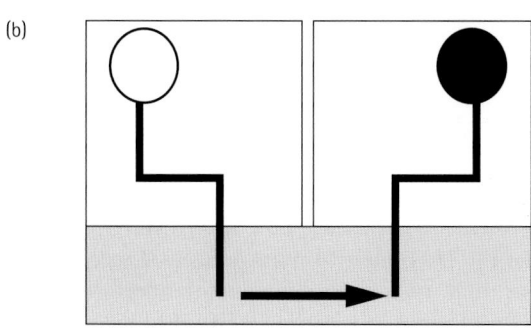

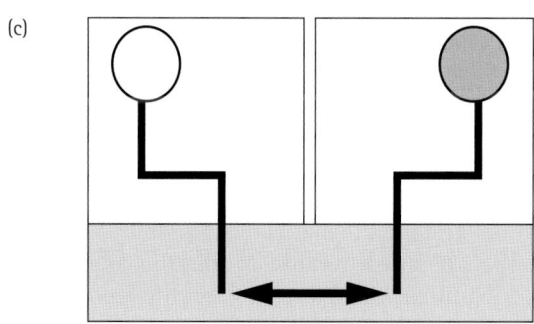

Figure 18.2 Effects of single fetal death on the survivor in MC twins. (a) The embolic theory. (b) The ischemic theory. (c) Bi-directional shunt between a fetus that would die in infancy and the survivor.

(1992), but not by data collected by Petterson et al (1993) and Nelson and Ellenberg (1995). In addition, using the Hardy–Weinberg rule to estimate zygosity, similar risks of CP were found in MZ and DZ (Petterson et al 1990). These discrepant observations might be explained by the proportion of like-sexed twins in a given twin population, which comprise all MZ twins and half of the DZ twins. This case-mix depends, in turn, on the proportion of iatrogenic twins in different populations as well as in different periods. For example, 50% of all like-sexed spontaneous twins are MZ (the Hardy–Weinberg rule) whereas only about 10% of like-sexed iatrogenic twins are assumed to be MZ. Thus, the higher the incidence of iatrogenic twins the lower the proportion of MZ sets among like-sexed twins. Moreover, and not the least important, the uncertainty is even greater con-

sidering the uncertain proportion of MC placentas among iatrogenic twins.

In the absence of population-based information regarding chorionicity and subsequent child development, hospital-based data should be interpreted with caution because of small sample size and case-mix of MC twins with and without TTTS, or those delivered at or before term. Adegbite et al (2004) determined the incidence of neurological morbidity in 76 MC and 78 DC twins born between 24 and 34 weeks' gestation. Overall, neurological morbidity in preterm MC infants was 7-fold higher than in DC infants because of chronic TTTS, discordant birth weight, and co-twin death in utero. MC infants had a higher incidence of CP (8% vs. 1%) and neurological morbidity (15% vs. 3%) than DC infants. Minakami et al (1999) examined the effects of chorionicity in 1-year-old infants from 44 MC and 164 DC sets and concluded that MC twins are at increased risk of adverse outcomes as compared with DC twins, mainly because of TTTS. Finally, Burguet and coworkers (1999) found a 6-fold increased risk for CP and severe disability in a group of prospectively examined preterm infants born from a MC twin gestation.

In this context, two additional points should be considered. First, albeit rarely, higher-order multiples (primarily triplets) might be MZ and even MC. However, the main problem is with the more frequent occurrence of DC triplets, i.e. MC twins and a singleton. In this construct, all the problems of MC twinning superimpose upon the risks of preterm birth associated with triplet gestations. The second point relates to the question why brain damage is also more frequent in the survivor when both twins were born alive but one dies in infancy (Pharoah 2005a, Scher et al 2002) when the theory suggests that damage to the survivor occurs because of an acute reduction of blood pressure following fetal death. The hypothesis proposed by Pharoah (2005b) is that hemodynamic instability (in the form of bi-directional shunts, Figure 18.2) with episodes of acute feto-fetal transfusion may produce ischemic damage in either or both twins with a resultant clinical abnormality depending on the severity, site or combination of the site and timing of observed damage. Thus, such an acute feto-fetal transfusion may cause non-fatal damage in both twins, but the severity of ischemic injury would cause infant death in one twin and CP in the survivor. The hypothesis goes on to suggest that a significant proportion of congenital anomalies and CP of unknown etiology might be attributable to MC placentation and that these anomalies, even in singletons, may be explained by early, unrecognized or unrecorded loss of one twin in these conceptions (Pharoah 2005b).

Finally, it seems that intertwin anastomoses might not be the only culprit for brain injury in MC twins. Because the presence of inflammation in the umbilical cord (funisitis) is highly associated with subsequent brain injury, Phung and coworkers (2002) evaluated the association between chorionicity and discordant chorioamnionitis and funisitis in twin gestations. In their meticulous retrospective analysis of

1156 twin placentas, the frequencies of chorioamnionitis in the non-presenting twin were significantly lower in DC compared with MC placentas and the frequency of advanced inflammation (i.e. chorioamnionitis with funisitis) was significantly lower in the non-presenting twin than in the presenting twin, but only in DC-separate placentas. The authors concluded that MC placentas are much more vulnerable to the spread of inflammation from the presenting to the non-presenting gestational sac.

It should be pointed out that it is currently unclear if preterm rupture of membranes is related to excess risk of CP among preterm twins irrespective of chorionicity (Livinec et al 2005).

THE EFFECT OF TTTS

TTTS is a relatively rare condition known for centuries. TTTS is expected to occur in 10–15% of the spontaneous MC twins, i.e. 2–4 per 10 000 births, but this number is unknown for iatrogenic twins. Regardless, TTTS attracts scientific attention for more than two decades mainly because the current prenatal diagnosis allows treatment of this complicated situation (Blickstein 1990).

Information about CP following pregnancies complicated by TTTS, with and without treatment, is available from numerous small series, whereas larger studies come primarily from referral centers and are flawed by inevitable selection bias. Moreover, until recently, studies were flawed by different diagnostic criteria, diverse severity staging and different management protocols. Irrespective of these caveats and irrespective of fetal death, it is generally accepted that the inter-fetal shunt through the transplacental anastomoses neatly explains the mechanism of neurological injury in TTTS.

In the case–control study of 17 cases, Cincotta et al (2000) found PVL and cerebral atrophy in 17% of the TTTS group, but none in the controls. Among survivors of the TTTS, 22% had CP and global developmental delay. The authors concluded that long-term neurodevelopmental morbidity in survivors of the TTTS is high. In contrast to these dismal figures, no major neurological injuries developed in any of the 33 infants, whose pregnancies were complicated by TTTS and treated with one or repeated amnioreduction, born alive after 27 weeks' gestation, without congenital malformations and survived the neonatal period (Mari et al 2001). More recently, Dickinson et al (2005) assessed 49 children from pregnancies complicated by TTTS in comparison to a contemporaneous regional cohort of preterm infants. These authors found that TTTS is associated with a significant reduction in IQ score in very preterm survivors, but there seems to be no increase in the prevalence of CP and no difference in the overall behavior and adaptive behavior scale scores. Lopriore and coworkers (2003) determined the neurodevelopmental outcomes in children after TTTS treated by either amnioreduction or no intervention. Abnormal cranial ultrasonographic findings were reported in 41% of the 29 TTTS survivors, as well as a high incidence (21%) of

CP, especially after intrauterine fetal demise of a co-twin. A similar observation was also reported by Seng et al (2000) in their series of 18 pairs of twins with TTTS. Frusca et al (2003) evaluated 32 MC pregnancies complicated by TTTS treated by amnioreduction. Eighteen out of 31 babies (58%) had a normal neurological development, 8 had major and 5 had minor neurological disabilities. Number of amnioreductions (>2) and birth weight <1000 g were both associated with abnormal neurological follow-up.

To exclude the potential confounder of birth weight, Hikino et al (2006) compared 33 newborns with TTTS and weight-matched singleton controls. Ten of the 12 (83%) TTTS patients who were diagnosed at <25 weeks and born at <28 weeks died in utero or in the neonatal period. However, CP, epilepsy and mental retardation did not differ between TTTS and control groups. The morbidity and severity of neurological deficits at school age were also similar in both groups.

At present, it is unclear how the treatment method may increase the likelihood of brain injury. A recent hypothesis suggests that radical amnioreduction performed after 24 weeks' gestation might cause a shift of blood from the fetus into the placenta and this shift might cause acute hypovolemia and explain some of the severe neurological outcomes, such as hypoxic–ischemic brain damage seen in these cases (Rodeck et al 2006). The most extensive study regarding treatment of TTTS comes from the Eurofetus randomized trial that compared the efficacy and safety of either serial amnioreduction or selective fetoscopic laser coagulation of the communicating vessels on the chorionic plate in severe TTTS at midgestation (Senat 2004). The study was concluded earlier than planned because an interim analysis demonstrated a significant benefit from laser therapy. As compared with the amnioreduction group, the laser group had (among other advantages) a lower incidence of cystic PVL and was more likely to be free of neurological complications at six months of age.

In summary, it appears that neurological damage in the TTTS is primarily gestational age-dependent and associated with syndrome-related death of one of the twins. The more severe the TTTS the more likely is that one twin will die in utero or that pregnancy will end at an earlier gestational age. The risk of CP might therefore be reduced when treatment is able to prolong pregnancy, avoid fetal death or at least interrupt between the two fetal circulations. At present, there is strong argument in favor of selective fetoscopic laser coagulation of the transplacental anastomoses.

THE EFFECT OF FETAL GROWTH

This limitation of the uterine environment to nurture two (or more) fetuses to the same extent as in singleton gestations increases with increasing gestational age and becomes evident in the third trimester when birth weights of multiples are lower than those of singletons. In addition, absolute intrauterine or relative (discordant) growth restriction is common and, at lower levels, may implicate an adaptive measure to promote an advanced gestational age at birth (Blickstein et al 2000). Williams and O'Brien (1998) suggest that phenotypic markers of asymmetric growth restriction are a better correlate of both mortality and CP in twins. In contrast, Rydhstroem (1995) concluded that birth weight discordance seems not to be related to neurological disability later in life because of similar distributions of birth weight discordance when twins with disability were compared with the population of all live-born twins weighing <2500 g. Disabled twins had a significantly lower birth weight for gestational age, but only 8.7% of the twins were considered as small for gestational age. More recently, Scher et al (2002) found that twins from growth-discordant pairs were at increased risk of both mortality and CP, a finding that is indirectly supported by the observation of Yinon et al (2005) who found that growth restriction in preterm discordant twins is associated with a 7.7-fold increased risk for major neonatal morbidity, including intraventricular hemorrhage.

It should be stressed that information related to genuine growth restriction in twins is largely not available because the required intrauterine follow-up to establish growth restriction is poorly documented and, in addition, the designation of small for gestational age frequently employs singleton standards rather than birth weight by gestational age ('growth curves') standards for twins and higher-order multiples. From a practical point of view, even population-based studies may be of insufficient sample-size to document a relationship between risk of CP and intrauterine growth (Gliniania et al 2006). To further explore this relationship, data from 9 European CP registers were examined (Gliniania et al 2006). Sex-specific fetal growth standards for twins were derived for each of the 373 twin cases. The authors found that for twins born at $\geqslant$32 weeks' gestation, an increased risk of CP is associated with deviations from optimal intrauterine growth at about 1 SD above mean weight, whereas for twins born at <32 weeks' gestation, this pattern is only demonstrable for babies weighing below the optimum weight-for-gestation.

Discordant growth among MC twins is an important subset of growth aberrations. This circumstance is currently considered to be distinct from TTTS and is related to unequal sharing of the placental territory and to the frequent velamentous cord insertion of the smaller twin. In some instances, one may wonder how the smaller twin survives despite sharing less than 10% of the placental surface. It is currently postulated that an arterio-arterial ('rescue') anastomosis supplies the smaller twin. The relation with cerebral palsy was studied by Gratacos et al (2004) who prospectively examined a cohort of 42 MC twins diagnosed with single growth restriction and managed expectantly. This cohort was compared to 29 DC and 32 MC twins without single growth restriction, delivered at 26–34 weeks during the study period. The incidence of fetal demise and PVL was significantly increased in MC twins complicated with single growth restriction as compared with the other study groups. The

incidence of fetal demise and parenchymal brain damage was significantly higher in pregnancies with intermittent absent or reversed end diastolic velocity measured by Doppler than in those without these Doppler findings. Brain damage usually occurred in the larger twin, irrespective of whether the smaller twin was born alive or not (Gratacos et al 2004).

In summary, the contribution of growth aberrations to neurological damage cannot be excluded, regardless of the conflicting data.

EMBRYONIC AND EARLY FETAL LOSS

Embryonic loss is relatively frequent among multiple gestations, creating the so-called 'vanishing twin' syndrome (Landy & Keith 1998). It has been hypothesized that the mechanism involved in brain damage in the survivor following single fetal demise in advanced pregnancies might also be implicated in the etiology of spastic cerebral palsy in singleton survivors of the vanishing twin syndrome (Pharoah & Cooke 1997). In simple terms, this hypothesis suggests that a significant proportion of congenital anomalies and CP of unknown etiology are attributable to a MC placentation and that these anomalies, even in singletons, may be explained by early, unrecognized or unrecorded loss of one conceptus in a MC conception (Pharoah 2005a). However, the main problem with this theory is that the 'classic' ultrasound image of the vanishing twin syndrome is more often suggestive of DC placentas that usually lack intertwin anastomoses (Blickstein 1998). It could be argued, however, that our knowledge about the DC placenta and the absence of transplacental vascular connections derives from the examination of placentas delivered at the second and third trimester. It may well be that some DC placentas do have anastomoses, but they disappear at the same time of the 'vanishing' of one twin.

Regardless of the hypotheses, it has been established that many early fetal deaths are frequently overlooked. Pahroah (2002) found significant errors in registration of fetal deaths, in the presence of a fetus papyraceous, and in correctly registering the gender of the demised fetus. The result of this miscoding and inconsistency in recording fetal sex is difficulty in assuming that different registered sex represents in fact, dizygotic multiple births. More recently, Pharoah (2006) reported on some improvement in registration of fetal deaths in multiple pregnancies, but noted a gray-zone where fetal death occurs before 24 weeks, and which causes national and international confusion whether or not registration is legally required.

In the absence of complete registration of embryonic and fetal deaths it is clearly impossible to relate any adverse outcome to the vanishing twin syndrome in the population at large. However, more complete registries exist for ART conceptions. Recently, Pinborg et al (2005) assessed the incidence rates of spontaneous reductions in in vitro fertilization/intracytoplasmic sperm injection (IVF/ICSI) twin gestations and compared short- and long-term morbidity in survivors of a vanishing co-twin with singletons and live born twins. Of all IVF singletons born, 10.4% come from a twin gestation in early pregnancy (i.e. survivors of the vanishing twin syndrome). After adjustments, survivors of the vanishing twin syndrome were more frequently born preterm and had a low birth weight. However, no excess risk of neurological complications in survivors of a vanishing co-twin compared to the singleton cohort was found. Similar results were obtained from an underpowered case-control study of maternities with evidence of a vanishing twin on ultrasound (Newton et al 2006).

Taken together, the association of embryonic and early fetal loss and CP cannot be disproved unless further research is done on this intriguing subject.

MODE OF DELIVERY

Multiple births might be associated with increased intrapartum asphyxia mainly because of frequent fetal malpresentation leading to potentially traumatic delivery. Moreover, intervention during labor for signs of fetal distress seems to be more difficult simply because intrapartum monitoring is more difficult in twins than in singletons. It is also generally accepted that the second-born is doing worse in terms of immediate neonatal outcome regardless of the mode of delivery (Scher et al 2002).

Whereas the vast majority of higher-order multiples are born by the abdominal route, the current practice is to recommend a cesarean section for all pairs with a non-vertex presenting twin and a vaginal delivery for vertex-vertex twin sets. The preferred mode of delivery for vertex-non-vertex pairs is still controversial and a subject for an ongoing international randomized trial. Irrespective of the presentation combination, the recent reports suggest that more than 60% of the twins are born by cesarean section.

In the context of this chapter, it seems pertinent to consider the mode of delivery of LBW infants. One epidemiological study (Rydhstrom 1990a) focused on the effect of cesarean section on CP and mental retardation in twins weighing <1500 g. The analysis did not reveal any significant impact of cesarean section on the CP rates for LBW twins, even when fetal presentation was considered. The same author (Rydhstrom 1990b) also examined the effect of cesarean delivery in twins with birth weight difference of ≥1.0 Kg and, again, no correlation was found between mode of delivery and CP and/or mental retardation at the age of 8 years or more. Shinwell and coworkers (2003) also reported no effect of the mode of delivery on adverse neurological findings among VLBW twins and triplets.

SPECIAL SITUATIONS

Some rare forms of multiple pregnancies are a true clinical challenge. These special situations exist in monoamniotic conceptions, when both twins are contained within the same sac and cord entanglement is the rule rather than the exception. In such circumstances, tightening of the cord may

cause double fetal death and not less important, it may cause single fetal death with the consequent risk of brain damage to the survivor. For this reason many clinicians will opt for an elective preterm cesarean delivery at 32–33 weeks' gestation. This gestational age is chosen as a compromise between the risk of intrauterine fetal death and the risk of extreme preterm birth.

In general, elective preterm delivery – that is, a prophylactic measure to avoid potential complications – is not unanimously accepted because of the associated risks of preterm birth. This management, exclusively suggested for monoamniotic twins, was recently suggested also for all MC twins. Barigye et al (2005) examined the prospective death in MC twins and found that the substantial prospective risk (4.3%) of single or double deaths was sufficiently high to consider an elective preterm delivery in uncomplicated MC pregnancies and also proposed a valid argument that even single deaths are a serious threat to the survivor. Another study, however, found a much lower prospective risk of 1.2% and questioned this recommendation (Simoes et al 2006). To date, there are insufficient data to compare between the risks of brain (and other organ) injury as a result of elective preterm births and the prospective risk of mortality in MC twins.

Another special circumstance is the heroic measure of delayed interval delivery carried out in extremely preterm births, i.e. intentionally increasing the interval between delivery of the first fetus and subsequent fetuses. Despite some favorable European reports of a significant latency, the American experience was different (Livingston et al 2004): a median latency of 2 days, 2 in utero deaths out of 19 retained fetuses, 10 neonatal deaths and 7 survived until hospital discharge, of which 6 had major sequelae from prematurity.

This chapter is incomplete without pointing out the increased risk of brain anomalies in multiple pregnancies. Data from the USA suggest that hydrocephaly and microcephaly were identified at birth in 5.0/10 000 and 5.9/10 000 live born twins, respectively (Ananth & Smulian 2005). After adjustment for potential confounders, these figures were significantly lower for the period 1998–2000 compared with 1989–1991, and possibly reflecting the advances in prenatal diagnosis and the feasibility of selective termination of the anomalous fetus.

EPILOGUE

The evidence suggests that brain injury and multiple births are causally related. This relationship emerges from the inherent inability of the uterine milieu to adequately nurture multiples. It follows that the primary cause of brain injury in multiples is preterm birth and not the relatively rare syndromes (Blickstein 2006a). However, this substantial risk of prematurity is frequently preceded (or superimposed) by additional risks that are associated with one of the many pathological twinning processes. In many instances it is unknown what the exact cause of brain injury is. For

Table 18.1 Factors that were attributed to the increased risk of brain injury in multiple pregnancies. Question mark denotes equivocal findings

Preterm and extremely preterm birth
Very and extremely low birth weight
Intrauterine growth restriction
Congenital brain anomalies
Preterm rupture of membranes (?)
MC twinning
Single fetal death in MC twins
Bi-directional shunt in MC twins (?)
Embryonic death (?)
Traumatic delivery (?)

example, consider the case of grade III TTTS complicated with discordant growth that was treated by laser photocoagulation of the inter-twin anastomoses at 21 weeks and delivered vaginally at 26 weeks because of preterm rupture of membranes and chorioamnionitis. In such a circumstance – which is not infrequently encountered – brain damage could possibly be attributed to preterm birth, to the inflammatory process that preceded amniorrhexis, to the TTTS per se, to intrauterine growth restriction and perhaps to the method of delivery.

Many of the attributed risk factors for brain injury during a multiple pregnancy are incompletely understood (Table 18.1). In some instances, evidence is lacking for an otherwise logical explanation. For example, the statement that twin pregnancies reach term early (i.e. at 37–38 weeks) is supported by several lines of circumstantial evidence. Thus, it

would be only logical to deliver all twins by this gestational period and avoid all the risks associated with post-term pregnancies. However, there is no evidence that such a policy is effective in reducing the risk of brain injury.

Finally, whereas elimination of perinatal brain injury is probably impossible, reduction of the incidence of brain damage is achievable and of primary importance to every clinician worldwide. Thus, in the context of multiple pregnancy, the first step is reduction of the number of iatrogenic high order multiples (Blickstein & Keith 2005). It is comforting to note that a trend toward a decrease in the incidence of triplets or more has been documented in the past 5 years in several developed countries (Blickstein & Keith 2005). However, at the same time, the number of twins continued to increase. The net effect of these different trends is a continuing increase in the number of preterm births at risk for brain damage. Thus, the ultimate goal would be a singleton pregnancy following assisted procreation. The second step is to better understand the natural history of twin gestations. Because, at present, the elimination of prematurity is not feasible, it is more important and certainly more realistic to look for practical methods to reduce the prevalence of extreme prematurity.

Finally, no doubt exists that multiple pregnancies are at high risk and, as such, deserve the closest observation possible. This sweeping statement does not imply that there is remedy for every complication of multiple pregnancies. Nevertheless, it suggests that consultation with specialized clinics and trained personnel should be sought as frequently as required. When indicated, transfer to a tertiary center – for both pregnancy surveillance and delivery – should be encouraged. The double or triple joy of having twins or triplets should not be clouded by potentially preventable brain injury.

REFERENCES

Adegbite A L, Castille S, Ward S, Bajoria R 2004 Neuromorbidity in preterm twins in relation to chorionicity and discordant birth weight. Am J Obstet Gynecol 190:156–163.

Ananth C V, Smulian J Cm 2005 Trends in congenital malformations, chromosomal anomalies, and infant mortality in twin births. In: Blickstein I, Keith LG (eds). Multiple pregnancy. 2nd edn. Taylor and Francis, Oxford, UK, pp. 246–251.

Barigye O, Pasquini L, Galea P et al 2005 High risk of unexpected late fetal death in monochorionic twins despite intensive ultrasound surveillance: a cohort study. PLoS Med 2:e172.

Blickstein I 1990 The twin-twin transfusion syndrome. Obstet Gynecol 76:714–722.

Blickstein I 1998 Reflections on the hypothesis for the etiology of spastic cerebral palsy caused by the 'vanishing twin' syndrome. Dev Med Child Neurol 40:358.

Blickstein I 2000 When does 'term' occur in twin gestations? Gemell Rev 1:116–117.

Blickstein I 2004 Do multiple gestations raise the risk of cerebral palsy? Clin Perinatol 31:395–408.

Blickstein I 2005 Estimation of iatrogenic monozygotic twinning rate following assisted reproduction:

Pitfalls and caveats. Am J Obstet Gynecol 192:365–368.

Blickstein I 2006a Monochorionicity in perspective. Ultrasound Obstet Gynecol 27:235–238.

Blickstein I 2006b Epidemiology of cerebral palsy in multiple pregnancies. In: Kilby M, Baker P, Critchley H, Field D (eds) Multiple pregnancy. RCOG, London, UK, pp. 245–254.

Blickstein I, Goldman R D, Mazkereth R 2000 Adaptive growth restriction as a pattern of birth weight discordance in twin gestations. Obstet Gynecol 96:986–990.

Blickstein I, Keith L G 2001 The spectrum of iatrogenic multiple pregnancy. In: Blickstein I, Keith L G (eds) Iatrogenic multiple pregnancy: Clinical implications. Parthenon, London, pp. 1–7.

Blickstein I, Keith L G 2005 The decreased rates of triplet births: temporal trends and biologic speculations. Am J Obstet Gynecol 193: 327–331.

Blickstein I, Weissman A 1999 Estimating the risk of cerebral palsy following assisted conceptions. N Eng J Med 341:313–314.

Bonellie S R, Currie D, Chalmers J 2005 Comparison of risk factors for cerebral palsy

in twins and singletons. Dev Med Child Neurol 47:587–91.

Burguet A, Monnet E, Pauchard J Y et al 1999 Some risk factors for cerebral palsy in very premature infants: importance of premature rupture of membranes and monochorionic twin placentation. Biol Neonate 75:177–186.

Cincotta R B, Gray P H, Phythian G et al 2000 Long term outcome of twin-twin transfusion syndrome. Arch Dis Child Fetal Neonatal Ed 83:F171–F176.

Derom C, Derom R 2005 The East Flanders prospective twin survey. In: Blickstein I, Keith L G (eds) Multiple pregnancy, 2nd edn. Taylor and Francis, Oxford UK, pp. 39–47.

Dickinson J E, Duncombe G J, Evans S F et al 2005 The long term neurologic outcome of children from pregnancies complicated by twin-to-twin transfusion syndrome. BJOG 112:63–68.

Dimitriou G, Pharoah P O, Nicolaides K H, Greenough A 2004 Cerebral palsy in triplet pregnancies with and without iatrogenic reduction. Eur J Pediatr 163:449–451.

Frusca T, Soregaroli M, Fichera A et al 2003 Pregnancies complicated by twin-twin transfusion syndrome: outcome and long-term neurological follow-up. Eur J Obstet Gynecol Reprod Biol 107:145–150.

Geva E, Lerner-Geva L, Stavorovsky Z et al 1998 Multifetal pregnancy reduction: a possible risk factor for periventricular leukomalacia in premature newborns. Fertil Steril 69:845–850.

Glinianaia S V, Jarvis S, Topp M et al 2006 SCPE Collaboration of European Cerebral Palsy Registers. Intrauterine growth and cerebral palsy in twins: a European multicenter study. Twin Res Hum Genet 9:460–466.

Gratacos E, Carreras E, Becker J et al 2004 Prevalence of neurological damage in monochorionic twins with selective intrauterine growth restriction and intermittent absent or reversed end-diastolic umbilical artery flow. Ultrasound Obstet Gynecol 24:159–163.

Grether J K, Nelson K B, Cummins S K 1993 Twinning and cerebral palsy: experience in four northern California counties, births 1983 through 1985. Pediatrics 92:854–858.

Helmerhorst F M, Perquin D A, Donker D, Keirse M J 2004 Perinatal outcome of singletons and twins after assisted conception: a systematic review of controlled studies. BMJ 328:261.

Hikino S, Ohga S, Kanda T et al 2006 Long-term outcome of infants with twin-to-twin transfusion syndrome. Fetal Diagn Ther 22:68–74.

Hvidtjorn D, Grove J, Schendel D E et al 2006 Cerebral palsy among children born after in vitro fertilization: the role of preterm delivery — a population-based, cohort study. Pediatrics 118:475–482.

Kiely J L, Kiely M, Blickstein I 2000 Contribution of the rise in multiple births to a potential increase in cerebral palsy. Pediat Res 47:314.

Landy H J, Keith L G 1998 The vanishing twin: a review. Hum Reprod Update 4:177–183.

Laplaza F J, Root L, Tassanawipas A, Cervera P 1992 Cerebral palsy in twins. Dev Med Child Neurol 34:1053–1063.

Liu J, Li Z, Lin Q et al 2000 Cerebral palsy and multiple births in China. Int J Epidemiol 29:292–299.

Livinec F, Ancel P Y, Marret S et al 2005 Prenatal risk factors for cerebral palsy in very preterm singletons and twins. Obstet Gynecol 105:1341–1347.

Livingston J C, Livingston L W, Ramsey R, Sibai B M 2004 Second-trimester asynchronous multifetal delivery results in poor perinatal outcome. Obstet Gynecol 103:77–81.

Lopriore E, Nagel H T, Vandenbussche F P, Walther F J 2003 Long-term neurodevelopmental outcome in twin-to-twin transfusion syndrome. Am J Obstet Gynecol 189:1314–1319.

Luke B, Bigger H R, Leurgans S, Sietsema D 1996 The cost of prematurity: a case-control study of twins vs singletons. Am J Public Health 86:809–814.

Luke B, Brown M B, Alexandre P K et al 2005 The cost of twin pregnancy: maternal and neonatal factors. Am J Obstet Gynecol 192:909–915.

Mari G, Detti L, Oz U, Abuhamad A Z 2001 Long-term outcome in twin-twin transfusion syndrome treated with serial aggressive amnioreduction. Am J Obstet Gynecol 183:211–217.

Martin J A, Hamilton B E, Sutton P D et al 2003 Births: final data for 2002. Natl Vital Stat Rep 52:1–113.

Minakami H, Honma Y, Matsubara S et al I 1999 Effects of placental chorionicity on outcome in twin pregnancies. A cohort study. J Reprod Med 44:595–600.

Minakami H, Sato I 1996 Reestimating date of delivery in multifetal pregnancies. J Am Med Assoc 275:1432–1434.

Nelson K B, Ellenberg J H 1995 Childhood neurological disorders in twins. Paediatr Perinat Epidemiol 9:135–145.

Newton R, Casabonne D, Johnson A, Pharoah P 2003 A case-control study of vanishing twin as a risk factor for cerebral palsy. Twin Res 6:83–84.

Petterson B, Nelson K B, Watson L, Stanley F 1993 Twins, triplets, and cerebral palsy in births in Western Australia in the 1980s. BMJ 307: 1239–1243.

Petterson B, Stanley F, Henderson D 1990 Cerebral palsy in multiple births in Western Australia: genetic aspects. Am J Med Genet 37:346–351.

Pharoah P O 2001 Cerebral palsy in the surviving twin associated with infant death of the co-twin. Arch Dis Child Fetal Neonatal Ed 84:F111–F116.

Pharoah P O 2002 Errors in birth registrations and coding of twins and higher order multiples. Twin Res 5:270–272.

Pharoah P O 2005a Risk of cerebral palsy in multiple pregnancies. Obstet Gynecol Clin North Am 32:55–67.

Pharoah P O 2005b Causal hypothesis for some congenital anomalies. Twin Res Hum Genet 8:543–550.

Pharoah P O 2006 Fetal death registration in multiple births: anomalies and clinical significance. Twin Res Hum Genet 9:587–590.

Pharoah P O D, Cooke T 1996 Cerebral palsy and multiple births. Arch Dis Child Fetal Neonatal ed 75: F174–F177.

Pharoah P O, Adi Y 2000 Consequences of in-utero death in a twin pregnancy. Lancet 355:1597–1602.

Pharoah P O, Cooke R W 1997 A hypothesis for the aetiology of spastic cerebral palsy — the vanishing twin. Dev Med Child Neurol 39:292–296.

Phung D T, Blickstein I, Goldman R D et al 2002 The Northwestern Twin Chorionicity Study: I. Discordant inflammatory findings that are related to chorionicity in presenting versus nonpresenting twins. Am J Obstet Gynecol 186:1041–1045.

Pinborg A, Lidegaard O, la Cour Freiesleben N, Andersen A N 2005 Consequences of vanishing twins in IVF/ICSI pregnancies. Hum Reprod 20:2821–2829.

Pinborg A, Loft A, Schmidt L et al 2004 Neurological sequelae in twins born after assisted conception: controlled national cohort study. BMJ 329:311.

Rodeck C H, Weisz B, Peebles D M, Jauniaux E 2006 Hypothesis: the placental 'steal' phenomenon — a possible hazard of amnioreduction. Fetal Diagn Ther 21:302–306.

Rydhstroem H 1995 The relationship of birth weight and birth weight discordance to cerebral palsy or mental retardation later in life for twins weighing less than 2500 grams. Am J Obstet Gynecol 173:680–686.

Rydhstrom H 1990a Prognosis for twins with birth weight less than 1500 gm: the impact of cesarean section in relation to fetal presentation. Am J Obstet Gynecol 163:528–533.

Rydhstrom H 1990b Prognosis for twins discordant in birth weight of 1.0 kg or more: the impact of cesarean section. J Perinat Med 18:31–37.

Scher A I, Petterson B, Blair E et al 2002 The risk of mortality or cerebral palsy in twins: a collaborative population-based study. Pediatr Res 52:671–681.

Senat M V, Deprest J, Boulvain M et al 2004 Endoscopic laser surgery versus serial amnioreduction for severe twin-to-twin transfusion syndrome. N Engl J Med 351:136–144.

Seng Y C, Rajadurai V S 2000 Twin-twin transfusion syndrome: a five year review. Arch Dis Child Fetal Neonatal Ed 83:F168–170.

Shinwell E S, Blickstein I, Lusky A, Reichman B 2003 Excess risk of mortality in very low birthweight triplets: a national, population based study. Arch Dis Child Fetal Neonatal Ed 88:F36–F40.

Simoes T, Amaral N, Lerman R et al 2006 Prospective risk of intrauterine death of monochorionic-diamniotic twins. Am J Obstet Gynecol 195:134–139.

Topp M, Huusom L D, Langhoff-Roos J et al 2004 Multiple birth and cerebral palsy in Europe: a multicenter study. Acta Obstet Gynecol Scand 83:548–553.

Touyama M, Ochiai Y, Touyama J 2000 Cerebral palsy in twins in Okinawa. No To Hattatsu 32:35–38.

Williams K, Hennessy E, Alberman B 1996 Cerebral palsy: effects of twinning, birthweight, and gestational age. Arch Dis Child Fetal Neonatal ed 75: F178–F182.

Williams M C, O'Brien W F 1998 Low weight/length ratio to assess risk of cerebral palsy and perinatal mortality in twins. Am J Perinatol 15:225–228.

Yinon Y, Mazkereth R, Rosentzweig N et al 2005 Growth restriction as a determinant of outcome in preterm discordant twins. Obstet Gynecol 105:80–84.

Yokoyama Y, Shimizu T, Hayakawa K 1995 Prevalence of cerebral palsy in twins, triplets and quadruplets. Int J Epidemiol 24:943–958.

Infection, inflammation and brain injury

Jimmy Espinoza, Roberto Romero, Francesca Gotsch, Juan Pedro Kusanovic, Offer Erez, Bo Hyun Yoon and Sonia S Hassan

INTRODUCTION

Fetal infection/inflammation has been implicated in the pathophysiology of preterm parturition and fetal and neonatal injury (Gomez et al 1998b, Romero et al 1998b), as well as long-term handicap including cerebral palsy (CP) (Yoon et al 2000a) and chronic lung disease (Yoon et al 1999b). Intrauterine infection/inflammation, now recognized as a frequent and important cause of preterm parturition (Brocklehurst 1999, Gibbs et al 1992, Goldenberg et al 2000, Gomez et al 1998b, Ledger 1989, Minkoff 1983, Naeye & Ross 1982, Romero & Mazor 1988, Romero et al 1988, 1998b), is the only pathologic process for which both a firm causal link with prematurity has been established and a defined molecular pathophysiology is known (Romero et al 1994). In this chapter, we review the role of maternal and fetal infection/inflammation as a mechanism of disease of brain injury in both term and preterm pregnancies.

INFLAMMATION AS A MECHANISM OF DISEASE

The traditional signs and symptoms of inflammation including heat, pain, redness, swelling and loss of function describe localized inflammation (Gallin & Snyderman 1999). However, the diagnosis of systemic inflammation includes a different set of criteria now referred to as the 'systemic inflammatory response syndrome' (SIRS). This term was introduced in 1992 by the American College of Chest Physicians and the Society of Critical Care Medicine to describe a complex set of findings that often involve cardiovascular abnormalities thought to be the result of systemic activation of the innate immune system in adults (American College of Chest Physicians/Society of Critical Care Medicine Consensus Conference 1992). The changes include fever, tachycardia, hyperventilation and an elevated white blood cell count (American College of Chest Physicians/Society of Critical Care Medicine Consensus Conference 1992), and have been attributed to the effects of cytokines and other pro-inflammatory mediators (Weiss et al 1999). More recently, the same organization reported that the elevation of circulating pro-inflammatory mediators, such as IL-6, may be associated with SIRS and that this observation may lead to a new definition of the syndrome in adult patients, as the clinical and laboratory findings originally proposed to characterize SIRS were non-specific (Levy et al 2003). The fetal counterpart of SIRS was first described in 1997 (Gomez et al 1997), using the same parameter now proposed for use in adults, namely an elevated plasma IL-6 concentration. The term 'fetal inflammatory response syndrome' (FIRS) was coined to refer to this entity (Gomez et al 1998b).

Inflammation is a host response to various insults, including infection, trauma, toxins, and neoplasia (Gallin & Snyderman 1999). In adults, an excessive inflammatory response has been implicated in the pathogenesis of diabetes, atherosclerosis, Alzheimer disease, cataracts, cancer, rheumatic fever, systemic lupus erythematosus, as well as rheumatoid arthritis (Gallin & Snyderman 1999). In contrast, the only described cause of systemic inflammation in the fetus is infection (Gomez et al 1998b).

THE FETAL INFLAMMATORY RESPONSE SYNDROME

The term 'fetal inflammatory response syndrome' was coined to define a subclinical condition originally described in fetuses of women presenting with preterm labor and intact membranes, as well as preterm premature rupture of membranes (PROM) (Gomez et al 1998b, Romero et al 1998b). The operational definition was a fetal plasma IL-6 concentration above 11 pg/mL (Romero et al 1998b). IL-6, a major mediator of the host response to infection and tissue damage, is capable of eliciting biochemical, physiologic and immunologic changes in the host, including stimulation of the production of C-reactive protein by liver cells, the acute phase plasma protein response, activation of T and natural killer cells, etc.

The original work describing FIRS was based on fetal blood samples obtained by cordocentesis (Gomez et al 1998b, Romero et al 1998b). Similar conclusions have been drawn by studying umbilical cord blood at birth including the elevation of pro-inflammatory cytokines and their relationship to the likelihood of clinical and suspected sepsis (Chaiworapongsa et al 2002b, Witt et al 2005, Yoon et al 1999b).

Pathological examination of the umbilical cord is a simple approach to determine whether fetal inflammation was present before birth. Funisitis and chorionic vasculitis are the histopathologic hallmark of FIRS (Pacora et al 2002). Funisitis is associated with endothelial activation, a key mechanism in the development of organ damage (D'Alquen et al 2005). Indeed, neonates with funisitis are at increased risk for neonatal sepsis (Yoon et al 2000b) and long-term handicaps, such as bronchopulmonary dysplasia (BPD) (Yoon et al 1999b) and CP (Yoon et al 2000a).

Another approach to detect FIRS is to measure the concentration of C-reactive protein in umbilical cord blood, which is elevated in patients with amniotic fluid infection, funisitis and congenital neonatal sepsis (Yoon et al 2003). In addition, intra-amniotic inflammation is a risk factor for impending preterm delivery and adverse perinatal outcome in women with preterm delivery; thus neutrophils in the amniotic fluid are predominantly of fetal origin (Sampson et al 1997) and the amniotic fluid white blood cell count can be used as an indirect index of fetal inflammation (Sampson et al 1997).

Fetal microbial invasion or other insults result in a systemic fetal inflammatory response that can progress to multiple organ dysfunction, septic shock and even death in the absence of timely delivery. Evidence of multi-systemic involvement in cases of FIRS includes increased concentrations of fetal plasma MMP-9 (Romero et al 1998a), an enzyme involved in the digestion of type IV collagen and in the pathophysiology of preterm PROM (Romero et al 2002). Moreover, several fetal organs (see below), including the brain, (see below), lungs, hematopoietic system, adrenals, heart, kidneys, thymus and skin, have been proposed to be target organs during FIRS (Fig. 19.1) (Berry et al 1995, 1998, Di Naro et al 2006, Espinoza et al 2003, Gomez et al 1998a, Heine et al 1998, Kim et al 2003, Romero et al 2004, Yoon et al 1998, 1999a).

WHY DOES THE FETUS MOUNT AN INFLAMMATORY RESPONSE?

The fetal inflammatory response syndrome was first described in the context of intrauterine infection. It was proposed that the onset of preterm labor would have survival value and that it would be part of the repertoire of host defense mechanisms against infection (Gomez et al 1998b, Romero et al 1998b). The fetus would use the effector limb of the immune response via the secretion of pro-inflammatory cytokines to signal the onset of labor and exit a hostile intrauterine environment. Evidence in support of this hypothesis has recently been provided by Lahra et al (Lahra & Jeffery 2004), who reported that infants who survived the neonatal period had a higher prevalence of histological chorioamnionitis (95% CI, 1.02–1.21; $P = 0.02$) and a higher rate of umbilical vasculitis/funisitis at 25 to 29 weeks of gestation (95% CI, 0.33–0.86; $P = 0.01$) and at 30 to 34 weeks of gestation (95% CI, 0.18–0.85; $P = 0.02$), when compared to those who died in the perinatal period.

CONTRIBUTION OF FETAL INFECTION/ INFLAMMATION TO WHITE MATTER DAMAGE AND CEREBRAL PALSY (see also p. 439)

WHITE MATTER DAMAGE

White matter lesions can be localized or diffuse; the localized form is characterized by localized necrosis of all cellular elements with subsequent cystic formation (Volpe 2001). In contrast, the diffuse form is characterized by a diffuse injury to oligodendroglial precursors (Volpe 2001). Recent neuroimaging studies indicate that the prevalence of periventricular white matter lesions is declining, whereas that of focal or diffuse non-cystic white-matter injury is increasing in the perinatal period (Back 2006). The conventional approach to diagnose the focal component of peri-

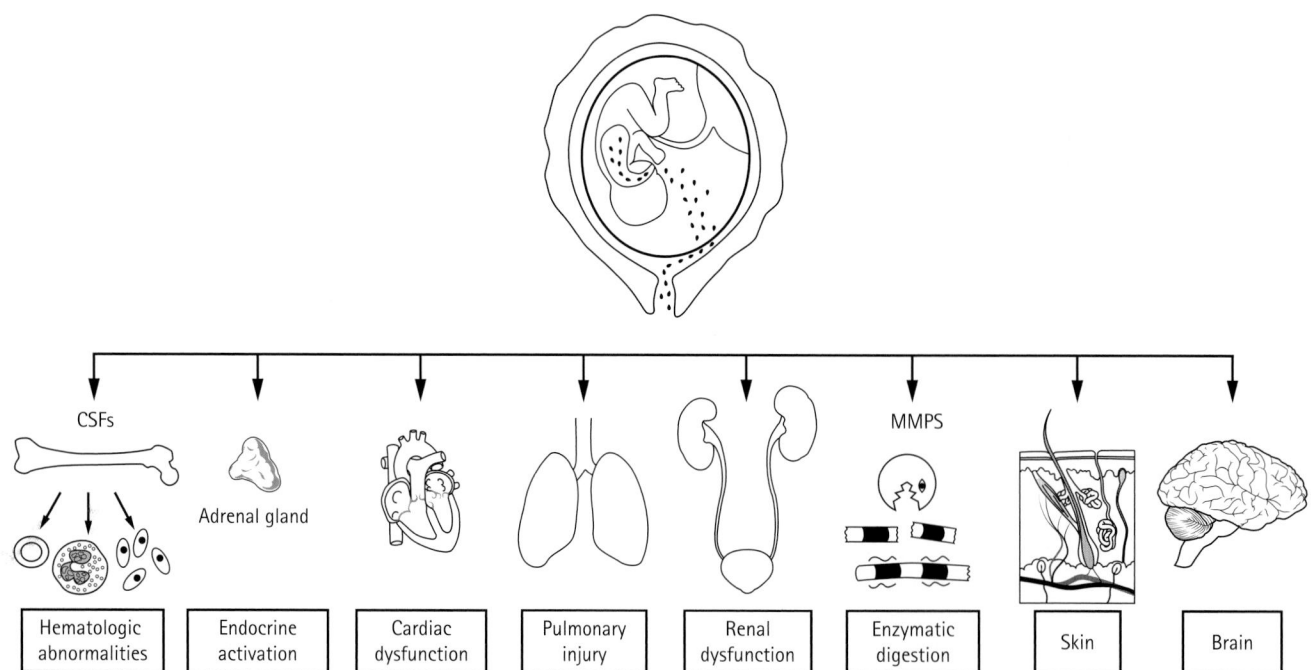

Figure 19.1 Fetal target organs during fetal inflammatory response syndrome (FIRS).

ventricular lesions is cranial ultrasonography in the neonatal period. However, the diffuse form of the white matter damage cannot be identified using this approach (Volpe 2001). Thus, diffusion-weighted magnetic resonance imaging (MRI) (Counsell et al 2003, Inder et al 1999) has been used to determine the presence of the diffuse white matter damage. However, the diagnostic indices of this method have not been reported (Volpe 2001). Additional imaging techniques include diffusion tensor (MRI) (Huppi et al 2001) and magnetic resonance spectroscopy (MRS) (Robertson et al 2000).

Initial reports using MRS indicate that the brains of neonates with white matter damage have different biochemical profiles than those of neonates without these lesions (Robertson et al 2000). The authors compared the peak area ratios of lactate/phosphocreatine (Cr), N-acetyl aspartate (NAA)/Cr, myo-inositol/Cr and choline/Cr using proton magnetic resonance spectroscopy, and reported that the mean peak area ratios of lactate/Cr and myo-inositol/Cr were significantly higher in infants with white matter lesions than that of infants without white matter lesions (Robertson et al 2000).

White matter damage (WMD) identified by neonatal brain ultrasound is currently the best predictor of long-term disability in preterm infants (Dammann et al 2005, de Vries & Groenendaal 2002). Adverse outcomes associated with WMD include cognitive limitations (Dammann et al 2002), behavioral problems (Hagberg et al 2001), visuospatial difficulties (Stewart et al 1999) and CP (Kuban & Leviton 1994). WMD is more common among children of pregnancies complicated by chorioamnionitis (Verma et al 1997) and purulent amniotic fluid (Bejar et al 1988), as well as among neonates with bacteremia (Leviton & Paneth 1990).

Experimental evidence indicates that intrauterine infection results in WMD and neuronal lesions (Bell & Hallenbeck 2002, Debillon 2003, Debillon et al 2000, Duncan et al 2002, Hagberg et al 2002, Mallard et al 2003, Yoon et al 1997b). Yoon et al (1997b) experimentally induced ascending intrauterine infection with *E. coli* in 31 pregnant rabbits and inoculated 14 controls with sterile saline solution. Histological evidence of WMD was identified in 12 fetuses born to 10 *E. coli*-inoculated rabbits, as opposed to none in the control group ($P < 0.05$). All cases with WMD had evidence of intra-uterine inflammation. Similar findings were reported by DeBillon et al (2000, 2003). Increased cytokine expression in the white matter (mainly TNF-α (Deguchi et al 1996, 1997, Kadhim et al 2001, Yoon et al 1997c) and, to a lesser extent, IL-6 (Yoon et al 1997c), IL-1β (Kadhim et al 2001, Yoon et al 1997c) and IL-2 (Kadhim et al 2002) has been demonstrated by immunohistochemistry studies performed in neonatal brains with periventricular leukomalacia (PVL), while increased immunoreactivity for TNF-α has been reported in the neocortex, hippocampus, basal ganglia and thalamus of neonatal brains with PVL (Kadhim et al 2003).

PROPOSED MECHANISMS OF WHITE MATTER DAMAGE DURING INFECTION/INFLAMMATION

1. *Pro-inflammatory cytokines:* The release of inflammatory cytokines (i.e. TNF-α) during the course of intrauterine infection could participate in the pathogenesis of PVL by four different mechanisms (Leviton 1993):
   (1) Induction of fetal hypotension and brain ischemia (Iida et al 1992).
   (2) Stimulation of the tissue factor production and release, which in turn activates the hemostatic system and contributes to coagulation necrosis of white matter (van der et al 1990).
   (3) Induction of the release of platelet activating factor, which could act as a membrane detergent causing direct brain damage (Camussi et al 1987).
   (4) A direct cytotoxic effect of TNF-α on oligodendrocytes and myelin (Robbins et al 1992, Selmaj & Raine 1988).

More recently, the same group (Dammann & Leviton 2000) proposed a conceptual framework by which an initiator (infectious or non-infectious) may induce maternal and/or fetal inflammatory responses which will in turn lead to intraventricular hemorrhage, white matter damage and long-term neurological disability (Fig. 19.2). Accumulating evidence indicates that the uterine cavity is not sterile in non-pregnant women (Andrews et al 2005, Ansbacher et al 1967, Cowling et al 1992, Moller et al 1995, Nelson & Nichols 1986). We have proposed that abnormal

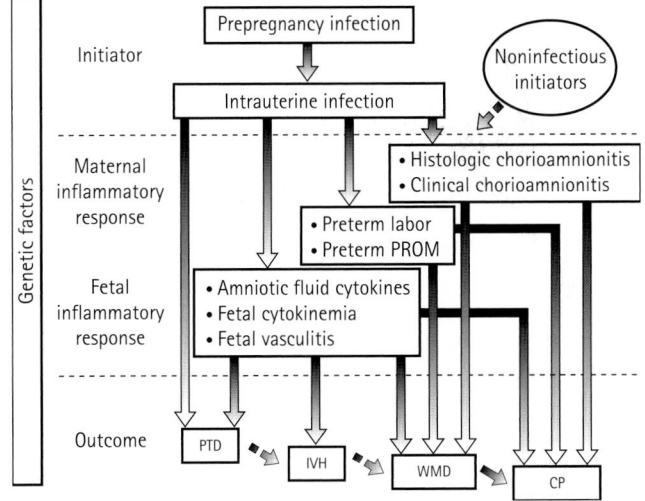

Figure 19.2 Conceptual framework by which before or during pregnancy, an initiator (infectious or non-infectious) may induce maternal and fetal inflammatory responses which will in turn lead to white matter damage and long-term neurological disability. (Modified from Dammann O, Leviton A 2000 Curr Opin Pediatr 12:99–104.)

microbial–host interaction in the endometrium before pregnancy may predispose to adverse pregnancy outcomes including intra-amniotic infection, preterm birth and long term handicap (Espinoza et al 2006).

Yoon et al (1997a) proposed a mechanism by which inflammatory cytokines could lead to WMD and CP. Microbial invasion of the amniotic cavity (which occurs in approximately 25% of preterm births) results in congenital fetal infection/inflammation that stimulates fetal mononuclear cells to produce IL-1β and TNF-α. These cytokines increase the permeability of the blood–brain barrier, thus facilitating the passage of microbial products and cytokines into the brain (Sharief & Thompson 1992, Wong et al 2004). Microbial products then stimulate the human fetal microglia to produce IL-1 and TNF-α, with subsequent activation of astrocyte proliferation and production of TNF-α. TNF-α damages oligodendrocytes, the cells responsible for the deposition of myelin. Interferon-γ and lipopolysaccharide (LPS) also increase the permeability of the blood–brain barrier and this increase in permeability is, at least in part, dependent on cGMP and nitric oxide (Wong et al 2004). For a detailed review of the evidence linking prenatal exposure to lipopolysaccharide and brain injury, the reader is referred to Hagberg and Mallard's excellent review (Hagberg & Mallard 2005).

2. *Adaptive immunity in the pathophysiology of white matter damage:* Evidence for involvement of the adaptive arm of the immune system in the pathogenesis of WMD comes from the study of Duggan et al (2001), who proposed that activated memory T cells may be involved in brain injury among neonates born between 23 and 29 weeks. The investigators reported that the percentage of CD45RO⁺ cells is higher among neonates with cerebral lesions detected by MRI when compared to neonates with normal MRI results. MRI abnormalities included germinal layer or intraventricular hemorrhage, discrete periventricular lesions and/or cystic lesions in the caudate nucleus. The authors proposed that the high concentration of fetal cytokines may be due to antigen exposure and is not secondary to the brain injury, hypoxia or parturition (Duggan et al 2001). In a recent review, Leviton et al proposed that the adaptive immune system contributes to the intensity and duration of the processes resulting in white matter damage (Leviton et al 2005). The authors provided the following evidence in support of this view:

   (1) Interleukin-2 protein expression and its receptor were detected in all brains (*n* = 10) of neonates with white matter lesions (Kadhim et al 2002). This cytokine is produced by activated T lymphocytes and is toxic to oligodendrocytes and myelin (Curatolo et al 1997).
   (2) Neonates with white matter damage tend to have lower thymus weight at autopsy and are more likely to have thymic atrophy histologically (Leviton et al 1978). Moreover, among preterm newborns who did

survive, those who developed cerebral white matter damage were more likely to have thymus involution as assessed on chest radiographs (Kuban et al 2006).
   (3) In an animal model of brain damage, the systemic administration of IL-9, a cytokine produced by activated T cells, exacerbates white matter damage (Dommergues et al 2000, Leviton et al 2005).

Elovitz et al (2006) harvested brain tissue from mice exposed to LPS and reported that in mice intrauterine exposure to LPS was associated with a reactive astrocytosis, a decline in pro-oligodendrocytes and a significant up-regulation of genes associated with Th1 and Th2 responses including: IL-6, IL-2, TNF, IL-1β, GM-CSF, IFN-γ, IL-15, IL10, IL-4, IL-13, T-cell receptor, CD28, interferon regulatory factor among others. Moreover, the authors reported that genes associated with cell death, specifically caspases 1, 3, 8 and 9 as well as apaf-1, were over-expressed in the brain of fetuses exposed to LPS, suggesting that cell death pathways are activated in fetal brains in response to intrauterine exposure to microbial products.

3. *Reactive oxygen species (ROS):* Evidence in support of the role of reactive oxygen species in white matter damage includes the observations that ROS generation is associated with periventricular white matter lesions in animal models of ischemia–reperfusion injury (Welin et al 2005) and the demonstration that protein nitration and lipid peroxidation are present in periventricular white matter lesions in humans (Haynes et al 2003). However, perhaps the most compelling evidence is that provided by Wang et al (2007), who demonstrated that the administration of *N*-acetylcysteine, a free radical scavenger agent, reduces LPS-sensitized hypoxic–ischemic brain injury in rats during the neonatal period (Wang et al 2007) (see Proposed Prophylactic Interventions section). Of note, reactive oxygen species are more toxic to oligodendroglial precursors than to mature oligodendroglia (Volpe 2001), and it has been speculated that this may be due to immaturity in the detoxification system including glutathione peroxidase and catalase (Volpe 2001).

4. *Hemodynamic disturbances:* In the context of FIRS, we proposed that the combination of inflammatory changes in the brain and fetal systemic hypotension may increase the likelihood of cerebral injury (Romero et al 2004). Evidence in support of this view is the observation by Yanowitz et al (2002) that neonates born with histologic chorioamnionitis had several hemodynamic abnormalities, including a decreased mean and diastolic blood pressure. Furthermore, these authors reported a negative correlation between mean blood pressure and umbilical cord IL-6 concentrations (Fig. 19.3) (Yanowitz et al 2002). Thus, it is possible that fetal hypotension and other hemodynamic changes may contribute to the pathophysiology of white matter

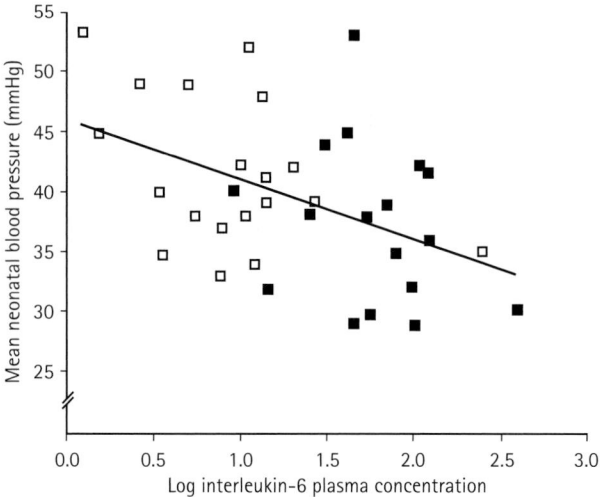

Figure 19.3 Relationship between neonatal mean arterial blood pressure and plasma IL-6 concentration in the cord blood. Solid and open squares represent cases with and without histologic chorioamnionitis, respectively. (Reproduced with permission Yanowitz T D et al 2002 Pediatr Res 51:310–316.)

damage and cerebral palsy (Garnier et al 2003). Experimental evidence in support of this view was reported by Eklind et al (2001), who administered bacterial endotoxin (LPS 0.3 mg/Kg) to 7-day-old rats 4 hours prior to unilateral hypoxia–ischemia induce by carotid occlusion. The pups were sacrificed on postnatal day 10 and the brain tissue was examined. The rectal temperature was recorded and cerebral blood flow measured using autoradiographic methods. The authors reported that the area of brain infarction induced by a combination of LPS and 20 or 30 minutes of ischemia was similar to that induced by 50 minutes of ischemia and vehicle injection. The investigators proposed that the innate immune system may be involved in the increased vulnerability of the neonatal brain following the combination of infection and hypoxia–ischemia. Collectively, this evidence suggests that fetal hemodynamic disturbances may contribute to brain damage in the context of fetal systemic inflammation.

5. *Other proposed mechanisms*: Hagberg et al proposed that hypoglycemia, hyperthermia and lactic acidosis may also contribute to brain damage induced by bacterial products (Hagberg et al 2002). An excess of extracellular glutamate (Volpe 2001) may also contribute to white matter injury since glutamate can lead to death of oligodendroglial precursors by both non-receptor and receptor-mediated mechanisms (Oka et al 1993). However, it is unclear whether this mechanism of disease may be operative in infection/inflammation-induced brain damage.

6. *Are Toll-like receptors involved in the mechanisms of brain injury?* Elovitz et al (2007) recently compared the gene expression of cytokine and chemokines in brain tissues after intrauterine injection with LPS between pups knockout for TLR-4 (TLR-4 –/–) and wild type animals. The authors reported that the IL-13 mRNA expression was significantly higher in brain tissues from knockout pups than wild type animals. However, there were no significant differences in the expression of IL-1, TNF, CCL3 and other chemokines. The authors concluded that targeting TLR-4 is unlikely to be effective at preventing adverse neurological outcomes from inflammation-induced preterm birth (Elovitz et al 2007).

Although prematurity and antenatal infection/inflammation are considered risk factors for both WMD and BPD, there is no evidence that BPD or other adverse neonatal respiratory outcomes are more common among infants with a sonographic diagnosis of WMD than those without such a diagnosis (Dammann et al 2004a, O'Shea et al 1996, Rojas et al 1995, Yoon et al 2002). In contrast, an association between BPD and CP has been reported in five of six studies (Dammann et al 2004a, 2004b, Gray et al 1995, Majnemer et al 2000, Skidmore et al 1990, Vohr et al 1991, Vrlenich et al 1995). Dammann and Leviton coined the term 'tip-of-the-iceberg' effect to describe this paradox that BPD is associated with CP, but not its predecessor (WMD) (Dammann et al 2004b). The hypothesis is that what is seen during brain ultrasonography represents only a small portion of all the WMD occurring in preterm infants. Specifically, ultrasound would not be sufficiently sensitive to detect all WMD lesions associated with later developmental disabilities (Dammann et al 2004a). For example, while ultrasound is capable of identifying gross necrotic lesions of the cerebral white matter, it does not perform as well as diffusion-weighted MRI in the identification of early diffuse WMD (Dammann et al 2004a).

CEREBRAL PALSY

Despite advances in obstetric and neonatal care, the overall prevalence of cerebral palsy has remained stable (Hoon 2005). White-matter damage, as determined by conventional magnetic resonance imaging, is the leading cause of cerebral palsy in children born preterm (Hoon 2005). Indeed, as many as 20% of very low birthweight infants have cystic and/or diffuse white-matter injury with evidence of associated pathology in other cortical and subcortical structures (Hoon 2005).

Cerebral palsy is characterized by aberrant control of movement or posture that appears early on and can lead to costly, life-long disability (Grether & Nelson 1997). The estimated annual prevalence of CP ranges from 1.5 to 2.5 per 1000 live births, depending on the studied cohort (Paneth & Kiely 1984, Stanley & Watson 1992).

There is strong evidence linking brain injury and infant exposure to perinatal infection and inflammation (Grether & Nelson 1997, Murphy et al 1995, Nelson et al 1998, Yoon et al 1997a, 1997b). In 1955, Eastman and DeLeon observed that intrapartum maternal fever was associated with a seven-fold increase in the risk of CP (Eastman & DeLeon 1955). In 1978, Nelson and Ellenberg (1978), using data from the Collaborative Perinatal Project, showed that among low-birth-weight infants, chorioamnionitis increased the risk of CP from 12 per 1000 to 39 per 1000 live births. These observations were independently confirmed by several other studies (Alexander et al 1998, Bejar et al 1988, Grether & Nelson 1997, Murphy et al 1995, O'Shea et al 1998, Verma et al 1997). The general view is that an initiating event (either pre-pregnancy infection or intrauterine infection) leads to maternal and fetal inflammatory responses, which, in turn, contribute to adverse outcomes such as preterm delivery, intraventricular hemorrhage (IVH), WMD and neurodevelopment disability (mainly CP) (Dammann & Leviton 2000). The following evidence supports this concept:

(1) a fetal inflammatory response precedes spontaneous preterm delivery (Gomez et al 1998b, Romero et al 1998b);

(2) chorioamnionitis is associated with an increased risk of CP (Alexander et al 1998, Bejar et al 1988, Grether & Nelson 1997, Murphy et al 1995, Nelson 2002, O'Shea et al 1998, Shea et al 1997, Verma et al 1997);

(3) white matter lesions are associated with spontaneous preterm labor (DeReuck et al 1972, Johnston et al 1995, Leviton & Paneth 1990, Tamisari et al 1986, Verma et al 1997, Yoon et al 1996);

(4) infection is causally linked to WMD (Bejar et al 1988, Leviton & Paneth 1990, Verma et al 1997, Yoon et al 1997b);

(5) fetal cytokinemia is associated with IVH, WMD, and CP (Benett 1996, Camussi et al 1987, Dammann & Leviton 2000, Iida et al 1992, Leviton 1993, Robbins et al 1992, Selmaj & Raine 1988, Yoon et al 1997a, 1997c); and

(6) chorionic and umbilical cord vessel inflammation (fetal vasculitis) is associated with an increased risk for IVH, WMD and CP (McGuire et al 1994, Monzon-Bordonaba et al 1998, Stuber et al 1996, Wilson et al 1997, Yoon et al 2000a).

Prematurity and CP are strongly associated (Leviton & Paneth 1990). Indeed, approximately one-third of all neonates who later have signs of CP weigh less than 2500 g at birth (Hagberg et al 1989). The CP rate of newborns whose birthweights are <1500 g is 25 to 31 times higher than that of those with a normal birthweight (Hagberg et al 1989). A possible mechanism contributing to the increased risk of CP among extremely premature infants is their inability to produce an adequate amount of proteins that modulate the synthesis of inflammatory cytokines (Blahnik et al 2001, Brus 1997, Brus et al 1994, Chheda et al 1996, Dammann et al 2005, Grether et al 1999, Jones et al 1996, Nelson et al 1998) or help to minimize oxidative stress (Dammann et al 2005, Rogers et al 2000). In addition, some fetuses may have an increased genetic susceptibility to develop CP in the setting of intrauterine infection/inflammation. Nelson et al (2005) have recently examined the association of genetic polymorphisms and CP in premature infants. In a case-control study of 96 infants with CP and 119 control children delivered before 32 weeks, an association with CP was observed in heterozygotes for the following single nucleotide polymorphisms (SNPs): endothelial nitric oxide synthase (eNOS) A-922G (OR: 3.0, 95% CI: 1.4–6.4), factor 7 (F7) arg353gln and del[-323]10bp-ins (OR: 2.7, 95% CI: 1.1–6.5), plasminogen activation inhibitor factor-1 (PAI-1) 4G(-675)5G and G11053T (OR: 3.2, 95% CI: 1.2–8.7) and lymphotoxin A (LTA) thr26asn (OR: 2.1, 95% CI: 1.0–4.6). These SNPs are related to nitric oxide, thrombosis or thrombolysis and cytokine function, respectively.

The association between chorioamnionitis and subsequent development of CP has been investigated extensively (Grether & Nelson 2000, Jacobsson et al 2000, Leviton et al 1999, Matsuda et al 2000, Ng et al 2000, O'Shea et al 1998, Redline et al 1998, Roland et al 1996, Yoon et al 1997a, 2000a). A recent meta-analysis reporting on the association of chorioamnionitis and CP concluded that clinical chorioamnionitis is associated with an increased risk of both CP and WMD, with respective relative risk ratios of 4.9 (95% CI: 4.5–2.5) and 2.6 (95% CI: 4.7–3.9) for each of these outcomes (Wu 2002). Evidence supporting a role for the fetus in the process of chorioamnionitis is derived from studies comparing IL-6 concentrations in umbilical venous blood obtained from pregnancies with ($n = 26$) and without ($n = 111$) clinical chorioamnionitis (Chaiworapongsa et al 2002b). The median concentration of venous plasma IL-6 was higher in neonates born to mothers with clinical chorioamnionitis than in those born to women in the control group. Sixty-two percent (16/26) of the neonates born to women with clinical chorioamnionitis had elevated plasma concentrations of IL-6 > 11 pg/mL in the umbilical vein. The observation that the concentration of IL-6 was higher in the blood from the umbilical artery than in the umbilical vein suggests a fetal origin of the excess plasma IL-6.

Further evidence that a fetal inflammatory response is involved in the pathophysiology of CP comes from the study of Yoon et al (2000a), who followed 123 preterm children to the age of three, observing that the odds of developing CP were higher in the presence of funisitis (OR: 5.5, 95% CI: 1.2–24.5), increased amniotic fluid IL-6 concentrations (OR: 6.4, 95% CI: 1.3–33.0) and increased amniotic fluid IL-8 concentrations (OR: 5.9, 95% CI: 1.1–30.7). All 14 children who subsequently developed CP had evidence of WMD, while 11 had evidence of intrauterine inflammation. Fifty percent (7/14) of the children had positive amniotic fluid cultures. Although histologic chorioamnionitis was associated with subsequent development of CP, this relationship disappeared after adjusting for gestational age at birth. The findings of this study suggest that it is the fetal, rather than the maternal inflammatory response, which predisposes to CP. Nonetheless, neither infection nor inflammation were considered sufficient causal factors for WMD or CP, as the latter did not develop in 82% (23/28) of fetuses with documented microbial invasion of the amniotic cavity and in 76% (34/45) of those with evidence of intrauterine inflammation. Other studies supporting a link between fetal inflammation and brain injury have documented higher concentrations of IL-6 (Duggan et al 2001, Viscardi et al 2004, Yoon et al 1996), TNF-α (Duggan et al 2001) and MMP-8 (Moon et al 2002) in the umbilical cord blood and amniotic fluid (Yoon et al 1997a, 2000a) of fetuses with WMD who subsequently developed CP. Recently, Kaukola et al (2004) performed a case-control study that included 19 children with CP and 19 controls matched by gestational age at birth. The serum concentrations of eight cytokines (ciliary neutrotrophic factor, IL-5, IL-12p40, IL-12p70, IL-13, IL-15, macrophage migration inhibitory factor and TNF-related apoptosis inducing ligand) were found to be higher in cord blood samples of neonates who subsequently developed CP. Similarly, serum concentrations of epidermal growth factor and three chemokines (B-lymphocyte chemoattractant, MCP-3 and monokine induced by interferon-γ) were higher in cord blood samples from infants with CP than in controls. Infants with CP born preterm had a different pattern of cytokines in the cord blood than infants with CP that delivered at term, suggesting that the pathophysiology of CP may vary according to the gestational age at birth.

PROPOSED PROPHYLACTIC INTERVENTIONS TO PREVENT OR REDUCE THE RISK OF BRAIN DAMAGE

The administration of antimicrobial agents may eradicate microbial invasion of the amniotic cavity in cases of preterm PROM (Ben Haroush et al 2002, Romero et al 1998a). The results of the ORACLE I trial suggest that antibiotic administration may not only delay the onset of labor, but improve neonatal outcome (Kenyon et al 2001) as well. These findings are supported by experimental evidence in pregnant rabbits inoculated with *Escherichia coli* (Fidel et al 2003). Antibiotic administration within 12 hours of microbial inoculation (but not after 18 hours) prevented maternal fever, reduced the rate of preterm delivery and improved neonatal survival.

Earlier reports indicated a possible association between antibiotic administration and cerebral palsy (Leviton et al 1999, O'Shea et al 1998). Indeed, antibiotic administration has been associated with an odds ratio 2.2 (95% CI: 1.0–4.7) for cerebral palsy in very low birthweight infants (O'Shea et al 1998). Moreover, Leviton et al (1999) reported that antibiotic administration in the index pregnancy was associated with white matter damage, as determined by the presence of echolucent images seen on cranial ultrasound, if birth occurred within one hour of membrane rupture. However, the authors speculated that antibiotic administration may serve merely as a marker of the infection for which it was administered, or that the antibiotic itself may

have a deleterious effect on white matter (Leviton et al 1999). However, in animals, minocycline, a semi-synthetic second generation tetracycline, has been reported to reduce LPS-induced neurological dysfunction and brain injury in neonatal rats (Fan et al 2005). This has been proposed to be due to its putative effect as an inhibitor of microglial activation (Fan et al 2005). Thus, the association of antibiotic administration and brain damage remains uncertain.

Agents that downregulate the inflammatory response, such as anti-inflammatory cytokines (i.e. IL-10) (Rodts-Palenik et al 2002, Terrone et al 2001), antibodies to macrophage migration inhibitory factor (MIF) (Calandra et al 2000, Chaiworapongsa et al 2002a) and antioxidants, may also play a role in preventing preterm delivery, neonatal injury and long-term perinatal morbidity (Ben Haroush et al 2002, Wang et al 2007). For example, a combination of antibiotics and immunomodulators (dexamethasone and indometacin) was effective in non-human pregnant primates to eradicate infection, suppress the inflammatory response and prolong gestation in experimental premature labor induced by intra-amniotic inoculation with group B streptococci (Gravett et al 2003).

Recently, *N*-acetylcysteine (NAC), a free radical scavenger agent, has been reported to reduce LPS-sensitized hypoxic-ischemic brain injury. The authors reported that *N*-acetylcysteine administration (200 mg/Kg) was associated with up to 78% reduction of brain injury in the group of animals that received NAC before and after the ischemic insult and 41% in the early post ischemic treatment group. Moreover, the authors reported that NAC administration was associated with:

(1) reduced isoprostane activation and nitrotyrosine formation;
(2) increased levels of the antioxidants glutathione, thioredoxin-2, and
(3) inhibition of caspase-3, calpain and caspase-1 activation.

The authors concluded that NAC provides substantial neuroprotection against brain injury in a model that combines infection/inflammation and hypoxia–ischemia, a protection that was associated with improvement of the redox state and inhibition of apoptosis, suggesting that these events play a role in the brain injury induced by a combination of hypoxia–ischemia and bacterial products.

Collectively, this evidence indicates that immunomodulation, and antioxidant treatment or a combination of them may constitute effective interventions in preventing fetal injury.

ACKNOWLEDGMENT

This research was supported by the Intramural Program of the National Institute of Child Health and Human Development, NIH, DHHS.

REFERENCES

Alexander J M, Gilstrap L C, Cox S M et al 1998 Clinical chorioamnionitis and the prognosis for very low birth weight infants. Obstet Gynecol 91:725–729.

American College of Chest Physicians/Society of Critical Care Medicine Consensus Conference: definitions for sepsis and organ failure and guidelines for the use of innovative therapies in sepsis 1992. Crit Care Med 20:864–874.

Andrews W W, Goldenberg R L, Hauth J C et al 2005 Endometrial microbial colonization and plasma cell endometritis after spontaneous or indicated preterm versus term delivery. Am J Obstet Gynecol 193:739–745.

Ansbacher R, Boyson W A, Morris J A 1967 Sterility of the uterine cavity. Am J Obstet Gynecol 99:394–396.

Back S A 2006 Perinatal white matter injury: the changing spectrum of pathology and emerging insights into pathogenetic mechanisms. Ment Retard Dev Disabil Res Rev 12:129–140.

Bejar R, Wozniak P, Allard M et al 1988 Antenatal origin of neurologic damage in newborn infants. I. Preterm infants. Am J Obstet Gynecol 159:357–363.

Bell M J, Hallenbeck J M 2002 Effects of intrauterine inflammation on developing rat brain. J Neurosci Res 70:570–579.

Ben Haroush A, Harell D, Hod M et al 2002 Plasma levels of vitamin E in pregnant women prior to the development of preeclampsia and other hypertensive complications. Gynecol Obstet Invest 54:26–30.

Benett J C 1996 Approach to the patient with immune disease. In: Benett J C, Plum F (eds) Cecil textbook of medicine. WB Saunders, Philadephila, pp. 1993–1998.

Berry S M, Gomez R, Athayde N et al 1998 The role of granulocyte colony stimulating factor in the neutrophilia observed in the fetal inflammatory response syndrome. Am J Obstet Gynecol 178:S202.

Berry S M, Romero R, Gomez R et al 1995 Premature parturition is characterized by in utero activation of the fetal immune system. Am J Obstet Gynecol 173:1315–1320.

Blahnik M J, Ramanathan R, Riley C R, Minoo P 2001 Lipopolysaccharide-induced tumor necrosis factor-alpha and IL-10 production by lung macrophages from preterm and term neonates. Pediatr Res 50:726–731.

Brocklehurst P 1999 Infection and preterm delivery. BMJ 318:548–549.

Brus F, Van Oeveren W, Okken A, Oetomo S B 1994 Activation of the plasma clotting, fibrinolytic, and kinin-kallikrein system in preterm infants with severe idiopathic respiratory distress syndrome. Pediatr Res 36:647–653.

Brus F, Van Oeveren W, Okken A, Oetomo S B 1997 Disease severity is correlated with plasma clotting and fibrinolytic and kinin-kallikrein activity in neonatal respiratory distress syndrome. Pediatr Res 41:120–127.

Calandra T, Echtenacher B, Roy D L et al 2000 Protection from septic shock by neutralization of macrophage migration inhibitory factor. Nat Med 6:164–170.

Camussi G, Bussolino F, Salvidio G, Baglioni C 1987 Tumor necrosis factor/cachectin stimulates peritoneal macrophages, polymorphonuclear neutrophils, and vascular endothelial cells to synthesize and release platelet-activating factor. J Exp Med 166:1390–1404.

Chaiworapongsa T, Espinoza J, Kim Y M et al 2002a A novel mediator of septic shock, macrophage migration inhibitory factor, is increased in intra-amniotic infection. Am J Obstet Gynecol 187:S73.

Chaiworapongsa T, Romero R, Kim J C et al 2002b Evidence for fetal involvement in the pathologic process of clinical chorioamnionitis. Am J Obstet Gynecol 186:1178–1182.

Chheda S, Palkowetz K H, Garofalo R et al 1996 Decreased interleukin-10 production by neonatal monocytes and T cells: relationship to decreased production and expression of tumor necrosis factor-alpha and its receptors. Pediatr Res 40:475–483.

Counsell S J, Allsop J M, Harrison M C et al 2003 Diffusion-weighted imaging of the brain in preterm infants with focal and diffuse white matter abnormality. Pediatrics 112:1–7.

Cowling P, McCoy D R, Marshall R J et al 1992 Bacterial colonization of the non-pregnant uterus: a study of pre-menopausal abdominal hysterectomy specimens. Eur J Clin Microbiol Infect Dis 11:204–205.

Curatolo L, Valsasina B, Caccia C et al 1997 Recombinant human IL-2 is cytotoxic to oligodendrocytes after in vitro self aggregation. Cytokine 9:734–739.

D'Alquen D, Kramer B W, Seidenspinner S et al 2005 Activation of umbilical cord endothelial cells and fetal inflammatory response in preterm infants with chorioamnionitis and funisitis. Pediatr Res 57:263–269.

Dammann O, Allred E N, Van Marter L J et al 2004a Bronchopulmonary dysplasia is not associated with ultrasound-defined cerebral white matter damage in preterm newborns. Pediatr Res 55:319–325.

Dammann O, Kuban K C, Leviton A 2002 Perinatal infection, fetal inflammatory response, white matter damage, and cognitive limitations in children born preterm. Ment Retard Dev Disabil Res Rev 8:46–50.

Dammann O, Leviton A 2000 Role of the fetus in perinatal infection and neonatal brain damage. Curr Opin Pediatr 12:99–104.

Dammann O, Leviton A, Bartels D B, Dammann C E 2004b Lung and brain damage in preterm newborns. Are they related? How? Why? Biol Neonate 85:305–313.

Dammann O, Leviton A, Gappa M, Dammann C E 2005 Lung and brain damage in preterm newborns, and their association with gestational age, prematurity subgroup, infection/inflammation and long term outcome. BJOG 112 Suppl 1:4–9.

de Vries L S, Groenendaal F 2002 Neuroimaging in the preterm infant. Ment Retard Dev Disabil Res Rev 8:273–280.

Debillon T, Gras-Leguen C, Leroy S et al 2003 Patterns of cerebral inflammatory response in a rabbit model of intrauterine infection-mediated brain lesion. Brain Res Dev Brain Res 145:39–48.

Debillon T, Gras-Leguen C, Verielle V et al 2000 Intrauterine infection induces programmed cell death in rabbit periventricular white matter. Pediatr Res 47:736–742.

Deguchi K, Mizuguchi M, Takashima S 1996 Immunohistochemical expression of tumor necrosis factor alpha in neonatal leukomalacia. Pediatr Neurol 14:13–16.

Deguchi K, Oguchi K, Takashima S 1997 Characteristic neuropathology of leukomalacia in extremely low birth weight infants. Pediatr Neurol 16:296–300.

DeReuck J, Chattha A S, Richardson E P, Jr 1972 Pathogenesis and evolution of periventricular leukomalacia in infancy. Arch Neurol 27:229–236.

Di Naro E, Cromi A, Ghezzi F et al 2006 Fetal thymic involution: a sonographic marker of the fetal inflammatory response syndrome. Am J Obstet Gynecol 194:153–159.

Dommergues M A, Patkai J, Renauld J C et al 2000 Proinflammatory cytokines and interleukin-9 exacerbate excitotoxic lesions of the newborn murine neopallium. Ann Neurol 47:54–63.

Duggan P J, Maalouf E F, Watts T L et al 2001 Intrauterine T-cell activation and increased proinflammatory cytokine concentrations in preterm infants with cerebral lesions. Lancet 358:1699–1700.

Duncan J R, Cock M L, Scheerlinck J P et al 2002 White matter injury after repeated endotoxin exposure in the preterm ovine fetus. Pediatr Res 52:941–949.

Eastman N J, DeLeon M 1955 The etiology of cerebral palsy. Am J Obstet Gynecol 69:950–961.

Eklind S, Mallard C, Leverin A L et al 2001 Bacterial endotoxin sensitizes the immature brain to hypoxic-ischaemic injury. Eur J Neurosci 13:1101–1106.

Elovitz M A, Chai J, Gonzales J, Richa J 2007 Preventing fetal brain injury in preterm birth: is targeting TLR-4 the answer? Reprod Sci 14(1):132A. Ref Type: Abstract

Elovitz M A, Mrinalini C, Sammel M D 2006 Elucidating the early signal transduction pathways leading to fetal brain injury in preterm birth. Pediatr Res 59:50–55.

Espinoza J, Chaiworapongsa T, Romero R et al 2003 Antimicrobial peptides in amniotic fluid: defensins, calprotectin and bacterial/permeability-increasing protein in patients with microbial invasion of the amniotic cavity, intra-amniotic inflammation, preterm labor and premature rupture of membranes. J Matern Fetal Neonatal Med 13:2–21.

Espinoza J, Erez O, Romero R 2006 Preconceptional antibiotic treatment to prevent preterm birth in women with a previous preterm delivery. Am J Obstet Gynecol 194:630–637.

Fan L W, Pang Y, Lin S et al 2005 Minocycline reduces lipopolysaccharide-induced neurological dysfunction and brain injury in the neonatal rat. J Neurosci Res 82:71–82.

Fidel P, Ghezzi F, Romero R et al 2003 The effect of antibiotic therapy on intrauterine infection-induced preterm parturition in rabbits. J Matern Fetal Neonatal Med 14:57–64.

Gallin J I, Snyderman R 1999 Inflammation: historical perspective. In: Fearon D T, Haynes B F, Nathan C (eds) Inflammation: basic principles and clinical correlates. Lippincott Williams & Wilkins, Philadelphia, pp. 5–12.

Garnier Y, Coumans A B, Jensen A et al 2003 Infection-related perinatal brain injury: the pathogenic role of impaired fetal cardiovascular control. J Soc Gynecol Investig 10:450–459.

Gibbs R S, Romero R, Hillier S L et al 1992 A review of premature birth and subclinical infection. Am J Obstet Gynecol 166:1515–1528.

Goldenberg R L, Hauth J C, Andrews W W 2000 Intrauterine infection and preterm delivery. N Engl J Med 342:1500–1507.

Gomez R, Berry S, Yoon B H et al 1998a The hematologic profile of the fetus with systemic inflammatory response syndrome. Am J Obstet Gynecol 178:S202.

Gomez R, Ghezzi F, Romero R et al 1997 Two thirds of human fetuses with microbial invasion of the amniotic cavity have a detectable systemic cytokine response before birth. Am J Obstet Gynecol 176:514.

Gomez R, Romero R, Ghezzi F et al 1998b The fetal inflammatory response syndrome. Am J Obstet Gynecol 179:194–202.

Gravett M G, Sadowsky D, Witkin M, Novy M 2003 Immunomodulators plus antibiotics to prevent preterm delivery in experimental intra-amniotic infection (IAI). Am J Obstet Gynecol 189:S56.

Gray P H, Burns Y R, Mohay H A et al 1995 Neurodevelopmental outcome of preterm infants with bronchopulmonary dysplasia. Arch Dis Child Fetal Neonatal Ed 73:F128–F134.

Grether J K, Nelson K B 1997 Maternal infection and cerebral palsy in infants of normal birth weight. JAMA 278:207–211.

Grether J K, Nelson K B 2000 Intrauterine infection and cerebral palsy in preterm children. Am J Obstet Gynecol 182:S95.

Grether J K, Nelson K B, Dambrosia J M, Phillips T M 1999 Interferons and cerebral palsy. J Pediatr 134:324–332.

Hagberg B, Hagberg G, Beckung E, Uvebrant P 2001 Changing panorama of cerebral palsy in Sweden. VIII. Prevalence and origin in the birth year period 1991–94. Acta Paediatr 90:271–277.

Hagberg B, Hagberg G, Olow I, von Wendt L 1989 The changing panorama of cerebral palsy in Sweden. V. The birth year period 1979–82. Acta Paediatr Scand 78:283–290.

Hagberg H, Mallard C 2005 Effect of inflammation on central nervous system development and vulnerability. Curr Opin Neurol 18:117–123.

Hagberg H, Peebles D, Mallard C 2002 Models of white matter injury: comparison of infectious, hypoxic-ischemic, and excitotoxic insults. Ment Retard Dev Disabil Res Rev 8:30–38.

Haynes R L, Folkerth R D, Keefe R J et al 2003 Nitrosative and oxidative injury to premyelinating oligodendrocytes in periventricular leukomalacia. J Neuropathol Exp Neurol 62:441–450.

Heine R P, Wiesenfeld H, Mortimer L, Greig P C 1998 Amniotic fluid defensins: potential markers of subclinical intrauterine infection. Clin Infect Dis 27:513–518.

Hoon A H, Jr 2005 Neuroimaging in cerebral palsy: Patterns of brain dysgenesis and injury. J Child Neurol 20:936–939.

Huppi P S, Murphy B, Maier S E et al 2001 Microstructural brain development after perinatal cerebral white matter injury assessed by diffusion tensor magnetic resonance imaging. Pediatrics 107:455–460.

Iida K, Takashima S, Takeuchi Y 1992 Etiologies and distribution of neonatal leukomalacia. Pediatr Neurol 8:205–209.

Inder T, Huppi P S, Zientara G P et al 1999 Early detection of periventricular leukomalacia by diffusion-weighted magnetic resonance imaging techniques. J Pediatr 134:631–634.

Jacobsson B, Hagberg G, Hagberg B et al 2000 Cerebral palsy in preterm infants: a population based analysis of antenatal risk factors. Am J Obstet Gynecol 182:S29.

Johnston M V, Trescher W H, Taylor G A 1995 Hypoxic and ischemic central nervous system disorders in infants and children. Adv Pediatr 42:1–45.

Jones C A, Cayabyab R G, Kwong K Y et al 1996 Undetectable interleukin (IL)-10 and persistent IL-8 expression early in hyaline membrane disease: a possible developmental basis for the predisposition to chronic lung inflammation in preterm newborns. Pediatr Res 39:966–975.

Kadhim H, Tabarki B, De Prez C et al 2002 Interleukin-2 in the pathogenesis of perinatal white matter damage. Neurology 58:1125–1128.

Kadhim H, Tabarki B, De Prez C, Sebire G 2003 Cytokine immunoreactivity in cortical and subcortical neurons in periventricular leukomalacia: are cytokines implicated in neuronal dysfunction in cerebral palsy? Acta Neuropathol (Berl) 105:209–216.

Kadhim H, Tabarki B, Verellen G et al 2001 Inflammatory cytokines in the pathogenesis of periventricular leukomalacia. Neurology 56:1278–1284.

Kaukola T, Satyaraj E, Patel D D et al 2004 Cerebral palsy is characterized by protein mediators in cord serum. Ann Neurol 55:186–194.

Kenyon S L, Taylor D J, Tarnow-Mordi W 2001 Broad-spectrum antibiotics for preterm, prelabour rupture of fetal membranes: the ORACLE I randomised trial. ORACLE Collaborative Group. Lancet 357:979–988.

Kim Y M, Kim G J, Kim M R et al 2003 Skin: An active component of the fetal innate immune system. Am J Obstet Gynecol 189(6), S74.

Kuban J D, Allred E N, Leviton A 2006 Thymus involution and cerebral white matter damage in extremely low gestational age neonates. Biol Neonate 90:252–257.

Kuban K C, Leviton A 1994 Cerebral palsy. N Engl J Med 330:188–195.

Lahra M M, Jeffery H E 2004 A fetal response to chorioamnionitis is associated with early survival after preterm birth. Am J Obstet Gynecol 190:147–151.

Ledger W J 1989 Infection and premature labor. Am J Perinatol 6:234–236.

Leviton A 1993 Preterm birth and cerebral palsy: is tumor necrosis factor the missing link? Dev Med Child Neurol 35:553–558.

Leviton A, Dammann O, Durum S K 2005 The adaptive immune response in neonatal cerebral white matter damage. Ann Neurol 58:821–828.

Leviton A, Gilles F H, Vawter G F 1978 The thymus in infants with perinatal telencephalic leukoencephalopathy. Arch Neurol 35:377–381.

Leviton A, Paneth N 1990 White matter damage in preterm newborns — an epidemiologic perspective. Early Hum Dev 24:1–22.

Leviton A, Paneth N, Reuss M L et al 1999 Maternal infection, fetal inflammatory response, and brain damage in very low birth weight infants. Developmental Epidemiology Network Investigators. Pediatr Res 46:566–575.

Levy M M, Fink M P, Marshall J C, Abraham E, Angus D, Cook D et al 2003 2001 SCCM/ESICM/ACCP/ATS/SIS International Sepsis Definitions Conference. Intensive Care Med 29:530–538.

McGuire W, Hill A V, Allsopp C E et al 1994 Variation in the TNF-alpha promoter region associated with susceptibility to cerebral malaria. Nature 371:508–510.

Majnemer A, Riley P, Shevell M et al 2000 Severe bronchopulmonary dysplasia increases risk for later neurological and motor sequelae in preterm survivors. Dev Med Child Neurol 42:53–60.

Mallard C, Welin A K, Peebles D et al 2003 White matter injury following systemic endotoxemia or asphyxia in the fetal sheep. Neurochem Res 28:215–223.

Matsuda Y, Kouno S, Hiroyama Y et al 2000 Intrauterine infection, magnesium sulfate exposure and cerebral palsy in infants born between 26 and 30 weeks of gestation. Eur J Obstet Gynecol Reprod Biol 91:159–164.

Minkoff H 1983 Prematurity: infection as an etiologic factor. Obstet Gynecol 62:137–144.

Moller B R, Kristiansen F V, Thorsen P et al 1995 Sterility of the uterine cavity. Acta Obstet Gynecol Scand 74:216–219.

Monzon-Bordonaba F, Parry S, Holder J et al 1998 A genetic marker for preterm delivery. J Soc Gynecol Investig 5:71A.

Moon J B, Kim J C, Yoon B H et al 2002 Amniotic fluid matrix metalloproteinase-8 and the development of cerebral palsy. J Perinat Med 30:301–306.

Murphy D J, Sellers S, MacKenzie I Z et al 1995 Case-control study of antenatal and intrapartum risk factors for cerebral palsy in very preterm singleton babies. Lancet 346:1449–1454.

Naeye R L, Ross S M 1982 Amniotic fluid infection syndrome. Clin Obstet Gynaecol 9:593–607.

Nelson K B 2002 The epidemiology of cerebral palsy in term infants. Ment Retard Dev Disabil Res Rev 8:146–150.

Nelson K B, Dambrosia J M, Grether J K, Phillips T M 1998 Neonatal cytokines and coagulation factors in children with cerebral palsy. Ann Neurol 44:665–675.

Nelson K B, Dambrosia J M, Iovannisci D M et al 2005 Genetic polymorphisms and cerebral palsy in very preterm infants. Pediatr Res 57:494–499.

Nelson K B, Ellenberg J H 1978 Epidemiology of cerebral palsy. Adv Neurol 19:421–435.

Nelson L H, Nichols S B 1986 Effectiveness of the Isaacs cell sampler for endometrial cultures. J Reprod Med 31:473–477.

Ng E, Asztalos E, Rose T et al 2000 The association of clinical and histologic chorioamnionitis (CA) with cystic periventricular leukomalacia (cPVL) and cerebral palsy (CP) in preterm infants. Pediatr Res 47:318A.

O'Shea T M, Goldstein D J, deRegnier R A et al 1996 Outcome at 4 to 5 years of age in children recovered from neonatal chronic lung disease. Dev Med Child Neurol 38:830–839.

O'Shea T M, Klinepeter K L, Dillard R G 1998 Prenatal events and the risk of cerebral palsy in very low birth weight infants. Am J Epidemiol 147:362–369.

O'Shea T M, Klinepeter K L, Meis P J, Dillard R G 1998 Intrauterine infection and the risk of cerebral palsy in very low-birthweight infants. Paediatr Perinat Epidemiol 12:72–83.

Oka A, Belliveau M J, Rosenberg P A, Volpe J J 1993 Vulnerability of oligodendroglia to glutamate: pharmacology, mechanisms, and prevention. J Neurosci 13:1441–1453.

Pacora P, Chaiworapongsa T, Maymon E et al 2002 Funisitis and chorionic vasculitis: the histological counterpart of the fetal inflammatory response syndrome. J Matern Fetal Neonatal Med 11:18–25.

Paneth N, Kiely J 1984 The frequency of cerebral palsy: a review of population studies in industrialized nations since 1950. In: Stanley F, Alberman E (eds) The epidemiology of the cerebral palsies. Blackwell Scientific, Oxford, pp. 46–56.

Redline R W, Wilson-Costello D, Borawski E et al 1998 Placental lesions associated with neurologic impairment and cerebral palsy in very low-birth-weight infants. Arch Pathol Lab Med 122:1091–1098.

Robbins D S, Shirazi Y, Drysdale B E et al 1992 Production of cytokine profile in plasma of baboons challenged with lethal and sublethal Escherichia coli. Circ Schock 33:84–91.

Robertson N J, Kuint J, Counsell T J et al 2000 Characterization of cerebral white matter damage in preterm infants using 1H and 31P magnetic resonance spectroscopy. J Cereb Blood Flow Metab 20:1446–1456.

Rodts-Palenik S, Barrilleaux P, Thgpen B et al 2002 Intravenous interleukin-10/antibiotic therapy prolongs gestation, improves birthweight, and reduces fetal wastage in E. coli-mediated preterm labor. Am J Obstet Gynecol 186:S65.

Rogers S, Witz G, Anwar M et al 2000 Antioxidant capacity and oxygen radical diseases in the preterm newborn. Arch Pediatr Adolesc Med 154:544–548.

Rojas M A, Gonzalez A, Bancalari E et al 1995 Changing trends in the epidemiology and pathogenesis of neonatal chronic lung disease. J Pediatr 126:605–610.

Roland E H, Magee J F, Rodriguez E et al 1996 Placental abnormalities: insights into pathogenesis of cystic periventricular leukomalacia. Ann Neurol 40:3213.

Romero R, Athayde N, Gomez R et al 1998a The fetal inflammatory response syndrome is characterized by the outpouring of a potent extracellular matrix degrading enzyme into the fetal circulation. Am J Obstet Gynecol 178:S3.

Romero R, Chaiworapongsa T, Espinoza J et al 2002 Fetal plasma MMP-9 concentrations are elevated in preterm premature rupture of the membranes. Am J Obstet Gynecol 187:1125–1130.

Romero R, Espinoza J, Goncalves L F et al 2004 Fetal cardiac dysfunction in preterm premature rupture of membranes. J Matern Fetal Neonatal Med 16:146–157.

Romero R, Gomez R, Ghezzi F et al 1998b A fetal systemic inflammatory response is followed by the spontaneous onset of preterm parturition. Am J Obstet Gynecol 179:186–193.

Romero R, Mazor M 1988 Infection and preterm labor. Clin Obstet Gynecol 31:553–584.

Romero R, Mazor M, Munoz H et al 1994 The preterm labor syndrome. Ann N Y Acad Sci 734:414–429.

Romero R, Mazor M, Wu Y K et al 1988 Infection in the pathogenesis of preterm labor. Semin Perinatol 12:262–279.

Sampson J E, Theve R P, Blatman R N et al 1997 Fetal origin of amniotic fluid polymorphonuclear leukocytes. Am J Obstet Gynecol 176:77–81.

Selmaj K W, Raine C S 1988 Tumor necrosis factor mediates myelin and oligodendrocyte damage in vitro. Ann Neurol 23:339–346.

Sharief M K, Thompson E J 1992 In vivo relationship of tumor necrosis factor-alpha to blood-brain barrier damage in patients with active multiple sclerosis. J Neuroimmunol 38:27–33.

Shea K G, Coleman S S, Carroll K et al 1997 Pemberton pericapsular osteotomy to treat a dysplastic hip in cerebral palsy. J Bone Joint Surg Am 79:1342–1351.

Skidmore M D, Rivers A, Hack M 1990 Increased risk of cerebral palsy among very low-birthweight infants with chronic lung disease. Dev Med Child Neurol 32:325–332.

Stanley F J, Watson L 1992 Trends in perinatal mortality and cerebral palsy in Western Australia, 1967 to 1985. BMJ 304:1658–1663.

Stewart A L, Rifkin L, Amess P N et al 1999 Brain structure and neurocognitive and behavioural function in adolescents who were born very preterm. Lancet 353:1653–1657.

Stuber F, Petersen M, Bokelmann F, Schade U 1996 A genomic polymorphism within the tumor necrosis factor locus influences plasma tumor necrosis factor-alpha concentrations and outcome of patients with severe sepsis. Crit Care Med 24:381–384.

Tamisari L, Vigi V, Fortini C, Scarpa P 1986 Neonatal periventricular leukomalacia: diagnosis and evolution evaluated by real-time ultrasound. Helv Paediatr Acta 41:399–407.

Terrone D A, Rinehart B K, Granger J P et al 2001 Interleukin-10 administration and bacterial endotoxin-induced preterm birth in a rat model. Obstet Gynecol 98:476–480.

van der P T, Buller H R, ten Cate H et al 1990 Activation of coagulation after administration of tumor necrosis factor to normal subjects. N Engl J Med 322:1622–1627.

Verma U, Tejani N, Klein S et al 1997 Obstetric antecedents of intraventricular hemorrhage and periventricular leukomalacia in the low-birth-weight neonate. Am J Obstet Gynecol 176:275–281.

Viscardi R M, Muhumuza C K, Rodriguez A et al 2004 Inflammatory markers in intrauterine and fetal blood and cerebrospinal fluid compartments are associated with adverse pulmonary and neurologic outcomes in preterm infants. Pediatr Res 55:1009–1017.

Vohr B R, Coll C G, Lobato D et al 1991 Neurodevelopmental and medical status of low-birthweight survivors of bronchopulmonary dysplasia at 10 to 12 years of age. Dev Med Child Neurol 33:690–697.

Volpe J J 2001 Neurobiology of periventricular leukomalacia in the premature infant. Pediatr Res 50:553–562.

Vrlenich L A, Bozynski M E, Shyr Y et al 1995 The effect of bronchopulmonary dysplasia on growth at school age. Pediatrics 95:855–859.

Wang X, Svedin P, Nie C et al 2007 N-acetylcysteine reduces lipopolysaccharide-sensitized hypoxic-ischemic brain injury. Ann Neurol 61(3):263–271.

Weiss M, Moldawer L L, Schneider E M 1999 Granulocyte colony-stimulating factor to prevent the progression of systemic nonresponsiveness in systemic inflammatory response syndrome and sepsis. Blood 93:425–439.

Welin A K, Sandberg M, Lindblom A et al 2005 White matter injury following prolonged free radical formation in the 0.65 gestation fetal sheep brain. Pediatr Res 58:100–105.

Wilson A G, Symons J A, McDowell T L et al 1997 Effects of a polymorphism in the human tumor necrosis factor alpha promoter on transcriptional activation. Proc Natl Acad Sci U S A 94:3195–3199.

Witt A, Berger A, Gruber C J et al 2005 IL-8 concentrations in maternal serum, amniotic fluid and cord blood in relation to different pathogens within the amniotic cavity. J Perinat Med 33:22–26.

Wong D, Dorovini-Zis K, Vincent S R 2004 Cytokines, nitric oxide, and cGMP modulate the permeability of an in vitro model of the human blood-brain barrier. Exp Neurol 190:446–455.

Wu Y W 2002 Systematic review of chorioamnionitis and cerebral palsy. Ment Retard Dev Disabil Res Rev 8:25–29.

Yanowitz T D, Jordan J A, Gilmour C H et al 2002 Hemodynamic disturbances in premature infants born after chorioamnionitis: association with cord blood cytokine concentrations. Pediatr Res 51:310–316.

Yoon B H, Jun J K, Romero R et al 1997a Amniotic fluid inflammatory cytokines (interleukin-6, interleukin-1beta, and tumor necrosis factor-alpha), neonatal brain white matter lesions, and cerebral palsy. Am J Obstet Gynecol 177:19–26.

Yoon B H, Kim C J, Romero R et al 1997b Experimentally induced intrauterine infection causes fetal brain white matter lesions in rabbits. Am J Obstet Gynecol 177:797–802.

Yoon B H, Kim Y A, Romero R et al 1999a Association of oligohydramnios in women with preterm premature rupture of membranes with an inflammatory response in fetal, amniotic, and maternal compartments. Am J Obstet Gynecol 181:784–788.

Yoon B H, Romero R, Jun J K et al 1998 An increase in fetal plasma cortisol but not dehydroepiandrosterone sulfate is followed by the onset of preterm labor in patients with preterm premature rupture of the membranes. Am J Obstet Gynecol 179:1107–1114.

Yoon B H, Romero R, Kim C J et al 1997c High expression of tumor necrosis factor-alpha and interleukin-6 in periventricular leukomalacia. Am J Obstet Gynecol 177:406–411.

Yoon B H, Romero R, Kim K S et al 1999b A systemic fetal inflammatory response and the development of bronchopulmonary dysplasia. Am J Obstet Gynecol 181:773–779.

Yoon B H, Romero R, Park J S et al 2000a Fetal exposure to an intra-amniotic inflammation and the development of cerebral palsy at the age of three years. Am J Obstet Gynecol 182:675–681.

Yoon B H, Romero R, Park J S et al 2000b The relationship among inflammatory lesions of the umbilical cord (funisitis), umbilical cord plasma interleukin 6 concentration, amniotic fluid infection, and neonatal sepsis. Am J Obstet Gynecol 183:1124–1129.

Yoon B H, Romero R, Shim J Y et al 2002 'Atypical' chronic lung disease of the newborn is linked to fetal systemic inflammation. Am J Obstet Gynecol 187:S129.

Yoon B H, Romero R, Shim J Y et al 2003 C-reactive protein in umbilical cord blood: a simple and widely available clinical method to assess the risk of amniotic fluid infection and funisitis. J Matern Fetal Neonatal Med 14:85–90.

Yoon B H, Romero R, Yang S H et al 1996 Interleukin-6 concentrations in umbilical cord plasma are elevated in neonates with white matter lesions associated with periventricular leukomalacia. Am J Obstet Gynecol 174:1433–1440.

Neonatal intracranial hemorrhage

Malcolm I. Levene and Linda S. de Vries

Key Points

- Germinal matrix hemorrhage–intraventricular hemorrhage (GMH–IVH) is the commonest form of intracranial hemorrhage in premature infants (30–40% of very low birth weight infants; 15% of these will involve the cerebral parenchyma)
- The most convincing drug shown to prevent GMH–IVH is antenatally administered corticosteroids and postnatal indometacin. No drugs have been definitely shown to reduce disability
- If the GMH–IVH does not involve the parenchyma and is not associated with ventricular dilatation the child is not at increased risk of disability compared with age matched children. The majority of those with parenchymal hemorrhage will develop cerebral palsy
- Subarachnoid hemorrhage is common in premature infants and the prognosis is generally good
- Cerebral sinus thrombosis is rarely diagnosed but has a relatively good prognosis. A thrombophilic tendency is often a causative factor

---

INTRODUCTION

Hemorrhages involving the neonatal brain are among the most frequent and important conditions affecting the newborn. Intracerebral hemorrhage is more common in the neonatal period than at any other time, but there is a wide spectrum of hemorrhagic lesions, with differing etiologies and varying prognostic significance. Table 20.1 lists the types of hemorrhage reported in the newborn brain and each will be discussed separately.

Table 20.1 Localization and site of origin of various types of intracranial hemorrhage

Type of hemorrhage	Site of origin
Subdural	—
Subarachnoid	Primary
	Secondary to intraventricular hemorrhage
	Subarachnoid hematoma
Intraventricular	Germinal matrix
	Choroid plexus
	Cerebral parenchyma
Intraparenchymal	Periventricular white matter
	Thalamus
	Arteriovenous malformation
Intracerebellar	—

With the introduction of modern imaging techniques in the late 1970s, intracranial hemorrhage could be studied in living infants and information on its pathogenesis and outcome in surviving children assessed. The incidence of intracranial hemorrhage in asymptomatic healthy full-term infants is 3.5–5% (Heibel et al 1993, Mercuri et al 1998). Before that, information could only be obtained from autopsy material which would bias the findings towards the more severe degrees of hemorrhage. Despite the obvious limitations of post-mortem studies, a definite trend can be observed over the last 60 years. In 1938, Craig analyzed 126 post-mortem examinations in which intracranial hemorrhage was discovered and found subdural hematoma to be common, occurring in almost half of the cases. A similar assessment 40 years later from Hammersmith Hospital, UK autopsies during the years 1978–1979 showed a considerable decline in the proportion of subdural hemorrhages, with a corresponding marked increase in the percentage of germinal matrix hemorrhage–intraventricular hemorrhage (GMH–IVH) (Levene et al 1985). This is due to a marked reduction in the number of fatal subdural hemorrhages associated with more careful obstetric management of the second stage of labor and the relative increase in cases of GMH–IVH associated with longer survival of very premature infants supported by neonatal intensive care who are most at risk of GMH–IVH. This is now the most frequent and important cause of intracranial hemorrhage in neonatal medicine.

GERMINAL MATRIX HEMORRHAGE AND INTRAVENTRICULAR HEMORRHAGE

The terminology used to describe hemorrhage in and around the lateral ventricles is confusing and lacks a clear consensus view. Intraventricular hemorrhage is an imprecise term used to describe bleeding within the ventricular cavities but arising from any site. It may be impossible to distinguish on ultrasound examination the presence of liquid phase blood in the lateral ventricle. Consequently, the distinction between unruptured GMH and IVH can often not be made confidently by this imaging technique alone. The generic term 'periventricular hemorrhage' is also widely used to refer to hemorrhage originating in the germinal matrix, often with involvement of the lateral ventricles and on occasions also involving the periventricular white matter. It is now clear that hemorrhage occurring de novo in the periventricular white matter, without germinal matrix bleeding, also occurs not infrequently, and this condition might be referred to more accurately as periventricular hemorrhage. For these semantic reasons we have chosen to use the term 'germinal matrix hemorrhage–intraventricular hemorrhage' (GMH–IVH) to refer to a common form of intracranial hemorrhage usually seen in premature infants. Throughout this section the term 'GMH–IVH' is used in a general sense to describe the condition that other authors have described by a variety of terms but which we believe to refer to the same condition. There is now growing evidence that a proportion of hemorrhagic lesions in the cerebral parenchyma has quite a different pathophysiologic basis from GMH–IVH and is ischemic in origin. This is discussed in detail in Chapter 21.

PATHOLOGY

Kowitz (1914) was the first to publish a report of IVH in the neonate and included 128 cases, but Ruckensteiner and Zollner (1929) were the first to recognize that, in premature infants, blood in the ventricles commonly occurred as the result of hemorrhage within the subependymal germinal matrix. The subependymal germinal matrix is a transient structure and is initially the site of vigorous neuroblast and glioblast mitotic activity. When cell division is complete and after the majority of the neurons have completed their migration, the relative size of the periventricular germinal matrix progressively decreases, but a conspicuous mass of cells persist over the head and body of the caudate nucleus until 33–34 weeks of gestation. Residual matrix tissue persists in the roof of the temporal horn and in the external wall of the occipital horn. These glial precursors develop into oligodendrocytes and astrocytes and migrate all over the cerebrum.

The arterial supply of the germinal matrix is from the recurrent artery of Heubner (a branch of the anterior cerebral artery), as well as terminal branches of the lateral striate arteries. These vessels divide to give the germinal matrix a rich bed of vascular afferents. Takashima and Tanaka (1978) have suggested that the germinal matrix represents a border zone between the striate and thalamic arteries and as such is particularly vulnerable to infarction (see below). Venous drainage of the germinal matrix is via many small veins into the terminal vein. These are joined anteriorly at the level of the foramen of Monro by the septal, choroidal and thalamostriate veins just before the terminal vein turns sharply back on itself (Takashima & Tanaka 1978). The terminal vein drains into the internal cerebral vein and then into the vein of Galen.

The site of GMH depends on the maturity of the infant. In the least mature infants (24–28 weeks), Hambleton and Wigglesworth (1976) found GMH to be larger and occur most frequently over the body of the caudate nucleus, and in more mature infants the lesion was seen over the head of the caudate nucleus.

Although some disagreement still exists concerning the vascular origin of GMH, the predominant view at present is that hemorrhage arises from the thin walled veins (Cole et al 1974, Ghazi-Birry et al 1997, Grontoft 1953, Moody et al 1994, Nakamura et al 1990). In a large number of cases examined histologically, blood from the GMH was seen tunneling along the perivenous space of a germinal matrix vein leading to compression of patent veins and secondary rupture of smaller connecting venous tributaries (Ghazi-Birry et al 1997). This in turn causes venous stasis, increased venous pressure and reduced perfusion pressure through this part of the brain.

Hambleton and Wigglesworth (1976), using post-mortem injection techniques, failed to show evidence of rupture of either veins or arteries, but reported hemorrhage to occur as the result of disruption of the capillary bed.

The immature veins are vulnerable to rupture as the result of under-developed basal lamina, incomplete glial support and poor matrix support. Ment et al (1995) have suggested that the immaturity is transient. They showed that the germinal matrix vessels change significantly over the first four days of life to greater continuity of the basement membrane, and by 10 days after birth the length and number of tight junctions had increased and the number of supporting cells surrounding the germinal matrix vessels had risen. This rapid maturation, presumably as a result of early birth, accounts for the frequency of GMH in the first few days of life.

In 80% of cases of GMH, blood ruptures through the ependyma into the lateral ventricles, causing IVH. GMH is bilateral in half of affected brains, with a slight left-sided preponderance (Donn & Bowerman 1985). In bilateral lesions the hemorrhages are usually asymmetrical (Fig. 20.1). Bleeding sites may be multiple and in some cases develop in the roof of the temporal horn and posteriorly in the germinal matrix of the external wall of the lateral ventricle. Involvement of different sites is now more often recognized with increased use of early MRI. Bleeding may also extend into the caudate nucleus and other adjacent structures. Blood may also extend into the ventricle from primary bleeding of the tela choroidea and from the choroid plexus.

Parenchymal hemorrhage

Parenchymal hemorrhage occurs in approximately 15% of infants with GMH–IVH and is usually unilateral and does not involve the cortical mantle. If the baby survives the lesion, a large porencephalic cavity may develop (see p. 412).

It has been thought in the past that parenchymal hemorrhage was due to direct extension of hemorrhage into the periventricular white matter, but this has now been discounted as a likely explanation for its development. Bleeding into an area of previously compromised periventricular white matter occurs as a result of periventricular leukomalacia (PVL) which may be confused with primary parenchymal hemorrhage. PVL is described in detail in the next chapter but is usually a symmetrical condition compared with the very asymmetrical appearance of parenchymal hemorrhage.

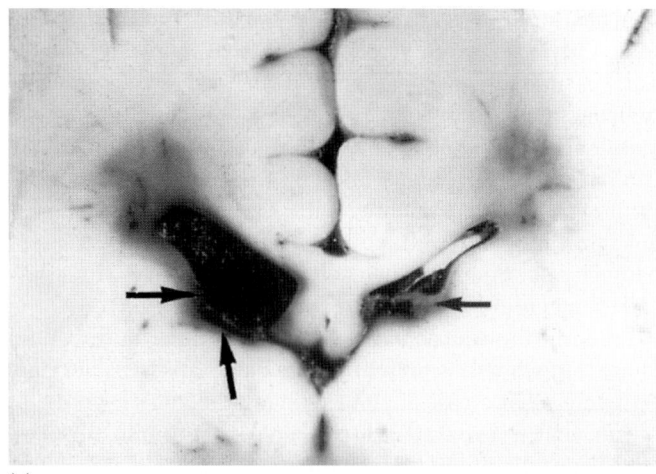

(a)

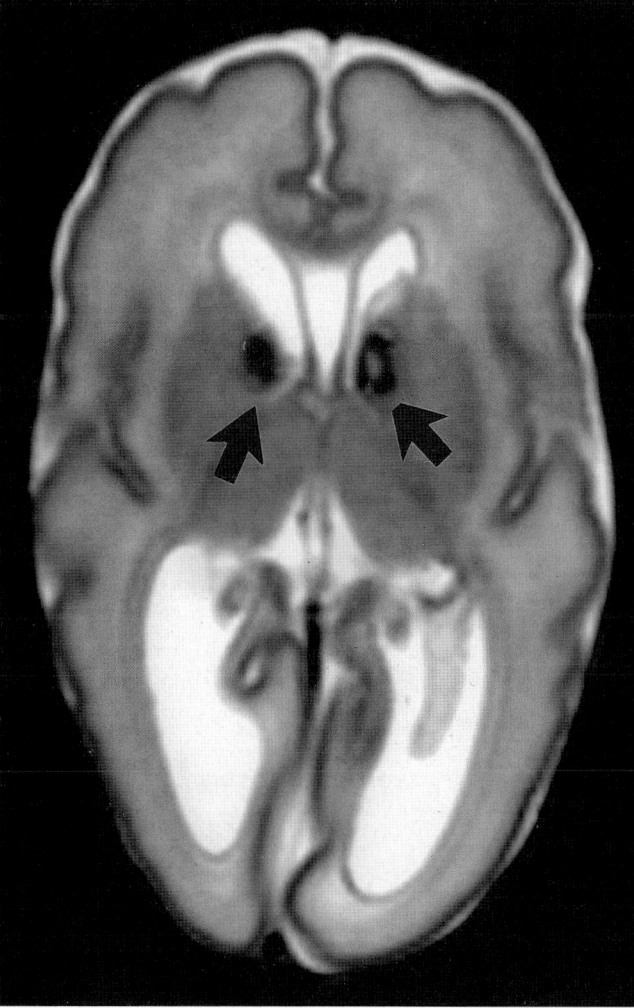

(b)

Figure 20.1 (a) Bilateral GMH (arrow) with rupture into the left lateral ventricle, which is filled with clot. (b) Appearances on T2-weighted MR axial scan (GMH arrow).

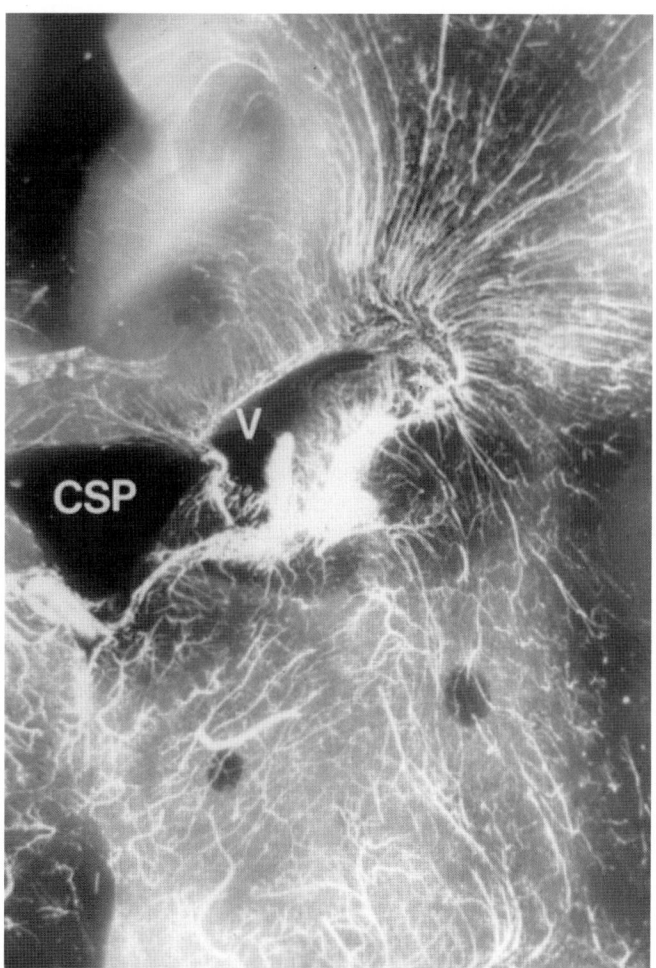

Figure 20.2 Microvenography showing the fan-shaped leash of veins in the deep periventricular white matter of a neonate of 28 weeks of gestation. V, ventricle; CSP, cavum septi pellucidi. (Reproduced with permission from Elsevier Science, from Takashima et al 1986.)

The cause of parenchymal hemorrhage is now thought to be due to venous infarction. The deep periventricular white matter is served by a fan-shaped leash of short and long medullary veins which flow vertically into subependymal veins (Takashima & Tanaka 1978, Takashima et al 1986) and this is illustrated in Figure 20.2. A careful pathologic study of infants dying with periventricular intraparenchymal cerebral hemorrhage showed that the ependyma remained intact, indicating that direct spread from the lateral ventricle could not have occurred (Gould et al 1987). These authors suggested that clot in the germinal matrix causes obstruction to the terminal vein with reduction in cerebral perfusion in the white matter drained by these veins. There is evidence for this mechanism from pathologic specimens (Pape & Wigglesworth 1979) and an example is shown in Figure 20.3. Histology showed that the hemorrhage is mainly perivascular and radiates outwards from the angle of the lateral ventricle, closely following the distribution of the medullary veins draining the white matter. Marked ischemic injury was not found (Gould et al 1987). Low cerebral blood flow in the periventricular region has been shown by positron emission tomography to occur on the side of GMH–IVH, which is most likely to reflect the low perfusion seen in venous infarction (Volpe et al 1983).

Venous infarction has also been reported to occur following intraventricular clot formation (Pape & Wigglesworth 1979). We have reported ultrasound evidence for extension of GMH–IVH in 15% of infants with this form of hemorrhage over a period of up to 48 hours (Levene & de Vries 1984). The initial lesion is one of distention of the ventricle with clot, and subsequently extension of echodensity into the periventricular white matter occurs (Fig. 20.4).

A recent report (Govaert et al 1999) suggests that a discrete unilateral hemorrhagic lesion in the temporal lobe (Fig. 20.5) or around the atrium of very premature infants is secondary to venous infarction of either the inferior ventricular vein or the lateral atrial veins. These lesions are suggested to occur as a result of GMH causing obstruction to these veins with eventual venous infarction.

It has been suggested that blood within the lateral ventricle liberates vasoactive compounds that induce local arterial spasm within the periventricular arteries to produce ischemia with subsequent infarction (Stutchfield & Cooke 1989). The time-scale for the evolution of this lesion will be similar to that of venous infarction (Edvinsson et al 1986, White et al 1975). Stutchfield and Cooke (1989) found that 45% of premature infants with ultrasound evidence of parenchymal infarction had cerebrospinal fluid (CSF) potassium concentrations above 2SD from the mean.

Blood in the ventricular system may remain in the liquid phase, but when it is present in large amounts clots develop. In severe cases a cast of clot involving the lateral, third and fourth ventricular system forms and, if the infant survives, ventricular dilatation is almost inevitable (see Ch. 42). Alternatively, multiple small clots may develop which are suspended in the liquid phase of the intraventricular blood, and these may also cause obstruction to CSF drainage. Blood commonly collects in the subarachnoid spaces of the posterior fossa and may extend into the basal cistern.

INCIDENCE

Although prenatal hemorrhage is well documented (see Ch. 18) it occurs rarely and GMH–IVH is essentially a postnatal event. The incidence of GMH–IVH is directly related to the maturity of the infant, and for infants weighing below 1500 g (approximating to 30 weeks of gestation) the current incidence is about 30%, although some centers report significantly lower figures (Allan et al 1997). The incidence of hemorrhage increases with reducing gestational age below 30 weeks (see Fig. 20.6) and conversely becomes progressively less common with advancing gestational age. Intraparenchymal hemorrhage was reported in the 1990s to be relatively uncommon with an average incidence of 5% (range 2–11%) (Allan et al 1997, Batton et al 1994, Claris et al 1996, Cooke 1994, Rademaker et al 1994). There is very considerable variation in the incidence of GMH–IVH in different NICUs over the same period of time. In Canada in 1996–1997 the overall incidence of any grade of hemor-

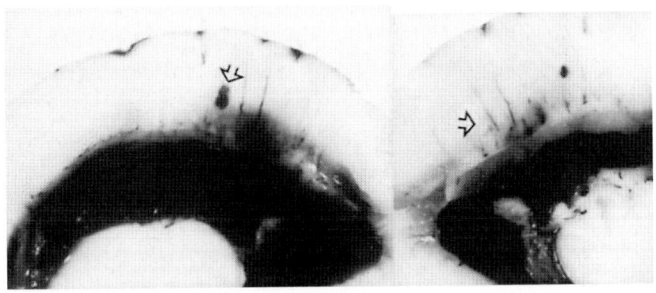

Figure 20.3 Close-up of the two hemispheres from an infant of 30 weeks of gestation showing distention of both lateral ventricles with clot. There is congestion of the veins draining the deep periventricular white matter. Note also the white spots of periventricular leukomalacia (arrow) and the secondary bleeding into the necrotic tissue.

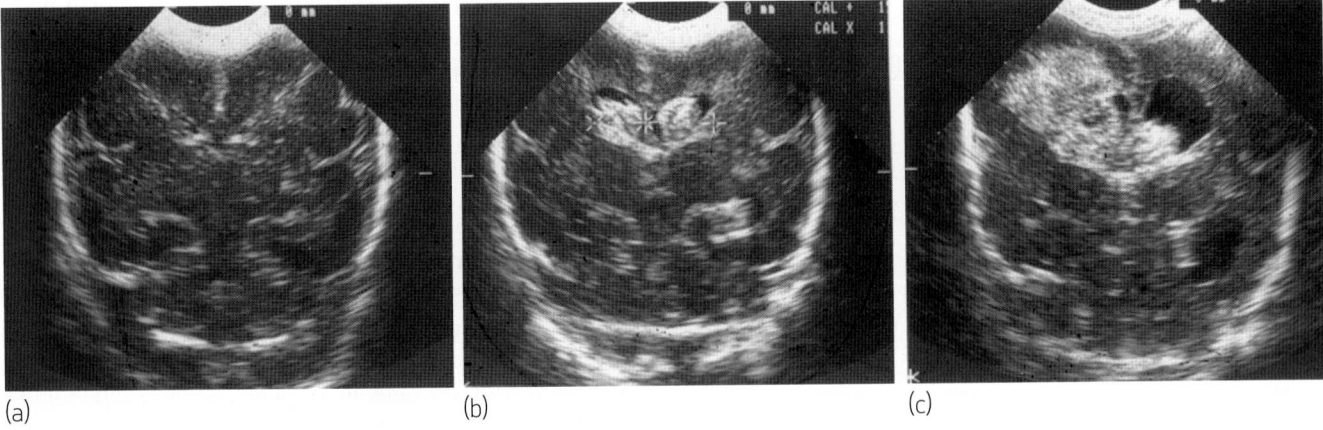

(a)   (b)   (c)

Figure 20.4 Evolution of GMH–IVH in an infant born at 27 weeks. (a) Normal scan on day 1. (b) Large bilateral intraventricular hemorrhage on day 2. (c) Right-sided parenchymal involvement on day 3.

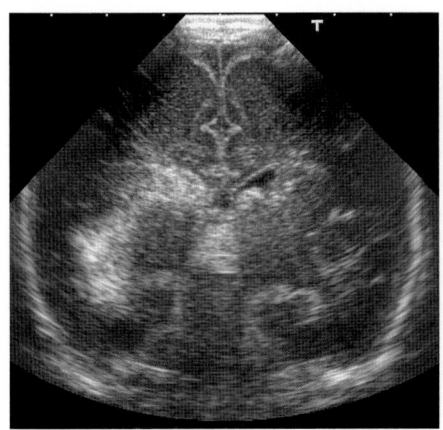 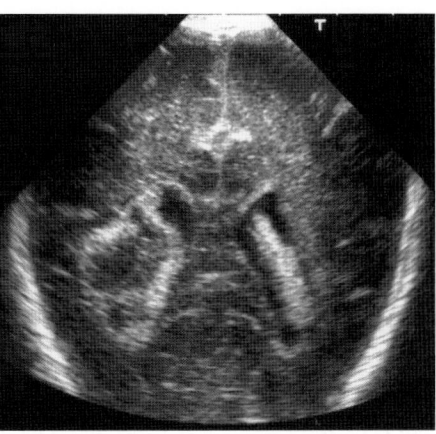

Figure 20.5 Focal atrial lobe infarction secondary to GMH–IVH seen on ultrasound coronal scan in the early and later cystic phase.

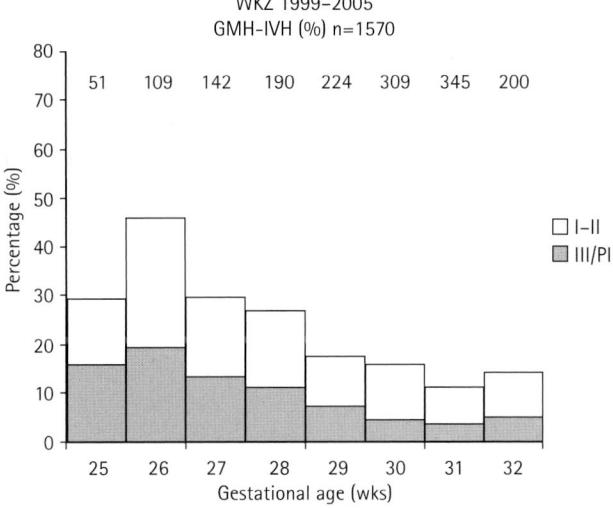

WKZ 1999–2005
GMH-IVH (%) n=1570

IVH I–II: 12,1%; III/PI:7.7%

Figure 20.6 Incidence of GMH–IVH in extremely premature infants by gestational age from Wilhelmina Children's Hospital, Utrecht (1999–2006). The number at the top of each column refers to the number of infants in each group; shaded areas represent proportion with parenchymal hemorrhage.

rhage was 48% for infants <27 weeks over 17 units, but this ranged between 27–89% for individual units (Synnes et al 2001). Avoidable factors to account for this variation were suggested to include route of delivery, outborn vs. inborn, use of antenatal steroids and early use of vasopressors.

In the last 15 years, with the introduction of high uptake of antenatal corticosteroids and surfactant therapy, the incidence of GMH–IVH appears to be falling. In the USA the incidence of GMH–IVH was 9% in 1990–1993 compared with 23% in 1982–1985 (Allan et al 1994). The decline in incidence is particularly marked for intraparenchymal lesions (Allan et al 1994, Cooke 1994, 1999) although this was not confirmed in a recent study by Hamrick et al (2004).

Incidence in mature infants

The true incidence in infants of 35 weeks of gestation and above is difficult to derive as most infants born at this

maturity are healthy and are not referred to neonatal units for intensive care or intracranial scanning. Those that are referred are clearly highly selected, and the incidence of GMH–IVH in this group will not be representative of the whole population. Although GMH–IVH is uncommon in mature infants it is well documented (Cartwright et al 1979, Fenichel et al 1984, Mitchell & O'Tuama 1980, Palma et al 1979, Scher et al 1982). By 35–36 weeks, involution of the subependymal germinal matrix is almost complete and bleeding in this area is uncommon. The overall incidence of GMH–IVH diagnosed by ultrasound is 2–5% of an unselected, asymptomatic group of full-term infants (Hayden et al 1985, Heibel et al 1993, Mercuri et al 1998). It was bilateral in approximately one-half of cases (Hayden et al 1985) and in a group of 1000 unselected low-risk full-term infants approximately 1% had associated IVH (Heibel et al 1993). IVH due to choroid plexus hemorrhage (see below) accounted for a further 1%.

Mature infants described in isolated case reports are likely to be symptomatic for the attending clinicians to perform scans, and it is not surprising that in these infants the majority of lesions are extensive and some involve the cerebral parenchyma. Asphyxia may precede the hemorrhage in mature infants, but this is not invariable, and often there are no obvious risk factors. IVH in full-term infants has been reported to be due to choroid plexus or tela choroidea hemorrhage, vascular malformations or extension of parenchymal hemorrhagic infarcts, and these are all discussed on page 418. Thalamic hemorrhage (see p. 420) is reported to be the commonest cause of IVH in full-term infants who present with acute onset of hemorrhage up to 1 month of age (Roland et al 1990). This may be related to sinovenous thrombosis as was recently shown by Wu et al (2003). Other causes in mature babies include blunt abdominal trauma (Wehberg et al 1992) and following aspiration of an intraventricular reservoir (Moghal et al 1992). The prognosis for a group of infants presenting at term with symptomatic IVH was mixed (Jocelyn & Casiro 1992). One-half were apparently normal at a mean age of 36 months, but one-third had severe handicaps. In general, extensive IVH occurring in full-term infants is very unusual.

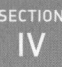

TIMING OF THE BLEED

As discussed above, GMH–IVH is generally a condition that occurs after birth. Initially, the age at onset of hemorrhage was inferred from autopsy material and reflected a bias towards the most severe cases. Indirect methods designed to time the onset of GMH–IVH have depended on analysis of the proportion of radioactively labeled red cells (Tsiantos et al 1974) or the proportion of mature erythrocytes in the intracerebral clot found at autopsy (Emerson et al 1977). These studies suggested that most bleeds occurred within the first 48 hours after birth.

The introduction of real-time ultrasound allowed frequent scanning of high-risk infants to accurately time the onset of GMH–IVH. Approximately 90% of these hemorrhages occur in the first week of life (Bejar et al 1980, de Crespigny et al 1982, Dolfin et al 1983, Levene et al 1982, Ment et al 1984a, Szymonowicz & Yu 1984a, Thorburn et al 1982) and the majority within the first 3 days of life. Approximately half of all cases of GMH–IVH occur in the first 24 hours of life (Beverley et al 1984a, Dolfin et al 1983, McDonald et al 1984b, Perlman & Volpe 1986).

Very early hemorrhage has been described. Anderson et al (1988) reported a group of infants with established GMH–IVH by 1 hour after birth, and infants with very early hemorrhage (<12 hours) have been considered to be an etiologically distinct group (Leviton et al 1988). Others have reported 19–27% of infants with GMH–IVH developed very early lesions, less than 12 hours from birth (Leviton et al 1991b, Ment et al 1992). Factors in labor may be particularly important in the development of these early lesions (see below).

Late-onset GMH–IVH is not uncommon, and in one study 15% of very low birth weight infants developed hemorrhage after 2 weeks of life (Trounce et al 1986). Hecht et al (1983) reported 17 infants with late onset of hemorrhage after 1 week of age, and all but two were confined to the region of the germinal matrix. Late onset GMH–IVH beyond the first week of life is reported to occur in the caudothalamic groove and be associated with the development of chronic lung disease (Smets et al 1997), but the pathophysiology of these lesions is unclear. If late GMH–IVH occurs, it is usually benign with little likelihood of serious adverse outcome.

Repeated ultrasound scans have shown that in 10–20% of infants, progression in the initial size of the GMH–IVH occurs over 24–48 hours, and this is illustrated in Figure 20.4 (Levene & de Vries 1984, Rademaker et al 1994, Shankaran et al 1982). Venous infarction is probably the most common mechanism by which this happens, and this is discussed on page 398.

ETIOLOGY

GMH–IVH is a condition of prematurity related to rupture of small vessels within the germinal matrix, and is most likely to occur in babies with respiratory distress syndrome (RDS). Many other factors have been described in the etiology of the condition, but in many studies the timing of the hemor-

rhage has not been established and, consequently, the cause and effect of hemorrhage may become confused. The most useful studies are those that have accurately timed the onset of GMH–IVH and analyzed risk factors only up until the time of hemorrhage. The following represents those risk factors that have been consistently reported to be important.

Prenatal factors

It has been suggested that early onset GMH–IVH before 12 hours of age represents a group of babies in whom prenatal factors are particularly important in the development of the condition (Anderson et al 1988, Leviton et al 1988).

Although prenatal factors are not a major factor in the etiology of GMH–IVH, they are increasingly recognized as being important in some cases. In a small group of babies known to have prenatal onset of parenchymal hemorrhage, pre-eclampsia, HELLP (Hemolysis, Elevated Liver enzymes, Low Platelets), fetal heart decelerations on the cardiotocograph and absent end-diastolic flow have all been described (de Vries et al 1998a). A number of reports have shown that maternal pre-eclampsia is associated with a significantly reduced risk of GMH–IVH (Ancel et al 2005, Developmental Epidemiology Network Investigators 1998, Kuban et al 1992, Spinillo et al 2007), even for large lesions (Shankaran et al 1996). Further analysis suggests that this effect may not be direct but reflects the more mature nature of babies born to mothers with pregnancy induced hypertension (Developmental Epidemiology Network Investigators 1998). Others have suggested that markers of a chronic hypoxic intrauterine environment may increase the risk of GMH–IVH, in particular, elevated uric acid as a marker of previous hypoxic-ischemic exposure (Perlman & Risser 1998) and total nucleated red blood cell count on day 1 of $>2.0 \times 10^9/l$ (Green et al 1995). Other protective factors for severe GMH–IVH include female sex (Heuchan et al 2002, Tioseco et al 2006) and African-American maternal race (Shankaran et al 1996).

A full course of antenatal corticosteroids is a very important factor in reducing the risk of GMH–IVH (Shankaran et al 1996), but it is not clear whether this is due to a direct effect on the brain or mediated through reduction in the severity of lung disease (see p. 401). Use of β-sympathomimetic tocolysis (Groome et al 1992) and magnesium sulfate administration to mothers in preterm labor (Mittendorf et al 2002) have both been suggested to significantly increase the risk of GMH–IVH developing in the infant, although this has not been reported by others (Anderson et al 1992, Levene et al 1982, Leviton et al 1991a).

One large study of the risk of GMH–IVH in multiple births treated with antenatal steroids showed no increased risk compared with singletons (Blickstein et al 2006) and others have shown no increased risk in the second born twin compared with the first (Gibson et al 1996).

Histological signs of amniotic infection have been reported to increase the risk of GMH–IVH in one study (Developmental Epidemiology Network Investigators 1998), but in another no increased risk was reported following histological chorioamnionitis (Sarkar et al 2005). Heavy maternal smoking may also be a factor for increasing risk of smaller hemorrhages (Spinillo et al 1995).

Intrapartum factors

In studies of monitoring in labor the fetuses that subsequently developed severe GMH–IVH with parenchymal involvement, there were significantly increased numbers of abnormal fetal heart rate patterns, although the numbers reported were small (Strauss et al 1985) or possibly the result of earlier fetal insult (de Vries et al 1998b). Others have shown no predictive benefit from cardiotocography in labor (Beverley et al 1984a, Levene et al 1982, Tejani et al 1984).

No report has found that cord blood gases predict the overall risk of GMH–IVH (Beverley & Chance 1984, Beverley et al 1984a, Ment et al 1992, Tejani & Verma 1989, Tejani et al 1984), but a low cord pH (<7.2) was a predictive factor for early onset GMH (Leviton et al 1991a). Low Apgar scores have been correlated with the development of hemorrhage (Beverley et al 1984a, D'Souza et al 1995, Heuchan et al 2002, Ment et al 1992, Strauss et al 1985, Tejani & Verma 1989). The majority of reports find no such association (Beverley & Chance 1984, de Crespigny & Robinson 1983, Hawgood et al 1984, Levene et al 1982, Leviton et al 1991a, Thorburn et al 1982). Szymonowicz et al (1984b) have found that severe facial bruising, a feature of birth trauma, was a strong predictor of infants likely to develop more severe forms of hemorrhage.

Condition at birth appeared to be associated with early onset GMH–IVH (Leviton et al 1991a), and exposure of the fetus to the active phase of labor (defined as commencing when the cervix reached 4 cm dilatation) also increased the risk of more severe hemorrhage (Anderson et al 1992). The importance of method of delivery on the development of GMH–IVH is controversial. Vaginal delivery and vertex delivery were considered to be important independent variables in the development of early hemorrhage (Ment et al 1992), but another five well-conducted studies have found no significant difference in the incidence of GMH–IVH between infants born vaginally and those presenting either by the breech or vertex (Bada et al 1984, de Crespigny & Levene et al 1982, Robinson 1983, Strauss et al 1985, Tejani et al 1984).

Most reports do not find that elective cesarean section, when the woman is not in labor, protects the infant from developing GMH–IVH (Bada et al 1984, Levene et al 1982, Malloy et al 1991, Morales et al 1989, Strauss et al 1985). Another study found cesarean section to lower the incidence of GMH–IVH compared with vaginal delivery, but neither reduced the severity of hemorrhage, nor reduced the mortality rate (de Crespigny & Robinson 1983). A protective effect of cesarean section has been claimed by others (Leviton et al 1991b, Tejani et al 1984, Thorburn et al 1982), but in the former study the majority of infants delivered by section was significantly more mature, thus reducing the likelihood of GMH–IVH occurring. There is no good evidence that cesarean section protects the premature infant against GMH–IVH.

Breech delivery is associated with higher risk of large GMH–IVH, but this effect is lost in multivariate analysis (Shakaran et al 1996). Vacuum extraction does not increase the risk of GMH–IVH in premature infants (Thomas et al 1997).

A recent study by Mercer et al (2006) suggested that delayed cord clamping led to a reduction in GMH–IVH, with five (14%) in the delayed clamping group vs. 13 (36%) in the nondelayed group; $P = 0.03$). The impact of cord-clamping group on IVH was evaluated adjusting for gestational age and cesarean section. The final model indicated that the IVH rate was >3 times higher in the ICC group (odds ratio [OR]: 3.5, 95% confidence interval [CI] 1.1–11.1).

It has been suggested that infants born outside a perinatal center and transported in have a higher incidence of GMH–IVH (Clark et al 1981, Hawgood et al 1984, Heuchan et al 2002, 2005, Levene et al 1982). The transported infants are highly selected, as those who are in good condition at birth may not be referred, thus biasing the group towards those with more severe illness and who are more likely to have intracerebral hemorrhage. Clark et al (1981) studied a group of very low birth weight infants in a geographically well-defined area. All infants born outside the perinatal center were referred in and there was no selection on the basis of severity of illness. Only 29% of the inborn infants had GMH–IVH compared with 79% of those outborn. Results from the NEOPAIN trial (Palmer et al 2005) showed that outborn babies were more likely to have severe IVH ($P = 0.0005$) and this increased risk persisted after controlling for severity of illness, but when adjustments were made for antenatal steroids the difference between in- and outborn was no longer significant.

Lung disease and its complications

Respiratory distress syndrome (RDS) is the most consistently recognized risk factor predisposing to GMH–IVH in premature infants. The association between massive intracranial hemorrhage (many of which were GMH–IVH in origin) and the presence of RDS was first made by Harrison et al (1968). They attributed the hemorrhage to severe hypoxia consequent on the lung disease. Subsequently, the association has been confirmed by other groups (Cooke 1981, D'Souza et al 1995, Levene et al 1982, Perlman et al 1983, Szymonowicz et al 1984b, Thorburn et al 1982), but there is probably not a causal relationship between RDS and hemorrhage. Infants with severe RDS require mechanical ventilation and are subject to complications associated with this form of treatment. It has been suggested that hypercapnia, pneumothorax and the fluctuating pattern of systemic blood pressure cause GMH–IVH, and these are discussed below.

Hypercapnia occurs commonly as a complication of severe RDS and is a potent vasodilator of newborn intracerebral arterioles (Archer et al 1986). This is thought to be an important factor in the development of GMH. A number of studies have reported hypercapnia to be an independent factor in the evolution of GMH–IVH (Cooke 1981, Dykes et al 1980, Levene et al 1982, Szymonowicz et al 1984b, Wallin et al

1990). Levene et al (1982) found that 81% of low birth weight infants who had both hypercapnia ($PaCO_2 > 6$ kPa) and severe acidosis (pH < 7.1) developed GMH–IVH and more than half of these infants had moderate or severe degrees of hemorrhage. One study analyzed the effect of hypercapnia on severe GMH–IVH (grade III–IV) and showed that there was an independent effect on risk of hemorrhage. A maximum $PaCO_2$ of 13.3 kPa (100 mmHg) doubled the risk of large hemorrhage compared to a baby with a maximum $PaCO_2$ of 6.7 kPa (50 mmHg) (Kaiser et al 2006).

Metabolic acidosis has also been reported to be an important independent variable in the development of GMH–IVH (Cooke 1981, Hawgood et al 1984, Levene et al 1982), although others have not confirmed this (Thorburn et al 1982). In the older literature infusion of sodium bicarbonate to treat metabolic acidosis has been claimed to be an important cause of GMH–IVH (Anderson et al 1976, Simmons et al 1974, Wigglesworth et al 1976). The rapid or large infusion of a hypertonic base induces osmotic gradients between blood and brain, causing cerebral shrinkage and subsequent hemorrhage. It has been calculated that an infusion of 10 mL of molar concentration sodium bicarbonate over less than 4 hours will produce such a gradient (Finberg 1977). Subsequent prospective studies also suggested that rapid infusion of hyperosmolar sodium bicarbonate was associated with a significantly increased incidence of GMH–IVH (Hawgood et al 1984, Papile et al 1978). Dykes et al (1980) found that administration of sodium bicarbonate after the first day of life was also a significant risk factor in the development of GMH–IVH. A controlled study of bicarbonate infusion in high-risk premature infants could not confirm this as a cause of GMH–IVH (Corbet et al 1977). These studies did not account for the timing of the hemorrhage and confusion between cause and effect is possible. There are no recent reports suggesting that sodium bicarbonate infusion is an important risk factor prior to the onset of GMH–IVH, but dosage of this agent is now considerably less than previously reported. Unless large volumes of sodium bicarbonate or other hyperosmolar solutions are used these substances are unlikely to produce GMH–IVH by a direct effect.

Pneumothorax has frequently been reported to cause or be an important factor in the development of GMH–IVH (Dykes et al 1980, Hill et al 1982, Lipscomb et al 1981, Peabody 1981, Szymonowicz et al 1984a, 1984b, Thorburn et al 1982, Wallin et al 1990), although a number of other equally careful studies have failed to substantiate this association (Cooke et al 1981, Levene et al 1982). In a prospective study, GMH–IVH was usually found to have developed within 6 hours of the clinical diagnosis of pneumothorax (Hill et al 1982). In each infant in whom blood pressure was measured, there was an increase in diastolic pressure and a fall in pH at the time of pneumothorax. Hill et al (1982) suggest that GMH–IVH occurs as the direct result of the increase in blood pressure consequent on the development of pneumothorax.

High frequency ventilation (HFV) has been reported to be associated with an increased risk of intracranial hemorrhage (HiFO Study Group 1993, Wiswell et al 1996). A meta-analysis of nine studies comparing HFV with conventional ventilation showed no excess of GMH–IVH or more severe forms of IVH (Clark et al 1996) and more recent Cochrane reviews show that high frequency jet or oscillation ventilation as elective treatment is not associated with an excess of GMH–IVH (Bhuta & Henderson-Smart 1999a, Henderson-Smart et al 1999). In a review of rescue high-frequency oscillatory ventilation versus conventional ventilation in preterm infants there was an increase in IVH of any grade compared with conventional ventilation (RR 1.77; CI 1.06, 2.96) and that there is a strong trend towards more severe forms of IVH (Bhuta & Henderson-Smart 2007).

Cardiovascular factors

It is generally thought that ill premature infants cannot regulate their cerebral blood flow (CBF) constant in the presence of changes in systemic blood pressure and, consequently, extremes of CBF predispose to either ischemia or hemorrhage in the vulnerable germinal matrix (Lou et al 1979, Pape & Wigglesworth 1979). A number of studies have attempted to relate loss of autoregulation to the development of hemorrhage (Ahmann et al 1983, Ment et al 1981, Milligan 1980), but all have major methodologic problems and do not prove the hypothesis.

Acute changes in blood pressure due to rapid infusions of blood or plasma and leading to GMH–IVH have been reported (Dykes et al 1980, Hawgood et al 1984, McDonald et al 1984b, Milligan 1980), but it is of considerable interest that most studies that have assessed the relationship between blood pressure and GMH–IVH have shown a strong relationship between periods of hypotension and the development of hemorrhage (Miall-Allen et al 1987, Watkins et al 1989), with occasional exceptions (D'Souza et al 1995). Mehrabani et al (1991) found that hypotension associated with pneumothorax increased the risk of more severe GMH–IVH by almost ten times compared with infants who had pneumothorax without hypotension. The explanation for this association may be that hypotension causes infarction of the germinal matrix as originally suggested by Towbin (1968). An alternative explanation is that hypotension causes a resetting of the vascular tone within the germinal matrix, and when the blood pressure increases to a more normal level (not necessarily hypertensive) GMH occurs. To support this, a Japanese group (Funato et al 1992) continuously scanned a group of infants at risk of GMH–IVH. They accurately timed the onset of hemorrhage in four cases, and in all four an increase of blood pressure was noted at the time of the hemorrhage compared with the lower blood pressure prior to the bleed. They suggest that GMH–IVH is due to a reperfusion injury. In support of this, Goddard-Finegold et al (1982) produced GMH–IVH in an animal model by rapid volume expansion in puppies that had been previously rendered hypotensive. This did not occur following infusion in untreated normotensive animals.

It has been reported that GMH–IVH occurs mainly in infants who are ventilated and show an unstable pattern of blood pressure characterized by rapid beat-to-beat fluctuations (Perlman et al 1983, Van Bel et al 1987). Perlman et al (1983) suggested that the fluctuating blood pressure pattern led to similar changes in CBF which caused rupture of the germinal matrix vessels. In contrast, Miall-Allen et al (1989) in a similar study assessed the coefficient of variation in systolic blood pressure prior to the onset of GMH–IVH and found that the percentage of time when this was greater than 5% was significantly higher in those infants who did not develop hemorrhage. They did not see the very large beat-to-beat variations reported by Perlman et al (1983). The risk of GMH–IVH may be related to the propagation of this blood pressure variability to the brain through an open ductus arteriosus (Mullaart et al 1994).

It has been observed that another important and common cause of sudden marked changes in systolic pressure is the handling of the infant (Perry et al 1990), but there was no correlation between attempts at reducing these responses and the subsequent development of GMH–IVH. In support of this, no difference in the incidence of GMH–IVH was found in a controlled study of premature babies who had a 'reduced manipulation' protocol compared with the standard 'frequent handling' management (Als et al 2004, Bada et al 1990), but there was an improvement in neurological outcome in the individualized developmental care group (Als et al 2004).

The role of increased intracerebral venous pressure has also been suggested to be an important cause of GMH–IVH (Reynolds et al 1979). Little is known of the relationship between RDS and venous pressure, but anatomical evidence exists for severe venous stasis in the right atrium, jugular veins and deep venous system of Galen in neonatal respiratory disease. Increased intracranial venous pressure observed during the course of mechanical ventilation has been reported by Vert et al (1975), and others have also reported increased pressure in the right atrium (Perlman & Volpe 1986) and major changes in perfusion pressure due to fluctuating venous pressure (Perlman & Volpe 1987). Toubas et al (1978) have described an increase in central venous pressure in hypothermic experimental animals.

It has been reported that infants with patent ductus arteriosus (PDA) are at increased risk of developing GMH–IVH due to hemodynamic disturbances associated with the ductal shunt (Martin et al 1982, Perlman et al 1981). Additionally, once the ductus has been surgically ligated there is a sudden increase in systemic blood pressure (Marshall et al 1982) which may cause GMH. Other studies have shown no correlation between GMH–IVH and PDA (Ment et al 1984a) or acute onset or extension of an existing GMH–IVH lesion after surgical ligation of the ductus (Strange et al 1985). A careful hemodynamic study of Doppler assessment of the ductal patency has suggested that larger PDA diameter and higher right ventricular output are significantly associated with the risk of subsequently developing a severe GMH–IVH (Evans & Kluckow 1996).

It is most likely that cardiovascular hemodynamic instability is a key risk factor for the development of GMH–IVH and it is the constellation of critical changes in CBF mediated by interaction between the baby's spontaneous respiratory activity and the ventilator via a PDA which is the critical factor in the development of hemorrhage of this type. Performing echocardiographic measurement of the superior vena cava (SVC) flow several times during the first day after birth, Osborn et al (2003) were able to show that late GMH–IVH was associated with antecedent low SVC flow during the first day.

Inflammation

There is much interest in the role of inflammation as a trigger to a number of neonatal diseases including PVL. This is discussed in detail in Chapter 19. Gopel et al (2005) showed that infants who developed IVH had a higher concentration of the pro-inflammatory cytokine IL-6 in umbilical cord blood although others have not been able to replicate these findings.

Extravascular pressure

The brain loses extracellular fluid over the first few days of life, and it has been suggested that shrinkage predisposes to vessel rupture due to a lower tissue hydrostatic pressure and an acute increase between intra- and extravascular pressure gradients (DeCourten & Rabinowicz 1981). Others have shown that prevention of postnatal water loss from the brain by prolactin injection prevents intracerebral hemorrhage (Coulter et al 1985). A high serum sodium concentration (>145 mmol/L), as a marker of reduced extravascular volume, was correlated with the development of GMH–IVH, but no significant association could be found (Lupton et al 1990).

Coagulation defects

It has been postulated by a variety of researchers that after capillary rupture has occurred, bleeding is more likely to continue in the presence of coagulation disturbances (Beverley et al 1984b, Chessels & Wigglesworth 1972, Foley & McNicol 1977, McDonald et al 1984a, Setzer et al 1982, Thorburn et al 1982). Few studies have examined clotting before the onset of hemorrhage and results are conflicting. Beverley et al (1984b) found no significant differences at birth in a variety of coagulation studies in infants who later developed GMH–IVH, but at 48 hours of age there were significant differences in activated partial thromboplastin time and the activity of some clotting factors between the non-hemorrhage and GMH–IVH groups, but they could not show a relationship between the timing of GMH–IVH and the severity of coagulopathy. Conversely, McDonald et al (1984a) found a significant association between coagulopathy in the first few hours of life and subsequent GMH–IVH or extension of intracranial hemorrhage. The use of heparin to maintain patency of intravascular catheters is an equivocal risk factor. A fourfold increased risk has been reported from a retrospective study (Lesko et al 1986), but a more recent randomized control study has shown no increased risk (Chang et al 1997). Petaja et al (2001) showed the risk of IVH was increased in preterm infants with thrombophilic abnormality. A more recent study among 595 very low birth weight infants however found that the frequency of intraventricular hemorrhage or periventricular leukomalacia was not significantly influenced by any of the genetic variants tested (Hartel et al 2006).

Indometacin, a potent prostaglandin synthetase inhibitor, is used widely in premature infants to close a PDA and has been suggested to be a risk factor for GMH. Corazza et al (1984) found that indometacin significantly prolonged the bleeding time within 2 hours of its administration, but they and others (Maher et al 1985) could find no convincing link between indometacin administration and the initiation or maximal size of hemorrhage. More recently indometacin has been convincingly shown to reduce the risk of GMH–IVH (see p. 407).

Other factors

Flush solutions containing benzyl alcohol as a preservative have been suggested to cause GMH–IVH (Hiller et al 1986, Menon et al 1984), and withdrawal of benzyl alcohol from clinical use was associated with a considerable reduction in the number of infants with moderate or severe hemorrhage (Jardine & Rogers 1989). Clearly, iatrogenic causes of GMH–IVH must always be suspected, as new treatments are commonly introduced into neonatal medicine in an uncontrolled manner. Placing an umbilical artery catheter at the level of T_6–T_{11} (a high position) has been suggested to cause retrograde flow in the cerebral circulation, and in a retrospective study, placement of the catheter in the high position compared with the low (L_3–L_5) was significantly associated both with the development of GMH–IVH and its severity (Schick et al 1989).

Vigorous and frequent physiotherapy has been described to be the cause of a particular type of intracranial hemorrhage that may be confused with GMH–IVH in extremely premature infants (Harding et al 1998). In survivors this lesion leads to encephaloclastic porencephaly. Its origin is thought to be hemorrhagic infarction and is similar pathologically to the findings seen in older infants with shaking injuries as a result of non-accidental injury caused by shearing of bridging vessels over the brain surface.

A unifying hypothesis

GMH–IVH may occur when the structural integrity of the vessel wall is compromised and then ruptures following subsequent changes in intravascular pressure or blood flow. An additional hypothetical factor may be alterations in extravascular pressure. Various factors may be associated with acute changes in intravascular pressure which can be either respiratory or cardiovascular in origin. Respiratory risk factors include mechanical ventilation and pneumothorax which induce vasodilatation secondary to hypercapnia. The most important cardiovascular factors are those that cause a change in CBF and hypotensive infants may be most vulnerable once the blood pressure is restored. The changes

in blood pressure, and consequently in blood flow through the germinal matrix, are most likely to occur in the presence of hypercapnia and hypoxia, as these factors maximally dilate the cerebral arterioles. Prostaglandins play an important role in the vascular tone of the germinal matrix vessels, and factors may act at this level to predispose the infant to changes in local blood flow and rupture of compromised vessels. Once rupture has occurred, coagulopathy will exacerbate bleeding, which may then become more extensive and rupture into the lateral ventricles. Further impaired flow as the result of venous congestion (p. 398) occurs in the periventricular white matter, leading to venous infarction. This mechanism is summarized in Figure 20.7.

DIAGNOSIS
Clinical

This is discussed in detail in Chapter 9, and will be summarized briefly here. Before the introduction of scanning techniques, GMH–IVH was thought to be a devastating condition with obvious clinical signs. Volpe (1977) described two clinical manifestations: a rapidly evolving catastrophic deterioration and, less commonly, a slower saltatory course. Lazzara et al (1978) reported the main physical signs associated with GMH–IVH diagnosed by computerized tomography (CT) to include a tense fontanelle and either increase or decrease in spontaneous activity. In another study,

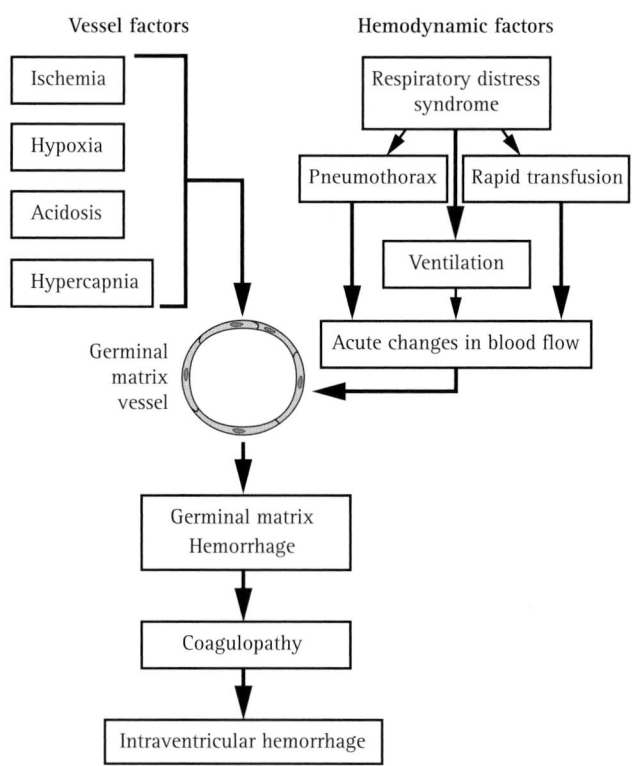

Figure 20.7 A model for the development of GMH and IVH which is dependent on both vessel and hemodynamic factors.

decerebrate posturing was seen in one-half of infants who were shown to have GMH–IVH on CT scans, but clonic seizures were seen equally frequently in the group of infants without hemorrhage (Krishnamoorthy et al 1977).

With the introduction of routine scanning techniques it was recognized that the majority of infants with GMH–IVH showed no overt symptoms. Burstein et al (1979) reported that the frequency of 'silent' hemorrhage was as high as 68% in a group of very low birth weight infants.

Comprehensive neurologic assessment methods have shown that a variety of clinical signs correlate with the presence of GMH–IVH, including impaired visual tracking, abnormal popliteal angle, later development of roving eye movements, decrease in tone and poor motility (Dubowitz et al 1981). Others have also found infants with GMH–IVH to have increased tone in the lower limbs (particularly popliteal angle) and hypotonia of the neck (particularly flexor muscles) and upper limb girdle muscles. In addition, those with GMH–IVH had brisker tendon reflexes and clonus of the ankle (Stewart et al 1983a).

Clinical assessment at full-term in prematurely born infants is useful in predicting outcome and has been shown to be a better predictor of poor outcome than neonatal ultrasound abnormalities (Dubowitz et al 1984). Of the 62 infants considered normal at 40 weeks, 91% were assessed as normal at 1 year. Abnormal movement patterns associated with intracranial pathology are discussed in detail in Chapter 9.

Imaging (see also Ch. 6)

CT was first used to diagnose GMH–IVH in 1976 (Pevsner et al 1976) but is inappropriate for routine clinical use. In 1979, ultrasound was shown to be a sensitive method for diagnosing GMH–IVH and has now become widely used as a convenient and safe method for detecting this condition. More recently, magnetic resonance imaging (MRI) has become widely used instead of CT scanning. The role of these three techniques in diagnosing hemorrhage is fully discussed in Chapter 6.

Electroencephalography (see also Ch. 12)

Cukier et al (1972) first described a specific EEG abnormality associated with GMH–IVH. This was referred to as a positive rolandic sharp wave, and the association has been confirmed subsequently by other workers (Blume & Dreyfus-Brisac 1982). Unfortunately, this abnormality appears not to be sensitive for uncomplicated GMH–IVH (Clancy et al 1984, Watanabe et al 1983) nor specific (Lombroso 1982). Positive rolandic sharp waves have also been reported in periventricular leukomalacia (Lombroso 1982, Marret et al 1986) and this particular EEG pattern is common when GMH–IVH is associated with severe leukomalacia. Therefore, the EEG may not be a useful method for diagnosing GMH–IVH alone but may be of value in prognosis because of frequently associated parenchymal lesions. The role of this technique is fully discussed in Chapter 12.

PREVENTION OF GMH–IVH

There is a large body of data investigating the role of vitamins and drugs in the prevention of GMH–IVH (Table 20.2) and a few studies have shown convincing data that GMH–IVH can be prevented when treatment is given either prenatally or postnatally. Figures 20.8 and 20.9 summarize this data where up-to-date systematic reviews are available.

Antenatal drug interventions

ANTENATAL CORTICOSTEROIDS (Fig. 20.8) To date 21 randomized controlled trials involving over 4000 babies have evaluated the role of corticosteroids in improving perinatal outcome when given antenatally to women in premature labor. A systematic review (Roberts & Dalziel 2007) of these trials has shown that corticosteroid administration is associated with a significant reduction in the risk of intraventricular hemorrhage (OR 0.54; CI 0.43, 0.69). There is also a strong trend towards improving long-term neurologic outcome in survivors (OR 0.64; CI 0.14, 2.98). It is not known whether the steroids reduce the incidence of GMH–IVH through the reduction in risk and severity of respiratory distress syndrome, stabilization of blood pressure or whether there is a direct cerebral protective effect. Studies of postnatal rescue corticosteroid administration to premature babies with severe lung disease within 96 hours of birth have shown no reduction in the risk of severe IVH.

ANTENATAL PHENOBARBITONE (Fig. 20.8) To date there have been 8 trials involving over 1600 babies of phenobarbitone given to mothers in preterm labor to prevent GMH–IVH and these have been systematically reviewed (Crowther & Henderson-Smart 1999a). When all 8 studies were compared there was a significant reduction in the rate of GMH–IVH of all grades of severity (RR 0.75; CI 0.65, 0.88) and in more severe grades of IVH (RR 0.49; CI 0.32, 0.74). There were few data on outcome of survivors, but no difference in the incidence of adverse outcome was found when the children between 18 and 36 months of age were assessed.

Table 20.2 Agents evaluated in preventing GMH–IVH

Postnatal administration	Antenatal administration
*Ethamsylate	*Corticosteroids
*Factor XIII concentrate	*Phenobarbitone
*Fresh frozen plasma	*Vitamin K
*Indometacin	
*Pancuronium	
*Phenobarbitone	
Surfactant	
Tranexamic acid	
*Vitamin A	
*Vitamin E	

*These have been shown on at least one randomized control study to significantly reduce the risk of hemorrhage. See the text for a detailed discussion.

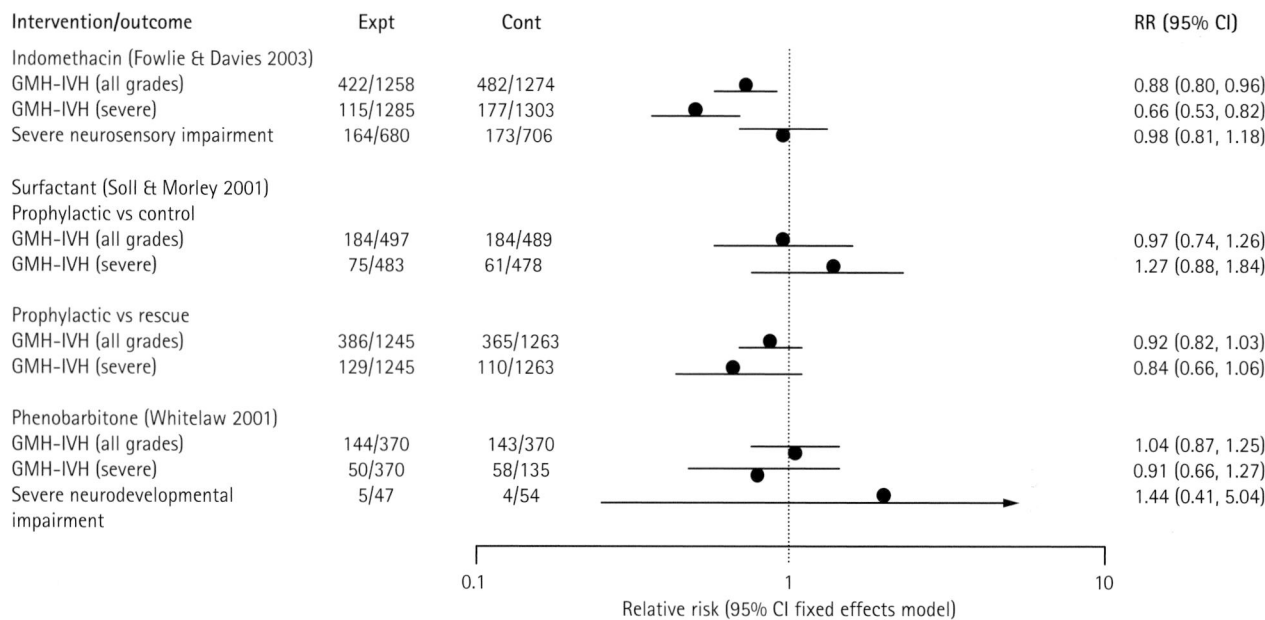

Intervention/outcome	Expt	Cont	RR (95%CI)
Prenatal corticosteroids			
GMH–IVH (diagnosed on U/S)	47 / 300	77 / 296	0.57 (0.41, 0.78)
Long term neurological abnormality	23 / 403	32 / 375	0.65 (0.39, 1.08)
Prenatal phenobarbital			
All GMH–IVH	196 / 762	252 / 741	0.75 (0.65, 0.88)
Severe (grades 3, 4) IVH	32 / 731	65 / 708	0.49 (0.32, 0.74)
Cerebral palsy	20 / 259	18 / 259	1.07 (0.58, 1.96)
Prenatal vitamin K			
All GMH–IVH	108 / 300	131 / 306	0.82 (0.67, 1.00)
Severe (grades 3, 4) IVH	23 / 300	32 / 306	0.75 (0.45, 1.25)
Prenatal TRH			
All GMH–IVH	282 / 1819	262 / 1826	1.08 (0.93, 1.26)
Severe (grades 3, 4) IVH	72 / 1647	64 / 1666	1.13 (0.82, 1.57)

Relative risk (95% CI fixed effects model)

Figure 20.8 Results of systematic reviews of prenatal drug interventions to prevent GMH–IVH or disability.

Intervention/outcome	Expt	Cont	RR (95% CI)
Indomethacin (Fowlie & Davies 2003)			
GMH-IVH (all grades)	422/1258	482/1274	0.88 (0.80, 0.96)
GMH-IVH (severe)	115/1285	177/1303	0.66 (0.53, 0.82)
Severe neurosensory impairment	164/680	173/706	0.98 (0.81, 1.18)
Surfactant (Soll & Morley 2001)			
Prophylactic vs control			
GMH-IVH (all grades)	184/497	184/489	0.97 (0.74, 1.26)
GMH-IVH (severe)	75/483	61/478	1.27 (0.88, 1.84)
Prophylactic vs rescue			
GMH-IVH (all grades)	386/1245	365/1263	0.92 (0.82, 1.03)
GMH-IVH (severe)	129/1245	110/1263	0.84 (0.66, 1.06)
Phenobarbitone (Whitelaw 2001)			
GMH-IVH (all grades)	144/370	143/370	1.04 (0.87, 1.25)
GMH-IVH (severe)	50/370	58/135	0.91 (0.66, 1.27)
Severe neurodevelopmental impairment	5/47	4/54	1.44 (0.41, 5.04)

Relative risk (95% CI fixed effects model)

Figure 20.9 Results of systematic reviews of postnatal interventions to prevent GMH–IVH.

The methodological quality of some of these reports was questioned (Crowther & Henderson-Smart 1999a). Some studies failed to randomize, others did not have a placebo arm, and the rates of exclusion of many of these studies were high. When these studies were excluded, the protective effect of antenatally administered phenobarbitone disappeared. Therefore the benefit of antenatal phenobarbitone in preventing disability has not been proven and if only high-quality randomized controlled trials are considered, there is no evidence that antenatally administered phenobarbitone has any effect.

ANTENATAL MAGNESIUM SULFATE There have been a number of retrospective reports of magnesium sulfate given either to terminate preterm labor or used as treatment for maternal hypertension in protecting the fetus against the subsequent development of cerebral palsy (Nelson & Grether 1995, Schendel et al 1996). The precise mechanism by which neuroprotection is apparently conferred is unknown, but a number of studies have investigated whether antenatal magnesium sulfate treatment reduces the incidence of GMH–IVH. In retrospective observational studies, the evidence that magnesium sulfate prevents GMH–IVH is equivocal, but a recent study of 799 babies with birthweight ≤1 Kg showed that it had no protective effect for the more severe types of IVH (Kimberlin et al 1998).

A systematic review of randomized controlled trials of magnesium sulfate in women in preterm labor described only two, both of poor quality. There was no difference in GMH–IVH in the only trial that reported neurologic complications in the newborn (Crowther & Moore 1999). It has been suggested that when magnesium sulfate is used in conjunction with indometacin to suppress preterm labor there is a significant excess of babies who develop severe IVH compared with the babies of mothers given magnesium sulfate alone (Iannucci et al 1996). There has also been a report that antenatal magnesium sulfate may increase neonatal mortality (Mittendorf et al 1997), although this is disputed and further prospective studies are still on-going. No reduction in the incidence of either a small or a large GMH–IVH was found in the recent Australian RCT (ACTOMg-Sop4) randomized multicenter study (Crowther et al 2003).

A retrospective study has suggested that premature infants exposed to antenatal magnesium sulfate were found to have a reduced risk of cystic PVL (FineSmith et al 1997), but there are no other studies to substantiate this.

ANTENATAL VITAMIN K (Fig. 20.8) A systemic review has compared 5 randomized studies involving 420 women to evaluate the role of vitamin K in the prevention of GMH–IVH, given to women in labor or very likely to deliver a premature infant (Crowther & Henderson-Smart 1999b). The rationale for giving vitamin K is to reduce the tendency to coagulopathy in the immature infant, which is probably an important factor in the subsequent development of hemorrhage. Despite initial enthusiasm for this therapy, the effects appear to be marginal. Antenatal vitamin K was associated with a strong, but non-significant trend towards reduction in the overall rate of GMH–IVH (RR 0.82; CI 0.67–1.00) as well as a somewhat less strong reduction in the more severe types of IVH (RR 0.75; CI 0.45, 1.25). Unfortunately, only one of these 5 studies was rated as of acceptable quality by the reviewers and this study showed a non-significant trend towards protection against GMH–IVH. Follow-up of babies enrolled into these studies was very poor and no differences were seen.

THYROTROPIN-RELEASING HORMONE (Fig. 20.8) Thyroid hormone has been postulated as an important factor in maturation of the developing lung and the immature CNS. Administration of thyrotropin-releasing hormone (TRH) together with corticosteroids to mothers in, or at high risk of, premature labor has been evaluated in its outcome on GMH–IVH. To date 13 trials have been published involving over 4500 women. In a systematic review of these studies (Crowther et al 1999) there was no difference in the incidence of either any GMH–IVH or of severe IVH between the two groups. Information on the outcome of survivors was available for only one of these studies (ACTOBAT 1995) and

there was an increased incidence of motor delay (RR 1.31; CI 1.09–1.56), motor impairment (RR 1.51; CI 1.01, 2.24) and social delay (RR 1.25; CI 1.03–1.51) in the TRH treated group. This is a worrying finding and suggests that TRH may have a negative effect on early brain development.

HYDROXYPROGESERONE 17 Alpha-hydroxyprogesterone has been shown in women at risk of premature delivery to significantly reduce the risk of delivery before 37 weeks (RR 0.66, CI 0.54, 0.91). The authors of the largest study (Meis et al 2003) also showed that in infants whose mothers had this treatment there was a significantly lower risk of GMH–IVH (RR 0.25, CI 0.9–0.92). It is not clear whether this effect is due to fewer preterm infants being born in the progesterone group or whether there is a direct cerebral effect. There is no data from 6 studies on whether this correlates with improved subsequent outcome in the children (Dodd et al 2007).

Postnatal drug interventions

POSTNATAL PHENOBARBITONE This was the first agent claimed to prevent GMH–IVH. Donn et al (1981) gave two loading doses of 10 mg/Kg intravenously 12 hours apart and adjusted the maintenance dose to achieve a serum level of 20–30 μg/mL by the third day of life. GMH–IVH occurred in only 4 of the 30 (13%) infants in the phenobarbitone group compared with 14 of the 30 (47%) control infants ($P = 0.01$). They reported their results again after studying a total of 105 babies and continued to show an impressive reduction in the incidence of GMH–IVH in the treated group (Donn et al 1982). This study was not performed blind and the neonatal staff knew which infants received the drug. Since this original report a meta-analysis of 9 RCTs involving 740 patients (Whitelaw & Odd 2007) showed no differences between the phenobarbitone and control groups for any size of GMH–IVH or in more severe hemorrhages (see Fig. 20.9).

There have been only 2 follow-up reports of infants from these phenobarbitone studies. There were no differences at 18 months in neurologic items (Krishnamoorthy et al 1990) or in neurodevelopmental impairment at a mean age of 27 months (Ruth et al 1988). In conclusion, there is no evidence that postnatally administered phenobarbitone has any benefit in the prevention of GMH–IVH.

POSTNATAL INDOMETACIN (Fig. 20.9) Indomethacin (now known as indometacin) is a potent prostaglandin synthetase inhibitor and inactivates prostaglandin and other prostaglandin-like compounds. In an animal study, Ment et al (1983) found in puppies that indometacin significantly reduced the incidence of GMH–IVH induced by a hypotension/hypertension technique. The pretreated puppies had significantly fewer fluctuations in blood pressure and indometacin appeared to ameliorate lability of blood pressure. This same group subsequently reported in a series of randomized controlled studies that indometacin significantly reduces the incidence of GMH–IVH in premature infants (Ment et al 1985b, 1988, 1994). These studies randomized 431 infants to receive indometacin 0.1 mg/Kg i.v. at 6 and 12 postnatal hours and every 24 hours for two more doses or placebo. The mechanism of action is unclear but may involve free-radical scavenging effect or inhibition of active calcium transport in vascular smooth muscle.

Indometacin in the prevention of GMH–IVH and subsequent brain injury has now been extensively investigated. Fowlie and Davis (2003) reported a systematic review of 19 randomized controlled studies using prophylactic indometacin in premature infants. The incidence of GMH–IVH of all grades was significantly reduced in indometacin treated groups (RR 0.88; CI 0.80, 0.96). When only more severe degrees of hemorrhage were reported (Papille grade 3 and 4) this effect was still present (RR 0.66; CI 0.53, 0.82).

Outcome measures of death or severe neurosensory impairment were reported in 4 studies, but no significant effect of indometacin could be found (RR 1.02; CI 0.90, 1.15) (Fowlie & Davis 2003). Two follow-up studies reported a trend towards less severe disability in the indometacin group (Bandstra et al 1988, Ment et al 1994). One study showed that there was a significant improvement in Stanford–Binet IQ scores at 36 months when both maternal education and infant birth weight were controlled for ($P = 0.044$) (Ment et al 1996). A recent post-hoc analysis of the original indometacin trial suggested that boys exposed to indometacin had significantly better outcome in verbal test scores than females (Ment et al 2006), suggesting a gender specific effect.

IBUPROFEN Ibuprofen is used as an alternative to indometacin in the medical management of patent ductus arteriosus and acts in a similar manner by prostaglandin synthase inhibition. A recent RCT has evaluated whether ibuprofen when given shortly after birth to a group of premature infants (<28 weeks gestation) reduces the incidence of GMH–IVH (Dani et al 2005). Ibuprofen did not reduce the incidence of any degree of GMH–IVH when compared to control (OR 0.96, CI 0.48, 2.03) or more severe GMH–IVH (grade 2–4) (OR 0.87, CI 0.25, 3.05) compared with controls.

POSTNATAL ETAMSYLATE As GMH–IVH occurs by capillary bleeding from the germinal matrix, Morgan et al (1981) suggested that ethamsylate (now known as etamsylate), a drug known to reduce capillary bleeding, may prevent this form of hemorrhage. They enrolled 70 very low birth weight infants in a double-blind controlled study using 0.1 mg/Kg of drug or placebo. There was a significantly reduced incidence of GMH–IVH in etamsylate treated infants, but the frequency of larger bleeds was no different between the two groups. They subsequently enrolled more infants (not in a randomized manner) and reported that there was a reduction in neurologic abnormalities at follow-up, as well as a reduc-

tion in the number of ventriculoperitoneal shunts needed to treat posthemorrhagic hydrocephalus (Cooke & Morgan 1984). It has been suggested that as well as the platelet effect etamsylate reduces the synthesis of prostaglandins (Ment et al 1984b), which may protect the germinal matrix from rapid fluctuations in CBF.

A multicenter trial assessing the effect of etamsylate in the prevention of GMH–IVH (Benson et al 1986) has also suggested that etamsylate has a protective effect in both reducing the incidence of IVH and limiting the size of the eventual lesion. A total of 330 very low birth weight infants were enrolled and only 18.5% of the treated group developed IVH or parenchymal hemorrhage compared with 29.8% of the controls. There was no difference in mortality between the two groups. Outcome on surviving infants has been described from two different cohorts treated in the newborn period with etamsylate as part of an RCT (Elbourne et al 2001, Schulte et al 2005). Neither study showed significant differences in outcome between the two groups. There is no support for the proposition that etamsylate reduces functional brain injury.

POSTNATAL VITAMIN E Chiswick et al (1983) from Manchester, UK have claimed that early treatment with vitamin E protects against IVH in premature infants. They attempted to distinguish, by ultrasound scanning, ruptured from unruptured GMH, and on this basis showed an apparent protective effect of vitamin E on the frequency of GMH–IVH. However, when the combined incidences of both GMHs and IVHs were compared there was no difference in the incidence of GMH–IVH between the two groups. It is not possible using ultrasound to make the distinction, Chiswick et al claim, but they subsequently reported the results of a larger prospective randomized trial (Sinha et al 1987). Unfortunately, this study was not carried out in a blind manner, but they found that both inborn and outborn babies pretreated with vitamin E had a lower incidence of IVH and parenchymal hemorrhage.

Two further studies have suggested that vitamin E has an effect in protecting against GMH–IVH (Fish et al 1990, Speer et al 1984). In a randomized control study of intramuscular vitamin E in neonates of birth weight 1 Kg or less, this agent was shown to significantly reduce the incidence of any type of intracranial hemorrhage as well as severe hemorrhage only in the group of infants with a birth weight of 750 g and below (Fish et al 1990). There appeared to be no complications of treatment in this study. Another study of infants weighing less than 1 Kg at birth (Phelps 1984) showed that 14 of 43 infants pretreated with vitamin E developed severe hemorrhage compared with only 4 of 42 given placebo.

In an overview of 4 vitamin E studies that assessed its effect on GMH–IVH, Law et al (1990) concluded that 'vitamin E supplementation might not prevent neurological disability (as the result of GMH–IVH), and at best it would do so in no more than 2.5 percent of all treated infants'.

It is suggested that vitamin E stabilizes endothelial membranes, thus limiting the extent of hemorrhage (Chiswick et al 1983, Speer et al 1984). Alternatively, prevention of mitochondrial damage by its activity in scavenging oxygen free-radicals has been proposed as its main mechanism of action (Ment 1985a). In addition, it has been shown that superoxide dismutase (a powerful oxygen free-radical scavenger) reduces the incidence of periventricular hemorrhage in an animal model (Ment et al 1985a).

Evidence has accumulated in the USA suggesting that a particular form of parenteral vitamin E (E-Ferol) causes thrombocytopenia, renal dysfunction and cholestatic liver failure (Bove et al 1985). It is not clear whether this is a direct effect of the vitamin preparation or occurs as a result of the vehicle in which the drug is administered. In view of the potential hazards of this agent and doubt as to its efficacy in preventing GMH–IVH, we cannot recommend it for routine use in premature infants.

POSTNATAL PANCURONIUM Pancuronium, a non-depolarizing neuromuscular blocker, has also been shown to prevent GMH–IVH in premature infants with marked beat-to-beat fluctuations in blood pressure (Perlman et al 1985). This pattern occurs in infants who actively expire against a positive-pressure inspiratory breath of the mechanical ventilator. Perlman et al (1985) recognized a group of infants with the fluctuating blood pressure pattern and paralyzed a randomly selected proportion of them. GMH–IVH developed in all ten spontaneously breathing infants, but only 5 of 14 given pancuronium developed hemorrhage and in 4 of the 5 GMH–IVH developed after the paralysis had worn off. On closer examination of their data only 20 of the 166 (12%) infants they studied actually developed GMH–IVH, an incidence well below that reported previously by Volpe in a population of very low birth weight infants (Tarby & Volpe 1982). This must raise the question of how representative of high-risk infants was their cohort.

Two previous studies of pancuronium failed to show any significant reduction in the incidence of GMH–IVH (Greenhough et al 1984, Pollitzer et al 1981). Further information must be obtained on the safety and efficacy of neuromuscular blockade in the prevention of GMH–IVH before it becomes routinely accepted.

POSTNATAL PLASMA EXPANSION Beverley et al (1985) reported a reduction in the incidence of GMH–IVH from 41 to 14% by means of early infusion of 10 mL/Kg of fresh frozen plasma (FFP) on admission to the neonatal unit and then again at 48 hours from birth. This was highly statistically significant ($P = 0.022$). The mechanism by which FFP prevents hemorrhage is unclear. They did not find that it reduced the frequency of clotting abnormalities in these infants, but did not report blood pressure data. It is possible that the reduction in incidence of severe GMH–IVH was related to the prevention of cerebral ischemia due to the effects of the FFP stabilizing the cerebral circulation.

More recently, a much larger study (Northern Neonatal Nursing Initiative Trial Group 1996) involving 776 babies compared early administration of 20 mL/Kg fresh frozen plasma (FFP) with 20 mL/Kg of a gelatin based plasma substitute (Gelofusin) and a control group with no bolus infusion. There was no difference in mortality or in IVH diagnosed at autopsy (ultrasound data was not reported). There was no difference in the number of disabled children alive at two years after birth (100% follow-up).

POSTNATAL VITAMIN A Low levels of vitamin A have been reported in a group of very low birth weight babies who sustained severe intracranial bleeding (Papagaroufalis et al 1988). Vitamin A has a role in the integrity of vascular endothelium and this may be important in the pathogenesis of GMH–IVH. This group organized a randomized control study to supplement a group of very immature infants with either intramuscular vitamin A (5000 IU within 12 hours and then 3750 IU daily) or placebo (Papagaroufalis et al 1991). There was a significant reduction in severe GMH–IVH in the vitamin A group and a trend towards reduction in all grades of hemorrhage.

POSTNATAL FACTOR XIII CONCENTRATE Premature infants with intracranial hemorrhage have been shown to have a markedly reduced platelet count and low fibrinogen and factor XIII activity (Shirahata et al 1990). Shirahata et al gave factor XIII concentrate within 6 hours of birth to a group of premature infants at risk of GMH–IVH and found a significant reduction in the incidence of hemorrhage in the group treated with factor XIII compared with controls. The role of recombinant activated factor VII in the prevention of GMH–IVH was also recently explored (Robertson 2006, Veldman 2006), but not enough data have so far been collected to suggest a protective effect.

POSTNATAL TRANEXAMIC ACID Another drug that reduces fibrinolytic activity of the germinal matrix is tranexamic acid and this has also been assessed for its ability to prevent GMH–IVH. In a double-blind controlled study of 100 very low birth weight infants, no reduction in either the incidence or severity of hemorrhage was found (Hensey et al 1984).

EXOGENOUS SURFACTANT (Fig. 20.9) Exogenous surfactant is a very effective agent in reducing mortality in premature infants with RDS. A number of studies have evaluated the role of surfactant in the prevention of GMH–IVH. A systematic review (Soll 1999) of prophylactic use of both synthetic and natural surfactants found no evidence that surfactant reduces the risk of GMH–IVH (any grade), or severe IVH, or the development of subsequent cerebral palsy. A second systematic review (Soll & Morley 2002) of prophylactic surfactant versus selective use in premature infants showed a non-significant trend towards reducing any grade of GMH–IVH (OR 0.92, CI 0.82, 1.03) and severe IVH (OR

0.84, CI 0.66, 1.06) in the surfactant compared with the control group.

The effects of rapid instillation of surfactant into the trachea on cerebral function and blood pressure have been examined. A short period of electrocerebral depression was reported lasting less than 10 minutes after instillation of the surfactant (Hellstrom-Westas et al 1992). The effect of surfactant on blood pressure has also been reported. A transient fall in mean arterial blood pressure of 6 mmHg (Cowan et al 1991) and 9.3 mmHg (Hellstrom-Westas et al 1992) immediately after giving the surfactant may be an important factor in the EEG changes and the later development of GMH–IVH.

GENERAL METHODS It has been noted that hypercapnia vasodilates cerebral arterioles and together with failure of autoregulation may predispose to GMH. Lou et al (1982) have retrospectively analyzed the $PaCO_2$ values following elective intubation and resuscitation in a group of very premature infants. They suggested that hyperventilation might re-establish autoregulation in these babies and consequently prevent GMH–IVH. No infant developed hemorrhage whose early $PaCO_2$ was less than 25 mmHg and hemorrhage tended to occur in the infants with the highest $PaCO_2$ levels measured in the first hour. All the infants with early GMH–IVH were born vaginally. The authors claim that the severity of the infants' lung disease was not the reason for the differences in $PaCO_2$ and the reduced incidence of GMH–IVH. These results must be treated with caution in view of the retrospective and uncontrolled nature of this study and the demonstration that hypocapnia is an important factor in the development of cystic PVL (p. 441).

Two controlled studies have been conducted to compare the neonatal outcome for elective versus selective cesarean section in the very premature baby (Zlatnik 1993). The results for reduction of the risk of intracranial pathology were contradictory, but taken together these studies were small and no significant effect was reported.

A group in Melbourne (Szymonowicz et al 1986) has attempted to modify early neonatal management in order to reduce the incidence of GMH–IVH in infants with a birth weight below 1250 g. They achieved significant improvement in measurements of pH, body temperature and blood pressure measured on admission to the neonatal unit and subsequently found significantly lower $PaCO_2$ tensions and higher blood pressure measurements. Infants treated by these methods had a 36% incidence of GMH–IVH compared with a 60% incidence in infants of the same birth weight treated by less aggressive means in a previous period. This was a highly significant reduction in the incidence of hemorrhage ($P < 0.001$). They claim that changes in neonatal management may account for an apparent reduction in the incidence of GMH–IVH in drug studies, particularly if these are not performed blind.

Handling of small, sick infants is known to be associated with large swings in systemic blood pressure (see p. 402).

Bada et al (1990) have attempted to assess whether a protocol of reduced manipulation of these babies reduces the incidence of GMH–IVH. There were no statistically significant differences between the standard management group and the reduced handling group. The differences in intervention time in the two groups were only significant for the first 48 hours, and even on the first day of life when the differences were greatest this amounted to an average of 2.4 hours (Als et al 2004). NIDCAP (Newborn Individualized Developmental Care) was assessed in an RCT for its role in altering brain function and structure. The incidence of IVH was small in both arms of the study but this form of management in the first 2 weeks of life did show better neurobehavioral functioning at 9 months of age (Als et al 2004).

PROGNOSIS

Determining the prognosis in infants who had sustained GMH–IVH is confused due to other confounding variables. GMH–IVH occurs in prematurely born infants, and it is known that very low birth weight infants have significantly lower scores of cognitive ability and motor adaptation than infants born at full-term. In a subgroup of very low birth weight babies without any evidence of brain pathology following repeated ultrasound examinations, in the newborn period, when compared with full-term control infants, they show significantly more clumsiness and lower IQ scores (Marlow et al 2005). Clearly the effect of very premature birth has its own long-term effects on brain function, quite apart from the effect of GMH–IVH. In addition to premature birth, other confounding variables include the general effects of severe prematurity on the developing brain, specific pathology such as periventricular leukomalacia (see Ch. 21) and later effects of socioeconomic class (Vohr & Ment 1996).

Mortality

Death in extremely premature infants may be due to a variety of causes including lung disease, sepsis, necrotizing enterocolitis and brain hemorrhage. At autopsy, cerebral hemorrhage may be found, but this may not be the primary cause of death and deciding what single insult killed the infant may be impossible. In general, it appears that the more severe the degree of hemorrhage, the higher is the mortality (Shankaran et al 1982, Smith et al 1983, Thorburn et al 1981). Hemorrhage confined to the region of the germinal matrix does not increase the risk of death, but intraparenchymal involvement has a high mortality. Approximately one-half (Ahmann et al 1983, de Vries et al 1998b, Martin et al 1984) to eighty-four percent (Larroque et al 2003, Thorburn et al 1981, Trounce et al 1986) of infants with intraparenchymal lesions die, although the staff and parental attitudes towards large IVH may influence the survival statistics.

Neurodevelopmental outcome

It is now recognized that about one third of babies born very premature and who subsequently develop cerebral palsy showed no abnormality on repeated cranial ultrasound scans performed throughout the neonatal period (Ancel et al 2006, Laptook et al 2005). Performing ultrasound on a more regular basis and for a longer period of time brought this number down to one fifth (de Vries et al 2004). Clearly ultrasound scans do not detect major neuropathology in these infants and white matter damage, which cranial ultrasound is poor at detecting, is missed. As a result neurodevelopmental disability may be misinterpreted as being due to more obvious lesions detected by ultrasound such as small GMH–IVH. Consequently caution must be used in interpreting outcome from ultrasound studies.

Early studies reporting outcome are biased towards those cases with the most obvious clinical presentation as it was only those who had CT scans performed (Kosmetatos et al 1980, Krishnamoorthy et al 1979). Studies in which all very premature infants had regular ultrasound scans provide more accurate follow-up data. There appears to be little increased risk of handicap in infants with grade I hemorrhage confined to the region of the germinal matrix, compared with similar infants without GMH–IVH (Papile et al 1983, Shankaran et al 1982, Stewart et al 1983b). Some authors have also suggested that moderate hemorrhage (clot in the lateral ventricles with no parenchymal extension) does not significantly increase the risk of adverse outcome compared with mild GMH–IVH (Dubowitz et al 1984, Papile et al 1983, Stewart et al 1983b). However, others have suggested a definite trend between the size of GMH–IVH and incidence of severe disability (Catto-Smith et al 1985). The latter authors report that two-thirds of infants with this form of hemorrhage had major disability, an incidence higher than most other follow-up studies. In summary, the prognosis for infants with uncomplicated GMH–IVH (no parenchymal extension or ventricular dilatation) is very likely to be good with respect to these infants not developing cerebral palsy.

Earlier studies relating the severity of GMH–IVH to outcome in school-age children agree that providing hemorrhage does not extend into the cerebral parenchyma and there is no significant ventricular dilatation the outcome is no different from infants born of the same degree of prematurity but without evidence of GMH–IVH (Levene et al 1992, Lowe & Papile 1990, Vohr et al 1992). At 5 years of age, 60% of children with Papile grade III and IV hemorrhage were normal on neurologic assessment and children with grade I and II GMH–IVH had no worse outcome than prematurely born children with no GMH–IVH (Vohr et al 1992). Lowe and Papile (1990) found that on a battery of tests the children with previous GMH–IVH (Papile grade I and II) did not perform significantly worse on any one test, but when all tests were combined together they did perform less well than a prematurely born group without hemorrhage. Similarly, when a group of very low birth weight infants were seen at 5 years and tests of motor impairment (degree of clumsiness) performed, although the presence of GMH–IVH did not impair performance, when those infants

who had 'prolonged flare' as well as GMH–IVH were considered, the 'double ultrasound abnormality' was associated with less good motor performance (Levene et al 1992). Motor coordination was impaired at 5 years in very low birth weight infants to the same degree whether or not the child had IVH in the neonatal period (Vohr et al 1992). There is a suggestion that language development at 3 years of age may be worse in infants with a birth weight below 1000 g if they had sustained GMH–IVH (Grunau et al 1990).

More recently recruited long-term follow up studies of very immature babies with less severe forms of GMH–IVH have shown an increase in the prevalence of cerebral palsy in grade 2 hemorrhage (24%) compared with only 6% for grade 1 or similar weight infants with no evidence of hemorrhage (Sherlock et al 2005). Surprisingly there were no such differences in dyspraxia or the incidence of major neurosensory disability at age 8 years when grade 2 was compared with similar infants <28 weeks of gestation without GMH–IVH. In another study, Patra et al (2006) found that when babies born weighing <1 Kg with either grade 1–2 GMH–IVH and who survived until the age of 20 months were compared with a similar cohort without hemorrhage they scored lower on Bailey subscores and had significantly more major neurologic abnormality and neurodevelopmental impairment. It is likely that these most recent studies are reporting increasingly immature infants who survived compared with earlier years and that relatively minor brain injury in these babies is an important factor in worse outcome.

INTRAPARENCHYMAL HEMORRHAGE

There may be difficulty in distinguishing the underlying pathology of 'parenchymal hemorrhage' as both venous infarction and PVL may cause bleeding into the white matter which makes predicting outcome problematic. In this section we refer to intraparenchymal hemorrhage as being unilateral with no evidence of involvement of the contralateral hemisphere. Follow-up studies agree that there is a high incidence of adverse neurodevelopmental outcome whatever the cause. Major handicap ranges from about 50% to 100% of infants with parenchymal involvement (Catto-Smith et al 1985, de Vries et al 1998b, 2001, Dubowitz et al 1984, Papile et al 1983, Shankaran et al 1982, Stewart et al 1983b, TeKoiste et al 1985). McMenamin et al (1984) have suggested that outcome following this form of hemorrhage is much worse in infants weighing less than 1000 g at birth compared with larger babies. Furthermore, they found that survivors of large parenchymal lesions all had more significant handicap than those surviving less extensive parenchymal involvement. Bassam et al (2006) used a three point scoring system and showed that a higher score (extensive, bilateral and associated with a midline shift) was associated with a worse outcome. The distinction between the ultrasound appearances of periventricular leukomalacia and parenchymal involvement due to venous infarction may be very difficult in the first week of life. Evolution to poren-cephaly or multiple cystic degeneration helps to clarify the pathology, and this is why early abnormal ultrasound appearances (those present in the first two weeks of life) are less good at predicting adverse outcome than those made later when the lesions have had time to evolve fully (Cooke 1987, Nwaesei et al 1988, Stewart et al 1987). MRI used to assess the degree of myelination predicts neurodevelopmental outcome at 3 years of age, but was found to be less accurate in its predictive ability than cranial ultrasound (van der Bor et al 1992).

In a study of 1636 premature infants born between 1990 and 1998, de Vries et al (2004) found that 12% of survivors with large IVH (blood distending the ventricle in the acute phase and clot filling >50% of the ventricle) developed cerebral palsy compared with 47% who developed it after surviving unilateral parenchymal hemorrhage. The most common form of cerebral palsy was spastic hemiplegia, contralateral to the side of the parenchymal hemorrhage. The location of the unilateral parenchymal hemorrhage also appears to predict risk of cerebral palsy. Nine of 10 babies with parenchymal lesions in the fronto-parietal region did not develop cerebral palsy, compared with all survivors of apparent hemorrhage in the occipital region who did so (Rademaker et al 1994). MR studies may show asymmetry of the myelination of the posterior limb of the internal capsule and cerebral peduncles when imaged at term and is thought to be due to Wallerian degeneration secondary to dying back of axons following parenchymal damage in some babies (Cowan and de Vries 2005, de Vries et al 2001).

Porencephaly

The prognosis for established porencephaly is also controversial. A bad prognosis with cerebral palsy (Cooke 1987, Guzzetta et al 1986) and developmental impairment (Cooke 1987) has been reported, but de Vries et al (1985, 2001) suggest that the outcome in infants with porencephaly is much more benign. It is important to note that despite extensive hemorrhage and early signs of cerebral palsy, the eventual disability may be mild and the child should be able to attend a normal school (Fawer et al 1983). The outcome of 16 prematurely born infants with posthemorrhagic porencephalic cavities was reviewed at a mean age of 33 months (Blackman et al 1991). They found that 81% of the children had cerebral palsy, but only 19% had moderate or severe cognitive deficits.

SEQUELAE OF GMH–IVH

Metabolic complications

A number of hormonal disturbances or metabolic problems are described in association with various types of intracranial hemorrhage. Some of these are also discussed on page 562 as they may occur as the result of birth asphyxia or other forms of intracranial pathology.

Inappropriate antidiuretic hormone secretion has been reported in a few premature infants with CT scan diagnosis of intracranial hemorrhage (Moylan et al 1978). Central diabetes insipidus has also been reported in a premature infant with GMH–IVH (Adams et al 1976). This was a transient condition and required short-term treatment with a vasopressin-like agent.

Hyperpyrexia following GMH–IVH is well recognized (Gomes & Weerasuriya 1975) and this is seen particularly in full-term infants and may occur following a variety of different forms of intracranial hemorrhage. Elevated body temperature may persist for weeks and may initially cause confusion with meningitis, particularly if there is a high CSF white cell count with low glucose.

Subependymal pseudocyst

Cyst formation is a relatively common finding in the subependymal region at the head of the caudate nucleus in the newborn (Fig. 20.10). Cavitation within the germinal matrix is referred to as a pseudocyst because it is not lined by epithelium (Larroche 1972). These commonly develop after a small hemorrhage in the region of the germinal matrix and are easily recognized on ultrasound. They may develop following a variety of insults including prenatal infection with rubella or cytomegalovirus (Shaw & Alvord 1974). They may also occur as a 'normal' event if the rapidly developing germinal matrix outgrows its blood supply. In some cases the pseudocysts may be more anterior and bilateral (Rademaker et al 1993) and care must be taken not to confuse them with cystic periventricular leukomalacia (see p. 21). When the pseudocyst occurs following GMH–IVH it has no prognostic significance and if it represents the only cerebral insult the prognosis is excellent.

Encephaloclastic porencephaly

Encephaloclastic porencephaly refers to a fluid-filled defect lying within the cerebral parenchyma and communicating with a lateral ventricle.

Porencephaly occurs relatively commonly in the perinatal brain due to a variety of insults. The pathology of porencephaly is discussed in Chapter 13 and the antenatal diagnosis and significance are discussed in Chapter 15. Porencephaly may occur as a result of intracranial hemorrhage or infarction.

Porencephaly is a common finding in premature infants at the site of a pre-existing venous infarct (see p. 398) and develops in approximately two-thirds of infants with parenchymal hemorrhage or hemorrhagic infarction (Pasternak et al 1980), and these can be detected by imaging techniques. The time interval between initial hemorrhage and its evolution through to porencephaly may be 6–8 weeks.

The prognosis for infants and children with porencephaly depends entirely on the underlying cause of the porencephalic lesion. Its prognosis in infants with porencephaly secondary to venous infarction is discussed on page 411. Rarely the porencephalic cavity progressively expands, and this may cause deterioration in cerebral function (Tardieu et al 1981). Although the measured CSF pressure is not elevated, ventriculoperitoneal shunting can result in remark-

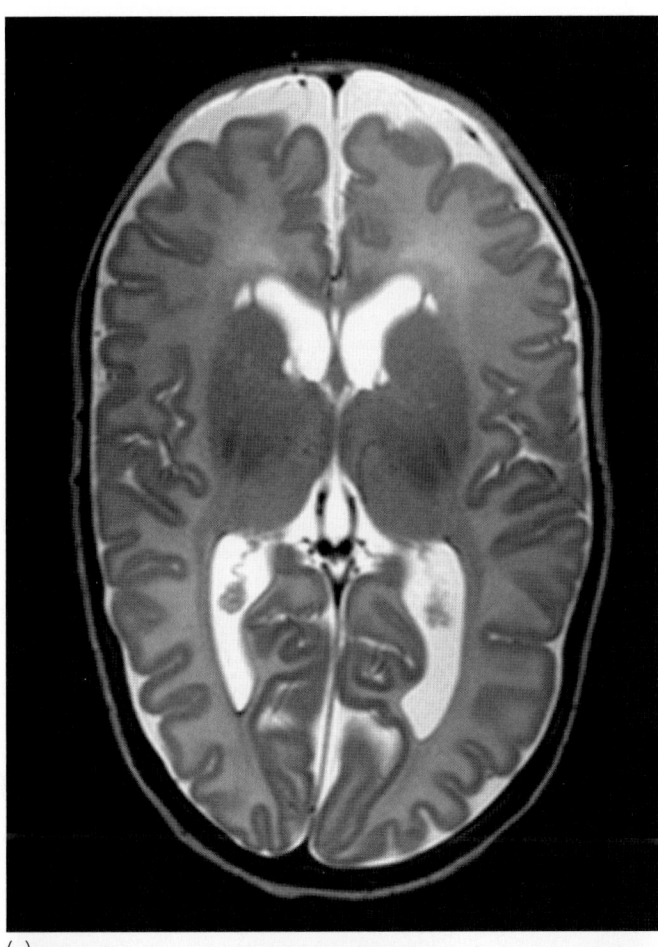

(a)

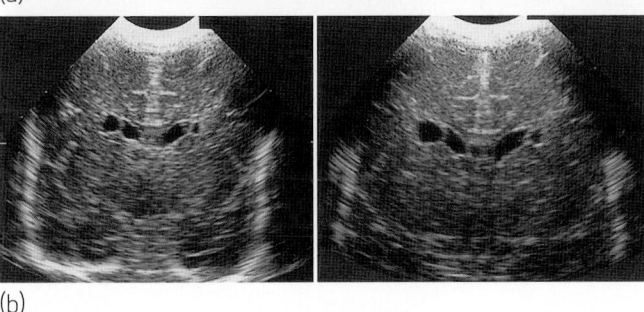

(b)

Figure 20.10 Subependymal pseudocysts. (a) Ultrasound scans showing bilateral pseudocysts. (b) MRI, T2SE at term equivalent age shows small germinal matrix cysts following germinal matrix hemorrhage and bilateral subependymal pseudocysts.

able improvement of focal motor deficits and intellectual development.

Posthemorrhagic hydrocephalus

This complication occurs relatively frequently following GMH–IVH, and is discussed in detail in Chapters 42 and 43.

SUBDURAL HEMORRHAGE

Fatal subdural hemorrhage is now rare but the incidence in surviving children is difficult to obtain. An epidemiological study in the UK and Republic of Ireland found that the incidence of subdural hematoma and effusion was 24.1 per 100 000 of infants 0–1 years (Hobbs et al 2005). The majority of these were thought to be due to non-accidental injury, but 14% were reported to result from either perinatal factors or 'birth trauma' and usually presented shortly after birth. In another recent study of causes of subdural hemorrhage diagnosed by CT brain scan only 1 of 74 were thought to be perinatal in origin (hemorrhagic disease of the newborn) but this study was heavily biased towards non-accidental injury (Datta et al 2005). The most relevant study with respect to perinatal subdural hemorrhages was from Sheffield (UK) where 111 unselected full-term infants were scanned with MR within 48 hours of birth. All were thought to be well babies who were neurologically normal (Whitby et al 2004). Nine of 111 (8%) had subdural hemorrhage and all had resolved by 4 weeks.

ETIOLOGY

Subdural hemorrhage may be due to a number of different underlying causes, but birth trauma is the most commonly recurring factor. In larger subdural hematoma expansion of the hemorrhagic mass occurs as fluid is osmotically drawn into the high protein clot over the first 3 weeks after the bleed. This is referred to as subacute hemorrhage or subdural hematoma (Minns 2005). If the lesion fails to resolve a chronic subdural collection develops, referred to as a subdural effusion. The subdural hemorrhage is usually small (<3 mm maximum transverse dimensions) and may be sub- or supratentorial in equal proportion involving both sites (Chamnanvanakij et al 2002). When supratentorial, bleeding was invariably in a posterior location over the occipital or parietal lobes (Whitby et al 2003).

Dural tear

This was usually associated with rapid delivery of the infant's head or trauma associated with difficult instrumental delivery. The dura mater divides the brain into three compartments: the two cerebral hemispheres and the cerebellum. The main folds are the falx cerebri and the tentorium cerebelli. The major venous sinuses are contained within these folds and dural tears are likely to cause extensive bleeding from the adjacent sinus. Welch and Strand (1986) have suggested that some extensive subdural hemorrhages are due to arterial bleeding, which is also likely to be due to trauma.

The fetal head withstands the compressive effects of labor well if the mechanical forces are applied evenly. With passage of the head through the birth canal the head molds to a long occipito-frontal diameter. If delivery is too rapid, then the mechanical forces are less well tolerated and there will be sudden changes in head shape. This causes stretching and possibly tearing of the dura. As long-axis stretching is most common, it is the vertical part of the tentorium that is most stressed and liable to rupture (Fig. 20.11). Subdural hemorrhage in the posterior fossa usually arises from rupture of the vein of Galen, straight or lateral sinuses. The most common site of hemorrhage appears to be at the falcotentorial junction near the incisura (Huang & Shen 1991). Tears of the falx cerebri are rare and occasionally subdural hemorrhage is associated with sinus thrombosis (Craig 1938).

Bridging vein rupture

In infancy non-accidental injury is the commonest cause of subdural hemorrhage which occurs as the result of rupture of bridging veins resulting from vascular shearing of these small veins between the cortical surface of the brain as they cross the subdural space. The shear stress results from the baby being violently shaken ('shaken baby injury'). In the neonate bridging vein rupture also occurs as a result of birth trauma due to rupture of the superior cerebral bridging veins (Pape & Wigglesworth 1979). These lesions occur most commonly over the cerebral convexity (Fig. 20.12) and may be seen in association with subarachnoid hemorrhage.

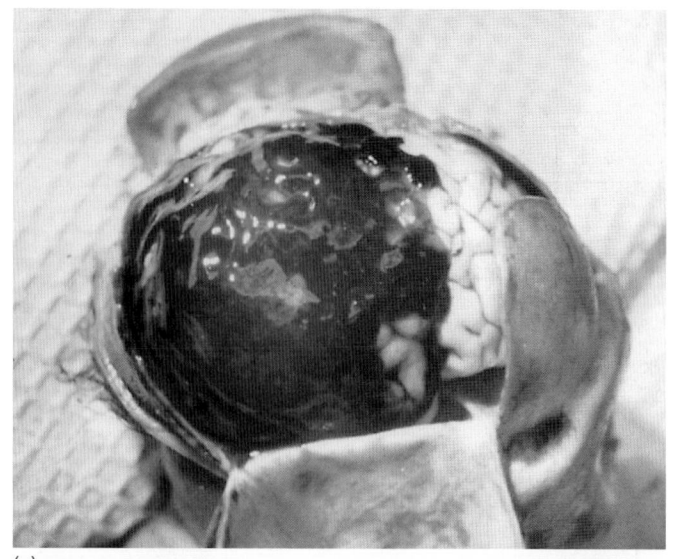

(a)

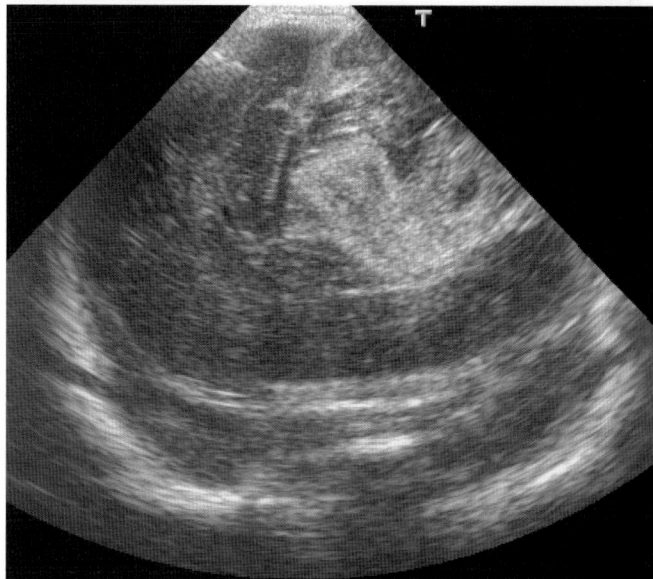

(b)

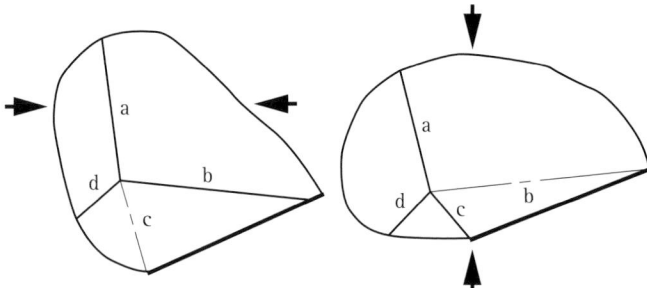

Figure 20.11 Dural tears associated with compressional stress to the neonatal head. The diagram on the left shows the effect of occipitofrontal compression with greatest strain on the vertical part of the tentorium (c). The diagram on the right shows the effect of compression between vault and base, with greatest strain on the horizontal part of the tentorium (b). Falx cerebri (a); line of junction of tentorium and falx (d). (Redrawn from Holland 1922.)

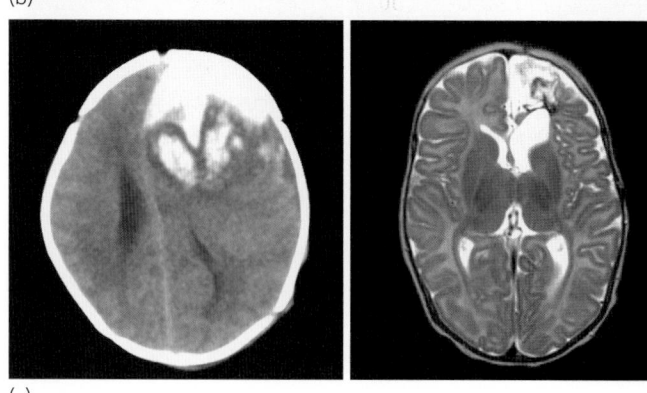

(c)

Figure 20.12 (a) Subdural hematoma over the right cerebral hemisphere. After reflection of the skull, thick blood clot remained over the cerebral convexity. (Reproduced, with permission, from Larroche 1984.) (b) Cranial ultrasound, coronal view showing a midline shift and a large left-sided parenchymal hemorrhage as well as a subdural hemorrhage. (c) CT scan prior to a surgical procedure to remove the subdural blood and the MRI (T2SE) performed at 3 months showing an area of cavitation and mild ex-vacuo dilatation.

Occipital osteodiastasis

Subdural hemorrhage may be associated with vaginal breech delivery in which there is excessive extension of the infant's neck. This causes separation of the squamous and lateral portions of the occipital bone (osteodiastasis) and direct injury to structures within the posterior cranial fossa, including the cerebellum and brainstem (Hemsath 1934, Wigglesworth & Husemeyer 1977). Exceptionally this may occur due to parietal diastasis. The prognosis is reported to be worse than in babies who have sustained subdural hemorrhage as the result of vacuum extraction (Odita & Hebi 1996).

Vacuum extraction

Vacuum extraction is well recognized to be associated with the development of subdural hemorrhage. This may be due to dural tears (Castillo & Fordham 1995, Hanigan et al 1990, Hayashi et al 1987, Huang & Shen 1991, Odita & Hebi 1996, Romodanov & Brodsky 1987), but in many cases the hemorrhage is small and causes few or no clinical signs. In one study 63% of babies with asymptomatic subdural hemorrhage had been born by actual or attempted vacuum delivery (Whitby et al 2004). The application of the vacuum cup to the vertex with longitudinal traction exerts vertical stresses on the tentorium with tearing and hemorrhage similar to that seen with forceps delivery. Hanigan et al (1990) described a distinctive pattern of hemorrhage due to vacuum extraction with extension over the superior surface of the cerebellum or inferior surface of the occipital lobe. Avrahami et al (1993) scanned ten babies born by the vacuum extractor who showed no clinical signs of either trauma or asphyxia and found that all of them showed evidence of hemorrhage representing a combination of subarachnoid, intradural tentorial bleeding and small juxtatentorial intracerebral hemorrhage, although in no cases were these bleeds thought to be severe. Other intracranial lesions including GMH–IVH, cerebellar hemorrhage and arterial infarction have also been reported as the result of vacuum extraction (Castillo & Fordham 1995). The reported prognosis from SDH due to vacuum extraction is generally good (Hayashi et al 1987, Odita & Hebi 1996). It must be noted that birth by cesarean section does not prevent subdural hemorrhage (Whitby et al 2004).

Convexity hemorrhage

The term 'convexity hemorrhage' is used because the precise origin of the bleeding is unclear and compression of the brain may occur with eventual infarction, thus making determination of the underlying lesion difficult. These lesions have also been referred to as lobar hemorrhages (Hanigan et al 1995). Convexity subdural hemorrhages may be more common in infants with coagulation disorders or those undergoing exchange transfusions (Morgan et al 1983).

Fetal subdural hematoma

There have been a number of reports of fetal subdural hematomas diagnosed either in utero or with chronic hematoma diagnosed shortly after an uneventful birth (for review see Arkman & Cracco 2000). A few cases are associated with blunt maternal trauma (Stephens et al 1997) or fetal coagulopathy, but the majority has no obvious antecedents. Prognosis was poor in the cases of larger hemorrhage, but normal outcome has been reported.

Other causes

Other causes can be considered under the following headings:

Bleeding disorders. Subdural hemorrhage in infants has been reported due to congenital bleeding disorders including factor V deficiency (Ehrenforth et al 1998, Salloja et al 2000) and factor VIII deficiency (Myles et al 2001), or a platelet function disorder (Hermansky–Pudlak disorder) (Russell-Eggitt et al 2000).

Post-meningitis. It may also be caused by meningitis (particularly *Haemophilus influenzae*), but is rarely seen in the neonatal period. A chronic subdural hemorrhage may be due to asymptomatic bleeding in the neonatal period which causes insidious symptoms some weeks or months after birth. In this case there is accumulation of fluid around the initial bleed due to an osmotic effect that creates a space occupying lesion. Determining the timing of the original bleed may be very difficult.

Rebleeding after the onset of subdural hemorrhage may occur up to four days later (Craig 1938). Rebleeding occurs as the result of resuscitation with restoration of blood pressure, or as the result of falling intracranial pressure in the few days after the original bleed.

CLINICAL FINDINGS

It is now known that many babies are asymptomatic with less severe forms of subdural hemorrhage. In those with symptoms they are often non-specific and depend on the severity and localization of the hemorrhage. In some cases symptoms may be delayed and only occur after a period of apparent neurologic normality (chronic subdural collection). This may be due to dural tear without damage to major vessels. More commonly, symptoms and signs are due to either raised intracranial pressure or associated asphyxial injury (Hayashi et al 1987). In a study of 26 near-term infants, CT diagnoses of subdural hemorrhage (and therefore symptomatic to demand a scan) were mainly non-specific including unexplained apnea, dusky episodes, subtle seizures, hypotonia or decreased limb movements (Chamnanvanakij et al 2002).

Massive hemorrhage may be associated with shock, coma and rapid demise. Posterior fossa hemorrhage has been reported to produce a recognizable symptom complex (Govaert et al 1990). This includes a tense fontanelle, decrease or absence of motor tone, lethargy, and reduced or absent primitive reflexes, apnea, irregular patterns of breathing, facial palsy and skew deviation of the eyes. A fixed bradycardia and sighing respiration are particular features of posterior fossa pathology. Although seizures are commonly seen, they are not necessary for the clinical diagnosis (Govaert et al 1990). Retinal hemorrhages have been reported in approximately 25% of cases (Hayashi et al 1987).

Convexity subdural hemorrhage may present with generalized or multifocal seizures. Occasionally, focal neurologic signs are seen, in particular a difference in tone between the two sides. Volpe (1977) suggests that the most distinctive sign of compression is a non-reactive or sluggish pupil due to third cranial nerve compression. It is likely that most infants with mild subdural bleeding have no symptoms or signs at all.

DIAGNOSIS

Ultrasound is not reliable in diagnosing or excluding small subdural lesions. Large convexity hemorrhages, particularly when causing displacement of midline structures, should be detected on ultrasound examination, or the echo-free subdural effusion may be seen. Scanning through the posterior fontanelle (Maertens 1989), mastoid fontanelle (Buckley et al 1997) or foramen magnum (Sudakoff et al 1993) may add precision to the diagnosis of tentorial abnormalities.

CT and MRI are more sensitive techniques for detecting smaller lesions, but even with these techniques distinction between small subdural hemorrhage and normal appearance may be impossible (Ludwig et al 1980). Subdural bleeding should be considered in all asphyxiated infants and, as its compressive effects are treatable, CT or MRI examination is recommended whenever this possibility is considered.

The features of subdural hemorrhage on CT scans have been described by Govaert et al (1990):

(1) Pericerebellar subdural hematoma. Intracerebellar hemorrhage may be present.
(2) Obvious hemorrhage in or around the tentorial apex, straight sinus and behind the third ventricle. These tend to coalesce to form a triangular area with its base against the occipital bone.
(3) Presence of hemorrhage between the posterior cerebral hemorrhages.

Infants with CT or MRI evidence of posterior fossa hemorrhage may have either subdural or cerebellar hemorrhage and distinction between the two may be difficult. The two conditions appear to occur with equal frequency in the neonate (Scotti et al 1981), but intracerebellar hemorrhage is more common in premature infants, and subdural hemorrhage is more likely in full-term infants (Menezes et al 1983). Figure 20.13 shows an example of subdural hemorrhage due to a tentorial tear diagnosed by CT.

TREATMENT

Most subdural hemorrhages require no treatment. In one study 25 of 26 babies with subdural hemorrhage diagnosed on CT imaging were managed expectantly and only one required surgical treatment for a depressed skull fracture. None required evacuation of the subdural hematoma (Chamnanvanakij et al 2002). Convexity hemorrhages causing a

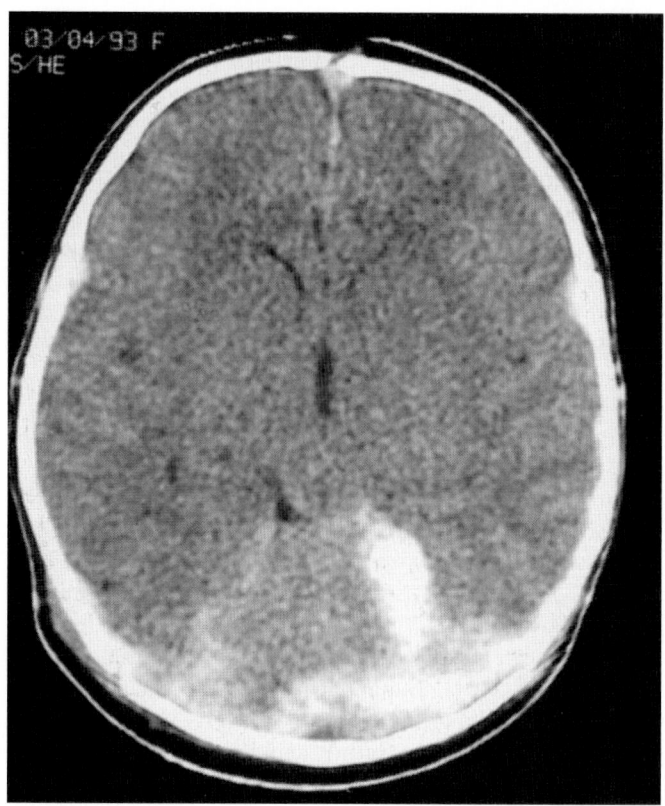

Figure 20.13 CT scan showing subdural hemorrhage associated with a tear of the left fold of the tentorium cerebelli.

midline shift should be decompressed by subdural tap (Vinchon et al 2005). Craniotomy may be necessary if the collection is not accessible to needling through the fontanelle. It is, however, important to distinguish clinical signs arising from diffuse cerebral involvement as occurs in asphyxia from focal abnormalities arising from hemorrhage. Treatment directed towards a minor collection will not improve the clinical signs or eventual prognosis in the presence of more diffuse cerebral injury.

The neurosurgical management of subdural hemorrhage is controversial. Massive subdural hemorrhage in the posterior cranial fossa may require aspiration of clot at craniotomy. Definite indications for craniotomy include signs of brainstem compression and raised intracranial pressure due to developing hydrocephalus (Huang & Shen 1991). In a review of 15 neonates referred for neurosurgical management for posterior fossa subdural hematomas only 8 required evacuation of clot and 7 apparently resolved spontaneously on serial imaging (Richard et al 1997). Neurosurgical management of hydrocephalus may be necessary.

PROGNOSIS

The prognosis for most subdural hemorrhages is good as the bleeding is usually relatively small (Castillo & Fordham 1995, Hayashi et al 1987, Odita & Hebi 1996), although those born by the breech, presumably with basal hemorrhage secondary to occipital osteodiastasis, are reported to have a worse prognosis (Odita & Hebi 1996). In one study almost 50% of survivors of subdural hematoma referred to a neurosurgical service were normal at 4.5 years, and one third were moderately to profoundly developmentally delayed (Richard et al 1997), presumably related to associated cerebral injury.

COMPLICATIONS

Hydrocephalus

Hydrocephalus may develop as the result of two mechanisms following subdural hemorrhage: obstructive and resorptive (Govaert & de Vries 1997). In the former the mass effect of the hemorrhage causes acute obstruction to CSF flow, particularly at the site of the aqueduct or fourth ventricle, with symptoms or signs developing a few days after the onset of the lesion. Later, a disturbance in CSF resorption at the arachnoid granulations may cause late onset of hydrocephalus in infancy some weeks after birth.

Secondary cerebral infarction

Govaert et al (1992b) have reported a series of seven cases of cerebral artery infarction in association with intracranial hemorrhage due to tentorial tears. They postulate that arterial compression occurs as the result of one of two mechanisms. First, supratentorial intracranial hypertension causes uncal herniation with occlusion of the ipsilateral posterior cerebral artery. Second, convexity subdural hemorrhage in the posterior fossa causes compression of the ipsilateral middle cerebral artery or its branches. Prolonged arterial compression leads to cerebral infarction in the distribution of that vessel (see also Ch. 21).

SUBARACHNOID HEMORRHAGE

Subarachnoid hemorrhage (SAH) may be primary or secondary to blood tracking through the ventricular system, usually from an IVH (see p. 395). Blood exits from the fourth ventricle through the foramina of Luschka and Magendie into the subarachnoid space. Primary hemorrhage is due to either leakage from the fine vessels of the leptomeningeal plexus, or to rupture of the larger veins within the subarachnoid space. It is quite unlike SAH seen in adults, which is a devastating condition caused by rupture of an arterial aneurysm.

Minor focal SAH is commonly seen in autopsy specimens, particularly in premature infants. These small lesions are probably clinically insignificant. It may be impossible to distinguish subpial hemorrhage microscopically from that confined to the subarachnoid space, and this distinction can only be made histologically (Friede 1972). The etiology of both conditions is probably hypoxic and develops owing to oozing from veins. SAH may occur in full-term babies owing to a congenital coagulopathy, or one that is secondary to vitamin K deficiency (Chaou et al 1984). The incidence of primary SAH diagnosed by CT scanning has been reported to be 7% of 118 infants of birth weight less than 1800 g

(Shinnar et al 1982). A large study of premature infants <2.0 Kg reported the incidence of SAH diagnosed by ultrasound to be 7% (Paneth et al 1994).

Larroche (1977) described 33 cases of a much more extensive form of primary SAH occurring over the cerebral convexity, often involving the temporal lobes (Figs 20.14 and 20.15) and these have also been referred to by Hanigan et al (1995) as lobar hemorrhages (see p. 456). This lesion has a sharply defined border and may be very extensive, causing severe hemorrhagic necrosis to underlying cortical and subcortical structures due to a compressive effect. The convexity lesion was mainly seen in infants with bleeding disorders and particularly those having an exchange transfusion. The

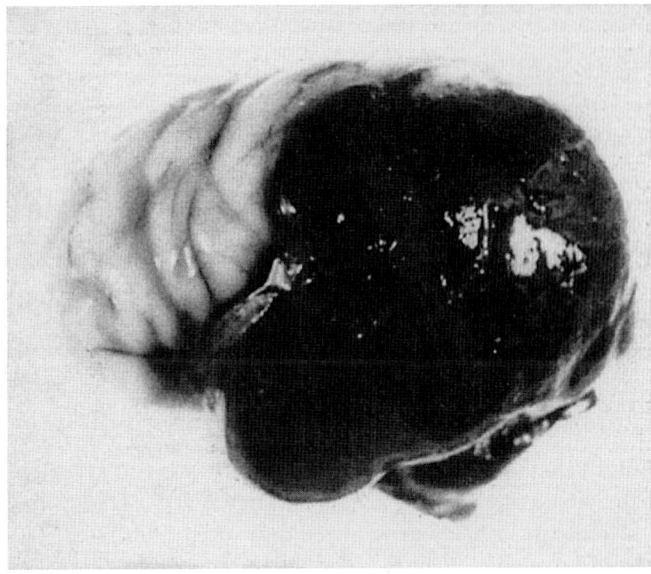

(a)

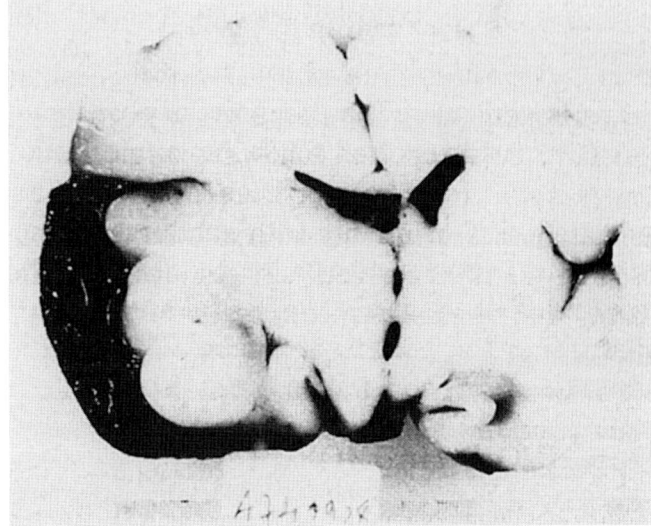

(b)

Figure 20.14 (a) SAH over the left temporal, parietal and occipital lobes. (b) Coronal section shows a small GMH-IVH with SAH compressing and displacing the left hemisphere. (Reproduced, with permission, from Larroche 1984).

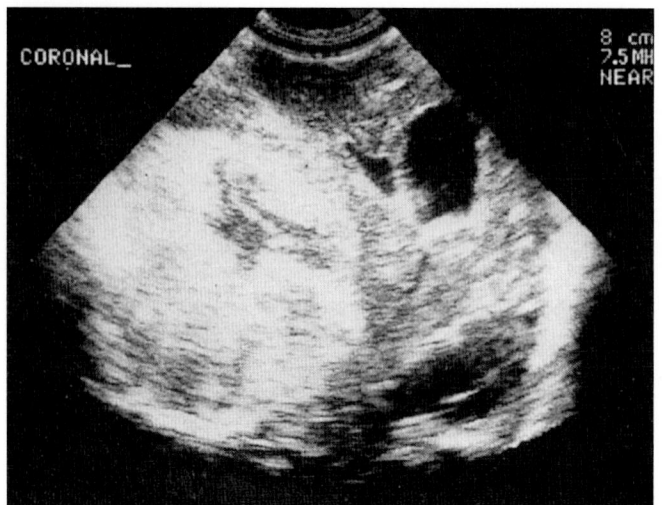

Figure 20.15 Ultrasound scan showing massive right-sided convexity hemorrhage in an infant born with severe allo-immune thrombocytopenia.

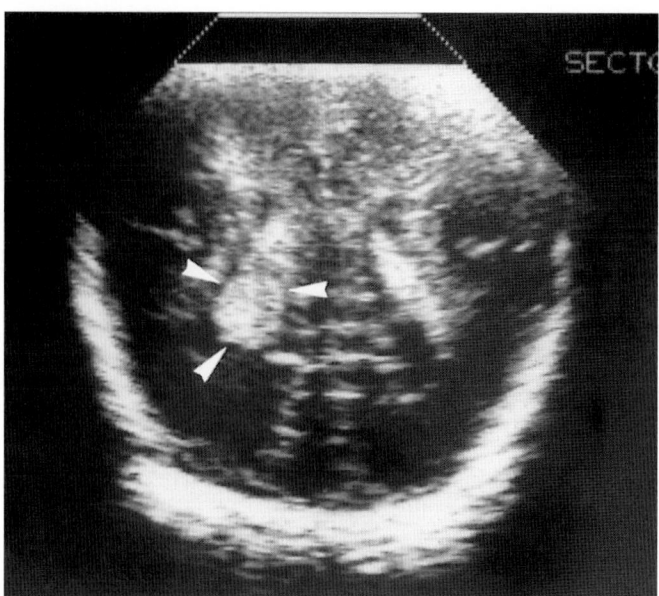

Figure 20.16 Choroid plexus hematoma (arrows) adherent to the left choroid plexus, diagnosed on ultrasound scanning. (Reproduced, with permission, from Levene et al 1985.)

underlying cause of this condition is unclear but arterial occlusion cannot be excluded (see also convexity hemorrhage, page 415).

CLINICAL FINDINGS

The majority of infants with SAH are asymptomatic. Massive convexity SAH may cause symptoms similar to large subdural hemorrhage with coma and shock. Large convexity lesions may also produce focal signs. The classic symptom associated with this type of hemorrhage is convulsion. Convulsions are usually generalized and often multifocal. The infants usually behave and feed remarkably normally between seizures. Nystagmus and apneic episodes have also been reported to be associated with SAH. Asphyxia often accompanies significant SAH and the symptoms may be related to this more generalized abnormality. In a study of 7 term infants in whom superficial parenchymal and leptomeningeal hemorrhage was detected by MR/CT scan the condition of all the babies at birth was good and all presented with seizures or apnea within 36 hours of birth. In 5 of the 7 there was decreased diffusion in the underlying parenchyma with overlying soft-tissue swelling (Huang & Robertson 2004).

DIAGNOSIS

Traditionally the diagnosis has been made by lumbar puncture. A non-traumatic tap with free flow of blood-stained CSF that does not clear in successive tubes strongly suggests the diagnosis of SAH, but this will not distinguish primary from secondary hemorrhage. Brain imaging by CT or MR is the most sensitive method for making the diagnosis, although SAH may be indistinguishable from subdural hemorrhage under certain conditions. Abnormal echogenicity in the intracerebral cisterns has been described as a sensitive ultrasound sign for SAH, but is poorly specific (Kazam et al 1994).

PROGNOSIS

The prognosis is generally thought to be good even in infants presenting with seizures (Rose & Lambroso 1970), but Fenichel et al (1984) reported that only five out of ten infants with the CT diagnosis of SAH were subsequently normal. The follow-up period in these infants was short, and further information is awaited. Posthemorrhagic hydrocephalus may occur following primary SAH, but this is not common.

CHOROID PLEXUS HEMORRHAGE

Bleeding from the choroid plexus is a common cause of IVH. Larroche (1977) has reported minor bleeding into the choroid plexus to be associated with, or to cause, IVH in 25% of cases. In another post-mortem study, Friede (1975) found choroid plexus hemorrhage in only 7% of neonatal brains. Heibel et al (1993) scanned the brain of 1000 consecutively born, clinically normal full-term infants on day 3 of life and found that 1.1% of these babies had choroid plexus hemorrhage; two were confined to the choroid plexus and nine had ruptured into the lateral ventricles. The most frequent site of bleeding is into the posterior tufts at the level of the glomus. Autopsy studies emphasize that choroid plexus hemorrhage occurs most commonly in full-term infants (Donat et al 1978, Lacey & Terplan 1982) and may arise following birth asphyxia.

DIAGNOSIS

There are no recognized clinical features of choroid plexus hemorrhage and the diagnosis can be made by ultrasound (Fig. 20.16), CT or MRI examination.

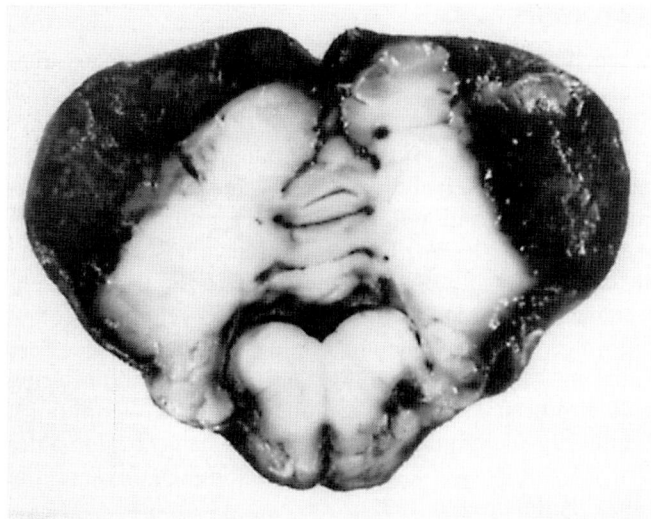

(a)

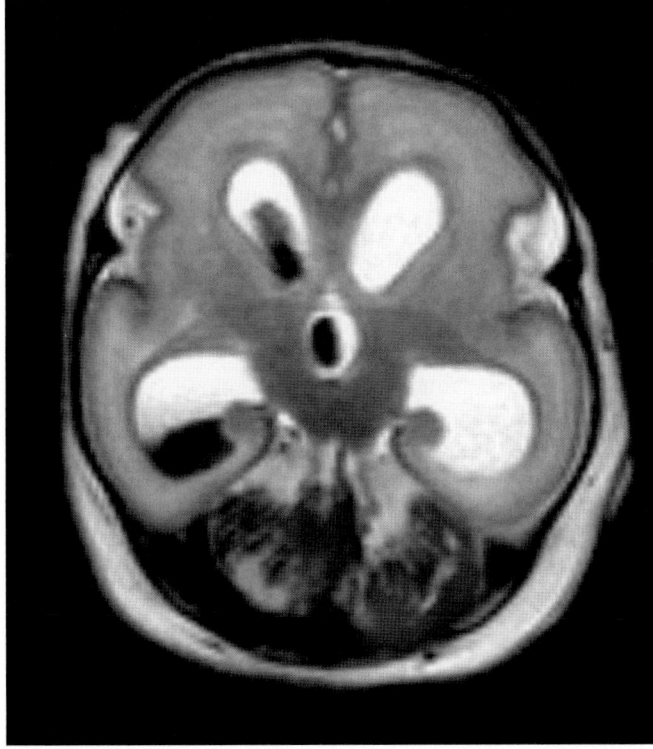

(b)

Figure 20.17 (a) Bilateral cerebellar hematoma in an infant born at 28 weeks of gestation. (b) MRI (T2SE) of an infant born at 27 weeks of gestation showing a large bilateral IVH as well as hemorrhages in both cerebellar hemispheres.

INTRACEREBELLAR HEMORRHAGE (ICBH)

Primary hemorrhage into the cerebellum is well recognized (Fig. 20.17) and has been reported to occur in 2.5% of a high-risk preterm population (Merrill et al 1998). Diffuse microscopic hemorrhages are seen in premature infants and not uncommonly in association with periventricular hemorrhage or, rarely, with meningoencephalitis (Larroche 1977). They usually arise either within the cerebellar cortex or, less commonly, in the subependymal layer of the roof of the fourth ventricle (Pape & Wigglesworth 1979). It has been suggested that bleeding into the cerebellar folia is related to poor vascularization of the cerebellar cortex (Pape & Wigglesworth 1979). Large primary cerebellar hematomata are much less common and have been diagnosed in life in both premature (Grunnet & Shields 1975, Martin et al 1976, Peterson et al 1984) and full-term infants (Fishman et al 1981, Ravenel 1979, Rom et al 1978). Massive cerebellar hemorrhage of prenatal onset has been described (Hadi et al 1994). Bleeding disorders or severe rhesus isoimmunization has been reported to be common etiological factors.

Secondary hemorrhages due to occipital osteodiastasis associated with breech delivery have been described (Wigglesworth & Husemeyer 1977) or a face-mask applied by a tight-fitting band around the back of the infant's head (Pape et al 1976). The tight band caused distortion of the occipital bone and probably mechanical trauma to the cerebellum with venous infarction.

A recent population study of very immature babies using MR imaging has reported the incidence of ICBH to be 7% and in 75% the hemorrhage was unilateral (Dyet et al 2006). Secondary cerebellar atrophy developed in two thirds of those with hemorrhage. An ultrasound study of over 1200 very low birth weight infants reported an incidence of ICBH to be 2.8% (Limperopoulos et al 2005a) and was considerably more commonly seen in the smallest infants <750 g compared with those >1.0 Kg. In this report 71% of the ICBH was unilateral and 23% was in the cerebellar vermis. Unilateral ICBH has been shown to be associated with subsequent contralateral decrease in supratentorial brain volume at term, presumably as the result of axonal degeneration or loss of transsynaptic stimulation (Limperopoulos et al 2005b)

DIAGNOSIS

Clinical features include apnea and bradycardia, seizures, fixed bradycardia, opisthotonus and nystagmus. These features are similar to those described for infants with subdural hemorrhage arising in the posterior cranial fossa, and these two conditions may be extremely difficult to distinguish even by imaging techniques (Scotti et al 1981). Merrill et al (1998) have described a clinically silent presentation in a group of premature infants with cerebellar hemorrhage.

Routine ultrasound scanning has a low detection rate for intracerebellar hemorrhage, but views through the posterior fontanelle have been reported to increase the detection rate significantly (Limperopoulos et al 2005a, Merrill et al 1998). Diagnosis is more accurate by CT or MRI examination.

MANAGEMENT

Suboccipital craniotomy has been performed successfully in a few full-term infants (Ravenel 1979, Rom et al 1978), but conservative management has also been advocated, apparently with good outcome (Fishman et al 1981).

THALAMIC HEMORRHAGE

This may be primary or due to extension of hemorrhage arising from the germinal matrix. Primary hemorrhage into the thalamus in the newborn has been described and there may be secondary rupture into the lateral ventricle (de Vries et al 1992, Govaert et al 1992a, Roland et al 1990, Trounce et al 1985). It is almost always unilateral and has been reported less commonly in preterm infants (De Vries et al 1992). Two recent cases with acute onset have been described in apparently healthy 8-week-old infants (Incorpora et al 1999). The cause of this type of lesion is unknown but does not appear to be due to an arterio-venous malformation, trauma or coagulopathy. Asphyxia is a predisposing factor in a number of unilateral cases (de Vries et al 1992). Cerebral vein thrombosis has been suggested to be a cause in two cases (Govaert et al 1992a) and hemorrhagic infarction in three cases (Roland et al 1990). Wu et al (23003) have reported that IVH in term infants and thalamic hemorrhage in particular is caused by pre-existing sinovenous thrombosis. Hemorrhagic infarction of the thalamus (Fig. 20.18) may be indistinguishable macroscopically from primary hemorrhage. Very rarely, hemorrhage into the basal ganglia may occur due to microangiomata. Alonso et al (1984) have reported two such cases occurring in neonates.

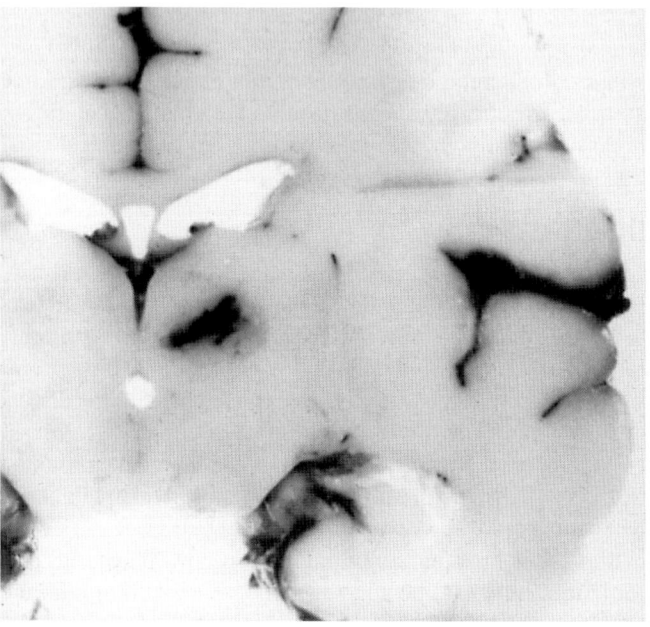

Figure 20.18 Hemorrhagic infarction within the right thalamus in a premature infant with congenital listeriosis. SAH is also visible in the sylvian fissure.

DIAGNOSIS

A specific clinical syndrome associated with primary thalamic hemorrhage has been described. The condition presents usually in previously well babies at about 7–14 days with acute onset of seizures and a bulging fontanelle. In the initial report, most had dramatic eye signs, including sunsetting and eye deviation downwards and outwards to the side of the thalamic lesion. The abnormal eye posture is due to the close proximity of the hemorrhage to the frontomesencephalic pathway of the optic tract. Later reports have not confirmed these ophthalmic findings (Roland et al 1990). Facial palsy, apnea, irritability and opisthotonic posturing have also been reported in a proportion of affected infants. A minority of infants had pre-existing asphyxia (de Vries et al 1992, Roland et al 1990) and meningitis (Govaert et al 1992a, Perlman et al 1992).

Diagnosis may be confirmed by ultrasound, CT or MRI examination (Fig. 20.19). Roland et al (1990) reported a minority of babies had decreased tissue attenuation adjacent to the hemorrhage on CT, suggestive of thalamic infarction. Evidence of venous thrombosis has been reported on CT (Roland et al 1990) and MRI (Govaert et al 1992a). In view of the association with sinovenous thrombosis, MR venography should form part of the routine workup of these babies. Cerebral angiography is necessary to exclude microangiomata, but this is rarely indicated. Confusion has arisen between this condition and infants with the appearance of bilateral 'bright' thalamic lesions, as illustrated on page 551 (Donn et al 1984, Kotagel et al 1983, Kreusser et al 1984, Shen et al 1986, Voit et al 1985). All these cases occurred in full-term infants sustaining severe asphyxia who were profoundly neurologically abnormal from birth. Autopsy showed these cases, reported as 'bright' thalamic appearances, to be due to hemorrhagic necrosis (Kreusser et al 1984). These case reports appear to be fundamentally different from the 'benign' intrathalamic hemorrhage originally reported by Trounce et al (1985).

PROGNOSIS

The infants with unilateral thalamic hemorrhage showed abnormal neurologic signs for some time. Initial reports suggested that the majority of infants had no neurodevelopmental abnormality at 18 months, but later follow-up suggests that approximately half have moderate-to-severe neurodevelopmental sequelae (personal observation on reported cases, Roland et al 1990). In contrast, all asphyxiated infants with a bilateral bright thalamic appearance are dead or severely handicapped.

PARENCHYMAL HEMORRHAGE

The distinction between a primary hemorrhagic process extending from an intraventricular bleed and bleeding into previously ischemic periventricular tissue is difficult and is discussed in detail on page 443. In addition, confusion between primary parenchymal hemorrhage and cerebral

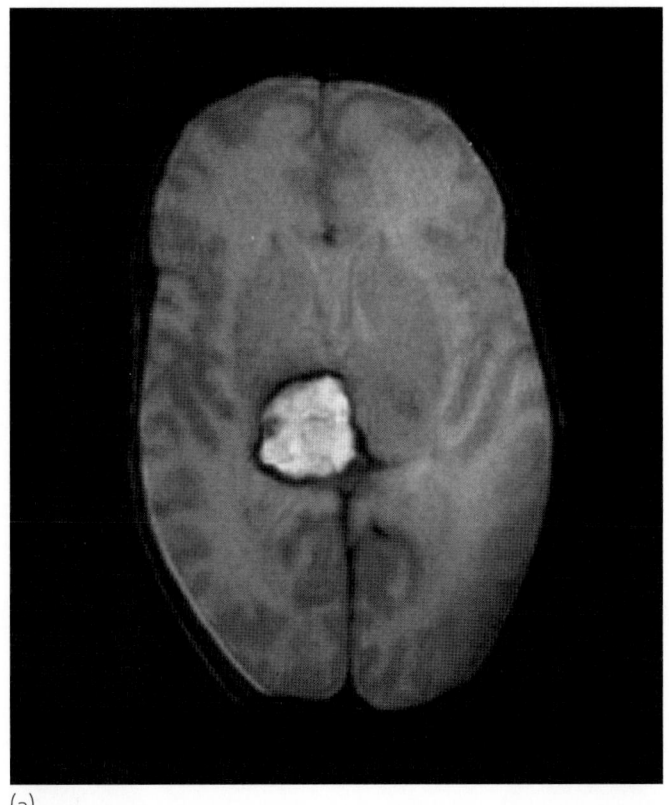

(a)

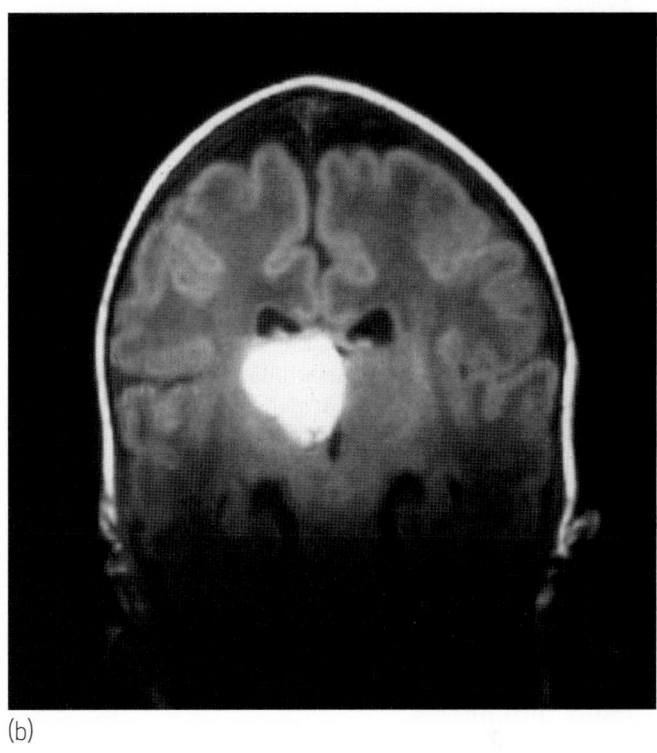

(b)

Figure 20.19 Unilateral thalamic hemorrhage seen on MRI in a preterm infant of 34 weeks gestational age. (a) Spin echo T1, 500/15 TR/TE. (b) T2, 2500/90 TR/TE.

artery infarction may easily occur. Distinction between these two conditions is possible, and cerebral artery infarction is discussed in Chapter 21.

ETIOLOGY

The causes of parenchymal hemorrhage in a term baby include the following:

- Coagulopathy
  - vitamin K deficiency
  - isoimmune thrombocytopenia
  - specific clotting factor deficiency
  - liver disorders
    - α_1-antitrypsin deficiency
    - Alagille syndrome
  - heparinization
  - protein C deficiency
- Venous thrombosis
  - sinus thrombosis
  - other vessels
- Arteriovenous malformation
- Others
  - ECMO
  - tumor

- aneurysm rupture
- blueberry muffin lesions
- cavernous hemangiomata

Coagulopathy

Most of the reported cases of primary intraparenchymal hemorrhage have been associated with fetal or neonatal coagulopathy (Bleyer & Skinner 1976, Chaou et al 1984, Matsuzaka et al 1989, Michaud et al 1991, Morales & Stroup 1985, Motohara et al 1984, Sadowitz & Balcom 1985, Sia et al 1985, Whitelaw et al 1984, Zalneraitis et al 1979). Prenatal intracranial hemorrhage is discussed in detail in Chapter 18. The most common cause for the bleeding disorder is vitamin K deficiency (Aydinli et al 1998). This occurs in solely breast-fed infants who are not given vitamin K at birth. Intracranial hemorrhage due to vitamin K deficiency is most likely to occur beyond the neonatal period and may be devastating in its severity. The median age of presentation was reported to be 46 (range 26–111) days and occurred almost exclusively in exclusively breast fed infants, not treated with vitamin K (Zengin et al 2006). In one study of 11 babies with intracranial hemorrhage due to vitamin K deficiency, 75% of them suffered long-term neurodisability (Aydinli et al 1998). It is now clear that a single prophylactic vitamin K injection will protect the full-term infant from significant, late intracranial hemorrhage due to vitamin K deficiency (Matsuzaka et al 1989).

Isoimmune thrombocytopenia is a cause of prenatal intracranial hemorrhage and is not prevented by cesarean section (van den Akker 2006). Specific clotting factor deficiency reported to cause early onset intraparenchymal hemorrhage in the neonatal period includes factor V (Lee et al 2001), VIII (Kulkarni & Lusher 1999) and X (Herrmann et al 2005). Protein C deficiency, a very rare cause of intravascular thrombosis and secondary coagulopathy, has been reported to be associated with severe intracranial hemorrhage (Voutsinas et al 1991), and periventricular leukomalacia (personal case), as has transplacental transfer of an acquired factor VII:C inhibitor (Ries et al 1995).

Liver disease due to α_1-antitrypsin deficiency may present with intracranial hemorrhage associated with coagulation disorders (Bussel et al 1997, Hope et al 1982, Jenkins et al 1982, Payne & Hasegawa 1984). Alagille syndrome is also reported to cause spontaneous intracranial bleeding as a result of a coagulation disorder (Vorstman et al 2003).

Venous thrombosis

Both intraventricular hemorrhage and intraparenchymal hemorrhage have increasingly been recognized to be secondary to sinovenous thrombosis (Wu et al 2003). They report that 31% of infants with these types of hemorrhage have sinovenous thrombosis in the deep venous system, the transverse sinus, the superior sagittal sinus and the medullary vein. Others have reported temporal lobe infarction appearing as a large hemorrhage due to thrombosis of the basal cerebral vein (Govaert et al 2001) or the vein of Labbe (Kalpatthi et al 2005).

Arteriovenous malformations

Intraparenchymal hemorrhage due to an arterio-venous malformation is rare but has been reported (Hamada et al 2001, Heck et al 2002, Jee et al 2002, Ozek et al 1996). An arterio-venous malformation of the choroid plexus is also rarely reported (Wakai et al 1990), as is rupture of a vein of Galen aneurysm (Meyers et al 2000). Another case report described a neonatal cavernous angioma located in the basal ganglia (Kon et al 2006).

Other

Intraparenchymal hemorrhage has been reported in 10% of infants undergoing extracorporeal membrane oxygenation (ECMO) therapy (Hardart & Fackler et al 1999). This is often the result of following heparinization for ECMO (Bowerman et al 1985, Watson et al 1990). Intracranial hemorrhage appears to be particularly common in premature infants treated with this technique (Cilley et al 1986, Hardart et al 2004).

Very rarely, parenchymal hemorrhage in infants may occur and be caused by an intracerebral tumor (Palma et al 1979), or an arterio-venous malformation of the choroid plexus. McLellan et al (1986) have reported a case of local-ized hematoma (Fig. 20.20) in the frontoparietal area caused by aneurysmal rupture of the middle cerebral artery. Blueberry muffin lesions (cutaneous hematopoiesis in severely anemic babies) have been reported to be associated with extensive intraparenchymal hemorrhage (Smets & van Aken

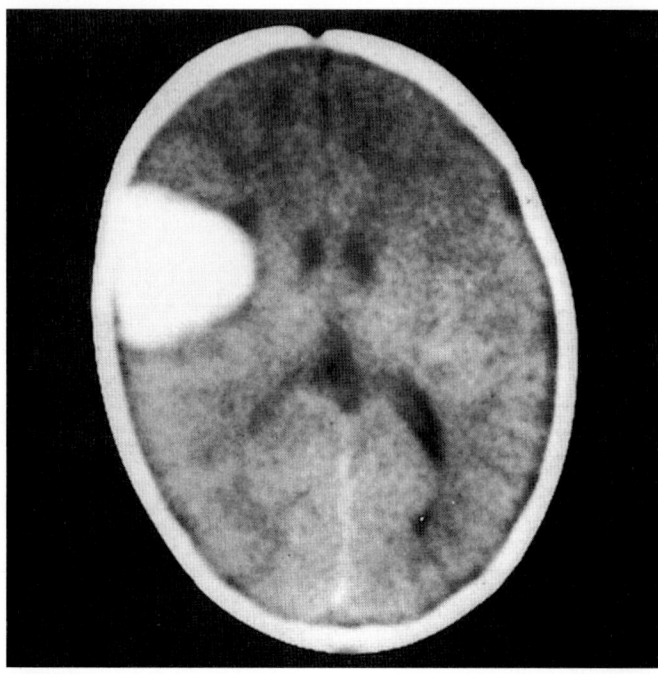

(a)

(b)

Figure 20.20 (a) Parenchymal hematoma in the right frontoparietal lobe seen on CT. (b) Angiography shows an arterial aneurysm (arrow) in an ascending branch of the right middle cerebral artery. (Reproduced, with permission, from McLellan et al 1986.)

1998). Diffuse neonatal hemangiomatosis has been reported to be the cause of multiple intracranial hemorrhages in one baby (Poirer et al 1990).

DIAGNOSIS

Clinical features usually suggest a bleeding disorder, as multiple petechial hemorrhages are present on the infant's skin. The infant may only show minor neurologic disturbances including lethargy and irritability. Seizures are common. Diagnosis is confirmed by ultrasound, CT and MRI examination (Fig. 20.21).

MANAGEMENT

Hemorrhage due to vitamin K deficiency is a preventable condition if synthetic vitamin K is given routinely to all infants at birth. Vitamin K should be given to infants with intracerebral hemorrhages and other clotting disorders

should be treated as appropriate. Platelet transfusions may be necessary in infants with severe thrombocytopenia. A history of allo-immune thrombocytopenia with intracranial hemorrhage in a sibling should alert the obstetrician to the high risk of prenatal bleeding in subsequent pregnancies. Measurement of fetal platelets with intrauterine platelet transfusion if necessary may reduce the risk of prenatal bleeding in subsequent pregnancies (Bussel et al 1997). Postnatally, specific neurologic treatment is only necessary if progressive ventriculomegaly occurs.

PROGNOSIS

From the case-reports published up to the present time it appears that approximately one-third of infants die, one-third are handicapped and one-third are subsequently neurologically normal.

OTHER CRANIAL HEMORRHAGES

EXTRADURAL (EPIDURAL) HEMORRHAGE

This has been very rarely reported in the neonatal literature and is usually due to trauma, often as a result of skull fracture with resultant underlying arterial bleeding. Skull fracture is rare in newborn infants owing to poor mineralization of the skull vault, but becomes progressively more common with trauma after 40 weeks of gestation. Extradural hemorrhage has been reported as the result of complicated breech delivery and difficult instrumental maneuvers. Takagi et al (1978) found extradural hemorrhage to account for only 1.5% of all intracranial hemorrhages discovered at autopsy.

An extradural hemorrhage is usually associated with a cephalhematoma over the fracture. The diagnosis is best made by CT or MR scanning. The imaging features are a biconvex mass adjacent to the inner table of the skull. Early liquefaction of the clot within 24–48 hours is seen on scanning and fluid levels within the clot may also be seen. Lam et al (1991) reported six cases in full-term infants diagnosed by ultrasound and confirmed on CT examination.

Infants in whom the diagnosis is made on imaging are usually relatively well and the major symptom is seizures, but between fits the babies are not neurologically abnormal (Lam et al 1991). Acute extradural hemorrhage may cause intracranial hypertension, uncal herniation and secondary infarction due to nipping of a major cerebral artery.

A large convexity extradural collection may require evacuation via a craniotomy if needle evacuation is not successful in relieving the intracranial mass effect. The prognosis is good in mild cases, but is poor in severe hemorrhage with arterial rupture.

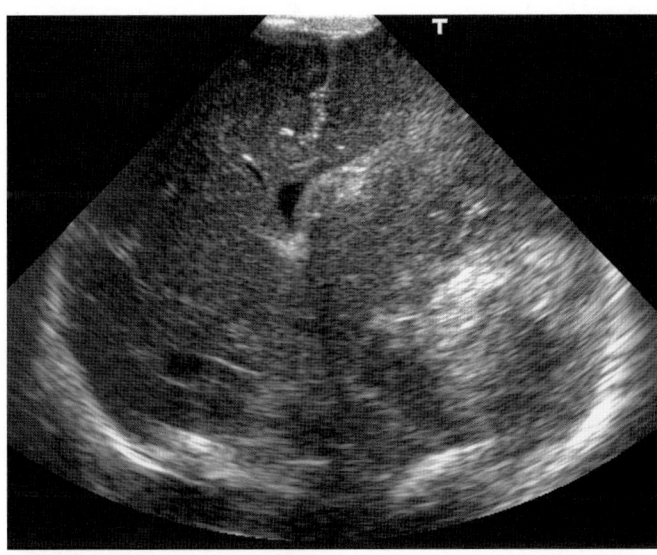
(a)

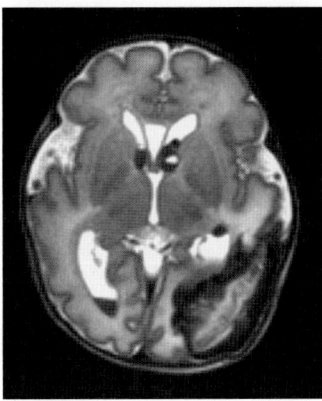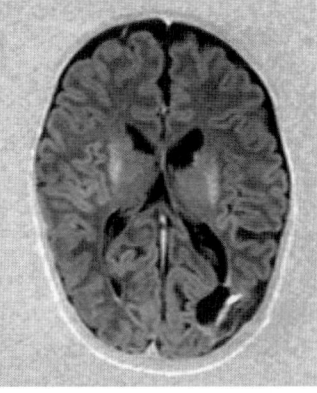
(b)

Figure 20.21 Evolution of a parenchymal hemorrhage associated with a subdural hemorrhage involving the left temporal lobe. (a) Ultrasound scans at 2 days. (b) (C) MRI scan in the same infant at 3 weeks at term equivalent age.

SUBAPONEUROTIC HEMORRHAGE

This is not an intracranial hemorrhage, but refers to bleeding over the infant's skull, but under the cranial aponeurosis (subgaleal space). It may occur spontaneously and has been reported particularly in babies of Afro-Caribbean origin and may also be associated with vitamin K deficiency, particularly in association with vacuum extraction (Ahuja et al 1969) and, less commonly, hemophilia. Ng et al (1995) describe an incidence of 0.8 per 1000 deliveries in a Chinese population and almost all were instrumental deliveries. They reported that vacuum extraction represented a 60-fold increase in risk for this condition.

Rapid and massive blood loss may occur into the subaponeurotic space with shock and hypotension and this may cause severe secondary cerebral ischemia. A fluctuant 'fluid filled' swelling is present over the scalp, usually in the occipital region. It may rapidly expand as active bleeding occurs into it and it becomes very tight and bluish in appearance. Rarely, the hemorrhage may not be obvious or not occur for up to 48 hours. The infant's hemoglobin level may fall, but in severe and acute cases the hemoglobin level remains normal as there has not been enough time for hemodilution to develop. Treatment involves careful observation and monitoring for signs of shock. Resuscitation must be undertaken early with plasma or blood. The reported mortality is 19–25% (Govaert et al 1992c, Ng et al 1995) and many of the babies who died had associated asphyxia, although it may be difficult to know whether the under-estimated hypovolemia as a result of the hemorrhage was a major factor in the asphyxial state.

CEPHALHEMATOMA

This refers to bleeding between the periosteum of the skull and the bone. The blood is confined by the periosteal membrane and therefore precisely overlies the affected bone. Because the bleeding is slow the hematoma may not be noticed on the first day of life and may appear to grow over the first few days. It usually remains for several weeks and may heal leaving a raised calcified edge. It usually affects the parietal bone and may be bilateral. Rarely, the occipital bone is affected when the cephalhematoma crosses the midline. Hemorrhage is due to the skull being buffeted either by the maternal pelvis or the trauma of instrumental delivery (forceps or vacuum extractor). There is rarely an underlying extradural hemorrhage (see above) and skull fracture should be considered.

SINOVENOUS THROMBOSIS

This is discussed in Chapter 21.

REFERENCES

Adams J M, Kenny J D, Rudolph A J 1976 Central diabetes insipidus following intraventricular hemorrhage. J Pediatr 88:292–294.

Ahmann P A, Dykes F D, Lazzara A et al 1983 Relationship between pressure passivity and subependymal/intraventricular hemorrhage as assessed by pulsed Doppler ultrasound. Pediatrics 72:665–669.

Ahuja G L, Willoughby M L N, Kerr M M, Hutchison K H 1969 Massive subaponeurotoic haemorrhage in infants born by vacuum extraction. Br Med J 3:743–745.

Allan W C, Vohr B, Makuch R W et al 1997 Antecedents of cerebral palsy in a multicenter trial of indomethacin for intraventricular hemorrhage. Arch Pediatr Adolesc Med 151:580–585.

Allan WC, Dransfield DA, Kessler DL 1994 Cerebral palsy in preterm infants. Lancet 343:1048.

Alonso A, Taboada D, Alvarez J A et al 1984 Spontaneous hematomas caused by microangiomatosis of the basal ganglia. Child Brain 11:202–211.

Als H, Duffy F H, McNulty G B et al 2004 Early experience alters brain function and structure. Pediatrics 113:846–857.

Ancel P Y, Marret S, Larroque B et al, 2005 Are maternal hypertension and small-for-gestational age risk factors for severe intraventricular hemorrhage and cystic periventricular leukomalacia? Results of the EPIPAGE cohort study. Am J Gynecol 193(1):178–184.

Anderson G D, Bada H S, Shaver D C et al 1992 The effect of Cesarean section on intraventricular hemorrhage in the preterm infant. Am J Obstet Gynecol 166:1091–1101.

Anderson G D, Bada H S, Sibai B M et al 1988 The relationship between labor and route of delivery in the preterm infant. Am J Obstet Gynecol 158:1382–1390.

Anderson J M, Bain A D, Brown J K et al 1976 Hyaline-membrane disease, alkaline buffer treatment, and cerebral intraventricular hemorrhage. Lancet i:117–119.

Archer LNJ, Evans DH, Patton JY, Levene MI 1986 Controlled hypercapnia and neonatal cerebral artery Doppler ultrasound wave form. Pediatr Res 20:218–221.

Avrahami E, Frishman E, Minz M 1993 CT demonstration of intracranial hemorrhage in term newborn following vacuum extractor delivery. Neuroradiology 35:107–108.

Aydinli N, Citak A, Caliskan C et al 1998 Vitamin K deficiency — late onset intracranial hemorrhage. Eur J Paediatr Neurol 2:199–203.

Bada H S, Korones S B, Anderson G D et al 1984 Obstetric factors and relative risk of neonatal germinal layer/intraventricular hemorrhage. Am J Obstet Gynecol 148:798–804.

Bada H S, Korones S B, Perry E H et al 1990 Frequent handling in the neonatal intensive care unit and intraventricular hemorrhage. J Pediatr 117:126–131.

Bandstra E S, Montalvo B M, Goldberg R N et al 1988 Prophylactic indomethacin for prevention of intraventricular hemorrhage in premature infants. Pediatrics 82:533–542.

Bassan H, Benson C B, Limperopoulos C et al 2006 Ultrasonographic features and severity scoring of periventricular hemorrhagic infarction in relation to risk factors and outcome. Pediatrics 117(6):2111–2118.

Batton Daniel G, Holtrop P, DeWitte D et al 1994 Current gestational age-related incidence of major intraventricular hemorrhage. J Pediatr 125:623–625.

Bedard M P, Shankaran S, Slovis T L et al 1984 Effect of prophylactic phenobarbital on intraventricular hemorrhage in high-risk infants. Pediatrics 73:435–439.

Bejar R, Curbelo V, Coen R W 1980 Diagnosis and follow-up of intraventricular and intracerebral hemorrhages by ultrasound studies of infant's brain through the fontanelles and sutures. Pediatrics 66:661–673.

Benson J W T, Drayton M R, Hayward C et al 1986 Multicentre trial of ethamsylate for prevention of periventricular hemorrhage in very low birthweight infants. Lancet ii:1297–1300.

Bergman I, Bauer R E, Barmada M A et al 1985 Intracerebral hemorrhage in the full-term neonatal infant. Pediatrics 75:488–496.

Beverley D W, Chance G 1984 Cord blood gases, birth asphyxia and intraventricular hemorrhage. Arch Dis Child 59:884–897.

Beverley D W, Chance G W, Inwood M J et al 1984a Intraventricular haemorrhage: timing of occurrence and relationship to perinatal events. Br J Obstet Gynaecol 91:1007–1013.

Beverley D W, Chance G W, Inwood M J et al 1984b Intraventricular hemorrhage and haemostasis defects. Arch Dis Child 59:444–448.

Beverley D W, Pitts-Tucker T J, Congdon P J et al 1985 Prevention of intraventricular hemorrhage by fresh frozen plasma. Arch Dis Child 60:710–713.

Bhuta T, Henderson-Smart D J 1999a Elective high frequency jet ventilation versus conventional ventilation for neonatal respiratory distress syndrome in preterm infants. Cochrane Database of Systematic Reviews. Issue 3. Oxford: Update.

Bhuta T, Henderson-Smart D J 2007 Rescue high frequency oscillatory ventilation versus conventional ventilation for pulmonary dysfunction in preterm infants. Cochrane Database of Systematic Reviews. Issue 4. Oxford: Update.

Blackman J A, McGuinness G A, Bale J F, Smith W L 1991 Large postnatally acquired porencephalic cysts: unexpected development outcomes. J Child Neurol 6:58–64.

Bleyer W A, Skinner A L 1976 Fatal neonatal hemorrhage after maternal anticonvulsant therapy. J Am Med Assoc 235:626–627.

Blume W T, Dreyfus-Brisac C 1982 Positive Rolandic sharp waves in neonatal EEG: types and significance. Electroencephalog Clin Neurophysiol 53:227–282.

Bove K, Kosmetatos N, Wedig K E et al 1985 Vasculopathic hepatotoxicity associated with E-Ferol syndrome in low-birthweight infants. J Am Med Assoc 254:2422–2430.

Bowerman R A, Zwischenberger J B, Andrews A F, Bartlett R H 1985 Cranial sonography of the infant treated with extracorporeal membrane oxygenation. Am J Roentgenol 145:161–166.

Buckley K M, Taylor G A, Estroff J A et al 1997 Use of the mastoid fontanelle for improved sonographic visualization of the neonatal midbrain and posterior fossa. Am J Roentgenol 168:1021–1025.

Burstein J, Papile L A, Burstein R 1979 Intraventricular hemorrhage in premature newborns: a prospective study with CT. Am J Roentgenol 132:631–635.

Bussel J B, Zabusky M R, Berkowitz R L, McFarland J G 1997 Fetal alloimmune thrombocytopenia. N Engl J Med 337:22–26.

Cartwright G W, Culbertson K, Schreiner R L, Garg B P 1979 Changes in clinical presentation of term infants with intracranial hemorrhage. Dev Med Child Neurol 21:730–737.

Castillo M, Fordham L A 1995 MR of neurologically symptomatic newborns after vacuum extraction delivery. AJNR Am J Neuroradiol 16:816–818.

Catto-Smith A G, Yu V Y H, Bajuk B et al 1985 Effect of neonatal periventricular hemorrhage on neurodevelopmental outcome. Arch Dis Child 60:8–11.

Chang G Y, Lueder F L, DiMichele D M et al 1997 Heparin and the risk of intraventricular hemorrhage in premature infants. J Pediatr 131:362–366.

Chaou W-T, Chou M-L, Eitzman D V 1984 Intracranial hemorrhage and vitamin K deficiency in early infancy. J Pediatr 105:880–884.

Chen J 1993 Ethamsylate in the prevention of periventricular-intraventricular hemorrhage in premature infants. J Formosan Med Assoc 92:889–893.

Chessells J M, Wigglesworth J S 1972 Coagulation studies in preterm infants with respiratory distress and intracranial hemorrhage. Arch Dis Child 47:564–570.

Chiswick M L, Johnson M, Woodhall C et al 1983 Protective effect of vitamin E (dl-alpha-tocopherol) against intraventricular hemorrhage in premature babies. Br Med J 287:81–84.

Cilley R E, Zwischenberger J B, Andrews A F et al 1986 Intracranial hemorrhage during extracorporeal membrane oxygenation in neonates. Pediatrics 78:699–704.

Clancy R R, Tharp B R, Enzman D 1984 EEG in premature infants with intraventricular hemorrhage. Neurology 34:583–590.

Claris O, Besnier S, Lapillonne A et al 1996 Incidence of ischemic-hemorrhage cerebral lesions in premature infants of gestational age ≤28 weeks: a prospective ultrasound study. Biol Neonate 70:29–34.

Clark C E, Clyman R I, Roth R S 1981 Risk factor analysis of intraventricular hemorrhage in low birth weight infants. J Pediatr 99:625–628.

Clark R H, Dykes F D, Bachman T E, Ashurst J T 1996 Intraventricular hemorrhage and high-frequency ventilation: A meta-analysis of prospective clinical trials. Pediatrics 98:1058–1061.

Cole V A, Durbin G M, Olaffson A et al 1974 Pathogenesis of intraventricular hemorrhage in newborn infants. Arch Dis Child 49:722–728.

Cooke R W 1981 Factors associated with periventricular hemorrhage in very low birth weight infants. Arch Dis Child 56:425–431.

Cooke R W I 1987 Early and late cranial ultrasonographic appearances and outcome in very low birthweight infants. Arch Dis Child 62:931–937.

Cooke R W I 1994 Survival and cerebral morbidity in preterm infants. Lancet 343:1578.

Cooke R W I 1999 Trends in incidence of cranial ultrasound lesions and cerebral palsy in very low birthweight infants 1982–93. Arch Dis Child Fetal Neonat Ed 80:F115–117.

Cooke R W I, Morgan I M, Coad N A G 1981 Pneumothorax, mechanical ventilation, and periventricular hemorrhage. Lancet i:555.

Cooke R W I, Morgan M E I 1984 Prophylactic ethamsylate for periventricular hemorrhage. Arch Dis Child 59:82–84.

Corazza M S, Davis R F, Merritt A et al 1984 Prolonged bleeding time in preterm infants receiving indomethacin for patent ductus arteriosus. J Pediatr 105:292–296.

Corbet A J, Adams J M, Kenny J D et al 1977 Controlled trial of bicarbonate therapy in high-risk premature newborn infants. J Pediatr 91:771–776.

Coulter D M, La Pine T R, Gooch M 1985 Treatment to prevent postnatal loss of brain water reduces the risk of intracranial hemorrhage in the beagle puppy. Pediatric Research 19:1322–1326.

Cowan F M, de Vries L S 2005 The internal capsule in neonatal imaging. Semin Fetal Neonatal Med,10(5):461–474.

Cowan F, Whitelaw A, Wertheim D, Silverman M 1991 Cerebral blood flow velocity changes after rapid administration of surfactant. Arch Dis Child 66:1105–1109.

Craig W S 1938 Intracranial hemorrhage in the new-born. Arch Dis Child 13:89–124.

Crowley P 1999 Prophylactic corticosteroids for preterm delivery (Cochrane Review). In: The Cochrane Library, Issue 2. Oxford: Update Software.

Crowther C A, Alfirevic Z, Haslam R R 1999 Prenatal thyrotropin-releasing hormone (TRH) for preterm birth. Cochrane Library Issue 2. Oxford, Update Software.

Crowther C A, Henderson-Smart D J 1999a Phenobarbital prior to preterm birth for the prevention of neonatal periventricular hemorrhage (PVH) (Cochrane Review). In: The Cochrane Library, Issue 2. Oxford: Update Software.

Crowther C A, Henderson-Smart D J 1999b Vitamin K prior to preterm birth for the prevention of periventricular hemorrhage (Cochrane Review). In: The Cochrane Library, Issue 2. Oxford: Update Software.

Crowther C A, Hiller J E, Doyle L W, Haslam R R, for the Australasian collaborative trial of magnesium sulphate 2003 Effect of magnesium sulfate given for neuroprotection before preterm birth. JAMA 290:2669—2676.

Crowther C A, Moore V 1999 Magnesium for preventing preterm birth after threatened preterm labour (Cochrane Review). In: The Cochrane Library, Issue 2. Oxford: Update Software.

Cukier F, Andre M, Monod N, Dreyfus-Brisac C 1972 Apport de l'EEG au diagnostic des hemorrhagies intra-ventriculaires du premature. Revue Electroencephalographie et Neurophysiologie Clinique 2:318–322.

D'Souza S W, Janakova H, Minors D et al 1995 Blood pressure, heart rate, and skin temperature in preterm infants: associations with periventricular hemorrhage. Arch Dis Child 72:F162–F167.

de Crespigny L Ch, Robinson H P 1983 Can obstetricians prevent neonatal intraventricular hemorrhage? Aust NZ J Obstet Gynaecol 23:146–149.

de Crespigny L, Mackay R, Muston L J et al 1982 Timing of neonatal cerebroventricular hemorrhage with ultrasound. Arch Dis Child 57:231–233.

de Vries L S et al 2000 Neuropediatrics (In press).

de Vries L S, Dubowitz L M S, Dubowitz V 1985 Predictive value of cranial ultrasound in the newborn baby: a reappraisal. Lancet ii:137–140.

de Vries L S, Eken P, Groenendaal F et al 1998a Antenatal onset of haemorrhagic and/or ischaemic lesions in preterm infants: prevalence and associated obstetric variables. Arch Dis Child Fetal Neonatal Edn 78:F51–F56.

de Vries L S, Rademaker K J, Groenendaal F et al 1998b Correlation between neonatal cranial ultrasound, MRI in infancy and neurodevelopmental outcome in infants with a large intraventricular hemorrhage with or without unilateral parenchymal involvement. Neuropediatrics 29:180–188.

de Vries L S, Smet M, Goemans N et al 1992 Unilateral thalamic hemorrhage in the pre-term and full-term newborn. Neuropediatrics 23:153–156.

de Vries LS, van Haastert IC, Rademaker KJ, Koopman C, Groenendaal F 2004 Ultrasound abnormalities preceding cerebral palsy in high-risk preterm infants. J Pediatrics 144, 815–820.

DeCourten G M, Rabinowicz T 1981 Intraventricular hemorrhage in premature infants: reappraisal and a new hypothesis. Dev Med Child Neurol 23:389–403.

Developmental Epidemiology Network Investigators 1998 The correlation between placental pathology and intraventricular hemorrhage in the preterm infant. Pediatr Res 43:15–19.

Dolfin T, Skidmore M B, Fong K W et al 1983 Incidence, severity and timing of subependymal and intraventricular hemorrhages in preterm infants born in a perinatal unit as detected by serial real-time ultrasound. Pediatrics 71:541–546.

Donat J F, Okazaki H, Kleinberg F, Reagan T J 1978 Intraventricular hemorrhages in full-term and premature infants. Mayo Clinic Proceedings 53:437–441.

Donn S M, Bowerman R A 1985 Unilateral germinal matrix hemorrhage in the newborn. J Ultrasound Med 4:251–253.

Donn S M, Bowerman R A, DiPietro M A, Gebarski S S 1984 Sonographic appearance of neonatal thalamic-striatal hemorrhage. J Ultrasound Med 3:231–233.

Donn S M, Roloff D W, Goldstein G W 1981 Prevention of intraventricular hemorrhage in preterm infants by phenobarbitone: a controlled trial. Lancet ii:215–217.

Donn S M, Roloff D W, Goldstein G W 1982 Phenobarbitone and neonatal intraventricular hemorrhage. Lancet i:1240–1241.

Dubowitz L M S, Dubowitz V, Palmer P G et al 1984 Correlation of neurologic assessment in the preterm newborn infant with outcome at one year. J Pediatr 105:452–456.

Dubowitz L M S, Levene M I, Morante A et al 1981 Neurologic signs in neonatal intraventricular hemorrhage: a correlation with real-time ultrasound. J Pediatr 99:127–133.

Dykes F D, Lazzara A, Ahmann P et al 1980 Intraventricular hemorrhage: a prospective evaluation of etiopathogenesis. Pediatrics 66:42–49.

Edvinsson L, Lou H C, Tvede K 1986 On the pathogenesis of regional cerebral ischaemia in intracranial hemorrhage: a causal influence of potassium? Pediatr Res 20:478–480.

Ehlers H, Courville C B 1936 Thrombosis of internal cerebral veins in infancy and childhood. J Pediatr 8:600–623.

Eick J J, Miller K D, Bell K A, Tutton R H 1981 Computed tomography of deep cerebral venous thrombosis in children. Neuroradiology 140:399–402.

Emerson P, Fujimura M, Howat P et al 1977 Timing of intraventricular hemorrhage. Arch Dis Child 52:183–187.

Evans N, Kluckow M 1996 Early ductal shunting and intraventricular hemorrhage in ventilated preterm infants. Arch Dis Child 75:F183–F186.

Fawer C-L, Levene M I, Dubowitz L M S 1983 Intraventricular hemorrhage in a preterm neonate: discordance between clinical course and ultrasound scan. Neuropediatrics 14:242–244.

Fenichel G M, Webster D L, Wong W K T 1984 Intracranial hemorrhage in the term infant. Arch Neurol 41:30–34.

Finberg L 1977 The relationship of intravenous infusions and intracranial hemorrhage — a commentary. J Pediatr 91:777–778.

Fine Smith R B, Roche K, Yellin P B et al 1997 Effect of magnesium sulfate on the development of cystic periventricular leukomalacia in preterm infants. Am J Perinatol 14:303–307.

Fish W H, Cohen M, Franzek D et al 1990 Effect of intramuscular vitamin E on mortality and intracranial hemorrhage in neonates of 1000 grams or less. Pediatrics 85:578–584.

Fishman M A, Percy A K, Cheek W R, Speer M E 1981 Successful conservative management of cerebellar hematomas in term neonates. J Pediatr 98:466–468.

Foley M E, McNicol G P 1977 An in vitro study of acidosis, platelet function, and perinatal cerebral intraventricular hemorrhage. Lancet i:1230–1232.

Fowlie P W 1999 Intravenous indomethacin for preventing mortality and morbidity in very low birth weight infants (Cochrane Review). In: The Cochrane Library, Issue 2. Oxford: Update Software.

Friede R L 1972 Subpial hemorrhage in infants. J Neuropathol Exp Neurol 31:548–556.

Friede R L 1975 Developmental neuropathology. Springer-Verlag, Vienna.

Funato M, Tamai H, Noma K et al 1992 Clinical events in association with timing of intraventricular hemorrhage in preterm infants. J Pediatr 121: 614–619.

Gebara B M, Goetting M G, Wang A M 1995 Dural sinus thrombosis complicating subclavian vein catheterization: treatment with local thrombolysis. Pediatrics 95:138–140.

Ghazi-Birry H S, Brown W R, Moody D M et al 1997 Human germinal matrix: Venous origin of hemorrhage and vascular characteristics. AJNR Am J Neuroradiol 18:219–229.

Goddard-Finegold J, Armstrong D, Zeller R S 1982 Intraventricular hemorrhage following volume expansion after hypovolaemic hypotension in the newborn beagle. J Pediatr 100:796–799.

Gomes W J, Weerasuriya N 1975 Hyperpyrexia in neonates: a sign of intraventricular hemorrhage. Indian Pediatrics 12:505–507.

Gopel W, Hartel C, Ahrens P et al 2006 Interleukin-6-174-genotype, sepsis and cerebral injury in very low birth weight infants. Genes Immun 7(1):65–68.

Gould S J, Howard S, Hope P L, Reynolds E O R 1987 Periventricular intraparenchymal cerebral hemorrhage in preterm infants: the role of venous infarction. J Pathol 151:197–202.

Govaert P, Achten E, Vanhaesebrouck P et al 1992a Deep cerebral venous thrombosis in thalamo-

ventricular hemorrhage of the term newborn. Pediatr Radiol 22:123–127.

Govaert P, Calliauw L, Vanhaesebrouck P et al 1990 On the management of neonatal tentorial damage. Eight case reports and a review of the literature. Acta Neurochirurg 106:52–64.

Govaert P, de Vries L S 1997 An atlas of neonatal brain sonography. Clinics in Developmental Medicine 141–142, pp. 109–126. Mac Keith, London.

Govaert P, Smets K, Matthys E, Oostra A 1999 Neonatal focal temporal lobe or atrial wall haemorrhagic infarction. Arch Dis Child Fetal Neonatal En 81: F211–F216.

Govaert P, Vanhaesebrouck P, de Praeter C 1992b Traumatic neonatal intracranial bleeding and stroke. Arch Dis Child 67:840–845.

Govaert P, Vanhaesebrouck P, De Praeter C et al 1992c Vacuum extraction, bone injury and neonatal subgaleal bleeding. Eur J Pediatr 151:532–535.

Green D W, Hendon B, Mimouni F B 1995 Nucleated erythrocytes and intraventricular hemorrhage in preterm neonates. Pediatrics 96:475–478.

Greenhough A, Wood S, Morley C J, Davis J A 1984 Pancuronium prevents pneumothoraces in ventilated premature babies who actively expire against positive pressure inflation. Lancet i:1–3.

Grontoft O 1953 Intracerebral and meningeal hemorrhages in perinatally deceased infants. I. Intracerebral hemorrhages. Acta Obstet Gynaecol Scand 32:308–324.

Groome L J, Goldenberg R L, Cliver S P et al 1992 March of Dimes Multicenter Study Group 1992 Neonatal periventricular-intraventricular hemorrhage after maternal sympathomimetic tocolysis. Am J Obstet Gynecol 167:873–879.

Grunau R V, Kearney S M, Whitfield M F 1990 Language development at 3 years in pre-term children of birth weight below 1000 g. Br J Disord Commun 25:173–182.

Grunnet M L, Shields W O 1975 Cerebellar hemorrhage in the premature infant. J Pediatr 88:605–608.

Guzzetta F, Shackelford G D, Volpe S et al 1986 Periventricular intraparenchymal echodensities in the premature newborn: critical determinant of neurologic outcome. Pediatrics 78:995–1006.

Hadi H A, Finley J, Mallette J W, Strickland D 1994 Prenatal diagnosis of cerebellar hemorrhage: medicolegal implications. Am J Obstet Gynecol 170:1392–1395.

Hambleton G, Wigglesworth J S 1976 Origin of intraventricular hemorrhage in the preterm infant. Arch Dis Child 51:651–659.

Hamrick S E, Miller SP, Leonard C et al 2004 Trends in severe brain injury and neurodevelopmental outcome in premature newborn infants: the role of cystic periventricular leukomalacia. Journal of Pediatrics145:593–599.

Hanigan W C, Morgan A M, Stahlberg L K, Hiller J L 1990 Tentorial hemorrhage associated with vacuum extraction. Pediatrics 85:534–539.

Hanigan W C, Powell F C, Palagallo G, Miller T C 1995 Lobar hemorrhages in full-term neonates. Child Nerv Syst 11:276–280.

Harding J E, Miles F K I, Becroft D M 1998 Chest physiotherapy may be associated with brain damage in extremely premature infants. J Pediatr 132:440–444.

Harrison V C, Heese H, Klein M 1968 Intracranial hemorrhage associated with hyaline membrane disease. Arch Dis Child 43:116–120.

Hartel C, Konig I, Koster S et al 2006 Genetic polymorphisms of hemostasis genes and primary outcome of very low birth weight infants. Pediatrics, 118(2):683–689.

Hawgood S, Spong J, Yu V Y H 1984 Intraventricular hemorrhage: incidence and outcome in a population of very low birth weight infants. Am J Dis Child 138:136–139.

Hayashi T, Hashimoto T, Fukuda S et al 1987 Neonatal subdural hematoma secondary to birth injury. Clinical analysis of 48 survivors. Child Nerv Syst 3:23–29.

Hecht S T, Filly R A, Callen P W, Wilson-Davis S L 1983 Intracranial hemorrhage: late onset in the preterm neonate. Radiology 149:697–699.

Heibel M, Heber R, Bechinger D, Kornhuber H H 1993 Early diagnosis of perinatal cerebral lesions in apparently normal full-term newborns by ultrasound of the brain. Neuroradiology 35:85–91.

Hellstrom-Westas L, Bell A H, Skov L et al 1992 Cerebroelectrical depression following surfactant treatment in preterm neonates. Pediatrics 89:643–647.

Hemsath F A 1934 Birth injury of the occipital bone with a report of thirty-two cases. Am J Obstet Gynecol 27:194–203.

Henderson-Smart D J, Bhuta T, Cools F, Offringa M 1999 Elective high frequency oscillatory ventilation versus conventional dysfunction in preterm infants. Cochrane Database of Systematic Reviews, Issue 3. Oxford: Update.

Hensey O J, Morgan M E I, Cooke R W I 1984 Tranexamic acid in the prevention of periventricular hemorrhage. Arch Dis Child 59:719–721.

Heuchan AM, Evans N, Henderson Smart DJ, Simpson JM 2002 Perinatal risk factors for major intraventricular haemorrhage in the Australian and New Zealand Neonatal Network, 1995–97. Arch Dis Child Fetal Neonatal Ed 86,F86–F90.

HiFO Study Group 1993 Randomized study of high-frequency oscillatory ventilation in infants with severe respiratory distress syndrome. J Pediatr 122:609–619.

Higashida R T, Helmer E, Halbach V V 1989 Direct thrombolytic therapy for superior sagittal sinus thrombosis. Am J Roentgenol 10:S4–S6.

Hill A, Perlman J M, Volpe J J 1982 Relationship of pneumothorax to occurrence of intraventricular hemorrhage in the premature newborn. Pediatrics 69:144–149.

Hiller J L, Benda G I, Rahatzad M et al 1986 Benzyl alcohol toxicity: impact on mortality and intraventricular hemorrhage among very low birthweight infants. Pediatrics 77:500–506.

Holland E 1922 Cranial stress in the foetus during labour and on the effects of excessive stress on the intracranial contents. J Obstetr Gynecol Br Empire 29:549–569.

Hope P L, Hall M A, Millward-Sadler G H, Normand I C S 1982 Alpha-1-antitrypsin deficiency presenting as a bleeding diathesis in the newborn. Arch Dis Child 57:68–79.

Horbar J D 1992 Prevention of periventricular-intraventricular hemorrhage. In: Sinclair J C, Bracken M B (eds) Effective care of the newborn infant. Oxford University Press, Oxford, pp. 562–589.

Huang C C, Shen E Y 1991 Tentorial subdural hemorrhage in term newborns: ultrasonographic diagnosis and clinical correlates. Pediatric Neurology 7:171–177.

Iannucci T A, Besinger R E, Fisher S G et al 1996 Effect of dual tocolysis on the incidence of severe intraventricular hemorrhage among extremely low-birth-weight infants. Am J Obstet Gynecol 175:1043–1046.

Incorpora G, Pavone P, Smilari P G et al 1999 Late primary unilateral thalamic hemorrhage in infancy: Report of two cases. Neuropediatrics 30:264–267.

Jardine D S, Rogers K 1989 Relationship of benzyl alcohol to kernicterus, intraventricular hemorrhage, and mortality in preterm infants. Pediatrics 83:153–160.

Jenkins H R, Leonard J V, Kay J D S et al 1982 Alpha-1-antitrypsin deficiency, bleeding diathesis, and intracranial hemorrhage. Arch Dis Child 57:722–723.

Jocelyn L J, Casiro O G 1992 Neurodevelopmental outcome of term infants with intraventricular hemorrhage. Am J Dis Child 146:194–197.

Kassal R, Anwar M, Kashlan F et al 2005 Umbilical vein interleukin-6 levels in very low birth weight infants developing intraventricular hemorrhage. Brain Develop 27,483–487.

Kazam E, Rudelli R, Monte W et al 1994 Sonographic diagnosis of cisternal subarachnoid hemorrhage in the premature infant. AJNR Am J Neuroradiol 15:1009–1020.

Keeney S E, Adcock E W, McArdle C B 1991 Prospective observations of 100 high-risk neonates by high-field (1.5 tesla) magnetic resonance imaging of the central nervous system: I. Intraventricular and extracerebral lesions. Pediatrics 87:421–430.

Kimberlin D E, Hauth J C, Goldenberg R L et al 1998 The effect of maternal magnesium sulfate treatment on neonatal morbidity in < or = 1000-gram infants. Am J Perinatol 15:635–641.

Kon T, Mori H, Hasegawa K, Nishiyama K, Tanaka R, Takahashi H 2006 Neonatal cavernous angioma located in the basal ganglia with profuse intraoperative bleeding. Childs Nerv Syst. [Epub ahead of print]

Kosmetatos N, Dinter C, Williams M L et al 1980 Intracranial hemorrhage in the premature: its predictive features and outcome. Am J Dis Child 134:855–859.

Kotagel S, Toce S, Kotagel P, Archer C 1983 Symmetrical bithalamic and striatal hemorrhage following perinatal hypoxia in a term infant. J Comput Assist Tomogr 7:353–355.

Kowitz H L 1914 Intrakranielle blutungen and Pachymeningitis Haemorrhagia chronica interna bis Neugeborensen und Sauglingen. Virchows Archiv. A. Pathological Anatomy and Physiology 215:233–246.

Kreusser K L, Schmidt R E, Shackelford G D, Volpe J J 1984 Value of ultrasound for identification of acute hemorrhagic necrosis of thalamus and basal ganglia in an asphyxiated term infant. Ann Neurol 16:361–363.

Krishnamoorthy K S, Fernandez R A, Momose K J et al 1977 Evaluation of neonatal intracranial hemorrhage by computerized tomography. Pediatrics 59:165–172.

Krishnamoorthy K S, Kuban K C K, Leviton A et al 1990 Periventricular–intraventricular hemorrhage sonographic localization, phenobarbital, and motor abnormalities in low birth weight infants. Pediatrics 85:1027–1033.

Kuban K C K, Leviton A, Krishnamoorthy K S et al 1986 Neonatal intracranial hemorrhage and phenobarbital. Pediatrics 77:443–450.

Kuban K C K, Leviton A, Pagano M et al 1992 Maternal toxemia is associated with reduced incidence of germinal matrix hemorrhage in premature babies. J Child Neurol 7:70–76.

Lacey D J & Terplan K 1982 Intraventricular hemorrhage in full-term neonates. Dev Med Child Neurol 24:332–337.

Lam A, Cruz G B, Johnson I 1991 Extradural hematoma in neonates. J Ultrasound Med 10:205–209.

Larroche J-C 1972 Sub-ependymal pseudocysts in the newborn. Biol Neonate 21:170–183.

Larroche J-C 1977 Developmental pathology of the neonate. Amsterdam: Excerpta Medica.

Larroche J-C 1984 Perinatal brain damage. In: Adams J H, Corsellis J, Duchen L W (eds) Greenfield's neuropathology. Edward Arnold, London pp. 451–489.

Larroque B, Marret S, Ancel PY et al 2003 White matter damage and intraventricular hemorrhage in very preterm infants: the EPIPAGE study J Pediatr,143(4):477–483.

Law M R, Wijewardene K, Wald N J 1990 Is routine vitamin E administration justified in very low-birthweight infants? Dev Med Child Neurol 32:442–450.

Lazzara A, Ahmann P A, Dykes T D et al 1978 Clinical predictability of intraventricular hemorrhage in preterm infants. Ann Neurol 4:187.

Le Blanc R, O'Gorman A M 1980 Neonatal intracranial hemorrhage: a clinical and serial computerized tomographic study. J Neurosurg 53:642–651.

Lesko S M, Mitchell A A, Epstein M F et al 1986 Heparin use as a risk factor for intraventricular hemorrhage in low-birth-weight infants. N Engl J Med 314:1156–1160.

Levene M I, de Vries S H 1984 Extension of neonatal intraventricular hemorrhage. Arch Dis Child 59:631–636.

Levene M I, Fawer C-L, Lamont R F 1982 Risk factors in the development of intraventricular hemorrhage in the preterm neonate. Arch Dis Child 57:410–417.

Levene M I, Williams J L, Fawer C-L 1985 Ultrasound of the infant brain. Clin Dev Med 92:4.

Levene M, Dowling S, Graham M 1992 Impaired motor function (clumsiness) in 5 year old children: correlation with neonatal ultrasound scans. Arch Dis Child 67:687–690.

Leviton A, Fenton T, Kuban K C, Pagano M 1991a Labor and delivery characteristics and the risk of germinal matrix hemorrhage in low birth weight infants. J Child Neurol 6:35–40.

Leviton A, Pagano M, Kuban K C K 1988 Etiologic heterogeneity of intracranial hemorrhages in preterm newborns. Pediatr Neurol 4:274–278.

Leviton A, Pagano M, Kuban K C K et al 1991b The epidemiology of germinal matrix hemorrhage during the first half-day of life. Dev Med Child Neurol 33:138–145.

Lipscomb A P, Thorburn R J, Reynolds E O R et al 1981 Pneumothorax and cerebral hemorrhage in preterm infants. Lancet i:414–416.

Lombroso C T 1982 Neonatal electroencephalography. In: Niedermeyer E, daSilva F L (eds) Electroencephalography. Urban & Schwarzenberg, Baltimore.

Lou H C, Lassen N A, Friis-Hansen B 1979 Is arterial hypertension crucial for the development of cerebral hemorrhage in premature infants? Lancet i:1215–1217.

Lou H C, Phibbs R H, Wilson S L, Gregory G A 1982 Hyperventilation at birth may prevent early periventricular hemorrhage. Lancet i:1407.

Lowe J, Papile L A 1990 Neurodevelopmental performance of very-low-birth-weight infants with mild periventricular intraventricular hemorrhage. Am J Dis Child 144:1242–1245.

Ludwig B, Brand M, Brockerhoff P 1980 Postpartum CT examination of the heads of full term infants. Neuroradiology 20:145–154.

Lupton B A, Roland E H, Whitfield M F, Hill A 1990 Serum sodium concentration and intravascular hemorrhage in premature infants. Am J Dis Child 144:1019–1021.

McDonald M M, Johnson M L, Rumack C M 1984a Role of coagulopathy in newborn intracranial hemorrhage. Pediatrics 74:26–31.

McDonald M M, Rumack C M, Johnson M L 1984b Timing and antecedents of intracranial hemorrhage in the newborn. Pediatrics 74:32–36.

McLellan N J, Prasad R, Punt J 1986 Spontaneous subhyaloid and retinal hemorrhages in an infant. Arch Dis Child 61:1130–1132.

McMenamin J B, Shackelford G D, Volpe J J 1984 Outcome of neonatal intraventricular hemorrhage with periventricular echodense lesions. Ann Neurol 15:285–290.

Maertens P 1989 Imaging through the posterior fontanelle. J Child Neurol 4(suppl):S62–S67.

Maher P, Lane B, Ballard R et al 1985 Does indomethacin cause extension of intracranial hemorrhages: a preliminary study. Pediatrics 75:497–500.

Malloy M H, Onstad L, Wright E 1991 The effect of cesarian delivery on birth outcome in very low birth weight infants. Obstet Gynecol 77:498–503.

Marret S, Parain D, Samson-Dollfus D et al 1986 Positive rolandic sharp waves and periventricular leukomalacia in the newborn. Neuropediatrics 17:199–202.

Marshall T A, Marshall F, Reddy P P 1982 Physiologic changes associated with ligation of the ductus arteriosus in preterm infants. J Pediatrics 101:749–753.

Martin C G, Snider A R, Katz S M et al 1982 Abnormal cerebral blood flow patterns in preterm infants with a large patent ductus arteriosus. Journal of Pediatrics 101:587–593.

Martin D J, Pape K E, Daneman A 1984 The site of neonatal periventricular hemorrhage: an important prognostic sign of mortality and morbidity. Ann Radiol 27:243–246.

Martin R, Roesmann U, Fanaroff A 1976 Massive intracerebellar hemorrhage in low birth weight infants. Journal of Pediatrics 89:290–292.

Matsuzaka T, Yoshinaga M, Tsuji Y et al 1989 Incidence and causes of intracranial hemorrhage in infancy: a prospective surveillance study after vitamin K prophylaxis. Brain Dev 11:384–388.

Mehrabani D, Gowen C W, Kopelman A E 1991 Association of pneumothorax and hypotension with intraventricular hemorrhage. Arch Dis Child 66:48–51.

Menezes A H, Smith D E, Bell W E 1983 Posterior fossa hemorrhage in the term neonate. Neurosurgery 13:452–456.

Menon P A, Thach B T, Smith C H et al 1984 Benzyl alcohol toxicity in a neonatal intensive care unit: incidence, symptomatology and mortality. Am J Perinatol 1:288–292.

Ment L R, Duncan C C, Ehrenkranz R A et al 1984a Intraventricular hemorrhage in the preterm neonate: timing and cerebral blood flow changes. J Pediatr 104:419–425.

Ment L R, Duncan C C, Ehrenkranz R A et al 1985b Randomized indomethacin trial for prevention of intraventricular hemorrhage in very low birthweight infants. J Pediatr 107:937–943.

Ment L R, Ehrenkranz R A, Lange R C 1981 Alterations in cerebral blood flow in preterm infants with intraventricular hemorrhage. Pediatrics 68:763–769.

Ment L R, Oh W, Ehrenkranz R A 1994 Low dose indomethacin and prevention of intraventricular hemorrhage: a multicenter randomized control trial. Pediatr 93:543–550.

Ment L R, OH W, Philip A G S et al 1992 Risk factors for early intraventricular hemorrhage in low birth weight infants. J Pediatr 121:776–783.

Ment L R, Stewart W B, Duncan C C 1984b Beagle puppy model of intraventricular hemorrhage: ethamsylate studies. Prostaglandins 27:245–256.

Ment L R, Stewart W B, Duncan C C 1985a Beagle puppy model of intraventricular hemorrhage: effect of superoxide dismutase on cerebral blood flow and prostaglandins. J Neurosurg 62:563–569.

Ment L R, Stewart W B, Scott D T, Duncan C C 1983 Beagle puppy model of intraventricular hemorrhage: randomized indomethacin prevention trial. Neurology 33:179–184.

Ment L R, Vohr B, Oh W et al 1996 Neurodevelopmental outcome at 36 months corrected age of preterm infants in the multicenter indomethacin intraventricular hemorrhage prevention trial. Pediatrics 98:714–715.

Ment L R, Westerveld M, Makuch R et al 1998 Cognitive outcome at 4 1/2 years of very low birth weight infants. Pediatr 102:159–160.

Ment LR, Stewart WB, Ardito TA, Madri JA 1995 Germinal matrix microvascular maturation correlates inversely with the risk period for neonatal intraventricular hemorrhage. Brain Res. Develop Brain Res 84,142–149.

Mercer J S, Vohr B R, McGrath M M et al 2006 Delayed cord clamping in very preterm infants reduces the incidence of intraventricular hemorrhage and late-onset sepsis: a randomized, controlled trial. Pediatrics, 117(4):1235–1242.

Mercuri E, Dubowitz L, Paterson Brown S, Cowan F 1998 Incidence of cranial ultrasound abnormalities in apparently well neonates on a postnatal ward: correlation with antenatal and perinatal factors and neurological status. Arch Dis Child Fetal Neonatal Edn 79:F185–F189.

Merrill J D, Piecuch R E, Fell S C et al 1998 A new pattern of cerebellar hemorrhages in preterm infants. Pediatrics 102:E62.

Miall-Allen V M, de Vries L S, Whitelaw A G L 1987 Mean arterial blood pressure and neonatal cerebral lesions. Arch Dis Child 62:1068–1069.

Michaud J L, Rivard G E, Chessex P 1991 Intracranial hemorrhage in a newborn with hemophilia following elective cesarean section. Am J Pediatr Hematol Oncol 13:473–475.

Milligan D W A 1980 Failure of autoregulation and intraventricular hemorrhage in preterm infants. Lancet i:896–898.

Mitchell W, O'Tuama L 1980 Cerebral intraventricular hemorrhages in infants: a widening age spectrum. Pediatrics 65:35–39.

Mittendorf R, Covert R, Boman J et al 1997 Is tocolytic magnesium sulphate associated with increased total paediatric mortality? Lancet 350:1517.

Moghal N E, Quinn M W, Levene M I, Puntis J W L 1992 Intraventricular hemorrhage after aspiration of ventricular reservoirs. Arch Dis Child 67:448–449.

Moody D M, Brown W R, Challa V R, Block S M 1994 Alkaline phosphatase histochemical staining in the study of germinal matrix hemorrhage and brain vascular morphology in a very-low-birth-weight neonate. Pediatr Res 35:424–430.

Morales W J, O'Brien W F, Knuppel R A et al 1989 The effect of mode of delivery on the risk of intraventricular hemorrhage in nondiscordant twin gestations under 1500 g. Obstet Gynecol 73:107–110.

Morales W J, Stroup M 1985 Intracranial hemorrhage in utero due to isoimmune neonatal thrombocytopenia. Obstet Gynecol 65:205–215.

Morgan M E I, Benson J W T, Cooke R W I 1981 Ethamsylate reduces the incidence of periventricular hemorrhage in very low birth weight babies. Lancet ii:830–831.

Morgan M E I, Hensey O J, Cooke R W I 1983 Convexity cerebral hemorrhage in the neonate: in vivo ultrasound diagnosis. Arch Dis Child 58:814–818.

Morgan M E I, Massey R F, Cooke R W I 1982 Does phenobarbitone prevent periventricular hemorrhage in very low birth weight babies? A controlled trial. Pediatrics 70:186–189.

Motohara K, Matsukura M, Matsuda I et al 1984 Severe vitamin K deficiency in breast-fed infants. J Pediatr 105:943–945.

Moylan F M, Herrin J T, Krishnamoorthy K et al 1978 Inappropriate antidiuretic hormone secretion in premature infants with cerebral palsy. Am J Dis Child 132:399–402.

Mullaart R A, Hopman J C W, Rotteveel J J et al 1994 Cerebral blood flow fluctuation in neonatal respiratory distress and periventricular hemorrhage. Early Hum Dev 37:179–185.

Nakamura Y, Okudera T, Fukuda S, Hashimoto T 1990 Germinal matrix hemorrhage of venous origin in preterm neonates. Hum Pathol 21:1059–1062.

Nelson K B, Grether J K 1995 Can magnesium sulfate reduce the risk of cerebral palsy in very low birthweight infants? Paediatr 95:263–269.

Ng P C, Siu Y K, Lewindon P J 1995 Subaponeurotic hemorrhage in the 1990s: a 3-year surveillance. Acta Paediatr 84:1065–1069.

Northern Neonatal Nursing Initiative Trial Group 1996 Randomised trial of prophylactic early fresh-frozen plasma or gelatin or glucose in preterm babies: outcome at 2 years. Lancet 348:229–232.

Nwaesei C G, Allen A C, Vincer M J 1988 Effect of timing of cerebral ultrasonography on the prediction of later neurodevelopmental outcome in high-risk preterm infants. J Pediatr 112:970–975.

Odita J C, Hebi S 1996 CT and MRI characteristics of intracranial hemorrhage complicating breech and vacuum delivery. Pediatr Radiol 26:782–785.

Osborn D A, Evans N, Kluckow M 2003 Hemodynamic and antecedent risk factors of early and late periventricular/intraventricular hemorrhage in premature infants. Pediatrics,112:33–39.

Palma P A, Miner M E, Morriss F H et al 1979 Intraventricular hemorrhage in the neonate born at term. Am J Dis Child 133:941–944.

Palmer K G, Kronsberg S S, Barton B A et al 2005 Effect of inborn versus outborn delivery on clinical outcomes in ventilated preterm neonates: secondary results from the NEOPAIN trial. J Perinatol 25(4):270–275.

Paneth N, Rudelli R, Kazam E, Monte W 1994 Brain damage in the preterm infant. Clinics in Developmental Medicine No 131. Cambridge University Press, Cambridge.

Papagaroufalis C, Megreli Ch, Hagjigeorgi Ch, Xanthou M 1991 A trial of vitamin A supplementation for the prevention of intraventricular hemorrhage in very low birth weight infants. J Perinatal Med 19(suppl 1):382–387.

Papagaroufalis C, Pantazatou E, Megreli Ch et al 1988 Low vitamin A plasma levels (VAPL) preceding massive intracranial bleeding (MIB) in very-low-birth-weight (VLBW) neonates. Pediatr Res 23:556A.

Pape K E, Armstrong D L, Fitzhardinge P M 1976 Central nervous system pathology associated with mask ventilation in the very low birth weight infant: a new etiology for intracerebellar hemorrhages. Pediatrics 58:473–483.

Pape K E, Wigglesworth J S 1979 Hemorrhage, ischaemia and the perinatal brain. Clin Dev Med 69/70.

Papile L-A, Burstein J, Burstein R et al 1978 Relationship of intravenous sodium bicarbonate infusions and cerebral intraventricular hemorrhage. J Pediatr 93:834–836.

Papile L-A, Munsick-Bruno G, Schaefer A 1983 Relationship of cerebral intraventricular hemorrhage and early childhood neurologic handicap. J Pediatr 103:273–277.

Pasternak J F, Mantovani J F, Volpe J J 1980 Porencephaly from periventricular intracerebral hemorrhage in a premature infant. Am J Dis Child 134:673–675.

Payne N R, Hasegawa D K 1984 Vitamin K deficiency in newborns. Pediatrics 73:712–716.

Peabody J L 1981 Mechanical ventilation of the newborn . . . good news . . . bad news. Crit Care Med 9:710–713.

Perlman J M, Goodman S, Kreusser K L, Volpe J J 1985 Reduction in intraventricular hemorrhage by elimination of fluctuating cerebral blood flow velocity in preterm infants with respiratory distress syndrome. N Engl J Med 312:1353–1357.

Perlman J M, Hill A, Volpe J J 1981 The effect of patent ductus arteriosus on flow velocity in the anterior cerebral arteries: ductal steal in the premature newborn infant. J Pediatr 99:767–771.

Perlman J M, McMenamin J B, Volpe J J 1983 Fluctuating cerebral blood flow velocity in respiratory distress syndrome: relation to the development of intraventricular hemorrhage. N Engl J Medicine 309:204–209.

Perlman J M, Risser R 1998 Relationship of uric acid concentrations and severe intraventricular hemorrhage/leukomalacia in the premature infant. J Pediatr 132:436–439.

Perlman J M, Volpe J J 1986 Are venous circulatory abnormalities important in pathogenesis of intraventricular hemorrhage in preterm infants? Ann Neurol 20:434–435.

Perlman J M, Volpe J J 1987 Are venous circulatory abnormalities important in the pathogenesis of hemorrhagic and/or ischemic cerebral injury? Pediatrics 80:705–711.

Perlman JM, Rollins N, Sanchez PJ 1992 Late-onset meningitis in sick, very-low-birthweight infants. Clinical and sonographic observations. Am J Dis Child 146;1297–1301.

Perry E H, Bada H S, Ray J D 1990 Blood pressure increases, birth weight-dependent stability boundary, and intraventricular hemorrhage. Pediatrics 85:727–732.

Peterson C M, Smith W L, Franklen E A 1984 Neonatal intracerebellar hemorrhage: detection by real-time ultrasound. Radiology 150:391–392.

Peysner P H, Garcia-Bunuel R, Leeds N, Finkelstein M 1976 Subependymal and intraventricular hemorrhage in neonates: early diagnosis by computed tomography. Radiology 119:111–114.

Phelps D L 1984 Vitamin E and CNS hemorrhage. Pediatrics 74:1113–1114.

Pollitzer M J, Reynolds E O R, Shaw D G, Thomas R M 1981 Pancuronium during mechanical ventilation speeds recovery of the lungs of infants with hyaline membrane disease. Lancet i:346–348.

Porter F L, Marshall R E, Moore J A, Miller H 1985 Effect of phenobarbital on motor activity and intraventricular hemorrhage in preterm infants with respiratory disease weighing less than 1500 grams. Am J Perinatol 2:63–66.

Rademaker K J, de Vries L S, Barth P G 1993 Subependymal pseudocysts: ultrasound diagnosis and findings at follow-up. Acta Paediatr Scand 82:394–399.

Rademaker K J, Groenendaal F, Jansen G H et al 1994 Unilateral haemorrhagic parenchymal lesions in the preterm infant: shape, site and prognosis. Acta Paediatr Scand 83:602–608.

Rao K C V G, Knipp H C, Wagner E J 1981 Computed tomographic findings in cerebral sinus and venous thrombosis. Radiology 140:391–398.

Ravenel S D 1979 Posterior fossa hemorrhage in the term newborn: report of two cases. Pediatrics 64:39–42.

Reynolds M L, Evans C, Reynolds E O R et al 1979 Intracranial hemorrhage in the preterm sheep fetus. Early Hum Dev 3/2:163–186.

Richard P, Rutka J T, Drake J M et al 1997 Management and outcomes of posterior fossa subdural hematomas in neonates. Neurosurgery 40;1190–1200.

Ries M, Wolfel D, Maier-Brandt B 1995 Severe intracranial hemorrhage in a newborn infant with transplacental transfer of an acquired factor VIII : C inhibitor. J Pediatr 127:649–650.

Rivkin M J, Anderson M L, Kaye E M 1992 Neonatal idiopathic cerebral venous thrombosis: an unrecognized cause of transient seizures or lethargy. Ann Neurol 32:51–56.

Robertson J D 2006 Prevention of intraventricular haemorrhage: a role for recombinant activated factor VII? J Paediatr Child Health.;42(6):325–331.

Roland E H, Flodmark O, Hill A 1990 Thalamic hemorrhage with intraventricular hemorrhage in the full-term newborn. Pediatrics 85:737–742.

Rom S, Serfontein G L, Humphreys R P 1978 Intracerebellar hematoma in the neonate. J Pediatr 93:486–488.

Romodanov A P, Brodsky Y S 1987 Subdural hematomas in the newborn: surgical treatment and results. Surg Neurol 28:253–258.

Rose A L, Lombroso C T 1970 Neonatal seizure states: a study of clinical, pathological, and electroencephalographic features in 137 full-term babies with a long-term follow-up. Pediatrics 45:404–425.

Ruckensteiner E, Zollner F 1929 Uber die Blutungen im Gebiete der Vena terminalis bei Neugeborenen. Frankfurt Zeitschrift für Pathologie 37:568–578.

Ruth V, Virkola K, Paetau R, Raivio K O 1988 Early high-dose phenobarbital treatment for prevention of hypoxic-ischemic brain damage in very low birth weight infants. J Pediatr 112:81–86.

Sadowitz P D, Balcom R 1985 Intrauterine intracranial hemorrhage in an infant with isoimmune thrombocytopenia. Clin Pediatr 24:655–657.

Schendel D E, Berg C J, Yeargin-Allsopp M et al 1996 Prenatal magnesium sulfate exposure and the risk for cerebral palsy or mental retardation among very low-birth-weight children aged 3 to 5 years. JAMA 276:1805–1810.

Scher M S, Wright F S, Lockman L A, Thompson T R 1982 Intraventricular hemorrhage in the full-term neonate. Arch Neurol 39:769–772.

Schick J B, Beck A L, DeSilva H N 1989 Umbilical artery catheter position and intraventricular hemorrhage. J Perinatol 9:382–385.

Scotti G, Fodmark O, Harwood-Nash D C, Humphries R P 1981 Posterior fossa hemorrhages in the newborn. J Comput Assist Tomogr 5:68–72.

Setzer E S, Webb I B, Wassenaar J W 1982 Platelet dysfunction and coagulopathy in intraventricular hemorrhage in the premature infant. J Pediatr 100:599–605.

Shankaran S, Bauer C R, Bain R et al 1996 Prenatal and perinatal risk and protective factors for neonatal intracranial hemorrhage. Arch Pediatr Adolesc Med 150:491–497.

Shankaran S, Slovis T L, Bedard M P, Poland R L 1982 Sonographic classification of intracranial hemorrhage: a prognostic indicator of mortality, morbidity and short-term neurologic outcome. J Pediatr 100:469–475.

Shaw C-M, Alvord E C 1974 Subependymal germinolysis. Arch Neurol 31:374–381.

Shen E Y, Huang C C, Chyou S C et al 1986 Sonographic finding of the bright thalamus. Arch Dis Child 61:1096–1099.

Shinnar S, Molteni R A, Gammon K et al 1982 Intraventricular hemorrhage in the premature infant: a changing outlook. N Engl J Med 306:1464–1468.

Shirahata A, Nakamura T, Shimono M et al 1990 Blood coagulation findings and the efficacy of factor XIII concentrate in premature infants with intracranial hemorrhages. Thrombosis Res 57:755–763.

Sia C G, Amigo N C, Harper R G et al 1985 Failure of cesarian section to prevent intracranial hemorrhage in siblings with isoimmune neonatal thrombocytopenia. Am J Obstet Gynecol 153:79–81.

Simmons M A, Adcock E W, Bard H, Battaglia F C 1974 Hypernatraemia and intracranial hemorrhage in neonates. N Engl J Med 291:6–10.

Sinha S, Davies J, Toner N et al 1987 Vitamin E supplementation reduces the incidence of periventricular hemorrhages in very preterm babies. Lancet i:466–471.

Smets K, De Kezel C, Govaert P 1997 Subependymal caudothalamic groove hyperechogenicity and neonatal chronic lung disease. Acta Paediatrica 86:1370–1373.

Smets K, Van Aken S 1998 Fetomaternal hemorrhage and prenatal intracranial bleeding: two more causes of blueberry muffin baby. Eur J Pediatr 157:932–934.

Smith W L, McGuinness G, Cavanaugh D, Courtney S 1983 Ultrasound screening of premature infants: longitudinal follow-up of intracranial hemorrhage. Radiology 147:445–448.

Soll R F, Morley C J 1999 Prophylactic versus selective use of surfactant for preventing morbidity and mortality in preterm infants (Cochrane Review). In: The Cochrane Library, Issue 2. Oxford: Update Software.

Speer M E, Blifeld C, Rudolph A J et al 1984 Intraventricular hemorrhage and vitamin E in very low birth weight infant: evidence for efficacy of early intramuscular vitamin E administration. Pediatrics 74:1107–1112.

Spinillo A, Gardella B, Preti E, Zanchi S,Tzialla C,Stronati M 2007 Preeclampsia and Brain Damage among Preterm Infants: A Changed Panorama in a 20-Year Analysis. Am J Perinatol. 2007 ePub.

Spinillo A, Ometto A, Stronati M et al 1995 Epidemiologic association between maternal smoking during pregnancy and intracranial hemorrhage in preterm infants. J Pediatr 127:473–479.

Stewart A L, Reynolds E O R, Hope P L 1987 Probability of neurodevelopmental disorders estimated from ultrasound appearance of brains of very preterm infants. Dev Med Child Neurol 29:3–11.

Stewart A L, Thorburn R J, Hope P L et al 1983b Ultrasound appearance of the brain in very preterm infants and neurodevelopmental outcome at 18 months of age. Arch Dis Child 58:598–604.

Stewart A L, Thorburn R J, Lipscomb A P, Amiel-Tison C 1983a Neonatal neurologic examinations of very preterm infants: comparison of results with ultrasound diagnosis of periventricular hemorrhage. Am J Perinatol 1:6–11.

Strange M J, Myers G, Kirklin J K et al 1985 Surgical closure of patent ductus arteriosus does not increase the risk of intraventricular hemorrhage in the preterm infant. J Pediatr 107:602–604.

Strauss A, Kirz D, Modanlou H D, Freeman R K 1985 Perinatal events and the very low-birth weight infant. Am J Obstet Gynecol 151:1022–1027.

Stutchfield P R, Cooke R W I 1989 Electrolytes and glucose in cerebrospinal fluid of premature infants with intraventricular hemorrhage: role of potassium in cerebral infarction. Arch Dis Child 64:470–475.

Sudakoff G S, Montazemi M, Rifkin M D 1993 The foramen magnum: the underutilized acoustic window to the posterior fossa. J Ultrasound Med 12:205–210.

Szymonowicz W, Yu V Y H 1984a Timing and evolution of periventricular hemorrhage in infants weighing 1250 g or less at birth. Arch Dis Child 59:7–12.

Szymonowicz W, Yu V Y H, Walker A, Wilson F 1986 Reduction in periventricular hemorrhages in preterm infants. Arch Dis Child 61:661–665.

Szymonowicz W, Yu V Y H, Wilson F E 1984b Antecedents of periventricular hemorrhage in infants weighing 1250 g or less at birth. Arch Dis Child 59:13–17.

Takagi T, Nagai R, Wakabayashi S et al 1978 Extradural hemorrhage in the newborn as a result of birth trauma. Child Brain 4:306–318.

Takashima S, Mito T, Ando Y 1986 Pathogenesis of periventricular white matter hemorrhages in preterm infants. Brain Devel 8:25–30.

Takashima S, Tanaka K 1978 Microangiography and vascular permeability of the subependymal matrix in the premature infant. Can J Neurol Sci 5:45–50.

Tarby T J, Volpe J J 1982 Intraventricular hemorrhage in the premature infant. Pediatr Clin North Am 29:1077–1089.

Tardieu M, Evrard P, Lyon G 1981 Progressive expanding congenital porencephalies: a treatable cause of progressive encephalopathy. Pediatrics 68:198–202.

Tejani N, Rebold B, Tuck S et al 1984 Obstetric factors in the causation of early periventricular-intraventricular hemorrhage. Obstet Gynecol 64:510–515.

Tejani N, Verma U L 1989 Correlation of Apgar scores and umbilical artery acid-base status to mortality and morbidity in the low birth weight neonate. Obstet Gynecol 73:597–600.

TeKoiste K A, Bennett F C, Mack L A 1985 Follow-up of infants receiving cranial ultrasound for intracranial hemorrhage. Am J Dis Child 139:299–303.

Thorburn R J, Lipscomb A P, Stewart A L 1982 Timing and antecedents of periventricular hemorrhage and of cerebral atrophy in very preterm infants. Early Hum Dev 7:221–238.

Thorburn R J, Lipscomb A P, Stewart A L et al 1981 Prediction of death and major handicap in very preterm infants by brain ultrasound. Lancet i:1119–1121.

Toubas P L, Hof R P, Heymann M, Rudolph A 1978 Effects of hypothermia and rewarming on the neonatal circulation. Archives Françaises Pediatrie (suppl) 35:84–92.

Towbin A 1968 Cerebral intraventricular hemorrhage and subependymal matrix infarction in the fetus and premature newborn. Am J Pathol 52:121–134.

Trounce J Q, Dodd K L, Fawer C-L et al 1985 Primary thalamic hemorrhage in the newborn: a new clinical entity. Lancet i:190–192.

Trounce J Q, Rutter N, Levene M I 1986 A prospective study of the incidence of periventricular leukomalacia and intraventricular hemorrhage in the preterm neonate. Arch Dis Child 61:1196–1202.

Tsiantos A, Victorin L, Relier J P et al 1974 Intracranial hemorrhage in the prematurely born infant. Timing of clots and evaluation of clinical signs and symptoms. J Pediatr 85:854–859.

Van Bel F, Van de Bor M, Stijnen T et al 1987 Aetiological role of cerebral blood-flow alterations in development and extension of peri-intraventricular hemorrhage. Dev Med Child Neurol 29:601–614.

van der Bor M, den Ouden L, Guit G L 1992 Value of cranial ultrasound and magnetic resonance imaging in predicting neurodevelopmental outcome in preterm infants. Pediatrics 90:196–199.

Veldman A, Josef J, Fischer D, Volk W R 2006 A prospective pilot study of prophylactic treatment of preterm neonates with recombinant activated factor VII during the first 72 hours of life. Pediatr Crit Care Med;7(1):34–39.

Vert P, Nomin P, Sibout M 1975 Intracranial venous pressure in the newborn: variations in physiological state and in neurologic and respiratory distress. In: Stern L (ed.) Intensive care in the newborn. Masson, New York.

Vinchon M, Pierrat V, Tchofo PJ, Soto-Ares G, Dhellemmes P 2005 Traumatic intracranial hemorrhage in newborns. Childs Nerv Syst. 21(12):1042–1048.

Vohr B, Coll C G, Flanagan P, Oh W 1992 Effects of intraventricular hemorrhage and socioeconomic status on perceptual, cognitive, and neurologic status of low birth weight infants at 5 years of age. J Pediatr 121:280–285.

Vohr B, Ment L R 1996 Intraventricular hemorrhage in the preterm infant. Early Hum Dev 44:1–16.

Voit T, Lemburg P, Stork W 1985 NMR studies in thalamic-striatal necrosis. Lancet ii:445.

Volpe J J 1977 Neonatal intracranial hemorrhage: pathophysiology, neuropathology and clinical features. Clin Perinatol 4:77–102.

Volpe J J, Herscovitch P, Perlman J M, Raichle M E 1983 Positron emission tomography in the newborn: extensive impairment of regional blood flow with intraventricular hemorrhage and hemorrhagic involvement. Pediatrics 72: 589–601.

Voutsinas L, Gorey M T, Gould R et al 1991 Venous sinus thrombosis as a cause of parenchymal and intraventricular hemorrhage in the full-term neonate. Clin Imaging 15:273–275.

Waanabe K, Hakamada S, Kuroyanagi M et al 1983 Electroencephalographic study of intraventricular hemorrhage in the preterm newborn. Neuropaediatr 14:225–230.

Wakai S, Andoh Y, Nagai M et al 1990 Choroid plexus arteriovenous malformation in a full-term neonate. Journal of Neurosurgery 72:127–129.

Wallin L A, Rosenfeld C R, Laptook A R et al 1990 Neonatal intracranial hemorrhage: II. Risk factor analysis in an inborn population. Early Hum Dev 23:129–137.

Watkins A M C, West C R, Cooke R W I 1989 Blood pressure and cerebral haemorrhage and ischaemia in very low birthweight infants. Early Hum Development 19:103–110.

Watson J W, Brown D M, Lally K P et al 1990 Complications of extracorporeal membrane oxygenation in neonates. South Med J 83:1262–1265.

Wehberg K, Vincent M, Garrison B et al 1992 Intraventricular hemorrhage in the full-term neonate associated with abdominal compression. Pediatrics 89:327–329.

Welch K & Strand R 1986 Traumatic parturitional intracranial hemorrhage. Dev Med Child Neurol 28:156–164.

Whitby EH, Griffirths PD, Rutter S et al 2003 Frequency and natural history of subdural haemorrhages in babies and relation to obstetric factors. Lancet 362:846–851.

White R P, Hagen A A, Morgan H et al 1975 Experimental study on the genesis of cerebral vasospasm. Stroke 6:52–57.

Whitelaw A G, Haines M E, Bolsover W, Harris E 1984 Factor V deficiency and antenatal intraventricular hemorrhage. Arch Dis Child 59:997–999.

Whitelaw A, Odd D 2007 Postnatal phenobarbital for the prevention of intraventricular hemorrhage in preterm infants. Cochrane Database of Systematic Reviews. 4.

Whitelaw A, Placzek M, Dubowitz L et al 1983 Phenobarbitone for prevention of periventricular hemorrhage in very low birth weight infants. Lancet ii:1168–1170.

Wigglesworth J S, Husemeyer R P 1977 Intracranial birth trauma in vaginal breech delivery: the continued importance of injury to the occipital bone. Br J Obstet Gynaecol 84:684–691.

Wigglesworth J S, Keith I H, Girling D J, Slade S A 1976 Hyaline membrane disease, alkali and intraventricular hemorrhage. Arch Dis Child 51:755–759.

Wiswell T E, Graziani L J, Kornhauser M S et al 1996 High-frequency jet ventilation in the early management of respiratory distress syndrome is associated with a greater risk for adverse outcome. Pediatrics 98:1035–1043.

Wu YW, Hamrick SE, Miller SP, Haward MF et al 2003 Intraventricular hemorrhage in term neonates caused by sinovenous thrombosis. Annals of Neurology; 54:123–126.

Zalneraitis E L, Young R S K, Krishnamoorthy K S 1979 Intracranial hemorrhage in utero as a complication of isoimmune thrombocytopenia. J Pediatr 95:611–614.

Zlatnik F J 1993 The Iowa premature breech trial. Am J Perinatol 10:60–63.

Zuerrer M, Martin E, Boltshauser E 1991 MR imaging of intracranial hemorrhage in neonates and infants at 2.35 tesla. Neuroradiology 33:223–229.

CHAPTER

21

Cerebral ischemic lesions

Linda S. de Vries, Serena J. Counsell and Malcolm I. Levene

Key Points

- The term periventricular white matter injury (PWMI) is preferred to periventricular leukomalacia (PVL)
- Diffuse PWMI appears to be a milder form of injury than PVL
- The incidence of cystic leukomalacia is declining
- Perinatal stroke is the second most common cause of neonatal seizures in the full-term infant
- Neonatal magnetic resonance imaging (MRI) and especially diffusion weighted imaging (DWI) plays an important role in early prediction of hemiplegia

---

INTRODUCTION

Brain ischemia occurs as the result of a variety of perinatal insults. During intrapartum asphyxia, cerebral hypoperfusion together with hypoxia produces a typical pathologic and clinical appearance which is discussed in Chapter 22. In this section we will refer to the more specific condition of cerebral ischemia associated to some extent with vascular compromise. This may develop in the watershed area between the vascular territory of two arterial beds, as occurs in a number of infants with leukomalacia, or following infarction of the whole or a branch of a major cerebral artery.

PERIVENTRICULAR WHITE MATTER INJURY

The term periventricular white matter injury (PWMI) is considered a spectrum of cerebral injury that ranges from focal cystic necrotic lesions, which is still referred to as periventricular leukomalacia (PVL) and a more diffuse form of white matter injury, referred to as PWMI. The latter term is now more often used than the term PVL. Periventricular leukomalacia was a term used to refer to necrotic lesions in the white matter, often seen as small cysts on histological examination or on cranial ultrasound. Leukomalacia literally means 'softening of the white matter'. The presence of cystic lesions in the white matter was well recognized to be an important cause of neurodevelopmental sequelae and is almost invariably related to the development of cerebral palsy later in infancy. Cystic necrotic lesions, which were still commonly seen a decade or so ago, have now become increasingly rare with advances in obstetric and neonatal care (Hamrick et al 2004). The more diffuse form of PWMI is especially common in the less mature preterm infants who are now surviving in ever increasing numbers and are often referred to as the ELGAN group (extremely low gestational age newborns). It should be emphasized that PWMI can also be seen in term infants, especially in those with congenital heart disease (Galli et al 2004, Wernovsky et al 2005). While the focal cystic form of white matter damage was considered to be basically ischemic, the more diffuse form of WMD is now considered to be especially associated with increased vulnerability of oligodendroglia to oxidative stress and to inflammatory processes. The diagnosis using cranial ultrasound is not very reliable in the non-cystic form, but the use of neonatal MRI is now increasing and will hopefully advance our understanding of this condition.

HISTORICAL REVIEW

Ischemic lesions in general and periventricular leukomalacia (PVL) in particular have commonly been diagnosed at autopsy, before the era of the newer imaging techniques. The necrotic cystic type of white matter injury (PVL) has been known to pathologists for over a century (Parrot 1873, Virchow 1867). It was pointed out by the latter that the problem was more common in premature infants and he therefore assumed that the immature white matter might be especially vulnerable in this age group. A major advance in understanding this condition occurred in 1962 when Banker and Larroche described the pathologic changes in 51 infants. They introduced the name 'periventricular leukomalacia' to describe their observation of the periventricular 'white spots' seen macroscopically (Fig. 21.1) and the softening (malacia) of the white matter (leukos). Perinatal anoxia was noted in the clinical history of all their cases, and they were the first to suggest that the condition was vascular in origin. Van den Bergh (1969) and De Reuck et al (1972) further stressed the vascular origin of these lesions and attributed the cause to hypoperfusion of the boundary zones between ventriculofugal and ventriculopetal arteries. This hypothesis was supported by Armstrong and Norman in 1974, which showed that hemorrhages could occur as a secondary process into these ischemic lesions (Fig. 21.2). Leech and Alvord (1974) reported that the lesions could extend beyond the periventricular region into the subcortical white matter. Takashima and Tanaka (1978) performed post-mortem cerebral angiography and showed that the boundary zones between the ventriculofugal and ventriculopetal arteries were affected in the infants with PVL. Takashima et al (1978) performed similar studies in more mature infants and showed a relatively avascular triangle in the white matter at the depths of the sulci. These areas corresponded well with the site of the subcortical lesions seen in more mature infants. They

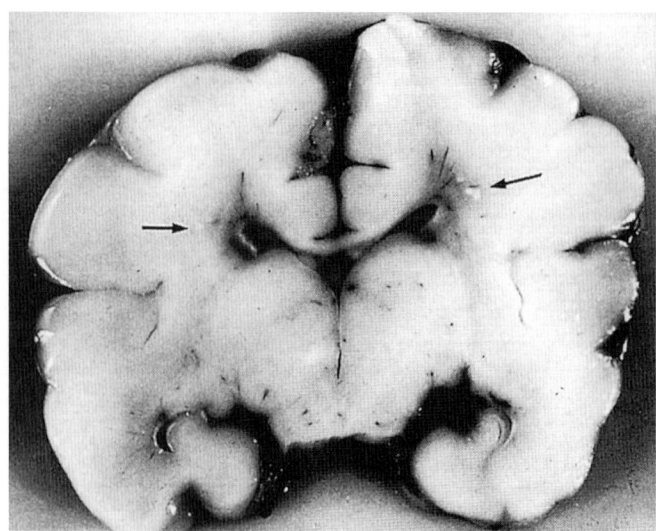

Figure 21.1 Bilateral 'white spots' (arrows) of PVL. Histologically, glial proliferation and calcification were present. Small bilateral germinal matrix hemorrhage is also present.

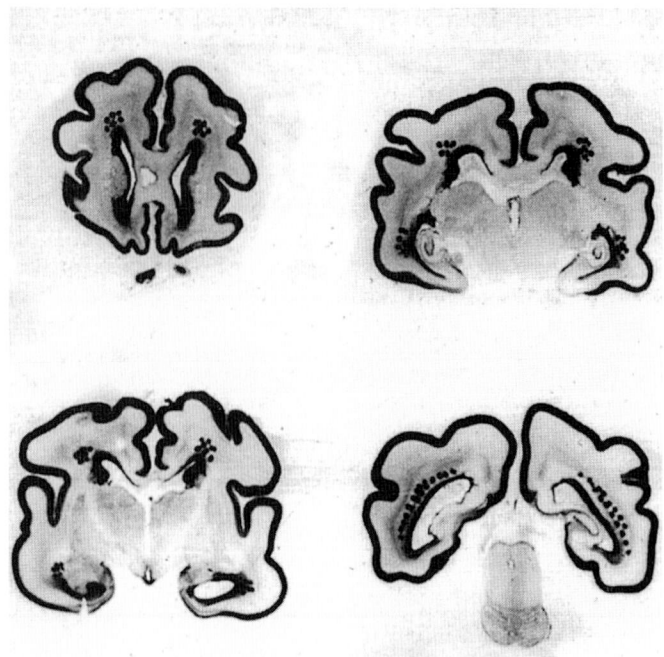

Figure 21.3 Distribution of PVL lesions. The sites of predilection of white matter lesions are superimposed on brain sections stained with cresyl violet. (Reproduced, with permission, from Larroche 1984.)

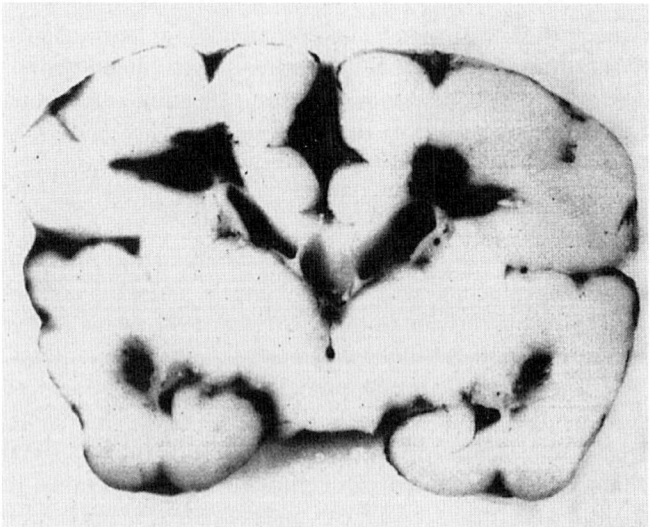

Figure 21.2 Hemorrhagic necrosis into bilateral PVL lesions.

therefore suggested that the distribution of these cystic lesions was related to the maturity of the vascular supply.

Kuban and Gilles (1985) and Nelson et al (1991) did not support the ventriculofugal/ventriculopetal periventricular white matter vascular border zone model, as they were not able to confirm the existence of ventriculofugal arteries described by van den Bergh and De Reuck. Kuban and Gilles (1985) injected the cerebral arteries of human fetal cadavers with silicone and looked at these specimens using high-power stereomicroscopic observations of thick specimens, and were unable to visualize ventriculofugal arteries. When they examined these specimens at low magnification and without stereoscopy they were able to reproduce the results of van den Bergh, and concluded that both van den Bergh as well as De Reuck mistook transcerebral channels within the periventric-

ular white matter, superimposed on the distal ends of striate arteries, for ventriculofugal arteries. Similar conclusions were drawn by Moody et al (1990) using different techniques. They suggested that the medullary veins, which converge in a radial fashion out of the centrum semiovale towards the ventricles, were mistaken for ventriculofugal arteries, and once again questioned the ventriculofugal/ventriculopetal vascular border zone model as the basis for PVL.

During more recent years, it has become clear that hypoperfusion may play a role but other, probably more important, factors are involved, such as excitatory amino acids, the vulnerability of immature oligodendrocytes to oxidative stress and the role of proinflammatory cytokines (see below).

PATHOLOGY

Using a morphological definition, a focal necrotic subtype (PVL) and a diffuse subtype can be recognized on histopathology. The necrotic foci evolve into cysts that will subsequently collapse and this will be followed by focal scar formation. The more diffuse type of injury involves preferential injury to the premyelinating oligodendrocytes (pre-OLs) extending beyond the periventricular white matter into the central white matter resulting in a global delay in myelination. Macroscopical examination of focal necrotic PVL shows a typical distribution of the periventricular lesions involving the external angle of the lateral ventricles (centrum semiovale), the corona radiata, the optic radiation (trigone and occipital horn) and the auditory radiation (temporal horn) (Fig. 21.3).

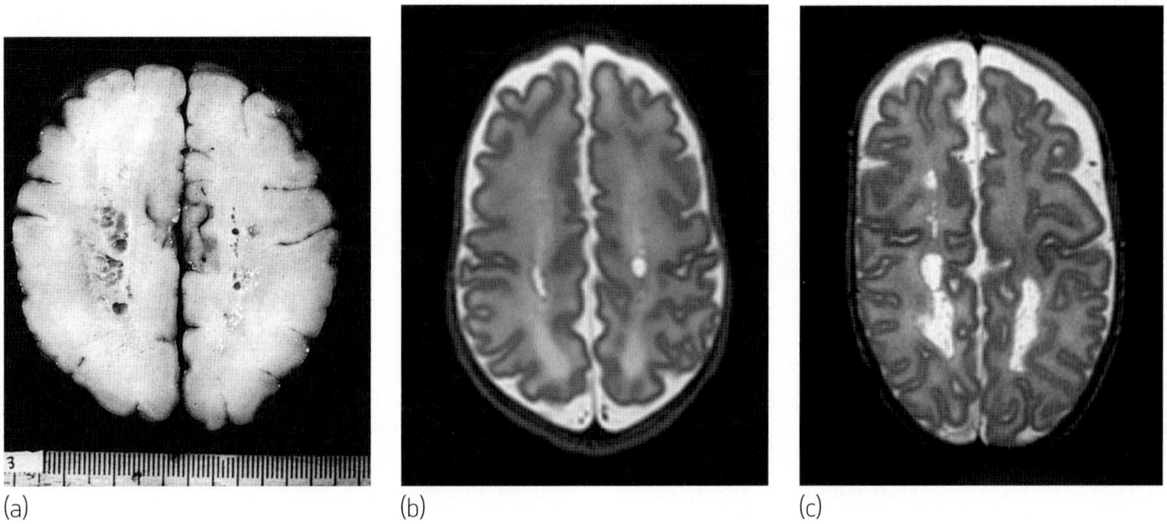

Figure 21.4 Cystic leukomalacia. (a) Horizontal section of brain from an infant of 29 weeks of gestation who survived for 5 weeks. (Reproduced, with permission, from Larroche 1984.) (b) MRI (T2SE) at term equivalent age showing localized cysts. (c) MRI (T2SE) showing extensive cystic leukomalacia.

Histologic findings depend on the duration between the insult and the time of death. The earliest changes consist of coagulation necrosis, characterized by loss of architecture, and this can be found within 5–8 hours following an insult. A few days later, nuclear debris, astrocytes and macrophages are noted to fill the periphery of the necrotic area. These macrophages can remain for months or years. The center of the necrotic area may liquefy, resulting in small cavities, usually not communicating with the lateral ventricles (Fig. 21.4a). Calcified capillaries can sometimes be noted in the periphery of these areas. Cavitation is not always observed, and gliosis and persisting macrophages may be noted instead. Thinning of the white matter with enlargement of the lateral ventricles is present in both cases.

Owing to the prolonged survival of severely ill very low birth weight (VLBW) infants, the morphologic expression of the brain insult has changed significantly from the histology originally described by Banker and Larroche (1962). Paneth et al (1990) reported autopsy findings of 22 preterm infants who died beyond 5 days of age. Of these infants, 15 had either acute or chronic white matter necrosis, but this was restricted to the periventricular white matter in only a minority of the cases. Only 3 infants had histologic findings as originally reported by Banker and Larroche in 1962. The other 12 infants either did not have the classic histologic features of PVL or, if they did, the lesions were not restricted to the periventricular white matter. They concluded that in the VLBW infant white matter necrosis need not be restricted to the periventricular region and can sometimes be histologically different from PVL as originally described. In the 33 infants studied by Back et al (2005), a mixture of preterm and full-term infants, two types of early

PWMI were identified. Diffuse white matter lesions were always present and contained hypertrophied/transforming microglias that were extensively localized within the deep white matter. By contrast, focal lesions were uncommonly seen and were restricted to the subventricular zone. The lesions located in the subventricular zone were regions of apparent focal coagulative necrosis, a common antecedent to PVL. They were characterized by focal collections of phagocytic macrophages.

The use of immunohistochemistry has improved our understanding of this condition considerably. Using this technique, Deguchi et al (1997, 1999) showed the distribution of PWMI in 85 infants (22–41 weeks gestation) to be more widespread in the most immature infants, involving the deep and intermediate white matter. It was shown that glial fibrillary acidic protein (GFAP) positive astrocytes were increased in the deep white matter, often also spreading to the intermediate white matter in all PVL cases. Cells positive for tumor necrosis factor-α (TNF-α) were present in 69% of PWMI cases and β-amyloid precursor protein (β-APP) in 76% of cases. β-APP is a membrane spanning glycoprotein generated in the neuronal cell body that is transported to axons and accumulates in damaged axons. It can either be a marker of axonal injury, or it may be upregulated in response to brain injury. Some studies have suggested that β-APP is a growth factor and a protector against excitotoxic or ischemic insults. It is an excellent marker for foci of necrosis and can readily identify the otherwise subtle morphologic features of white matter necrosis in the immature brain. Ninety-four percent of the infants with a gestational age below 29 weeks showed widespread distribution of PWMI, whereas most of those with a gestational age greater than 34 weeks developed focal PWMI.

GFAP, TNF-α or β-APP positive cells were not found in any of the controls. β-APP positive axons proved to be a useful marker for demonstrating the type of PWMI. In a subsequent study they pointed out that β-APP positive cells were only seen in the early stages of prenatal PWMI (Meng et al 1997). The same group (Meng & Takashima 1999) also studied the expression of transforming growth factor-β1 in PWMI, a factor considered to be synthesized in response to brain injury. This factor was observed in glial cells around necrotic foci in the white matter and was only present in the subacute stage of PWMI, in those with focal stages and in the more mature infants (gestational age >32 weeks). They suggested that transforming growth factor-β1 might contribute to tissue remodeling and healing after ischemic injury.

The incidence of PWMI in these pathologic studies varies between 7 and 34% (Armstrong & Norman 1974, Pape & Wigglesworth 1979), but increases to over 80% by taking only those infants who required ventilation and survived beyond the first 7 days of life (Shuman & Selednik 1980). In a more recent study, 68% of the 22 VLBW infants who survived at least 6 days were diagnosed as having some degree of white matter necrosis (Paneth et al 1990).

The data by Back et al (2005) showed that early PWMI was related to oxidative damage that particularly targeted the oligodendrocyte lineage, whereas other neuronal and glial cell types were markedly more resistant. From this study they were able to conclude that the predilection of preterm infants for PWMI is related to selective lipid peroxidation-mediated injury of cerebral white matter and targeted death of oligodendrocyte progenitors.

Prenatal onset of leukomalacia was also noted by pathologists when studying stillbirths or infants who died within the first few days of life. The incidence varied from 1.1% (Sims 1985) to 20% in stillbirths and 16.4% of infants who died within the first 3 days of life. Of the preterm infants, 14.3% had prenatal onset PWMI which consisted of widespread necrosis (Iida 1993).

PATHOPHYSIOLOGY

There is no generally accepted pathophysiologic mechanism to explain the development of PWMI and a number of different theories exist (Back 2006).

The vascular theory

The historical concept that PVL is caused by hypoperfusion is supported by only a few animal studies. Abramovicz (1964) obliterated the basilar artery and ligated one or both common carotid arteries in mature cats. Subsequently, he was able to show patchy infarcts close to the ventricular wall in the centrum semiovale.

Other groups have used dogs as animal models. Young et al (1982) produced systemic hypotension either by withdrawal of blood or by injection of *E. coli* into the perito-

neum, and showed a significant reduction of cerebral blood flow (CBF) in the periventricular white matter while the blood flow to the cortical and deep gray matter was preserved. Ment et al (1985a) induced hemorrhagic hypotension in beagle puppies and found similar results. Yoshioka et al (1992) performed bilateral carotid artery occlusion in 7 mongrel puppies and found that 6 of the 7 brains had uni- or multiloculated cysts in the periventricular white matter and significantly reduced myelination compared with controls. Using bilateral carotid artery occlusion in 5-day-old rats, Uehara et al (1999) were able to induce white matter changes in 91% of the animals. Matsuda et al (1999) induced systemic hemorrhagic hypotension in fetal sheep by rapid withdrawal of 35% of the fetoplacental blood volume and produced periventricular white matter lesions, consisting of coagulation necrosis and/or diffuse axonal swelling in 5 out of 6 fetuses. An interesting observation was made by Ohyu et al (1999) who performed repeated umbilical cord occlusion in near-term fetal sheep and subsequently detected multiple necrotic foci predominantly in the periventricular white matter.

In a more recent elegant animal experiment, using instrumented 0.65 gestation fetal sheep, where cerebral blood flow was interrupted by bilateral carotid occlusion, it was found that the *duration* of cerebral ischemia was a critical factor required to generate a graded spectrum of PWMI. Ischemia of shorter duration (30 or 37 minutes) only affected the frontal and parietal periventricular white matter, whereas a duration of 45 minutes of ischemia led to extensive damage also affecting cortical and subcortical gray matter and an even longer duration led to extensive cystic necrotic encephalomalacia (Riddle et al 2006). It was of interest that the extent of white matter damage depended on the presence of susceptible populations of late oligodendrocyte progenitors.

A reduction in CBF after hypocarbia due to vasoconstriction was noted in animal experiments (Saphiro et al 1980). Reuter and Disney (1986) have shown that there is a nonlinear positive correlation between $PaCO_2$ and regional CBF in the white matter of newborn dogs. Hypocarbia ($PaCO_2$ 2.67 kPa) of only 1 hour duration has been shown to reduce brain energy levels and increase cerebral cortex disruption in neonatal piglets compared with control normocarbic animals (Fritz et al 2001).

In different types of animal experiments, the periventricular white matter has appeared to be more susceptible than other areas of the brain. Ment et al (1985a) noted a regional increase in glucose utilization in the periventricular white matter and therefore assumed uncoupling between local CBF and glucose metabolism in the periventricular white matter. This uncoupling was also noted by Cavazutti and Duffy (1982), who looked at hyperemia following hypoxia. They found that the compensatory hyperemia was less pronounced in the periventricular white matter, while an extremely high rate of glycolysis was found in this area compared with other regions of the brain. Prostaglandin E_2, a potent vasodilator, was also carefully studied by Ment et al (1985b) in beagles subjected to hypotension. The concentration of prostaglandin E_2 was shown to increase to a lesser extent in the periventricular white matter than in the cortex and gray matter.

The excitotoxic theory

Animal studies suggest that hypoperfusion alone could be an oversimplification in explaining the pathophysiology of PVL, and an increasing number of these studies are looking at the role of excitatory amino acids in relation to neuronal damage (see Chapters 22 and 27). Gressens et al (1999) were able to induce cystic PVL by injecting the glutaminergic analog ibotenate intracerebrally into newborn mice. By simultaneously injecting a trophic factor, vasoactive intestinal peptide (VIP), a reduction up to 87% of these excitotoxic lesions was obtained. Using the same model, this group also showed a protective effect of a glycine antagonist and NO synthase inhibitor (Marret et al 1999). Meng and Takashima (1999) also suggested that exogenous transforming growth factor-β1 could have a therapeutic effect, being involved in a delayed glial response. They studied 25 neonates with PVL using immunohistochemistry and found this growth factor to be present in 16 cases, especially in the subacute stage of PVL and only in the more mature infants (greater than 32 weeks gestation). The expression was more obvious in focal PVL. In a recent study by Medja et al (2006) thiorphan, a neutral endopeptidase inhibitor, administered into the peritoneum of newborn mice was found to reduce ibotenate induced cortical lesions up to 57% and cortical caspase-3 cleavage up to 59%. The window for therapeutic intervention was long, as the drug was still effective when administered 12 hours after the insult. The protective effect was seen in the gray, but not in the white matter. Leroux et al (2007) studied the role of tissue-plasminogen activator (t-PA) in a mouse model for white matter injury, using ibotenic acid. Intracerebral hrt-PA induced WM cystic lesions in t-PA$^{-/-}$ mice and had an additive effect when co-injected with high-dose ibotenic acid. Welin et al (2007) used melatonin in fetal sheep who were subjected to umbilical cord occlusion. The production of 8-isoprostanes following umbilical cord occlusion was attenuated and there was a reduction in the number of activated microglia cells and TUNEL-positive cells in melatonin treated fetuses, suggesting a protective effect of melatonin.

The oligodendroglial theory

Following the work of Oka et al (1993) who showed that cultured oligodendroglial cells were highly vulnerable to glutamate induced cell death, Back et al (1998) extensively studied maturation dependent vulnerability of oligodendrocytes (OLs) to oxidative stress. They were able to develop an in vitro system to study two distinct OL maturational stages: the preOL and the mature-OL, the preOL being the mitotically active premyelinating precursor to the mature myelin basic protein positive OL. They examined whether OLs display maturation dependent survival in response to cystine deprivation, the latter being a form of oxidative stress that involves depletion of intracellular glutathione. PreOLs in contrast to OLs indeed displayed increased susceptibility to death associated with free radical mediated injury, induced by glutathione depletion or exogenous reactive oxygen species. Maturation of OLs correlated with increased resistance to oxidative stress. The increased vulnerability of the preOLs to oxidative stress correlated with a greater dependence on intracellular glutathione for survival. The toxicity of glutathione depletion was prevented by glutathione replacement. Glutathione depletion caused a marked rise in reactive oxygen species, whose toxicity could be prevented by antioxidants α-tocopherol and idebenone. Increased susceptibility of preOLs to oxidative stress may be due to delayed maturational expression of genes that suppress apoptosis.

Alternatively, the death of preOLs may be regulated by a specific pathway triggered by oxidative stress that is downregulated in mature OLs. Jelinski et al (1999) used 7-day-old rats for a hypoxic–ischemic model, exposing them to 8% oxygen with temporary occlusion of the carotid arteries. Oligodendroblasts were identified using the O4 antibody. They suggest that the vulnerable glial cell type that makes a contribution to the development of PVL is the oligodendroblast, as a decrease of these cells was seen within 24 hours after the insult. Another group studied the distribution and development of ferritin-containing cells by immunohistochemistry and found that the OL was the predominant cell type. Ferritin-positive cells were present in the periventricular and subcortical white matter from 25 weeks onwards. They suggested that ferritin-positive glia were related to the process of myelination and maturation of the OL (Ozawa et al 1994). More recent data by Back (2006) and Riddle et al (2006) further support this theory.

The inflammation theory

Many recent experimental as well as human studies have provided strong evidence for a causal relationship between ascending intrauterine infection, the production of proinflammatory cytokines and white matter damage (see reviews by Dammann & Leviton 1997a, 1998, 1999 and Rothwell et al 1997). The first animal study suggesting the importance of infection was by Gilles et al in 1976. They administered intraperitoneal *E. coli* endotoxin to neonatal kittens for 6 days and found telencephalic leukoencephalopathy at post-mortem. The severity of the lesions appeared to be related to the dose of the endotoxin. More recently, Yoon et al (1997a) performed hysteroscopy in rabbits at 20–21 days of gestation and inoculated either *E. coli* ($n = 31$) or saline ($n = 14$), treating both groups with ampicillin-sulbactam. The rabbits were killed 5–6 days later. They noted histologic evidence of white matter damage in 12 of the *E. coli* inoculated group compared with none in the saline group ($P < 0.005$). A more recent study was performed in the preterm ovine fetus (Duncan et al 2002). At 0.7 of gestation, six catheterized fetuses received three to five intravenous injections of LPS (1 micro g/Kg) over 5 days; seven fetuses served as controls. Brain tissue was examined 10–11 d after the initial LPS injection. After LPS on day 1 and 2, fetuses became transiently hypoxemic and hypotensive and blood IL-6 levels were increased, but these responses were smaller or absent after subsequent LPS exposures. Neural injury was observed in all LPS-exposed fetuses, most prominently in the cerebral white matter. Injury ranged from diffuse subcortical damage to PWMI and in the brainstem the cross-sectional area of the corticospinal tract was reduced by 30%.

In a similar experiment, also using 0.7 gestation ovine fetuses, profound reductions in placental blood flow and cerebral O_2 delivery were seen, which could contribute to fetal brain injury. Reduced O_2 delivery to white matter was similar to that in other brain regions. Mechanisms that enable fetal CBF to increase in hypoxemic conditions were apparently ineffective in the presence of LPS. Garnier et al (2006) also studied the preterm fetal sheep following intravenous application of endotoxin and found that this caused focal periventricular brain white matter injury, inflammation and an increase in S100B protein release.

Levels of endotoxin measured in a clinical setting were measured by Okumura et al (1999a). They were unable to show a correlation between raised endotoxin levels and the presence of PVL and, unfortunately, were unable to perform simultaneous cytokine measurements.

Many bacterial products besides endotoxin can stimulate the production of cytokines. Deguchi et al (1996) and Yoon et al (1997b) used immunohistochemical staining on brain sections having histologic evidence of PVL, and compared them with brain sections without leukomalacia. Expression of TNF-α and interleukin-6 was found significantly more often in brain sections that showed evidence of leukomalacia. Interleukin-6 has been reported to play a role in guiding the developing bipotential oligodendrocyte precursor cell, O-2A, towards the astrocyte and away from the pathway leading to a mature oligodendrocyte (Kahn & de Vellis 1994). Deguchi et al (1996) noted that TNF-α was mainly expressed in glial cells in the deep white matter. It is of interest that TNF-α expression was also present in the controls during the late fetal period, but later than in the leukomalacia cases. These two studies provided further support for the hypothesis that proinflammatory cytokines play a role in the genesis of PVL. Even more convincing is the study by Dommergues et al (2000) who pretreated pups with interleukin 1-β, IL-6, IL-9 or TNF-α. They were able to show that the pretreated pups developed significantly larger cortical and white matter damage than controls when later exposed to the neurotoxin ibotenate. Induction of TNF-α and inducible nitric oxide synthase was, however, also detected following fetal hypoxia induced by repetitive umbilical cord occlusion (Ohyu et al 1999). Kadhim et al

(2006) explored potential TNF-α signaling pathways in 12 human brains with PVL and conducted in situ immunohistochemical investigations to search for possible expression of cytokine receptors in these brains. Six infants were 34 weeks or more and 4 of these had a congenital heart defect. TNF-α overexpression was associated with immune reactivity for p75TNFalphaR2 and p55TNFalphaR1 receptors in affected PVL areas.

Several groups have subsequently measured cytokines in the amniotic fluid, in fetal plasma, and cord blood. TNF-α, interleukin-1 and interleukin-6 all play a role in normal pregnancy (Opsjln et al 1993), but levels have been shown to be elevated in the amniotic fluid of pregnant women with chorioamnionitis (Yoon et al 1997c). Baud et al (1999a) were able to find an association between the amniotic fluid level of interleukin-1β and the degree of vascular extension of chorioamnionitis. TNF-α best predicted the development of severe early neonatal infection. In this study, the cytokines were unable to predict the development of PVL, but Yoon et al (1997c) did show a significant relationship between raised interleukin-1β and interleukin-6 levels in the amniotic fluid with white matter lesions. Gomez et al (1998) measured interleukin-6 levels in both the amniotic fluid as well as the fetal plasma in women with preterm labor and premature prolonged rupture of membranes and found interleukin-6 in fetal plasma to be significantly higher in the fetus who went on to develop severe neonatal morbidity, which also included PVL. In another study by Yoon's group interleukin-6 concentrations greater than 400 pg/mL in umbilical cord plasma were associated with a sixfold increase in white matter disease (Yoon et al 1996). Goepfert et al (2004) studied umbilical cord plasma IL-6 levels and neonatal outcomes in 309 infants born between 24 weeks and 32 weeks gestation. IL-6 levels beyond the 90th percentile (> or = 516.6 pg/mL) were significantly associated with periventricular leukomalacia (PVL; odds ratio [OR] 15, 95% CI 2–149) and necrotizing enterocolitis (NEC; OR 6, 95% CI 1.1–33). In the multivariate analysis, an IL-6 level 107.7 pg/mL or greater (determined by receiver operating curve analysis) remained a significant independent risk factor for PVL (OR 30.3, 95% CI 4.5–203.6). Hansen-Pupp et al (2005) analyzed pro-inflammatory [tumor necrosis factor-alpha (TNF-α), interferon-gamma (IFN-γ), IL-1β, IL-2, IL-6, IL-8, IL-12] and modulatory (IL-4, IL-10) cytokines from cord blood, and at 6, 24 and 72 hours postnatal age. Levels of IFN-γ at 6, 24, and 72 hours were increased in infants developing white matter brain damage (WMD) compared with those without WMD. The same group found increased levels of cord IL-1ra levels to be associated with neonatal morbidity and adverse outcome in preterm infants, with a better prediction for female infants (Elsman et al 2006). Ellison et al (2005) compared CSF and plasma cytokine levels and were unable to find a significant correlation between paired CSF and plasma concentrations for any cytokine. They were able to study 146 preterm infants and found that preterm infants with MRI-defined cerebral white matter injury had higher levels of IL-6, IL-10, and TNF-α in the CSF than infants without such injury. Harding et al (2004) looked at a functional polymorphism in the IL-6 gene promoter: a C > G change at position -174, as it was shown that in vitro IL-6 production in lipopolysaccharide-stimulated neonatal monocytes is higher among those of CC genotype than among G-allele carriers. Compared with children with CG + GG genotype, children who were homozygous for the C allele had higher frequency of severe neonatal hemorrhagic lesions (large IVH or hemorrhagic parenchymal injury) and images consistent with WMD. CC genotype increased the risk of the development of severe hemorrhagic lesions (odds ratio [OR]: 3.5; 95% confidence interval [CI]: 1.0–12.2; $P = 0.038$) and WMD (OR: 4.1; 95% CI: 1.4–12.2; $P = 0.008$).

CLASSIFICATION

Unfortunately there is no agreement on classification of lesions of the brain parenchyma. Following the introduction of the term 'periventricular leukomalacia' by Banker and Larroche in 1962, many groups of pathologists have used this term, but others have identified more widespread white matter damage, consisting of hypertrophic astrocytes, amphophilic globules, necrotic foci, and acutely damaged glia which were widespread in the cerebral white matter. This condition has been referred to as 'leukoencephalopathy' (Gilles & Murphy 1969). Kuban et al (1999) prefer to describe echodensities and echolucencies as one condition, even in cases with a classic unilateral parenchymal hemorrhage. Paneth (1999) proposed the term 'white matter damage'.

The majority of papers based on cranial ultrasound still use the term periventricular leukomalacia (PVL) and we have also used it in this context. We have been using a grading system for PVL (Table 21.1) that is now quite commonly employed by other groups (de Vries et al 1992). More recent papers using MRI use the term 'periventricular white matter damage' or 'punctate white matter lesions' and we have used these terms in this context as well.

Table 21.1 Classification of periventricular and subcortical leukomalacia based on cranial ultrasound findings (de Vries et al 1992)

• Grade I	Periventricular echodense area, present for 7 days or more
• Grade II	Periventricular echodense areas evolving into localized frontoparietal cysts
• Grade III	Periventricular echodense areas evolving into multiple cysts in the parieto-occipital white matter
• Grade IV	Echodense areas in the deep white matter, with evolution into multiple subcortical cysts

INCIDENCE

The first reports of PVL described the ultrasound findings in a small number of cases only. However, several population studies have been performed, reporting an incidence of between 2.3 and 17.8% (Levene et al 1983, Perlman et al 1996, Sinha et al 1985, Spinillo et al 1998, Stevenson et al 1998, Trounce et al 1986b, Weindling et al 1985a, Zupan et al 1996). The lowest incidence of less than 1% was recently reported by Hamrick et al (2004) who also found a significant decrease in the incidence over a 15 year period. The incidence will vary with the type of patient admitted to the intensive care unit (Larroche et al 1986), the type of transducer used (5 or 7.5 MHz), the number of ultrasound examinations performed, the number of weeks during which the examinations were done and the definition used to describe PVL. Those authors who find a low incidence have restricted the term 'PVL' to apply to infants who developed extensive cystic lesions, while those giving a higher incidence have also included localized cystic lesions restricted to the centrum semiovale (Fawer et al 1985b). Trounce et al (1986b) reported a 9.5% incidence of cystic PVL. If prolonged flares were included in the PVL category, the incidence increased to 26%. The incidence of flares (echodensities seen in two planes and lasting more than 2 weeks) was found to be 12.5%. Extensive cystic lesions, both in the trigone and in the centrum semiovale, were noted in only 2.7% of all the infants. Stevenson et al (1998) studied a very large inborn cohort with a birth weight <1500 g. PVL was noted in 6% of the 2771 infants who had ultrasound examinations after 2 weeks, but no distinction for cystic PVL was made. We feel that this distinction is of significance, in relation to later outcome (see below).

TIMING

The onset of PVL usually occurs in the perinatal period, but any severe deterioration in the condition of the infant, such as occurs with necrotizing enterocolitis or septicemia, up until 40 weeks of postmenstrual age, can still lead to this condition (Andre et al 2001, de Vries et al 1986, Perlman et al 1996, Rushton et al 1985, Zupan et al 1996). Repeated ultrasound examinations beyond the first 2 weeks of life are therefore of importance (Townsend et al 1999). This is in contrast to germinal matrix hemorrhage—intraventricular hemorrhage (GMH-IVH), which is known to occur rarely beyond the first week of life (Fawer et al 1984, Partridge et al 1983). PVL may also be due to insults occurring in utero (Baetmann et al 1996, Barth 1984, Bejar et al 1988, 1990, Larroche 1986, Szymonowicz et al 1986), and this is discussed in more detail in Chapter 18. A study by Hayakawa et al (1999) used EEG recordings within 72 hours of life to determine the time of onset in 26 infants with cystic PVL. Acute stage abnormalities were present in 14 of these infants, suggestive of a perinatal onset. The EEG was initially normal in 7 infants who were considered to have a postnatal onset, and chronic stage abnormalities were recognized in the remaining 5, suggestive of antenatal onset PVL.

ETIOLOGY

A relatively small number of studies have been carried out to identify risk factors for leukomalacia. Early on, the risk factors identified for PVL in these studies were based on small numbers of cases and were not as uniform as those previously identified for germinal matrix hemorrhage–intraventricular hemorrhage (GMH–IVH), but this has changed over the last few years. In some studies, infants with extensive cystic leukomalacia were compared with controls or infants with GMH–IVH while in others infants with prolonged flares also formed part of the PVL study group. Infants with associated GMH–IVH were included in some studies and excluded in others, which complicated interpretation and comparison of the results.

Prenatal factors

In contrast to GMH–IVH, prenatal risk factors have been identified by several groups.

Multiple gestation

Bejar et al (1988) identified a condition referred to as antenatal white matter necrosis in 13 out of 127 (10.3%) preterm infants with a gestational age below 36 weeks. This was defined as cystic lesions present at birth or developing during the first 3 days of life. Placental vascular anastomoses in multiple pregnancies, funisitis and purulent amniotic fluid were identified as independent risk factors. A second study from the same group (Bejar et al 1990) identified antenatal white matter necrosis in 14 out of 101 (13.8%) infants who were members of twin or triplet sets. Using logistic regression analysis, antenatal white matter necrosis was predicted by the presence of artery-to-artery or vein-to-vein anastomoses and by intrauterine fetal death of a co-twin. The incidence of antenatal white matter necrosis in infants of multiple gestation was reported to be 13.8%, and this was not significantly higher than the same condition occurring in singletons. Monochorionic infants, however, had an incidence of antenatal white matter necrosis of 30% which was significantly higher ($P < 0.005$) than the 3.3% incidence reported in singletons or dichorionic infants. Burguet et al (1999) also found monochorionic twin placentation to be an important risk factor for cerebral palsy. The relation between death of a co-twin and severe neurologic sequelae has been reported previously (Rydhstrom & Ingemarsson 1993, Szymonowicz et al 1986) (see Ch. 18). Multifetal pregnancy reduction was also shown to be an additional risk factor for PVL (Geva et al 1998).

Tocolysis

Baerts et al (1990) reported the possible adverse role of indometacin, used during pregnancy as a tocolytic agent. Using multivariate analysis they identified indometacin as an independent and significant risk factor for cystic PVL ($P = 0.001$).

In a recent meta-analyis by Amin et al (2007) antenatal indometacin was associated with an increased risk of periventricular leukomalacia (odds ratio (OR), 2.0; 95% confidence interval (CI), 1.3–3.1), but not associated with intraventricular hemorrhage, patent ductus arteriosus, respiratory distress syndrome, bronchopulmonary dysplasia, and mortality. Spinillo et al (1998) found that the long-term use of ritodrine increased the risk for transient echodense lesions.

Fetal heart rate patterns

Okamura et al (1997) examined fetal heart rate tracings for base line heart rate, variability and decelerations. They also described a specific pattern, 'the flip flop' pattern, which is an oscillatory tracing pattern with increased baseline variability and tachycardia with superimposed deceleration. This 'flip flop pattern' was significantly more common in the fetuses that went on to develop cystic PVL.

Infection (see p. 386)

More than a decade ago, several groups noted an association between bacterial contamination or infection and antenatal white matter necrosis (Bejar et al 1988, Leviton & Gilles 1984, Sims et al 1985). Bejar et al (1988) identified funisitis and purulent amniotic fluid as independent risk factors for antenatal white matter necrosis. Leviton and Gilles (1984) showed that 85% of infants who died with white matter lesions had a gram-negative bacteremia. Sims et al (1985) found that brain lesions of prenatal onset were associated with amnionitis and acute intrauterine infection.

Several studies have looked at obstetric antecedents of PVL. Perlman et al (1996) studied 632 preterm infants, each weighing 1750 g or less and identified preterm rupture of membranes and chorioamnionitis to be significant predictors of cystic PVL, using univariate analysis. Zupan et al (1996) showed that 19% of the infants who had abnormal white cell count/C-reactive protein, or positive bacterial cultures, or whose mothers had signs of infection, developed PVL compared with 6% of those without these signs. Verma et al (1997) studied 745 preterm infants with birth weights below 1750 g. They made a distinction between cases with preterm rupture of membranes, refractory preterm labor with intact membranes, and delivery initiated by the physician for maternal or fetal indications. They noted that the incidence and severity of both IVH as well as PVL significantly increased in both preterm rupture of membranes and preterm labor. Alexander et al (1998) looked at an even larger group of preterm infants with birth weights of 1500 g or less and found that 7% of them had been exposed to chorioamnionitis. Using multiple regression analysis and adjusting for preterm rupture of membranes, a significant association was found with the development of cystic PVL (OR 3.4; 95% CI 1.6–7.3).

In several studies identifying risk factors for cerebral palsy, chorioamnionitis and prolonged rupture of membranes were found to be major predictors of cerebral palsy (Burguet et al 1999, Grether et al 1996, Murphy et al 1996, Nelson & Ellenberg 1985, O'Shea et al 1998a, 1998b), but this was not confirmed in some more recent studies (Grether et al 2003, Kaukola et al 2006, Nelson et al 2003). In a recent retrospective study maternal antibiotics administered prior to delivery were associated with a decreased risk of cystic PVL, while there was no effect on mortality, or severe IVH (Paul et al 2003).

Antepartum hemorrhage

Three groups identified antepartum hemorrhage as a risk factor for PVL (Calvert et al 1986, Sinha et al 1985, Weindling et al 1985a). Other groups were unable to confirm this (Trounce et al 1988, Tzogalis et al 1988). Gibbs and Weindling (1994) reported placental abruption to be associated with a fourfold increased incidence of PVL and large hemorrhages; 10 out of 29 cases developed cystic PVL compared with 10% of their matched controls.

In utero methamphetamine exposure was recently associated with development of c-PVL in a preterm infant born at 30 weeks gestation, 3 days following methamphetamine exposure (Murphy et al 2007).

Intrapartum factors

Place of birth

Being outborn was identified as an independent risk factor for PVL by de Vries et al (1988b) but not others (Trounce et al 1988, Tzogalis et al 1988). As those infants who are transported to a neonatal intensive care unit are highly selected, care should be taken to interpret data collected in a tertiary intensive care unit. Grether et al (1996) found that being born in a level I facility was significantly associated with the development of cerebral palsy.

Mode of delivery

To date, the mode of delivery has not been consistently found to be of importance in the development of PVL Ikonen et al (1988) reported that infants who developed PVL were delivered significantly more often by the vaginal route ($P < 0.003$). Emergency cesarean section was associated with an increased risk for PVL in one study by de Vries et al 1988b who found the need for an emergency cesarean section significantly higher in infants with extensive cystic PVL than those who developed a large GMH–IVH. Baud et al (1998a) showed a significant reduction in PVL when the infant was delivered by cesarean section in the presence of chorioamnionitis (OR 0.15; 95% CI 0.04–0.57). Hansen and Leviton (1999) found vaginal delivery to be associated with white matter disease, but only on univariate analysis; the strength of this relationship was markedly reduced on multivariate analysis when inflammation was taken into account. This suggests that vaginal delivery is only a marker for antecedent inflammation and/or infection. In a recent study Deulofeut et al (2005), who studied a cohort of 397 infants, found that in infants weighing less than less 1251 g and who survived, vaginal delivery had a strong association with PVL (5% versus 1%; OR 11.53, 95% CI 1.66–125).

Condition at birth

Both cord blood gases as well as Apgar scores have been reported by some groups to predict the risk of developing PVL (Calvert et al 1986, de Vries et al 1988b, Sinha et al 1985, Tzogalis et al 1988, Weindling et al 1985a) but not in other careful studies (Ikonen et al 1988, 1992, Perlman et al 1996, Trounce et al 1988).

Gestational age

Immaturity has been shown to be inversely related to the frequency and degree of GMH–IVH (Trounce et al 1988). This is not a consistent finding for PVL, and it appears that the infant's brain may remain susceptible to PVL for a longer period of gestation. In some studies (Calvert et al 1986, Ikonen et al 1988) infants with PVL were matched with controls that had a similar gestational age, making it impossible to identify gestational age as a risk factor. It should also be taken into account that the gestational age at birth may not bear much relationship to the age at which a baby develops PVL following an acute clinical deterioration many weeks after birth (de Vries et al 1986, Perlman et al 1996, Zupan et al 1996). No relationship between the gestational age and PVL was found by several groups (de Vries et al 1988b, Ikonen et al 1992, Trounce et al 1988, Weindling et al 1985a). Tzogalis et al (1988) did find, however, that infants who developed PVL were significantly less mature than their normal controls (29.8 vs. 31.9 weeks). In a study by Ikonen et al (1988), 12 infants with extensive cystic PVL were all noted to have a gestational age of 31 or 32 weeks. de Vries et al (1988b) noted that infants with extensive cystic PVL were significantly more mature than infants who developed large hemorrhages (30.1 vs. 28.3 weeks) (Fig. 21.5), a finding supported by Perlman et al (1996) (gestational age 29.4 weeks for PVL compared with 26.6 weeks for large GMH–IVH, $P < 0.01$). In the study by Stevenson et al (1998), PVL

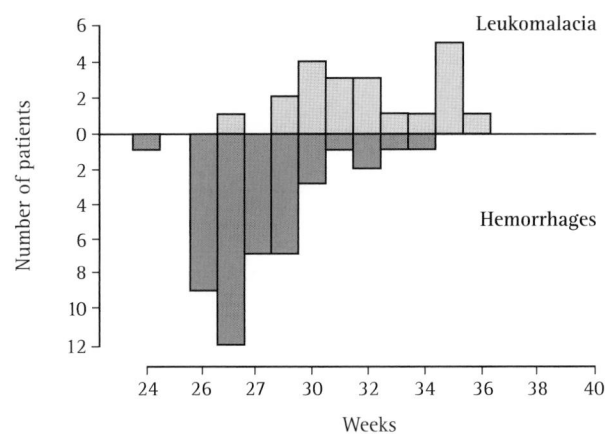

Figure 21.5 Age in postmenstrual weeks at the onset of hemorrhagic and ischemic lesions.

varied between 6 and 7% for those infants weighing 500–1500 g. Bejar et al (1988) found antenatal white matter necrosis to be inversely related to the birth weight, and was more frequent in infants weighing more than 1000 g (19%). Dyet et al (2006) also did not find relationship with GA for MRI confirmed DEHSI.

Lung disease and its complications

While respiratory distress syndrome is the most consistently recognized risk factor predisposing to GMH–IVH in preterm infants, this is not the case for PVL. Mechanical ventilation has, however, been identified by most groups to have a significant association with PVL (de Vries et al 1988b, Sinha et al 1985, Trounce et al 1988, Weindling et al 1985a). Sinha et al (1990) compared babies with early onset PVL to infants with late-onset PVL (days 4–70), and noted that hyaline membrane disease was associated with the latter group, while a history of intrauterine growth restriction and recurrent apnea was more common in the early onset group. Complications associated with mechanical ventilation, such as pneumothorax, hypocarbia and hypercapnia, have all been identified as risk factors for PVL, and these are discussed below.

Hypocarbia

A recent review of 15 reports of the development of cystic PVL or cerebral palsy arising in babies who had been subjected to inadvertent hypocarbia highlighted the strong circumstantial link between hypocarbia and brain damage (Levene 2007). In the study by Okumura et al (2001) the time-averaged carbon dioxide (CO_2) index, was larger, the time-averaged CO_2 lower and the time-averaged pH higher in infants with PVL than in those with normal development on the third day of life. Shankaran et al (2006) studied 21 preterm infants with cPVL and found that a cumulative exposure to hypocarbia and not hyperoxia was independently related to risk of cPVL. In addition infants found to be hypocarbic on day 1 showed increased cerebral fractional oxygen extraction, higher serum lactate and a slower EEG signal than a group of normocapnic babies (Victor et al 2005).

It appears that those infants with only mild respiratory distress are especially at risk of experiencing periods of hyperventilation. With the introduction of high frequency oscillation, there has been concern about an increase in the number of cases with cystic PVL. Wiswell et al (1996a) have pointed out that high frequency jet ventilation may produce substantial hypocapnia: 18 out of 52 surviving infants developed cystic PVL. Logistic regression analysis revealed that infants with cystic PVL were significantly more likely to have greater cumulative hypocarbia below a threshold of 3.3 kPa (25 mmHg) during the first day of life. In another study, Wiswell et al (1996b) randomized 73 preterm infants to receive high frequency jet ventilation or conventional ventilation and found that those being treated with high frequency jet ventilation were significantly more likely to

develop cystic PVL ($P = 0.022$), but a meta-analysis was unable to relate an increased risk of cystic-PVL with high frequency ventilation (Cools & Offringa 1999). Vannucci et al (1995, 1997) studied the effect of hyper- and hypocarbia in an immature hypoxia–ischemia rat model and noted an adverse effect of hypocarbia as well as a protective effect of mild hypercarbia. The increased successful use of nasal CPAP, sometimes with intubation only for the administration of surfactant, may further reduce the incidence in cPVL, but so far there are no randomized studies to support this.

The data as it stands is suggestive that hypocarbia in premature infants, particularly in the first few days of life, may cause critical under-perfusion of white matter resulting in white matter damage. Hypocarbia in ventilated babies should be avoided.

Pneumothorax

Several studies have identified pneumothorax as a risk factor for PVL (de Vries et al 1988b, Sinha et al 1985, Trounce et al 1988).

Cardiovascular factors

As PVL is considered by some to be related to hypoperfusion of the boundary zones between ventriculofugal and ventriculopetal arteries, hypotension was expected to be an important risk factor of the occurrence of PVL, but this could not be confirmed in some of the earlier studies (Trounce et al 1988, Watkins et al 1989, Weindling et al 1985a). Iida et al (1992) did find hypotension to be significantly related to the development of PVL in a small group of infants. It should be stressed that other factors identified as risk factors, such as septicemia, surgery and apneic spells, may all be associated with fluctuations in blood pressure. Lou et al (1979) performed radioactive xenon studies in sick preterm infants and showed a marked reduction in CBF coinciding with hypotension. Using NIRS Tsuji et al (2000) found that concordant changes (coherence scores >5) in HbD and MAP, consistent with impaired cerebrovascular autoregulation, were observed in 17 of the 32 infants (53%). Eight of the 17 infants (47%) developed severe GMH–IVH or PVL or both, suggesting that impaired cerebrovascular autoregulation is relatively common and that the presence of this impairment is associated with a high likelihood of occurrence of severe GMH–IVH/PVL.

Patent ductus arteriosus

An association between a patent ductus arteriosus and PVL has been reported in two studies (de Vries et al 1988b, Sinha et al 1985). Infants with a patent ductus arteriosus may have reduced CBF as measured by Doppler ultrasound. Following administration of indometacin, a further reduction in CBF velocity has been shown in Doppler studies (Cowan 1986, Evans et al 1987), but no data have been published showing an association between postnatal treatment with indometacin and the development of PVL.

Hyperbilirubinemia

In some of the early studies hyperbilirubinemia was identified as an independent variable for PVL (Ikonen et al 1988, Trounce et al 1988). Ikonen et al (1992) performed a second study, looking prospectively at a cohort of 103 infants with gestational age below 33 weeks. They once again were able to identify the mean levels of total serum bilirubin as a significant independent risk factor. The hyperbilirubinemia usually coincided with prolonged hypocarbia (<4 kPa), identified as the second independent risk factor. Their hypothesis was that the toxic effects of a high bilirubin concentration may be especially deleterious to brain tissue that has already been underperfused due to prolonged hypocarbia. This finding would fit in with data from van de Bor et al (1989), who showed that there is an increasing prevalence of cerebral palsy in preterm infants with increasing total serum bilirubin levels. In a study by Graziani et al (1992), however, there was no evidence to suggest that hyperbilirubinemia was causally related to cerebral palsy or periventricular cysts.

Hypothyroxinemia

Leviton et al (1999) studied 1414 preterm infants with birth weights of 1500 g or less, and were able to show that the preterm infants with a thyroxine level below 67.8 nmol/L had twice the risk of 'echolucencies' as their peers with higher thyroxine levels. The multicenter antenatal TRH study noted a trend toward more motor impairment in the TRH treated group (Crowther et al 1997). Antenatal treatment, however, combined TRH with corticosteroids.

Postnatal dexamethasone treatment

There is concern about the (early) use of dexamethasone and its effect on neurodevelopmental outcome. Yeh et al (1998) randomized 133 infants within the first 12 hours after birth and treatment was continued for 4 weeks. They showed a significant increase in neuromotor dysfunction at 2 years of age (25/63 vs. 12/70). O'Shea et al (1999) showed that more infants treated with dexamethasone developed cerebral palsy (25% vs. 9%) at 1 year of age. Papile et al (1998) showed poor head growth following dexamethasone treatment. Shinwell et al (2000) performed a randomized multicenter study in which dexamethasone or a placebo was given within 12 hours of age and continued for 3 days. Long term follow-up on 159 infants showed a significantly higher incidence of cerebral palsy (49 compared to 15%; OR 4.62; 95% CI 2.38–8.98) in those treated with dexamethasone. Infants treated with dexamethasone had more cystic PVL but this did not reach statistical significance (22% compared with 13%). It is of interest that 22% of their cerebral palsy cases did not have any ultrasound abnormalities. Shinwell and colleagues propose the possibility of a direct neurotoxic effect of dexamethasone in the neonatal period. As the study involved 18 centers, it cannot also be excluded that the standard of neonatal ultrasonography was not of the same level in all centers and that some of the infants with cystic

PVL were missed. Halliday et al (2006a, 2006b, 2006c) published 3 meta-analyses to assess the effect of steroids used postnatally to treat chronic lung disease and report the risk of brain injury. They found postnatal corticosteroids to be neurotoxic when given in high dose or when administered in the first 96 hours of life. The mechanism for the neurotoxic effect is not known and variations in the design of various studies together with the differing dosage regimens and the high proportion of babies treated with off label steroid in the control group makes interpretation of these studies difficult, but caution is urged in the use of high-dose steroids for chronic lung disease, particularly in the first week of life.

Pyruvate carboxylase deficiency

Brun et al (1999) have suggested that this metabolic disorder can present on ultrasound scan with appearance similar to cystic PVL. They however confused subependymal pseudocysts with 'frontal cystic-PVL.'

UNIFYING HYPOTHESIS

Although PVL/PWMI can still be considered an ischemic lesion, the vulnerability of the white matter to other factors also appears to play an important role. First, the increased vulnerability of the immature oligodendrocyte to glutamate was shown by Back et al (1998) using cultured oligodendroglia. Second, the proinflammatory cytokines play a role, probably even before delivery. An association of raised interleukins 1 and 6 and TNF-α which has been studied in the amniotic fluid as well as in the cord blood, and white matter disease is now well established, with data coming from both animal experiments as well as from human clinical studies. Cytotoxic cytokines can, however, also be released during ischemia. After delivery, complications related to mechanical ventilation can occur and we are now well aware that vasoconstriction due to hypocarbia is a rather common risk factor. Care should be taken to avoid this, especially when using high frequency ventilation.

PREVENTION

The first results about possible prevention of PVL are now being published, but their clinical utility is still very limited.

Antenatal drug intervention

Nelson and Grether (1995) showed a reduction in cerebral palsy cases after in utero exposure to magnesium sulfate. Another retrospective study (FineSmith et al 1997) even showed a significant reduction in the incidence of cystic PVL among 492 infants each weighing less than 1750 g. Canterino et al (1999), however, were unable to show a protective effect of this drug on the development of severe ultrasound abnormalities in 918 infants with birth weights below 1750 g. The large randomized trial also did not show a protective effect (Crowther et al 2003). There are no convincing data available at present to suggest that magnesium sulfate prevents antenatal PVL.

Antenatal steroids lead to a significant reduction in the incidence of PVL in appropriate for gestational age preterm infants delivered following preterm labor with or without ruptured membranes, but not in those with fetal growth restriction (Elimian et al 1999). Baud et al (1999b) showed a reduced risk of cystic PVL with antenatal administration of betamethasone, but not with dexamethasone (4.4% vs. 11%, compared with 8.4% when no corticosteroids were given at all). Betamethasone and dexamethasone differ by only one methyl group, but betamethasone has a longer half life. It has been suggested that sulfating agents present in dexamethasone may be neurotoxic. The study was, however, retrospective and uncontrolled.

Russell and Cooke (1995) randomly allocated 400 infants with gestational ages between 24 and 32 weeks to receive either allopurinol or a placebo for the first 7 days of life. They were unable to show a protective effect for the development of cystic PVL, bronchopulmonary dysplasia, or retinopathy of prematurity. Hypoxanthine levels at birth were, however, significantly higher in infants who went on to develop cystic PVL. These data are in agreement with recent findings by Perlman and Risset (1998) who found significantly higher uric acid concentrations on day 1 in those who went on to develop severe intraventricular hemorrhages or cystic PVL.

DIAGNOSIS AND EVOLUTION OF PVL

With the use of newer imaging techniques it is now well recognized that many infants with PVL survive. Performing sequential ultrasound studies, valuable information about the timing, the evolution of the ultrasound changes, and the possible risk factors have been reported in the mid-1980s (Chow et al 1985, Dolfin et al 1984).

Ultrasound

Correlation with autopsy findings has varied a lot in the literature, with mostly a low sensitivity when infants died in the echogenic stage (Baarsma et al 1987, Carson et al 1990, Hope et al 988, Paneth et al 1990, Szymonowicz et al 1984). The data of Hope et al (1988) were especially disappointing, with a sensitivity of only 28% and a specificity of 86%. The sensitivity was very good once cystic lesions had developed during life (de Vries et al 1988, Fawer et al 1985a, Trounce et al 1986). The frequency of the ultrasound transducers (5 vs. 7.5 MHz), the interval between serial ultrasound examinations, and the time that elapsed between the last scan and the postmortem studies should all be taken into account when interpreting these data. Instead of comparing ultrasound data with autopsy findings, several recent studies have now compared ultrasound findings with neonatal MRI findings and also found a low sensitivity (40–50%) (Debillon et al 2003, Inder et al 2003, Maalouf et al 2001, Miller et al 2003).

Timing the onset of the lesion can be deduced from the evolution of the ultrasound changes. Areas of increased echogenicity are usually seen within 24–48 hours following an acute clinical episode (Fig. 21.6a). This increase in echogenicity was initially thought to be due to hemorrhages occurring in the ischemic areas, following restoration of the circulation. Several authors have shown that non-hemorrhagic infarction is also able to give this echogenic appearance (Delaporte et al 1985, Martin et al 1983, Trounce et al 1986a). This can be confirmed at autopsy or by the use of MRI.

It is assumed that severe congestion may cause this increase in echogenicity. The densities can resolve but usually persist until the dense areas break down into cystic lesions 2–4 weeks later. The cysts appear in clusters in the area of previous echogenicity. They vary in diameter between a few millimeters to over a centimeter and do not usually communicate with the ventricles (Fig. 21.6B). When PVL occurs together with a large intraventricular hemorrhage (IVH) and posthemorrhagic ventricular dilatation, communication of the cystic lesions with the ventricular system does occur and is referred to as pseudoventricle formation (Grant et al 1986). The cysts remain for several weeks, but tend to become smaller and are usually not visible on ultrasound examination once the infant is 2–3 months old (Fig. 21.6c, Fig. 21.7). When the cysts become less apparent, exvacuo dilatation of the lateral ventricles can be noted (Bozynski et al 1985). The outline of the cysts may disappear completely and histologic examination will show gliosis, delayed myelination and mild ventricular dilatation (Rodriguez et al 1990, Trounce et al 1986a). Most reports concerning cystic PVL have described the development of cysts in the periventricular white matter. Tsuru et al (1995) described the evolution of cysts in the cerebellar folia in three premature infants, and Coley and Hogan (1997) reported one preterm infant who developed cysts in the corpus callosum.

While extensive cystic lesions have now become rare in modern neonatal intensive care units, smaller cysts can be seen to develop (Fig. 21.8). These cysts can be unilateral and few in number and can only be visualized with a high resolution (7.5 MHz) transducer. Pierrat et al (2001) found that in more than 50% of the infants with localized cystic lesions, these cysts were first diagnosed beyond day 28. de Vries et al (2004) found a similar number of infants developing cysts beyond the end of the first month, i.e. 53% for those with localized cystic lesions, compared to 38% among those with extensive cystic lesions. Both studies stress the importance of repeated ultrasound studies beyond the first month of age.

In a study by Boxma et al (2005) increased echogenicity was noted in the para-atrial area in 84% of their normal infants, situated bilaterally between the inner end of the lateral fissure and the upper third of the choroid plexus. The localization of the hyperechoic band suggested that it represents part of the optic radiation. This band of increased

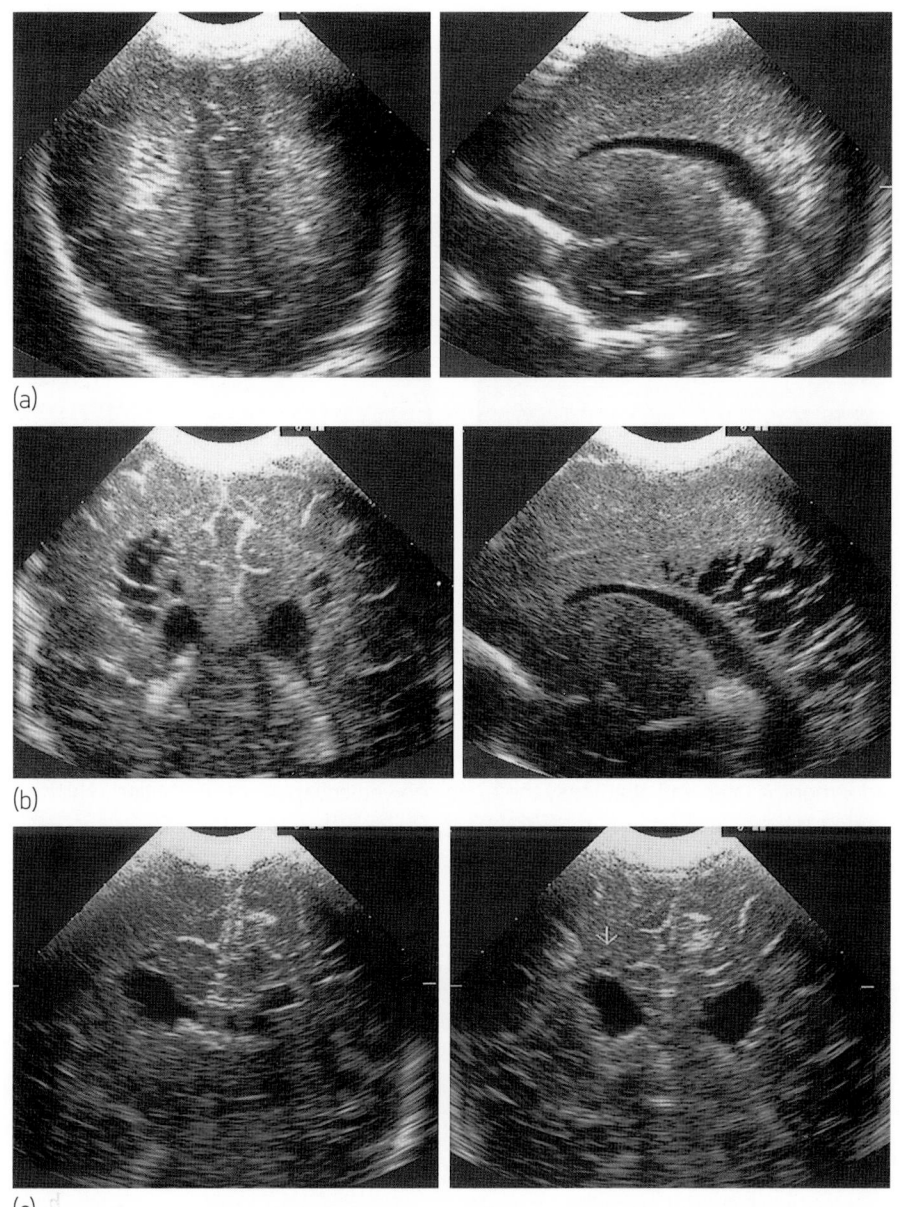

(a)

(b)

(c)

Figure 21.6 Cranial ultrasound performed on day 10 in a preterm infant (gestational age 28 weeks; birth weight 800 g) showing increased echogenicity, more marked on the right than on the left on the coronal view (a, left) and the right parasagittal view (a, right). Same views in the same child, shown 6 weeks later (b), showing extensive cystic evolution. The cysts are separate from the lateral ventricles and are more extensive than would have been expected on the basis of the preceding echogenicity. At 6 months of age mild ex-vacuo dilatation is shown as well as only one remaining cyst (arrow) (c).

echogenicity was not present in nine infants diagnosed with PVL and could therefore be an early marker of PWMI.

While it is relatively uncommon for a child to develop cystic lesions, many infants develop increased echogenicity at the external angle of the lateral ventricle without, or with less, apparent echogenicity around the occipital horns (Di Pietro et al 1986, Guzzetta et al 1986, McMenamin et al 1984). Trounce et al (1986b) defined the periventricular echodensities as prolonged 'flares' if they persisted for at least 14 days (Fig. 21.9). Such flares subsequently resolve, but mild ventricular dilatation can be observed in some of these infants when they are scanned again between 6 and 9 months of age, and this can be asymmetrical where the periventricular echodensities were asymmetrical to start with. Subsequent widening of the interhemispheric fissure has also been recorded in a few infants with flares in the

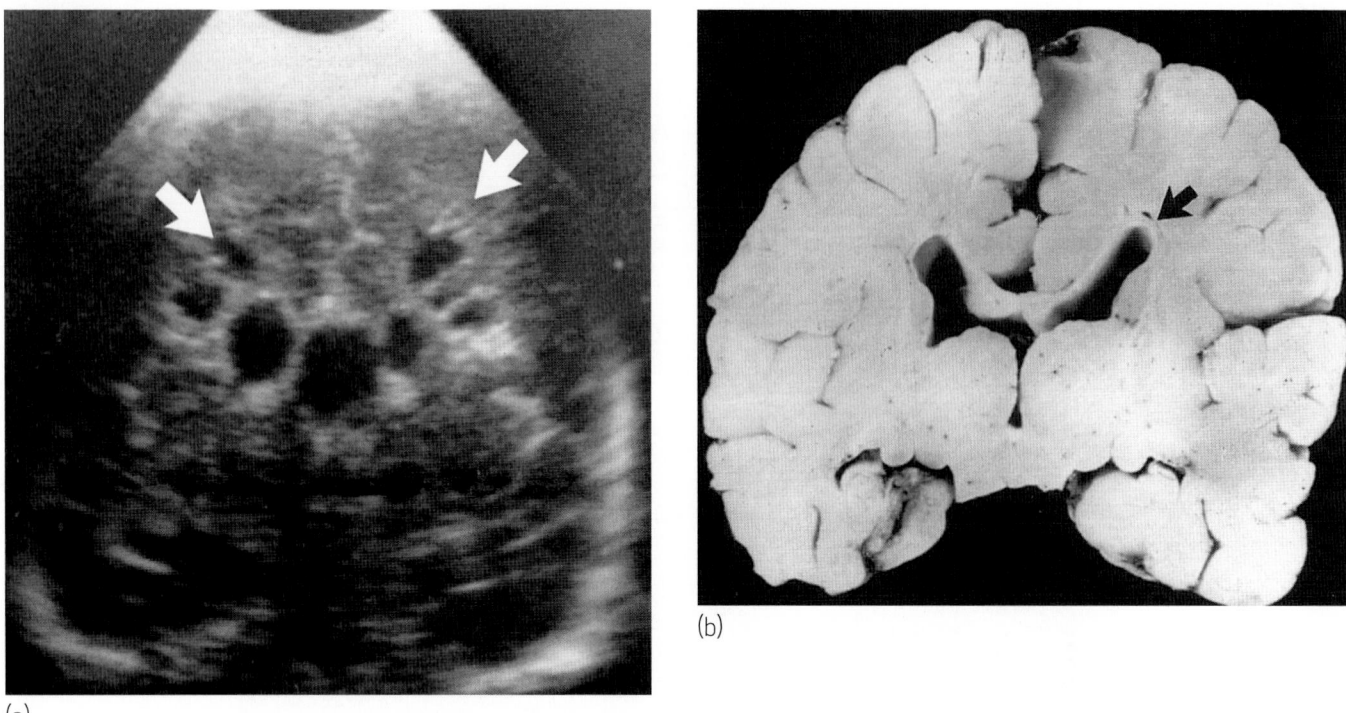

(a)

(b)

Figure 21.7 Evolution of cystic PVL lesions. (a) Coronal ultrasound scan showing multiple echo-free cavities (arrows) in the white matter. (b) The infant died 3 months later, and at autopsy the brain showed collapse of the cavities, which were only just visible (arrow).

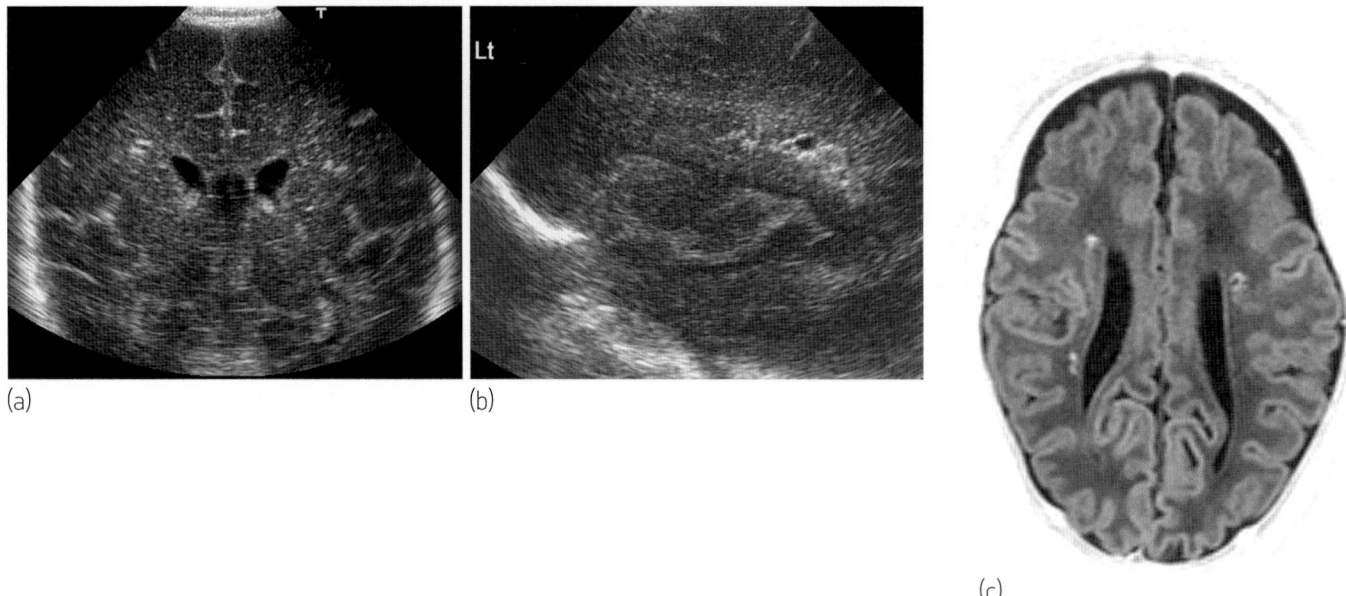

(a)   (b)

(c)

Figure 21.8 (a) Coronal and persagittal ultrasound, performed at 5 weeks of age showing bilateral localized cystic lesions. (b) MRI of the same infant at term equivalent age showing small cystic lesions surrounded by a rim of increased signal intensity, suggestive of gliosis.

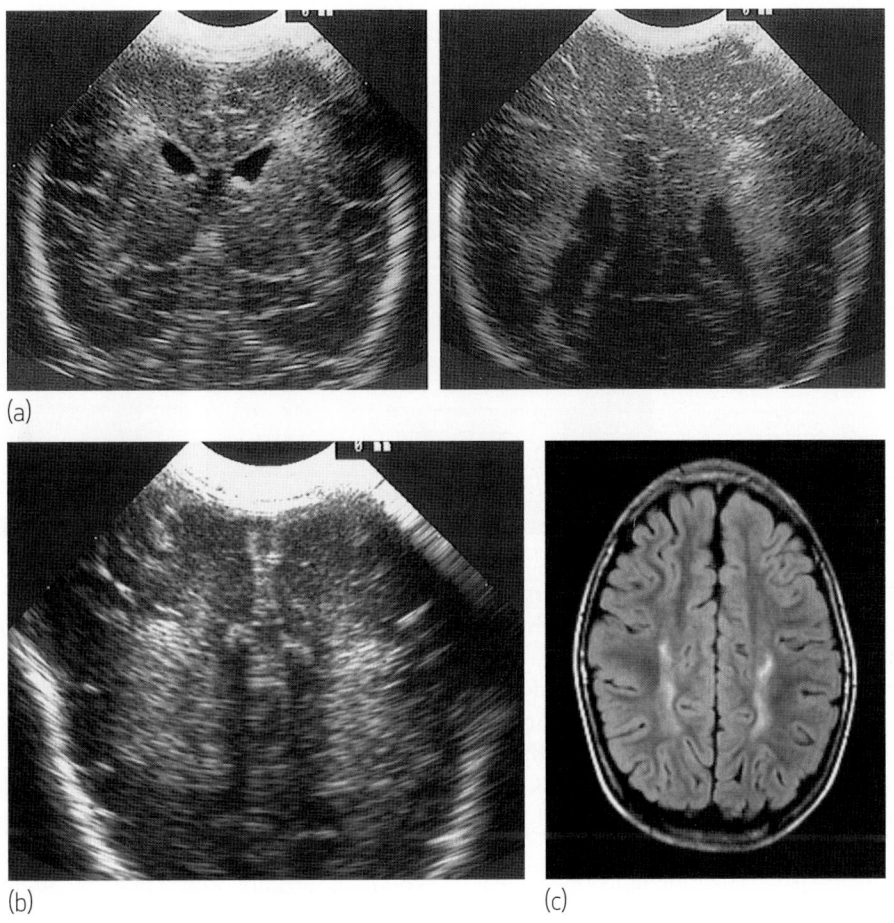

(a)

(b)

(c)

Figure 21.9 (a) Cranial ultrasound, coronal views, performed on day 14 in a preterm infant (gestational age 28 weeks; birth weight 1100 g). Increased echogenicity is noted, especially at the level of the external angle of the lateral ventricles. (b) Cranial ultrasound, coronal view angling backwards, performed on day 14 in a preterm infant (gestational age 28 weeks; birth weight 1250 g) showing increased echogenicity. (c) MRI correlate, FLAIR sequence at the age of 8 years. The child outgrew her mild diplegia.

neonatal period, possibly indicating some degree of atrophy and this was recently shown to correlate well with outcome at 3 years of age (Horsch et al 2005). In a few infants who died, gliosis has been observed at autopsy, and it is therefore likely that these flares represent a milder degree of PVL (de Vries et al 1988a, Fawer et al 1985a, McMenamin et al 1984, Trounce et al 1986a). It still needs to be seen whether these flares also correlate well with diffuse excessive high signal intensity (DEHSI) diagnosed at the term equivalent age MRI.

Magnetic resonance imaging (see also Ch. 6)
The use of MRI plays an important role in the early stage of PVL, when it is still uncertain whether cysts will evolve. It has been reported that many infants with areas of increased periventricular echogenicity on ultrasound show small petechial hemorrhages within a larger area of abnormal signal intensity but these can also be present in those infants without subsequent cystic evolution (Schouman-Claeys et al

1993, van Wezel-Meijler et al 1998). Cysts are sometimes seen at an earlier stage, with more anatomical detail and can be more numerous and extensive than seen on ultrasound (Sie et al 2000). Petechial or more extensive hemorrhages within the areas recognized as 'flares' on ultrasound were present in 50% of their 50 infants studied using early MRI. Early detection of the diffuse component of PVL can possibly be detected at a very early stage using diffusion-weighted MRI. Inder et al (1999a) reported one case showing marked restriction of water diffusion on day 5 in the absence of abnormal signal on conventional MRI and without increased echogenicity on ultrasound. The infant went on to develop extensive cystic PVL. The same group was also able to show the postmigrational development of polymicrogyria by performing MRI at 31 and at 40 weeks postmenstrual age in an infant with cystic PVL (Inder et al 1999b). In a preterm infant who underwent MRI soon after cysts were identified on cranial ultrasound, hyperintense regions on diffusion weighted imaging (DWI) adjacent to the

Figure 21.10 MRI (T2SE) at the level of the centrum semiovale of two preterm infants at term equivalent age, showing normal signal intensity of the white matter (left) and severe DEHSI (right).

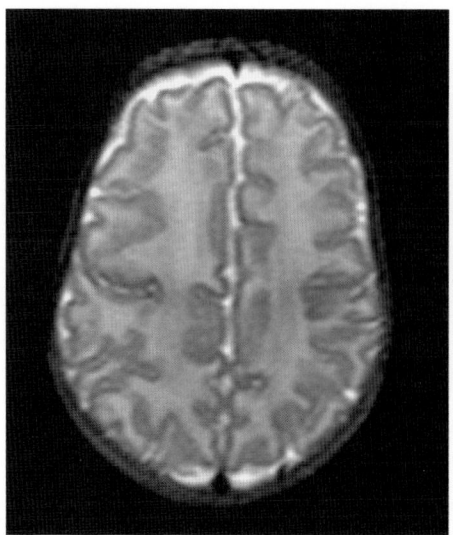
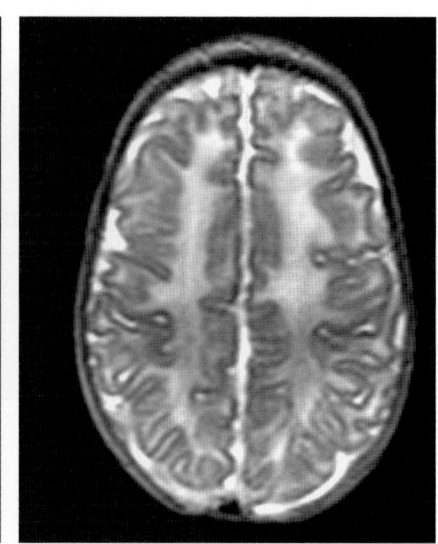

cystic lesions correlated with areas that were undergoing active degeneration with cytotoxic edema, apoptosis and macrophage infiltration (Roelants-Van Rijn et al 2001). In the infants with localized cysts, neonatal MRI tended to show more extensive changes in signal intensity throughout the periventricular white matter and MRI performed during the second year of life showed more extensive gliosis than would be expected on the basis of the few localized cysts seen in the neonatal period (de Vries et al 1993).

Recent MRI studies have also shed some light on the significance of transient echodensities seen on ultrasound. Van Wezel-Meijler et al (1998) showed a strong positive correlation between presence of echodensities on ultrasound and the degree of signal change of the periventricular white matter on MRI, suggesting that echodensities on ultrasound and signal intensity changes in the periventricular white matter on MRI are due to the same lesion. Signal changes were often still present on MRI following disappearance on ultrasound and sometimes these were more extensive than the echodensities had been. In a small number of cases signal changes were seen on MRI in the absence of (previous) echodensities on ultrasound, suggesting that MRI is more sensitive than ultrasound. Follow-up of these 42 infants until 12 months corrected age (van Wezel-Meijler et al 1999) showed that abnormalities found with both imaging techniques were associated with a high incidence of transient motor problems during infancy. It was of interest, however, that the degree of echogenicity had the highest predictive value, compared with duration of the echodensities and signal changes on MRI.

The myelinated posterior limb of the internal capsule is clearly identified as high signal intensity at term equivalent age on T1 weighted MRI. Absence of the normal high signal intensity in this region at term equivalent age in PVL is associated with motor impairment at 2 years corrected age and bilateral signal abnormalities are associated with the subsequent development of spastic diplegia or quadriplegia (Roelants-van Rijn 2001).

Conventional MRI has demonstrated non-focal white matter abnormality in the majority of preterm infants at term equivalent age (Fig 21.10). In a study of 100 infants, born between 23 and 32 weeks GA, common imaging findings in the preterm brain were enlarged ventricles, white matter atrophy, delayed cortical development and an enlarged subarachnoid space. This imaging pattern was observed in 10 out of 11 infants born less than 26 weeks GA (Inder et al, 2003). In another consecutive cohort study, ventriculomegaly and enlarged subarachnoid space were observed in 75% and 38% of infants respectively. In addition, around 75% of preterm infants appeared to have areas of DEHSI within the white matter on T2 weighted MRI, with a correspondingly low signal on T1 weighted imaging (Maalouf et al 1999). In the absence of pathologic correlation, it is unclear what the signal intensity changes in DEHSI represent, but they are not observed in term born control infants and probably represent diffuse white matter abnormality associated with preterm birth. The ultrasound correlate of DEHSI is not well defined and it is not clear whether it represents the consequence of prolonged 'flares' or white matter echogenicity without cyst formation or whether it represents different or additional pathological processes. It has been suggested that DEHSI may be the neuroimaging correlate of diffuse PVL or telencephalic leukoencephalopathy (Volpe 2003), however this has not been confirmed histologically. Indeed, DEHSI may not reflect a specific injury but rather abnormal development as a result of premature delivery into the extrauterine environment of the neonatal intensive care unit, with a cessation in normal placental growth factors and nutrients normally transferred to the fetus in the third trimester.

In a recent large cohort study, no association was found between the observation of DEHSI and gestational age at birth, birth weight, mode of delivery, chorioamnionitis or postnatal steroid exposure. However, there was a lower incidence of DEHSI among infants with IUGR (risk ratio: 0.74; 95% confidence interval: 0.5–0.94; $P = 0.018$) (Dyet et al 2006). Importantly, the observation of DEHSI at term equivalent age is correlated with significantly lower developmental quotient scores at 18–36 months corrected age (no DEHSI: 111 ± 20; DEHSI: 94 ± 11.6; severe DEHSI: 92 ± 7.5; $P = 0.027$) (Dyet et al 2006). Of course, follow-up studies at school age and older are required to determine the long term neurodevelopmental outcome of preterm infants who have DEHSI at term. The visual assessment of DEHSI on MR images is subjective, as contrast depends on the window and contrast levels chosen to view the images. Quantitative MR techniques, such as diffusion weighted MR imaging, allow white matter to be assessed objectively and have been used to study white matter in the preterm brain. In diffusion-weighted MRI, the three-dimensional brownian motion of water in tissue is the dominant contrast mechanism in the image. In a medium that has no restrictive boundaries, diffusion is equal in all directions and is called isotropic diffusion. However, in tissue with ordered microstructure, such as the cerebral white matter, water diffuses preferentially along the course of white matter tracts and diffusion across axons is hindered. Diffusion tensor imaging (DTI) provides information regarding the mean displacement of water molecules, the apparent diffusion coefficient (ADC) and the directional dependence of diffusion due to intrinsic microstructural barriers that is diffusion anisotropy.

A number of studies have investigated the white matter in the preterm brain using DWI/DTI. Huppi et al (1998) found that ADC values in the central white matter are higher and relative anisotropy (RA) values are lower in both the central white matter and posterior limb of the internal capsule in preterm infants at term compared to term-born infants. Miller et al. (2002) reported a significant increase in ADC values with increasing GA in the frontal white matter and visual association areas in infants with moderate white matter injury (Miller et al 2002). In addition, the authors observed an absence of the normal maturational increase in RA in a number of white matter regions in infants with moderate white matter injury and in the frontal region in infants with only minimal white matter injury (Miller et al 2002). Using a voxel based analysis approach, termed tract base spatial statistics (TBSS) (Smith et al 2006), reduced fraction anisotropy (FA) in the white matter in preterm infants at term compared to term born controls has been identified in the centrum semiovale, frontal white matter and genu of the corpus callosum. These regions were more extensive in preterm infants who were born ≤ 28 weeks GA and regions of abnormality in these infants included the posterior aspect of the posterior limb of the internal capsule, the external capsule and the isthmus and the middle portion of the body of the corpus callosum (Anjari et al 2007).

DEHSI has also been assessed using diffusion weighted imaging (DWI) (Counsell et al 2003) and diffusion tensor imaging (DTI) (Counsell et al 2006). Elevated ADC values have been demonstrated in the white matter at the level of the centrum semiovale in preterm infants with DEHSI at term equivalent age (Counsell et al 2003). In a more recent

study, elevated radial diffusivity was found in many white matter regions, including the splenium of the corpus callosum and the posterior aspect of the posterior limb of the internal capsule (Counsell et al 2006). Increased diffusivity suggests an increase in water content, a reduction in viscosity or increased membrane permeability. Myelination and premyelination changes result in a decrease in diffusivity radial to white matter tracts. Increased radial diffusivity has been observed in mature animal models of dysmyelination (Song et al 2003) and so, in regions that are myelinating at this age, such as the posterior portion of the posterior limb of the internal capsule and the central white matter at the level of the centrum semiovale, these findings may be indicative of delayed myelination in preterm infants with DEHSI. As diffusivity perpendicular to fibres decreases with increasing gestational age (Mukherjee et al 2002, Partridge et al 2004, Suzuki et al 2003) the diffusion characteristics observed in DEHSI may be due to delayed maturation of white matter. The elevated ADC values observed in infants with DEHSI appear to be associated with reduced volume of central grey matter. Using deformation based morphometry, Boardman et al (2006) demonstrated that regional tissue contraction was evident in the thalamus and lentiform nucleus in preterm infants at term equivalent age when compared to term controls. This diminished central gray matter volume was most marked in infants with elevated ADC values in white matter, suggesting a link between abnormalities in white matter and in central gray matter (Boardman et al 2006).

It is now possible to assess connectivity using diffusion tensor tractography. These studies have demonstrated involvement of the sensory and motor pathways, corpus callosum, posterior limb of the internal capsule and superior longitudinal fasciculus (Counsell et al 2007, Fan et al 2006, Hoon et al 2002, Staudt et al 2006, Thomas et al 2005) and disrupted thalamo-cortical connections (Counsell et al 2007) in children and adolescents with PVL and hemorrhagic parenchymal involvement (HPI). One elegant study, which combined diffusion tractography and transcranial magnetic stimulation (TMS), has shown that axons of the somatosensory projection curve around the focal lesion yet still connect to postcentral sulcus (Staudt et al 2006). However, in a single case with unilateral HPI and bilateral PVL, connections between the somatosensory cortex and thalamus were severely disrupted on the side ipsilateral to the HPI (Counsell et al 2007).

MRI studies have identified non-specific focal, punctate lesions in the cerebral white matter of the preterm brain (Childs et al 2001, Maalouf et al 2001). These lesions are high signal intensity on T1 weighted imaging and frequently, but not always, low signal on T2 weighted imaging. In the early neonatal period these punctate lesions probably represent small petechial hemorrhages, which are frequently no longer apparent at term equivalent age. Lesions that are still evident at term equivalent age, however, may be indicative of gliosis (Childs et al 2001). Punctate white matter lesions are often observed in a linear pattern; however, their distribution varies and is not restricted to the immediate periventricular white matter. In a consecutive cohort study of over 100 preterm infants who were serially imaged from soon after birth up to term equivalent age, punctate white matter lesions were observed in 22% of infants (Dyet et al 2006). Whilst in another study of infants from a cohort of 60 babies imaged at 36 weeks GA, these lesions were identified in 13% of infants (Arthur 2006). The difference in incidence reported in these two studies is probably due to the age of the infants at scanning as these lesions become less obvious with increasing post menstrual age. The correlation between the observation of these punctate white matter lesions on MRI and cranial ultrasound is poor (Childs et al 2001, Debillon et al 2003, Maalouf et al 2001). To date, no correlation between clinical variables such as gestational age, birth weight, mode of delivery, chorioamnionitis or intra-uterine growth restriction (IUGR) and the presence of punctate white matter lesions within the white matter has been identified (Dyet et al 2006).

In a recent MRI study, preterm infants with punctate white matter lesions on MRI at term equivalent age were found to have delayed myelination and diminished cortical folding compared to preterm infants with no evidence of lesions on MRI, suggesting that these lesions impact on overall brain development, perhaps through impaired synaptogenesis and aberrant connectivity (Ramenghi et al 2007). It appears that isolated punctate lesions are associated with a good prognosis at early neurodevelopmental assessment (Cornette et al 2002, Dyet et al 2006). However, in the light of these recent MRI findings (Ramenghi et al 2007), longer term studies are required to determine the consequence of these lesions on later neurodevelopment.

Magnetic resonance spectroscopy (see Ch. 11)

This has been shown to be of value in predicting the importance of these early echodensities. Hamilton et al (1986) showed that all infants with periventricular echodensity who had a PCr/Pi ratio below the normal range either died or developed extensive cystic lesions, while most of those with normal ratios did not develop extensive cystic lesions (p. 174). Groenendaal et al (1997) studied 19 infants with cystic PVL, using proton magnetic resonance spectroscopy and were able to show that this test predicted neurodevelopmental outcome (Fig. 21.11). N-acetyl aspartate:choline ratios significantly related to the grade of PVL and also showed a correlation with developmental quotients at 12 months or more.

Neurophysiology

Other techniques have recently become available to aid early prediction as to the significance of these areas of increased echogenicity. Connell et al (1987) used continuous 24-hour, four-channel EEG recordings and noted marked abnormalities (seizures, low amplitude) in those infants who had densities that subsequently evolved into extensive cystic lesions, while the EEG findings of those with transient periventricu-

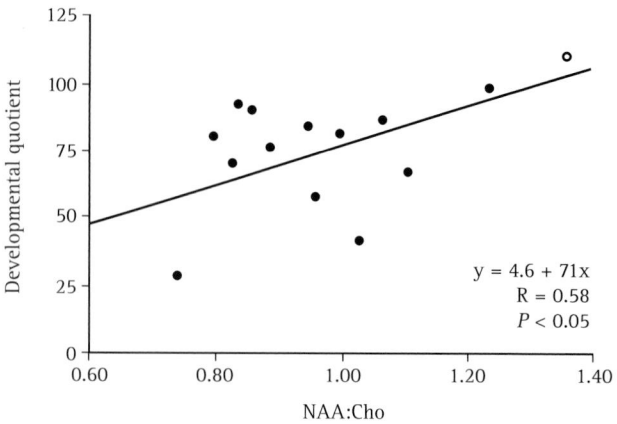

Figure 21.11 Correlation between developmental quotients and NAA:Cho ratio in 15 preterm infants with cystic PVL, studied using proton magnetic resonance spectroscopy at 40 weeks postmenstrual age. C, normal; c handicap. (Reproduced with permission from Dev Med Child Neurol 39:1997, Groenendaal et al Fig. 3.)

lar densities and subsequently normal development were normal (Ch. 12). The importance of positive rolandic sharp waves has been recognized by several groups (Baud et al 1998b, Marret et al 1986, 1992, 1997, Okumura et al 1999b). A retrospective study by Baud et al (1998b) showed the presence of positive rolandic sharp waves to be very specific markers of PVL. The sensitivity was, however, only 32.4% for the less mature infants (<28 weeks gestation) compared to 87.8% for those with a gestational age between 28 and 32 weeks, with a specificity of 100% and 99.8% respectively. Kubota et al (2001) used the EEG to more precisely define the onset of PVL.

The value of evoked responses is discussed in detail in Chapter 12. Abnormalities of both visual as well as somatosensory evoked potentials are still of limited value in the infants with PVL (de Vries et al 1987, Ekert et al 1997, Pierrat et al 1993). Visual evoked responses and somatosensory evoked potentials performed at 40 weeks of postmenstrual age were, however, absent in infants having subcortical lesions, and EEG recordings were severely abnormal in the acute stages. Abnormalities were still present at 40 weeks in infants with subcortical leukomalacia, while abnormalities seen in the infants with PVL were only present in the acute phase, with complete recovery at 40 weeks of postmenstrual age in most infants. Kato et al (2005) found visual evoked potentials (VEPs) to be 'absent', in 13 of their 14 infants (93%). 'Delayed latency' was seen in two infants and 'abnormal waveform' was seen in one infant. It was of interest that the flash VEPs changed from normal to abnormal within 10 days after birth in most cases. The study was restricted to data obtained within the first 3 weeks and it was not reported whether recovery was seen at term equivalent age.

OUTCOME

In the 1980s there were many follow-up studies of infants who had developed GMH–IVH in the neonatal period (Catto-Smith et al 1985, Thorburn et al 1981). These studies suggested that the size of the hemorrhages and the presence of ventricular dilatation were of prognostic significance (Palmer et al 1982, Stewart et al 1983). Ultrasound examinations were often still performed with linear array equipment utilizing a 5 or 3.5 MHz transducer. It is therefore likely that cases of PVL were missed, or that densities seen in the acute phase were interpreted as parenchymal hemorrhages. Stewart et al (1983) stressed the predictive value of cerebral atrophy, diagnosed when irregular ventricular dilatation was noted in association with normal or delayed head growth. They assumed this to be due to ischemia and cerebral infarction. de Vries et al (1985a) were the first to compare the neurodevelopmental outcome of infants with a large IVH (with or without intraparenchymal involvement) with infants who developed extensive cystic PVL. At early follow-up (9–24 months) they noted that 43% of the infants with large hemorrhages were functioning at a normal level, compared with none of those with extensive cystic lesions. Only 3 of the 23 infants with large hemorrhages, who also showed associated ischemic lesions on their ultrasound scans, were severely handicapped with quadriplegia and severe mental retardation. The presence of ischemic lesions was thus of more predictive value than the size of the hemorrhage.

Transient periventricular echodensities (PVE)

The outcome of infants with transient periventricular echodensities has so far been reported in several studies (Appleton et al 1990, Chen et al 2004, de Vries et al 1988c, Fazzi et al 1994, Levene et al 1992, McMenamin et al 1984, Resch et al 2006, Ringelberg & van de Bor 1993). Dammann and Leviton (1997b) reviewed the studies that mentioned transient densities and proposed to make a distinction between brief flares (1–6 days), intermediate flares (7–13 days) and prolonged flares (14 or more days). Most studies would suggest that the duration of the PVE is important and a duration of more than 10–14 days is more likely to be associated with a worse neurodevelopmental outcome.

de Vries et al (1988b) studied 59 infants with transient periventricular echodensities. The neurodevelopmental outcome of 53 of these infants was compared with 92 infants with normal ultrasound scans. Four of the 53 infants with periventricular echodensities developed spastic diplegia and 24 developed transient dystonia, whereas only 8 of the 92 infants with normal ultrasound scans demonstrated this finding ($P < 0.001$) (Fig. 21.12). The persistence of the echodensities was important, as it was noted that densities remaining for more than 10 days were most likely to be associated with subsequent problems. The site of the densities was also important, as both infants with densities in the trigone were noted to develop cerebral palsy. When re-examining 44 of these infants at the age of 6 years and comparing them to 62 infants with normal ultrasound scans,

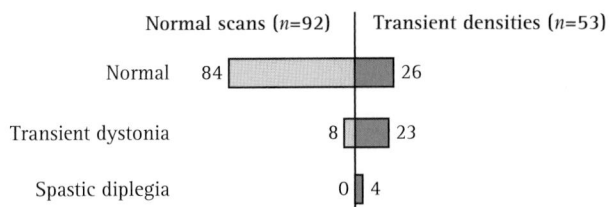

Figure 21.12 Neurodevelopmental outcome of infants without ultrasound abnormalities and infants with transient periventricular echodensities.

no differences in cognitive abilities were found between the groups, but the results of standardized motor assessment showed that performance decreased significantly with increasing duration of periventricular densities (Jongmans et al 1993). Fawer et al (1987) studied 24 infants with PVL, 5 of whom had densities present for more than 2 weeks without subsequent evolution into cystic lesions. Three of these infants with frontal densities were found to be normal at follow-up while the other two infants who were noted to have densities in the frontoparietal or frontoparieto-occipital white matter developed spastic diplegia. In a subsequent study by Fawer and Calame (1991), children were assessed at 5 years of age. Children with small focal PVL (tiny cysts or persistent echodensities) had lower cognitive abilities on the McCarthy scale and were noted to have more abnormal neuromotor signs and more attention deficits when compared with children giving normal scans or having isolated hemorrhage.

Similar data were collected by Appleton et al (1990), who looked at the neurodevelopmental outcome of 15 infants who had periventricular echodensities in the absence of associated IVH. At follow-up, 4 infants had neurologic abnormalities (spastic diplegia in 2 infants with densities persisting for 21 and 35 days, respectively). On the other hand, Pidcock et al (1990), using a 5 or 7.5 MHz transducer, were unable to confirm this. In another follow-up study of VLBW infants at 5 years, the presence of transient periventricular echodensities (referred to as prolonged flare) on the neonatal scans predicted motor impairment (clumsiness), but only when GMH–IVH occurred in the same baby (Levene et al 1992). In the group of infants studied by Ringelberg and van de Bor (1993) only 10 infants with flares persisting beyond the first week of life were included and 1 of these (10%) developed cerebral palsy. Fazzi et al (1994) studied 12 infants with 'prolonged flares,' which they defined as present for more than 14 days. Of these, 6 developed cerebral palsy, 4 had mild neurologic signs, and only 2 were normal. It is possible that the long duration of the flares explains the high incidence of cerebral palsy in this study. The importance of the duration was recently supported by Resch et al (2006) who noted a significant increase in adverse neurodevelopmental outcome with increasing duration of PVE. Of 33 infants with duration of PVE < 7 days, 1 (3%) had an adverse neurodevelopmental outcome, compared to 6 (24%) of 25 infants with a duration of PVE of 7–14 days, and 6

(43%) of 14 infants with a duration of PVE > 14 days ($P < 0.002$, RR 7.920, 95% CI 1.017–61.661; $P < 0.001$, RR 14.143, 95% CI 1.871–106.895, respectively). Similar observations were made by Pisani et al (2006) who studied 164 preterm infants who were divided into three groups with normal ultrasound findings, transient periventricular echodensities (less than 14 days) and preterm infants with persistent echodensities. Developmental outcome was assessed at up until 12 months corrected age using the Griffiths Mental Developmental Scale. The infants with persistent PVE only showed a favorable outcome in 22.2% which was significantly different from the other two groups ($P < 0.001$). The exact duration of flares will, however, not always be known as this requires sequential scans after the first week of life.

de Vries et al (1993) reported MRI data of 15 infants with PVL, diagnosed using cranial ultrasound in the neonatal period, who all developed cerebral palsy, 6 of whom had extensive cystic PVL and none was able to walk. Four infants had localized small cysts in the frontoparietal periventricular white matter and one of them was walking independently. Five had transient periventricular echodensities and three learned to walk at 20 and 26 months, respectively. All infants with extensive cystic PVL on neonatal ultrasound had an irregular ventricular enlargement, a decrease in peritrigonal white matter and extensive gliosis as shown by MRI. In the other two groups, gliosis was present in all, but tended to be less extensive, especially in those with transient periventricular echodensities only. Ventricular enlargement was present in only one of the five infants with transient echodensities on ultrasound. When comparing the MRI data with the initial ultrasound data, there was, in general, good agreement between neonatal ultrasound data and later changes on MRI, but in some cases extensive MRI abnormalities were seen in spite of apparently localized abnormalities on cranial ultrasound. Van Wezel-Meijer et al (1999) performed both neonatal MRI scans and repeats at 12 months corrected age in a group of infants with transient densities on ultrasound. Transient tone abnormalities during the first year were common, but none developed cerebral palsy. On the repeat MRI scan at 1 year corrected age, gliosis was noted in 10 infants. The lack of cerebral palsy cases can probably be explained by the fact that infants with severe and inhomogeneous echodensities were not eligible for this study.

Bos et al (1998) combined ultrasound data with general movement studies and noted the latter to be of better predictive value, especially when these abnormal general movements persisted for longer.

All these studies would imply that transient periventricular echodensity or non-cavitating parenchymal density is less predictive, but they should not be disregarded as they probably represent mild PVL.

Extensive cystic leukomalacia

At present follow-up studies dealing with PVL can be divided into four main categories described below:

- Reports of infants with the ultrasound diagnosis of (cystic) PVL with the inherent variation in the definition of the condition.
- Populations of preterm infants in which attempts are made to identify specific ultrasound abnormalities with outcome. In these studies there are often uncertainties about both the quality of the imaging as well as the number of scans performed.
- Populations of preterm infants who had MRI at term equivalent age and where attempts have been made to correlate different degrees of white matter abnormalities with outcome.
- Selection of ex-preterm infants with established spastic diplegia in whom the diagnosis of PVL is made by MRI in childhood (Fig. 21.13).

Category 1

The number of infants in this category are usually small (Bowerman et al 1984, Bozynski et al 1985, Calvert et al 1986, Rogers et al 1994, Weindling et al 1985b). Most infants developed cerebral palsy, with or without associated seizures, visual impairment and a variable degree of mental retardation. Rogers et al (1994) performed measurements of the periventricular region where the cysts were seen and found the antero-posterior extent on parasagittal view, a measurement that helped to predict the type and severity of motor and cognitive disabilities. Bilateral cystic PVL with a width of greater than 2 cm was always associated with the development of quadriplegia.

In four other studies, infants with PVL were studied and follow-up data reported. Monset-Couchard et al (1988) studied 30 infants with a spectrum of cystic PVL. While 8 out of 11 infants with minor cystic lesions were normal at follow-up, all infants with severe cystic lesions had neurologic sequelae. Cases including posterior lesions or presenting solely with such lesions had a worse outcome. Fazzi et al (1994) described neurodevelopmental outcome at 5–7 years in 37 infants with PVL. All infants with large cysts (>5 mm) developed cerebral palsy, compared with 2 out of 11 with small cysts. A further 7 had mild neurologic signs. Prognosis was related to site and number of cysts. They also noted that the cognitive profiles were disharmonic, with a better verbal than performance IQ.

The study of Fujimoto et al (1994) is one of the few not to find either the size or the site of the cysts as predicting the development of cerebral palsy. They studied 24 infants (25–37 weeks gestation) with cystic-PVL, 14 with symmetrical parieto-occipital cysts and 10 with asymmetrical cysts. Those with symmetrical cysts all developed cerebral palsy compared with 60% of those with asymmetrical cysts.

Bennett et al (1990) were unable to confirm the predictive value of cystic lesions. Only 4 out of 15 (26.7%) infants with cystic PVL developed cerebral palsy compared with 4 out of 9 infants (44.4%) with severe intracranial hemorrhage. Their data may be criticized, as infants having localized cystic lesions were grouped together with infants having extensive

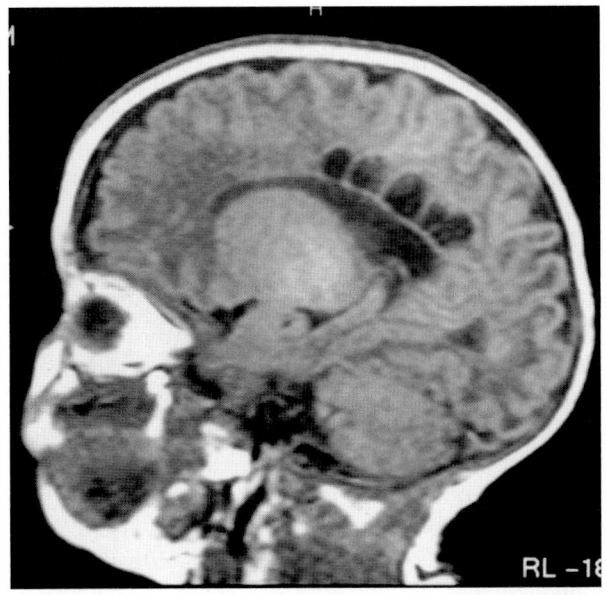

(a)

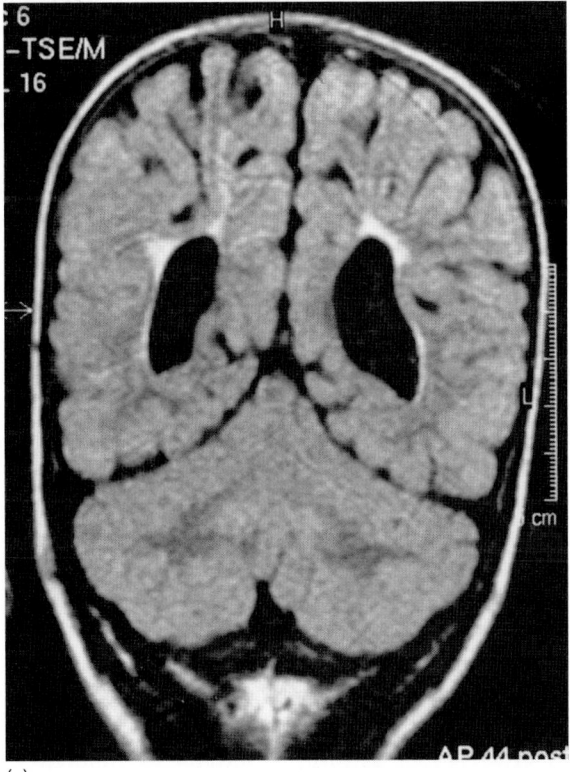

(c)

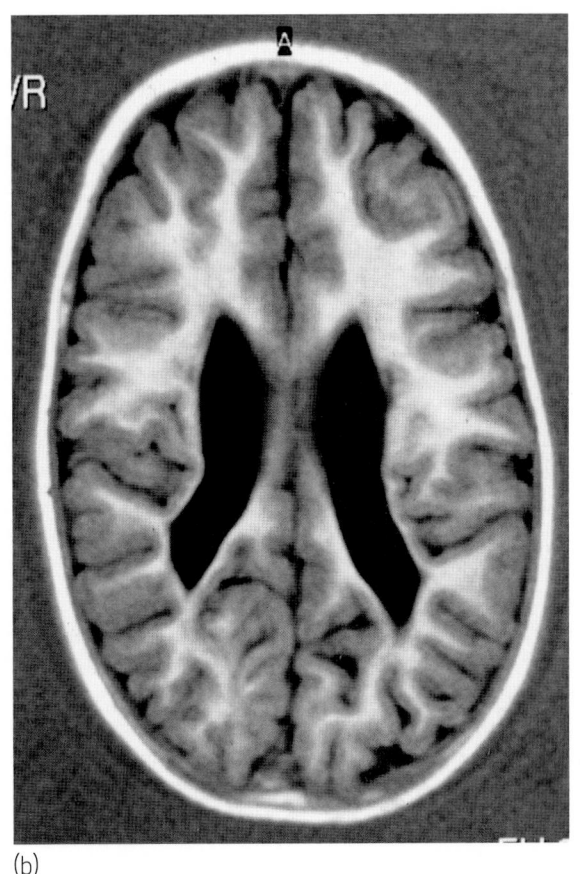

(b)

Figure 21.13 MR scan at 40 weeks postmenstrual age of a child who developed extensive cystic PVL following necrotizing enterocolitis. (a) A T1-weighted sequence shows multiple cysts separate from the lateral ventricle on this parasagittal view. A repeat MR scan was done at 20 months. (b) The inversion recovery scan at mid-ventricular level shows delay in myelination, particularly around the irregularly dilated occipital horns. (c) The FLAIR sequence shows moderate irregular ventricular dilatation and high signal intensity suggestive of gliosis.

cysts. Ricci et al (2006a) used the Hammersmith Infant Neurological Examination at 6–9 months in 24 infants with cystic PVL. Neck and trunk extensor tone, and a posture of flexed arms and extended legs between 6 and 9 months were always associated with the inability to sit unsupported at 2 years, whilst truncal hypotonia and extended arms and legs were associated with unsupported sitting but not walking. Optimality scores between 41 and 60 were generally associated with sitting but not walking at 2 years while scores below 40 were always associated with the inability to sit independently at 2 years. All infants who did not develop cerebral palsy at 2 years had scores >60.

Category 2

These are largely population based studies (Aziz et al 1995, Bennett et al 1990, Fazzi et al 1992, Graham et al 1987, Graziani et al 1987, Pidcock et al 1990, Zorzi et al 1988). Graham et al (1987) described the correlation between ultrasound findings and neurodevelopmental outcome at 18 months in 156 survivors of a cohort of infants each weighing 1500 g or less. All infants with PVH alone or GMH–IVH confined to the lateral ventricle were normal at follow-up. The presence of cysts accurately predicted abnormal outcome (94%) and was highly specific (96%). Of the 12 infants with cerebral palsy, 10 had ultrasound evidence of PVL. No infants with cysts confined to the frontal region or the centrum semiovale developed cerebral palsy, while cysts in the occipital region were always associated with a poor outcome.

Zorzi et al (1988) studied 154 preterm infants of 32 weeks or less. Of these, 24 (15.5%) had intraparenchymal cystic lesions related to intraparenchymal hemorrhage in 8 cases and to PVL in a further 16 cases. The 8 infants with one large cyst developed cerebral palsy and a severe deficit was present in 4 of them. All infants with extensive cystic PVL developed cerebral palsy, while 1 out of 4 with localized cystic PVL and 3 out of 4 with unilateral localized cystic PVL were normal at follow-up. The site of the cystic lesions was taken into account and cysts were present in the occipital region in the majority of the infants studied.

Pidcock et al (1990) studied 127 infants of 32 weeks or less who had some degree of periventricular echodensity, classified as mild, moderate or severe. The evolution of cysts was also taken into account and cysts were divided into three groups, depending on their size. Of the 127 infants, 26 developed cerebral palsy and all had cystic lesions. In 8 infants, moderate to severe periventricular echodensity with cysts of less than 2 mm were present, and in the other 18, cysts were over 3 mm in size. It is of interest that 19 out of 36 infants with cystic lesions did not develop cerebral palsy and in 5 of these 19 infants cystic lesions were large. These authors explained that the absence of cerebral palsy in these infants was related to the site of the cysts, being either anterior or posterior to the caudothalamic notch, suggesting sparing of the corticospinal tracts. The absence of cerebral palsy in the presence of diffuse cysts had been previously noted by the same group in three infants (Graziani et al 1987).

Pinto-Martin et al (1995) published 2-year follow-up data of 777 infants each weighing 501–2000 g. They found brain lesions diagnosed by ultrasound to be powerful predictors of cerebral palsy, especially the disabling form. Parenchymal echolucencies and ventricular enlargement were the most powerful predictors in a multivariate logistic regression analysis (OR 15.4, 95% CI 7.6–31.1) but the presence of a GMH–IVH also carried a risk (OR 3.5, 95% CI 1.7–6.9). This study can however be criticized, as only 47% of their cases had an ultrasound examination beyond the first week of life and no information is given about the type of transducer used.

Category 3
A few important recent studies have reported a large cohort of preterm infants, who had both neonatal ultrasound

imaging as well as MRI at term equivalent age. It was first of all noted that cystic PVL has nowadays become a rare disorder with only 4 out of 100 infants showing cystic PVL (Inder et al 2003). In a recent study by the same group (Woodward et al 2006) 167 preterm infants had an MRI at term equivalent age and moderate-to-severe cerebral white-matter abnormalities, present in 21% of the infants, were predictive of the following adverse outcomes at two years of age: cognitive delay (odds ratio, 3.6; 95% confidence interval, 1.5 to 8.7), motor delay (odds ratio, 10.3; 95% confidence interval, 3.5 to 30.8), cerebral palsy (odds ratio, 9.6; 95% confidence interval, 3.2 to 28.3), and neurosensory impairment (odds ratio, 4.2; 95% confidence interval, 1.6 to 11.3). Even after adjustment for major ultrasound lesions including cystic PVL, moderate-to-severe white-matter abnormalities on MRI still predicted severe motor delay and cerebral palsy. In another cohort study by Dyet et al (2006), 119 (80%) infants were studied with both ultrasound and term equivalent age MRI and 80% was noted to have diffuse excessive high signal intensity within the white matter on T2-weighted scans. Adverse outcomes were associated with major destructive lesions, which were only seen in two surviving infants, diffuse excessive high signal intensity within the white matter, cerebellar hemorrhage and ventricular dilation after intraventricular hemorrhage but not with punctate white matter lesions, hemorrhage or ventricular dilation without intraventricular hemorrhage.

Category 4
An increasing number of recent follow-up studies have selected babies on the basis of their history (preterm birth) and the type of cerebral palsy (spastic diplegia). A relation between abnormalities and sensorimotor outcome has been established, often with special attention to visuo-perceptual impairment. Koeda and Takeshita (1992) reported that the volume of the peritrigonal white matter of the parietal and occipital lobes was significantly correlated with visuo-perceptual impairment in diplegic children following preterm delivery. Goto et al (1994) found thinning of the parietal and/or occipital white matter in diplegic children with visuo-spatial cognitive deficit. Ito et al (1996) measured the ratio of the areas of the posterior horns to the anterior horns and found a negative correlation with visuo-perceptual ability. Fedrizzi et al (1996) performed MRI in 30 children with spastic diplegia, when they were 6–14 years old. They studied the relation between the pattern of cognitive impairment and their MRI features. They noted a significant difference between verbal and performance IQ, indicating a specific failure in the visuo-spatial function, as indeed they had shown previously at 3 years of age (Fedrizzi 1993). The severity of abnormalities on MRI (ventricular dilatation, white matter reduction or involvement and thinning of the posterior part of the corpus callosum) correlated with the full scale and performance IQ but not with the verbal IQ. Several other studies (Cioni et al 1997a) also found a strong correlation between the degree of MRI abnormalities and

sensorimotor outcome. Melhem et al (2000) showed a significant association between lateral ventricular volumes and the degree of motor and cognitive impairment. Only Yokochi et al (1991) reported that neither the degree of ventricular dilatation nor the amount of white matter loss correlated with the degree of mental impairment.

The works of Marin-Padilla (1997) and Inder et al (1999a) have helped to foster a better understanding of the cognitive problems that arise following damage to the white matter, by showing that destruction of axonic fibers can cause input deprivation and output isolation on the overlying gray matter, thus affecting its subsequent development. The gray matter 'survives' but is deprived of incoming inputs (corticopetal fibers) and is unable to establish connections with distant cortical regions (cortico-fugal fiber destruction). This can result in ex vacuo dilatation due to antero- and retrograde degeneration of damaged axis cylinders, causing a generalized reduction of white matter fibers. Inder et al (1999b) used a quantitative three-dimensional volumetric MRI technique and were able to show a reduction in cortical gray matter volume at term.

Performing MRI later in infancy has led to two interesting observations. Iai et al (1994) measured several ratios of the corpus callosum in 43 infants with spastic diplegia and found a significant correlation between the ratio of the thickness of the splenium to the length of the corpus callosum and the level of motor impairment. Yokochi (1997) performed MRI in 44 preterm infants with spastic cerebral palsy. All had changes on MRI compatible with PVL. In 22 of these infants, abnormalities were seen in the pulvinar (posterior part of the thalamus) and the posterior part of the internal capsule in addition to the abnormalities in the periventricular white matter. The gestational age at delivery of these infants had been significantly greater compared with those not having thalamic involvement. Mental retardation and paroxysmal ocular downward deviation were also more common in these infants.

Ventriculomegaly

Ventriculomegaly or ventricular enlargement should be mentioned as a separate entity. This finding can be seen in the absence of excessive head growth and has therefore also been referred to as ex vacuo dilatation, related to a decrease in white matter. This phenomenon appears to be especially common in the less mature premature infants without any preceding GMH–IVH or transient echodensities. Leviton and Gilles (1996) reviewed this condition and hypothesized that this is a well recognized form of 'neonatal white matter disease'. Diffuse astrocytosis is recognized at post-mortem, poor head growth and delayed myelination on MRI are seen in survivors. They relate these findings to oligodendrocyte demise and dysfunction.

Several follow-up studies have found that ventriculomegaly is associated with a poor outcome. Whitaker et al (1996) noted a poorer cognitive function at 6 years of age in those with ventriculomegaly and parenchymal involvement. Ventriculomegaly was recently identified as the most important predictor for a IQ of less than 70 (OR 19; 95% CI 4.5–80.6) by Ment et al (1999). They did not find an association with PVL, but this condition had a very low incidence in their population. Kuban et al (1999) found a clear association of white matter disorders with intraventricular hemorrhage (IVH) and ventriculomegaly. Infants with both were at 18–29-fold greater risk of white matter damage. In this study no distinction was made between an echolucency following a unilateral parenchymal hemorrhage or bilateral echodensities characteristic of early stage PWMI.

Cerebral visual impairment (see also Ch. 37)

Several groups have paid special attention to associated visual impairment (Calvert et al 1986, Cioni et al 1996, 1997b, de Vries et al 1985b, 1987, Eken et al 1994, 1996, Fedrizzi et al 1996, Gibson et al 1990, Jacobsen et al 1996, Scher et al 1989). In a prospective longitudinal study of 51 preterm infants, Eken et al (1994) have again noted the risk of associated visual impairment in infants with cystic leukomalacia. No ultrasound abnormalities were present in 18 infants: 17 had a variety of GMH–IVH and 16 had PVL (non-cystic in 5). From 40 weeks of postmenstrual age until 18 months of age, visual acuity and visual evoked potentials were performed at regular intervals. None of the infants without ultrasound abnormalities or with GMH–IVH had impaired visual acuity beyond 3 months of corrected age. Impaired visual acuity was noted only in infants with extensive cystic PVL. Of the 11 infants with cystic lesions, acuity estimates were unrecordable or more than one octave below the tenth centile in 4 children and on the tenth centile in 3. The visual problems were especially severe in the more mature preterm infants (35–37 weeks of gestation) with cysts extending into the deep white matter. The authors stress the importance of early visual testing, as this enables us to identify infants with visual impairment at an early age. When these children were tested again at 5½ years of age, none of the 7 with cerebral visual impairment at 18 months had improved. Good correlations were found both for visual acuity as well as cognition for the whole group (van den Hout et al 1998).

Cioni et al (1997b) investigated visual outcome in 96 preterm infants who had a normal ultrasound scan (18 cases), prolonged transient echodensities (34 infants) or severe cystic-PVL (44 infants). MRI was available in 12 of the cystic-PVL cases, 6 of the moderate PVL group and none of the controls. They found a high incidence of cerebral visual impairment, consisting mainly of low visual acuity, severe oculomotor disorders and reduced visual field in the infants with cystic PVL. These findings were less common in the moderate PVL group. Abnormalities of the optic radiation on MRI correlated with visual outcome (specificity 82%, sensitivity 69%). MRI abnormalities in the visual cortex were highly specific (100%) but had a very low sensitivity (15%). A very similar study was performed in 38 preterm infants by Lanzi et al (1998). Cerebral visual impairment was present in 66% of these infants and once again there was a good correlation between the degree of visual impairment and abnormalities on MRI, consisting mainly of an abnormal MR signal in the optic radiation and atrophy of the calcarine cortex in the most severe cases. In 6 of the 9 blind patients optic atrophy was also noted. In an earlier study they also noted abnormalities in the lateral geniculate body in 2 of their blind cases (Uggetti et al 1996). Ricci et al (2006b) studied 12 infants with cystic PVL and found that six of the 12 infants who also had obvious associated signs of atrophy of the thalami had severe and wide-ranging abnormalities of visual function in all testing domains.

Subcortical leukomalacia

Leech et al first reported in 1974 that white matter lesions can extend into the deep white matter. Involvement of the subcortical white matter appears to be more common in neonates with a gestational age above 34 weeks. This is supported by post-mortem angiography studies by Takashima et al (1978) who showed a triangular, watershed area at the depth of the sulci in the full-term infant (Fig. 21.14). The development of extensive cystic lesions in the subcortical white matter is not at all common (Fig. 21.15) and in its most extensive form may be described as multicystic leuko-encephalomalacia (MCLE), which is discussed on page 551. The appearance of these cystic lesions was first shown in living infants using pneumoencephalography by Taboada et al (1980), who found rounded dilated lateral and third ventricles in nine microcephalic infants. In an attempt to explain the apparent conservation of the thickness of the cerebral parenchyma they performed pneumoencephalographic studies, needling the anterior fontanelle. Using this method they were able to show separate subcortical cysts.

CT scans of these infants merely showed areas of decreased attenuation and dilatation of the ventricles.

Ultrasonography can show the evolution of subcortical leukomalacia non-invasively, as was first described by Pfister-Goedeke and Boltshauser (1982). The evolution of the ultrasound changes is as follows. The cysts occur within 2–3 weeks after the insult and tend to be larger in diameter than in the infants with PVL (see Fig. 21.16). The cysts are noted to persist far beyond 40 weeks of postmenstrual age and can be recognized by ultrasonography as long as the fontanelle permits this form of examination to be performed. de Vries et al (1985b, 1987) and Eken et al (1994) especially noted associated visual problems in infants with extensive cystic PVL and especially in those with cysts extending into the subcortical white matter. So far, no distinction has been made between infants with lesions restricted to the periventricular white matter and infants with subcortical lesions, but as most of the studies were looking at infants with a gestational age of 32 weeks or less, the majority of the studies mentioned above would have included infants mainly with lesions in the periventricular white matter. Lutschg et al (1983) reported on 8 full-term and 2 preterm infants who suffered birth asphyxia and subsequently developed subcortical leukomalacia as diagnosed by CT. All infants were hypo- or hypertonic at 3 months of age, with microcephaly in 7 and infantile spasms in 9. Trounce and Levene (1985) and de Vries et al (1987) noted a marked difference between the outcome in infants with periventricular lesions and those with subcortical lesions. de Vries et al (1987) noted that while eight survivors with cystic PVL all developed diplegia and a squint, quadriplegia was found in the seven survivors with cysts extending into the deep white matter. Associated

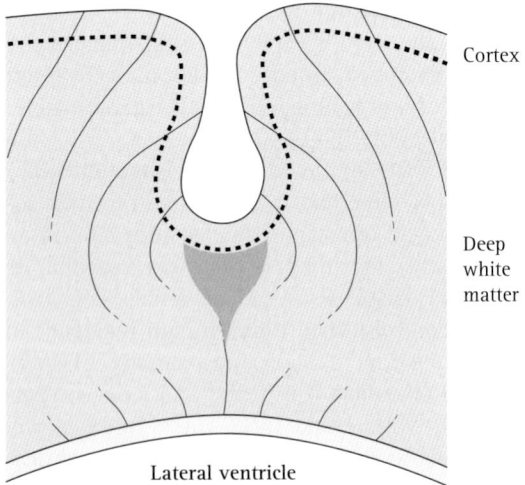

Figure 21.14 A coronal section through cortex, white matter and lateral ventricle. There is a watershed area of subcortical white matter (stippled) exposed to ischemic injury. (Redrawn from Takashima et al 1978 © American Medical Society.)

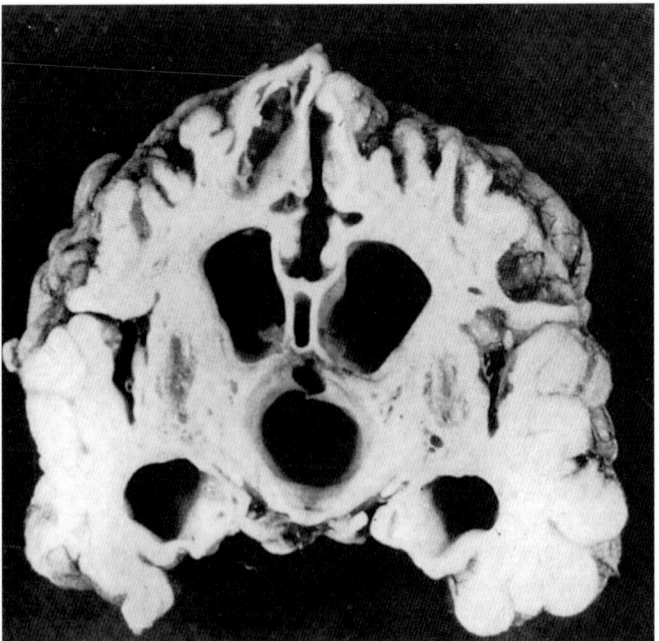

Figure 21.15 Cystic subcortical leukomalacia. There is an irregular cavity in the subcortical region on the left side.

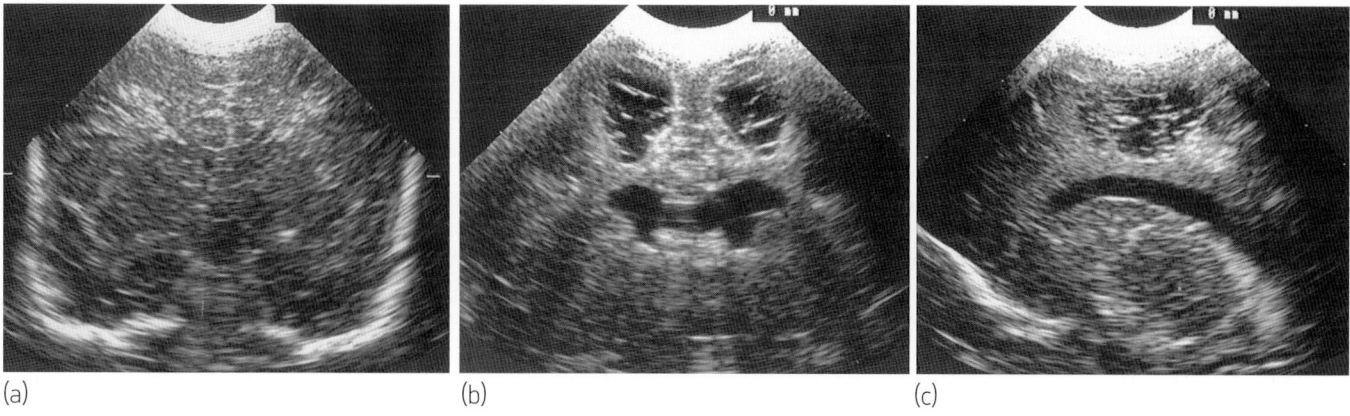

(a)　　　　　　　　　　　(b)　　　　　　　　　　　(c)

Figure 21.16 Evolution of subcortical leukomalacia on ultrasound scans. (a) Coronal scan showing a 'fuzzy' brain with slit-like ventricles. (b) Same infant 5 days later showing increased echodensity around the lateral ventricles. (c) Scan at 7 months of age showing multiple subcortical cysts and ventricular dilatation.

problems, such as cortical blindness, microcephaly, severe mental retardation and seizures, were also commonly seen in most of the infants with subcortical lesions.

This marked difference in later outcome fitted in well with MRI findings, performed between 9 and 18 months of age. Infants with PVL showed delayed myelination, especially around the irregularly dilated occipital horns. On the short T_2 spin echo sequence, areas of high signal intensity, suggestive of gliosis, were noted in areas where the cystic lesions were initially seen on cranial ultrasound (see Fig. 21.8). Subsequent scans did, however, show progression of myelination. The children with subcortical lesions, however, showed persistence of the cystic lesions and little or no myelination. There was also evidence of marked cortical atrophy, indicating that the initial lesions were much more extensive than could be visualized by ultrasonography in the neonatal period. At follow-up very little, if any, progression of myelination was noted (Fig. 21.17). Yokochi (1998) performed MRI in 13 children with subcortical leukomalacia and border zone infarction. Mental retardation was more marked in these cases than motor impairment, which consisted mainly of truncal swaying and ataxia.

PERINATAL STROKE

Two types of stroke occur in the newborn period: arterial ischemic, which is usually referred to as 'perinatal arterial stroke (PAS)' or 'neonatal stroke' and venous thrombotic, best known as 'sinovenous thrombosis (SVT).' Both subtypes are now increasingly being recognized, as more newborn infants, presenting with neonatal seizures, now routinely have MRI. Several stroke registers exist, collecting data of newborn infants as well as children (Deveber et al 2001, Steinlin et al 2005).

SINOVENOUS THROMBOSIS (SVT)

The incidence of SVT is reported as 41 per 100 000 live births, considerably less than the 1 per 4000 reported for

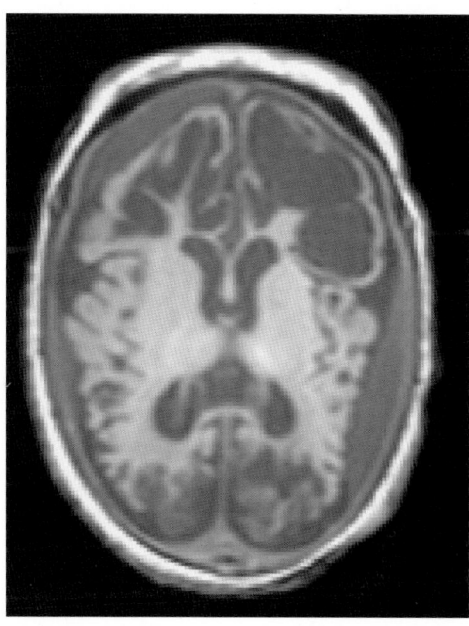

Figure 21.17 MRI scans of an infant born at 40 weeks with an examination at 8 weeks. Axial T1-weighted image showing extensive cysts in the subcortical white matter. No myelination of the posterior limb of the internal capsule is seen.

PAS. It should however be taken into account that 43 per cent of all children with SVT are newborns (deVeber et al 2001, Wu et al 2002).

Anatomy

The venous drainage of the brain can be considered as an internal and an external system. The external system drains the cerebral cortex and much of the white matter via the dural sinuses and external cortical veins. The internal system drains the basal ganglia, pons, and medulla via the internal cerebral veins and vein of Galen. Thrombosis of the internal cerebral veins is thought to be less common than dural sinus thrombosis and may extend from primary dural sinus thrombosis (Ehlers & Courville 1936).

Timing and presentation
In a large study of 42 newborn infants, time of onset was around the time of birth in 23 infants (55%) and later during the first week after birth in an additional eleven infants (Fitzgerald et al 2006). Presentation was usually with seizures (57–71%) in the three largest studies reported so far. Respiratory distress (19%) or apnea (19%) was present, while other symptoms, such as poor feeding, weight loss, acidosis and meningitis (10–12%) were less common in the study of Fitzgerald et al (2006). In another population of 30 infants, 57% presented with seizures and 17% received ECMO treatment (Wu et al 2002).

Etiology
Data from the Canadian Stroke register showed an association of sepsis including septicemia, meningitis, otitis media and brain abscess (16%) and dehydration (30%) with neonatal SVT (deVeber et al 2001). In a study by Wu et al (2002) a variety of risk factors during gestation or delivery were noted (82%). Chorioamnionitis was the most common maternal risk factor (20%), not confirmed in the study by Fitzgerald et al (2006). Pre-eclampsia/hypertension is reported to be a common maternal complication in babies who develop SVT (Fitzgerald et al 2006, Hunt et al 2001, Wu et al 2002). Numbers in these studies remain small and so far there is no study with matched case controls. Other reported causes include birth or postnatal trauma (particularly skull fracture) and impaired blood flow through the sinuses and veins (dehydration particularly associated with gastroenteritis and polycythemia and sepsis). Cardiac defects have also been described as a predisposing factor (Fitzgerald et al 2006). Impairment in venous drainage leading to sinus thrombosis may occur secondary to placement of a thin catheter in the internal jugular or subclavian veins (Gebara et al 1995).

A proportion of the infants studied by Fitzgerald et al (2006) have been studied for prothrombotic risk factors with Factor V Leiden and MTHFR C677T mutation found in 13 and 40% respectively.

Clinical features
There are no specific neurologic signs that suggest neonatal cerebral venous thrombosis, but this condition should be suspected in dehydrated infants or those with pre-existing neurologic disease if exacerbation of neurologic features occurs. General signs include features of raised intracranial pressure, convulsions, hypertonia and opisthotonus. Rivkin et al (1992) have reported lethargy and unexplained seizures to be the main symptoms in a group of seven infants with cerebral venous thrombosis. We have seen this condition on MRI in asymptomatic, routinely scanned babies. Associated intracranial and intraventricular hemorrhage have been reported with cerebral venous thrombosis (Ehlers & Courville

1936, Govaert et al 1992, Roland et al 1990) and it has been suggested that sinovenous thrombosis is an important cause of thalamic hemorrhage (p. 420) and intraventricular hemorrhage in term infants (Wu et al 2003).

Diagnosis
Ultrasound is unlikely to diagnose thrombosis in superficial sinuses because the vessels are too close to the skull. Color flow Doppler has not been reported to reliably diagnose this condition. CT scans may suggest the diagnosis by increased density along the course of the vein of Galen and straight sinus (Eick et al 1981) or a high-density thrombus in a cerebral cortical vein. CT enhancement may reveal specific abnormalities (Rao et al 1981), including gyral or tentorial enhancement, and a filling defect in the straight sinus ('empty delta sign').

Diagnosis is now usually made using MRI or CT, although more extensive disease was recognized on MR than suspected by CT examination (Rivkin et al 1992). Wu et al (2003) reported on 29 infants born >36 weeks gestation, who presented with an IVH, showing that SVT should always be considered in these children as 31% was diagnosed to have a SVT. This was especially common when the IVH was associated with a thalamic hemorrhage (p. 420). Twenty-six of the 29 infants had a CT or MRI and it was shown that 4/5 with a thalamic hemorrhage versus 5/21 without thalamic hemorrhage had an SVT ($P = 0.03$) (Fig. 21.18).

In the population studied by Fitzgerald et al (2006), 50% had involvement of a single sinus, most commonly the sagittal sinus (67%), similar to the 61% noted by Deveber et al (2001). The transverse sinus was affected in 55% and the straight sinus in 33%. About half of the infants had more than one sinus occluded.

Management
General management includes attention to the state of hydration and management of seizures. In recent years it has become more common to use antithrombotic therapy in neonates with SVT, but there are no evidence based guidelines. Current recommendations are to use low molecular weight heparin if there is no evidence of major intracranial hemorrhage. Therapy is given for 6–12 weeks depending on the extent of recanalization after 6 weeks (Monagle et al 2004). If heparinization is not used initially, a second MR scan after 5 days is recommended to assess propagation of the initial thrombus. If there has been progression use of heparin may be indicated at that stage.

Prognosis
Information about long term outcome is still limited. DeVeber et al (2001) reported a mortality of 7% and neurological deficit in 37% of their infants and a recurrence risk of symptomatic thrombosis of 8%. In the study by Fitzgerald et al (2006) only one infant (2%) died, but 79% had some sort of impairment at last follow-up, with 41% having at least moderate to severe motor impairment and 33% moder-

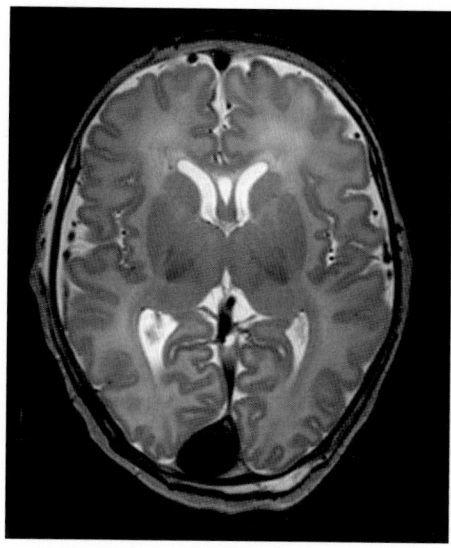
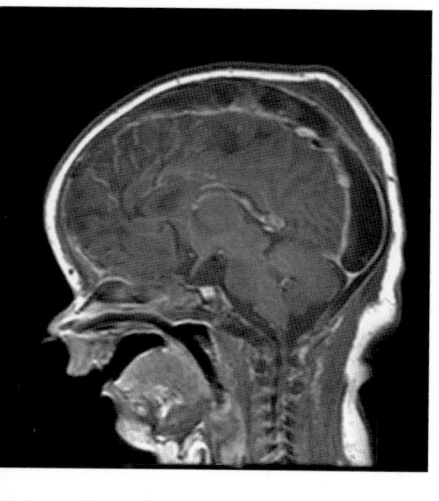

Figure 21.18 MRI, transverse T2SE (a) and midsagittal T1 with gadolinium enhancement showing extensive sinovenous thrombosis with severe dilatation of the occluded superior sagittal sinus.

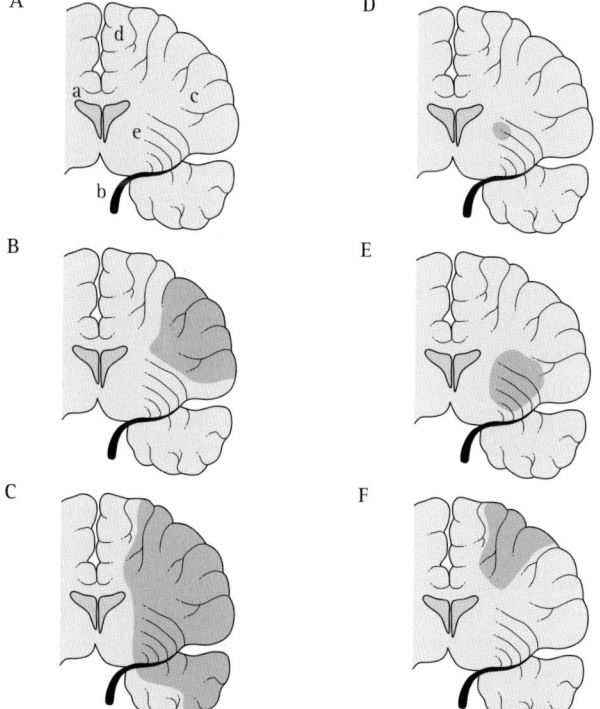

Figure 21.19 Schematic drawing, showing (A) the different branches of the middle cerebral artery, with (B) involvement of a cortical branch; (C) involvement of the main branch; (D) involvement of one or (E) more lenticulostriate branches and (F) the boundary zone between the anterior and middle cerebral artery. (Adapted from Kappelle et al 1991, with permission, Neuropediatrics 28:1997, de Vries et al, Fig. 1 © by the Lancet Ltd.)

ate to severe cognitive impairment. The subsequent development of infantile spasms has also been reported in some surviving infants at the age of 7–11 months (Soman et al 2006).

PERINATAL ARTERIAL STROKE (PAS)

Infarction of a major artery or a branch arising from it is now recognized in an increasing number of newborn infants, with an incidence of approximately 1 per 3000–4000 live births (Lynch et al 2001, Nelson & Lynch 2004).

Lesions involving the left hemisphere are three to four times more common than those of the right hemisphere. This is suggested to be due to either hemodynamic differences between right and left carotid arteries arising as the result of a patent ductus arteriosus or preferential flow of placental emboli into the left side vessels rather than the right. Middle cerebral artery infarction occurs twice as commonly as involvement of any other artery. The anterior cerebral artery is rarely recognized to be affected, but this may reflect the silent nature of symptoms related to involvement of this vessel.

Both de Vries et al (1997) as well as Mercuri et al (1999) used a classification according to the main artery involved. Infarcts in the territory of the middle cerebral artery were further subdivided into main branch, cortical branch and lenticulostriate branch infarctions (Fig 21.19).

Pathology

Cerebral artery infarction in the neonate has been defined as a severe disorganization or even complete disruption of both gray and white matter caused by embolic, thrombotic or ischemic events (Barmada et al 1979). The term perinatal arterial stroke (PAS) is nowadays most commonly used. The five cases described by Friede in 1975 were all wedge-shaped hemorrhagic lesions involving cortical, subcortical and deep periventricular white matter. Friede (1975) could only positively identify these lesions as infarctive histologically. This is different from the experience that we have nowadays in infants who mostly survive and have early neuro-imaging, showing purely ischemic lesions in the majority of the cases.

Larroche (1977) described the pathologic appearance of cerebral artery infarction in six cases. In those infants dying in the acute stage of the condition, the hemisphere was swollen and deeply congested. There was involvement of both white matter and cortex, with secondary hemorrhagic infarction in some cases. In those infants who survived for longer, contraction of the affected area was seen with softening and multiple cystic degeneration, giving a honeycomb appearance on sectioning (Fig. 21.20). The extent of the atrophic process was thought to reflect the level of arterial infarction. In some cases, infarction occurred very early in fetal life, and these brains showed extensive porencephalic cyst formation. This is discussed in more detail in Chapter 13. More recently, Aso et al (1990) performed autopsies in nine cases and found that all but one of these had one or more additional lesions, such as PVL, pontosubicular necrosis, and anoxic–ischemic neuronal necrosis.

Incidence

The introduction of modern imaging techniques has confirmed the pathologist's impression that PAS occurs commonly. Several hundreds of cases have been reported where the diagnosis was made in life (Benders et al 2007, Billard et al 1982, Chasnoff et al 1986, Clancy et al 1985, de Vries et al 1997, Filipek et al 1987, Fujimoto et al 1992, Hill et al 1983, Jan & Camfield 1998, Koelfen et al 1995, Lee et al 2005, Levene 1987, Levy et al 1985, Mannino & Trauner 1983, Mantovani & Gerber 1984, Ment et al 1984, Mercuri et al 1999, Nanni et al 1984, Perlman et al 1994, Roodhooft et al 1987, Trauner & Mannino 1986, Voorhies et al 1984, Wulfeck et al 1991). Data concerning the incidence are scarce and reflect the population from which the data are drawn. Barmada et al (1979) reported PAS in over 5% of infants examined at autopsy. More recent studies have looked at newborn infants admitted to a neonatal unit with seizures and/or apneas. Lien et al (1995) found a prevalence of 0.01% (1 : 10 000). Estan and Hope (1997) studied a 7-year cohort and reported a prevalence of 0.025% (1 : 4000), which is rather similar to the findings of Perlman et al (1994) who found a prevalence of 0.02% (1 : 5000). Several groups found neonatal stroke to be the second most common cause for neonatal seizures (Estan & Hope 1997, Levy et al 1985, Lien et al 1995). In the latter study, 49% of the infants had seizures due to hypoxic–ischemic encephalopathy and 12% due to unilateral cerebral infarction. Little data is available about focal infarction in preterm infants except for the pathologic study by Paneth et al (1994), who found lesions in the thalami or basal ganglia in 17% of the post-mortem cases belonging to a cohort born in the New Jersey counties between 1984 and 1987. In a recent hospital based study we found an incidence of 7 per 1000 preterm infants with a gestational age less than 35 weeks (Benders et al 2007).

Timing of the infarction

PAS can occur both before, as well as in the immediate, perinatal neonatal period. Before the era of widespread use of neuroimaging techniques, it was a common belief that a prenatal stroke was more common, but at present there is little data in the literature to support this. A distinction is nowadays made between 'early neonatal stroke' with symptoms on day 1–3 and 'late neonatal stroke' with symptoms up until 28 days. As the infants are often well enough to go to the postnatal ward, subtle seizures, occurring during the first few days, may go unnoticed and the child may first present at 4–6 months of age with an asymmetrical grasp, which is now often referred to as 'presumed perinatal stroke' (Lee et al 2005). Mercuri et al (1995), however, showed that when the threshold to perform neonatal imaging, and in particular MRI, is low in infants with neonatal seizures, focal infarction will be identified in the majority of these infants. Using ultrasound or conventional MRI, the lesions only become apparent during the first week of life (Cowan et al 2005). Diffusion-weighted imaging always clearly showed the area of infarction on the initial scan. It is reported that acute diffusion-weighted changes are maximal between 1 and 5 days after the acute lesion and normalize between 1 and 2 weeks (de Vries et al 2005, Mercuri & Cowan 1999). These findings suggest a perinatal onset, as diffusion-weighted imaging abnormalities become less obvious within 2 weeks after the onset (Cowan et al 1994) (Fig. 21.21).

Etiology

Stroke in the newborn does not appear to be the same condition as seen in older children and adults. In children the

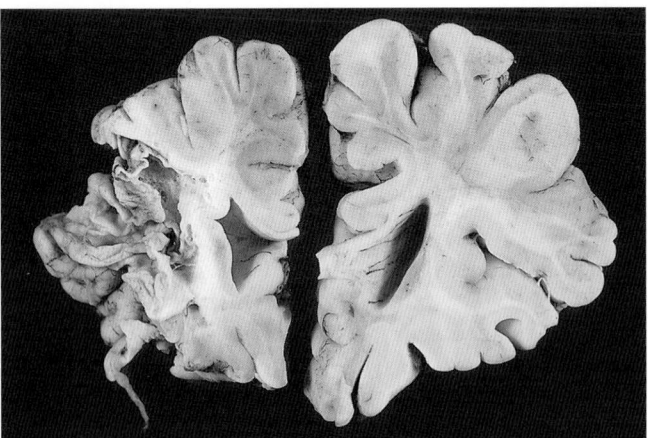

Figure 21.20 Infarction involving cortex and white matter in the distribution of the middle cerebral artery. The infant developed following cardiac surgery and the infarction may have been due to an embolus during this procedure. (Courtesy of Dr. P. Nikkels, Department of Paediatric Pathology, Utrecht.)

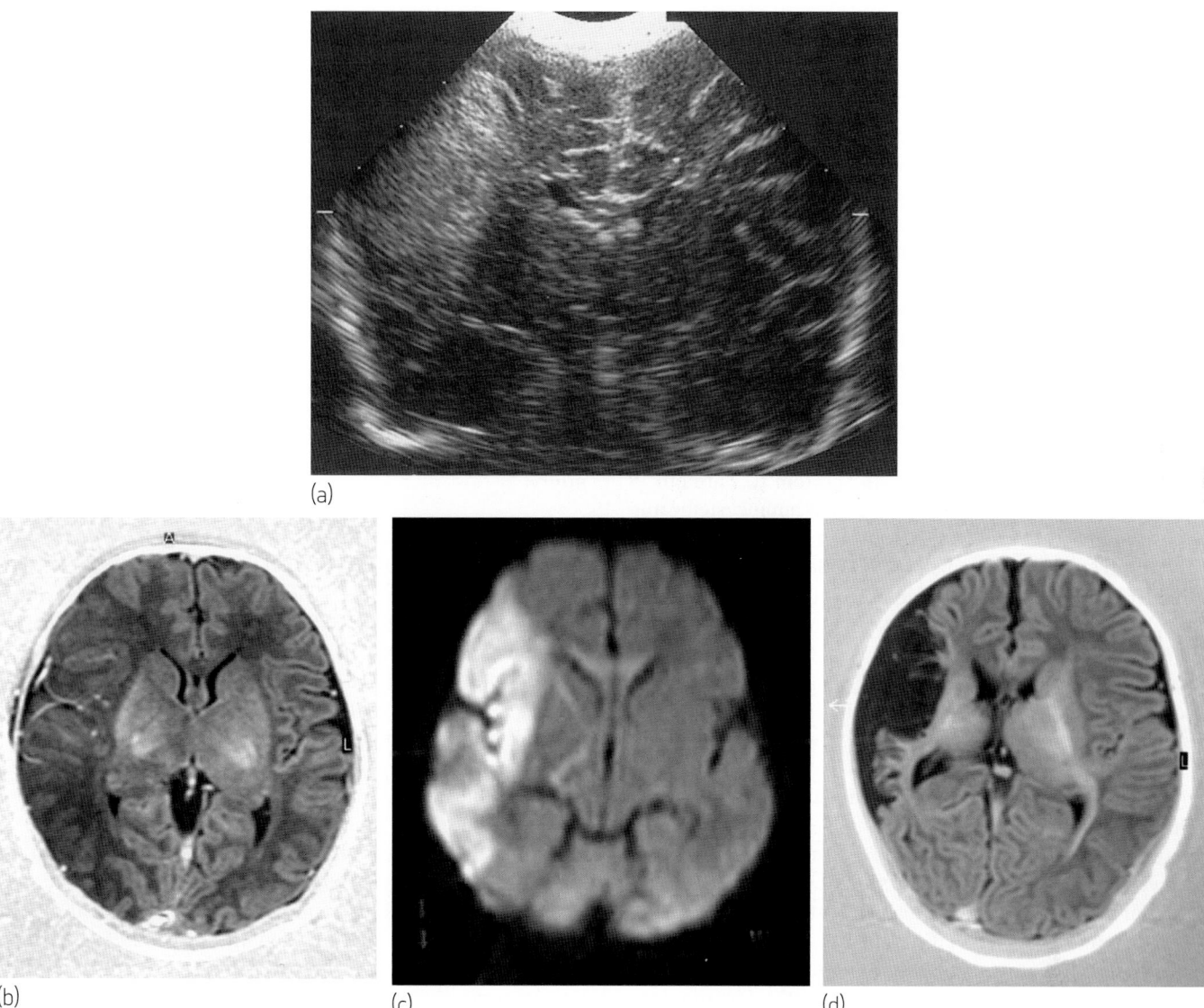

(a)

(b)   (c)   (d)

Figure 21.21 Middle cerebral artery infarction in a full-term infant. (a) Cranial ultrasound, coronal view, day 7, showing areas of increased echogenicity in the distribution of the main branch of the left middle cerebral artery. (b) MRI, IR sequence of the same infant performed on day 5, shows a large area of low signal intensity in the same region. (c) Diffusion weighted imaging shows an increased signal in the same distribution as well as the internal capsule. (d) Repeat MRI, IR sequence at 3 months of age shows cystic evolution in the affected area. Also note the absence of the normal myelination of the posterior limb on the affected side and involvement of the basal ganglia. (Reproduced, with permission, from de Vries et al, Archives Disease of Childhood 2005.)

most common cause of stroke is hemorrhage (whether arteriovenous malformation, aneurysm or tumor), and arterial occlusion occurs less frequently (Eeg-Olofsson & Ringheim 1983). Hemorrhagic stroke is less common in the newborn; although venous infarction due to sinus thrombosis is well recognized it is less frequently seen at autopsy than cerebral artery occlusion.

The causes of neonatal stroke fall into three groups: embolization, thrombosis and ischemia (Mannino & Trauner 1983). Embolic causes are the most commonly reported

(Barmada et al 1979) and twin-to-twin transfusion as well as congenital heart disease are well recognized (Benders et al 2007). Emboli arising from a patent ductus arteriosus or the placenta (Cocker et al 1965) have also been reported. Temporal artery catheterization has been related to ipsilateral cerebral infarction (Bull et al 1980), and disseminated intravascular coagulation and sepsis have also been associated with the development of thrombotic arterial infarction. Clancy et al (1985) reported that asphyxia and polycythemia were additional important predisposing factors, and described one infant who had sustained severe and prolonged hypertension before the stroke.

In some reports, infarction of watershed areas between cerebral artery vascular distributions are included with descriptions of single artery infarction (Mercuri & Cowan 1999). These watershed infarctions are most probably due to severe partial intermittent asphyxia, which is discussed in detail in Chapter 26, and are probably best considered separately from single vessel infarction.

Maternal cocaine abuse has also been considered to cause stroke (Chasnoff et al 1986, Dominguez et al 1991, Hoyme et al 1990, Volpe 1992). In a study of 43 women who abused crack cocaine during pregnancy, 17% of their infants had evidence of cortical infarction (stroke) compared with only 2% of the matched control group (Heier et al 1991).

Others have emphasized the association with coagulation abnormalities (decreased levels of protein C, protein S and antithrombin III and elevated levels of homocysteine and Lp(a), protein Z) as well as certain genetic mutations and polymorphisms (such as factor V Leiden G1691A, factor IIG20210A and methylenetetrahydrofolate reductase C677T) have been identified as possible risk factors (Debus et al 1988, Gunther et al 2000, Kurnik et al 2003, Thorarensen et al 1997, Varelas et al 1998). Association with elevated maternal cardiolipin and antiphospholipid antibodies has also been occasionally reported (Akanli et al 1998, de Klerk et al 1997, Silver et al 1992).

More recently population based studies, using case matched controls have been looking at etiological factors responsible for PAS in term infants and these were noted to be diverse. A few reports found several maternal, pre- and perinatal risk factors to be independently associated with the development of PAS (Golomb et al 2001, Lee et al 2005). Infertility, pre-eclampsia, prolonged rupture of membranes and chorioamnionitis were recently identified as independent maternal risk factors (Lee et al 2005). Neonatal risk factors, such as congenital heart disease, infection, dehydration, polycythemia, prothrombotic factors and others, have also been found to be associated with PAS (Kurnik et al 2003, Nelson & Lynch 2004). PAS was found to be more common in boys in a recent study by Golomb et al (2004).

Arterial dissection should be especially considered when more than one arterial territory is affected and has been reported in a minority of the infants (Lequin et al 2004).

Adverse perinatal events were present in 11 of the 24 infants studied by Mercuri et al (1999). However, none of these had a pH < 7.0 and only 5 infants had a 1 min Apgar score below 5. Other studies also did not find significant perinatal asphyxia among their cases (Jan et al 1998, Levy et al 1985, Perlman et al 1994). A more recent study by Ramaswamy et al (2004) found only six cases with neonatal stroke among 124 infants admitted with neonatal encephalopathy.

The majority of the children reported are born at or near term age. It has however been our experience that focal infarction also occurs in the preterm infant (Amato et al 1990, Barmada et al 1979, Benders et al 2007, de Vries et al 1988d), but is then often a chance finding on routine ultrasound imaging (Abels et al 2006, de Vries et al 1997). Using case matched controls (3 controls per case, matched for GA) we have looked at etiological factors responsible for PAS in our preterm infants and noted these to be different from those born at term. TTTS (19% vs 3%; OR 31.2 (CI 2.9–340.0), $P = 0.005$), fetal heart rate abnormality (58% vs 26%; OR 5,2 (CI 1.5–17.6), $P = 0.008$) and hypoglycemia (42% vs. 18%; OR 3,9 (CI 1.2 − 12.6), $P = 0.02$) were identified as independent risk factors for preterm PAS. Involvement of the main branch was less common in the preterm population, who more often present with cortical infarction or infarction of one or more lenticulostriate branches of the middle cerebral artery.

Diagnosis

Acute onset of seizures is the most common presenting feature. Billard et al (1982) reported the onset of seizures between 8 and 60 hours after birth in all 8 of their cases, and seizures occurred in 10 out of 11 reported by Clancy et al (1985). In the 16 infants studied by Mercuri et al (1995), 6 presented with seizures occurring within the first 24 hours and 8 between 24 and 48 hours. In the largest group of infants reported so far (Kurnik et al 2003), 156 (73%) of the 215 infants presented with focal seizures and a further 4% with generalized seizures. Hypotonia (10%) and apneas (13%) were the other most common presenting symptoms. Apneas were more common in 2 small studies. Three of the 18 infants reported by Fujimoto et al (1992) and 5 out of 16 studied by Mercuri et al (1995) presented with apneas, requiring a short period of mechanical ventilation in some. Among full-term infants presenting with seizures, cerebral infarction is recognized to be the second most common cause (Estan & Hope 1997) with hypoxic-ischemic encephalopathy being the most common one. The convulsions are usually of the focal clonic variety, but multifocal tonic or subtle seizures may all be seen. Many of the infants show no major clinical neurologic abnormality between seizures. In most studies, treatment with only phenobarbitone was sufficient, but among the 7 infants reported by Filipek et al (1987), 5 required more than one drug to control the seizures. In an infant who presents with hemiconvulsions, the diagnosis of PAS is most likely and always warrants MR imaging also when cranial ultrasound is considered normal. Presentation with clinical seizures is less common in preterm infants. Only 2 of the 17 preterm infants studied by de Vries et al (1997) did have clinical seizures. In our more recent study of 31 preterm infants, 8 presented with apneas/seizures. Routine cranial ultrasound will usually lead to the diagnosis in this age group (Benders et al 2007).

Infants with middle cerebral artery infarction may show asymmetry or hypotonia on early neurologic examination, but Mercuri et al (1999) did not find these early neurologic abnormalities to be predictive of an adverse neurologic outcome. Infants with posterior cerebral artery infarction may develop abnormal eye signs, which later can be shown to be due to homonymous hemianopia.

In the infants with 'presumed perinatal stroke' presentation is usually with a hand preference at an age of 2 months or above (Lee et al 2005).

Imaging
Ultrasonography

Diagnosis by ultrasound is possible, but this modality is not always reliable. If hemorrhagic infarction is present the focal increased echodensity is obvious, but Hill et al (1983) have reported increased echoes from non-hemorrhagic infarcted areas. Sometimes, extensive stroke may show none or relatively subtle changes on ultrasound and especially smaller superficially located cortical infarcts will be missed. A wedge-shaped increase in echogenicity tends to become more apparent by the end of the first week (Cowan et al 2005, Golomb et al 2003) (Fig. 21.21a). Hernanz-Schulman et al (1988) noted the absence of gyral definition, absence of vascular pulsations, altered parenchymal echogenicity and territorial distribution as characteristic sonographic findings. Absence of arterial pulsations were also noted by Messer et al (1991) and Perlman et al (1994). Taylor (1994) however, studied 8 infants using color Doppler sonography and noted an increase in size and number of visible vessels in the periphery of the infarct, and increased mean blood flow velocity in vessels supplying or draining the infarcted areas in 4 infants. A diminished vessel size number was found in one case. Repeat studies showed the development of multiple small irregular blood vessels in the periphery of the infarct in two cases.

Although ultrasound may not always detect cerebral artery infarction in its early stages, it may be useful later when the honeycomb cystic lesions have developed. At this stage some ex vacuo dilatation of the ipsilateral ventricle can also be noted.

Computerized tomography

As the lesion extends into the cortex, its full extent can be better identified using CT or MRI (Fig. 21.20b). CT is of more value than ultrasound in establishing the diagnosis, but a normal scan within 48 hours of birth does not exclude this condition and with easier access to MRI in most neonatal centres, the latter technique is a better option. At least two CT scans over 1 week are necessary before the condition can be excluded. The classic appearance is a wedge-shaped area of low attenuation with irregular margins. If bleeding occurs into the infarcted region, areas of high attenuation may be seen on CT scan examination. A mass effect may be seen due to severe edema surrounding the infarcted area. Rescanning some months later shows full-thickness loss of cerebral tissue in the same distribution. Thalamic atrophy can also be found later during the first

year and is regarded to be due to retrograde degeneration (Giroud et al 1995).

Magnetic resonance imaging

The more widespread use of MRI has been especially useful in the diagnosis of focal infarction, but some hours at least must pass before conventional MR images can show abnormality after an acute stroke event (Mercuri & Cowan 1999). At a very early stage (24–48 hours), when CT scans or even conventional MRI may fail to detect a focal infarction, diffusion-weighted imaging does identify the lesion within hours after its onset. In diffusion-weighted MRI (DWI), image contrast depends mainly on differences in the molecular motion of water rather than changes in T1 or T2. Increases in T1 or T2 appear later and probably require the presence of vasogenic edema. Cowan et al (1994) were the first to use this technique in neonatal infarction and showed that the diffusion-weighted changes were most marked on the initial scan, at a stage that the changes were not or less clearly seen on conventional MRI. Even when only conventional MR sequences are used, more anatomical detail is obtained compared with ultrasound or CT. Mercuri et al (1995) reported on 16 infants with neonatal seizures who had early MRI, of whom 10 had evidence of focal infarction. Although the lesion was also identified using ultrasound in 9, MRI provided much better anatomical definition of the extent of the lesions. Focal white matter hemorrhages were found in a further 4 cases and only 2 infants presenting with seizures did not show any abnormalities on MRI. Similar data were reported by Rollins et al (1994). A repeat scan can show thalamic atrophy (Giroud et al 1995) and asymmetry at the level of the mesencephalon, which can be seen as early as 6 weeks after the onset (Bouza et al 1994). Smith and Baumann (1991) found ipsilateral atrophy of the pons or midbrain to be strongly associated with congenital lesions. These changes are referred to as wallerian degeneration due to transaxonal neuronal degeneration. Using DWI during the first week after onset of PAS may show 'pre-wallerian degeneration,' seen as abnormal signal intensity descending into the corticospinal tracts. Abnormal signal intensity of the cerebral peduncles was noted to be a strong predictor of subsequent development of wallerian degeneration and hemiplegia (de Vries et al 2005, Kirton et al 2007). Using MRI in preterm infants with unilateral thalamic echogenicities, de Vries et al (1997) identified areas of focal infarction, which looked very similar to lacunar infarcts in children and adults (Fig. 21.22). These lesions occur following occlusion or spasm of one or more of the lenticulostriate branches of the middle cerebral artery.

Performing MRI enables us to perform proton spectroscopy and MR angiography (MRA) during the same session. Groenendaal et al (1995) described three infants with a middle cerebral artery and one with a posterior cerebral artery infarction. Lactate resonances were present and confined to the area of infarction in the two infants who were scanned within the first two weeks of life and in one of them lactate was still present on a repeat scan at 3 months of age. All four showed a decrease in *N*-acetyl aspartate to choline ratios in the area of infarction. MRA can sometimes show a decreased flow in the middle cerebral artery on the affected side (Fig. 21.23) which can resolve and be no longer present on a follow-up scan suggesting transient vasospasm. Koelfen et al (1993) performed MRA on 8 infants with a middle cerebral artery infarct aged 1.5–8.4 years. MRA studies still showed abnormalities corresponding to the expected vascular distribution of the parenchymal lesion. MRA was normal in one case and showed a hypoplastic middle cerebral artery main stem with or without visible flow in the secondary branches in the other 7 infants.

Radionuclide brain scanning

This technique is no longer being used in diagnosing cerebral artery infarction. It has in the past been shown that γ-emitting technetium is retained only in areas of damaged blood–brain barrier and thus will delineate the area of vascular damage (Fig. 21.24). O'Brien et al (1979) performed technetium scans on 85 asphyxiated full-term infants and found uptake in the region of the middle cerebral artery in 20% of cases.

Cerebral arteriography

This is a highly invasive procedure in infancy and unnecessary in most cases (Roodhooft et al 1987), especially now that MRA has become more widely available. Less invasive digital intravenous angiography has been used in the diagnosis of neonatal occlusive vascular disease (Voorhies et al 1984). Contrast medium is injected via an umbilical venous catheter that has been advanced to lie near the right atrium. This technique, although relatively safe, is probably not necessary, as surgical treatment to remove an embolus is not feasible.

Electroencephalography

EEG has also been used in the diagnosis of neonatal stroke (Billard et al 1982, Clancy et al 1985, Levy et al 1985, Mantovani & Gerber 1984, Mercuri et al 1999). This investigation revealed focal abnormalities in almost all patients. These included persistent localized voltage reduction, focal slowing, sharp waves and focal seizure activity. Mercuri et al (1999) found an abnormal background pattern, even when only recorded on two channels, to be the best predictor of adverse neurologic outcome.

PROGNOSIS

The outlook in most cases is relatively good. Spastic hemiplegia is the most important sequel, particularly following infarction of the main branch of the middle cerebral artery. Two-thirds of children with hemiplegia, however, are of normal intelligence. Homonymous hemianopia may follow posterior cerebral artery infarction. Outcome is very much dependent on the threshold to perform MRI and on the artery involved and whether the main branch is involved or only a cortical branch or one of the lenticulostriate branches. de Vries et al (1997) and Benders et al (2007) noted that involvement of the lenticulostriate branches was more common in preterm infants. Only 3 out of 16 infants with involvement of a cortical branch or one or more lenticulostriate branches developed cerebral palsy in contrast to all 5 survivors with main branch involvement. Govaert et al (2000) suggested that cranial ultrasound was important in the prediction of hemiplegia. In the parasagittal view attention should be paid to involvement of the central groove, which is usually present in those with involvement of the main branch and those with involvement of the anterior trunk of the middle cerebral artery. Published follow-up data from case reports suggest that over half of all infants surviving neonatal stroke are entirely normal at 12–18 months of age. Trauner and Mannino (1986) found that 8 out of 10 infants with neonatal cerebral infarction were normal at 2–5 years. The two children in whom neurologic deficits were found were only mildly affected. In a later study, the same group (Wulfeck et al 1991) reported that a hemiplegia initially noted in 11 out of 14 cases had resolved in 5 of these 11 cases by 2 years of age. A subsequent study by the same group (Trauner et al 1993) noted some degree of hemiparesis in 21 of their 29 cases, but a very favorable prognosis in terms of intellectual outcome. Seizures were a common

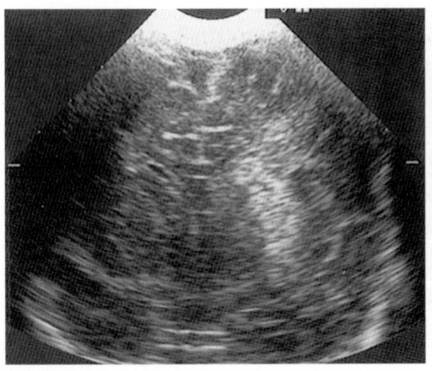
(a)

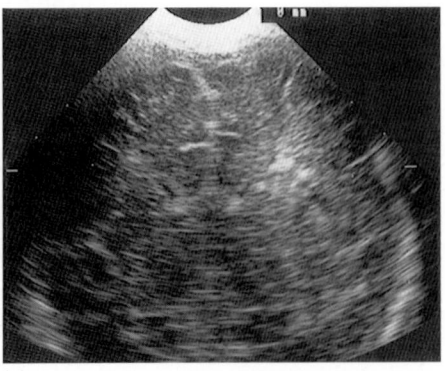
(b)

Figure 21.22 Cranial ultrasound, coronal views, showing (a) a giant lacunar infarction, seen as a wedge shaped echogenic area at the level of the caudate nucleus and the striate on day 1 with (b) associated periventricular echogenicity in a more posterior coronal view, in a monozygous twin, following the death of the co-twin at 35 weeks.

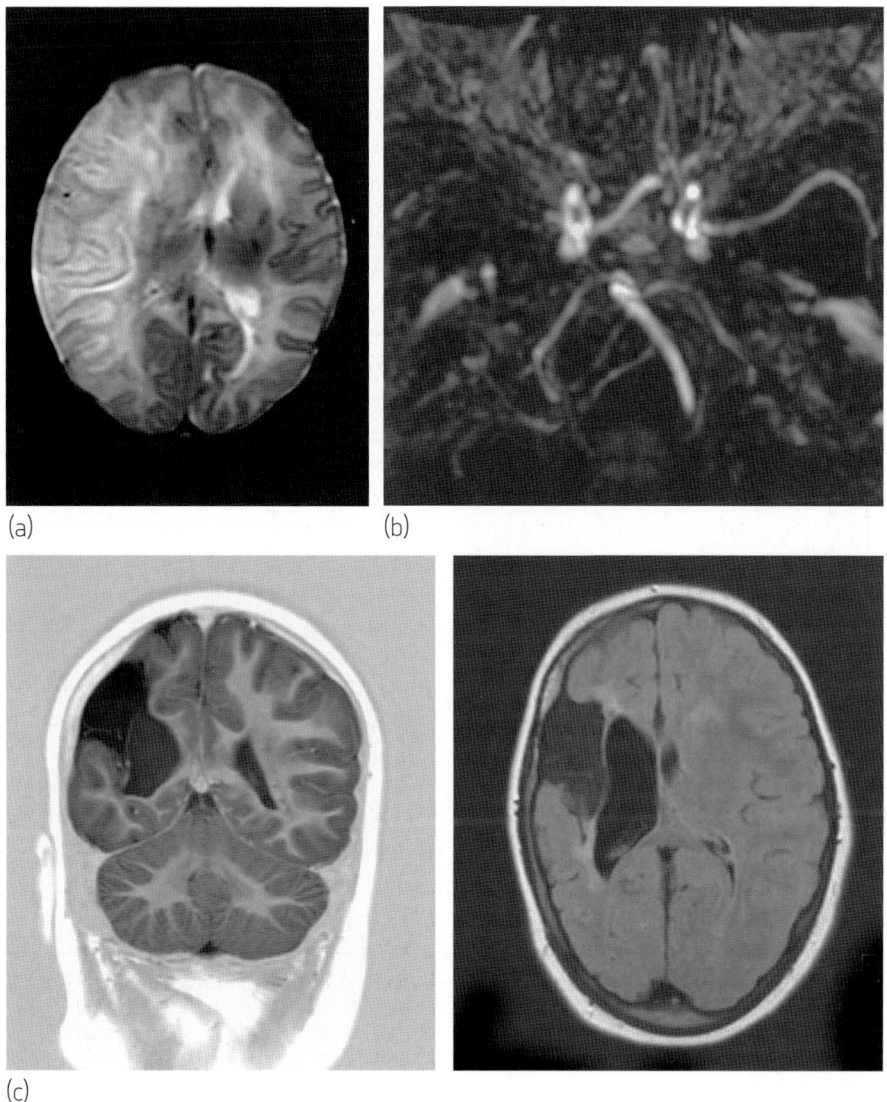

(a)   (b)

(c)

Figure 21.23 Middle cerebral artery infarction in a full-term infant. (a) MRI, a T2 weighted SE sequence, performed on day 7, shows increased signal intensity in the distribution of the right middle cerebral artery. (b) MR angiography, performed during the same examination. A difference in signal intensity is seen between the right and left middle cerebral artery, suggestive of decreased flow on the right side. (c) A repeat MRI at 8 years shows an area of large cavitation on the axial FLAIR sequence (left) and also loss of white matter on the coronal inversion recovery sequence.

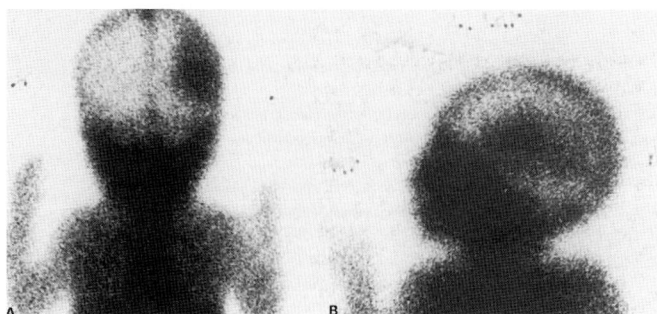

Figure 21.24 Radionuclide technetium scan of an infant with middle cerebral artery infarction. There is retention of radionuclide tracer in the region supplied by the left middle cerebral artery on (A) coronal and (B) sagittal planes.

complication and occurred beyond the neonatal period in 52% of their infants.

In the study of Fujimoto et al (1992) only 5 of the 28 infants (28%) developed hemiplegia and 11 of the 16 infants studied by Sran and Baumann (1988) were also making apparently normal developmental progress. In the cohort studied by Mercuri et al (1999) only 5 of the 24 infants (20%) developed a hemiplegia. A further 2 had mild asymmetry and 2 had mild global delay. Only those cases with involvement of the hemisphere, basal ganglia as well the internal capsule on their first scan tended to develop a hemiplegia or an asymmetry of tone. The same group of infant was assessed again at school age (Mercuri et al 2004). The number of infants with a hemiplegia had slightly increased to 30% and a further 7 (30%) showed some neu-romotor abnormality such as asymmetry on the neurologic examination (*n* = 4) or poor scores on the neuromotor test without any sign of asymmetry (*n* = 3). The remaining 9 children had a normal motor outcome. Hemiplegia was found only in children who had concomitant involvement of hemisphere, internal capsule, and basal ganglia on brain MRI. Children with involvement of the internal capsule, associated either with basal ganglia or hemispheric lesions, did not show hemiplegia but still had motor difficulties. In another report that assessed visual function, sequential studies were performed on 12 babies with focal infarction (Mercuri et al 1996). A relatively high incidence of abnor-malities was reported on at least one of their battery of tests.

Goodman and Graham (1996) noted that half of all chil-dren with hemiplegia have psychiatric disorders including problems with behavior, emotions or relationships severe enough to interfere with the child's everyday life. They usually present with irritability, anxiety and hyperactivity/inattention.

Evidence of modified organization was shown by Lewine et al (1994) combining magnetoencephalography and MRI in an adult who had suffered a left-sided middle cerebral artery infarction as a neonate. More recently several impor-tant studies have been performed, combining transcranial magnetic stimulation (TMS), functional MRI and DTI (Guzetta et al 2007, Seghier et al 2005, Staudt et al 2006). Patients with congenital unilateral brain lesions may reorganize their primary motor function in the contralesional hemisphere as a result of the preservation of ipsilateral corticospinal pro-jections, normally withdrawn within the first year after birth (Eyre 2003, Staudt et al 2002, 2004). Staudt et al (2004) showed that when a lesion abolishes the normal contralat-eral corticospinal control over the paretic hand, the contra-lesional hemisphere develops (or maintains) fast-conducting ipsilateral corticospinal pathways to the paretic hand. This reorganization with ipsilateral corticospinal tracts can mediate a useful hand function. Normal hand function however, seemed only possible with preserved crossed cor-ticospinal projections from the contralateral hemisphere. Guzzetta et al (2007) also recently suggested that ipsilesional reorganization is more effective in the restoration of a good motor function as opposed to the contralesional reorganization.

In summary and based on the estimated incidence of perinatal cerebral vascular infarction, it might be expected that this condition is the cause of the neurologic deficit in up to 20% of children with cerebral palsy (Levene 1987). This is further supported by recent data by Wu et al (2006) who noted that 22% of 377 infants with cerebral palsy showed focal arterial infarction on head imaging.

REFERENCES

Abels L, Lequin M, Govaert P 2006 Sonographic templates of newborn perforator stroke. Pediatr Radiol 36:663–669.

Abramovicz A 1964 The pathogenesis of perinatal brain damage and their conditions of occurrence in primates. Adv Neurol 27:85–95.

Akanli L F, Trasi S S, Thuraisamy K et al 1998 Neonatal middle cerebral artery infarction: association with elevated maternal anticardiolipin antibodies. Am J Perinatol 15:399–402.

Alexander J M, Gilstrap L C, Cox S M et al 1998 Clinical chorioamnionitis and the prognosis for very low birth weight infants. Obstet Gynecol 91:725–729.

Amato M, Huppi P, Herschkowitz N, Huber P 1991 Prenatal stroke suggested by intrauterine ultrasound and confirmed by magnetic resonance imaging. Neuropediatrics 22:100–102.

Amin S B, Sinkin R A, Glantz J C 2007 Meta-analysis of the effect of antenatal indometacin on neonatal outcomes. AM J Obstet Gynecol 197:486.e1–486.e10.

Andre P, Thebaud B, Delavaucoupet J et al 2001 Late-onset cystic periventricular leukomalacia in premature infants: a threat until term. Am J Perinatol 18(2):79–86.

Anjari M, Srinivasan L, Allsop J M et al 2007 Diffusion tensor imaging with tract-based spatial statistics reveals local white matter abnormalities in preterm infants. NeuroImage (in press).

Appleton R E, Lee R E J, Hey E N 1990 Neurodevelopmental outcome of transient neonatal intracerebral echodensities. Arch Dis Child 65:27–29.

Armstrong D, Norman M G 1974 Periventricular leukomalacia in neonates: complications and sequelae. Arch Dis Child 49:367–375.

Arthur R 2006 Magnetic resonance imaging in preterm infants. Pediatr Radiol 36:593–607.

Aso K, Scher M, Barmada M A 1990 Cerebral infarcts and seizures in the neonate. J Child Neurol 5:224–228.

Aziz K, Vickar D B, Sauve R S et al 1995 Province-based study of neurologic disability of children weighing 500 through 1249 grams at birth in relation to neonatal cerebral ultrasound findings. Pediatrics 95:837–844.

Baarsma R, Laurini R N, Baerts W, Okken A 1987 Reliability of sonography in non-haemorrhagic periventricular leukomalacia. Pediatric Radiology 17:189–191.

Back S A 2006 Perinatal white matter injury: the changing spectrum of pathology and emerging insights into pathogenetic mechanisms. Ment Retard Dev Disabil Res Rev 12(2):129–140.

Back S A, Gan X, Li Y, Rosenberg P A, Volpe J J 1998 Maturation-dependent vulnerability of oligodendrocytes to oxidative stress-induced death caused by glutathione depletion. J Neurosci 18:6241–6253.

Back S A, Luo N L, Mallinson R A et al 2005 Selective vulnerability of preterm white matter to oxidative damage defined by F2-isoprostanes. Ann Neurol 58(1):108–120.

Baerts W, Fetter W P F, Hop W C J et al 1990 Cerebral lesions in preterm infants after tocolytic indomethacin. Dev Med Child Neurol 32:910–918.

Baetmann M, Kahn T, Lenard H-G, Voit T 1996 Fetal CNS damage after exposure to maternal trauma during pregnancy. Acta Paediatr 85:1331–1338.

Banker B Q, Larroche J-C 1962 Periventricular leukomalacia of infancy: a form of neonatal anoxic encephalopathy. Arch Neurol 7:386–410.

Barmada M A, Moossy J, Shuman R M 1979 Cerebral infarcts with arterial occlusion in neonates. Ann Neurol 6:495–502.

Barth P G 1984 Prenatal clastic encephalopathies. Clin Neurol Neurosurg 86:65–75.

Baud O, d'Allest A-M, Lacaze-Masmonteil T et al 1998b The early diagnosis of periventricular leukomalacia in premature infants with positive Rolandic sharp waves on serial electroencephalography. J Pediatr 132:813–817.

Baud O, Emilie D, Pelletier E et al 1999a Amniotic fluid concentrations of interleukin-1 beta, interleukin-6 and TNF-alpha in chorioamnionitis before 32 weeks of gestation: histological associations and neonatal outcome. Br J Obstet Gynaecol 106:72–77.

Baud O, Foix-L'Helias L, Kaminski M et al 1999b Antenatal glucocorticoid treatment and cystic periventricular leukomalacia in very premature infants. N Engl J Med 341:1190–1196.

Baud O, Ville Y, Zupan V et al 1998a Are neonatal brain lesions due to intrauterine infection related to mode of delivery? Br J Obstet Gynecol 105:121–124.

Bejar R, Vigliocco G, Gramajo H et al 1990 Antenatal origin of neurologic damage in newborn infants. II. Multiple gestations. Am J Obstet Gynecol 162:1230–1236.

Bejar R, Wozniak P, Allard M et al 1988 Antenatal origin of neurologic damage in newborn infants. I. Preterm infants. Am J Obstet Gynecol 159:357–363.

Benders M J N L, Groenendaal F, Uiterwaal C S P M et al 2007 Maternal and infant characteristics associated with perinatal arterial stroke in the preterm infant. Stroke (in press).

Bennett F C, Silver G, Leung E J, Mack L A 1990 Periventricular echodensities detected by cranial ultrasonography: usefulness in predicting neurodevelopmental outcome in low-birth weight, preterm infants. Pediatrics 85:400–404.

Billard C, Dulac O, Diebler R 1982 Ramollissement cérébral ischemique du nouveau-né: une étiologie possible des états de mal convulsifs neonatale. Arch Françaises de Pediatrie 39:677–683.

Boardman J P, Counsell S J, Rueckert D et al 2006 Abnormal deep grey matter development following preterm birth detected using deformation based morphometry. NeuorImage 32:70–80.

Bos A F, Martijn A, Okken A, Prechtl H F 1998 Quality of general movements in preterm infants with transient periventricular echodensities. Acta Paediatrica 87:328–335.

Bouza H, Rutherford M, Acolet D et al 1994 Evolution of early hemiplegic signs in full-term infants with unilateral brain lesions in the neonatal period: a prospective study. Neuropediatrics 25:201–207.

Bowerman R A, Donn S M, DiPietro M A et al 1984 Periventricular leukomalacia in the preterm infant: sonographic and clinical features. Radiology 151:383–388.

Boxma A, Lequin M, Ramenghi LA et al 2005 Sonographic detection of the optic radiation. Acta Paediatr 94(10):1455–1461.

Bozynski M E, Nelson M N, Matalon T A S et al 1985 Cavitary periventricular leukomalacia: incidence and short term outcome in infants weighing <1200 grams at birth. Dev Med Child Neurol 27:572–577.

Brun N, Robitaille Y, Grignon A et al 1999 Pyruvate carboxylase deficiency: prenatal onset of ischemia-like brain lesions in two sibs with the acute neonatal form. Am J Med Genet 84:94–101.

Bull M J, Schreiner R L, Garg B P et al 1980 Neurologic complications following temporal artery catheterization. J Pediatr 96:1071–1073.

Burguet A, Monnet E, Pauchard J Y et al 1999 Some risk factors for cerebral palsy in very premature infants: importance of premature rupture of membranes and monochorionic twin placentation. Biol Neonate 75:177–186.

Calvert S A, Hoskins E M, Fong K W, Forsyth S C 1986 Periventricular leukomalacia: ultrasonic diagnosis and neurological outcome. Acta Paediatr Scand 75:489–496.

Carson S C, Hertzberg B S, Bowie J D, Burger P C 1990 Value of sonography in the diagnosis of intracranial haemorrhage and periventricular leukomalacia: a postmortem study of 35 cases. Am J Neuroradiol 11:677–683.

Catto-Smith A G, Yu V Y H, Bajuk B et al 1985 Effect of neonatal periventricular haemorrhage on neurodevelopmental outcome. Arch Dis Child 60:8–11.

Cavazutti M, Duffy T E 1982 Regulation of cerebral blood flow in normal and hypoxic newborn dogs. Ann Neurol 11:247–257.

Chasnoff I J, Bussey M E, Savich R, Stack C M 1986 Perinatal cerebral infarction and maternal cocaine use. J Pediatr 108:456–459.

Chen C C, Huang C B, Chung M Y et al 2004 Periventricular echogenicity is related to delayed neurodevelopment of preterm infants. Am J Perinatol 21(8):483–489.

Childs A M, Cornette L, Ramenghi LA et al 2001 Magnetic resonance and cranial ultrasound characteristics of periventricular white matter abnormalities in newborn infants. Clin Radiol 56:647–655.

Chow P P, Morgan J G, Taylor K J W 1985 Neonatal periventricular leukomalacia: a real-time sonographic diagnosis with CT correlation. Am J Radiol 145:155–160.

Cioni G, Di Paco M C, Bertucelli B et al 1997a MRI findings and sensorimotor development in infants with bilateral spastic cerebral palsy. Brain Dev 19:245–253.

Cioni G, Fazzi B, Coluccini M et al 1997b Cerebral visual impairment in preterm infants with periventricular leukomalacia. Pediatr Neurol 17:331–338.

Cioni G, Fazzi B, Ipata A E et al 1996 Correlation between cerebral visual impairment and magnetic resonance imaging in children with neonatal encephalopathy. Dev Med Child Neurol 38:120–132.

Clancy R, Malin S, Laraque D et al 1985 Focal motor seizures heralding stroke in fullterm neonates. Am J Dis Child 139:601–606.

Cocker J, George S W, Yates P O 1965 Perinatal occlusion of the middle cerebral artery. Dev Med Child Neurol 7:235–243.

Coley B D, Hogan M J 1997 Cystic periventricular leukomalacia of the corpus callosum. Pediatr Radiol 27:583–585.

Connell J A, Oozeer R C, Regev R et al 1987 Continuous 4 channel EEG monitoring in the evaluation of echodense ultrasound lesions and cystic leukomalacia. Arch Dis Child 62:1019–1024.

Cools F, Offringa M 1999 Meta-analysis of elective high frequency ventilation in preterm infants with respiratory distress syndrome. Arch Dis Child 80: F15–F20.

Cornette L G, Tanner S F, Ramenghi L A et al 2002 Magnetic resonance imaging of the infant brain: anatomical characteristics and clinical significance of punctate lesions. Arch Dis Child Fetal Neonatal Ed. 86:F171–177.

Counsell S J, Allsop J M, Harrison M C et al 2003 Diffusion weighted imaging of the brain in preterm infants with focal and diffuse white matter abnormality. Pediatrics 112:1–7.

Counsell S J, Dyet L E, Larkman D J et al 2007). Thalamo-cortical connectivity in children born preterm mapped using probabilistic magnetic resonance tractography. Neuroimage 34:896–904.

Counsell S J, Shen Y, Boardman J P et al 2006 Axial and radial diffusivity in preterm infants who have diffuse white matter changes on conventional magnetic resonance imaging at term equivalent age. Pediatrics 117:376–386.

Cowan F 1986 Indomethacin, patent ductus arteriosus, and cerebral blood flow. J Pediatr 109:341–344.

Cowan F M, Pennock J M, Hanrahan J D et al 1994 Early detection of cerebral infarction and hypoxic-ischemic encephalopathy in neonates using diffusion-weighted magnetic resonance imaging. Neuropediatrics 25:172–175.

Cowan F, Mercuri E, Groenendaal F et al 2005 Does cranial ultrasound imaging identify arterial cerebral infarction in term neonates? Arch Dis Child Fetal Neonatal Ed. 90:F252–F256.

Crowther C A, Hiller J E, Doyle LW, Haslam RR 2003 Effect of magnesium sulfate given for neuroprotection before preterm birth: a randomized controlled trial. JAMA 290(20):2669–2676.

Crowther C A, Hiller J E, Haslam R R et al 1997 Australian Collaborative Trial of Antenatal Thyrotropin-Releasing Hormone: adverse effects at 12-month follow-up. ACTOBAT Study Group 99:311–317.

Dammann O, Leviton A 1997a Maternal intrauterine infection, cytokines, and brain damage in the preterm newborn. Pediatr Res 42:1–8.

Dammann O, Leviton A 1997b Duration of transient hyperechoic images of white matter in very-low-birthweight infants: a proposed classification. Dev Med Child Neurol 39:2–5.

Dammann O, Leviton A 1998 Infection remote from the brain, neonatal white matter damage, and cerebral palsy in the preterm infant. Semin Pediatr Neurol 5:190–201.

Dammann O, Leviton A 1999 Brain damage in preterm newborns: might enhancement of developmentally regulated endogenous protection open a door for prevention? Pediatrics 104:541–550.

De Klerk O L, de Vries T W, Sinnige L G F 1997 An unusual cause of neonatal seizures in a newborn infant. Pediatrics 100:E8.

De Reuck J, Chattha A S, Richardson E P 1972 Pathogenesis and evolution of leukomalacia in infancy. Arch Neurol 27:229–236.

de Vries L S, Connell J C, Pennock J M et al 1987 Neurological, electrophysiological and MRI abnormalities in infants with extensive cystic leukomalacia. Neuropediatrics 18:61–66.

de Vries L S, Dubowitz L M S 1985b Cystic leukomalacia in preterm infants: site of lesion in relation to prognosis. Lancet ii:1075–1076.

de Vries L S, Dubowitz L M S, Dubowitz V et al 1985a Predictive value of cranial ultrasound: a reappraisal. Lancet ii:137–140.

de Vries L S, Eken P, Dubowitz L M S 1992 The spectrum of leukomalacia using cranial ultrasound. Behav Brain Res 49:1–6.

de Vries L S, Eken P, Groenendaal F et al 1993 Correlation between the degree of periventricular leukomalacia diagnosed using cranial ultrasound and MRI later in infancy in children with cerebral palsy. Neuropediatrics 24:263–268.

de Vries L S, Groenendaal F, Eken P et al 1997 Infarcts in the vascular distribution of the middle cerebral artery in preterm and fullterm infants. Neuropediatrics 28:88–96.

de Vries L S, Regev R, Connell J A et al 1988d Localised cerebral infarction in the premature infant: ultrasound diagnosis and correlation with CT and MRI. Pediatrics 81:31–34.

de Vries L S, Regev R, Dubowitz L M S 1986 Late onset cystic leukomalacia. Arch Dis Child 61: 298–299.

de Vries L S, Regev R, Dubowitz L M S et al 1988b Perinatal risk factors for the development of extensive cystic leukomalacia. Am J Dis Child 142:732–735.

de Vries L S, Regev R, Pennock J M et al 1988c Ultrasound evolution and later outcome of infants with periventricular densities. Early Hum Dev 16:225–233.

de Vries L S, Van der Grond J, Van Haastert I C, Groenendaal F 2005 Prediction of outcome in new-born infants with arterial ischaemic stroke using diffusion–weighted magnetic resonance imaging. Neuropediatrics 36:12–20.

de Vries L S, Van Haastert I L, Rademaker K J et al 2004 Ultrasound abnormalities preceding cerebral palsy in high-risk preterm infants. J Pediatr 144(6):815–820.

de Vries L S, Wigglesworth J S, Regev R, Dubowitz L M S 1988a Evolution of periventricular leukomalacia during the neonatal period and infancy: correlation of imaging and postmortem findings. Early Hum Dev 17:205–219.

Debillon T, N'Guyen S, Muet A et al 2003 Limitations of ultrasonography for diagnosing white matter damage in preterm infants. Arch Dis Child Fetal Neonatal Ed 88:F275–F279.

Debus O, Koch H G, Kurlemann G et al 1998 Factor V Leiden and genetic defects of thrombophilia in childhood porencephaly. Arch Dis Child 78:F121–F124.

Deguchi K, Mizuguchi M, Takashima S 1996 Immunohistochemical staining of tumor necrosis factor-alpha in neonatal leukomalacia. Pediatr Neurol 14:13–14.

Deguchi K, Oguchi K, Matsuura N et al 1999 Periventricular leukomalacia: relation to gestational age and axonal injury. Pediatr Neurol 20:370–374.

Deguchi K, Oguchi K, Takashima S 1997 Characteristic neuropathology of leukomalacia in extremely low birth weight infants. Paediatr Neurol 16:296–300.

Delaporte B, Labrune M, Imbert M C, Dahan M 1985 Early echographic findings in non-haemorrhagic periventricular leukomalacia in the premature infant. Pediatr Radiol 15:82–84.

Deulofeut R, Sola A, Lee B et al 2005 The impact of vaginal delivery in premature infants weighing less than 1,251 grams.Obstet Gynecol 105(3):525–531.

deVeber G, Andrew M, Adams C et al Canadian Pediatric Ischemic Stroke Study Group 2001 Cerebral sinovenous thrombosis in children. N Engl J Med 9,345:417–423.

Di Pietro M A, Brody B A, Teele R L 1986 Peritrigonal echogenic 'blush' on cranial sonography: pathologic correlates. Am J Radiol 146:1067–1072.

Dolfin T, Skidmore M B, Fong K W et al 1984 Diagnosis and evolution of periventricular leukomalacia: a study with real-time ultrasound. Early Hum Dev 9:105–109.

Dominguez R, Vila-Coro A A, Slopis J M, Bohan T P 1991 Brain and ocular abnormalities in infants with in utero exposure to cocaine and other street drugs. Am J Dis Child 145:688–695.

Dommergues M A, Patkai J, Renauld J C et al 2000 Proinflammatory cytokines and interleukin-9 exacerbate excitotoxic lesions of the newborn murine neopallium. Ann Neurol 47:54–63.

Duncan J R, Cock M L, Scheerlinck J P et al 2002 White matter injury after repeated endotoxin exposure in the preterm ovine fetus. Pediatr Res 52(6):941–949.

Dyet L, Kennea N, Counsell S J et al 2006 The natural history of brain lesions in extremely preterm infants investigated by MR imaging. Pediatrics 118:536–548.

Eeg-Olofsson O, Ringheim Y 1983 Stroke in children: clinical characteristics and prognosis. Acta Paediatr Scand 72:391–395.

Ehlers H, Courville C B 1936 Thrombosis of internal cerebral veins in infancy and childhood. J Pediatr 8:600–623.

Eick J J, Miller K D, Bell K A, Tutton R H 1981 Computed tomography of deep cerebral venous thrombosis in children. Neuroradiology 140:399–402.

Eken P, de Vries L S, van Nieuwenhuizen O et al 1996 Early predictors of cerebral visual impairment in infants with cystic leukomalacia. Neuropediatrics 27:16–25.

Eken P, van Nieuwenhuizen O, van der Graaf Y et al 1994 Relation between neonatal cranial ultrasound abnormalities and cerebral visual impairment in infancy. Dev Med Child Neurol 36:3–15.

Ekert P G, Taylor M J, Keenan N K et al 1997 Early somatosensory evoked potentials in preterm infants: their prognostic utility. Biol Neonate 71:83–91.

Elimian A, Verma U, Canterino J et al 1999 Effectiveness of antenatal steroids in obstetric subgroups. Obstet Gynecol 93:174–179.

Ellison V J, Mocatta T J, Winterbourn C C et al 2005 The relationship of CSF and plasma cytokine levels to cerebral white matter injury in the premature newborn. Pediatric Research 57(2):282–286.

Elsmen E, Ley D, Cilio C M et al 2006 Umbilical cord levels of interleukin-1 receptor antagonist and neonatal outcome. Biology of the Neonate 89(4):220–226.

Estan J, Hope P 1997 Unilateral neonatal cerebral infarction in full term infants. Arch Dis Child 76: F88–F93.

Evans D M, Levene M I, Archer L N J 1987 The effect of indomethacin on cerebral blood-flow velocity in premature infants. Dev Med Child Neurol 29:776–782.

Eyre J A 2003 Development and plasticity of the corticospinal system in man. Neural Plast 10:93–106.

Fan G G, Yu B, Quan S M et al 2006 Potential of diffusion tensor MRI in the assessment of periventricular leukomalacia. Clinical Radiology 61:358–364.

Fawer C-L, Calame A 1991 Significance of ultrasound appearances in the neurological development and cognitive abilities of preterm infants at 5 years. Eur J Pediatr 150:515–520.

Fawer C-L, Calame A, Anderegg A 1984 Real-time ultrasonography in the neonate: a systematic study of high risk infant population. Helvet Acta Paediatr 39:34–45.

Fawer C-L, Calame A, Furrer M-T 1985b Neurodevelopmental outcome at 12 months of age related to cerebral ultrasound appearances of high risk preterm infants. Early Hum Dev 11:123–132.

Fawer C-L, Calame A, Perentes E, Anderegg A 1985a Periventricular leukomalacia: a correlation study between real-time ultrasound and autopsy findings. Neuroradiology 27:292–300.

Fawer C-L, Diebold P, Calame A 1987 Periventricular leukomalacia and neurodevelopmental outcome in preterm infants. Arch Dis Child 62:30–36.

Fazzi E, Lanzi G, Gerardo A et al 1992 Neurodevelopmental outcome in very-low-birth-weight infants with or without periventricular haemorrhage and/or leukomalacia. Acta Paediatr 81:808–811.

Fazzi E, Orcesi S, Caffi L et al 1994 Neurodevelopmental outcome at 5–7 years in preterm infants with periventricular leukomalacia. Neuropediatrics 25:134–139.

Fedrizzi E, Inverno M, Botteon G et al 1993 The cognitive development of children born preterm and affected by spastic diplegia. Brain Dev 15:428–432.

Fedrizzi E, Inverno M, Bruzzone M G et al 1996 MRI features of cerebral lesions and cognitive functions in preterm spastic diplegic children. Paediatr Neurol 15:207–212.

Filipek P A, Krishnamoorthy K S, Davis K R, Kuehnle K 1987 Focal cerebral infarction in the newborn: a distinct entity. Paediatr Neurol 3:141–147.

FineSmith R B, Roche K, Yellin P B et al 1997 Effect of magnesium sulfate on the development of cystic periventricular leukomalacia in preterm infants. Am J Perinatol 14:303–307.

Fitzgerald K C, Williams L S, Garg B P et al 2006 Cerebral sinovenous thrombosis in the neonate. Arch Neurol 63:405–409.

Friede R 1975 Developmental neuropathology. Springer-Verlag, Vienna..

Fritz K I, Ashraf Q M, Mishra O P et al 2001 Effect of moderate hypocapnic ventilation on nuclear DNA fragmentation and energy metabolism in the cerebral cortex of newborn piglets. Pediatr Res 50:586–589.

Fujimoto S, Yamaguchi N, Togari H et al 1994b Cerebral palsy of cystic periventricular leukomalacia in low-birth-weight infants. Acta Paediatr 83:397–401.

Fujimoto S, Yokochi K, Togari H et al 1992 Neonatal cerebral infarction: symptoms, CT findings and prognosis. Brain Dev 14:48–52.

Galli K K, Zimmerman R A, Jarvik G P et al 2004 Periventricular leukomalacia is common after neonatal cardiac surgery. J Thorac Cardiovasc Surg 127(3):692–704.

Garnier Y, Berger R, Alm S et al 2006 Systemic endotoxin administration results in increased S100B protein blood levels and periventricular brain white matter injury in the preterm fetal sheep. Eur J Obstet Gynecol Reprod Biol 1,124(1):15–22.

Garnier Y, Berger R, Alm S et al 2006 Systemic Gebara B M, Goetting M G, Wang A R 1995 Dural sinus thrombosis complicating subclavian vein catheterization: treatment with local thrombolysis. Pediatrics 95:138–140.

Geva E, Lerner-Geva L, Stavorovsky Z et al 1998 Multifetal pregnancy reduction: a possible risk factor for periventricular leukomalacia. Fertil Steril 69:845–850.

Gibbs J M, Weindling A M 1994 Neonatal intracranial lesions following placental abruption. Eur J Pediatr 153:195–197.

Gibson N A, Fielder A R, Trounce J Q, Levene M I 1990 Ophthalmic findings in infants of very low birthweight. Dev Med Child Neurol 32:7–13.

Gilles F H, Leviton A, Kerr C S 1976 Endotoxin leukoencephalopathy in the telencephalon of the newborn kitten. J Neurol Sci 27:183–191.

Gilles F H, Murphy S F 1969 Perinatal telencephalic leucoencephalopathy. J Neurosurg Psychiatry 32:404–413.

Giroud M, Fayolle H, Martin D et al 1995 Late thalamic atrophy in infarction of the middle cerebral artery territory in neonates. Child Nerv Syst 11:133–136.

Goepfert A R, Andrews W W, Carlo W et al 2004 Umbilical cord plasma interleukin-6 concentrations in preterm infants and risk of neonatal morbidity. Am J Obstet Gynecol 191(4):1375–1381.

Golomb M R, Dick P T, MacGregor D L et al 2003 Cranial ultrasonography has a low sensitivity for detecting arterial ischemic stroke in term neonates. J Child Neurol 18(2):98–103.

Golomb M R, Dick P T, MacGregor D L et al 2004 Neonatal arterial ischemic stroke and cerebral sinovenous thrombosis are more commonly diagnosed in boys. J Child Neurol 19(7):493–497.

Golomb M R, MacGregor D L, Domi T et al 2001 Presumed pre- or perinatal arterial ischemic stroke: risk factors and outcomes. Ann Neurol 50(2):163–168.

Gomez, Romero R, Ghezzi F et al 1998 The fetal inflammatory response syndrome. Am J Obstet Gynecol 179:194–202.

Goodman R, Graham P 1996 Psychiatric problems in children with hemiplegia: cross sectional epidemiological survey. BMJ 312:1065–1069.

Goto M, Ota R, Iai M et al 1994 MRI changes and deficits of higher brain functions in preterm diplegia. Acta Paediatr 83:506–511.

Govaert P, Achten E, Vanhaesebrouck P et al 1992 Deep cerebral venous thrombosis in thalamo-ventricular hemorrhage of the term newborn. Pediatr Radiol 22:123–127.

Govaert P, Matthys E, Zecic A et al 2000 Perinatal cortical infarction within middle cerebral artery trunks. Arch Dis Child 82:F59–F63.

Graham M, Levene M I, Trounce J Q, Rutter N 1987 Prediction of cerebral palsy in very low birth weight infants: prospective ultrasound study. Lancet ii:593–596.

Grant E G, Schellinger D, Smith Y, Uscinski R H 1986 Periventricular leukomalacia in combination with intraventricular hemorrhage; sonographic features and sequelae. Am J Neuroradiol 7:443–447.

Graziani L J, Mitchell D G, Kornhauser M et al 1992 Neurodevelopment of preterm infants: neonatal neurosonographic and serum bilirubin studies. Pediatrics 89:229–234.

Graziani L J, Pasto M, Stanley C et al 1987 Neonatal neurosonographic correlates of cerebral palsy in preterm infants. Pediatrics 78:88–95.

Gressens P, Besse L, Robberecht P et al 1999 Neuroprotection of the developing brain by systemic administration of vasoactive intestinal peptide derivatives. J Pharmacol Exp Ther 288:1207–1213.

Grether J K, Nelson K B, Emery III E S, Cummins S K 1996 Prenatal and perinatal factors and cerebral palsy in very low birth weight infants. J Pediatr 128:407–414.

Grether J K, Nelson K B, Walsh E et al 2003 Intrauterine exposure to infection and risk of cerebral palsy in very preterm infants. Arch Pediatr Adolesc Med 157(1):26–32.

Groenendaal F, van der Grond J, van Haastert I 1997 Early cerebral proton MRS and neurodevelopmental outcome in infants with cystic leukomalacia. Dev Med Child Neurol 39:373–379.

Groenendaal F, van der Grond J, Witkamp T D, de Vries L S 1995 Magnetic resonance spectroscopic imaging in neonatal stroke. Neuropediatrics 26:243–248.

Gunther G, Junker R, Strater R et al 2000 Childhood Stroke Study Group. Symptomatic ischemic stroke in full-term neonates: role of acquired and genetic prothrombotic risk factors. Stroke 31(10):2437–2441.

Guzzetta A, Bonanni P, Biagi L et al (2007 Reorganisation of the somatosensory system after early brain damage. Clin Neurophysiol 118(5):1110–1121.

Guzzetta F, Shackelford G D, Volpe S et al 1986 Periventricular intraparenchymal echodensities in the premature newborn: critical determinant of neurologic outcome. Pediatrics 78:995–1006.

Halliday H L, Erenkranz R A, Doyle L W 2006a Early postnatal corticosteroids (<96 hours) for preventing chronic lung disease in preterm infants [review]. Cochrane Library, Issue 1. Oxford: Update Sodtware.

Halliday H L, Erenkranz R A, Doyle L W 2006b Moderately early postnatal corticosteroids (7–14 days) for preventing chronic lung disease in preterm infants [review]. Cochrane Library, Issue 1. Oxford: Update Sodtware.

Halliday H L, Erenkranz R A, Doyle L W 2006c Delayed (>3 weeks) postnatal corticosteroids for chronic lung disease in preterm infants [review]. Cochrane Library, Issue 1. Oxford: Update Sodtware.

Hamilton P A, Hope P L, Cady F B et al 1986 Impaired energy metabolism in brains of newborn infants with increased cerebral echodensities. Lancet i: 1242–1246.

Hamrick S E, Miller S P, Leonard C et al 2004 Trends in severe brain injury and neurodevelopmental outcome in premature newborn infants: the role of cystic periventricular leukomalacia. J Pediatrics 145(5):593–599.

Hansen A, Leviton A 1999 Labor and delivery characteristics and risks of cranial ultrasonographic abnormalities among very-low-birth-weight infants. The Developmental Epidemiology Network Investigators. Am J Obstet Gynecol 181:997–1006.

Hansen-Pupp I, Harling S, Berg A C et al 2005 Circulating interferon-gamma and white matter brain damage in preterm infants. Pediatr Res 58(5):946–952.

Harding D R, Dhamrait S, Whitelaw A et al 2004 Does interleukin-6 genotype influence cerebral injury or developmental progress after preterm birth? Pediatrics 114(4):941–947.

Hayakawa F, Okumura A, Kato T et al 1999 Determination of timing of brain injury in preterm infants with periventricular leukomalacia with serial neonatal electroencephalography. Pediatrics 104:1077–1081.

Heier L A, Carpanzano C R, Mast J 1991 Maternal cocaine abuse: the spectrum of radiologic abnormalities in the neonatal CNS. Am J Neuroradiol 12:951–956.

Hernanz-Schulman M, Cohen W, Genieser N B 1988 Sonography of cerebral infarction in infancy. Am J Radiol 150:897–902.

Hill A, Martin D J, Danemann A, Fitz C R 1983 Focal ischemic cerebral injury in the newborn: diagnosis by ultrasound and correlation with computed tomographic scans. Pediatrics 71:790–793.

Hoon A H, Lawrie W T, Melhelm E R et al 2002 Diffusion tensor imaging of periventricular leukomalacia shows affected sensory cortex white matter pathways. Neurology 59:752–756.

Hope P J, Gould S J, Howard S et al 1988 Ultrasound diagnosis of pathologically verified lesions in the brains of very preterm infants. Dev Med Child Neurol 30:457–471.

Horsch S, Muentjes C, Franz A, Roll C 2005 Ultrasound diagnosis of brain atrophy is related to neurodevelopmental outcome in preterm infants. Acta Paediatr 94(12):1815–1821.

Hoyme H E, Jones K L, Dixon S D et al 1990 Prenatal cocaine exposure and fetal vascular disruption. Pediatrics 85:743–747.

Hunt R W, Badawi N, Laing S et al 2001 Pre-eclampsia: a predisposing factor for neonatal venous sinus thrombosis? Pediatr Neurol 25:242–246.

Iai M, Tanabe Y, Goto M et al 1994 A comparative magnetic resonance imaging study of the corpus callosum in neurologically normal children and children with spastic diplegia. Acta Paediatr 83:1086–1090.

Iida K 1993 Neuropathologic study of newborns with prenatal-onset leukomalacia. Paediatr Neurol 9:45–48.

Iida K, Takashima S, Takeuchi Y 1992 Etiologies and distribution of neonatal leukomalacia. Pediatr Neurol 8:205–209.

Ikonen R S, Janas M O, Koivikko M J et al 1992 Hyperbilirubinaemia, hypocarbia and periventricular leukomalacia in preterm infants: relationship to cerebral palsy. Acta Paediatr Scand 81:802–807.

Ikonen R S, Kuusinen E J, Janas M O 1988 Possible etiological factors in extensive periventricular leukomalacia of preterm infants. Acta Paediatr Scand 77:489–495.

Inder T E, Wells S J, Mogridge N B et al 2003 Defining the nature of the cerebral abnormalities in the premature infant: a qualitative magnetic resonance imaging study. J Pediatr 143:171–179.

Inder T, Hüppi P, Zientara G P et al 1999a Early detection of periventricular leukomalacia by diffusion-weighted magnetic resonance imaging techniques. J Pediatr 134:631–634.

Inder T, Hüppi P, Zientara G P et al 1999b The postmigrational development of polymicrogyria documented by magnetic resonance imaging from 31 weeks' postconceptional age. Ann Neurol 45:798–801.

Ito J, Saijo H, Araki A et al 1996 Assessment of visuoperceptual disturbance in children with spastic diplegia using measurements of the lateral ventricles on cerebral MRI. Dev Med Child Neurol 38:496–502.

Jacobsen L, Ek U, Fernell et al 1996 Visual impairment in preterm children with periventricular leukomalacia – visual, cognitive and neuropaediatric characteristics related to cerebral imaging. Dev Med Child Neurol 38:724–735.

Jan M M, Camfield P R 1998 Outcome of neonatal stroke in full-term infants without significant birth asphyxia. Eur J Pediatr 157:846–848.

Jelinski S E, Yager J Y, Juurlink B H J 1999 Preferential injury of oligo-dendroglioblasts by a short hypoxic-ischemic insult. Brain Res 815:150–153.

Jongmans M, Henderson S, de Vries L S, Dubowitz L M S 1993 Duration of periventricular densities in preterm infants and neurological outcome at six years. Arch Dis Childhood 69:9–13.

Kadhim H, Khalifa M, Deltenre P et al 2006 Molecular mechanisms of cell death in periventricular leukomalacia. Neurology 25,67(2):293–299.

Kahn M A, De Vellis J 1994 Regulation of an oligodendrocyte progenitor cell line by the interleukin-6 family of cytokines. Glia 12:87–98.

Kato T, Okumura A, Hayakawa F et al 2005 The evolutionary change of flash visual evoked potentials in preterm infants with periventricular leukomalacia. Clin Neurophysiol 116(3):690–695.

Kaukola T, Herva R, Perhomaa M et al 2006 Population cohort associating chorioamnionitis, cord inflammatory cytokines and neurologic outcome in very preterm, extremely low birth weight infants. Pediatric Research 59(3):478–483.

Kirton A, Shroff M, Visvanathan T, deVeber G 2007 Quantified corticospinal tract diffusion restriction predicts neonatal stroke outcome. Stroke 38(3):974–980.

Koeda T, Takeshita K 1992 Visuo-perceptual impairment and cerebral lesions in spastic diplegia with preterm birth. Brain Devel 14:239–244.

Koelfen W, Freud M, Varnholt V 1995 Neonatal stroke involving the middle cerebral artery in term infants: clinical presentation, EEG and imaging studies, and outcome. Dev Med Child Neurol 37:204–212.

Koelfen W, Freund M, Koming S et al 1993 Results of parenchymal and angiographic magnetic resonance imaging and neuropsychological testing of children after stroke as neonates. Eur J Pediatr 152:1030–1035.

Kuban K C K, Gilles F H 1985 Human telencephalic angiogenesis. Ann Neurol 17:539–548.

Kuban S, Sanocka U, Leviton A et al 1999 White matter disorders of prematurity: association with intraventricular hemorrhage and ventriculomegaly. J Pediatr 134:539–546.

Kubota T, Okumura A, Hayakawa F et al 2001 Relation between the date of cyst formation observable on ultrasonography and the timing of injury determined by serial electroencephalography in preterm infants with periventricular leukomalacia. Brain Dev 23(6):390–394.

Kurnik K, Kosch A, Strater R et al 2003 Childhood Stroke Study Group. Recurrent thromboembolism in infants and children suffering from symptomatic neonatal arterial stroke: a prospective follow-up study. Stroke 34(12):2887–2892.

Lanzi G, Fazzi E, Uggetti C et al 1998 Cerebral visual impairment in periventricular leukomalacia. Neuropediatrics 29:145–150.

Larroche J-C 1977 Developmental pathology of the neonate. Excerpta Medica, Amsterdam.

Larroche J-C 1984 Perinatal brain damage. In: Adams J H, Corsellis J A N, Duchen L W (eds) Greenfield's neuropathology, 4th edn. Edward Arnold, London.

Larroche J-C 1986 Fetal encephalopathies of circulatory origin. Biol Neonate 50:61–74.

Larroche J-C, Bethmann O, Beadoin M, Couhard M 1986 Brain damage in the premature infant: early lesions and new aspects of sequelae. Italian J Neurol Sciences (suppl) 5:43–52.

Lee J, Croen L A, Backstrand K H et al (2005 Maternal and infant characteristics associated with perinatal arterial stroke in the infant. JAMA 293:723–729.

Leech R W, Alvord E C 1974 Morphologic variation in periventricular leukomalacia. Am J Pathol 74:591–600.

Lequin MH, Peeters EA, Holscher HC et al 2004 Arterial infarction caused by carotid artery dissection in the neonate. Eur J Paediatr Neurol 8(3):155–160.

Leroux P, Hennebert O, Legros H et al 2007 Role of tissue-plasminogen activator (t-PA) in a mouse model of neonatal white matter lesions: Interaction with plasmin inhibitors and anti-inflammatory drugs Neuroscience. Epub

Levene M 2007 Minimising neonatal brain injury: how research in the past five years has changed my clinical practice. Arch Dis Child 92:261–265.

Levene M I 1987 Neonatal neurology. Churchill Livingstone, Edinburgh.

Levene M I, Dowling S, Graham M et al 1992 Impaired motor function (clumsiness) in 5 year old children: correlation with neonatal ultrasound scans. Arch Dis Child 67:687–690.

Levene M I, Trounce J Q 1986 Cause of neonatal convulsions: towards more precise diagnosis. Arch Dis Child 61:78–79.

Levene M I, Wigglesworth J S, Dubowitz V 1983 Hemorrhagic periventricular leukomalacia: a real-time ultrasound study. Pediatrics 71:794–797.

Leviton A, Gilles F 1996 Ventriculomegaly, delayed myelination, white matter hypoplasia, and 'periventricular' leukomalacia: how are they related? Pediatr Neurol 15:127–136.

Leviton A, Gilles F H 1984 Acquired perinatal leukoencephalopathy. Ann Neurol 16:1–8.

Leviton A, Paneth N, Reuss M L et al 1999 Hypothyroxinaemia of prematurity and the risk of cerebral white matter damage. J Pediatr 134:706–711.

Levy S R, Abrams I F, Marshall P C, Rosquette E E 1985 Seizures and cerebral infarction in the full-term newborn. Ann Neurol 17:366–370.

Lewine J D, Stur R S, Davis L E et al 1994 Cortical organization in adulthood is modified by neonatal infarct: A case study. Radiology 190:93–96.

Lien J M, Towers C V, Quilligan E J et al 1995 Term early-onset neonatal seizures: obstetric characteristics, etiologic classifications, and perinatal care. Obstet Gynecol 85:163–169.

Lou H C, Lassen N A, Friis-Hansen B 1979 Impaired autoregulation of cerebral blood flow in the distressed newborn infant. J Pediatr 94:118–121.

Lutschg J, Hanggeli C, Huber P 1983 The evolution of cerebral hemispheric lesions due to pre- or perinatal asphyxia (clinical and neuroradiological correlation). Helvet Paediatr Acta 38:245–254.

Lynch J K, Nelson K B 2001 Epidemiology of perinatal stroke. Curr Opin Pediatr 13:499–505.

Maalouf E F, Duggan P J, Counsell S J et al 2001 Comparison of findings on cranial ultrasound and magnetic resonance imaging in preterm infants. Pediatrics 107:719–727.

Maalouf E F, Duggan P J, Rutherford M A et al 1999 Magnetic resonance imaging of the brain in a cohort of extremely preterm infants. J Pediatr 135:351–357.

McMenamin J B, Shackelford G D, Volpe J J 1984 Outcome of neonatal IVH with periventricular echodense lesions. Ann Neurol 15:285–290.

Mannino F L, Trauner D A 1983 Stroke in neonates. J Pediatr 102:605–610.

Mantovani J F, Gerber G J 1984 'Idiopathic' neonatal cerebral infarction. Am J Dis Child 138:359–362.

Marin-Padilla M 1997 Developmental neuropathology and impact of perinatal brain damage. II: White matter lesions of the neocortex. J Neuropathol Exp Neurol 56:219–235.

Marret S, Bonnier C, Raymackers J M et al 1999 Glycine antagonist and NO synthase inhibitor protect the developing mouse brain against neonatal excitotoxic lesions. Pediatr Res 45:337–342.

Marret S, Parain D, Jeannot E et al 1992 Positive rolandic sharp waves in the EEG of the premature newborn: a five year prospective study. Arch Dis Child 67:948–951.

Marret S, Parain D, Ménard J F et al 1997 Prognostic value of neonatal electroencephalography in premature newborns less than 33 weeks of gestational age. Electroencephalogr Clin Neurophysiol 102:178–185.

Marret S, Parain D, Samson-Dollfus D et al 1986 Positive rolandic sharp waves and periventricular leukomalacia in the newborn. Neuropediatrics 17:199–202.

Martin D J, Hill A, Fitz C R et al 1983 Hypoxic/ischemic cerebral injury in the neonatal brain: a report of monographic features with computed tomographic correlation. Pediatr Radiol 13:307–312.

Matsuda T, Okuyama K, Cho K et al 1999 Induction of antenatal periventricular leukomalacia by hemorrhagic hypotension in the chronically instrumented fetal sheep. Am J Obstet Gynecol 181:725–730.

Medja F, Lelievre V, Fontaine R H et al 2006 Thiorphan, a neutral endopeptidase inhibitor used for diarrhoea, is neuroprotective in newborn mice. Brain 129(Pt 12):3209–3223.

Melhem E R, Hoon A H, Ferrucci J T et al 2000 Periventricular leukomalacia: relationship between lateral ventricular volume on brain MR images and severity of cognitive and motor impairment. Radiology 214:199–204.

Meng S Z, Arai Y, Deguchi K, Takashima S 1997 Early detection of axonal and neuronal lesions in prenatal-onset periventricular leukomalacia. Brain Dev 19:480–484.

Meng S Z, Takashima S 1999 Expression of transforming growth factor-beta 1 in periventricular leukomalacia. J Child Neurol 14:377–381.

Ment L R, Duncan C C, Ehrenkrantz R A 1984 Perinatal cerebral infarction. Ann Neurol 16:559–568.

Ment L R, Stewart W B, Duncan C C et al 1985a Beagle puppy model of perinatal cerebral infarction: acute changes in cerebral blood flow and metabolism during hemorrhagic hypotension. J Neurosurg 63:441–447.

Ment L R, Stewart W B, Duncan C C et al 1985b Beagle puppy model of perinatal cerebral infarction: acute changes in cerebral prostaglandins during hemorrhagic hypotension. J Neurosurg 63:899–904.

Ment L R, Vohr B, Allan W et al 1999 The etiology and outcome of cerebral ventriculomegaly at term in very low birth weight preterm infants. Pediatrics 104:243–248.

Mercuri E, Atkinson J, Braddick O et al 1996 Visual function and perinatal focal cerebral infarction. Arch Dis Child 75:F76–F81.

Mercuri E, Barnett A, Rutherford M et al 2004 Neonatal cerebral infarction and neuromotor outcome at school age. Pediatrics 113:95–100.

Mercuri E, Cowan F 1999 Cerebral infarction in the newborn infant: review of the literature and personal experience. Eur J Paediatr Neurol 3:255–263.

Mercuri E, Cowan F, Rutherford M A et al 1995 Ischaemic and haemorrhagic brain lesions in newborns with seizures and normal Apgar scores. Arch Dis Child 73:F67–F74.

Mercuri E, Rutherford M A, Cowan F et al 1999 Early prognostic indicators of outcome in infants with neonatal cerebral infarction: a clinical, electroencephalogram, and magnetic resonance imaging study. Pediatrics 103:39–44.

Messer J, Haddad J, Casanova R 1991 Transcranial Doppler evaluation of cerebral infarction in the neonate. Neuropediatrics 22:147–151.

Miller S P, Cozzio C C, Goldstein R B et al 2003 Comparing the diagnosis of white matter injury in premature newborns with serial MR imaging and transfontanel ultrasonography findings. AJNR Am J Neuroradiol 24(8):1661–1669.

Miller S P, Ferriero D M, Leonard C et al 2005 Early brain injury in premature newborns detected with magnetic resonance imaging is associated with adverse early neurodevelopmental outcome. J Pediatr 147(5):609–616.

Miller S P, Vigneron D B, Henry R G et al 2002 Serial quantitative diffusion tensor MRI of the premature brain: development in newborns with and without injury. J Magn Reson Imaging 16(6):621–632.

Monagle P, Chan A, Massicotte P et al 2004 Antithrombotic therapy in children: the Seventh ACCP Conference on antithrombotic and thrombolytic therapy. Chest 126 (3 Suppl):645S–687S.

Monset-Couchard M, de Bethmann O, Radvyani-Bouvet M-F et al 1988 Neurodevelopmental outcome in cystic periventricular leukomalacia (CPVL) (30 cases). Neuropediatrics 19:124–131.

Moody D M, Bell M A, Challa V R 1990 Anatomic features of the cerebral vascular pattern that predict vulnerability to perfusion or oxygenation deficiency. Am J Neuroradiol 11:431–439.

Mukherjee P, Miller J H, Shimony J S et al 2002 Diffusion-tensor MR imaging of gray and white matter development during normal human brain maturation. AJNR Am J Neuroradiol 23, 9:1445–1456.

Murphy C R, Bell E F, Sato Y, Klein J M 2007 Periventricular leukomalacia and prenatal methamphetamine exposure: a case report. Am J Perinatol 24(2):123–126.

Murphy D J, Squier M V, Hope P L et al 1996 Clinical associations and time of onset of cerebral white matter damage in very preterm babies. Arch Dis Child 75:F27–F32.

Nanni G S, Kaude J V, Reeder J D 1984 Ischemic brain infarct in a neonate: ultrasound diagnosis and follow-up. J Clin Ultrasound 12:229–231.

Nelson K B, Ellenberg J H 1985 Antecedents of cerebral palsy. I. Univariate analysis of risk factors. N Engl J Med 315:81–86.

Nelson K B, Grether J K 1995 Can magnesium sulfate reduce the risk of cerebral palsy in very low birthweight infants? Pediatrics Feb, 95(2):263–269.

Nelson K B, Grether J K, Dambrosia J M et al 2003 Neonatal cytokines and cerebral palsy in very preterm infants. Pediatr Res 53(4):600–607.

Nelson K B, Lynch J K 2004 Stroke in newborn infants. Lancet Neurol 3:150–158.

Nelson M D, Gonzalez-Gomez I, Gilles F H 1991 The search for human telencephalic ventriculofugal arteries. Am J Neuroradiol 12:215–222.

O'Brien M J, Ash J M, Gilday D L 1979 Radionucleide brain scanning in perinatal hypoxia. Dev Med Child Neurol 21:161–168.

O'Shea T M, Klinepeter K L, Dillard R G 1998b Prenatal events and the risk of cerebral palsy in very low birth weight infants. Am J Epidemiol 147:362–369.

O'Shea T M, Klinepeter K L, Meis P J, Dillard R G 1998a Intrauterine infection and the risk of cerebral palsy in very low-birth weight infants. Paediatr Perinat Epidemiol 12:72–83.

O'Shea T M, Kothadia J M, Klinepeter K L et al 1999 Randomized placebo-controlled trial of a 42 day tapering course of dexamethasone to reduce the duration of ventilator dependency in very low birth weight infants: outcome of study participants at 1-year adjusted age. Pediatrics 104:15–21.

Ohyu J, Marumo G, Ozawa H et al 1999 Early axonal and glial pathology in fetal sheep brains with leukomalacia induced by repeated umbilical cord occlusion. Brain Dev 21:248–252.

Oka A, Belliveau M J, Rosenberg P A, Volpe J J 1993 Vulnerability of oligodendroglia to glutamate: pharmacology, mechanisms and prevention. J Neurosci 13:1441–1453.

Okamura M, Itakura A, Kurauchi O et al 1997 Fetal heart rate patterns associated with periventricular leukomalacia. Int J Gynecol Obstet 56:13–18.

Okumura A, Hayakawa F, Kato T et al 1999a Correlation between the serum level of endotoxin and periventricular leukomalacia in preterm infants. Brain Dev 21:378–381.

Okumura A, Hayakawa F, Kato T et al 1999b Positive Rolandic sharp waves in preterm infants with periventricular leukomalacia: their relation to background electroencephalographic abnormalities. Neuropediatrics 30:278–282.

Okumura A, Hayakawa F, Kato T et al 2001 Hypocarbia in preterm infants with periventricular leukomalacia: the relation between hypocarbia and mechanical ventilation. Pediatrics 107(3):469–475.

Opsjln S L, Wathen N C, Tingulstad S et al 1993 Tumor necrosis factor, interleukin-1, and interleukin-6 in normal human pregnancy. Am J Obstet Gynecol 169:397–404.

Ozawa H, Nishida A, Mito T, Takashima S 1994 Development of ferritin-positive cells in cerebrum of human brain. Pediatr Neurol 10:44–48.

Palmer P, Dubowitz L M S, Levene M I, Dubowitz V 1982 Developmental and neurological progress of preterm infants with intraventricular haemorrhage and ventricular dilatation. Arch Dis Child 57:748–753.

Paneth N 1999 Classifying brain damage in preterm infants. J Pediatr 134:527–529.

Paneth N, Rudelli R, Kazam E et al 1994 Associated pathological lesions: cerebellar haemorrhage, pontosubicular necrosis, basal ganglia necrosis. Clin Dev Med 131:163–174.

Paneth N, Rudelli R, Monte W et al 1990 White matter necrosis in very low birth weight infants: neuropathologic and ultrasonographic findings in infants surviving six days or longer. J Pediatr 116:975–984.

Pape K E, Wigglesworth J S 1979 Haemorrhage, ischaemia and the perinatal brain. Clin Dev Med 69/70.

Papile L-A, Tyson J E, Stoll B J et al 1998 A multicenter trial of two dexamethasone regimens in ventilator-dependent premature infants. N Engl J Med 333:1112–1118.

Parrot J 1873 Etude sur la ramollissement de l'encephale chez la nouveau-né. Arch Physiol Norm Pathol 5:59–73, 176–195, 283–330.

Partridge J C, Babcock D S, Steichen J J, Bokyung K H 1983 Optimal timing for diagnostic ultrasound in low birth weight infants for detection of intracranial haemorrhage and ventricular dilatation. J Pediatr 102:281–287.

Partridge S C, Mukherjee P, Henry R G et al 2004 Diffusion tensor imaging: serial quantitation of white matter tract maturity in premature newborns. Neuroimage 22, 3:1302–1314.

Paul D A, Coleman M M, Leef K H et al 2003 Maternal antibiotics and decreased periventricular leukomalacia in very low-birth-weight infants. Arch Pediatr Adolesc Med 157(2):145–149.

Perlman J M, Risser R 1998 Relationship of uric acid concentrations and severe intraventricular haemorrhage/leukomalacia in the premature infant. J Pediatr 132:436–439.

Perlman J M, Risser R, Broyles R S 1996 Bilateral cystic periventricular leukomalacia in the premature infant: associated risk factors. Pediatrics 97:822–827.

Perlman J M, Rollins N K, Evans D 1994 Neonatal stroke: clinical characteristics and cerebral blood flow velocity measurements. Pediatr Neurol 11:281–284.

Pfister-Goedeke L, Boltshauser E 1982 Postnatale Entwicklung einer multilokularen zystischen Enczephalopathie beim Neugeborenen. Helvet Paediatr Acta 37:59–65.

Pidcock F S, Graziani L J, Stanley C et al 1990 Neurosonographic features of periventricular echodensities associated with cerebral palsy in preterm infants. J Pediatr 116:417–422.

Pierrat V, Duquennoy C, van Haastert I C et al 2001 Ultrasound diagnosis and neurodevelopmental outcome of localised and extensive cystic periventricular leucomalacia. Arch Dis Child Fetal Neonatal Ed 84(3):F151–F156.

Pierrat V, Eken P, Duquennoy C et al 1993 Prognostic value of early somatosensory evoked potentials in neonates with cystic leukomalacia. Dev Med Child Neurol 35:683–690.

Pinto-Martin J, Riolo S, Cnaan A et al 1995 Cranial ultrasound prediction of disabling and non-disabling cerebral palsy at age two in a low birth weight population. Pediatrics 95:249–254.

Pisani F, Leali L, Moretti S et al 2006 Transient periventricular echodensities in preterms and neurodevelopmental outcome. J Child Neurol 21(3):230–235.

Ramaswamy V, Miller S P, Barkovich A J et al 2004 Perinatal stroke in term infants with neonatal encephalopathy. Neurology 8,62(11):2088–2091.

Ramenghi L A, Fumagalli M, Righini A et al 2007 Magnetic resonance imaging assessment of brain maturation in preterm neonates with punctate white matter lesions. Neuroradiology 49(2):161–167.

Rao K C V G, Knipp H C, Wagner E J 1981 Computed tomographic findings in cerebral sinus and venous thrombosis. Radiology 140:391–398.

Resch B, Jammernegg A, Perl E et al 2006 Correlation of grading and duration of periventricular echodensities with neurodevelopmental outcome in preterm infants. Pediatr Radiol,36(8):810–815.

Reuter J H, Disney T A 1986 Regional cerebral blood flow and cerebral metabolic rate of oxygen during hyperventilation in the newborn dog. Pediatric Research 20:1102–1106.

Ricci D, Anker S, Cowan F et al 2006b Thalamic atrophy in infants with PVL and cerebral visual impairment. Early Hum Dev 82(9):591–595.

Ricci D, Cowan F, Pane M et al 2006a Neurological examination at 6 to 9 months in infants with cystic periventricular leukomalacia. Neuropediatrics 37(4):247–252.

Riddle A, Luo N L, Manese M et al 2006 Spatial heterogeneity in oligodendrocyte lineage maturation and not cerebral blood flow predicts fetal ovine periventricular white matter injury. J Neurosci 26(11):3045–3055.

Ringelberg J, van der Bor M 1993 Outcome of transient periventricular echodensities in preterm infants. Neuropediatrics 24:269–273.

Rivkin M J, Anderson M L, Kaye E M 1992 Neonatal idiopathic cerebral venous thrombosis: an unrecognized cause of transient seizures or lethargy. Ann Neurol 32:51–56.

Rodriguez, Claus D, Verellen G, Lyon G 1990 Periventricular leukomalacia: ultrasonic and neuropathological correlations. Dev Med Child Neurol 32:347–355.

Roelants-van Rijn A M, Groenendaal F, Beek F J et al 2001 Parenchymal brain injury in the preterm infant: comparison of cranial ultrasound, MRI and neurodevelopmental outcome. Neuropediatrics 32:80–89.

Roelants-van Rijn A M, Nikkels P G J, Groenendaal F et al 2001 Neonatal diffusion weighted MR imaging: relation with histopathology or follow-up MR examination. Neuropediatrics 32:286–294.

Rogers B, Msall M, Owens T et al 1994 Cystic periventricular leukomalacia and type of cerebral palsy in preterm infants. J Pediatr 125:S1–S8.

Roland E H, Flodmark O, Hill A 1990 Thalamic hemorrhage with intraventricular hemorrhage in the full-term newborn. Pediatrics 85(5):737–742.

Rollins N K, Morriss M C, Evans D, Perlman J M 1994 The role of early MR in the evaluation of the term infant with seizures. Am J Neuroradiol 15:239–248.

Roodhooft A M, Parizel P M, Van Acker K J et al 1987 Idiopathic cerebral arterial infarction with paucity of symptoms in the full-term neonate. Pediatrics 80:381–385.

Rothwell N J, Loddick S A, Stroemer P 1997 Interleukins and cerebral ischaemia. Int Rev Neurobiol 40:281–298.

Rushton D I, Preston P R, Durbin G M 1985 Structure and evolution of echodense lesions in the neonatal brain. Arch Dis Child 60:798–808.

Russell G A, Cooke R W 1995 Randomised controlled trial of allopurinol prophylaxis in very preterm infants. Arch Dis Child Fetal Neonatal Edn 73: F27–F31.

Rydhstrom H, Ingemarsson I 1993 Prognosis and long-term follow-up of a twin after antenatal death of the co-twin. J Reprod Med 38:142–146.

Saphiro H M, Greenberg J H, Van Horn Naughton K, Reivich M 1980 Heterogeneity of local cerebral blood flow — p_aCO_2 sensitivity in neonatal dogs. J App Physiol 49:113–118.

Scher M S, Dobson V, Carpenter N A, Guthrie R D 1989 Visual and neurological outcome of infants with periventricular leukomalacia. Dev Med Child Neurol 31:353–365.

Schouman-Claeys E, Henry-Feugeas M C, Roset F et al 1993 Periventricular leukomalacia: correlation between MR imaging and autopsy findings during the first 2 months of life. Radiology 189:59–64.

Seghier M L, Lazeyras F, Zimine S et al 2005 Visual recovery after perinatal stroke evidenced by functional and diffusion MRI: case report. BMC Neurol 26,5:17.

Shankaran S, Langer JC, Kazzi SN et al 2006 Cumulative index of exposure to hypocarbia and hyperoxia as risk factors for periventricular leukomalacia in low birth weight infants. Pediatrics. 118:1654–1659.

Shinwell E S, Karplus M, Reich D et al 2000 Early postnatal dexamethasone therapy is associated with increased incidence of cerebral palsy. Arch Dis Child Fetal and Neonat Ed 83:F177–F186.

Shuman R M, Selednik L J 1980 Periventricular leukomalacia: a one year autopsy study. Arch Neurol 37:231–235.

Sie L T L, van der Knaap M S, van Wezel-Meyler G et al 2000 Early magnetic resonance imaging compared to ultrasound in neonates with periventricular leukomalacia. Am J Neurorad 21:852–861.

Silver R K, MacGregor S N, Pasternak, Neely S E 1992 Fetal stroke associated with elevated maternal anticardiolipin antibodies. Obstet Gynecol 80:497–499.

Sims M E, Beckwitt Turkel S et al 1985 Brain injury and intrauterine death. Am J Obstet Gynecol 151:721–723.

Sinha S K, D'Souza S W, Rivlin E, Chiswick M L 1990 Ischaemic brain lesions diagnosed at birth in preterm infants: clinical events and developmental outcome. Arch Dis Child 65:1017–1020.

Sinha S K, Davies J M, Sims D G, Chiswick M L 1985 Relation between periventricular haemorrhage and ischaemic brain lesions diagnosed by ultrasound in very preterm infants. Lancet ii:1154–1155.

Smith C D, Baumann R J 1991 Clinical features and magnetic resonance imaging in congenital and childhood stroke. J Child Neurol 6:263–272.

Smith S M, Jenkinson M, Johansen-Berg H et al 2006 Tract-based spatial statistics: voxel-wise analysis of multi-subject diffusion data. NeuroImage 31(4):1487–1505.

Soman T B, Moharir M, DeVeber G et al 2006 Infantile spasms as an adverse outcome of neonatal cortical sinovenous thrombosis. J Child Neurol 21(2):126–131.

Song S K, Sun S W, Ramsbottom M J et al 2003 Dysmyelination revealed through MRI as increased radial (but unchanged axial) diffusion of water. Neuroimage 17:1429–1436.

Spinillo A, Capuzzo E, Stronati M et al 1998 Obstetric risk factors for periventricular leukomalacia among preterm infants. Br J Obstet Gynaecol 105:865–871.

Sran S K, Baumann R J 1988 Outcome of neonatal strokes. Am J Dis Child 142:1086–1088.

Staudt M, Braun C, Gerloff C et al 2006 Developing somatosensory projections bypass periventricular brain lesions. Neurology 67:522–525.

Staudt M, Gerloff C, Grodd W et al 2004 Reorganization in congenital hemiparesis acquired at different gestational ages. Ann Neurol 56:854–863.

Staudt M, Grodd W, Gerloff C, 2002 Two types of ipsilateral reorganization in congenital hemiparesis: a TMS and fMRI study. Brain 125:2222–2237.

Steinlin M, Pfister I, Pavlovic J et al The Swiss Societies of Paediatric Neurology and Neonatology 2005 The first three years of the Swiss Neuropaediatric Stroke Registry (SNPSR): a population-based study of incidence, symptoms and risk factors Neuropediatrics 36:90–97.

Stevenson D K, Wright L L, Lemons J A et al 1998 Very low birth weight outcomes of the National Institute of Child Health and Human Development Neonatal Research Network, January 1993 through December 1994. Am J Obstet Gynecol 179:1632–1639.

Stewart A L, Thorburn R J, Hope P L et al 1983 Ultrasound appearance of the brain in very preterm infants and neurodevelopmental outcome at 18 months of age. Arch Dis Child 58:598–604.

Suzuki Y, Matsuzawa H, Kwee IL,, Nakada T 2003 Absolute eigenvalue diffusion tensor analysis for human brain maturation. NMR Biomed 16:257–260.

Szymonowicz W, Preston H, Yu V Y H 1986 The surviving monozygotic twin. Arch Dis Child 61:454–458.

Szymonowicz W, Yu V Y H, Wilson F E 1984 Antecedents of periventricular haemorrhage in infants weighing 1250 grams or less at birth. Arch Dis Child 59:13–17.

Taboada D, Alonso A, Olague R et al 1980 Radiological diagnosis of periventricular and subcortical leukomalacia. Neuroradiology 20:33–41.

Takashima J, Armstrong D, Becker L E 1978 Subcortical leukomalacia: relationship to development of the cerebral sulcus and its vascular supply. Arch Neurol 35:470–472.

Takashima J, Tanaka K 1978 Development of cerebral architecture and its relationship to periventricular leukomalacia. Arch Neurol 35:11–16.

Takashima S, Iida K, Deguchi K 1995 Periventricular leukomalacia, glial development and myelination. Early Hum Dev 43:177–184.

Taylor G A 1994 Alterations in regional cerebral blood flow in neonatal stroke: preliminary findings with color Doppler sonography. Pediatr Radiol 24:111–115.

Thomas B, Eyssen M, Peeters R et al 2005 Quantitative diffusion tensor imaging in cerebral palsy due to periventricular white matter injury. Brain 128:2562–2577.

Thorarensen O, Ryan S, Hunter J et al 1997 Factor V Leiden mutation: an unrecognized cause of hemiplegic cerebral palsy, neonatal stroke and placental thrombosis. Ann Neurol 42:372–375.

Thorburn R J, Lipscomb A P, Stewart A L et al 1981 Prediction of death and major handicap in very preterm infants by brain ultrasound. Lancet i:1119–1121.

Townsend S F, Rumack C M, Thilo E H et al 1999 Late neurosonographic screening is important to the diagnosis of periventricular leukomalacia and ventricular enlargement in preterm infants. Pediatr Radiol 29:347–352.

Trauner D A, Chase C, Walker P, Wulfeck B 1993 Neurologic profiles of infants and children after perinatal stroke. Pediatr Neurol 9:383–386.

Trauner D A, Mannino F L 1986 Neurodevelopmental outcome after neonatal cerebrovascular incident. J Pediatr 108:459–461.

Trounce J Q, Fagan D, Levene M I 1986b Intraventricular haemorrhage and periventricular leukomalacia: ultrasound and autopsy correlation. Arch Dis Child 62:1203–1207.

Trounce J Q, Levene M I 1985 Diagnosis and outcome of subcortical cystic leukomalacia. Arch Dis Child 60:1041–1044.

Trounce J Q, Rutter N, Levene M I 1986a Periventricular leucomalacia and intraventricular haemorrhage in the preterm neonate. Arch Dis Child 61:1196–1202.

Trounce J Q, Shaw O E, Levene M I, Rutter N 1988 Clinical risk factors and periventricular leucomalacia. Arch Dis Child 63:17–22.

Tsuji M, Saul J P, du Plessis A, Eichenwald E et al 2000 Cerebral intravascular oxygenation correlates with mean arterial pressure in critically ill premature infants. Pediatrics 106(4):625–632.

Tsuru A, Mizuguchi M, Takashima S 1995 Cystic leukomalacia in the cerebellar folia of premature infants. Acta Neuropathologica 90:400–402.

Tzogalis D, Fawer C L, Wong Y, Calame A 1988 Risk factors associated with the development of peri-intraventricular haemorrhage and periventricular leukomalacia. Helvetica Paediatrica Acta 43:363–376.

Uehara H, Yoshioka H, Kawase S et al 1999 A new model of white matter injury in neonatal rats with bilateral carotid artery occlusion. Brain Res 837:213–220.

Uggetti C, Egitto M G, Fazzi E et al 1996 Cerebral visual impairment in periventricular leukomalacia: MR correlation. Am J Neuroradiol 17:979–985.

Van de Bor M, van Zeben-van der A T M, Verloove-Vanhoorick S P et al 1989 Hyperbilirubinemia in preterm infants and neurodevelopmental outcome at 2 years of age: results of a national collaborative survey. Pediatrics 83:915–920.

Van den Bergh R 1969 The periventricular intracerebral blood supply. In: Meyer J, Lechner H, Eichhorn O (eds) Research of the cerebral circulation. Charles C Thomas, Springfield, IL, pp. 52–65.

Van den Hout B M, Eken P, van der Linden D et al 1998 Visual, cognitive and neurodevelopmental outcome at 5½ years in children with perinatal haemorrhagic- ischaemic brain lesions. Dev Med Child Neurol 40:820–828.

Van Wezel-Meijler G, van der Knaap M S, Oosting J et al 1999 Predictive value of neonatal MRI as compared to ultrasound in premature infants with mild periventricular white matter changes. Neuropediatrics 30:231–238.

Van Wezel-Meijler G, van der Knaap M S, Sie L T L et al 1998 Magnetic resonance imaging of the brain in premature infants during the neonatal period. Normal phenomena and reflection of mild ultrasound abnormalities. Neuropediatrics 129:89–96.

Vannucci R C, Brucklacher R M, Vannucci S 1997 Effect of carbon dioxide on cerebral metabolism during hypoxia-ischemia in the immature rat. Pediatric Res 42:24–29.

Vannucci R C, Towfighi J, Heitjan D F, Brucklacher R M 1995 Carbon dioxide protects the perinatal brain from hypoxic-ischemic damage: an experimental study in the immature rat. Pediatrics 95:868–874.

Varelas P N, Sleight B J, Rinder H M et al 1998 Stroke in a neonate heterozygous for factor V Leiden. Pediatr Neurol 18:262–264.

Verma U, Tejani N, Klein S et al 1997 Am J Obstet Gynecol 176:275–281.

Victor S, Appleton R E, Beirne M et al 2005 Effect of carbon dioxide on background cerebral electrrical activity and fractional oxygen extraction in very low birth weight infants just after birth. Pediatr Res 58:579–585.

Virchow R 1867 Zur pathologishen Anatomie des Gehirns. I. Congenitale Enzephalitis und Myelitis. Virchows Archiv 38:129–142.

Volpe J J 1992 Effect of cocaine use on the fetus. N Engl J Med 327:399–407.

Volpe J J 2003 Cerebral white matter injury of the premature infant – more common than you think. Pediatrics 112:176–180.

Voorhies T M, Lipper E G, Lee B C P et al 1984 Occlusive vascular disease in asphyxiated newborn infants. J Pediatr 105:92–96.

Watkins A M C, West C R, Cooke R W I 1989 Blood pressure and cerebral haemorrhage and ischaemia in very low birthweight infants. Early Hum Dev 19:103–110.

Weindling A M, Rochefort M J, Calvert S A et al 1985b Development of cerebral palsy after sonographic detection of periventricular cysts in the newborn. Dev Med Child Neurol 27:800–806.

Weindling A M, Wilkinson A R, Cook J et al 1985a Perinatal events which precede periventricular haemorrhage and leukomalacia in the newborn. Br J Obstet Gynaecol 92:1218–1223.

Welin A K, Svedin P, Lapatto R et al 2007 Melatonin reduces inflammation and cell death in white matter in the mid-gestation fetal sheep following umbilical cord occlusion. Pediatric Research 61(2):153–158.

Wernovsky G, Shillingford A J, Gaynor J W 2005 Central nervous system outcomes in children with complex congenital heart disease. Curr Opin Cardiol 20(2):94–99.

Whitaker A H, Feldman J F, Van Rossem R et al 1996 Neonatal cranial ultrasound abnormalities in low birth weight infants: relation to cognitive outcomes at six years of age. Pediatrics 98:719–729.

Wiswell T E, Graziani L J, Kornhauser M S et al 1996a Effects of hypocarbia on the development of cystic periventricular leukomalacia in premature infants treated with high-frequency jet ventilatation. Pediatrics 98:918–924.

Wiswell T E, Graziani L J, Kornhauser M S et al 1996b High-frequency jet ventilatation in the early management of respiratory distress syndrome is associated with a greater risk for adverse outcomes. Pediatrics 98:1035–1043.

Woodward L J, Anderson P J, Austin N C et al 2006 Neonatal MRI to predict neurodevelopmental outcomes in preterm infants. N Engl J Med 355(7):685–694.

Wu Y W, Croen L A, Shah S J et al 2006 Cerebral palsy in a term population: risk factors and neuroimaging findings. Pediatrics 118:690–697.

Wu Y W, Hamrick S E G, Miller S P et al 2003 Intraventricular hemorrhage in term neonates caused by sinovenous thrombosis. Ann Neurol 54:123–126.

Wu Y W, Miller S P, Chin K et al 2002 Multiple risk factors in neonatal sinovenous thrombosis. Neurology 59:438–440.

Wulfeck B B, Trauner D A, Tallal P A 1991 Neurologic, cognitive and linguistic features of infants after early stroke. Paediatr Neurol 7:266–269.

Yeh T F, Lin Y J, Huang C C et al 1998 Early dexamethasone therapy in premature infants: a follow-up study. Pediatrics 101:e7.

Yokochi K 1997 Thalamic lesions revealed by MR associated with periventricular leukomalacia and clinical profiles of subjects. Acta Paediatrica 86:493–496.

Yokochi K 1998 Clinical profiles of subjects with subcortical leukomalacia and border zone infarction revealed by MRI. Acta Paediatrica 87:879–883.

Yokochi K, Aiba K, Horie M et al 1991 Magnetic resonance imaging in children with spastic diplegia: correlation with the severity of their motor and mental abnormality. Dev Med Child Dev 33:18–25.

Yoon B H, Jun J K, Romero R et al 1997c Amniotic fluid inflammatory cytokines (interleukin-6, interleukin-1 beta and tumor necrosis factor-alpha), neonatal brain white matter lesions and cerebral palsy. Am J Obstet Gynecol 177:19–26.

Yoon B H, Kim C J, Romero R et al 1997a Experimentally induced intrauterine infection causes fetal brain white matter lesions in rabbits. Am J Obstet Gynecol 177:797–802.

Yoon B H, Romero R, Ha Yang S et al 1996 Interleukin-6 concentrations in umbilical cord plasma are elevated in neonates with white matter lesions associated with periventricular leukomalacia. Am J Obstet Gynecol 174:1433–1440.

Yoon B H, Romero R, Kim C J et al 1997b High expression of tumor necrosis factor-alpha and interleukin-6 in periventricular leukomalacia. Am J Obstet Gynecol 177:406–411.

Yoshioka H, Goma H, Ochi M et al 1992 Experimental periventricular leukomalacia in the puppy: neurology, ^{31}P-MRS and neuropathology. Biol Neonate 62:303.

Young R S K, Hernandez M J, Yagel S K 1982 Selective reduction of blood flow to white matter during hypotension in newborn dogs: a possible mechanism of periventricular leukomalacia. Ann Neurol 12:445–448.

Zorzi C, Angonese I, Zaramella P et al 1988 Periventricular intraparenchymal cystic lesions: critical determinant of neurodevelopmental outcome in preterm infants. Helvet Paediatr Acta 43:195–202.

Zupan V, Gonzalez P, Lacaze-Masmonteil T et al 1996 Periventricular leukomalacia: risk factors revisited. Dev Med Child Neurol 38:1061–1067.

CHAPTER
22

Pathophysiology of asphyxia

Laura Bennet, Jennifer A. Westgate, Peter D. Gluckman and Alistair J. Gunn

---

Key Points

- Acute onset of asphyxia is associated with bradycardia, increased systemic blood pressure, but no increase in cerebral blood flow (CBF)
- Progressive moderate asphyxia is associated with a doubling of CBF with no hypotension
- In the primary phase of asphyxial neuronal injury, depolarization occurs leading to Na$^+$ and Ca^{++} entry with cell swelling (cytotoxic edema) and extracellular accumulation of excitatory amino acid neurotransmitters
- In the delayed phase, neuronal necrosis and/or apoptosis occur as the result of a number of intraneuronal biochemical events

---

INTRODUCTION

For most of the 20th century the concept of perinatal brain damage centered on cerebral palsy and intrapartum asphyxia. It is only in the last 20 years that this view has been seriously challenged by clinical and epidemiologic studies which have demonstrated that approximately 70–90% or more of cerebral palsy is unrelated to intrapartum events (MacLennan 1999). Many term infants who subsequently develop cerebral palsy are believed to have sustained asphyxial events in mid-gestation. In some cases, prenatal injury may lead to chronically abnormal heart tracings and impaired ability to adapt to labor which may be confounded with an acute event.

In those infants who do have evidence of an acute, perinatal event, the key link between exposure to asphyxia and subsequent neurodevelopmental impairment is the early onset of neonatal encephalopathy (MacLennan 1999). Newborns with mild encephalopathy are completely normal to follow-up, while all of those with severe (stage III) encephalopathy die or have severe handicap. In contrast, only half of those with moderate (stage II) hypoxic–ischemic encephalopathy develop handicap; however, even those who do not develop neurologic impairment are at risk of future academic failure (Robertson & Finer 1993).

At the same time it has become clear that the predictive value for cerebral palsy of various markers for potentially injurious asphyxia, such as abnormal fetal heart rate tracings, is consistently weak (Nelson et al 1996). For example, more than half of babies born with severe acidosis (base deficit >16 mmol/L and pH < 7.0) do not develop encephalopathy, while conversely encephalopathy can still occur, although at low frequency, in association with relatively modest acidosis (Low 1997). These data contrast with the presence of (very) non-reassuring fetal heart rate tracings and severe metabolic acidosis in those infants who do develop neonatal encephalopathy (Westgate et al 1999).

CHARACTERISTICS OF PERINATAL ASPHYXIAL ENCEPHALOPATHY

Perinatal asphyxial encephalopathy has a number of distinct characteristics that limit extrapolation from studies of the neonatal or adult brain. First, the etiology of the insult is generally global, affecting the whole fetus. Thus the fetal systemic and cardiovascular responses are critical to understanding the pathogenesis of injury. Second, the insult is generally reversible, whether spontaneously or therapeutically (e.g. delivery and resuscitation) and so can be associated with an evolving pattern of cerebral dysfunction and delayed injury after the insult. Third, although the injury may be a single acute episode, it is commonly due to repeated insults. Fourth, many of the insults occur in the stable and warmer thermal environment of the uterus. Finally, the maturity of the brain has a considerable effect on how neurons and glia respond to asphyxia.

It is now understood that the fetal response to asphyxia is not stereotypical, but rather depends upon both the nature of the insult and the condition of the fetus (Fig. 22.1). In fact, it appears that the fetus is spectacularly good at defending itself against such insults, and injury occurs only in a very narrow window between intact survival and death. This chapter focuses on recent developments in our understanding of the factors that determine whether the brain is damaged after an asphyxial insult. We will review the systemic adaptations of the fetus to asphyxia, the underlying cellular mechanisms of cerebral damage and the factors modulating neuronal death.

SYSTEMIC AND CARDIOVASCULAR ADAPTATION TO ASPHYXIA

The systemic adaptations of the fetus to whole body asphyxia are critical to outcome. Although the focus of most of the classic studies in this area was to delineate the cardiovascular and cerebrovascular responses, more recently the relationship between particular patterns of asphyxia and neural outcome has been examined, as summarized in Table 22.1. The great majority of studies of the pathophysiology of asphyxia have been performed in the chronically instrumented fetal sheep, studied in utero.

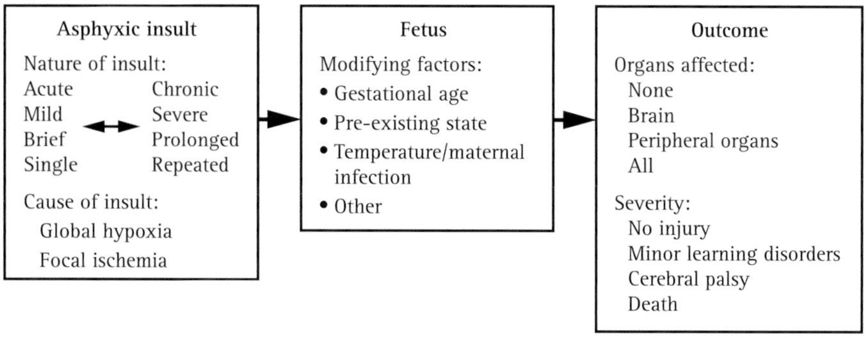

Figure 22.1 Flow diagram of the determinants of cerebral injury after perinatal asphyxia.

ADAPTATIONS TO FETAL LIFE

The fetus is highly adapted to intrauterine conditions, which include low partial pressures of oxygen and relatively limited supply of other substrates compared with postnatal life. The fetus cannot store oxygen and is wholly dependent on a steady supply, but the fetus normally exists with a surplus of oxygen relative to its metabolic needs. This surplus provides a significant margin of safety when oxygen delivery is impaired. For the fetus hypoxia is perhaps the greatest challenge to its wellbeing in utero and consequently the fetus has several adaptive features, some unique to the fetus, which help it to defend itself from injury. These adaptive features include: higher blood flow to organs; left shift of the oxygen dissociation curve which increases the capacity to carry oxygen and oxygen extraction at typical oxygen tensions; the capacity to significantly reduce energy-consuming processes; greater anaerobic capacity in many tissues, and the capacity to redistribute blood flow towards essential organs away from the periphery. During hypoxia the fetus can maintain normal oxygen consumption until oxygen delivery is reduced by half. Additional structural features of the fetal circulation also augment these adaptive features including the systems of 'shunts,' such as the ductus arteriosus and preferential blood flow streaming in the inferior vena cava to avoid intermixing of oxygenated blood from the placenta and deoxygenated blood in the fetal venous system. These features ensure maximal oxygen delivery to essential organs such as the brain and heart. The preferential streaming patterns may be augmented during hypoxia to help maintain oxygen delivery to these organs.

These adaptations work sufficiently well in the majority of cases that even the concept of 'birth asphyxia' itself has been controversial. However, from recent studies where cerebral function has been monitored from birth in infants with clinical evidence of birth asphyxia, it is clear that many such children did have a precipitating episode in the immediate peripartum period, with evidence of acute evolving cerebral injury (Hellström Westas et al 1995, Roth et al 1997, Westgate et al 1999). Follow-up of these children has shown a significant number to have long-term cognitive or functional sequelae, demonstrating that birth asphyxia is a true syndrome (Roth et al 1997).

Table 22.1 Summary of cardiovascular and cerebrovascular adaptations to asphyxia

The healthy fetus has considerable aerobic and anaerobic reserves to cope with transient or mild hypoxia

The fetal defenses against hypoxia depend on the type and severity of the insult, maturation and fetal wellbeing

During moderate hypoxia blood flow is redirected to key organs and flow is also redirected within the brain towards the structures important for autonomic function such as the brainstem

During severe asphyxia of rapid onset the adaptations are similar but more extreme. Blood flow to the brain as a whole may not be increased, but appears to be maintained so long as blood pressure is normal or raised

Progression of severe asphyxia results in failure of adaptation and progressive hypotension and hypoperfusion

VARIABLE DECELERATIONS

Intermittent or repeated insults as seen during labor allow partial recovery and adaptation between periods of hypoxia, but eventually hypotension begins to develop during hypoxia and becomes progressively more severe

The initial changes in the fetal heart rate (FHR) during acute asphyxia are reflex mediated. Thus FHR changes during variable decelerations poorly reflect the development of fetal hypotension or acidosis

In previously healthy fetuses, late recovery from severe variable decelerations is seen only in a subgroup of profoundly compromised fetuses

ETIOLOGY OF ASPHYXIA

Systemic fetal asphyxia may be of fetal, placental or maternal origin. Fetal causes include decreased fetal hemoglobin (e.g. hemolysis or feto-maternal hemorrhage), cord prolapse, cord compression, cord entanglements and true knots in the cord. Placental causes include placenta previa, vasa previa and placental abruption. Maternal causes include systemic hypoxia (for example anemia or hemorrhage), and reduced utero-placental blood flow due to hypotension, vasospasm accompanying hypertension and uterine hyperactivity.

Clearly, the different etiological factors lead to different patterns of asphyxia, which may be acute, chronic or acute on the background of chronic impairment. In labor, fetal asphyxia will most commonly be brief, but frequently repeated. Perfusion of the placenta has been shown to be inversely proportional to the rise in intrauterine pressure during contractions (Janbu & Nesheim 1987). Conversely, catastrophic events such as cord prolapse or abruption will cause a single profound immediate insult. After placental abruption fetal blood loss with volume contraction further potentiates the direct effects of hypoxia on the fetus.

HYPOXIA

The response of the fetal sheep to moderate, stable hypoxia has been extensively characterized (Giussani et al 1994). Fetal isocapnic hypoxia is typically induced by reduction of maternal inspired oxygen fraction to 10%. In the late gestation fetus, this is associated with an initial transient, moderate bradycardia followed by tachycardia and a rise in blood pressure (Fig. 22.2). There is an overall increase in combined ventricular output (CVO) and increased flow to essentially all organs (Giussani et al 1994, Hanson 1997). As hypoxia becomes greater there is a rapid transition in the distribution of CVO, with further increases in blood flow to vital organs, such as the brain, heart and adrenals, at the expense of peripheral organs which show a decrease in flow (Giussani et al 1994, Jensen 1996). This phenomenon is termed 'centralization' of the circulation.

Cerebral oxygen consumption is little changed, even if arterial oxygen content falls as low as 1 mmol/L thanks to the compensating increases in both cerebral blood flow (CBF) and oxygen extraction (Jones et al 1977, Sheldon et al 1979). Within the brain there is a greater increase in blood flow to the brainstem compared with the cerebrum, such that oxygen delivery is fully maintained to the brainstem, but not to the cerebrum (Jensen 1996). Nitric oxide (NO) has been shown to play a role in mediating the local increase in CBF (Hanson 1997).

Components of these changes in fetal heart rate (FHR) and CVO are reflexly mediated and the afferent limbs are in part mediated by muscarinic (parasympathetic) pathways and by α-adrenergic stimulation (Giussani et al 1994, Hanson 1997). The adrenergic input is derived partly from the sympathetic neural system and partly by circulating catecholamines released from the adrenal medulla. The rise in blood pressure during asphyxia is at least partly mediated by increased release of vasopressors, including the catecholamines, arginine vasopressin and angiotensin II (Giussani et al 1994, Hanson 1997). There are also large adrenocorticotropic and cortisol responses to hypoxia. Their role in the cardiovascular response to hypoxia is unclear, but cortisol has been shown to modulate the actions of other vasopressors (Tangalakis et al 1992).

Prolonged hypoxia

The effect of prolonged hypoxemia on cerebral metabolism in near-term fetal sheep has been studied during stepwise reductions of the maternal inspired oxygen concentration from 18% to 10–12% over four successive days (Richardson & Bocking 1998). Until the fetal arterial oxygen saturation was reduced to less than 30% of baseline, cerebral oxidative metabolism remained stable. At the lowest inspired oxygen concentration (with 3% CO_2) a progressive metabolic acidemia was induced. Initially, CBF increased, thus maintaining cerebral oxygen delivery as seen in acute studies. Eventually, when the pH fell below 7.00, cerebral oxygen consumption fell to less than 50% of control values.

If mild-to-moderate hypoxia is continued the fetus may be able to fully adapt, as measured by normalization of FHR, blood pressure, the incidence of fetal breathing and body movements, although redistribution of blood flow is maintained (Richardson & Bocking 1998) by a sustained increase in peripheral tone (Danielson et al 2005). These fetuses can improve tissue oxygen delivery to near baseline levels by increasing hemoglobin synthesis, mediated by greater erythropoietin release (Kitanaka et al 1989). This is consistent with the clinical situation of 'brain sparing' in growth retardation.

Maturational changes in responses to hypoxia

The cardiovascular response to fetal hypoxia appears to be age related. In the premature fetal sheep before 100 days (0.7) gestation, isocapnic hypoxia and hemorrhagic hypotension are not associated with hypertension, bradycardia or peripheral vasoconstriction. Thus it has been suggested that peripheral vasomotor control starts to develop at 0.7 gestation, coincident with maturation of neurohormonal regulators and chemoreceptor function (Hanson 1997, Jensen 1996). However, when interpreting these results it is also important to consider the degree of hypoxia in relation to the much greater anaerobic capacity of the premature fetus. This is discussed below in the section on premature fetal asphyxia. It is likely that the degree of hypoxia attained in these studies did not reduce tissue oxygen availability below the critical threshold for this developmental stage.

ASPHYXIA

Studies of asphyxia by definition involve both hypoxia and hypercapnia with metabolic acidosis. The complex relationship between severity of metabolic acidosis and outcome is summarized in Table 22.1. It is important to appreciate that in these studies of asphyxia a greater depth of hypoxia is typically attained than is possible using maternal inhalational hypoxia. Further, asphyxia can be induced relatively abruptly, limiting the time available for adaptation. Brief, total clamping of the uterine artery or umbilical cord leads to a rapid reduction of fetal oxygenation within a few minutes, and this is associated with massive hemodynamic changes and rapid metabolic deterioration (Parer 1998). In

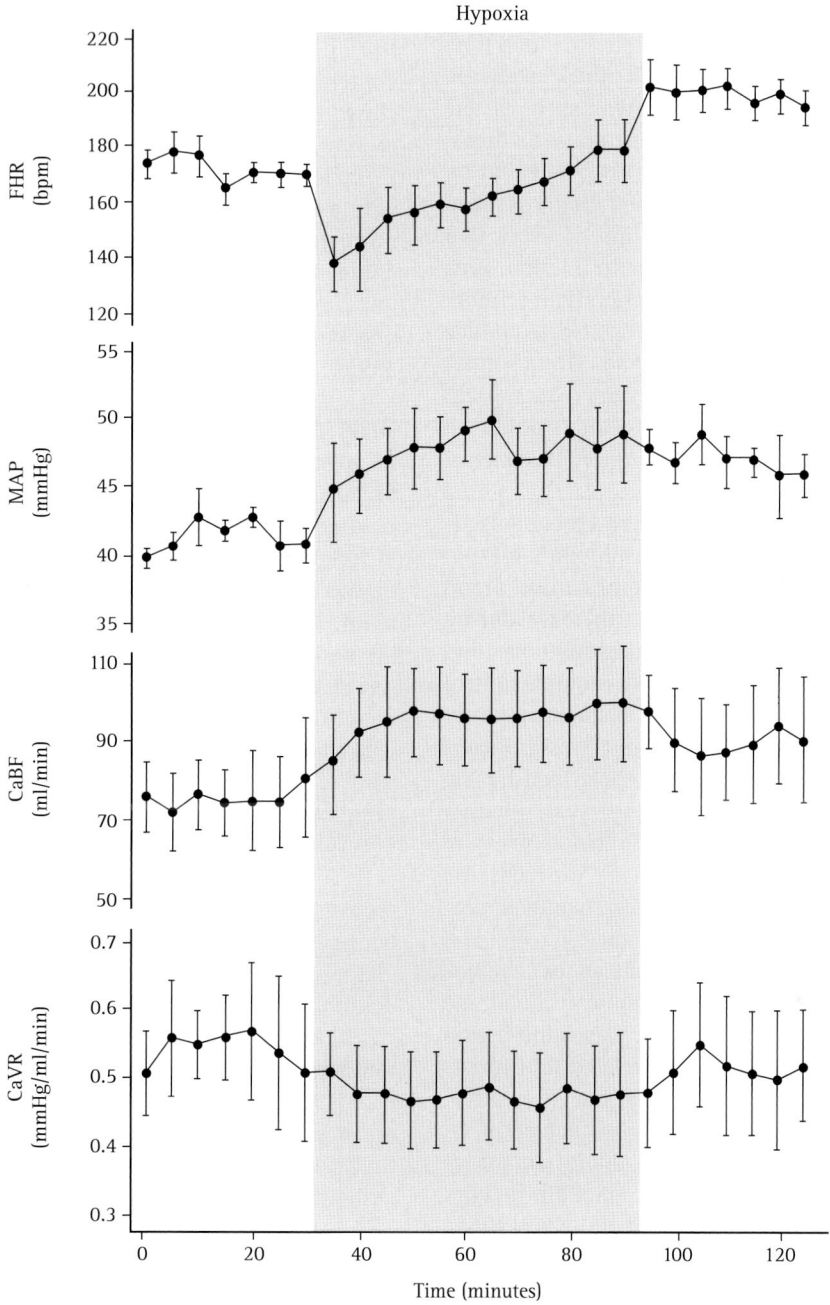

Figure 22.2 The responses in the near-term fetal sheep to moderate isocapnic hypoxia for 60 minutes, induced by altering the maternal inspired gas mixture, showing changes in fetal heart rate (FHR), mean arterial blood pressure (MAP), carotid blood flow (CaBF) and carotid vascular resistance (CaVR). Moderate hypoxia is associated with a sustained redistribution of blood flow away from peripheral organs to essential organs such as the brain (see Giussani et al 1994 for review). (Data derived from Bennet et al 1998.)

contrast, gradual partial occlusion induces a slow fetal metabolic deterioration without the acute fetal cardiovascular responses of bradycardia and hypertension; this is a function of the relative hypoxia attained (de Haan et al 1993).

The responses to moderate asphyxia are similar to those described above for hypoxia, with redistribution of blood flow to essential organs (Bennet et al 1998). During pro-

found asphyxia, corresponding with a severe reduction of uterine blood flow to 25% or less and a fetal arterial oxygen content of less than 1 mmol/L, the cardiovascular responses of the normal fetus are substantially different. Bradycardia is sustained and there is a generalized peripheral vasoconstriction involving essentially all organs (Bennet et al 1998). CBF does not increase or may even fall despite initially increased fetal blood pressure, due to significantly increased cerebral vasoconstriction. In the near-term sheep, blood flow within the brain, is preferentially redirected during asphyxia to protect structures important for survival such as the brainstem. Speculatively this redirection may maintain autonomic function at the expense of the cerebrum (Jensen 1996). Further, the reduced oxygen content limits oxygen extraction from the blood. The combination of these two factors, restricted CBF and reduced oxygen extraction, profoundly restricts cerebral oxygen consumption (Parer 1998). Partial cord compression for 90 minutes, titrated to induce severe asphyxia in near-term fetal sheep, had effects similar to those following a correspondingly severe reduction of uterine perfusion (Ikeda et al 1998). Both methods produced similar levels of asphyxia and cerebral injury (Ikeda et al 1998).

Figure 22.3 shows the cardiovascular and cerebrovascular responses of a near-term fetus to asphyxia of rapid onset. This figure demonstrates the failure of carotid blood flow (CaBF, used as an index of CBF) to increase during asphyxia in contrast to the rise seen during hypoxia (Fig. 22.2). CaBF is instead briefly maintained around control values before falling. The failure of CBF to increase is not due to hypotension but rather is a function of a significant rise in cerebral vascular resistance as demonstrated by the increase in carotid vascular resistance (Fig. 22.3) (Bennet et al 1998, Parer 1998). During asphyxia blood pressure initially increases markedly but as asphyxia proceeds the fetus becomes hypotensive (Fig. 22.3). The sustained bradycardia and increased peripheral resistance in the late gestation fetus during asphyxia are mediated by chemoreflexes; a logarithmic rise in circulating catecholamine levels further augments the peripheral vasoconstriction (Hanson 1997). Hypotension is primarily related to asphyxial impairment of myocardial contractility, due to a direct inhibitory effect of profound acidosis and depletion of myocardial glycogen stores (Rosen et al 1986). Once glycogen is depleted, there is rapid loss of high energy metabolites such as ATP in mitochondria (Shelley 1961). During a shorter episode, e.g. 5 min of asphyxia, the fetus may not become hypotensive. If the insult is repeated before myocardial glycogen can be replenished, successive periods of asphyxia will be associated with increasing duration of hypotension.

Another possible factor leading to impaired contractility during asphyxia is myocardial injury, which has been found after severe birth asphyxia and with congenital heart disease in limited case series (Donnelly 1987). Studies in adult animals have shown that there may be a significant delay in recovery of cardiac contractility after reperfusion from brief ischemia in the absence of necrosis. This delayed recovery has been termed 'myocardial stunning,' and this may contribute to progressive myocardial dysfunction and to delayed recovery of heart rate after repeated umbilical cord occlusions in the fetal lamb (Gunn et al 2000).

Progressive asphyxia

During gradually induced asphyxia, even to arterial oxygen contents of less than 1 mmol/L, fetal adaptation may be closer to that seen with hypoxia. Progressive reduction of uterine perfusion over a 3–4 h period in near-term fetal sheep led to a mean pH < 7.00, serum lactate levels >14 mM, with a fetal mortality of 53%. Surviving animals remained normotensive and normoglycemic and CBF was more than doubled. Interestingly however, in surviving fetuses neuronal damage was limited to selective loss of the very large, metabolically active cerebellar Purkinje cells (De Haan et al 1993).

Brief repeated asphyxia

In normal human labor, uterine contractions are relatively brief (typically less than one or two minutes). Total umbilical cord occlusions have been studied in fetal lambs near-term at frequencies consistent with active labor, either 1 min out of every 2.5 min or 2 min out of every 5 min, continued for many hours until fetal hypotension (<20 mmHg) occurred (de Haan et al 1997a, 1997b). There was an initial sustained rise in blood pressure during early occlusions followed after 15 min by the appearance of a biphasic pattern. This pattern was characterized by an initial rise in blood pressure at the start of each occlusion, followed by a fall. From then on a progressive fall in the nadir of fetal arterial blood pressure occurred with each occlusion.

At a pH between 7.04 and 6.85 in individual fetuses, the recovery of arterial blood pressure after each occlusion became markedly delayed. The rapid decompensation associated with this sustained hypotension was associated with delayed recovery of the fetal heart rate in only a third of cases, illustrating the poor diagnostic value of fetal heart rate monitoring to identify the compromised fetus (de Haan et al 1997a). Histologic analysis demonstrated the presence of focal neuronal damage in the parasagittal cortex, the thalamus and the cerebellum, while the hippocampus and striatum were almost wholly spared (de Haan et al 1997b).

Maturational changes in fetal responses to asphyxia

The preterm fetal sheep at 90 days gestation, prior to the onset of cortical myelination, can tolerate extended periods of up to 20 minutes of umbilical cord occlusion without neuronal loss (George et al 2004, Keunen et al 1997, Mallard et al 1994). The very prolonged cardiac survival (up to 30 minutes) (Fig. 22.4) (Bennet et al 1999, George et al 2004) corresponds with the attainment of maximal levels of cardiac glycogen at this gestation (Shelley 1961). Interestingly, while the premature fetal response to hypoxia appears to be different to that seen at term, the response during asphyxia was similar to that seen in more mature fetuses, with sustained bradycardia, accompanied by circulatory centralization, initial hypertension, then a progressive fall in pressure (Bennet et al 1998, 1999). Similarly to the term fetus, there was no increase in blood flow to the brain and again this

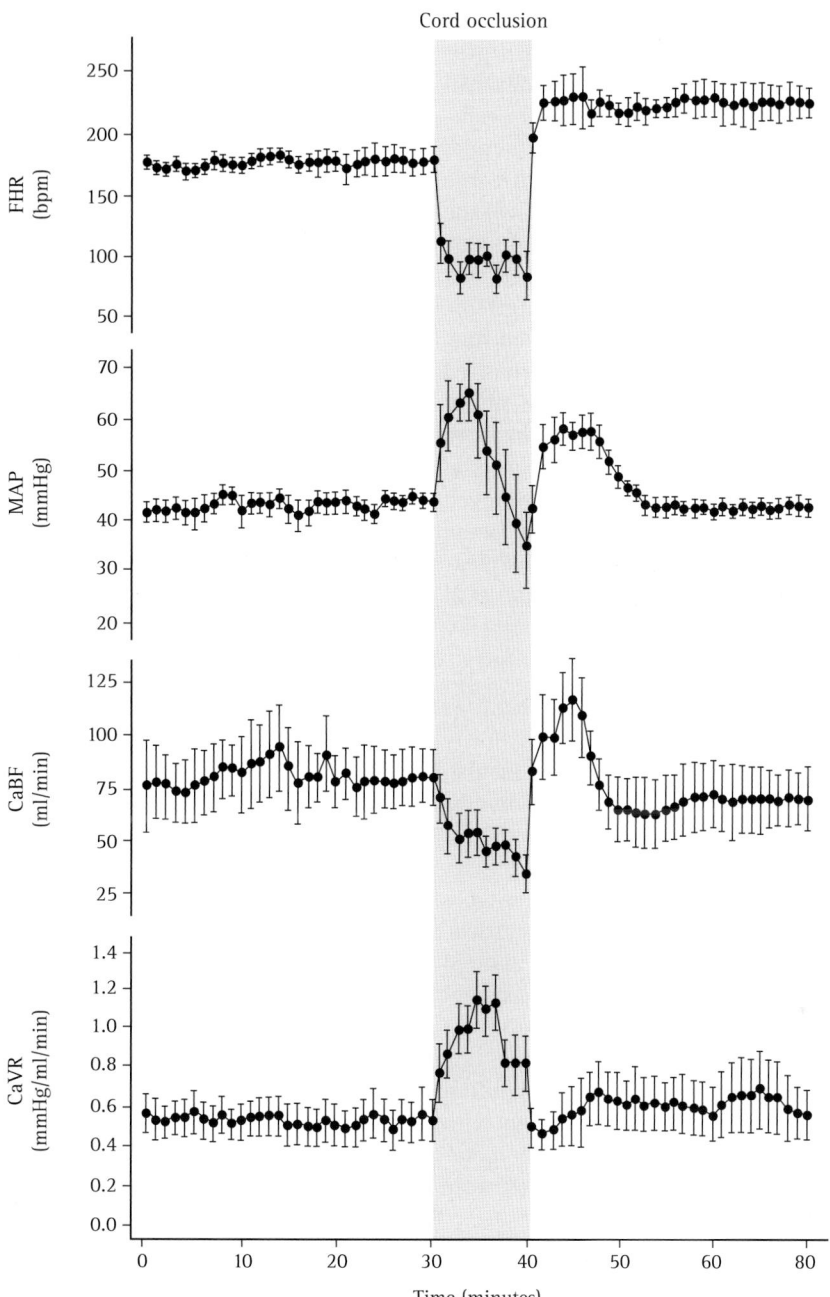

Figure 22.3 The responses in the near-term fetal sheep to complete umbilical cord occlusion for 10 minutes. In contrast to the response to moderate hypoxia, the profound fall in fetal heart rate (FHR) is maintained throughout the occlusion. Fetal mean arterial blood pressure (MAP) was initially elevated but then fell to below normal just prior to release. Carotid blood flow (CaBF) did not increase, and this was associated with a large increase in carotid vascular resistance (CaVR). Hypotension and hypoperfusion develop in the second half of the occlusion. (Data derived from Bennet et al 1998.)

was due to a significant increase in vascular resistance rather than to hypotension (Bennet et al 1999). The mechanism mediating this remains speculative. As shown in Figures 22.4 and 22.5, once blood pressure begins to fall CaBF falls in parallel. The fall in pressure is partly a function of the loss of redistribution of blood flow as seen in Figure 22.5 with a rise in femoral blood flow. The mechanisms

mediating this loss of redistribution are unknown, but may relate to changes in sympathetic nerve activity. A similar phenomenon is also seen at term (Jensen 1996).

In the latter half of a maximal interval of asphyxia in the preterm fetus, there is progressive failure of CVO, with a fall in both central and peripheral perfusion. This phase is much less likely to be seen for any significant duration in the term fetus as glycogen stores in the term fetus are depleted more quickly. The near-term fetus is unable to survive such prolonged periods of sustained hypotension, and typically will recover from a maximum of 10–12 minutes of cord occlusion compared with up to 25 minutes at 0.7 gestation (Bennet et al 2007a, 2007b) and 30 minutes at 0.6 gestation (George et al 2004). As a consequence of this extended survival the premature fetus is exposed to profound and prolonged hypotension and hypoperfusion. It may be speculated that during this final phase of asphyxia in the premature fetus there is a catastrophic failure of redistribution of blood flow within the fetal brain, which places previously protected areas of the brain, such as the brainstem, at risk of injury (Myers 1977), consistent with clinical reports (Barkovich & Sargent 1995). Post-asphyxia, a brief period of arterial hypertension and hyperperfusion is followed by a prolonged period of hypoperfusion, despite normalization of blood pressure, with a reduction in cerebral oxygenation as measured by near-infrared spectroscopy (Fig. 22.6) (Bennet et al 1999).

Chronic asphyxia

In addition to its potential impact on neurodevelopment (as outlined below, p. 483), chronic asphyxia may also adversely affect the ability of the fetus to adapt to acute insults. Chronic placental insufficiency leads to fetal arterial hypertension and myocardial hypertrophy, with increased umbilical artery resistance. Experimentally growth retarded fetuses exhibit sustained elevation of plasma catecholamines, cortisol and prostaglandin E_2, with a significant fall in corticotrophin, and when challenged with hypoxia have a blunted rise in plasma catecholamines (Hanson 1998). Consistent with this, whereas normoxic fetuses were able to tolerate brief occlusions of the umbilical cord repeated at a rate consistent with early labor for at least 4 hours, without exhibiting hypotension, twin and triplet fetal sheep with pre-existing hypoxia developed severe, progressive metabolic acidosis and hypotension and in many cases were

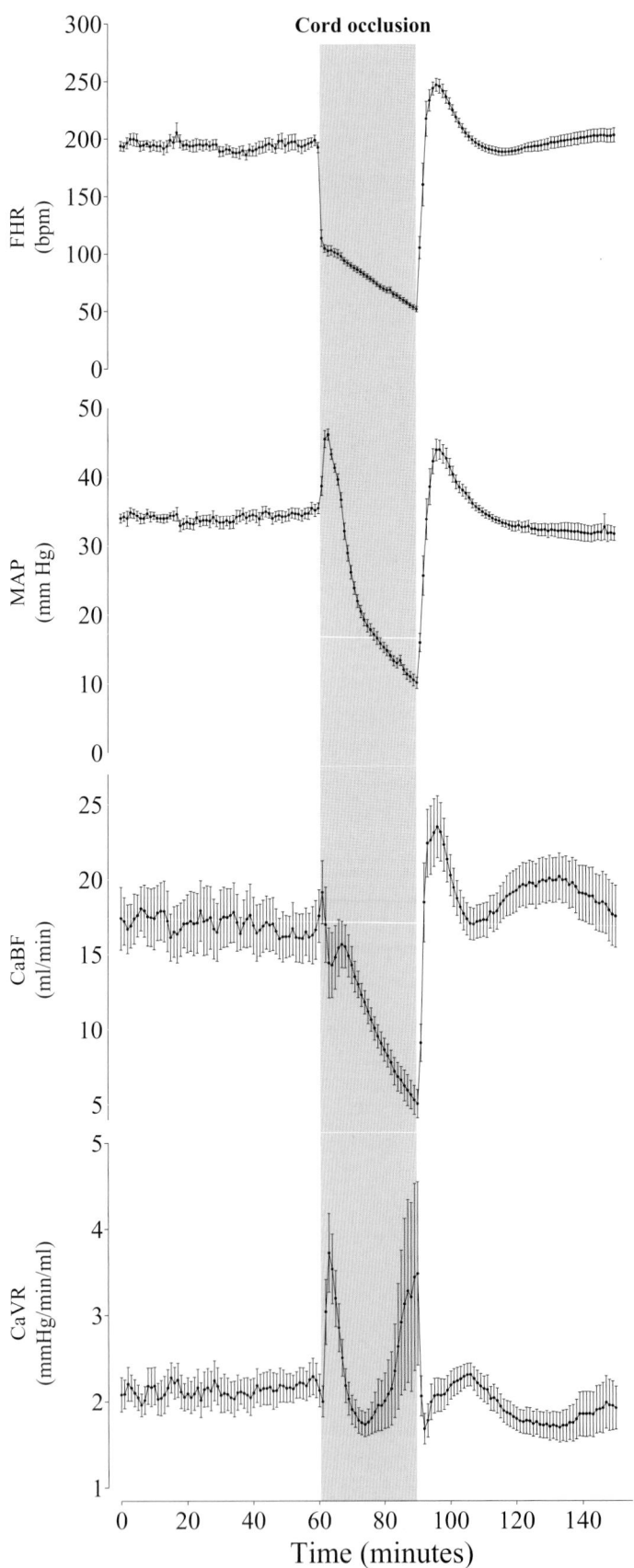

Figure 22.4 The responses of the mid-gestation (0.6 gestation) fetal sheep to complete umbilical cord occlusion for 30 minutes, showing fetal heart rate (FHR), mean arterial blood pressure (MAP), carotid blood flow (CaBF) and carotid vascular resistance (CaVR). Contrary to early reports, the overall response of the premature fetus was similar to that of the near-term fetus, with sustained bradycardia, redistribution of blood flow away from the periphery to essential organs with initial hypertension. With continued asphyxia there was failure of adaptation with profound hypotension and hypoperfusion. The major difference with the near-term fetus (Fig. 22.3) was that the premature fetus was able to survive such a prolonged period of cord occlusion. (Data derived from Bennet et al 1999.)

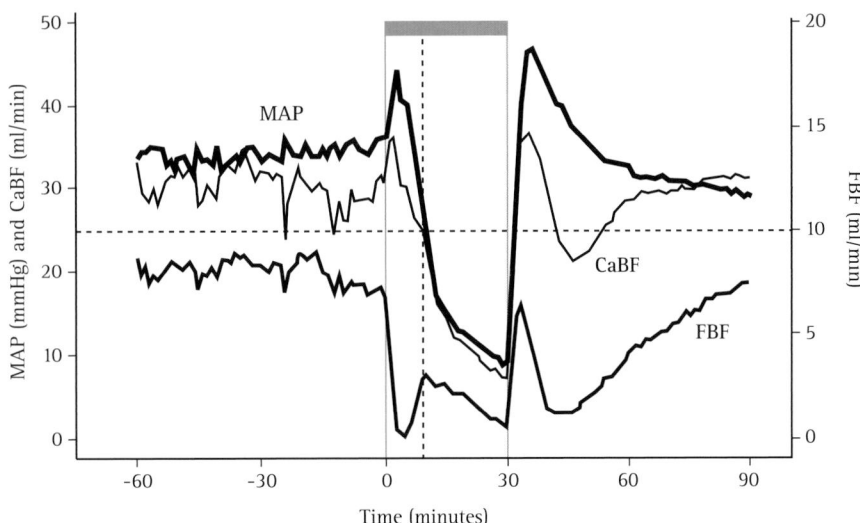

Figure 22.5 An example of the relationship between hypotension and carotid and femoral blood flow (CaBF and FBF) during cord occlusion in a 0.6 gestation fetal sheep. The start and end of occlusion are shown by the solid lines and the bar. Note that the CaBF began to fall only when mean arterial blood pressure (MAP) was below baseline levels (shown by the dotted horizontal line), and thereafter paralleled the changes in MAP very closely. It is interesting that this also corresponded with failure of peripheral vasoconstriction (increased FBF, shown by the vertical dotted line). Similar changes are seen near-term, but with earlier onset of hypotension and hypoperfusion.

unable to survive the full series of occlusions (Westgate et al 2005).

PATHOGENESIS OF CELL DEATH

WHAT INITIATES NEURONAL INJURY?

At the most fundamental level, injury requires a period of insufficient delivery of oxygen and substrates such as glucose (and other substances such as lactate in the fetus) such that neurons (and glia) cannot maintain homeostasis. If oxygen is reduced but substrate delivery is effectively maintained (i.e. pure or nearly pure hypoxia), the cells adapt in two ways. First, they can use anaerobic metabolism to support their production of high-energy metabolites for a time. The use of anaerobic metabolism is of course very inefficient since anaerobic glycolysis produces lactate and only 2 ATP, whereas aerobic glycolysis produces 38 ATP. Thus glucose reserves are rapidly consumed, and a metabolic acidosis develops with local and systemic consequences. Second, they can to some extent reduce non-obligatory energy consumption. This is clearly seen in neurons, where moderate hypoxia typically induces a switch to lower frequency states requiring less oxygen consumption. As an insult becomes more severe, neuronal activity will then cease completely, at a threshold above that which causes actual neuronal depolarization. This reduced activity is actively mediated by inhibitory neuromodulators such as adenosine (Hunter et al 2003).

In contrast, under conditions of combined reduction of oxygen and substrate the neuron's options are much more

limited, as not only is there less oxygen, but there is also much less glucose available to allow anaerobic metabolism. This may occur during either pure ischemia (reduced tissue blood flow) and even more critically during conditions of hypoxia–ischemia, i.e. both reduced oxygen content and reduced total blood flow. In the fetus, hypoxia–ischemia commonly occurs due to hypoxic cardiac compromise. Under these conditions depletion of high energy metabolites will occur much more rapidly and profoundly, while at the same time, there may actually be less acidosis both because there is much less glucose available to be metabolized to lactate, and because the insult is evolving more quickly (Table 22.2).

These concepts help to explain the consistent observation, discussed later in this chapter, that most cerebral injury after acute insults occurs in association with hypotension and consequent tissue hypoperfusion or ischemia. Technically, asphyxia is defined as the combination of impaired respiratory gas exchange (i.e. hypoxia and hypercapnia) accompanied by the development of metabolic acidosis. When we think about the impact on the brain of clinical asphyxia it will be critical to keep in mind that this definition tells us much about things that can be measured relatively easily (blood gases and systemic acidosis) and essentially nothing about blood pressure or perfusion of the brain.

CEREBRAL INJURY: AN 'EVOLVING' PROCESS

The seminal concept to emerge from both experimental and clinical studies is that brain cell death does not necessarily occur during hypoxia or ischemia (the 'primary' phase of

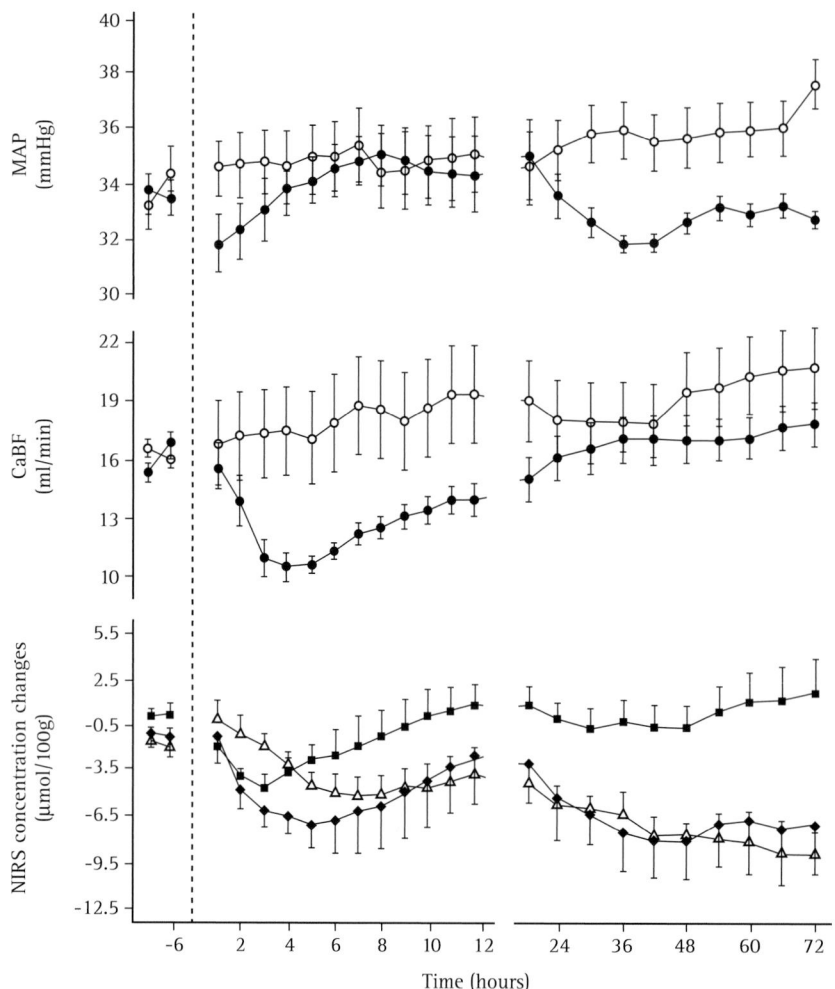

Figure 22.6 The recovery of the near mid-gestation (0.6 gestation) fetal sheep following 30 minutes of complete umbilical cord occlusion (denoted by the heavy dashed line; for occlusion data see Figure 22.4). In the top and middle panels, open symbols are control fetuses and closed symbols are asphyxiated fetuses. Post-asphyxia carotid blood flow (CaBF) showed a secondary fall, with a nadir after 4–6 h. This secondary change was not due to a fall in mean arterial blood pressure (MAP). The near-infrared spectroscopy (NIRS) data (bottom panel) include only the asphyxia group. A similar secondary fall was seen in total cerebral hemoglobin (diamonds), which is the sum of oxyhemoglobin (closed squares) and deoxyhemoglobin (open triangles), and provides an index of total cerebral blood volume. This fall was mainly due to a significant reduction in cerebral oxyhemoglobin around 2–4 hours post-asphyxia suggesting a true impairment of cerebral perfusion that may have contributed to the final injury. (Data derived from Bennet et al 1999.)

injury), but rather they may precipitate a cascade of biochemical processes leading to delayed cell death hours or even days afterwards (the 'secondary' phase), as summarized in Table 22.3. The sequence is illustrated in Figure 22.7. Experimental studies have demonstrated the existence of both a primary phase of energy failure during hypoxia-ischemia, a 'latent' phase during which oxidative metabolism normalizes, followed by secondary failure of oxidative metabolism in piglets (Lorek et al 1994) and immature rats (Blumberg et al 1997). Clinically, neural injury with no initial recovery of oxidative metabolism is seen after sufficiently severe or prolonged asphyxia (Azzopardi et al 1989), but in many other cases infants show initial, transient recov-

ery of cerebral oxidative metabolism followed by a secondary deterioration, with cerebral energy failure from 6 to 15 hours after birth (Azzopardi et al 1989, Roth et al 1997). In asphyxiated infants there is a close correlation between the degree of secondary energy failure and neurodevelopmental outcome at 1 and 4 years of age (Roth et al 1997).

A critical aspect of these findings is that a single 'subthreshold' insult that causes either minor or no neural injury can lead to a phase of increased vulnerability to further insults. Conversely, the delayed evolution of cell death after more severe insults suggests the potential for the prevention of brain cell death by interrupting the events which lead to secondary cell death (Gunn 2000).

Table 22.2 Acidosis and the pathogenesis of cell death

There is no intrinsic, physiologic relationship between the amount of systemic anaerobic metabolism (as reflected by metabolic acidosis) and the development of neuronal injury. The crude clinical correlation between the two is simply consistent with the fact that hypoxic–ischemic damage occurs under anaerobic conditions

Systemic acidosis during asphyxia is primarily related to peripheral vasoconstriction, acting to redistribute blood flow to essential organs. Even when a proportion of whole body anaerobic metabolism is central, so long as sufficient glucose is available to neurons to support basal energy metabolism, injury will not occur. Thus profound arterial metabolic acidosis may still accompany successful protection of the brain, with a normal outcome

During very prolonged periods of asphyxia with ongoing lactic acidosis, very severe acidosis may compromise fetal adaptation, including blood flow redistribution and cardiac contractility, promoting hypotension and thus causing cerebral hypoxia–ischemia

Conversely during more acute insults, with impaired tissue perfusion, less glucose is delivered to neurons and so less lactate is produced. Thus, injury may occur despite relatively modest levels of acidosis

Acute-on-chronic insults where there is reduced fetal metabolic reserve also have the potential to lead to injury after relatively short periods of acute asphyxia and moderate acidosis

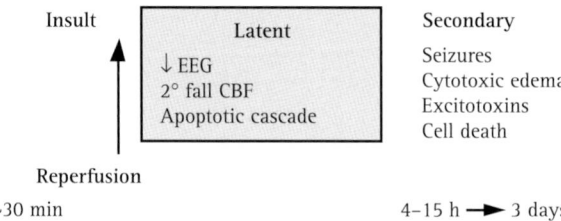

Figure 22.7 Flow chart illustrating the relationship between the mechanisms active in the pathophysiologically defined phases of cerebral injury after a severe reversible hypoxic–ischemic insult. During the immediate reperfusion period, lasting approximately 30 minutes, cellular energy metabolism is restored, with resolution of the acute hypoxic depolarization and cell swelling. This is followed by a latent phase, with near-normal oxidative cerebral energy metabolism as shown by magnetic resonance spectroscopy, but depressed electroencephalogram (EEG) activity and often a delayed period of reduced cerebral blood flow (CBF). The latent phase is believed to be associated with the intracellular components of the apoptotic cascade. This may be followed by secondary deterioration with delayed seizures and cytotoxic edema, extracellular accumulation of potential cytotoxins (such as the excitatory neurotransmitters), and 4–15 h after the asphyxia, failure of oxidative metabolism and damage. The changes in the secondary phase may take 3 days or more to resolve.

Table 22.3 Summary: the evolution of neural injury

Neuronal death does not necessarily occur at the time of the insult. Hypoxia–ischemia may activate pre-existing cell death pathways leading to evolving cell death

The different stages of evolution of delayed cell death are reflected in characteristic pathophysiologic changes. Experimentally successful intervention has been shown in the reperfusion and latent phases. To date no successful treatment has been shown for interventions delayed until after the onset of secondary deterioration

During recovery from a mild 'threshold' insult the fetus may be more vulnerable to any further insult or to environmental factors such as hyperthermia or impaired cardiovascular function

acquired or genetic thrombophilias (Nelson 2007). The evolution of injury is quite different from that seen after global insults with reperfusion. In a focal ischemic injury, such as adult stroke, there is a dense ischemic core characterized by primary cell death with pannecrosis. This core is surrounded by an ischemic 'penumbra' which has some residual blood supply. Damage extends from the core out to the penumbra over a few hours under experimental conditions. The evolution of damage in the penumbra has been associated with waves of depolarization which deplete remaining cellular energy reserves (Lipton 1999).

PATHOPHYSIOLOGIC CORRELATES OF THE PHASES OF NEURAL INJURY

Many of the pathophysiologic events associated with evolution of injury have been characterized in a model of reversible cerebral ischemia in the chronically instrumented fetal sheep, studied in utero (Williams et al 1991). The primary and secondary phases of injury seen in this paradigm are shown in Figure 22.8. During carotid artery occlusion, the EEG shows an immediate loss of amplitude, becoming isoelectric after 30 seconds, and remains so until the end of occlusion. After 30 minutes of occlusion, the EEG remains suppressed for 5–9 hours (George et al 2004, Gunn et al 1997). During this period of reduced neural activity, a secondary hypoperfusion develops, which reflects depressed

FOCAL INSULTS

Post-asphyxial encephalopathy is typically associated with global, reversible hypoxia–ischemia. Purely focal lesions can occur in the newborn, typically in infants with no evidence of exposure to asphyxia, and are often associated with

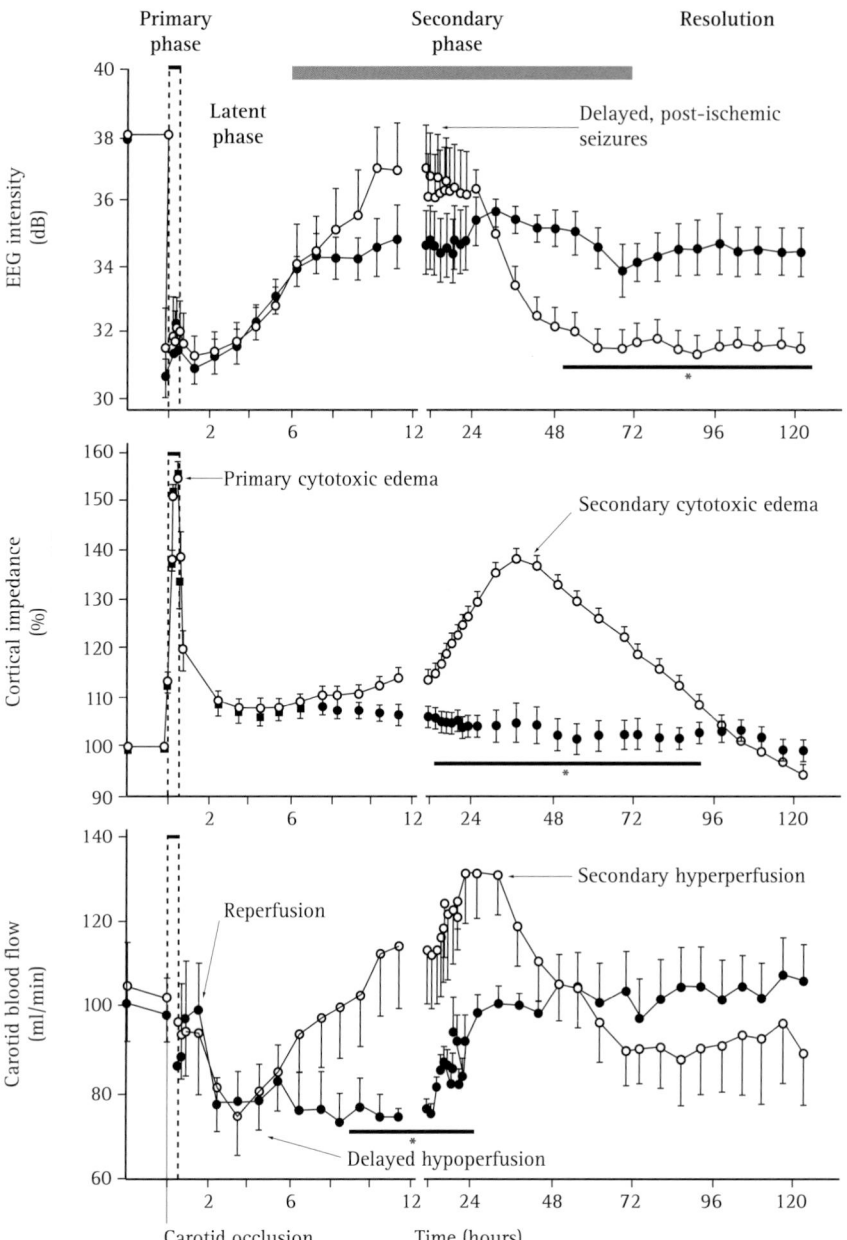

Figure 22.8 The relationship between the phases of neural injury and changes in the fetal electroencephalogram (EEG), impedance and carotid blood flow after 30 minutes of global cerebral ischemia in the near-term fetal sheep. Impedance is a measure of cytotoxic edema in the parietal cortex. Fetuses received either sham cooling (○) or cerebral hypothermia (●) started 5.5 h after reperfusion, and continued until 72 h. The hypothermia group shows better recovery of EEG intensity after resolution of delayed seizures and complete suppression of the secondary rise in impedance. The phase of secondary hypoperfusion is extended by hypothermia but resolves spontaneously despite continued cooling for 72 h. (Data derived from Gunn et al 1998. Mean ± SEM, *$P < 0.05$.)

cerebral metabolism (Gunn et al 1997, Jensen et al 2006). The significance of this remains elusive, as this is also seen after 'threshold' insults which do not cause cell death. In the adult, the duration, but not the depth, of the secondary reduction in CBF has been correlated with the severity of the insult (Michenfelder & Milde 1990). The secondary phase is marked by an abrupt onset of seizure activity, with an increase in CBF (Gunn et al 1997) and cytotoxic edema. The

delayed seizure activity peaks rapidly at approximately 12 hours, then progressively resolves over 1–2 days. The residual EEG intensity after resolution of seizures is related to the amount of neuronal death in the underlying cortex.

The development of cytotoxic edema can be monitored using cortical impedance (Williams et al 1991). This is a technique whereby the electrical resistance (impedance) to a low amplitude alternating current is measured; the impedance of a tissue rises concomitantly as cells depolarize and fluid shifts from the extracellular to the intracellular space. Thus a rise in impedance reflects cell swelling. As shown in Figure 22.8, there is a rapid rise in impedance during ischemia, which almost completely resolves over 30–60 minutes of reperfusion. The secondary evolution of cytotoxic edema, initiated after the onset of seizures, peaks much later and takes 2–3 days to resolve. Even if seizures are abolished by infusion of a selective glutamate antagonist, the secondary rise is only delayed (Tan et al 1992), suggesting that the edema is not a direct consequence of seizures but rather primarily reflects ongoing encephalopathic processes. The timing of secondary edema is consistent with that of secondary energy failure after perinatal asphyxia, as measured by magnetic resonance spectroscopy (MRS) in the infant (Reynolds et al 1991) and piglet (Lorek et al 1994). Interestingly, studies in fetal sheep using near infrared spectroscopy also suggest that mitochondrial failure occurs in this delayed phase (Bennet et al 2006, Marks et al 1996), consistent with clinical data (Toet et al 2006).

Histologic analysis after 3 days' recovery shows that 30 minutes of ischemia causes consistent injury of the parasagittal cortex and dorsal hippocampus, with macroscopically visible laminar necrosis. Our group has shown that microscopically there is at least 75–90% neuronal death in the parasagittal cortex, with lesser loss in other areas (Gunn et al 1997) and this is illustrated in Figure 22.9. The depths of the sulci tend to show greater damage than the adjacent gyri. This pattern of injury with predominant parasagittal and sulcal injury, is a classic 'watershed' distribution which is commonly seen in asphyxiated term neonates (Volpe 1995).

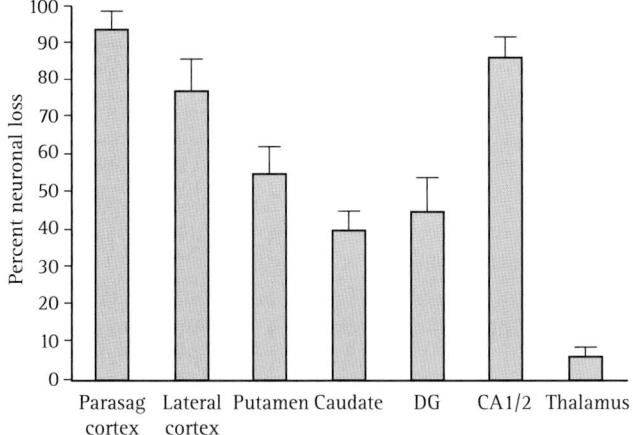

Figure 22.9 Comparison of neuronal loss (mean ± SEM) in different brain regions 5 days after severe ischemia (bilateral carotid artery occlusion for 30 minutes) in the near-term fetal sheep. Injury is greatest in the parasagittal cortex and in the underlying dorsal horn of the hippocampus. In contrast, the granule cells of the dentate gyrus (DG) of the hippocampus and the nuclei of the striatum and thalamus (putamen and caudate) are relatively spared. This pattern of injury is in the classic 'watershed' distribution (see Gunn et al 1997, 1998).

THE PRIMARY PHASE

Once the neuron's supply of high-energy metabolites such as ATP can no longer be maintained during hypoxia–ischemia, there is failure of the energy dependent mechanisms of intracellular homeostasis such as the Na^+/K^+ ATP-dependent pump. Neuronal depolarization occurs and leads to sodium and calcium entry into cells. This in turn favors further cation and water entry, leading to cell swelling (cytotoxic edema). If sufficiently severe this may cause immediate neuronal lysis, but before this stage the swollen neurons may still recover if hypoxia is stopped or if the osmotic environment is manipulated (in vitro) to prevent cell swelling (Goldberg & Choi 1993). Finally, re-uptake of excitatory amino acid neurotransmitters (EAAs) such as glutamate is also energy dependent. Thus typically, ischemia is associated with extracellular accumulation of the EAAs. Receptor mediated binding by these neurotransmitters further favors both immediate swelling, by opening receptor linked Na^+/K^+ channels (e.g. the *N*-methyl D-aspartate, NMDA, subtype of glutamate receptor) as well as calcium entry (e.g. the NMDA and the α-amino-3-hydroxy-5-methyl-4-isoxazolepropionic acid, AMPA, subtype of glutamate receptor) (Choi 1995).

Ionic calcium is normally actively maintained at very low concentrations in the cell (10 000-fold lower than in extracellular fluid). This gradient allows calcium to be used by the cell as an intracellular signaling mechanism. Although the rise in intracellular calcium during hypoxia does not cause immediate cell death, it can inappropriately activate enzymes and signal transduction systems that favor free radical production, kinase activities and hydroxyapatite precipitation which are all potentially damaging (Choi 1995). Oxygen free radicals are derived partially from such calcium activated enzymatic processes and partly from excess purine production as ATP is exhausted. It is generally believed that oxygen free radicals play a particular role in damaging essential cell membrane components during the immediate recovery from asphyxia (the reperfusion phase), when tissue oxygen levels abruptly recover (Fellman & Raivio 1997).

THE DELAYED PHASE

Although neurons (and glia) may initially recover from the primary injury, processes initiated by exposure to hypoxia–ischemia may lead to cell death hours or days later. The longer and more severe the insult, generally, the greater proportion of primary neural death (Beilharz et al 1995). Delayed appearance of histologically defined cell death has been directly demonstrated after asphyxial brain injury from clinical and experimental studies (Gunn 2000).

Necrosis and apoptosis

Two morphologic patterns of delayed cell death have been described: necrosis and apoptosis (Raff 1992). Necrosis is defined by loss of plasma membrane integrity associated with a random pattern of DNA degradation. Typically there is swelling of the cytoplasm and organelles, with little change initially to the nucleus. Apoptosis is defined by shrinkage of the cell, 'karyohexis,' associated with specific endonuclease mediated DNA degradation. Eventually, the shrunken cell breaks into small fragments. Karyohexis is the classic microscopic picture of condensation of chromatin (i.e. a dark shrunken nucleus) with loss of the reticular formation in the cytoplasm (leading to eosinophilia on light microscopy). The active degradation of DNA by endonucleases, which cleave the chromatin at internucleosomal points, leads to fragments of fixed size, with a characteristic laddered appearance on chromatography.

By analogy with the active process of developmental loss of excess cells (including neurons) it is suggested that an apoptotic morphology reflects active cell death, involving a cascade of 'suicide' processes (Raff 1992). In contrast, necrosis is suggested to reflect biophysical damage to the cell (cell membrane instability, ion shifts, etc.), particularly lysis in the primary phase. Both are clearly described in infants dying after perinatal asphyxia (Edwards et al 1997, Scott & Hegyi 1997). Apoptosis may be initiated by several intracellular pathways, but the final events involve alterations in the ratio of various intracellular factors such as Bcl (which inhibits apoptosis) and Bax which promotes apoptosis, and to activation of a family of proteases related to interleukin converting enzyme, known as caspases (Lipton 1999). The final events involve endonuclease mediated DNA fragmentation (Beilharz et al 1995).

Although a greater proportion of necrotic cell death is seen with increasing severity of the primary insult (Beilharz et al 1995), it has become clear that the underlying processes may not be as clearly separated as originally thought. Even slowly evolving, treatable cell death can occur by necrosis (Colbourne et al 1999), and hypoxic cell death in vitro appears to include a combination of both apoptotic and necrotic processes, with one or the other being more prominent depending on factors such as maturity (Gottron et al 1997, Porteracailliau et al 1997). Furthermore, there is evidence that mitochondrial calcium overload is a critical event in both apoptotic and necrotic cell death and that 'antiapoptotic' nuclear proteins such as Bcl can also inhibit necrotic cell death (Lipton 1999).

The concept remains an important one, considering that if neuronal and glial cell death is an active response, mediated by activation of second and third messenger events after an acute event (whether specifically due to a preset 'death program' or to less specific pathways initiated by excess free calcium, inflammatory pathways and/or cytotoxins), then it should logically be possible to interrupt these events.

Intracellular calcium accumulation

The events promoting or sustaining delayed cell death after reperfusion are not known. Mitochondrial calcium overload during hypoxia–ischemia appears to be one of the critical steps initiating delayed death (Choi 1995), and therapeutic strategies to reduce calcium induced neuronal death are discussed in Chapter 27. Other proposed damaging factors include loss of trophic growth factor support, free radical release during reperfusion, and abnormal glutaminergic receptor activity.

Microglial activation

There is a close temporal association between microglial activation and the development of apoptosis, and thus this has been proposed to be a causal relationship (Lees 1993). Microglia are the macrophages resident in the brain, but other macrophages may also cross from the circulation and play a role in the activation of the neuroimmune system after asphyxial injury. Activated microglia express a number of cytotoxic cytokines such as tumor necrosis factor alpha (TNF-α) as well as the cytotoxic radicals NO and H_2O_2. This neuroimmune system has probably evolved as a protective response to viral and bacterial infection at the cost of retaining a potential neurotoxic role (Lees 1993).

Seizures and excitotoxins

In the human neonate, seizure activity is a bad prognostic indicator (Hellström Westas et al 1995). In vivo microdialysis after ischemia in the fetal sheep shows that both glutamate and NO are induced in the secondary phase (Tan et al 1996). The elevation in extracellular glutamate is closely associated with the onset of post-asphyxial seizures, and treatment with a specific antagonist of the NMDA type of glutamate receptor potently abolishes the seizures. However, this treatment had no effect on the most severely affected region (the parasagittal cortex) and had a modest effect in more peripheral regions, suggesting that these post-ischemic seizures only have a partial role in extending the area of brain injury (Tan et al 1992).

ENDOGENOUS PROTECTIVE MECHANISMS

A number of endogenous protective responses of the brain act to limit injury. These responses include release of neuromodulators/inhibitory neurotransmitters, induction of neurotrophic factors and intracellular anti-apoptotic systems, and postnatally, spontaneous cerebral hypothermia. An illustration of the potential protective effects of endogenous cellular responses is that a single, subthreshold insult that does not cause damage may markedly increase resistance to a subsequent more severe insult. Several hours must elapse for preconditioning to be seen, and its effect then attenuates after several days, consistent with the time course of a wide range of stress gene responses to ischemia (Massa et al 1996). Several of the mechanisms discussed below may be involved, including induction of anti-apoptotic genes such as *BCL-2*, growth factors such as insulin-like growth factor or fibroblast growth factor, free radical scavengers, adenosine and the heat shock proteins.

Inhibitory neuromodulators

Ischemia and asphyxia are typically associated with a large increase in inhibitory neuromodulators such as γ-amino butyric acid (GABA), adenosine and cerebral opioids (Shuaib & Kanthan 1997). Microdialysis studies in the fetal lamb suggest that compared with postnatal studies, there is a disproportionately large release of GABA relative to that of the excitotoxins during ischemia (Tan et al 1996). Interestingly, adult species such as the turtle that are very tolerant to hypoxia also show a very elevated GABA and adenosine response to anoxia (Nilsson & Lutz 1991). In contrast with the acute increase in GABA, in the fetal lamb, there was no elevation of GABA during the secondary phase (Tan et al 1996). This loss of GABA release during the secondary phase may be one contributor to the development of very intense seizures that are difficult to manage. The period of reduced cerebral blood flow and metabolism in the early recovery phase after asphyxia also appears to be actively mediated through different inhibitory neuromodulators such as the alpha2 adrenoreceptor (Dean et al 2006).

It has been proposed that endogenous release of these inhibitory factors helps limit cerebral injury by reducing neural activity (Hunter et al 2003) and, thus, that increasing cerebral inhibitory responses may be a logical treatment (Shuaib & Kanthan 1997). However, the results of many studies using this approach have been contradictory with, for example, evidence of protection both with agonists and antagonists to the adenosine receptors (Bona et al 1997, Shuaib & Kanthan 1997). This is discussed in detail in Chapter 28.

Endogenous neurotrophic factors

Cerebral injury is associated with increased neurotrophic activity (defined by the ability to support neuronal survival in vitro), which is considerably greater in the immature brain than later in life (Guan et al 2003). Studies suggest that neuronal injury is associated with rapid, transient activity dependent expression of neurotrophins (such as nerve growth factor-β, brain derived growth factor, neurotensin 3 and activin A) in neurons, contrasting with a delayed and more persistent injury induced expression of certain growth factors (insulin-like growth factor 1 (IGF-1) and transforming growth factor beta (TGF-β) within glia (Guan et al 2003). For example, the broadly anti-apoptotic agent IGF-1 and two of its binding proteins (IGFBP-2 and IGFBP-3) are intensely induced 3–5 days after hypoxic–ischemic injury in the developing brain. The binding proteins may perhaps act to transport and target IGF-1 to particular cell types. Endogenous administration of growth factors such as IGF-1 can reduce loss of both neurons and oligodendrocytes after ischemia (Guan et al 2003).

Cerebrovascular responses in the delayed phase

A delayed period of hyperperfusion or 'luxury perfusion' is well described after perinatal asphyxia (Ilves et al 1998). There is evidence that this hyperperfusion in the delayed phase may in part protect marginally viable tissue (Abi Raad et al 1999). Putatively neuroprotective agents such as the calcium antagonists that depress blood pressure, and thus impair CBF in the post-asphyxial period, may aggravate brain injury (Gunn & Gluckman 1998). Factors that may mediate the hyperperfusion phase include NO (Marks et al

1996) and prostacyclin (Walton et al 1997). NO is a volatile, rapidly regulated, neuromodulator that can be produced by NO synthases (NOS) in endothelial cells (eNOS), neurons (nNOS) and by neutrophils or microglia (inducible NOS, or iNOS). Citrulline, a degradation production of NO, is induced in extracellular brain fluid in the secondary phase after ischemia, which may suggest a role for NO in delayed injury (Tan et al 1996).

It is vital to take into consideration the multiple roles of NO in order to interpret its effects on neural injury. The endothelial NO is a vasodilator which under physiological conditions plays an important role in the regulation of cerebral blood flow (CBF), cerebral autoregulation, blood flow–metabolism coupling and the control of platelet aggregation and adhesion (Faraci & Heistad 1998). NO has also been shown to play a role in regulating fetal CBF (Hanson 1997). Thus, it is perhaps not surprising that as most NO production derives from induction of endothelial NOS, non-specific inhibition of NO production following ischemia has been associated with increased cerebral injury, probably due to impairment of cerebral perfusion (Marks et al 1996).

nNOS is Ca^{2+} dependent and thus activated by intracellular calcium accumulation during ischemia, and nNOS expression in the developing brain correlates with regions of selective neuronal loss in the developing rat brain. iNOS is inducible by cytokines and released by activated macrophages in very highly concentrated killing bursts. Macrophage activation occurs in the delayed phase of injury, and thus it is a likely mediator of cytotoxicity in that phase. Selective inhibition of nNOS or iNOS is suggested to be neuroprotective (Bolanos & Almeida 1999). However, recent data suggest that this protection is dependent on gender (Nijboer et al 2007). Much more work is required to dissect their contribution to brain damage.

Acidosis: friend or foe?

The systemic acidosis caused by asphyxia is both associated with and can exacerbate fetal compromise, for example by impairing cardiac contractility. The direct effect on neural injury, however, is complex. In vitro, acidosis limits both hypoxic and excitotoxic neuronal injury in hippocampal neurons (Giffard et al 1990, Tombaugh 1994). It is a striking observation that in experimental studies in the fetal sheep, the dorsal horn of the hippocampus is very vulnerable to short periods of dense ischemia or asphyxia, but has been reported to be spared after both brief repeated asphyxia and prolonged partial asphyxia (de Haan et al 1997b). Consistent with the hypothesis that local acidosis may actually protect this region, a very profound acidosis developed during brief repeated cord occlusions (pH 6.83 ± 0.03) (de Haan et al 1997b), whereas there was only a mild metabolic acidosis after 10 minutes of umbilical cord occlusion with severe selective loss in the cornu ammonis fields of the hippocampus (5 minutes after reperfusion the mean pH was >7.10) (Mallard et al 1992).

PATHOPHYSIOLOGIC DETERMINANTS OF ASPHYXIAL INJURY

Recent studies using well defined experimental paradigms of asphyxia in the near-term fetal sheep have explored the relationship between the distribution of neuronal damage and the type of insult. These studies suggest that the key factor precipitating and localizing injury is local cerebral hypoperfusion due to hypotension. In addition, a number of factors modify the impact of asphyxia on the brain, including the pattern of repetition of insults as well as fetal factors such as gestational age, pre-existing metabolic state and cerebral temperature (see Fig. 22.1 and Table 22.4).

HYPOTENSION AND THE 'WATERSHED' DISTRIBUTION OF NEURONAL LOSS

The development of hypotension appears to be the critical factor precipitating neural injury after acute insults. This is readily understood as reduced perfusion will reduce the supply of glucose for anaerobic metabolism, compounding the reduction of oxygen delivery and content. The real life importance of hypotension is supported by both the pattern of neural damage, and the correlation of injury with arterial blood pressure across multiple paradigms.

Table 22.4 Summary of the determinants of acute asphyxial neural injury

Cerebral perfusion is linearly compromised by hypotension during asphyxia. The combination of reduced perfusion with hypoxia (i.e. hypoxia–ischemia) not only further reduces the amount of oxygen delivered to the brain but also compounds this by reducing the supply of glucose for anaerobic metabolism. This commonly leads to a 'watershed' distribution of injury

Increased spacing between relatively prolonged episodes of ischemia or asphyxia is associated with a relative increase in striatal injury

The brain matures from caudal to rostral. Thus, in the premature brain the cortex is relatively immature, particularly in the superficial layers, and is less susceptible to hypoxic–ischemic injury than subcortical white and gray matter

The dominant neuropathologic correlate of handicap in surviving premature infants is the distinctive white matter lesion, periventricular leukomalacia (PVL), which occurs before oligodendrocyte maturation, and is strongly associated with evidence of maternal infection, with a fetal systemic inflammatory response and with exposure to asphyxia (p. 19)

Environmental conditions during recovery from asphyxia can critically affect outcome. Experimentally, moderate cerebral hypothermia initiated in the latent phase and continued until resolution of secondary changes can dramatically reduce neural injury

The close relationship between changes in CaBF and blood pressure during asphyxia is shown by Figures 22.3–22.5. In these fetuses, mean arterial blood pressure (MAP) initially rose with intense peripheral vasoconstriction. At this time CaBF was maintained. As cord occlusion was continued MAP eventually fell, probably as a function of impaired cardiac contractility and failure of peripheral redistribution. When MAP fell below baseline, carotid blood flow fell in parallel. It appeared that there was a small window during which flow was maintained as pressure was falling (Fig. 22.5), suggesting that autoregulation was intact. This is consistent with the normal relatively narrow range of fetal cerebrovasculature autoregulation (Parer 1998).

In the term fetus, neural injury has been commonly reported in areas such as the parasagittal cortex, the dorsal horn of the hippocampus and the cerebellar neocortex after a range of insults including pure ischemia, prolonged single complete umbilical cord occlusion, prolonged partial asphyxia and repeated brief cord occlusion (Figs 22.9, left panel and 22.10) (de Haan 1993, 1997b, Gunn et al 1992, 1997, Mallard et al 1992). These areas are 'watershed' zones within the borders between major cerebral arteries, where perfusion pressure is least, and, clinically, lesions in these areas in adults and children are typically seen after systemic hypotension (Torvik 1984).

Some data suggest that limited or localized white or gray matter injury may occur even when significant hypotension is not seen (de Haan et al 1993, Ikeda et al 1998), particularly when hypoxia is very prolonged (Rees et al 1998). Clearly there may have been some relative hypoperfusion in these studies. Nevertheless, there is a strong correlation between either the depth or duration of hypotension and the amount of neuronal loss within individual studies of acute asphyxia (de Haan et al 1997b, 1997c, Gunn et al 1992, Ikeda et al 1998).

This is also seen between similar paradigms causing severe fetal acidosis that have been manipulated to either cause fetal hypotension (Gunn et al 1992, Ikeda et al 1998) or not (de Haan et al 1993). In fetal lambs exposed to prolonged severe partial asphyxia, as judged by the degree of metabolic compromise, neuronal loss occurred only in those in whom one or more episodes of acute hypotension occurred (Ikeda et al 1998). In contrast, in a similar study where an equally 'severe' insult was induced gradually and titrated to maintain normal or elevated blood pressure throughout the insult, no neuronal loss was seen outside the cerebellum (de Haan et al 1993).

PATTERN OF INJURY: REPEATED INSULTS

The one apparent exception to a general tendency to a 'watershed' distribution after global asphyxial insults near-term is the selective neuronal loss in striatal nuclei (putamen and caudate nucleus; Fig. 22.10, right panel) which is seen when relatively prolonged periods of asphyxia or ischemia are repeated (de Haan et al 1997c, Mallard et al 1993). Whereas 30 minutes of continuous cerebral ischemia leads

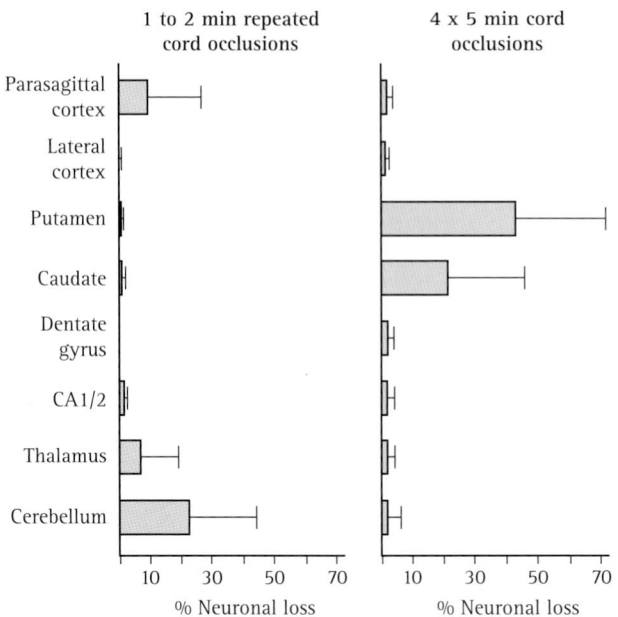

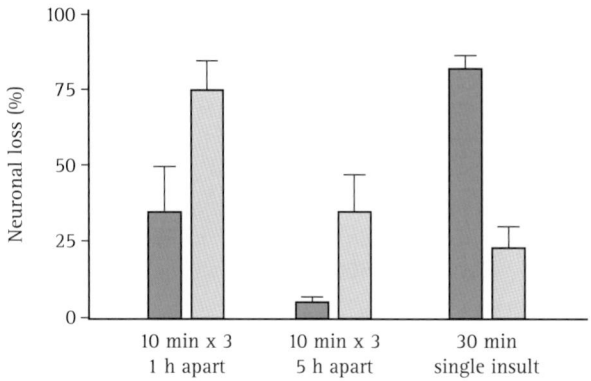

Figure 22.10 The distribution of neuronal loss assessed after 3 days recovery from two different patterns of prenatal asphyxia in near-term fetal sheep. The left panel shows the effects of brief (1 or 2 min) cord occlusions repeated at frequencies consistent with established labor. Occlusions were terminated after a variable time, when the fetal blood pressure fell below 20 mmHg for two successive occlusions. This insult led to damage in the watershed regions of the parasagittal cortex and cerebellum (de Haan et al 1997b). The right hand panel shows the effect of five minute episodes of cord occlusion, repeated four times, at intervals of 30 minutes. This paradigm is associated with selective neuronal loss in the putamen and caudate nucleus, which are nuclei of the striatum. CA 1/2 and the dentate gyrus are regions of the hippocampus. Mean ± SD. (Data derived from de Haan et al 1997c.)

to predominantly parasagittal cortical neuronal loss, with only moderate striatal injury, when the insult was divided into three separate episodes of ischemia, a greater proportion of striatal injury was seen relative to cortical neuronal loss (Figs 22.9 and 22.11) (Mallard et al 1993). Intriguingly, significant striatal involvement was also seen after prolonged partial asphyxia in which distinct episodes of bradycardia and hypotension occurred (Gunn et al 1992).

It is thus likely that the pathogenesis of striatal involvement in the near-term fetus is related to the precise timing of episodic asphyxia and not to more severe local hypoperfusion, since the striatum is not in a watershed zone but rather within the territory of the middle cerebral artery. The vulnerability of the medium sized neurons of the striatum to this type of insult may be related to a greater release of glutamate into the striatal extracellular space after repeated insults compared with a single insult of the same cumulative duration. Consistent with this speculation, immunohistochemical techniques have shown that inhibitory striatal neurons were primarily lost (Mallard et al 1995).

Figure 22.11 The effects of different intervals between insults on the distribution of cerebral damage after ischemia in the near-term fetal sheep. Cerebral ischemia was induced by carotid occlusion for 10 minutes and repeated three times, at intervals of either 1 h or 5 h, compared with a single continuous episode of 30 minutes occlusion. The divided insults were associated with a preponderance of striatal injury, whereas a single episode of 30 minutes of carotid occlusion was associated with severe cortical neuronal loss. Increasing the interval to 5 h nearly completely abolished cortical injury, but was still associated with significant neuronal loss in the striatum. Light bars are results for striatum and dark bars are those for parasagittal cortex. (Data derived from Mallard et al 1993.)

PREMATURE BRAIN INJURY: THE EFFECT OF MATURATION

Surprisingly little work has been done to resolve the effect of maturation on sensitivity to injury. This is of critical importance, for two reasons. First, in recent years improvements in obstetric and pediatric management have resulted in significantly increased survival of preterm infants from 24 weeks of gestation, with an associated increase in later handicap (Kiely & Susser 1992). Second, many infants may sustain neural injuries well before birth, including a significant number of infants with cerebral palsy (Stanley 1992) (see also Chapters 18 and 46). The characteristic patterns of cerebral injury in the preterm fetus differ from those seen at term or after birth. Key features include preferential injury of subcortical structures and white matter.

Cortical resistance to injury

Clinical imaging data suggest that profound asphyxia before 32 weeks gestation is associated with injury to subcortical structures, particularly the diencephalon (including the thalamus), basal ganglia and brainstem (Barkovich & Sargent 1995). In contrast, overt cortical injury is uncommon. This is consistent with the patterns observed in infants with cerebral palsy of prenatal origin who show predominantly diencephalic lesions, variably associated with periventricular leukomalacia (PVL), cortical or subcortical lesions and ventricular dilatation (Volpe 1995). Similarly, fetal sheep at 0.6 to 0.7 gestation (96 to 102 days), maturations comparable to the 26 to 32 week gestation human fetus, show the same pattern of damage to the periventricular white matter and subcortical gray matter, with sparing of the cortex (Bennet et al 2007b, George et al 2004).

This difference is consistent with the normal caudal to rostral pattern of myelination and anatomical maturation, and the much greater anaerobic reserves and lower overall cerebral aerobic requirements of preterm fetuses compared with term (Gunn et al 2001). This is an area requiring considerably greater attention.

Pathogenesis of white matter injury

In the very low birth weight infant the distinctive white matter lesion, PVL, is the major pathologic associate of later developmental handicap. Key factors that have been identified include vascular development, the intrinsic vulnerability of the oligodendrocyte to neurotoxic factors and exposure to maternal/chorionic membrane infection. PVL characteristically occurs in areas that represent arterial end zones or border zones (Perlman 1998). Prolonged hypoperfusion owing to hypotension, or associated with hypocapnia, potentially exposes these areas to greater ischemia, as discussed above.

The immaturity of oligodendrocyte precursors is clearly critical, as the period of greatest risk for PVL is before myelination has begun, at a time when oligodendrocyte precursors are actively proliferating and differentiating. Such actively differentiating cells have an increased metabolic demand and are sensitive to substrate limitation. It has been suggested that developing oligodendroglia are very sensitive to the excitatory neurotransmitter glutamate and to free radical toxicity because of a developmental lack of antioxidant enzymes to mediate oxidative stress (Back et al 2007).

Finally, compelling evidence has recently linked prenatal inflammation or infection to later cerebral palsy (Nelson et al 1998). Exposure to maternal or placental infection is associated both with increased risk of preterm birth and also with brain lesions predictive of cerebral palsy (Dammann & Leviton 1997). It is likely that the effect of infection is mediated by systemic inflammation since fetal plasma interleukin levels including interleukins 1, 8, 9, TNF-α and the interferons are strongly and independently associated with PVL (Nelson et al 1998) (see also Chapter 21).

Intraventricular hemorrhage (IVH) and white matter injury

The pathogenesis of these disorders is discussed in detail in Chapters 19 and 21. IVH with extension into the periventricular regions is also associated with adverse outcome. The white matter injury appears to be a venous infarction with hemorrhage occurring as a secondary phenomenon. Further, there is evidence of prolonged loss of cerebrovascular autoregulation post-asphyxia which may leave the fetal brain vulnerable to factors causing fluctuations in blood pressure and thus CBF; this is proposed to be a key mechanism in the pathogenesis of IVH. Other factors that may contribute to IVH include the fragility of immature germinal matrix capillaries, deficient vascular support and a limited vasodi-

latory capacity impairing perfusion during asphyxia. In this regard, the antenatal administration of glucocorticoids has been associated with a significant reduction in the sonographic incidence of severe IVH and the associated white matter involvement (p. 405).

PRE-EXISTING METABOLIC STATUS AND CHRONIC HYPOXIA

While the original studies of factors influencing the degree and distribution of brain injury, primarily by Myers (Myers 1977), focused on metabolic status, the issue remains controversial. It has been suggested, for example, that hyperglycemia is protective against hypoxia-ischemia in the infant rat (Vannucci et al 1997) but not in the piglet (LeBlanc et al 1993). The extreme differences between these neonatal species in the degree of neural maturation and activity of cerebral glucose transporters may underlie the different outcomes (Vannucci et al 1997). The most common metabolic disturbance to the fetus is intrauterine growth retardation associated with placental dysfunction. Although there is reasonable clinical information that this condition is usually associated with a greater risk of brain injury, recent studies have suggested a marked fall in the rate of encephalopathy in growth restricted babies over time (Westgate et al 1999). This would suggest that the apparently increased sensitivity to injury is mostly due to reduced aerobic reserves, leading to early onset of systemic compromise during labor (Westgate et al 2005).

Neural maturation is markedly altered in intrauterine growth retardation with some aspects delayed and others advanced (Cook et al 1988, Stanley et al 1989). This is likely to influence the response to asphyxia but also to introduce a confounding independent effect on neural development. Severe growth retardation has been associated with altered neurotransmitter expression, reduced cerebral myelination, altered synaptogenesis and smaller brain size (Kramer et al 1990). The effect of the timing and severity of placental restriction has been examined in a range of studies in fetal sheep (Rees et al 1998). Chronic mild growth retardation due to peri-conceptual placental restriction was associated with delayed formation of neuronal connections in the hippocampus, cerebellum and visual cortex, but did not alter neuronal migration or numbers. In contrast, in studies in the near mid-gestation fetus, hypoxia induced by a variety of methods was associated with a reduction in numbers of Purkinje cells in the cerebellum and delayed development of neural processes. With more severe hypoxia the cortex and hippocampus were also affected and there was reduced subcortical myelination. The cerebellum develops later in gestation than the hippocampus, and thus appears to be more susceptible to the effects of chronic hypoxia (Rees et al 1998). Intriguingly, a recent study suggested that rat pups with moderate growth restriction showed reduced white matter injury after an excitotoxic insult, whereas those with severe growth restriction had increased damage, pointing to a complex balance between protective and sensitizing effects of placental restriction (Olivier et al 2007).

CEREBRAL TEMPERATURE

There is now good evidence from a range of species and paradigms that small, clinically relevant changes in post-ischemic cerebral temperature can critically modulate encephalopathic processes that are initiated during hypoxia-ischemic insults, and which extend into the secondary phase of neuronal loss (Gunn 2000). Conversely, prolonged mild hyperthermia during the secondary phase increases injury. The role of therapeutic hypothermia in neonatal brain protection is discussed on page 569.

While asphyxia may not be preventable, experimental data make it clear that cerebral injury is an evolving process, which can be modified by numerous external factors such as blood pressure management, infection and temperature.

This means that the opportunity exists to provide effective treatment for asphyxia. However, considerable research still needs to be done to refine our understanding of the mechanisms of injury and to develop appropriate therapeutic strategies for different clinical situations, including the very premature infant.

ACKNOWLEDGMENTS

The authors' work reported in this review has been supported by grants from the Health Research Council of New Zealand, the March of Dimes Birth Defects Trust, the Lottery Health Board of New Zealand and the Auckland Medical Research Foundation.

REFERENCES

Abi Raad R, Tan W K, Bennet L et al 1999 Role of the cerebrovascular and metabolic responses in the delayed phases of injury after transient cerebral ischemia in fetal sheep. Stroke 30:2735–2742.

Azzopardi D, Wyatt J S, Cady E B et al 1989 Prognosis of newborn infants with hypoxic-ischemic brain injury assessed by phosphorus magnetic resonance spectroscopy. Pediatr Res 25:445–451.

Back S A, Riddle A, McClure M M 2007 Maturation-dependent vulnerability of perinatal white matter in premature birth. Stroke 38:724–730.

Barkovich A J, Sargent S K 1995 Profound asphyxia in the premature infant: imaging findings. AJNR Am J Neuroradiol 16:1837–1846.

Beilharz E J, Williams C E, Dragunow M et al 1995 Mechanisms of delayed cell death following hypoxic-ischemic injury in the immature rat: evidence for apoptosis during selective neuronal loss. Brain Res 29:1–14.

Bennet L, Peebles D M, Edwards A D et al 1998 The cerebral hemodynamic response to asphyxia and hypoxia in the near-term fetal sheep as measured by near-infrared spectroscopy. Pediatr Res 44:951–957.

Bennet L, Roelfsema V, Dean J et al 2007a Regulation of cytochrome oxidase redox state during umbilical cord occlusion in preterm fetal sheep. Am J Physiol Regul Integr Comp Physiol 292:R1569–R1576.

Bennet L, Roelfsema V, George S et al 2007b The effect of cerebral hypothermia on white and grey matter injury induced by severe hypoxia in preterm fetal sheep. J Physiol 578:491–506.

Bennet L, Rossenrode S, Gunning M I et al 1999 The cardiovascular and cerebrovascular responses of the immature fetal sheep to acute umbilical cord occlusion. J Physiol (Lond) 517:247–257.

Blumberg R M, Cady E B, Wigglesworth J S et al 1997 Relation between delayed impairment of cerebral energy metabolism and infarction following transient focal hypoxia-ischaemia in the developing brain. Exp Brain Res 113:130–137.

Bolanos J P, Almeida A 1999 Roles of nitric oxide in brain hypoxia-ischemia. Biochim Biophys Acta 1411:415–436.

Bona E, Aden U, Gilland E et al 1997 Neonatal cerebral hypoxia-ischemia — the effect of adenosine receptor antagonists. Neuropharmacology 36:1327–1338.

Choi D W 1995 Calcium: still center-stage in hypoxic-ischemic neuronal death. Trends Neurosc 18:58–60.

Colbourne F, Sutherland G R, Auer R N 1999 Electron microscopic evidence against apoptosis as the mechanism of neuronal death in global ischemia. J Neurosci 19:4200–4210.

Cook C J, Gluckman P D, Williams C E, Bennet L 1988 Precocial neural function in the growth retarded fetal lamb. Pediatr Res 24:600–605.

Dammann O, Leviton A 1997 Maternal intrauterine infection, cytokines, and brain damage in the preterm newborn. Pediatr Res 42:1–8.

Danielson L, McMillen I C, Dyer J L, Morrison J L 2005 Restriction of placental growth results in greater hypotensive response to alpha-adrenergic blockade in fetal sheep during late gestation. J Physiol 563:611–620.

de Haan H H, Gunn A J, Gluckman P D 1997a Fetal heart rate changes do not reflect cardiovascular deterioration during brief repeated umbilical cord occlusions in near-term fetal lambs. Am J Obstet Gynecol 176:8–17.

de Haan H H, Gunn A J, Williams C E et al 1997c Magnesium sulfate therapy during asphyxia in near-term fetal lambs does not compromise the fetus but does not reduce cerebral injury. Am J Obstet Gynecol 176:18–27.

de Haan H H, Gunn A J, Williams C E, Gluckman P D 1997b Brief repeated umbilical cord occlusions cause sustained cytotoxic cerebral edema and focal infarcts in near-term fetal lambs. Pediatr Res 41:96–104.

de Haan H H, Van Reempts J L, Vles J S et al 1993 Effects of asphyxia on the fetal lamb brain. Am J Obstet Gynecol 169:1493–1501.

Dean J M, Gunn A J, Wassink G et al 2006 Endogenous alpha(2)-adrenergic receptor-mediated neuroprotection after severe hypoxia in preterm fetal sheep. Neuroscience 142:615–628.

Donnelly W H 1987 Ischemic myocardial necrosis and papillary muscle dysfunction in infants and children. Am J Cardiovasc Pathol 1:173–188.

Edwards A D, Cox P, Hope P L et al 1997 Apoptosis in the brains of infants suffering intrauterine cerebral injury. Pediatr Res 42:684–689.

Faraci F M, Heistad D D 1998 Regulation of the cerebral circulation: role of endothelium and potassium channels. Physiol Rev 78:53–97.

Fellman V, Raivio K O 1997 Reperfusion injury as the mechanism of brain damage after perinatal asphyxia. Pediatr Res 41:599–606.

George S, Gunn A J, Westgate J A et al 2004 Fetal heart rate variability and brainstem injury after asphyxia in preterm fetal sheep. Am J Physiol Regul Integr Comp Physiol 287:R925–R933.

Giffard R G, Monyer H, Christine C W, Choi D W 1990 Acidosis reduces NMDA receptor activation, glutamate neurotoxicity, and oxygen-glucose deprivation neuronal injury in cortical cultures. Brain Res 506:339–342.

Giussani D A, Spencer J A D, Hanson M A 1994 Fetal cardiovascular reflex responses to hypoxaemia. Fetal Matern Med Rev 6:17–37.

Goldberg M P, Choi D W 1993 Combined oxygen and glucose deprivation in cortical cell culture — calcium-dependent and calcium-independent mechanisms of neuronal injury. J Neurosci 13:3510–3524.

Gottron F J, Ying H S, Choi D W 1997 Caspase inhibition selectively reduces the apoptotic component of oxygen-glucose deprivation-induced cortical neuronal cell death. Mol Cell Neurosci 9:159–169.

Guan J, Bennet L, Gluckman P D, Gunn A J 2003 Insulin-like growth factor-1 and post-ischemic brain injury. Prog Neurobiol 70:443–462.

Gunn A J 2000 Cerebral hypothermia for the prevention of neural injury after perinatal asphyxia. Curr Opin Paediatr 12:111–115.

Gunn A J, Gluckman P D 1998 Pharmacologic strategies for the prevention of perinatal brain damage. Semin Perinatol 3:87–101.

Gunn A J, Gunn T R, de Haan H H et al 1997 Dramatic neuronal rescue with prolonged selective head cooling after ischemia in fetal lambs. J Clin Invest 99:248–256.

Gunn A J, Gunn T R, Gunning M I et al 1998 Neuroprotection with prolonged head cooling started before postischemic seizures in fetal sheep. Pediatrics 102:1098–1106.

Gunn A J, Maxwell L, de Haan H H et al 2000 Delayed hypotension and sub-endocardial injury after repeated umbilical cord occlusion in near-term fetal lambs. Am J Obstet Gynecol 183:1564–1572.

Gunn A J, Parer J T, Mallard E C et al 1992 Cerebral histological and electrophysiological changes after asphyxia in fetal sheep. Pediatr Res 31:486–491.

Gunn A J, Quaedackers J S, Guan J et al 2001 The premature fetus: not as defenseless as we thought, but still paradoxically vulnerable? Dev Neurosci 23:175–179.

Hansen A 1977 Extracellular potassium concentration in juvenile and adult rat brain cortex during anoxia. Acta Physiol Scand 99:412–420.

Hanson M A 1997 Do we now understand the control of the fetal circulation? Eur J Obstet Gynecol Reprod Biol 75:55–61.

Hanson M A 1998 Role of chemoreceptors in effects of chronic hypoxia. Comparative Biochem Physiol A Mol Integr Physiol 119:695–703.

Hellstrom Westas L, Rosen I, Svenningsen N W 1995 Predictive value of early continuous amplitude integrated EEG recordings on outcome after severe birth asphyxia in full term infants. Arch Dis Child Fetal Neonat Edn 72:F34–F38.

Hunter C J, Bennet L, Power G G et al 2003 Key neuroprotective role for endogenous adenosine A1 receptor activation during asphyxia in the fetal sheep. Stroke 34:2240–2245.

Ikeda T, Murata Y, Quilligan E J et al 1998 Physiologic and histologic changes in near-term fetal lambs exposed to asphyxia by partial umbilical cord occlusion. Am J Obstet Gynecol 178:24–32.

Ilves P, Talvik R, Talvik T 1998 Changes in Doppler ultrasonography in asphyxiated term infants with hypoxic-ischaemic encephalopathy. Acta Paediatr Scand 87:680–684.

Janbu T, Nesheim B I 1987 Uterine artery blood velocities during contractions in pregnancy and labour related to intrauterine pressure. Br J Obstet Gynaecol 94:1150–1155.

Jensen A 1996 The brain of the asphyxiated fetus — basic research. Eur J Obstet Gynecol Reprod 65:19–24.

Jones M, Jr, Sheldon R E, Peeters L L et al 1977 Fetal cerebral oxygen consumption at different levels of oxygenation. J Appl Physiol 43:1080–1084.

Keunen H, Blanco C E, Van Reempts J L, Hasaart T H 1997 Absence of neuronal damage after umbilical cord occlusion of 10, 15, and 20 minutes in midgestation fetal sheep. Am J Obstet Gynecol 176:515–520.

Kiely J L, Susser M 1992 Preterm birth, intrauterine growth retardation and perinatal mortality. Am J Public Health 82:343–344.

Kitanaka T, Alonso J G, Gilbert R D et al 1989 Fetal responses to long-term hypoxemia in sheep. Am J Physiol 256:R1348–R1354.

Kramer M S, Olivier M, McLean F H et al 1990 Impact of intrauterine growth retardation and body proportionality on fetal and neonatal outcome. Pediatrics 86:707–713.

LeBlanc M H, Huang M, Vig V et al 1993 Glucose affects the severity of hypoxic-ischemic brain injury in newborn pigs. Stroke 24:1055–1062.

Lees G J 1993 The possible contribution of microglia and macrophages to delayed neuronal death after ischemia. J Neurol Sci 114:119–122.

Lipton P 1999 Ischemic cell death in brain neurons. Physiol Rev 79:1431–1568.

Lorek A, Takei Y, Cady E B et al 1994 Delayed ('secondary') cerebral energy failure after acute hypoxia-ischemia in the newborn piglet: continuous 48-hour studies by phosphorus magnetic resonance spectroscopy. Pediatr Res 36:699–706.

Low J A 1997 Intrapartum fetal asphyxia: definition, diagnosis, and classification. Am J Obset Gynecol 176:957–959.

MacLennan A, The International Cerebral Palsy Task Force, Gunn A J et al 1999 A template for defining a causal relation between acute intrapartum events and cerebral palsy: international consensus statement. BMJ 319:1054–1059.

Mallard E C, Gunn A J, Williams C E et al 1992 Transient umbilical cord occlusion causes hippocampal damage in the fetal sheep. Am J Obstet Gynecol 167:1423–1430.

Mallard E C, Waldvogel H J, Williams C E et al 1995 Repeated asphyxia causes loss of striatal projection neurons in the fetal sheep brain. Neuroscience 65:827–836.

Mallard E C, Williams C E, Gunn A J et al 1993 Frequent episodes of brief ischemia sensitize the fetal sheep brain to neuronal loss and induce striatal injury. Pediatr Res 33:61–65.

Mallard E C, Williams C E, Johnston B M, Gluckman P D 1994 Increased vulnerability to neuronal damage after umbilical cord occlusion in fetal sheep with advancing gestation. Am J Obstet Gynecol 170:206–214.

Marks K A, Mallard E C, Roberts I et al 1996 Nitric oxide synthase inhibition attenuates delayed vasodilation and increases injury following cerebral ischemia in fetal sheep. Pediatr Res 40:185–191.

Massa S M, Swanson R A, Sharp F R 1996 The stress gene response in brain. Cerebrovasc Brain Metab Rev 8:95–158.

Michenfelder J D, Milde J H 1990 Postischemic canine cerebral blood flow appears to be determined by cerebral metabolic needs. J Cereb Blood Flow Metab 10:71–76.

Myers R E 1977 Experimental models of perinatal brain damage: relevance to human pathology. In: Gluck L (ed) Intrauterine asphyxia and the developing fetal brain. Year Book Medical, Chicago, IL, p 37–97.

Nelson K B 2007 Perinatal ischemic stroke. Stroke 38:742–745.

Nelson K B, Dambrosia J M, Grether J K, Phillips T M 1998 Neonatal cytokines and coagulation factors in children with cerebral palsy. Ann Neurol 44:665–675.

Nelson K B, Dambrosia J M, Ting T Y, Grether J K 1996 Uncertain value of electronic fetal monitoring in predicting cerebral palsy. N Engl J Med 334:613–618.

Nijboer C H, Groenendaal F, Kavelaars A et al 2007 Gender-specific neuroprotection by 2-iminobiotin after hypoxia-ischemia in the neonatal rat via a nitric oxide independent pathway. J Cereb Blood Flow Metab 27:282–292.

Nilsson G E, Lutz P L 1991 Release of inhibitory neurotransmitters in response to anoxia in turtle brain. Am J Physiol 261:R32–R37.

Olivier P, Baud O, Bouslama M et al 2007 Moderate growth restriction: deleterious and protective effects on white matter damage. Neurobiol Dis 26:253–263.

Parer J T 1998 Effects of fetal asphyxia on brain cell structure and function: limits of tolerance. Comp Biochem Physiol A Mol Integr Physiol 119:711–716.

Perlman J M 1998 White matter injury in the preterm infant: an important determination of abnormal neurodevelopment outcome. Early Hum Dev 53:99–120.

Porteracailliau C, Price D L, Martin L J 1997 Excitotoxic neuronal death in the immature brain is an apoptosis — necrosis morphological continuum. J Comp Neurol 378:70–87.

Raff M C 1992 Social controls on cell survival and cell death. Nature 356:397–400.

Rees S, Mallard C, Breen S et al 1998 Fetal brain injury following prolonged hypoxemia and placental insufficiency: a review. Comp Biochemi Physiol A, Mol Integr Physiol 119:653–660.

Reynolds E O, McCormick D C, Roth S C et al 1991 New non-invasive methods for the investigation of cerebral oxidative metabolism and haemodynamics in newborn infants. Ann Med 23:681–686.

Richardson B S, Bocking A D 1998 Metabolic and circulatory adaptations to chronic hypoxia in the fetus. Comp Biochem Physiol A Mol Integr Physiol 119:717–723.

Robertson C M, Finer N N 1993 Long-term follow-up of term neonates with perinatal asphyxia. Clin Perinatol 20:483–500.

Rosen K G, Hrbek A, Karlsson K, Kjellmer I 1986 Fetal cerebral, cardiovascular and metabolic reactions to intermittent occlusion of ovine maternal placental blood flow. Acta Physiol Scand 126:209–216.

Roth S C, Baudin J, Cady E et al 1997 Relation of deranged neonatal cerebral oxidative metabolism with neurodevelopmental outcome and head circumference at 4 years. Dev Med Child Neurol 39:718–725.

Scott R J, Hegyi L 1997 Cell death in perinatal hypoxic-ischaemic brain injury. Neuropathol Appl Neurobiol 23:307–314.

Sheldon R E, Peeters L L, Jones M D, Jr et al 1979 Redistribution of cardiac output and oxygen delivery in the hypoxemic fetal lamb. Am J Obstet Gynecol 135:1071–1078.

Shelley H J 1961 Glycogen reserves and their changes at birth and in anoxia. Br Med Bull 17:137–143.

Shuaib A, Kanthan R 1997 Amplification of inhibitory mechanisms in cerebral ischemia: an alternative approach to neuronal protection. Histol Histopathol 12:185–194.

Stanley F J 1992 Survival and cerebral palsy in low birthweight infants: implications for perinatal care. Paediatr Perinat Epidemiol 6:298–310.

Stanley O, Fleming P, Morgan M 1989 Abnormal development of visual function following intrauterine growth retardation. Early Hum Dev 19:87–101.

Tan W K M, Williams C E, During M J et al 1996 Accumulation of cytotoxins during the development of seizures and edema after hypoxic-ischemic injury in late gestation fetal sheep. Pediatr Res 39:791–797.

Tan W K M, Williams C E, Gunn A J et al 1992 Suppression of postischemic epileptiform activity with MK-801 improves neural outcome in fetal sheep. Ann Neurol 32:677–682.

Tangalakis K, Lumbers E R, Moritz K M et al 1992 Effect of cortisol on blood pressure and vascular reactivity in the ovine fetus. Exp Physiol 77:709–717.

Toet M C, Lemmers P M, van Schelven L J, van Bel F 2006 Cerebral oxygenation and electrical activity after birth asphyxia: their relation to outcome. Pediatrics 117:333–339.

Tombaugh G C 1994 Mild acidosis delays hypoxic spreading depression and improves neuronal recovery in hippocampal slices. J Neurosci 14:5635–5643.

Torvik A 1984 The pathogenesis of watershed infarcts in the brain. Stroke 15:221–223.

Vannucci S J, Maher F, Simpson I A 1997 Glucose transporter proteins in brain: delivery of glucose to neurons and glia. Glia 21:2–21.

Volpe J J 1995 Hypoxic-ischemic encephalopathy: neuropathology and pathogenesis. In: WB Saunders (ed) Neurology of the newborn, 3rd edn. WB Saunders, Philadelphia, PA, pp. 279–313.

Walton M, Sirimanne E, Williams C et al 1997 Prostaglandin H synthase-2 and cytosolic phospholipase A(2) in the hypoxic-ischemic brain — role in neuronal death or survival. Mol Brain Res 50:165–170.

Westgate J A, Gunn A J, Gunn T R 1999 Antecedents of neonatal encephalopathy with fetal acidaemia at term. Br J Obstet Gynaecol 106:774–782.

Westgate J, Wassink G, Bennet L, Gunn A J 2005 Spontaneous hypoxia in multiple pregnancy is associated with early fetal decompensation and greater T wave elevation during brief repeated cord occlusion in near-term fetal sheep. Am J Obstet Gynecol 193:1526–1533.

Williams C E, Gunn A J, Gluckman P D 1991 The time course of intracellular edema and epileptiform activity following prenatal cerebral ischemia in sheep. Stroke 22:516–521.

CHAPTER

23

Antenatal prediction of asphyxia

K. A. Sorem, James F. Smith and Maurice L. Druzin

Key Points

- Perinatal asphyxia is a hypoxic–ischemic insult that may occur antepartum, intrapartum or after birth
- Perinatal asphyxia was thought to be associated with brain damage and cerebral palsy, yet it is unlikely to be the cause for cerebral palsy unless the severity of the asphyxial insult is nearly lethal
- Recent analysis of cerebral palsy and birth asphyxia indicates that only 10% of cases of cerebral palsy (1–2 per 10 000) were associated with birth asphyxia
- Fetal asphyxia occurs as a result of absent or insufficient placental blood flow due to acute or chronic events
- The terms 'perinatal asphyxia' and 'hypoxic–ischemic injury' imply a specific cause and effect which may be difficult to determine clinically
- Hypoxic–ischemic damage begins during the injury (impaired placental exchange) and extends into the period of resuscitation or reperfusion
- Although meconium may indicate that fetal stress has occurred, it does not predict fetal neurological impairment
- Later evidence for hypoxic–ischemic brain injury in the neonate is available from a variety of imaging modalities, including computed tomography (CT), single photon emission computed tomography (SPECT), magnetic resonance imaging (MRI), positron emission tomography (PET) and cranial sonography
- Fetal wellbeing is currently evaluated using several antepartum tests including the non-stress test, contraction stress test, ultrasonographic evaluation of the fetal biophysical state and fetal Doppler ultrasound
- Significant advances in obstetrical and neonatal care have contributed to the observed decline in perinatal morbidity and mortality over the last half-century

INTRODUCTION

Perinatal asphyxia is a hypoxic–ischemic insult that may occur antepartum, intrapartum or after birth. Historically, perinatal asphyxia was thought to be associated with brain damage and cerebral palsy (Little 1862), yet it is unlikely to be the cause of cerebral palsy unless the asphyxial insult is near lethal (Winkler et al 1991). Recent analysis of cerebral palsy and birth asphyxia indicates that only 10% of cases of cerebral palsy (1–2 per 10 000) were associated with birth asphyxia (Nelson & Ellenberg 1986). Conversely, 2% of newborns have 'asphyxial exposure,' and the majority of these recover without neurologic sequelae (Low 1993). While improvements in perinatal and neonatal care have resulted in an overall reduction of morbidity and mortality, long-term studies investigating cerebral palsy show the incidence of this significant condition to have remained largely unchanged in the last 50 years (Low 2004). Nevertheless, asphyxial brain injury remains a significant cause of peri-natal morbidity and mortality, and continues to contribute to the incidence of cerebral palsy (Bracci et al 2006). Identification of the fetus at risk for asphyxia remains a clinical challenge.

DEFINITION OF PERINATAL ASPHYXIA

A task force of the World Federation of Neurology Group has defined asphyxia as a condition of impaired gas exchange which, if it persists, leads to progressive hypercapnia and hypoxemia (Bax & Nelson 1993). Fetal asphyxia occurs as a result of absent or insufficient placental blood flow due to acute or chronic events. These include umbilical cord occlusion, altered placental gas exchange (placental abruption, insufficiency or previa), inadequate perfusion of the maternal side of the placenta (maternal hypotension, vasospasm or abnormal contractions) and impaired maternal oxygenation (severe anemia, cardiac or pulmonary disease). Newborn asphyxia may result from cardio-respiratory complications after delivery, including respiratory distress syndrome, apnea and birth trauma. Hypoxic–ischemia is defined as tissue damage resulting from inadequate oxygen and substrate delivery. If blood flow and oxygenation are restored, the tissue damage is minimal; however, with prolonged asphyxia irreversible cell loss may occur.

The terms 'perinatal asphyxia' and 'hypoxic–ischemic injury' imply a specific cause and effect which may be difficult to determine clinically. Furthermore, the terms 'fetal distress' and 'birth asphyxia,' which have been common in the medical vernacular, are non-specific and imprecise. Specific criteria to define an acute intrapartum hypoxic event sufficient to cause cerebral palsy have been promoted and include: (1) profound umbilical artery metabolic or mixed acidemia (pH < 7.00), (2) persistence of an Apgar score of 0–3 for longer than 5 minutes, (3) neonatal neurologic sequelae, (4) multi-organ system dysfunction, e.g. cardiovascular, gastrointestinal, hematologic, pulmonary or renal (ACOG 1996 and ACOG 2005).

Complete assessment of the neonate at risk for neurologic sequelae includes evaluation of CNS dysfunction, including seizures, abnormal respiration, altered activity states (such as hyperalertness or somnolence), impaired reflexes (such as suck and gag), abnormal ocular responses or a bulging anterior fontanelle. Additionally, abnormal EEGs may be observed in newborns with hypoxic–ischemic encephalopathy. Clinical features of neonatal hypoxic–ischemic encephalopathy are shown in Table 23.1 (Carter et al 1993).

Although multiple organ systems may be affected by hypoxic–ischemic injury, including cardiovascular, respiratory, renal, metabolic, gastrointestinal and hematologic, only CNS involvement has residual sequelae at long term follow-up (Shankaran et al 1991). One clinical classification of intrapartum fetal asphyxia described by Low is shown in Table 23.2.

PATHOPHYSIOLOGY OF PERINATAL ASPHYXIA

Hypoxic–ischemic damage begins during the injury (impaired placental exchange) and extends into the period of resuscitation or reperfusion. At the biochemical level, cellular injury within the CNS initiates a cascade of molecular events which leads to accumulation of excitatory amino acids, increased intracellular calcium and increased free radical production (Delivoria-Papadapoulos & Mishra 1998). Oxidative metabolism is replaced by anaerobic metabolism, resulting in the accumulation of nicotinamide-adenine dinucleotide (NADH), flavin-adenine dinucleotide (FADH) and lactic acid. ATP is depleted as glycolysis fails to keep up with cellular demands, and transcellular ionic pumps fail, leading to the disruption of sodium, chloride, calcium and cellular water. Cytotoxic edema evolves. Free fatty acids accumulate as membrane phospholipids break down and undergo peroxidation by oxygen free-radicals. Glutamate is generated from axon terminals, along with nitric oxide, both of which may be directly toxic to adjacent neuronal cells. Cell death may follow due to the effects of acidosis, energy failure and lipid peroxidation (Vannucci & Palmer 1997, Vannucci & Perlman 1997). Furthermore, depletion of growth factors and inflammatory cells may lead to extensive cellular damage within the CNS (Gluckman & Williams 1992).

Following prolonged hypoxic–ischemic injury, some cells within the CNS may not recover function, resulting in regional or global infarction. In adults and experimental animals, the therapeutic window of intervention and recovery is longer than that of the fetus and newborn because the process of cellular destruction is much more rapid in the perinatal period (Vannucci & Palmer 1997). In the human fetus and neonate, the therapeutic window is estimated to be less than 2 hours (Vannucci & Perlman 1997).

Infant laboratory primates subjected to hypoxic–ischemic injury demonstrate distinct patterns of CNS damage, depending on the nature of the asphyxial insult. Brief total asphyxia damages subcortical nuclei in the thalamus and brainstem, whereas prolonged partial asphyxia damages cerebral white matter, beginning in parasagittal areas (Meyers 1975). Pasternak reported a study of 11 term human infants who sustained an acute near total intrauterine asphyxia and demonstrated a similar pattern of brain damage, depending on the magnitude and timing of the hypoxic–ischemic insult. On postnatal MRI, acute near total asphyxia appeared to damage the thalamus, brainstem and basal ganglia, presumably because of the relatively high basal metabolic rate, whereas subacute partial asphyxia led to damage primarily in the cerebral hemispheres owing to shunting of blood to the brainstem and cerebellum (Pasternak & Gorey 1998).

After brief episodes of asphyxia, restoration of blood flow may lead to re-oxygenation and end organ survival. However, reperfusion of ischemic brain tissue after a severe insult may deliver harmful reactive oxygen metabolites causing further tissue damage. In addition to damaging the cell directly, reactive oxygen metabolites delivered by reperfusion also promote the expression of adhesion molecules on endothelial or parenchymal cells. This leads to accumulation of neutrophils that cause necrosis of cortical brain cells

Table 23.1 Clinical features of neonatal hypoxic-ischemic encephalopathy	
Time after birth (hours)	Clinical features
12–24	Hyperalertness; hyper-excitability; seizures; apnea; jitteriness; weakness
24–72	Obtundation or coma; ataxic respirations with respiratory arrest; abnormal oculomotor reflexes; impaired papillary response; intracranial hemorrhage (premature neonates) with subsequent deterioration
>72	Persistent stupor; abnormal or absent sucking, swallowing, and gag reflexes; generalized hypotonia; weakness

Source: Modified from Volpe J J 1987 Hypoxic ischemic encephalopathy: clinical aspects. In: Neurology of the newborn, 2nd edn. WB Saunders, Philadelphia, PA, p. 236, with permission.

Table 23.2 Classification of intrapartum fetal asphyxia			
Asphyxia	Metabolic acidosis at delivery	Encephalopathy	Cardiovascular, respiratory, or renal complication
Mild	+	±	±
Moderate	+	++	±
Severe	+	+++	+++

Source: Modified from Low J A 1997 Intrapartum fetal asphyxia: definition, diagnosis, and classification. Am J Obstet Gynecol 176:957–959, with permission.

or delayed neuronal death through apoptosis. Pathologic evidence of cellular damage includes cell shrinkage, membrane blebbing, chromatin concentration and DNA fragmentation (Tominaga et al 1993). Therefore, it appears that cell damage occurs during both the ischemic and reperfusion phase of an asphyxial insult (Fellman & Raivio 1991).

After a severe asphyxial event, neonates often enter a phase of neurologic depression characterized by suppressed EEG and abnormal activity level. Oxygen free-radicals may induce prolonged cerebral hypoperfusion, reducing cerebral metabolism, protein synthesis and electrical activity (Leffler et al 1989). Post-asphyxial seizures in the neonate lasting more than 30 minutes are associated with poor neurologic outcome and cerebral infarction (Mellits et al 1982, Williams et al 1992). Seizures that are primarily multifocal clonic type may add additional insult to the injured brain by increasing metabolic demands on cortical cells.

FETAL RESPONSE TO ASPHYXIA (see also Ch. 22)

A fetal asphyxial insult may vary from hypoxia (decreased oxygenation) to anoxia (absent oxygenation). The fetus may not tolerate complete anoxia for more than 10 minutes, and survivors of complete total cord occlusion generally show multiple cerebral lesions, primarily in the brain stem. Through physiologic compensatory mechanisms, experimental fetal sheep have been shown to be capable of surviving an 80% decrease in cerebral oxygen uptake (Field et al 1991), indicating that the healthy fetus may tolerate even extreme hypoxia. Conversely, fetal sheep exposed to long term hypoxic stress by restricted umbilical cord blood flow demonstrate elevated nitric oxide activity and diminished cardiovascular defense to acute hypoxia (Gardner et al 2002). During a hypoxic event, blood flow is reduced to the pulmonary, renal and splanchnic areas with preferential perfusion of the heart, brain and adrenal glands (Peeters et al 1979). Furthermore, recent regional blood flow studies in fetal sheep using radioactive microspheres confirm that perfusion of the myocardium appears to be preferentially preserved over the cerebral cortex following episodes of hypoxic stress (Ley et al 2004). Within the brain, hypoxia leads to preferential blood flow to the brain stem, with decreased blood flow to white matter and the cerebral cortex. Blood oxygen level dependent signal intensity by magnetic resonance imaging appears to decrease more prominently in the fetal sheep cerebellum, compared to the cerebrum, during induced hypoxia, suggesting that the cerebellum may be more prone to effects of hypoxic stress (Wedegartner et al 2005). Experimental evidence suggests that fetal compensatory mechanisms may allow intact survival following hypoxia in the normal fetus, but chronic hypoxic stress may diminish adequate compensatory response. The fetal cerebral cortex, cerebellum, brainstem and myocardium appear to have differing responses and tolerance to hypoxic insult. The relevance of these experimental findings to the human fetus and its responses remains to be elucidated.

The fetal heart rate response to hypoxia has been intensively investigated experimentally and in the human fetus for many years. One fetal response to hypoxia, bradycardia, results from chemoreceptor stimulation of the vagus nerve. Increased sympathetic activity and peripheral vasoconstriction increase fetal blood pressure and maintain bradycardia (Hanson 1988). In addition to CNS regulation of fetal heart rate via sympathetic and parasympathetic neurons, catecholamines released from the adrenal glands directly depress the myocardium, leading to late cardiac decelerations observed on fetal heart rate monitoring. Although anaerobic glycolysis and the accumulation of pyruvate and lactate lead ultimately to metabolic acidosis, brain injury appears to be associated more strongly with fetal hypotension than with the degree of hypoxia or acidosis (De Haan et al 1997, Mallard et al 1992). Loss of fetal heart rate variability may accompany fetal hypoxia (Paul et al 1975) as well as other conditions that indicate CNS depression, such as drug exposure and structural CNS anomalies. In a 10-year study of antepartum fetal heart rate monitoring, Ayodeji and Kuhn reported that 19% of fetuses with 'critical reserve patterns' (late decelerations and loss of variability) had major structural malformations, suggesting that some fetuses may have inappropriate responses to hypoxia based on pre-existing CNS abnormalities (Ayodeji & Kuhn 1986). Genetics may also influence the fetal response to asphyxia, as demonstrated in animal models, which show that factors that mediate the response to induced hypoxia are genetically determined (Labudova et al 1999). Recently, complete cord occlusion for 20 versus 30 minutes was compared in fetal sheep (George et al 2004). In the 20-minute group, an increase in heart rate variability in the first 5 minutes after occlusion, followed by a decrease in variability for the remainder of the occlusion, was noted. The decrease in variability gradually resolved over 4 hours, with return to baseline and normal EEG patterns and movements. However, in the last 10 minutes of occlusion in the 30-minute group, increased variability in the heart rate was noted associated with abnormal atrial activity. After reperfusion, abnormal EEG findings and associated abnormal fetal movements were noted and persisted, and decreased variability remained. Histologic exam at 72 hours demonstrated severe brain stem injury in the 30-minute group, but not the 20-minute group. This suggests that epileptiform activity related to neural injury may confound interpretation of heart rate variability, mimicking normal recovery in the presence of profound injury.

Changes in fetal activity include decreased gross body movements and cessation of fetal breathing (Vintzileos et al 1991). Koos et al demonstrated in studies on fetal sheep that decrease in fetal breathing movements is evident after a decrease in fetal PO_2 of 6 mmHg (Koos et al 1987). This effect appears to be gestational age-dependent, with immature fetuses exhibiting less hypoxic inhibition than fetuses close to term. The biochemical mechanisms of the hypoxic inhibition of fetal breathing movements may result from

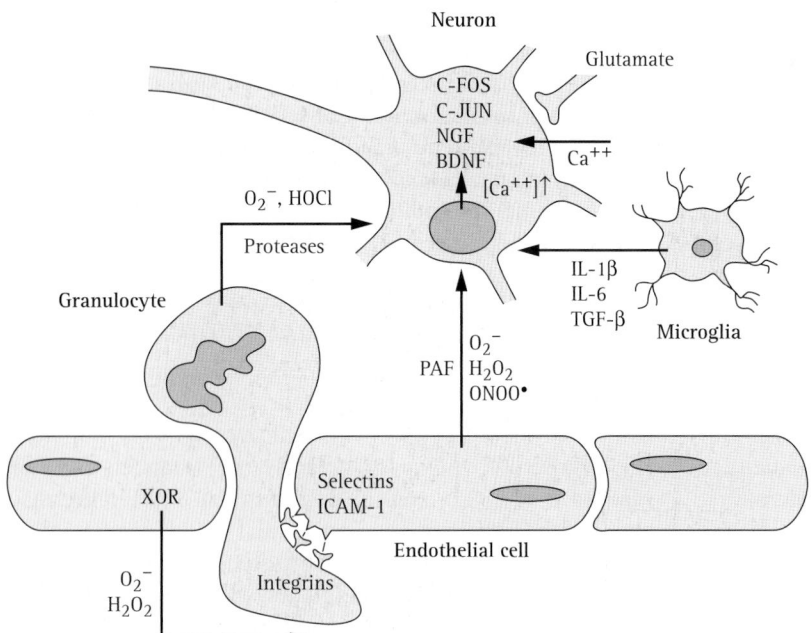

Figure 23.1 Reperfusion injury and neuronal damage following hypoxic insult. Reactive oxygen metabolites generated by endothelial and parenchymal cells lead to cell necrosis and end organ damage. NGF, nerve growth factor; BDNF, brain derived neurotrophic factor; TGF, transforming growth factor; PAF, platelet-activating factor; ONOO•, peroxynitrite. (From Fellman V, Raivio K 1997 Reperfusion injury as the mechanism of brain damage after perinatal asphyxia. Pediatr Res 41:600, with permission.)

changing brain stem concentrations of adenosine, which may be mediated by local levels of prostaglandin E_2 (Kitterman et al 1983). Both the severity and duration of hypoxia contribute to the effect on fetal breathing movements, as well as to the decreased eye movements and gross body movements observed with hypoxemia.

MARKERS FOR PERINATAL ASPHYXIA

Fetal meconium in the amniotic fluid is a relatively common finding in labor, occurring in 18% of deliveries. Although meconium may indicate that fetal stress has occurred, it does not predict neurologic impairment in the normal term fetus (Nelson & Ellenberg 1984). Prior to the widespread use of electronic fetal monitoring, the Collaborative Perinatal Study (1966) reported that 64% of the cases of amniotic fluid meconium were attributable to chorioamnionitis and only 0.2% to recognized intrapartum hypoxemic disorders (Anonymous 1966). Katz and Bowes suggest that among some fetuses with asphyxial exposure, it is the underlying asphyxia, rather than the observed meconium, that is responsible for the pulmonary pathology (Katz & Bowes 1992). However, the phenomenon of meconium aspiration syndrome in neonates born by Cesarean section in the absence of known adverse antepartum or intrapartum events indicates that meconium may also have direct effects on pulmonary vasculature. In vitro studies have demonstrated that macrophages may transport meconium directly from the amniotic fluid into the umbilical cord (Altschuler et al 1992), where it stimulates the release of vasoconstrictors within the placenta and fetus. Whether the vasoconstrictive effect of meconium contributes to damage within vulnerable cerebral vessels is speculative. In one study of 43 children with spastic quadriplegia, staining of the amniotic fluid was the only identified risk factor for cerebral palsy. Although all of the children had neuroimaging studies which identified lesions consistent with the type of severe brain damage produced by hypoxic–ischemia, not all of the newborns had abnormal umbilical artery pH or elevated base deficit (Naeye 1995). Amnioinfusion, initially thought to protect against meconium aspiration sequelae by 'dilution' of meconium, has recently been shown to be ineffective in reducing injury related to the presence of meconium (Fraser et al 2005). This further suggests that although meconium may be associated with hypoxic stress, its presence in the amniotic fluid merely indicates a fetus at risk for the potentially damaging physiologic responses, and not direct toxicity from the material itself.

Apgar scores, long used to quantify clinical depression in the first minutes of life (Apgar 1953), reflect several variables including gestational age, muscular disorders, CNS abnormalities, cardiorespiratory problems and maternal medication, in addition to antepartum or intrapartum hypoxia. Whereas moderately and briefly low Apgar scores are not related to subsequent neurologic outcome, severely low, late and very late Apgar scores are much better predictors of cerebral palsy. Although a 5-minute Apgar score of 0–3 is associated with a slight increased risk of cerebral palsy in term infants, the increase is from 0.3% to 1% (ACOG 1996). However, if such a score is associated with a 10-min Apgar of 4 or greater, there is a 99% chance of normal development. A 10-min Apgar score that does not improve (0–3) may indicate persistent hypoperfusion or hypoxia and is associated with a 16.7% risk of cerebral palsy (Freeman & Nelson 1988). A score of 0–3 at 20 minutes after delivery is associated with a 59% mortality rate and cerebral palsy in 57% of survivors (Nelson & Ellenberg 1981).

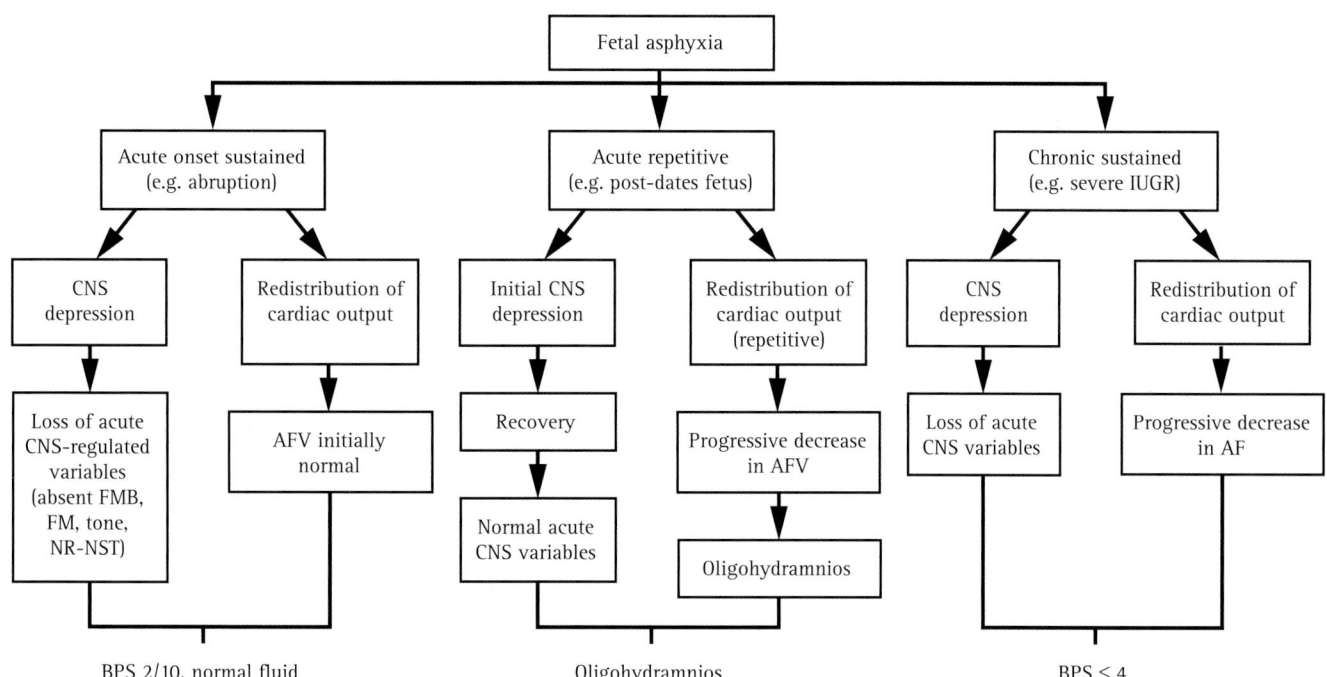

Figure 23.2 Schematic representation of the mechanisms by which the fetal response to hypoxic insult may affect the biophysical score. The fetal responses may vary with acute versus chronic hypoxia and will be affected by the duration, severity, rate of onset and repetitive frequency of the insult. CNS, central nervous system; IUGR, intrauterine growth restriction; FBM, fetal breathing movements; FM, fetal movement; NR-NST, non-reactive non-stress test; AFV, amniotic fluid volume; BPS, biophysical profile score. (From Tsang H H, Manning F A Biophysical profile scoring. In: Druzin M L (ed.) Antepartum fetal assessment. Blackwell Scientific, Boston, MA, p. 33, with permission.)

Evaluation of the acid–base status of the fetus and neonate has improved identification of newborns at risk for neurologic complications associated with antepartum or intrapartum asphyxia. The normal umbilical artery pH for term newborns is 7.2 (SD ± 0.08) and the mean base deficit is 8.3 mmol/L (SD ± 4.0 mmol/L) (Skyes & Johnson 1982), indicating that all newborns respond to the relative hypoxia of labor with a mixed metabolic and respiratory acidosis. This is not surprising, given the repetitive interruption of uteroplacental blood flow occurring with uterine contractions. In the normal term fetus with an intact CNS these episodes of intermittent hypoxia are well tolerated. The level of fetal acidemia that is considered pathologic or associated with increased morbidity and mortality is controversial. For such neonatal outcomes as intensive care unit admission and need for assisted ventilation, there appears to be a progressive risk beginning with near normal values for pH and base excess and positively associated with increasing pathologic values (Victory et al 2004). For more serious neonatal sequelae such as permanent neurologic damage, umbilical artery pH less than 7.0 is a better predictor (Hauth 1996), and ACOG has included an umbilical artery pH of 7.00 as a cut-off for clinically relevant acidemia in its definition of perinatal asphyxia. In a study of 3506 newborns, 87 of whom had pH less than 7.00, Goldaber suggests that the level of pathologic fetal acidemia is even lower (Goldaber

et al 1991). Factors such as prematurity, fetal growth restriction, infection, hypertension, collagen vascular diseases and prolonged pregnancy may all contribute to both a decreased tolerance to labor and a diminished fetal response.

Interpretation of umbilical artery blood gases requires examination of the PO_2, PCO_2 and bicarbonate, as well as the base deficit. According to Low, a base deficit of greater than 12 to 16 (occurring in 2% and 0.5% of newborns, respectively) represents the threshold for significant metabolic acidosis (Low 1997). Others have proposed the threshold of 15 mmol/L, with a compensatory calculation for severe hypercarbia (PCO_2 greater than 66 mmHg), indicating a mixed respiratory and metabolic acidosis (Goldaber et al 1991). Kruger et al have reported a threshold of 4.8 mmol/L for clinically significant lactate levels in fetal scalp blood, correlating with an increased risk of hypoxic–ischemic encephalopathy (Kruger et al 1999). All of these measurements, however, reflect a cumulative fetal response and do not indicate the timing or duration of the asphyxial exposure. As with Apgar scores, only extremely abnormal values of pH and base deficit are associated with abnormal neurologic outcome, as 80% of infants with umbilical cord pH less than 7.0 at birth will have normal neurologic development (Goodwin et al 1992).

Other markers for hypoxemia and asphyxia, such as neonatal lymphocyte count, nucleated red blood cells (NRBC) and urinary lactate to creatinine ratios have been investigated for their utility in determining the timing of an asphyxial event. In 1941, Anderson reported that chorionic capillaries within the placentas of fetuses with intrauterine asphyxia had an increase in NRBCs (Anderson 1941). Phelan and Korst subsequently observed that an NRBC count greater than 10 per 100 white blood cells was significantly higher in infants who were neurologically impaired as a result of hypoxic–ischemia (Korst et al 1996, Phelan et al 1995). In one study of 46 neurologically impaired infants, lower NRBC counts were observed in intrapartum asphyxial events closer to the birth than those with presumed asphyxial events more remote from delivery. Infants whose identified hypoxemic events were uterine ruptures had lower numbers of NRBCs than those whose asphyxial exposures were described by abnormal fetal heart rate tracings (non-reactive EFM tracings or tachycardia) (Phelan et al 1995). In Naeye's study of 16 neonates with hypoxic–ischemic encephalopathy, lymphocyte counts of greater than 10000/mm^3 were significantly higher than those observed in control groups consisting of infants with low Apgar scores and without cerebral palsy. Elevated lymphocyte counts in the affected neonates were also observed compared with infants with cerebral palsy from developmental delays unrelated to antepartum and intrapartum events (Naeye & Localio 1995).

Other biomarkers for neonatal brain injury have been investigated. In a report of 40 newborns with asphyxial exposure and 58 control infants, Huang et al reported a significantly elevated urinary lactate to creatinine ratio in infants with hypoxic exposure who developed encephalopathy (16.75), compared with both normal infants (0.09) and infants with asphyxial exposure who did not develop encephalopathy (0.19) (Huang et al 1999). Rapid measures for serum lactate exist (studies on cord blood following adverse perinatal events were carried out by Bracci et al (2006)). Non-protein-bound iron appears to be a reliable marker for brain injury (Buonocore et al 2003). The contribution of the inflammatory response to the development of neurologic injury is further supported by elevations of inflammatory protein mediators found in the cord blood of infants subsequently diagnosed with cerebral palsy (Kaukola et al 2004). Astroglial calcium binding protein S100, which is a marker for brain injury in adults, has been investigated in preterm and term neonates with and without brain injury, and may be a useful marker (Bracci 2006). Activin A, a protein produced by the placenta, decidua and fetal membranes, increases in response to hypoxia, and correlates with other markers and biochemical features of perinatal hypoxia (Bracci 2006). Important in all of the investigations of biochemical markers is timing of injury in the human fetus, which is largely determined by history and clinical assessments. Because of the high number of false positive rates of any abnormal findings on fetal heart rate monitoring, and the impossibility of excluding antenatal causes, the exact timing of subcatastrophic asphyxial events in human studies cannot be accurately determined. This limits the clinical application of assessments of NRBCs, neonatal lymphocytes and other biomarkers of perinatal asphyxia. Because of advances in potential therapies for infants exposed to hypoxic–ischemic events (Palmer & Vannucci 1993), recognition of neonates at risk and understanding the timing of the insult remain critical clinical research goals.

NEUROIMAGING AND PERINATAL HYPOXIC–ISCHEMIC BRAIN INJURY (see also Ch. 6)

Later evidence for hypoxic–ischemic brain injury in the neonate is available from a variety of imaging modalities, including computed tomography (CT), single photon emission computed tomography (SPECT), magnetic resonance imaging (MRI), positron emission tomography (PET) and cranial sonography. Recent advances in the application and accessibility of fetal MRI have led to increasing use of this modality in many aspects of fetal medicine, including the potential diagnosis of congenital and acquired brain lesions. Protocols have been developed that help systematize the application of fetal MRI (Prayer et al 2004), and several reports now describe normal embryonic and fetal neurodevelopment as assessed by fetal MRI (Grossman et al 2006, Prayer et al 2006, Rados et al 2006). One case of in utero fetal cerebral intra-parenchymal ischemia diagnosed by MRI has been reported in a severely growth restricted fetus (Sibony et al 1998). MRI has been used to assess fetal brain injury related to abnormal pregnancies presumably complicated by chronic stress (Borowska-Matwiejczuk K et al 2003), and in hypoxic and infectious insults (Girard et al 2003).

In term infants with neuroimaging abnormalities following asphyxial events, the ischemic injury results in diffuse infarctions in the parasagittal cortex and parieto-occipital cortex. Thromboembolic multifocal infarcts, thalamic, and basal ganglia infarcts and middle cerebral artery infarcts may also be observed. In one study of 11 infants who suffered acute near-total intrauterine asphyxia, imaging studies reported a consistent pattern of injury in the subcortical brain nuclei with relative sparing of the white matter. Seven of the 11 infants with hypoxic–ischemic encephalopathy and this pattern of brain injury had good cognitive outcomes; however, long-term neurologic deficits included spastic quadriplegia, mild cerebral palsy, deafness, behavioral abnormalities and dystonia. Although 10 of the 11 patients did not have significant multiorgan system failure, the one infant who died in the neonatal period had evidence of hepatic abnormality (Pasternak & Gorey 1998). In another study of 20 term infants with moderate-to-severe hypoxic–ischemic encephalopathy, decreased tissue attenuation in the central gray matter (thalami and basal ganglia) was observed in the absence of cortical changes. This pattern of injury indicated an extremely poor prognosis, with 35% of infants expiring in the neonatal period and the remaining survivors all affected with neurologic abnormalities including spastic quadriplegia, microcephaly and seizures (Roland et al 1998).

In preterm infants with hypoxic–ischemic encephalopathy, brain injuries usually result from hemorrhage, either in the vascular subependymal areas, within the cerebral ventricles, or within the parenchyma. Infrequently, the periventricular white matter region is affected bilaterally and periventricular leukomalacia (PVL) results. The specific pattern of perinatal CNS damage in the preterm infant is demonstrated primarily in the deep strata of the cerebellum, germinal tissue, periventricular white matter and basal ganglia, in contrast to mainly cortical damage in the term infant. This distinction is influenced by three gestational age-dependent factors: (1) presence or absence of germinal matrix tissue, (2) the underlying process of CNS organogenesis and (3) the degree of development of neurovasculature (Towbin 1986). Neurodevelopmental prognoses among preterm infants with asphyxial exposure and abnormal neuroimaging studies vary widely, with factors such as infection and developmental immaturity contributing to possible CNS damage from asphyxial exposure.

Neuropathologic studies confirm the findings of neuroimaging and have shown that both the gray matter and the white matter of the brain may undergo necrosis as a result of lethal hypoxic–ischemia. In one post-mortem study of 120 perinatal deaths attributed to perinatal asphyxia, CNS necrosis was observed in 16 infants, including lesions that occurred in the antepartum period as well as intrapartum (Low et al 1989). In the first half of pregnancy, ischemic CNS insults may lead to porencephalic cysts, multicystic encephalomalacia and hydrencephaly. In this study of term infants, two infants with antenatal hypoxic–ischemia had evidence of PVL. In five infants remote from term, the hypoxic–ischemic insult occurred in the 12-hour period before the onset of labor, presumably due to antepartum hemorrhage. The pattern of CNS pathology in this group showed neuronal necrosis of the cerebral cortex, and the inferior olive and dorsal nucleus of the vagus nerve of the brain stem, large germinal matrix hemorrhage and intraventricular hemorrhage. The four neonates in the intrapartum asphyxia group delivered with clinical evidence of asphyxia as well as abnormal pH and acid–base status. The observed neuropathology in the intrapartum asphyxia group included extensive neuronal necrosis of the basal ganglia and thalamus, with limited necrosis in the cerebellar cortex and brain stem.

In summary, establishing the temporal relationship between an asphyxial event and the associated findings on neuroimaging and neuropathology is difficult and imprecise. Term and preterm infants exhibit different patterns of brain injury after asphyxial events, and the pattern associated with asphyxial injury remote from delivery may occasionally be distinct. Neonates who expire of sudden cardiorespiratory failure as a result of catastrophic asphyxia may not demonstrate any neuropathologic findings because of rapid demise. Furthermore, as mentioned earlier, findings consistent with an acute intrapartum event do not rule out pre-existing subclinical subacute lesions that may enhance fetal susceptibility to the intermittent hypoxia of normal and abnormal labors. Nevertheless, MRI remains a promising tool in understanding of perinatal brain injury, and likely will see an expanding role in this area in the future (Gressens & Luton 2004).

ANTEPARTUM ASPHYXIA

In the United States, perinatal mortality, which includes late fetal deaths (after 28 weeks) as well as early neonatal deaths (less than 6 days of life), has been declining steadily since 1965, reaching 8.7 per 1000 in 1991 and 7.3 per 1000 in 1997 (CDC 1998, US Department of Health and Human Services 1995). Antepartum deaths may be due to a variety of causes including congenital malformations, pregnancy complications and infection, as well as to chronic or acute hypoxic–ischemia. Of the 70–90% of fetal deaths that occur prior to the onset of labor, approximately one-third are due to hypoxia (Lammer et al 1989). In contrast, intrapartum fetal deaths are primarily asphyxial, in some cases due to severe hypoxia or anoxia and in some cases due to abnormal fetal response.

Reducing the rate of lethal antepartum asphyxia remains a difficult clinical task, not only because of the unpredictable nature of the underlying causes but also because of the relatively long period of time over which it may occur (Grant & Elborne 1989). Identifying subcatastrophic hypoxial insults that may lead to long-term neurologic morbidity is yet more complex. One strategy to reduce antepartum fetal deaths is to identify pregnancies that are at increased risk for decreased uteroplacental blood flow, such as those complicated by hypertension, collagen vascular diseases and diabetes, and to subject these patients to a schedule of antepartum evaluation or testing. Fetuses at risk for antenatal acute and chronic asphyxia, including those with intrauterine fetal growth restriction (Soothill et al 1987) and prolonged pregnancy, may also benefit from antepartum surveillance.

ANTEPARTUM FETAL TESTING

Fetal wellbeing is currently evaluated using several antepartum tests including the non-stress test, contraction stress test, ultrasonographic evaluation of the fetal biophysical state and fetal Doppler. Of the tests that involve observations of fetal heart rate by cardiotocography, the non-stress test is the most widely used. The use of the non-stress test evolved from observations of fetal heart tracings in labor as well as in experimental animal models. Whereas late decelerations and loss of variability on electronic fetal monitoring (EFM) have been linked with fetal acidosis (Murata et al 1982), accelerations of the fetal heart in response to fetal activity, contractions, or external stimulation, have been associated with adequate fetal oxygenation and neurologic response. To produce a normal (reactive) fetal heart rate tracing on EFM, the fetal heart must demonstrate intact electrical conduction pathways involving myocardial, neurologic and hormonal receptors as well as intact sympathetic and parasympathetic reflexes and normal myocardial contractility (Dalton et al 1983).

The normal fetal heart baseline is between 110 and 160 bpm. The healthy term fetus demonstrates an average of 34 heart rate accelerations per hour, averaging 20 to 25 bpm above baseline and lasting up to 40 seconds (Patrick et al 1984). At term, fetal heart rate accelerations are associated with fetal movement more than 85% of the time and more than 90% of fetal body movements are accompanied by accelerations. The association of fetal heart rate accelerations and fetal movement increases with advancing gestational age, representing neurologic maturation and integration of reflex responses and autonomic tone.

The most common cause for absent fetal heart rate accelerations is fetal sleep, although other factors such as maternal narcotics, CNS depressants, maternal smoking or β-blockers may reduce fetal heart rate variability as well (Keegan et al 1979, Margulis et al 1984, Phelan 1979). Episodes of decreased fetal movement associated with diminished fetal heart rate variability indicate a quiet fetal sleep cycle and may last from 20 to 120 minutes in the term fetus. Active sleep cycles in the fetus occur throughout most of a 24-hour day and involve increased fetal breathing, increased fetal heart rate variability, rapid eye movements and occasional body movements. Brief periods of 'wakefulness' occur approximately 15–20% of the day and are associated with increased gross body movements and maximal fetal heart rate variability.

NON-STRESS TEST

The non-stress test (NST) is usually performed in an outpatient setting, with the patient in a reclining chair or bed with left lateral tilt to avoid supine hypotension. The fetal heart rate is monitored using the Doppler ultrasound transducer,

and the tocodynamometer is used to detect uterine contractions. During the test the patient reports fetal activity, although the record of these fetal movements does not affect the interpretation of the test. As with intrapartum fetal monitoring, acute fetal hypoxemia in the antepartum period may cause profound decreases in fetal movement and heart rate accelerations. Chronic hypoxia, however, may yield a more gradual decline in fetal function and response as compensatory circulatory shunting occurs.

Guidelines for interpretation of fetal heart rate (FHR) monitoring have been developed by the Research Planning Workshop for the National Institute of Child Health and Human Development (1996) (Anonymous 1997). These guidelines apply to interpretation of antepartum as well as intrapartum EFM. First, any patterns of the fetal heart rate are reported as baseline, periodic or episodic. Second, the following five components of fetal heart rate patterns must be described qualitatively and quantitatively: (1) baseline rate, (2) baseline variability, (3) presence of accelerations, (4) periodic or episodic decelerations and (5) changes or trends in fetal heart rate patterns over time. An acceleration of the fetal heart rate is defined as a visually abrupt increase in the FHR above baseline. The peak is to be greater than or equal to 15 bpm over the baseline and lasting 15 seconds or more. Prior to 32 weeks gestation, accelerations are defined as 10 bpm over baseline for duration of 10 seconds or greater. The most widely applied definition of a normal or reactive non-stress test involves two accelerations meeting the above criteria in a 20-minute period.

On initial testing, 85% of NSTs will be reactive and 15% will be non-reactive (Lavery 1982). The NST is most predictive when it is normal or reactive. A reactive NST has been associated with a perinatal mortality of approximately 5 per 1000 (Phelan 1981). Although the rate of perinatal demise after a non-reactive NST is considerably higher, up to 40 per 1000, this group contains a large number of false positive tests, as high as 75–90% (Lavery 1982). The majority of fetuses with a non-reactive NST will not suffer death or morbidity following the test; however, follow-up testing is generally indicated, whether by prolonged NST, contraction stress test or biophysical profile.

Vibroacoustic stimulation (VAS) has been used to stimulate the fetus that may be in a quiet sleep state. The artificial larynx, which generates a sound pressure of 82 dB measured at 1 meter of air, is the most commonly used device (Gagnon et al 1989). VAS has been shown to increase the mean duration of heart rate accelerations, the mean amplitude of accelerations and total time spent in accelerations. FHR variability and gross body movements are also increased. Using VAS in the setting of non-reactive NSTs, the incidence of non-reactivity is reduced from 14 to 9%, and the time spent in testing is reduced. In one study by Druzin et al, the incidence of non-reactive NSTs in fetuses after 26 weeks was significantly decreased with the use of VAS (Druzin et al 1989), obviating the need for further testing to follow up a non-reactive test.

Table 23.3 Indications for antepartum fetal testing	
• Asthma	• Polyhydramnios
• Abnormal fetal heart tones	• Poor obstetric history
• Cardiac disease	• Prolonged pregnancy
• Cholestasis of pregnancy	• Pre-eclampsia
• Chronic hypertension	• Preterm labor
• Collagen vascular disease	• Preterm premature rupture
• Congenital anomalies	of membranes
• Decreased fetal movement	• Prior stillbirth
• Diabetes	• Renal disease
• Fetal growth restriction	• Rh disease
• Intrauterine procedure	(isoimmunization)
• Multiple gestation	• Sickle cell disease
• Oligohydramnios	• Substance abuse
• Placenta previa	• Third trimester bleeding
	• Thyroid disease

Significant bradycardia, defined as a fetal heart rate of less than 90 bpm or a fall in the fetal baseline more than 40 bpm (ACOG 1984, Druzin et al 1981), has been observed in 1–2% of all NSTs. Bradycardia on NST has been associated with increased perinatal morbidity and mortality, including intrauterine fetal demise, structural malformations and fetal growth restriction (Bourgeois et al 1984, Druzin 1989). Moreover, the incidence of abnormal intrapartum FHR tracing and subsequent Cesarean delivery is higher in those with bradycardia on antepartum heart tracing on NST compared with those who have reactive NSTs without significant bradycardia. Although a non-reactive NST is also associated with an abnormal intrapartum FHR tracing and increased intervention rate, the positive predictive value of the tracing with bradycardia leading to Cesarean delivery is higher (Dashow & Read 1984). Because perinatal mortality rates may be as high as 25% in fetuses with spontaneous significant bradycardias, delivery is generally indicated for the term fetus, but management of the preterm fetus may be more complex. Presence or absence of variability in the setting of significant bradycardia may not be helpful in distinguishing fetuses at increased risk for perinatal hypoxia. Corticosteroid administration and conservative management may follow assessment of the amniotic fluid index and targeted ultrasound for fetal anomalies, with continuous fetal monitoring for the early preterm fetus.

In high-risk pregnancies, increasing the interval of testing to twice per week can reduce the false negative rate of the NST. Boehm et al (1986) reported an overall decrease in the fetal death rate from 6.1/1000 to 1.9/1000 when twice weekly testing was used. Because the fetal death rate is increased in pregnancies with diabetes, hypertension and fetal growth restriction, these pregnancies should be monitored with twice weekly NSTs. The incidence of fetal death following a normal NST in prolonged pregnancies is not significantly increased over the general tested pregnant population (2.7/1000) (Barss et al 1981); however, the risk–benefit ratio of intervention on behalf of the term mature fetus may favor induction of labor in some cases.

CONTRACTION STRESS TEST

The contraction stress test (CST), also known as the oxytocin challenge test, was the first antepartum test used for fetal surveillance. When contractions produce decreased blood flow in the intervillous spaces of the placenta, varying degrees of hypoxia may lead to signs of stress in the fetus. On FHR monitoring, the fetus with diminished placental respiratory reserve may respond to the stress of contractions with late decelerations. Interpretation of the presence or absence of late decelerations and the pattern of decelerations form the basis for interpretation of the CST.

Prior to the test, which is generally performed on a labor and delivery suite or specialized antepartum testing unit, maternal blood pressure is monitored periodically while uterine contractions and FHR are recorded using external monitors. Oxytocin is administered by intravenous infusion,

beginning at 0.5 mU/min. The infusion is doubled every 15 minutes until three contractions in 10 minutes are achieved. After the CST is achieved, FHR monitoring should continue until contractions cease. As an alternative to oxytocin infusion, the nipple stimulation test may be used. Using self-nipple massage, over 85% of patients can achieve adequate uterine contractions for evaluation (Oki et al 1987) with no difference in the incidence of positive and negative tests compared with the CST. Absolute contraindications to the CST include premature preterm rupture of the membranes, third trimester bleeding and cervical incompetence. Relative contraindications include preterm labor, polyhydramnios, prior cesarean section and multiple gestation.

Interpretation of the CST follows the definitions described by Freeman (1975). A positive (abnormal) test is defined as a 10-minute segment of the FHR tracing which includes at least three contractions, each followed by late decelerations. A negative (normal) test is one with no late decelerations after three uterine contractions. A CST with negative windows and occasional late decelerations is read as suspicious, and equivocal describes the tracing with occasional late decelerations and no negative window. A CST with both negative and positive windows is interpreted as positive. A suspicious or equivocal CST should be repeated in 24 hours, and most of these tests will become negative. Bruce et al (1978) observed that 5 of 67 patients with initial CSTs read as suspicious were subsequently positive.

Although a negative CST has been consistently associated with a good outcome (perinatal mortality less than 1/1000 within 1 week of the test), the relatively high false positive rate (up to 30%) limits the utility of the test (Evertson et al 1978, Freeman et al 1982). Furthermore, Druzin et al (1980) reported that a non-reactive NST with a negative contraction stress test did not have the same predictive accuracy as the reactive NST. Overall, the rate of perinatal death following a positive CST is elevated at 7–15%. Although a positive CST is an indication for delivery, it is not necessarily an indication for cesarean section, as labor may proceed safely with continuous FHR monitoring. The positive CST had been associated not only with an increased incidence of fetal death, but also with an increased incidence of perinatal morbidity as detected by low 5-minute Apgar scores, fetal growth restriction, and meconium stained amniotic fluid, intrapartum fetal distress and neonatal depression.

No prospective randomized trials with sufficient numbers of risk-matched gravidas have been reported for either the CST or the NST. Evaluation of the current literature shows a wide range of testing standards and thresholds yielding a yet wider range of test sensitivity, specificity and positive predictive values. Because the positive predictive value depends on the incidence of fetal compromise in a given population, the application of these tests to low-risk patients will decrease the performance of the test. For both the NST and the CST the specificity is relatively high (>90%), with sensitivities of 45–55%. Most evaluations of the CST use perinatal mortality as a primary outcome measure with few conclusions regarding the impact of abnormal tests on perinatal morbidity and neurologic outcome. Because of the low sensitivity of these tests (i.e. high number of false positives), additional fetal testing may be performed prior to intervention (delivery), especially when the fetus is known or suspected to be immature.

BIOPHYSICAL PROFILE

Fetal hypoxemia has been shown to alter biophysical activities such as fetal breathing and movement, as well as tone and heart rate patterns. Fetal biophysical profile (BPP) scoring was therefore developed using dynamic ultrasound examination to assess the wellbeing of the fetus. Ultrasound examination of the fetus is also used to detect abnormalities of amniotic fluid, fetal size, placental location and umbilical cord insertion site. Fetal biophysical responses to asphyxia include both acute and chronic responses. The acute fetal response to hypoxia includes changes in CNS regulated activities, such as breathing and movement. Chronic responses to decreased oxygenation include low levels of amniotic fluid and restricted fetal growth.

The BPP method as described by Manning et al (1985) uses real time ultrasound for scored evaluation of fetal breathing movements, fetal tone, gross body movements and amniotic fluid volume. An NST may follow the ultrasound examination of the fetus. The longitudinal scan plane is used to view the fetus with simultaneous evaluation of upper and lower extremities, as well as the fetal thorax. The test continues for 30 minutes or until all the parameters have been observed. Two points are scored for each of the above variables for a maximum score of 8 out of 8. If the NST is generally performed if one of more of the other four variables is abnormal, two points are scored for a reactive NST and the total for a normal test is then scored as 10 out of 10. All of the components are assumed to be of equal significance, and therefore are each assigned two points. In one analysis of 342 abnormal tests, Manning demonstrated that the distribution of score variables is almost equal among possible combinations (Manning et al 1990).

According to Vintzileos et al (1983), fetal biophysical activities that appear earliest in fetal development are the last to disappear with fetal hypoxia. The fetal tone center in the cortex begins to function at approximately 8 weeks. Fetal tone, therefore, would be the last parameter to be lost with deteriorating fetal condition. The fetal movement center, which functions at approximately 9 weeks, would be more sensitive than fetal tone. Fetal breathing, which develops at approximately 20 weeks, may be lost sooner than movement and tone. Finally, fetal heart rate reactivity, which relies on development of the posterior thalamus and medulla as well as intact CNS reflexes, may not reliably appear until the late third trimester (>28 weeks). Using this hypothesis, the BPP may be used to evaluate the preterm fetus in which FHR reactivity has not been established.

Like the reactive NST, a normal BPP is highly predictive of a non-asphyxiated fetus with intact CNS responses. In one prospective blinded study of 216 high-risk pregnancies, Manning found no perinatal deaths when all five variables of the test were normal (Manning et al 1980). However, unlike the NST, several aspects of fetal response are evaluated using the BPP, and the resulting proportion of normal tests is higher (97.5%). A false negative rate of the BPP is also lower than that of the NST alone (2–5/1000). Similar to the NST, the use of vibroacoustic stimulation of the fetus with an abnormal or equivocal BPP has been shown to improve the biophysical score without decreasing the false negative rate (Inglis et al 1993), and shortens the testing time when applied at the beginning of an exam (Pinette et al 2005). Moreover, the scoring system for the BPP (see Table 23.4) may reveal a spectrum of fetal asphyxial response. Good obstetric management mandates interpretation of the individual components as well as consideration of obstetric factors, such as gestational age, underlying fetal and maternal disease, maternal drug exposure and prematurity. According to a summary of data in eight studies of BPP for fetal evaluation, involving 23 780 patients and 54 337 tests, the overall corrected perinatal mortality of the BPP was calculated at 0.726/1000 (Manning 1992).

To evaluate the effect of fetal assessment by BPP on the risk of perinatal morbidity, Manning evaluated the incidence of cerebral palsy in fetuses that were evaluated by BPP compared with those who were not. In a retrospective study of 84 947 live births over a 5-year period, the overall incidence of cerebral palsy was 3.68/1000. The incidence of cerebral palsy in 26 290 referred high risk patients who had antenatal testing with BPP was 1.33/1000 live births compared with 4.74/1000 in 58 657 untested patients (Manning et al 1998). In another study examining the relationship between abnormal BPP and cerebral palsy, Manning reported that the fetuses with abnormal BPP were more likely to develop fetal distress in labor (88.8%), acidosis (77.7%) and neonatal seizures (88.8%). Antenatal asphyxia as predicted based on BPP appears to be associated with cerebral damage in 29.6% of cases (Manning et al 1997).

A combined strategy of non-stress testing, evaluation of amniotic fluid index (AFI), biophysical profile, umbilical velocimetry and contraction stress testing may be used in the antepartum assessment of the fetus at risk for hypoxic stress. One general algorithm for fetal evaluation is represented in Figure 23.3. The specific indication for testing, the gestational age, and other compounding maternal and fetal factors may influence the testing interval as well as the combined number of tests required to raise the suspicion of fetal jeopardy to the point of delivery. When abnormal antepartum testing indicates the need for delivery, this may be accomplished by either the vaginal or abdominal route, depending on the fetal response to the stress of labor and other obstetric indications. The ease and acceptability of NST and BPP, compared to the CST, have led to decreasing use of CST in favor of these other two tests in current practice (Huddleston 2002).

Table 23.4 Biophysical profile scoring and interpretation

Biophysical variable	Normal (score = 2)	Abnormal (score = 0)
Fetal breathing movements	At least one episode of fetal breathing movement of at least 30 seconds duration in 30 minutes	Absent fetal breathing or no episode of greater than 30 seconds in 30 minutes
Gross body movements	At least three discrete body or limb movements in 30 minutes	Two or fewer body or limb movements in 30 minutes
Fetal tone	At least one episode of active extension with return to flexion of fetal limbs or trunk, includes opening and closing the hand	Either slow extension with return to partial flexion, or movement of the limb in full extension or no fetal movement
Reactive non-stress test	At least two episodes of fetal heart rate acceleration of greater than or equal to 15 bpm and of at least 15 seconds duration associated with fetal movement in 30 minutes	Less than two episodes of acceleration of fetal heart rate greater than or equal to 15 bpm, and of at least 15 seconds in duration associated with fetal movement in 30 minutes
Amniotic fluid volume	At least one pocket of amniotic fluid that measures 2 cm by 2 cm in two perpendicular planes	Either no amniotic fluid pocket or a pocket less than 2 cm in two perpendicular planes

Source: From Tsang H H, Manning F A Biophysical profile scoring. In: Druzin M L (ed.) Antepartum fetal assessment. Blackwell Scientific, Boston, MA, p. 33, with permission.

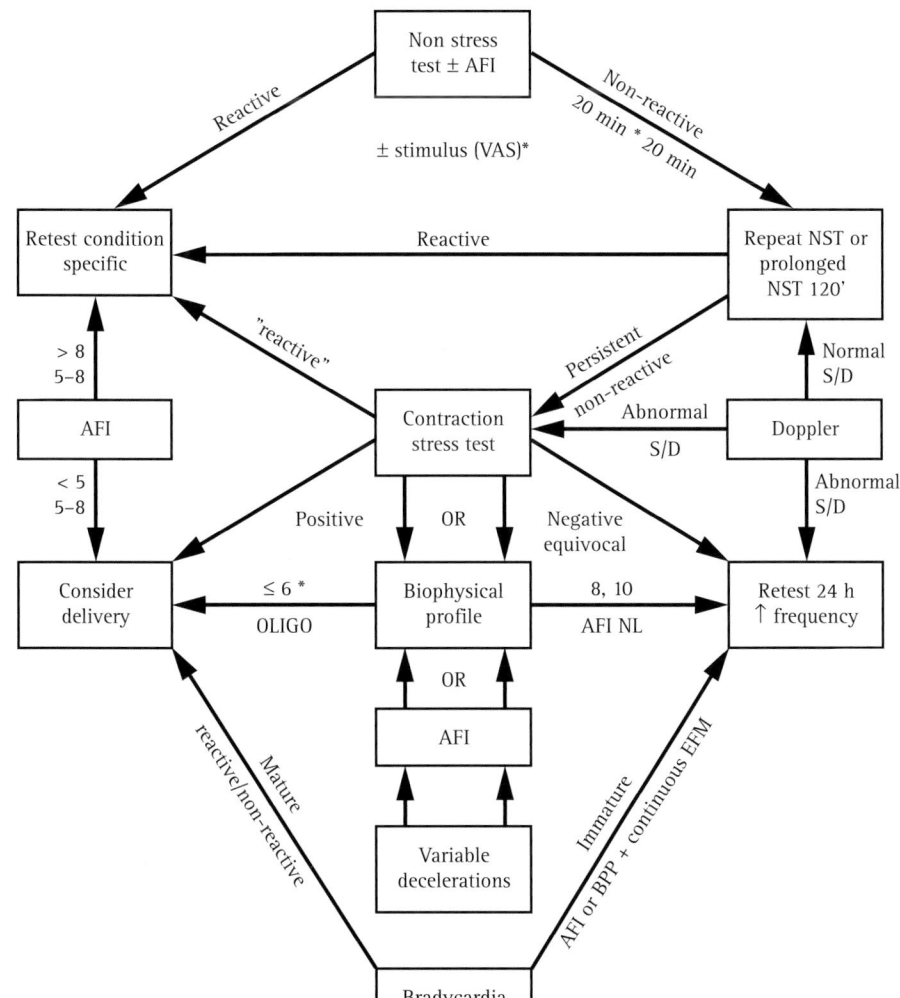

Figure 23.3 Fetal antepartum testing scheme. The most commonly used antepartum test is the non-stress test (NST). Depending on abnormalities of testing, other follow-up tests may be indicated; the contraction stress test is less commonly used in current practice. AFI, amniotic fluid index; VAS, vibroacoustic stimulation; BPP, biophysical profile; S/D; systolic to diastolic ratio.

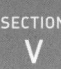

DOPPLER VELOCIMETRY OF THE UMBILICAL VESSELS (see also Ch. 10)

Because of the need for better antenatal tests to reduce unnecessary intervention in pregnancies with false positive tests, umbilical artery Doppler velocimetry has been widely investigated. The principle upon which Doppler testing of the fetus may be useful relies on an incomplete understanding of the physiology of uteroplacental blood flow. Continuous wave Doppler systems generate flow velocity waveforms that reflect the distribution and intensity of the Doppler frequency shifts over time. Provided the angle of insonation and the transmitted frequency of the ultrasound beam are constant, these frequency shifts are proportional to changes in flow velocity within the umbilical vessels.

Clinically, the most commonly used fetal Doppler evaluation is reported as the ratio of the peak systolic velocity waveform to the nadir at diastole (S/D). The greater the diastolic flow, the lower the ratio. As the peripheral resistance increases, the diastolic flow falls, resulting in an elevated S/D. At various gestational ages the fetal circulation demonstrates characteristic Doppler waveforms. In the first trimester of pregnancy, the umbilical artery has high pulsatility and consequently generates a Doppler waveform with reduced diastolic flow (elevated S/D). This pattern results from elevated downstream resistance in the umbilical and placental vessels. As resistance in the placental vessels drops in the second trimester from growth of small muscular arteries in the tertiary stem villi of the placenta, diastolic flow increases and the S/D decreases. This pattern of decreasing pulsatility and increasing diastolic flow continues throughout normal gestation. By 30 weeks gestation, the S/D in the umbilical artery should be less than 3.0. Absent or reverse diastolic flow reflects an abnormally elevated level of fetal peripheral resistance that may indicate fetal jeopardy.

Other methods of reporting fetal arterial Doppler waveforms include the pulsatility index and the resistance index. The pulsatility index is calculated as the systolic minus the diastolic values divided by the mean of the velocity waveform profile (S – D/mean). The resistance index (Pourcelot ratio) is expressed as S – D/S. These indices are useful in statistical analyses when there is absent (the S/D is infinity) or reversed end diastolic flow.

Several studies have suggested that umbilical artery Doppler provides a reasonable estimation of umbilical cord blood flow. Decreases in the S/D ratio, therefore, reflect placental abnormalities in flow and resistance, rather than hypoxia or asphyxia per se. Using a sheep model, Trudinger et al (1987) embolized the umbilical placental circulation with microspheres each day for nine days and observed the resulting Doppler waveforms. The umbilical S/D ratio increased steadily with increasing vascular resistance in the placental bed. However, umbilical blood flow did not fall significantly until the placental resistance was maximal. Morrow and Ritchie (1989) used a similar model of progressive embolization and likewise observed a progressive

increase in the S/D ratio, followed by absent end diastolic flow, then reversed diastolic flow. In this study, increasing the blood viscosity 100% by increasing the fetal hematocrit had minimal effect on the S/D ratio, indicating that umbilical blood flow, not necessarily hypoxia, induced abnormal Doppler waveforms in the umbilical artery. Because decreased umbilical artery flow may not produce hypoxemia in the well compensated fetus, abnormal Doppler velocimetry neither reliably predicts antenatal hypoxic–ischemic conditions nor demonstrates chronic asphyxia, but may help determine the 'at-risk' fetus. Five central and peripheral vessels of fetuses with IUGR were serially investigated by Ferrazzi et al (2002) in an attempt to determine temporal and sequential changes and their correlation with fetal heart rate monitoring and BPP scoring. The vessels included the umbilical artery, middle cerebral artery, ductus venosus, pulmonary artery and aorta. Early changes were identified in the umbilical and middle cerebral arteries, and late changes in the pulmonary artery and aorta. However, 60% of fetuses demonstrated abnormal fetal heart rate changes prior to abnormal late changes in the pulmonary artery and aorta. Furthermore, concordance for abnormal BPP scores and Doppler assessments in fetuses with IUGR could be found in only 44% of cases in a study by Baschat et al (2006).

In assessing placental function and umbilical blood flow, Doppler velocimetry has been investigated as an antenatal predictor of fetal condition. In one study by Devoe et al (1990), Doppler velocimetry was used along with NST and amniotic fluid evaluation to determine the predictive value in predicting poor perinatal outcome as determined by fetal distress in labor, low 5-minute Apgar scores, neonatal acidosis and perinatal mortality. The overall perinatal mortality using all three techniques was 2.1 per 1000. Although each method had a specificity of approximately 90%, sensitivities for the NST and Doppler velocimetry were 69% and 21%, respectively. The positive predictive value of all three tests combined in predicting abnormal outcome was 100%. In a meta-analysis of 12 randomized controlled trials of Doppler velocimetry in high risk pregnancies, Alfirevic and Nielson (1995) detected a significant decrease in perinatal deaths and cesarean deliveries for fetal distress among pregnancies in which Doppler velocimetry was used for antenatal surveillance.

Although Doppler velocimetry has not been shown to be predictive of poor pregnancy outcome in low risk pregnancies (Mason et al 1993), this antenatal test performs better in pregnancies at risk for intrauterine growth restriction, including hypertension and collagen vascular diseases. An elevation of the S/D may precede the identification of fetal growth restriction, and may be more predictive of neonatal morbidity than the NST alone (Trudinger et al 1986). Because the absence of diastolic flow in pregnancies complicated by fetal growth restriction has been associated with increased perinatal mortality, these fetuses may require either intense on-going fetal surveillance or delivery. Abnormal Doppler velocimetry appears to be associated with abnormal fetal conditions including aneuploidy (Martinex-Crespo et al 1996), and major structural malformations (Tannirandorn et al 1993), indicating a possible need for a combination of antenatal tests in evaluating the wellbeing of these high risk fetuses.

SUMMARY

Overall, significant advances in obstetric and neonatal care, along with improvements in the antenatal prediction and prevention of fetal asphyxia, have contributed to the observed decline in perinatal morbidity and mortality over the last half-century. Ultrasound and other imaging techniques have allowed clinicians to observe fetal anatomy, biophysical status, the intrauterine environment and fetal response to stress. The etiologies of congenital and acquired fetal and neonatal brain disorders are diverse. The detection and prevention of neurologic damage, therefore, remain a continual challenge. Early identification of risk factors for neurologic sequelae as well as advancements in understanding neonatal response to hypoxia has been crucial to the development of strategies to limit further injury.

Identification and timely delivery of the fetus exposed to hypoxic stress may improve the neurologic outcomes in some cases. However, this strategy could lead to avoidable complications of prematurity if the diagnosis of hypoxia is in error. The ideal antenatal strategy would include reliable, easy and cost effective testing to identify fetuses at risk for neurologic impairment, prior to the time of irreversible damage. For benefit, the strategy would need to exist in a system allowing for identification and prevention of intrapartum asphyxial injury, and effective neonatal therapies to reduce the morbidity of injury once it has occurred. Investigation in antenatal determinants of neurologic injury continues, and will assist in advancing understanding of the pathophysiology, timing and prevention of congenital and acquired neurologic impairment.

REFERENCES

ACOG (American College of Obstetrics and Gynecology) 1996 Use and abuse of the Apgar score. ACOG Committee Opinion Number 174, July 1996.

ACOG (American College of Obstetrics and Gynecology) 2005 Inappropriate us of the terms fetal distress and birth asphyxia. ACOG Committee Opinion Number 326, December 2005.

Alfirevic Z, Nielson J P 1995 Doppler ultrasonography in high-risk pregnancies: systematic review with meta-analysis. Am J Obstet Gynecol 172:1379–1387.

Altschuler G, Arizawa M, Molnar-Nadasdy G 1992 Meconium induced umbilical cord vascular necrosis and ulceration. A potential link between placenta and poor pregnancy outcome. Obstet Gynecol 79:760–766.

AMCOG 1992 Fetal and neonatal injury. American College of Obstetricians and Gynecologists Technical Bulletin 163.

Anderson G W 1941 Studies on the nucleated red blood cell count in the chronic capillaries and cord blood of various ages of pregnancy. Am J Obstet Gynecol 42:1–12.

Anonymous 1966 The collaborative study on cerebral palsy, mental retardation and other neurological and sensory disorders of infancy and childhood manual. Public Health Service, Bethesda, MD.

Anonymous 1997 Electronic fetal heart rate monitoring: research guidelines for interpretation. National Institute of Health Research Planning Workshop. Am J Obstet Gynecol 177:1385–1390.

Apgar V 1953 A proposal for a new method of evaluation of the newborn infant. Current Res Anesth Analg 32:260–267.

Ayodeji O, Kuhn R 1986 Abnormal antepartum cardiotocography and major fetal abnormalities. Aust NZ J Obstet Gynaecol 26:120–123.

Barss V A, Frigoletto F D, Diamond F 1981 Stillbirth after nonstress testing. Obstet Gynecol 65:541–544.

Baschat A A, Galan H L, Bhide A et al 2006 Doppler and biophysical assessment in growth restricted fetuses: distribution of test results. Ultrasound Obstet Gynecol 27:41–47.

Bax M, Nelson K B 1993 Birth asphyxia: a statement. Dev Med Child Neurol 35:1022–1024.

Boehm F H, Salyer S, Shah D M et al 1986 Improved outcome of twice-weekly nonstress testing. Obstet Gynecol 67:566–570.

Borowska-Matwiejczuk K, Lemancewicz A, Tarasow E et al 2003 Assessment of fetal distress based on magnetic resonance examinations: preliminary report. Acad Radiol 10:1274–1282.

Bourgeois F J, Thiagarajah S, Harbert G M 1984 The significance of fetal heart rate decelerations during nonstress testing. Am J Obstet Gynecol 150:213–216.

Bracci R, Perrone S, Buonocore G 2006 The timing of neonatal brain damage. Biol Neonate 90:145–155.

Bruce S L, Petrie R H, Yeh S Y 1978 The suspicious contraction stress test. Obstet Gynecol 51:415–418.

Buonocore G, Perrone S, Longini M et al 2003 Non protein bound iron as a predictive marker of neonatal brain damage. Brain 126:1–7.

Carter B S, Haverkamp A D, Merenstein G B 1993 The definition of acute perinatal asphyxia. Clin Perinatol 20:287–304.

CDC (Centers for Disease Control and Prevention) 1998 NCHS, National Vital Statistics System: vital statistics of the United States, vol. II, mortality, Part A; Infant mortality rates, fetal mortality rates, and perinatal mortality rates according to race: United States, selected years 1950–1998. Public Health Service, Washington, DC, U.S. Govt Printing Office.

Dalton K J, Dawes G S, Patrick J E 1983 The autonomic nervous system and fetal heart rate variability. Am J Obstet Gynecol 146:456–462.

Dashow E E, Read J A 1984 Significant fetal bradycardia during antepartum fetal heart rate testing. Am J Obstet Gynecol 148:187–190.

De Haan H H, Gunn A J, Gluckman P D 1997 Fetal heart rate changes do not reflect cardiovascular deterioration during brief repeated umbilical cord occlusions in near-term fetal lambs. Am J Obstet Gynecol 176:8–17.

Delivoria-Papadopoulos M, Mishra O P 1998 Mechanisms of cerebral injury in perinatal asphyxia and strategies for prevention. J Pediatr 132:S30–S34.

Devoe L D, Gardner P, Dear C et al 1990 The diagnostic value of concurrent nonstress testing, amniotic fluid measurement, and doppler velocimetry in screening a general high-risk population. Am J Obstet Gynecol 163:1040–1047.

Dildy G A, Clark S L, Garite T J et al 1999 Current status of the multicenter randomized clinical trial on fetal oxygen saturation monitoring in the United States. Eur J Obstet Gynecol Reprod Biol 72:S43–S50.

Dildy G A, Clark S L, Louks C A 1993 Preliminary experience with intrapartum fetal pulse oximetry in humans. Obstet Gynecol 81:630–635.

Druzin M L 1989 Fetal bradycardia during antepartum testing. J Reprod Med 34:47–51.

Druzin M L, Edersheim T G, Hutson J M et al 1989 The effect of vibroacoustic stimulation on the nonstress test at gestational ages of thirty two weeks or less. Am J Obstet Gynecol 166:1476–1478.

Druzin M L, Gratacos J, Keegan K et al 1981 Antepartum fetal heart rate testing VII. The significance of bradycardia. Am J Obstet Gynecol 139:194–198.

Druzin M L, Gratacos J, Paul R H 1980 Antepartum fetal heart rate testing: predictive reliability of 'normal' tests in the prevention of antepartum death. Am J Obstet Gynecol 137:746–747.

Evertson L R, Gauthier R J, Collea J L 1978 Fetal demise following negative contraction stress test. Obstet Gynecol 51:671–673.

Fellman V, Raivio K 1991 Reperfusion injury as the mechanism of brain damage after perinatal asphyxia. Pediatr Res 41:599–606.

Field D R, Parer J T, Baker B W et al 1991 Fetal heart rate variability and cerebral oxygen consumption in fetal sheep during asphyxia. Eur J Obstet Gynecol Reprod Biol 42:145–153.

Fraser W D, Hofmeyr J, Lede R et al 2005 Amnioinfusion for the prevention of the meconium aspiration syndrome. N Engl J Med 353:909–917.

Freeman J M, Nelson K 1988 Intrapartum asphyxia and cerebral palsy. Pediatrics 82:240–249.

Freeman R K 1975 The use of the oxytocin challenge test for antepartum clinical evaluation of uteroplacental respiratory function. Am J Obstet Gynecol 121:481–489.

Freeman R, Anderson G, Dorchester W 1982 A prospective multi-institutional study of antepartum fetal heart rate monitoring. I. Risk of perinatal mortality according to antepartum fetal heart rate results. Am J Obstet Gynecol 143:771–777.

Gagnon, Foreman J, Hunse C et al 1989 Effects of low frequency vibration on human term fetuses. Am J Obstet Gynecol 161:1479–1485.

Gardner D S, Fowden A L, Giussani D A 2002 Adverse intrauterine conditions diminish the fetal defense against acute hypoxia by increasing nitric oxide activity. Circulation 106:2278–2283.

George S, Gunn A J, Westgate J A et al 2004 Fetal heart rate variability and brain stem injury after asphyxia in preterm fetal sheep. Am J Physiol Regul Integr Comp Physiology 287:R925–R933.

Girard N, Gire C, Sigaudy S et al 2003 MR imaging of acquired fetal brain disorders. Childs Nerv Syst 19:490–500.

Gluckman P D, Williams C E 1992 When and why do brain cells die? Dev Med Child Neurol 34:1010–1014.

Goldaber K G, Gilstrap L C, Leveno K J et al 1991 Pathologic fetal acidemia. Obstet Gynecol 78:1103–1107.

Goodwin T M, Belai I, Hernandez P et al 1992 Asphyxial complications in the term newborn with severe umbilical acidemia. Am J Obstet Gynecol 167:1506–1512.

Grant A, Elbourne D 1989 Fetal movement counting to assess fetal well being. In: Chalmers I, Enkin M, Keirse MJNC (eds) Effective care in pregnancy and childbirth. Oxford University Press, Oxford, p. 440.

Gressens P, Luton D 2004 Fetal MRI: obstetric and neurologic perspectives. Pediatr Radiol 34:682–684.

Grossman R, Hoffman C, Mardor Y et al 2006 Quantitative MRI measurements of human fetal brain development in utero. Neuroimage 33:463–470.

Hanson M A 1988 The importance of baro- and chemoreflexes in the control of the fetal cardiovascular system. J Dev Physiol 10:491–511.

Hauth J C 1996 Fetal monitoring: Utility and interpretation of umbilical cord gases and fetal blood sampling. In: Acute perinatal asphyxia in term infants. National Institutes of Health, Bethesda, MD, pp. 63–72.

Huang C-C, Wang S-T, Chang Y-C et al 1999 Measurement of urinary lactate: creatinine ratio for the early identification of newborn infants at risk for hypoxic–ischemic encephalopathy. N Engl J Med 341:328–335.

Huddleston E F 2002 Continued utility of the contraction stress test? Clin Obstet Gynecol 45:1005–1014.

Inglis S R, Druzin M L, Wagner W E, Kogut E 1993 The use of vibroacoustic stimulation during the abnormal or equivocal biophysical profile. Obstet Gynecol 82:371–374.

Katz V L, Bowes W A Jr 1992 Meconium aspiration syndrome: reflections on a murky subject. Am J Obstet Gynecol 166:171–183.

Kaukola T, Satyraj E, Patel D D et al 2004 Cerebral palsy is characterized by protein mediators in the cord serum. Ann Neurol 55:186–194.

Keegan K, Paul R, Broussard P et al 1979 Antepartum fetal heart rate testing. III. The effect of phenobarbitol on the nonstress test. Am J Obstet Gynecol 133:579–582.

Kitterman J A, Liggins G C, Fewell J E et al 1983 Inhibition of breathing movements in fetal sheep by prostaglandins. J Appl Physiol 54:687–692.

Koos B J, Matsuda K, Power G G 1987 Fetal breathing, sleep state, and cardiovascular responses to graded hypoxia in sheep. J Appl Physiol 62:1033–1039.

Korst L M, Phelan J P, Ahn M O, Martina G I 1996 Nucleated red blood cells: an update on the marker for fetal asphyxia. Am J Obstet Gynecol 175:843–846.

Kruger K, Hallberg B, Blennow M et al 1999 Predictive value of fetal scalp blood lactate concentrations and pH as markers of neurologic disability. Am J Obstet Gynecol 181:1072–1078.

Labudova O, Schuller E, Yeghiazarjan et al 1999 Genes involved in the pathophysiology of perinatal asphyxia. Life Sciences 64:1831–1838.

Lammer E J, Brown L E, Anderka M T, Guyer B 1989 Classification and analysis of fetal deaths in Massachusetts. JAMA 261:1757–1762.

Lavery J P 1982 Nonstress fetal heart rate testing. Clin Obstet Gynecol 25:689–705.

Leffler C W, Busija D W, Mirro R et al 1989 The effects of ischemia on brain blood flow and oxygen consumption in newborn pigs. Am J Physiol 257: H1917–H1926.

Ley D, Oskarsson G, Bellander M et al 2004 Different responses of myocardium and cerebral blood flow to cord occlusion in exteriorized fetal sheep. Pediatr Res 55:568–575.

Little W J 1862 On the influence of abnormal parturition, difficult labors, premature birth, and asphyxia neonatorum on the mental and physical condition of the child, especially in relation to deformities. Trans Obstet Soc Lond 2:293.

Low J 1997 Intrapartum fetal asphyxia: definition, diagnosis and classification. Am J Obstet Gynecol 176:957–959.

Low J A 1993 The relationship of asphyxia in the mature fetus to long-term neurologic function. Clin Obstet Gynecol 36:82–90.

Low J A 2004 Reflections on the occurrence and significance of antepartum fetal asphyxia. Best Pract Res Clin Obstet Gynecol 18(3):375–382.

Low J A, Robertson D M, Simpson L L 1989 Temporal relationship of neuropathologic conditions caused by perinatal asphyxia. Am J Obstet Gynecol 160:608–614.

Luttkus A, Fengler T W, Friedman W et al 1995 Continuous monitoring of fetal oxygen saturation by pulse oximetry. Obstet Gynecol 85:183–186.

Mallard E C, Gunn A J, Williams E C et al 1992 Umbilical cord occlusion causes cerebral damage in the fetal sheep. Am J Obstet Gynecol 167:1423–1430.

Manning F A 1992 Biophysical profile scoring. In: Nijhuis J (ed) Fetal behavior. Oxford University Press, New York, p. 241.

Manning F A, Bondagji N, Harman C R et al 1997 Fetal assessment based on the fetal biophysical score: Relationship of last BPS to subsequent cerebral palsy. Journal de Gynecologie, Obstetrique et Biologie de la Reproduction 26:720–729.

Manning F A, Bondagji N, Harman C R et al 1998 Am J Obstet Gynecol 178:696–706.

Manning F A, Morrison I R, Harman C R, Menticoglou S M 1990 The abnormal biophysical profile: analysis of distribution of abnormal variables. Am J Obstet Gynecol 162:918–927.

Manning F A, Morrison I, Lange I R et al 1985 Fetal assessment based on fetal biophysical profile scoring: Experience in 12 620 referred high-risk pregnancies. Am J Obstet Gynecol 151:343–350.

Manning F A, Platt L D, Sipos L 1980 Antepartum fetal evaluation: development of a fetal biophysical profile. Am J Obstet Gynecol 136:787–795.

Margulis E, Binder D, Cohen A et al 1984 The effect of propranolol on the nonstress test. Am J Obstet Gynecol 148:340–341.

Martinex-Crespo J M, Comas C, Ojuel H et al 1996 Umbilical artery pulsatility index in early pregnancies with chromosomal anomalies. Br J Obstet Gynaecol 103:330–334.

Mason G C, Lilford R J, Porter J, Tyrell S 1993 Randomized comparison of routine versus highly selective use of doppler ultrasound in low risk pregnancies. Br J Obstet Gynaecol 100:130–133.

Mellits E, Holden K, Freeman J 1982 Neonatal seizures: II. A multivariate analysis of factors associated with outcome. Pediatrics 70:177–185.

Meyers R E 1975 Four patterns of perinatal brain damage and their conditions of occurrence in primates. Adv Neurol 10:223–234.

Morrow R, Ritchie K 1989 Doppler ultrasound velocimetry and its role in obstetrics. Clin Perinatol 16:771–778.

Murata Y, Martin C B, Ikenoue T et al 1982 Fetal heart rate accelerations and late decelerations during the course of intrauterine death in chronically catheterized Rhesus monkeys. Am J Obstet Gynecol 144:218–223.

Naeye R 1995 Can meconium in the amniotic fluid injure the fetal brain? Obstet Gynecol 86:720–724.

Naeye R L, Localio A R 1995 Determining the time before birth when ischemia and hypoxemia initiated cerebral palsy. Obstet Gynecol 86:713–719.

Nelson K B, Ellenberg J H 1981 Apgar scores as predictors of chronic neurologic disability. Pediatrics 68:36–64.

Nelson K B, Ellenberg J H 1984 Obstetric complications as risk factors for cerebral or seizure disorders. JAMA 251:1843–1848.

Nelson K B, Ellenberg J H 1986 Antecedents of cerebral palsy. Multivariate analysis of risk. N Engl J Med 315:81–86.

Oki E Y, Keegan K A, Freeman R D, Dorchester W 1987 The breast-stimulated contraction stress test. J Reprod Med 32:919–923.

Palmer C, Vannucci R C 1993 Potential new therapies for perinatal cerebral hypoxia–ischemia. Clin Perinatol 20:411–432.

Pasternak J F, Gorey M T 1998 The syndrome of acute near total intrauterine asphyxia in the term infant. Pediatr Neurol 18:391–398.

Patrick J, Carmichael L, Chess L, Staples C 1984 Acceleration of the human fetal heart at 38 to 40 weeks gestational age. Am J Obstet Gynecol 148:35–41.

Paul R H, Suidan A K, Yeh S et al 1975 Clinical fetal monitoring: VII. The evaluation of and significance of intrapartum baseline FHR variability. Am J Obstet Gynecol 123:206–210.

Peeters L L, Sheldon R D, Jones M D et al 1979 Blood flow to fetal organs as a function of arterial oxygen content. Am J Obstet Gynecol 135:637–646.

Phelan J 1981 The nonstress test: a review of 3000 tests. Am J Obstet Gynecol 139:7–10.

Phelan J P 1979 Diminished fetal reactivity with smoking. Am J Obstet Gynecol 136:230–233.

Phelan J P, Ahn M O, Korst L M, Martin G I 1995 Nucleated red blood cells: a marker for fetal asphyxia? Am J Obstet Gynecol 173:1380–1384.

Pinette M G, Blackstone J, Wax J R, Cartin A 2005). Using fetal acoustic stimulation to shorten the biophysical profile. J Clin Ultrasound 33:223–225.

Prayer D, Brugger PC, Prayer L 2004 Fetal MRI: techniques and protocols. Pediatr Radiol 34:685–693.

Prayer D, Kasprian G, Krampl E et al 2006 MRI of normal fetal brain development. Eur J Radiol 57:199–216.

Rados M, Judas M, Kostovic I 2006 In vitro MRI of brain development. Eur J Radiol 57:187–198.

Roland E H, Poskitt K, Rodrigues E et al 1998 Perinatal hypoxic ischemic injury: clinical features and neuroimaging. Ann Neurol 44:161–166.

Shankaran S, Woldt E, Koepke T et al 1991 Acute neonatal morbidity and long-term central nervous system sequelae of perinatal asphyxia in term infants. Early Hum Dev 25:135–148.

Sibony O, Stempfle N, Luton D et al 1998 In utero fetal cerebral intraparenchymal ischemia diagnosed by nuclear magnetic resonance. Dev Med Child Neurol 40:122–123.

Skyes G S, Johnson P 1982 Do Apgar scores indicate asphyxia? Lancet 1:494–496.

Soothill P W, Nicolaides K H, Campbell S 1987 Perinatal asphyxia, hyperlacticaemia, hypoglycemia, and ethyroblastosis in growth retarded fetuses. BMJ 294:1051–1053.

Tannirandorn Y, Witoonpanich P, Phaosavasdi S 1993 Doppler umbilical artery flow velocity waveforms in pregnancies complicated by major fetal malformations. J Med Assoc Thai 76:494–500.

Tominaga T, Kure S, Narisawa K, Yoshimoto T 1993 Endonuclease activation following focal ischemic injury in the rat brain. Brain Res 608:21–26.

Towbin A 1986 Obstetric malpractice litigation: The pathologist's view. Am J Obstet Gynecol 155:927–935.

Trudinger B J, Cook C M, Jones L et al 1986 A comparison of fetal heart rate monitoring and umbilical artery waveforms in the recognition of fetal compromise. Br J Obstet Gynaecol 93:171–175.

Trudinger B J, Stevens D, Connelly A et al 1987 Umbilical artery flow velocity waveforms and placental resistance: The effects of embolization of the umbilical circulation. Am J Obstet Gynecol 157:1443–1448.

US Department of Health and Human Services 1995 Childbirth USA '94. US Government Printing Office, Washington, DC.

Vannucci R C, Palmer C 1997 Hypoxic ischemic encephalopathy: pathogenesis and neuropathology. In: Farnoff A A, Martin R J (eds) Neonatal and perinatal medicine. Mosby-Yearbook, Philadelphia, PA, pp. 856–877.

Vannucci R C, Perlman J M 1997 Interventions for perinatal hypoxic ischemic encephalopathy. Pediatrics 100:1004–1014.

Victory R, Penava D, da Silva O et al 2004 Umbilical cord pH and base excess values in relation to adverse outcome events for infants delivering at term. Am J Obstet Gynecol 191:2021–2028.

Vintzileos A M, Campbell W A, Ingardia C J, Nochimson D J 1983 The fetal biophysical profile and its predictive value. Obstet Gynecol 62:271–278.

Vintzileos A M, Fleming A D, Scorza W E et al 1991 Relationship between fetal biophysical profile and umbilical cord gas values. Am J Obstet Gynecol 165:707–713.

Wedegartner U, Tchirikov M, Schafer S et al 2005 Fetal sheep brains: findings at functional blood oxygen level-dependent 3-T MR imaging-relationship to maternal oxygen saturation during hypoxia. Radiology 237(3):919–926.

Williams C E, Gunn A J, Mallard E C et al 1992 Outcome after ischemia in the developing sheep brain: an electroencephalographic and histological study. Ann Neurol 31:14–21.

Winkler C L, Hanth J C, Tucker J M et al 1991 Neonatal complications at term as related to the degree of umbilical artery acidemia. Am J Obstet Gynecol 164:637–641.

CHAPTER
24

Intrapartum monitoring for asphyxia
David A. Miller

Key Points

- Fetal heart rate decelerations (late, variable or prolonged) signal interruption of the pathway of oxygen transfer from the environment to the fetus
- Acute intrapartum interruption of oxygen transfer does not result in neurologic injury unless the fetal response progresses at least to the stage of significant metabolic acidemia (umbilical artery pH < 7.0 and base deficit ⩾ 12 mmol/L)
- Moderate variability and/or acceleration reliably predict the absence of metabolic acidemia

---

INTRODUCTION

When electronic fetal heart rate monitoring was introduced into clinical practice, many believed it would have a significant impact on perinatal mortality and cerebral palsy. In the decades that followed, the limitations of the technology have become clearer and the original optimism has been replaced by more realistic expectations. Research has helped clarify the physiology and pathophysiology of fetal heart rate changes. Standardized terminology has been introduced and new methods of intrapartum monitoring are showing promise. This chapter will review the evolution of electronic fetal heart rate monitoring and the relationship between fetal heart rate patterns, fetal physiology and newborn outcome.

FETAL HEART RATE AUSCULTATION

Auscultation of the fetal heart, described as early as the 17th century in Le Goust's 'Humani Foetus Historia' (Philippeaux: Notice biographique et bibliographique sur Philippe Le Goust 1879), was first reported in Western medical literature by Mayor (1818) in 1818. In 1822, Le Jumeau (1822) reported his observations of the fetal heart sounds using Laennec's stethoscope and proposed that auscultation of the fetal heart could be useful in confirming pregnancy, diagnosing multiple pregnancy, determining fetal position and judging the state of fetal health or disease by changes in strength and frequency of the heart tones. Later, Kennedy (1833), Schwartz (1870), Winckel (1893) and others described fetal heart rate (FHR) changes associated with umbilical cord compression, head compression and 'fetal distress.' Kilian (1888) and Winckel (1893) proposed indications for forceps delivery based upon FHR abnormalities such as tachycardia, bradycardia, 'irregularity' and 'impurity of tone.' Schwartz (1870) and Seitz (1903) speculated upon the relationship between

FHR changes and fetal oxygenation. Remarkably, these observations were made using only the stethoscope (mediate auscultation), or the ear of the examiner placed directly upon the maternal abdomen (immediate auscultation). In 1917, Hillis described the modified stethoscope known today as the DeLee-Hillis fetoscope (DeLee 1922, Hillis 1917).

ELECTRONIC FETAL MONITORING

In 1906, Cremer (1906) recorded the first fetal electrocardiograph (ECG). Placing one electrode on the maternal abdomen above the fundus and another in the vagina, he observed small fetal electrical impulses among the higher-voltage maternal signals. Despite technological improvements, the quality of abdominal fetal ECG tracings has remained unreliable, and the clinical usefulness of the technique is limited.

The concept of direct application of the ECG electrode to the fetus in utero was introduced in the 1950s (Kaplan & Toyama 1958, Smyth 1953, Sureau 1956), with results clearly superior to those obtained abdominally. During the 1960s, Hon (1966) in the United States, Caldeyro-Barcia et al (1966) in Uruguay and Hammacher (1967) in Germany pioneered the development of electronic monitoring. The first practical clinical electronic fetal monitor became available in the United States in 1968 and throughout the 1970s fetal monitoring became increasingly incorporated into obstetric management (Williams & Hawes 1979). The introduction of Doppler ultrasound technology permitted FHR monitoring in patients with intact membranes. By 2002, electronic FHR monitoring was used in approximately 85% of all births in the United States (Martin et al 2003).

'FETAL DISTRESS' AND 'FETAL ASPHYXIA'

Historically, the objective of EFM was to identify the fetus in 'distress' so that measures could be taken in time to avert permanent brain damage or death. However, the assumptions underlying this objective have been called into question. At the most fundamental level, there has never been a consensus in the medical literature regarding the definition of the term 'fetal distress'. Kirschbaum described it as 'a condition in which fetal physiology is so altered as to make death or permanent injury a probability within a relatively short period of time' (Kirschbaum 1969). Some have based the definition on FHR abnormalities (Haesslein & Niswander 1980, Haverkamp et al 1979), while others have focused on abnormal fetal blood gas values or low Apgar scores. In

2005, the Committee on Obstetric Practice of the American College of Obstetricians and Gynecologists expressed concern about the continued use of the term 'fetal distress', noting that the term is imprecise, non-specific and has a low positive predictive value even in high-risk populations (ACOG 2005a). Further complicating the situation, the evolution of non-standardized FHR terminology led many to equate 'fetal distress' with 'fetal asphyxia', yet another term for which no consensus definition exists. For example, the term 'asphyxia' is derived from a Greek word meaning 'a stopping of the pulse'. Webster defines it as 'a lack of oxygen or excess carbon dioxide that is usually caused by interruption of breathing' (Webster's Ninth New Collegiate Dictionary 1985). The World Federation of Neurology Group defined asphyxia as a condition of impaired gas exchange, which, if it persists, leads to progressive hypoxemia and hypercapnia (Bax & Melson 1993). Low defined asphyxia as a combination of hypoxia, hypercapnia and metabolic acidosis (Low et al 1997). Historically, a clinical diagnosis of 'birth asphyxia' was assigned on the basis of a variety of observations, including meconium passage, 'abnormal' FHR patterns, low Apgar scores and 'abnormal' blood gases. In 1989, Gilstrap et al (1989) recommended that the diagnosis of 'birth asphyxia' be reserved for infants who are severely depressed (5' Apgar <3) and acidemic (pH <7.00) at birth, require resuscitation, and have seizures in the first day of life. In 1995, the American College of Obstetricians and Gynecologists defined asphyxia as a combination of hypoxia and metabolic acidosis (ACOG 1995). However, in 2005, the Committee on Obstetric Practice of the American College of Obstetricians and Gynecologists stated unequivocally that 'birth asphyxia' is a non-specific diagnosis and should not be used (ACOG 2005a). Because of a lack of consensus regarding definitions, the terms 'fetal distress' and 'asphyxia' will be replaced in this chapter by more specific terms whenever possible. These terms are summarized in Table 24.1.

At the cellular level, hypoxia, acidosis and ischemia trigger a cascade of events, including membrane depolarization, disruption of normal energy metabolism, altered release and re-uptake of neurotransmitters, ion shifts, protease activation, free radical production and phospholipid degradation (Johnson 1993). If prolonged, this may lead to cell death, and eventually, death of the organism. Levels of hypoxia, acidosis and ischemia that are sublethal to the organism may result in clinical evidence of cellular dysfunc-

tion. Clinical manifestations of myocardial injury include conduction abnormalities, myocardial dysfunction and congestive heart failure. Manifestations in the gastrointestinal tract include hypoxic–ischemic mucosal injury, stress ulcers, hepatic injury and necrotizing enterocolitis. In the lungs, sequelae of hypoxia and acidosis include impaired surfactant production, respiratory distress syndrome, meconium aspiration syndrome and persistent pulmonary hypertension. Renal injury may lead to renal insufficiency or acute renal failure. Hematologic manifestations include thrombocytopenia, neutropenia and disseminated intravascular coagulation. In the central nervous system, hypoxia, acidosis and ischemia can trigger multiple biochemical cascades involving excitatory amino acids, calcium, free radicals, nitric oxide, proinflammatory cytokines and bioactive lipids.

Impaired neuronal water-regulatory mechanisms and disruption of the blood–brain barrier may lead to cerebral edema and neuronal necrosis. Disruption of normal membrane depolarization, neurotransmission and receptor stimulation may lead to seizures and respiratory depression. One of the most publicized consequences of fetal central nervous system injury is cerebral palsy.

CEREBRAL PALSY (see also Ch. 46)

Cerebral palsy (CP) is 'a chronic disability, characterized by aberrant control of movement and posture, appearing early in life and not the result of recognized progressive disease' (Nelson & Ellenberg 1978). It may be accompanied by mental retardation and seizures (Alberman 1978, Nelson & Ellenberg 1986) as well as cortical visual impairment. The insult responsible for the later development of CP may occur at any time during the prenatal, perinatal or postnatal periods (NIH 1985). Cerebral palsy is classified, along with mental retardation, learning disorders, autism and epilepsy, as a major disorder of neurodevelopment. Unlike mental retardation, learning disorders, autism and epilepsy, the relationship between CP and abnormal or difficult birth has long been recognized. However, the correlation is much weaker than originally assumed.

In 1862, William Little (1862), a British orthopedic surgeon, presented to the Obstetrical Society of London a treatise, 'On the influence of abnormal parturition, difficult labours, premature birth and asphyxia neonatorum, on the mental and physical condition of the child, especially in relation to deformities'. He reviewed the birth histories of children with spastic rigidity and found a high incidence of preterm delivery, breech presentation, prolonged labor, late onset of crying and respiration, neonatal convulsions and stupor. Little concluded that infantile spastic palsies could be caused by virtually nothing other than abnormalities of the birth process. Schreiber (1938), in 1938, reviewed the birth records of 500 patients with cerebral symptoms, and noted a 70% incidence of birth apnea. In 1951, Lilienfeld (Lilienfeld & Parkhurst 1951, Lilienfeld & Pasamanick 1955) reported

---

Table 24.1 Definitions

Hypoxemia — Decreased oxygen content in the blood

Hypoxia — Decreased oxygen content in the tissues

Acidemia — Increased concentration of hydrogen ions in the blood

Acidosis — Increased concentration of hydrogen ions in the tissue

Ischemia — Decreased blood supply to tissues

higher incidences of placenta previa, malpresentation, prematurity and abruptio placentae in children with CP than in controls. In 1955, Eastman and DeLeon (1955) reviewed the obstetrical histories of 96 patients with CP and noted that the immediate neonatal condition was described as 'poor' (abnormal respiratory behavior, flaccidity, cyanosis) in 41% of the cases compared to only 2% of controls. In addition, they reported higher incidences of third trimester bleeding, prematurity, breech delivery, mid-forceps delivery, shoulder dystocia, prolonged second stage, fetal distress, prolonged neonatal apnea, intrapartum fever and prolonged neonatal fever in infants later diagnosed with CP. Of note, there were also significantly more congenital anomalies (polydactyly, facial clefts) in the CP group. In 1962, Eastman et al (1962) reviewed 753 cases of CP and found significantly more cases of prematurity, multiple gestation, malpresentation, resuscitation requirement, hemolytic disease, hypoxia due to cord prolapse, abruption and pre-eclampsia than in controls. In this series, as well, there was a significantly higher incidence of congenital anomalies in the CP group. In the same year, Steer and Bonney (1962) studied the histories of 317 patients with CP and found that 41 (13%) were attributable to kernicterus and other neurological disease. Among the remaining 276, 116 (43%) had no historical evidence of anoxia and 160 (57%) had evidence of possible anoxia. In 92 of the latter, anoxia was suspected solely on the basis of neonatal incubator requirement. 'Possible anoxia' was diagnosed in the remaining 68 cases by a range of criteria including severe toxemia, tight nuchal cord, cord prolapse and intrapartum maternal death. In 1985, using data from the Collaborative Perinatal Project, Nelson and Ellenberg (1985) reported an increased incidence of CP in low birth weight infants. In term neonates, prolonged depression of Apgar scores was significantly associated with CP.

Data in animals further implicated abnormalities of labor as a cause of neurologic injury. Windle and Becker (1943) demonstrated clinical and histopathologic evidence of neuronal damage in fetal guinea-pigs that were deprived of oxygen. Windle later studied fetal rhesus monkeys (Faro & Windle 1969, Ranck & Windle 1959) and reported clinical and histopathologic changes associated with prolonged total anoxia, hypercapnia, severe acidosis and hypotension. Total anoxia for less than 8 minutes did not result in consistent neuronal injury, whereas anoxia for more than 10 minutes invariably produced neuropathology. There were no survivors beyond 20–25 minutes of total anoxia. In animal models, total anoxia produced a pattern of neural necrosis in the brainstem, thalamus and basal ganglia, with relative sparing of the cerebral cortex. These injuries manifested clinically as seizures, ataxia and athetosis, consistent with the dyskinetic subtype of CP-related brain injury. They were not consistent with the more common spastic quadriplegic subtype of CP, which involves injury to the cerebral cortex. In the late 1960s and early 1970s, Myers (1969, 1972) demonstrated that, unlike total anoxia, repeated partial interruption of fetal oxygenation in monkeys produced acidosis, late

FHR decelerations and neuropathologic abnormalities consistent with the clinical and histopathologic findings in the spastic quadriplegic subtype of CP. In addition to lesions in the thalamus and basal ganglia, repeated partial interruption of fetal oxygenation resulted in generalized cerebral necrosis or focal necrosis in the parasagittal regions and the border zones between the parietal and occipital lobes.

Although the conclusions of early epidemiologic studies have been called into question (Blair & Stanley 1988, Freud 1957, Haddow & Gage 1960, Nelson & Ellenberg 1986), they created and fostered the belief that birth-related insults were the primary cause of CP. In reality, these studies demonstrated that an insult during labor might be one cause of CP. More recently, attention has been focused upon the relative contributions of possible prenatal factors, including congenital CNS abnormalities, infections, mercury toxicity, in-utero strokes, maternal hyperthyroidism and maternal proteinuria (Nelson & Ellenberg 1986, Paneth 1993). Nelson and Ellenberg (1986) performed a multivariate analysis of risk in 189 cases of cerebral palsy from the Collaborative Perinatal Project. After accounting for major non-CNS congenital malformations, birthweight <2000 g, microcephaly and alternative explanations for CP, they reported that only 9% of CP cases were associated with birth asphyxia (defined as one or more of the following: lowest FHR <60 beats per minute, five-minute Apgar score <3, time to first cry >5 minutes). In 1988, Blair and Stanley (1988) analyzed 183 CP cases and 549 matched controls, reaching very similar conclusions. A diagnosis of 'birth asphyxia' was assigned to all infants with 'fetal distress' and a one-minute Apgar <7 or a spontaneous respiration time of >2 minutes. Fetal distress was defined as any of the following: (1) meconium, (2) FHR >160 or <120 beats per minute, (3) 'abnormal' FHR tracing or (4) documentation of 'fetal distress' – not otherwise specified. Using these criteria, they demonstrated that 'birth asphyxia' nearly tripled the odds of developing CP (odds ratio 2.84, 95% confidence interval 1.85 to 4.37). However, the vast majority of these infants did not develop CP. Furthermore, among 183 cases of CP, only 13 had evidence of a birth related injury on the basis of the above criteria. They concluded that only 8.2% of CP was attributable to 'birth asphyxia'.

The prevalence of CP has not decreased appreciably over several decades (Stanley & Blair 1991). In fact, some reports suggest that the prevalence of CP has increased in Japan (Takesita et al 1989), Australia (Stanley 1992), Finland (Riikonen et al 1989) and the United Kingdom (Riikonen et al 1989, Pharoah et al 1990), possibly due to improved survival of low birthweight infants at increased risk for CP (Ellenberg & Nelson 1979). Although the cause in most cases of CP is unknown, adverse events before labor appear to play a greater role than previously recognized. Imaging modalities such as ultrasound, computed tomography, magnetic resonance imaging and technetium scanning are providing new insights into the prenatal origins of neurologic injury. Following hypoxic–ischemic injury, neuronal necrosis produces characteristic changes that evolve over the course of days to weeks. These changes frequently are detectable with imaging techniques and can aid in establishing the timing of the injury. The location of the abnormality appears to play a role in the timing of the injury as well. Periventricular leukomalacia is associated with injuries occurring before 34 weeks of gestation. Parasagittal neuronal damage appears to be associated more frequently with hypoxic–ischemic injury in term infants. Greater understanding of the etiologic factors involved in the development of CP should help to rectify the persistent misconception that intrapartum events are the sole cause of the disorder. This, in turn, should lead to more realistic expectations of the possible benefits of intrapartum fetal monitoring.

HISTORY OF FHR PATTERNS AND FETAL CONDITION

As early as the 19th century, researchers using auscultation recognized that certain FHR patterns were associated with poor perinatal outcome. In 1833, Kennedy (1833) related Bodson's description of fetal distress in association with a FHR pattern exhibiting 'slowness of its return when a contraction is passing on'. In 1838, Schwartz (1838) recommended frequent counting of the fetal heart tones in labor, and implicated 'asphyxic intoxication' as a cause of alterations in their 'individual normal frequency', noting that 'in those cases in which the heart sounds returned slowly to their earlier rhythm, or when the attenuations persisted or deteriorated during the pauses, the result would be a weak, moribund or dead fetus' (Gültekin-Zootzmann 1975). Seitz (1903), in 1903 described three progressively ominous stages of FHR deceleration. He attributed the first two stages to irritation and paralysis of the vagal centers, and the third to paralysis of all extracardiac nerve centers, concluding that it was possible to detect early signs of compromise before the fetus was actually in danger. The introduction of EFM and fetal scalp blood sampling in the 1960s provided additional tools to evaluate the fetus. In 1967, Hon and Quilligan (1967) proposed a system for classification of FHR decelerations and in 1969 Kubli et al (1969) demonstrated the relationship between the type and severity of FHR deceleration and the fetal scalp pH. They reported that fetuses with no decelerations, early decelerations or mild variable decelerations had average scalp pH values >7.29, while those with severe variable or late decelerations had pH values <7.15. Many investigators have demonstrated the importance of FHR variability and FHR accelerations as indicators of the absence of metabolic acidemia (Clark et al 1984, Hammacher et al 1968, Hon & Lee 1963, Krebs et al 1979, Martin 1982, Paul et al 1975, Smith et al 1986). More recently, fetal pulse oximetry and fetal ECG analysis have added to our understanding of the complex relationship between fetal biochemistry and the neurologic regulation of FHR. Fetal pulse oximetry and fetal ST segment analysis (STAN) will be reviewed later in this chapter.

ELECTRONIC FETAL MONITORING VS. TRADITIONAL AUSCULTATION

When EFM replaced the traditional practice of intermittent intrapartum FHR auscultation in the 1970s, a series of studies (Amato 1977, Chan et al 1973, Edington et al 1975, Hamilton et al 1978, Johnstone et al 1978, Kelly & Kulkarni 1973, Koh et al 1975, Lee & Baggish 1976, Paul et al 1977, Shenker et al 1975, Tutera & Newman 1975) reported significantly lower perinatal mortality rates in electronically monitored patients. These studies were non-randomized and employed non-concurrent controls. Critics have cited rapidly improving neonatal care and falling perinatal mortality rates as possible sources of bias. MacDonald (MacDonald & Grant 1987) pointed out that, over the time period of these studies, hospitals not using EFM experienced rates of improvement in perinatal outcome similar to those seen in hospitals that were using EFM. Despite the inevitable shortcomings of non-randomized trials, these studies had the effect of validating the use of EFM.

In 1976, the first of a series of randomized, controlled trials was published, comparing EFM to intermittent auscultation of the FHR during labor. To date, ten such studies have been published: five in high-risk populations (Haverkamp et al 1976, 1979, Luthy et al 1987, Renou et al 1976, Vintzileos et al 1993), three in low-risk populations (Kelso et al 1978, Leveno et al 1986, Wood et al 1981) and two in combined low- and high-risk populations (MacDonald et al 1985, Neldam et al 1986). These trials are summarized in Table 24.2.

RANDOMIZED CONTROLLED TRIALS OF EFM VS. AUSCULTATION

In 1976, Haverkamp and associates (Haverkamp et al 1976) in Denver reported the first prospective, randomized study of 483 high-risk obstetric patients, comparing electronic fetal monitoring with intermittent FHR auscultation in labor. A point-rating system (Goodwin et al 1969) was used to assess risk status. In the EFM group, a scalp electrode was placed as soon as possible. Auscultation in the control group was performed every 15 minutes in the first stage of labor and every 5 minutes in the second stage, for 30 seconds after uterine contractions. Electronic monitoring was employed in both groups, but was blinded in the control group. In the EFM group, FHR patterns were evaluated using the criteria of Kubli and Hon (Kubli et al 1969). In patients with late decelerations or severe variable decelerations that persisted after 15 minutes of corrective measures (oxygen, positional changes, correction of hypotension), delivery was accomplished. Fetal distress in the control group was diagnosed by the presence of bradycardia to 100 beats per minute after three or more consecutive contractions. Delivery was accomplished if fetal distress was not relieved within 15 minutes. There were no significant differences in outcome as measured by perinatal mortality, Apgar scores, cord blood

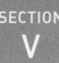
Table 24.2 Prospective randomized clinical trials of EFM vs. intermittent FHR auscultation

Authors	Year	N (total)	Risk status	Perinatal mortality	Neonatal neurologic signs	Cesarean section rate
Haverkamp et al	1976	483	High	ND	ND	↑
Renou et al	1976	350	High	ND	↓	↑
Kelso et al	1978	504	Low	ND	ND	↑
Haverkamp et al	1979	690	High	ND	ND	↑
Wood et al	1981	989	Low	ND	ND	ND
MacDonald et al	1985	12964	Combined	ND	↓	ND
Leveno et al	1986	14618	Low	ND	ND	↑*
Neldam et al	1986	969	Combined	ND	ND	ND
Luthy et al	1987	246	High	ND	ND	ND
Vintzileos et al	1993	1428	High	↓	ND	ND

ND = No difference, ↓ = Lower in EFM group, ↑ = Higher in EFM group, ↑* = Higher in EFM group (cesarean for 'fetal distress' increased (9% vs. 4%). Overall cesarean rate not reported).

pH values, neurological signs in the neonate or neonatal nursery morbidity between the EFM and control groups. The monitored group, however, had significantly higher rates of cesarean section overall (16.5% vs. 6.8%), and cesarean section for fetal distress (7.4% vs. 1.2%). Questions have been raised concerning the comparability of the two groups. For instance, review of the monitor tracings revealed more abnormal FHR patterns early in labor in the study group. Furthermore, the study group had a higher rate of maternal postpartum infectious morbidity (13.2% vs. 4.6%) which was not explained by the increased rate of cesarean birth. These findings suggest that the study group may have represented a higher-risk population than did the control group and that effective randomization was not achieved.

The second study, by Renou et al (1976) in Melbourne, Australia in 1976, randomized 350 high-risk patients into EFM and auscultation groups. High-risk patients were defined as those with a poor obstetric history, a medical or obstetric complication, an abnormal FHR detected by auscultation, or meconium in the amniotic fluid. Continuous EFM was performed in the study group and scalp pH was measured if the FHR tracing was judged to be abnormal. Abnormalities were defined as a slowing of the FHR in relation to the contraction cycle, a baseline FHR less than 100 beats per minute or loss of normal beat-to-beat variability (Renou & Wood 1974). The protocol for auscultation in the control group was not reported. Criteria for intervention were not specified in either group. There were no significant differences between the groups with respect to perinatal mortality, Apgar scores or maternal or neonatal infection. Patients in the monitored group, however, had significantly higher cord blood pH values and significantly lower incidences of neonatal intensive care unit (NICU) admission, neonatal neurologic signs and/or symptoms and neonatally diagnosed brain damage (not further defined). The cesarean section rate was significantly higher in the monitored group than in the control group (22.3% vs. 13.7%); however the indications for intervention were not specified, making this

difference difficult to interpret. The authors commented that the difference in cesarean section rates was not statistically significant after removal of six patients in the monitored group who had had a previous cesarean birth. The rationale for removing these patients on the basis of their previous operations was unclear since, presumably, the initial decision had been made to allow them a trial of labor. The rates of cesarean section for fetal distress were not reported.

In 1978, Kelso et al (1978) in Sheffield, England, published the first randomized, controlled trial comparing EFM and intermittent auscultation in 504 low-risk patients. High-risk patients were excluded according to listed criteria, including multiple gestation, breech presentation, hypertension and diabetes, among other medical and obstetrical complications. Continuous EFM was employed in study patients, with a fetal scalp electrode placed as early as possible. Auscultation in the control group was performed at least every 15 minutes for one minute during and immediately following a contraction. Crossover was not permitted and scalp pH determination was not utilized. The dip area (Shelley & Tipton 1971) was used as a measure of fetal distress in the EFM group; however criteria for intervention were not specified. In the control group, a FHR higher than 160 beats per minute or lower than 120 beats per minute was considered indicative of fetal distress. There were no significant differences between the groups with respect to perinatal mortality, low Apgar scores, cord blood pH values, NICU admissions or lengths of stay, neonatal or maternal infections, or abnormal neonatal neurologic findings. The only significant difference between the groups was an increase in the incidence of cesarean birth in the monitored group (9.5% vs. 4.4%). There was no statistical difference, however, in the incidence of cesarean section for fetal distress (EFM 1.6%, control 1.2%).

In 1979, Haverkamp and associates (Haverkamp et al 1979) published a second randomized, controlled trial in high-risk patients which was similar in design to the first, but included additional measures of infant status as well as the option to perform fetal scalp pH determination during labor. Blinded EFM in the control group was not performed in this trial. A total of 690 high-risk patients were randomized into three groups. In the first group, fetal assessment during labor was accomplished by intermittent auscultation. The second group had continuous EFM alone and the third group had continuous EFM with the option to measure scalp blood pH as needed. Risk assessment guidelines, auscultation protocols and criteria for the diagnosis of fetal distress were the same as in their previous study. Among the three groups, no significant differences were found in perinatal mortality, Apgar scores, cord blood pH values, maternal or neonatal infectious morbidity, NICU admissions or neonatal neurological abnormalities. A significant increase in the incidence of cesarean birth was demonstrated in the group with EFM alone (EFM alone–18%, EFM with the option to scalp sample–11%, auscultation–6%). The option to perform scalp sampling resulted in an intermediate cesarean section rate that was not significantly different from either of the other groups. When analyzed together, electronically monitored patients had a significantly higher incidence of cesarean section for fetal distress than did controls (5.2% vs. 0.43%).

The fifth trial was published in 1981 by Wood et al in Melbourne, Australia. A total of 989 low-risk patients (890 at one hospital and 99 at another) were randomized to receive EFM or intermittent auscultation. High-risk pregnancies were excluded based upon listed criteria including previous preterm delivery, meconium stained amniotic fluid, fetal tachycardia or bradycardia, maternal renal disease, hypertension, diabetes and other medical and obstetric complications. Monitored patients had placement of a fetal scalp electrode as early as possible. The protocol for auscultated patients was not described. Scalp pH measurements were made as needed. Fetal distress was diagnosed as in the previous study by Renou (Renou & Wood 1974, Renou et al 1976). The criteria for operative intervention were not specified. No significant differences between the groups were seen in perinatal mortality, Apgar scores, cord blood pH values, NICU admissions or neonatal neurologic abnormalities. In this study, the cesarean section rates were not significantly different between the groups (4% in the monitored group and 2% in the auscultated group), although the overall rate of operative intervention (including forceps) was significantly higher in the monitored group. Rates of cesarean section for fetal distress were not reported. It should be noted that the randomization process was compromised at the larger study hospital, requiring subsequent data manipulation.

In 1985, MacDonald et al (1985), in Dublin and Oxford, published a randomized, controlled trial comparing EFM with intermittent FHR auscultation in 12964 pregnancies. It was the first study to calculate prospectively the sample size needed to demonstrate statistically significant differences between the groups. Prior to initiation of the study, estimates were made of the anticipated frequencies of intrapartum stillbirths, neonatal deaths, neonatal seizures in survivors and other severe abnormal neurological characteristics. They calculated that 13000 patients would be needed to demonstrate a 50% reduction in the combined incidence of intrapartum stillbirths, neonatal deaths and neonatal seizures in survivors (power 75%, $P < 0.05$). A trial of that size would have a 50% chance of detecting a 50% reduction in the rate of seizures, alone. Risk status was determined according to listed criteria, and 22.5% of the study participants were identified as high-risk. Amniotomy was performed within one hour of admission in all patients and those with either no fluid or moderate to dense meconium were excluded from participation in the study. In the EFM group, a fetal scalp electrode was applied as early as possible and scalp pH measurements were used as needed. Criteria for evaluation of the FHR tracings were similar to those of Kubli and Hon (Kubli et al 1969). Suspicious or ominous tracings were those with marked tachycardia or bradycardia, moderate tachycardia or bradycardia with decreased variability, absent-minimal variability, late decelerations, moderate to severe variable decelerations and other difficult-to-interpret patterns. In the first stage of labor, a scalp pH was performed if such patterns persisted for at least 10 minutes. A scalp pH <7.20 was an indication for delivery. If the fetal scalp pH was between 7.20 and 7.25 with persistent suspicious or ominous FHR patterns, or <7.20 regardless of the FHR pattern, delivery was accomplished. If the scalp pH was >7.25, but the tracing remained suspicious or ominous, the scalp pH was repeated within 30 to 60 minutes. In the second stage of labor, delivery was accomplished if FHR abnormalities persisted for at least 10 minutes. In the control group, FHR auscultation was performed every 15 minutes for 60 seconds in the first stage of labor and between each contraction during the second stage. If the FHR was <100 beats per minute or >160 beats per minute during three contractions and could not be corrected with conservative measures, a scalp pH was measured and managed as above, or delivery was expedited, depending on the stage of labor. Blood sampling also was performed at unspecified intervals in the control group when labor exceeded 8 hours. There were no significant differences between the groups in perinatal mortality, low Apgar scores, neonatal trauma, resuscitation requirement, NICU admissions or infectious morbidity. Among the 28 perinatal deaths, asphyxia was considered to be the primary cause in 7 cases in each group. There were significantly more cases of neonatal seizures and persistent neurologic abnormalities (>1 week) in the control group, however no differences with respect to neurologic abnormality remained at one-year and four-year follow-up (3 cases in each group). Labor was significantly shorter in the EFM group and analgesia (meperidine) was required less often. Twice as many fetuses with low scalp pH (<7.20) were identified in the EFM group and scalp sampling was used more frequently (EFM 4.4%, control 3.5%). The cesarean section rate in the EFM group (2.4%) was not significantly different from the auscultated group (2.2%). Overall rates of operative delivery were higher in the EFM group (10.6% vs. 8.5%) due to an increased incidence of forceps delivery (8.2% vs. 6.3%). Rates of cesarean section for fetal distress were not significantly different (EFM 0.4%, control 0.2%). In the control group, the allocated method of auscultation was used throughout labor in 97.7%. The remaining 2.3% crossed over and underwent EFM secondary to prolonged labor (1.3%), meconium (0.2%), FHR abnormality (0.4%) and other reasons (0.4%). In patients randomized to EFM, only 80.7% used it throughout labor.

The overall frequency of seizures in the 22.5% who were classified as high-risk was 4.3/1000. This was significantly higher than in the low-risk group (2.6/1000). The incidence of seizures in surviving neonates was the same in both groups (2.3/1000). Electronic monitoring did not reduce the seizure incidence to a greater extent in high-risk patients than in low-risk patients. In this study, the largest to date, EFM was associated with no increase in maternal morbidity.

In 1986, Neldam and associates (Neldam et al 1986) in Copenhagen, Denmark, reported a randomized, controlled trial of EFM vs. intermittent auscultation in 969 combined low- and high-risk patients. The study excluded women with pregestational diabetes mellitus. In the EFM group, monitoring was initiated when patients no longer desired to ambulate. A scalp electrode was placed as soon as possible thereafter. In the control group, fetal heart tones were auscultated twice an hour for at least 15 seconds at cervical dilatation <5 cm, every 15 minutes from 5 cm until the second stage of labor and for 30 seconds after each contraction, or at least every five minutes during the second stage. Scalp pH sampling was optional and was performed only 5 times (EFM 3, control 2). In the EFM group, intervention was considered if FHR abnormalities remained unresolved after 15 minutes of corrective measures. These abnormalities included bradycardia <120 beats per minute, tachycardia >160 beats per minute, late decelerations, variable decelerations (not further specified), silent FHR pattern (beat-to-beat variability <5 beats per minute) and saltatory pattern (variability >25 beats per minute). Intervention was considered in the control group if the FHR was <100 beats per minute following three or more consecutive contractions. No statistical differences were detected between the groups with respect to perinatal mortality, low Apgar scores, seizures, NICU admissions or lengths of stay. Significantly more pathological FHR patterns were detected in the EFM group, however there was no difference in the incidence of cesarean delivery.

In 1986, Leveno and colleagues published a randomized trial comparing universal monitoring with 'selective' monitoring in 34 995 pregnancies (Leveno et al 1986). Among these, 14 618 were considered 'low risk' and were randomized to EFM or to intermittent auscultation during alternate months. Perinatal mortality, 5-minute Apgar scores, NICU admissions, ventilator requirement and neonatal seizures

were similar in the two groups. There were more cases of 'abnormal fetal heart rate' in the monitored group leading to significantly more cesarean sections for 'fetal distress' (9% vs. 4%). However, overall cesarean rates were not reported, making it difficult to compare these results with those of other randomized trials.

The ninth study, by Luthy et al (1987), in Seattle and Vancouver, compared EFM and auscultation in 246 high-risk patients with preterm labor. Inclusion criteria were preterm labor, singleton gestation, cephalic presentation, estimated gestational age 26–32 weeks and estimated fetal weight 700–1750 grams. Patients with preterm premature rupture of the membranes were not excluded. In the EFM group, external monitoring was used until advanced cervical dilatation (7 cm), at which time amniotomy was performed and a scalp electrode was placed. In those with ruptured membranes, a scalp electrode was placed once delivery was inevitable. Ominous FHR patterns were those with persistent late decelerations with at least three successive contractions in the absence of correctable cause, FHR greater than 180 beats per minute with total loss of variability persisting more than 15 minutes, FHR less than 100 beats per minute for more than three minutes, or severe variable decelerations persisting for more than 30 minutes. An ominous FHR pattern lasting for more than 30 minutes, or a scalp pH of <7.20 was an indication for delivery. In the control group, auscultation was performed for at least 30 seconds, at least every 15 minutes in the first stage of labor and at least every 5 minutes in the second stage. Ominous patterns were those with FHR less than 100 beats per minute for more than 30 seconds after three or more consecutive contractions, baseline FHR greater than 180 beats per minute for more than 15 minutes or less than 100 beats per minute for more than 60 seconds. Scalp pH was used as clinically indicated in both groups. Fetal scalp pH <7.20 or ominous FHR patterns in the absence of a correctable cause were considered indications for delivery. The groups did not differ with respect to the use of tocolytics, corticosteroids, oxytocin or regional anesthesia. There were no differences in perinatal mortality, low Apgar scores, cord pH values, neonatal seizures, respiratory distress syndrome or intracranial hemorrhage. Cesarean section rates were similar (EFM 15.6%, controls 15.2%). There was no difference in the incidence of cesarean section for 'fetal distress' (EFM 8.2%, controls 5.6%).

The most recent randomized trial, published in 1993 by Vintzileos et al (1993), was conducted in Athens, Greece, and compared EFM and intermittent auscultation in 1428 patients in a population with high baseline perinatal mortality rates of 20.4–22.6 per 1000. The relatively high incidence of the outcome measure to be studied (perinatal death) markedly improved the likelihood of detecting a statistically significant effect of EFM. Using an average incidence of 21 perinatal deaths per 1000, they prospectively calculated that a sample of 2210 patients would have an 80% chance of detecting a 67% reduction in perinatal mortality at the 0.05

level of significance. Reviews were conducted every three months, and the study was ended after the third review in light of a statistically significant five-fold decrease in perinatal mortality in the EFM group. The study included women with singleton living fetuses with estimated gestational ages >26 weeks. Fetuses with known congenital or chromosomal anomalies were excluded. In the EFM group, external monitoring was used as long as satisfactory tracings were obtained. Scalp electrodes were placed as needed. In the control group, FHR auscultation was performed every 15 minutes during the first stage of labor and every 5 minutes during the second stage. The FHR was counted during contractions and for at least 30 seconds immediately afterward. Non-reassuring patterns in the EFM group included late decelerations, prolonged decelerations <80 beats per minute for >2 minutes, severe variables <70 beats per minute for >60 seconds, variable decelerations with a rising baseline and loss of variability, tachycardia with decreased variability (<5 beats per minute), persistent decreased variability or a sinusoidal pattern. In the auscultated group, 'non-reassuring' patterns included a FHR <100 beats per minute during and immediately after a contraction, a persistent FHR <100 beats per minute or >160 beats per minute. Fetal scalp blood sampling was not used in either group and crossover was not permitted. In both groups, delivery was accomplished if non-reassuring FHR patterns failed to resolve after 20 minutes of conservative measures. There were significantly fewer perinatal deaths in the EFM group than in the controls (2.6/1000 vs. 13/1000). Furthermore, there were no 'hypoxia-related' perinatal deaths in the EFM group, whereas 6 such deaths occurred in the auscultation group (0.9%). This difference was statistically significant. The groups did not differ significantly with respect to low Apgar scores, NICU admissions or lengths of stay, ventilator requirements, neonatal hypoxic-ischemic encephalopathy, intraventricular hemorrhage, seizures, hypotonia, necrotizing enterocolitis or respiratory distress syndrome. Although the incidence of cesarean section for fetal distress was significantly higher in the EFM group (5.3% vs. 2.3%), the overall incidence of cesarean birth was not significantly different between the EFM and control groups (9.5% vs. 8.6%).

POTENTIAL BENEFITS OF ELECTRONIC FETAL MONITORING

When EFM was introduced in the 1960s, proponents anticipated marked reductions in perinatal mortality and neurologic injury. Regarding the former, nine out of ten randomized clinical trials conducted since 1976 failed to detect a statistically significant difference in perinatal mortality between EFM and intermittent FHR auscultation (Table 24.2). However, it is crucial to point out that many non-randomized trials (Amato 1977, Chan et al 1973, Edington et al 1975, Hamilton et al 1978, Johnstone et al 1978, Kelly & Kulkarni 1973, Koh et al 1975, Lee & Baggish 1976, Paul et al 1977, Shenker et al 1975, Tutera & Newman 1975)

demonstrated significant reductions in intrapartum death rates when electronic monitoring was introduced and that only one of the ten randomized trials (Vintzileos et al 1993) had sufficient statistical power to demonstrate a reduction in perinatal death. In that trial, electronically monitored patients had a statistically significant 5-fold improvement in perinatal mortality compared to those followed in labor with intermittent auscultation. In comparison to the high perinatal mortality rates (20.4–22.6/1000) in the study by Vintzileos (Vintzileos et al 1993), MacDonald (MacDonald et al 1985) calculated the combined anticipated frequencies of intrapartum stillbirths and neonatal deaths in the Dublin trial to be 3 per 1000. In such a population, a study with an 80% likelihood of detecting a 50% reduction in perinatal mortality ($P < 0.5$) would require more than 34 000 patients (Fleiss 1981). The total number of patients in all ten studies, combined, was 33 241. A meta-analysis of nine published randomized trials by Vintzileos et al (1995) reported a significantly lower incidence of perinatal mortality due to fetal hypoxia in monitored patients. However, 'fetal hypoxia' was not defined specifically in this study. Moreover, if there had been one fewer case of perinatal death in the intermittent auscultation group, the study results would not have reached statistical significance.

With respect to neonatal neurologic injury, the problem of sample size is the same. Seven of the ten trials (Haverkamp et al 1976, 1979, Kelso et al 1978, Leveno et al 1986, Luthy et al 1987, Vintzileos et al 1993, Wood et al 1981) showed no benefit of EFM (Table 24.2). Two trials (MacDonald et al 1985, Renou et al 1976) reported fewer neonatal seizures in the EFM groups. Thacker conducted a meta-analysis in 2001 and concluded that continuous EFM resulted in fewer neonatal seizures but no change in the incidence of CP (Thacker & Stroup 1999). The cesarean delivery rate was increased by 41%. Vintzileos et al (1995) reported that electronic monitoring was superior to intermittent auscultation in detecting fetal acidemia at birth in 1419 patients who had umbilical cord blood acid–base measurements. The only study to examine long-term neurodevelopment (MacDonald et al 1985, Grant et al 1989) found no difference between the groups in the incidence of neurologic abnormality at one or four years of age. Assuming that incidence of CP is approximately 2 per 1000, and that approximately 10% of CP is attributable to birth-related hypoxia, acidosis and ischemia, the anticipated incidence of birth-related CP is approximately 0.2 per 1000. A study large enough to detect a 50% reduction in the incidence of birth-related CP (power 80%, $P < 0.05$) would require more than 500 000 patients (Fleiss 1981). It is not surprising that the randomized trials to date have been unable to detect a statistically significant reduction in CP with the use of EFM.

No randomized trials have investigated possible associations between specific FHR patterns and long-term neurologic outcome. However, Nelson et al (1996), reported a population-based study of the association of CP with specific intrapartum FHR patterns. Multiple late decelerations, (odds ratio 3.9; 95 percent confidence interval, 1.7 to 9.3), and decreased variability (odds ratio 2.7; 95 percent confidence interval, 1.1 to 5.8) were associated with an increased risk of CP. The risk persisted after correction for multiple other risk factors. However, because of the low prevalence of CP in the population, the false-positive rate of these FHR abnormalities for predicting CP was 99.8%, clearly demonstrating the poor predictive value of these observations. According to this study, multiple late decelerations and decreased FHR variability correctly predicted brain injury in only 1 out of 500 cases.

POTENTIAL RISKS OF ELECTRONIC FETAL MONITORING

Early concerns regarding the potential for maternal or neonatal bacterial infections in electronically monitored patients appear to have been unfounded. One randomized trial (Haverkamp et al 1976) demonstrated an increased risk of maternal infectious morbidity in patients randomized to EFM. However, these results are difficult to interpret in light of the fact that fetal scalp electrodes were used in both the EFM and control groups (FHR tracings were recorded in the control group, but clinicians did not have access to them). The largest randomized trial to date (MacDonald et al 1985) revealed no increased infectious morbidity in electronically monitored patients. Nevertheless, disruption of the integrity of fetal skin with a fetal scalp electrode should be avoided in patients at risk for vertical perinatal transmission of viral infections, including HIV and hepatitis.

Meta-analyses of the randomized trials of EFM versus intermittent auscultation identify a higher risk of operative intervention in the monitored group compared to controls (Thacker & Stroup 1999, Vintzileos et al 1995). Data from the most recent randomized trials, however, suggest that the effect of EFM on cesarean section rates is minimal. While four early randomized trials (Haverkamp et al 1976, 1979, Kelso et al 1978, Renou et al 1976) reported significantly more cesarean deliveries in electronically monitored patients, five more recent studies (Luthy et al 1987, MacDonald et al 1985, Neldam et al 1986, Vintzileos et al 1993, Wood et al 1981) revealed no such difference and one (Leveno et al 1986) reported data only on rates of cesarean delivery for 'fetal distress,' not overall cesarean section rates. It is possible that the early impact of EFM on cesarean section rates has been mitigated by more recent changes in interpretation and management that have accompanied decades of clinical experience with the technique.

Despite a lack of consensus on many points, EFM has been demonstrated to be at least as effective in preventing perinatal morbidity and mortality as is frequent FHR auscultation with intensive, one-on-one nursing. While this level of individualized nursing care may be available in some settings, most delivery units will find the personnel requirements to be impractical and cost-prohibitive.

OTHER METHODS OF FETAL MONITORING

One of the major shortcomings of electronic fetal monitoring is a high rate of false-positive results. Even the most abnormal patterns are poorly predictive of neonatal morbidity (Banta & Thacker 1979, Clark et al 1996, Nelson et al 1996, Tejani et al 1975). This has led to exploration of alternative methods of evaluating fetal status.

INTRAPARTUM FETAL SCALP PH DETERMINATION

Intermittent sampling of scalp blood for pH determination was described in the 1960s and studied extensively in the 1970s. However, its use has been limited by many factors, including the requirements for cervical dilation and membrane rupture, technical difficulty of the procedure, the need for serial pH determinations and uncertainty regarding interpretation and application of results. In one study, a scalp pH = 7.2 correctly predicted an umbilical artery pH <7.0 in 9% of cases and correctly predicted hypoxic-ischemic encephalopathy in only 3% of cases (Kruger et al 1999). Moreover, a review from a large obstetric center revealed no increase in the rates of fetal distress, cesarean section for fetal distress, low Apgar scores, meconium aspiration or 'perinatal asphyxia' when scalp pH sampling was eliminated from clinical practice (Goodwin et al 1994).

The applicability of continuous intrapartum monitoring of fetal scalp pH was explored in the 1970s (Bloch 1978, Lauersen et al 1979, Stamm et al 1976, Sturbois et al 1977). Lauersen et al (1979) reported 76.9–87% correlation between the readings of a continuous fetal scalp tissue pH electrode and intermittent fetal scalp pH determinations. The technique was considered to be clinically useful in 65% of 40 patients studied. Complications included inflammation at the electrode site in one case and breakage of the electrode during application in one case with retention of a fragment of the electrode in the fetal scalp. The authors reported good correlation between continuous pH readings and immediate neonatal outcome. Others have reported no correlation between pH values and outcome (Huch et al 1980). Inconsistent correlation with outcome and technical obstacles have limited the usefulness of this technique in clinical practice.

Investigators exploring the potential of fetal transcutaneous pO_2 and pCO_2 monitoring during labor have demonstrated correlation with umbilical artery blood gas values and FHR patterns (Aarnoudse et al 1985, Baxi et al 1988, Bergmans et al 1993, Huch et al 1980, Okane et al 1989, Schmidt et al 1985, Willcourt & Queenan 1981). However, technical obstacles have limited the usefulness of this technique as well.

COMPUTER ANALYSIS OF FHR

Subjective interpretation of FHR tracings by visual analysis is hampered by inconsistency and imprecision. In an attempt to overcome this limitation, Dawes and others derived a system of numeric analysis of FHR (Dawes 1991). Computer analysis of intrapartum FHR records has been reported to be more precise than visual assessment (Dawes et al 1992, Pello et al 1991). However, intrapartum computer analysis has not been shown to improve prediction of neonatal outcome. Keith et al (1995) reported the results of a multicenter trial of an intelligent computer system using clinical data in addition to FHR data. In 50 cases analyzed, the system's performance was indistinguishable from that of 17 expert clinicians. The authors reported that the system was highly consistent, recommended no unnecessary intervention and performed better than all but two of the experts.

FETAL PULSE OXIMETRY

Intrapartum reflectance fetal pulse oximetry is a modification of transmission pulse oximetry that indirectly measures the oxygen saturation of hemoglobin in fetal blood (Dildy et al 1996a). An intrauterine sensor placed in contact with fetal skin uses the differential absorption of red and infrared light by oxygenated and deoxygenated fetal hemoglobin to provide continuous estimation of fetal oxygen saturation. Sensors have been reported to obtain reliable signals 45 to 60% of the time (Dildy et al 1993). In fetal sheep, normal aerobic metabolism is maintained at oxygen saturations above 30% (Nijland et al 1995, Oeseburg et al 1992). Below that level, metabolic acidosis, and eventually metabolic acidemia, may develop. In 1994 Dildy et al (1994) reported a multicenter experience with 291 human subjects. A wide range of SpO_2 values was noted; however during the second stage of labor, SpO2 values of 33% were 2 standard deviations below the mean, consistent with the lower limit of normal in animal studies. In 122 patients, Seelbach-Gobel et al (1994) reported that SpO_2 values less than 30% for >10 minutes predicted postpartum pH values <7.2 in more than 50% of cases. Dildy et al (1996b) later reported 1101 paired umbilical artery and vein specimens. An umbilical arterial blood SaO_2 >30% was associated with an umbilical arterial blood pH <7.13 in only 1% of cases while an umbilical arterial blood SaO_2 <30% was associated with an umbilical arterial blood pH <7.13 in 8.6% of cases.

A German multicenter study (Kuhnert et al 1998) including 46 fetuses validated the critical threshold SpO_2 of 30% and concluded that SpO_2 values below this level for more than 10 minutes correlated with decreased intrapartum scalp pH and decreased postpartum cord blood pH values. These results suggested that continuous intrapartum fetal pulse oximetry might improve the predictive value of standard EFM by providing additional information on fetal oxygenation and acid–base status in cases of abnormal or confusing FHR tracings. Improved ability to determine the fetal status in these cases might reduce the rate of cesarean section for presumed fetal compromise. To investigate this possibility, Garite et al (2000) conducted a multicenter randomized controlled trial of fetal pulse oximetry in 1010 patients with abnormal intrapartum FHR patterns. Patients

with FHR patterns demonstrating absence of accelerations, presence of late or variable decelerations, minimal FHR variability, marked FHR variability, bradycardia, tachycardia or sinusoidal pattern were randomized to undergo monitoring with standard EFM alone ($n = 502$) or EFM plus fetal pulse oximetry ($n = 508$). The groups were comparable with respect to most demographic characteristics. Labor induction (56% vs. 49%) and prostaglandin use (31% vs. 25%) were more frequent in the study group. The authors reported a statistically significant 50% reduction in the incidence of cesarean delivery for 'nonreassuring fetal status' (5% vs. 10%) in patients monitored with EFM plus pulse oximetry. However, the overall cesarean rate was not different in the two groups because of a statistically higher rate of cesarean delivery for 'dystocia' in the study group. In May 2000, fetal pulse oximetry was approved provisionally by the United States Food and Drug Administration. In September of 2001, the American College of Obstetricians and Gynecologists Committee on Obstetric Practice issued a Committee Opinion stating that it could not at that time endorse the adoption of the device in clinical practice because of concerns that its introduction could further escalate the cost of medical care without necessarily improving clinical outcome (ACOG 2001). The committee recommended further prospective, randomized clinical trials of the technology. Since that time, several randomized trials have been published that tend to confirm the findings of Garite et al (2001).

A prospective, randomized controlled trial from Australia compared EFM alone to EFM plus pulse oximetry in 600 patients with abnormal intrapartum FHR tracings (East et al 2006). The authors reported a significantly lower rate of cesarean section for 'nonreassuring fetal status' in the study group (24.9% vs. 32.2%). However, more cesareans were performed for 'dystocia' and other indications in the study group, resulting in a cesarean rate of 45.9% in the group monitored with EFM plus pulse oximetry compared to a rate of 48.1% in the group monitored with EFM alone. These differences were not statistically significant (RR 0.95, 95% CI 0.80–1.13, $P = 0.478$).

In 2005, Klauser and colleagues published a prospective, randomized, controlled trial comparing EFM alone to EFM plus fetal pulse oximetry in 327 patients with abnormal FHR patterns (Klauser et al 2005). This study demonstrated no significant difference in overall cesarean rates between the two groups. Cesarean rates for 'nonreassuring FHR tracing' (29% vs. 32%) and 'dystocia' (22% vs. 23%) were statistically similar in the study and control groups, respectively.

In 2006, the NICHD Maternal-Fetal Medicine Units Network published a multicenter, randomized, controlled trial of fetal oxygen saturation monitoring in 5341 patients (Bloom et al 2006). In those randomized to the 'open' group ($n = 2629$), continuous pulse oximetry information was available to the birth attendants. Patients randomized to the 'masked' group ($n = 2712$) had fetal pulse oximetry monitors

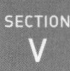

placed; however the information was not available to the birth attendants. The cesarean section rate in the 'open' group was not statistically different from that in the 'masked' group (26.3% vs. 27.5%). Moreover, there were no significant differences in the rates of cesarean for fetal heart rate abnormalities (7.1% vs. 7.9%) or for dystocia (18.6% vs. 19.2%). The authors concluded that knowledge of intrapartum fetal oxygen saturation had no significant effect on the rates of cesarean delivery or with improvement in the condition of the newborn.

The results of a number of randomized trials led the manufacturer of the fetal pulse oximeter to announce that it would no longer distribute the sensors needed for the monitors, effectively withdrawing it from the market.

ST SEGMENT ANALYSIS

Study of the fetal electrocardiogram (ECG) has produced some promising results. In sheep, FHR decelerations that accompanied hypoxemia were associated with characteristic changes in the fetal P–R interval. In 2000, Strachan et al compared standard EFM with EFM plus P–R interval analysis in 1038 women (Strachan et al 2000). The groups demonstrated statistically similar rates of operative intervention for presumed fetal distress and no differences in newborn outcomes.

The S–T segment of the fetal ECG represents myocardial repolarization. Myocardial hypoxia can lead to elevation of the S–T segment and T wave secondary to catecholamine release, β-adrenoceptor activation, glycogenolysis and tissue metabolic acidosis (Hökegård et al 1981, Rosén et al 1984, Widmark et al 1991). These observations have led to the development of technology to analyze the fetal ECG plus the S–T waveform (STAN) (Arulkumaran et al 1990, Lilja et al 1989). One randomized trial in 2434 patients demonstrated a 46% reduction in operative intervention for fetal distress when S–T segment analysis was added to standard EFM (Westgate et al 1993). Operative interventions for dystocia and other indications were not increased. Fewer cases of metabolic acidemia and low 5-minute Apgar scores were observed in the group with EFM plus S–T segment analysis, however these differences did not reach statistical significance.

Another trial using newer technology included 4966 women randomized to EFM alone versus EFM plus S–T segment analysis (Amer-Wåhlin et al 2001). When analyzed according to intention to treat, the incidence of umbilical artery acidemia was 53% lower in the EFM plus S–T segment analysis group. In the EFM plus S–T segment analysis group, the incidence of cesarean section for fetal distress was 8%, compared to 9% in the group monitored with EFM alone ($P = 0.047$). After excluding patients with inadequate FHR recordings and fetal malformations, these differences were slightly more pronounced.

A recent meta-analysis of four studies, including 9829 women, concluded that adjunctive S–T segment analysis was associated with significantly fewer cases of severe metabolic acidemia at birth, fewer cases of neonatal encephalopathy and fewer operative vaginal deliveries (Neilson 2006). However, there were no significant differences in cesarean delivery rates, low 5-minute Apgar scores or NICU admissions. This meta-analysis suggests that S–T segment analysis might prove to be a useful adjunct to standard EFM. While initial results are promising, further research is needed to define the role of this technology in clinical practice.

INTRAPARTUM FHR INTERPRETATION AND MANAGEMENT

Since the introduction of EFM into clinical practice, it has become increasingly apparent that a lack of standardized terminology has critically hindered systematic evaluation of the technology. In an attempt to address this shortcoming, the National Institute of Child Health and Human Development (NICHD) convened a panel of experts in the area of fetal monitoring. Meetings were held between 1995 and 1996 with the goals of establishing 'standardized and unambiguous definitions' of FHR patterns and developing recommendations for research in intrapartum FHR monitoring so that the technique could be studied more systematically and meaningfully. In 1997, the NICHD group published recommendations for interpretation of FHR monitoring and standardization of nomenclature (Electronic fetal heart rate monitoring: research guidelines for interpretation. National Institute of Child Health and Human Development Research Planning Workshop 1997). These recommendations have since been endorsed by ACOG and the Association of Women's Health, Obstetric and Neonatal Nursing (AWHONN) (ACOG 2005b). The NICHD panel emphasized that the primary objective was to establish standardized definitions, not to address the putative etiologies of the various FHR patterns or their relationship to fetal hypoxemia or metabolic acidemia. The standardized definitions apply to the interpretation of patterns produced from a direct fetal electrode detecting the fetal ECG or from an external Doppler device detecting fetal cardiac motion using the autocorrelation technique. Patterns are defined as baseline, periodic or episodic. Periodic patterns are those associated with uterine contractions and episodic patterns are those not associated with uterine contractions. Periodic and episodic patterns are defined as 'abrupt' if the onset to nadir (or peak) is <30 seconds and 'gradual' if the onset to nadir (or peak) is ≥30 seconds. Although terms such as 'beat-to-beat' variability, 'short-term' variability and 'long-term' variability are used frequently in clinical practice, the panel recommended that no distinction be made between short-term variability (or beat-to-beat variability) and long-term variability because in actual practice they are visually determined as a unit. Finally, the panel emphasized that fetal heart rate patterns do not occur alone and generally evolve over time. Therefore, a full description of a FHR tracing requires a qualitative and quantitative description of each of the characteristics summarized in Table 24.3.

Table 24.3 Full description of a FHR tracing requires a qualitative and quantitative description of each of the following

1. Baseline rate
2. Baseline FHR variability
3. Presence of accelerations
4. Periodic or episodic decelerations
5. Changes or trends of FHR patterns over time

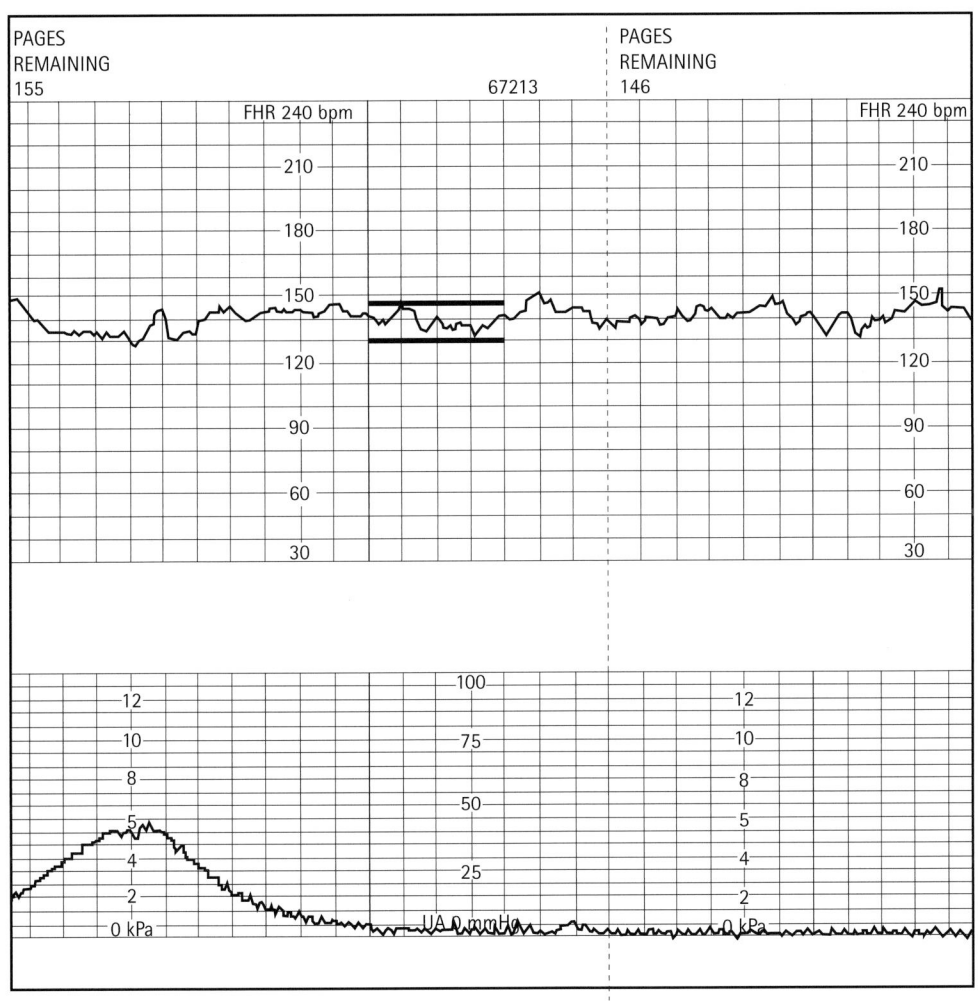

Figure 24.1 Moderate FHR variability.

DEFINITIONS OF FHR PATTERNS

BASELINE FETAL HEART RATE

Baseline FHR is defined as the approximate mean FHR rounded to increments of 5 beats per minute during a 10-minute segment, excluding periodic or episodic changes, periods of marked FHR variability and segments of the baseline that differ by >25 beats per minute. In any 10-minute window the minimum baseline duration must be at least 2 minutes or the baseline for that period is deemed indeterminate. In this case, it may be necessary to refer to the previous 10-minute segment(s) for determination of the baseline. Normal FHR baseline ranges from 110 to 160 beats per minute. A FHR baseline below 110 beats per minute is defined as bradycardia and a rate in excess of 160 beats per minute is defined as tachycardia. Bradycardia and tachycardia are quantitated by the actual FHR in beats per minute, or the visually determined range if the FHR is not stable at one rate.

BASELINE FETAL HEART RATE VARIABILITY

Baseline FHR variability is defined as fluctuations in the baseline FHR of two cycles per minute or greater. The fluctuations are irregular in amplitude and frequency. Variability is quantitated in beats per minute and is measured from the peak to the trough of a single cycle. The categories of FHR variability are defined as summarized in Table 24.4. Figure 24.1 depicts moderate FHR variability (6–25 beats per

Table 24.4 Categories of FHR variability
1. Absent FHR variability: Amplitude range undetectable
2. Minimal FHR variability: Amplitude range detectable but ≤5 beats per minute
3. Moderate FHR variability: Amplitude range 6 to 25 beats per minute
4. Marked FHR variability: Amplitude range >25 beats per minute

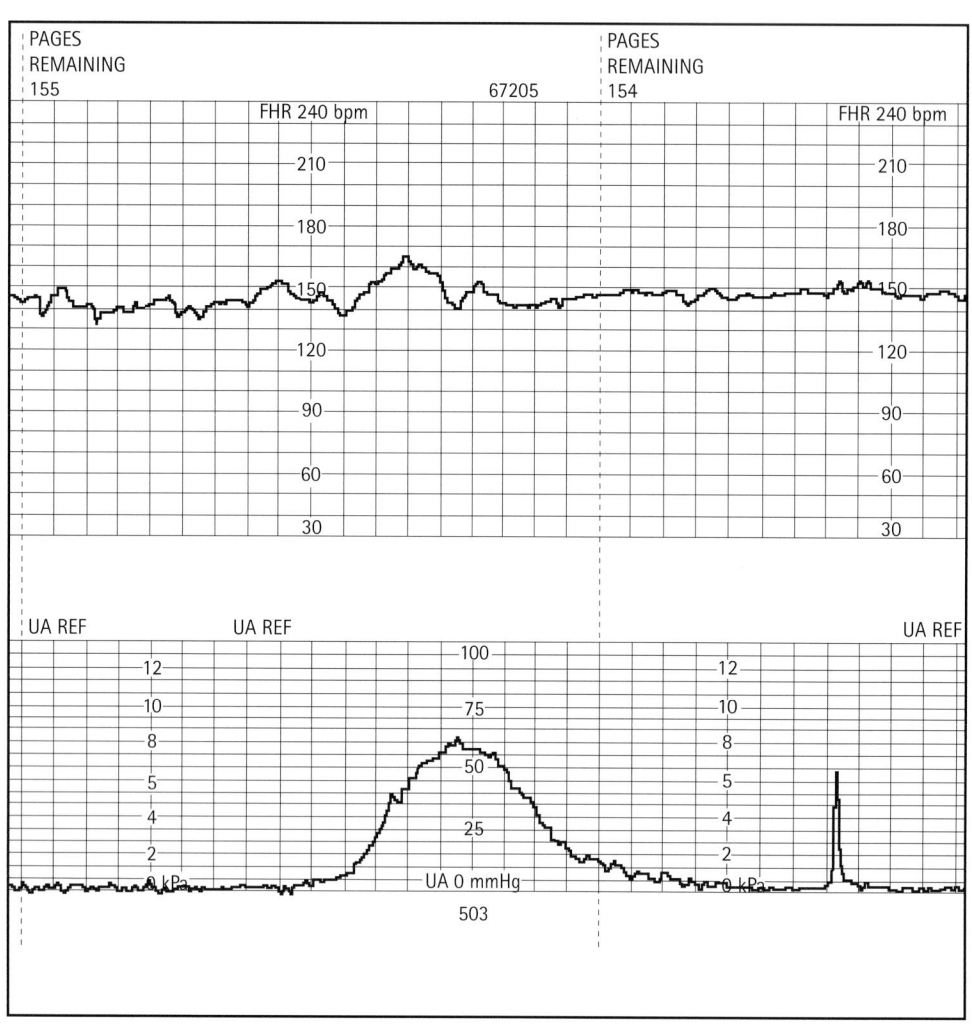

Figure 24.2 Acceleration.

minute). No distinction is made between 'short-term' ('beat-to-beat') variability and 'long-term' variability because in actual practice they are visually determined as a unit. There is no consensus whether 'beat-to-beat' variability alone is interpretable to the unaided eye. The sinusoidal pattern has a smooth, sine wave-like pattern of regular frequency and amplitude. It is not included in the definition of FHR variability.

ACCELERATION

Acceleration is as an abrupt (onset to peak <30 seconds) increase in FHR above the baseline, calculated from the most recently determined portion of the baseline. The peak is at least 15 beats per minute above the baseline and the acceleration lasts at least 15 seconds from the onset to return to baseline. Figure 24.2 depicts a FHR acceleration. Before 32 weeks of gestation, acceleration is defined as having a peak at least 10 beats per minute above the baseline and a duration of at least 10 seconds. An acceleration lasting ≥2 minutes but less than 10 minutes is defined as a prolonged acceleration. An acceleration lasting 10 minutes or longer is defined as a baseline change. The amplitude of an acceleration is quantitated in beats per minute above the baseline excluding transient spikes or electronic artifact. The duration is quantitated in minutes and seconds. Decelerations are quantitated similarly.

DECELERATION

LATE DECELERATION

Late deceleration of the FHR is defined as a gradual (onset to nadir ≥30 seconds) decrease of the FHR from the baseline and subsequent return to the baseline associated with a uterine contraction. The decrease is calculated from the most recently determined portion of the baseline. In most cases the onset, nadir and recovery of the deceleration occur after the beginning, peak and ending of the contraction, respectively. Figure 24.3 depicts a late deceleration. Late decelerations are defined as recurrent if they occur with at least 50% of uterine contractions in any 20-minute segment.

EARLY DECELERATION

Early deceleration is defined as a gradual (onset to nadir ≥30 seconds) decrease of the FHR from the baseline and subsequent return to the baseline associated with a uterine contraction. In most cases the onset, nadir and recovery of the deceleration occur at the same time as the beginning, peak and ending of the contraction, respectively. Early decelerations are defined as recurrent if they occur with at least 50% of uterine contractions in any 20-minute segment.

VARIABLE DECELERATION

Variable deceleration of the FHR is defined as an abrupt (onset to nadir <30 seconds) decrease in FHR below the baseline, calculated from the most recently determined portion of the baseline. The decrease in FHR below the baseline is at least 15 beats per minute and the deceleration lasts at least 15 seconds from onset to return to baseline. Figure 24.4 depicts a variable deceleration. Variable decelerations are not necessarily associated with uterine contractions. If they are, variable decelerations are defined as recurrent if they occur with at least 50% of uterine contractions in any 20-minute segment.

PROLONGED DECELERATION

Prolonged deceleration of the FHR is defined as a decrease (either gradual or abrupt) in FHR at least 15 beats per minute below the baseline lasting at least 2 minutes from onset to

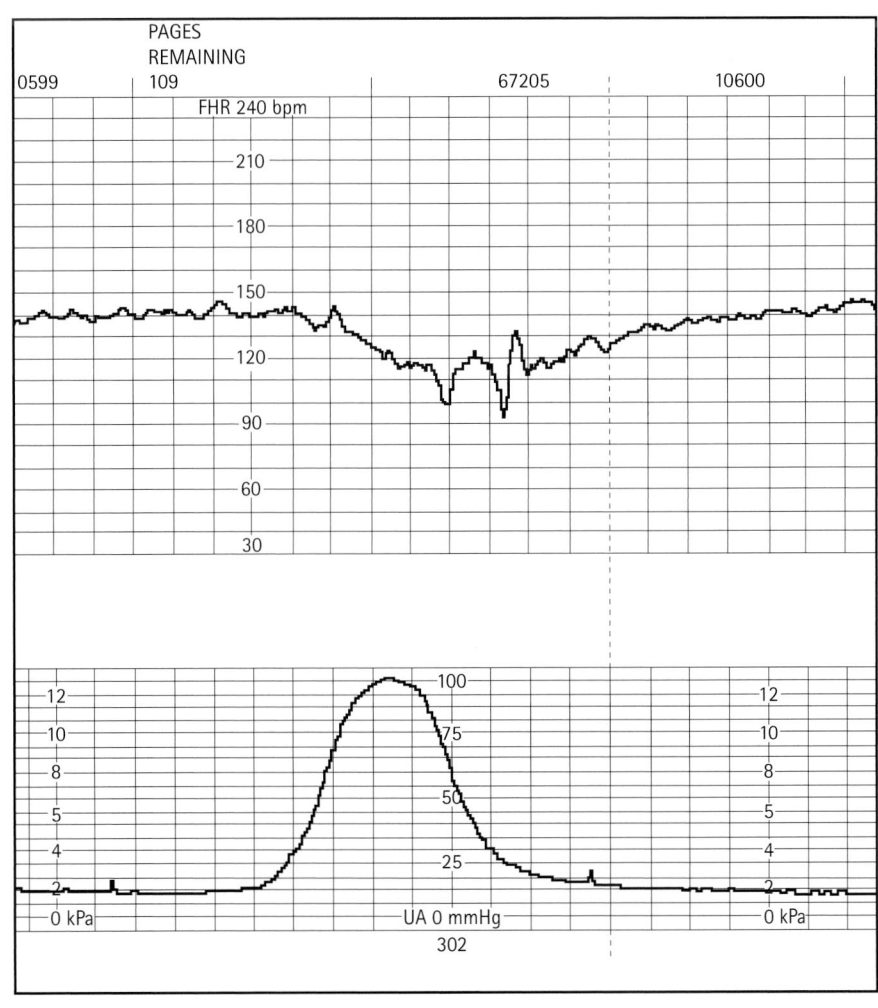

Figure 24.3 Late deceleration.

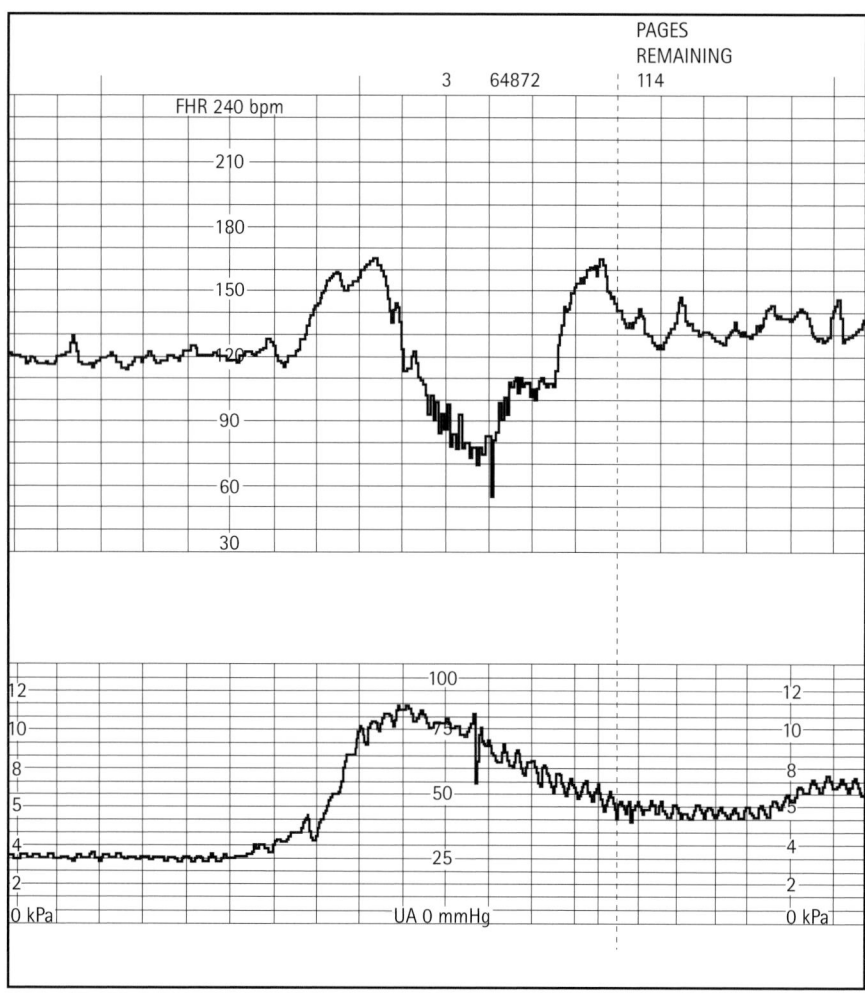

Figure 24.4 Variable deceleration.

return to baseline. If the deceleration lasts 10 minutes or longer, it is defined as a baseline change.

CHANGES OR TRENDS IN THE FHR PATTERNS OVER TIME

A full description of a FHR tracing should include an assessment of the changes and trends in the baseline FHR, variability and frequency of FHR accelerations over time. In addition, the description should include any changes or trends in the frequency, depth, duration and type of FHR deceleration. These changes should be described and evaluated in the context of gestational age, maternal medical conditions, medications, uterine activity, prior results of fetal assessment and other factors that might influence the FHR.

MANAGEMENT OF INTRAPARTUM FHR PATTERNS

A FHR tracing demonstrating a normal baseline rate (110–160 beats per minute), moderate FHR variability (6–25 beats per minute), accelerations and no decelerations is highly predictive of the absence of fetal metabolic acidemia. By extension, it is highly predictive of normal fetal tissue oxygenation and the absence of tissue acidosis. On the other end of the spectrum, a FHR tracing demonstrating absent FHR variability, absent FHR accelerations and recurrent or prolonged decelerations is associated with an increased risk of fetal metabolic acidemia (ACOG 2003). However, when the FHR tracing demonstrates patterns between these two extremes, consensus is more difficult to achieve. Nevertheless, understanding of the physiology and pathophysiology of FHR changes can provide a window into the fetal environment and help guide management. Anytime a FHR pattern suggests an interruption of normal fetal oxygenation, it is appropriate for the clinician to evaluate the pathway of oxygen delivery from the environment to the fetus and to institute appropriate corrective measures. Oxygen travels down a predictable pathway from the environment to the fetal tissues. Inhalation carries oxygen to the maternal lungs. From there it is carried by maternal blood to the heart, the vascular tree, the uterus, placenta, umbilical cord and finally to the fetus (Fig. 24.5). Table 24.5 summarizes the assessment and appropriate corrective measures at each step.

Table 24.5 Assessment and management of interrupted fetal oxygenation

Step	Assessment	Management considerations
Lungs	Airway and breathing Auscultation Pulse oximetry or blood gas analysis if needed	Oxygen if needed
Heart	Heart rate and rhythm Auscultation Blood pressure	Treat hypotension, hypertension, arrhythmia if needed
Vasculature	Heart rate Blood pressure Assess volume status	Treat hypotension, hypertension if needed Position change, intravenous fluid bolus
Uterus	Contraction frequency, strength and baseline tone Intrauterine pressure catheter if needed Exclude uterine rupture	Discontinue or reduce dose of uterine stimulant Administer uterine relaxant If uterine rupture suspected, prepare for delivery
Placenta	Exclude placental abruption Exclude bleeding placenta previa	If placental abruption or bleeding placenta previa suspected, prepare for delivery
Umbilical cord	Vaginal exam Exclude umbilical cord prolapse	Position change Consider amnioinfusion if cord compression suspected If cord prolapse is documented, prepare for delivery

Environment
Maternal lungs
Maternal heart
Vasculature
Uterus
Placenta
Umbilical cord
Fetus

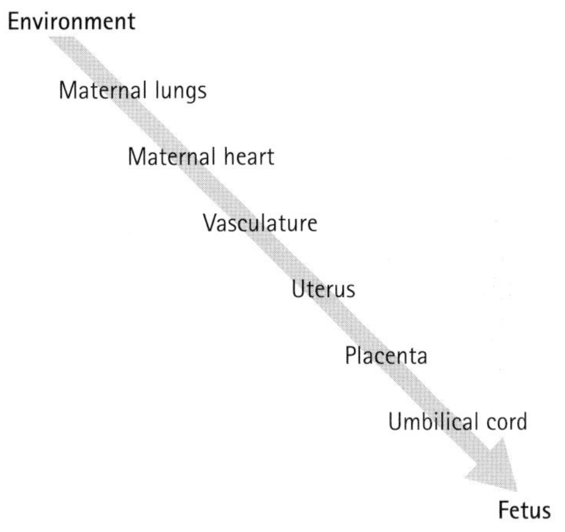

Figure 24.5 Pathway of oxygen from the environment to the fetus.

BASELINE FETAL HEART RATE

BRADYCARDIA

Bradycardia is defined as an abnormally low baseline FHR (<110 beats per minute), and must be differentiated from the FHR changes characteristic of decelerations. Although FHR decelerations are very common, true fetal bradycardia is not. A FHR baseline between 90 and 110 beats per minute in association with moderate variability and accelerations most likely represents a normal variant. Rarely, fetal bradycardia may be seen in association with maternal beta-blocker therapy, hypothermia, hypoglycemia, hypothyroidism or fetal heart block. Documentation of fetal heart block should prompt a search for structural fetal cardiac abnormalities,

which may be observed in as many as 20% of cases. Other possible causes of heart block include viral infections (i.e. cytomegalovirus) and maternal systemic lupus erythematosus with anti-Ro (SSA) antibodies. Most congenital causes of intrapartum fetal bradycardia do not present as acute changes in the FHR and rarely require emergency intervention. During labor, an abrupt drop in the FHR more likely represents a deceleration than a change in the baseline and should be managed as a deceleration until proven otherwise. The clinician should assess the oxygen pathway from the environment to the fetus and institute appropriate corrective measures.

TACHYCARDIA

Fetal tachycardia has many possible etiologies. The underlying cause should be identified and treated, when possible. Often, it is associated with infection and fever. The source of any maternal fever must be aggressively sought and intra-amniotic infection excluded. The diagnosis of chorioamnionitis requires intrapartum antibiotic therapy. Possible causative medications should be discontinued and maternal hyperthyroidism should be excluded. Fetal cardiac arrhythmias may require ultrasonographic evaluation to rule out structural lesions and cardiac failure. Anti-arrhythmic therapy may be instituted if deemed necessary. Tachycardia alone does not confirm the presence of metabolic acidemia. However, tachycardia may be observed in association with other FHR patterns suggestive of metabolic acidemia, including absent FHR variability, absent accelerations and recurrent or prolonged FHR decelerations. If reduced fetal oxygenation is suspected, the oxygen pathway should be assessed and appropriate corrective measures instituted. If the FHR tracing cannot reliably exclude metabolic acidemia, and if corrective measures are not successful, consideration should be given to delivery.

BASELINE FHR VARIABILITY

Variability in the FHR results from autonomic regulation of fetal cardiac activity in response to changes in blood pressure, pO2 and pCO2. Fluctuations in fetal blood pressure are detected by aortic arch baroreceptors while changes in pO2 and pCO2 are detected by chemoreceptors. Chemoreceptors and baroreceptors communicate with the medullary vasomotor center, which in turn modulates sympathetic and parasympathetic outflow. The parasympathetic arm of the fetal autonomic nervous system, by way of the vagus nerve, is thought to be primarily responsible for FHR variability. Moderate (normal) variability reflects normal autonomic regulation of the cardiac conduction system and is highly predictive of the absence of fetal metabolic acidemia (Hammacher et al 1968, Hon & Lee 1963, Krebs et al 1979, Martin 1982, Paul et al 1975). Variability that is ≤5 beats per minute most often reflects decreased fetal CNS activity associated with a fetal sleep state. Other possible causes include medications (magnesium sulfate, nalbuphine), fetal anomalies and prematurity (ACOG 2005b). If minimal or absent FHR variability is persistent, fetal metabolic acidemia should be excluded. The oxygen pathway should be assessed and appropriate corrective measures instituted. Fetal scalp stimulation or vibroacoustic stimulation may provoke FHR accelerations and improve FHR variability. If present, these observations are highly predictive of the absence of metabolic acidemia.

SINUSOIDAL PATTERN

The sinusoidal FHR pattern is an uncommon FHR baseline abnormality. The pattern presents as a smooth sine wave with an amplitude of 5–15 beats per minute and a frequency of 2–5 cycles per minute. Although the pathophysiologic mechanism is not known, this pattern characteristically is associated with severe fetal anemia. It may also occur in association with chorioamnionitis (Gleicher et al 1980), fetal sepsis or administration of narcotic analgesics. In the setting of a persistent sinusoidal pattern, delivery may be necessary.

ACCELERATIONS

Accelerations in FHR occur in association with fetal movement, probably as a result of increased catecholamine release and decreased vagal stimulation of the heart. Starting at approximately 30–32 weeks gestation, they normally occur during the fetal wake state at a rate of 15–20 per hour. Like moderate variability, FHR accelerations are highly predictive of the absence of metabolic acidemia. The persistent absence of spontaneous accelerations, on the other hand, is abnormal and may reflect fetal acidemia. Absent FHR accelerations must be interpreted carefully in the context of the clinical presentation and other FHR characteristics. During labor,

the frequency and amplitude of FHR accelerations may be diminished by fetal sleep state, common medications (magnesium sulfate, morphine) or fetal metabolic acidemia. If decreased fetal oxygenation is suspected, the oxygen pathway should be assessed and appropriate corrective measures instituted. In the absence of spontaneous accelerations, fetal scalp stimulation or vibroacoustic stimulation often provokes fetal movement and FHR accelerations that are associated with normal scalp pH values (Clark et al 1986, Irion et al 1996, Spencer 1991). If these measures fail to provoke FHR accelerations, and if other FHR characteristics are suggestive of developing acidemia, delivery may be necessary.

DECELERATIONS

LATE DECELERATION

A late deceleration is a reflex fetal response to transient hypoxemia during a uterine contraction. Myometrial contractions compress maternal blood vessels traversing the uterine wall and can interrupt maternal perfusion of the intervillous space of the placenta. Reduced delivery of oxygenated blood to the intervillous space can reduce the diffusion of oxygen into the fetal capillary blood in the chorionic villi, leading to a decline in fetal pO_2 below the normal range of approximately 15–25 mmHg. If the fetal pO_2 falls below a critical threshold, chemoreceptors signal the medullary vasomotor center to initiate a protective reflex response (Martin et al 1979). Sympathetic outflow causes peripheral vasoconstriction and centralization of blood volume to perfuse the brain, heart and adrenal glands. The resulting increase in peripheral resistance causes a rise in mean arterial blood pressure and a baroreceptor-mediated reflex slowing of the heart rate to reduce cardiac output and return the blood pressure to normal. Isolated late decelerations within an otherwise normal tracing usually have little clinical consequence. However, recurrent episodes of transient hypoxemia eventually may lead to tissue hypoxia. If sustained, tissue hypoxia can initiate a cascade of metabolic events leading to fetal injury or even death. Initially, reduced tissue oxygen may force the peripheral tissues to convert from aerobic to anaerobic metabolism to meet their energy needs. This relatively inefficient process results in the production of lactic acid. Unlike carbon dioxide, generated from aerobic metabolism, lactic acid crosses the placenta slowly and can accumulate in the tissues, leading to metabolic acidosis. Accumulation of lactic acid in excess of the fetal buffering capacity can lead to metabolic acidemia, blunting of vagal regulation of the FHR and consequent loss of accelerations, loss of variability and rising baseline rate. Furthermore, persistent hypoxia and acidosis in the peripheral tissues can disrupt energy production and impair the function of peripheral vascular smooth muscle cells. Failure of peripheral vasoconstriction reduces systemic vascular resistance and results in hypotension, compromising the pressure-dependent perfusion of the fetal brain and coronary arteries. As the cascade continues, cardiac hypoxia–ischemia results in FHR deceleration, reducing cardiac output and further exacerbating hypoperfusion of the brain, heart and other organs. Hypoxia, acidosis and hypoperfusion can result in hypoxic–ischemic injury to multiple organ systems. The goal in treating late decelerations is to prevent the initiation of this cascade of events by improving the delivery of oxygen from the environment to the fetus and correcting the hypoxemia that provides the initial trigger. Even in the setting of recurrent late decelerations, it is critical to note that a normal baseline FHR, moderate variability and accelerations are highly predictive of the absence of metabolic acidemia. The oxygen pathway should be assessed thoroughly and appropriate corrective measures initiated. Usual corrective measures include administration of supplemental oxygen, left lateral decubitus positioning to improve maternal venous return and cardiac output, intravenous fluid bolus of 250–500 cc of crystalloid to restore the maternal intravascular volume and improve cardiac output, discontinuation of uterine stimulants and administration of uterine relaxants. If these measures are not successful or if the FHR tracing does not provide reliable evidence of the absence of metabolic acidemia, delivery should be considered.

EARLY DECELERATIONS

Early decelerations probably result from fetal head compression and reflex augmentation of vagal tone. Perinatal outcome is not adversely impacted by these decelerations and they are considered clinically benign.

VARIABLE DECELERATIONS

Variable decelerations result from umbilical cord compression and have a variable temporal relationship to uterine contractions. Initially, umbilical vein compression decreases fetal venous return and causes reflex FHR elevation. Subsequent umbilical arterial compression increases fetal peripheral resistance and produces a rapid-onset baroreceptor-mediated slowing of the heart rate. Maximum vagal tone may result in a junctional or idioventricular rhythm that appears as a relatively stable rate of 60–70 beats per minute at the base of the deceleration. As the cord is decompressed, this sequence of events occurs in reverse. Isolated variable decelerations usually have little clinical consequence. During variable decelerations, the fetal pO_2 may decline, at times below the normal range of 15–25 mmHg. Recurrent variable decelerations may result in sufficient hypoxemia to cause tissue hypoxia. If sustained, tissue hypoxia may initiate the same cascade of metabolic derangements triggered by recurrent late decelerations. When recurrent variable decelerations are present, prolapse of the umbilical cord must be excluded. Maternal positional changes may relieve cord compression. Excessive uterine activity may be relieved by discontinuing uterine stimulants, administering uterine relaxants or both. Intrapartum amnioinfusion is a procedure by which saline is infused through an intrauterine catheter

into the amniotic cavity in an attempt to restore the amniotic fluid volume to normal. The goal of these corrective measures is to relieve the intermittent umbilical cord compression that results in variable FHR decelerations, transient fetal hypoxemia and eventual tissue hypoxia. Even in the setting of recurrent variable decelerations, it is important to note that a normal baseline rate, moderate variability and accelerations are highly predictive of the absence of metabolic acidemia. In most cases, this provides assurance that tissue hypoxia, if present, has not yet initiated the cascade of metabolic events leading to failure of peripheral vasoconstriction, hypotension and hypoxic–ischemic injury. However, there is some evidence in animal models that frequent episodes of hypoxemia, produced by umbilical cord occlusion over a period of hours, can result in fetal injury even in the absence of metabolic academia (Clapp et al 1988). When recurrent variable decelerations are present, appropriate corrective measures should be undertaken. If these measures are not successful in relieving the decelerations within a reasonable time or if the FHR tracing cannot reliably exclude metabolic acidemia, delivery should be considered.

PROLONGED DECELERATIONS

Prolonged decelerations reflect acute interruption of oxygen delivery from the environment to the fetus. The oxygen pathway should be assessed and appropriate intervention initiated. As summarized in Figure 24.5, this pathway consists of the lungs, heart, vasculature, uterus, placenta and umbilical cord. Maternal and fetal oxygen carrying capacity should be considered as well. Prolonged decelerations frequently are caused by umbilical cord compression or prolapse, excessive uterine activity, maternal hypotension, placental abruption or uterine rupture. However, each step in the pathway must be evaluated to exclude all possibilities. Maternal positional changes and/or manual elevation of the fetal head may relieve cord compression, if present. Documentation of separate maternal and fetal heart rates is necessary. Uterine rupture and placental abruption should be excluded clinically if possible. Acute maternal hypotension may respond to positional changes, fluids and ephedrine, if necessary. Discontinuing uterine stimulants and/or administering uterine relaxants may relieve excessive uterine activity. Oxygen is administered to the mother by facemask. If the above measures fail to result in resolution of the prolonged deceleration within minutes, delivery should be expedited.

ACUTE INTRAPARTUM EVENTS AND CEREBRAL PALSY

Neonatal encephalopathy and CP result from intrapartum events in approximately 1–2 per 10 000 deliveries. Yet, despite the rarity of birth-related CP, there has been significant controversy in the literature regarding the link between FHR patterns, neonatal encephalopathy and brain injury. In 2003, ACOG and the American Academy of Pediatrics jointly

Table 24.6 Essential criteria that define an acute intrapartum event sufficient to cause cerebral palsy (must meet all four)
1. Evidence of a metabolic acidosis in umbilical cord arterial blood obtained at delivery (pH <7 and base deficit ≥12 mmol/L)
2. Early onset of severe or moderate neonatal encephalopathy in infants born at 34 or more weeks of gestation
3. Cerebral palsy of the spastic quadriplegic or dyskinetic type
4. Exclusion of other identifiable etiologies such as trauma, coagulation disorders, infectious conditions or genetic disorders

Table 24.7 Criteria that collectively suggest the event occurred within 48 hours of birth
1. A sentinel (signal) hypoxic event occurring immediately before or during labor
2. A sudden and sustained fetal bradycardia or the absence of fetal heart rate variability in the presence of persistent, late, or variable decelerations, usually after a hypoxic sentinel event when the pattern was previously normal
3. Apgar scores of 0–3 beyond 5 minutes
4. Onset of multisystem involvement within 72 hours of birth

published a monograph entitled 'Neonatal Encephalopathy and Cerebral Palsy: Defining the Pathogenesis and Pathophysiology' (ACOG 2003). One goal of the publication was to summarize the world literature regarding the relationship between intrapartum FHR monitoring, hypoxic–ischemic events and the subsequent development of CP. The task force identified specific criteria that define an acute intrapartum event sufficient to cause cerebral palsy (Table 24.6) and recommended that all four be present in order to attribute cerebral palsy to an acute intrapartum hypoxic event. It is important to note that spastic quadriplegia and, less commonly, dyskinetic cerebral palsy are the only types of cerebral palsy associated with acute hypoxic intrapartum events. Hemiparetic cerebral palsy, hemiplegic cerebral palsy, spastic diplegia and ataxia are unlikely to result from acute intrapartum hypoxia. The task force identified additional criteria that collectively suggest the event occurred within 48 hours of birth. These criteria are summarized in Table 24.7.

CONCLUSION

Significant changes in intrapartum management have taken place over the last four decades, highlighted by the rapid proliferation of electronic fetal monitoring, the decline in maternal and perinatal mortality and the rising utilization of cesarean section. Many widely held beliefs have been challenged. Large case-control studies have demonstrated the limited contribution of 'birth asphyxia' to the incidence of CP. Randomized trials have dampened the early enthusiasm regarding the potential benefits of EFM. Nevertheless, the objective of intrapartum management remains the same: to optimize the outcome for both mother and fetus by (1) preventing intrapartum fetal hypoxemia, hypoxia, metabolic acidosis, metabolic acidemia and possible long-term sequelae, and (2) avoiding unnecessary operative deliveries. To that end, the most effective resource available to the obstetrician is a thorough understanding of the FHR patterns associated with normal and abnormal fetal physiologic states.

REFERENCES

Aarnoudse J G, Huisjes H J, Gordon H et al 1985 Fetal subcutaneous scalp pO₂ and abnormal heart rate during labor. Am J Obstet Gynecol 153:565–566.

ACOG (American College of Obstetricians and Gynecologists) 1995 Fetal heart rate patterns: monitoring, interpretation and management. ACOG Technical Bulletin No 207. ACOG, Washington, DC.

ACOG (American College of Obstetricians and Gynecologists) 2001 Committee on Obstetric Practice Fetal Pulse Oximetry. ACOG Committee Opinion No. 258, September.

ACOG (American College of Obstetricians and Gynecologists) 2003 Task Force on Neonatal Encephalopathy and Cerebral Palsy, American College of Obstetricians and Gynecologists, American Academy of Pediatrics Neonatal encephalopathy and cerebral palsy: Defining the pathogenesis and pathophysiology. American College of Obstetricians and Gynecologists, Washington.

ACOG (American College of Obstetricians and Gynecologists) 2005a ACOG Committee Opinion No. 326. Inappropriate use of the terms fetal distress and birth asphyxia. Obstet Gynecol 106:1469–1470.

ACOG (American College of Obstetricians and Gynecologists) 2005b Intrapartum fetal heart rate monitoring ACOG Practice Bulletin No.70 American College of Obstetricians and Gynecologists. Obstet Gynecol 106:1453–1461.

Alberman E 1978 Main causes of major mental handicap: prevalence and epidemiology. In: DIBA Foundation Symposium 59: Major mental handicap: methods and costs of prevention. Elsevier-Excerpta Medica, Amsterdam.

Amato J L 1977 Fetal monitoring in a community hospital: a statistical analysis. Obstet Gynecol 50:269–274.

Amer-Wåhlin I, Hellsten C, Norén H et al 2001 Cardiotocography only versus cardiotocography plus ST analysis of fetal electrocardiogram for intrapartum fetal monitoring: a Swedish randomised controlled trial. Lancet 358:534–538.

Arulkumaran S, Lilja H, Lindecrantz K et al 1990 Fetal ECG waveform analysis should improve fetal surveillance in labour. J Perinatal Med 18:13–22.

Banta H D, Thacker S B 1979 Costs and benefits to electronic fetal monitoring: a review of the literature. Rockville (MD): National Center for Health Services Research. Report No.: DHEW-PHS-79-3245.

Bax M, Melson K B 1993 Birth asphyxia: A statement. Dev Med Child Neurol 35:1022–1024.

Baxi L V, Petrie R H, James L S 1988 Human fetal oxygenation (tcPo2), heart rate variability and uterine activity following maternal administration of meperidine. J Perinat Med 16:23–30.

Bergmans M G M, van Geijn H P, Weber T et al 1993 Fetal transcutaneous PCO2 measurements during labor. Eur J Obstet Gynecol 51:1–7.

Blair E, Stanley F J 1988 Intrapartum asphyxia: A rare cause of cerebral palsy. J Pediatr 112:515–519.

Bloch B 1978 Measurement of fetal scalp pH by continuous-recording scalp electrode and correlation with capillary blood pH. S Afr Med J 54:448–550.

Bloom S L, Spong C Y, Thom E et al 2006 Fetal pulse oximetry and cesarean delivery. N Engl J Med 355:2195–2202.

Caldeyro-Barcia R, Mendez-Bauer C, Posiero J J et al 1966 Control of the human fetal heart rate during labor. In: Cassels D E (ed.) The heart and circulation of the newborn and infant. Grune and Stratton, New York, p. 7–36.

Chan W H, Paul R H, Toews J 1973 Intrapartum fetal monitoring: Maternal and fetal morbidity and perinatal mortality. Obstet Gynecol 41:7–13.

Clapp J F, Peress N S, Wesley M, Mann L I 1988 Brain damage after intermittent partial cord occlusion in the chronically instrumented fetal lamb. Am J Obstet Gynecol 159:504–509.

Clark S L, Gimovsky M L, Miller F C 1984 The scalp stimulation test: A clinical alternative to fetal scalp blood sampling. Am J Obstet Gynecol 148:274–277.

Cremer M V 1906 Ueber die direckte Ableitung der Aktionsstrome des menchlichen Herzens vom Oesophagus und ueber das Elektrokardiogramm des Fetus. Munch Med Wochenschr 53:811.

Dawes G S 1991 Computerised analysis of the fetal heart rate. Eur J Obstet Gynecol Reprod Biol 42(Suppl):S5–S8.

Dawes G S, Moulden M, Sheil O, Redman C W G 1992 Approximate entropy, a statistic of regularity, applied to fetal heart rate data before and during labor. Obstet Gynecol 80:763–768.

DeLee J B 1922 Ein nues Stethoskopf fur die Geburtshilfe besonders geeignet. Zentralbl Gynaekol 46:1688.

Dildy G A, Clark S L, Loucks C A 1993 Preliminary experience with intrapartum fetal pulse oximetry in humans. Obstet Gynecol 81:630–635.

Dildy G A, Clark S L, Loucks C A 1996a Intrapartum fetal pulse oximetry: Past, present, and future. Am J Obstet Gynecol 175(1):1–9.

Dildy G A, Thorp J A, Yeast J D, Clark S L 1996b The relationship between oxygen saturation and pH in umbilical blood: implications for intrapartum fetal oxygen saturation monitoring. Am J Obstet Gynecol 175(3 Pt 1):682–687.

Dildy G A, van den Berg P P, Katz M et al 1994 Intrapartum fetal pulse oximetry: fetal oxygen saturation trends during labor and relation to delivery outcome. Am J Obstet Gynecol 171:679–684.

East C E, Brennecke S P, King J F et al 2006 The effect of intrapartum fetal pulse oximetry, in the presence of a nonreassuring fetal heart rate pattern, on operative delivery rates: A multicenter, randomized, controlled trial (the FOREMOST trial). Am J Obstet Gynecol 194:606.e1–606.e16.

Eastman N J, DeLeon M 1955 The etiology of cerebral palsy. Am J Obstet Gynecol 69:950–961.

Eastman N J, Kohl S G, Maisel J E, Kavaler F 1962 The obstetrical background of 753 cases of cerebral palsy. Obstet Gynecol Survey 17:459–500.

Edington P T, Sibanda J, Beard R W 1975 Influence on clinical practice of routine intra-partum fetal monitoring. Br Med J 3:341–343.

Electronic fetal heart rate monitoring: research guidelines for interpretation. National Institute of Child Health and Human Development Research Planning Workshop 1997 Am J Obstet Gynecol 177:1385–1390.

Ellenberg J H, Nelson K B 1979 Birth weight and gestational age in children with cerebral palsy or seizure disorders. Am J Dis Child 133:1044.

Faro M D, Windle W F 1969 Transneuronal degeneration in brains of monkeys asphyxiated at birth. Exp Neurol 24:38–53.

Fleiss J L 1981 Statistical methods for rates and proportions, 2nd edn. Wiley, pp. 38–45.

Freud S 1957 Die Infantile Cerebrallähmung. Nothnagels Spez Path u Therapie. Wien IX:2.

Garite T J, Dildy G A, McNamara H et al 2000 A multicenter controlled trial of fetal pulse oximetry in the intrapartum management of nonreassuring fetal heart rate patterns. Am J Obstet Gynecol 183:1049–1058.

Gilstrap L C, Leveno K J, Burris J et al 1989 Diagnosis of birth asphyxia on the basis of fetal pH, Apgar score, and newborn cerebral dysfunction. Am J Obstet Gynecol 161:825–830.

Gleicher H, Runowicz C, Brown B 1980 Sinusoidal fetal heart rate patterns in association with amnionitis. Obstet Gynecol 56:109.

Goodwin J W, Dunne J T, Thomas R W 1969 Antepartum identification of the fetus at risk. Can Med Assoc J 101:458.

Goodwin T M, Milner-Masterson L, Paul R H 1994 Elimination of fetal scalp blood sampling on a large clinical service. Obstet Gynecol 83(6):971–974.

Grant A, O'Brien N, Joy M et al 1989 Cerebral palsy among children born during the Dublin randomized trial of intrapartum monitoring. Lancet 2:1233–1236.

Gültekin-Zootzmann B 1975 The history of monitoring the human fetus. J Perinat Med 3:135–144.

Haddow K M, Gage R P 1960 Neurologic lesions in relation to asphyxia of the newborn and locators of pregnancy: long-term follow-up. Pediatrics 26:616–622.

Haesslein H C, Niswander K R 1980 Fetal distress in term pregnancies. Am J Obstet Gynecol 137:245–253.

Hamilton L A, Gottschalk W, Vidyasagar D et al 1978 Effects of monitoring on perinates. Int J Gynaecol Obstet 15:483–490.

Hammacher K 1967 The diagnosis of fetal distress with an electronic fetal heart monitor. In: Horsky J, Stembera Z K (eds) Intrauterine dangers to the fetus. Excerpta Medica, Amsterdam.

Hammacher K., Huter K A, Bokelmann J, Werners P H 1968 Foetal heart frequency and perinatal condition of the foetus and newborn. Gynaecologia 166:439–460.

Haverkamp A D, Orleans M, Langendoerfer S et al 1979 A controlled trial of the differential effects of intrapartum fetal monitoring. Am J Obstet Gynecol 134:399–408.

Haverkamp A D, Thompson H E, McFee J G, Cetrullo C 1976 The evaluation of continuous fetal heart rate monitoring in high-risk pregnancy. Am J Obstet Gynecol 125:310–320.

Hillis D S 1917 Attachment for the stethoscope. JAMA 68:910.

Hökegård K H, Eriksson B O, Kjellemer I et al 1981 Myocardial metabolism in relation to electrocardiographic changes and cardiac function during graded hypoxia in the fetal lamb. Acta Physiol Scand 113:1–7.

Hon E H 1966 The human fetal circulation in normal labor. In: Cassels D E (ed.) The heart and circulation of the newborn and infant. Grune and Stratton, New York, pp. 37–52.

Hon E H, Lee S T 1963 The electronic evaluation of the fetal heart rate. VIII. Patterns preceding fetal death: further observations. Am J Obstet Gynecol 87:814–826.

Hon E H, Quilligan E J 1967 The classification of fetal heart rate. Conn Med 31:779.

Huch A, Huch R, Schneider H, Peabody J 1980 Experience with transcutaneous PO2 (tcPO2) monitoring of mother, fetus and newborn. J Perinat Med 8:51–72.

Irion O, Stuckelberger P, Moutquin J M et al 1996 Is intrapartum vibratory acoustic stimulation a valid alternative to fetal scalp pH determination? Br J Obstet Gynaecol 103:642–647.

Johnson M V 1993 Cellular alterations associated with perinatal asphyxia. Clin Invest Med 16–2:122–132.

Johnstone F D, Campbell D M, Hughes G J 1978 Antenatal care: has continuous intrapartum monitoring made any impact on fetal outcome? Lancet 1:1298–1300.

Kaplan S, Toyama S 1958 Fetal electrocardiography: Utilizing abdominal and intrauterine leads. Obstet Gynecol 11:391.

Keith R D F, Beckly S, Garibaldi J M et al 1995 A multicentre comparative study of 17 experts and an intelligent computer system for managing labour using the cardiotocogram. Br J Obstet Gynaecol 102(9):688–700.

Kelly V C, Kulkarni D 1973 Experiences with fetal monitoring in a community hospital. Obstet Gynecol 41:818–824.

Kelso I M, Parsons R J, Lawrence G F et al 1978 An assessment of continuous fetal heart rate monitoring in labor: a randomized trial. Am J Obstet Gynecol 131:526–532.

Kennedy E. Observations of obstetrical auscultation. Hodges and Smith, Dublin, 1833.

Kilian: quoted by Jaggard W W 1888 In: Hirst B C (ed.) A system of obstetrics. Lea Broth, Philadelphia.

Kirschbaum T H 1969 Editorial: Diagnosis of fetal distress. Obstet Gynecol 34:721–728.

Klauser C K, Christensen E E, Chauhan S P et al 2005 Use of fetal pulse oximetry among high-risk women in labor: A randomized clinical trial. Am J Obstet Gynecol 192:1810–1819.

Koh K S, Greves D, Yung S et al 1975 Experience with fetal monitoring in a university teaching hospital. Can Med Assoc J 112:455–462.

Krebs H B, Petres R E, Dunn L J et al 1979 Intrapartum fetal heart rate monitoring. 1. Classification and prognosis of fetal heart rate patterns. Am J Obstet Gynecol 133:762–772.

Kruger K, Hallberg B et al 1999 Predictive value of fetal scalp blood lactate concentration and pH markers of neurologic disability. Am J Obstet Gynecol 181:1072.

Kubli F W, Hon E H, Khazin A F, Takemura H 1969 Observations on heart rate and pH in the human fetus during labor. Am J Obstet Gynecol 104:1190–1206.

Kuhnert M, Seelbach-Goebel G, Butterwegge M 1998 Predictive agreement between the fetal arterial oxygen saturation and fetal scalp pH: results of the German multicenter study. Am J Obstet Gynecol 178(2):330–335.

Lauersen N H, Miller F C, Paul R H 1979 Continuous intrapartum monitoring of fetal scalp pH. Am J Obstet Gynecol 133:44–50.

Le Jumeau J A (de Kergaradec) 1822 Mémoire sur l'Auscultation appliquée à l'Etude de la Grossesse ou Recherches sur deux nouveaux signes propres à faire reconnaître plusieurs circonstances de l'Etat de Gestation, lu à l'Académie royale de médecine, dans sa séance générale du 26 décembre 1821, Paris.

Lee W K, Baggish M S 1976 The effect of unselected intrapartum fetal monitoring. Obstet Gynecol 47:516–520.

Leveno K J, Cunningham F G, Nelson S et al 1986 A prospective comparison of selective and universal electronic fetal monitoring in 34,995 pregnancies. N Engl J Med 315:615–619.

Lilienfeld A M, Parkhurst E 1951 Study of association of factors of pregnancy and parturition with development of cerebral palsy: preliminary report. Am J Hyg 53:262–270.

Lilienfeld A M, Pasamanick B P 1955 The association of maternal and fetal factors with the development of cerebral palsy and epilepsy. Am J Obstet Gynecol 70:93–101.

Lilja H, Karlsson K, Lindecrantz K, Rosén K G 1989 Microprocessor based waveform analysis of the fetal electrocardiogram during labor. Int J Gynecol Obstet 30:109–116.

Little W J 1862 On the influence of abnormal parturition, difficult labours, premature birth and asphyxia neonatorum, on the mental and physical condition of the child, especially in relation to deformities. Trans Obstet Soc London 3:293.

Low J A, Lindsay B G, Derrick E J 1997 Threshold of metabolic acidosis associated with newborn complications. Am J Obstetr Gynecol 177:1391–1394.

Luthy D A, Kirkwood K S, van Belle G et al 1987 A randomized trial of electronic fetal monitoring in preterm labor. Obstet Gynecol 69:687–695.

MacDonald D, Grant A 1987 Fetal surveillance in labour — the present position. In: Bonnar J (ed.) Recent advances in obstetrics and gynaecology, Vol. 15. Churchill Livingstone, London, pp. 83–100.

MacDonald D, Grant A, Sheridan-Pereira M et al 1985 The Dublin randomized controlled trial of intrapartum fetal heart rate monitoring. Am J Obstet Gynecol 152:524–539.

Martin C B 1982 Physiology and clinical use of fetal heart rate variability. Clin Perinatol 9:339–352.

Martin C B Jr, de Haan J, van der Wildt B et al 1979 Mechanisms of late decelerations in the fetal heart rate. A study with autonomic blocking agents in fetal lambs. Eur J Obsatet Gynecol Reprod Biol 9:361–373.

Martin J A, Hamilton B E, Sutton P D et al 2003 Births: final data for 2002. Natl Viatal Stat Rep 52:1–113.

Mayor H (1818) Biblioth Univ. de Genève, Nov 9, quoted by Thomas H 1935 Classical contributions to obstetrics and gynecology. Charles C Thomas, Springfield, Illinois.

Myers R E 1969 Fetal asphyxia and perinatal brain damage affecting human development. Publ No 185, Pan American Health Organization, Washington, pp. 205–214.

Myers R E 1972 Two patterns of perinatal brain damage and their conditions of occurrence. Am J Obstet Gynecol 122:246–276.

Neilson J P 2006 Fetal electrocardiogram (ECG) for fetal monitoring during labour. Cochrane Database of Systematic Reviews 2006, Issue 3. Art. No.: CD000116. DOI: 10.1002/14651858.CD000116.pub2.

Neldam S, Osler M, Hansen P K et al 1986 Intrapartum fetal heart rate monitoring in a combined low- and high-risk population: a controlled clinical trial. Eur J Obstet Gynecol Reprod Biol 23:1–11.

Nelson K B, Dambrosia J M, Ting T Y, Grether J K 1996 Uncertain value of electronic fetal monitoring in predicting cerebral palsy. N Engl J Med 334(10):613–618.

Nelson K B, Ellenberg J H 1978 Epidemiology of cerebral palsy. In: Schoenberg B S (ed.) Advances in neurology, Vol. 19. Raven Press, New York, pp. 421–435.

Nelson K B, Ellenberg J H 1985 Antecedents of cerebral palsy I. Univariate analysis of risks. Am J Dis Child 139:1031–1038.

Nelson K B, Ellenberg J H 1986 Antecedents of cerebral palsy: multivariate analysis of risk. N Engl J Med 315:81–86.

NIH (National Institutes of Health) on Causes of Mental Retardation and Cerebral Palsy 1985 Task force on joint assessment of prenatal and perinatal factors associated with brain disorders 1985. Pediatrics 76:457.

Nijland R, Jongsma H W, Nijhuis J G et al 1995 Arterial oxygen saturation in relation to metabolic acidosis in fetal lambs. Am J Obstet Gynecol 172:810–819.

Oeseburg B, Ringnalda B E M, Crevels J et al 1992 Fetal oxygenation in chronic maternal hypoxia: what's critical? Adv Exp Med Biol 317:499–502.

Okane M, Shigemitsu S, Inaba J et al 1989 Non-invasive continuous fetal transcutaneous pO_2 and pCO_2 monitoring during labor. J Perinat Med 17:399–410.

Paneth N 1993 The causes of cerebral palsy. Recent evidence. Clin Invest Med 16:95–102.

Paul R H, Huey J R, Yaeger C F 1977 Clinical fetal monitoring – its effect on cesarean section rate and perinatal mortality: five-year trends. Postgrad Med 61:160–164.

Paul R H, Suidan A K, Yeh S, Hon E H 1975 The evaluation and significance of intrapartum baseline FHR variability. Am J Obstet Gynecol 123:206–210.

Pello L C, Rosevear B M, Dawes G S et al 1991 Computerized fetal heart rate analysis in labor. Obstet Gynecol 78:602–610.

Pharoah P O D, Cooke T, Cooke R W I et al 1990 Birthweight specific trends in cerebral palsy. Arch Dis Child 65:602–606.

Philippeaux: Notice biographique et bibliographique sur Philippe Le Goust. Archives de tocologie des maladies des femmes, Paris 1879,6:304.

Ranck J B, Windle W F 1959 Brain damage in the monkey, Maccaca mulatta, by asphyxia neonatorum. Exp Neurol 1:130–154.

Renou P, Chang A, Anderson I, Wood C 1976 Controlled trial of fetal intensive care. Am J Obstet Gynecol 126:470–476.

Renou P, Wood C 1974 Interpretation of the continuous fetal heart rate record. Clin Obstet Gynaecol 1:191–215.

Riikonen R, Raumavirta S, Sinivuori E et al 1989 Changing pattern of cerebral palsy in the south-west region of Finland. Acta Paed Scant 78:581–587.

Rosén K G, Dagbjartsson A, Henriksson B A et al 1984 The relationship between circulating catecholamine and ST waveform in the fetal lamb electrocardiogram during hypoxia. Am J Obstet Gynecol 149:190–195.

Schmidt S, Langner K, Dudenhausen J W, Saling E 1985 Measurement of transcutaneous pCO_2 and pO_2 in the fetus during labor. Arch Gynecol 236:145–151.

Schreiber F 1938 Apnea of the newborn and associated cerebral injury: a clinical and statistical study. JAMA 111:1263.

Schwartz H 1870 Arch Gynaekol 1:361.

Schwartz H. Die vorzeitgen Athembewegungen. Leipzig 1838.

Seelbach-Gobel B, Butterwegge M, Kuhnert M, Heupel M 1994 Fetal reflectance pulse oximetry sub partu. Experiences — prognostic significance and consequences — goals. Zeitschr Geburtshilfe Perinatol 198:67–71.

Seitz L 1903 Die fetalen Herztöne unter der Geburt. Habil-Schrift, Munchen.

Shelley T, Tipton R H 1971 Dip Area: A quantitative measure of fetal heart rate patterns. J Obstet Gynecol Br Commonw 78:694–701.

Shenker L, Post R C, Seiler J S 1975 Routine electronic monitoring of fetal heart rate and uterine activity during labor. Obstet Gynecol 46:185–189.

Small M L, Beall M, Platt L D et al 1989 Continuous tissue pH monitoring in the term fetus. Am J Obstet Gynecol 161(2):323–329.

Smith C V, Nquyen H N, Phelan J P, Paul R H 1986. Intrapartum assessment of fetal well-being: A comparison of fetal acoustic stimulation with acid-base determinations. Am J Obstet Gynecol 155:726–728.

Smyth C N 1953 Experimental electrocardiography of the foetus. Lancet 2:1124–1126.

Spencer J A 1991 Predictive value of a fetal heart rate acceleration at the time of fetal blood sampling in labour. J Perinat Med 19(3):207–215.

Stamm O, Latscha U, Janecek P, Campana A 1976 Development of a special electrode for continuous subcutaneous pH measurement in the infant scalp. Am J Obstet Gynecol 124:193–195.

Stanley F 1992 Survival and cerebral palsy in low birthweight infants, implications for perinatal care. Paed Perinat Epidemiol 6:298–310.

Stanley F J, Blair E 1991 Why have we failed to reduce the frequency of cerebral palsy? Med J Aust 154:623.

Steer C W, Bonney W 1962 Obstetric factors in cerebral palsy. Am J Obstet Gynecol 83:526–531.

Strachan B K, van Wijngaarden W J et al 2000 Cardiotocography only verus cardiotocography plus PR-interval analysis in intrapartum surveillance: a randomized, multicentre trial. Lancet 355:456–459.

Sturbois G, Uzan S, Rotten D et al 1977 Continuous subcutaneous pH measurement in human fetuses: correlations with scalp and umbilical blood pH. Am J Obstet Gynecol 128:901–903.

Sureau C L 1956 Recherches electrocardiographiques foetal au cours de la gestation et du travail: premiers resultat d'une nouvelle technique d'enregistrement par electrodes endouterines. Gynecol Obstet 55:21.

Takesita K, Ando Y, Ohtani K et al 1989 Cerebral palsy in Tottori, Japan. Neuroepidemiol 8:184–192.

Tejani N, Mann L, Bhakthavathsalan A et al 1975 Correlation of fetal heart rate–uterine contraction patterns and fetal scalp blood pH. Obstet Gynecol 46:392–396.

Thacker S B, Stroup D F 1999 Continuous electronic heart rate monitoring versus intermittent auscultation for assessmend during labor. Cochrane Review. In: The Cochrane Library, 3. Oxford: Update Software.

Tutera G, Newman R L 1975 Fetal monitoring: its effect on the perinatal mortality and caesarean section rates and its complications. Am J Obstet Gynecol 122:750–754.

Vintzileos A M, Antsaklis A, Varvarigos I et al 1993 A randomized trial of intrapartum electronic fetal heart rate monitoring versus intermittent auscultation. Obstet Gynecol 81:899–907.

Vintzileos A M, Nochimson D J, Antsaklis A et al 1995 Comparison of intrapartum electronic fetal heart rate monitoring versus intermittent ausculatation in detecting fetal acidemia at birth. Am J Obstet Gynecol 173:1021–1024.

Vintzileos A M, Nochimson D J, Guzman E R et al 1995 Intrapartum electronic fetal heart rate monitoring versus intermittent auscultation: a meta-analysis. Obstet Gynecol 85:149–155.

Webster's Ninth New Collegiate Dictionary 1985 Merriam-Webster, Springfield Massachusetts.

Westgate J, Harris M, Curnow J S, Greene K R 1993 Plymouth randomized trial of cardiotocogram only versus ST waveform plus cardiotogram for intrapartum monitoring in 2400 cases. Am J Obstet Gynecol 169:1151–1160.

Widmark C, Jansson T, Lindecrantz K, Rosén KG 1991 ECG waveform, short term heart rate variability and plasma catecholamine concentrations in response to hypoxia in intrauterine growth retarded guinea pig fetuses. J Dev Physiol 15:161–168.

Willcourt R, Queenan J T 1981 Fetal scalp blood sampling and transcutaneous pO_2. Clin Perinatol 8:87–99.

Williams R L, Hawes W E 1979 Cesarean section, fetal monitoring and perinatal mortality in California. Am J Public Health 69:864.

Winckel F 1893 Lehrbuch der Geburtshilfe. Veit, Leipzig.

Windle W F, Becker R F 1943 Asphyxia neonatorum: An experimental study in the guinea pig. Am J Obstet Gynecol 45:183–199.

Wood C, Renou P, Oats J et al 1981 A controlled trial of fetal heart rate monitoring in a low-risk obstetric population. Am J Obstet Gynecol 141:527–534.

Prediction of asphyxia with fetal gas analysis

Medhat Alberry, Sergio de la Fuente and Peter W. Soothill

Key Points

- The terms asphyxia, hypoxemia, acidosis and acidemia are often used in a confusing and sometimes interchangeable way, which leads to confusion and misunderstanding
- Asphyxia is defined as a condition of impaired gas exchange, which if persistent, will lead to progressive hypoxemia and hypercapnia — about 2% of neonates are born with the condition
- The effect of asphyxia on the individual neonate is variable and difficult to predict. Outcome depends on the severity of the asphyxia, its duration, the gestational age at which it occurred and the mechanisms that led to its development
- It is important to distinguish between acute (hours) and chronic (weeks) asphyxia as the mechanisms and effects are different
- Less than 20% of cerebral palsy may be the result of events which occur in labor or delivery
- Fetal scalp blood sampling remains the standard technique to assess acid/base status in labor although other techniques, such as pulse oximetry, are being evaluated as direct estimates of oxygen status
- It is important to apply the criteria that aid in the diagnosis of cerebral palsy (CP) secondary to acute intrapartum asphyxia which will help identify the cases where the pathophysiology of brain injury may be prevented or arrested

---

INTRODUCTION

'Asphyxia' originates from the Greek word for 'pulse-less,' which we equate to 'death,' and so in our view, the general usage of this term is so poorly defined as to be useless. It is used to mean a sick baby at birth, which, for many years, has been recognized as being associated with long-term neurological lesions in infants (Little 1862). Major recent advances in obstetric and neonatal care have led to greater expectations by doctors and patients for excellent pregnancy, delivery and newborn outcomes. Perinatal mortality has fallen so substantially that reducing preventable neurological handicap has now become the priority; consequently, death is no longer an adequate end-point with which to assess obstetric care.

Despite the widely recognized association between poor condition at birth and long-term damage, the diagnosis of asphyxia has been confused not only because of the lack of an adequate definition but also because there is no simple direct linear relationship between the severity of asphyxia and the amount of damage that results. Further confounding factors include the duration and frequency of the asphyxial events and the gestational age at which they occur. Moreover, animal studies, which have attempted to describe the effects of 'chronic asphyxia,' have tended to study hypoxia

over several hours rather than the more clinically relevant time period, which is weeks. Finally, the inevitable lack of experimental studies in humans has led to notorious differences of opinion in interpreting the relationship between cause, timing, chronicity and effect of asphyxia on one hand and neurological handicaps on the other.

The complexity described above is reflected in the consensus reached for the clinical definition of fetal asphyxia. This requires three criteria to be met: a lack of oxygen in the blood, an abnormal acid–base status and a pathophysiological effect on the neonate. By these criteria, at least 2% of all neonates experience asphyxia during labor and delivery and some of them are damaged as a result (Low 1997). However, in many of these cases, the damage will have occurred before the labor started (e.g. as a result of chronic placental dysfunction) and it has become increasingly clear that this has often been under-recognized due to the difficulty in obtaining objective criteria of measurement.

In this chapter, we will review the methods of assessing fetal blood gases and acid–base status and evaluate them as predictors of 'asphyxia,' whilst clearly distinguishing between acute and chronic disease. Moreover, we will focus on cerebral palsy, particularly the proportion of cases attributed to acute birth asphyxia in children born at term.

DEFINITIONS

HYPOXIA, ACIDOSIS, ASPHYXIA AND HYPOXIC–ISCHEMIC ENCEPHALOPATHY

The World Federation of Neurology Group defined asphyxia as 'a condition of impaired gas exchange leading, if it persists, to progressive hypoxemia and hypercapnia' (Bax & Nelson 1993). Significant hypoxemia in the fetus is usually followed by metabolic acidosis, so some authors feel that any definition must also include this aspect to meet the pathophysiological process (Low 1997). For the word asphyxia to have any meaning other than hypoxia and/or acidosis, the reader should consider its links to clinical consequences, and so in addition to blood gas and acid–base balance analysis, pathological effects shortly after birth may be considered. Central nervous system, cardiac, respiratory and renal complications are usually associated with severe asphyxia and can be readily identified. The neurological features are often described as hypoxic–ischemic encephalopathy (HIE) which is a common disease of the newborn and has traditionally been considered to have a strong association with chronic disability in childhood (Sarnat & Sarnat

1976). However, this has been challenged by several studies in the 1980s and 1990s. In neonatal medicine, this term has come to replace the diagnosis of birth asphyxia.

Although HIE is helpful in neonatal medicine, because it includes postnatal information, the term cannot be used prospectively in fetal medicine, and the word 'asphyxia' is often taken to be synonymous with fetal hypoxia and/or acidosis (Soothill et al 1989). However, these measurements should be interpreted only as a very rough identifier of a group at high risk for asphyxia at birth rather than being diagnostic.

PO_2 and PCO_2 are terms that refer to the partial pressure of a gas. They can be defined as the tension required to maintain the same amount of a gas dissolved in the water phase of plasma, which, under normal conditions, is not greater than 2% of the total oxygen contained in the blood.

Hypoxemia means a decreased oxygen content in blood and can be produced either because of reduced PO_2 or reduced hemoglobin concentration (Soothill et al 1989). Hypoxia refers to reduced use of oxygen by the tissues. This can be caused either by impaired supply from hypoxemia, impaired blood flow or reduced uptake of oxygen by the tissues (e.g. metabolism failure from cyanide poisoning). A low PO_2 should be defined as a partial pressure of oxygen more than 2 standard deviations (2 SD) below the normal mean for gestational age in the blood, and before labor, this measurement is relatively simple to define, because gestational age-dependent charts are available (Nicolaides et al 1989, Soothill et al 1986). After the onset of delivery, it is not always clear what range should apply because the 'normal' values are changed by the duration of labor, the use of anesthetics and the mode of delivery.

Acidosis refers to a high hydrogen ion concentration in the tissues. While fetal tissue pH is relatively stable, its measurement is not realistically possible. Acidemia refers to a high H^+ ion concentration in the blood, which can be easily measured, and it usually reflects the levels in the tissues. In adults, acidemia is defined as a pH of 7.35 or less in arterial blood. In the fetus, the cut-off values to define acidemia are less clear and are dependent on the site of blood sampling. Traditionally, the definition was a pH of less than 7.20 for fetal scalp blood or 2 SDs below the mean (pH 7.10–7.18) in the umbilical artery after delivery (Gilstrap 1998). However, this approach is still not clear because to produce complications in the newborn, in the absence of other problems such as trauma or sepsis, umbilical arterial acidosis must be more severe. The American College of Obstetricians and Gynecologists has recommended considering a pH less than 7.00 as pathological or severely acidemic in the umbilical artery at birth. pH values less than 6.61 in the umbilical arterial blood have been described as probably incompatible with life (Belai et al 1998). Before delivery, interpretation is simpler because normal reference ranges for fetal gases have been established throughout the pregnancy by cordocentesis (Nicolaides et al 1989).

NORMAL OXYGEN DELIVERY TO THE FETUS

OXYGEN CARRIAGE IN THE BLOOD

As shown in Figure 25.1, gases are transported from the mother to the fetus and vice versa by a double circulatory system through the placenta. Oxygen diffuses down a decreasing gradient of partial pressure from air in the lungs (PO_2 150 mm Hg), pulmonary capillary vessels (105 mm Hg), arterial blood (95 mm Hg), placental vessels (30–40 mm Hg), umbilical venous fetal blood (20–30 mm Hg) to finally equilibrate PO_2 with the fetal tissues at a PO_2 of around 10–20 mm Hg in a term fetus (Towell 1976).

Despite the low PO_2 levels, fetal blood has a high oxygen content due to both the high affinity of fetal hemoglobin and its high concentration; the latter increases in a linear fashion from the second trimester throughout pregnancy (Nicolaides et al 1988b). Not only is the blood oxygen content quite high, but normally the organs, especially the heart and brain, are well perfused because of the high fetal cardiac output. Indeed, when under stress, there are physiological compensatory mechanisms including blood redistribution and a further increase in fetal oxygen extraction (see below). For all of these reasons, oxygen delivery to some organs per gram of tissue is actually greater in the fetus than to the same organ in the adult.

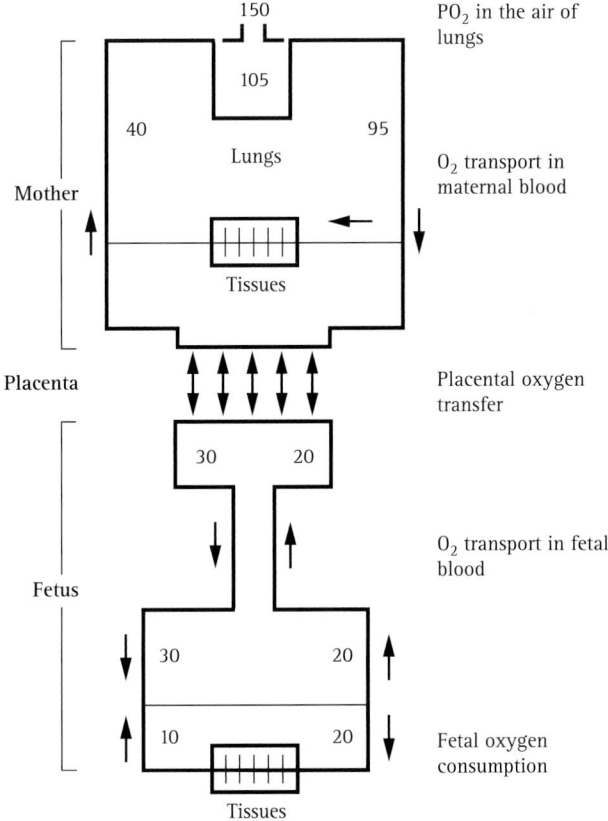

Figure 25.1 Oxygen gradient between the maternal lungs and the fetal tissues. (Modified from Towell 1976.)

The flow of oxygen to the tissues is known as oxygen delivery, which is the product of the volume of blood flow to a tissue and its oxygen content. The latter is dependent on the hemoglobin concentration and oxygen saturation. The ability of hemoglobin to carry oxygen varies in different physiological conditions and is affected by the hemoglobin oxygen affinity. This property correlates the amount of oxygen bound to hemoglobin for a given PO_2 in a sigmoid curve known as the hemoglobin dissociation curve (Fig. 25.2). The oxygen saturation is the percentage of hemoglobin that is oxygenated and accounts for about 98% of the total oxygen in blood. The affinity for oxygen is dependent on the type of hemoglobin and fetal hemoglobin has a greater affinity for oxygen than the adult type, so its curve is shifted to the left. This means that at the same PO_2, fetal hemoglobin will be more saturated than adult. This is described by the $P50$, which is the partial pressure of oxygen at which the hemoglobin is 50% saturated; for fetal hemoglobin, this level is 21 mm Hg, whereas for the adult, it is 27 mm Hg. Due to this property, at the levels of PO_2 in the fetus, 13 mL of oxygen are carried by 100 mL of blood. This is very similar to the 15 mL per 100 mL carried by the maternal blood, and so the fetus is not hypoxemic despite the lower PO_2 (Willcourt 1987). It is therefore not surprising that the saturation of fetal hemoglobin is on average about 60% in the umbilical vein at term (Bozzetti et al 1987, McNamara et al 1992, Richardson et al 1998).

In the fetus, the hemoglobin dissociation curve can be affected by pH and perhaps temperature. By increasing temperature or decreasing pH the hemoglobin molecule becomes less bound to oxygen, and the dissociation curve is shifted to the right. 2,3-Diphosphoglycerate (2,3-DPG), a product of glycolysis, causes a right shift of the adult dissociation curve, but it has little effect with fetal hemoglobin (Soothill et al 1988).

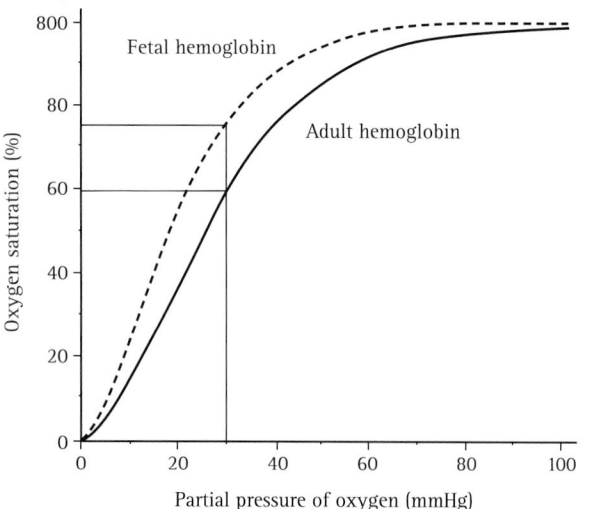

Figure 25.2 PO_2 dissociation curve of adult and fetal hemoglobin.

At term, the uterine blood flow is 1200 mL/min with a PO_2 of about 95 mm Hg. It leaves the uterine veins with a PO_2 of about 40 mm Hg, and this difference is due to fetal, uterine and placental oxygen extraction. Fetal oxygen extraction is the ratio between fetal oxygen consumption and oxygen delivery, and it also can be expressed in mathematical terms as:

$$\text{Oxygen extraction} = (CvO_2 - CaO_2)/CvO_2,$$

where Cv and Ca represent the venous and arterial oxygen content, respectively.

Using cord blood gases from normal vaginal deliveries and cesarean sections (CS) at term, Rurak estimated that, at a fetal umbilical artery PaO_2 of 20 mm Hg, the human fetus extracts about 47% of the available oxygen (Rurak et al 1987). Because the umbilical artery flow, estimated from Doppler studies, is about 120 mL/min/kg fetus (Gill et al 1984) and the venous–arterial oxygen difference is 6–7 vol/100 mL, it has been calculated that the fetus consumes at term roughly 20–30 mL of oxygen per minute. This changes during the pregnancy, and the umbilical arterial PO_2 falls significantly with gestational age (Soothill et al 1986), suggesting an increased fractional oxygen extraction in the human fetus as the gestation progresses (Richardson et al 1998). Oxygen extraction has been found to be increased under some conditions where oxygen delivery is reduced, such as cord compression or CS after labor (Richardson et al 1998).

CIRCULATION

When the oxygenated blood comes back to the fetus from the placenta through the umbilical vein, it enters the fetal liver where it joins the umbilical segment of the left portal vein (Callen 1994). This vessel, before reaching the main portal stem, divides into small branches supplying the hepatic parenchyma and a thin muscular vein, the ductus venosus. The majority of blood goes through the liver to the inferior vena cava, but a proportion (which can vary) will bypass this organ through the ductus. Color Doppler studies have shown two streams, the left and the right, and these have been seen to extend into the inferior vena cava before the right atrium (Kiserud et al 1992). The right stream carries the less oxygenated blood from the liver and the inferior part of the body to the right atrium and ventricle. The left pathway transports the more oxygenated blood directly from the placenta through the ductus venosus to the left atrium. This differential flow is facilitated by the eustachian valve and septum primum, which conduct the blood through the foramen ovale to the left chambers.

From the left ventricle, the blood goes to the aortic arch and through the neck vessels to the brain. Soon after the division of the vessels to the head and neck, the aortic arch joins the ductus arteriosus, which shunts blood from the pulmonary artery into the aorta, and so a mixture of oxygenated and deoxygenated blood is distributed to the rest of the fetal body. Finally the umbilical arteries, which arise from the internal iliac arteries, reach the placenta and complete the circulatory cycle.

NORMAL GAS EXCHANGE ACROSS THE PLACENTA — DIFFUSION VS. PERFUSION LIMITATION

Fetal vessels in the placenta are distributed into 15–20 cotyledons. Here, the vessels divide to form the villous tree, which is bathed by maternal blood in the intervillous space. The human placenta is consequently classified as the hemochorial type and feto-maternal exchange occurs across the syncytial-vascular membrane in an area that varies from 4 to 14 m^2 (Sadler 1995). Comparing the placenta with the lung, it appears to be a less efficient organ, because despite their similar weight, the oxygen transfer rate at term is about 24 mL of oxygen per minute, which is about 10–20 times less than the oxygen exchanged by the lungs (Longo 1981).

The circulation of the fetal blood in the villi permits the exchange of gases by diffusion, favored by the high partial pressure gradients between the maternal and fetal blood flow. The exchange is restricted by diffusion of the molecules across the membrane but also by the blood flow in both fetal and maternal compartments (Longo 1981). In other words, if the blood flow is slow enough, and if the membrane is sufficiently permeable to O_2, maternal and fetal blood could exit the exchanger with similar pO$_2$ values.

FETAL RESPIRATION

Normal respiration in fetal cells requires oxygen and glucose to produce energy. Glucose is transformed into pyruvate in the cytoplasm from where it enters into the mitochondria and is metabolized by the Krebs cycle. As a consequence, carbon dioxide and high-energy electrons are produced, which are carried by NADH and FADH$_2$ into a complex system of electron carriers in the mitochondrial inner membrane (respiratory chain). Here, they combine with molecular oxygen to produce water in a series of redox reactions that lead to a net production of 36 molecules of ATP at the end of the cycle.

IMPAIRED OXYGEN DELIVERY TO THE FETUS

Under conditions of abnormally low oxygen levels, the process of metabolizing glucose occurs in a less efficient way than when there is sufficient oxygen. Pyruvate cannot enter the Krebs cycle to be oxidized but is instead transformed into lactate by accepting H$^+$ from NADH. The overall net energy production of the process is only two molecules of ATP compared with 36 released by the aerobic pathway. With anaerobic respiration, the fetal cells can continue to work for a while but at the expense of increasing the H$^+$ ion concentration in the cytoplasm and subsequently in the blood. When the oxygen supply is restored, the accumulated lactate is converted back to pyruvate and NADH hydrogen is transferred to the flavoprotein cytochrome chain.

When placental gas exchange is significantly impaired (at any step of the oxygen transport pathway) and the compensatory mechanisms have become insufficient, the fetus develops hypoxemia. Also, progressive hypercapnia will occur, and so respiratory acidosis will be developed. This is reflected in an umbilical artery PCO_2 of 75 mm Hg or more at birth (Low 1994) with a correspondingly low pH. Such a respiratory acidosis can occur in a variety of clinical conditions, such as in a sudden decrease of placental or umbilical perfusion or maternal hypoventilation. If the situation persists, anaerobic metabolism will eventually lead to metabolic acidosis where base will be consumed (buffer base <30 mmol/L); the umbilical artery base deficit may fall to as low as 12–16 mmol/L and the pH will decrease.

By strict definition, respiratory acidosis occurs when there is an increased PCO_2 with a low pH but a normal bicarbonate (HCO_3^-) and metabolic acidosis is a low pH with a normal PCO_2 but decreased HCO_3^-. Mixed acidosis is when there is an increased PCO_2 as well as a decreased HCO_3. In severe respiratory acidosis, HCO_3^- will be increased by 1 mEq/L for each 10 mm Hg increased PCO_2, but it is important to realize that HCO_3 is not measured in blood by most blood gas machines but calculated from the PCO_2 and pH measurements.

Chronic fetal hypoxemia from placental dysfunction leads to hypoxia, hypercapnia, hyperlacticemia and acidosis, and so mixed respiratory and metabolic acidosis (Nicolaides et al 1989). Such a mixed chronic acidemia in small for gestational age (SGA) fetuses has been shown to be associated with somewhat reduced subsequent neurodevelopment (Soothill et al 1995). In contrast, a short-term, acute, mixed acidosis can be severe, and no abnormal outcome would be expected, as long as the fetus was well before this event. It can show a high degree of tolerance to such hypoxic events through physiological compensatory mechanisms. These factors make the distinction between respiratory and metabolic acidosis no longer useful, and the terms chronic or acute acidosis are preferred (Bobrow & Soothill 1999).

In studies by cordocentesis in normal pregnancies, the umbilical vein lactate concentration was higher than in the artery towards the end of pregnancy, suggesting that the normoxemic human fetus consumes lactate of placental origin (Soothill et al 1986). In anemic human fetuses, it has been possible to study the arteriovenous lactate difference, and it has been shown that the placenta clears lactate from the fetal circulation as a result of transfer to the mother or metabolism. As shown in Figure 25.3, the placental capacity to clear lactate is exceeded when anemia is severe, and as a consequence, the lactate venous concentration rises (Soothill et al 1987c) (see below). Also, in hypoxic SGA fetuses, lactic acid is increased (Soothill et al 1987a), probably due to reduced oxidative metabolism, and here, the origin of lactate seems to be fetal (Nicolaides et al 1989). Therefore, it has been suggested that the placenta can repay a fetal oxygen debt, which is analogous to the liver repaying such a deficiency for the muscles in the heavily exercising adults.

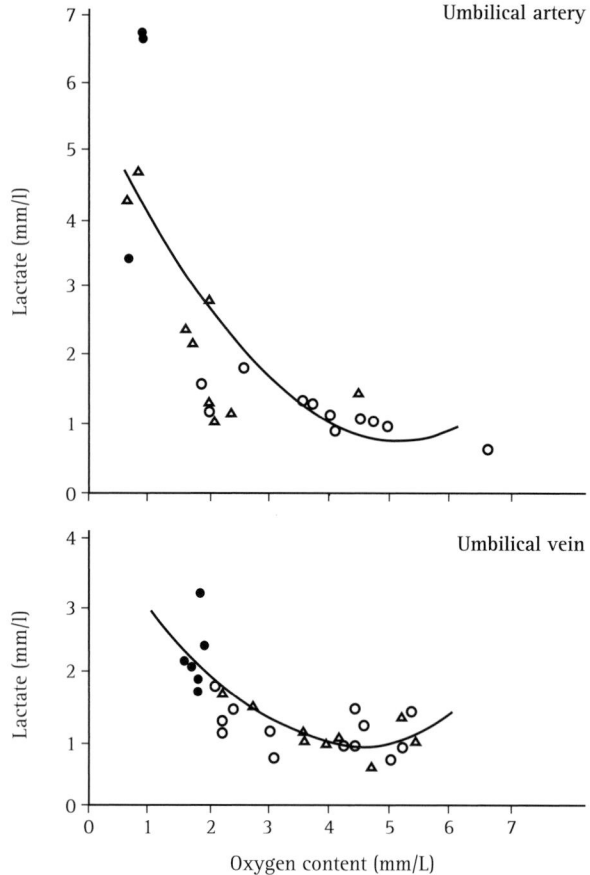

Figure 25.3 Relationship between fetal plasma lactate concentration to blood oxygen content in 32 rhesus-affected pregnancies. (Adapted from Soothill et al 1987a.) Open circles indicate the values before transfusion, open triangles indicate the values from subsequent transfusions, and solid circles indicate values from hydropic fetuses.

ASPHYXIA

The predictive value of cord blood acidemia at birth for poor subsequent neonatal outcome, particularly brain damage, is very weak (Fee et al 1990, Ruth & Raivio 1988). Although this may be partly explained by variation between individuals, it is clear that the mechanism leading to asphyxia, the gestational age at which it occurred as well as its severity and duration are all important elements when determining the predictive value of blood gases for prognosis. Furthermore, not only is the prediction of damage in a population weak, but the severity of damage in an individual patient depends on many other factors, such as the previous metabolic and cardiovascular states, the presence of predisposing factors antenatally and the repetition or pattern of any previous hypoxic insults.

Asphyxial events, either 'acute' or 'chronic,' can have different causes, characteristics and consequences. Therefore, the way to distinguish acute from chronic is not only based on duration, and a time cut-off, but also the nature

of the disease and its cause. However, in general events lasting hours are classified as acute and those acting over weeks, chronic (Bobrow & Soothill et al 1999). This fundamental distinction has not been adequately appreciated in the past, especially when counseling the parents of children asphyxiated at birth, and so these different groups are described separately in the rest of this section.

ACUTE ASPHYXIA

Pathophysiology (see also Ch. 22)

Acute asphyxia is usually followed by a number of changes in the fetal circulation mediated by the autonomic nervous system (Jensen & Lang 1992). The initial response is an increase in the systemic blood pressure due to a rapid and profound vasoconstriction and consequently a decrease in the blood flow to peripheral organs (Jensen et al 1987). Although the total umbilical blood flow is maintained, in hypoxia, the proportion of blood passing through the ductus venosus to the inferior vena cava is increased, thereby reducing the oxygen delivery to the liver (Paulick et al 1990, Rudolph 1983).

A redistribution process tends to facilitate delivery of the most oxygenated blood to the heart, brain and adrenal glands at the expense of the lungs, kidneys, gastrointestinal tract and carcass (Ball et al 1994a, 1994b, Bocking et al 1988, Peeters et al 1979). Blood flow to the heart and brain is maintained overall, but redistribution occurs within the brain, favoring the brainstem at the expense of cerebrum and choroid plexuses. Also, a good blood supply to the adrenals seems to be vital for fetal sheep survival, and vasodilatation leads to almost a doubling of oxygen delivery in hypoxia (Jensen et al 1987). The redistribution responses do not occur in medically sympathectomized fetal sheep (Jensen & Lang 1992), and so seem to be mediated by a chemoreflex (Jensen & Hanson 1995) and possibly modulated by endogenous opioids (Espinoza et al 1989).

During acute hypoxia, cerebral and myocardial oxidative metabolism is maintained due to an increased blood flow, increased cerebral oxygen extraction and decreased myocardial work (Low et al 1994, Richardson 1989). Fetal oxygen consumption is maintained by increased oxygen extraction when fetal oxygen delivery is mildly or moderately reduced for as long as 24 hours. With a more severe episode of hypoxia, where oxygen delivery is reduced to over 50%, these mechanisms become inefficient and decompensation occurs. The fetus develops severe metabolic acidosis, hypotension and variable degrees of damage influenced by individual levels of tolerance (Ball et al 1994a).

Causes

Oxygen delivery to the uterus can be acutely affected by many conditions that result in maternal hypotension, impairment of utero-placental blood supply, placental abruption or obstruction of umbilical blood flow. Very severe maternal hypotension can be caused by many conditions such as massive maternal hemorrhage, an exaggerated response to hypotensive drugs or after epidural anesthesia. The latter can occur due to the loss of sympathetic tone in the legs, which leads to vasodilatation when epidural or spinal anesthesia is undertaken without adequate intra-vascular volume preload. Hypertonic uterine contractions can cause a reduction of the maternal blood supply due to a high intrauterine pressure and high tension in the uterine wall, which is crossed by branches of the uterine artery to reach the placenta. Placental abruption occurs when the placenta is partly or completely detached from the uterine wall, so losing part or the entire gas exchange surface. This is usually a sudden phenomenon, which occurs more frequently in some obstetric conditions such as pre-eclampsia. Finally, cord compression can also interrupt fetal gas exchange. This can be intermittent with uterine contractions in labor, when the umbilical cord is around the neck or in oligohydramnios, but also sustained as seen in true knots or cord prolapse.

Diagnosis with blood gases

The blood gas and acid–base state have been used to assess fetal wellbeing during labor or following birth. The American College of Obstetricians and Gynecologists has stated that a plausible link between perinatal asphyxia and a subsequent neurological deficit cannot be made unless the umbilical artery pH is less than 7.00, accompanied by both a significant metabolic component as well as an abnormal clinical newborn course (ACOG 1992). The latter refers to persistently low Apgar scores (e.g. 0–3 for longer than 5 min), signs of newborn encephalopathy and other organ compromises such as in the cardiovascular, respiratory and renal systems.

Due to the heterogeneity of factors related to the nature and severity of the exposure to asphyxia, it is still not possible to predict the occurrence or extent of damage in an individual fetus (Parer 1998). As mentioned above, acidosis does not predict neurologic dysfunction (Fee et al 1990, Ruth & Raivio 1988), and also a very wide range of acid–base values are found in babies with a normal condition, as indicated by Apgar scores (Helwig et al 1996). However data suggest that the metabolic component of fetal acidemia (i.e. base deficit and bicarbonate) is the most important variable in subsequent neonatal morbidity. On the other hand the umbilical artery PO_2 has no apparent clinical utility (Andres et al 1999).

At present, the long-term outcome is better predicted by classifying the severity of the intrapartum asphyxia combined with consideration of the short-term neonatal events rather than blood gases alone (Low 1997). Although it is not possible to predict asphyxia at birth or its future consequences with fetal blood gases only, normal results may help to exclude intrapartum hypoxia as a cause of brain damage (Winkler et al 1991). However, it has to be considered that a fetus could have been damaged by an earlier acute asphyxial event that was corrected before labor started such that the blood gases at delivery would not necessarily be abnormal. In the same way, gas analysis can be affected by

attempting to improve the condition of an asphyxiated fetus during labor with the use of maternal oxygen therapy or tocolysis (Burke et al 1989, McNamara et al 1993, Tejani et al 1983).

Scalp blood gases

Cardiotocography (CTG) is a good tool for detecting fetal acidosis, but the specificity of a non-reassuring test is poor, giving an unacceptably high false positive rate. One study reported a 99.8% false positive rate in a group of 155 636 children over 2500 g and estimated that according to CTG criteria, 2324 non-beneficial CS would have been done to avoid one child with cerebral palsy (Nelson et al 1996).

Intrapartum scalp blood samples to improve fetal assessment in the presence of ominous CTG patterns have been effective in reducing the increased intervention rate (Ayromlooi & Garfinkel 1980, Katz et al 1981, Young et al 1980, Zalar & Quilligan 1979), but the technique is only possible after cervical dilatation and rupture of the membranes. After a small incision in the scalp, a capillary blood sample can be obtained for testing. It provides only a single 'snapshot' of fetal acid–base status and so gives no information about the previous fetal condition or the trend of change. There are some devices for continuous tissue pH measurement (Small et al 1989), but more recently, the trend has been to replace these with non-invasive techniques. A scalp blood pH between 7.24 and 7.20 is considered borderline and less than 7.2 as acidotic (Bretscher & Saling 1967). It is important to keep in mind that scalp blood pH may be influenced by the maternal acid–base status and perhaps caput succedaneum (O'Connor et al 1979).

Although scalp sampling has been very useful for many years, there are some concerns about the technique. It is relatively invasive and so could increase the transmission rate of infectious diseases such as HIV. The necessity of repeated sampling and the technical difficulties involved in obtaining adequate samples can be a problem. The equipment used is relatively expensive and may be required infrequently. Also, the poor correlation between pH and predictable neurologic consequences in the child has led some to rely on fetal heart rate monitoring and propose that scalp pH sampling should be removed from standards of care (Perkins 1997).

Optical spectroscopy

In the last few years, there has been a trend towards non-invasive devices to continuously monitor fetal oxygenation, especially of the brain. Optical spectroscopy is a technique that estimates blood oxygen saturation based on the different absorption properties of oxyhemoglobin and deoxyhemoglobin to red and near infrared light (Benaron et al 1995). This wavelength can penetrate through the fetal skull and brain, from where it is scattered in a constant way. Differences detected in diffused or transmitted light intensity can be attributed to the different absorption coefficient of oxygenated to deoxygenated hemoglobin (Benaron et al 1995, Kurth et al 1993). There are two optical spectroscopy-based techniques to monitor fetal hemoglobin oxygen saturation in labor, cerebral optical spectroscopy and fetal pulse oximetry. Cerebral optical spectroscopy uses a transmission device, with light-emitting diodes and a photo-detector positioned on opposite sides of the vascular bed. This allows the measurement of light absorption of the entire cerebral vascular bed, which is mainly venous blood (Wahr et al 1996).

Pulse oximetry was introduced to medicine in the late 1970s, and thereafter, it has been used in several medical disciplines such as anesthetics, adult and neonatal intensive care. It uses a reflectance system, where the light-emitting diode and photo-detector are positioned adjacent to one another, on the same skin surface, with a pulsed signal to detect changes in the pulsatile arterial bed. A recent validation of the technique in human fetuses has included comparisons with umbilical vein oxygen saturation and cord blood pH at birth (McNamara et al 1992). An oxygen saturation of less than 30% is a useful threshold to define a risk of fetal acidosis (Carbonne et al 1997, East et al 1997, Goffinet et al 1997, Kuhnert et al 1993), but acidosis follows only when a low oxygen saturation is maintained for long periods. In one study of 400 labors, the fetal pH fell by 0.02 pH units/10 min, while the fetal saturation was less than or equal to 30%. Acidosis was never found when the saturation was under 30% for less than 10 min in a previously non-acidemic fetus (Seelbach-Gobel et al 1999).

Currently, the optical devices are being used in association with CTG and fetal scalp blood analysis, but in view of the problems with both mentioned above, the role of the non-invasive oximetry techniques may increase in the future. Randomized trials comparing CTG and fetal scalp sampling with CTG and pulse oximetry are being considered, but to the knowledge of the authors, none has been reported at the time of writing. However, several randomized controlled trials evaluating CTG and pulse oximetry versus CTG alone have reported that the addition of fetal pulse oximetry in fetal wellbeing assessment during labor resulted in a statistically significant reduction in the operative intervention for non-reassuring fetal status, compared with the use of conventional CTG monitoring alone. However, there was no significant difference in the overall operative delivery rates or neonatal outcomes (East et al 2006, Garite et al 2000).

Cord blood gases

Blood samples can be easily obtained from the umbilical artery and vein after delivery from a section of the cord clamped before the neonate takes a first breath. This is a very useful technique to assess retrospectively the condition of the fetus, and its results can give a valuable guide to immediate neonatal care. Cord blood gases have helped us to understand many aspects of the pathophysiology and incidence of asphyxia at birth and to evaluate both our management of labor and the efficacy of new methods of fetal assessment (Gordon & Johnson 1985). However, unless acidemia is severe its correlation with neurologic dysfunction is quite poor (see above).

Attempts to improve the prediction of asphyxia include determination of the origin of acidosis (maternal or fetal) to distinguish between respiratory and metabolic acidosis (Goodwin et al 1992, Ingemarsson & Arulkumaran 1986, Low et al 1994) and to assess differences in arteriovenous pH, PCO_2 and PO_2 (Belai et al 1998, Westgate et al 1994). Since the duration of the insult is usually not known, Low has theorized that the umbilical arterio-venous buffer base difference may help, because it varies inversely with the duration of the acute asphyxia (<6 mmol/L indicating long-term and >6 mmol/L short-term). A small arterial-venous difference is also expected in placental dysfunction (Low et al 1994).

It is very important that appropriate normal ranges are used to interpret cord blood pH. Often, a low normal pH is interpreted as abnormal – some published values are shown in Table 25.1. Even when these ranges are used, values below the normal range (–2 SD) are usually associated with a normal outcome.

Acute asphyxia and cerebral palsy

Cerebral palsy (CP) is one of the commonest causes of long term neurological deficits in children, affecting 2–3 per 1000 school aged children. It is a non-progressive motor disorder of early onset and predominantly presented as movement disorders which may be spastic, ataxic or dyskinetic. It may be accompanied by seizures and/or mental

Table 25.1 Normal pH values for umbilical artery at birth (vaginal delivery vs. CS)

Authors	Vaginal delivery (mean ± SD)	–2SD	Cesarean section (mean ± SD)
Helwig et al 1996	7.26 ± 0.08	7.10	—
Ruth & Raivio 1988	7.29 ± 0.07	7.15	7.31 ± 0.03
Loh et al 1998	7.21 ± 0.08	7.05	7.22 ± 0.07
Yeomans et al 1985	7.28 ± 0.05	7.18	—
Yoon and Kim 1994	7.24 ± 0.07	7.10	No labor 7.27 ± 0.05
			Labor 7.26 ± 0.05

The lower limit of normal (–2 SD) is shown for normal vaginal deliveries.

retardation. However, around 50% of the children with CP will have normal intelligence (Paneth & Stark 1983, Perlman 1997).

The causes of CP are often unknown but may be secondary to antepartum events, intrapartum acute hypoxia or postpartum causes. Traditionally, intrapartum asphyxia was considered as the primary cause of CP. There is a vast amount of evidence supporting the view that approximately 70%–80% of CP cases are antepartum in origin while 10%–20% are related to birth asphyxia (Blair & Stanley 1988, Perlman 2006a, Stanley & Alberman 1984, Torfs et al 1990). However, accurate determination of the cause and timing of the hypoxic injury is extremely challenging. Therefore the International Cerebral Palsy Task Force suggested certain criteria to relate CP to intrapartum events: (1) metabolic acidosis in umbilical artery or early neonatal blood samples (pH < 7.00 and base deficit = 12 mmol/L); (2) early onset of severe or moderate encephalopathy in infants born at = 34 weeks; and (3) spastic quadriplegia or dyskinetic CP (MacLennan 1999). Other suggestive criteria include a sentinel hypoxic event occurring immediately before or during labor, sudden, rapid and sustained deterioration of the fetal heart rate pattern usually after the hypoxic sentinel event where the pattern was previously normal, Apgar scores of 0–6 for longer than 5 minutes, early evidence of multi-system involvement and early imaging evidence of acute cerebral abnormality (MacLennan 1999).

The European Cerebral Palsy Study correlated brain MRI images with the timing of ischemic injury in CP cases and found that only about 20% of people with CP might be assessed as having some type of obstetric substandard care as the cause of their brain damage (Bax et al 2006). However, the work by Cowan et al (2003) quoted a significantly higher percentage of cases (about 80%) caused by acute birth asphyxia. We noted that in the latter study cases with proven viral or bacterial infection were not excluded from allocation to an intrapartum cause and the data did not exclude the possibility that antenatal factors could have predisposed to or initiated a pathway for brain injury. Also the Swedish study of a population of live-births between 1995 and 1998 (Himmelmann et al 2005) concluded that 35% of CP in children born at term was considered to be peri- or neonatal hypoxia/acidosis in origin although a higher proportion (about 70%) of the dyskinetic type of CP. However in that report the criteria used to diagnose acute perinatal asphyxia were clinical and imaging without reference to cord blood, and so normal pH results might have excluded a proportion of the cases thought to be due to acute acidosis. Moreover evidence of multi-system organ involvement was not reported. Had these criteria also been applied the number of the cases of CP ascribed to acute perinatal asphyxia would have been less and then perhaps the results would have been similar to the 10–20% reported in the previously mentioned studies.

Another way to assess the proportion of CP caused by acute events in labor is to measure the importance of other causes/antenatal predisposing factors. Many have been identified including fetal growth restriction secondary to placental insufficiency, multiple pregnancy, fetal infection, in vitro fertilization treatment, maternal bleeding, and maternal drug use or thyroid disease. Genetic causes, epidemiological factors and several other pregnancy complications such as pre-eclampsia can be relevant (Badawi et al 1998a, Lidegaard et al 2005). Intrapartum factors suggested to increase the risk on neonatal encephalopathy include maternal pyrexia and persistent occipito-posterior position. Moreover, operative vaginal delivery and emergency cesarean section were both associated with an increased risk, whereas it was lower with elective cesarean section (Badawi et al 1998b). Another contributing factor which should be added to the equation is that a significant proportion of CP is acquired post-neonatally mainly due to non-hypoxic causes and this will be an especially significant proportion in the very pre-term (Reid et al 2006).

Usually the fetal brain is well protected from hypoxia due to the cardiovascular compensatory responses but when hypoxic myocardial failure has developed, multi-organ compromise will eventually lead to fetal or neonatal death. Moreover experimentation in primates has shown that in order to cause disability, acute asphyxia must be prolonged, severe and nearly fatal (Beller 1995). This could explain why acute asphyxia rarely causes neurological handicap but when severe enough to change the outcome often results in death. When chronic conditions are excluded, intrapartum asphyxia, although associated with an increased mortality, is very rarely associated with permanent damage (Goodwin et al 1992). In a study done by Nelson and Ellenberg (1986), where they examined 189 children with CP, they studied the potential prenatal and perinatal risk factors predicting CP and the percentage of cases that can be attributed to these factors. They included that, on clinical bases only, 9% of the studied population was secondary to birth asphyxia. Furthermore, the proportion of CP identified after including the data related to birth events was only slightly higher than when the antenatal factors were considered alone.

Multiple causes may interact through toxic, oxidative or other pathophysiological mechanisms. A single factor may often be insufficient to produce cerebral damage, unless present to an extensive degree, whereas two or three interacting pathogenic assaults may overcome natural defences and produce irreversible brain injury. The more the potential causes, timing and predisposing factors of brain injury leading to CP are explored, the more we realize the complexity of the diagnosis of this condition.

Despite marked improvement in perinatal care over the last three decades, the incidence of CP due to peripartum asphyxia remains unchanged. This could be due to several factors: The current neonatal management protocols are supportive rather than aiming at the arrest of the ongoing brain pathology (Perlman 2006b), which may result in improved survival of very low birth weight neonates who are at greatest risk of acquiring ischemic brain injury. Also we are often unable to identify fetuses at highest risk of developing hypoxic brain injury during labor. However, several therapeutic modalities are being investigated for the management of moderate or severe hypoxic–ischemic encephalopathy and whole-body hypothermia has shown a reduction in the risk of death or disability (Shankaran et al 2005). Moreover, selective head cooling has shown a decrease in the severity of both neurodevelopmental disability and EEG changes (Gluckman et al 2005). Also phenobarbital, oxygen radical scavengers, NO inhibitors, growth factors and anti-cytokines are promising lines of management. They all target cases secondary to acute hypoxic–ischemic brain injury aiming at the reversal of the acute pathophysiological mechanisms underlying brain cell damage (Shalaka & Perlman 2004). The availability of treatment options for cases caused by acute events is making better future identification methods of the timing and etiology of brain injury in hypoxic–ischemic encephalopathy even more important. However since most HIE cases will not develop CP such approaches can only have a limited impact on the prevalence of CP.

CHRONIC ASPHYXIA

Pathophysiology (see also Ch. 22)

The animal models of chronic asphyxia do not completely resemble human placental dysfunction, so care must be taken when trying to use these data to understand the process in the human fetus (Soothill et al 1989). Also, animal experiments described as 'chronic' have often referred to hours or, at most, days of study, so the results may be more relevant to acute rather than chronic asphyxia in humans. However, some data are available, and in the sheep fetus, when hypoxia is prolonged over several days, oxygen consumption is no longer sustained and starts to fall with diminishing oxygen delivery (Anderson et al 1986). With chronic oxygen restriction over several days, redistribution of blood flow to vital organs becomes less pronounced than with acute asphyxia (Richardson et al 1998). A considerable reduction in oxygen consumption can be tolerated because of adaptive mechanisms such as reduced fetal activity and a lowered metabolic rate: therefore, the growth-restricted fetus can become less active (Richardson et al 1998). In the human, the hypoxemic small-for-gestational-age (SGA) fetus further compensates by increasing oxygen transport in the blood by increasing the manufacture of hemoglobin (Soothill et al 1987c) as a result of increased plasma erythropoietin (Snijders et al 1993).

Fetal growth restriction (FGR) has been induced experimentally in several species using maternal under-nutrition, chronic hypoxia, prolonged reduction in uterine blood flow, reduction in placental size and endocrine alterations. A sheep model, using the pre-conceptual removal of endometrial caruncles, has been able to produce fetal growth restriction by reducing placental size. The study showed

that the fetuses were chronically starved, hypoxemic, polycythemic and hypoglycemic (Robinson et al 1979), so mimicking the findings in human chronic placental dysfunction. The effects of chronic hypoxia on the fetus, particularly the brain, have been investigated in a large number of studies. When intrauterine hypoxia was induced in piglets, the FGR piglets showed a significantly higher rate of cerebral apoptosis than the normal weight ones, suggesting an increased vulnerability to apoptosis in the FGR piglets (Burke et al 2006). Furthermore, Doppler studies in human (uterine artery, umbilical artery and middle cerebral artery) have shown a clear relationship between the degree of placental vascular resistance and brain sparing in hypoxic fetuses (Cheema et al 2006).

Severe fetal anemia can also reduce fetal oxygen content and cause acidemia when the hemoglobin concentration has dropped to about one-third of the normal value for the gestational age (4–6 g/dL) with an oxygen content below 2 mmol/L (Soothill et al 1987c) (Fig. 25.3). The fetus reacts by increasing the blood-flow velocity and redistributing oxygen delivery in favor of the most vital organs (Fumia et al 1984), as in placental insufficiency, thus leading to a decrease in pH and HCO_3 and an increase in umbilical artery lactate concentration. The terminal state of fetal hydrops, which is the presence of fluid in at least two serous cavities in addition to skin edema, is interpreted as the inability of the fetus to sustain the increased cardiac output in hypoxic conditions (Soothill et al 1987b).

Causes

Maternal

Sustained reduction in fetal oxygen availability throughout the pregnancy can occur as a consequence of severe maternal disease causing maternal hypoxemia, including cardiac and respiratory diseases. However, in order to produce significant fetal effects, the maternal disease may be sufficiently severe to produce infertility. Other maternal diseases, particularly those affecting the uteroplacental vascular bed (pre-eclampsia, vasculopathies, connective tissue diseases, diabetes, chronic hypertension) may reduce fetal oxygenation. In general, maternal anemia does not affect fetal oxygenation, because the determining factor for placental oxygen transfer is the PO_2 difference, which is not affected by maternal anemia. Since maternal oxygen supply to the placenta is usually maintained by increased maternal blood flow and the fetal hemoglobin concentration is normal (Soothill 1994), the fetal blood oxygen content will be normal. This has been confirmed in animal studies when chronically anemic pregnant ewes have shown that the fetus is not hypoxemic or acidemic (Mostello et al 1991).

Placental

Variable grades of hypoxemia and metabolic acidosis may occur in placental dysfunction (Pardi et al 1987, Soothill et al 1987a). The most established cause is when the normal cytotrophoblast invasion of the distal segments of the spiral arteries during the late first and early second trimester is incomplete (Pijnenborg et al 1980). This process has been shown to occur incompletely in women who develop pre-eclampsia and when there is growth restricted fetuses probably due to an abnormal interaction between trophoblast and the spinal arteries (Khong et al 1986), which leads to a dysfunctional placenta. Others have postulated that the origin of fetal hypoxia in these FGR fetuses is due to a failure of oxygen transport from the intervillous space to the umbilical vein. If this were so, the intervillous PO_2 would be very close to maternal arterial PO_2. This 'chronic intra-placental hyperoxia' may be the cause of a reaction in the trophoblast and the villous core responsible for the impairment of oxygen transport (Kingdom & Kaufmann 1997).

Whatever the site of the problem, many other abnormal nutrient and hormonal findings also occur in FGR fetuses and probably relate to impaired placental function. These results have been reviewed previously and they are beyond the scope of this chapter (Soothill 1994, Soothill et al 1992b).

Fetal

Diseases of the fetus can occasionally lead to hypoxia and also acidosis, particularly severe fetal anemia (Soothill et al 1987b) as a result of hemolysis (Rhesus immunization), infections (Parvovirus B-19), feto-maternal hemorrhage or hemoglobinopathies (alpha-thalassemia major). Structural heart abnormalities can produce abnormal organ perfusion due to reduced cardiac output. This is also seen in some fetal cardiac arrhythmias, especially in congenital heart block or supraventricular tachycardia, where the high heart rate prevents a normal filling of the main cardiac chambers, consequently reducing the ventricular ejection volume. Finally, another cause of abnormal gases in the fetus is cardiac failure due to a hyperdynamic circulation resulting from intra- (hemangioma, arterio-venous malformation) or extra-fetal shunts (twin-to-twin transfusion, TRAP sequence, placental and cord arteriovenous malformations).

Diagnosis with blood gases

In contrast to acute asphyxia, in which acidemia is caused by acute changes in a previously healthy child, with rapidly changing blood-gas results, in chronic situations, fetal blood gases are more representative of the fetal condition and reflect better the underlining pathology. In these situations, hypoxemia is usually sustained and almost always progressive. When acidemia has developed, a cause-effect relationship with neurological damage seems more likely (Soothill et al 1992a).

Cordocentesis allows fetal blood to be obtained directly from cord vessels during pregnancy from about 18 weeks onwards. Initially, the procedure was done with fetoscopic guidance (Rodeck & Campbell 1978), but more recently, it

was simplified to ultrasound guidance (Daffos et al 1983). The needle is directed under ultrasound control to the vessels at about 1 cm from the placental insertion of the cord, ideally targeting the vein. This is the safest place to sample, and the procedure-related risk of pregnancy loss is no higher than 2% as long as a free loop of the cord is avoided. Nevertheless, on some rare occasions, the sample has to be obtained from the right ventricle of the fetal heart or the intrahepatic portion of the umbilical vein, but fetal paralysis or analgesia might be considered in these cases (Montemagno & Soothill 1997). Due to the difference in the gas composition, it is important to identify the vessel sampled as artery or vein to accurately establish the fetal acid–base status. In this sense, perhaps cardiac samples would not be ideal since this blood does not exactly match with 'arterial' or 'venous' composition, because it is incompletely mixed (foramen ovale, ductus arteriosus).

Fetal blood sampling has shown that severe acidosis can occur in non-laboring high-risk fetuses (Nicolaides et al 1986). Normal reference ranges of umbilical venous and arterial blood PO_2, PCO_2, pH and lactate have been obtained for appropriate gestational age fetuses (Nicolaides et al 1989, Soothill et al 1986); see Table 25.2.

The demonstration of chronic intrauterine hypoxia and acidosis in some growth-retarded fetuses (Soothill et al 1987a) has led some to attempt maternal oxygen therapy, aimed at improving fetal blood gases, while waiting for fetal viability (Nicolaides et al 1987). Although this led to an increased fetal PO_2 and improved Doppler flow patterns, no improvements were seen in fetal weight (Battaglia et al 1992) or fetal oxygen consumption (Harding et al 1992). Furthermore, artificial supplements of oxygen and nutrients in theory could be harmful (Harding et al 1992), making this therapy difficult to recommend. Therefore, at present, no in utero treatment is possible, and the prognosis depends on the gestational age at which chronic hypoxia and acidosis develop.

Table 25.2 Blood gases, pH and lactate in 208 AGA and 196 SGA fetuses obtained by cordocentesis at 18–38 weeks gestation

Parameter	AGA fetuses Mean ± SD	SGA fetuses Mean ± SD
U artery PO_2	28.0 ± 4.2	20.8 ± 8.0
U vein PO_2	42.7 ± 7.4	31.5 ± 10.0
U artery PCO_2	35.0 ± 2.0	47.3 ± 10.1
U vein PCO_2	34.9 ± 3.8	41.0 ± 9.9
U artery pH	7.37 ± 0.03	7.32 ± 0.07
U vein pH	7.41 ± 0.03	7.35 ± 0.08

Only figures for 25 weeks are shown. Since the normal values change with gestational age, the figures shown must not be used to assess results at any gestational age other than 25 weeks. Source: Nicolaides et al 1989.

Even chronically severely acidotic fetuses may survive and appear well if they can be delivered above 32 weeks gestation, although they might be damaged by chronic oxygen deficiency (Soothill 1994). The mode of delivery in these babies is almost always by CS, because they have achieved a point where placental function is so poor that there is no margin of safety or fetal reserve to withstand even the uterine contractions of normal labor.

A very important advance was when it was shown that hypoxic fetuses can be identified by the non-invasive test of Doppler. Indeed, some have claimed that after knowing the Doppler study results, fetal blood gases have little further value in predicting perinatal death (Nicolini et al 1990). Nevertheless, there is some evidence that infants who were chronically acidemic as fetuses may have lower developmental quotients (Soothill et al 1992a), and although this does not establish acidemia as necessarily causative, it appears that this is quite likely. It has been hypothesized that if the fetuses with placental dysfunction are delivered when they are hypoxemic, but before they become acidemic, neurological damage might be avoided (Soothill 1994).

Other methods

Nowadays, the only direct clinical method to identify chronic fetal acidemia is cordocentesis, but because it is not free of risk, its use has been limited. Indirect methods to search for chronic asphyxia have been developed, such as CTG and biophysical profile score (BPS), but these are ineffective because of a high false positive rate (Low et al 1986) and a weak association with neonatal morbidity (Soothill et al 1993) and because they do not usually become abnormal until a pre-terminal stage (Ribbert et al 1993).

Currently, Doppler ultrasound is the only non-invasive method that is able to predict with acceptable specificity the existence of chronic asphyxia in the fetus (Nicolaides et al 1988a) by detecting the hemodynamic changes that occur in response to fetal hypoxemia and acidemia. Studies in pregnancies with growth-retarded fetuses have shown that altered fetal gases at cordocentesis are associated with an increased impedance to flow in umbilical arteries, descending thoracic aorta, and decreased impedance in common carotids and cerebral arteries (Bilardo et al 1990). Umbilical artery pulsatility index (PI) progressively increases as chronic hypoxemia develops, and the end diastolic flow (EDF) often becomes absent or reversed when acidemia is present (Steiner et al 1995). In advanced acidemia, venous Doppler flow also becomes abnormal, probably reflecting myocardial failure due to hypoxia and ischemia (Hecher et al 1995, Rizzo et al 1995).

When abnormal umbilical arterial Doppler results are obtained in a fetus with normal anatomy, it is possible to classify these SGA fetuses as growth-restricted as a consequence of dysfunctional placenta. This diagnosis makes an active management approach essential. Alternatively, normal Dopplers with a SGA fetus at the end of the pregnancy virtually exclude placental insufficiency as causing the small

fetal size. These babies can be regarded merely as SGA (Holmes & Soothill 1999). It appears that the obstetric management of these cases does not need to be any different from the normal population (Soothill et al 1999). Nevertheless, screening with umbilical artery Dopplers in a low-risk population has proven to be of limited value (Beattie & Dornan 1989), and at the moment, it is only recommended if the fetus is small for the date. Moreover, several markers in maternal blood have demonstrated the relation between FGR and chronic hypoxia secondary to placental dysfunction. Changes in maternal serum level of activin A, inhibin A, insulin-like growth factor-I and increased circulating levels of fetal DNA were shown to relate to poor placental transfer42. Yet all these markers are still under investigation and have not been employed clinically (Alberry in press, Bobrow et al 2002, Holmes et al 1998). Although antenatal estimation of the fetal weight is possible by ultrasound, it has an error of 10–15% (Chauhan et al 1998), but this varies with the use of different formulae and is increased at both ends of the gaussian distribution. We opted to use the measurement of the abdominal circumference and classify the fetus as SGA if this is below 2 SD for the gestation.

CONCLUSIONS

Asphyxia is a poor term, which everyone involved in the care of newborns and fetuses should now try to avoid. The word is probably best replaced with 'acidemia,' but this has to be used with a very clear understanding of the difference between acute and chronic as described above. The title of this chapter therefore becomes something of a self fulfilling prophecy, but certainly, normal blood gases can be extremely useful in excluding acidosis as a cause of brain damage.

When looked at from the view of a doctor caring for a child with brain damage, obstetric data may give an indication of whether chronic acidosis is likely to have been the cause. The first is the birth weight. If this was less than 2 SD for the gestational age, a chronic in utero cause of the brain damage becomes much more likely. This opinion would be supported by oligohydramnios on ultrasound scan but above all by an abnormal umbilical artery Doppler assessment. If the Dopplers were abnormal (umbilical artery PI > 2 SD) in a baby with a birth weight less than 2 SD, then chronic placental insufficiency is almost certain (Bobrow & Soothill 1999) and so should be seriously considered as the cause of any brain damage.

Normal blood gases make previous chronic acidosis very unlikely. Acidosis at birth is very common and, when acute, is very rarely a cause of brain damage. This has been supported by a large number of studies over the past twenty years: many of them have examined several antenatal causes and predisposing factors of brain damage. Therefore acidosis at birth in a baby with the other features of chronic placental insufficiency is important and may be a valuable predictor of outcome.

REFERENCES

ACOG (American College of Obstetricians and Gynecologists) 1992 Fetal and neonatal neurologic injury. Washington, DC: American College of Obstetricians and Gynecologists, ACOG technical bulletin no. 163.

Alberry M, Soothill P W 2007 Management of FGR. Arch Dis Childhood 92(1):62–67.

Anderson D F, Parks C M, Faber J J 1986 Fetal O_2 consumption in sheep during controlled long-term reductions in umbilical blood flow. Am J Physiol 250: H1037–H1042.

Andres R L, Saade G, Gilstrap LC et al 1999 Association between umbilical blood gas parameters and neonatal morbidity and death in neonates with pathologic fetal acidemia. Am J Obstet Gynecol 181(4):867–871

Ayromlooli J, Garfinkel R 1980 Impact of fetal scalp blood pH on the incidence of caesarean section performed for fetal distress. Int J Gynaecol Obstet 17:391–392.

Badawi N, Kurinczuk J J, Keogh J M et al 1998a Antepartum risk factors for newborn encephalopathy: the Western Australian case control study. BMJ 317:1549–1553

Badawi N, Kurinczuk J J, Keogh J M et al 1998b Intrapartum risk factors for newborn encephalopathy: the Western Australian case-control study. BMJ 317:1554–1558.

Ball R H, Espinoza M I, Parer J T et al 1994a Regional blood flow in asphyxiated fetuses with seizures. Am J Obstet Gynecol 170:156–161.

Ball R H, Parer J T, Caldwell L E et al 1994b Regional blood flow and metabolism in ovine fetuses during severe cord occlusion. Am J Obstet Gynecol 171:1549–1555.

Battaglia C, Artini P G, D'Ambrogio G et al 1992 Maternal hyperoxygenation in the treatment of intrauterine growth retardation. Am J Obstet Gynecol 167:430–435.

Bax M, Nelson K B 1993 Birth asphyxia: a statement. Dev Med Child Neurol 35:1002–1004.

Bax M, Tydeman C, Flodmark O 2006 Clinical and MRI correlates of cerebral palsy. JAMA 296:1602–1608.

Beattie R B, Dornan J C 1989 Antenatal screening for intrauterine growth retardation with umbilical artery Doppler ultrasonography. BMJ 298(6674):631–635.

Belai Y, Goodwin T M, Durand M et al 1998 Umbilical arteriovenous pO_2 and pCO_2 differences and neonatal morbidity in term infants with severe acidosis. Am J Obstet Gynecol 178:13–19.

Beller F K 1995 The cerebral palsy story: a catastrophic misunderstanding in obstetrics. Obstet Gynecol Surv 50:83.

Benaron D A, Kurth C D, Steven J M et al 1995 Transcranial optical path length in infants by near–infrared phase-shift spectroscopy. J Clin Monit 11:109–117.

Bilardo C M, Nicolaides K H, Campbell S 1990 Doppler measurements of fetal and uteroplacental circulations: relationship with umbilical venous blood gases measured at cordocentesis. Am J Obstet Gynecol 162:115–120.

Blair E, Stanley F J 1988 Intrapartum asphyxia — a rare cause of cerebral palsy. J Pediatr 112:515–519.

Bobrow C S, Holmes R P, Muttukrishna S et al 2002 Maternal serum activin A, inhibin A, and follistatin in pregnancies with appropriately grown and small-for-gestational-age fetuses classified by umbilical artery Doppler ultrasound. Am J Obstet Gynecol 186(2):283–287.

Bobrow C S, Soothill P W 1999 Causes and consequences of fetal acidosis. Arch Dis Child Fetal Neonatal 80:F246–F249.

Bocking A D, Ganong R, White S E et al 1988 Circulatory response to prolonged hypoxemia in fetal sheep. Am J Obstet Gynecol 159:1418–1424.

Bozzetti P, Buscaglia M, Cetin I et al 1987 Respiratory gases, acid-base balance and lactate concentrations of the midterm human fetus. Biol Neonate 52:188–197.

Bretscher J, Saling E 1967 pH values in the human fetus during labor. Am J Obstet Gynecol 97:906–911.

Burke C, Sinclaira K, Cowinc G et al 2006 Intrauterine growth restriction due to uteroplacental vascular insufficiency leads to increased hypoxia-induced cerebral apoptosis in newborn piglets. Brain Res 1098:19–25.

Burke M S, Porreco R P, Day D et al 1989 Intrauterine resuscitation with tocolysis. An alternate month clinical trial. J Perinatol 9:296–300.

Callen P W 1994 Ultrasound evaluation of normal fetal anatomy. In: Callen P W (ed.) Ultrasonography in obstetrics and gynecology, 2nd edn. WB Saunders, Philadelphia, PA, pp. 144–188.

Carbonne B, Langer B, Goffinet F et al 1997 Multicenter study on the clinical value of fetal pulse oximetry. II. Compared predictive values of pulse oximetry and fetal blood analysis. The French Study Group on Fetal Pulse Oximetry. Am J Obstet Gynecol 177:593–598.

Chauhan S P, Charania S F, McLaren R A et al 1998 Ultrasonographic estimate of birth weight at 24 to 34 weeks: a multicenter study. Am J Obstet Gynecol 179:909–916.

Cheema R, Dubiel M, Gudmundsson S 2006 Fetal brain sparing is strongly related to the degree of increased placental vascular impedance. J Perinat Med 34(4):318–322

Cowan F, Rutherford M, Groenendaal F et al 2003 Origin and timing of brain lesions in term infants with neonatal encephalopathy. Lancet 1361(9359):736–742.

Daffos F, Capella-Pavlovsky M, Forestier F 1983 Fetal blood sampling via the umbilical cord using a needle guided by ultrasound. Report of 66 cases. Prenat Diagn 3:271–277.

East C E, Brennecke S P, King J F et al (On behalf of The FOREMOST Study Group) 2006 The effect of intrapartum fetal pulse oximetry, in the presence of a nonreassuring fetal heart rate pattern, on operative delivery rates: A multicenter, randomized, controlled trial (the FOREMOST trial). Am J Obstet Gynecol 194:606.e1–606.e16.

East C E, Dunster K R, Colditz P B et al 1997 Fetal oxygen saturation monitoring in labour: an analysis of 118 cases. Aust NZ J Obstet Gynaecol 37:397–401.

Espinoza M, Riquelme R, Germain A M et al 1989 Role of endogenous opioids in the cardiovascular responses to asphyxia in fetal sheep. Am J Physiol 256:R1063–R1068.

Fee S C, Malee K, Deddish R et al 1990 Severe acidosis and subsequent neurologic status. Am J Obstet Gynecol 162:802–886.

Fumia F D, Edelstone D I, Holzman I R 1984 Blood flow and oxygen delivery to fetal organs as functions of fetal hematocrit. Am J Obstet Gynecol 150:274–282.

Garite T J, Dildy G A, McNamara H et al 2000 A multicenter controlled trial of fetal pulse oximetry in the intrapartum management of nonreassuring fetal heart rate patterns. Am J Obstet Gynecol 183(5):1049–1058.

Gill R W, Kossoff G, Warren P S et al 1984 Umbilical venous flow in normal and complicated pregnancy. Ultrasound Med Biol 10:349–363.

Gilstrap L C 1998 In: Creasy R, Resnik R (eds) Maternal-fetal medicine, 4th edn. Saunders, Philadelphia, PA, Ch 22, pp. 331–339.

Gluckman P D, Wyatt J S, Azzopardi D et al 2005 Selective head cooling with mild systemic hypothermia after neonatal encephalopathy: multicentre randomised trial. Lancet 19–25,365(9460):663–670.

Goffinet F, Langer B, Carbonne B et al 1997 Multicenter study on the clinical value of fetal pulse oximetry. I. Methodologic evaluation. The French Study Group on Fetal Pulse Oximetry. Am J Obstet Gynecol 177:1238–1246.

Goodwin T M, Belai I, Hernandez P et al 1992 Asphyxial complications in the term newborn with severe umbilical acidemia. Am J Obstet Gynecol 167:1506–1512.

Gordon A, Johnson J W 1985 Value of umbilical blood acid-base studies in fetal assessment. J Reprod Med 30:329–336.

Harding J E, Owens J A, Robinson J S 1992 Should we try to supplement the growth retarded fetus? A cautionary tale. Br J Obstet Gynaecol 99:707–709.

Hecher K, Campbell S, Doyle P et al 1995 Assessment of fetal compromise by Doppler ultrasound investigation of the fetal circulation. Arterial, intracardiac, and venous blood flow velocity studies. Circulation 91:129–138.

Helwig J T, Parer J T, Kilpatrick S J et al 1996 Umbilical cord blood acid-base state: what is normal? Am J Obstet Gynecol 174:1807–1812.

Himmelmann K, Hagberg G, Beckung E et al 2005 The changing panorama of cerebral palsy in Sweden. IX. Prevalence and origin in the birth-year period 1995–1998. Acta Paediatr 94(3):287–294.

Holmes R P, Holly J M, Soothill P W 1998 A prospective study of maternal serum insulin-like growth factor-I in pregnancies with appropriately grown or growth restricted fetuses. Br J Obstet Gynaecol 105(12):1273–1278.

Holmes R, Soothill P W 1999 Small fetuses with normal Dopplers are appropriately grown with normal pregnancy outcome. Presented at BMFMS 1999. J Obstet Gynecol 19:S23.

Ingemarsson I, Arulkumaran S 1986 Fetal acid-base balance in low-risk patients in labour. Am J Obstet Gynecol 155:66–69.

Jensen A, Hanson M A 1995 Circulatory responses to acute asphyxia in intact and chemodenervated fetal sheep near term. Reprod Fertil Dev 7:1351–1359.

Jensen A, Hohmann M, Kunzel W 1987 Dynamic changes in organ blood flow and oxygen consumption during acute asphyxia in fetal sheep. J Dev Physiol 9:543–559.

Jensen A, Lang U 1992 Foetal circulatory responses to arrest of uterine blood flow in sheep: effects of chemical sympathectomy. J Dev Physiol 17:75–86.

Katz M, Meizner I, Mazor M et al 1981 Fetal heart rate patterns and scalp blood pH as predictors of fetal distress. Isr J Med Sci 17:260–265.

Khong T Y, De Wolf F, Robertson W B et al 1986 Inadequate maternal vascular response to placentation in pregnancies complicated by pre-eclampsia and by small-for-gestational age infants. Br J Obstet Gynaecol 93:1049–1059.

Kingdom J C, Kaufmann P 1997 Oxygen and placental villous development: origins of fetal hypoxia. Placenta 18:613–621, 623–666.

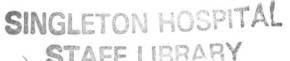

Kiserud T, Eik-Ness S H, Hellevik L R et al 1992 Ductus venosus: a longitudinal Doppler velocimetric study of the human fetus. J Matern Fetal Invest 2:5–11.

Kuhnert M, Seelbach-Goebel B, Butterwegge M 1998 Predictive agreement between the fetal arterial oxygen saturation and fetal scalp pH: results of the German multicenter study. Am J Obstet Gynecol 178:330–335.

Kurth C D, Steven J M, Benaron D et al 1993 Near-infrared monitoring of the cerebral circulation. J Clin Monit 9:163–170.

Lidegaard O, Pinborg A, Andersen A N 2005 Imprinting diseases and IVF: Danish National IVF cohort study. Hum Reprod 20:950–954.

Little W J 1862 On the influence of abnormal parturition, difficult labour, premature birth and asphyxia neonatorum on the mental and physical condition of the child, especially in relation to deformities. Trans London Obstet Soc 3:293–325.

Loh S F, Woodworth A, Yeo G S 1998 Umbilical cord blood gas analysis at delivery. Singapore Med J 39:151–155.

Longo L D 1981 The interrelations of maternal-fetal transfer and placental blood flow. In: Young M, Boyd R D H, Longo L D et al (eds) Placental transfer methods and interpretations. Placenta supplement 2. WB Saunders, Philadelphia, PA, pp. 45–64.

Low J A 1997 Intrapartum fetal asphyxia: Definition, diagnosis, and classification. Am J Obstet Gynecol 176:957–959.

Low J A, McGrath M J, Marshall S J et al 1986 The relationship between antepartum fetal heart rate, intrapartum fetal heart rate, and fetal acid-base status. Am J Obstet Gynecol 154:769–776.

Low J A, Panagiotopoulos C, Derrick E J 1994 Newborn complications after intrapartum asphyxia with metabolic acidosis in the term fetus. Am J Obstet Gynecol 170:1081–1087.

MacLennan A 1999 A template for defining a causal relation between intrapartum events and cerebral palsy: international consensus statement. BMJ 319(7216):1054–1059.

McNamara H, Chung D C, Lilford R et al 1992 Do fetal pulse oximetry readings at delivery correlate with cord blood oxygenation and acidaemia? Br J Obstet Gynaecol 99:735–738.

McNamara H, Johnson N, Lilford R 1993 The effect on fetal arteriolar oxygen saturation resulting from giving oxygen to the mother measured by pulse oximetry. Br J Obstet Gynecol 100:446–449.

Montemagno R, Soothill P W 1997 Invasive procedures. In: Fisk N, Moise K (eds) Fetal therapy, invasive and transplacental. Cambridge University Press, Cambridge, pp. 9–26.

Mostello D, Chalk C, Khoury J et al 1991 Chronic anemia in pregnant ewes: maternal and fetal effects. Am J Physiol 261:R1075–R1083.

Nelson K B, Dambrosia J M, Ting T Y et al 1996 Uncertain values of electronic fetal monitoring in predicting cerebral palsy. N Engl J Med 334:613–618.

Nelson K B, Ellenberg J H 1986 Antecedents of cerebral palsy. N Engl J Med 315:81–86.

Nicolaides K H, Bilardo C M, Soothill P W et al 1988a Absence of end diastolic frequencies in umbilical artery: a sign of fetal hypoxia and acidosis. Br Med J 297:1026–1027.

Nicolaides K H, Campbell S, Bradley R J et al 1987 Maternal oxygen therapy for intrauterine growth retardation. Lancet 1:942–945.

Nicolaides K H, Economides D L, Soothill P W 1989 Blood gases, pH and lactate in appropriate- and small-for-gestational-age fetuses. Am J Obstet Gynecol 161:996–1001.

Nicolaides K H, Soothill P W, Clewell W H et al 1988b Fetal haemoglobin measurement in the assessment of red cell isoimmunisation. Lancet 1(8594):1073–1075.

Nicolaides K H, Soothill P W, Rodeck C H et al 1986 Ultrasound-guided sampling of umbilical cord and placental blood to assess fetal wellbeing. Lancet 1:1065–1067.

Nicolini U, Nicolaidis P, Fisk N M et al 1990 Limited role of fetal blood sampling in prediction of outcome in intrauterine growth retardation. Lancet 336:768–772.

O'Connor M C, Hytten F E, Zanelli G D 1979 Is the fetus 'scalped' in labour? Lancet 2:947–949.

Paneth N, Stark R I 1983 Cerebral palsy and mental retardation in relation to indications of perinatal asphyxia. Am J Obstet Gynecol 47:960–966.

Pardi G, Buscaglia M, Ferrazzi E et al 1987 Cord sampling for the evaluation of oxygenation and acid-base balance in growth-retarded human fetuses. Am J Obstet Gynecol 157:1221–1228.

Parer J T 1998 Effects of fetal asphyxia on brain cell structure and function: limits of tolerance. Comp Biochem Physiol A Mol Integr Physiol 119:711–716.

Paulick R P, Meyers R L, Rudolph C D et al 1990 Venous responses to hypoxemia in the fetal lamb. J Dev Physiol 14:81–88.

Peeters L L H, Sheldon R E, Jones M D et al 1979 Blood flow to fetal organs as a function of arterial oxygen content. Am J Obstet Gynecol 135:637–646.

Perkins R P 1997 Requiem for a heavyweight: the demise of scalp blood pH sampling. J Matern Fetal Med 6:298–300.

Perlman J M 1997 Intrapartum hypoxic-ischemic cerebral injury and subsequent cerebral palsy: medicolegal issues. Pediatrics 99:851–859.

Perlman J M 2006a Intrapartum asphyxia and cerebral palsy: is there a link? Clin Perinatol 33(2):335–353.

Perlman J M 2006b Summary Proceedings from the Neurology Group on Hypoxic-Ischemic Encephalopathy. Pediatrics 117(3).

Pijnenborg R, Dixon G, Robertson W B et al 1980 Trophoblastic invasion of human decidua from 8 to 18 weeks of pregnancy. Placenta 1:3–19.

Reid S M, Lanigan A, Reddihough D S 2006 Post-neonatally acquired cerebral palsy in Victoria, Australia, 1970–1999. J Paediatr Child Health 42(10):606–611.

Ribbert L S, Visser G H, Mulder E J et al 1993 Changes with time in fetal heart rate variation, movement incidences and haemodynamics in intrauterine growth retarded fetuses: a longitudinal approach to the assessment of fetal well being. Early Hum Dev 31:195–208.

Richardson B S 1989 Fetal adaptive responses to asphyxia. Clin Perinatol 16:595–611.

Richardson B, Nodwell A, Webster K et al 1998 Fetal oxygen saturation and fractional extraction at birth and the relationship to measures of acidosis. Am J Obstet Gynecol 178:572–579.

Rizzo G, Capponi A, Arduini D et al 1995 The value of fetal arterial, cardiac and venous flows in predicting pH and blood gases measured in umbilical blood at cordocentesis in growth retarded fetuses. Br J Obstet Gynaecol 102:963–969.

Robinson J S, Kingston E J, Jones C T et al 1979 Studies on experimental growth retardation in sheep. The effect of removal of a endometrial caruncles on fetal size and metabolism. J Dev Physiol 1:379–398.

Rodeck C H, Campbell S 1978 Sampling pure fetal blood by fetoscopy in second trimester of pregnancy. Br Med J 2:728–730.

Rudolph A M 1983 Hepatic and ductus venosus blood flows during fetal life. Hepatology 3:254–258.

Rurak D, Selke P, Fisher M et al 1987 Fetal oxygen extraction: Comparison of the human and sheep. Am J Obstet Gynecol 156:360–366.

Ruth V J, Raivio K O 1988 Perinatal brain damage: predictive value of metabolic acidosis and the Apgar score. BMJ 297:24–27.

Sadler T W 1995 Fetal membranes and placenta. In: Sadler T W (ed.) Medical embryology, 7th edn. Williams & Wilkins, Baltimore, MD, pp. 101–121.

Sarnat H B, Sarnat M S 1976 Neonatal encephalopathy following fetal distress. Arch Neurol 33:696–705.

Seelbach-Gobel B, Heupel M, Kuhnert M et al 1999 The prediction of fetal acidosis by means of intrapartum fetal pulse oximetry. Am J Obstet Gynecol 180:73–81.

Shalaka L, Perlman J M 2004 Hypoxic-ischemic brain injury in the term infant — current concepts. Early Hum Dev 80:125– 141.

Shankaran S, Laptook A, Ehrenkranz R et al 2005 Whole-body hypothermia for neonates with hypoxic-ischemic encephalopathy. N Engl J Med 353:1574–1584.

Small M I, Beall M, Platt L D et al 1989 Continuous tissue pH monitoring in the term fetus. Am J Obstet Gynecol 161:323–329.

Snijders R J, Abbas A, Melby O et al 1993 Fetal plasma erythropoietin concentration in severe growth retardation. Am J Obstet Gynecol 168:615–619.

Soothill P W 1994 Diagnosis of intrauterine growth retardation and its fetal and perinatal consequences. Acta Paediatr Suppl 399:55–59.

Soothill P W, Ajayi R A, Campbell S et al 1992a Relationship between fetal acidaemia at cordocentesis and subsequent neurodevelopment. Ultrasound Obstet Gynecol 2:80–83.

Soothill P W, Ajayi R A, Campbell S et al 1993 Prediction of morbidity in small and normally grown fetuses by fetal heart rate variability, Biophysical profile score and umbilical artery Doppler studies. Br J Obstet Gynaecol 100:742–745.

Soothill P W, Ajayi R A, Campbell S et al 1995 Fetal oxygenation at cordocentesis, maternal smoking and childhood neuro-development. Eur J Obstet Gynecol Reprod Biol 59:21–24.

Soothill P W, Ajayi R A, Nicolaides K N 1992b Fetal biochemistry in growth retardation. Early Hum Dev 29:91–97.

Soothill P W, Bobrow C S, Holmes R 1999 Small for gestational age is not a diagnosis. Ultrasound Obstet Gynecol 13:225–228.

Soothill P W, Lestas A N, Nicolaides K H et al 1988 2,3-Diphosphoglicerate in normal, anaemic and transfused human fetuses. Clin Sci 74:527–530.

Soothill P W, Nicolaides K H, Campbell S 1987a Prenatal asphyxia, hyperlacticaemia, hypoglycaemia, and erythroblastosis in growth retarded fetuses. BMJ (Clin Res Ed) 294:1051–1053.

Soothill P W, Nicolaides K H, Rodeck C H 1987b Effect of anaemia on fetal acid-base status. Br J Obstet Gynaecol 94:880–883.

Soothill P W, Nicolaides K H, Rodeck C H 1989 Fetal blood gas and acid-base parameters. In Rodeck C H (ed.) Fetal medicine 1. Blackwell Scientific, Oxford, pp. 57–89.

Soothill P W, Nicolaides K H, Rodeck C H et al 1986 Effects of gestational age on fetal and intervillous blood gas and acid-base values in human pregnancy. Fetal Ther 1:168–175.

Soothill P W, Nicolaides K H, Rodeck C H et al 1987c Relationship of fetal haemoglobin and oxygen content to lactate concentration in Rh isoimmunized pregnancies. Obstet Gynecol 69:268–271.

Stanley F, Alberman E 1984 The epidemiology of cerebral palsy. JB Lippincott, Philadelphia, PA.

Steiner H, Staudach A, Spitzer D et al 1995 Growth deficient fetuses with absent or reversed umbilical artery end-diastolic flow are metabolically compromised. Early Hum Dev 41:1–9.

Susan M, Lanigan A, Reddihough D 2006 Post-neonatally acquired cerebral palsy in Victoria, Australia 1970–1999. J Paediatr Child Health 42:606–611.

Tejani N A, Verma U L, Chatterjee S et al 1983 Terbutaline in the management of acute intrapartum fetal acidosis. J Reprod Med 28:857–861.

Torfs C P, Van der berg B J, Oeschali F W 1990 Prenatal and perinatal factors in the etiology of cerebral palsy. J Pediatr 116:615–619.

Towell M E 1976 Fetal respiratory physiology. In: Goodwin J W, Godden J O, Chance G W (eds) Perinatal medicine. Longman: Canada, Toronto, pp. 171–186.

Wahr J A, Tremper K K, Samra S et al 1996 Near-infrared spectroscopy: theory and applications. J Cardiothorac Vasc Anesth 10:406–418.

Westgate J, Garibaldi J M, Greene K R 1994 Umbilical cord blood gas analysis at delivery: a time for quality data. Br J Obstet Gynaecol 101:1054–1063.

Willcourt R F 1987 Fetal blood gases and pH: current application. In Studd J (ed.) Progress in obstetric and gynecology, Vol. 6. Churchill Livingstone, Edinburgh, pp. 155–174.

Winkler C L, Hauth J C, Tucker J M et al 1991 Neonatal complications at term as related to the degree of umbilical artery acidaemia. Am J Obstet Gynecol 164:637–641.

Yeomans E R, Hauth J C, Gilstrap L C 3rd et al 1985 Umbilical cord pH, PCO_2, and bicarbonate following uncomplicated term vaginal deliveries. Am J Obstet Gynecol 151:798–800.

Yoon B H, Kim S W 1994 The effect of labor on the normal values of umbilical blood acid-base status. Acta Obstet Gynecol Scand 73:555–561.

Young D C, Gray J H, Luther E R et al 1980 Fetal scalp blood pH sampling: Its value in an active obstetric unit. Am J Obstet Gynecol 136:276–281.

Zalar R W, Quilligan E J 1979 The influence of scalp sampling on the caesarean section rate for fetal distress. Am J Obstet Gynecol 135:239–246.

CHAPTER

26

The asphyxiated newborn infant

Luc Cornette and Malcolm I. Levene

> ### Key Points
>
> - There is no single or generally agreed diagnosis of 'birth asphyxia'. The diagnosis can be assessed retrospectively by attention to seven clinical features
> - Cerebral pathology resulting from a hypoxic–ischemic insult depends on gestational age of the infant when the insult occurred as well as the severity and duration of the insult
> - Access to expert and rapid resuscitation immediately after birth is essential for asphyxiated newborn infants
> - There are few proven evidence based interventions in the management of the asphyxiated newborn infant. Postnatal corticosteroid treatment and hyperventilation are potentially hazardous
> - There is no evidence that suppressing all seizure activity with anticonvulsant drugs improves the subsequent outcome of the baby
> - The best clinical predictor of adverse outcome is severity of hypoxic–ischemic encephalopathy (HIE): moderate and severe HIE has a 25% and 80% risk of adverse outcome respectively

INTRODUCTION

In the developed world, birth asphyxia is arguably the most common cause of perinatally acquired severe brain injury in full-term infants. Annually, about 4 million neonates are affected world wide. Approximately one million will die and an equal number will develop serious sequelae (WHO 2003). It is a tragedy for a normally developed fetus to sustain cerebral injury during the last hours of prenatal life and then to survive for many more years with a major disability.

For pediatricians, birth asphyxia remains a frustrating condition to treat as prevention of the condition is outside their control, and there have been few or no improvements in clinical management in the last 20 years. The antenatal and intrapartum aspects of detection and prevention are discussed in Chapters 23 and 24. Potentially effective new brain protection therapy for birth asphyxia is discussed in Chapter 27.

DEFINITION

Apnea at birth is a relatively common feature, particularly in premature infants. This may cause the Apgar score to be depressed and require the infant to be resuscitated. There may be little evidence that the baby has suffered the hypoxic–ischemic pathophysiological insult inherent to the term 'birth asphyxia'. Because of the fundamental differences in the definition and neuropathological sequelae of asphyxia between preterm and full-term infants, this chapter only discusses perinatal asphyxia with reference to the mature infant. The neuropathological insults seen in premature infants are predominantly hemorrhagic or ischemic, and intrapartum events only rarely precipitate these conditions. They are discussed in detail in Section IV.

The term asphyxia refers to impairment of placental or pulmonary gas exchange resulting in three biochemical components: hypoxemia, hypercapnia and acidosis (Low 1997a). 'Birth asphyxia' is widely used as a clinical diagnosis, but there is little consensus as to what is meant by it. Hypoxic–ischemic insult better describes the pathophysiology of intrapartum asphyxia and stresses the two major components of the condition. Cerebral ischemia, i.e. blood flow below the level necessary to support normal function, is not well tolerated, and pure ischemic lesions may occur as the result of sudden hypovolemia. Hypoxia on its own is well tolerated by the immature brain, providing that minimum quantities of metabolic substrate (mainly glucose) are delivered to the brain. Regardless of the cause, cardiac failure ultimately occurs when hypoxia is prolonged, resulting in hypotension, ischemia and lactic acidosis. Thus, ischemia is both a cause and a result of hypoxia and compounds the complications of hypoxia by impairing the removal of metabolic and respiratory by-products (e.g. lactic acid).

The cerebral lesions that develop following an episode of intense ischemia are different to those seen when hypoxia and ischemia act together, as occurs as the result of intrapartum asphyxia. Pure ischemic lesions in premature and full-term infants are discussed in Chapter 21. A diagnosis of an asphyxiating event should not be made without some evidence of an interruption of oxygen (O_2) supply or blood flow to the fetus. These events can be secondary to problems within the mother (e.g. hypotension, toxemia, uterine tetany, uterine rupture), the placenta or umbilical cord (e.g. abruption, infection or inflammation, or umbilical cord compression or occlusion), or the fetus or infant (e.g. central nervous system depression, anomalies, infection) (Nelson 2003).

The fetus is well adapted to the rigors of labor, and these protective mechanisms are discussed in Chapter 22. A severe hypoxic–ischemic insult may overwhelm these adaptive mechanisms and cause the vital organs to be compromised. The determinants of whether the insult is severe enough to cause dysfunction are its intensity and duration. An intense insult such as cord prolapse or massive placental abruption causes the fetus to be rapidly compromised, whereas a less intense insult such as intermittent placental insufficiency associated with hypertonic uterine contractions will need a longer duration to have a similarly severe effect on the fetus. It is often not possible to know clinically either the degree of intensity or the duration of the intrapartum insult.

PRECONDITIONING

It has recently been recognized in animal studies that a period of hypoxia prior to a more severe hypoxic–ischemic insult protects the immature brain from hypoxic–ischemic injury compared with the animal that was not exposed to the preceding hypoxia (Brucklacher et al 2002). This has been referred to as 'preconditioning' and is probably due to increased expression of a variety of genes which contribute to the development of hypoxia-induced tolerance (Bernaudin et al 2002).

THE 'ASPHYXIA SYNDROME'

There is no universally accepted clinical definition of asphyxia, and all the following features are used as possible markers of the condition; indeed some recommended that the term 'birth asphyxia' should not be used (Bax & Nelson 1993). There are many conditions in medicine that cannot be diagnosed accurately with a blood test or radiological procedure. In these cases, a careful clinical history, together with exclusion of alternative diagnoses, usually suffices to make the diagnosis. There is no single test to diagnose birth asphyxia, and it is necessary to adopt a similar approach to that for the diagnosis of migraine or epilepsy. This will involve considering asphyxia as a syndrome, or collection of features, with the exclusion of alternative conditions (Levene 1995). To adopt this approach, it is necessary for three aspects to be considered:

1. assessment of diagnostic criteria;
2. exclusion of alternative possible diagnoses;
3. consideration of results from contributory diagnostic tests.

Each of these is considered below.

Assessment of diagnostic criteria

None of the features listed below on their own are diagnostic, but the more that are present, the more likely it is that asphyxia has occurred. The presence of four out of six items should make the diagnosis of moderate probability, providing that the exclusion criteria are met, and five or six out of six gives a good probability of the diagnosis being generally accepted.

The most common time for a baby to be acutely asphyxiated is at the end of labor, with birth releasing the fetus from a hostile intrauterine environment. In these cases, there is likely to be evidence of increasing fetal distress, poor adaptation to birth and hypoxic–ischemic encephalopathy with evidence of transient impairment in other organ systems. Less commonly, a severe asphyxial event may occur several hours or even days prior to delivery such as prolonged, but reversible, uterine hypertonus due to excess pharmacological stimulation or transient severe maternal hypotension. Under these conditions, the baby may not show fetal distress immediately prior to birth, as cardiovascular recovery from the acute event has occurred (autoresuscitation), and the baby may be born in relatively good condition. The baby may, nevertheless, show signs of hypoxic–ischemic encephalopathy (HIE), although the sequence may be altered (e.g. very early convulsions) by the interval between insult and delivery.

Fetal distress

Fetal asphyxia during labor occurs as the result of placental compromise or, rarely, umbilical cord compression. These conditions affect the entire fetus, and methods to detect fetal distress usually monitor the effects of these insults on the cardiovascular system. Chapters 24 and 25 discuss these methods. There is no clinically reliable method for assessing central nervous system function during labor, and evidence of fetal distress does not necessarily indicate that the fetal brain has been compromised. Intrapartum electronic fetal heart rate monitoring, i.e. cardiotocography (CTG), is not good at distinguishing fetal stress (a normal reaction to the rigors of labor) from fetal distress. Consequently, abnormalities on a CTG are relatively poorly sensitive to intrapartum asphyxia (high number of false positives). While fetal heart rate patterns will not discriminate all asphyxial exposures, CTG supplemented by fetal blood gas and acid–base assessment can be a useful fetal assessment paradigm for intrapartum fetal asphyxia (Low et al 2001). The CTG is, however, more likely to be a relatively specific test, as a normal CTG probably indicates that the fetus is not suffering from acute intrapartum asphyxia at the time that the CTG is being registered. Continuous measurement of fetal O_2 saturation during labor, i.e. fetal pulse oximetry, as an adjunct to electronic fetal monitoring, does not seem to provide additional information, as there is no difference in condition of the newborn compared to using CTG alone (Bloom et al 2006). More recently fetal ECG monitoring has been shown to reduce the high false positive rate of standard CTG monitoring. Automatic ST-waveform analysis appears to be a better predictor of fetal acidosis than standard CTG monitoring (Amer-Wahlin 2001).

Passage of meconium

Meconium is passed prior to delivery in 10–20% of full-term infants. Heavy contamination of the amniotic fluid has been suggested to be a feature of fetal distress (Meis et al 1978). The passage of meconium is, however, a very weak marker of those babies likely to sustain irreversible cerebral injury as the result of intrapartum asphyxia. Nelson and Ellenberg (1984) reported that only 0.4% of infants weighing more than 2500 g who had meconium-stained liquor were later found to have cerebral palsy.

Metabolic acidosis

Anaerobic metabolism is a normal physiological response during episodes of hypoxemia with generation of lactic acid. Fetal acid–base balance can be assessed through antepartum umbilical cord blood sampling, fetal scalp blood assessment, or umbilical cord blood sampling immediately after delivery. Fetal acidosis may be measured by blood pH or by the base deficit. Metabolic acidosis results in excess production of acid and decreased buffer base, which is referred to as the base deficit or negative base excess. The major buffers utilized by the fetus for neutralizing hydrogen ion production are plasma bicarbonate and hemoglobin. When adequate fetal oxygenation does not occur, complete oxidative metabolism of carbohydrates to carbon dioxide (CO_2) and water is impaired and metabolism proceeds along an anaerobic pathway with production of organic acids, such as lactate, which are not readily excreted or metabolized. Accumulation of lactate can deplete the buffer system and result in decreased buffer base. The severity of the metabolic acidosis may reflect either the duration or the intensity of the asphyxial event, but metabolic acidosis does not correlate with those infants who later are shown to have sustained neurological deficit (see Ch. 25). Although fetal acidosis is widely taken to be pH < 7.20, a more reliable value indicating the possibility of neurological compromise is pH = 7.05 or pH = 7.0.

Base deficit values have a significantly greater usefulness than umbilical cord pH values (Ross & Gala 2002), because base excess does not change significantly with respiratory acidosis and demonstrates a linear, rather than logarithmic, correlation to the degree of metabolic acidosis. The normal fetal base deficit entering labor is −1 to −2 mmol/L. It is generally assumed that asphyxial injury does not occur until the fetal base deficit is ≤12 mmol/L (Ross & Gala 2002). Notably, most newborns with a base deficit of ≤12 mmol/L do not demonstrate neurologic injury. The risk of moderate or severe complications in newborns with umbilical artery base deficit greater than 16 mmol/L was fourfold higher than in those at 12 to 16 mmol/L (40 and 10 percent, respectively) (Low 1997b).

Loss of buffer base is unlikely to occur in the neonatal period, unless there is continued neonatal severe hypoxemia, hypotension or sepsis. Therefore, if no sodium bicarbonate was administered, one may assume minimal acute changes in the buffer base among infants who are appropriately resuscitated and oxygenated in the immediate newborn period. Conversely, continued severe hypoxemia (e.g. inadequate ventilation) during the neonatal period may result in base excess losses similar to severe intrapartum asphyxia (i.e. 1 mmol/L per 2 min) (Ross & Gala 2002).

Maladaptation at birth

This refers to the baby who is born in a less than optimal condition, and this can be measured as a low Apgar score or delay in establishing spontaneous respiration. Failure of adaptive mechanisms is most likely to occur in preterm infants and does not imply that the baby has suffered a significant hypoxic–ischemic event immediately prior to birth.

Dr. Virginia Apgar, an obstetrical anesthesiologist, first described the scoring system which now bears her name (Apgar 1953). She developed a simple scoring system based on a sum of five numbers, aimed at assessing the effect of obstetrical practice on the clinical condition immediately after birth, i.e. at 60 seconds of life. An additional score obtained at 5 min of age gained universal acceptance after the report from the Collaborative Study on Cerebral Palsy showed a stronger relation between the 5 min score and neonatal mortality than the 1 min score (Drage et al 1964). While the Apgar score is effective for describing the infant's condition shortly after birth, and while it will remain a valid method to assess the effectiveness of resuscitative efforts and the vitality of the infant, it was never intended to be a measure of perinatal asphyxia. The 5-minute score has the inherent problem of poor inter-observer variability (O'Donnell et al 2006) and it may also be influenced by non-asphyxial factors such as prematurity and maternal drug (opiate) depression. Donald (1959) defined 'asphyxia neonatorum' as failure to establish spontaneous ventilation at birth, but there may be many causes for this, including depression of ventilation due to drugs, trauma and, rarely, neuromuscular disorders affecting the onset of spontaneous breathing. Delay in spontaneous respiratory activity is not a good predictor of neurological disability (Ergander et al 1983).

It is therefore not surprising that the score is a very weak predictor of those infants who are later identified as having neurodevelopmental deficits caused by perinatal asphyxia (see p. 573). Nevertheless, depression of the Apgar score has been widely used in diagnosing perinatal asphyxia, and a score of 3 or less at 5 min is often taken as indicating a severe asphyxial insult (Ergander et al 1983, Nelson & Ellenberg 1981).

Attempts have been made to identify babies at high risk of neonatal seizures on the basis of very early neonatal markers. Poor condition, as measured by the combination of three factors at birth (Apgar score of 5 at 5 min, the need for intubation and a cord blood pH of 7.00), has been reported to increase the risk of neonatal seizures (and presumably disability) 340-fold (Perlman & Risser 1996).

Hypoxic–ischemic encephalopathy

Disturbances in the neurological behavior of the infant following birth may be a sensitive indicator of significant cerebral asphyxial insult. Hypoxic–ischemic encephalopathy (HIE) is a term used to describe a consistent pattern of neurological signs that progress in a regular manner. The clinical features of HIE are described on page 552. HIE is not the only cause of encephalopathy in the newborn period (Nelson & Leviton 1991), and alternative causes must be considered and excluded before HIE can be reliably used as a feature of neurological deficit. In particular, neonatal convulsions alone with clinical interseizure normality are not a feature of HIE, nor is the baby who shows an unchanging pattern of neurological abnormalities in the newborn period. It has been suggested that in the majority of cases, 'neonatal encephalopathy' in full-term babies may not be due to intrapartum events, but may originate in the antepartum period (Adamson et al 1995).

It is likely that intrapartum asphyxia severe enough to cause neurodevelopmental handicap will be associated with clinical neurological dysfunction, and if no abnormalities occur, the infant appears to be at little risk. Unfortunately, HIE must be a retrospective diagnosis and does not appear to correlate well with the Apgar score (Levene et al 1986).

Multiorgan involvement

There is consensus of opinion amongst representative obstetric and pediatric associations that multiorgan dysfunction (MOD) is a constant feature in infants with post-asphyxial HIE (Shah et al 2004). The scope of organ involvement in perinatal asphyxia varies among series, depending in part upon the definitions used for asphyxia and organ dysfunction. Shah et al (2004) report a retrospective study of 130 term infants with asphyxia, in which dysfunction was present in the following organ systems: pulmonary (86%), hepatic (85%), renal (70%) and cardiovascular (62%). The kidneys and myocardium are particularly vulnerable. Evidence of acute and transient compromise to more than one organ suggests that an acute asphyxial event in labor was the common pathway by which these organs were affected.

Series have been described of babies who developed HIE with the later development of cerebral palsy and who had no, or only a minor, multiorgan system dysfunction (Pasternak & Gorey 1998, Phelan et al 1998). In most of these cases, intrapartum asphyxia was documented to be of short duration (mean 32 min) and was severe and unexpected, such as occurs with uterine rupture and cord prolapse (Phelan et al 1998).

Nucleated red blood cells (nRBCs, also called normoblasts) in the peripheral blood film have been suggested to be a marker of asphyxia (see p. 560). The fetus responds to O_2 deprivation by diverting blood to the vital organs and by stimulating production and release of erythropoietin, which speeds up erythropoiesis as a means of improving fetal oxygenation. This process results in an increased proportion of immature nRBCs. Asphyxiated full-term infants have a significantly higher nRBC count than non-asphyxiated babies of the same gestational age (Phelan et al 1995). There is no statistically significant difference in the numbers of asphyxiated babies with evidence of a more prolonged asphyxial insult as opposed to a terminal severe asphyxial event. In one study nRBC counts were highest when antenatal bradycardia had lasted longer than 25 min and dropped by 50% 14.8 h after birth (Naeye & Shaffer 2005). Newborn nRBC counts should however not be relied on as the sole determinant of the severity or duration of intra-uterine asphyxia: there is a large overlap between the nRBC values after acute, subacute and chronic asphyxia; asphyxia of any duration does not always cause an increased nRBC count, and extreme increases may be found in normal non-asphyxiated neonates (Hermansen 2001).

Combination of markers

It becomes clear that a single marker of in utero stress provides little useful information regarding the 'asphyxial process,' and thus, the relationship to neonatal brain injury or subsequent cerebral palsy (Perlman 2006). A constellation of markers carries greater value in identifying infants who are at greatest risk for evolving neonatal brain injury.

Exclusion of alternative possible diagnoses

All the individual features of 'asphyxia' discussed above may occur as the result of alternative causes. Failure to establish spontaneous respirations immediately after birth may be due to maternal opiate administration or, more rarely, neuromuscular disorders. Later-onset encephalopathy may be due to a number of conditions, which can be relatively easily excluded (Table 26.1). Hypoglycemia occurs more commonly in asphyxiated infants and may not be severe enough to cause encephalopathy. Severe and persistent hypoglycemia suggests that the abnormal neurological behavior is more likely to be due to hypoglycemia rather than it being an associated factor. The three groups of conditions that are most commonly misdiagnosed as HIE are the following and should be considered in every case with appropriate investigations if necessary. Investigations for these are described elsewhere in this book.

- Central nervous system infection (Ch. 32).
- Inborn errors of metabolism presenting with early encephalopathy (Ch. 33).
- Congenital brain malformations (Ch. 13).

Routine lumbar puncture, brain imaging, biochemical screening (urine and blood) for inborn errors of metabolism and careful examination for subtle dysmorphic features should be part of the assessment of all infants in whom the diagnosis of asphyxia is suspected.

Contributory diagnostic tests

There are three important diagnostic tests that help to determine whether an acute asphyxial insult has occurred prior to delivery: EEG, imaging and Doppler assessment. Each of these is discussed in detail below. A hypoxic–ischemic event usually causes a consistent abnormality in these tests and this may change with time from the insult. These diagnostic tests may also help with prognosis.

Table 26.1 Exclusion criteria in consideration of the birth asphyxia syndrome

Meningitis
Cerebral hemorrhage
Perinatal stroke
Brain malformation
Dysmorphic or chromosomal conditions
Inborn errors of metabolism
Severe hypoglycemia

Accurate serial head-circumference measurements are simple and important assessments of cerebral injury. Secondary microcephaly is an important sign of acute cerebral injury. If the occipitofrontal head circumference was in the normal range at birth, with rapid slowing in head (brain) growth after birth, then this is an important indicator that an insult had occurred around the time of birth. It is not possible to define the cause of the insult and its timing may have been several days or even weeks prior to delivery.

INCIDENCE

The incidence of birth asphyxia in full-term infants has been variously reported from the USA, Sweden and Britain to be between 1.8 and 9.0 cases per 1000 deliveries (Brown et al 1974, Ergander et al 1983, Finer et al 1981, Levene et al 1985a, MacDonald et al 1980, Nelson & Ellenberg 1981, Thornberg et al 1995a). The incidence of low Apgar scores in babies with birth weights of less than 1500 g is 15-fold higher than infants weighing over 3000 g (Palme-Kilander 1992). In two studies, asphyxia was defined as an Apgar score of 3 or less at 5 min (Ergander et al 1983, Nelson & Ellenberg 1981) and another included all infants who required intermittent positive-pressure ventilation for more than 1 min (MacDonald et al 1980). In a cohort of all babies born in Sweden in 1985, 1.6 per 1000 live-born infants did not breathe spontaneously within 20 min of delivery (Palme-Kilander 1992). In another more recent Swedish study, 6.9 per 1000 live-born term babies had an Apgar score <7 at 5 min (Thornberg et al 1995a).

Three studies reported the incidence of HIE. Brown et al (1974) found that 5.9 per 1000 full-term deliveries showed clinical signs due to intrapartum asphyxia, and in Leicester, Levene et al (1985a) reported an incidence of 6.0 per 1000 inborn infants. Moderate and severe HIE occurred in 1.1 and 1.0 per 1000 infants, respectively. One-quarter of the infants with HIE born in Leicester showed intrauterine growth retardation, which is comparable to the 29% reported by Finer et al (1981). A third study (Sweden) reported 'birth asphyxia with HIE' to occur in 1.8 per 1000 of term births from 1985 to 1991 (Thornberg et al 1995a). Intrauterine growth retardation was six times more common in the asphyxiated than the control group. A recent study from a region in France reported a prevalence of birth asphyxia of 0.86 per 1000 term live births. 56% were thought to arise intrapartum and 13% antepartum (Pierrat et al 2005). In the rest no accurate timing was possible.

The incidence of perinatal asphyxia is much more common in the developing world than in developed countries. The World Health Organization estimates that nearly 4 million newborn infants suffer moderate or severe asphyxia with 'at least 800 000 dying and an equal number developing sequelae such as epilepsy, mental retardation, cerebral palsy and learning disabilities' (WHO 1991). In India, the incidence of death due to birth asphyxia in mature infants was estimated to be 10 per 1000 (Costello & Manandhar 1994). In Nigeria, the incidence of HIE is reported to be 26.5 per 1000 live births (Airedale 1991), i.e. four to five times higher than in Britain and the USA. There is a trend towards a higher prevalence of asphyxia in Africa than Asia (Ellis & Manandhar 1999).

In the West, there appears to have been a reduction in the incidence of asphyxia in full-term infants over recent years. In California, the incidence of birth asphyxia for normal birth weight infants has fallen from 14.8 in 1991 to 1.3 per 1000 live births in 2000 (Wu et al 2004). The incidence of infants with convulsions apparently due to severe asphyxia, born in Montreal in Canada, and weighing more than 2500 g at birth, fell from 1.8 per 1000 in 1960 to 0.7 per 1000 in 1978–1980 (Cyr et al 1984). Figures from Paris (Amiel-Tison 1979) have shown a dramatic fall in the incidence of mild and moderate encephalopathy in full-term infants over a 4-year period. In 1974, the incidence of this condition was 18.9 per 1000 and for the years 1976–1978 it had fallen to 3.9 per 1000. There was, however, no change in the proportion of infants who were stillborn due to intrapartum asphyxia or who had the most severe form of encephalopathy. Two cohorts of full-term infants born in England in 1976–1980 and 1984–1988 showed that there has been a decline in the incidence of HIE from 7.7 per 1000 to 4.6 per 1000 in the intervening 4-year period (Hull & Dodd 1992).

PATHOLOGY

Although we once thought that there was a simple relationship between energy failure and tissue necrosis, we now know that a complex web of biochemical cascades can result in distinct modes of cell death, as well as specific patterns of pathology. Consistent pathological features associated with birth asphyxia have been recognized since the 19th century. Ulegyria, i.e. a mushroom-like gyrus, was first described by Bressler (1899) and status marmoratus or état marbré involving the basal ganglia was reported by Anton (1893). Despite these observations, no single distinct or uniform pathological appearance is recognized following severe hypoxic–ischemic injury. The brain may be globally affected with extensive swelling and necrosis, or pathological lesions may be more focal and discrete. These heterogeneous and clinically unpredictable appearances are related to the variety of pathophysiological insults to which the fetus is exposed. The majority of pathological lesions seen in the brain following asphyxia have been explained either as ischemic injury based on a vascular etiology or as the vulnerability of certain regions of the brain to metabolic injury.

The major factors affecting the development of particular pathological lesions include:

1. *Developmental age at which the insult occurs.* Insults in the first half of pregnancy will lead to disruption of neuronal migration and pachygyria (see p. 238).

Involvement of the white matter occurs commonly in immature infants (periventricular leukomalacia) and often in conjunction with periventricular hemorrhage. This condition, together with subcortical leukomalacia, is discussed in detail in Chapter 21, and this section will deal mainly with neuronal necrosis, which is commonly seen in full-term infants following asphyxia.

2. *The duration between the onset of the insult and the age at which the brain is examined.* Within hours of the insult, the brain may appear grossly normal. In the first 48 h, histological examination may be unremarkable, but later, acidophilic staining of the cytoplasm with pyknosis or nuclear fragmentation is seen (Pape & Wigglesworth 1979). Electron microscopy reveals a diffuse change involving both vascular endothelium and neurons. Hemorrhage may be present on removing the brain from the skull. Subdural bleeding due to tentorial tears may be seen, and subarachnoid hemorrhage is particularly common.

3. *Duration of the insult.* This is discussed in detail in Chapter 22. A very short, but intense insult may cause a different pattern of cerebral injury than a more protracted partial intermittent form of asphyxial compromise. Acute and total asphyxia produced a totally different type of injury involving thalamus, brainstem and spinal cord structures (Myers 1972). When episodes of total asphyxia are superimposed upon episodes of partial asphyxia, mixed lesions may develop.

4. *Partial intermittent asphyxia* has been produced in animal studies by a variety of means, but in all, there has been maintenance of some blood flow despite very low O_2 concentrations. In these studies, brain injury affects primarily the cerebral cortex with severe brain swelling. The distribution of injury is described mainly in areas of brain between the end branches of two vascular territories, i.e. the so-called watershed zones. These regions are extremely vulnerable to decreases in cerebral perfusion pressure. The watershed regions lie anteriorly between the anterior and middle cerebral arteries, primarily in the parasagittal region of the anterior frontal and parietal lobes, and posteriorly between the middle and posterior cerebral arteries in the parasagittal region of the posterior parietal and occipital lobes (Zimmerman et al 2005). There is also an inferior watershed zone in the region of the posterior inferior temporal lobes. Deeper structures in the brain are either spared or significantly less badly affected. Human post-mortem studies have shown a similar distribution of lesions, and imaging studies on surviving children have supported these findings. Watershed territory injuries of the supratentorial brain occur in term fetuses and neonates when there is a gradual reduction in blood flow and oxygenation (e.g.

oligohydramnios producing cord compression, or placental insufficiency, or in the postpartum perinatal period when there are difficulties in resuscitation of the infant). A series of such events occurring over 1 or more hours, or even longer, results in variable injury to either or both the gray and white matter at the site of the watershed zone. Prolongation of the insult can produce a pattern of injury beyond the usual watershed region, including elements of both a partial prolonged asphyxia and profound asphyxia (Zimmerman et al 2005). Over time, severe partial prolonged asphyxia may result in subcortical cystic encephalomalacia, in addition to the finding of a global supratentorial cortical and subcortical atrophy.

Cerebral edema

Within 24–48 h, gross swelling with marked flattening and widening of the gyri and obliteration of the sulci may occur. The brain at this time is soft and very friable. In some cases, cerebral herniation may have occurred with grooving of the uncus and partial cerebellar displacement through the foramen magnum, but this is infrequent. On cutting the brain, the ventricles are slit-like and little cerebrospinal fluid drains out. Protrusion of the infundibulum into the interpeduncular cistern may occur (Larroche 1984).

Brain swelling and intracranial hypertension do not occur in all severely asphyxiated full-term infants (Levene et al 1987, Pryse-Davies & Beard 1973), and the factors involved in their development are not clear. Klatzo (1967) has classified brain edema into two types: vasogenic and cytotoxic. In vasogenic edema, there is an increase in leakiness of the blood–brain barrier, allowing entry of serum proteins into the cerebral parenchyma. The resulting increase in intracerebral osmotic pressure leads to the accumulation of fluid within the extracellular compartment of the brain. Cytotoxic edema is due to the failure of cellular membrane pumps with entry of Na^+ and swelling of the cells. Cytotoxic edema probably occurs earlier and in response to the initial hypoxic–ischemic insult and may affect the gray matter in preference to the white matter (Klatzo 1985). Later, and in response to a less clearly defined insult, the blood–brain barrier opens to proteins. The swollen brain seen at autopsy probably results predominantly from vasogenic edema, and this does not reach a maximum effect until 48 h after birth (Anderson & Belton 1974). In a fetal lamb model, vasogenic edema did not appear to be a significant feature following hypoxic–ischemic insult, at least in the first 24 h (Tweed et al 1981).

Injury to gray matter

It is rare for isolated lesions to occur in only one area of the brain, and multiple or focal sites of involvement are usual, but for the sake of clarity, neuropathological features will be described under separate subheadings. MR studies have recognized two major forms of gray matter brain injury arising as a result of HIE in term infants; the parasagittal (watershed lesion) and basal ganglia involvement. Miller et al (2005) described a total of 173 term newborns with neonatal encephalopathy and reported watershed injury predominant in 45% and basal ganglia/thalamus injury in 25%.

Cortex

In the acute stages following asphyxia, the cerebral cortex may appear normal, but within a week or two, it may become fluctuant to touch and occasionally cystic. On a cut section, the cortex may show a gray-brown discoloration (Larroche 1984). Ulegyria, a macroscopic appearance of gyral sclerosis with widening of the sulci (mushroom-like gyrus), is seen in some infants who have survived the asphyxial event by months or years (Fig. 26.1). This change represents a post-swelling phenomenon in which the vasculature to the base of the gyrus has been compromised by the swelling to a greater extent than at the apex, leading to more severe tissue loss within the gyrus at the depth of

the sulcus (Villani et al 2003). Ulegyria thus most likely is a watershed insult (see below). Microscopically, cortical involvement may be focal or diffuse and may preferentially involve certain cortical layers, notably III and V, with II being well preserved (Larroche 1984). This may be due to relative differences in metabolic rate (Farkas-Bargeton & Diebler 1978). The hippocampus is particularly vulnerable to hypoxic insults, and partial or total destruction of pyramid cells within this area is almost invariable following significant cerebral asphyxic injury (Larroche 1977). Other particularly vulnerable areas include the pre- and postcentral gyri and the visual cortex around the calcarine fissure.

Parasagittal (watershed) injury

Progressive periods of asphyxial insult cause increased neuronal loss as the duration of insult lengthens (Williams et al 1992), but the cerebrum is not uniformly affected. Severe asphyxia in mature fetal sheep produces selective

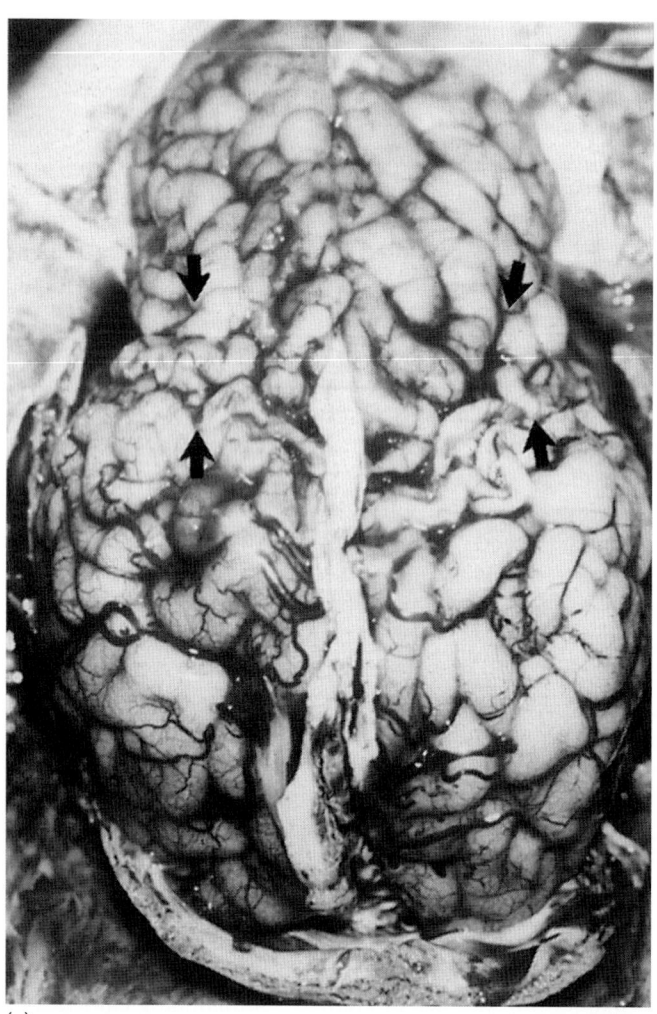

(a)

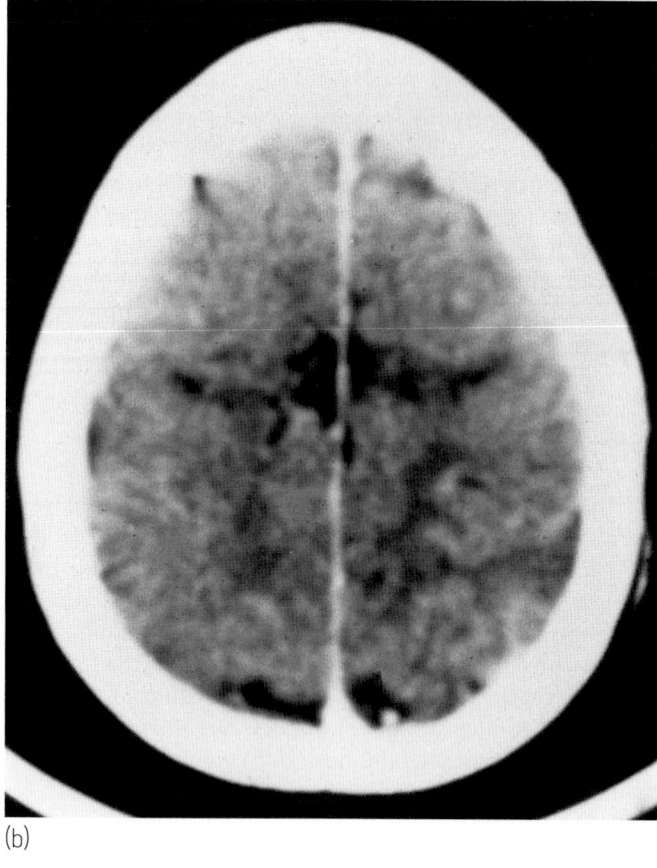

(b)

Figure 26.1 Ulegyria. (a) There is sclerosis and cortical atrophy of the brain in the region between the anterior and middle cerebral arteries (arrows). (b) Computerized tomography scan showing areas of low attenuation representing ulegyria in the central corticosubcortical area.

damage in the regions of the parasagittal cortex and striatum (Gunn et al 1992). Volpe (1977) has drawn particular attention to the parasagittal injury seen in full-term asphyxiated infants. Cortical necrosis occurring at the junction between the territories of the anterior, middle and posterior cerebral arteries (i.e. watershed zones) has been produced experimentally in animals (Brierley et al 1969) and recognized at autopsy in the brains of children (Adams et al 1966). These authors have related this boundary zone injury to hypotension affecting the region between major arterial distribution. Similar lesions (Fig. 26.2) have been produced in fetal monkeys by inducing maternal hypotension for 1–5 h (Brann & Myers 1975). Parasagittal cerebral injury thus refers to bilateral cortical and adjacent subcortical white matter necrosis that involves the superior medial, and particularly, the posterior aspects of the cerebral convexities (Perlman 2006).

This lesion has been diagnosed during life by means of technetium brain scans (Volpe & Pasternak 1977) or positron emission tomography (Volpe et al 1985). Seventeen infants with evidence of significant postasphyxial encephalopathy were studied within the first 5 days. There was a consistent, symmetrical decrease in cerebral blood flow (CBF) of up to 50% to the parasagittal regions that was more marked posteriorly than anteriorly.

The upper extremities are affected more severely than are the lower extremities, since the injury predominantly involves the cortex that subserves proximal extremity motor function (Volpe 2001). Spastic quadriplegia is the most frequent long-term consequence of injury to the watershed region.

Subcortical structures

The region immediately below the cortical ribbon is particularly vulnerable to the effects of perinatal asphyxia due to the temporary vascular watershed exposed in full-term infants. As ventriculofugal arteries develop between 32 and 44 weeks gestational age, such development is believed to shift the watershed region from periventricular at preterm to cortical at term, explaining a centrifugal shift of injury with brain maturity (Grant & Yu 2006). In the term infant, cortical and subcortical structures at the depths of sulci are particularly likely to develop infarction (Fig. 26.3) and may evolve to subcortical leukomalacia (see p. 454) or multicystic leukoencephalopathy (MCLE, see below).

Barth et al (1984) have described a pattern of injury that occurs as the result of asphyxia in the central corticosubcortical area (Figs 26.1b and 26.4). This is the primary motor and sensory cortical areas. The distribution of this injury cannot be explained on the basis of a watershed distribution, and it is thought that infarction occurs as a result of the increased metabolic rate of these neurons during asphyxia. This lesion gives a typical appearance on computerized tomography (CT) (Barth et al 1984).

Basal ganglia

Pathological studies of term neonates who succumbed to a profound hypoxic–ischemic event show relative cortical sparing and deep gray matter injury, particularly involving hippocampi, lateral geniculate nuclei, putamen, ventrolateral thalami and dorsal mesencephalon. These regions have high concentrations of excitatory amino acids (glutamate,

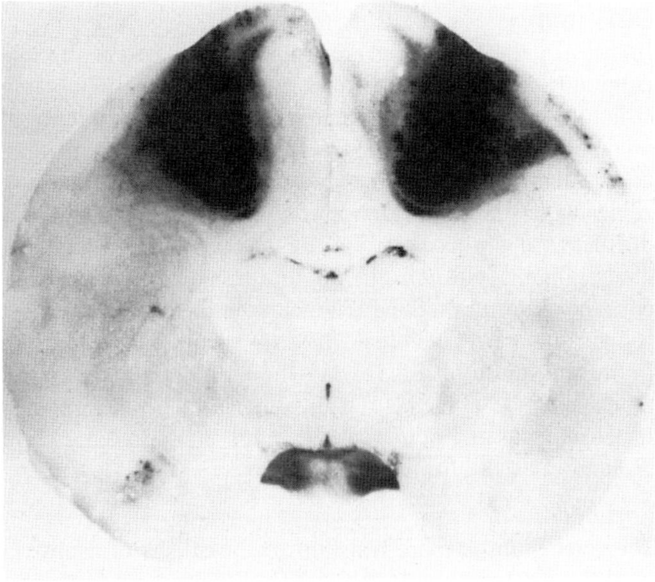

Figure 26.2 Parasagittal injury. Coronal section through a fetal monkey brain showing an asphyxial injury similar to the parasagittal watershed lesion. (Reproduced, with permission, from Brann and Myers 1975.)

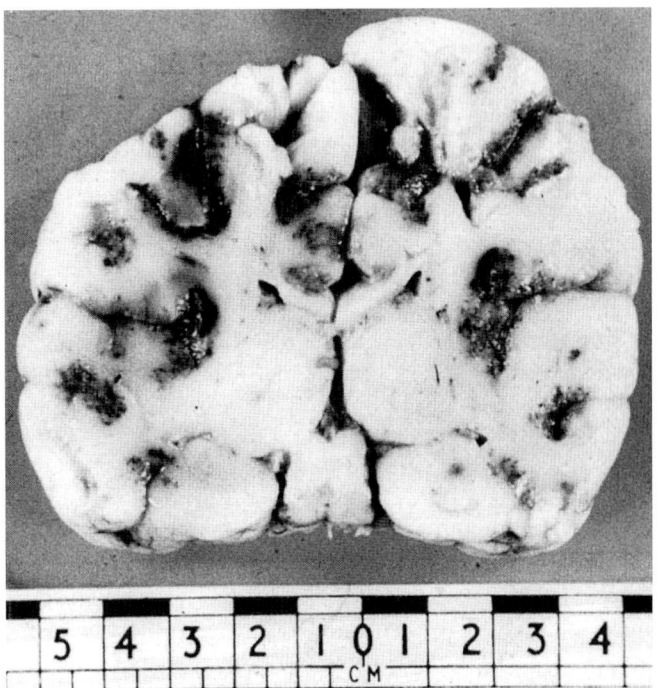

Figure 26.3 Deep cortical and subcortical hemorrhagic necrosis. The depths of the sulci are most severely involved.

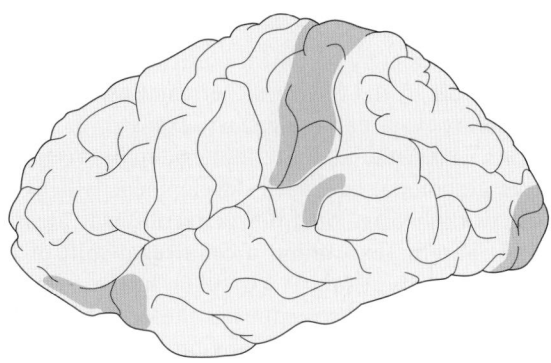

Figure 26.4 Distribution of vulnerable cortical and subcortical injury. (Redrawn, with permission, from Barth et al 1984 © Masson Editeur.)

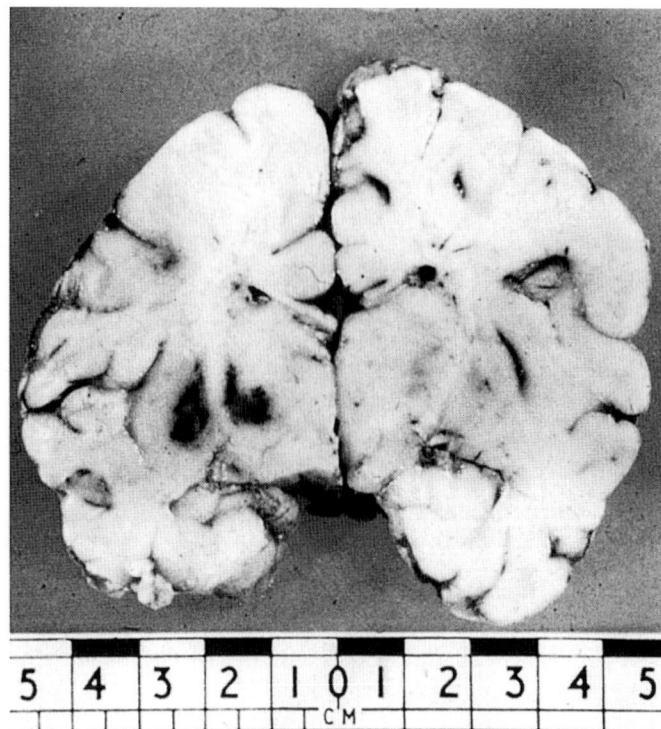

Figure 26.5 Hemorrhagic infarction of the left basal ganglion. Both the lentiform nucleus and lateral thalamus are involved, with the white matter or the internal capsule being spared.

aspartate) and corresponding NMDA receptors. Excessive stimulation of these receptors results in depolarization of neuronal membranes, excessive calcium influx, activation of lipases and proteases, generation of free fatty acids and free radicals, mitochondrial dysfunction, depletion of energy stores and ultimate neuronal death (Grant & Yu 2006).

Status marmoratus is the classic neuropathological lesion affecting the basal ganglia and is seen only in infants who survive the asphyxia by many months. This is a visible marble-like appearance of the thalamus and basal ganglia and is due to abnormal myelination. Rorke (1982) states that this is a rare condition and is uncommonly seen even in infants who survive for many years after severe asphyxial insults. Rorke found lesions confined to the basal ganglia in only 3% of perinatal autopsies, but these lesions were relatively commonly seen together with more extensive cerebral injury. The majority of infants with selective damage to the thalamus had frank infarction with or without hemorrhage. Cystic infarction is also seen, and in some cases has been related to maternal drug addiction (Rorke 1982). Lesions apparent in the thalamus usually indicate more extensive involvement throughout the central nervous system.

Hemorrhage or hemorrhagic infarction involving the basal ganglia is seen frequently following birth asphyxia in full-term infants (Fig. 26.5). Such consistent abnormality involving the thalamus and basal ganglia has been reported in surviving severely asphyxiated newborn infants (Kotagel et al 1983, Morimoto et al 1985) and is especially associated with acute, near total intrauterine asphyxia at the end of labor (Pasternak & Gorey 1998). These lesions have been recognized on ultrasound, CT and magnetic resonance imaging (MRI) (Barkovich 1992, Eken et al 1994, Miller et al 2005 Pasternak & Gorey 1998, Voit et al 1987). Autopsy correlation suggests that this may be due to capillary proliferation and microcalcification. This may reflect evolving status marmoratus and, when these appearances are seen, the prognosis is very poor. They should not be confused with a unilateral thalamic hemorrhage (see p. 420). Scanning children at a later stage may reveal symmetrical bi-thalamic

calcification (Colamaria et al 1988), and this also appears to be a good marker of previous severe asphyxial injury (Fig. 26.6). MR scans in infancy may show these characteristic abnormalities of the basal ganglia (Fig. 26.7).

Brainstem

Injuries to the brainstem are usually associated with concomitant lesions to the basal ganglia. The most vulnerable structure is the inferior colliculus, probably due to its high metabolic rate, but the reticular formation, lateral geniculate bodies and pontine nuclei may also be involved. Leech and Alvord (1977) found evidence of brainstem lesions in 15 out of 16 (93%) brains that they examined. Lesions from the diencephalon, through the midbrain, pons, medulla and cord, have been described (Schneider et al 1975). Brainstem lesions are rarely evident on macroscopic examination. Brainstem injury also involving the basal ganglia has been reported to be associated with abnormal eye movements, facial diplegia and poor sucking reflex in a surviving child (Roland et al 1988).

Cerebellum

The cerebellum is more resistant to the effects of asphyxia than the cerebrum, and pathological involvement following perinatal asphyxia has been reported infrequently. The dentate nuclei, Purkinje cells and internal granular layers appear to be most vulnerable. Interestingly, the external granular layer is usually normal (Larroche 1977). Bilateral

CHAPTER
26

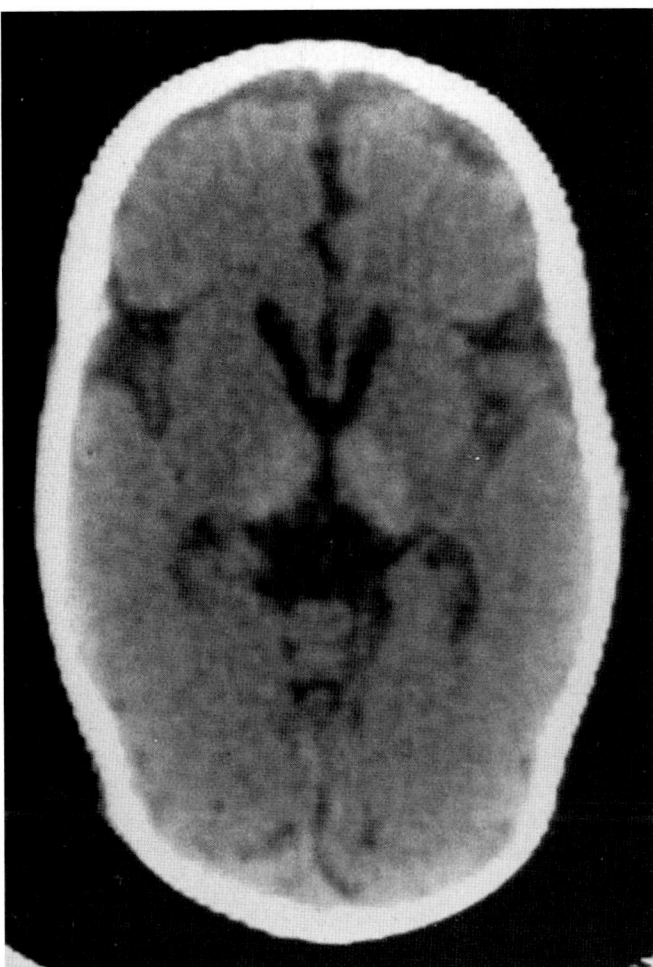

Figure 26.6 Bright thalami seen on a CT scan in an infant who had suffered from severe birth asphyxia some months earlier. The high attenuation was due to calcification. Note also the generalized cerebral atrophy.

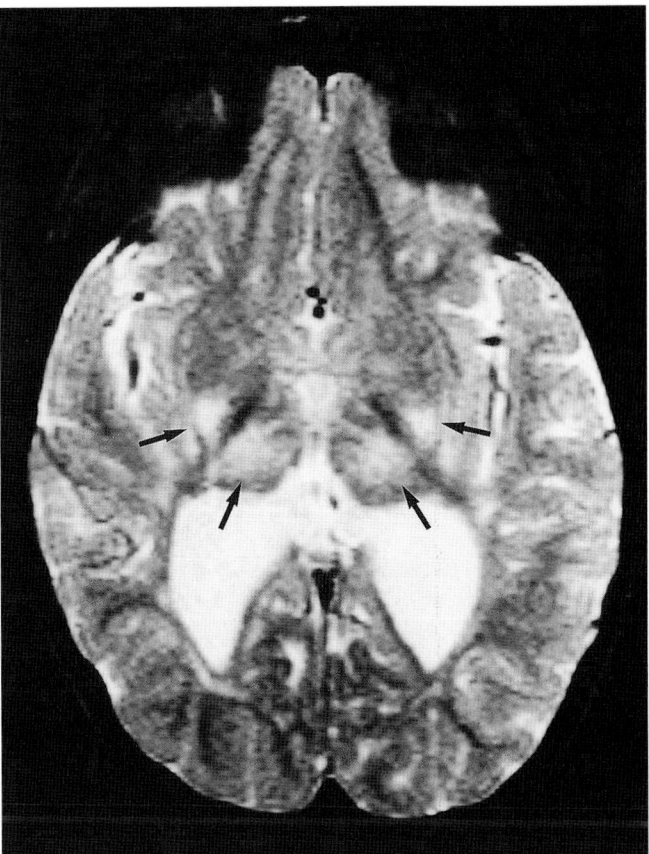

Figure 26.7 Axial MR scan showing abnormal T2 signal in the thalami and the lentiform nuclei (arrows) in a 2-year-old child with a dystonic form of cerebral palsy.

lesions may occur in the watershed region between the two superior and inferior cerebellar arteries (Friede 1975). Occipital diastasis may cause local trauma to the cerebellum and is described in Chapter 20. One-third of infants found at post-mortem to have obvious brain swelling showed cerebellar herniation (Pryse-Davies & Beard 1973).

Spinal cord

Lesions within the cord are rarely obvious on macroscopic examination, but evidence of asphyxial injury is present microscopically. The gracile and cuneate nuclei, nuclei of the medulla oblongata and the anterior horn cells are particularly vulnerable. Trauma to the spinal cord may be associated with intrapartum asphyxia (see Ch. 39).

Multicystic leukoencephalopathy (MCLE)

Multicystic leukoencephalopathy (MCLE) is a rare, but well-recognized, form of pathology that is seen as the end result of severe hypoxic–ischemic insult. MCLE occurs in mature babies and is very rarely reported to occur below 35 weeks

of gestational age. In an MR study of 65 surviving term infants with perinatal asphyxia and brain injury, 15% showed MCLE (Tekgul et al 2004). Multiple areas of cavitation form a honeycomb appearance of the cortex and subcortical white matter. The gyral shape is usually not distorted and is maintained by the molecular layer and leptomeninges. Cavitation is most common in the distribution of the carotid arterial supply (frontal, parietal and temporal lobes), and the occipital region is severely involved less commonly. The brainstem and cerebellum are spared. Imaging studies (Keeney et al 1991) have shown a similar distribution of cavities to autopsy studies (Fig. 26.8).

The babies have usually sustained clear evidence of intrapartum asphyxial insult, although the type of insult is variable. Acute compromise such as placental abruption, more sustained partial intermittent asphyxia and severe fetomaternal hemorrhage have all been implicated in its causation. MCLE has also been reported as the result of very severe insults in the neonatal period including cardiovascular collapse and meningitis (Frigieri et al 1996). The babies show markedly abnormal neurological behavior with grade III (severe) encephalopathy.

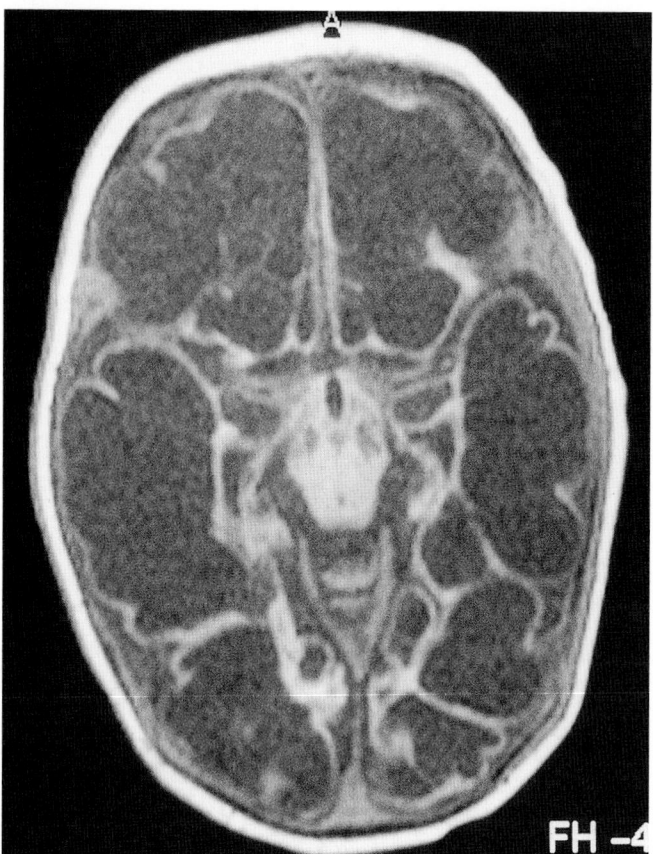

Figure 26.8 Multicystic leukoencephalopathy. Axial MR T1 weighted image showing extensive cavitation with destruction of most of the cerebral tissue in this section.

It is not clear what the underlying pathophysiology is that results in MCLE, and its evolution is unpredictable. Two explanations have been advanced. In the first, it is suggested that severe edema and the high water content of the immature brain cause a further impairment of cerebral blood flow (Friede 1975). We have anecdotally recognized clinical evidence of severe brain swelling preceding the development of extensive cavitation in a number of cases. An alternative hypothesis is that it is due to intense vasospasm in the distribution of the carotid vasculature rather than the vertebrobasilar vessels that are devoid of sympathetic innervation (Sheth et al 1995). This accounts for the distribution of the cavitation.

CLINICAL FEATURES

Mature infants exposed to a period of asphyxia usually show a definite and predictable sequence of neurological symptoms and signs. The relationship between an acute hypoxic-ischemic event and a sequence of abnormal signs has been described in infants who have sustained 'near-miss sudden infant death syndrome' and who had previously been normal. A number of these babies showed a consistent progression of signs, including an initial period of near normality fol-

lowed by seizures, deterioration in conscious level and deepening coma (Constantinou et al 1989). This sequence is very similar to that seen in severely asphyxiated infants. Premature babies may also show a similar sequence of neurological abnormalities (Niijima & Levene 1989), but this is uncommon, and HIE is only reliably seen in the full-term neonate.

The severity and progression of symptoms depend on the intensity of the hypoxic–ischemic event. The reason for the regular progression is not clear but certainly reflects pathophysiological changes in terms of CBF, cerebral metabolism and increase in brain swelling. Some of the clinical features, such as differential tone between upper and lower limbs, can be explained on the basis of parasagittal vascular injury (Volpe 2001). Chapter 9 details the clinical assessment and the features seen in infants with birth asphyxia. In this section, discussion is confined to the progression and clinical grading of HIE.

Sarnat and Sarnat (1976) were the first to devise a method describing the progression of symptoms in asphyxiated full-term infants and combined it together with EEG activity. The clinical stages are shown in Table 26.2. Subsequently, a number of methods based on the Sarnat scheme have been described that can be used to refer to the maximum level of neurological abnormality in mature infants (Amiel-Tison 1979, Amiel-Tison & Ellison 1986, Fenichel 1983, Finer et al 1981, Levene et al 1985a). All these methods utilize a three-point grading system referring to mild, moderate and severe abnormality.

Mild encephalopathy

These infants show no alteration in conscious level but appear to be 'hyperalert'. They spend more time in an awake and restless state, often with staring eyes. They show excessive response to stimulation and are jittery with spontaneous or exaggerated Moro reflexes. The infant's passive limb tone is normal, but there is usually some mild increase on assessment of active tone. When held in a sitting position, some head lag is noticeable, but the tone in the neck extensors is relatively increased compared with the flexors. Limb reflexes are normal or slightly increased, but sustained ankle clonus may be elicitable. Clinically apparent seizures do not occur. The sucking reflex is often weak and the infants need encouragement to complete feeds. Sarnat and Sarnat (1976) found the duration of mild encephalopathy to range between 1.5 and 18 h, but we allow up to 48 h for complete recovery to occur (Levene et al 1985a). Amiel-Tison and Ellison (1986) allow up to 7 days for complete recovery in mild encephalopathy.

Moderate encephalopathy

The main features of this condition are seizures and lethargy with a reduction in spontaneous movements. These infants are slower to react to stimuli and their responses may be incomplete. A somewhat higher threshold is usually necessary before a reaction is seen. The infants lie in a more hypotonic posture with abducted arms and legs. A consistent

Table 26.2 Clinical grading system for post-asphyxial encephalopathy (Sarnat & Sarnat 1976 © American Medical Society)

	Mild (1)	Moderate (2)	Severe (3)
LEVEL OF CONSCIOUSNESS	Hyperalert	Lethargic	Stuporose
NEUROMUSCULAR CONTROL			
Muscle tone	Normal	Mild hypotonia	Flaccid
Posture	Mild distal flexion	Strong distal flexion	Intermittent decerebration
Stretch reflexes	Overactive	Overactive	Decreased or absent
SEGMENTAL MYOCLONUS	Present	Present	Absent
COMPLEX REFLEXES			
Suck	Weak	Weak or absent	Absent
Moro	Strong: low threshold	Weak: incomplete; high threshold	Absent
Oculovestibular	Normal	Overactive	Weak or absent
Tonic neck	Slight	Strong	Absent
Autonomic function	Generalized sympathetic	Generalized parasympathetic	Both systems depressed
Pupils	Mydriasis	Miosis	Variable; often unequal; poor light reflex
Heart rate	Tachycardia	Bradycardia	Variable
Bronchial and salivary secretions	Sparse	Profuse	Variable
Gastrointestinal motility	Normal or decreased	Increased; diarrhoea	Variable
Seizures	None	Common; focal or multifocal	Uncommon (excluding decerebration)

feature is differential tone between upper and lower limbs. The arms show much less spontaneous movement and are relatively hypotonic compared with the legs (Volpe & Pasternak 1977). Tendon jerks are exaggerated and the Moro reflex incomplete. Autonomic function is largely parasympathetic with relative bradycardia and constricted pupils. The sucking reflex is poor and feeding incomplete; tube feeding is usually necessary. Onset of convulsions is most common after 12 h from birth but may be seen earlier. They may be subtle or fragmentary and relatively easy to control pharmacologically. Sarnat and Sarnat (1976) found that these infants showed abnormal behavior for a mean of 4.7 days. Complete recovery (if it occurs) may take several weeks, but some improvement is usually seen by the end of the first week.

Severe encephalopathy

These infants are comatose with severe hypotonia and usually require respiratory support from birth. They are profoundly hypotonic with no spontaneous movements. Seizures are frequent and may be prolonged. The most severely asphyxiated infants of this group may have no seizure activity associated with an iso-electric EEG. Tendon jerks and primitive reflexes are usually absent. The infants have no

suck reflex but may show abnormal sucking-like seizure movements. Pupils are fixed and dilated or react only sluggishly to light. Infants who die due to asphyxia all have severe encephalopathy. With recovery, the infants may show a progression from hypotonia to extensor hypertonicity (Brown et al 1974). Some infants can recover fully, but this may take up to 6 weeks.

Both moderate and severe encephalopathies follow a progression of clinical signs. In the first few hours, the infant may breathe spontaneously and show increasing tone and movement activity. Seizures initially appear to be subtle and then become more overt and last for a longer time with progression of the encephalopathy. The infant later becomes more hypotonic and enters a period of stabilization, although seizures may continue to be a problem. Subsequently, signs of clinical recovery occur in some infants. Others show changes in their pattern of neurological abnormality predictive of severe neurodevelopmental sequelae.

The timing and distribution of abnormal neurological signs may correlate with the type of asphyxial insult and the distribution of ensuing brain injury. Infants in whom HIE developed after severe acute asphyxial insult and who were shown to have permanent brain impairment tended to have earlier seizure onset (mean 6.6 h) compared with a mean onset of 11.1 h in infants with evidence of a more protracted aspyhxial insult (Ahn et al 1998). Specific patterns of abnormal neurological signs have been reported in babies with differing distribution of anatomical brain lesions due to asphyxia. Full-term infants with predominantly basal ganglia involvement on MR imaging are reported to show persistent and diffuse neurological abnormalities compared with those who sustain injury mainly in the white matter who show a different clinical pattern with improved sucking reflex and less severe abnormalities in tone (Mercuri et al 1999).

INVESTIGATIONS

The diagnosis of birth asphyxia is usually made on clinical criteria. Evidence for intrapartum compromise such as fetal bradycardia, passage of meconium, CTG abnormalities, low Apgar scores, or delay in establishing respiration will alert the clinician to the condition, and the subsequent evolution of clinical signs and symptoms is usually sufficient to make a firm diagnosis of HIE. Early assessment of the degree of HIE can provide prognostic information for both clinical management and the potential use of cerebroprotective strategies. However, some infants present late to the clinician, information on intrapartum events may be absent or incomplete, and clinical assessment may prove difficult because the neurological state of the infant may be altered by pharmacological interventions such as sedation, muscle relaxation or anti-convulsant treatment. Further investigations may thus be necessary to elucidate the cause of the neurological abnormalities, or to monitor an asphyxiated infant who receives neuromuscular paralysis, or to provide prognostic information in the acute stages of HIE. This is further discussed in the section on outcome.

It is important to consider alternative causes for encephalopathy in every baby thought to have been asphyxiated. Since meningitis is the most common treatable condition that may cause similar symptoms to HIE, a lumbar puncture should be considered in all infants who are encephalopathic. Asphyxia and neonatal meningitis may occur in the same infant.

Imaging

Imaging techniques such as ultrasound, CT and MR imaging have been used to study the neonatal brain following birth asphyxia. Details of these techniques together with examples of pathology are discussed in Chapter 6.

In practice, all infants with moderate or severe postasphyxial encephalopathy should have a routine ultrasound scan performed within 48 h of birth. Clinically significant and treatable lesions should be suspected by this technique, particularly if a midline shift is present. A convexity subdural or subarachnoid hemorrhage will require CT or MR scanning to delineate its precise position and its response to treatment if this is undertaken (Fig. 26.9). Note that ultrasound is of limited value in evaluating watershed injuries in the term infant. When performed through the anterior

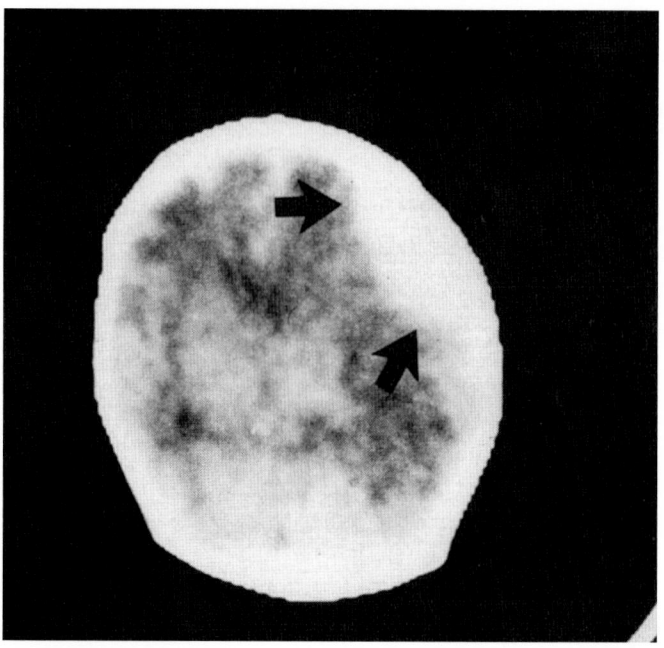

Figure 26.9 CT scan showing convexity left-sided hemorrhage (arrow) present in a severely asphyxiated infant. Note the midline shift and extensive areas of low attenuation.

fontanel, significant portions of the most common sites for watershed infarction can be missed, i.e. the anterosuperior frontal lobes, the superior posterior parietal and occipital lobes. In addition, cranial sonography is an insensitive tool for identifying milder white matter abnormalities that can be appreciated on head MR imaging (Miller et al 2003).

MR (spectroscopy and imaging) has shown, through serial studies, that brain injury evolves over days after a hypoxic-ischemic insult (Azzopardi et al 1989, Ferriero 2004, Martin & Barkovich 1995, Penrice et al 1996). The precise sequence depends on the type of asphyxial insult and the region of brain most compromised.

- Using MR imaging, in the first 2–3 days, a low signal on T1-weighted images and a high signal on T2-weighted images is seen. In acute total asphyxia, signal changes may be particularly present in the lentiform nucleus as well as other parts of the basal ganglia and along the corticospinal tracts. Following severe partial intermittent asphyxia, the abnormal signal may be particularly obvious in the vascular boundary zones.
- By 4–5 days, T1 shortening becomes evident in the abnormal area.
- At about 7 days, T1 shortening becomes most pronounced and may persist for 4 weeks or more.
- A low signal on T2-weighted images slowly develops over the first month and may persist for 2–3 months. In babies with the most severe form of asphyxia, MR abnormalities tend to occur in areas of developing or established myelination (Martin & Barkovich 1995).

Cowan et al (2003) used conventional MR imaging or post-mortem examination in 351 full-term infants with neonatal encephalopathy and/or early seizures to distinguish between lesions acquired antenatally and those that developed in the immediate perinatal period (i.e. intra- and early post-partum). Infants were divided into those with neonatal encephalopathy (with or without seizures) plus evidence of perinatal asphyxia (group 1), versus those who presented with seizures within 3 days of birth without other evidence of encephalopathy (group 2). The data strongly suggest for both groups that events in the immediate perinatal period are most important in neonatal brain injury.

Diffusion-weighted MR imaging (DWI) has further improved our ability to time the onset of brain lesions, as the technique can identify injury at early stages, owing to its ability to detect subtle alterations in brain water (Bydder & Rutherford 2001). In most cases, neonatal hypoxic–ischemic brain injury can be detected on DWI within 23 h of life, but the sensitivity of DWI changes over time (Barkovich et al 2001). The apparent diffusion coefficient (ADC) decreases with an acute injury, possibly due to (1) a decrease in extracellular fluid caused by cellular swelling (cytotoxic edema), swelling of mitochondria, reduction of cytoplasmic diffusion, (2) axonal swelling, and (3) other mechanisms, such as membrane changes caused by fatty acid peroxidation (Hüppi 2002). The reduction in ADC that occurs with brain injury in the term newborn evolves over the initial days of life and normalizes over the second week. Diffusion MRI therefore provides a dynamic window on evolving neonatal brain injury. In addition, serial diffusion tensor imaging can detect differences in the maturation of white matter, providing detailed and quantifiable data regarding brain development in injured newborns (Miller 2002b).

MR imaging with calculation of DWI should thus be done as soon as clinically possible (see also Ch. 6 for sequence of changes seen on MR). The role of DWI and MR spectroscopy is to provide early detection of injury (usually by day 1), to determine the pattern of injury, and to assess the severity and extent of the injury. DWI is the most sensitive and successful technique for detection of the earliest changes of parasagittal injury owing to partial prolonged asphyxia (Wolf et al 2001). Often a second MR between day 5 and 8 is helpful to rule out progression and determine the evolution of injury, as white matter injury may not be evident until this time (Grant 2006). After day 8, DWI is often insensitive but in neonates with HIE, T1 and T2 weighted abnormalities are typically easily identified.

Using MR imaging and acute neonatal diffusion-weighted MR imaging (DWI) there are primarily three patterns of brain injury that can be identified (Grant & Yu 2006).

1. The central pattern involves the ventrolateral thalamus, posterior putamen, hippocampi, corticospinal tract or perirolandic cortex. This pattern is thought to result when there is profound hypoxia and ischemia lasting for a relatively short period (minutes) ('near total

asphyxia') in brain regions with high energy demand. Very severe near total asphyxia (e.g. fetal bradycardia of 30 min) can show the classic profound pattern of injury, but with a cortical involvement beyond the perirolandic cortex.

2. A peripheral pattern involves the cortex and white matter, however with sparing of the ventrolateral thalamus, corticospinal tract or perirolandic cortex. This pattern is thought to result from a more global brain hypoxia and ischemia, that is more prolonged (hours) but less profound ('partial prolonged asphyxia'). It involves parasagittal lesions, i.e. lesions at the vascular border zones between anterior, middle and posterior cerebral arteries (watershed pattern). Watershed injuries may be predominantly one sided; the reasons for this asymmetry in a setting of a global hypoxic–ischemic injury are unknown.

3. Finally one can observe a focal pattern, i.e. also called vascular territory lesions.

Cerebral edema

Generally, in a newborn term infant with a large enough injury, edema becomes visible on ultrasound, CT and T2-weighted MR imaging by 24 h post-event and increases to peak edema by 72 h. Cerebral edema may be recognized on ultrasound imaging as a generalized increase in echodensity throughout the brain, loss of normal anatomical landmarks and slit-like ventricles after 24 h of life (Babcock & Ball 1983, Martin et al 1983, Skeffington & Pearse 1983).

The CT appearance of cerebral edema includes extensive areas of low attenuation, which appears to be related to the severity of the asphyxial insult (for examples, see p. 554). However, the white matter in a term newborn brain contains high water content, and therefore milder degrees of edema and white matter injury can be difficult to appreciate on head CT. Moderate or severe involvement affecting white matter or cortex occurs in approximately 40% of asphyxiated full-term infants examined by CT (Adsett et al 1985, Finer et al 1983, Fitzhardinge et al 1981, Flodmark et al 1980, Lipp-Zwahlen et al 1985a, Magilner & Wertheimer 1980, Schrumpf et al 1980). This represents a high-risk group of infants who were selected for scanning in view of the severity of their neurological involvement.

Signs of brain swelling on an MR scan were seen in almost all infants scanned within 5 days of life with HIE and disappeared rapidly after this time (Rutherford et al 1995). Abnormalities include small extracerebral space, loss of the sylvian fissures, narrowing of the interhemispheric fissure and slit-like anterior horns of the lateral ventricles. Diffusion-weighted MR imaging can detect, but may overestimate, areas of cytotoxic edema, in which cystic changes may gradually develop (Roelants-van Rijn, 2001a).

Basal ganglia

The basal ganglia show a variety of abnormalities following birth asphyxia, including echodensity confined to the region of the basal ganglia (Levene et al 1985b, Shen et al 1986).

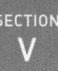

This latter condition (see p. 92) has been reported only rarely and has been assumed to be due to edema, but Shen et al (1986) report that the increase in echoes persists for over 6 months in some cases; this is far too long to be due to edema. CT and MRI have shown local lesions apparently confined to the thalamus (Morimoto et al 1985, Rutherford et al 1995, Shewman et al 1981, Voit et al 1985) (see Figs 26.6 and 26.7). These appearances may be due to infarction, edema, calcification or hemorrhage (Kotagel et al 1983). Shewman et al (1981) have reported that the high-attenuation thalamic lesions show considerable enhancement on infusion of radiopaque dye, suggesting that they are due to postischemic hypervascularity. The distinction between the bilateral thalamic density and thalamic hemorrhage is discussed in detail in Chapter 6.

DWI abnormalities in central patterns of injury caused by profound insults may underestimate the degree of injury on follow-up, but typically brainstem involvement on acute DWI or markedly decreased ADCs in the posterior limb internal capsule involve a poorer prognosis (Hunt et al 2004).

Posterior limb of the internal capsule (PLIC)

Since the PLIC is the first area to myelinate in the immature brain, loss of T1-weighted signal in this region is a reliable and early indicator of severe hypoxic–ischemic injury (Rutherford et al 1998). A second early MR marker of post-asphyxial injury is the abnormal high T1-weighted signal in the deep portions of the pre- and postcentral gyri.

Cortical abnormality

Cortical abnormality is seen on ultrasound imaging only if a very high frequency (10-MHz transducer) is routinely used. These changes occur between 48 and 72 h (Eken et al 1994) and correlate with laminar necrosis on histology. Cortical/subcortical changes are well recognized also on MR imaging and may represent a breakdown of deep white matter (Rutherford et al 1995). Often loss of gray-white distinction can be seen by 2 days on T2-weighted images in areas with cortical involvement (Grant & Yu 2006). Regions of bright DWI signal in peripheral patterns of injury involve both white matter and cortex.

Multicystic leukomalacia

Multicystic leukomalacia, involving the periventricular region, and subcortical leukomalacia (see p. 454) have also been diagnosed by ultrasound following severe birth asphyxia (Babcock & Ball 1983, Frigieri et al 1996, Levene et al 1985b, Martin et al 1983, Tekgul et al 2004, Trounce & Levene 1985).

Intracranial hemorrhage

Asphyxiated infants show a high incidence of intracranial hemorrhage diagnosed by various imaging techniques. Their incidence ranges from 19 to 73% of at-risk infants (Adsett et al 1985, Finer et al 1983, Fitzhardinge et al 1981, Flodmark et al 1980, Gerard et al 1981, Lipp-Zwahlen et al 1985a, Magilner & Wertheimer 1980). Analysis of cumula-tive data gives an overall risk of hemorrhage of approximately 30% in infants showing clinical evidence of significant asphyxia. More than half of the lesions are due to subarachnoid hemorrhage. Also, watershed infarctions may become reperfused by blood flow within arterioles. In the reperfusion situation, the blood vessels involved at the site of watershed damage are injured. As a result, rupture of the wall of the damaged arterioles occurs, leading to bleeding within the brain tissue located in the watershed zone (Zimmerman et al 2005).

Infarction

Infarction of a major cerebral artery occurs relatively commonly in asphyxiated babies (Voorhies et al 1983) and should be apparent on brain imaging. This condition is discussed fully in Chapter 21. Imaging detects an abnormality in the distribution of the affected vessel. Ultrasound may be a useful screening test for this condition, but infarction of a major cerebral artery may occur in the presence of a normal ultrasound scan, so it is important to perform CT or MR scans on all full-term infants in whom cerebral artery infarction is suspected. Clinical suspicion should be aroused by focal convulsions or the presence of asymmetrical neurological signs. The tissue supplied by the infarcted vessel usually becomes necrotic and is replaced by a porencephalic cyst, again seen in the vascular distribution of the affected vessel. This is a useful marker in the older child with this particular lesion.

Measurement of intracranial pressure

Cerebral edema may occur as the result of a hypoxic-ischemic insult and leads to intracranial hypertension in some cases. Direct assessment of intracranial pressure by means of a subarachnoid catheter has shown that only 50% of asphyxiated infants actually develop intracranial hypertension, and monitoring may not significantly alter the outcome in the majority of infants (Levene et al 1987).

Attempts have been made to measure intracranial pressure (ICP) both directly and indirectly across the anterior fontanelle. The latter has the obvious advantage of being non-invasive but may also be less accurate. Unfortunately, indirect transfontanel methods are unreliable and inaccurate.

Direct methods

Doubts about the accuracy of indirect methods have prompted a number of attempts at invasive measurement of ICP in infants. Goitein and Amit (1982) described placement through the fontanel of a 22-gauge Quick-Cath into the subdural space, and found no complications associated with this technique. Levene and Evans (1983) used a fine subarachnoid catheter inserted percutaneously to monitor ICP and have used this successfully in over 30 infants without complications associated with the technique. McWilliam and Stephenson (1984) published a method for monitoring ICP directly from the anterior horn of the lateral ventricle. To date, this has not been described in the neonate.

Methods to measure ICP directly using devices inserted into the skull are more accurate and reliable, and all appear to be remarkably safe in clinical practice.

Normal ICP

Normal ICP in full-term infants is derived from indirect measurement using transfontanellar devices and is probably inaccurate and unreliable. For obvious reasons, there are no data from direct measurement techniques in normal babies. Kaiser and Whitelaw (1987) have reported normal lumbar cerebrospinal fluid pressure to range from 0 to 5.5 mmHg measured at lumbar puncture. In practice, we estimate normal ICP in mature normal neonates to be <6 mmHg.

Cerebral perfusion pressure

This concept has been used in adults and children to describe the resistance to cerebral perfusion due to elevations in ICP. Cerebral perfusion pressure (CPP) is calculated by subtracting ICP from the mean arterial blood pressure (MAP):

$$CPP = MAP - ICP.$$

In essence, the driving force of blood through the cerebral arterioles will be reduced by increments in ICP if the MAP remains unchanged.

A critically low CPP has been associated with poor outcome in adults (Rowan et al 1972) and infants (Raju et al 1983). The normal range for CPP in infants has been prone to the same methodological problems inherent in the measurement of ICP.

Electrodiagnostic tests

These methods include electroencephalography and evoked responses and are discussed in detail in Chapter 12. They are important investigations that help to strengthen the clinical diagnosis of birth asphyxia.

Polygraphic electroencephalography is a widely available technique applicable to the newborn infant. This technique has been shown to be a good prognostic indicator following birth asphyxia (Takeuchi & Watanabe 1989, Watanabe et al 1980), but it requires considerable skill and experience in the interpretation of the tracings. It is limited to short recordings lasting only minutes in time. For this reason, methods to continuously monitor cerebral electrical activity have been developed. The techniques of continuous EEG, cerebral function monitoring (CFM) or amplitude integrated EEG (aEEG) have at least a three-fold role in asphyxiated infants (see p. 201). Firstly, the techniques may provide useful prognostic information, especially in the first hours after birth, e.g. when investigating the speed of recovery of an initially poor CFM trace (Van Rooij et al 2005). Secondly, it may aid the diagnosis of seizures. Thirdly, aEEG is also of value in the selection of infants who might benefit from neuroprotective therapy.

Doppler assessment

Consistent changes in Doppler signals from major cerebral arteries following birth asphyxia have been described (Levene et al 1989), and these changes occur in a particular sequence (see p. 167). Doppler ultrasound has also been shown to be a useful prognostic indicator following birth asphyxia (Levene et al 1989), and this is discussed on page 577. Doppler ultrasound has not been shown to have a role in the acute management of birth asphyxia.

Near-infrared spectroscopy

Near-infrared spectroscopy (NIRS) was introduced in 1977 as a technology that is capable of non-invasive monitoring of oxygenation in living tissue. NIRS operates on the principle that near-infrared (NIR) light (700–1000 nm) passes easily through tissue and is absorbed in an O_2-dependent manner by chromophores that include hemoglobin and cytochrome aa3 (Jobsis 1977). This technique is described in detail in Chapter 11. The technique permits cotside measurement of cerebral hemodynamics in babies undergoing intensive care. Without interrupting the routine care of the infant, NIRS can measure the absolute changes in oxyhemoglobin and deoxyhemoglobin concentrations directly, and can be used to derive additional hemodynamic variables of clinical interest (CBV, CBF).

An increase in cerebral blood volume (CBV) on the first day of life is a sensitive predictor of adverse outcome (Meek et al 1999). In addition, abnormal regional cerebral O_2 saturation (rSO$_2$) and fractional cerebral tissue O_2 extraction (FTOE) reflect secondary energy failure, the former (rSO$_2$) correlating well with outcome after severe asphyxia (Toet et al 2006).

However, the relationships between flow, oxygenation and function remain weak (Greisen 2006). Several practical problems with the technology have led for this technique to remain almost exclusively a research instrument, likely to provide important new insights into the complex interrelationships among physiologic and pathologic conditions that contribute to brain injury in infants with HIE (Wolfberg & du Plessis 2006).

Biochemical methods

As indicated in the section on the pathophysiology of birth asphyxia, a cascade of biochemical reactions occurs during and after an asphyxial event, and so, changes in biochemical markers are potentially useful methods for monitoring the progress of the condition. Table 26.3 lists the biochemical markers reported in the literature to assess the diagnosis or progress of an asphyxial insult. These methods focus on changes in the body or brain's energy states, hormonal response or markers of brain-based proteins usually accessible only at lumbar puncture.

The problem with many of these markers is that they assess total body effects of asphyxia rather than just those affecting the brain. It is suggested that as the blood–brain barrier in neonates is less functionally competent, aerobically derived enzymes may cross more readily into the systemic circulation, thus enabling cerebral pathology to be monitored reliably on blood specimens in older patients. Recent studies have assessed these markers in CSF that reflect the brain condition more closely. The main purpose

Table 26.3 Biochemical markers reported to be used in the diagnosis of birth asphyxia and/or prediction of outcome following a hypoxic–ischemic event

Energy metabolism	Hormones	Brain derived proteins
Fetal blood pH	Vasopressin	Aspartate/glutamate
Cord blood pH (A–V) difference	Erythropoietin	GFAP
Cord blood PCO_2 (A–V) difference	Norepinephrine	Myelin basic protein
Buffer base	Insulin	BDNF
Lactate (blood, brain)	Prolactin	Nestin
Urinary lactate/pyruvate ratio	Growth hormone	
Lactate/pyruvate ratio	Catecholamines	
Lactate dehydrogenase and isoenzymes	ACTH	Brain enzymes
Hydroxybutyrate dehydrogenase	Endorphins	Creatine kinase (CK-BB)
Hypoxanthine (blood, CSF)	Somatostatin	Neuron specific enolase
Cyclic AMP	Aldosterone	
Adenosine		
Uric acid/creatinine ratio		Cytokines
		TNFα
		IL-1β
		IL-6

of these biochemical markers is in the prediction of outcome, and this is discussed on page 559.

Energy metabolism

Anaerobic metabolism, a precursor of asphyxia, causes both respiratory and metabolic acidosis with fall in blood pH and increase in lactate. Acidosis has been proposed as a marker of duration and/or severity of a hypoxic–ischemic insult. Cord-blood pH varies depending on whether an artery or vein is sampled; the pH of arterial blood is normally lower than venous blood. Severe cord-blood acidosis (arterial pH < 7.05) occurs in about 2.5% of unselected full-term infants (Westgate 1993), but few of these babies show major signs of 'asphyxia'. In one study, 61% of all babies with a pH < 7.00 did not require admission to a neonatal unit (Goldaber et al 1991), and in another study, only 22% of babies with a similar degree of cord-blood acidosis developed seizures (Perlman & Risser 1996). A normal arterial cord-blood level may be useful in suggesting that anaerobic metabolism has not occurred immediately prior to delivery.

In an acidotic fetus, the size of the difference may indicate whether the acidosis has occurred acutely or not. Chronic anaerobic metabolism will produce a smaller difference as the placenta will have had time to equilibrate the difference. A large difference suggests acute onset of acidosis usually with cord compression. Low et al (1993) found a significantly poorer neurodevelopmental outcome in babies with metabolic acidosis who had a narrow artery-to-vein difference (<6 mmol/L) compared with those with similar metabolic acidosis, but a large artery-to-vein difference

(>6 mmol/L). Marked elevation of urinary lactate:creatinine ratio predicted an increased risk of HIE in term asphyxiated babies (Huang et al 1999).

Lactate production as the result of anaerobic metabolism is an important component of metabolic acidosis detected at birth. Intracerebral lactic acid accumulation may be responsible for the development of cerebral edema, but it is suggested that there is poor correlation between blood lactic acidemia and intracerebral levels. Acidemia as the result of fetal compromise usually resolves spontaneously (Farkas et al 1995), but cerebral lactate levels in white and gray matter remain elevated for a considerably longer time after resolution of systemic blood lactate levels (Thoresen et al 1988). ^{1}H MRS has shown that high levels of intracerebral lactate occur shortly after acute asphyxia in full-term human neonates (Groenendaal et al 1994, Hanrahan et al 1996, Leth et al 1996, Penrice et al 1996) and that high levels or prolonged detection of lactate predict bad outcome. The somewhat counter intuitive findings of Robertson et al (2001), who measured intracellular brain pH (pH_i) with MRS, reported the worst prognosis for outcome in babies with the most alkaline pH_i measurement, particularly where this persisted for more than 2 weeks.

The energy state within the brain can be assessed in a number of ways, both directly and indirectly. The high-energy molecule ATP is necessary for normal cellular function, and this can be directly assessed by measuring the PCr/P_i ratio using ^{31}P MRS (see Ch. 11). Wyatt et al (1989) produced a series of phosphorus spectra from asphyxiated babies and showed that there is a delayed deterioration in the brain energy state suggestive of a slowly progressive disruption of oxidative phosphorylation in brain tissue (Figs 11.3 and 26.10). In the hours after a severe hypoxic–ischemic insult, the PCr/P_i ratio falls, indicating a continuing degradation of high-energy substrate to inorganic phosphorus. This degradation in ATP is associated with a poor outcome (Lorek et al 1994, Martin et al 1996, Roth et al 1997). It is, however, unlikely that MRS will ever be available as a routine technique for monitoring cerebral function following birth asphyxia, but it provides invaluable insight into the pathophysiology of this condition.

During hypoxia, ATP is degraded to AMP and hence to hypoxanthine (Hx). Hx acts as a substrate for the formation of O_2 derived free radicals during reoxygenation. This is discussed in detail in Chapter 22. Cyclic AMP is synthesized in mitochondria from ATP and has been shown to be very low in CSF samples in term asphyxiated infants, and such infants have been shown to have a very poor outcome (Pourcyrous et al 1999). Saugstad (1975) suggested that Hx is a sensitive and specific measure of energy state following perinatal asphyxia. Various studies have shown a wide overlap between Hx in normal control and asphyxiated fetuses (O'Connor et al 1981). In a study of cord-blood Hx measurements, Thiringer (1983) found a poor correlation between Hx and low Apgar scores, but abnormal clinical findings correlated better. Hx therefore is not a specific measure of cerebral energy breakdown but reflects whole-body changes. The liver and brain appear to contribute most to total Hx following severe fetal hypoxia, and consequently, Hx is of little value in the prediction of neurological outcome.

Brain enzymes

Creatine kinase (CK) is derived from brain, heart and skeletal muscle in response to tissue injury. Attempts have been made to separate the three isoenzymes chemically in order to study changes in the brain-derived enzyme (CK-BB) following asphyxia. Worley et al (1985) have shown CK-BB to be derived from both neurons and astrocytes. A variety of methods, including electrophoretic separation (Cuestas 1980, Walsh et al 1982) and radioimmunoassay (Thompson et al 1980, Worley et al 1985), have been used to measure CK-BB. These methods, particularly electrophoresis, have been criticized because they do not separate the component CK-BB accurately from cardiac enzyme CK-MB (Hoo & Goedde 1982). The measurements of CK-BB can be badly contaminated by CK-MB, thus rendering results unreliable.

Studies have shown that low levels of CK-BB predict a subsequent normal outcome reasonably well, and significantly elevated levels found during the first 12 h of life predict a later neurological abnormality in a relatively high proportion of asphyxiated newborn infants (Fernandez et al 1987, Walsh et al 1982). Others could not, however, find any correlation between the levels of CK-BB isoenzyme in cord blood and depressed Apgar scores or cord-blood pH

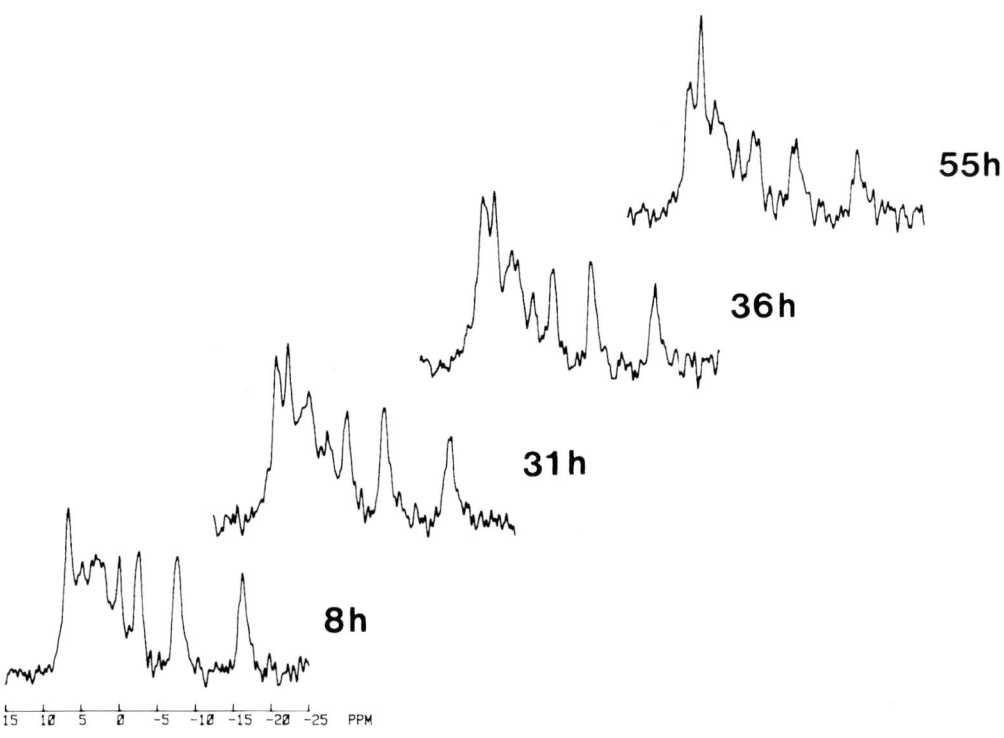

Figure 26.10 A series of MRS phosphorus spectra from a severely asphyxiated full-term infant scanned at varying times from birth (ages indicated in hours) showing a progressive deterioration of the PCr/P_i ratio with time. (Reproduced, with permission, from Wyatt et al 1989.)

(Amato et al 1986, Ruth 1989). In addition, there was no correlation between CK-BB activity and developmental quotient at 2 years (Ruth 1989). The role of the CK-BB isoenzyme in quantifying cerebral injury is thus not clear. Certainly, earlier techniques have failed to separate accurately the various isoenzymes.

Lactate and hydroxybutyrate dehydrogenase (LDH and HBDH) have been used as indicators of neurological damage in asphyxiated newborn infants. Isoenzyme studies have suggested that LDH originated from neuronal tissue, but studies have not suggested that blood enzyme levels are good discriminators of at-risk infants (Hall et al 1980). Elevated levels of LDH and its isoenzymes LDH2 and LDH3 in CSF have been suggested to be better predictors of death and disability (Dalens et al 1981, Fernandez et al 1986).

Neuron-specific enolase (NSE) is released into both CSF and serum following damage to the brain. Studies have shown that babies with HIE have higher levels of NSE than controls and that those with the most severe grades of HIE had the highest NSE levels in CSF (Thornberg et al 1995b). Infants who died or sustained motor deficit as the result of an asphyxial insult were found to have the highest levels of NSE in CSF (Garcia-Alix et al 1994).

S100B protein is concentrated mainly in neurons and glial cells of the central nervous system. Its concentration in peripheral blood and cerebrospinal fluid is increased as a result of brain damage in adults, infants and fetuses. However, animal studies indicate S100B serum increases may occur out of the 'window of opportunity' to initiate neuronal rescue therapy, as the increase does not occur before 48 hours after the insult (Kecskes et al 2005).

Whereas the predictive value on neurological outcome of aEEG has been published to be 91.5% (Hellström-Westas 1995), serum concentrations of brain-specific proteins sampled on the first day of life seem to have limited value in predicting severe brain damage after birth asphyxia, since recent literature produces conflicting results. Elevated concentrations of serum protein S100B, NSE and CK-BB studied on day 1 in 29 asphyxiated infants compared to 20 control infants did not correlate with neurodevelopmental delay at the age of 20 months (Nagdyman et al 2001, 2003). On the other hand, longitudinal S100B protein measurements in urine soon after birth have been suggested as a useful tool to identify which asphyxiated infants are at risk for long-term neurological sequelae (Gazzolo et al 2003). It may well be that longitudinal protein measurements during days after the asphyxiating insult are necessary to predict neurological outcome. Indeed, a recent study involving 18 months follow-up in 62 term infants with HIE indicates that determination of serum S100B on postnatal days 1 to 4 inversely correlates with a good outcome (Thorngren-Jerneck et al 2004).

Brain-derived proteins

A number of brain-derived proteins have been found to be elevated in the CSF of neonates who have sustained a hypoxic–ischemic insult. These include glial fibrillary acidic protein (GFAP), a structural protein of intermediate filaments in astroglia (Blennow et al 1995), myelin basic protein (Garcia-Alix et al 1994), brain-derived neurotrophic factor (BDNF) (Korhonen et al 1998), and nestin, an intermediate filament protein derived from reactive astrocytes (Grigelioniene et al 1996).

The CSF concentration of the excitatory neurotransmitter amino acids, glutamate and aspartate, have been shown to increase by over 250% in asphyxiated infants (Hagberg et al 1993). The highest increase was reported in the infants with the most severe forms of HIE.

Recently, nitrotyrosine, a reaction product of peroxynitrite and proteins, was found in the postmortem examination of brain tissue of full-term neonates, suggesting that nitric oxide toxicity might have a role in hypoxic–ischemic brain injury at term (Groenendaal 2006). This may be relevant for neuroprotective strategies in full-term neonates with perinatal asphyxia.

Hormones

Asphyxia is a potent stimulator of a wide endocrine response. There is a massive catecholamine release in response to birth, and this is even greater in asphyxia (Hagberg et al 1993). Inappropriately high insulin levels are reported in a group of asphyxiated babies, and these babies are reported to have a worse outcome (Davis et al 1999). Elevated growth hormone and depressed prolactin values have been reported in asphyxiated neonates (Varvarigou et al 1996), and this may reflect pituitary compromise. Hypoxia is also known to stimulate release of arginine vasopressin from the pituitary, and high levels of vasopressin have been found in the cord plasma of asphyxiated babies (De Vane & Porter 1980), but this did not correlate with neurodevelopmental outcome at 2 years (Ruth et al 1988).

Erythropoietin (Epo) is produced by the fetal kidney within a few hours of a hypoxic insult. In a group of infants with apparent acute asphyxia, those infants with definite adverse outcome had significantly higher cord blood Epo levels than asphyxiated controls without abnormal outcome (Ruth et al 1988). Epo deserves further attention as a sensitive biochemical marker of intrapartum hypoxia, but it is not a specific marker of a cerebral injury. Excess nRBCs in peripheral blood may occur as a result of abnormal Epo production and may be a marker of chronic hypoxia (see p. 545).

Cytokines

Cytokines are a group of chemical messengers with both pro- and anti-inflammatory actions and are released as the result of tissue injury. A number of specific cytokines including TNFα, IL-1β, IL-6, and IL-8 have been shown to be elevated in the CSF of asphyxiated babies compared with controls (Martin-Ancel et al 1997, Oygur et al 1998, Savman et al 1998). The magnitude of response to IL-6 has also been shown to correlate with neurodevelopmental outcome (Martin-Ancel et al 1997, Savman et al 1998).

Complement

In human neonates, the development of HIE is associated with complement activation, manifested by increased serum concentrations of the complement anaphylatoxins C3a and C5a, coincident with depletion/consumption of C1q and Factor B (Sonntag et al 1998). Whether complement activation participates in post-asphyxial cerebral injury in human neonates is not known. Since the complement system, although downregulated in the fetus and newborn infant, contributes significantly to antibacterial host defense, clinical application of complement inhibition must await proof that the benefits of inhibiting the complement activation exceed the risks of blocking the anti-infectious and other adaptive functions of complement (Lassiter 2004).

Complications

During the acute hypoxic–ischemic insult, changes occur in the distribution of blood flow in order to preserve circulation to the most vital organs, as described in Chapter 22. In summary, blood flow to the brain, myocardium, and adrenal glands increases in inverse proportion to the arterial O_2 content and at the expense of blood flow to the kidneys, muscle, liver and gastrointestinal tract (i.e. the so-called diving reflex). This accounts for the increased vulnerability of some organs to acute asphyxial events, and anticipation of complications is important in the appropriate management of such infants. The criteria for determining the appropriate timing for evaluation of infants for multiorgan dysfunction have not been fully studied. Data indicate that 24–72 h after birth is most likely to capture biochemical and electrocardiographic abnormalities associated with asphyxia (Shah et al 2004).

Kidney

The presentation and course of renal dysfunction depend upon the severity and duration of the hypoxic–ischemic event. A mild insult may cause a transient loss of renal concentrating ability, whereas severe asphyxia results in diffuse tubular dysfunction with impaired reabsorption of sodium and water and decreased glomerular filtration rate.

Prerenal failure must be distinguished from intrinsic renal disease, using a fluid challenge of 10 to 20 mL/Kg of isotonic saline over 30 to 60 min. If urine output remains less than 1 mL/Kg/h and intravascular volume is adequate, furosemide (1 mg/Kg i.v.) must be given. Lack of response usually indicates intrinsic renal disease. Alternatively, calculation of the fractional excretion of sodium may help to distinguish between prerenal and renal failure.

Asphyxia in fetal or newborn animals causes a marked reduction in renal blood flow (Rudolph 1969) with a significant increase in the vascular resistance of the kidney (Alward et al 1978, Dauber et al 1976). Doppler studies of renal hemodynamics after birth asphyxia have shown an increase in apparent renal vascular resistance (Akinbi et al 1994) and a reduction in renal systolic flow velocity, which predicts the development of acute renal failure (Luciano et al 1998). Renal failure may also occur due to myoglobinuria following tissue breakdown in asphyxiated infants (Kojima et al 1985).

The incidence of renal impairment, as defined by oliguria (<1 mL/Kg/h), following birth asphyxia has been reported to vary between 23 and 55% (Fernandez et al 1989, Perlman & Tack 1988). A recent prospective case controlled study of 70 asphyxiated infants indicated renal failure in 33 patients (47 percent), of which 7 were oliguric and 26 were non-oliguric (Gupta et al 2005). Acute renal failure (defined as a plasma creatinine level >130 µmol/L for at least 2 consecutive days) was reported in 19% of a group of asphyxiated infants born at 34 weeks of gestational age and above (Roberts et al 1990). There was a relatively poor concordance in these studies between renal impairment and HIE. A more sophisticated assessment of renal tubular function has shown that urinary concentrations of N-acetyl-glucosaminidase (NAG) was significantly higher in a group of full-term asphyxiated neonates compared to controls (Willis et al 1997). There was also a significant increase in urinary NAG excretion with increasing severity of perinatal asphyxia, as indicated by the HIE grade.

Gastrointestinal tract

Asphyxiated babies have been shown to be more likely to have abnormalities in intestinal motility with intolerance of enteral feeds (Berseth & McCoy 1992). Necrotizing enterocolitis (NEC) is the major complication affecting the bowel in asphyxiated infants, although this is rare amongst cohorts of full-term asphyxiated infants (Perlman et al 1989). Fitzhardinge (1977) reported one-third of infants with NEC to have suffered asphyxia before its onset. In contrast to the presentation in premature infants, NEC in term infants typically presents within the first few days after birth and predominantly affects the colon (Andrews 1990). Asphyxiated infants also show an apparent increase in resistance of mesenteric vessels (Akinbi et al 1994), which may predispose them to post-asphyxial bowel problems.

Hepatic dysfunction is also described in asphyxiated infants (Goldberg et al 1983, Zanardo et al 1985). One of the fetal responses to hypoxia is increased shunting of blood through the ductus venosus, with subsequent hepatic hypoxia and elevations of serum glutamic-oxaloacetic transaminase (SGOT) and glutamic-pyruvic transaminase (SGPT). Fetuses who suffer acute injury may not proceed with the physiologic process of centralizing their circulation, and thus SGOT and SGPT levels may still be normal.

Cardiovascular system

Cardiac output

Asphyxia can cause myocardial ischemia, which usually is transient. Myocardial dysfunction and tricuspid insufficiency result in decreased stroke volume, reduced cardiac output and subsequent systemic hypotension (Bucciarelli et al 1977). In addition, some infants have signs of respiratory distress, heart failure or shock. Rarely myocardial dysfunction results in cardiogenic shock and death (Burnard & James 1961, Cabal et al 1980). The diagnosis is confirmed by echocardiography, which should be obtained in all infants in whom myocardial ischemia is suspected. In a group of infants with low Apgar scores and acidosis (pH < 7.10), their blood pressure, cardiac output, and stroke volume were found to be lower than a similar, but non-acidotic, group. Myocardial dysfunction detected by Doppler ultrasound studies has been reported in 28–50% of asphyxiated infants (Bennhagen et al 1998, Perlman et al 1989, van Bel & Walther 1990). Dopamine is valuable in increasing blood pressure in asphyxiated infants by its inotropic effect (Di Sessa et al 1981), which improves cardiac output and stroke volume (Walther et al 1985).

Myocardial infarction

Ischemic necrosis of the papillary muscle following severe birth asphyxia has been found in a high proportion of autopsy specimens (De Sa & Donnelly 1984, Donnelly et al 1980). Evidence for myocardial ischemia is often present on ECG assessment (Daga et al 1983, Primhak et al 1985). Cardiac troponin T levels were suggested as a useful marker for myocardial necrosis (Szymankiewicz et al 2005).

Lung

Several pulmonary disorders can be associated with perinatal asphyxia, such as meconium aspiration syndrome, persistent pulmonary hypertension, acute respiratory distress syndrome (RDS) and pulmonary edema due to myocardial dysfunction.

Meconium aspiration is a common accompaniment of HIE. Hypoxia induces fetal gasping during labor as well as passage of meconium, and meconium aspiration occurs before the infant is born. Pulmonary hypertension is a common complication of meconium aspiration, and the ensuing systemic hypoxemia may further compromise cerebral function. Pulmonary hypertension has been reported to be a specific complication of birth asphyxia and may be severe (Perlman et al 1989). It has been suggested that in some asphyxiated infants, the pulmonary hypertension may be due to pulmonary embolism (Arnold et al 1985). RDS appears to be due to increased pulmonary capillary permeability to plasma proteins, which leads to inactivation of surfactant.

The breathing pattern of asphyxiated full-term infants shows a variety of abnormal patterns compared with controls. There are more apneic periods and longer duration of apneic episodes when they occur. The duration of time spent in periodic breathing is also prolonged (Sasidharan 1992).

Metabolism

A variety of metabolic problems may arise in asphyxiated infants, including hyponatremia, hypoglycemia, hypocalcemia, metabolic acidosis and hyperammonemia. Hyponatremia may occur due to fluid retention as a result of renal compromise or due to inappropriate antidiuretic hormone secretion (IADHS). Perinatal asphyxia causes high levels of circulating ADH (Daniel et al 1978, Speer et al 1984) and fluid retention occurs as a result of this (see above). IADHS

is recognized by the combination of dilute plasma and concentrated urine.

Transient hyperammonemia, in association with severe perinatal asphyxia, has been described (Goldberg et al 1979). Some of the clinical features seen in these infants and thought to be due to asphyxia, including hyperthermia, hypertension and lack of beat-to-beat variability, may have been caused by the hyperammonemia. The reason for the transient elevation in serum ammonia levels is not known.

Hematological complications

If the bone marrow itself had an ischemic injury, the first sign of marrow suppression would be thrombocytopenia (platelet count <100 000/μL) at approximately 5 to 7 days of age, because platelets have the shortest half-life of the marrow products (Hankins 2002). The marrow recovers over time.

Disseminated intravascular coagulation (DIC) occurs commonly following intrapartum asphyxia (Anderson et al 1974, Chadd et al 1971, Chessells & Wigglesworth 1970, Suzuki & Morishita 1998). Bleeding due to DIC may cause severe secondary complications including intracranial hemorrhage. Anderson et al (1974) could find no evidence that DIC was associated with significant intracerebral thrombus deposition.

In a group of asphyxiated babies, there was a marked abnormality in a number of variables suggestive of DIC (Suzuki & Morishita 1998). These included significantly low levels of factor XIII, and elevated thrombin-antithrombin (TAT) complexes, D-dimer, fibrin and fibrinogen degradation products (FDP), and soluble fibrin monomer complexes (SFMC).

MANAGEMENT

The immediate management of birth asphyxia is directed first towards rapid and efficient resuscitation and then stabilization of the infant's condition (Cornette & Levene 2001). Asphyxia may compromise the functions of a variety of immature organ systems (see p. 22), and anticipation of such complications with appropriate management is essential. The management of the asphyxiated infant must be considered in relation to general systemic complications as well as directing therapy towards the brain. Brain-oriented management (Ch. 27) is misplaced if complications such as systemic hypotension are unrecognized or inadequately treated. Severely asphyxiated infants must be treated in the same manner as the very-low-birth-weight infant, with adequate monitoring and the provision of cerebrally oriented intensive care, should this be necessary.

RESUSCITATION

Dawes (1968) has described the sequence of events that occur during experimental asphyxia of fetal rhesus monkeys. Immediately following the asphyxial insult, there is an episode of regular small-volume breaths followed by a fall in the heart rate and cessation of breathing. This is termed primary apnea, and the animal looks cyanosed as a result of these changes. With no intervention, the period of primary apnea lasts for up to a minute and is followed by spontaneous gasping, which is maintained for a further 4–5 min before a second period of apnea develops. If resuscitation is not undertaken at the stage of secondary apnea, then the animal will die. This sequence of events is similar to those that have been observed to occur in the human newborn. These stages are summarized in Figure 26.11. The need for resuscitation can be anticipated in many cases, and risk factors are listed in Table 26.4. Despite this, in a national Swedish survey, 19% of all babies who required resuscitation were not anticipated prior to delivery (Palme-Kilander 1992).

Immediate measures

At birth, the newborn baby's condition should be rapidly assessed and priority given to three major aspects of resuscitation in the following order:

1. A – Airway. Establish a safe and secure airway.
2. B – Breathing. Establish adequate and appropriate ventilation.
3. C – Circulation. Ensure that the heart rate and cardiac output are appropriate.

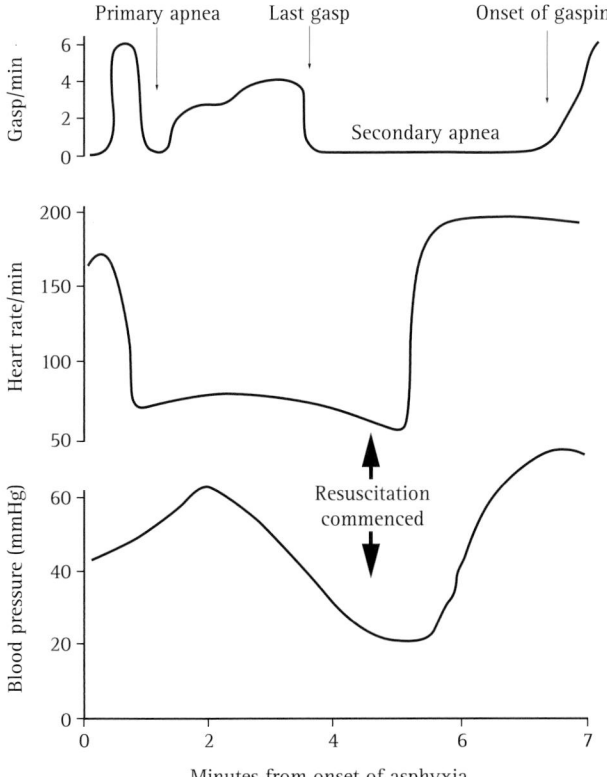

Figure 26.11 Physiological effects of acute asphyxia and the response to resuscitation. (Redrawn, with permission, from Dawes 1968.)

This section is not intended to act as a guide to resuscitation methods, but it is most important that all professional personnel working in an environment where it is planned to deliver babies must be trained and regularly retrained in appropriate resuscitation techniques. All equipment must be regularly checked to ensure that it is in working order. It has been shown in China that the introduction of neonatal resuscitation program guidelines developed by the American Academy of Pediatrics and the American Heart Association produced a threefold reduction in perinatal mortality (Zhu et al 1997).

Babies who fail to rapidly adapt to birth by establishing spontaneous breathing and become pink should be quickly dried and transferred to a resuscitation trolley. The type of resuscitation depends on the infant's degree of depression. This can be summarized as:

1. Apneic with a heart rate above 100 beats per minute (bpm). This represents primary apnea, and the infant requires little more than vigorous cutaneous stimulation and O_2 blown across his or her nostrils.
2. Apneic with a heart rate below 100 bpm. This may represent the stage of secondary apnea. Suction of the mouth and nares should be applied followed by 5 inflation breaths by means of a bag and a tight-fitting face-mask. The heart rate should pick up, and the color should improve. The baby will then usually rapidly develop spontaneous respirations. Some babies may be apneic because their mothers have recently been given an opiate for pain relief. Naloxone is a specific opiate antagonist and should be given (0.1 mg/Kg by deep intramuscular injection) if the mother has received opiates within 4 h of delivery.
3. Persistent failure to breathe and/or persistent bradycardia. The baby should be intubated and given intermittent positive-pressure ventilation (IPPV).
4. Persistent bradycardia or asystole. IPPV and cardiac massage should be rapidly started. Vascular access should be quickly established, and intravenous drugs

Table 26.4 Factors indicating a significantly increased risk that an infant may need resuscitation at birth
Prematurity
Diagnosis of fetal distress
Heavy meconium staining of the liquor
Fetal acidosis (pH < 7.2) measured from a scalp sample
Known major congenital malformation
Twins
Any delivery under general anesthesia
Mid-cavity or rotational forceps
Rhesus disease
Significant antepartum hemorrhage

such as epinephrine (adrenaline) and calcium gluconate should be given. Epinephrine appears to be as effective if given down the endotracheal tube.

It has been the practice in many delivery rooms to resuscitate babies with 100% O$_2$. This has recently been questioned as leading to a number of potential risks including reduction of cerebral blood flow (Lundstrom et al 1995) and excessive free-radical release (Saugstad 1998). A large, randomized control trial of the effects of newborn resuscitation with ambient air compared to 100% O$_2$ (Resair 2 trial) has shown that babies who received room-air resuscitation had fewer postnatal problems than those who received 100% O$_2$, although none of the differences were statistically significant (Saugstad et al 1998). In particular, mortality in the first 7 days, overall neonatal mortality, and death from moderate or severe HIE were all less in the room air group. The follow-up of 213 infants recruited to the Resair 2 showed no significant differences in somatic growth or neurologic handicap at an age of 18 to 24 months in infants resuscitated with either 21% or 100% O$_2$ at birth (Saugstad et al 2003). Neonates resuscitated with 100% O$_2$ exhibit biochemical findings reflecting prolonged oxidative stress (e.g. lower reduced-to-oxidized-glutathione ratio, increased activities of superoxide dismutase and catalase in erythrocytes), present even after 4 weeks of postnatal life, which do not appear in the ambient air group (Vento et al 2001). Based on these data, there appears to be little justification for routinely resuscitating asphyxiated newborn babies in high O$_2$ concentrations, but neither the Resuscitation Council (UK) nor the American Academy of Pediatrics currently recommends routine resuscitation in room air. Adjustable O$_2$ supply (O$_2$ blenders) as a back-up for treatment failure with air must be available at any time (Hansmann 2004). Also, special neonatal emergencies commonly associated with impaired lung function and persistent pulmonary hypertension of the newborn, such as severe asphyxia, fulminant sepsis, meconium aspiration and congenital diaphragmatic hernia, might require O$_2$ concentrations up to 100% immediately after birth.

Approximately 20 to 30% of meconium-stained infants require resuscitation in the delivery room. Routine intrapartum oropharyngeal suctioning of all infants delivered with meconium-stained amniotic fluid has been questioned by a recent randomized study that showed no benefit from this routine intervention with regard to the development of meconium aspiration syndrome (Vain et al 2004). Direct laryngeal suctioning to remove meconium from the airway should be conducted only on depressed infants (absent respirations, heart rate less than 100 beats per minute or poor muscle tone). A meta-analysis of four randomized, controlled trials does not support the use of endotracheal intubation in vigorous, meconium-stained infants (Halliday 2000). Saline lavage, aimed at loosening intrapulmonary meconium and improving its retrieval from the airway, may be detrimental since surfactant can be washed out together with meconium. Tracheal lavage with dilute surfactant may have some benefit (Lam & Yeung 1999).

There is no documented benefit in keeping core temperature above normal at birth for asphyxiated infants (Gunn & Bennet 2001). Perinatal hyperthermia should thus be avoided in the delivery room and during transport to a perinatal center. In the animal model, hyperthermia during resuscitation and reperfusion causes increased neuronal injury and release of O$_2$ free radicals and excitatory amino acids (Suehiro et al 1999). Maternal temperature should be monitored and fever should be treated. Since maternal fever has been associated with neonatal seizures, increased mortality and cerebral palsy, the aim should also be to avoid iatrogenic hyperthermia in newborns who have required resuscitation. The promising results of therapeutic hypothermia in the term infant are discussed on page 569.

Early assessment of arterial pH is helpful as a baseline, and a further measure should be made 1 h later. It is usually unnecessary to correct metabolic acidosis as a routine procedure during resuscitation. If the baby has a good circulation and adequate ventilation, then he or she should be able to correct his or her own metabolic acidosis. Bicarbonate (1 to 2 mEq/Kg of a 0.5 mEq/mL solution) should be administered by slow intravenous infusion only if the acidemia is persistent despite adequate ventilation and oxygenation, and only if blood gas values are available to monitor the response. There are no randomized controlled trials that evaluate the efficacy of bicarbonate in neonatal resuscitation.

If volume expansion is needed acutely in the delivery room, an isotonic crystalloid solution (e.g. normal saline) should be administered, using slow intravenous administration of 10 mL/Kg as an initial dose. O-negative blood may be used if there is evidence of intrapartum blood loss (e.g. placenta previa, ruptured cord). The routine use of albumin in neonatal resuscitation is controversial, but there is no evidence that this practice is beneficial for the baby, as it may be associated with additional myocardial compromise (Roberton 1997).

The role of intravenous glucose during resuscitation is discussed on page 566.

SYSTEMIC MANAGEMENT

Once adequate ventilation and circulation have been established, the newborn should be transferred to an environment in which close monitoring of systemic and cerebral function and anticipatory care can be provided. Thorough documentation of all observations and actions is essential for good clinical care, communication and medico-legal considerations.

Respiratory support

Following immediate resuscitation, respiratory support may be necessary for comatose infants with severe encephalopathy and those with coincident lung disease, of which meconium aspiration is the most common. Spontaneously breathing infants should be electively intubated and ventilated if they develop hypercapnia due to depression of respiratory drive or lung disease [$PaCO_2$ > 7 kPa (53 mmHg)]. While in the mature animal model, gentle ventilation with permissive hypercapnia is neuroprotective, currently no data are available about the role of hypercapnia in term infants after a hypoxic–ischemic insult. A meta-analysis of permissive hypercapnia in the prevention of morbidity and mortality of mechanically ventilated, newborn infants did not show any benefit from this strategy (Woodgate & Davies 2001).

It is often difficult to immediately achieve and maintain the correct balance between hyperoxemia, hypoxemia, hypercapnia and hypocapnia. Due to a variable cardiorespiratory postnatal adaptation to therapeutic interventions, episodes of hyperoxemia and hypocapnia can easily and unintentionally occur in ventilated asphyxiated infants during the first postnatal hours, and may be associated with adverse outcome (Klinger et al 2005). Hyperoxemia results in the release of toxic free O_2 radicals, whilst hypocapnia in animals is known to decrease cerebral blood flow, but not consistently in human newborns (Rosenberg 1992). O_2 supplementation and ventilation should therefore be rigorously controlled by careful assessment of post-resuscitation arterial blood gas estimates. Although there are no clear guidelines, and although the desired PaO_2 may vary depending on the co-existence of pulmonary hypertension, normoxia and normocapnia would appear to be proper therapeutic goals in mature infants (PaO_2 to be maintained in the range of 10–12 kPa [75–90 mmHg] and $PaCO_2$ to be maintained in the range of 4.5–5.1 kPa (36–40 mmHg). Hyperventilation in the management of suspected cerebral edema is discussed on page 568.

The post-asphyxiated infant with respiratory failure should be closely monitored for the development of pulmonary hypertension, and the need for inhaled nitric oxide. A recent meta-analysis showed that surfactant administration decreased the number of infants treated with extracorporeal membrane oxygenation in those with meconium aspiration syndrome that led to moderate or severe respiratory failure (Soll & Dargaville 2000).

Infants with frequent and prolonged convulsions may also need to be supported by mechanical ventilation, and this may become necessary as a result of their anticonvulsant management. The fear of inducing respiratory arrest by adequate dosage of anticonvulsants is irrational. The effects of prolonged or frequent seizures make the need to treat this complication adequately essential (see Ch. 34). If fear of the infant requiring mechanical ventilation is a factor in avoiding adequate anticonvulsant therapy, then the infant should be referred to a center where this can be safely and rapidly undertaken.

Fluids

Hypertension, hypoxemia, hypovolemia, activation of the renin–angiotensin–aldosterone system and intra-renal-adenosine system, as well as stimulation of catecholamines and increased vasopressin, all contribute to the development of renal dysfunction in the asphyxiated newborn (Toth-Heyn et al 2000). Oliguria due to renal compromise is managed by careful maintenance of the fluid balance and daily measurement of plasma creatinine levels. Assessment of the state of hydration in severely oliguric patients may be facilitated by measuring the central venous pressure. A bladder catheter should be inserted to measure urine volume and to exclude lower urinary tract obstruction. Intake and output, daily weight and concentrations of serum creatinine, electrolytes, calcium and phosphorus should be monitored. Sodium, potassium and phosphorus intake should be restricted. Medications should be adjusted according to the extent of renal dysfunction.

When hypovolemia is the primary cause of renal dysfunction, the urinary output should normalize within a few hours, after rapid volume replacement with normal saline. When no diuresis occurs, fluid administration should be repeated, unless the neonate has signs of myocardial dysfunction. In the absence of hypovolemia, fluid restriction is widely used to prevent brain swelling, but the evidence that fluid intake contributes to cerebral edema is lacking. The baby should be given only the volume of fluid necessary to keep him or her just adequately hydrated. This requires at least daily measurement of serum osmolality and urinary concentration (specific gravity), aiming to maintain the serum osmolality in the region of 290 mOsm/L and the urinary specific gravity at 1010.

Fluid restriction to insensible losses plus urine output is also important in asphyxiated infants who have complications such as inappropriate antidiuretic hormone (ADH) secretion and renal compromise. Inappropriate ADH secretion is suspected in the event of increase in body weight, decrease in serum sodium and increase in urine osmolarity. The fluid intake should be restricted until the serum osmolality and serum sodium levels return to normal. A renal vasodilator and diuretic response to dopamine is seen with low doses (0.5–2 µg/Kg/min) and results from stimulation of dopaminergic receptors. Fluid restriction is also recommended in the presence of acute tubular necrosis. Temporary peritoneal dialysis treatment may be necessary in the case of persistent oliguria/anuria, azotemia and other complications (e.g. hyperkalemia).

Renal adenosine acts as a vasoconstrictive metabolite in the kidney after hypoxia–ischemia and contributes to a fall in glomerular filtration rate. Hence, increasing renal blood flow is one important method of improving a renal imbalance. A recent study suggests that blocking the effects of renal adenosine with a single dose of theophylline (8 mg/Kg), a non-specific adenosine antagonist, may have beneficial effects on reducing renal dysfunction when given in the first postnatal hour to asphyxiated full-term infants (Jenik et al 2000). Larger studies are warranted before the use of theophylline in asphyxiated term newborns can be considered for clinical practice.

Blood pressure

Acutely asphyxiated infants may develop severe post-resuscitative myocardial depression, cardiomegaly, tricuspid regurgitation, reduced cardiac output and hypotension (Kern et al 1997). Volume load is contraindicated in such infants since a further increase in preload may further compromise cardiac function. Hypotension thus occurs frequently in severely asphyxiated infants, and continuous monitoring of arterial blood pressure is essential (Diprose et al 1986). Volume expansion is often ineffective in restoring normotension, and dopamine (5–15 μg/Kg/min) or dobutamine (2.5–15.0 μg/Kg/min) is usually necessary to raise the blood pressure to the normal range. It is important to maintain systemic blood pressure in the normal range because cerebral autoregulation is often absent in term infants after a major hypoxic–ischemic insult (Boylan et al 2000).

Hemostasis

Disturbances in blood clotting are most commonly due to disseminated intravascular coagulation. Management is supportive, and there is no place for systemic heparinization. The infant should receive additional vitamin K and may require either fresh frozen plasma for replacement of clotting factors or platelet transfusions, or both. Regular hematological checks of clotting function should be performed in all infants with severe birth asphyxia.

Infection

A high index of suspicion for infection must be maintained in all ill infants. Routine use of antibiotics cannot be recommended and should be used only for clinical indications or suspected infection. Early neonatal meningitis may present clinically in a manner similar to birth asphyxia, and if there is any doubt, a lumbar puncture must be performed.

Other

Calcemia and magnesemia levels are frequently low in the infant with birth asphyxia and these parameters should be closely monitored and treated as clinically indicated. Provision of adequate nutritional support is important. The primary purpose is to reduce tissue catabolism, causing excessive production of nitrogenous wastes, acids and potassium. Finally, the team caring for the newborn should inform the parents of the infant's condition at the earliest opportunity. Parents should be informed of resuscitative procedures undertaken and their indications. Parents need to be encouraged to ask questions and to have a maximum of contact with the newly born infant.

STANDARD BRAIN-ORIENTED MANAGEMENT

Traditionally, the standard management of the asphyxiated infant has been directed towards achieving a stable condition, adequate treatment of seizures and preventing or controlling cerebral edema. Increased awareness of subtle fits or asymptomatic electroconvulsive seizure activity in infants given neuromuscular relaxing agents has led to a wider use of continuous EEG monitoring (see Ch. 12). Adequate control of seizures is essential, and this is discussed in Chapter 34.

When analyzing the effect of drugs in hypoxic–ischemic injury, the pathogenesis of the injury must be considered in relation to the pharmacological action of the drug. Following perinatal asphyxia, both the primary and the secondary cerebral insults may vary in severity and, although interdependent, they may not necessarily be sequential. Ideally, in order to predict the likelihood of acute intracerebral sequelae, it is necessary to know for how long the fetus or infant has suffered significant cerebral underperfusion and whether there was a period of complete anoxia (cardiac arrest). Once resuscitation has been achieved, further variables include whether or not cerebral hypoperfusion (the 'no reflow phenomenon') has developed and whether intracranial hypertension intervened to impede cerebral perfusion further. The measurement of cerebral blood flow is fundamental to understanding these events, but this is not possible in the routine management of the asphyxiated newborn infant (see Ch. 11). Uncertainty concerning the duration of intrapartum asphyxia is common in the clinical setting, and this makes assessment and management of birth asphyxia largely empirical.

Glucose

Transmission of electric impulses and biosynthetic reactions within the neurons require a continuous source of energy, produced by the breakdown of glucose into pyruvate, which enters the citric acid cycle in order to produce adenosine triphosphate (ATP). Glucose metabolism during hypoxia-ischemia has been studied extensively. Transport from glucose into the brain is mediated by a diffusion-type transport system composed by several membrane proteins (e.g. GLUT-1 and GLUT-3). A reduction in CBF below a critical ischemic threshold leads to neuronal death due to reduced O_2 and glucose delivery. Using [18]FDG-positron emission tomography (PET) during the subacute period after perinatal asphyxia in 20 term infants, it was demonstrated that CMRgl (i.e. total and regional cerebral glucose metabolism) was inversely correlated with the severity of HIE. CMRgl is thus highly correlated with the severity of HIE and short-term outcome (Thorngren-Jerneck et al 2001).

The basic pathophysiologic knowledge for a final understanding of the contribution of brain glucose levels to brain damage has not been provided yet. The decision as to whether or not to give asphyxiated infants glucose therefore remains unresolved. The deleterious effects of high levels of glucose on asphyxial cerebral injury in the adolescent or mature animal have been reviewed by Myers et al (1983). This has been extended by some to the fetus and newborn, but the evidence to support this is very limited.

More recent data have shown conclusively that there is a fundamental difference in the way the immature and mature brain responds to glucose infusion. The immature brain appears to be protected by elevated blood glucose levels immediately prior to asphyxia compared with animals that were not exposed to additional glucose (Vannucci & Mujsce 1992). The evidence that administration of glucose after asphyxia in immature animals is beneficial remains controversial. Hattori and Wasterlain (1990) have shown that glucose treatment following hypoxic–ischemic insult in 7-day-old rat pups protects against neuropathological damage compared to controls. Another study also using 7-day-old rat pups found that treatment with glucose immediately after a hypoxic–ischemic insult caused more severe neuronal damage than in animals exposed to a similar insult without glucose infusion (Sheldon et al 1992).

It is clear that hypoglycemia following asphyxia must be avoided. In the human situation, it is not possible to give clear advice about the use of additional glucose following a severe asphyxial event, and we must await a controlled study in the context of birth asphyxia. For the time being, we adhere to the principle of maintaining normoglycemia in clinical practice following hypoxia–ischemia, i.e. a continuous infusion of glucose at a rate of 4–6 mg/Kg/min until enteral feeding is carefully started.

Anticonvulsants

It is now thought on the basis of animal studies that frequent short-lived convulsions occurring in the neonatal period result in morphological changes involving cortical neuronal activation and density when the brain is examined in adult life (Holmes et al 1998) as well as significant functional adverse effects on subsequent learning and memory. Early convulsions may also increase the susceptibility to further brain damage if subsequent prolonged convulsions develop in later childhood (see Levene 2002 for review). Seizures may cause further neuronal compromise through increased metabolic demands, excitatory amino acid release and disturbances in ventilation and perfusion. This understanding has caused the clinical approach to neonatal convulsions as a result of HIE to shift more in favor of anticonvulsant treatment. Unfortunately currently used anticonvulsants are relatively ineffective in controlling neonatal seizures. The management of neonatal convulsions is considered in detail in Chapter 34.

Barbiturates

This group of drugs has multiple actions on the central nervous system and is still the mainstay of brain-oriented management of the asphyxiated newborn infant. The main benefit of barbiturates in the management of hypoxic–ischemic injury has been demonstrated in human and animal studies but only when the drug was given before the asphyxial event (Campbell et al 1968, Cockburn et al 1969, Goodlin & Lloyd 1970). There have been a number of randomized clinical trials assessing the cerebral protective effects of a barbiturate (phenobarbitone or thiopentone) in neonates following birth asphyxia. There were no significant differences in outcome, but 14 of the 17 infants given thiopentone treatment required inotropic support for hypotension compared with only seven of 15 controls (Goldberg et al 1986). Eyre and Wilkinson (1986) have reported the use of thiopentone in six severely asphyxiated neonates. The dosage was sufficient to produce an iso-electric EEG. In two infants, the infusion was stopped because of hypotension, and in all six, the outcome was death or severe handicap.

More recently, a randomized (non-blinded) controlled study of phenobarbitone (40 mg/Kg over 1 h) prior to the onset of seizures in 20 severely asphyxiated babies showed that the outcome at 3 years was significantly better than in a similar group of babies where phenobarbitone was only given after onset of seizures (Hall et al 1998). A Cochrane review of anticonvulsants in the neonatal period in the prevention of mortality and morbidity did not confirm this benefit (Evans & Levene 2001).

In an important study Painter et al (1999) performed a randomized controlled trial comparing phenobarbitone with phenytoin in the management of EEG diagnosed neonatal convulsions. In less than 50% of either group were the convulsions completely controlled and this proportion was only marginally increased to 59% when both drugs were used together.

Phenobarbitone has been reported to have adverse effects on the developing brain, including inhibition of brain growth, neuronal toxicity and adverse cognitive and behavioral effects when administered to young animals (Levene 2002). However, despite concerns about phenobarbitone toxicity, this drug remains the first-line anticonvulsant (20 mg/Kg loading dose followed by 3 mg/Kg 12-hourly). The dosage of phenobarbitone should be carefully monitored in asphyxiated infants as toxicity may easily occur. Gal et al (1984) have shown that asphyxiated neonates require about half the maintenance dose compared with non-asphyxiated infants to achieve a similar plasma concentration.

Other anticonvulsants

If frequent or prolonged convulsions continue, then a second half loading dose of phenobarbitone can be given (10 mg/Kg). Phenytoin is also widely used to treat post-asphyxial convulsions. A loading dose of 20 mg/Kg may be used to achieve control of frequent seizures. However, phenytoin shows unpredictable plasma levels during maintenance therapy, as well as cardiotoxicity. Phenytoin is contraindicated with lidocaine (see below). Its efficacy in stopping neonatal convulsions is no better than phenobarbitone (Painter et al 1999). Clonazepam has been used as a second-line anticonvulsant (100 µg/Kg loading dose) followed by an intermittent dosage regimen every 24 hours.

More recently, two other anticonvulsants have been used to treat asphyxiated newborn infants; midazolam (0.05 mg/Kg as a loading dose followed by a continuous infusion of 0.15 mg/Kg/h) and lidocaine (lignocaine) (2 mg/Kg as a loading dose followed by 6 mg/Kg/h). There may be synergism between these drugs, and they may be a useful combination in babies with refractory seizures. Further randomized clinical trial data are needed to confirm that midazolam is effective for neonatal seizures, especially since midazolam has not always been effective in published trials

(Boylan et al 2004). The potentially cardiotoxic effects of lidocaine are rarely seen, but are more common if phenytoin has been given prior to the infusion of lidocaine having been started.

It remains unclear for how long anticonvulsants should be continued for post-asphyxial convulsions. As anticonvulsant therapy is based on limited data, and taking into account the potential toxicity of some anticonvulsant drugs, we recommend to discontinue the anticonvulsants once the infant is thought to be neurologically normal on clinical examination.

Cerebral edema

There is some dispute as to the role of cerebral edema in contributing to acute cerebral injury following asphyxia. Brann and Myers (1975) have shown evidence of cerebral edema both macroscopically and microscopically within 2 hours of severe asphyxia in a fetal monkey. In our experience, the median time for severe intracranial hypertension (i.e. intracranial pressure >15 mmHg) to develop in the human neonate following asphyxia is 26 h (unpublished data). These data are not of course incompatible, but the implication that early cerebral edema has a role in the primary pathogenesis of brain injury following intrapartum hypoxic–ischemic injury is unsubstantiated. Cerebral edema severe enough to cause secondary cerebral hypoperfusion is a potential complication of asphyxia, and adequate treatment of intracranial hypertension will not per se prevent brain injury. Levene et al (1987) have analyzed the results of monitoring and treating raised intracranial pressure in full-term asphyxiated infants. In less than 10% of the babies studied could intervention to control intracranial hypertension have had any significant beneficial effect on outcome.

There is no evidence that the routine monitoring of intracranial pressure and appropriate management makes any improvement in outcome.

Corticosteroids

The role of steroids in the management of asphyxia is controversial, with few data available for either newborn humans or experimental animals. Studies on 5-day-old rats, whose brains at that age are at a comparable state of development to the full-term human brain, showed that treatment with dexamethasone before asphyxiation resulted in less severe cerebral effects than in untreated animals (Adlard & De Souza 1976). The use of steroids following neonatal asphyxia was ineffective in treating or preventing cerebral edema (De Souza & Dobbing 1973).

It has been suggested that dexamethasone has its main benefit in treating vasogenic edema and is less effective in cytotoxic edema (Yamaguchi et al 1976), but in clinical practice, both types of brain swelling probably occur together. Corticosteroids have their major role in the treatment of focal cerebral edema associated with tumor or abscess, neither of which bears a close resemblance to the generalized brain swelling that occurs following perinatal asphyxia. In addition, there is a body of evidence on the adverse effects of steroids on the developing brain even when used over a short period of time (Weichsel 1977). Fitzhardinge et al (1974) found measurable differences in neurological function of children who had received hydrocortisone only in the first 24 h of life, compared with untreated controls. Levene and Evans (1985) found no improvement in cerebral perfusion pressure within 6 hours of giving dexamethasone. There is no good evidence for the beneficial effect of using steroids after a hypoxic–ischemic insult in the newborn and their use is not recommended.

Hyperventilation

There is a predictable relationship between $PaCO_2$ and cerebral blood flow. Increasing carbon dioxide tension induces cerebral arteriolar vasodilatation with increase in cerebral blood flow and vice versa (see Fig. 26.12). In adults, for every 0.13 kPa (1 mmHg) change in $PaCO_2$, there is approximately a 3% change in cerebral blood flow over the physiological range for $PaCO_2$ (Bruce 1984). This proportional change diminishes for levels of $PaCO_2$, below 2.7 kPa (20 mmHg). Following perinatal asphyxia, the arteriolar response may be less sensitive to changes in $PaCO_2$, and in some, there may be a paradoxical increase in cerebral blood flow with controlled hyperventilation (Sankaran 1984). Cerebral ischemia is an important component of the pathophysiology of postasphyxial injury in cerebral hypoperfusion, and it is possible that severe hyperventilation may exacerbate impaired reperfusion to the compromised brain. This is strongly implicated in PVL in premature infants (see p. 441).

There have been no clinical trials of hyperventilation in asphyxiated newborn infants. In practice, we attempt to maintain the $PaCO_2$ in asphyxiated infants who are mechanically ventilated at about 4.5 kPa (34 mmHg). A high positive end-expiratory pressure (PEEP) level is likely to produce a higher $PaCO_2$ (Stewart et al 1981), and PEEP should be kept as low as possible in asphyxiated infants who are mechanically ventilated. Hyperventilation should be avoided.

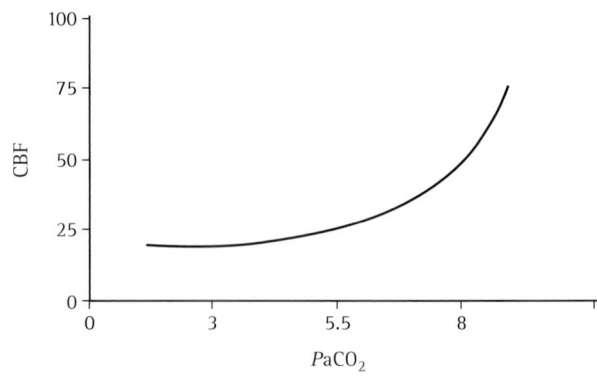

Figure 26.12 Relationship between $PaCO_2$ and cerebral blood flow (CBF). (Redrawn from Bruce 1984.)

Osmotic agents

A variety of agents, including mannitol, glycerol and urea, have been used to shrink the swollen neonatal brain. These agents act by inducing a higher osmotic pressure across the blood–brain barrier, thereby causing intracerebral shrinkage. A theoretical hazard is the entry of the osmotic agent into the brain through the damaged blood–brain barrier, causing a rebound effect of brain swelling. In a neonatal animal model, mannitol significantly reduced the brain water content when given immediately after an asphyxial event (Mujsce et al 1988), but it did not reduce the severity or distribution of brain damage in treated versus untreated animals. Mannitol is the only osmotic agent where published data exist on its use in the newborn. Marchal et al (1974) in an uncontrolled study gave mannitol to 225 babies with the diagnosis of asphyxia, although the precise indications for treatment varied. Early treatment was defined as mannitol infusion (1 g/Kg) before the baby was 2 h of age. There were significantly fewer deaths ($P = 0.005$), and the survivors had a better neurological outcome ($P = 0.014$) in the early treatment group compared with those treated after 2 hours. A fall in intracranial pressure and an improvement in cerebral perfusion pressure were found on each occasion when mannitol (1 g/Kg over 20 min) was infused intravenously in a group of severely asphyxiated babies (Levene & Evans 1985). This appears to be the only agent which is of proven value in treating intracranial hypertension in the asphyxiated newborn. Despite the reduction in ICP in many babies, our follow-up data did not suggest that this made any difference to long-term outcome.

Barbiturates

As mentioned above, barbiturates increase cerebral vascular resistance, thereby reducing cerebral blood flow, and it is this action that contributes to the lowering of intracranial pressure in the swollen brain. It is unlikely that this will improve cerebral perfusion pressure.

New modalities in brain management

There is considerable interest and ongoing research into neuroprotection following hypoxic–ischemic insults and this is reviewed in Chapter 27. Much of this work is speculative and a long way from clinical trials. Three treatment modalities have been assessed in human asphyxiated neonates and these will be discussed here.

Hypothermia

There have been many studies in animal models evaluating the neuroprotective effect of hypothermia and these experiments have shown that cooling during hypoxia–ischemia, even with relatively mild hypothermia, results in long-term neuroprotection in immature animals. The mechanisms for the apparent neuroprotective effects of hypothermia are unclear, but multiple mechanisms have been proposed. These include:

- reduction in neurotransmitter release, including glutamate;

- reduction in metabolic rate with reduced brain O_2 consumption;
- reduction in number of seizures;
- attenuation of changes in some of the protein kinases;
- inhibition in the production of free radicals, particularly hydroxyl possibly by inhibiting NO production;
- reduction in inflammatory mediators such as IL-1β;
- inhibition of apoptosis;
- reduction in the disruption of the blood-brain barrier with inhibition of cerebral edema.

Clinical studies of therapeutic hypothermia have been encouraging. Two studies of global cerebral asphyxial injury following cardiac arrest in adults have shown a significant improvement in outcome following cardiac arrest (Bernard et al 2002, Hypothermia after Cardiac Arrest Study Group 2002). In the neonate, therapeutic hypothermia has been shown to reduce brain injury evident on MR when cooled babies were compared with non-cooled but similarly asphyxiated infants (Inder et al 2004).

A number of randomized controlled studies have been conducted comparing mild therapeutic hypothermia (33.5°C) for 72 hours with normothermia (37°C). The two largest studies reported to date compared brain cooling using a cooling cap (Gluckman et al 2005) and total body cooling (Shankaran et al 2005) and both have shown that this form of treatment instituted within 6 hours of birth in severely asphyxiated infants reduces adverse outcome (death or moderate or severe disability). Therapeutic hypothermia conducted in specialized centers appears to be a safe technique and to date is not associated with a significant risk of complications. A third even larger European study (TOBY) has completed enrollment of 325 babies without any evidence of significant harm during the hypothermic management period or in the immediate rewarming stage. Outcome of this study will not be available until 2008. A recent meta-analysis (Table 26.5) of the three published studies to date shows a significant reduction in death or disability in the hypothermic group compared with the normothermic group (Edwards & Azzopardi 2006).

The role of therapeutic hypothermia following severe birth asphyxia is as yet unproven although the preliminary results are encouraging. An executive summary of the US National Institute of Child Health and Human Development workshop (Higgins et al 2006) has concluded that although hypothermia appears to be a potentially promising therapy for HIE, long-term efficacy and safety is yet to be established and its future use should be restricted to those babies where parents have been appropriately counseled about the uncertainty of long-term benefit. All babies subjected to therapeutic hypothermia should be registered with national or international hypothermia registries.

Allopurinol

Post hypoxic–ischemic injury is thought to be in part due to free-radical damage to both brain and heart. Allopurinol reduces free radical production by inhibition of xanthine

Table 26.5 Meta-analysis of three published studies of outcome following hypothermia vs. normothermia (with permission). Coolcap (Gluckman et al 2005, Eicher et al 2005a, 2005b), NICHD (Shankaran et al 2005). Reproduced from Edwards and Azzopardi 2006

Review: Hypothermia
Comparison: Hypothermia versus normothermia
Outcome: Death or disability

Study or sub-category	Hypothermia n/N	Control n/N	RR (fixed) 95% CI	Weight %	RR (fixed) 95% CI
Coolcap	59/108	73/110		46.10	0.82 (0.66 to 1.02)
Eicher	14/27	21/25		13.90	0.62 (0.41 to 0.92)
NICHD	45/102	64/106		40.00	0.73 (0.56 to 0.95)
Total (95% CI)	237	241		100.00	0.76 (0.65 to 0.89)

Total events: 118 (hypothermia), 158 (control)
Test for heterogeneity: $\chi^2 = 1.63$, df = 2 (p = 0.44), $I^2 = 0\%$
Test for overall effect: z = 3.48 (p = 0.0005)

0.1 0.2 0.5 1 2 5 10

oxidase and by possibly scavenging hydroxyl free radicals. In immature rat pups, post-treatment with allopurinol reduces hypoxic–ischemic brain damage (Palmer et al 1993) and improves electrocortical activity in newborn asphyxiated sheep (Shadid et al 1998). A double-blind randomized controlled trial of allopurinol in Holland enrolled 32 term infants with severe birth asphyxia to receive either intravenous allopurinol (40 mg/Kg) or placebo. Despite early indications that it improved neonatal EEG function, further experience showed that allopurinol did not reduce mortality and morbidity which remained high despite treatment (Benders et al 2006).

Hyperbaric oxygen

In China hyperbaric O_2 is widely used to treat babies with HIE and is thought to reverse local hypoxia, inhibit post-ischemic vasoconstriction and promote the formation of collagen matrix essential for angiogenesis and restoration of cerebral blood flow (Liu et al 2006). A recent meta-analysis of 20 mainly Chinese trials of hyperbaric O_2 used to treat HIE in term infants compared with 'usual care' showed that there was a reduction in mortality (OR 0.26 95%, CI 0.14–0.46) and neurological sequelae (OR 0.41, 0.27–0.61) (Liu et al 2006). Unfortunately the quality of these trials was considered to be poor by Western standards and cannot be relied on for evidence of beneficial effect.

OUTCOME

Prediction of outcome in asphyxiated infants is of obvious importance for the parents, as they will ask 'will my baby be handicapped?' An accurate and honest answer may be available from the results of good follow-up studies. Another important aspect of predicting outcome is the question of when it is appropriate to abandon resuscitative efforts or

withdraw intensive care in infants likely to be severely handicapped. The answers to these questions are beginning to emerge, but a critical review of the assessment methods is necessary, and this is discussed in detail below. A major problem in the evaluation of follow-up studies is the failure to distinguish whether the data refer to full-term babies only or a mixture of mature and immature infants. In addition, the problem of defining what is asphyxia influences outcome statistics. For the purpose of this review, only reports from full-term infants will be considered, and the outcome from different assessment techniques will be discussed separately. The utility of any test can be evaluated from its sensitivity, specificity and positive predictive value. Sensitivity refers to the percentage of handicapped infants detected by the test, and specificity is the percentage of normal infants detected by a normal test. Positive predictive value is the proportion of times a positive test predicts adverse outcome. To evaluate any assessment of outcome, all these variables should be considered. Wherever it has been possible to calculate these figures, they are given in the text.

There is some evidence that the prognosis following intrapartum asphyxia has improved over recent years (Finer et al 1983). A Swedish study reported that 50% of infants surviving asphyxia between 1973 and 1976 had significant neurodevelopmental sequelae, in contrast to a 17% incidence of handicap in those born between 1976 and 1979 (Svenningsen et al 1982). Svenningsen et al related the improved outcome to the introduction of brain-oriented intensive care, but there has been no single therapeutic innovation that has improved the outcome for asphyxiated babies over recent years.

Few data are available for the outcome of asphyxiated term babies born in developing countries. One recent study from Kathmandu in Nepal reports that the overall risk of death or major disability at 1 year of age in a group of term babies with signs of neonatal encephalopathy was 62% compared with only 4% of normal controls (Ellis et al 1999). This is considerably higher than in the developed world. The relative risk of impairment in survivors of grade I neonatal encephalopathy was 5.3 (95% CI 0.9, 30), and for grade II neonatal encephalopathy, 32.1 (95% CI 7.9, 131).

MORTALITY

The mortality rate of live-born asphyxiated infants depends on the severity of the insult and the intensity of treatment. If asphyxia is defined by depression of the Apgar score, then mortality increases inversely to gestational age and birth weight.

MacDonald et al (1980) report an overall mortality of 46% in severely asphyxiated infants of all gestational ages, and the presence of intrauterine growth retardation, respiratory distress syndrome and hypothermia were all associated with a significantly higher risk of death. In another study, over half of the infants died, if born with an Apgar score of 0 at birth, or delay in establishing respiration until 20 minutes after birth (Scott 1976). In the well-known study of Nelson and Ellenberg (1981) over 40 000 infants had an accurate assessment of the Apgar score. Those with a birth weight below 2500 g with severe depression of the Apgar score at 15 and 20 min had approximately a 90% chance of dying, but this was considerably less in infants weighing more than 2500 g. Casey et al (2001) demonstrated that the association between low 5 min Apgar scores and an increased risk of neonatal death remains pertinent almost 50 years after the introduction of the scoring system: for 132 228 infants born at term, the mortality rate was 244 per 1000 for infants with 5 min Apgar scores of 0–3, as compared with 0.2 per 1000 for infants with 5 min scores of 7–10 (Table 26.6). In addition, the study demonstrates that the Apgar score predicts neonatal death more accurately than the umbilical-artery pH, as the risk of neonatal death in term infants with 5 min Apgar scores of 0–3 was eight times the risk in term infants with umbilical-artery blood pH values of 7.00 or less.

Delay in establishing spontaneous respiration also seems to predict the risk of death. Steiner and Nelligan (1975) have shown that infants who have not established regular breathing 30 minutes after return of the heartbeat subsequently have a very poor outcome. They suggest that resuscitation under these circumstances should not be continued for longer than this time. By contrast, a Swedish study found that 25% of babies who had not breathed spontaneously by 20 min were without significant handicap (Ergander et al 1983). Peliowski and Finer (1992) have reviewed the literature and report the outcome of only 35 full-term babies who did not breathe spontaneously by 30 min and 24 (80%) died or were significantly handicapped.

When to abandon resuscitation
1. If an infant has no cardiac output after 10 min of effective resuscitation, then treatment should be abandoned.
2. If a baby is not breathing spontaneously by 30 min, then the value of further resuscitation should be seriously questioned. Other causes for failure to breathe spontaneously should be considered, such as opiate depression and neuromuscular disorders. The final decision to abandon resuscitation should be made by the most senior neonatologist/pediatrician available.

DISABILITY

At present, there is no single measure of fetal or neonatal condition that accurately predicts later neurodevelopmental disability. It has been suggested that a diagnosis of encephalopathic perinatal asphyxia requires the evidence of neonatal neurologic abnormalities and multi-system organ dysfunction, in addition to both a low 5 min Apgar score and neonatal acidosis (ACOG 1996).

Babies born apparently dead, but resuscitated rapidly, may subsequently be neurologically normal (Jain et al 1991, Scott 1976, Steiner & Nelligan 1975). Casalaz et al (1998) described 29 babies of gestational age 36 weeks and above, born with a zero 1 min Apgar score and who were success-

Table 26.6 Risk of death according to Apgar scores at 5 minutes for preterm and term infants (from Casey et al 2001). The Apgar scores 7–10 represent the reference group

Five minute Apgar score	No of live births	Neonatal deaths (rate per 1000 births)	Relative risk (95% CI)
Preterm births (26–36 weeks of gestation)			
0–3	92	315	59 (40–87)
4–6	556	72	13 (9–20)
7–10	12 751	5	1
Term births (≥37 weeks)			
0–3	86	244	1460 (835–2555)
4–6	561	9	53 (20–140)
7–10	131 581	0.2	1

fully resuscitated. Forty-five percent of these babies were subsequently described as normal, and a further 34% died prior to discharge from hospital. Of those who went home, only 31.5% were disabled. Disability probably depends on the duration and severity of the asphyxial insult as well as the development of cardiovascular complications.

Asphyxia has been described as having an all or none effect. The majority of very severely asphyxiated babies die, and the majority of the remainder are without major neurological deficit and are often reported as being 'normal' at follow-up. Only a very small proportion are disabled. This effect may be illusory as there are very few good long-term follow-up studies to assess the children for less severe forms of disability such as clumsiness, attention deficit disorders and learning problems.

Finer et al (1983) in Canada have regularly assessed a group of full-term asphyxiated infants at 27 months, 3.5 years (Robertson & Finer 1985) and 8 years (Robertson et al 1989). They showed that there is a gradation of effect on the intelligence quotient (IQ) for different degrees of severity of the asphyxial insult. At 3.5 years, the children with moderate HIE had a median Stanford Binet IQ of 92.3 compared with 101.5 in babies with mild HIE (Robertson & Finer 1985). At 8 years, there was a difference in IQ of 11 points between children with moderate HIE and mild HIE and 17 points between moderate HIE and a non-asphyxiated control group (Robertson et al 1989). Children who survived severe HIE had a median IQ of 48 at 8 years. Cognitive impairment as measured by the IQ therefore appears to represent a continuum of disability reflecting the severity of the initial asphyxial insult.

The classic disability suffered by the survivors of severe asphyxia is cerebral palsy. This may be associated with intellectual impairment, blindness and epilepsy, but the motor deficit is invariably present with these other disabilities. Mental retardation alone is not a recognized sequel to intrapartum asphyxia. Two distinct forms of cerebral palsy occur as the result of birth asphyxia at full term: spastic quadriplegia and choreoathetosis, or a combination of these two. These two patterns of motor deficit presumably reflect the regions of the brain predominantly affected by the asphyxial process (see p. 546).

The late onset of dystonia (including athetosis) with normal intelligence has been described many years following perinatal asphyxia (Saint Hilaire et al 1991, Scott & Jankovic 1996). The mean age of onset in these studies was over 10 years, with progression over a further 7–10 years. In one study, the latency in neonates with a hypoxic–ischemic etiology was 27.6 years (Scott & Jankovic 1996). In another study, none of the subjects were severely disabled by the dystonia (Saint Hilaire et al 1991).

Fetal assessment
Passage of meconium
Thick meconium present in the liquor at the onset of labor carries a sevenfold increased risk of perinatal death (MacDonald et al 1985). Meconium staining of the liquor does not, however, predict the risk of subsequent disability. Ninety-nine percent of all babies born with meconium-stained liquor do not have cerebral palsy (Freeman & Nelson 1988).

Acidosis
Low et al (1978a) defined fetal acidosis as an umbilical artery buffer base of less than 34 mmol/L, and these infants had on average a lower 1- and 5-min Apgar score than a control, non-acidotic group. However, they could find no differences in neurological outcome between the acidotic and control groups at 12 months of age. During the course of normal labor, the PaO_2 drops, the $PaCO_2$ rises, and the base deficit rises. In most centers, a pH of more than 7.2 is considered normal and a pH of 7.0 to 7.2 is considered mild or moderate acidemia. Severe acidemia is when the pH is below 7.0. Just as the Apgar score alone is a poor predictor of outcome, metabolic acidosis in isolation also proves to be a poor predictor of significant perinatal brain injury. Ruth and Raivio (1988) assessed umbilical arterial acid-base values on 982 live-born (mainly full-term) infants and correlated these measurements with neurodevelopmental outcome at 12 months of age. The positive predictive value for low pH (<7.16) and high lactate (>5.4 mmol/L) with reference to abnormal outcome was only 8 and 5%, respectively. Of 314 infants who had severe umbilical artery acidosis with long-term follow-up that were identified in the world literature, 27 (8.6%) children subsequently were found to be brain-damaged (Kirkendall & Phelan 2001). Murray et al (2006) recently used early continuous electroencephalographic monitoring after perinatal asphyxia in term infants. It was demonstrated that the degree of metabolic acidosis (whether measured as base deficit, lactate or pH) could not reliably predict neonatal seizures. Only the 5 min Apgar score was significantly associated with both Sarnat grade and electroencephalographic abnormalities. Therefore, acidosis at birth does not appear to predict adverse outcome and cannot be used as a measure of potential compromise to the fetal brain. In addition, whilst measurements of umbilical-artery blood gases provide an accurate assessment of the immediate neonatal condition, their usefulness is limited because the results are often not available until after decisions regarding the treatment of the infant have been made (Papile 2001). In contrast, the absence of severe acidosis does not ensure a favorable neurologic outcome.

Hermansen (2003) suggested there even may exist a beneficial effect of a mild to moderate acidosis, i.e. an acidosis paradox. Firstly, hypercarbia may result in cerebral vasodilatation and increased cerebral blood flow. Secondly, acidosis has been shown to decrease cerebral metabolism and lower the oxidative needs of the brain. Finally, acidosis promotes the unloading of O_2 from the fetal hemoglobin by shifting the O_2 dissociation curve. These three mechanisms theoretically lead to an adequate amount of O_2 delivery to the brain tissue, which potentially limits damage. These protective effects would be lost, however, with severe acidosis.

Cardiotocography (CTG)

The fetal condition is assessed widely by means of measuring the fetal heart rate (see Ch. 24). This can be done intermittently by means of a stethoscope or by an electronic device. Continuous electronic fetal heart rate monitoring and evaluation of changes in heart rate with contractions (cardiotocography) have become very widely used in recent years, but there are relatively few data on the long-term prediction of outcome. Despite a near 3-decade experience with intensive fetal heart rate monitoring, aimed at the early detection of intrapartum fetal distress in sufficient time to prevent fetal brain injury, the impact on subsequent neurologic outcome has been minimal (Perlman 2006).

Grant (1989) has reviewed the literature on fetal monitoring and performed meta-analyses on the published data. When electronic fetal monitoring with scalp blood sampling for fetal pH is compared with intermittent auscultation, there is no significant reduction in perinatal deaths (odds ratio 0.81, 95% CI 0.22–2.98). Cardiotocogram (CTG) monitoring increases the risk of Cesarean section fourfold compared with intermittent auscultation. When the effect of electronic fetal monitoring and scalp sampling was compared with intermittent auscultation on neonatal seizures, there was a significant reduction in the number of infants with convulsions in those fetuses continuously monitored (odds ratio 0.49, 95% CI 0.29–0.82).

There are limited data on the correlation with CTG monitoring and subsequent disability. Painter et al (1978) followed up 38 full-term infants with 'ominous' fetal heart-rate patterns. These infants showed moderate to severely variable patterns with or without late decelerations. Of the 38 infants, five were neurologically abnormal at 1 year of age, and four in the group had patterns showing severe variability. Surprisingly, few of these infants had depressed Apgar scores. A subsequent report stated that none of these children were abnormal in later childhood (Paneth & Stark 1983). Ingemarrson et al (1981) showed that fewer infants were born with depressed Apgar scores over three time periods following the introduction of CTG monitoring, but in the high-risk full-term pregnancies, there was no statistically significant reduction in neurological sequelae at 2 years, although there was a trend towards improvement. This study was undertaken over a period of time when many changes were introduced in both obstetric and neonatal management, and no firm conclusions on the prognostic value of abnormal CTGs can be made.

In a limited follow-up study from Dublin of electronic fetal heart rate monitoring versus intermittent auscultation, there were no differences in the number of children with cerebral palsy in the two groups (Grant et al 1989).

In conclusion, CTG monitoring increases the rate of operative deliveries, but does not reduce the risk of perinatal death. There is good evidence that the number of neonatal convulsions is reduced in the group that are electronically monitored but that there is no reduction in the risk of cerebral palsy.

Apgar score

Whilst the 10-point Apgar score was not intended to be a measure of perinatal asphyxia, depression of the score has traditionally been widely used as a method for determining asphyxia and predicting outcome. The score does not reflect how long the infant suffered from intrapartum asphyxia and, therefore, is, in most cases, a blunt instrument for predicting outcome.

The risk of handicap following depression of the Apgar score is best estimated from the data of Nelson and Ellenberg (1981). In full-term infants, the risk only becomes significant if the Apgar score remains 0–3 at 20 minutes. Depression of the Apgar score to this degree at 15 minutes is associated with less than a 10% risk of subsequent cerebral palsy in surviving infants. In another study, 93% of infants with severely depressed Apgar scores (0 at 1 min and/or 0–3 at 5 min) were normal at follow-up (Thomson et al 1977).

An overview of three studies investigating the outcome of full-term babies with depressed Apgar scores of 3 or less at 5 min showed that this carried an overall risk of mortality of 16% but only a 3% risk of handicap in surviving infants (Peliowski & Finer 1992). Levene et al (1986) identified a group of infants at risk of handicap following intrapartum asphyxia and assessed the sensitivity of various degrees of Apgar score depression (Table 26.7). They found an Apgar score of 5 or less at 10 min to be the most sensitive predictor of outcome, and this was also highly specific.

Onset of spontaneous respiration

The time to the onset of spontaneous breathing or the first breath, or, alternatively, the need for intubation has been used by many as an alternative marker of immediate neonatal condition that might be more useful than the Apgar score in assessing the severity of asphyxia. Unfortunately, these markers are likely to be even less discriminatory, as they measure only one characteristic and may be influenced

Table 26.7 Sensitivity and specificity of six different grades of Apgar depression (Levene et al 1986)

Depression of Apgar score	N	Sensitivity (%)	Specificity (%)
<3 at 1 min: >5 by 5 min	42	13	38
<5 at 5 min: >5 by 10 min	35	17	67
<3 at 5 min: >5 by 10 min	10	13	90
<5 at 10 min: >5 by 20 min	15	43	95
<3 at 10 min: >5 by 20 min	5	17	99
<5 at 20 min: or more	3	13	100

by other factors that cause depression of respiration, such as the administration of maternal drugs and neuromuscular disease of the newborn.

Failure to establish spontaneous respiration by 30 min carries a very high risk of handicap or death (see above). Scott (1976) reported a remarkably low risk of handicap in a group of surviving infants who had shown no spontaneous respiration by 20 min from birth. Ergander et al (1983) reported that 71% of babies who had established spontaneous respiration by 20 min were normal or only had minimal handicap. In another study, almost 70% of mature infants who had required IPPV for more than 1 min were normal (Mulligan et al 1980). Fysh et al (1982) reported an infant who did not establish regular respiration for 25 min and who had an arterial pH of 6.6 at 1 h. This infant was entirely normal at 3 years of age, and it is interesting to note that the infant had neither convulsions nor any other neurological abnormality in the newborn period, supporting the contention that the severity of clinical neurological abnormality is the more important predictor of adverse outcome.

Presence of multiorgan dysfunction

There seems to be little association between the presence/absence of multiorgan dysfunction (MOD) and outcome in infants with severe post-asphyxial HIE. Whilst Shah et al (2004) confirmed evidence of MOD in all infants with severe intra-partum asphyxia, no relation was observed between individual or combinations of organ involvements and long term outcome. Inconsistencies in organ involvement are also observed in animal experiments under controlled conditions (Jensen 1999), suggesting variation in individual vulnerability and variable activation of the diving reflex, dependent on the cause of asphyxia.

Hypoxic–ischemic encephalopathy

Moderate or severe encephalopathy following intrapartum asphyxia has been shown to be a more sensitive predictor of death or severe neurodevelopmental sequelae than depression of the Apgar scores (Levene et al 1986). Different studies have reported an outcome related to the severity of HIE (Amiel-Tison & Ellison 1986, Dixon et al 2002, Finer et al 1981, 1983, Levene et al 1986, Low et al 1985, Robertson & Finer 1985, Sarnat & Sarnat 1976), and these methods are discussed in Chapter 9. Although some vary slightly in their definition of the grades of encephalopathy, there is remarkable consensus when predicting adverse outcome. Results from six of these studies are shown in Table 26.8. No infant with mild HIE developed a significant neurodevelopmental handicap. The one handicapped infant in the study of Levene et al (1986) had congenital myopathy. The incidence of severe handicap or death in the moderate encephalopathy group varied between 15 and 27%. Robertson and Finer (1985) found all infants with severe encephalopathy to have a poor outcome, but this was not the case in the majority of studies. Surprisingly, up to 25% of infants comatose due to asphyxia, but who survived, were without any significant handicap.

Peliowski and Finer (1992) have reported a meta-analysis of five published studies reporting outcome by severity of HIE. The risk of death for babies with severe, moderate, and mild HIE is 61, 5.6, and less than 1%, respectively.

The duration of time that infants show clinical neurological abnormalities following asphyxia correlates well with the risk of handicap. Sarnat and Sarnat (1976) reported that a good outcome was seen in infants with moderate encephalopathy (lethargy, hypotonia and seizures) if abnormal clinical signs had disappeared within 5 days of life. In another study, only infants with neurological signs persisting for more than 6 weeks developed cerebral palsy (Scott 1976). Recovery to a normal neurological score by 7 days after birth was found by Thompson et al (1997) to be a very good prognostic marker.

Badawi et al (2005) reported from Western Australia a follow-up study of 251 survivors of moderate or severe neonatal encephalopathy (NE), but not all cases were due to birth asphyxia. CP was diagnosed in 8% in the moderate NE group at a minimum age of 5 years. Amongst survivors at 5 years in the severe NE group, CP was diagnosed in 23%.

Table 26.8 Proportion of disabled children depending on their degree of HIE (only full-term infants included)

Reference	n	Proportion severely abnormal or dead (%)			
		Mild (1)	Moderate (2)	Severe (3)	Duration of follow-up (years)
Sarnat & Sarnat (1976)	21	—	25	100	1
Finer et al (1981)	89	0	15	92	3.5
Robertson & Finer (1985)	200	0	27	100	3.5
Low et al (1985)	42	—[a]	27	50	1
Levene et al (1986)	122	1[b]	25	75	2.5 (median)
Dixon et al (2002)	195	—[c]	25	62	1–2

[a]Mild and moderate HIE considered together
[b]Handicap due to congenital myopathy
[c]Not included in study

Those children with CP were more likely to have spastic quadriplegia or dyskinetic (athetoid) forms of the condition and in addition to CP, cognitive impairment and epilepsy were other common disabilities in the group of survivors.

In a British study (Marlow et al 2005) reported outcome at a mean of 7 years in 68 survivors of neonatal encephalopathy was graded as either moderate or severe. Fifteen (22%) had CP of whom all but two were in the severe NE group. Eight had quadriplegia, 1 diplegia, and 6 had hemiplegia. None were reported to have a dyskinetic form. Of the children with CP two also had sensorineural hearing impairment and one had cortical blindness.

Subtle disabilities

Most studies reporting outcome of babies with NE or HIE have concentrated on hard neurological disability such as cerebral palsy and intellectual impairment. More recently reports have appeared reporting outcome in asphyxiated babies who did not have such severe abnormalities. One such study reported motor and cognitive outcome at 5½–6½ years in a group of 34 children with NE, but no subsequent evidence of CP. Abnormalities in subtle motor function were shown in 5/32 (15.6%). In all 5 cases there were abnormalities on the MR brain scan (Barnett et al 2002). These cases are sometimes labeled as 'clumsy children' but more recently the term development coordination disorder (DCD) has been used.

Marlow et al (2005) reported that there was a reduction in cognitive scores in children without disability, but only in those with severe NE (11.3 points below a control group and 9.6 points below the moderate NE group). Testing showed that children surviving with severe or moderate NE, but without major disability also showed worse language, attention/executive and memory scores. They also showed higher overall behavioral scores in the severe NE group. They found that if children with motor disability were excluded, then 67% of the severe NE group had special educational needs.

Scoring systems

Various scoring systems to summarize the extent of neurological abnormalities after asphyxia have been developed (Bao et al 1993, Carter et al 1998, Ekert et al 1997, Lipper et al 1986, Perlman & Risser 1996, Thompson et al 1997). Lipper et al's postasphyxial score (PAS) was assigned within the first 24 hours, based on 17 items, six of which are related to tone. The optimal (maximum) score was 39, and no infants with a score of 6 or less survived without a severe handicap. The PAS correctly predicted abnormal outcome (sensitivity) at 1 year in 95% of infants and showed a specificity of 83%. Thompson et al (1997) devised a score based on nine signs (two based on tone or posture) with a maximum abnormality score of 22. They showed that babies with a maximum score of >15 had a positive predictive value of 92% with sensitivity and specificity of 71 and 96% respectively. Levene et al (1986) found a moderate or severe encephalopathy to have a positive predictive value for adverse outcome (handicap or death) of 96% and a specificity of 78%.

Three further systems have attempted to look at very early markers of neonatal complications that fall short of neurodevelopmental outcome (Perlman & Risser 1996). The aim of these studies was to identify a group of babies soon after birth who were at risk of permanent injury and in whom timely intervention may improve outcome (see Ch. 28). Table 26.9 shows the sensitivity, specificity and positive predictive value of these scoring systems. Caution must be exercised in interpreting the predictive value of these tests as neurodevelopmental outcome was not assessed, but rather variables that may or may not be good markers of the risk of adverse outcome.

A recent large retrospectively designed study evaluated 365 infants with HIE and found three clinical parameters to be predictors of severe adverse outcome (death or severe disability): administration of chest compression for >1 min, onset of regular respirations >30 min after birth, and base deficit value of >16 mmol/L on any blood gas analysis within

Table 26.9 Comparison of four scoring systems for prediction of term infants at risk of poor outcome following asphyxia

Author	Scoring system	Outcome variable	Sensitivity (%)	Specificity (%)	PPV (%)
Perlman & Risser (1996)	pH ≥7.00 Delivery room intubation Apgar ≤5 at 5 min	Neonatal seizures	80	98.8	80
Ekert et al (1997)	Spontaneous respiration ≥10 min Onset seizures ≤4 h	HIE	71	73	69
Carter et al (1998)	Score ≥6[a]	Multiorgan failure	—	—	73
Miller et al (2004)	Encephalopathy scores[a] day 1 day 1–3	Development at 30 months	72 73	94 96	84 89

[a]See text for scoring system
PPV = positive predictive value

the first 4 h from birth (Shah et al 2006). Severe outcome rates with none, one, two, or all three predictors were 46, 64, 76, and 93% respectively. Miller et al (2004) developed an encephalopathy score based on six items (feeding, alertness, tone, respiratory status, reflexes and seizures) with a maximum score of 6 (worst) whilst 0 represents optimality. A maximum score on day 1 with seizures predicted abnormal outcome at 30 months with a sensitivity of 72%, specificity of 94% and positive predictive value of 84%.

The type of abnormal neurological signs may also predict poor outcome. Brown et al (1974) recognize two clinical categories that are particularly associated with death or handicap. In the group with persistent hypotonia, only 16% were normal, and in those in whom hypotonia evolved to extensor hypertonia, only 23% were normal. Among infants with a predominant extensor type of abnormality, 56% were normal on follow-up. Apathy in the newborn period had also been reported to occur more frequently in infants with abnormal outcome, but no children were found to be severely handicapped in this group (De Souza & Richards 1978). Convulsions may predict outcome to some extent. Approximately half of the asphyxiated infants with neonatal seizures have some functional handicap (see Ch. 34).

It is clear that the severity of abnormal neurological behavior occurring after birth in infants who have suffered intrapartum asphyxia is an excellent predictor of subsequent outcome.

The pattern of abnormal neurological signs in asphyxiated babies may correlate with the distribution of brain injury. Full-term infants with predominantly basal ganglia involvement on MR imaging have persistent and diffuse neurological abnormalities compared with those who sustain injury mainly in the white matter. These latter show a different clinical pattern with an improved sucking reflex and less severe abnormalities in tone (Mercuri et al 1999). Rosenbloom (1994) has described a group of severely asphyxiated babies with later development of dyskinetic (choreoathetoid) cerebral palsy to have relatively little evidence of HIE in the neonatal period presumably because of cortical sparing.

Interesting data is emerging from current hypothermia trials in term asphyxiated newborns. For instance, Ambalavanan et al (2006) recently performed a secondary analysis of data from the multicenter, randomized, controlled trial of hypothermia in HIE ($n = 205$ newborns) (Shankaran 2005), identifying predictor variables and developing scoring systems and classification trees to predict death/disability or death in infants with HIE. If validated, scoring systems and classification trees may help in the assessment of prognosis and may prove useful for risk identification in future neuroprotection intervention trials.

Brain imaging

Computerized tomography (CT) is reported to be a good predictor of bad neurodevelopmental outcome in asphyxiated babies when extensive areas of hypodensity are seen in scans taken at 7–14 days after birth (Adsett et al 1985, Fitzhardinge et al 1981, Lipper et al 1986). The sensitivity and specificity of abnormal scans (diffuse or global decrease in density) in the prediction of major handicap or subsequent death are reported to be 90–91 and 60–80%, respectively (Adsett et al 1985, Lipper et al 1986). In contrast, others have shown no correlation between abnormal CT scans and outcome, but these studies were performed within 7 days from birth (Finer et al 1983, Lipp-Zwahlen et al 1985b). In summary, CT appears to be a good predictor of subsequent outcome in asphyxiated full-term infants, but only if the scan is done after the first week of life. This limits the value of this technique in the acute management of the severely asphyxiated infant in whom withdrawal of care is considered.

Distribution of MR signal abnormalities can be subdivided according to the severity of hypoxia–ischemia (Barkovich et al 1995). Cases of mild to moderate hypoperfusion are characterized by parasagittal lesions, involving vascular border zones between anterior, middle and posterior cerebral arteries (watershed pattern), whereas profound hypotension involves primary lateral thalami, posterior putamen, hippocampi and perirolandic gyri (cortical highlighting) (Aida et al 1998, Barkovich et al 1998, Rutherford et al 1996). It is clear that the risk of an abnormal neurodevelopmental outcome increases with the severity of the injury; however the pattern of injury also conveys important prognostic information. Newborns with a predominantly watershed pattern suffer from cognitive impairments that often occur without functional motor deficits (Miller et al 2004). In contrast, a basal ganglia-thalamus predominant pattern (Miller et al 2004) as well as an abnormal signal intensity in the posterior limb of the internal capsule (PLIC) on MRI are associated with severely impaired motor and cognitive outcomes (Rutherford et al 1998). Indeed, the best predictor of bad outcome in MR scans taken in the first 10 days of life is abnormality of signal intensity within the PLIC (Rutherford et al 1998). This is best seen on IR sequences and often associated with more extensive abnormalities within the basal ganglia. An abnormal or equivocal signal intensity within the PLIC predicted abnormal outcome with a sensitivity of 90%, specificity of 100% and positive predictive value of 100%. Given the frequent co-occurrence of watershed injury (Miller et al 2004) and cerebellar injury (Le Strange et al 2004) with the basal ganglia-thalamus predominant pattern, cognitive deficits may result from damage to areas outside the deep gray nuclei themselves.

Advanced brain imaging, i.e. quantitative morphometric MR techniques, MR spectroscopy and DWI (see Ch. 6), is emerging as a powerful tool to correlate the location and severity of brain lesions with neurodevelopmental outcome. The techniques can now be applied to measure subtle brain injuries, such as white matter injuries, and determine their association with long-term cognitive deficits (Miller et al 2002a, Nagy et al 2005). For example, in a recent case series, five patients with delayed recall, in the setting of intact semantic memory and motor function between 8 and 14 years, were found to have bilateral hippocampal atrophy using advanced MR techniques (Gadian et al 2000).

Two scoring systems have been described, which rate abnormalities seen on early MR scans in term asphyxiated infants (Barkovich et al 1998, Rutherford et al 1995). In MR studies performed before the seventh day after birth, higher scores as the result of basal ganglia abnormalities were most highly predictive of adverse outcome at 12 months (Barkovich et al 1998).

Electroencephalography

These techniques are discussed fully in Chapter 12. The EEG abnormalities seen in mature asphyxiated infants and associated with a poor prognosis include iso-electric recordings and periodic patterns (Holmes et al 1982, Sarnat & Sarnat 1976, Selton & Andre 1997, Wertheim et al 1994) and persistent low-voltage states (Holmes et al 1982). Holmes et al (1983) have shown that some infants with a burst suppression pattern can be stimulated to produce continuous activity, and in these infants, the prognosis is better. A normal EEG in asphyxiated infants is usually associated with an excellent prognosis (Rose & Lombroso 1970, Sarnat & Sarnat 1976, Selton & Andre 1997, Watanabe et al 1980, Wertheim et al 1994).

Peliowski and Finer (1992) have performed a meta-analysis on four studies where early EEG assessment could be correlated with outcome in groups of asphyxiated mature neonates. Severe EEG abnormalities included burst suppression, low-voltage, or iso-electric EEGs, and moderate EEG abnormality included slow wave activity. The overall risk of death or handicap derived from these studies is 95% for a severely abnormal EEG, 64% for a moderately abnormal EEG, and 3.3% for a normal or mildly abnormal EEG. Further studies published since this meta-analysis have confirmed these findings (Selton & Andre 1997, Wertheim et al 1994).

Cerebral function monitoring, a single channel compressed EEG signal (also referred to as amplitude integrated EEG–aEEG) is now widely used in neonates and is discussed in detail in Chapter 12. Several studies aim to determine the natural course of aEEG patterns during the first days of life in severely asphyxiated term infants, this in relation to neurologic outcome at 24 months or later (Shalak et al 2003). Normal voltage patterns (continuous and discontinuous normal voltage) up to 48 h of life seem predictive for normal neurologic outcomes (Ter Horst et al 2004). Burst suppression or paroxysmal activity has been reported to be associated with a poor outcome (Thornberg & Ekstrom-Jodal 1994), and these abnormalities may be present within 4 h of birth (Eken et al 1995). Spontaneous recovery of severely abnormal aEEG patterns is not uncommon; the sooner the abnormalities on aEEG disappear, the better the prognosis.

Evoked response EEGs such as visual, auditory and somatosensory evoked potentials may also provide accurate prognostic information in asphyxia, and the role of these techniques in the prediction of outcome following birth asphyxia is discussed in Chapter 12.

Intracranial pressure

Continuous measurement of intracranial pressure by a sub-arachnoid catheter gives some prognostic information (Levene et al 1987). No infant with a sustained rise in intracranial pressure of 15 mmHg or more lasting for an hour or more survived without major handicap. Infants with sustained elevations in intracranial pressure above 10 mmHg generally had a worse prognosis than those without a rise to this level, but a cut-off of 10 mmHg was not as sensitive for handicap as a sustained elevation to 15 mmHg.

Interestingly, low cerebral perfusion pressure did not predict outcome as well as intracranial hypertension (Levene et al 1987). This is probably because hypotension can cause a low cerebral perfusion pressure without any significant cerebral edema. The hypotension reflects cardiovascular injury with a good prognosis rather than cerebral compromise.

Doppler assessment

The use of Doppler ultrasound to assess cerebral hemodynamics has been shown to be a useful prognostic indicator in term asphyxiated newborns (Archer et al 1986, Ilves et al 1998, Levene et al 1989, Liao & Hung 1997, Low et al 1994). The measurement of PRI (Pourcelot's resistance index; see p. 557) predicts outcome in asphyxiated full-term infants with an 86% accuracy (Archer et al 1986). A low PRI (<0.55) predicts adverse outcome with a sensitivity and a specificity of 100 and 81%, respectively. In a more recent study using duplex Doppler that allows calculation of cerebral blood flow velocity (CBFV) within the anterior cerebral artery, Levene et al (1989) showed that a CBFV value 3SDs above the mean had a positive predictive value for adverse outcome (death or handicap) of 94% compared with 83% for a PRI < 0.55. The sensitivity for high CBFV was 57%, and the specificity 88%. The advantage of Doppler assessment is that abnormalities become apparent within 12–60 h after birth (Archer et al 1986, Ilves et al 1998, Levene et al 1989).

Magnetic resonance spectroscopy (see also Ch. 11)

Magnetic resonance spectroscopy (MRS) allows for the non-invasive detection of tissue metabolism and in vivo biochemistry, i.e. the separation of a variety of biochemical compounds within the brain, such as lactate, N-acetyl aspartate, choline and creatine, providing functional data regarding metabolic integrity in specific regions of the brain (Vigneron et al 2001). Using MRS, changes related to asphyxia have been studied in full-term newborn infants. The technique, especially three-dimensional MRS, can be used to define the injury at its inception and can possibly be linked to future neurodevelopmental outcome measures, to determine which newborns are at high risk for adverse neurologic sequelae and should receive therapy (Miller et al 2002a).

Two techniques have been used, based on ^{31}P and ^{1}H proton spectroscopy. The former provides information on phosphorylated energy states within the brain. The phosphorus metabolites ATP, phosphocreatine (PCr) and inorganic phosphorus (P_i) can be measured, and the PCr/P_i ratio has been used to assess the state of degradation of the cerebral energy state. Degradation in ATP is associated with a poor outcome (Lorek et al 1994, Martin et al 1996, Moorcroft et al 1991, Roth et al 1997). A PCr/P_i ratio below the range of values from normal infants predicted an adverse outcome after asphyxia with a sensitivity and a specificity of 88 and 83%, respectively. The positive predictive value was 64% (Moorcroft et al 1991).

^{1}H proton spectroscopy has also been evaluated in a group of severely asphyxiated and encephalopathic infants, and high levels of intracerebral lactate and low *N*-acetylaspartate predict adverse outcome (Groenendaal et al 1994, Hanrahan et al 1999, Kadri et al 2003, Leth et al 1996, Peden et al 1993, Penrice et al 1996, Roelants-van Rijn 2001b). The role of ^{1}H proton spectroscopy in neonates that are not encephalopathic is less clear: when lactate is present in the acute stages, it suggests that anaerobic metabolism is occurring. However, absence of lactate does not exclude anaerobic metabolism, because rebound hyperperfusion can decrease tissue lactate levels (Grant 2006). Myo-inositol among other metabolites (betaine, taurine) regulates cell volume during osmotic stress. Preliminary data showed that early increases in myo-inositol/Cr in infants with neonatal encephalopathy are associated with increased lactate/Cr, MR imaging changes of severe injury, and a poor neurodevelopmental outcome at one year of age (Robertson et al 2001). Finally, as MRS made it possible to study the underlying metabolic mechanisms that define the pathophysiologic events taking place in neonatal brain injury, it emerges that proton spectroscopy may well be an important tool to guide and monitor interventions aimed at brain protection (Hüppi 2002).

NEONATAL BRAIN DEATH

The concept of brain death is now well established in children, and guidelines on diagnosis have been published in both the USA (Task Force 1987) and Britain (British Paediatric Association 1991). These criteria are compared in Table 26.10. Both documents agree that brain death cannot be diagnosed in premature infants, but there is some disagreement as to the diagnosis of brain death in the mature neonate. The British Paediatric Association document states that in infants of 37 weeks' gestation to 2 months of age, 'given the state of knowledge it is rarely possible to diagnose confidently brain stem death at this age,' and in infants below 37 weeks' gestation, 'the concept of brain stem death is inappropriate for infants of this age group'. In the USA, the Special Task Force of the American Academy of Pediatrics concludes that 'in term newborns (>38 weeks' gestation), the criteria (for diagnosing brain death) are useful seven days after the neurologic insult'.

These differences revolve around the rapid developmental changes seen in the later stages of gestation and the early weeks of life. This means that there cannot be absolute reliance placed on the presence or absence of brainstem reflexes at this developmental age. Volpe (1987) describes two infants with apparent brain death including coma, absent respiration, loss of pupillary responses to light and loss of other brainstem responses who survived. One, a 35-week-old infant, showed near-normal development at 1 year of age, and the other, a full-term infant, regained brainstem reflexes 24 hours following the first examination and left hospital alive, albeit in a persistent vegetative state.

Another difference between the American and British criteria is the inclusion of laboratory data (EEG and radionuclide angiography) in the American guidelines. Indeed, because of the limitations on the clinical examination of neonates, an observation period of 48 hours is recommended, as well as a confirmatory test, such as electroencephalography or a study of cerebral blood flow (Wijdicks 2001). The natural history of the iso-electric EEG in the neonatal period is now well established in terms of predicting bad outcome, but many babies with this abnormality survive despite irreversible brain injury (see p. 12). Limited experience of radionuclide angiography in the neonatal period in confirming brain death makes its routine use questionable.

Ashwal and Schneider (1989) described the clinical course of 18 premature and full-term infants whom they felt showed the features of brain death including coma, apnea and absent brainstem reflexes. Additional information including EEG and radionuclide scanning was performed in most. Nine of the 18 infants with clinical signs of brain death had an iso-electric EEG on the first examination, and 11 of the 17 in whom radionuclide scanning was performed showed no evidence of cerebral blood flow. Serum levels of phenobarbitone greater than 25 µg/mL were thought to suppress the EEG and make this investigation unreliable. They conclude that in full-term infants, the persistence of clinical signs of brainstem death was inconsistent with survival, and in premature infants, the persistence of the signs for 3 days was inconsistent with survival off the ventilator. They also report that an isoelectric EEG in the absence of factors known to suppress the EEG was associated with inevitable death if the clinical signs of brain death persisted for 24 hours. Although all the babies in this study died, some survived for some time in a persistent vegetative state. This underlines the difficulty in neonates of diagnosing 'brain death' in the context of brainstem death. It is not unusual for some brainstem functions, such as respiratory activity, to persist despite the fact that the brain has been massively and irreparably damaged.

Some investigations are helpful in the evaluation of irreversible and massive cerebral injury. These include severe EEG abnormalities as described on p. 557, abnormal Doppler values (low PRI or high CBFV; see p. 557) and MRS if this

Table 26.10 Comparison of the British and US (American Academy of Pediatrics) criteria for the diagnosis of brain death

Criteria	British Paediatric Association	AAP Special Task Force
Preconditions	Comatose and apneic Clear diagnosis	Comatose and apneic Clear diagnosis Flaccid tone and absence of spontaneous movements
Exclusions	Drug, endocrine and metabolic causes excluded Neuromuscular blockade has been demonstrably reversed No hypothermia	Toxic and metabolic disorders excluded Sedative, hypnotic and paralytic drugs excluded No hypotension No hypothermia
Absence of brainstem function	No pupillary response No corneal reflex No vestibulo-ocular reflex (Caloric test) No doll's eyes reflex No motor response to pain in cranial nerve V distribution No gag reflex to suction of trachea Apnea persists despite a rise in $PaCO_2 >$ 50 mmHg (6.6 kPa) against a background of normoxia	Absence of movement of bulbar musculature including facial and oropharyngeal muscles No corneal reflex No vestibular-ocular reflex or spontaneous eye movements No cough reflex No smiling or rooting reflex No gag reflex on suction of trachea Respiratory movements absent with patient off ventilator Apnea using standardized methods after other criteria met
Laboratory tests	Not necessary	EEG — electrocerebral silence over 30 min CBF — cerebral radionuclide angiogram demonstrating arrest of carotid circulation at base of skull and absence of intracranial arterial circulation
Observation period	Two examinations 12–24 h apart by two separate clinicians, one of whom is a pediatrician and one not primarily involved in the child's care	Two examinations and EEGs separated by: in infants 7 days to 2 months –48 h apart; in infants 2–12 months –24 h apart

is available. A sequence of changes within the anterior cerebral artery detected by Doppler ultrasound have been described as a feature of neonatal brain death. These include initially a decrease and subsequent loss of the diastolic component, followed by the appearance of retrograde flow and, finally, loss of both systolic and diastolic flow in the cerebral vessel with preservation of flow in the common carotid artery (McMenamin & Volpe 1983). In our experience, this is a very rare sequence of events and cannot be relied on to make the diagnosis of brain death in the neonatal period.

INDICATIONS FOR WITHDRAWAL OF CARE

During resuscitation, the following recommendations have been made (Neonatal Resuscitation Program) (Perlman 2006):

1. a consistent and coordinated approach by the obstetric and neonatal teams in conjunction with the parents is imperative;
2. when the possibility of survival is very low and the likelihood of severe morbidity is high, the parents' wishes about resuscitation or withdrawal of support should be respected;
3. discontinuation of resuscitation should be considered after 10 minutes of effective resuscitation in infants with asystole from birth. The 10 minute timing should not be confused with the time from birth, because it may take several minutes to establish an effective and coordinated resuscitation.

During the post-resuscitative phase, it is our belief that the criteria for brain death in the neonate are not helpful, and the clinical decision as to when to withdraw care should be made after full evaluation of all the laboratory information and repeated clinical assessment of the child. In our view, the best early predictors of adverse outcome are the severity of the clinical examination, i.e. moderate to severe encephalopathy coupled with a sustained iso-electric, low voltage state and discontinuous activity on electro-encephalogram (EEG), appearing by 6 hours. Our practice is therefore to assess severely asphyxiated infants with EEG (or CFM) at 6 hours and to reassess EEG together with a Doppler study at the age of 24 hours. If these tests at 6 hours and 24 hours are all abnormal, the term 'irreversible brain injury' is used and the parents are advised that the prognosis is extremely poor. When speaking to the parents, the terms 'irreversible' and 'massive brain injury' are more honest than 'brain death,' with its implications that the child will not survive off the mechanical ventilator. Many of these babies do breathe once disconnected from the ventilator, and this may cause considerable distress to the parents if they are not warned about this in advance.

REFERENCES

Adams J H, Brierley J B, Connor R C R 1966 The effects of systemic hypotension upon the human brain: clinical and neuropathological observations in 11 cases. Brain 89:235–268.

Adamson S J, Alessandra L M, Badawi B et al 1995 Predictors of neonatal encephalopathy in full term infants. BMJ 311:598–602.

Adlard B P F, De Souza S W 1976 Influence of asphyxia and of dexamethasone on ATP concentrations in the immature rat brain. Biol Neonate 24:82–88.

Adsett D B, Fitz C R, Hill A 1985 Hypoxic-ischaemic cerebral injury in the term newborn: correlation of CT findings with neurological outcome. Dev Med Child Neurol 27:155–160.

Ahn M O, Korst L M, Phelan J P et al 1998 Does the onset of neonatal seizures correlate with the timing of fetal neurologic injury? Clin Pediatr 37:673–676.

Aida N, Nishimura G, Hachiya Y et al 1998 MR imaging of perinatal brain damage: comparison of clinical outcome with initial and follow-up MR findings. Am J Neuroradiol 19:1909–1921.

Airedale A I 1991 Birth asphyxia and hypoxic-ischaemic encephalopathy: incidence and severity. Ann Trop Paediatr 11:331–335.

Akinbi H, Abbasi S, Hilpert P L et al 1994 Gastrointestinal and renal blood flow velocity profile in neonates with birth asphyxia. J Pediatr 125:625–627.

Alward C T, Hook J B, Helmrath T A 1978 Effects of asphyxia on renal function in the newborn piglet. Pediatr Res 12:225–228.

Amato M, Gambon R C, von Muralt G 1986 Accuracy of apgar score and arterial cord-blood pH in diagnosis of perinatal brain-damage assessed by CK-BB isoenzyme measurement. J Perinatal Med 14:335–338.

Ambalavanan N, Carlo WA, Shankaran S et al 2006 Predicting outcomes of neonates diagnosed with hypoxemic-ischemic encephalopathy. Pediatrics 118:2084–2093.

American College of Obstetricians and Gynecologists 1996 Use and abuse of the apgar score. Pediatrics 98:141–142.

Amer-Whalin I, Hellsten C, Noren H, Hagberg H 2001 Cardiotocography only versus cardiotocography plus ST analysis of fetal electrocardiogram for intrapartum fetal monitoring. Lancet 358:534–438.

Amiel-Tison C 1979 Birth injury as a cause of brain dysfunction in full-term newborns. In: Korobkin R, Guilleminault L (eds) Advances in perinatal neurology. Spectrum, New York, Vol. 1.

Amiel-Tison C, Ellison P 1986 Birth asphyxia in the fullterm newborn: early assessment and outcome. Dev Med Child Neurol 28:671–682.

Anderson J M, Belton N R 1974 Water and electrolyte abnormalities in the human brain after severe intrapartum asphyxia. J Neurol Neurosurg Psychiatry 37:514–520.

Anderson J M, Brown J K, Cockburn F 1974 On the role of disseminated intravascular coagulation in the pathology of birth asphyxia. Dev Med Child Neurol 16:581–591.

Andrews D A, Sawin R S, Ledbetter D J et al 1990 Necrotizing enterocolitis in term neonates. Am J Surg 159:507–509.

Anton G 1893 Uber die Betheiligung der basalen Gehringaglien bei Bewegungsstorungen und insbesondere bei der Chorea; nut Demonstrationen von Gehirnschaitten. Wiener Klinische Wochenschrift 6:859–861.

Apgar V 1953 A proposal for a new method of evaluation of the newborn infant. Curr Res Anesthesia Analgesia 32:260–267.

Archer L N J, Levene M I, Evans D H 1986 Cerebral artery Doppler ultrasonography for prediction of outcome after perinatal asphyxia. Lancet ii:1116–1118.

Arnold J, O'Brodovich H, Whyte R et al 1985 Pulmonary thromboemboli after neonatal asphyxia. J Pediatr 106:806–809.

Ashwal S, Schneider S 1989 Brain death in the newborn. Pediatrics 84:429–437.

Azzopardi D, Wyatt J S, Cady E B et al 1989 Prognosis of newborn infants with hypoxic-ischemic brain injury assessed by phosphorus magnetic resonance spectroscopy. Pediatr Res 25:445–451.

Babcock D S, Ball W 1983 Postasphyxial encephalopathy in full-term infants: ultrasound diagnosis. Radiology 148:417–423.

Badawi N, Felix J F, Kurinczuk J J et al 2005 cerebral palsy following term newborn necephalopathy: a population-based study. Dev Med Child Neurol 47:293–298.

Bao X L, Yu R J, Li Z S 1993 20 item neonatal behavioural neurological assessment used in predicting prognosis of asphyxiated newborn. Chin Med J 106:211–215.

Barkovich A J 1992 MR and CT evaluation of profound neonatal and infantile asphyxia. Am J Neuroradiol 13:950–972.

Barkovich A J, Hajnal B L, Vigneron D et al 1998 Prediction of neuromotor outcome in perinatal asphyxia: evaluation of MR scoring systems. Am J Neuroradiol 19:143–149.

Barkovich A J, Westmark K D, Bedi H S et al 2001 Proton spectroscopy and diffusion imaging on the first day of life after perinatal asphyxia: preliminary report. AJNR Am J Neuroradiol 22(9):1786–1794.

Barkovich A, Westmark K, Partridge C et al 1995 Perinatal asphyxia: MR-findings in the first 10 days. Am J Neuroradiol 16:427–438.

Barnett A, Mercuri E, Rutherford M et al 2002 Neurological and perceptual-motor outcome at 5–6 years of age in children with neonatal encephalopathy: relationship with neonatal brain MRI. Neuropediatrics 33(5):242–248.

Barth P G, Valk J, Olislagers-de Slegte R 1984 Aspect scanographique des zones corticales et sous-corticales centrales dans les paralysies cerebrales. J Neuroradiol 11:65–71.

Bax M, Nelson K B 1993 Birth asphyxia: a statement. Dev Med Child Neurol 35:1023–1024.

Benders M J, Bos A F, Rademater C M et al 2006 Early postnatal allopurinol does not improve short term outcome after severe birth asphyxia. Arch Dis Child Fetal Neonatal Ed 91:163–165.

Bennhagen R G, Weintraub R G, Lundstrom N R et al 1998 Hypoxic-ischaemic encephalopathy is associated with regional changes in cerebral blood flow velocity and alterations in cardiovascular function. Biol Neonate 73:275–286.

Bernard S A, Gray T W, Buist M D et al 2002 Treatment of comatose survivors of out-of-hospital cardiac arrest with induced hypothermia. N Engl J Med 346(8):557–563.

Bernaudin M, Tang Y, Reilly M et al 2002 Brain genomic response following hypoxia and re-oxygenation in the neonatal rat. Identification of genes that might contribute to hypoxia-induced ischemic tolerance. J Biol Chem 277(42):39728–39738.

Berseth C L, McCoy H H 1992 Birth asphyxia alters neonatal intestinal motility in term neonates. Pediatrics 90:669–673.

Blennow M, Hagberg H, Rosengren L 1995 Glial fibrillary acidic protein in the cerebrospinal fluid: a possible indicator of prognosis in full-term asphyxiated newborn infants? Pediatr Res 37:260–264.

Bloom S L, Spong C Y, Thorn E et al 2006 Fetal pulse oximetry and cesarean delivery. N Engl J Med 355:2195–2202.

Boylan G B, Rennie J M, Chorley G et al 2004 Second-line anticonvulsant treatment of neonatal seizures: a video-EEG monitoring study. Neurology 62:486–488.

Boylan G B, Young K, Panerai R B et al 2000 Dynamic cerebral autoregulation in sick newborn infants. Pediatr Res 48:12–17.

Brann A W, Myers R E 1975 Central nervous system findings in the new born monkey following severe in utero partial asphyxia. Neurology 25:327.

Bressler J 1899 Klinische und pathologisch-anatomische Beitrage zur Mikrogyrie. Archiv für Psychiatrie 31:566–573.

Brierley J B, Brown A W, Excell B J et al 1969 Brain damage in the rhesus monkey resulting from profound arterial hypotension. 1. Its nature, distribution and general physiological correlates. Brain Res 13:68–100.

British Paediatric Association 1991 Diagnosis of brain stem death in infants and children. A working party report of the British Paediatric Association. British Paediatric Association, London.

Brown J K, Purvis R J, Forfar J O et al 1974 Neurological aspects of perinatal asphyxia. Dev Med Child Neurol 16:567–580.

Bruce D A 1984 Effects of hyperventilation on cerebral blood flow and metabolism. Clin Perinatol 11:673–680.

Brucklacher R M, Vannucci R C, Vannucci S J 2002 Hypoxic preconditioning increases brain glycogen and delays energy depletion from hypoxia-ischemia in the immature rat. Dev Neurosci 24(5):411–417.

Bucciarelli R L, Nelson R M, Egan E A et al 1977 Transient tricuspid insufficiency of the newborn: a form of myocardial dysfunction in stressed newborns. Pediatrics 59:330–334.

Burnard E D, James L A 1961 Failure of the heart after undue asphyxia at birth. Pediatrics 28:545–547.

Bydder G M, Rutherford M A 2001 Diffusion-weighted imaging of the brain in neonates and infants. Magn Reson Imaging Clin N Am 9:83–98.

Cabal L A, Devaskar U, Siassi B et al 1980 Cardiogenic shock associated with perinatal asphyxia in preterm infants. J Pediatr 4:705–710.

Campbell A G M, Milligin J E, Talner N S 1968 The effect of pretreatment with pentobarbital, meperidine or hyperbaric oxygen on the response to anoxia and resuscitation in newborn rabbits. J Pediatr 72:518–527.

Carter S, McNabb F, Merenstein G B 1998 Prospective validation of a scoring system for predicting neonatal morbidity after acute perinatal asphyxia. J Pediatr 132:619–623.

Casalaz D M, Marlow N, Speidel B D 1998 Outcome of resuscitation following unexpected apparent stillbirth. Arch Dis Childhood 78:F112–F115.

Casey B M, McIntire D D, Leveno K J 2001 The continuing value of the Apgar score for the assessment of newborn infants. N Engl J Med 344:467–471.

Chadd M A, Elwood P C, Gray O P et al 1971 Coagulation defects in hypoxic full-term newborn infants. Br Med J iv:516–518.

Chessells J M, Wigglesworth J S 1970 Secondary haemorrhagic disease of the newborn. Arch Dis Childhood 45:539–543.

Cockburn F, Daniel S S, Dawes G S et al 1969 The effect of pentobarbital anesthesia on resuscitation and brain damage in fetal rhesus monkeys asphyxiated on delivery. J Pediatr 75:281–291.

Colamaria V, Curatolo P, Cusmai R et al 1988 Symmetrical bithalamic hyperdensities in asphyxiated full-term newborns: an early indicator of status marmoratus. Brain Dev 10:57–59.

Constantinou J E C, Gillis J, Ouvrier R A et al 1989 Hypoxic-ischaemic encephalopathy after near miss sudden infant death syndrome. Arch Dis Child 64:703–708.

Cornette L, Levene M I 2001 Post-resuscitative management of the asphyxiated term and preterm infant. Semin Neonatol 6:271–282.

Costello A M, Manandhar D S 1994 Perinatal asphyxia in less developed countries.

Cowan F, Rutherford M, Groenendaal F et al 2003 Origin and timing of brain lesions in term infants with neonatal encephalopathy. Lancet 361:736–742.

Cuestas R A 1980 Creatine kinase isoenzymes in high-risk infants. Pediatr Res 14:935–938.

Cyr R M, Usher R H, McLean F H 1984 Changing patterns of birth asphyxia and trauma over 20 years. Am J Obstet Gynecol 48:490–498.

Daga S R, Prabhu P G, Chandrashekhar L et al 1983 Myocardial ischemia following birth asphyxia. Ind Pediatr 20:567–571.

Dalens B, Viallard J-L, Raynauld E-J et al 1981 CSF levels of lactate and hydroxybutyrate dehydrogenase as indicators of neurological sequelae after neonatal brain damage. Dev Med Child Neurol 23:228–233.

Daniel S S, Husain M K, Milliez J et al 1978 Renal response of the fetal lamb to complete occlusion of the umbilical cord. Am J Obstet Gynecol 131:514–519.

Dauber I M, Krauss A N, Symchych P S et al 1976 Renal failure following perinatal asphyxia. J Pediatr 88:851–855.

Davis D J, Creery W D, Radziuk J 1999 Inappropriately high plasma insulin levels in suspected perinatal asphyxia. Acta Paediatr 88:76–81.

Dawes G 1968 Fetal and neonatal physiology. Year Book, Chicago, IL.

De Sa D J, Donnelly W H 1984 Myocardial necrosis in the newborn. Perspec Pediatr Pathol 8:295–311.

De Souza S W, Dobbing J 1973 Cerebral oedema in developing brain. III. Brain water and electrolytes in immature asphyxiated rats treated with dexamethasone. Biol Neonate 22:388–397.

De Souza S W, Richards B 1978 Neurological sequelae in newborn babies after perinatal asphyxia. Arch Dis Childhood 53:564–569.

De Vane G W, Porter J C 1980 An apparent stress-induced release of arginine vasopressin by human neonates. J Clin Endocrinol Metab 51:1412–1416.

Di Sessa T G, Leitner M, Ti C C et al 1981 The cardiovascular effects of dopamine in the severely asphyxiated neonate. J Pediatr 99:772–776.

Diprose G K, Evans D H, Archer L N J et al 1986 Dinamap fails to detect hypotension in very low birthweight infants. Arch Dis Childhood 61:771–773.

Dixon G, Badawi N, Kurinczuk J J et al 2002 Early developmental outcomes after newborn encephalopathy. Pediatrics 109(1):26–33.

Donald I 1959 Birth: adaptation from intrauterine to extrauterine life. In: Holland E, Bourne A (eds) British obstetric practice. Heinemann, London.

Donnelly W H, Bucciarelli R L, Nelson R M 1980 Ischemic papillary muscle necrosis in stressed newborn infants. J Pediatr 96:295–300.

Drage J S, Kennedy C, Schwarz B K 1964 The Apgar score as an index of neonatal mortality: a report from the collaborative study of cerebral palsy. Obstet Gynecology 24:222–230.

Edwards A D, Azzopardi D V 2006 Therapeutic hypothermia following perinatal asphyxia. Arch Dis Child Fetal Neonatal Ed 91(2):F127–F131.

Eicher D J, Wagner C L, Katikaneni L P et al 2005a Moderate hypothermia in neonatal encephalopathy: safety outcomes. Pediatr Neurol 32(1):18–24.

Eicher D J, Wagner C L, Katikaneni L P et al 2005b Moderate hypothermia in neonatal encephalopathy: efficacy outcomes. Pediatr Neurol 32(1):11–17.

Eken P, Jansen G H, Groenendaal F et al 1994 Intracranial lesions in the full term infant with hypoxic ischaemic encephalopathy: ultrasound and autopsy correlation. Neuropediatrics 25:301–307.

Eken P, Toet M C, Groenendaal F et al 1995 Predictive value of early neuroimaging, pulsed Doppler and neurophysiology in full term infants with hypoxic-ischaemic encephalopathy. Arch Dis Childhood 73:F75–F80.

Ekert, Perlman M, Steinlin M et al 1997 Predicting the outcome of postasphyxial hypoxic-ischaemic encephalopathy within 4 hours of birth. J Pediatr 131:613–617.

Ellis M, Manandhar D 1999 Progress in perinatal asphyxia. Semin Neonatol 4:183–191.

Ellis M, Manandhar N, Shrestha P S et al 1999 Outcome at 1 year of neonatal encephalopathy in Kathmandu, Nepal. Dev Med Child Neurol 41:689–695.

Ergander U, Eriksson M, Zetterstrom R 1983 Severe neonatal asphyxia: incidence and prediction of outcome in the Stockholm area. Acta Paediatr Scand 72:321–325.

Evans D J, Levene M I 2001 Anticonvulsants for preventing mortality and morbidity in full term newborns with perinatal asphyxia. The Cochrane Database of Systematic Reviews 1:review.

Eyre J A, Wilkinson A R 1986 Thiopentone-induced coma after severe birth asphyxia. Arch Dis Childhood 61:1084–1089.

Farkas A G, Robson S C, Kyei-Mensah A et al 1995 Acid-base changes after severe birth acidaemia. J Perinatal Med 23:249–255.

Farkas-Bargeton E, Diebler M F 1978 A topographical study of enzyme maturation in human cerebral neocortex: a histological and biochemical study. In: Brazier M A B, Petsche H (eds) Architectonics and the cerebral cortex. Raven, New York, NY.

Fenichel G M 1983 Hypoxic-ischemic encephalopathy in the newborn. Arch Neurol 40:261–266.

Fernandez F, Barrio V, Guzman J et al 1989 Beta-2-microglobulin in the assessment of renal function in full term newborns following perinatal asphyxia. J Perinatal Med 17:453–459.

Fernandez F, Quero J, Verdu A et al 1986 L D H isoenzymes in CSF in the diagnosis of neonatal brain damage. Acta Neurol Scand 74:30–33.

Fernandez F, Verdu A, Quero J et al 1987 Serum CPK-BB isoenzyme in the assessment of brain damage in asphyctic term infants. Acta Paediatr Scand 76:914–918.

Ferriero D M 2004 Neonatal brain injury. N Engl J Med 351:1985–1995.

Finer N N, Robertson C M, Peters K L et al 1983 Factors affecting outcome in hypoxic-ischemic encephalopathy in term infants. Am J Dis Children 137:21–25.

Finer N N, Robertson C M, Richards R T et al 1981 Hypoxic-ischemic encephalopathy in term neonates: perinatal factors and outcome. J Pediatr 98:112–117.

Fitzhardinge P M 1977 Complications of asphyxia and their therapy. In: Gluck L (ed.) Intrauterine asphyxia and the developing fetal brain. Year Book, Chicago, IL.

Fitzhardinge P M, Eisen E, Lejtonyi C et al 1974 Sequelae of early steroid administration to the newborn infant. Pediatrics 53:877–883.

Fitzhardinge P M, Flodmark O, Fitz C R et al 1981 The prognostic value of computed tomography as an adjunct to assessment of the term infant with postasphyxial encephalopathy. J Pediatr 99:777–781.

Flodmark O, Becker L E, Harwood-Nash D C et al 1980 Correlation between computed tomography and autopsy in premature and full-term neonates that have suffered perinatal asphyxia. Radiology 137:93–103.

Freeman J, Nelson K 1988 Intrapartum asphyxia and cerebral palsy. Pediatrics 82:240–249.

Friede R L 1975 Developmental neuropathology. Springer, Berlin.

Frigieri G, Guidi B, Costa Zaccarelli S et al 1996 Multicystic encephalomalacia in term infants. Child's Nerv Syst 12:759–764.

Fysh W J, Turner G M, Dunn P M 1982 Neurological normality after extreme birth asphyxia: case report. Br J Obstet Gynaecol 89:24–26.

Gadian D G, Aicardi J, Watkins K E et al 2000 Developmental amnesia associated with early hypoxic-ischaemic injury. Brain 123:499–507.

Gal P, Toback J, Erkan N V et al 1984 The influence of asphyxia on phenobarbital dosing requirements in neonates. Dev Pharmacol Ther 7:145–152.

Garcia-Alix A, Cabanas F, Pellicer A et al 1994 Neuron-specific enolase and myeline basic protein: relationship of cerebrospinal fluid concentrations to the neurologic condition of asphyxiated full-term infants. Pediatrics 93:234–240.

Gazzolo D, Marinoni E, Di Iorio R et al 2003 Measurement of urinary S100B protein concentrations for the early identification of brain damage in asphyxiated full-term infants. Arch Pediatr Adolesc Med 157:1163–1168.

Gerard P, Verheggen P, Bachy et al 1981 Interet de la tomodensitometrie cerebrale chez les enfants nes asphyxies. Archives Françaises de Pediatrie 38:591–596.

Gluckman P D, Wyatt J S, Azzopardi D, 2005 Selective head cooling with mild systemic hypothermia after neonatal encephalopathy: multicentre randomised trial. Lancet 365(9460):663–670.

Goitein K J, Amit Y 1982 Percutaneous placement of subdural catheter for measurement of intracranial pressure in small children. Crit Care Med 10:46–48.

Goldaber K G, Gilstrap L C, Leveno K J et al 1991 Pathological fetal acidemia. Obstet Gynaecol 78:1103–1107.

Goldberg R N, Cabal L A, Sinatra F R et al 1979 Hyperammonemia associated with perinatal asphyxia. Pediatrics 64:336–341.

Goldberg R N, Thomas D W, Sinatra F R 1983 Necrotizing enterocolitis in the asphyxiated full-term infant. Am J Perinatol 1:40–42.

Goldberg R, Moscoso P, Bauer C et al 1986 Use of barbiturate therapy in severe perinatal asphyxia: a randomized controlled trial. J Pediatr 109:851–856.

Goodlin R C, Lloyd D 1970 Use of drugs to protect against fetal asphyxia. American J Obstet Gynaecol 107:227–231.

Grant A 1989 Monitoring the fetus during labour. In: Chalmers I, Enkin M, Keirse M J N C (eds) Effective care in pregnancy and childbirth. Oxford University Press, Oxford, vol 2, pp. 846–882.

Grant P E, Yu D 2006 Acute injury to the immature brain with hypoxia with or without hypoperfusion.

Greisen G 2006 Brain monitoring in the neonate-the rationale. Clin Perinatol 33:613–618.

Grigelioniene G, Blennow M, Torok C et al 1996 Cerebrospinal fluid of newborn infants contains a deglycosylated from of the intermediate filament nestin. Pediatr Res 1996;40:809–814.

Groenendaal F, Lammers H, Smit D et al 2006 Nitrotyrosine in brain tissue of neonates after perinatal asphyxia. Arch Dis Child Fetal Neonatal Ed 91:F429–F433.

Groenendaal F, Veenhoven R H, van der Grond J et al 1994 Cerebral lactate and N-acetyl-aspartate/choline ratios in asphyxiated full-term neonates demonstrated in vivo using proton magnetic resonance spectroscopy. Pediatr Res 35:148–151.

Gunn A J, Bennet L 2001 Is temperature important in delivery room resuscitation? Semin Neonatol 6:241–249.

Gunn A J, Parer J T, Mallard E C et al 1992 Cerebral histologic and electrocorticographic changes after asphyxia in fetal sheep. Pediatr Res 31:486–491.

Gupta B D, Sharma P, Bagla J et al 2005 Renal failure in asphyxiated neonates. Indian Pediatr 42:928–934.

Hagberg H, Thornberg E, Blennow M et al 1993 Excitatory amino acids in the cerebrospinal fluid of asphyxiated infants: relationship to hypoxic-ischemic encephalopathy. Acta Paediatr 82:925–929.

Hall R T, Hall F K, Daily D K 1998 High-dose phenobarbital therapy in term newborn infants

with severe perinatal asphyxia: A randomized, prospective study with three year follow up. J Pediatr 345–348.

Hall R T, Kulkarni P B, Sheehan M B et al 1980 Cerebrospinal fluid lactate dehydrogenase in infants with perinatal asphyxia. Dev Med Child Neurol 22:300–307.

Halliday H L 2000 Endotracheal intubation at birth for preventing morbidity and mortality in vigorous, meconium-stained infants born at term. Cochrane Library Disk Issue 1 2000.

Hankins G D V, Koen S, Gei A F et al 2002 Neonatal organ system injury in acute birth asphyxia sufficient to result in neonatal encephalopathy. Obstet Gynecol 99:688–691.

Hanrahan J D, Cox I J, Azzopardi D et al 1999 Relation between proton magnetic resonance spectroscopy within 18 hours of birth asphyxia and neurodevelopment at 1 year of age. Dev Med Child Neurol 41:76–82.

Hanrahan J D, Sargentoni J, Azzopardi D et al 1996 Cerebral metabolism within 18 hours of birth asphyxia: a proton magnetic resonance spectroscopy study. Res 39:584–590.

Hansmann G 2004 Neonatal resuscitation on air: it is time to turn down the oxygen tanks. Lancet 364:1293–1294.

Hattori H, Wasterlain C G 1990 Posthypoxic glucose supplement reduces hypoxic-ischemic brain damage in the neonatal rat. Ann Neurol 28:122–128.

Hellström-Westas L, Rosén I, Svenningsen N W 1995 Predictive value of early continuous amplitude integrated EEG recordings on outcome after severe birth asphyxia in full term infants. Arch Dis Child 72:F34–F38.

Hermansen M C 2001 Nucleated red blood cells in the fetus and newborn. Arch Dis Child Fetal Neonatal Ed 84:211–215.

Hermansen M C 2003 The acidosis paradox: asphyxial brain injury without coincident acidemia. Dev Med Child Neurol 45:353–356.

Holmes G L, Gairsa J L, Chevassus–Aui-Louis N et al 1998 Consequences of neonatal seizures in the rat: morphological and behavioural effects. Ann Neurol 44:845–857.

Holmes G L, Rowe J, Hafford J 1983 Significance of reactive burst suppression following asphyxia in full term infants. Clin Electroencephalog 14:138–141.

Holmes G, Rowe J, Hafford J et al 1982 Prognostic value of the electroencephalogram in neonatal asphyxia. Electroencephalog Clin Neurophysiol 53:60–72.

Hoo J J, Goedde H W 1982 Determination of brain type creatine kinase for diagnosis of perinatal asphyxia — choice of method. Pediatr Res 16:806.

Huang C C, Wang S T, Chang Y C et al 1999 Measurement of the urinary lactate : creatinine ratio for the early identification of newborn infants at risk for hypoxic-ischemic encephalopathy. N Eng J Med 341:328–335.

Hull J, Dodd K L 1992 Falling incidence of hypoxic-ischaemic encephalopathy in term infants. Br J Obstet Gynaecol 9:386–391.

Hunt R W, Neil J J, Coleman L T et al 2004 Apparent diffusion coefficient in the posterior limb of the internal capsule predicts outcome after perinatal asphyxia. Pediatrics 114:999–1003.

Hüppi P 2002 Advances in postnatal neuroimaging: relevance to pathogenesis and treatment of brain injury. Clin Perinatol 29:827–856.

Hypothermia after Cardiac Arrest Study Group 2002 Mild therapeutic hypothermia to improve the neurologic outcome after cardiac arrest. N Engl J Med 346(8):549–556. Erratum in: N Engl J Med 2002 346(22):1756.

Ilves P, Talvik R, Talvik T 1998 Changes in Doppler ultrasonography in asphyxiated term infants with hypoxic-ischaemic encephalopathy. Acta Paediatr 87:680–684.

Inder T E, Hunt R W, Morley C J et al 2004 Randomized trial of systemic hypothermia selectively protects the cortex on MRI in term hypoxic-ischemic encephalopathy. J Pediatr 145(6):835–837.

Ingemarsson E, Ingemarsson I, Svenningsen N W 1981 Impact of routine fetal monitoring during labor on fetal outcome with long-term follow-up. Am J Obstet Gynecol 141:29–38.

Jain L, Ferre C, Vidyasagar D et al 1991 Cardiopulmonary resuscitation of apparently stillborn infants: survival and long-term outcome. J Pediatr 118:778–782.

Jenik A G, Ceriani Cernadas J M, Gorenstein A et al 2000 A randomized, double-blind, placebo-controlled trial of the effects of prophylactic theophylline on renal function in term neonates with perinatal asphyxia. Pediatrics 105:E45.

Jensen A, Garnier Y, Berger R 1999 Dynamics of fetal circulatory responses to hypoxia and asphyxia. Eur J Obstet Gynecol Reprod Biol 84:155–172.

Jobsis F F 1977 Noninvasive, infrared monitoring of cerebral and myocardial oxygen sufficiency and circulatory parameters. Science 198:1264–1267.

Kadri M, Shu S, Holshouser B et al 2003 Proton magnetic resonance spectroscopy improves outcome prediction in perinatal CNS insults. J Perinatol 23:181–185.

Kaiser A M, Whitelaw A G L 1987 Noninvasive monitoring of intracranial pressure — fact or fancy? Dev Med Child Neurol 29:320–326.

Kecskes Z, Dunster K R, Colditz P B 2005 NSE and S100 after hypoxia in the newborn pig. Pediatr Res 58:953–957.

Keeney S E, Adcock E W, McArdle C B 1991 Prospective observations of 100 high-risk neonates by high-field (1.5 Tesla) magnetic resonance imaging of the central nervous system. II. Lesions associated with hypoxic-ischemic encephalopathy. Pediatrics 87:431–438.

Kern K B, Hilwig R W, Berg R A et al 1997 Post-resuscitation left ventricular systolic and diastolic dysfunction. Treatment with dobutamine. Circulation 95:2610–2613.

Kirkendall C, Phelan J P 2001 Severe acidosis at birth and normal neurologic outcome. Prenat Neonatal Med 6:267–270.

Klatzo I 1967 Neuropathological aspects of brain damage. J Neuropathol Exp Neurol 26:1–5.

Klatzo I 1985 Brain oedema following brain ischaemia and the influence of therapy. Br J Anaesthesia 57:18–22.

Klinger G, Beyene J, Shah P et al 2005 Do hyperoxaemia and hypocapnia add to the risk of brain injury after intrapartum asphyxia? Arch Dis Child Fetal Neonatal Ed 90:49–52.

Kojima T, Kobayashi T, Matsuzaki S et al 1985 Effects of perinatal asphyxia and myoglobinuria on development of acute neonatal renal failure. Arch Dis Childhood 60:908–912.

Korhonen L, Riikonen R, Nawa H et al 1998 Brain derived neurotrophic factor is increased in cerebrospinal fluid of children suffering from asphyxia. Neurosci Lett 240:151–154.

Kotagel S, Toce S S, Kotagel P et al 1983 Symmetric bithalamic and striatal hemorrhage following perinatal hypoxia in a term infant. J Comput Assist Tomogr 7:353–355.

Lam B C C, Yeung C Y 1999 Surfactant lavage for meconium aspiration syndrome: a pilot study. Pediatrics 103:1014–1018.

Larroche J-C 1977 Developmental pathology of the neonate. Amsterdam: Excerpta Medica.

Larroche J-C 1984 Perinatal brain damage. In: Adams J H, Corsellis J A N, Duchen L W (eds) Greenfield's neuropathology. Arnold, London.

Lassiter H A 2004 The role of complement in neonatal hypoxic-ischemic cerebral injury. Clin Perinatol 31:117–127.

Le Strange E, Saeed N, Cowan F M et al 2004 MR imaging quantification of cerebellar growth following hypoxic-ischemic injury to the neonatal brain. Am J Neuroradiol 25:463–468.

Leech R W, Alvord E C 1977 Anoxic-ischemic encephalopathy in the human neonatal period: the significance of brain stem involvement. Arch Neurol 34:109–113.

Leth H, Toft P B, Peitersen B et al 1996 Use of brain lactate levels to predict outcome after perinatal asphyxia. Acta Paediatr 85:859–864.

Levene M I 1995 Birth asphyxia. In: David T J (ed.) Recent advance in paediatrics. Churchill Livingstone, Edinburgh, pp. 13–27.

Levene M I 2002 The clinical conundrum of neonatal seizures. Arch Dis Child Fet Neonatal Ed 86:F75–F77.

Levene M I, Evans D H 1983 Continuous measurement of subarachnoid pressure in the severely asphyxiated newborn. Arch Dis Childhood 58:1013–1015.

Levene M I, Evans D H 1985 Medical management of raised intracranial pressure after severe birth asphyxia. Arch Dis Childhood 60:12–16.

Levene M I, Evans D H, Forde A et al 1987 The value of intracranial pressure monitoring in asphyxiated newborn infants. Dev Med Child Neurol 29:311–319.

Levene M I, Fenton A C, Evans D H et al 1989 Severe birth asphyxia and abnormal cerebral blood-flow velocity. Dev Med Child Neurol 31:427–434.

Levene M I, Kornberg J, Williams T H C 1985a The incidence and severity of post-asphyxial encephalopathy in full-term infants. Early Human Dev 11:21–28.

Levene M I, Sands C, Grindulis H et al 1986 Comparison of two methods of predicting outcome in perinatal asphyxia. Lancet i:67–91.

Levene M I, Williams J L, Fawer C-L 1985b Ultrasound of the infant brain, No. 92. Spastics International Medical, Oxford.

Liao H T, Hung K L 1997 Anterior cerebral artery Doppler ultrasonograpy for prediction of outcome after perinatal asphyxia. Chung-Hua Min Kuo Hsiao Erh Ko I Hsueh Tsa Chih 38:208–212.

Lipper E G, Voorhies T M, Ross G et al 1986 Early predictors of one-year outcome for infants asphyxiated at birth. Dev Med Child Neurol 28:303–309.

Lipp-Zwahlen A E, Deonna T, Chrzanowski R et al 1985a Temporal evolution of hypoxic-ischaemic brain lesions in asphyxiated full-term newborns assessed by computerized tomography. Neuroradiology 27:138–144.

Lipp-Zwahlen A E, Deonna T, Micheli J L et al 1985b Prognostic value of neonatal C T scans in asphyxiated term babies: low density score compared with neonatal neurological signs. Neuropediatrics 16:209–217.

Liu Z, Xiong T, Meads C 2006 Clinical effectiveness of treatment with hyperbaric oxygen for neonatal hypoxic–ischemic encephalopathy: systematic review of Chinese literature. Br Med J 333:374.

Lorek A, Takei Y, Cady E B et al 1994 Delayed ('secondary') cerebral energy failure after acute hypoxia-ischemia in the newborn piglet: continuous 48-hour studies by phosphorus magnetic resonance spectroscopy. Pediatr Res 36:699–706.

Low J A 1993 The relationship of asphyxia in the mature fetus to long-term neurologic function. Clin Obstet Gynecol 36:82–90.

Low J A 1997a Intrapartum fetal asphyxia: definition, diagnosis, and classification. Am J Obstet Gynecol 100:1004–1014.

Low J A, Galbraith R S, Muir D et al 1978a Intrapartum fetal asphyxia: a preliminary report in regard to long-term morbidity. Am J Obstet Gynecol 130:525–533.

Low J A, Galbraith R S, Muir D W et al 1985 The relationship between perinatal hypoxia and newborn encephalopathy. Am J Obstet Gynecol 152:256–260.

Low J A, Galbraith R S, Raymond M J et al 1994 Cerebral blood flow velocity in term newborns following intrapartum fetal asphyxia. Acta Paediatr 83:1012–1016.

Low J A, Lindsay B G, Derrick E J 1997b Threshold of metabolic acidosis associated with newborn complications. Am J Obstet Gynecol 177:1391–1394.

Low J A, Pickersgill H, Killen H et al 2001 The prediction and prevention of intrapartum fetal asphyxia in term pregnancies. Am J Obstet Gynecol 184:724–730.

Luciano R, Gallini F, Romagnoli C et al 1998 Doppler evaluation of renal blood flow velocity as a predictive index of acute renal failure in perinatal asphyxia. Eur J Pediatr 157:656–660.

Lundstrom K, Pryds O, Greisen G 1995 Oxygen at birth and prolonged cerebral vasoconstriction in preterm infants. Arch Dis Childhood 73:F81–F84.

MacDonald D, Grant A, Sheridan-Pereira M et al 1985 The Dublin randomised trial of intrapartum fetal heart monitoring. Am J Obstet Gynecol 152:524–539.

MacDonald H M, Mulligan J C, Allan A C et al 1980 Neonatal asphyxia. 1. Relationship of obstetric and neonatal complications to neonatal mortality in 38 405 consecutive deliveries. J Pediatr 96:898–902.

McMenamin J B, Volpe J J 1983 Doppler ultrasonography in the determination of neonatal brain death. Ann Neurol 14:302–307.

McWilliam R C, Stephenson J B P 1984 Rapid bedside technique for intracranial pressure monitoring. Lancet ii:73–75.

Magilner A D, Wertheimer I S 1980 Preliminary results of a computed tomography study of neonatal brain hypoxia-ischemia. J Comput Assist Tomogr 4:457–463.

Marchal C, Costagliola P, Leveau Ph et al 1974 Traitement de la souffrance cerebrale neonatale d'origine anoxique par le mannitol. Revue de Pédiatrie 9:581–589.

Marlow N, Wolke D, Bracewell M A et al 2005 Neurologic and developmental disability at six years of age after extremely preterm birth. N Engl J Med 352(1):9–19.

Martin D J, Hill A, Fitz C R et al 1983 Hypoxic/ischemic cerebral injury in the neonatal brain. Pediatric Radiology 13:307–312.

Martin E, Barkovich A J 1995 Magnetic resonance imaging in perinatal asphyxia. Arch Dis Child Fetal Neonatal Ed 72(1):F62–F70.

Martin E, Buchli R, Ritter S et al 1996 Diagnostic and prognostic value of cerebral ^{31}P magnetic resonance spectroscopy in neonates with perinatal asphyxia. Pediatr Res 40:749–748.

Martin-Ancel A, Garcia-Alix A, Pascual-Salcedo D et al 1997 Interleukin-6 in the cerebrospinal fluid after perinatal asphyxia is related to early and late neurological manifestations. Pediatrics 100:789–791.

Meek J H, Elwell C E, McCormick D C et al 1999 Abnormal cerebral haemodynamics in perinatally asphyxiated neonates related to outcome. Arch Dis Child Fetal Neonatal Ed 81:F110–F115.

Meis P J, Hall M, Marshall J 1978 Meconium passage: a new classification for risk assessment during labor. Am J Obstet Gynecol 131:509.

Mercuri E, Guzzetta A, Haataja L et al 1999 Neonatal neurological examination in infants with hypoxic ischaemic encephalopathy: correlation with MRI findings. Neuropaediatrics 30:83–89.

Miller S P, Cozzio C C, Goldstein R B et al 2003 Comparing the diagnosis of white matter injury in premature newborns with serial MR imaging and transfontanel ultrasonography findings. Am J Neuroradiol 24:1661–1669.

Miller S P, Newton N, Ferriero D M et al 2002a Predictors of 30-month outcome after perinatal depression: role of proton MRS and socioeconomic factors. Pediatr Res 52:71–77.

Miller S P, Ramaswamy V, Michelson D et al 2004 Patterns of brain injury in term neonatal encephalopathy. J Pediatr 146:453–460.

Miller S P, Ramaswamy V, Michelson D et al 2005 Patterns of brain injury in term neonatal encephalopathy. J Pediatrics 146(4):453–460.

Miller S P, Vigneron D B, Henry R G et al 2002a Serial quantitative diffusion tensor MRI of the premature brain: development in newborns with and without injury. J Magn Reson Imaging 16(6):621–632.

Miller S P, Vigneron D B, Henry R G et al 2002b Serial quantitative diffusion tensor MRI of the premature brain: development in newborns with and without injury. J Magn Reson Imaging 16:621–632.

Moorcroft J, Bolas N M, Ives N K et al 1991 Global and depth resolved phosphorus magnetic resonance spectroscopy to predict outcome after birth asphyxia. Arch Dis Childhood 66:1119–1123.

Morimoto K, Sumita Y, Kitajima H et al 1985 Bilateral, asymmetrical hemorrhagic infarction of the basal ganglia and thalamus following neonatal asphyxia. No To Shinkei 37:133–137.

Mujsce D J, Stern D R, Vannucci R C et al 1988 Mannitol therapy in perinatal hypoxic-ischemic brain damage. Ann Neurol 24:338.

Mulligan J C, Painter M J, O'Donoghue P A et al 1980 Neonatal asphyxia. II. Neonatal mortality and long-term sequelae. J Pediatr 96:903–907.

Murray D M, Ryan C A, Boylan G B et al 2006 Prediction of seizures in asphyxiated neonates: correlation with continuous video-electroencephalographic monitoring. Pediatrics 118:41–46.

Myers R E 1972 Two patterns of perinatal brain damage and their conditions of occurrence. Am J Obstet Gynecology 112:246–276.

Myers R E, Wagner K R, Courten-Myers G M et al 1983 Brain metabolic and pathologic consequences of asphyxia. In: Milunsky A, Haddow R, Alpert E (eds) Advances in perinatal medicine. Plenum, New York, NY, vol. 3.

Naeye R L, Shaffer M L 2005 Postnatal laboratory timers of antenatal hypoxemic-ischemic brain damage. J Perinatol, 25(10):664–668.

Nagdyman N, Grimmer I, Scholz T et al 2003 Predictive value of brain-specific proteins in serum for neurodevelopmental outcome after birth asphyxia. Pediatr Res 54:270–275.

Nagdyman N, Komen W, Ko H K et al 2001 Early biochemical indicators of hypoxic-ischemic encephalopathy after birth asphyxia. Pediatr Res 49:502–506.

Nagy Z, Lindstrom K, Westerberg H et al 2005 Diffusion tensor imaging on teenagers, born at term with moderate hypoxic-ischemic encephalopathy. Pediatr Res 58:936–940.

Nelson K B 2003 Defining hypoxic-ischemic birth events. Dev Med Child Neurol 45:71–72.

Nelson K B, Ellenberg J H 1981 Apgar scores as predictors of chronic neurological disability. Pediatrics 68:36–44.

Nelson K B, Ellenberg J H 1984 Obstetric complications as risk factors for cerebral or seizure disorders. JAMA 251:1843–1848.

Nelson K B, Leviton A 1991 How much of neonatal encephalopathy is due to birth asphyxia? Am J Dis Children 145:1325–1331.

Niijima S, Levene M I 1989 Post-asphyxial encephalopathy in a preterm infant. Dev Med Child Neurol 31:395–397.

O'Connor M C, Harkness R A, Simmonds R J et al 1981 The measurement of hypoxanthine, xanthine, inosine and uridine in umbilical cord blood and fetal scalp blood samples as a measure of fetal hypoxia. Br J Obstet Gynaecol 88:381–390.

Oygur N, Sonmez O, Saka O et al 1998 Predictive value of plasma and cerebrospinal fluid tumour necrosis factor-α and interleukin-1β concentrations on outcome of full term infants with hypoxic-ischaemic encephalopathy. Arch Dis Childhood 79:F190–F193.

Painter M J, Depp R, O'Donogue P D 1978 Fetal heart rate patterns and development in the first year of life. Am J Obstet Gynecol 132:271–277.

Painter M J, Scher M S, Stein A D et al 1999 Phenobarbital compared with phenytoin for the treatment of neonatal seizures. N Eng J Med 341:485–489.

Palme-Kilander C 1992 Methods of resuscitation in low-Apgar-score newborn infants — A national survey. Acta Paediatr Scand 81:739–744.

Palmer C, Towfighi J, Roberts R, Heitjan DF 1993 Allopurinol administered after inducing hypoxic-ischemia reduces brain injury in 7-day-old rats. Pediatr Res 33:405–411.

Paneth N, Stark R I 1983 Cerebral palsy and mental retardation in relation to indicators of perinatal asphyxia. Am J Obstet Gynecol 147:960–966.

Pape K E, Wigglesworth J S 1979 Haemorrhage, ischaemia and the perinatal brain. Spastics International, London.

Papile L A 2001 The Apgar score in the 21st century. N Engl J Med 344:519–520.

Pasternak J F, Gorey M T 1998 The syndrome of acute near-total intrauterine asphyxia in the term infant. Pediatr Neurol 18:391–398.

Peden C J, Rutherford M A, Sargentoni J et al 1993 Proton spectroscopy of the neonatal brain following hypoxic-ischaemic injury. Dev Med Child Neurol 35:502–510.

Peliowski A, Finer N N 1992 Birth asphyxia in the term infant. In: Sinclair J C, Bracken M B (eds) Effective care of the newborn infant. Oxford University Press, Oxford, pp. 249–279.

Penrice J, Cady E B, Lorek A et al 1996 Proton magnetic resonance spectroscopy of the brain in normal preterm and term infants, and early changes after perinatal hypoxia-ischemia. Pediatr Res 40:6.

Perlman J M 2006 Intrapartum asphyxia and cerebral palsy: is there a link? Clinics in Perinatology 33:335–353.

Perlman J M, Kattwinkel J 2006 Delivery Room resuscitation. Past, present and the future. Clin Perinatol 33:1–9.

Perlman J M, Risser M S 1996 Can asphyxiated infants at risk for neonatal seizures be rapidly identified by current high-risk markers? Pediatrics 97:456–462.

Perlman J M, Tack E D 1988 Renal injury in the asphyxiated newborn infant: relationship to neurologic outcome. J Pediatr 113:875–879.

Perlman J M, Tack E D, Martin T et al 1989 Acute systemic organ injury in term infants after asphyxia. Am J Dis Childhood 143:617–620.

Phelan J P, Ahn M O, Korst L et al 1998 Intrapartum fetal asphyxial brain injury with absent multiorgan system dysfunction. J Maternal-Fetal Med 7:19–22.

Phelan J P, Myoung O A, Korst L M et al 1995 Nucleated red blood cells: a marker for fetal asphyxia? Am J Obstet Gynaecol 173:1380–1384.

Pierrat V, Haouari N, Liska A et al 2005 Prevalence, causes, and outcome at 2 years of age of newborn encephalopathy: population based study. Arch Dis Child Fetal Neonatal Ed 90(3):F257–F261.

Pourcyrous M, Bada H S, Yang W et al 1999 Prognostic significance of cerebrospinal fluid cyclic adenosine monophosphate in neonatal asphyxia. J Pediatr 134:90–96.

Primhak R A, Jedeikin R, Ellis G et al 1985 Myocardial ischaemia in asphyxia neonatorum. Acta Paediatr Scand 74:595–600.

Pryse-Davies J, Beard R W 1973 A necropsy study of brain swelling in the newborn with special reference to cerebellar herniation. J Pathol 109:51–73.

Raju T N, Doshi U, Vidyasagar D 1983 Low cerebral perfusion pressure: an indicator of poor prognosis in asphyxiated term infants. Brain Dev 5:478–482.

Roberton N R 1997 Use of albumin in neonatal resuscitation. Eur J Pediatr 156:428–431.

Roberts D S, Haycock G B, Dalton R N et al 1990 Prediction of acute renal failure after birth asphyxia. Arch Dis Childhood 65:1021–1028.

Robertson C M T, Finer N N, Grace M G A 1989 School performance of survivors of neonatal encephalopathy associated with birth asphyxia at term. J Pediatr 114:753–760.

Robertson C, Finer N 1985 Term infants with hypoxic-ischaemic encephalopathy: outcome at 3.5 years. Dev Med Child Neurol 27:473–484.

Robertson N J, Lewis R H, Cowan F M et al 2001 Early increases in brain myo-inositol measured by proton magnetic resonance spectroscopy in term infants with neonatal encephalopathy. Pediatr Res 50:692–700.

Roelants-Van Rijin A M, van der Grond J, de Vries L S et al 2001b Value of (1)H-MRS using different echo times in neonates with cerebral hypoxia-ischemia. Pediatr Res 49:356–362.

Roelants-van Rijn A M, Nikkels P G, Groenendaal F et al 2001a Neonatal diffusion-weighted MR imaging: relation to histopathology or follow-up MR examination. Neuropediatrics 32:286–294.

Roland E H, Hill A, Norman M G et al 1988 Selective brainstem injury in an asphyxiated newborn. Ann Neurol 23:89–92.

Rorke L B 1982 Pathology of perinatal brain injury. Raven, New York, NY.

Rose A L, Lombroso C T 1970 A study of clinical, pathological and electroencephalographic features in 137 full-term babies with a long term follow up. Pediatrics 111:133–141.

Rosenberg A A 1992 Response of the cerebral circulation to hypocarbia in postasphyxia newborn lambs. Pediatr Res 32:537–541.

Rosenbloom L 1994 Dyskinetic cerebral palsy and birth asphyxia. Dev Med Child Neurol 36:285–289.

Ross M G, Gala R 2002 Use of umbilical artery base excess: Algorithm for the timing of hypoxic injury. Am J Obstet Gynecol 187:1–9.

Roth S C, Baudin J, Cady E et al 1997 Relation of deranged neonatal cerebral oxidative metabolism with neurodevelopmental outcome and head circumference at 4 years. Dev Med Child Neurol 39:718–725.

Rowan J O, Johnston H, Harper A M et al 1972 Perfusion in intracranial hypertension. In: Borck M, Dietz H (eds) Intracranial pressure. Springer, New York, NY.

Rudolph A M 1969 The course and distribution of the fetal circulation. In: Wolstenholme G, O'Connor M J A (eds) Foetal autonomy. Churchill, London.

Ruth V J 1989 Prognostic value of creatine kinase BB-isoenzyme in high risk newborn infants. Arch Dis Childhood 64:563–568.

Ruth V J, Raivio K O 1988 Perinatal brain damage: predictive value of metabolic acidosis and the Apgar score. BMJ 297:24–27.

Ruth V, Autti-Ramo I, Granstrom M-L et al 1988 Prediction of perinatal brain damage by cord plasma vasopressin, erythropoietin, and hypoxanthine values. J Pediatr 113:800–815.

Rutherford M A, Pennock J M, Counsell S J et al 1998 Abonormal magnetic resonance signal in the internal capsule predicts poor neurodevelopmental outcome in infants with hypoxic ischemic encephalopathy. Pediatrics 102:323–329.

Rutherford M A, Pennock J M, Schwieso J E et al 1995 Hypoxic ischaemic encephalopathy: early magnetic resonance imaging findings and their evolution. Neuropediatrics 26:183–191.

Rutherford M A, Pennock J, Schwieso J et al 1996 Hypoxic-ischaemic encephalopathy: early and late magnetic resonance imaging findings in relation to outcome. Arch Dis Childhood 75:F145–F151.

Saint Hilaire M-H, Burke R E, Bressman S B et al 1991 Delayed-onset dystonia due to perinatal or early childhood asphyxia. Neurology 41:216–222.

Sankaran K 1984 Hypoxic-ischemic encephalopathy: cerebrovascular carbon dioxide reactivity in neonates. Am J Perinatol 1:114–117.

Sarnat H B, Sarnat M S 1976 Neonatal encephalopathy following fetal distress. Arch Neurol 33:696–705.

Sasidharan P 1992 Breathing pattern abnormalities in full term asphyxiated newborn infants. Arch Dis Childhood 67:440–442.

Saugstad O D 1975 Hypoxanthine as a measurement of hypoxia. Pediatr Res 9:158–161.

Saugstad O D 1998 Resuscitation with room-air or oxygen supplementation. Clin Perinatol 25:741–756.

Saugstad O D, Ramji S, Irani S F et al 2003 Resuscitation of newborn infants with 21% or 100% oxygen: follow-up at 18 to 24 months. Pediatrics 112:296–300.

Saugstad O D, Rootwelt, Aalen O 1998 Resuscitation of asphyxiated newborn infants with room air or oxygen: an international controlled trial: the Resair 2 study. Pediatrics 102.

Savman K, Blennow M, Gustafson K et al 1998 Cytokine response in cerebrospinal fluid after birth asphyxia. Pediatr Res 43:746–751.

Schneider H, Ballowitz L, Schachinger H et al 1975 Anoxic encephalopathy with predominant involvement of basal ganglia, brain stem and spinal cord in the perinatal period. Report on seven newborns. Acta Neuropathol 32:287–298.

Schrumpf J D, Sehring S, Killpack S et al 1980 Correlation of early neurologic outcome and CT findings in neonatal brain hypoxia and injury. J Comput Assist Tomogr 4:445–450.

Scott B L, Jankovic J 1996 Delayed-onset progressive movement disorders after static brain lesions. Am Acad Neurol 46:68–74.

Scott H 1976 Outcome of very severe birth asphyxia. Arch Dis Childhood 51:712–716.

Selton D, Andre M 1997 Prognosis of hypoxic-ischaemic encephalopathy in full term newborns — value of neonatal electroencephalography. Neuropediatrics 28:276–280.

Shadid M, Moison R, Steendijk P et al 1998 The effect of anitoxidative combination therapy on post hypoxic-ischemic perfusion, metabolism, and electrical activity of the newborn brain. Pediatr Res 44:119–124.

Shah P S, Beyene J et al 2006 Postasphyxial hypoxic-ischemic encephalopathy in neonates: outcome prediction rule within 4 hours of birth. Arch Pediatr Adolesc Med 160:729–736.

Shah P, Riphagen S, Beyene J et al 2004 Multiorgan dysfunction in infants with post-asphyxial hypoxic-ischaemic encephalopathy. Arch Dis Child Fetal Neonatal Ed 89:F152–F155.

Shalak L F, Laptook A R, Velaphi S C et al 2003 Amplitude-integrated electroencephalography coupled with an early neurologic examination enhances prediction of term infants at risk for persistent encephalopathy. Pediatrics 111:351–357.

Shankaran S, Laptook A R, Ehrenkranz R A et al 2005 Whole-body hypothermia for neonates with hypoxic-ischemic encephalopathy. N Engl J Med 353:1574–1584.

Sheldon R A, Partridge C, Ferriero D M 1992 Postischemic hyperglycemia is not protective to the neonatal rat. Pediat Res 32:489–493.

Shen E Y, Huang C C, Chyou S C et al 1986 Sonographic finding of the bright thalamus. Arch Dis Childhood 61:1096–1099.

Sheth R J, Bodensteiner J B, Riggs J E 1995 Differential involvement of the brain in neonatal asphyxia: a pathogenic explanation. J Child Neurol 10:463–466.

Shewman D A, Fine M, Masdeu J C et al 1981 Postischemic hypervascularity of infancy: a stage in the evolution of ischemic brain damage with characteristic CT scan. Ann Neurol 9:358–365.

Skeffington F S, Pearse R G 1983 The 'bright brain'. Arch Dis Childhood 58:509–511.

Soll R F, Dargaville P 2000 Surfactant for meconium aspiration syndrome in full term infants. Cochrane Library Disk Issue 2000.

Sonntag J, Wagner M H, Strauss E et al 1998 Complement and contact activation in term neonates after fetal acidosis. Arch Dis Child Fetal Neonatal Ed 78:F125–F128.

Speer M E, Gormon W A, Kaplan S L et al 1984 Elevation of plasma concentrations of arginine vasopressin following perinatal asphyxia. Acta Paediatr Scand 73:610–614.

Steiner H, Nelligan G 1975 Perinatal cardiac arrest: quality of the survivors. Arch Dis Childhood 50:696–702.

Stewart A R, Finer N N, Peters K L 1981 Effects of alterations of inspiratory and expiratory pressures and inspiratory/expiratory ratios on a mean airway pressure, blood gases and intracranial pressure. Pediatrics 67:474–481.

Suehiro E, Fujisawa H, Ito H et al 1999 Brain temperature modifies glutamate neurotoxicity in vivo. J Neurotrauma 16:285–297.

Suzuki S, Morishita S 1998 Hypercoagulability and DIC in high-risk infants. Semin Thrombosis Hemostasis 24:463–466.

Svenningsen N W, Blennow G, Lindroth M et al 1982 Brain-orientated intensive care treatment in severe neonatal asphyxia: effects of phenobarbitone protection. Arch Dis Childhood 57:176–183.

Szymankiewicz M, Matuszczak-Wleklak M, Hodgman J E et al 2005 Usefulness of cardiac troponin t and echocardiography in the diagnosis of hypoxic myocardial injury of full-term neonates. Biol Neonate 88:19–23.

Takeuchi T, Watanabe K 1989 The EEG evolution and neurological prognosis of perinatal hypoxia in neonates. Brain Dev 11:115–120.

Task Force 1987 Guidelines for the determination of brain death in children. Pediatrics 80:298–300.

Tekgul H, Yalaz M, Kutukculer N et al 2004 Value of biochemical markers for outcome in term infants with asphyxia. Pediatr Neurol 31(5):326–332.

ter Horst H J, Sommer C, Bergman K A et al 2004 Prognostic significance of amplitude-integrated EEG during the first 72 hours after birth in severely asphyxiated neonates. Pediatr Res 55:1026–1033.

Thiringer K 1983 Cord plasma hypoxanthine as a measure of foetal asphyxia: comparison with clinical assessment and laboratory measures. Acta Paediatr Scand 72:231–237.

Thompson C M, Puterman A S, Linley L L et al 1997 The value of a scoring system for hypoxic ischaemic encephalopathy in predicting neurodevelopmental outcome. Acta Paediatr 86:757–761.

Thompson R J, Graham J G, McQueen I N F et al 1980 Radio immunoassay of brain type creatine kinase-BB isoenzyme in human tissues and in serum of patients with neurological disorders. J Neurol Sci 47:241–254.

Thomson A J, Searle M, Russell G 1977 Quality of survival after severe birth asphyxia. Arch Dis Childhood 52:620–626.

Thoresen M, Hallstrom A, Whitelaw A et al 1988 Lactate and pyruvate changes in the cerebral gray and white matter during posthypoxic seizures in newborn pigs. Pediatr Res 44:746–754.

Thornberg E, Ekstrom-Jodal B 1994 Cerebral function monitoring: a method of predicting outcome in term neonates after severe perinatal asphyxia. Acta Paediatr 83:596–601.

Thornberg E, Thiringer K, Hagberg H et al 1995b Neuron specific enolase in asphyxiated newborns: association with encephalopathy and cerebral function monitor trace. Arch Dis Childhood 72:F39–F42.

Thornberg E, Thiringer K, Odeback A et al 1995a Birth asphyxia: incidence, clinical course and outcome in a Swedish population. Acta Paediatr 84:927–932.

Thorngren-Jerneck K, Alling C, Herbst A et al 2004 S100 protein in serum as a prognostic marker for cerebral injury in term newborn infants with hypoxic ischemic encephalopathy. Pediatr Res 55:406–412.

Thorngren-Jerneck K, Ohlsson T, Sandell A et al 2001 Cerebral glucose metabolism measured by positron emission tomography in term newborn infants with hypoxic ischemic encephalopathy. Pediatr Res 49:495–501.

Toet M C, Lemmers P M, van Schelven L J et al 2006 Cerebral oxygenation and electrical activity after birth asphyxia: their relation to outcome. Pediatrics 117:333–339.

Toth-Heyn P, Drukker A, Guignard J P 2000 The stressed neonatal kidney: from pathophysiology to clinical management of neonatal vasomotor nephropathy. Pediatr Nephrol 14:227–239.

Trounce J Q, Levene M I 1985 The diagnosis and outcome of subcortical cystic leukomalacia. Arch Dis Childhood 60:1041–1044.

Tweed W A, Pash M, Doig G 1981 Cerebrovascular mechanisms in perinatal asphyxia: the role of vasogenic brain edema. Pediatr Res 15:44–46.

Vain N E, Szyld E G, Prudent LM et al 2004 Oropharyngeal and nasopharyngeal suctioning of meconium-stained neonates before delivery of their shoulders: multicentre, randomised controlled trial. Lancet 364:597–602.

Van Bel F, Walther F J 1990 Myocardial dysfunction and cerebral blood flow velocity following birth asphyxia. Acta Paediatrica Scandinavica 79:756–762.

Van Rooij L G, Toet M C, Osredkar D et al 2005 Recovery of amplitude integrated electroencephalographic background patterns within 24 hours of perinatal asphyxia. Arch Dis Child Fetal Neonatal Ed 90:F245–F251.

Vannucci R C, Mujsce D J 1992 Effect of glucose on perinatal hypoxic-ischemic brain damage. Biol Neonate 62:215–224.

Varvarigou A, Vagenakis A G, Makri M et al 1996 Prolactin and growth hormone in perinatal asphyxia. Biol Neonate 69:76–83.

Vento M, Asensi M, Sastre J et al 2001 Resuscitation with room air instead of 100% oxygen prevents oxidative stress in moderately asphyxiated term neonates. Pediatrics 107:642–647.

Vigneron D B, Barkovich A J, Noworolski S M et al 2001 Three-dimensional proton MR spectroscopic imaging of premature and term neonates. Am J Neuroradiol 22:1424–1433.

Villani F, D'Incerti L, Granata T et al 2003 Epileptic and imaging findings in perinatal hypoxic–ischemic encephalopathy with ulegyria. Epilepsy Res 55:235–243.

Voit T, Lemburg P, Neuen E et al 1987 Damage of thalamus and basal ganglia in asphyxiated full-term neonates. Neuropediatrics 18:176–181.

Voit T, Lemburg P, Stork W 1985 NMR studies in thalamic-striatal necrosis. Lancet ii:445.

Volpe J J 1977 Observing the infant in the early hours after asphyxia. In: Gluck L (ed.) Intrauterine asphyxia and the developing fetal brain. Year Book, Chicago, IL.

Volpe J J 1987 Brain death determination in the newborn. Pediatrics 80:293–297.

Volpe J J 2001 Neurology of the newborn. 4th edition. WB Saunders, Philadelphia.

Volpe J J, Herscovitch P, Perlman J M et al 1985 Positron emission tomography in the asphyxiated term newborn: parasagittal impairment of cerebral blood flow. Ann Neurol 17:287–296.

Volpe J J, Pasternak J F 1977 Parasagittal cerebral injury in neonatal hypoxic-ischemic encephalopathy: clinical and neuroradiologic features. J Pediatr 91:472–476.

Voorhies T M, Ehrlich M E, Frayer W et al 1983 Occlusive vascular disease in perinatal cerebral hypoxia-ischemia. Am J Perinatol 1:1–5.

Walsh P, Jedeikin R, Ellis G et al 1982 Assessment of neurologic outcome in asphyxiated term infants by use of serial CK-BB isoenzyme measurement. J Pediatr 101:988–992.

Walther F J, Siassi B, Ramadan N A et al 1985 Cardiac output in newborn infants with transient myocardial dysfunction. J Pediatr 107:781–785.

Watanabe K, Miyazaki S, Hara K et al 1980 Behavioural state cycles, background EEGs and prognosis of newborns with perinatal hypoxia. Electroencephalogr Clin Neurophysiol 49:618–625.

Weichsel M E 1977 The therapeutic use of glucocorticoid hormones in the perinatal period: potential neurological hazards. Ann Neurology 2:364–366.

Wertheim D, Mercuri E, Faundez J C et al 1994 Prognostic value of continuous electroencephalographic recording in full term infants with hypoxic ischaemic encephalopathy. Arch Dis Childhood 71:F97–F102.

Westgate J 1993 The assessment of acid-base status at birth. DM thesis 114–143, University of Plymouth.

WHO (World Health Organization) 1991 Child health and development: health of the newborn. World Health Organization, Geneva.

WHO (World Health Organization) 2003 World Health Report 2002. World Health Organization, Geneva.

Wijdicks E F 2001 The diagnosis of brain death. N Engl J Med 344:1215–1221.

Williams C E, Gunn A J, Mallard C et al 1992 Outcome after ischemia in the developing sheep brain: an electroencephalographic and histological study. Ann Neurol 31:14–21.

Willis F, Summers J, Minutillo C et al 1997 Indices of renal tubular function in perinatal asphyxia. Arch Dis Childhood 77:F57–F60.

Wolf R I, Zimmerman R A, Clancy R et al 2001 Quantitative ADC measurements in term neonates for early detection of hypoxic-ischemic brain injury: initial experience. Radiology 218:825–833.

Wolfberg A J, du Plessis A J 2006 Near-Infrared Spectroscopy in the Fetus and Neonate. Clin Perinatol 33:707–728.

Woodgate P G, Davies M W 2001 Permissive hypercapnia for the prevention of morbidity and mortality in mechanically ventilated newborn infants. Cochrane Library Disk Issue 200l.

Worley G, Lipman B, Genolb I M et al 1985 Creatine kinase brain isoenzyme: relationship of cerebrospinal fluid concentration to the neurologic condition of newborns and cellular localization in the human brain. Pediatrics 76:15–21.

Wu Y W, Backstrand K H, Zhao S et al 2004 Declining diagnosis of birth asphyxia in California: 1991–2000. Pediatrics 114:1584–1590.

Wyatt J S, Edwards A D, Azzopardi D et al 1989 Magnetic resonance and near infrared spectroscopy for investigation of perinatal hypoxic-ischaemic brain injury. Arch Dis Childhood 64:953–963.

Yamaguchi M, Shirakata S, Yamasaki S et al 1976 Ischemic brain edema and compression brain edema. Stroke 7:77–83.

Zanardo V, Bondio M, Pesini G et al 1985 Serum glutamic-oxaloacetic transaminase and glutamic-pyruvic transaminase activity in premature and full-term asphyxiated newborns. Biol Neonate 47:61–69.

Zhu X Y, Fang H Q, Zeng S P et al 1997 The impact of the neonatal resuscitation programme guidelines (NRPG) on the neonatal mortality in a hospital in Zhuhai, China, Singapore. Med J 38:485–487.

Zimmerman R A, Wong AM-C, Bilaniuk L T 2005 Hypoxic and ischaemic brain insults in newborns and infants. In: Carty H, Brunelle F, Stringer D A, Kao S C S (eds) Imaging children. 2nd edition. Elsevier Churchill Livingstone, Edinburgh, pp. 1807–1862.

CHAPTER
27

Neuroprotection of the fetal and neonatal brain

Vincent Degos, Vincent Lelièvre and Pierre Gressens

> **Key Points**
>
> - Perinatal brain lesions have a multifactorial pathophysiology involving hypoxic–ischemic insults, excitotoxicity, inflammation, oxidative stress and growth factor deficiencies
> - A multi target approach might be necessary to achieve significant neuroprotection
> - Pathophysiological pathways are also involved in development
> - The adult is not a model for the newborn
> - Some potentially protective drugs are already used in humans
> - Neuroprotective strategies require early predictors of brain damage
> - Ethical issues need to be addressed

Injury to the perinatal brain is a leading cause of death and disability in children. Of major concern, neurological handicap of perinatal origin is not significantly decreasing in Western countries (Hagberg et al 1996, Vincer et al 2006). The major brain lesions associated with cerebral palsy and cognitive impairment are periventricular white matter damage (PWMD) mostly occurring in preterm infants (born below 32 weeks of gestation) and cortico-subcortical lesions mostly observed in term infants. For financial, technical and ethical reasons, the pharmaceutical industry has difficulties in making substantial investments in this area, which has left perinatologists with a limited therapeutic arsenal. At the present time, despite major improvements in neonatal care, there are no established therapeutic regimens that are successful for the treatment of perinatal brain lesions. Nevertheless, epidemiological and experimental data have allowed the identification of potential targets for neuroprotection. New animal models clearly show the pharmacology involved in neurodegeneration and neuroprotection (Dammann & Leviton 1997, Inder et al 1999, 2002, Nelson & Grether 1999, Pharoah et al 1989). Furthermore, some clinical trials using magnesium sulfate in preterm newborns or hypothermia in term newborns have been completed or are still in progress (Dommergues et al 2000, Hagberg et al 2002). One important difficulty is ethical, in whether society and regulatory bodies wish to help the pharmaceutical industry take the risk in working in this area.

PATHOPHYSIOLOGY OF PERINATAL BRAIN DAMAGE

During the last 15 years, the etiology of perinatal brain injury has been considered by many to be multifactorial rather than solely linked to cardiovascular instability and hypoxia–ischemia (Dammann & Leviton 1997, Nelson & Grether 1999).

Several prenatal, perinatal and postnatal factors have been implicated in the pathophysiology of brain lesions associated with cerebral palsy (Fig. 27.1), including hypoxic–ischemic insults, maternal infection yielding excess cytokines and other pro-inflammatory agents, excess release of glutamate initiating the excitotoxic cascade, and oxidative stress, growth factor deficiency, exposure to some drugs and maternal stress (Dammann & Leviton 1997, Dommergues 2000, Follett et al 2000, 2004, Gressens et al 1997, Hagberg et al 2002, Haynes et al 2003, Inder et al 2002, Laudenbach et al 2001, Loeliger et al 2003, Plaisant et al 2003, Tahraoui et al 2001, Volpe 2001). In addition, recent clinical studies support the existence of genetic factors of susceptibility (Harding et al 2004, Kerk et al 2006).

Although some of the potentially noxious factors are present in utero and were shown to be sufficient to cause permanent injury to the developing brain prior to neonatal life, several groups have hypothesized that some of these factors act as predisposing or sensitizing factors ('pro-damage conditions'), increasing the susceptibility to injury when a second unfavorable event occurs (Dammann et al 2002, Dommergues 2000, Eklind et al 2001, Gressens et al 2002, Nelson & Willoughby 2000). The understanding of this multiple-hit mechanism might be the key when designing a neuroprotective strategy.

Different animal models of perinatal brain damage have been produced (Hagberg et al 2002), allowing dissecting out of the underlying molecular and cellular mechanisms, and testing various neuroprotective strategies. PWMD of the preterm infant are usually mimicked by inducing infectious, inflammatory, excitotoxic or hypoxic–ischemic insults in mammals (newborn rodents, rabbits and cats, or fetal rats, rabbits and sheep) (Hagberg et al 2002). In addition, a model of preterm delivery (by cesarean section) has been developed in the baboon (Antonow-Schlorke et al 2003, Loeliger 2006), allowing determination of the impact of preterm birth and different strategies of ventilation on the developing white matter in a non-human primate species. Gray matter lesions of full term neonates are generally mimicked by hypoxic–ischemic or excitotoxic insults (newborn rodents, rabbits, piglets and dogs) (Derrick 2004, Hagberg et al 2002, Johnson 1987).

PATHOPHYSIOLOGY OF PWMD

Animal models have allowed successful identification of specific cell populations within the white matter that are

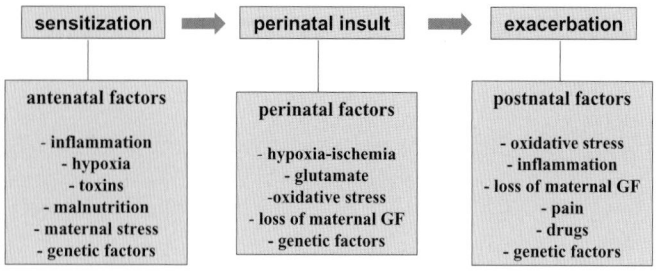

Figure 27.1 Schematic representation of the multiple-hit hypothesis in which a combination of two or more environmental or genetic factors occurring during the prenatal, perinatal or postnatal period induces or modulates brain lesions in human preterm neonates. GF, growth factors.

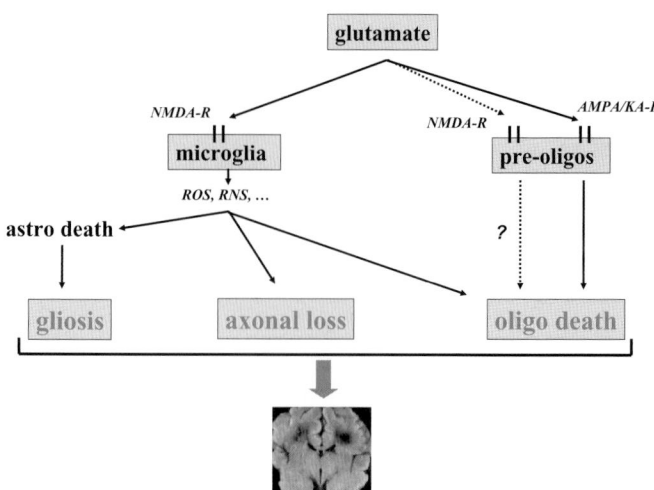

Figure 27.2 Schematic representation of the identified cellular and molecular pathways by which excess release of glutamate and pro-inflammatory cytokines may lead to PWMD in preterm newborns. Astro, astrocyte; KA, kainate; oligo(s), oligodendrocyte(s); R, receptors; RNS, reactive nitrogen species; ROS, reactive oxygen species.

critically involved in the pathophysiology of PWMD, including preoligodendrocytes (Follett et al 2000, 2004, Volpe 2001b) and microglia-macrophages (Dommergues et al 2003, Mesples et al 2005, Tahraoui et al 2001). Preoligodendrocytes, the precursors of myelinating oligodendrocytes which are a major glial population of the white matter, are highly vulnerable to oxidative stress due to a shortage of anti-oxidative defenses and to excess glutamate due to the high expression of alpha-3-amino-hydroxy-5-methyl-4-isoxazole propionic acid (AMPA) and kainate glutamatergic receptors (Follett 2000, 2004, Volpe 2001a). In addition, recent studies have identified the presence of functional N-methyl-D-aspartate (NMDA) glutamatergic receptors on oligodendroglial processes (Micu 2006, Salter & Fern 2005). Besides oligodendrocytes, brain macrophages-microglia can be rapidly activated in response to several stimuli or insults including inflammation, excess release of glutamate or hypoxia–ischemia. The microglial-macrophagic activation following excess release of glutamate seems to be linked to the transient expression of NMDA glutamatergic receptors by developing white matter microglia-macrophages (Dommergues et al 2003, Mesples et al 2005, Tahraoui et al 2001). Once activated, these microglia-macrophages can release a large array of toxic factors including reactive oxygen and nitrogen species. Figure 27.2 summarizes the major cellular and molecular elements identified so far in glutamate-induced excitotoxic PWMD. Of interest, human data obtained on post-mortem tissues support these experimental data (Kadhim et al 1988, Monier et al 2006, Volpe 2001a).

Furthermore, supporting previous hypotheses (Volpe 2001a), recent experimental studies have shown selective subplate neuronal cell death in models of PWMD (McQuillen 2003, Sfaello 2005). These subplate neurons play several important roles during brain development including axonal guidance and cortical organization. The molecular mechanisms by which these subplate neurons die are still poorly understood, not yet permitting design of specific neuroprotective strategies.

Finally, these animal models have also permitted further strengthening of the multiple-hit hypothesis. For example,

in a mouse model of excitotoxic PVL, simple exposure to pro-inflammatory cytokines (such as IL-1beta, IL-6 or TNF-alpha) did not actually produce brain lesions while a similar cytokine pre-treatment followed by a mild excitotoxic insult induced severe PWMD (Dommergues et al 2000).

PATHOPHYSIOLOGY OF NEURONAL CELL DEATH

Following exposure to hypoxia–ischemia (Fig. 27.3) (Hamrick & Ferriero 2003, Shalak & Perlman 2004), owing to the oxygen-glucose deprivation, there is a dramatic drop in ATP content leading to the failure of the sodium-potassium-ATP pump that maintains the polarity of the neuronal membrane. Membrane depolarization induces an excess release of glutamate leading to a massive sodium and calcium influx in neurons through the N-methyl-D-aspartate (NMDA) receptor. The increase in intracellular calcium excessively activates different enzymes including phospholipases, proteases and endonucleases as well as neuronal nitric oxide synthase (nNOS). This deleterious cascade is further exacerbated at the reperfusion phase due to excess superoxide formation (which will damage mitochondria and complex with NO to produce peroxynitrite) and the generation of free radicals. Reactive oxygen species will lead to lipid and protein oxidation and DNA alterations. Neuronal cell death has been shown in animal models to be a combination of necrosis, apoptosis and intermediate mechanisms. Mitochondrial damage, caspase activation and apoptosis inducing factor (AIF) play key roles in perinatal neuronal cell death (Hagberg 2004). Of particular interest, the delayed phase of neuronal cell death has been shown in rodents to be very protracted, lasting over weeks after the initial insult (Nakajima et al 2000).

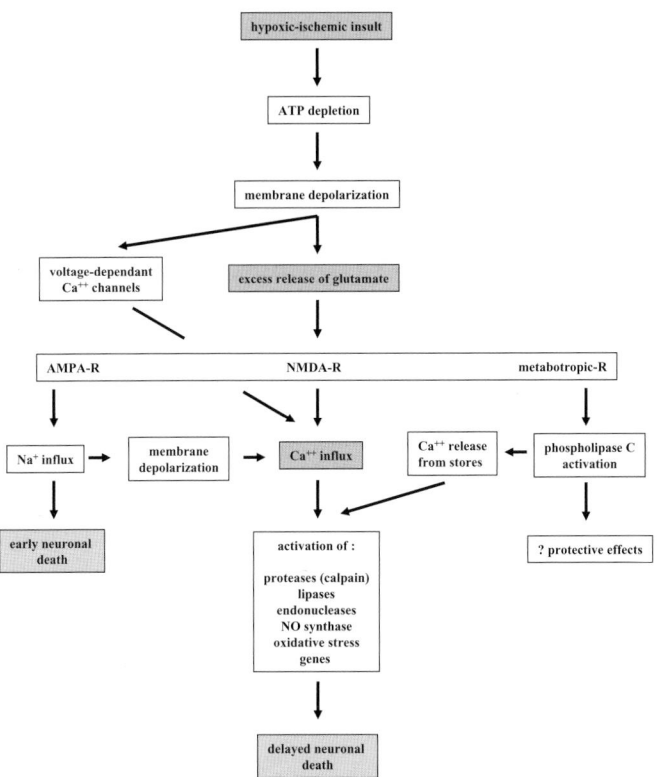

Figure 27.3 Schematic representation of the molecular cascade leading to neuronal cell death following perinatal hypoxic–ischemic insult in term newborns. R, receptors. (Adapted and modified from Hamrick et al 2003.)

POTENTIAL TARGETS FOR NEUROPROTECTION

GLUTAMATE RECEPTORS

Antagonists of the NMDA receptors for glutamate have been shown to be highly neuroprotective in different animal models of perinatal brain lesions (Johnston et al 2002). However, NMDA receptors play key roles in successive steps of brain development, including neuronal proliferation, neuronal migration, neuronal survival and neuronal differentiation (Lujan et al 2005). Therefore, blocking NMDA receptors at specific stages of brain development might be deleterious for normal brain development. Accordingly, Ikonomidou and Turski (2002) have shown that transient blockade of NMDA receptors with MK-801, a potent and noncompetitive antagonist, during postnatal growth spurt in rats leads to a severe apoptotic cell death. These experimental data of Ikonomidou and Turski (2002) likely preclude the use of potent NMDA receptor antagonists during brain development.

In contrast, blockade of AMPA and kainate receptors by drugs such as topiramate did not produce such devastating effects on neuronal survival (Glier et al 2004), although its effects on other steps of brain development like synapto-

genesis have not been evaluated. Topiramate is currently in use as a well-tolerated anti-epileptic drug in adults and children over two years of age (Elterman et al 1999). No data are available yet in human preterm or term infants. Topiramate was recently shown to protect pre-oligodendrocytes against excitotoxic or hypoxic–ischemic death (Follett et al 2004, Sfaello et al 2005), an important phenomenon in the pathophysiology of white matter lesions in the preterm infant, as well as to protect the periventricular white matter against damage induced by an AMPA-kainate agonist in newborn mice (Sfaello et al 2005).

Magnesium sulfate has multiple cellular effects including potential blockade of NMDA receptors. It has been used for decades as a tocolytic agent and in eclamptic mothers without any reported side effects for the fetus or newborn. However, studies precisely addressing the consequences of magnesium exposure on brain development and neuronal apoptosis are still lacking. Magnesium sulfate was shown to be neuroprotective in a mouse model of neonatal white matter damage (Marret et al 1995). The first multicenter controlled clinical trial where mothers at risk of preterm birth before 30 weeks of gestation were given magnesium has been recently completed. Results show the lack of significant perinatal side effects and some benefit for neurodevelopment of survivors examined at the age of two (Crowther et al 2003). Other similar clinical trials are in progress.

Other drugs potentially interfering with the glutamatergic neurotransmission, such as riluzole (which inhibits glutamate release and interferes with the activity of some proteins activated upon NMDA receptor activation) and amantadine or memantine (NMDA receptor antagonists deprived of the psychotomimetic and neurotoxic effects of phencyclidine or MK-801 when administered to adults), are neuroprotective in adult conditions where excitotoxicity is a key pathophysiological event. Their efficacy and safety in preterm newborns still need to be determined.

INFLAMMATION AND CYTOKINES

The role of pro-inflammatory cytokines and activated microglia-macrophages appears to be deleterious in extending neuronal injury and/or by sensitizing the developing brain to a second insult, and thus interference with their action would be expected to reduce subsequent neurological deficits. However, cytokines such as IL-1beta or IL-6 have been shown to have trophic effects on neurons at least in cell culture (Otten et al 2000). Similarly, activated microglia-macrophages, in addition to their toxic effects, can display protective properties such as excess glutamate scavenging through increased expression of glutamate transporters (Vallat-Decouvelaere et al 2003).

Tianeptine (Stablon®) has been shown to block the deleterious effects of inflammatory cytokines on neonatal excitotoxic PWMD in a mouse model (Plaisant et al 2003). Although its precise mechanism of action is unknown, tianeptine displays trophic properties and blocks the deleterious effects of inflammatory cytokines in several models, without interfering directly with glutamate receptors (Castanon et al 2001). This latter characteristic could limit the negative effect of tianeptine on normal brain development. Tianeptine is a well-tolerated antidepressant drug used in human adolescents and adults. No data are available in human newborns.

IL-10 is a Th2 anti-inflammatory cytokine which has marked suppressive effects on the production of proinflammatory cytokines by macrophages and downregulates the expression of activating molecules on these cells and dendritic cells (de Waal Malefyt et al 1991, Dziedzic et al 2002). Clinical trials based on IL-10 administration to adult patients suffering from auto-immune diseases such as psoriasis are currently in progress. Such studies may provide some preliminary information on the safety profile of IL-10 in humans. Similarly, TNF-alpha soluble receptor (Etanercept®), a TNF-alpha neutralizing agent, is currently used in human adults and children with Crohn disease and in other inflammatory diseases in adults (Akobeng & Zachos 2004). Like tianeptine, IL-10 and Etanercept® were shown to block the deleterious effects of inflammatory cytokines on murine neonatal excitotoxic brain damage (Mesples et al 2003) (Aden U and Gressens P, personal communication).

Several substances are known to inhibit microglia-macrophage function and/or activation in vitro and in vivo. Chloroquine alone or in combination with colchicine inhibits endocytosis, secretion and phagocytosis by blood-derived monocytes and macrophages. Tetracyclines are broad-spectrum antibiotics that display anti-inflammatory effects independent from their antimicrobial activity. Minocycline (a semi-synthetic second-generation tetracycline) inhibits microglial activation and protects neurons against ischemia in adult and developing rats (Arvin et al 2002, Fan et al 2006, Yrjanheikki et al 1999), although another study showed that minocycline can exacerbate hypoxic–ischemic cortical insult in neonatal mice (Tsuji et al 2004). Similarly, these drugs (chloroquine, chloroquine + colchicine or minocycline) were recently shown to reduce excitotoxic microglial-macrophagic activation and accompanying brain damage in newborn mice (Dommergues et al 2003). Although these drugs are rarely used in clinical pediatrics because of their side effects, drugs that modulate microglial activation could be proposed as candidate therapeutic agents in neonates at risk to develop brain damage.

Non-specific anti-inflammatory agents such as steroids or non-steroid anti-inflammatory drugs (NSAIDs, including indometacin and ibuprofen) could potentially have beneficial effects on perinatal brain damage. They are already largely used in human preterms for other indications including lung maturation and patent ductus arteriosus. However, the neuroprotective profile of NSAID against brain damage remains to be demonstrated both in animal models and in human studies specifically designed to test this neuroprotective hypothesis. Recently it was shown that cyclooxigenase-2 (cox-2) blockade by indometacin (a cox-1 and cox-2 inhibitor) or by nimesulide (a specific cox-2 inhibitor) abrogates the sensitizing effect of IL-1-beta on excitotoxic brain lesions in newborn mice (Favrais et al 2007). Experimental and epidemiological studies support a potential neuroprotective role of antenatal steroids against PWMD (O'Shea & Doyle 2001, Whitelaw & Thoresen 2000) but this benefit has to be balanced against the potential side effects of steroids on normal brain development when administered postnatally (Baud et al 2001, 2005, Baud 2004, Finer et al 2000).

OXIDATIVE STRESS

Neonates, and especially preterm infants, are highly vulnerable to oxidative or nitrosative stresses as they are relatively deficient in the cellular machinery required to detoxicate reactive oxygen and nitrogen species (Ferriero 2004). Oxidative and nitrosative stresses have been implicated in the animal models of perinatal brain damage (Grow & Barks 2002, McQuillen & Ferriero 2004). Therefore, the classic means of reducing oxidative and nitrosative stresses may be considered as potential therapeutic strategies. Some of these compounds have been successfully tested in animal models of perinatal brain damage (Largeron et al 2001, Marret et al 1999, Plaisant et al 2003, Vamecq et al 2003). Based on these experimental studies, allopurinol has been tested in human neonates with asphyxia without demonstrating any clinical benefit (Benders et al 2006).

Of note, while oxidative and nitrosative stresses have long been considered to be only produced during pathological processes, more recent data strongly suggest that low levels of NO and reactive oxygen species are also involved in physiological events such as control of gene transduction (Kroncke 2003).

Another way to minimize oxidative stress in neonates is to reduce the amount of pro-oxidative molecules given in the neonatal period, which include oxygen and iron. Oxygen can be a major source of oxidative stress especially during reperfusion phases and several studies have clearly identified the risk of excess inhaled oxygen for the preterm brain (Saugstad et al 2005). Similarly free iron induces the formation of reactive oxygen species and exogenous iron has been shown to significantly exacerbate excitotoxic PWMD in newborn mice (Dommergues et al 1998). However, this toxic effect of exogenous iron might be compensated in the clinical settings by the co-administration of erythropoietin which displays trophic properties (Siren et al 2001). Further experimental and clinical studies will be necessary to clarify this point.

PREVENTION OF DELAYED NEURONAL CELL DEATH

Proton MR spectroscopy has identified an early and a late phase of brain energy failure after perinatal asphyxia in term newborns or corresponding animal models (Hüppi 2002). These phases of energy failure are accompanied by periods of neuronal cell death (Shankaran 2002). As previously mentioned, the delayed phase of neuronal cell death has been shown in rodents to be very protracted, lasting over weeks after the initial insult (Nakajima et al 2000).

Hypothermia was shown to be highly neuroprotective in several experimental settings mimicking brain lesions of term neonates (McQuillen et al 2003, Thoresen 2000). Although hypothermia prevents the secondary energy failure occurring after asphyxia, its mechanism of action most likely involves multiple targets. Of potential concern, the effects of neonatal hypothermia on normal brain development have not been studied so far. However, multicenter controlled clinical trials have been completed (Gunn et al 1998, Hagberg et al 2002), showing a significant reduction of neurological handicap at 18 months of age in infants with a moderate neonatal insult, without any significant clinical side effects during the neonatal procedure. Other trials are still in progress.

Growth factors, such as IGF-1, nerve growth factor (NGF), or brain-derived neurotrophic factor (BDNF), which have anti-apoptotic properties, can prevent asphyxic or excitotoxic neuronal death in animal models of perinatal damage (Cheng et al 1997, Johnston et al 1996, 2002, Sfaello et al 2005, Sizonenko et al 2003). Interestingly, BDNF neuroprotective effects against excitotoxic neuronal cell death in the neonatal murine neocortex are highly stage-dependent (Husson et al 2005): at P5, BDNF was neuroprotective through TrkB receptors, MAPK pathway and reduced apoptosis, mimicking protective effects observed in the P7 rat model. In contrast, BDNF exacerbated neuronal death produced by ibotenate at P0 through increased apoptosis and p75^{NTR} receptors (another type of receptor for neurotrophins often associated with cell death), while BDNF had no detectable effect on lesions induced at P10.

In humans, and in several animal models, mutations in mitochondrial genes are known to be involved in neurological deficits and mitochondria are clearly involved in many apoptotic processes, including in perinatal brain damage. However, there are no therapies yet aimed at these major targets. Recent studies suggest that some trophic factors might, through an unknown mechanism, target mitochondrial function. Indeed, in vitro, BDNF, but not NGF, increases rat and mouse brain mitochondrial respiratory coupling at complex I (Markham et al 2004). Further studies will be necessary to confirm in vivo this effect on mitochondrial function and to determine the relevance of this mitochondrial effect in the overall neuroprotective effects of BDNF.

Neuropeptides are modulators of neuronal activity and could therefore modulate glutamate-induced neuronal cell death. Neuropeptides are subjected to enzymatic proteolysis leading to their inactivation and an inhibition of this degradation is a potential alternate therapeutic approach. Among the different identified peptidases, neutral endopeptidase (NEP or neprilysin) is the prototypical member of the M13 family of metalloproteinases and is widely distributed in various tissues. NEP is involved in the regulation and metabolism of a variety of biologically active peptides including tachykinins/neurokinins (Roques et al 1993).

Interestingly, racecadotril (Tiorfan®), an NEP inhibitor, is used in clinical practice for diarrhea with a remarkable safety profile (Schwartz 2000). Racecadotril is rapidly and entirely metabolized to its active metabolite thiorphan. A recent study showed that systemic administration of thiorphan was neuroprotective against excitotoxic neuronal cell death in newborn mice (Medja et al 2006). This neuroprotective effect was long-lasting and was still observed when thiorphan was administered 12 hours after the insult, showing a remarkable window for therapeutic intervention.

Caspases are effectors of apoptotic cell death and caspase inhibitors may be an attractive approach to preserve neuronal function by extending the therapeutic window and providing long-term neuroprotection. Currently, several inhibitors are in preclinical drug development (Legos 2001).

PLASTICITY AND REPAIR

Animal models have revealed a major area for therapeutic advances. Neuroprotective strategies can clearly stop lesions from getting worse, but agents which have neurotrophic properties can also affect repair in a developing brain. Although prevention and treatment at early stages of brain lesions are mostly desirable, post-lesion plasticity is the only affordable target in many cases, due to the lack of early detectors of perinatal brain lesions (Fig. 27.4).

This point has been highlighted in excitotoxic models of neonatal PWMD for melatonin (Husson et al 2002). Although melatonin did not prevent the initial appearance of PWMD, it did promote secondary lesion repair with axonal regrowth and/or sprouting. Behavioral studies support the hypothesis that melatonin-induced white matter histological repair is accompanied by improved learning capabilities. Melatonin is a safe compound (Penev & Zee 1997), including in term newborns (Gitto et al 2001), although its use has not often been evaluated in controlled trials. Therefore, melatonin derivatives which are under development (Valdoxan®) or already on the market (Roserem®) could be tested in controlled clinical trials.

In a similar excitotoxic model of neonatal PWMD, post-lesion plasticity was also induced by brain-derived neurotrophic factor (BDNF) (Husson et al 2005). However, the clinical use of BDNF is actually limited by its low capacity to cross the blood–brain barrier and by its central role in multiple steps of brain development, raising legitimate concerns about its direct use in newborns. Potential alternatives

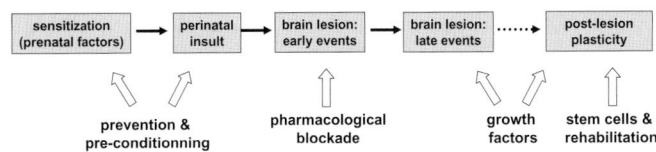

Figure 27.4 Schematic representation of the timeframe of potential strategies for neuroprotection of perinatal brain damage.

are either agents, such as ampakines (positive allosteric modulators of AMPA receptors) (Lauterborn et al 2000) or vasoactive intestinal peptide (VIP) (Moody et al 2003), which can cross the blood–brain barrier and increase BDNF production, or BDNF-expressing viral vectors which can increase BDNF production over a protracted period of time following a single intracerebral injection. These agents were shown experimentally to mimic the neuroprotective properties of BDNF (Dicou et al 2003, Gressens et al 1997, 1998, Husson et al 2005). Although promising these data require to be confirmed in other preclinical models and to be accompanied by data showing a gain of function.

In the last decade, numerous reports have demonstrated successful in vitro culture of stem cells and their subsequent differentiation in many specific cell populations (McKay 2004). Recent studies also showed potential for stem cell therapy in degenerative brain pathologies (Lindvall et al 2004), raising the possibility of being able to graft, at distance from the insult, these stem cells in a damaged brain in order to replace the missing neural cells.

Two major stem cell sources have been proven suitable to generate neuronal and glial cell subpopulations, multipotent embryonic stem cells (ES cells derived from the inner mass of early stage embryos) and neural stem cells (derived from early embryonic neural tissues). In vitro, ES cells are capable to spontaneously differentiate into various cell lineages. Addition of specific soluble factors in the culture medium resulted in enrichment in specific cell populations, including neural lineages. For instance, addition of VIP in the culture medium of murine ES cells enhanced the neuronal differentiation of these ES cells (Cazillis et al 2004). Similarly, in vitro, neural stem cells can differentiate into various neuronal and glial lineages, according to the culture conditions.

Despite the great hopes raised by cell therapy in various brain disorders, to our knowledge, there is not yet any report addressing experimentally the feasibility and the potential benefits of grafting stem cells following perinatal brain damage.

A potential alternative to grafting exogenous stem cells is to stimulate the endogenous production of neural progenitors from resident stem cells. Indeed, it was recently shown that an enhanced proliferation of neural stem/progenitor cells occurs in response to neonatal hypoxia–ischemia in newborn rats (Felling et al 2006). Although very promising, this approach requires (i) the demonstration that these newly formed neural cells survive and integrate into existing neuronal network and improve brain function, and (ii) the ability to pharmacologically stimulate the proliferation and/or survival of newly produced neural cells.

ETHICAL ISSUES

It is evident that there is an enormous medical and societal need – newborn children with brain lesions will carry the handicap all their lives. Thus any reduction of damage will have a major impact on the person and on potential carers. However, drugs may leave markers in development which are not necessarily due to the drug, but due to the combination of the reduced lesion and the developmental stage at which a drug is given. Thus there is the possibility of adolescents suing drug makers, where their lives have been saved, but certain developmental markers remain which might be, rightly or wrongly, ascribed to the drug. It is for this type of reason that the pharmaceutical industry has difficulties in engaging in this area. This is a debate for our litigious society and its willingness to accept benefit associated with some risk.

CONCLUSIONS

Neuroprotection of the perinatal brain is a health care priority both in terms of suffering and economy. Promising neuroprotective strategies are emerging. However, some factors prevent a major boom of this field:

(i)   lessons acquired from brain damage in the adult are not applicable to the premature infants without further evaluation;

(ii) neuroprotective drugs can disturb normal brain development which is very active at the time of birth;

(iii) setting up clinical trials in newborns immediately calls for ethical issues, which are for understandable reasons an obstacle for a larger implication of the pharmaceutical industry and which urgently requires an open and in-depth society debate;

(iv) the economically limited market of newborns in Western societies is an additional potential limitation for investment of pharmaceutical companies.

In addition, several important questions are still the focus of debate:

(i)   Do we need to combine several drugs to target the major underlying mechanisms?

(ii) In a given human preterm infant, can we determine the major pathophysiological mechanism(s) which is (are) at play?

(iii) Are the mechanisms at play in diffuse PWMD (which are more frequent in extremely preterm infants) similar to those described in classic PVL?

(iv) Can we design a strategy which can block brain damage without interfering with normal development?

(v)   Although brain lesions occurring in preterm and term infants share multiple risk factors and molecular mechanisms, can we identify the key differences in order to design the most appropriate therapeutic strategy for each developmental age?

ACKNOWLEDGMENTS

This work was supported by the Inserm, the Université Paris 7, the Fondation Motrice, the Fondation pour la Recherche Médicale, and the Fondation Grace de Monaco.

REFERENCES

Akobeng A K, Zachos M 2004 Tumor necrosis factor-alpha antibody for induction of remission in Crohn's disease. Cochrane Database Syst Rev CD003574.

Antonow-Schlorke I, Schwab M, Li C et al 2003 Glucocorticoid exposure at the dose used clinically alters cytoskeletal proteins and presynaptic terminals in the fetal baboon brain. J Physiol 547:117–123.

Arvin K L, Han B H, Du Y et al 2002 Minocycline markedly protects the neonatal brain against hypoxic-ischemic injury. Ann Neurol 52:54–61.

Baud O 2004 Antenatal corticosteroid therapy: benefits and risks. Acta Paediatr Suppl 93:6–10.

Baud O, Laudenbach V, Evrard P et al 2001 Neurotoxic effects of fluorinated glucocorticoid preparations on the developing mouse brain: role of preservatives. Pediatr Res 50:706–711.

Baud O, Verney C, Evrard P et al 2005 Injectable dexamethasone administration enhances cortical GABAergic neuronal differentiation in a novel model of postnatal steroid therapy in mice. Pediatr Res 57:149–156.

Benders M J, Bos A F, Rademaker C M et al 2006 Early postnatal allopurinol does not improve short term outcome after severe birth asphyxia. Arch Dis Child Fetal Neonatal Ed 91:F163–F165.

Castanon N, Bluthe R M, Dantzer R 2001 Chronic treatment with the atypical antidepressant tianeptine attenuates sickness behavior induced by peripheral but not central lipopolysaccharide and interleukin-1beta in the rat. Psychopharmacology (Berl) 154:50–60.

Cazillis M, Gonzalez B J, Billardon C et al 2004 VIP and PACAP induce selective neuronal differentiation of mouse embryonic stem cells. Eur J Neurosci 19:798–808.

Cheng Y, Gidday J M, Yan Q et al 1997 Marked age-dependent neuroprotection by brain-derived neurotrophic factor against neonatal hypoxic-ischemic brain injury. Ann Neurol 41:521–529.

Crowther C A, Hiller J E, Doyle L W et al 2003 Effect of magnesium sulfate given for neuroprotection before preterm birth: a randomized controlled trial. Jama 290:2669–2676.

Dammann O, Kuban K C, Leviton A 2002 Perinatal infection, fetal inflammatory response, white matter damage, and cognitive limitations in children born preterm. Ment Retard Dev Disabil Res Rev 8:46–50.

Dammann O, Leviton A 1997 Maternal intrauterine infection, cytokines, and brain damage in the preterm newborn. Pediatr Res 42:1–8.

de Waal Malefyt R, Abrams J, Bennett B et al 1991 Interleukin 10(IL-10) inhibits cytokine synthesis by human monocytes: an autoregulatory role of IL-10 produced by monocytes. J Exp Med 174:1209–1220.

Derrick M, Luo N L, Bregman J C et al 2004 Preterm fetal hypoxia-ischemia causes hypertonia and motor deficits in the neonatal rabbit: a model for human cerebral palsy? J Neurosci 24:24–34.

Dicou E, Rangon C M, Guimiot F et al 2003 Positive allosteric modulators of AMPA receptors are neuroprotective against lesions induced by an NMDA agonist in neonatal mouse brain. Brain Res 970:221–225.

Dommergues M A, Gallego J, Evrard P et al 1998 Iron supplementation aggravates periventricular cystic white matter lesions in newborn mice. Eur J Paediatr Neurol 2:313–318.

Dommergues M A, Patkai J, Renauld J C et al 2000 Proinflammatory cytokines and interleukin-9 exacerbate excitotoxic lesions of the newborn murine neopallidum. Ann Neurol 47:54–63.

Dommergues M A, Plaisant F, Verney C et al 2003 Early microglial activation following neonatal excitotoxic brain damage in mice: a potential target for neuroprotection. Neuroscience 121:619–628.

Dziedzic T, Bartus S, Klimkowicz A et al 2002 Intracerebral hemorrhage triggers interleukin-6 and interleukin-10 release in blood. Stroke 33:2334–2335.

Eklind S, Mallard C, Leverin A L et al 2001 Bacterial endotoxin sensitizes the immature brain to hypoxic-ischaemic injury. Eur J Neurosci 13:1101–1106.

Elterman R D, Glauser T A, Wyllie E et al 1999 A double-blind, randomized trial of topiramate as adjunctive therapy for partial-onset seizures in children. Topiramate YP Study Group. Neurology 52:1338–1344.

Fan L W, Lin S, Pang Y et al 2006 Minocycline attenuates hypoxia-ischemia-induced neurological dysfunction and brain injury in the juvenile rat. Eur J Neurosci 24:341–350.

Favrais G S L, Gressens P, Lelièvre V 2007 Cyclooxygenase-2 mediates the sensitizing effects of systemic IL-1-beta on excitotoxic brain lesions in newborn mice. Neurobiology of Disease 25:496–505.

Felling R J, Snyder M J, Romanko M J et al 2006 Neural stem/progenitor cells participate in the regenerative response to perinatal hypoxia/ischemia. J Neurosci 26:4359–4369.

Ferriero D M 2004 Neonatal brain injury. N Engl J Med 351:1985–1995.

Finer N N, Craft A, Vaucher Y E et al 2000 Postnatal steroids: short-term gain, long-term pain? J Pediatr 137:9–13.

Follett P L, Deng W, Dai W et al 2004 Glutamate receptor-mediated oligodendrocyte toxicity in periventricular leukomalacia: a protective role for topiramate. J Neurosci 24:4412–4420.

Follett P L, Rosenberg P A, Volpe J J et al 2000 NBQX attenuates excitotoxic injury in developing white matter. J Neurosci 20:9235–9241.

Gitto E, Karbownik M, Reiter R J et al 2001 Effects of melatonin treatment in septic newborns. Pediatr Res 50:756–760.

Glier C, Dzietko M, Bittigau P et al 2004 Therapeutic doses of topiramate are not toxic to the developing rat brain. Exp Neurol 187:403–409.

Gressens P, Marret S, Hill J M et al 1997 Vasoactive intestinal peptide prevents excitotoxic cell death in the murine developing brain. J Clin Invest 100:390–397.

Gressens P, Marret S, Martin J L et al 1998 Regulation of neuroprotective action of vasoactive intestinal peptide in the murine developing brain by protein kinase C and mitogen-activated protein kinase cascades: in vivo and in vitro studies. J Neurochem 70:2574–2584.

Gressens P, Rogido M, Paindaveine B et al 2002 The impact of neonatal intensive care practices on the developing brain. J Pediatr 140:646–653.

Grow J, Barks J D 2002 Pathogenesis of hypoxic-ischemic cerebral injury in the term infant: current concepts. Clin Perinatol 29:585–602.

Gunn A J, Gluckman P D, Gunn T R 1998 Selective head cooling in newborn infants after perinatal asphyxia: a safety study. Pediatrics 102:885–892.

Hagberg B, Hagberg G, Olow I et al 1996 The changing panorama of cerebral palsy in Sweden. VII. Prevalence and origin in the birth year period 1987–90. Acta Paediatr 85:954–960.

Hagberg H 2004 Mitochondrial impairment in the developing brain after hypoxia-ischemia. J Bioenerg Biomembr 36:369–373.

Hagberg H, Peebles D, Mallard C 2002 Models of white matter injury: comparison of infectious, hypoxic-ischemic, and excitotoxic insults. Ment Retard Dev Disabil Res Rev 8:30–38.

Hamrick S E, Ferriero D M 2003 The injury response in the term newborn brain: can we neuroprotect? Curr Opin Neurol 16:147–154.

Harding D R, Dhamrait S, Whitelaw A et al 2004 Does interleukin-6 genotype influence cerebral injury or developmental progress after preterm birth? Pediatrics 114:941–947.

Haynes R L, Folkerth R D, Keefe R J et al 2003 Nitrosative and oxidative injury to premyelinating oligodendrocytes in periventricular leukomalacia. J Neuropathol Exp Neurol 62:441–450.

Hüppi P S 2002 Advances in postnatal neuroimaging: relevance to pathogenesis and treatment of brain injury. Clin Perinatol 29:827–856.

Husson I, Mesples B, Bac P et al 2002 Melatoninergic neuroprotection of the murine periventricular white matter against neonatal excitotoxic challenge. Ann Neurol 51:82–92.

Husson I, Rangon C M, Lelievre V et al 2005 BDNF-induced white matter neuroprotection and stage-dependent neuronal survival following a neonatal excitotoxic challenge. Cereb Cortex 15:250–261.

Ikonomidou C, Turski L 2002 Why did NMDA receptor antagonists fail clinical trials for stroke and traumatic brain injury? Lancet Neurol 1:383–386.

Inder T E, Hüppi P S, Warfield S et al 1999 Periventricular white matter injury in the premature infant is followed by reduced cerebral cortical gray matter volume at term. Ann Neurol 46:755–760.

Inder T, Mocatta T, Darlow B et al 2002 Elevated free radical products in the cerebrospinal fluid of VLBW infants with cerebral white matter injury. Pediatr Res 52:213–218.

Johnson D L, Getson P, Shaer C et al 1987 Intraventricular hemorrhage in the newborn beagle puppy. A limited model of intraventricular hemorrhage in the premature infant. Pediatr Neurosci 13:78–83.

Johnston B M, Mallard E C, Williams C E et al 1996 Insulin-like growth factor-1 is a potent neuronal rescue agent after hypoxic-ischemic injury in fetal lambs. J Clin Invest 97:300–308.

Johnston M V, Nakajima W, Hagberg H 2002 Mechanisms of hypoxic neurodegeneration in the developing brain. Neuroscientist 8:212–220.

Kadhim H J, Gadisseux J F, Evrard P 1988 Topographical and cytological evolution of the glial phase during prenatal development of the human brain: histochemical and electron microscopic study. J Neuropathol Exp Neurol 47:166–188.

Kerk J, Dordelmann M, Bartels D B et al 2006 Multiplex measurement of cytokine/receptor gene polymorphisms and interaction between interleukin-10 (–1082) genotype and chorioamnionitis in extreme preterm delivery. J Soc Gynecol Investig 13:350–356.

Kroncke K D 2003 Nitrosative stress and transcription. Biol Chem 384:1365–1377.

Largeron M, Mesples B, Gressens P et al 2001 The neuroprotective activity of 8-alkylamino-1,4-benzoxazine antioxidants. Eur J Pharmacol 424:189–194.

Laudenbach V, Calo G, Guerrini R et al 2001 Nociceptin/orphanin FQ exacerbates excitotoxic white-matter lesions in the murine neonatal brain. J Clin Invest 107:457–466.

Lauterborn J C, Lynch G, Vanderklish P et al 2000 Positive modulation of AMPA receptors increases

593

neurotrophin expression by hippocampal and cortical neurons. J Neurosci 20:8–21.

Legos J J, Lee D, Erhardt J A 2001 Caspase inhibitors as neuroprotective agents. Expert Opin Emerg Drugs 6:81–94.

Lindvall O, Kokaia Z, Martinez-Serrano A 2004 Stem cell therapy for human neurodegenerative disorders–how to make it work. Nat Med 10 Suppl: S42–S50.

Loeliger M, Inder T, Cain S et al 2006 Cerebral outcomes in a preterm baboon model of early versus delayed nasal continuous positive airway pressure. Pediatrics 118:1640–1653.

Loeliger M, Watson C S, Reynolds J D et al 2003 Extracellular glutamate levels and neuropathology in cerebral white matter following repeated umbilical cord occlusion in the near term fetal sheep. Neuroscience 116:705–714.

Lujan R, Shigemoto R, Lopez-Bendito G 2005 Glutamate and GABA receptor signalling in the developing brain. Neuroscience 130:567–580.

McKay R D 2004 Stem cell biology and neurodegenerative disease. Philos Trans R Soc Lond B Biol Sci 359:851–856.

McQuillen P S, Ferriero D M 2004 Selective vulnerability in the developing central nervous system. Pediatr Neurol 30:227–235.

McQuillen P S, Sheldon R A, Shatz C J et al 2003 Selective vulnerability of subplate neurons after early neonatal hypoxia-ischemia. J Neurosci 23:3308–3315.

Markham A, Cameron I, Franklin P et al 2004 BDNF increases rat brain mitochondrial respiratory coupling at complex I, but not complex II. Eur J Neurosci 20:1189–1196.

Marret S, Bonnier C, Raymackers J M et al 1999 Glycine antagonist and NO synthase inhibitor protect the developing mouse brain against neonatal excitotoxic lesions. Pediatr Res 45:337–342.

Marret S, Gressens P, Gadisseux J F et al 1995 Prevention by magnesium of excitotoxic neuronal death in the developing brain: an animal model for clinical intervention studies. Dev Med Child Neurol 37:473–484.

Medja F, Lelievre V, Fontaine R H et al 2006 Thiorphan, a neutral endopeptidase inhibitor used for diarrhoea, is neuroprotective in newborn mice. Brain 129:3209–3223.

Mesples B, Plaisant F, Fontaine R H et al 2005 Pathophysiology of neonatal brain lesions: lessons from animal models of excitotoxicity. Acta Paediatr 94:185–190.

Mesples B, Plaisant F, Gressens P 2003 Effects of interleukin-10 on neonatal excitotoxic brain lesions in mice. Brain Res Dev Brain Res 141:25–32.

Micu I, Jiang Q, Coderre E et al 2006 NMDA receptors mediate calcium accumulation in myelin during chemical ischaemia. Nature 439:988–992.

Monier A, Evrard P, Gressens P et al 2006 Distribution and differentiation of microglia in the human encephalon during the first two trimesters of gestation. J Comp Neurol 499:565–582.

Moody T W, Hill J M, Jensen R T 2003 VIP as a trophic factor in the CNS and cancer cells. Peptides 24:163–177.

Nakajima W, Ishida A, Lange M S et al 2000 Apoptosis has a prolonged role in the neurodegeneration after hypoxic ischemia in the newborn rat. J Neurosci 20:7994–8004.

Nelson K B, Grether J K 1999 Causes of cerebral palsy. Curr Opin Pediatr 11:487–491.

Nelson K B, Willoughby R E 2000 Infection, inflammation and the risk of cerebral palsy. Curr Opin Neurol 13:133–139.

O'Shea T M, Doyle L W 2001 Perinatal glucocorticoid therapy and neurodevelopmental outcome: an epidemiologic perspective. Semin Neonatol 6:293–307.

Otten U, Marz P, Heese K et al 2000 Cytokines and neurotrophins interact in normal and diseased states. Ann N Y Acad Sci 917:322–330.

Penev P D, Zee P C 1997 Melatonin: a clinical perspective. Ann Neurol 42:545–553.

Pharoah P O, Cooke T, Rosenbloom L 1989 Acquired cerebral palsy. Arch Dis Child 64:1013–1016.

Plaisant F, Clippe A, Vander Stricht D et al 2003 Recombinant peroxiredoxin 5 protects against excitotoxic brain lesions in newborn mice. Free Radic Biol Med 34:862–872.

Plaisant F, Dommergues M A, Spedding M et al 2003 Neuroprotective properties of tianeptine: interactions with cytokines. Neuropharmacology 44:801–809.

Roques B P, Noble F, Dauge V et al 1993 Neutral endopeptidase 24.11: structure, inhibition, and experimental and clinical pharmacology. Pharmacol Rev 45:87–146.

Salter M G, Fern R 2005 NMDA receptors are expressed in developing oligodendrocyte processes and mediate injury. Nature 438:1167–1171.

Saugstad O D, Ramji S, Vento M 2005 Resuscitation of depressed newborn infants with ambient air or pure oxygen: a meta-analysis. Biol Neonate 87:27–34.

Schwartz J C 2000 Racecadotril: a new approach to the treatment of diarrhoea. Int J Antimicrob Agents 14:75–79.

Sfaello I, Baud O, Arzimanoglou A et al 2005 Topiramate prevents excitotoxic damage in the newborn rodent brain. Neurobiol Dis 20:837–848.

Sfaello I, Daire J L, Husson I et al 2005 Patterns of excitotoxin-induced brain lesions in the newborn rabbit: a neuropathological and MRI correlation. Dev Neurosci 27:160–168.

Shalak L, Perlman J M 2004 Hypoxic-ischemic brain injury in the term infant-current concepts. Early Hum Dev 80:125–141.

Shankaran S 2002 The postnatal management of the asphyxiated term infant. Clin Perinatol 29:675–692.

Siren A L, Fratelli M, Brines M et al 2001 Erythropoietin prevents neuronal apoptosis after cerebral ischemia and metabolic stress. Proc Natl Acad Sci U S A 98:4044–4049.

Sizonenko S V, Sirimanne E, Mayall Y et al 2003 Selective cortical alteration after hypoxic-ischemic injury in the very immature rat brain. Pediatr Res 54:263–269.

Tahraoui S L, Marret S, Bodenant C et al 2001 Central role of microglia in neonatal excitotoxic lesions of the murine periventricular white matter. Brain Pathol 11:56–71.

Thoresen M 2000 Cooling the newborn after asphyxia — physiological and experimental background and its clinical use. Semin Neonatol 5:61–73.

Tsuji M, Wilson M A, Lange M S et al 2004 Minocycline worsens hypoxic-ischemic brain injury in a neonatal mouse model. Exp Neurol 189:58–65.

Vallat-Decouvelaere A V, Chretien F, Gras G et al 2003 Expression of excitatory amino acid transporter-1 in brain macrophages and microglia of HIV-infected patients. A neuroprotective role for activated microglia? J Neuropathol Exp Neurol 62:475–485.

Vamecq J, Maurois P, Bac P et al 2003 Potent mammalian cerebroprotection and neuronal cell death inhibition are afforded by a synthetic antioxidant analogue of marine invertebrate cell protectant ovothiols. Eur J Neurosci 18:1110–1120.

Vincer M J, Allen A C, Joseph K S et al 2006 Increasing prevalence of cerebral palsy among very preterm infants: a population-based study. Pediatrics 118:1621–1626.

Volpe J J 2001a Neurobiology of periventricular leukomalacia in the premature infant. Pediatr Res 50:553–562.

Volpe J J 2001b Perinatal brain injury: from pathogenesis to neuroprotection. Ment Retard Dev Disabil Res Rev 7:56–64.

Whitelaw A, Thoresen M 2000 Antenatal steroids and the developing brain. Arch Dis Child Fetal Neonatal Ed 83:F154–F157.

Yrjanheikki J, Tikka T, Keinanen R et al 1999 A tetracycline derivative, minocycline, reduces inflammation and protects against focal cerebral ischemia with a wide therapeutic window. Proc Natl Acad Sci U S A 96:13496–13500.

CHAPTER
28

Medico-legal issues: the United Kingdom perspective

Roger V. Clements and Lewis Rosenbloom

Key Points

- Civil Procedure Rules, introduced following the Woolf reforms, now exercise strict control over the conduct of experts
- The House of Lords has qualified to some extent the Bolam principle in the case of Bolitho v. City and Hackney Health Authority
- Damages continue to increase, not only because of inflation but also because of changes in the law
- Errors leading to malpractice litigation in obstetrics are almost always the result of system failures and a cascade of error

---

THE SOCIAL CLIMATE

It is perhaps inevitable that one of the responses to being informed that a child has sustained brain damage or other mishap either in the perinatal period or indeed at any other time is that fault is perceived and a process of enquiry is commenced. It is beyond our remit in this chapter to discuss the NHS complaints machinery. For details of this an appropriate source is /www.dh.gov.uk/en/Policyandguidance/Organisationpolicy/Complaintspolicy/NHScomplaintsprocedure.

Rather here we focus on the process in which blame is perceived or attached to hospital units or individual practitioners and parents consider the possibility of litigation leading to compensation. It is unsurprising that towards the end of the last century the number of claims seemed to be escalating out of control. It is also outside our remit to speculate whether this was a North American import, a component of what is termed 'the compensation culture,' a reflection of the size of published settlements for individual children with brain damage or a combination of each of these together with other factors. As a consequence there can be few if any midwives, obstetricians or neonatologists in the UK who have not had some involvement in a claim for damages brought on behalf of a brain-damaged infant. More recent figures from the NHS Litigation Authority now suggest that at least in England, if not actually falling, the number of claims has leveled out.

THE LEGAL CLIMATE

In the late 1970s, three major events altered significantly the legal climate of clinical negligence litigation in the United Kingdom. Firstly, procedure in the Civil Courts in England and Wales (but not in Scotland) has been radically altered by the introduction of the Civil Procedure Rules 1998 which, notwithstanding their title, came into force in April 1999. Secondly, the common law in this area has been advanced by two landmark cases in the House of Lords (Bolitho v. City and Hackney Health Authority, 1998; Wells v. Wells 1999). Thirdly, during the same period, there have been landmark decisions in the Court of Appeal concerning consent for cesarean section (Re M B 1997; St. George's Healthcare NHS Trust v. S 1999). A fourth and more recent venture that may have significance in the future is the NHS Redress Scheme.

PROCEDURAL CHANGES

In his report on the Civil Justice System in England and Wales 'Access to Justice', Lord Woolf (1996) suggested a wide ranging reform of the system and proposed a new set of rules to bring those reforms into force. On 26 April 1999, the Civil Procedure Rules 1998 (CPR) came into effect in England and Wales. The purpose of the rules (Gumbel 1999a) was not only to effect the substantive reforms proposed but to simplify and reduce the size of the rules, simplifying the language and eliminating Latin. Part 1 of the New Rules states the overriding objective 'of enabling the courts to deal with cases justly', ensuring that the parties are on an equal footing, saving expense and dealing with cases in ways that are proportionate to the amount of money involved, the importance of the case, the complexity of the issues and the financial position of each party.

The Rules impose upon the courts the duty to manage cases, a radical reform, taking the pace and control of litigation out of the hands of the parties.

The language of the Rules is simplified; amongst the changes, the instigator of a civil action is no longer called a plaintiff – but a claimant. The result of the reforms has been a radical reduction of cases coming to trial; the pre-action exchange of letters and the improvements in pleading have resulted in much more open litigation; the exchange of evidence (both lay and expert) means that each side knows exactly what the other side's case will be. Now less than 1% of all proceedings issued end in trial. One of the most powerful instruments for settlement has been the discussions between experts on opposing sides to identify points of agreement and to explain areas of disagreement.

DEVELOPMENTS IN THE COMMON LAW

The House of Lords' judgment in Wells v. Wells (1999) has had a significant influence on the quantum of damage recovered by successful litigants. The judgment has had its more dramatic effects upon the damages awarded to cerebral palsy victims. The result of this judgment (Gumbel 1999b) was to reduce the discount rate (the rate at which the successful litigant could be expected to receive interest on his lump sum award) from 4.5 to 3% (Gumbel 1999b). Following the introduction of the Damages Act 1996 the Lord Chancellor reduced the rate further to 2.5%.

In professional negligence cases, the way in which the courts in the United Kingdom assess expert evidence has for more than 50 years been based on the landmark cases of Hunter (Hunter v. Hanley 1954) in Scotland and Bolam (Bolam v. Friern Hospital Management Committee 1957) in England and Wales. In December 1997 (Bolitho v. City and Hackney Health Authority 1998), the House of Lords considered the Bolam test for the first time in 9 years (Watt 1999). Whilst sustaining the principle upon which expert evidence is assessed by the courts, the House of Lords added an important reservation, Lord Browne-Wilkinson expressing the view that a court is not bound to hold that a defendant doctor escapes liability for negligent treatment and diagnosis just because he pleads evidence from a number of medical experts genuinely of the opinion that the defendant's treatment or diagnosis accords with sound medical practice. The court must be satisfied that the exponents of the body of opinion relied upon can demonstrate that such opinion had a logical basis and that by informing those views, the experts had directed their minds to the questions of comparative risk and benefits and reached a defensible conclusion. A judge might be entitled to the view that professional opinion was not capable of withstanding logical analysis and that the body of opinion relied upon was not reasonable or responsible.

In dealing with matters of consent, courts in the British Isles, almost alone in the developed world, have traditionally applied the responsible doctor test rather than the test applied throughout North America and Europe, the test of the prudent patient. That principle has now been eroded by recent judgments, somewhat indirectly in Bolitho (Bolitho v. City and Hackney Health Authority 1998; Watt 1999), and more recently in Chester v. Afshar (Chester v. Afshar [2004] UKHL 41) concerning warnings before surgery (Craggs & Hackett 2006, Shaw 2005).

The courts have on several occasions been asked to intervene in circumstances involving the refusal of treatment by a pregnant woman, refusal that might have threatened the life and wellbeing of her fetus and herself. In every case at the first instance, and in the only case to come before the Court of Appeal in advance of the event, the courts have ruled in favor of intervention and have declared lawful cesarean section notwithstanding the refusal of the mother. In Re M B (1997), Lady Justice Butler-Sloss, giving the leading judgment:

> rejected the submission that the rights of the unborn child should be weighed in the balance and upheld the principle that the competent mother has the

unqualified right to decide whether or not to accept surgical intervention in childbirth. However on the facts the court upheld the decision of the first instance judge who had held that the mother's phobia of the injection needle rendered her incompetent.

(Lord Justice Thorpe 1999a)

The only occasion on which the courts took a different view was in the case of St. George's Healthcare NHS Trust ex. Parte S (1999) in which, long after the event, the Court of Appeal was able to say that the autonomy of the woman is sacrosanct and must be preserved in future cases. In that case, the Court of Appeal laid down guidelines for the future conduct for cases, both by doctors and by lawyers, where maternal consent to intervention in pregnancy is refused. These matters, the absolute right of any adult to choose, to accept or refuse treatment and the rights of the fetus in law are discussed in detail elsewhere (Grace 1999, Lord Justice Thorpe 1999a).

THE NHS REDRESS SCHEME

In what may be perceived as a reaction to the increasing costs of settlements and the superficial attractions of no-fault compensation, draft legislation has recently been introduced in which a tariff for low value claims, irrespective of liability, is proposed. The scheme is not without its problems and it remains to be seen how it will eventually be enacted. High value claims such as those that relate to brain damage at birth are currently excluded from these proposals.

LITIGATION AND RISK MANAGEMENT

There is no doubting that the impetus for clinical risk management was provided by the increasing costs of malpractice litigation. The sums of money involved are significant. The Auditor General (1999) estimates that in total, potential liabilities within the National Health Service in England are £1.8 billion (£394 million of provisions and £1.4 billion assistance from departmental schemes), but this excludes the additional liabilities relating to incidents incurred but not yet reported and the cases where the NHS considers that there is less than 50% likelihood of a successful claim. However, these figures relate of course only to damages and legal costs. The true cost to the community is incalculable. Clinical risk management (Vincent & Clements 1995, 2006) is not primarily about the avoidance of litigation: it is about the avoidance of harm to patients. The Harvard Medical Practice Study (Brennan et al 1991) and the subsequent Australian Studies (Wilson et al 1995) have demonstrated that only a small proportion of negligent events result in litigation; if the focus remains with litigation, the majority of occasions on which patients are harmed will go unobserved and uncorrected.

In June 2000 the Department of Health published a study by an expert group 'An Organisation with a Memory' concluding that adverse health care events cannot be eliminated from complex modern health care but made recommendations designed to ensure that lessons from the past are used to reduce the risk to patients in the future. That process is still in its infancy.

The focus of clinical risk management therefore must be on the analysis of adverse events with the aim of reducing and, as far as possible, eliminating harm to the patient and dealing with the injured patient by continuity of care and swift compensation for the justified claimant. Clinical risk management is about the avoidance of harm to patients: it is not about the evasion of responsibility for that harm.

In an attempt to improve standards and reduce harm, there has been a flood of advice, in the form of guidelines; originally issued by various learned bodies such as Royal Colleges, these have now been adopted by NICE (the National Institute for Clinical Excellence). It is at present unclear how the courts will view these guidelines, but one view is that:

> With the law as it now stands, it is open to a judge to make finding of negligence even if the practitioner has carefully and conscientiously followed published guidelines – if subsequent research were, for example, to provide evidence that an accepted practice of the time was unsound, illogical, and based merely on convention and consensus.
>
> *(Leigh & James 1998)*

In addition the Confidential Enquiry into Stillbirths and Deaths in Infancy and the Confidential Enquiry into Maternal Death are two important national audits, looking at specific bad outcomes in maternity services.

EXPERT EVIDENCE

Part 35 of the CPR (White Book 1999), dealing with experts and assessors, has two principal themes:

- the overriding duty of the expert to the court;
- the proportionality of cost to the value of the claim.

Following the implementation of the New Rules, it may be expected that there will be less experts, less money available for experts, less time for experts to respond and less oral evidence. The Rules favor single experts, require a standard format for expert reports, provide for written questions to experts, encourage expert discussions and give the expert the right to ask the court for directions. Much of this is new. The practice direction to Part 35 (White Book 1999) sets out in detail the form and content of experts' reports. Perhaps the most important change for the medical expert is the requirement that 'where there is a range of opinion on the matters dealt with in the report', the expert must summarize the range of that opinion and give reasons for his own opinion.

The practice Direction associated with Part 35 of the CPR requires that within the report, the expert must give 'details of any literature or other material which the expert has relied on in making the report'. In some jurisdictions, text-book authorities are not much favored, but in the United Kingdom courts, the expert for the claimant will be expected to support his view of the standard of care required to be supported by standard textbooks current at the time.

The report must also include a summary of the conclusions reached and a statement that the expert understands his duty to the court and has complied with that duty. The report must contain a statement of truth, the precise wording of which is set out in the practice direction. The expert must also 'state the substance of all material instructions, whether written or oral, on the basis of which the report was written'. Once the report has been disclosed, questions may be put to the expert in writing within 28 days but 'must be for the purpose only of clarification of the report'. Part 35 provides the court with the power to direct that evidence on a particular issue shall be given by one expert only. The 'single joint expert' may be appointed by agreement between the parties, but if the parties cannot agree, the Rules provide for the court to 'direct that the expert be selected in such a . . . manner as the court may direct'. The reality is that the courts will not, at least for the foreseeable future, impose single experts on main issues of liability in medical negligence cases. They will, however, expect the parties to agree on single joint experts in many peripheral issues, and it is not unusual now in a cerebral palsy case for a single jointly instructed expert in neuroradiology to be appointed by mutual consent. Many issues concerning quantum will be increasingly delegated to a single expert.

The practice direction has been supplemented by the publication by the Civil Justice Council of a Protocol for the Instruction of Experts to give evidence in the civil courts in June 2005.

Part 35 encourages discussion between experts of opposing parties, to identify the issues in the proceedings and, where possible, to reach an agreement on an issue. The Clinical Disputes Forum, a body set up in the wake of the Woolf Inquiry, has issued guidelines on experts' discussions in the context of clinical disputes (Guidelines 2000); most of the recommendations have been incorporated into the model direction of the Queens Bench Masters for the conduct of Experts' Discussions. A useful and authoritative guide to expert evidence has recently been published by the Expert Witness Institute (Blom-Cooper 2006).

ESTABLISHING LIABILITY

A disproportionately large percentage of the NHS liability for malpractice claims results from birth injury. When, in the early 1990s the Legal Aid regulations changed so that the infant plaintiff was assessed on his/her own financial position, there was a flood of old cerebral palsy claims released into the system. Old claims continue to surface, for there is effectively no time limit. Parents are increasingly inclined, in the present climate, to seek financial remedy for an imperfect child. There is an overall increase in cerebral palsy because of the increased survival of low-birthweight infants. All of these facts make it likely that cerebral palsy claims will continue to grow and, since the judgment in Wells v. Wells, will be increasingly expensive for defendants.

For liability to be established it is necessary for there to be demonstrated breach of duty and for it next to be shown that this breach of duty has had a causative effect. *It is not enough to show, for instance, that care in labor was substandard unless it can also be demonstrated that the injuries sustained by the child are, on the balance of probabilities, the direct result of that substandard care.*

BREACH OF DUTY

The principal errors of obstetric management associated with claims for cerebral palsy are set out in Table 28.1.

CAUSATION

The brain damaging pathologies that can occur following appropriate or inappropriate standards of care are prematurity, hypoxic–ischemic infarction, hemorrhage, cytokine induced change and trauma. The effects on the brain are usually to produce cerebral palsy but less frequently there can be evidence of hydrocephalus and generalized brain damage.

It is neither possible nor appropriate to consider these comprehensively: instead a number of the clinical scenarios that occur frequently in medico-legal practice and are illustrative of the issues that require to be addressed are considered.

PRETERM LABOR

Preterm delivery and low birthweight are major risk factors for cerebral palsy (Dite et al 1998). The usual brain damaging pathologies under these circumstances are periventricular leukomalacia (Ch. 21) and intraventricular hemorrhage (Ch. 20) that extends into the brain and these can occur in combination. Preterm babies who develop respiratory distress syndrome (RDS) are at particular risk because of the combination of hypoxemia and mixed acidosis that result from this condition (Dear 1999). There is little convincing evidence that labor can be delayed significantly by the use of tocolytic drugs (Thornton 1999). However, for some time, there has been some convincing evidence that the administration of glucocorticoids to the mother in preterm labor before 34 weeks has a beneficial effect in reducing the incidence and severity of respiratory distress syndrome. The initial work by Liggins and Howie (1972) was published in the early 1970s, but it was not until 1989 (Crowley 1989) that a meta-analysis, bringing together a number of large studies, provided convincing statistical evidence of the effectiveness of this treatment.

From the publication of that review, it could be supposed that it would be easy for a claimant to demonstrate breach of duty if glucocorticoids were not administered in appropriate circumstances after that date. Even after 1989, there were those who feared maternal complications, particularly in the

Table 28.1

ANTENATAL
Failure to detect or to take account of:
— fetal abnormality
— intra-uterine infection, e.g. rubella, toxoplasmosis, herpes
— maternal hypertension including pre-eclampsia
— maternal diabetes
— special investigations (including ultrasound scans)
— intra-uterine growth restriction
— twins
— abnormal and/or unstable presentations
— cephalopelvic disproportion
— placental abruption
— placenta praevia
— the need to monitor fetal wellbeing
— preterm labor

LABOR
Failure to detect or to take account of:
— the abuse of oxytocin
— malpresentation
— disproportion
— umbilical cord complications
— CTG abnormalities
— fetal scalp blood samples
— dysfunctional labor and the secondary arrest of labor
— the need to avoid difficult vaginal delivery especially in the presence of fetal distress
— trial of labor
— previous injury to the uterus (VBAC)
— trial of forceps
— use of the ventouse
— the conduct and timing of cesarean section
— the need to conduct delivery in an appropriate environment
— the need to have the necessary pediatric and anesthetic assistance available
— the management of shoulder dystocia

POSTNATAL
Failure to detect or to take account of:
— the need to reverse the effect of narcotic drugs given to the mother
— the need to have the necessary pediatric assistance available
— the need to intubate or otherwise effectively resuscitate and provide proper respiratory support for the baby
— the appropriate surroundings and expertise required and necessary for the further care of the baby

presence of hypertension or when tocolytic drugs were being employed. There is ample evidence of the reluctance of the clinicians to use steroids in preterm labor in the published results of the open study of infants at high risk of, or with, respiratory insufficiency – the role of the surfactant (OSIRIS

Collaborative Group 1992). Of the premature infants entered into the trial (all of them by definition at high risk of RDS), 15.5–23.3% had had antenatal steroids. In some cases, there may have been anecdotal reasons for the withholding of steroids but even allowing for that, it is difficult to show that even the majority of hospitals in the United Kingdom were employing antenatal corticosteroids in the pre-delivery management of babies at high risk of RDS.

In infants born prematurely brain damage may occur as a consequence of inappropriate standards of neonatal care; failure competently to resuscitate, hypocapnia in association with overventilation, avoidable hypoxic episodes and inappropriate treatment of infections have all been the subject of litigation.

Hypoxic–ischemic brain damage at term (Ch. 26)

This subject is well reviewed, from the medicolegal aspect, by Dear and Newell (2001). Among other points they make clear that some permanent neurodisability which is not always identifiable as cerebral palsy is the result of hypoxic–ischemic injury to the fetal brain during the course of labor and delivery.

CEREBRAL PALSY — THE INTERNATIONAL CONSENSUS STATEMENT

In October 1999 the British Medical Journal (McLelland 1999) published 'A template for defining a causal relationship between acute intrapartum events and cerebral palsy: International Consensus Statement'. There were 49 authors from seven countries; similar articles had previously appeared elsewhere. Only 6 representatives from the British Isles took part and only one UK organization is listed amongst the supporters of the Consensus Statement, The Royal College of Obstetricians and Gynaecologists (RCOG). Involvement of the Royal College was somewhat informal: the document was shown to a few senior members of the College with an interest in feto-maternal medicine (but none with any great medico-legal experience), but did not pass through council or through the joint standing committee of the RCOG and the Royal College of Paediatrics and Child Health (RCPCH). Of the four obstetricians from the British Isles, three are past or present members of council of one of the medical defense organizations. No UK pediatric neurologist took part, although several were invited and declined. The RCPCH is not on the list of supporting bodies. So much for consensus! The article set out to review the literature on the link between cerebral palsy and birth events but contained no new research. Its shortcomings, both in terms of science (Dear et al 2000) and law (Pickering 2000), were subsequently demonstrated elsewhere. The statement attempts to set standards for expert evidence but appears to have a poor understanding of the law, the standard of proof required by the courts or the proper conduct of expert witnesses. The consensus statement seems to have had little influence on litigation in the courts in the United Kingdom.

HYPOXIC–ISCHEMIC DAMAGE BEFORE LABOR

Whilst the cause of the majority of cerebral palsy remains unknown, the commonest allegations in malpractice litigation surround hypoxia. Whilst a prenatal origin for neurological fetal injury is thought to be common, litigation is relatively infrequent. It is difficult for the claimant to establish a causative breach of duty because the markers for this condition are somewhat imprecise.

PROLONGED PARTIAL HYPOXIA–ISCHEMIA

Most actions coming before the courts alleging hypoxic cause for cerebral palsy relate to intrapartum events. Spastic tetraplegia and dyskinetic cerebral palsy are the conditions most commonly associated with an asphyxial cause (Rosenbloom 1996) (see Ch. 26). Tetraplegic cerebral palsy, the consequence of prolonged partial hypoxic–ischemia, is the condition most likely to lead to a successful action by an infant claimant with cerebral palsy. Several hours of abnormal cardiotocograph trace (CTG) with no intervention by medical staff provide sufficient ammunition to establish both breach of duty and causation. But what if there is no CTG? Save only in 'high risk' labor there is at present no consensus amongst experts that CTG monitoring is mandatory. The notion persisted for several years, supported by the Dublin Study (McDonald et al 1985), that listening to the baby some of the time is as effective as listening all of the time! In the absence of a CTG, the claimant has not only the difficulty of establishing that the trace would have demonstrated abnormality had it been in place but also that the defendant had a duty of care to monitor electronically. The argument cannot of course be maintained when uterotropic drugs, whether prostaglandin or oxytocin, are part of management. The abuse of Syntocinon® causing excessive uterine activity and intermittent chronic hypoxia is one of the most disturbing and frequent causes of successful litigation in this field.

Failure on the part of midwives and junior doctors to recognize clear CTG abnormalities is another cause for concern. With the drastic reduction in junior doctors' working hours, resident staff is exposed to much less clinical experience than in previous years. If levels of competence are to be maintained, formal teaching programs have to be introduced to compensate for this lack of experience. The NHS Litigation Authority set up a Clinical Negligence Scheme (CNST), a pooling arrangement for the costs of litigation in 1995; over the past decade they have introduced standards for participating Trusts (every Trust in England is now included) and have published separate standards for maternity services, regularly updated (www.NHSLA.com).

The involvement of consultants in the labor ward is widely acknowledged as the most effective solution to this difficulty, but at present, only lip service is paid to the notion. It is now the requirement of most consultant contracts that one or two sessions per week are dedicated to labor ward duties. Unfortunately, as might be expected, the use made of these sessions varies widely. There are examples of good practice throughout the country but any real change is unlikely until the nettle is grasped and consultant presence guaranteed on site throughout the 24 hours in all major obstetric departments.

Another area of concern is the relationship between the junior doctor and the midwife. Where senior house officers are training as general practitioners, they seldom achieve levels of competence and experience that exceed those of an experienced midwife. Yet, in many labor wards, the midwife is required to call the senior house officer, no matter how junior, if she is concerned about a CTG or any other aspect of the management of her patient. This is a recipe for delay and indecision. The senior house officer on the labor ward should be regarded as supernumerary until he/she has demonstrated a level of competence and experience appropriate for decision making.

Prolonged partial hypoxia in labor leading to brain damage does not necessarily produce a severe degree of cardiorespiratory depression with low Apgar scores at the time of delivery as there is preferential maintenance of brain stem perfusion under these circumstances. Affected infants, nevertheless, demonstrate features of hypoxic–ischemic encephalopathy in the neonatal period.

The timing of injury during prolonged partial hypoxia would appear to be variable; this is discussed by Dear and Newell (2001) who suggest that in clinical and medico-legal practice brain damage is frequently seen after periods of prolonged partial hypoxia in labor that exceed one hour.

ACUTE AND PROFOUND/NEAR-TOTAL HYPOXIA–ISCHEMIA

Dyskinetic cerebral palsy is associated with brief periods of acute near-total hypoxia–ischemia (Ch. 26). It may occur as the end result of a chronic asphyxial process but is more commonly seen as a result of one of the disasters of labor such as cord compromise, placental abruption, rupture of the uterus, acute maternal hypotension or shoulder dystocia.

The claimant is more likely to succeed if it can be argued on his/her behalf that the disaster should never have been allowed to occur. In placental abruption, the claimant seeking to bring an action on the grounds of lack of expedition is usually in great difficulty, for the defendants will argue cogently that the damage was achieved within minutes of the major abruption occurring. Any subsequent culpable delay was irrelevant to causation. Famously, one plaintiff (Murphy v. Wirral Health Authority 1996) was able to persuade the judge that the mother should not have been in labor at the time the abruption occurred, and, given the competent management of desultory labor requiring augmentation, should have delivered much earlier.

When the cord prolapses without prior warning soon after admission to the delivery suite, successful litigation is unlikely, but on many occasions, the accident is not fore-seeable. The presence of variable decelerations on the CTG often provides warning of an impending cord disaster, whilst the footling breech allowed to labor is, the claimant will argue, to invite a cord accident.

Amongst the handful of cases that have come to trial in the last three years, two have concerned the conduct of (Purver v Winchester & Eastleigh Healthcare HNS Trust [2007] EWHC 34 (QB); LS Law Medical[2007] 4 193–211), or failure to, conduct a trial of forceps (Kingsberry v. Greater Manchester Strategic Health Authority [2005] EWHC 2253 (QB); (2005) 87 BMLR 73) with consequent delay in cesarean rescue. Others have settled in similar circumstances. Failure of operative vaginal delivery should not result in hypoxic injury if the attempt is made in the appropriate circumstances.

Acute asphyxial injury in the vaginal delivery of a second twin frequently gives rise to complaints. For many years, the courts have taken the view that both an experienced obstetrician (Bull and Another v. Devon Area Health Authority 1993) and a competent anesthetist (Kralj v. McGrath 1986) should be present for twin delivery.

Rupture of the uterus in the context of vaginal birth after cesarean section (VBAC) is a common cause for litigation, but few cases get as far as the courts. The majority are settled at an early stage, for, in truth, the accident can seldom be defensible. The textbooks (Dickinson 1999) would suggest that any woman with one previous cesarean section and no other adverse features is eligible for VBAC. In this regard, neither twins nor breech nor non-diabetic macrosomia count as adverse features. More than one previous cesarean section remains controversial, and the authors concede that patient preference may influence choice. Generally accepted contra-indications include previous classic cesarean section and the diabetic macrosomic fetus.

Within this context it may be that the textbooks do not give adequate prominence to the question of consent. Since all series of VBAC report an incidence of scar rupture, it is no longer acceptable to recommend this form of management to a woman without explanation of the risk of rupture and its possible consequences. Most textbooks accept that oxytocin can be used in the conduct of VBAC, but Dickinson warns that caution should be exercised. So often it is the abuse of Syntocinon® in such circumstances that leads to disaster.

Amniotic fluid embolism (AFE) as a cause of cerebral palsy is rare. In recent years, the definition has become somewhat fudged with the introduction of the concept of an 'anaphylactoid syndrome' rather than true embolus. AFE figures too frequently in the defense of cases of unanticipated maternal collapse, probably because of its acknowledged appalling prognosis, and seems to have become again the refuge of the diagnostically destitute.

Shoulder dystocia with resulting anoxic injury or peripheral nerve injury (p. 785) has increasingly become a subject of litigation. A number of cases have come before the courts with varying success but a much greater number have settled. The textbooks in the United Kingdom were not all clear on the optimum management before about 1994, and for babies delivered before that date successful cases are difficult to bring. There is a potential defense to brachial plexus injury depending on a poorly understood theory of maternal 'propulsive forces' (Clements 2006); since many of these injuries occur in the context of operative vaginal delivery (when maternal propulsive forces have self-evidently failed), the defense is particularly difficult to maintain.

Both the animal studies of Myers (1972) and clinical experience – and also judicial interpretation of these data (Purver v Winchester & Eastleigh Healthcare HNS Trust [2007]EWHC 34 (QB); LS Law Medical[2007] 4 193–211) – suggest that the otherwise healthy fetal brain at term can cope with in the order of 10 minutes of profound hypoxia before brain damage begins. Thereafter brain damage increases progressively over the course of the next 10–20 minutes ultimately leading either to profound and extensive disability or to death of the infant.

Intracranial hemorrhage (see Ch. 20)

Intracranial hemorrhage, causing neurologic injury, may be the result of operative vaginal delivery. The potential for injury occurs with all manipulation of the fetal head whether by the obstetric forceps and ventouse or during delivery of the aftercoming head of the breech, by whatever means (Drife 1998). In these days of diminishing skills amongst junior doctors, the ventouse has gained in popularity because it is perceived to require less operative dexterity and to

be capable of causing less harm to the fetus. Nevertheless, the instrument is capable of producing subgaleal bleeding, cephalhematoma and primary subarachnoid or subarachnoid hemorrhage (Ch. 20).

Rotational operative vaginal delivery, particularly in inexpert hands, has the potential for inflicting severe cerebral damage. Head level is critical in such deliveries and often poorly documented. Since 1983 (Cardozo et al 1983), the advice has been quite clear that Kjelland forceps should not be applied to any head that is more than one-fifth palpable by abdominal palpation.

RECURRING THEMES

Throughout obstetric malpractice litigation, certain themes recur:

- communication failure;
- delay;
- cascade of events.

The junior doctor makes an error in the context of a busy labor ward, often in the middle of the night, but the fault lies only partly with that individual; to a greater extent, the fault lies with his senior colleagues who made poor decisions (or often, no decisions at all) in the antenatal clinic, the antenatal ward, or earlier in the labor. It often lies in the delay of the midwives or senior house officer (SHO) in failing to seek help earlier. The proximal cause of the accident is easy to identify and to blame; the remote cause – the system failure which set it up – is the real target of risk management.

REFERENCES

Access to Justice: Final Report to the Lord Chancellor on the Civil Justice System of England and Wales 1996 HMSO, London.

Blom-Cooper L 2006 Experts in the Civil Courts. OUP, Oxford.

Bolam v. Friern Hospital Management Committee 1995 (1957) 1WLR 582; (1957) 2 All ER 118. Clin Risk 1:84.

Bolitho v. City and Hackney Health Authority 1998 AC 232 HL (1997) 4 All ER 771 (1997) 3WLR 1151.

Brennan T A, Leape L L, Laird N et al 1991 Incidence of adverse events and negligence in hospitalised patients: results of the Harvard Medical Practice Study 1. N Engl J Med 324:370–386.

Bull and Another v. Devon Area Health Authority 1993 4 Med LR.

Cardozo L D, Gibb D M F, Studd J W W et al 1983 Should we abandon Kjelland's forceps? BMJ 287:315–319.

Clements R C 2006 Obstetric brachial plexus injury. Clin Risk 12:3–11.

Craggs A, Hackett R 2006 Healthcare providers need to guard against a new surge of clinical negligence claims spawned by the Chester v. Afshar, the claimant-friendly ruling of the House of Lords in October 2004. Clin Risks 12:123–124.

Crowley P 1989 Promoting pulmonary maturity. In: Chalmers I, Enkin M, Mark J N C (eds) Effective care in pregnancy and childbirth. Oxford University Press, Oxford, Ch. 45.

Dear P R F 1999 The preterm infant. Clin Risk 5:7–13.

Dear P R F, Newell S J 2001 Cerebral palsy and intrapartum events. In: Clements R V (ed.) Risk management and litigation in obstetrics and gynaecology. RCOG and RSM, London, Ch. 14.

Dear P, Rennie J, Newell S, Rosenbloom L 2000 Response to proposal of a template for defining a causal relation between acute intrapartum events and cerebral palsy. Clin Risk 6:137–142.

Dickinson J E 1999 Previous caesarean section. In: James D K, Steer P J, Weiner C P et al (eds) High risk pregnancy management options, 2nd edn. W B Saunders, Philadelphia, PA, Ch. 67.

Dite G S, Bell R, Reddihough D S et al 1998 Ante-natal and peri-natal antecedents of moderate and severe spastic cerebral palsy. Austral N Z J Obstet Gynaecol 38:377–383.

Drife J 1998 Intracranial haemorrhage in the newborn: obstetric aspects. Clin Risk 4:71–74.

Grace J 1999 Should the foetus have rights in law? Medico-Legal J 67:57–67.

Guidelines 2000 Guidelines on experts' discussions in the context of clinical disputes. Clin Risk 6:149–152.

Gumbel E A 1999a The new civil procedure rules: a first impression. Clin Risk 5:86–89.

Gumbel E A 1999b Damages in obstetric negligence cases: Part IV – Calculation of damages following the House of Lords' decision in Wells v. Wells. Clin Risk 5:14–16.

Hunter v. Hanley 1954 SC200. Clin Risk 5:59, 60.

Kingsberry v. Greater Manchester Strategic Health Authority 2005 EWHC 2253 (QB); (2005) 87 BMLR 73.

Kralj v. McGrath 1986 1 All ER 54.

Leigh T H, James C E 1998 Medico-legal commentary: shoulder dystocia. Br J Obstet Gynaecol 105:815–817.

Liggins G C, Howie R N 1972 A controlled trial of antepartum glucocorticoid treatment for prevention of the respiratory distress syndrome in premature infants. Paediatrics 50:515–525.

McDonald D, Grant A, Sheridan-Pereira M et al 1985 The Dublin randomized controlled trial of intrapartum fetal heart rate monitoring. Am J Obstet Gynaecol 152:524–539.

McLelland A 1999 A template for defining a causal relation between acute intrapartum events and cerebral palsy: international consensus statement. BMJ 319:1054–1059.

Murphy v. Wirral Health Authority 1996 7 Med LR 99–107.

OSIRIS Collaborative Group 1992 Early versus delayed neonatal administration of synthetic surfactant — the judgement of OSIRIS: the OSIRIS Collaborative Group (Open study of infants at High Risk or with Respiratory Insufficiency — the role of surfactant). Lancet 340:1363–1369.

Pickering J 2000 Legal comment on the internal consensus statement on causation of cerebral palsy. Clin Risk 6:143–144.

Purver v. Winchester & Eastleigh Healthcare HNS Trust 2007 EWHC 34 (QB); LS Law Medical [2007] 4 193–211.

Re M B 1997 2FCR 541 AC. 38 BMLR 175–194.

Rosenbloom L 1996 Perinatal asphyxial injury: clinical sequelae. Clin Risk 2:43–46.

Shaw M 2005 Is Chester v. Afshar the new Donoghue v. Stephenson? Clin Risk 11:47–50.

St George's Healthcare NHS Trust v. S, R v. Collins, ex pS 1999 Fam 26 CA (1998) 3WLR 936. 44 BMLR 160–196.

Thornton J M 1999 Preterm labour: obstetric aspects. Clin Risk 5:1–6.

Thorpe L J 1999a Consent for Caesarean section: Part 1 — development of the Law. Clin Risk 5:173–176.

Thorpe L J 1999b Consent for Caesarean section: Part 2 — autonomy, capacity, best interest, reasonable force and procedural guidelines. Clin Risk 5:209–212.

Vincent C, Clements R V 1995 Clinical risk management — why do we need it? Clin Risk 1:1–4.

Vincent C, Clements R V 2006 Making healthcare safer: the continuing challenge. Clin Risk 12:85–86.

Watt J 1999 Bolitho v. City and Hackney Health Authority. Clin Risk 5:17–20.

Wells v. Wells, Thomas v. Brighton Health Authority & Page v. Sheerness Steel plc 1999 1AC 345 HL (1998) 3 WLR 329. 43 BMLR 99–142.

White Book 1999 Civil procedure: the civil procedure rules. A White Book Service. Sweet & Maxwell, London.

Wilson R M, Runciman W B, Gibberd R W et al 1995 The Quality in Australian Healthcare Study. Med J Austral 163:458–471.

CHAPTER 29

Malpractice issues in perinatal medicine: the United States perspective

Barry S. Schifrin, Marc R. Lebed and Jay McCauley

INTRODUCTION

It was probably inevitable that the law and medicine would come into conflict irrespective of the fact that despite some obviously different approaches, these learned professions share more than they conflict. While medicine is fundamentally deductive and law inductive, both fields are centered in advocacy for the client. When it comes to medicine, the law tries to reconcile a body of science with the art of clinical practice. When it comes to the law, medicine tries to reconcile a body of laws with notions of fault and accountability. The relationship is abetted when the goals of better, more efficient care and prompt and effective methods of dealing with error and adverse outcome are agreed upon. On the other hand, when their paths cross, and each profession deems the other side to hold some unscrupulous advantage, when the 'playing field is perceived to be not level,' and when myth and misdirection are rampant and malpractice premiums have become excessive or insurance coverage unavailable, then the worst of the relationship comes to the fore and political and legislative resources are recruited to help control the dialog and the invective and define or create new rules of engagement. In the end, care is compromised as are notions of justice and access to the law.

HISTORIC PERSPECTIVE OF MALPRACTICE IN THE UNITED STATES

Malpractice suits were unheard of until the 1840s. Prior to that there were few quality controls over the medical practitioners or its numerous schools of practice. Malpractice suits became an issue after that time when allopathic physicians, to eliminate other 'schools of medicine,' created objective, national standards of practice and national medical societies and supported litigation to adjudicate allegations of negligence under tort law rather than contract law. Those medical factors that have sustained the movement include the innovative pressures on American medicine, the spread of uniform standards, and the advent of the 'deep pockets' of medical malpractice liability insurance. Three legal factors, contingent fees, citizen juries, and the nature of tort pleading in the United States, have also contributed to the present malpractice climate (Mohr 2000).

At the beginning of the 1960s more educated, informed and assertive patients began to question their physicians in the same manner that they evaluated their other goods and services. In general, this was poorly accepted by physicians, who for the most part maintained a traditional authoritarian stance in the care of their patients. The legislative crises of the 1970s, and the subsequent 'crises' of the 1980s, 1990s and 2000s brought with them tort reform, health maintenance organizations (HMOs), increasing regulation, decreasing autonomy, strained relations between physicians, hospital administrations and allied health care providers, and decreased physician and patient satisfaction.

MALPRACTICE LAW

Malpractice law is part of tort, or personal injury, law that affects large segments of society, including product liability, automobile accidents, airplane crashes and other examples of unintended harm. The objectives of malpractice litigation are straight forward: (1) to resolve disputes fairly with equal opportunity for 'justice' on both sides, (2) to compensate persons injured through negligence and (3) to prevent unsafe practices – i.e. raise the standard of care – all without resorting to armaments or fisticuffs. A plaintiff prevails in a lawsuit by proving the four Ds: that the defendant (1) owed a Duty of care to the plaintiff, (2) that there was a Deviation from an acceptable standard of care and (3) that there was a non-trivial injury to the plaintiff (Damages) that was (4) Directly caused by the deviation from the standard of care. A failure to demonstrate any one of the four means that the requirements, under the law, are not met. To begin the process, a patient approaches a lawyer. The reasons patients sue are many.

For patients and family members, the physical and emotional devastation of medical error cannot be easily overcome. As a rule, however, this circumstance has been made even more difficult because there has been no satisfactory explanation to the patient of the reason for the adverse outcome, no admission of negligence, no opportunity for questions and no consolation for loss. In reality, the patients want a forthright explanation of what happened, and want to understand if they had played a role in it. And if, just if, a mistake had been made, they expect an apology and an offer to compensate for the expense and aggravation. Patients undertaking a lawsuit are real people and whether the injury was the result of negligence or not, they, not the physicians burdened with a lawsuit, are the real victims. When asked, 'What was wrong with the care you or your child received?' or 'What complaints do you have about physicians?' patients respond rather specifically (Table 29.1). (See also Beckman et al 1994.)

The attorney is often the last person who is contacted, not the first. Most often patients are directed to an attorney by a member of the medical community. Indeed, many are amazed, when looking at medical malpractice cases, by the cold-blooded attitude so many defendants have taken toward patients who have been seriously, and sometimes grotesquely, harmed. Inhumanity and indifference to the suffering of others is in itself another form of injury.

When patients file suit, they are often made to feel as though they had done something wrong, as if seeking legal redress and compensation was in some sense an affront to the system, a personal assault on the physician. Many plaintiffs feel pressured by all the parties involved to agree to a settlement. In some instances, such advice may come from the plaintiff attorney or even the sitting judge. Indeed, on occasion extraordinary amounts of offered settlement are turned down, not because of the size of the award, but because all the details of their case would then come out publicly – they would have their day in court.

Physicians believe themselves to be operating in an environment of zero tolerance for error. It is embedded in their oath and dedication to 'do no harm,' in their professed desires to help others, and magnified by a historic paternalistic tendency to extend unrealistic expectations to their patients. The physician who has erred is wounded, and suffers the consequences of guilt, fear of reprisal (from the patient, hospital, regulatory agencies), embarrassment (peer) and sorrow for having harmed someone. Because medicine, for centuries, has been loath to identify negligent care (even in closed, protected settings), this system of justice has enfranchised the plaintiff's attorney, not especially trained for the purpose, to determine the medical and the legal merits of the case (they are not the same!). Under the contingency-fee relationship prevalent in the United States, the attorney takes a percentage of the award as a fee (often around 35%) to compensate for the costs, expenses and time absorbed in pursuing the case irrespective of the outcome; they take nothing if the defendant prevails. These expenses are not trivial; bringing a 'damaged child' case to court, for example, may easily cost $100 000 of up front expenses. It is not undertaken lightly.

But before the attorney can proceed, one of his first expenses will involve consultation with a medical expert (a physician) to determine whether the potential case satisfies the two most critical criteria of the four Ds: was there a Deviation from a reasonable standard of care and was there a Direct causal relationship between that failure and the adverse outcome? Damages and Duty, generally, are self-evident. Traditionally, the 'standard of care' is defined as the quality of care (customs and behavior) that would be expected of a reasonable practitioner in similar circumstances. These standards are drawn from members of the profession itself as well as documents that reflect a consensus on appropriate standards (plural) of care.

It should be emphasized that there is no single standard of care. Satisfying the need to do something reasonable under the circumstances, indeed, may permit mutually exclusive choices to be within the standard of care. Because the law holds the arcane nature of medicine, 'a learned profession,' to be beyond the grasp of common citizens, it requires the testimony of experts in the same field as the defendant. Neither the courts nor the legislatures can reasonably establish detailed conduct for professional practice without 'practicing medicine'.

Ideally, medical witnesses will be readily available and forthright and medical standards will be determinable from readily available medical records that are well documented, readable and responsive to questions of whether or not the medical conduct met a reasonable standard of care. The medical consultant/potential expert witness will possess both current knowledge and experience with the issues at hand, but, at any time in the review process, is honor bound to use all available relevant information and to apply broadly understood, minimal, standards of care – not their own personal standards. An expert witness must elaborate the standard for medical care at the time of the plaintiff's injury and give an opinion on whether the defendant's conduct met this standard. The standard is not unique to the expert, but rather must reflect general principles applicable to all practitioners, but at the same time, specific to the individual patient's circumstances. Ideally, it should be supported by scholarly literature. While it need not prescribe a single

Table 29.1 Why patients sue (Hickson et al)		
CITED DEFICIENCIES OF CARE		
Recognizing fetal distress		53%
Managing fetal distress		57%
Timely cesarean section		35%
Physician unavailable		29%
Birth injury (forceps)		28%
Consultation or transfer		10%
WHAT PROMPTED THE LAWSUIT?		
Person outside family		33%
Medical personnel	23/41	(56%)
Lawyer	8/41	(20%)
Money for long-term care		24%
Physician deception		24%
Child would have no future		20%
Find out what happened		20%
Prevent malpractice/revenge		19%
COMPLAINTS ABOUT PHYSICIANS		
Not informed about injury potential		70%
Misled patient		48%
Would not talk or answer questions		32%
Would not listen		13%

course of action, it must either (for the plaintiff) proscribe the defendant's conduct or (for the defense) endorse the defendant's conduct as an acceptable alternative. Therein lies the conflict (Meadow 2005, Meadow & Lantos 1996).

While the courts expect that medicine, as a learned, science-based discipline, will have articulated standards for practice in most circumstances, they also recognize that not all standards are formalized or even well defined, not all clinical circumstances can be circumscribed in some obvious standard of care, and there is 'art' to the practice of medicine. To overcome these hurdles the courts, using their own legal (not medical) standards of witness acceptability, allow appropriately qualified expert witnesses to express expert opinions. Indeed, the expert witness is the only party in the lawsuit who may express opinions; everyone else is only entitled to the 'facts' of the case. Ideally, the expert will not be an advocate, except perhaps of his own opinion, and will honestly present his or her understanding of the applicable standards without tailoring his responses to serve the single-minded ends of the lawyer engaging the expert.

Obtaining expert testimony has always been the most difficult part of medical malpractice litigation. Historically, experts were readily available to testify against competing medical disciplines, including homeopathic physicians and chiropractors, although they were expected to remain silent about the misconduct of members of their own profession (omerta). To abolish these vituperative, economic rivalries, the courts established the doctrines of 'school of practice' and 'locality rule' as the bases for qualifying expert witnesses.

The school of practice rule permits the differentiation of physicians into self-designated specialties depending on whether the case concerns procedures and expertise that are intrinsic to the specialty or general medical knowledge and techniques that are common to all physicians. Thus, obstetrical cases may involve family practitioners, midwives, obstetrician-gynecologists, as well as members in training; the potentially significant differences in their individual standards may indeed require expert witnesses from each of these specialties.

Before the standardization of medical training and certification that prevails today, there was a tremendous gulf between the skills and abilities of university-trained physicians and the graduates of 'less reputable' schools issuing diplomas. Thus, in many parts of the country, a physician's ability to serve as an expert would be determined by comparison with the other physicians in the community, or at least in similar neighboring communities. For obvious reasons, this rule essentially precluded injured patients from finding supportive expert testimony, effectively preventing most medical malpractice litigation. Reasonably, there is no longer a justification for any rule that impedes evaluation of what have become national standards of care on the sole basis that it is the norm for a given community. While most states have explicitly abolished the locality rule, it is being reinvigorated in some states as a tort reform measure (and

omerta) to deal with the problems of access to care and facilities in rural areas.

A national standard of care implies that the rural and urban physicians will have the same training and exercise the same level of judgment and diligence. The rule does not require that the rural physician have the same medical facilities, consultants, or other resources available. If the community does not have facilities for an emergency cesarean section, for example, the physician cannot be found negligent for failing to do this surgery within the 15 minutes that might be the standard in a well-equipped urban hospital. The physician, however, to comply with the standard of care, must inform the patient of the limitations of the available facilities and recommend prompt transfer if indicated. He must also make reasonable efforts to deal with the inevitability of requiring an emergency section – even in a rural community. Proper informed consent allows patients to balance the convenience of local care against the risks of inadequate facilities.

At trial, judges and jurors (the triers of fact) have no alternative but to judge the testimony of witnesses whether expert or percipient (fact) on the personal credibility of the witness. For the experts and the defendants, positive factors such as academic degrees, specialty board certification and publications enhance credibility. So do such factors as physical appearance, race, gender, command of English and personality. Previous participation in legal activities is also fair subject matter for the expert. At least in Federal Court the expert's legal activities over the last 5 years must be listed with the court prior to his appearance. For the expert witness, the foremost requirements are effective presentation and teaching ability. The expert must educate the judge and jury on the technical matters at hand. Irrespective of these considerations, the objective is to be believed.

The defendant also has to be believed but his/her role is much more focused; he/she has but one chore: to convince anyone who will listen (judge, juror, attorney, stenographer, bailiff, passerby) that he/she is a thoughtful, caring, concerned human being who did what was professionally reasonable under the circumstances. The defendant has no other job. Performing research, providing expert opinion, or combating the opinions of the opposing expert are all, we believe, someone else's function. As mentioned above, the defendant's demeanor in deposition or trial (as well as with patients) has a great deal to do both with the likelihood of lawsuit and its resolution.

Until 1993, federal courts had used the 'general acceptance' test, set forth in Frye v. United States, to assess the admissibility of expert scientific testimony. In 1993, the United States Supreme Court modified the standard for determining the admissibility of expert scientific testimony in federal trials. In Daubert, the court stated that the Frye test did not comport with the Federal Rules of Evidence and that a rigid 'general acceptance' requirement would be at odds with the 'liberal thrust' of the Federal Rules and their 'general approach to relaxing the traditional barriers to opinion testimony'. Accordingly, the court emphasized that a trial judge must screen the proposed scientific testimony to ensure that the testimony is relevant and reliable before allowing it to be presented at trial. If scientific, technical or other specialized knowledge will assist the trier of fact to understand the evidence or to determine a fact in issue, a witness qualified as an expert by knowledge, skill, experience, training or education may testify thereto in the form of an opinion or otherwise. It is a judicial decision, not a medical one.

The court set forth four factors that may be used to assist the trial judge in determining 'whether the expert is proposing to testify to scientific knowledge that will assist the trier of fact to understand or determine a fact in issue'. The factors that may be considered when determining the validity of a scientific theory or technique are: (1) whether the theory or technique can be tested, (2) whether the theory has been subject to peer review and publication, (3) the rate of error and (4) the acceptance of the theory or technique within the community. The court cautioned that '[t]he focus must be solely on principles and methodology, not on the conclusions that they generate'. The court emphasized that these factors are not exclusive. Thus, under Daubert, a defendant doctor may be considered negligent for treatment and diagnosis even though he presents evidence from a number of medical experts genuinely of the opinion that the defendant's care followed customary medical practice. The court must determine for itself the appropriateness and the logic of the professional opinion and find reassurance that the body of opinion relied upon was not created for defensive purposes (see below).

It is a curiosity that an expert's position may fail a Daubert challenge in one case but may continue to be offered in other cases! It seems counterintuitive that a lay judge is qualified to be asked to determine the qualifications and credibility of an expert. Some believe that the selection of medical experts should be the purview of medically trained peers. Indeed, there is an argument to be made that the specialty societies develop a list of 'true' experts that are available to either side or the judge himself.

Federal rules also give a judge the authority to (1) limit cumulative evidence, i.e. more than one expert testifying to the same issues unrelated to qualifications, (2) retain experts to assist the court or (3) with mutual consent appoint a single expert witness. Despite these available options, especially in 'damaged child' cases, there is an increasing tendency to line up a broad array of qualified experts on both sides, including an obstetrician, perinatologist, placental pathologist, neonatologist, neurologist, nurse, economist, neuroradiologist, etc. There is at least some evidence that this proliferation of experts (and costs), more likely driven by the defense, is counterproductive. Bors-Koefoed et al found that the use of multiple defense expert witnesses decreased the chances of a successful defense.

Many jurisdictions have attempted to insinuate the expert witness into the proceedings prior to the case being filed. In several states a report or affidavit of merit from the expert is required to launch the suit, in others only the testimony by the lawyer that he has contacted an expert is required. By and large there is no standard format for expert reports. While they are often quite minimal and non-specific there is an increasing trend to make them more substantive and even to limit in some states the allegations to those specifically identified in the report. There is also no requirement that the 'expert' who gave an affirmative opinion to the attorney, whether he signed the letter of merit or not, will subsequently be involved in the case, a deplorable circumstance as will be discussed below. Even if he/she were later involved, there are no mechanisms short of deposition or interrogatory to amplify on the experts' allegations. In some states, the expert cannot be deposed before trial and indeed his identity is unknown to the opposing side until he is called to the stand – widely referred to as 'trial by ambush'.

While the expert's opinion is normally protected by the doctrine of witness immunity, this does not protect the witness from fraud or from professional malpractice liability or from other forms of harassment. 'The goal to insuring that the path to truth is unobstructed and the judicial process is protected, by fostering an atmosphere where the expert witness will be forthright and candid in stating his or her opinion, is not advanced by immunizing the expert witness from . . . negligence in forming the opinion.' In one instance, a consulting expert was sued for failing to testify on behalf of the plaintiff in trial. The expert believed that causation could not be satisfactorily proven.

Increasingly, expert testimony has come under the scrutiny of the medical societies, especially ACOG which has been quick to associate expert testimony surrounding CTG with the high prevalence of allegations of obstetrical malpractice in brain-injured baby cases: 'Testimony regarding the cause of CP is a particular problem because it is commonly based on erroneous assumptions and obsolete science' (Scott 2005). Further, '(ACOG) members not registered to give opinions or who give rogue opinions not supported by the college should receive a warning, with loss of college membership if they are found guilty again'. In CP litigation, any expert asserting that a CP outcome was preventable, e.g. by earlier delivery, should have to produce evidence of good medical quality that the advocated policy has reduced rates of CP. To date, such evidence exists for very few available interventions (Hankins et al 2006, MacLennan et al 2005). These assaults have probably increased the reluctance of potential experts to participate on the plaintiff side. Nevertheless, censure or other administrative sanction is generally excluded from trial deliberation.

Because its value has been disparaged in various articles and editorials, the CTG has become a focus of legal attention. Its highly credentialed critics have emphasized the amount of inter- and intra-observer error and that it offers *no* benefit in terms of prevention of neurological injury or perinatal mortality (Alfirevic et al 2006, Hankins et al

2006, MacLennan & Robinson 2004, MacLennan 2001, MacLennan et al 2005). These statements, in turn flow from notions that, 'in most cases of CP the cause cannot be determined' and that 'few cases of fetal neurological injury occur during labor'. Given the above, it is commonplace in obstetrical malpractice cases to encounter questions about the validity of the interpretation of CTG patterns and their relationship to the management and the outcome. It was also inevitable that in a medico-legal case the defense attorneys, assisted by the testimony of board-certified obstetricians, would request a 'Frye hearing' in an attempt to exclude the CTG tracing from the trial, because, as the defense claimed, the evidence shows that CTG is 'junk science' and that the interpretation of patterns is 'unscientific'. The motion was denied and tracing and its interpretation were permitted.

It is perhaps instructive here to deal with the terms 'meritorious' and 'frivolous' as applied to malpractice cases. In brief, whether the case is meritorious or not is a function not of the result, but of whether there is a substantive question about the standard of care and its relationship to the outcome. In a frivolous case, there is no substantive question, the four Ds cannot be shown or linked, or any question of negligence is readily answered in the negative simply with the most cursory examination of the evidence.

Critics of the medical malpractice system charge that frivolous litigation is common and costly. In a study of 1452 closed malpractice claims from five liability insurers only 3 percent of the claims had no verifiable medical injuries. Most of the claims that were not associated with errors (370 of 515 (72 percent)) or injuries (31 of 37 (84 percent)) did not result in compensation; most that involved injuries due to error did (653 of 889 (73 percent)). Payment of claims not involving errors occurred less frequently than did the converse form of inaccuracy — non-payment of claims associated with errors. When claims not involving errors were compensated, payments were significantly lower on average than were payments for claims involving errors (313 205 dollars vs. 521 560 dollars, $P = 0.004$). Overall, claims not involving errors accounted for 13 to 16 percent of the system's total monetary costs. For every dollar spent on compensation, 54 cents went to administrative expenses (including those involving lawyers, experts and courts). Claims involving errors accounted for 78 percent of total administrative costs. *Conclusions*: Claims that lack evidence of error are not uncommon, but most are denied compensation. The vast majority of expenditures go toward litigation over errors and payment of them. The overhead costs of malpractice litigation are exorbitant (Studdert et al 2006).

Often, the complaints that prompt the visit to the attorney derive from actual or perceived slights by the physician related to a poor 'bedside manner', a disputed bill, a lack of timely response, etc. In this respect, it is important to understand how, given the unrequited emotional needs associated with adverse outcomes, malpractice litigation serves the purpose of emotional vindication. Such complaints are usually dismissed out of hand by the attorney in the first

interview with the patient or secondarily on the basis of the review by the consulting expert (Studdert et al 2006). It is not widely appreciated but the vast majority of patients who approach lawyers with complaints about their physicians are turned down (probably greater than 90%). Some patients are actually grateful to know that they did not receive substandard care and, equally important, that they themselves did not contribute to the adverse outcome. Despite any anger or frustration they may have with the conduct or deportment of the physician they often harbor notions of their own complicity in an adverse outcome, especially when there has been a brain-damaged baby. If they had only not skipped an appointment, not used the hot tub, not gained so much weight, etc. Being turned down in a request to sue a physician may have positive benefits of closure. It may indeed help them to forgive themselves. While it is quite uncommon to pursue a lawsuit based solely on an emotional misdemeanor by the physician, it becomes a powerful incentive to bring a lawsuit if the care has also been negligent. As will be seen in the statistics below, many negligent physicians are exculpated or avoid lawsuits entirely, not because of the facts of the case, but by a becoming demeanor to the patient or to the jury. Other physicians have been found negligent, not because of their care, but by their indifference toward the patient. It is this author's experience that the minute the jury perceives that the physician does not care vindication of his medical conduct is not possible.

Thus, to label as 'frivolous,' as many physicians have, all cases that plaintiffs lose, or are settled 'for economic reasons' or are dismissed, trivializes the tort system, the lawyers, the patients, the opposing expert witness and, in its way, impedes the solution of the malpractice problem and foments more error. This posture reveals an inadequate understanding of the dynamics of expert allegations, settlements, jury verdicts and even the process of peer review.

Given the affirmative report by his expert, the attorney is legally obligated to pursue discovery — the accession of all the relevant clinical data from the medical records or other sources. To flesh out the records and to understand something of the personality of the defendants, depositions are taken of the relevant treating or factual witness — sometimes including the custodian of records, etc. — and the various medical experts.

The defense against the allegation of failing to meet the standard of care of a malpractice case centers around issues of customary practice, clinical practice guidelines, informed consent and differentiating error from complication. In judging the conduct of the physician in a court of law, the court is guided by a notion called 'reasonable conduct'. Indeed, it is sufficiently vague as to require the participation of an expert witness to state what is and what is not 'reasonable conduct'. At least theoretically, the creation of clinical practice guidelines would simplify and implement broadly understood practices subscribing to a quality of care that could be objectively measured. At the same time, the quality of care would be improved and iatrogenic injury diminished.

There has been a broad implementation of 'clinical practice guidelines' from various hospitals, professional organizations and the government itself. A clinical practice guideline is any guide to the clinical management of a patient. These guidelines vary widely according to the purpose for which they are written and who has been selected to write them. They may be driven by medico-legal issues, by the cost of care or by the quality of care. While great emphasis has now been placed on the process of writing guidelines, many providers have become concerned with the basic precepts of guidelines, including the possible emergence of 'cookbook' medicine, the effect of patient variability, and the need to keep guidelines flexible, current and credible.

Clearly, one impetus for the creation of clinical practice guidelines for specific medical conditions and their treatment was the notion that they would help avoid or defend malpractice claims. Indeed, some day they might replace the 'reasonable conduct' standards and their dependence on expert testimony in medical cases and thereby discourage both defensive medical practices and spurious claims – after all, it is the medical profession and not the juries that establish the standard of care; the jury just attempts to find out what were the standards that the medical profession had set for itself in any given situation and then to determine whether those guidelines were appropriately and reasonably followed. There are several problems with the use of 'guidelines'. First, they may not be usable (admissible in evidence) at all. Because of the wide range of reasons for creating guidelines (care, costs, medico-legal protection) in many states, such guidelines constitute 'hearsay' in great measure because their author is not in court to be cross-examined. Finally, having followed the guidelines may not mean malpractice was not committed. Scrupulous adherence to the relevant guidelines for an amputation, for example, avails nothing if the wrong leg has been amputated. Thus it is that the notion that compliance with guidelines renders the clinician immune from lawsuit has not been upheld. Consensus, after all, is not necessarily wisdom, or applicable in all cases! As suggested above, the practice guidelines surrounding CTG and fetal neurological injury have created incompatible definitions and drawn fire as being dedicated to the defense of the physician rather than improving care. When the opinions of the opposing experts conflict irreconcilably over this issue, the jury comes face-to-face with the logical conundrum. Is the disagreement related to lack of awareness of the standards or is one of the experts lying? The jury assesses the credentials and the credibility and various other sources of information, to help them decide which expert is more credible in relating the individual patient's care to the prevailing standards.

One of the most widely quoted and misunderstood guidelines requires that institutions be capable of instituting an emergency cesarean section within 30 minutes of decision. Some institutions cannot meet these guidelines reliably while others maintain a standard that can result in an emer-

gency cesarean section in 10 minutes or less. While several studies have attempted to determine the reasonableness of 'the 30 min rule,' neither the studies nor the guidelines take into account certain realities or certain remedies (Althaus et al 2005, Chauhan et al 2003, Lavery et al 1999). The 30-minutes rule is shorthand designation for a more encompassing principle that, under certain conditions, performance of a cesarean section should be carried out as quickly as possible consistent with concern for the health and well-being of the mother and fetus, preferably within 30 minutes. But what is the standard if there is already one cesarean section in progress, or two? Under these circumstances, a delay becomes 'reasonable under the circumstances,' notwithstanding the fact that the standard of care required an earlier cesarean section. However, if a physician is late in realizing the need for cesarean section or is ready to operate within 20 minutes but fritters away 10 minutes beforehand, his conduct cannot possibly comport with a reasonable standard of care, even if the patient is delivered within 30 minutes. Further, it stands to reason that institutions normally unable to consistently meet the 30-minutes rule must modify their practices and exhibit a willingness to prepare for cesarean section early (even if it proves unnecessary) in anticipation of problems and make special arrangements for unique situations such as vaginal birth after cesarean (VBAC). Thus, the failure to meet the 30-minutes rule is rarely by itself a telling plaintiff's allegation. Much more frequently, the plaintiff's allegation is that the failure to properly interpret the fetal monitoring tracing or to properly estimate the feasibility of safe vaginal delivery hopelessly delayed the decision in the first place, irrespective of the 'decision to incision' interval.

There is frequent debate over whether 'official' pronouncements such as the 30-minutes rule are to be construed as monolithic 'standards of care'. More reasonably, it seems, that irrespective of whether these writings are entitled practice parameters, guidelines, standards, apocrypha, hints, clues, etc., the imprimatur of an official body gives any statement about care the force of a 'standard'. Indeed, during litigation, both sides are apt to offer these professional publications as standards to support their case irrespective of the disclaimer that these recommendations are guidelines rather than standards of care. Thus, guidelines, whatever their provenance, are never 'medico-legally binding' and can be directly and reasonably contravened by a thoughtful, alternative choice of care – that is annotated!

INFORMED CONSENT

Similarly, the patient has rights, no matter how appropriately they may be exercised, to influence decisions about her care. In dealing with matters of informed consent, most courts in the United States look to what a reasonable patient would want to know, not what a 'reasonable physician' would have said. The courts have on several occasions been asked to intervene in circumstances involving the refusal of treatment by a pregnant woman, refusal that nominally threatens the life and wellbeing of her fetus and herself. While the courts' responses have been varied, there is general consensus among the specialties that these ethical (not legal) issues should not be resolved in court and that considerable ethical weight should be given to the mother's decision as long as the consent has been proper and there has been no coercion. Lawsuits based entirely on informed consent are quite uncommon, but most such cases in obstetrics seem to involve VBAC, the use of operative delivery and the decision to induce labor with a previous history of shoulder dystocia. If the consent document signed by the potential VBAC patient, for example, is to truly represent that her consent is truly 'informed,' it must reveal the patient's understanding that she may either undergo an elective repeat cesarean section or, if she is a suitable candidate, attempt a VBAC. She must understand that not all patients are candidates for VBAC and that not all VBAC attempts will result in successful vaginal delivery. She must be aware that some of the determinable clinical factors that affect the success of VBAC become apparent only in labor. The patient must also understand that all pregnancies carry a small risk to both mother and fetus, whether or not the mother has had a previous cesarean section. In patients with a previous cesarean section, the risk of uterine rupture during a VBAC is approximately 1% and this occasionally may result in serious, potentially life-threatening complications for the mother or the baby.

In a search over the past 10 years of over 2100 articles for four major categories of neonatal morbidity and mortality Hankins et al (2006) found that elective cesarean significantly reduced the risk of permanent brachial plexus injury, of significant fetal injury and of neonatal encephalopathy and stillbirth. The prevalence of moderate to severe neonatal encephalopathy was estimated to be reduced by 83%, a statistic that seemingly indicts for the events of labor and delivery in the genesis of neonatal encephalopathy and contradicts the notions that intrapartum care has no preventative value. In maintaining respect for the patient's autonomy and decision-making capabilities the authors advocate informing the pregnant woman of the risk of each of the above categories when considering route of delivery. The fetal outcome in the present pregnancy, however, is not the only consideration. The patient must also receive counseling regarding the potential risks of a cesarean section for the current and especially for any subsequent pregnancies where the risks increase in direct relationship to the number of previous cesarean deliveries (Zimmerman 2004).

If the patient initially agrees to attempt VBAC, she needs to understand that she is entitled to an updating of the likelihood of success and to change her mind at any reasonable time and to obtain a cesarean section even during labor. Finally, the patient should understand that no decision, however thoughtfully made, or however reasonably pursued, guarantees a normal outcome for the mother or the infant.

The reader may now compare this approach with the deliberations in an informed consent case that was decided by the Wisconsin Supreme Court and that stretched the limits to which some physicians would go to reduce their cesarean delivery rate. In this case a patient presented with a history of two previous cesarean sections, the first undertaken for arrest of labor after 17 hours (the second was elective); she had agreed prior to labor to attempt VBAC. During labor, in the face of slow progress and severe abdominal pain, she changed her mind and repeatedly requested a cesarean section. Just as often the obstetrician maintained that it was unnecessary. The obstetrician commented, '. . . if I performed cesarean section on every woman who wanted one then all deliveries would be by cesarean section'. Intimidated, the patient no longer requested cesarean section. Ultimately, the uterus ruptured and the child was hopelessly injured despite delivery within 30 minutes. The physician defended his conduct on the ground that the original informed consent should prevail throughout the labor and that the standard of care had been met by the 'timely' delivery within 30 minutes. He noted that the patient had reaffirmed upon admission her earlier willingness to undergo a trial of labor and he maintained that labor continued 'without objection'.

The court (inviting the implication that the patient had been coerced) rejected the defense position that the patient's resignation implied acceptance of a continued trial of labor. The court did not comment on the change in the medical situation (dysfunctional labor, unexplained abdominal pain) that required medical reconsideration of the case and updating of the informed consent. The court did, however, conclude that the legal situation had changed:

Where two or more medically acceptable options for treatment are present, the competent patient has the absolute right to select from among those treatment options after being informed of the relative risks and benefits of each approach. But consent, once given, is not categorically immutable and the patient was entitled to withdraw her consent to VBAC. That indisputable withdrawal placed the patient and her physician in their original position – a blank slate on which the parties must again diagram their plan which in this case would have resulted in cesarean section. It was foreseeable that as a backlash to the alarm generated by this verdict along with other reports and settlements, many hospitals no longer permit VBAC deliveries and an increasing number of malpractice insurers are limiting their indemnification of physicians performing VBAC deliveries!

COMPLICATION OR ERROR?

The 'recognized risk defense' asserts that the undesirable outcome or injury in question is nothing more than an unavoidable complication – an understandable and acceptable risk of a properly considered and provided treatment. Accordingly, so long as the patient is reasonably apprised of the more serious and the commonplace risks and participates in the decision, in theory there can be no issue of negligence. A typical example is subgaleal or intracranial hemorrhage in the newborn following vacuum-assisted delivery. Indeed, every obstetrical text devotes significant space to such complications but only rarely do they include a full discussion about preventability or even the distinction between complication and negligence. Is intracranial/subgaleal hemorrhage following vacuum extraction, for example, an unavoidable risk or, in some instances, the result of negligence and how would that be determined? Similarly, is brachial plexus injury after shoulder dystocia a foreseeable event related to excessive lateral traction on the fetal neck, anticipated by multiple risk factors, or is it a totally unpredictable, unpreventable injury always unrelated to the care of the physician during delivery? In the courtroom, the plaintiff's attorney will use the statistics on complications as follows. A 'recognized complication' does not preclude that the complication was caused by negligence. Indeed, none, all or only some of these complications may represent negligence. For example, if 2% of all drivers run red lights, running red lights is a known complication of driving, but it is also a case of negligence. The most likely situation is that some of the injury is potentially avoidable. Thus, that a given adverse outcome is a known complication of a procedure tells an attorney nothing. The attorney wants to know why the complication occurs and, more importantly, why it occurred in this particular case.

PURSUING THE CASE

If the case is pursued, it may be settled by an agreement of the parties or may go to trial. While the physician believes himself disadvantaged in this system of finding fault, in reality the law gives health care providers considerable advantage. They are advantaged by the presumption of non-negligence. They do not have to be right in their care, just reasonable. The law denies the jury the right to decide medical issues and even requires expert witnesses from the profession itself. After an agreement to settle the case or after an adjudication that finds the defendant negligent, his insurance company bears the costs of both economic losses (lost earnings and medical bills) and non-economic losses, so-called 'pain and suffering'. The system is maintained in balance by the provision of insurance for both hospitals and physicians based on a pooling of risk, historically through separate lines of insurance. This minimizes the risk of bankruptcy by a single large payout and because resources are available to compensate patients. The cost of insurance coverage for hospitals is typically linked to the history of claims from year to year, an arrangement known as 'experience rating'. Physicians, on the other hand, unless their experience is extreme, are generally not risk rated, a potentially contrived actuarial practice.

In practice, this theoretically balanced system falls short of its objectives, as illustrated in the 'ire and angst' of contemporary malpractice litigation. This chapter, written at the end of 2006, will therefore attempt to review some of the competing, nay dueling, agendas that are being brought to bear in the medical, legal and political arenas. The enterprise redounds with myth and divisive and often contradictory data – sometimes of dubious provenance. The dust of the latest in these, increasingly disagreeable, epochal skirmishes for the malpractice 'high road' has not yet settled and is unlikely to be settled to everyone's satisfaction in the near future. In the authors' view, this situation prevails because each side, for its particular reasons, is unwilling to make the tort system work as it was designed to. Indeed some of the issues raised are ethical in nature, beyond the purview of the courts and the legislature.

MALPRACTICE MYTHOLOGY — THE FAILURE OF MEDICO-LEGAL EDUCATION

An enduring feature of the malpractice upheaval in the United States (and almost nowhere else) is the ignorance of malpractice doctrine in the medical community and beyond. Not only is there widespread fear of being sued, but there is also a great misperception about the requirements for proof of malpractice, the outcomes of lawsuits, the reasons patients sue and the influence of the insurance industry on the problem. There is also little appetite to deal with a major litogen (a factor promoting lawsuit) – physician behavior (Woods 2004).

Some current mythology: 'Malpractice relates to the incompetence of a few bad physicians'; 'Anyone can sue, everyone wins'; 'Every case resulting in CP will come to lawsuit'; 'The system is unfair and favors the plaintiff'; 'Patients who sue are greedy, ingrates'; 'Judges and juries cannot understand medicine'; 'Losing a lawsuit raises premiums and besmirches the physician's name in the community'; 'The plaintiff's attorney and the expert are the enemy, along with the judge, jury, insurance company'; 'Malpractice doesn't make care better'; 'The majority of suits in medicine are frivolous whether they are settled, dropped, go to jury trial, or lose'; 'We're living in a time when people have a higher expectation from physicians – that until proven otherwise, it's the doctor's fault'; 'The system is overrun with runaway juries and jackpot justice, with sinister lawyers and opportunistic plaintiffs preying on virtuous corporations, hospitals, and doctors in search of that big payout from the lawsuit lottery'. 'Medical malpractice lawsuits are a greater threat to public good than is medical malpractice itself' (Baker 2005). There is almost a universal belief that the injured child's appearance in the courtroom elicits sufficient sympathy from the jury for the plaintiff to win the case. As a result of lawsuits, patients cannot find doctors who are leaving the practice of medicine. Fear of lawsuits and high premiums are wasting huge amounts of money on defensive medicine and depriving Americans of access to health care.

There is broad publicity of these myths. Indeed, President Bush has asked Congress to cap damage awards for victims of medical malpractice on the assumption that capping awards will reduce those 'frivolous lawsuits' responsible for increasing doctors' insurance premiums and driving them out of business. Bush also has said that high malpractice rates drive up the cost of health care (Baker 2005).

Research in this area is so clearly to the contrary that the more interesting question is why it has so little traction (Baker 2005). There is abundant data to show that the frequency of medical malpractice is far greater than the number of lawsuits alleging malpractice, but it is not growing and the awards of lawsuits are tracking inflation. In fact, there is no explosion of lawsuits and runaway verdicts to blame for insurance crisis (Baker 2005). It is not widely understood that investment cycles influence both profitability and premiums. Indeed, there is a 'boom and bust cycle' in the insurance industry to blame for profits (Baker 2005). There are also poor underwriting practices that are not amenable to tort reform. While physicians need to be protected from the vicissitudes of the cycles, they need to improve their care.

The amount of money spent because of 'defensive medicine,' one of the main reasons why health care is believed to be so expensive, is not easily quantified. It seems far more productive to focus on wasteful procedures and poor-quality care unrelated to lawsuits (Baker 2005). Baker makes a plea not for more lawsuits as the Harvard study suggested; rather he attempts to deal with the failure of the medical profession, and others, to find any rehabilitative value in them. The suits, he believes, do some good. They are the reason we know more about the extent of medical malpractice than we would have had they been suppressed. It has been claimed they keep physicians honest and in some general way, may improve patient safety and outcome, but this will remain an elusive statistic. The system has provided compensation for some and they promote traditional values of fairness and access to legal resources (Baker 2005).

It seems that we are unlikely to eliminate error. Perhaps the biggest failure of malpractice lawsuits is not the error, but the failure to learn from error. We have more doctors than ever before and regional disparities have existed for some time. Limiting high risk procedures may be a beneficial effect – at least for some high-risk practitioners. If, in fact there were a need for more obstetricians, insurance reforms could easily solve it.

Physicians, after all, win about 80% of lawsuits that do go to court. It is naïve to believe that these were the cases in which the plaintiff's attorney forgot to bring the affected child into the courtroom. More reasonably, it is the thoughtful, compassionate physician, who manifests his sympathy and compassion, who most easily obtains the jury's favor and a favorable verdict.

The defendant is often unaware of the statistics that about 40% of cases are dropped and about 50% settle, sometimes as befitting the merits of the case and sometimes as a calculated strategy that limits exposure of assets. The physician who is terrified by an ad damnum clause (demand for damages) that greatly exceeds his insurance policy limits is

rarely in our experience reassured by his own attorney that the risk to his/her assets is essentially nil. The authors are unaware of any malpractice suit involving an obstetrician who was covered by a reasonable policy and who, despite a verdict that exceeded the policy limits, had to pay any money out of his own pocket. Despite counseling, the frightened obstetrician does 'not want to be the first one'. To some extent the defense attorney may be excused for failing to understand how impoverished the physician's medico-legal education is. As one American physician put it:

I fought in the battle of the bulge in World War II. We were trained, we were fighting a good cause and we were armed. I felt safer then than I do in a malpractice suit.

Education and reliable data are the antidotes to disabling myth. Medical and legal organizations have long recognized the importance of legal medicine and have repeatedly recommended its study by physicians in training – with minimal success. In 1952, the American Medical Association (AMA) advised that 'No medical student should be permitted to receive his medical degree without instruction in legal duties'. Four decades later, less than 50% of medical schools had medico-legal courses, considering the subject too unimportant to teach. Even fewer schools have any formal instruction on communication and dispute management skills. Many medical schools feel that the intense curriculum leaves no room for such instruction, and that the ability to communicate and deal with conflict is part of the student selection process, which is to be refined following their didactic medical school training, during their apprentice/mentor training of internship and residency.

Kollas, in 1997, studied the medico-legal knowledge base of senior residents in internal medicine. Only 28% felt they had been adequately trained in the subject. Only 26% could list the requirements for proof of malpractice, i.e. the four Ds.

A national survey of physicians in 1999 revealed that 58% had faced malpractice charges and that more than 20% had been sued at least three times. Almost 70% expected to be sued during their career. Despite the fact that physicians win the vast majority of cases that go to court, more than 75% of physicians polled felt that lay juries were not capable of deciding malpractice cases! While ready to admit that everyone makes mistakes and that they had made mistakes in other cases, virtually all physicians believe that the cases filed against them had no merit. Something (read tort reform) must be done, physicians cry, to stem the tide, to eliminate the reign of terror by the plaintiff's attorneys. Plaintiff's attorneys and some consumer groups also want to stem the tide as they see it – the tide of medical error, the tide of unsympathetic, unapologetic and ill-informed physicians.

When all of these myths are wiped away, the most devastating myth or fiction about malpractice, the one that resides deepest beneath the surface, is that the allegation of malpractice represents the allegation of incompetence, or misanthropy or malice. In fact, it simply represents an allegation of fallibility – being human and being capable of error. Imagine the response of the physician who believes that he or she is being accused of malice – the intention to do harm. The allegation of malice is precluded by the precepts of tort law and is rendered improper by the Hippocratic Oath by which the physician swears to 'First, do no harm' and, by implication, to 'intend no harm,' i.e. malice. Judges and jurors understand that the physician, like the speeding driver, did not intend harm. But the physician's good intentions are not the test of reasonable performance and the profession will be unlikely to regulate itself without fundamental understanding that the legal rules of evidence in negligence cases, including malpractice, exclude the accusation of the intent to harm. When misunderstanding about the law is combined with an appreciable incidence of medical error and a high resistance among physicians to report errors, then it seems that the 'culture of secrecy' derives in part from a 'culture of fear'. Thus, despite the attention to the subject of medical error and the formation of organizations devoted to patient safety, there has been little demonstrable evidence of a reduction in medical error. The solution will involve changes not only in the conduct of care but also in the educational, ethical and emotional components associated with medical errors.

We will attempt, in passing, to deal with these notions, but perhaps the following experiences will assist the reader to focus on the issue of patients' expectations of a perfect outcome. The senior author delivered his first baby as a medical student about 1963. After the delivery, the first words out of the mother's mouth were, 'Is my baby alright?' He would deliver his last baby about 40 years later and the first question this mother asked was exactly the same as the question asked by the mother 40 years earlier. In the intervening 40 years, the ultrasounds, computers and monitors of every description have allowed us to visualize the fetus, characterize its genetic composition, and determine its behavior, its growth and its tolerance to hypoxia. As a result, there has been a dramatic reduction in the risk of fetal anomaly or death, especially during labor. Labor rooms have become intensive care suites with remote surveillance capabilities. Indeed, it has never in history been safer to deliver a baby, or perversely, to be sued for negligent care. Everyone, patients and physicians included, understands that there are no guarantees with pregnancy and under the best of circumstances, considering the stakes, not all outcomes are perfect. As with all medical care, there is always an element of uncertainty – about care and about outcome. Are lawsuits generated by those patients who fail to understand this principle or by physicians who, confronted with a bad outcome, fail to educate their patients or respond compassionately?

With regard to the notion that the presentation of the handicapped child in the courtroom dooms the defense case because of sympathy for the child, the author has witnessed the following situation in the courtroom in the case of a neurologically handicapped infant. After their deliberations, the jury returned to the courtroom to announce their verdict before the judge and the various parties. When the judge asked for the decision of the jury, the foreman arose and asked the judge if he could first make a preliminary statement on behalf of each of the jury. With tears in his eyes, the foreman acknowledged that over the course of the trial the members of the jury felt that they had come to know and care for the parents and the afflicted child. He further stated that he wanted to extend from each member of the jury both their best wishes for the future and their considerable concern about the future support of the child. They did not find the physician negligent.

In medicine today there is considerable enthusiasm for 'evidence-based medicine,' epidemiologically driven decisions and structured reimbursement. There seems much less appetite for 'evidence-based law'. The initiatives derived from evidence-based medicine seem driven as much by motives of cost control as by the hope for better health care services. Similarly, the avoidance of error, such as the use of automated medication ordering and dispensing, and the efforts of risk management (safeguarding assets) while contributory may not directly enhance the quality of care. The extraordinary response to the Institute of Medicine study has led to a nationwide movement to find ways to reduce error and increase patient safety. The foundation of these efforts is based on increasing the ease and confidentiality of error reporting, as well as the facilitation of root cause analysis systems, team approach techniques, improved communication and dispute management techniques, all with the goal of improving patient care.

In this way, the avoidance of error and the efforts of risk management (safeguarding assets) have become as important as, if not more important than, ensuring the quality of care. The breadth of malpractice mythology and the detestation and fear of the malpractice system by the physicians and organized medicine have distracted our attention from the public's concern about the ineffectual efforts to improve outcome whether by the failure to adopt higher standards, failure to improve educational processes, or make meaningful the activities of peer review committees and professional societies.

PEER REVIEW

In 1973, the US Congress enacted legislation requiring physicians to initiate Peer Review Organizations to monitor the utilization and the quality of hospital and physician services in the federally funded Medicare program. Now more than 30 years later we must acknowledge the lack of a gold standard, medical or legal, for reviewing allegations of negligence and dealing meaningfully with medical error. Peer reviews produce inconsistent agreement and operate without formal rules or guidelines for review. They are left to the local hospital, and although the American College of Obstetricians and Gynecologists (ACOG) has attempted to provide outside review to individual hospitals, there is no analysis of such efforts. The majority of 'true' peer review exercises are driven by adverse outcomes and do not represent systemic reviews of the numerous latent processes promoting adverse outcome. These are left to the occasional review of a 'sentinel event'. With peer review the rules for reviewing records and for obtaining agreement about either the severity of any departure or the impact on the offending physician are inconstantly applied and haphazardly administered. Peer review requires the presence of the physician — an overt acknowledgment of the fact that medical records are often silent about important questions whose understanding is necessary to determine the standard of care. Despite the physician's presence, the deliberations of the peer review committee are not backed up by systemic reviews of the physician's conduct in similar cases. While matters of apology appear to be changing, the system was not designed to promote either patient education or an apology (Finkelstein et al 1997, Gallagher et al 2003, Woods 2004, Zimmerman 2004).

Peer review in obstetrics is especially problematic. The medical records of the infant may not be present, and there may not be anyone (neonatologists/pediatrician) present to discuss the infant's course and the impact of the obstetrical care on that course. The patient, moreover, is rarely, if ever, questioned about her perceptions of the care! Invariably, there is no long-term follow-up, especially if the infant is transferred to another hospital. The initiatives of the profession in confounding the timing of injury and the interpretation of CTG tracings almost certainly has an inhibiting influence on peer review and expert testimony. Imagine, therefore, a discussion at a Peer Review Meeting of the medical conduct in a case of shoulder dystocia and brachial plexus injury. The medical record is silent about the use of fundal pressure — as it should be: fundal pressure should not be used to relieve shoulder dystocia. As a result, the physician who had carefully documented a normal sequence of maneuvers was exonerated. During the malpractice case, however, incontrovertible evidence was produced that the 263 lb anesthesiologist was exerting sufficient force on top of the patient's abdomen to produce considerable pain and broad ecchymoses. The case was settled on behalf of the plaintiff!

Other complaints of lack of due process, poor reproducibility, and motivation by non-medical/non-scientific considerations plague discussions of the peer review process whether involving the practicing physician by a hospital department, the review of a manuscript submitted for publication, the funding of grants submitted for research, or the evaluation of expert testimony by professional societies (Judson, Cohen, Pegalis, American College of Physicians).

Peer reviews are conducted by people from the same department of the hospital and in many states are safeguarded from legal scrutiny under the common law privilege of self-critical analysis, a privilege that protects and encourages quality assessment, but that secrecy, in the final analysis, may be counterproductive for the ultimate objective of improved patient care and better transparency of medicines self-governance. At its most collegial, colleagues of the physician being reviewed are likely to minimize error on the notion that when their turn comes, similar cordiality and extenuation will prevail. After all, the objective of the process of review is not to find fault or apportion blame, but to improve outcomes for the future. The greatest failure of error is the failure to learn from it.

Gawande in an article in The New Yorker describes a surgical peer review exercise and the limitations of this process. He admits that he had made a serious medical error, but he was not obligated to face the peer review committee directly and the committee did not deal directly with the error itself in any remedial way. Under the heading of 'the banality of injury,' Gawande acknowledges that medial error is ubiquitous and makes the point that medical error is not the province of a select few culprits as common wisdom suggests. He avers, 'There are no "incompetent, unethical, negligent few," no basket of "bad apples" that conspire to taint all of medicine'.

Sometimes, however, peer review meetings may not be cordial and the meeting may become the venue for limitation of privileges or dismissal. Here, the purpose is not educational or remedial but political or economic, described under such appellations as 'economic credentialing' or 'sham peer review'. At these times, generally, hostility may prevail, the physician will have a lawyer present, and the battle will be joined. It is the law, not medicine that must safeguard due process in these cases. If it can be shown that the peer review process was being used for purposes other than those related to medical care, the deliberations of the committee may no longer be protected. In either circumstance, it is an expensive, unsatisfying experience for which physicians have little appetite — whatever the outcome.

There is evidence that the knowledge of an adverse outcome (hindsight bias) may cause the peer review committee, like the expert in a malpractice case, to criticize retrospectively the decisions of the treating doctor. While it might be better to withhold outcome information in both circumstances, it seems neither practical nor enforceable. There would seem to be no plausible basis for the ACOG Practice Bulletin that CTG patterns 'should not be subsequently reinterpreted,' an approach to communications, peer review, quality improvement and allegations of negligence that seems unique among medical specialties (ACOG 2005).

While a 1988 study of anesthetic mishaps from a national database found strong agreement among anesthesiologist reviewers, a later study about agreement among anesthesiologists assessing 12 actual malpractice cases whose verdict was known has implications both for malpractice and peer review. Here, the intraobserver agreement among observers was high (>80%). Of the eight cases with complete or virtually complete agreement between respondent anesthesiologists, three (37.5%) disagreed with the verdict rendered by the actual juries. In addition, anesthesiologists showed significant disagreement (>30%) among themselves in four of the case scenarios, indicating there may not be agreement regarding the standard of care in these clinical circumstances. Finally, anesthesiologists predicted jury verdicts poorly, with success rates of 50% or less in 7 of the 12 case scenarios. It should be pointed out that these reviews are usually parochial matters for only rarely does the peer review evaluation benefit from information obtained from the patient or in the hospital review, from bona fide experts in the field. These potential sources of enlightenment are available in the courtroom.

While there are correlations between the risk of lawsuit and such features of character as medical school prestige, physician intuition, gender, and even the apparently perverse inverse relationship between current medical knowledge and the likelihood of being sued, the fact is that most obstetricians are sued at least once in their professional life. Repeat offenders may sometimes occur, but are not a common problem. As Gawande poignantly asks, 'How do we keep good physicians from harming patients?' He and others invite the inference that it is not the peer review process that can accomplish this, in part because of the dynamics mentioned above, but also because the contributing causes to adverse events are often not detected by current medical review processes. We may also ask, what is the value of either peer review or even malpractice suits in improving care?

A study (generally known as the Harvard study) commissioned by New York State in 1986, and released in 1990, showed that although actual malpractice is relatively rare, it is nevertheless underreported. If anything, the study group believed that there were too few lawsuits. Further, they wrote:

> Physicians tended to equate a finding of negligence with a judgment of incompetence. Thus, although willing to admit that 'all doctors make mistakes,' physicians were often unwilling to label substandard care as negligent and were opposed to compensation for iatrogenic injury. Given medicine's delayed response to the problem of medical error, including the limitations of peer review, the public's only alternative therefore was for individual patients to try to hold individual practitioners, one at a time, to whatever medical standards could be upheld by lawyers and expert witnesses. It may be true that to address the problem of iatrogenic injuries seriously, we must reform the system of malpractice litigation.

What seems equally true is that the problems of iatrogenic injury and physician conduct cannot be contingent on changing the tort system alone.

THE ROLE OF THE PHYSICIAN

These complaints about the system also serve to camouflage the physician's role in the genesis of malpractice suits. 'It

has been estimated that, the risk of lawsuit "seems not to be predicted by patient characteristics, illness complexity, or even physicians" technical skills.' Instead, risk appears related to patients' dissatisfaction with their physicians' ability to establish rapport, develop trust, provide access, administer care and treatment consistent with reasonable expectations, deal effectively with conflict and communicate effectively. In an article by Hickson et al, patients who saw physicians with the highest number of lawsuits were more likely to complain that their physicians 'would not listen or return telephone calls,' were 'rude' and 'did not show respect'. Such complaints, furthermore, were similar to those documented in interviews with families who sued their physicians. Patients are less likely to sue (about 50% less) even for moderate and severe mistakes if the physician informs them of the mistake (basically, apologizes).

For the reasons mentioned above, physicians are untrained in the art of apology. It may seem counterintuitive for many physicians that one can accept responsibility for an outcome without admitting blameworthiness. In an analysis of 500 claims in obstetrics and gynecology, Lynch et al showed that 46% were misguided allegations and about half were due to incompetent care, an error of judgment, lack of expertise, poor supervision or inadequate staffing. The other half were due to poor communication and 'misguided allegations,' for which they recommend an alternative course of dispute resolution combined with improved communication. Parenthetically, the more time the physician spends with a patient the greater is the satisfaction of both patient and physician. In a survey reported by the ACOG, physicians reported wholesale changes in their practices (Table 29.2) and their fees as a result of malpractice suits – including greater consultation with the patient.

In 1997, a highly publicised article recommended that when doctors make a mistake that harms a patient, they should tell the patient what happened, apologize and do whatever it takes to repair the damage. Basic professional ethics aver that patients have a right to know what happened to them. It seems like the right thing to do as part of the physician's responsibility to his patient and it may be

Table 29.2 Malpractice-induced activities (from ACOG 1990)	
Modality	Percentage
Testing	76.2
Monitoring	73.3
Documenting	72.2
Informed consent	61.6
Consulting MDs	58.0
Patient information	51.2
Referrals	47.2
Staff presence	21.8

therapeutic for the physician who may feel guilt and distress. Telling the truth may also strengthen the patient's faith in the doctor while a cover-up that fails, as many do, may anger the patient and make him/her more inclined to sue. Cover-ups also antagonize juries. Medicine is a human enterprise and error (i.e. fallibility) is part of being human. 'We are programmed for error.'

Understandably, the notion of admitting error has drawn skeptical review from the medical community, the insurance companies and the defense bar. They fear that admitting mistakes will 'open the floodgates' to lawsuits and hurt their reputations and careers. They fear also that without tort reform to decrease the number of malpractice suits and large settlements, and to reduce the punitive implications of existing reporting, few doctors could risk owning up to errors. The notion that telling the truth, apologizing and reaching out to a family in grief can defuse some of the anger and polarization that characterize a typical lawsuit becomes hostage to the notion that every word you utter in consolation or contrition is an admission that can be used against you in a court of law. On top of that, defense lawyers then order doctors to say nothing until all the facts are in, and then to say nothing. It seems obvious to state that until legislative protections maintaining such admissions are enacted, it is very likely that lawyers will continue to order doctors to say nothing until all the facts have been ascertained through discovery, and then to say nothing. But is this a medico-legal problem, or is it an ethical problem? Baldwin suggests that increased levels of moral reasoning may diminish the risk of malpractice suit, making legislative protection unnecessary.

The Joint Commission on Hospital Accreditation (JCAHO) standards require the disclosure of sentinel events and other unanticipated outcomes of care to patients and to their family members when appropriate. Hospital administrators, fearing medical liability suits, are reluctant to comply with this standard. If disclosure is taken a step further to the offer of an apology, hospitals and physicians are even more likely to gravitate to traditional 'defend and deny' behaviors. Apology as it turns out is yet one more control that physicians exert over the risk of lawsuit. Thus, a prompt explanation of what is understood about what happened and its probable effects; assurance that an analysis will take place to understand what went wrong; follow-up based on the analysis to make it unlikely that such an event will happen again; and an apology will likely reduce the risk of lawsuit and heal, rather than harm, the physician–patient relationship. In fact, a growing number of hospitals, doctors and insurers have come to accept that genuine disclosure and apology may reduce error-related payouts and the frequency of litigation. Further, a growing number of states are passing ('I'm sorry') laws that protect an apology from being used against a doctor in court. Despite the ethical imperatives underlying such disclosure, it seems likely that more such fundamental protections will be needed before these practices become commonplace.

COMMON AREAS OF LITIGATION DURING LABOR (see Simpson & Knox 2003)

General problems relating to litigation in medicine include:

- Documentation, communication, institution of a chain of command or internal systems conflicts; when there are unresolved disagreements between physicians, nurses or midwives, or other health care providers arise. Of most concern are the attitudinal problems involving the interaction of nurses and physicians, which receive too little emphasis and are particularly difficult to change. Their potential serious impact on the ability of an obstetrical unit to provide 'high-reliability care' has been discussed at length by Simpson and Knox (2003).
- Discharge or transfer of a woman in active labor without proper medical evaluation or with an unstable medical complication of pregnancy or based on her inability to pay (also known as 'dumping'); according to Federal Law (EMTALA) medical personnel have obligations to provide an adequate medical screening exam (MSE) and stabilization treatment within the capabilities of the hospital to every patient with an emergency medical condition (EMC); and either transfer/ discharge the patient within guidelines. Transfers must be affected through qualified personnel. The transferring hospital, not the receiving hospital, has the responsibility to determine the mode, equipment and attendants for transfer.

Of the many specific types of cases, only some will be briefly discussed here: (1) the failure to properly interpret fetal monitoring tracings, (2) the poor conduct of operative vaginal delivery, (3) the management of the large infant and shoulder dystocia resulting in either brain damage with death or subsequent CP, or (4) the infant with brachial plexus injury (sometimes both).

Along with the measures taken by physicians in response to the threat of malpractice (Table 29.2), the profession, especially obstetrics, has embarked upon a series of defensive 'scientific' initiatives to modify its vocabulary and its accountability. Defensive medicine is a practice designed not for the purpose of answering clinical questions or directing therapy, but for the purpose of preventing lawsuits or counteracting plaintiff testimony in court. The ACOG, for example, has recommended the elimination of such universally applied terms of art as 'fetal distress,' 'perinatal asphyxia' and 'stat cesarean section' and have modified the definitions of 'low-' and 'midforceps'. Further articles have created definitive, unyielding requirements for the diagnosis of birth-related injury and suggest that labor related injury is rare and perhaps irreducible.

Irrespective of motivation, these publications have not been accompanied by any decrease in lawsuits, any improvement in outcome or any less defensive posture on the part of the obstetrical community. These efforts to make our specialty 'fair of speech' and litigation-proof discount important mechanisms of injury, diminish notions of medical judgment, inhibit scientific inquiry into the timing and mechanism of fetal injury, and delay the testing of new paradigms for dealing with adverse outcome. These articles attempt to influence the defense in these cases in several ways. An inexperienced lawyer may turn down a meritorious case because, as the guideline states, 'It is not possible to ascertain retrospectively whether earlier obstetric intervention could have prevented injury or cerebral damage in any individual case where no detectable sentinel hypoxic event occurred,' or because the umbilical artery pH was >7.0 despite obvious injury during labor or delivery. In addition, by insisting that extreme derangements in pH values are required to begin to make the correlation between labor events and subsequent neonatal injury, these criteria modify the level of proof normally required in malpractice suits. The burden of proof in these suits requires that the level of confidence in the relationship between the events and the outcome be more probable than not. It is well to compare these pronouncements with a widely respected authority of neonatal brain injury.

> Brain injury in the intrapartum [period] does occur, [it] effects a large absolute number of infants worldwide and represents a large source of potentially preventable neurological morbidity. Among the many adverse consequences of the explosion in obstetrical litigation has been a tendency in the medical profession to deny the importance or even existence of intrapartum brain injury (Volpe 1995).

These issues have also been discussed at some length for the brain-damaged infant and for brachial plexus injury.

Excessive doses of oxytocin or prostaglandins during induction or augmentation of labor resulting in excessive uterine activity with fetal distress or uterine rupture are very common allegations in malpracticed suits. A clear definition of excessive uterine activity is essential along with protocols to deal with it promptly when it occurs. While hyperstimulation of uterine activity can be the result of endogenous maternal oxytocin and prostaglandins, most hyperstimulation is the result of administration of oxytocin or prostaglandins. To avoid the recognized liability inherent in using the term hyperstimulation, many defendants, their attorneys and experts are quick to reserve the term hyperstimulation for excessive contractions that result in a non-reassuring CTG pattern (Simpson & Knox 2003). From the perspective of maternal–fetal safety, the only reasonable approach is to avoid prolonged periods of excessive uterine activity – irrespective of its designation or the response of the fetus.

Failure to appreciate deteriorating fetal status as a result of coached pushing efforts during the second stage of labor. In some cases, it is the maternal heart rate and not the fetal heart rate that is being monitored (Murray 2004, Schifrin et al 2001). In the presence of repetitive decelerations prolonged maternal breath holding (greater than 6–8 seconds)

or more than 3 pushing efforts per contraction during pushing should be avoided: pushing is stopped temporarily, pushing with every other contraction or every third contraction. It is crucial that normal baseline rate and variability should be identifiable between contractions. In the presence of an epidural, coached pushing does not significantly decrease the length of the second stage.

FETAL CARDIOTOCOGRAPHY (CTG)

In part, because of the pivotal role it plays in malpractice cases, there have been attacks on fetal monitoring that have come both from within the profession and from without. In an article in the Stanford University Law Review, Margaret Lent, a defense lawyer, argues that the widespread use of electronic fetal monitoring (CTG) is both medically and legally unsound. Ms Lent points to selected clinical trials to demonstrate that CTG does not reduce fetal mortality, morbidity or CP rates. She argues that because CTG has a very high false-positive rate and its usage correlates strongly with a rise in cesarean section rates it offers no medical advantage over auscultation. and provides no protection in the courtroom. She further argues that auscultation, at least as safe and effective as CTG, is also more likely to protect physicians from liability. Ms Lent concludes that obstetricians have an obligation to their patients and to themselves to adopt auscultation as the new standard of care. She finds 'no excuses left to defend the continued use of CTG'. The medical literature can be used to justify any position on monitoring, including those of Ms Lent (Alfirevic et al 2006, Graham et al 1997).

While failure on the part of the health care provider to recognize clear fetal heart rate abnormalities is frequently alleged in malpractice cases, to isolate the CTG tracing under these circumstances frequently oversteps its permissive role in obstetrical care. A normal CTG pattern permits ongoing labor only as long as safe vaginal delivery is a reasonable option. If the pattern turns abnormal (rising baseline, decreasing variability along with variable/late decelerations), especially in the second stage, then the questions are several. Can the pattern be ameliorated (by reducing the oxytocin, moderating the pushing efforts)? If the pattern cannot be ameliorated what is the feasibility of safe vaginal delivery given the estimated fetal weight, previous obstetrical history, position, presentation of the fetal head and progress in labor to this point? Experience suggests that the vast majority of cases hinge far more on the reasonableness of the conduct of obstetrical care (especially the second stage) than on the interpretation of the fetal monitor. Regardless, reviewers of malpractice cases consistently find that the CTG tracing has been frequently misinterpreted in allegations of negligence.

THE LEGAL CLIMATE

Most changes in both the medical and the legal professions are evolutionary and it is often difficult to define any sea change. The last three decades, however, have witnessed a number of remarkable and epochal changes in the medico-legal climate in the United States, with doubtless more to come. Many of the changes derive from periodic surges in malpractice premiums, reduced availability of insurance coverage and the exodus of major insurers from the market first in the early 1970s, again in the mid1980s, a lesser event in the 1990s and more recently in the new millennium. In each epoch, affected providers clamored for policy changes to inhibit litigation. In the 1970s, legislatures established joint underwriting associations to serve as insurers of last resort, special state patient compensation funds were introduced to absolve commercial insurers of responsibility for specified dollar portions of malpractice payments and public reinsurance mechanisms were established to fill gaps in the underwriting market. By the late 1970s, the malpractice crisis had abated – only to recur less than a decade later. In Washington State between 1984 and 1986, for example, malpractice premiums for obstetrics jumped approximately 100%. As a consequence, obstetricians marched on legislatures or joined many family physicians and midwives in an exodus from obstetric practice. Those remaining in practice became more reluctant to care for high-risk obstetric patients and less willing to accept indigent patients and reduced fees, irrespective of the fact that indigent patients, in fact, appear less likely to sue. In many rural areas across the United States obstetric care became virtually unobtainable. Periodically, these circumstances galvanized legislative activity in virtually every state and led to further far-reaching reforms of existing tort and insurance law with some stabilization of premiums – at least initially. After almost a decade of essentially flat premiums, premiums are rising exponentially, which is said to be due to the increasing size of awards and insurers leaving the medical malpractice business because of diminishing returns on investment. This has been aggravated by rising health care costs ($1.6 trillion in 2002 and increasing yearly) and efforts to control physician income. The average annual increase in health care costs from 2000 to 2004 was 12–16% with predictions that, whether or not the result of negligent care, they will rise by a further 8% in 2005, with likely little containment beyond that.

It is important to emphasize that premium levels are responsive to a variety of factors besides litigation dynamics, including previous losses, past and expected investment returns, business strategies and the degree of state regulation of rate changes. A January 2004 study found that nationwide, average premiums for all physicians between 2000 and 2002 rose by 15% – a rate of rise almost twice as fast as per capita total health care spending. Certain specialties had even greater increases, including obstetricians/gynecologists (22%) and internists and general surgeons (33%). Neurosurgeons, obstetricians, orthopedists and emergency room physicians are particularly likely to have premium rate increases. The rates for obstetricians/gynecologists vary nationally, but according to ACOG, between 2002 and 2003 about half of obstetricians/gynecologists were experiencing increases of 10–49% in their insurance premiums.

Premiums may influence physicians' decisions to join and leave the labor force, their choice of a medical specialty and their decision of where to locate, creating the potential for undeserved patient populations in certain specialties or geographic areas. Rising malpractice premiums may also encourage physicians to practice 'defensive medicine,' performing more tests and procedures than necessary in order to reduce exposure to lawsuits. Parenthetically, however, defensive medicine (ordering a test not for the purpose of furthering patient care, but for the legal protection of the physician) is indefensible in court. Imagine the physician-defendant responding to a question about the indication for a certain test with the answer: 'I didn't want to get sued'. Both rising malpractice premiums and defensive medicine practices may contribute to the rising health care costs and thus to an increase in health insurance premiums.

The choices for the obstetricians – short of some windfall protection scheme – are leave practice, move to a 'more compliant' state, give up obstetrics, obtain employment where malpractice insurance is provided, raise fees, discontinue seeing patients with restrictive payment structures or go bare, i.e. do not obtain any malpractice insurance. For many, there is no good option and their future will hinge on the least inimical choice. Beyond physicians, these rapidly rising medical malpractice premiums have again become an issue of increasing concern about the health care system for policy makers and the general public.

UNDERWRITER DATA CLAIMS PAYMENTS

The insurance industry also has its problems. In 2003, insurers were paying out in claims and expenses $1.38 for every medical malpractice premium dollar collected. (National Underwriter Data Services). Results have deteriorated steadily from 1998, when the rate of return was −7.6. Medical malpractice insurers' return on net worth was −7.4% in 2002, down from −4.7% in 2001. Results in 2002 were the worst in the following states: Arkansas, Nevada, Montana, Mississippi, Illinois and Missouri, with a return on net worth ranging from −33.7% in Arkansas −24.4% in Missouri. In reality, even in the good years, premiums rarely cover payouts. The system works in part because premiums are invested and with at least a modest return permit the insurance company to make a profit. This is abetted by the fact that malpractice suits, especially, take a long time to resolve – about 4 years on average.

The average claim payment rose almost 8% per annum from $95 000 in 1986 to $320 000 in 2002 despite the fact that the frequency of claims per 100 doctors has remained more or less constant. Only about 30% of claims result in insurance payouts, but expenses for cases, especially obstetrical (brain-injured baby cases), where there is no payout are considerable. Concurrently, insurance companies, along with the population at large, faced reduced income from investments to help offset underwriting losses.

Another study in 2004 found that hospital professional liability and physician liability claims costs have increased at a steady 9.7% since 2000 and are likely to rise at the same rate in 2004. Frequency, or the number of claims, is growing at 3% a year; claim severity (the dollar amount) is increasing by 6.5% annually. Hospital liability claim costs for 2004 are expected to reach almost $150 000 per claim, compared with $79 000 per claim in 1996. The average claim against a physician is expected to reach $178 000, compared with $120 000 in 1996.

JURY AWARDS AND SETTLEMENTS

In early 2005, a Towers Perrin study found that over the 28 years since 1975, when they were first identified separately, medical malpractice cost increases have outpaced those in other tort areas, rising at an average of 11.8% a year, compared with 9.2% for all other tort costs. In 2003, medical malpractice, at almost $27 billion, cost each American an average of $91 a year. This compares with $5 a year in 1975. Recent data suggest that while jury awards are stabilizing and the frequency of claims may be decreasing, the severity of malpractice claims is increasing and the range of awards is moving upward, in keeping with inflation (Baker 2005). Median medical malpractice jury awards have held steady at about $1 million over the 3 years 2000–2002. Awards ranged from a low of $11 000, almost double the amount of the previous year, to a high of $95 million. The average award in 2002 hit $6.25 million, up from $3.91 million in 2001. However, only a small fraction of cases go to trial and very large awards are frequently reduced after the fact and after the publicity.

The costs of perinatal injury are quite high, relative not only to the costs of settlement and defense but also to personal and professional upheaval for all concerned. As Simpson and Knox have pointed out, the perspective of human and system factors reveals themes, context, and conditions common to accidental injury in other high-risk domains. According to the Jury Verdict Research, in 2000 the median jury award for neonatal neurological injury had increased to $5 million compared to $725 000 in 1994, with 76% of the jury awards valued at greater than $1 million (compared to 40% in 1994). Higher awards were more likely to occur when the hospital was the sole defendant than when both were defendants.

Conventional wisdom holds several contributing factors to account for the increased incidence of malpractice claims. (1) People are more litigious; it is part of our culture and extends everywhere from lawyers themselves to city governments. (2) Given the media coverage and watchdog groups, there has been an increasing understanding by the public of the fallibility of physicians. The Public Citizen Health Research Group, and the more recently formed groups emphasizing both medical error and the need to improve

care as part of tort reform, have also helped fuel the public's demand for change. (3) Another factor is the diminishing intimacy of the patient–doctor relationship fomented in part by larger changes in the way health care is distributed (HMOs), by increasing overheads and by deteriorating reimbursement schedules. (4) Then, there is the increasing availability of medical experts to testify in malpractice cases (the breakdown of omerta). (5) Also, there is the increasing assertiveness of the courts and the increasing sophistication of the plaintiff's bar with more careful selection of meritorious suits. (6) Last, there is the need for assistance with financing medical bills. Indeed, there is a seeming increase in the frequency of lawsuits for the 'damaged child,' in part due to the large verdicts sometimes realized but also due to the increasing incidence of CP related to the increasing survival of low birth weight infants and the costs thereof.

Several clinical practices and media attention would seem also to be impacting on the frequency and type of lawsuit. As an example, the United States Food and Drug Administration (FDA) issued a national advisory on the risks of vacuum extractors. This was rapidly followed by a nationwide television program emphasizing some of the disastrous results with vacuums. In turn, there has been a dramatic increase both in the reporting of adverse events associated with vacuum deliveries to the FDA and in the number of lawsuits alleging negligent care in the use of vacuums. Similarly, the methods undertaken to lower the cesarean section rate in the United States have perhaps been accomplished at the expense of an increased risk of ruptured uterus, shoulder dystocia and lawsuit. While all authorities would agree that any woman with one previous cesarean section and no other adverse features may be eligible for an attempt at VBAC, if she chooses to do so after being carefully explained the options, some HMOs have refused to accede to the mother's choice and have required that every patient with a previous cesarean be given a trial of labor; a horrific, medically indefensible recommendation. One institution in California that adopted this policy was assessed almost $25 million as a result of 48 women who first suffered adverse outcome as a result of this policy.

PREVALENCE OF MEDICAL MALPRACTICE

A study (generally known as the Harvard study) commissioned by New York State in 1986, and repetition released in 1990, showed that although actual malpractice is relatively rare, it is nevertheless underreported. If anything, the study group believed that there were too few lawsuits (Brennan 1991). When hospital medical records from New York State were examined, the incidence of adverse events or injuries resulting from medical 'interventions' or treatment was 3.7%. The percentage of adverse events due to what the physician team characterized as 'negligence' (not necessarily a legal definition) was 1%. However, only one in eight who suffered from an adverse event due to negligence filed a medical malpractice claim, and only 1 in 15 received compensation. Most adverse events resulted in only minimal and transient disability and most of the patients' medical care expenses were paid for by health insurance. This helps to explain why only a small percentage of patients who are injured as a result of negligence file medical malpractice claims. However, a significant proportion (22%) of patients who did not file medical malpractice claims suffered moderate or greater incapacity. In the second phase of the study, researchers confirmed that some of the tort claims filed provided little or no evidence of medical malpractice or even an adverse event, suggesting that the tort system is 'very error-prone,' at least in its initial stages (related to the expert). This inefficiency in both the medical and the legal systems notwithstanding, the study noted that 'if anything, there are too few lawsuits'. The inference here is that more patients with adverse outcomes related to negligence should be suing.

Despite the allegations of ACOG regarding the lack of value of intrapartum care in the prevention of fetal injury or death, there are several studies of closed claims in obstetrics and their relationship to negligence or their adherence to guidelines. Julian et al reviewed the files of 220 obstetric closed-claim cases to identify common factors predisposing to claims and to suggest preventative measures. Identification of common obstetric risks and correct management of these risks were poor in these cases. Only 54% of the risks were recognized; of these, only 32% were correctly managed. A high percentage of risks were thought to be directly related to the obstetric outcome leading to the claim (66%). The authors feel obstetric closed claims can be studied and suggestions made to aid obstetricians in providing care. They concluded that obstetric malpractice closed claims are amenable to study; physicians and their patients would benefit from better data collection systems to identify risks in individual pregnancies, along with available resources to aid their management of patients. They felt that suits can be avoided through modification of physician behavior.

In 1989, Rosenblatt and Hurst reviewed all closed obstetric claims in the records of a major physician-sponsored malpractice insurer from 1982 to 1989. Of the 54 files closed during the 6.5-year period covered by this study, 21 (39%) involved physician reports of bad outcomes that did not lead to a formal claim. Of the 33 formal claims, 14 (42%) were dismissed, either by the plaintiff's attorney or by the courts. Eighteen of the remaining 19 claims were settled before trial, with an average payment to the plaintiff of $185000. The one suit that went to trial resulted in a defense verdict. A review of the case histories demonstrated that in the majority of cases when a payment was made, probable medical negligence had taken place. Non-meritorious claims were not compensated. For those cases in which a payment was made, the size of the settlement was commensurate with the seriousness of the injury, which almost always involved damage to the infant. Poor physician judgment was the most common source of error.

The surviving, handicapped infant continues to represent the highest payout/case. There are numerous representative reviews of closed cases (Table 29.3). An analysis of 353 closed claims involving obstetrician-gynecologists revealed that the 40 highest-paid claims (11.3%) accounted for 88.7% of the total dollars spent. The majority of these 23 (57.5%) were obstetrical, including the five highest claims and 17 of the first 20 highest-paid awards. Obstetrical negligence represented over $5 million (76.5%) of the total expense. Of the 40 cases, 23 (60%) were resolved with a compromise settlement, 9 claims (22.5%) were resolved with indemnity payment on the basis of verdict or pretrial compromise; 7 (17.5%) had no indemnity payment because of a jury verdict or voluntary dismissal. These seven were in the highest-paid claims group only because of expenses.

Table 29.3 Operative delivery notes

OP DEL NOTE: (A)

MF, OP OA, mid epis, no lac Apgar 8, 9 P and M intact EBL 400, M and B left DR in good cond.

Signature

Translation: Operative delivery note: Midforceps, occiput posterior (OP) to occiput anterior (OA), midline episiotomy, no lacerations Apgar scores 8, 9 at 1, 5 minutes. Placenta and membranes expressed intact. Estimated blood loss 400 mL. Mother and infant left the delivery room in good condition

OPERATIVE DELIVERY NOTE (B)

Procedures: Trial of forceps, midforceps rotation, episiotomy repaired

Findings: Gynecoid pelvis, normal active phase, +3 station, minimal molding, direct OP, epidural anesthesia, second stage 2.5 hours, pushing inadequate, patient tired EFW 3000. Prev. baby 2800 Indications: Persistent occiput posterior, prolonged second stage, secondary arrest of descent, tired patient

Informed consent: Discussed options with patient and husband, who agree and understand that if any difficulty is encountered, the forceps will be abandoned and cesarean section undertaken. The operating room has been alerted

Methods: Midline episiotomy Kielland forceps. Direct application to OP without difficulty Gentle rotation: ROT to OA. Kiellands removed, Simpson forceps applied. Gentle traction — delivered as OA

Fetal outcome: 3200-g male infant, APGAR 8, 9 (see individual features in chart)

Resuscitation: Oxygen only, no evidence of trauma to skull forceps, marks reveal appropriate placement

Maternal outcome: Perineum intact, episiotomy repaired, no lacerations

Placenta and membranes intact

Estimated blood loss: 300 cc

Mother left delivery room in good condition

Of the 40 cases, none were considered frivolous, 28 (70%) were judged to be meritorious, and 12 (30%) were judged to be non-meritorious. Seven of the latter settled without indemnity costs, including four that went to trial with a defense verdict and three that were dismissed, leaving five others in this group with proper treatment and indemnity costs. Expenses to defend all 12 cases of proper treatment totaled over $500 000. Irrespective of the absence of strict negligence, each of these 'non-meritorious claims' illustrated substantial deficits with the medical record or system failures – inviting the allegation of negligence and lawsuit (making the case appear meritorious). These analyses clearly reveal that bad outcomes may not be the fault of the physician, but that physician behavior in the conduct of the case and the conduct of the medical record contribute heavily to successful allegations of malpractice.

Ogburn et al reviewed 153 closed claims involving perinatal injury or death filed from 1980 through 1982 with the St. Paul Fire and Marine Insurance Company. The claims included were those in which an indemnity was paid or $1000 or more was expended on the legal defense. Cases were classified according to the presence or absence of medical negligence. Most of the complications leading to claims arose during labor and delivery. Many claims resulted from the failure to evaluate or treat in a manner consistent with accepted standards of care. Many lacked documentation of the physician's recognition of the risk factors involved. In the opinion of the reviewers, medical negligence occurred in 47% of the cases. Indemnity payment occurred with most (but not all!) of the claims judged to be associated with medical negligence. Payment to the claimant was also made in a number of cases in which the reviewer thought no malpractice had occurred. The authors concluded that these results suggest that improvements are needed in prenatal and perinatal health care as well as in the legal system used to address the problem of perinatal medical negligence.

In a study published in 2003, Ransom et al, tried to estimate whether guideline compliance affected medico-legal risk in obstetrics and whether malpractice claims data can provide useful information about compliance. From the claims experience of a large health system delivering approximately 12 000 infants annually, they retrospectively identified 290 delivery-related (diagnosis-related groups 370–374) malpractice claims and 262 control deliveries between 1988 and 1998. Clinical pathways for vaginal delivery and cesarean section, implemented in 1998, were used as a standard of care. They compared rates of non-compliance with the pathways in the claims and control groups. They found that non-compliance with the clinical pathways was significantly more common among claims than controls (43.2% vs. 11.7%, $P < 0.001$; odds ratio 5.76, 95% CI 3.59, 9.2). In 81 (79.4%) of the claims involving non-compliance with the pathway, the main allegation in the claim related directly to the departure from the pathway. The excess malpractice risk attributable to non-compliance explained approximately one-third (104 of 290) of the claims

filed (attributable risk 82.6%). They concluded that malpractice data are a useful resource in understanding breakdowns in processes of care and that adherence to clinical pathways might (1) reduce clinical variation, (2) improve the quality of care, and (3) protect clinicians and institutions against malpractice litigation. A study by Greenwood et al from the National Perinatal Epidemiology Unit, Oxford, United Kingdom compared the prevalence of criteria suggesting acute intrapartum hypoxia in children with CP according to whether a lawsuit was brought alleging obstetrical negligence. The subjects were singleton children with CP born between 1984 and 1993, excluding cases with a recognized postnatal cause for CP. Only one-fifth (27/138) of all singleton CP children were the subject of a lawsuit. The greater the number of criteria suggesting intrapartum insult the more likely was a legal claim ($P < 0.01$), but 36% (4/11) of those satisfying all required criteria did not make a claim. Of the 27 claims, 12 were discontinued, 8 were settled and in 7 the legal process was still pending at the time of the article. Furthermore, the presence of the three essential criteria for acute intrapartum hypoxia did not increase the likelihood of a legal claim being settled.

JCAHO has recently published a study of adverse perinatal outcome finding many examples of substandard care and communication in the genesis of adverse perinatal outcome (JCAHO 2004). Other studies have focused on the costs and outcomes of litigation but not on culpability. Closed claims provide valuable data, but because, on average, a medical liability case takes 3–5 years to come to closure, opportunities for timely intervention in unsafe practices are lost. The research value is further compromised when the details of cases that reach settlement are suffocated by 'gag clauses' that mandate silence not only on the amount of award, but also on the allegations and the admission or even acknowledgment of wrong-doing, thereby removing an obvious incentive to make care better. Hatlie and Sheridan have suggested that gag orders are counterproductive.

MEDICAL RECORDS

Unfortunately, the opinions that serve to launch medical or medico-legal proceedings are most often based on a review of medical records that are frequently silent on the intentions of the provider or their exercise of 'medical judgment'. They may be silent, as well, on fundamental details of the obstetrical care. As a result, medical records, which represent both a medical document and a legal document, often promote or perpetuate cases and confound their defense. A cost analysis of 3205 multispecialty claims showed an average cost per claim of $22 584. Deficits in the medical record, e.g. inadequate instructions, delayed entries, inadequate notes and consent-form issues, more than double the average cost. System failures nearly triple the average cost. Thus, while an erroneous decision may be defensible if the reasons leading to it are recorded in the chart, the changed record and the contradictory record are almost impossible to defend. Until medical records objectively communicate the findings, the attention paid, the comprehension that was achieved and offer a reasonable plan followed by appropriate and consistent action, their appearance in court will continue to be an uphill battle for the physician and he/she will get little credit for the thought process or use to his/her advantage the testimony of 'a witness whose memory never dies'.

As an aside, the reader is invited to compare the two enclosed notes regarding a midforceps procedure (Table 29.3). In the first example, the note invites lawsuit if there is an adverse outcome. The note provides no indication for, or details about, the procedure. It is more a personal memorandum than a responsible medical description relevant for decisions about care in future pregnancies for example. The second note, on the other hand, would seem to protect against lawsuit in several ways. The note (1) clearly bespeaks thoughtfulness, (2) bespeaks understanding of the medical issues and alternatives and (3) underscores the physician's efforts to provide a forthright explanation to the patient and her husband – all powerful disincentives to lawsuit. Naked may be the best disguise!

One can readily blame the plaintiff's attorney for bringing to suit an apparently frivolous case, but who is to blame (i.e. what has been learned?) for the negligent care and adverse outcome in situations where no suit is brought despite negligent care or where no award is made despite a suit and the physician's care is vindicated? Should the plaintiff's attorney be blamed for pursuing a case that his expert has told him, based on a review of the medical records only, is negligent care? Each of the articles that evaluated closed cases found appreciable amounts of agreed upon negligent care. Each emphasizes (1) the need for better data, (2) the inculpating role of physician behavior and (3) the importance of the review of malpractice claims to identify problem-prone clinical processes and suggest interventions that may improve outcome and reduce negligence.

It must be readily apparent from even these limited studies that not all meritorious suits succeed and not all non-meritorious suits (not the same as frivolous) lose. These articles leave it open to speculation why patients victimized by obvious medical negligence do not sue or why they are not compensated by the system in the face of agreed upon negligence. Clearly, patients without demonstrable evidence of negligence bring suit and sometimes they are rewarded in the system. The system does not work perfectly, but these studies from various specialties and perspectives strongly suggest that it is not a lottery.

In a study of 36 malpractice cases involving cervical spine surgery, for example, the authors found a common basis for suits included failure to diagnose and treatment (56%), lack of informed consent (64%), new neurologic deficits (64%), and pain and suffering (72%). All of the six plaintiff verdicts (average, $4.42 million) and four of the nine settlements (average, $1.6 million) involving surgery that resulted in new postoperative quadriplegia appeared to be appropriate. However, the author could discern 'no fault' in cases five

defendants had settled. On the other hand, the author found 'fault' in five defense verdicts rendered to three newly quadriplegic patients and two with new postoperative root injuries. These patients deserved monetary awards, but received no compensation whatsoever (Epstein 2002).

Given the non-medical issues that incite or color a case, physicians squander much of the advantage they have in the system! Thus, it is with some justification that critics of malpractice litigation point out that it is unrealistic to expect that increased levels of litigation will make compensation for injuries more 'just' or health care better. A reductio ad absurdum argument suggests that immunity from lawsuit, perhaps the true goal behind physicians' notion of tort reform, will, by eliminating lawsuits, achieve these goals. Some conventional tort reforms appear to be effective in reducing litigation costs and stabilizing insurance markets; they are not, however, designed to remedy the fundamental failings of the malpractice system – making care better and making the physician–patient relationship better. Fulfillment of these objectives may not require more sweeping tort reform; perhaps more sweeping 'thought reform' may be required or, alternatively, trying to make the system work as it was supposed to. These reforms can only come from the medical community.

LEGAL VULNERABILITY

The last several decades have also witnessed the development of new bases for lawsuit in reproductive matters, including wrongful birth and wrongful life. In the former, the parents with an injured child may bring suit alleging that negligent treatment or advice deprived them of the opportunity to avoid conception or terminate a pregnancy. The latter, brought on behalf of the child born with birth defects, alleges that the child would not have been born but for negligent advice to, or negligent treatment of, the parents. It should be emphasized that such allegations are actionable in some states but not in others. While not strictly related to malpractice, a mother who pleaded with her hopelessly premature infant's caretakers to discontinue resuscitation was not heeded, resulting in the survival of a severely handicapped child and a provisional $42 million verdict for the plaintiff.

TORT REFORM MEASURES

Most liability reform acts have four major components: (1) reforms directly addressing the size of awards – under the heading of caps on damages; (2) reforms intended to modify liability rules, to control the number of claims and size of payouts by eliminating joint and several liability for cases in which a plaintiff found to be partially at fault becomes responsible for a disproportionate share of the damages; (3) reforms limiting access to the courts, through shortening statutes of limitation – a reduction in the length of time during which lawsuit can be brought; and (4) periodic payments – the latitude to pay future economic damages over time. Some initiatives have legislated review panels to pass on the merit of a case prior to the institution of suit, while others have attempted to remove the infant who is brain damaged during birth from the medico-legal arena by the institution of no-fault insurance. Still other initiatives have attempted to increase the percentage of any award that goes to the patient by limiting the attorney's fees. The most popular of these, caps on premiums, have had the benefit of moderating the increases in insurance payments. A publication from the Rand Corporation has emphasized that in cases with modest claims there is indeed a reduction in indemnity payouts, but they cast doubt on the likely benefit of caps on the high-award cases where economic damages are large and 'pain and suffering' may be much smaller. It seems axiomatic that caps should not apply to frivolous suits where the cap should be zero.

In the 1970s 22 states legislated some form of prelitigation processes, including screening panels and mandatory binding and non-binding arbitration: only two remain active and neither has been effective. The costs of constitutional battles over due process rights for binding processes and the failed reduction of litigated cases in non-binding processes led to further soaring legal costs, rather than reductions. The only lasting 'tort reform,' although, as discussed later, with questionable material impact on malpractice frequency and awards, has been caps on non-economic damages, with the gold standard being that of California's Medical Injury Compensation Reform Act of 1975 (MICRA).

Tort reform, the mantra of the ACOG, the Bush administration, the Chamber of Commerce, the American Manufacturers Association and other business organizations to deal with high medical malpractice costs, makes sense only from the political aspect (Baker 2005). Capping awards on malpractice suits may offend trial lawyers, but it helps or holds harmless special interests in the insurance, drug and health care industries. It provides no assistance to patients who suffer grievous harm as a result of negligent care nor does it improve the delivery of medical care. To many, a $250 000 cap (the cap placed on non-economic damages in California) is poor acknowledgment indeed for the physical and emotional damage done to people who have suffered total paralysis, permanent blindness or severe brain injury because of medical errors. Indeed, many states burdened with high premiums have already set their own caps, but generally at more reasonable levels. It would seem more useful to consider making it harder for insurance companies to gain rate increases.

Guidelines for judges and juries might be enacted to help determine what compensation is reasonable in a given circumstance. Similar guidelines could help ensure that punitive damages, sometimes masquerading as non-economic damages, are high enough to deter bad conduct; $250 000 would hardly amount to a slap on the wrist.

The problem with frivolous lawsuits is best addressed by raising the hurdles for filing a malpractice suit, for example,

requiring an expert judgment on the merits of a case before it can proceed through the courts. As mentioned above, there seems to be no place for the expert witness to certify a case as meritorious if that same expert will not appear on the record for (public) report, deposition and trial if necessary.

The notion that the crisis of escalating malpractice insurance premiums is forcing doctors out of business remains murky. Insurance companies have substantially raised premiums for malpractice coverage for doctors in high-risk specialties like obstetrics and neurosurgery in some states, leading at least some doctors to curtail their services, retire or move. But when the Government Accountability Office visited five of the hardest hit states in 2003, it found only scattered problems and was unable to document wide-scale lack of access to medical care.

None of the tort reform proposals deal with the underlying need to diminish malpractice and to identify harmed patients and provide them with fair, prompt compensation, or provide tools for health care providers to properly prepare patients and deal effectively with unanticipated outcomes. Although they do resolve the desire of the health care industry and the insurance companies for fewer big court awards, they do not materially impact the frequency of suit. But they do act as a rollback of the legal rights of patients who are injured.

The Center for Justice and Democracy, a consumer advocacy group, recently commented that:

> It may be hard to understand why 'tort reform' is even on the national agenda at a time when insurance industry profits are booming, tort filings are declining, only 2% of injured people sue for compensation, punitive damages are rarely awarded, liability insurance costs for businesses are minuscule, medical malpractice insurance and claims are both less than 1% of all health care costs in America, and premium-gouging underwriting practices of the insurance industry have been widely exposed.

(See also Baker 2005.) Despite claims by the insurance industry, there is no evidence that malpractice premiums are the result of sharp increases in the amounts of money paid out for malpractice claims. And, tellingly, industry executives have carefully acknowledged that tort reforms will not result in substantial premium reductions – only an improvement in care can do that (Baker 2005).

Caps do not limit lawsuits. More reasonably, caps are intended to increase the hurdles to a lawsuit by diminishing the economic value of a suit. In cases where there is little economic loss (irrespective of negligence), victims may not be able to find lawyers to take their cases (www.saynotocaps.org/) because malpractice cases can cost plaintiff's lawyers hundreds of thousands of dollars out of pocket to prosecute, with no guarantee of recouping those expenses. As pointed out by the Rand Corporation study, caps have little impact on lawsuits where there are substantial economic losses, e.g. brain-damaged infant, maternal death. A one-size-fits-all cap cannot encompass the unique facts in any case and, in fact, more reasonably creates a system of 'one-size-fits-none'. It unfairly discriminates against victims with no economic losses, such as children, stay-at-home moms, the elderly, the poor and the mentally handicapped. The media unflinchingly promulgates numerous cases of tragic, ineffable medical error where such arbitrary limits (originally set in 1979) seem inadequate and, if not inadequate, arbitrary. Caps will not lower doctors' malpractice insurance premiums. (www.saynotocaps.org/reports/Premium Deceit.pdf: The Failure of Tort 'Reform' to Cut Insurance Rates) Average premiums are actually 16% higher in states with caps. In states that have recently adopted caps, most notably Texas and Florida, insurance rates are continuing to increase. Indeed the only thing keeping rates down in California – a state often cited as a model for caps – is insurance industry regulation provided by Proposition 103.

The amount of money awarded on pain and suffering is not known. In the majority of awards, those reached by settlement out of court, there is no distinction between economic and non-economic damages. In jury trials economic and non-economic damages are awarded separately, but there appears to be no calculation of either the amount or the propriety. Nor has there been any compilation of those extreme awards that are reduced, sometimes drastically, by judicial review. In three cases where the jury awarded over $220 million, the total cumulative amount received was $14 million (6 cents on the dollar!). There was no publication of the reduction! When adjusted for the skyrocketing rate of health care inflation, total payouts in malpractice cases remained flat until 2001. In the 3 years since, total payouts have declined each year.

Many states have enacted legal reforms that have effectively eliminated any lawsuits that could be construed as 'frivolous' by requiring a 'certificate of merit' from a physician certified in the same medical specialty as the doctor being sued. There have also been laws enacted to prevent 'venue shopping' for a more favorable jury. Indeed, a Republican state senator from Pennsylvania declared that 'There is no such thing as a frivolous lawsuit any more' in Pennsylvania. In addition, again in Pennsylvania, one of the 'red alert states,' there has been a significant increase in the number of physicians over the past several years, prompting one state legislator to call such claims of a doctor exodus as 'scare tactics'.

It is far from clear that malpractice costs are driving up the costs of health care. Malpractice costs account for less than 2% of the US health care budget. The Congressional Budget Office, in a report released in January 2004, found that legislation to cap damages in medical malpractice lawsuits would 'do little to hold down health care spending' or eliminate the practice of 'defensive medicine'. There is little evidence that the threat of malpractice lawsuits contributes to the practice of defensive medicine. Rather, it has been suggested that doctors order additional tests because it is good medical practice; doctors make money from additional testing; and managed care discourages unnecessary testing, or 'bad' defensive medicine.

Faulty underwriting and misfeasance by malpractice underwriters are additional factors contributing to the rise in premiums; they cannot be relieved by tort reform. In Pennsylvania in the late 1990s, six major malpractice insurers became insolvent because of risky premium underpricing, poor investment strategies and Enron-style malfeasance, leaving doctors to pay for their mismanagement. There is no basis for the notion that insurance companies routinely settle lawsuits just to make them go away. This seems more like a strategy for self-destruction and is contradicted by the closed-claims data presented above.

There can be little doubt that there is an immediate question of affordability that must be dealt with acutely. Indeed, several states have contributed significant amounts of public money to subsidize insurance premiums. Physicians remain the highest-paid professionals in the state, according to US Census data. Indeed, the incomes of obstetricians – the physicians most affected by higher premiums – are rising. For many, on average, doctors spend 1–5% of their gross revenues on medical malpractice insurance. It seems obvious also that many doctors supplement their incomes with fees from attorneys for providing 'independent medical evaluations' in malpractice cases.

ALTERNATIVE SYSTEM REFORMS

Experts have suggested a number of approaches, including special health courts with judges trained to deal with malpractice issues, required mediation, mandatory reporting of errors by doctors and prompt offers of compensation. Some of these will be reviewed briefly here. Not strictly a part of tort reform, alternative dispute resolution has much to recommend it.

The strict liability (no-fault) administrative system supports creation of a just patient safety culture and encourages reporting (and prevention) of adverse events. It has the advantages of dispensing with trial and supports open disclosure to the patient (not the public) as the deliberations are administrative. In this system the provider is accountable for all avoidable medically related losses and the matter can be resolved promptly. It eliminates the requirement of proving negligence, but the patient must establish that their injury was actually caused by the treatment. As a generalization, eligibility is based on avoidability rather than providers being strictly responsible for medically related losses. There is, unfortunately, the common perception that 'no-fault' means 'no accountability'. Examples include the Neurological Injury Compensation Association (NICA) in Florida and Virginia.

Although, the system of No-Fault is modeled after that of Workers Compensation and Automobile No-Fault claims, the complexity of determining causal and avoidable injury medical injury claims is very different. And although it removes negligence as a basis for the claim, it does not replace the regulatory system of reporting and the resultant physician fear, nor does it address the inbred philosophy of 'do no harm,' 'zero tolerance'. Since premiums in any no-fault system are based on injury rates, this creates an incentive to conceal injuries and reduce the admission of high-risk specialists to medical staffs. It may also discriminate against patients at high risk for injury. It is uncertain how the establishment of a no-fault system will impact cost. Some test programs have demonstrated that costs of a general no-fault system would exceed those of the present tort system. Finally, the introduction and administration of a no-fault medical injury system, whether public or private, will be complicated and likely politically encumbered.

Preventable events (ACEs) represents consensus on what constitutes an avoidable event. These are predetermined events that should not occur in quality health care delivery. They encourage prevention of avoidable events that can trigger eligibility for an early compensation offer. ACEs make 'avoidability,' and therefore eligibility for compensation, transparent to providers and patients alike. They standardize eligibility for compensation and provide quicker identification of eligible cases. There is, however, no comprehensive ACE list currently available, and there is concern as to who is to develop the categories of avoidable events. Brain-damaged infants, for example, would not be covered. Development of the list will, of course, require an array of expert consensus (selected by whom?). The use of ACEs provides a basis to determine eligibility for alternative and conventional compensation systems. It can also be paired with a standardized compensation fee schedule.

MEDIATION

Mediation represents a highly efficient option for non-adversarial resolution of health care conflicts. It is a process in which the parties to the conflict themselves, not lawyers, craft their own unique resolution to a conflict. Mediation is essentially facilitated communication and negotiation using a neutral third party. The process itself is non-binding and does not prevent the patient from moving forward to litigation. However, if a resolution is reached, it becomes binding under contract law and may even be brought as an order of the court. Mediation is highly cost-efficient and time sparing, in that it makes response to adverse events and their resolution more timely and boasts a greater than 90% resolution rate. It is widely accepted and highly successful in many 'industries' such as real estate and education, but has met with much resistance in the health care industry, especially in medical malpractice. It intensifies the pressure on patients to settle, thus reducing or avoiding litigation. Because confidentiality has been stripped from the mediation process in medical malpractice disputes by medical regulatory boards and reporting agencies, the successful application of the mediation process in physician–patient conflicts has therefore been crippled. Although confidentiality in error reporting is the foundation of most of the proposed legislation, it

has not been extended to the resolution of conflicts arising from alleged medical errors. The statutory obligation physicians have to report settlements of disputes involving quality of care issues creates a perverse incentive for physicians to move forward in litigation, especially when one considers the high attrition rate of malpractice claims and the likelihood of a physician prevailing in those cases that persist. It is likely that even in the face of tort reform mediation will remain an infrequently used medium for the resolution of physician–patient disputes.

ARBITRATION

As with mediation, arbitration provides economical and prompt adjudication of adverse events. Like mediation, it provides prompt, private settlement and compensation, yet is also subject to reporting requirements and regulatory oversight. The processes differ, however, in a few major factors. With arbitration the decision maker is a third party, the arbitrator(s) and the process is highly formalistic and adversarial.

There are two forms of arbitration, binding and non-binding. The latter is similar to mediation in that if either party disagrees with the arbitrator's decision, they may move on to litigation. The former, however, is a binding decision that cannot be appealed. Binding arbitration for malpractice claims has met with considerable legal opposition and non-binding arbitration has met with low utilization and increased litigation costs. Such systems intensify the pressure on patients to settle, thus reducing or avoiding litigation. They may be used with the current tort system — as well as with no-fault and ACEs. Kaiser Permanente, for example, requires enrollees to sign a 'willingness to arbitrate' agreement. With this approach, the health plan undertakes to resolve disputes through arbitration rather than go through the courts. This of course is not the same as a waiver of liability.

SPECIALIZED MEDICAL MALPRACTICE COURTS

There are three types of specialized courts under consideration: the Health Court, the Medical Board Administrative Adjudication System and the Tripartite Panel.

Health Court: This involves the creation of an alternative court system within the federal court system. This proposal will, as touted by the consumer advocate group Common Good, presumably make judgments more reliable and provide clearer lessons for deterrence of adverse outcome. In theory, it can provide more timely access, faster resolution of claims, along with more reliable and standardized compensation. It requires appointment of special expert courts to hear medical cases or administer compensation based on avoidable events. Health courts also make the system more transparent by providing public access to settlement and adjudication findings. It will require judges who have special knowledge or training in medicine. Although proponents believe that this form of adjudication will offer more consistent and informed decisions than the traditional trier of fact, a lay jury, many studies find that in comparison with expert's reviews, the present jury system is quite consistent.

Health courts may be paired with ACEs and a standardized compensation schedule – and may even add a trial option to an administrative system. There are precedents for these types of courts in certain tax and patent infringement and workers' compensation laws.

Medical Board Administrative Adjudication System: In 1988, the AMA, 31 medical specialty associations, the Physician Insurer's Association of America (PIAA), and the Counsel of Medical Specialty Societies created the Medical Liability Project to develop an equitable and efficient method to handle malpractice claims. They proposed a claims adjudication process based on fault and suggested that the states' medical boards act as the trier of fact in addition to their regulatory and disciplinary roles. This system would initially screen cases, offer free legal counsel for cases passing review and offer limited judicial review. In a parallel development, the AMA considers that the provision of expert testimony constitutes 'the practice of medicine' and that it should be subject to peer review by state medical boards. The AMA encourages the state medical associations to work with the licensing boards to develop effective disciplinary measures for fraudulent testimony.

Tripartite Panel: Also in 1988, the PIAA proposed an administrative system similar to that used for workers' compensation in the hope that patients would elect this more speedy system through the offer of incentives. The panel would consist of a judge, a physician and a lay person and function much like the few state screening panels that remain active. In cases where malpractice was found, all medical expenses would be paid under a specific method of computation, all non-economic awards would be based on a fixed schedule of benefits, and there would be a limit on attorney's fees.

PRETRIAL SCREENING PANELS

This is a system that is modeled after state programs that are presently functioning, with those of Maine and Vermont the most recognized. To enlist the Panel, the patient provides written notice to the physician and with the superior court to be acted upon within 90 days. The superior court selects a Panel Chair from a pool of retired judges and/or mediators with judicial or legal experience. The Chair selects from a court issued list one attorney and one physician panelist, of the same or relevant specialty. The parties may challenge the selection for cause. There is a Prehearing Discovery, then a Pretrial Screening Hearing that follows the format of an arbitration. Depositions are admissible, but expert testimony is unusual. The panel has prior access to written briefs, complete medical records, deposition transcripts. The panel then acts as the trier of both fact and law, under the standard used by lay juries, 'preponderance of the evidence'. It evaluates the case on the basis of the four Ds of negligence. Unanimous decisions by the panel on negligence and causation are admissible in court, in favor of either the patient or the provider. The decision of the panel, like in non-binding arbitration, does not bind either party from pursuing litigation and trial. Some systems allow recovery of costs by the losing party, but as stated previously, if it is the plaintiff, actual recovery is unlikely.

ENTERPRISE LIABILITY

Enterprise liability provides an incentive for prioritization of enterprise-wide safety. It shifts liability from the individual provider to a provider organization such as an integrated medical staff, IPO, large group practice, or hospital capable of influencing care across the systems. Enterprise liability essentially makes these organizations 'strictly liable' in both a legal and an economic sense by their responsibility for liability premiums for all staff involved in the organization, which could potentially impact the present punitive reporting system and allow for a freer flow of error reporting. Such a system would promote institutional safety and potentially stabilize liability insurance fees. Legal provisions (Stark laws) may prohibit liability insurance coverage of non-employee physicians. It works equally well with alternatives as well as the current tort system. The Department of Health and Human Services Office of Inspector General (OIG) historically has been concerned that a hospital's subsidy of malpractice insurance premiums for potential referral sources, including hospital medical staff, may implicate the antikickback statute, because the payments may be used to influence referrals. 'There is a particular concern where subsidies are offered in a conditional or selective manner that reflects current or anticipated referrals from the subsidized practitioners.' Hospitals may be able to subsidize the malpractice insurance of local obstetricians without triggering antikickback sanctions, according to an advisory opinion issued by the OIG. In this opinion, OIG outlines a specific case in which it would not impose antikickback sanctions against a medical center that provides subsidies to four community-based obstetricians who hold staff privileges at the medical center but are not employees of the facility.

Tort reform in many of its guises, however, has historically not been universally 'friendly' to the physician. In 1988, the US Congress established a National Practitioner Data Bank authorizing the collection of data about physicians and dentists from malpractice settlements, awards and disciplinary actions; these data were to be supplied by insurers, hospitals and HMOs. Queries of the Data Bank might be made by hospitals and physicians, but there is to be no access by the public or actual or prospective litigants including patients and attorneys although expanded access to this information is the subject of much debate. This tracking by the Data Bank has probably decreased the willingness of physicians to settle cases, but has probably not decreased the frequency of malpractice. The non-departmental public body (NDPB) reporting system is primarily based on the reporting of any formal written claim of malpractice that results in even one penny changing hands, regardless of admission of blame or severity of injury. Such reports carry great weight in considerations for staff privileges, provider contracts, and malpractice premium rates. Hatlie and Sheridan have argued that the NDPB should be abandoned.

Even more recently, there has been increasing attention on the amount of medical error that has heretofore gone unnoticed and undocumented. The AMA has created a Patient Safety Initiative and the Federal Government is considering legislation that will likely reorient the approach to error. Indeed, since the publication of the prestigious IOM's 'To Err is Human,' which claims that between 44 000 and 98 000 hospitalized patients die per year as a result of medical error, and subsequent studies such as that of Chaudhry and coworkers, patient safety has become the mantra of the Joint Commission on Accreditation, which has now embellished the requirements for disclosure of error. Programs for the evaluation of root cause analyses of reported errors and the resulting error reducing actions have become, as they should, a national priority.

Also potentially threatening to the physician are those tort reforms that are linked (politically) to the establishment of enhanced physician review panels, the creation of 'three strikes and you are out' rules, etc. In Texas, for example, along with a stringent tort reform bill passed in 2003, the Texas legislature gave the Texas State Board of Medical Examiners new authority to regulate medical practice through the passage of S.B. This bill gave the board increased funding for expert consultants and staff. These resources were used to assess the approximately 6000 complaints the board receives each year. As a result, Board enforcements have increased dramatically. Before the augmentation, cases were filed against physicians immediately, which immediately affected their records. The new system provides more due process, but is more far wide-ranging. Opponents of this feature of Texas Health litigation argue that standard of care issues should be left to local community medical societies or hospital peer review and credentialing societies. But when the boot is on the other foot and these organizations engage in sham peer review or economic credentialing, physicians complain about their unfair practices (see below). Physician groups complaining about S.B. want the presumption of innocence, the right to access details of the complaints against them, the right of discovery, the right to present witnesses and cross-examine witnesses and the right to appeal. How seductive is the illusion of a new idea – all of these features are present in current malpractice law, the beneficiary of 200 years of accumulated jurisprudence. Public Citizen's Health Research Group ranked Texas 23 out of the 50 states.

Reviews of the impact of tort reform on premiums suggest that while premiums do respond to increases in payments, they do not increase dollar for dollar (http://www.nber.org/papers/w10709). This suggests that other factors may also be important in explaining the recent jump in malpractice premiums, such as a less competitive insurance industry or a decline in insurers' investment income. There is little evidence that changes in malpractice premiums are linked to changes in either the total number of physicians or the number of physicians working in obstetrics/gynecology, surgery or internal medicine. There is weak evidence to suggest that the entry decisions of young physicians and the exit decisions of older physicians may be affected by malpractice premiums. There is stronger evidence to suggest that rural physicians are more sensitive to a change in premiums – a 10% increase in premiums results in a 1% decrease in rural physicians per capita and a 2% decrease in older rural MDs (http://www.nber.org/papers/w10709). Although there is no change in the frequency of most treatments, some data suggest that physicians may increase the use of screening procedures in response to higher premiums. Such practices however have had little effect on total Medicare expenditures, suggesting that the costs associated with defensive medicine practices may be small, at least for this age group. Thus, it is far from clear that state tort reforms will avert local physician shortages or lead to greater efficiencies in care. The stabilization of premiums, the initial response to most rounds of tort reform, may not indeed be the result of the tort reform legislation. Normally, it takes years before legislative tort reform has a direct impact on malpractice premiums and several, but not all, state courts have invalidated the cap on damages, the component of the law with the greatest potential to reduce premiums. Malpractice premiums are affected by a constellation of additional factors, including the general investment climate, interest rate cycles and insurance regulations.

Whether driven by legislation or not, it seems reasonable that stable malpractice insurance premiums offered by experienced, reputable companies are important reasons for maintaining physician availability and equilibrium.

There is no evidence that tort reform has resulted in better care or more realistic confrontation of error. Tort reform simply 'tinkers with certain aspects of the system in a piece-meal fashion without having to grapple with fundamental reform of either the health care delivery system, the reimbursement system or physician behavior'.

TORT REFORM AND FINANCES — LITIGATION AND RISK MANAGEMENT

There is universal agreement that the medical needs of those with adverse outcome require more attention, whether they are related to negligence or not. There is also universal agreement that the present functioning of the medico-legal system is an anachronism — neither is it efficient or error-free in reaching a settlement nor is the distribution of money equitable. In the United States, only about 28 cents of every premium dollar goes to injured patients after an average delay of 4.9 years to dispose of a case.

Is no-fault insurance better? To determine whether Florida's implementation of a no-fault system for birth-related neurological injuries reduced lawsuits and the total spending associated with such injuries, and whether no-fault was more efficient than customary tort procedures in distributing compensation, Sloan et al compared claims and payments before and after implementation of a no-fault system in 1989. They found that the number of tort claims for permanent labor-delivery injury and death indeed fell by about 16–32%. However, when no-fault claims were added to tort claims, the total frequency of claims rose by 11–38%. Further, of the estimated 479 children who suffered birth-related injuries annually, only 13 were compensated under no-fault. The total combined payments to patients and all lawyers did not decrease, but under no-fault, a much larger portion of the total went to patients. Thus, less than 3% of the total payments went to lawyers under no-fault versus 39% under tort – a new equilibrium. Some claimants with birth-related injuries were winners, taking home a larger percentage of their awards than their tort counterparts. Lawyers clearly lost under no-fault, but so did many children with birth-related neurologic injuries who did not qualify for coverage because of the narrow statutory definition.

SOLVING THE MALPRACTICE PROBLEM

While the focus of clinical risk management intuitively rests on the analysis of adverse events, it seems clear that this is the most inefficient way of reducing or eliminating harm to the patient. In the current climate, risk management tends to deal more with avoidance of blame and litigation than with the avoidance of harm to patients.

One of health care's principal patient safety success stories is anesthesiology. In the 1980s, in the midst of a separate medical liability crisis, the rate of anesthesia-related deaths was one in 10 000; 6000 people per year who had undergone anesthesia died or suffered brain damage, and anesthesiologists' liability insurance premiums had sharply escalated. Following a national news magazine broadcast that pilloried the field for these outcomes, the American Society of Anesthesiologists (ASA) decided to seize the opportunity presented by the crisis to improve anesthesiology safety. It started with the hiring of a systems engineer. Through close scientific examination of 359 anesthesia errors, every aspect of anesthesia care – equipment, practices, and caregivers – was analyzed. Eventually, with the commitment of leadership and resources toward the task, the many system failures revealed by the study were re-engineered, and anesthesia-related death rates fell dramatically.

The ASA uses case analysis to identify liability risk areas, monitor trends in patient injury, and design strategies for prevention. Today, the ASA Closed Claims Project – created in 1985 – contains 6448 closed insurance claims. Analyses of these claims have, for example, revealed patterns in patient injury in the use of regional anesthesia, in the placement of central venous catheters and in chronic pain man-

agement. Results of these analyses are published in the professional literature to aid practitioner learning and promote changes in practices that improve safety and reduce liability exposure.

Closed claims data analysis is the one way in which the current medical liability system helps to inform improvements in care delivery. However, reliance on closed claims for information related to error and injury is cumbersome at best. It may take years for an insurance or malpractice claim to close. These are years in which potentially vital information on substandard practices remains unknown. Providing patient safety researchers with access to open claims, now protected from external examination, could vastly improve efforts aimed at identifying worrisome patterns in care and designing appropriate safety interventions.

In addition to anesthesiology's early work in identifying the human factors and system failures that cause error, anesthesiology has also promoted reliance on standards and guidelines to support optimal anesthesiology care. Anesthesiology has also been at the forefront in the use of patient simulation for research, training and performance assessment. With simulation, no patients are at risk of exposure to novice caregivers or unproven technologies. Anesthesiology is still far from perfect, but its 'institutionalization of safety' continues to serve the field well as it tackles the continuing threats to patient safety that are endemic to modern medicine.

Medicine is different from industry in that the medical system has not adjusted to the realities of human fallibility. The circumstances of the contemporary malpractice situation continue to compromise both the provision and the safety of health care as well as our notions of justice, of access to the law and to health care.

Defensive statements over the value of obstetrical care cited above, notwithstanding, there is broad agreement that improvement in perinatal outcome is possible, that the events of labor do contribute significantly and that reviewing adverse outcomes and making obstetrical units more reliable in terms of communication and interpretation of tracings will enhance outcome (Knox et al 1999, Simpson & Knox 2000). Irrespective, we do not yet know the totality of injury related to the intrapartum period – irrespective of the mechanism. The estimates of the role of hypoxia vary widely, in great measure due to incompatible definitions and limited follow up. We have some estimates of the role of obvious trauma due to forceps or vacuum, but there are no reliable estimates of the toll of the other factors, nor are there universally agreed upon techniques for reliably determining the precise timing and mechanism of injury (Towner et al 1999).

This state of affairs benefits neither the patient nor, in the long run, the physician. While in some instances the fear of lawsuit has increased the amount of surveillance and may have even had a salutary effect on outcome, there is little argument that the present format for dealing with allegations of negligence provides any incentive to the profession to practice better medicine, provide better peer review, or, in the occasional instance, restrict the future practice of the physician whatever his conduct. True reform will require a systemic approach to error in medicine as elsewhere and some refinement of our ethics and an appreciation of the paradoxes of contemporary malpractice. To lower the risk of malpractice we must continue to attempt to raise the standards of care. We need this more than we need the identification of the 'bad apples' of our specialty. We must increase communication with the patient and remain their advocate. We must address the formal teaching of communication skills, conflict management and team development techniques throughout medical school and residency. We must construct effective error reporting and systems analysis programs that promote error reduction, while protecting physicians from being punished by arbitrary and ineffective reporting systems. We must not squander our greatest asset – the medical record – and we must stop playing the role of victim. Often the ultimate failure is often not the individual provider but the latent, systemic errors, errors for which our systems are programmed, but which are functionally immune from lawsuit. A lawsuit cannot make 'the system' a defendant. Finally, we must be willing to participate in the process of uncovering error and make the patients our allies in these efforts.

NOTE 1

The medical malpractice business, as with the property and casualty industry as a whole, has been characterized by a 'boom and bust' cyclicity since the mid-1970s. History would tell us that profitability can be restored in time, perhaps with tort reform and pricing structures (Martin & Bade 2002), or, more persuasively, by an 'increased emphasis on improving patient safety and elimination of all preventable medical errors' (Weinstein 2006). It seems that realizing these desiderata will require a national electronic medical record and the availability of rapid response teams in most hospitals. Most 'privileged communications' and 'peer review' are counterproductive and should be eliminated. There is benefit for patient and physician alike for full and prompt disclosure of any medical error or injury abetted, if necessary, by outside consultants. Physicians must be taught proper teamwork and communication skills, including how to give 'bad news' and how to learn from error. Frequent patient, nursing or medical staff complaints against providers must be critically, and constructively reviewed. The objectives of risk management and patient safety need to be aligned and proactive. Our science and research should support improved outcomes not defensive postures. Claims management should offer the patient early compensation when appropriate and pursue a vigorous defense when medical care is adequate. Experts should be identified who will render fair, unbiased reviews of medical care for either side with all of their findings being disclosed.

Similar experts need to devise clear, concise, evidence-based standards of care for common medical conditions' (Weinstein 2006).

NOTE 2

For the past decade, Radiology Associates of Albuquerque has provided physician expert testimony to plaintiff and defense attorneys. Initially, the business was confined to radiology consultation only. The division has expanded; it now includes more than 35 specialties and a national client base. This article will include a history of the division's growth and lessons learned as well as a look at the future of expert testimony in light of increasing emphasis on standards of care. Medical marketing in the present as well as in the future will also be addressed (Stevenson 1999).

NOTE 3

Using 36 malpractice cases involving cervical spine surgery. Queries included who sued, who was sued, who won, who lost and why? Six different tort reform models also were identified and explored. RESULTS: Common bases for suits included failure to diagnose and treatment (56%), lack of informed consent (64%), new neurologic deficits (64%), and pain and suffering (72%). All of the six plaintiff verdicts (average, $4.42 million) and four of the nine settlements (average, $1.6 million) involving surgery that resulted in new postoperative quadriplegia appeared to be appropriate. However, the author could discern 'no fault' in cases five defendants had settled and the surgeons did not deserve to lose. On the other hand, the author found 'fault' in five defense verdicts rendered to three newly quadriplegic patients and two with new postoperative root injuries. These patients deserved monetary awards, but received no compensation whatsoever. There currently are two models that would work better than the system in place in most states. These include the American Medical Association National Specialty Societies Medical Liability Project with the Alternative Dispute Resolution Model (SSMLP), and the Selective No Fault Models. Among the advantages shared by one or more of these models is their ability to reimburse injured patients while eliminating physician liability, to use malpractice panels rather than trials and to put a cap on damages. CONCLUSIONS: To solve the medical malpractice crisis, Congress, the individual states, or both should adopt tort reform. Two tort reform models, compensating injured patients and eliminating physician liability, appear to be not only effective but also fair to all concerned parties (Epstein 2002).

NOTE 4

Caps won't help patients by substantially lowering or stabilizing health-care costs. Malpractice-insurance premiums account for less than 2 percent of the nation's health-care spending.

REFERENCES

ACOG 2005 Practice Bulletin #70. Intrapartum fetal heart rate monitoring. Obstet Gynecol 106(6):1453–1460.

Alfirevic Z, Devane D, Gyte G M 2006 Continuous cardiotocography (CTG) as a form of electronic fetal monitoring (EFM) for fetal assessment during labour. Cochrane Database Syst Rev 3:CD006066.

Althaus J E, Petersen S M, Fox H E et al 2005 Can electronic fetal monitoring identify preterm neonates with cerebral white matter injury? Obstet Gynecol 105(3):458–465.

Baker T 2005 The medical malpractice myth. The University of Chicago Press, Chicago.

Beckman H B, Markakis K M, Suchman A L et al 1994 The doctor–patient relationship and malpractice. Lessons from plaintiff depositions. Arch Intern Med 154(12):1365–1370.

Chauhan S P, Martin J N, Henrichs C E et al 2003 Maternal and perinatal complications with uterine rupture in 142,075 patients who attempted vaginal birth after Cesarean delivery: A review of the literature. Am J Obstet Gynecol 189(2):408–417.

Epstein N E 2002 It is easier to confuse a jury than convince a judge: the crisis in medical malpractice. Spine 27(22):2425–2430.

Finkelstein D, Wu A W, Holtzman N A 1997 When a physician harms a patient by a medical error: ethical, legal, and risk-management considerations. J Clin Ethics 8(4):330–335.

Gallagher T H, Waterman A D, Ebers A G et al 2003 Patients' and physicians' attitudes regarding the disclosure of medical errors. JAMA 289(8): 1001–1007.

Graham E M, Forouzan I, Morgan M A 1997 A retrospective analysis of Erb's palsy cases and their relation to birth weight and trauma at delivery. J Matern Fetal Med 6(1):1–5.

Hankins G D, MacLennan A H, Speer M E et al 2006 Obstetric litigation is asphyxiating our maternity services. Obstet Gynecol 107(6):1382–1385.

JCAHO 2004 Sentinel Event Alert Issue # 30. Preventing infant death and injury during delivery. USA.

Knox G E, Simpson K R, Garite T J 1999 High reliability perinatal units: an approach to the prevention of patient injury and medical malpractice claims. J Healthc Risk Manag 19(2):24–32.

Lavery J P, Janssen J, Hutchinson L 1999 Is the obstetric guideline of 30 minutes from decision to incision for Caesarean delivery clinically significant? J Healthc Risk Manag 19(1):11–20.

MacLennan A H 2001 A guest editorial from abroad: medicolegal opinion-time for peer review. Obstet Gynecol Surv 56(3):121–123.

MacLennan A, Nelson K B, Hankins G et al 2005 Who will deliver our grandchildren? Implications of cerebral palsy litigation. JAMA 294(13):1688–1690.

MacLennan A, Robinson J 2004 Cerebral palsy and clinical negligence litigation: a cohort study. BJOG 111(1):92–93.

Martin T, Bade D 2002 Professional liability insurance rates — some history & solutions. Mo Med 99(10):532–534.

Meadow W 2005 Evidence-based expert testimony. Clin Perinatol 32(1):251–275, ix.

Meadow W, Lantos J D 1996 Expert testimony, legal reasoning, and justice. The case for adopting a data-based standard of care in allegations of medical negligence in the NICU. Clin Perinatol 23(3):583–595.

Mohr J C 2000 American medical malpractice litigation in historical perspective. JAMA 283(13):1731–1737.

Murray M L 2004 Maternal or fetal heart rate? Avoiding intrapartum misidentification. J Obstet Gynecol Neonatal Nurs 33(1):93–104.

Schifrin B, Harwell R, Rubinstein T et al 2001 Maternal heart rate pattern — a confounding factor in intrapartum fetal surveillance. Prenat Neonat Med 6:75–82.

Scott J R 2005 Expert witnesses: perpetuating a flawed system. Obstet Gynecol 106(5 Pt 1):902–903.

Simpson K R, Knox G E 2000 Risk management and electronic fetal monitoring: decreasing risk of adverse outcomes and liability exposure. J Perinat Neonatal Nurs 14(3):40–52.

Simpson K R, Knox G E 2003 Common areas of litigation related to care during labor and birth: recommendations to promote patient safety and decrease risk exposure. J Perinat Neonatal Nurs 17(2):110–125; quiz 126–127.

Stevenson J R 1999 An expert experiment — medico-legal expert testimony. Med Law 18(1):47–53.

Studdert D M, Mello M M, Gawande A A et al 2006 Claims, errors, and compensation payments in medical malpractice litigation. N Engl J Med 354(19):2024–2033.

Towner D, Castro M A, Eby-Wilkens E et al 1999 Effect of mode of delivery in nulliparous women on neonatal intracranial injury. N Engl J Med 341(23):1709–1714.

Volpe J, Neurology of the newborn, 3rd edn, 2001, Saunders, New York.

Weinstein L 2006 A multifaceted approach to improve patient safety, prevent medical errors and resolve the professional liability crisis. Am J Obstet Gynecol 194(4):1160–1165; discussion 1165–1167.

Woods M M D 2004 'Healing Words: The Power of Apology in Medicine': info@doctorsintouch.com

Zimmerman R 2004 Doctors' new tool to fight lawsuits: saying 'I'm sorry.' Malpractice insurers find owning up to errors soothes patient anger. 'The risks are extraordinary'. J Okla State Med Assoc 97(6):245–247.

CHAPTER

30

Toxoplasmosis

J. Nizard, Guillaume Benoist and Yves G. Ville

MODES OF CONTAMINATION

PARASITOLOGY

Toxoplasma gondii is a single-cell parasite protozoon. The oocyst form is excreted in the feces of cats, the definitive hosts in nature. Toxoplasmosis is spread by ingestion of oocysts or of cysts in their host-tissue either by ingestion of undercooked meat or by congenital vertical transmission. Ingestion of oocysts or tissue cysts will result in the spreading of organisms which will invade the intestinal mucosa and disseminate widely. *Toxoplasma* can infect, replicate and form cysts in all tissues. Tissue cysts persist for the host's lifetime and are considered the most likely cause of recrudescence of disease under particular circumstances such as immunosuppression (Desmonts et al 1990, Pons et al 1995).

MATERNAL INFECTION

Primary infection of the mother is usually asymptomatic, which justifies universal screening during pregnancy in some countries. When symptomatic, fever, malaise, fatigue and lymphadenopathy are the most frequent signs. However, persistent dysphagia and hepatitis can also reveal maternal toxoplasmosis.

CONGENITAL TOXOPLASMOSIS

Congenital transmission of toxoplasmosis occurs when *Toxoplasma* infects the fetus, most probably after having infected the placenta. There seems to be a close correlation between *Toxoplasma* isolation in the placenta and congenital toxoplasmosis (Desmonts & Couvreur 1974). However, the placenta acts as a barrier as well as a reservoir for *Toxoplasma*. Daffos (Daffos et al 1988) reported that in as much as 8% of the cases with an infected placenta, the fetuses and neonates did not show any evidence of seroconversion and remained asymptomatic by ten months after birth. These findings suggest that there must be a placentitis preceding fetal congenital infection (Desmonts & Couvreur 1984). This placentitis may evolve independently from the fetal infection. In up to 27% of cases, fetuses were found to be infected with non-infected placentae (Daffos et al 1988).

The fetus can theoretically only become infected if the mother acquires the infection during pregnancy or when the mother is immunosuppressed, mainly by long-term glucocorticoids treatments, Hodgkin disease, AIDS or systemic lupus erythematosus. Materno-fetal transmission has also been reported to occur in immunocompetent mothers, in whom the toxoplasmosis could be dated to have happened a few weeks prior to the beginning of pregnancy (Desmonts et al 1990, Marty et al 1991, Pons et al 1995, Velin et al 1991). These cases should lead us to advise women to wait at least 6 months before starting a new pregnancy after toxoplasmosis (Couvreur 1999). Nevertheless, there are reported cases of vertical transmission in immunocompetent mothers with a proven proper immunization long before pregnancy (Couvreur 1999, Fortier et al 1991, Gavinet et al 1997, Hennequin et al 1997, Lebas et al 2004). It is suspected that these cases are the consequence of either massive reinfection, or of infection with a different strain.

The vertical transmission rate of the parasite varies from 15% at 13 weeks of gestation, to 44% at 26 weeks and 71% at 36 weeks (Thiebaut et al 2007) (Fig. 30.1a). Desmonts (Desmonts & Couvreur 1974) in 1974 reports that, in all severe cases or fetal deaths, fetal infection was likely to have occurred between the 10th and the 28th week of gestation. On the contrary, in documented cases where infection developed during the third trimester of pregnancy they described subclinical symptoms in 56% and clinical symptoms in 5% of infected neonates (Desmonts & Couvreur 1974) (Fig. 30.1b). It seems that the rate of chorioretinitis is independent of gestational age at infection (Thiebaut et al 2007).

IMMUNOLOGY

IN THE MOTHER

Since maternal infection by *Toxoplasma gondii* is rarely diagnosed clinically, the diagnosis relies almost exclusively on biological and immunological findings to document infection and subsequent seroconversion. The parasitemia seems to occur very early after the infection and resume shortly after. It is therefore likely that placental infection, secondary to maternal parasitemia, also occurs very early after maternal acute infection. Thus, placenta infection occurs before any treatment is started.

Some cases of chronic parasitemia have however been described. It is uncertain whether chronic parasitemia is responsible for congenital toxoplasmosis, and whether it can disappear after appropriate treatment (Miller et al 1969).

A large number of different immunological tests can be used. *Toxoplasma* infection can be detected by the appearance of specific antibodies. The real challenge is to date precisely maternal seroconversion.

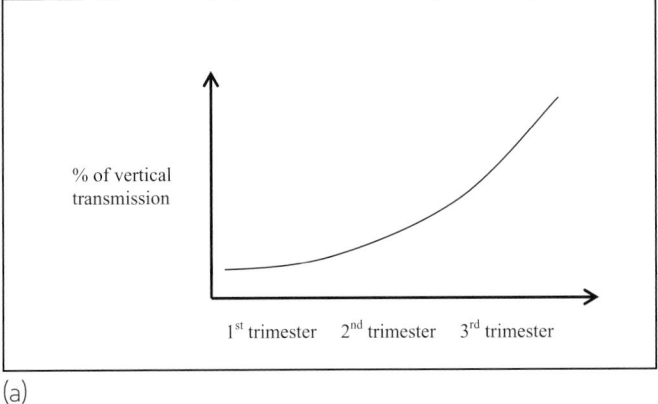

(a)

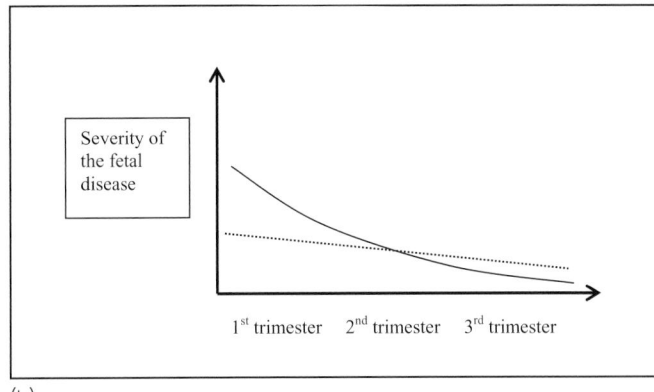

(b)

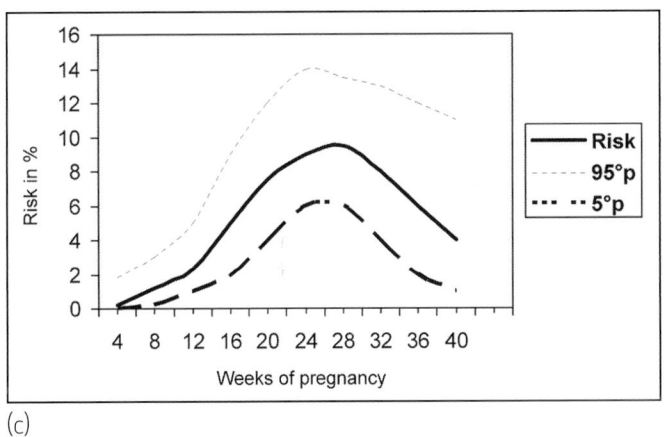

(c)

Figure 30.1 (a) Schematic representation of the vertical transmission of toxoplasmosis depending on the trimester of maternal seroconversion. (b) Schematic representation of the severity of the fetal affection depending on the trimester of maternal seroconversion (intracranial lesions; chorioretinitis). (c) Estimate risk of clinical signs before age 3 years according to the term of maternal seroconversion, when fetal infectious status is known (Dunn et al 1999).

The Sabin–Feldman dye test is one of the first to have been used on a large epidemiological scale. It is testing the presence of specific anti-*Toxoplasma* antibodies in the mother using the lytic capacity of the tested serum on live *Toxoplasma*. Sabin–Felman test is expressed in international units (IU) per milliliter of serum and is said to be high above 300 UI/mL. Indirect hemagglutination test (IHA) uses the agglutination of red blood cells expressing *Toxoplasma* antigens when exposed to serum containing anti-*Toxoplasma* IgG or IgM antibodies. Agglutination test is sensitive to IgM antibodies and can be used on a large scale in pregnant women. Conventional indirect fluorescent antibody test (IFA) detects specific antibodies using fluorescent-tagged specific *Toxoplasma* antigens and serum gammaglobulins. IFA is considered to be as specific as the dye test, provided it is not used in the serum of women with connective tissue disorder. IFA is considered high above a titer of 1:1000 (Dannemann et al 1990, Thulliez et al 1986). The conventional or capture enzyme-linked immunosorbent assay (ELISA) can be used independently to detect specific anti-*Toxoplasma* IgG, IgM or IgA (Stepick-Biek et al 1990). Immunosorbent agglutination assay (ISAGA) can detect anti-*Toxoplasma* IgG, IgM and IgE. Other specific tests can be used to detect selectively anti-*Toxoplasma* IgM antibodies such as the IgM fluorescent antibody test or the IgM enzyme-linked immunosorbent assay (Naot et al 1981). Finally, IgG

avidity for *Toxoplasma* antigens has become an essential step in difficult circumstances. This test can separate low-affinity IgG antibodies, which are produced at an early stage of the infection (<4 months), from higher binding affinity IgG antibodies that reflect past immunity (>4 months) (Jenum et al 1997, Lappalainen et al 1993).

A conventional single-serum assay does not make a clear distinction between a primary and a chronic infection, it only makes the diagnosis of toxoplasmosis. Specific IgM can persist for a long time, even at high levels. Elements in favor of a recent seroconversion (primary infection) are: the rise from negative or low titers to high titers at two different serum samples for the dye test, IHA or IFA and/or the rise from negative or low titers to high titers of specific IgM tests in two different serum samples 2–3 weeks apart. It is only when this does not support clearly the scenario of seroconversion that testing for IgG affinity or using specific assay for IgA and IgE can be helpful and is required (Lappalainen et al 1993).

IN THE FETUS AND THE NEWBORN

All these tests can be applied to fetuses and neonates, provided the serum sample is available. However the diagnosis of congenital toxoplasmosis in fetuses and newborns is more often based on the finding of toxoplasmosis DNA in the amniotic fluid rather than on immunological criteria. It is not clear whether the antibody response of the fetus/neonate is aimed at the same antigens. Low-molecular weight IgG can cross the placenta and therefore a fetus/neonate immunological answer to *Toxoplasma* will be detected by the presence of specific IgM, IgA or IgE in fetal/neonatal blood (Fortier et al 1997, Pinon et al 1996, Pratlong et al 1996).

EPIDEMIOLOGY

Seroprevalence for *Toxoplasma* among pregnant women varies widely not only from country to country but also from region to region within a given country. The relevance of a universal screening program for pregnant women to detect seronegative women, and perform subsequent serial screening of seronegative women for *Toxoplasma* through pregnancy depends on the seroprevalence and the incidence of seroconversion during pregnancy. It is therefore important to know the differences in different countries for these parameters. Table 30.1 shows a non-exhaustive list of recent studies on seroprevalence and incidence of toxoplasmosis in different countries.

Seroprevalence for toxoplasmosis increases with maternal age and parity (Ades & Nokes 1993, Allain et al 1998, Jenum et al 1998, Ljungstrom et al 1995, Valcavi et al 1995). It also depends upon ethnicity, influenced by cooking and eating habits (Gilbert et al 1993).

The incidence of toxoplasmosis among seronegative women depends primarily upon the prevalence in the general population. It ranges from 0.03% to 2.6% among seronegative women (Allain et al 1998, Ljungstrom et al 1995).

PREVENTION

Primary prevention is derived from the different modes of contamination: ingestion of oocysts from cat feces either directly by contact with cats or indirectly by contact with objects or food contaminated by cat feces, or by ingestion of meat containing cysts. Prevention should target seronegative pregnant women. This is therefore only possible in countries where serologic status is known, ideally before pregnancy.

Primary prevention of maternal toxoplasmosis, as well as that of immunodeficient patients, is based on education. The following recommendations should be given: meat should be cooked well done. Hands must be washed after handling raw meat and must not touch the eyes or mouth. Fruits and

Table 30.1 Seroprevalence and incidence of toxoplasmosis in different countries from recent studies	
Country	Seroprevalence and incidence if available
Sweden	Seroprevalence from 12 to 26% with a declining gradient from south to north. The estimated incidence of maternal toxoplasmosis ranges from 0.2% to 2.6% of susceptible pregnancies (Ljungstrom et al 1995).
Italy	Area of Parma: seroprevalence of 48.7% with an observed incidence of 0.27 to 0,69% (Valcavi et al 1995). Area of Naples: seroprevalence of 39% of pregnant women and 1.2% probably recently infected before the pregnancy (Buffolano et al 1996)
Norway	Seroprevalence of 10.9% among pregnant women with a decline from south to north (Jenum et al 1998)
UK	Eastern England: seroprevalence of 7.7% among pregnant women with 0.4% recent seroconversions. The estimated incidence of seroconversion ranges from 0.03–0.16% of pregnancies (Allain et al 1998). South Yorkshire: seroprevalence in a general population aged 20–40 years of age from 22.2% in 1969–1973 to 7.8% in 1988–1990 (Ades & Nokes 1993) West London: seroprevalence from 7.6 to 71.4%, with an average of 18.8%, these variations depend on the country of birth and ethnic group (Gilbert et al 1993)
Switzerland	Seroprevalence of 46.7% of pregnant women with an estimated incidence of 2.4% (Zuber & Jacquier 1995)
France	Paris: seroprevalence of 71% among French pregnant women and 52.4% among immigrant pregnant women with an estimated incidence of 1.6% seroconversion in susceptible pregnant women similar in French and non-French subpopulation (Jeannel et al 1988). Thirty years ago the incidence was estimated to be 6.3% among seronegative immigrant women in Paris and 1‰ in the general population (Desmonts & Couvreur 1974)
Bangladesh	Seroprevalence of 38.5% of pregnant women with wide variations according to socioeconomic status (Ashrafunnessa et al 1998)
Denmark	Seroprevalence of 27.8% with an estimated incidence of 0.2% of seroconversion among seronegative women (Lebech et al 1999)
Germany	Seroprevalence of 41.6% of pregnant women, the incidence of toxoplasmosis was 0.52% (Roos et al 1993)
Belgium	Brussels: seroprevalence of 53%, with an incidence of 1.4% to starting a program of counseling seronegative mothers. It was reduced to 0.53% after (Foulon et al 1984)
Greece	Seroprevalence estimated at 52.3% of pregnant women (Decavalas et al 1990)

vegetables must be washed before consumption and hands must be washed after handling them. Women should avoid contact with cats and cat litter boxes and finally avoid gardening or wear gloves when gardening (Foulon et al 1988, McCabe & Remington 1988).

Prevention of congenital toxoplasmosis is based on the identification of women at risk (i.e. seronegative women), treatment of women with seroconversion during pregnancy to reduce the risk of vertical transmission of the parasite, and termination of severely affected fetuses according to parents' wish after extensive counseling if the legislation of the country allows (Foulon et al 1988, McCabe & Remington 1988). Freezing meat seems to be efficient if it can be done for long enough (>24 hours) and at a temperature below −20°C. If these conditions cannot be met, freezing should not be proposed as a method of prevention of toxoplasmosis (McCabe & Remington 1988).

With these measures of primary prevention of maternal seroconversion, Foulon et al (1988) found a decrease of seroconversion during pregnancy among initially seronegative women from 1.43% (20 of 1403) over 1979 to 1982 when women had no particular recommendations concerning prevention to 0.95% (15 of 1571) over 1983 to 1986 following preventive measures. This reduction in the seroconversion rate of 34% was not statistically significant. When the same authors continued their study and included seronegative women who were given recommendations during pregnancy up to 1990, they found a reduction rate of seroconversion of 63%, going from 1.43% (20 of 1403) to 0.53% (19 of 3605). This reduction was found to be statistically significant and thus suggests that primary prevention can reduce the number of seroconversions during pregnancy.

Another way of prevention is acting on the parasite before it can directly or indirectly contaminate humans. This has been tried by vaccination of sheep against *Toxoplasma gondii* (Buxton 1998, Buxton et al 1993, Wastling et al 1994). Vaccination seems to be effective in sheep and could reduce the prevalence in humans in countries like France or Austria in the not too distant future.

CONGENITAL TOXOPLASMOSIS

The aim of diagnosing maternal toxoplasmosis is the prevention of materno-fetal transmission. The aim of diagnosis of fetal toxoplasmosis is to evaluate the severity of the disease in order to either treat the mother to reduce the severity of the disease in the fetus or terminate the pregnancy where applicable.

IN THE FETUS

The diagnosis of congenital toxoplasmosis may be attempted in utero when the mother develops primary toxoplasmosis either during the months preceding pregnancy (arbitrarily 6 months) or during pregnancy. To affect the fetus, the parasite first infects the placenta. The rate of transmission from the mother to the fetus is known and depends on gestational age (Fig. 30.1a,b). Overall, the rate of maternal–fetal transmission seems to be influenced by the delay between maternal seroconversion and initiation of treatment. There seems to be a benefit in vertical transmission when the treatment is initiated within 3 weeks compared to after 8 weeks after maternal seroconversion (Thiebaut et al 2007). The probability of transmission increases with gestation, whereas the severity of fetal infection decreases with gestation. Therefore, there are fewer cases of very early congenital toxoplasmosis, but they tend to be more severe. On the other hand, there are more congenital infections acquired at the end of the pregnancy but they tend to be less symptomatic. Thus, the largest number of severe cases occurs during the second trimester of pregnancy (Mombro et al 1995). It is important to consider that chorioretinitis rate is stable through gestational age (Thiebaut et al 2007). It is the rate of intracranial lesions that diminishes with gestational age at seroconversion.

The diagnosis of congenital toxoplasmosis in the fetus can be made using a combination of ultrasound examination and detection of the *Toxoplasma* in the amniotic fluid directly or by using polymerase-chain-reaction (PCR). Fetal blood sampling is feasible after 20 weeks of gestation. Fetal blood sampling after 20 weeks of gestation for *Toxoplasma* isolation or measuring specific *Toxoplasma* IgM and IgA and non-specific biological markers are no longer used for diagnostic purposes. The detection of *Toxoplasma* is done by intraperitoneal inoculation of the tested sample to the mouse. The drawback of this method is the 4 to 6 weeks delay to prove the isolation of the parasite. Before the development of PCR amplification of the parasite's DNA from amniotic fluid, the use of fetal blood sampling and ultrasound examination detected 83 to 92% of infected fetuses (Daffos et al 1988, Pratlong et al 1994).

PCR on amniotic fluid seems to have better results than the conventional method alone, with a sensitivity of 97.4% (95% CI 86.1–99.9) compared with 89.5% (95% CI 75.2–97.0%) and the same 100% specificity (95% CI 98.8–100) (Hohlfeld et al 1994). This technique, as the former ones, is dependent upon the experience of the laboratory and therefore pleads for processing all samples in a reference laboratory which will be able to control for technical pitfalls and provide with the most reliable interpretation of the tests.

For non-specific blood test, the main parameters are elevated eosinophils, thrombocytopenia, elevated gamma-GT and elevated LDH (Pratlong et al 1996). Asymptomatic infected fetuses would only show at most some degree of growth retardation as a marker of placental infection which can also typically show increased placental width which may also contain areas of calcifications or necrosis (Fig. 30.2A). When PCR on amniotic fluid is positive for *Toxoplasma* DNA, the diagnosis of an affected fetus is usually made by a combination of the following signs (Pratlong et al 1994): evidence of liver or other systemic failure with hepatomegaly (Fig. 30.2B) and ascites (Fig. 30.2F);

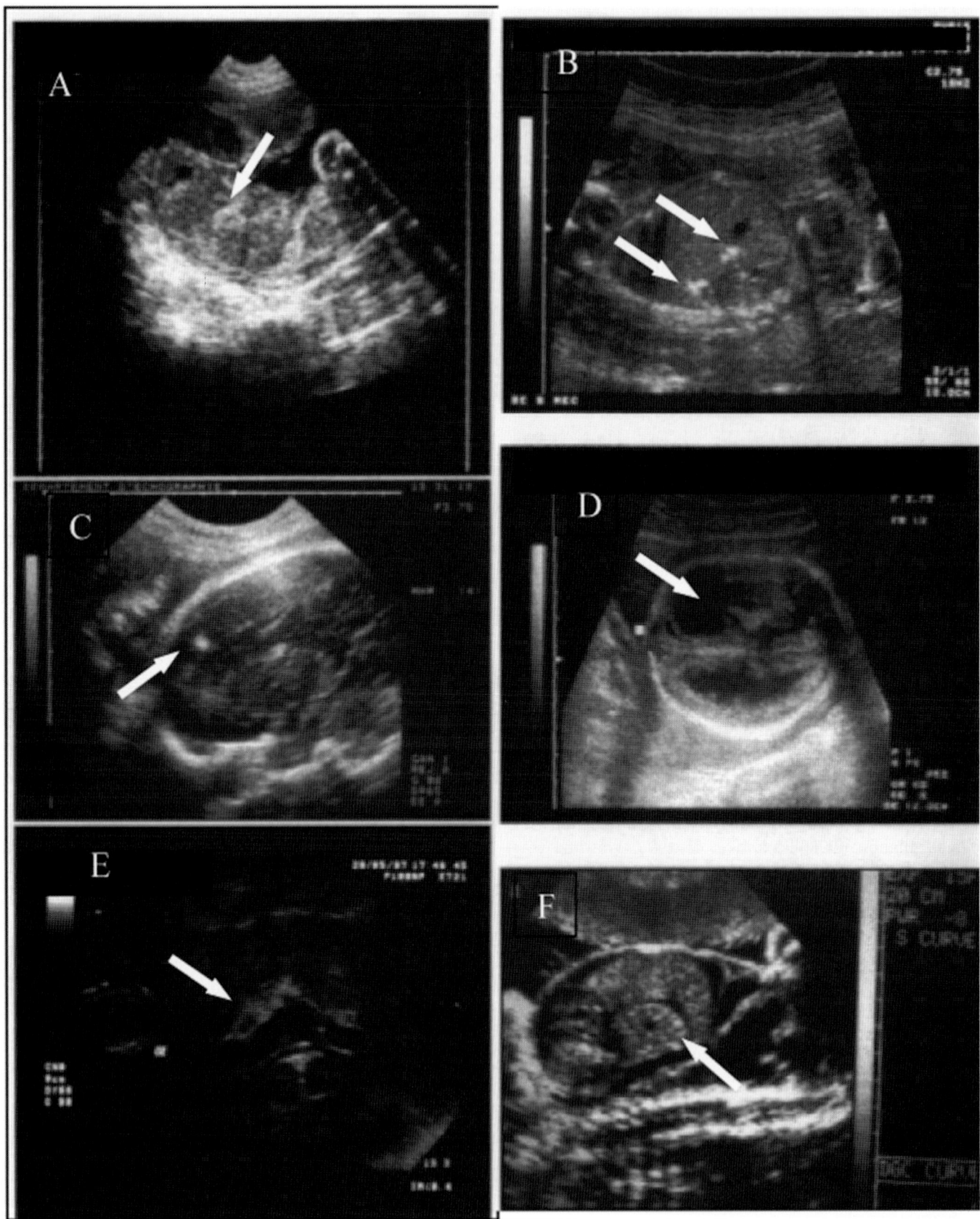

Figure 30.2 Pathological ultrasound findings during congenital toxoplasmosis. Arrows represent: in (A) a placentitis; in (B) hepatic calcifications; in (C) cerebral calcifications; in (D) destructive bilateral ventriculomegaly; in (E) another type of destructive ventriculomegaly; in (F) hyperechoic bowel with ascites.

hyperechogenic bowel (Fig. 30.2F) and/or intrauterine growth retardation that can be severe with normal Doppler, which should raise suspicion towards an infection. The neurological signs are both the most evocative and severe. Microcephaly is a major but late sign of severe affection. Unilateral or bilateral dilatation of the lateral ventricles of the brain with or without hydrocephaly are the most classic features (Fig. 30.2D,E), whereas intracranial calcifications or patchy hyperechogenic areas featuring areas of necrosis within the white matter are the most specific features for toxoplasmosis (Fig. 30.2C). Toxoplasmosis could be responsible for foci of necrotic encephalitis even if the ultrasound examination is normal, but these studies are now old (Desmonts et al 1985).

Most importantly, one should be aware that transplacental infection is dependent upon the ability of the placenta to prevent the passage of the parasite which can therefore be delayed as can also be the development of the fetal lesions. It is therefore mandatory to follow up the infected fetuses by serial targeted ultrasound examination every fortnight in a referral center. Indeed, subtle changes such as eye lesions (Lakhanpal et al 1983, Rothova et al 1993) could only be picked up by trained sonographers and would mandate appropriate counseling and other investigations such as intrauterine MRI in order to refine the prognosis. When PCR for *Toxoplasma* DNA is positive, ultrasound examination should be carried out every month. When maternal seroconversion occurs during the first trimester of pregnancy and subsequent ultrasound follow-up is normal, prognosis seems good with 78% subclinical toxoplasmosis and 19% chorioretinitis without major vision loss (Berrebi et al 2006). In this series, one child in 38 developed severe congenital toxoplasmosis. All mothers were treated.

IN THE NEONATE

When congenital toxoplasmosis is diagnosed in utero, clinical disease represents that approximately 25% of the cases will be asymptomatic (Daffos et al 1988, Desmonts et al 1985, Hohlfeld et al 1989, Pratlong et al 1996).

This rate may be dependent upon treatment of the mother during pregnancy. Up to recently, it was assumed that the percentage of infected neonates from mothers who seroconverted during the pregnancy was likely to be lower if the treatment was adequate, than if is inadequate or absent (Desmonts & Couvreur 1984, Mombro et al 1995). The Syrocot Study Group published a meta-analysis on individual patients' data showing that there seems to be no evidence that prenatal treatment significantly reduces the risk of clinical manifestations. These findings were consistent irrespective of the treatment sequence used (Thiebaut et al 2007).

Infected neonates are not always symptomatic at birth. Clinical symptoms can sometimes appear several years after birth and in some cases be severe (Wilson et al 1980). The consequences of congenital toxoplasmosis are:

Neurological: the most commonly described abnormalities, although rare, are mental retardation, microcephalus, hydrocephalus and its complications, motor disabilities, with sometimes hemiplegia and epilepsy (McAuley et al 1994). Roizen (Roizen et al 1995) described cases with seizures and motor abnormalities that resolve under treatment. He also described discontinuation of anticonvulsant therapy after adequate treatment of the neonate. These same children, that were treated for a year and followed up for 10 years, had cognitive functions mildly impaired when compared to non-infected children, but above the cognitive function of infected children with only a short course or no treatment. Radiologically, intracranial calcifications are very common signs that can be seen with or without symptoms. Patel showed that these calcifications were not stable and that their evolution depended upon treatment given to the child (Patel et al 1996). Children with at least one year of treatment after birth tend to have less intracranial calcifications, as opposed to children with short or no treatment who had calcifications that remained stable or even progressed further.

Ophthalmological: chorioretinitis is the most frequent complication of congenital toxoplasmosis. *Toxoplasma* invades the retina of the fetus, where it may change into the cyst form. Chorioretinitis and its most adverse consequences, severe visual loss and blindness, are thought to happen when cysts rupture and release parasites that multiply in the surrounding cells. Lesions are not always present at birth and most of them will appear during the first year of life. The occurrence of chorioretinitis is independent of the timing of maternal seroconversion and maternal–fetal transmission (Thiebaut et al 2007). Lesions may appear only after several years, justifying long-term treatment and follow-up even when the child is asymptomatic at birth (Guerina et al 1994, Koppe et al 1986, Peyron et al 1996, Wilson et al 1980). The probability of recurrence of acute episodes of chorioretinitis is around 50% (Rothova et al 1993).

Others: intrauterine death or spontaneous abortion, severe disseminated parasitemia that can result in death or serious handicap. It is estimated that the probability of intrauterine fetal demise or termination of pregnancy is 2% in a population of infected pregnancies (Thiebaut et al 2007). Neonatal complications also include hypoxia and hypoglycemia that can also cause neurological disabilities.

TREATMENT

In utero treatment includes the prevention of transmission of *Toxoplasma* from the mother to the fetus when the mother presents with acute infection and the reduction of the severity of the symptoms in the fetus and in the neonate.

Postnatal treatment aims at reducing the number of acute phases of infection and at decreasing the severity of the symptoms.

Treatment is ineffective on the cyst form within tissues. The aim of the treatment is to stop the replication of the parasite during the invasive phase of the infection.

Treatment does not seem to reduce the inflammation in chorioretinitis, which is more dependent upon the initial severity of the lesion (Rothova et al 1993). However, it is unclear whether early treatment of congenital toxoplasmosis can decrease the incidence of lesions in neonates (Couvreur et al 1984, Thiebaut et al 2007). Ideally, treatment should be used during the acute phase of disease in mothers. However, when maternal seroconversion is diagnosed, the acute phase is resumed, thus limiting the efficacy of any treatment.

Treatment usually combines different drugs. Some can cross the placenta and reach the fetus, some only get to the maternal circulation.

- Pyrimethamine is a folic acid antagonist. It can therefore depress the bone marrow and give most often only a macrocytic anemia, neutropenia or thrombopenia. It should therefore be associated to folinic acid that only the human cells can use. Folinic acid does not reduce the efficacy of pyrimethamine against *Toxoplasma*.
- Sulfonamide, associated to pyrimethamine and folinic acid, is the treatment of reference of an active infection.
- Spiramycin is the most commonly used macrolide to prevent placental passage of *Toxoplasma* in mothers who seroconverted. It is probably not effective in fetuses already infected and does not prevent for example neurotoxoplasmosis in immunosuppressed patients (Leport et al 1986).
- Corticosteroids are used in chorioretinitis to limit the inflammatory process.
- Clindamycin is commonly used instead of spiramycin in cases with proven allergy (Lakhanpal et al 1983).
- Trimethoprim associated with sulfamethoxazole (cotrimoxazole).
- Azithromycin and clarithromycin, both recent macrolides, are effective against *Toxoplasma gondii* and increase the effectiveness such as associations like pyrimethamine-sulfonamide at least in vitro (Alder et al 1994, Araujo et al 1988, Cantin & Chamberland 1993, Derouin 1995, Derouin et al 1992). Moreover, azithromycin was found effective on the cyst form in vitro (Huskinson-Mark et al 1991).

PREVENTION OF FETAL INFECTION IN ACUTE MATERNAL INFECTION JUST BEFORE OR DURING THE FIRST OR SECOND TRIMESTER OF PREGNANCY (Fig. 30.3)

If the vertical transmission occurs during the first or second trimester, the risk of severe fetal affection is important. Transmission is however rare. It is therefore important to make the diagnosis of fetal infection. It is best done by PCR amplification of the *Toxoplasma* genome in amniotic fluid after amniocentesis.

If the fetus is not infected (i.e. PCR negative or before amniocentesis)

Spiramycin is the drug most widely used. It seems to reduce the frequency of placentitis thus hopefully reducing the number of infected fetuses. Studies support that there were less infected fetuses with treatment, in each trimester of the pregnancy (Desmonts & Couvreur 1974). In this study, using prevention by spiramycin, only 24% of the fetuses from infected mothers were infected and a total of 11% of fetuses had a clinical disease. Spiramycin is said not to be curative for the fetus. The prevention of fetal toxoplasmosis by spiramycin, or other drugs, is not well established for all. Wallon (Wallon et al 1999), reviewing several studies, concludes that there are 'no good comparative data measuring the potential harms and benefits of antiparasitic drugs used for presumed antenatal *Toxoplasma* infection'. This statement was confirmed by Foulon (Foulon et al 1999) in a large multicenter study who found that the maternal–fetal transmission depended more upon gestational age at which the infection occurred than upon any treatment given to the mother. This is probably because placentitis occurs very early after maternal infection, hence before any treatment is given. Once more, by meta-analysis the Syrocot Study Group showed that only treatment given less than three weeks from maternal seroconversion seems to reduce the risk of vertical transmission.

If the fetus is infected (i.e. PCR positive on amniotic fluid), there are two possibilities

If monthly ultrasound examination is normal, the risk of severe congenital toxoplasmosis after birth is estimated to be less than 5% (Berrebi et al 2006). These patients are commonly switched from spiramycin to pyrimethamine-sulfonamide.

If ultrasound examination is abnormal, parents opt for either treatment by pyrimethamine-sulfonamide or termination of pregnancy following extensive counseling when applicable. It is nevertheless important to explain that up to now, there is no evidence that any treatment reduces the incidence of clinical manifestations in infancy (Thiebaut et al 2007). Termination of pregnancy is a possibility in severely affected cases, when legally and ethically possible. It is mainly done when fetal infection occurs during the first or second trimester of pregnancy, in 30 to 50% of the cases of infected fetuses (Daffos et al 1988, Hohlfeld et al 1989). Looking at recent and well documented studies, 60% of children born with congenital toxoplasmosis had no clinical or laboratory abnormality, and within the remaining 40% only 4% had symptoms at follow-up (Berrebi et al 1994). It is therefore very difficult to asses the risk of handicap in an infected fetus and to justify a termination of pregnancy.

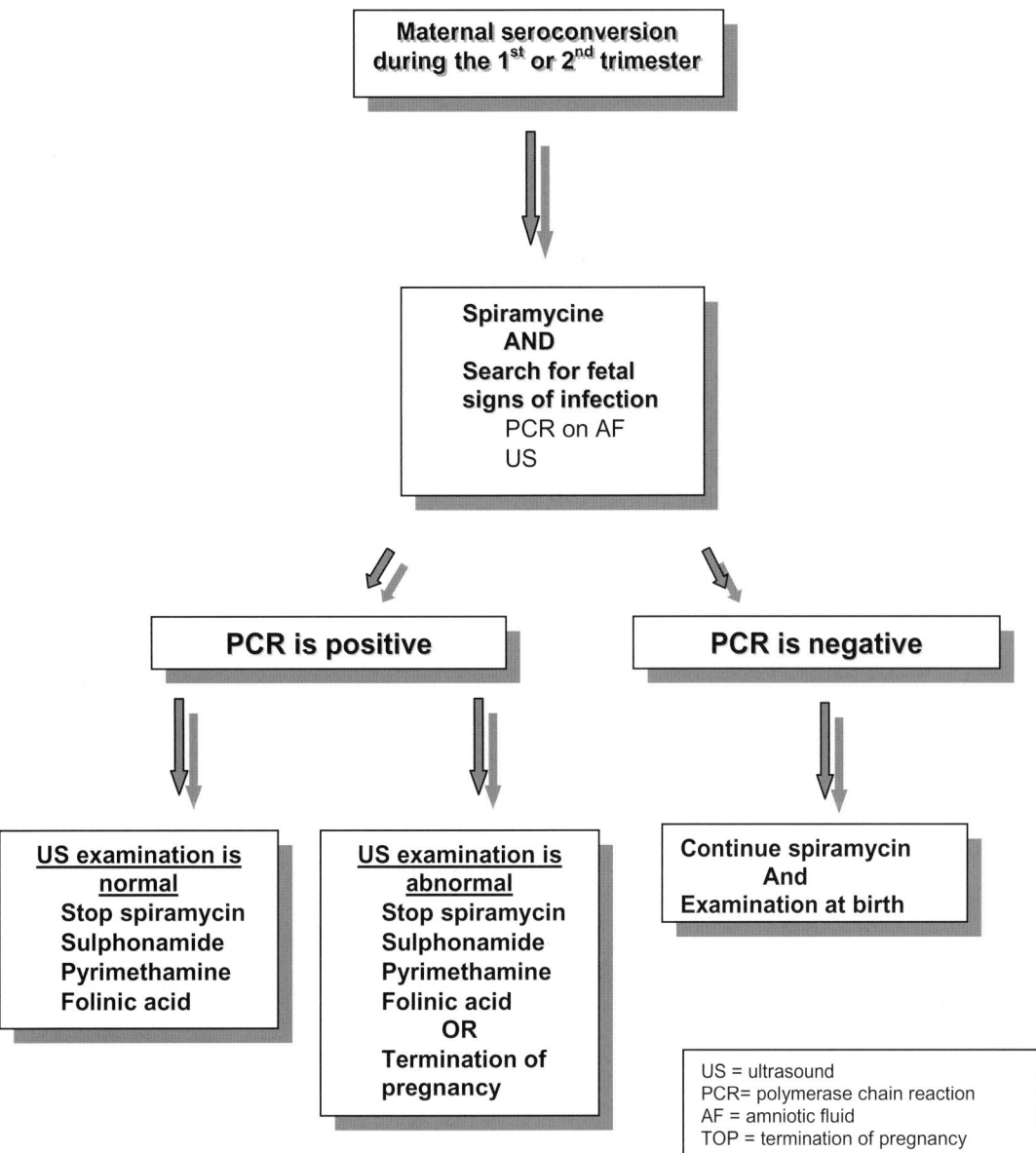

Figure 30.3 Management of maternal seroconversion during the first or second trimesters.

PREVENTION OF FETAL INFECTION WHEN THE MOTHER DEVELOPS ACUTE INFECTION JUST BEFORE OR DURING THE THIRD TRIMESTER OF PREGNANCY (Fig. 30.4)

The incidence of vertical transmission is very high here. The probability of severe neurological affection is rare but the risk of chorioretinitis is constant both in utero and after birth. The diagnosis of fetal infection is also made by combining PCR on amniotic fluid and ultrasound findings, but there is a risk of false negative results. We can either treat these fetuses as if they were infected or perform amniocentesis and serial ultrasound examination after starting spiramycin treatment. This will be continued up to delivery and placenta and cord blood will be examined for infection.

AT BIRTH

The attitude depends on the infectious status of the fetus and the results of the neonatal examination.

If the diagnosis of fetal infection was negative, investigations that should be performed after birth include:

- Parasitology of the placenta and the fetal blood.
- Neurological and ophthalmological examination.
- Ultrasound examination of the central nervous system.
- Neonatal immunological status.

It is important to be cautious with false negative results on amniotic fluid in the third trimester of pregnancy. An infected neonate, whether symptomatic or asymptomatic,

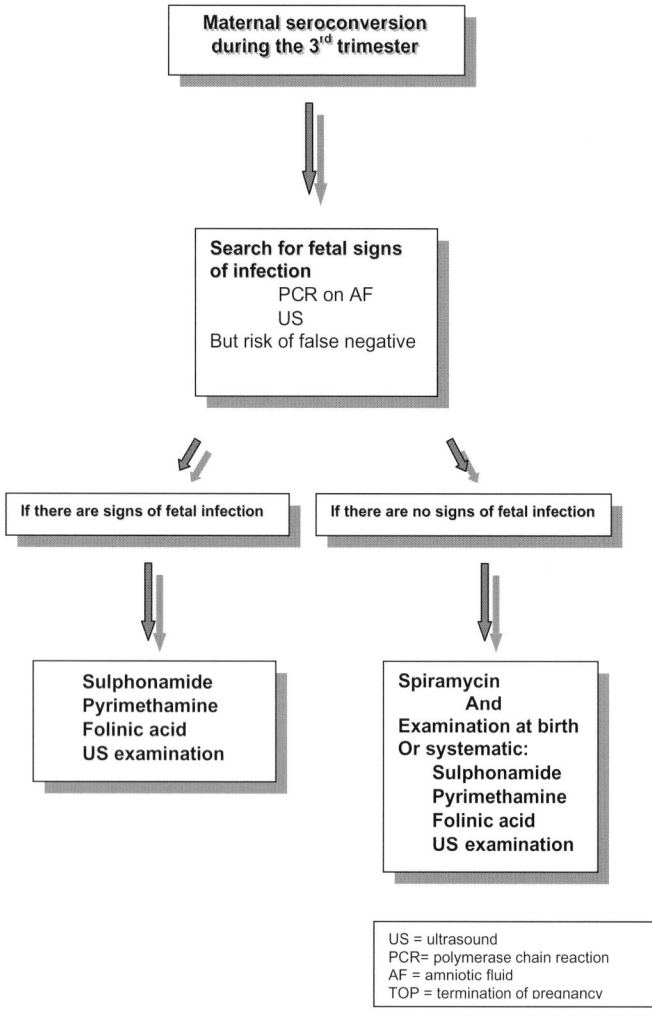

Figure 30.4 Management of maternal seroconversion during the third trimester.

will be treated by alternate treatment of pyrimethamine-sulfonamide-folinic acid for 3–4 weeks, followed by 4 to 6 weeks of spiramycin and so on for at least a year. Pyrimethamine-sulfonamide-folinic acid can also be used alone for a year. New lesions of chorioretinitis seem to develop less often during the first year of life in children receiving several courses of treatment (Couvreur et al 1984). The long term follow-up study of the Chicago Collaborative Treatment Trial (McAuley et al 1994), up to 10 years, suggested that after one year of treatment up to 70% of infants with severe central nervous system and ophthalmologic involvement at birth developed normally. Delay in diagnosis and therapy is indicative of a poor prognosis. It is noteworthy that only one infant was diagnosed with congenital toxoplasmosis in utero and all others after birth. Treatment is also known to decrease the occurrence and the development of intracranial calcifications.

The association of pyrimethamine-sulfonamide during pregnancy when the fetus is infected decreases the fetal immunological reaction to infection in the first year of life more than spiramycin alone (Fortier et al 1997). The association of pyrimethamine, sulfonamide and corticosteroids seems to be more efficient than the association of clindamycin-corticosteroids, cotrimoxazole-corticosteroids or no treatment in chorioretinitis (Rothova et al 1993). The treatment should be followed for at least one year and the follow-up continued until adolescence.

If the diagnosis of fetal infection was positive:

The most important thing here is not the diagnosis but the prognosis. Neonatal examination is usually easy:

- neurological and ophthalmological examination
- ultrasound examination of the central nervous system

The treatment started in utero should be continued and there will be a long-term follow-up.

REFERENCES

Ades A E, Nokes D J 1993 Modeling age- and time-specific incidence from seroprevalence: toxoplasmosis. Am J Epidemiol 137(9): 1022–1034.

Alder J, Hutch T, Meulbroek J A, Clement J C 1994 Treatment of experimental *Toxoplasma gondii* infection by clarithromycin-based combination therapy with minocycline or pyrimethamine. J Acquir Immune Defic Syndr 7(11):1141–1148.

Allain J P, Palmer C R, Pearson G 1998 Epidemiological study of latent and recent infection by *Toxoplasma gondii* in pregnant women from a regional population in the U.K. J Infect 36(2):189–196.

Araujo F G, Guptill D R, Remington J S 1988 Azithromycin, a macrolide antibiotic with potent activity against *Toxoplasma gondii*. Antimicrob Agents Chemother 32(5):755–757.

Ashrafunnessa, Khatun S, Islam M N, Huq T 1998 Seroprevalence of *Toxoplasma* antibodies among

the antenatal population in Bangladesh. J Obstet Gynaecol Res 24(2):115–119.

Berrebi A, Bardou M, Bessieres M H et al 2006 Outcome for children infected with congenital toxoplasmosis in the first trimester and with normal ultrasound findings: a study of 36 cases. Eur J Obstet Gynecol Reprod Biol (in press).

Berrebi A, Kobuch W E, Bessieres M H et al 1994 Termination of pregnancy for maternal toxoplasmosis. Lancet 344(8914):36–39.

Buffolano W, Gilbert R E, Holland F J et al 1996 Risk factors for recent toxoplasma infection in pregnant women in Naples. Epidemiol Infect 116(3):347–351.

Buxton D 1998 Protozoan infections (*Toxoplasma gondii*, *Neospora caninum* and *Sarcocystis* spp.) in sheep and goats: recent advances. Vet Res 29(3–4):289–310.

Buxton D, Thomson K M, Maley S, 1993 Experimental challenge of sheep 18 months after vaccination with

a live (S48) *Toxoplasma gondii* vaccine. Vet Rec 133(13):310–312.

Cantin L, Chamberland S 1993 In vitro evaluation of the activities of azithromycin alone and combined with pyrimethamine against *Toxoplasma gondii*. Antimicrob Agents Chemother 37(9):1993–1996.

Couvreur J 1999 Problems of congenital toxoplasmosis. Evolution over four decades. Presse Med 28(14):753–757.

Couvreur J, Desmonts G, Aron-Rosa D 1984 Ocular prognosis in congenital toxoplasmosis: the role of treatment. Preliminary communication. Ann Pediatr (Paris) 31(10):855–858.

Daffos F, Forestier F, Capella-Pavlovsky M et al 1988 Prenatal management of 746 pregnancies at risk for congenital toxoplasmosis. N Engl J Med 318(5):271–275.

Dannemann B R, Vaughan W C, Thulliez P, Remington J S 1990 Differential agglutination test for diagnosis of recently acquired infection with *Toxoplasma gondii*. J Clin Microbiol 28(9):1928–1933.

Decavalas G, Papapetropoulou M, Giannoulaki E et al 1990 Prevalence of *Toxoplasma gondii* antibodies in gravidas and recently aborted women and study of risk factors. Eur J Epidemiol 6(2):223–226.

Derouin F 1995 New pathogens and mode of action of azithromycin: *Toxoplasma gondii*. Pathol Biol (Paris) 43(6):561–564.

Derouin F, Almadany R, Chau F et al 1992 Synergistic activity of azithromycin and pyrimethamine or sulfadiazine in acute experimental toxoplasmosis. Antimicrob Agents Chemother 36(5):997–1001.

Desmonts G, Couvreur J 1974 Congenital toxoplasmosis. A prospective study of 378 pregnancies. N Engl J Med 290(20):1110–1116.

Desmonts G, Couvreur J 1984 Congenital toxoplasmosis. Prospective study of the outcome of pregnancy in 542 women with toxoplasmosis acquired during pregnancy. Ann Pediatr (Paris) 31(10):805–809.

Desmonts G, Couvreur J 1984 Natural history of congenital toxoplasmosis. Ann Pediatr (Paris) 31(10):799–802.

Desmonts G, Couvreur J, Thulliez P 1990 Congenital toxoplasmosis. 5 cases of mother-to-child transmission of pre-pregnancy infection. Presse Med 19(31):1445–1449.

Desmonts G, Daffos F, Forestier F et al 1985 Prenatal diagnosis of congenital toxoplasmosis. Lancet 1(8427):500–504.

Dunn D, Wallon M, Peyron F et al 1999 Mother-to-child transmission of toxoplasmosis: risk estimates for clinical counselling. Lancet 353(9167):1829–1833.

Fortier B, Ajana F, Pinto de Sousa M I et al 1991 Prevention and treatment of materno-fetal toxoplasmosis. Presse Med 20(29):1374–1383.

Fortier B, Coignard-Chatain C, Dao A et al 1997 Study of developing clinical outbreak and serological rebounds in children with congenital toxoplasmosis and follow-up during the first 2 years of life. Arch Pediatr 4(10):940–946.

Foulon W, Naessens A, Lauwers S et al 1988 Impact of primary prevention on the incidence of toxoplasmosis during pregnancy. Obstet Gynecol 72(3 Pt 1):363–366.

Foulon W, Naessens A, Volckaert M et al 1984 Congenital toxoplasmosis: a prospective survey in Brussels. Br J Obstet Gynaecol 91(5):419–423.

Foulon W, Villena I, Stray-Pedersen B et al 1999 Treatment of toxoplasmosis during pregnancy: a multicenter study of impact on fetal transmission and children's sequelae at age 1 year. Am J Obstet Gynecol 180(2 Pt 1):410–415.

Gavinet M F, Robert F, Firtion G et al 1997 Congenital toxoplasmosis due to maternal reinfection during pregnancy. J Clin Microbiol 35(5):1276–1277.

Gilbert R E, Tookey P A, Cubitt W D et al 1993 Prevalence of toxoplasma IgG among pregnant women in west London according to country of birth and ethnic group. BMJ 306(6871):185.

Guerina N G, Hsu H W, Meissner H C et al 1994 Neonatal serologic screening and early treatment for congenital *Toxoplasma gondii* infection. The New England Regional *Toxoplasma* Working Group. N Engl J Med 330(26):1858–1863.

Hennequin C, Dureau P, N'Guyen L et al 1997 Congenital toxoplasmosis acquired from an immune woman. Pediatr Infect Dis J 16(1):75–77.

Hohlfeld P, Daffos F, Costa J M et al 1994 Prenatal diagnosis of congenital toxoplasmosis with a polymerase-chain-reaction test on amniotic fluid. N Engl J Med 331(11):695–699.

Hohlfeld P, Daffos F, Thulliez P et al 1989 Fetal toxoplasmosis: outcome of pregnancy and infant follow-up after in utero treatment. J Pediatr 115(5 Pt 1):765–769.

Huskinson-Mark J, Araujo F G, Remington J S 1991 Evaluation of the effect of drugs on the cyst form of *Toxoplasma gondii*. J Infect Dis 164(1):170–171.

Jeannel D, Niel G, Costagliola D et al 1988 Epidemiology of toxoplasmosis among pregnant women in the Paris area. Int J Epidemiol 17(3):595–602.

Jenum P A, Kapperud G, Stray-Pedersen B et al 1998 Prevalence of *Toxoplasma gondii* specific immunoglobulin G antibodies among pregnant women in Norway. Epidemiol Infect 120(1):87–92.

Jenum P A, Stray-Pedersen B, Gundersen A G 1997 Improved diagnosis of primary *Toxoplasma gondii* infection in early pregnancy by determination of antitoxoplasma immunoglobulin G avidity. J Clin Microbiol 35(8):1972–1977.

Koppe J G, Loewer-Sieger D H, de Roever-Bonnet H 1986 Results of 20-year follow-up of congenital toxoplasmosis. Lancet 1(8475):254–256.

Lakhanpal V, Schocket S S, Nirankari V S 1983 Clindamycin in the treatment of toxoplasmic retinochoroiditis. Am J Ophthalmol 95(5):605–613.

Lappalainen M, Koskela P, Koskiniemi M et al 1993 Toxoplasmosis acquired during pregnancy: improved serodiagnosis based on avidity of IgG. J Infect Dis 167(3):691–697.

Lebas F, Ducrocq S, Mucignat V et al 2004 Congenital toxoplasmosis: a new case of infection during pregnancy in a previously immunized and immunocompetent woman. Arch Pediatr 11(8):926–928.

Lebech M, Andersen O, Christensen N C et al 1999 Feasibility of neonatal screening for toxoplasma infection in the absence of prenatal treatment. Danish Congenital Toxoplasmosis Study Group. Lancet 353(9167):1834–1837.

Leport C, Vilde J L, Katlama C et al 1986 Failure of spiramycin to prevent neurotoxoplasmosis in immunosupposed patients. JAMA 255(17):2290.

Ljungstrom I, Gille E, Nokes J et al 1995 Seroepidemiology of *Toxoplasma gondii* among pregnant women in different parts of Sweden. Eur J Epidemiol 11(2):149–156.

McAuley J, Boyer K M, Patel D et al 1994 Early and longitudinal evaluations of treated infants and children and untreated historical patients with congenital toxoplasmosis: the Chicago Collaborative Treatment Trial. Clin Infect Dis 18(1):38–72.

McCabe R, Remington J S 1988 Toxoplasmosis: the time has come. N Engl J Med 318(5):313–315.

Marty P, Le Fichoux Y, Deville A, Forest H 1991 Congenital toxoplasmosis and preconceptional maternal ganglionic toxoplasmosis. Presse Med 20(8):387.

Miller M J, Aronson W J, Remington J S 1969 Late parasitemia in asymptomatic acquired toxoplasmosis. Ann Intern Med 71(1):139–145.

Mombro M, Perathoner C, Leone A et al 1995 Congenital toxoplasmosis: 10-year follow up. Eur J Pediatr 154(8):635–639.

Naot Y, Desmonts G, Remington J S 1981 IgM enzyme-linked immunosorbent assay test for the diagnosis of congenital *Toxoplasma* infection. J Pediatr 98(1):32–36.

Patel D V, Holfels E M, Vogel N P et al 1996 Resolution of intracranial calcifications in infants with treated congenital toxoplasmosis. Radiology 199(2):433–440.

Peyron F, Wallon M, Bernardoux C 1996 Long-term follow-up of patients with congenital ocular toxoplasmosis. N Engl J Med 334(15):993–994.

Pinon J M, Chemla C, Villena I et al 1996 Early neonatal diagnosis of congenital toxoplasmosis: value of comparative enzyme-linked immunofiltration assay immunological profiles and anti-*Toxoplasma gondii* immunoglobulin M (IgM) or IgA immunocapture and implications for postnatal therapeutic strategies. J Clin Microbiol 34(3):579–583.

Pons J C, Sigrand C, Grangeot-Keros L et al 1995 Congenital toxoplasmosis: transmission to the fetus of a pre-pregnancy maternal infection. Presse Med 24(3):179–182.

Pratlong F, Boulot P, Issert E et al 1994 Fetal diagnosis of toxoplasmosis in 190 women infected during pregnancy. Prenat Diagn 14(3):191–198.

Pratlong F, Boulot P, Villena I et al 1996 Antenatal diagnosis of congenital toxoplasmosis: evaluation of the biological parameters in a cohort of 286 patients. Br J Obstet Gynaecol 103(6):552–557.

Roizen N, Swisher C N, Stein M A et al 1995 Neurologic and developmental outcome in treated congenital toxoplasmosis. Pediatrics 95(1):11–20.

Roos T, Martius J, Gross U, Schrod L 1993 Systematic serologic screening for toxoplasmosis in pregnancy. Obstet Gynecol 81(2):243–250.

Rothova A, Meenken C, Buitenhuis H J et al 1993 Therapy for ocular toxoplasmosis. Am J Ophthalmol 115(4):517–523.

Stepick-Biek P, Thulliez P, Araujo F G, Remington J S 1990 IgA antibodies for diagnosis of acute congenital and acquired toxoplasmosis. J Infect Dis 162(1):270–273.

Thiebaut R, Leproust S, Chene G, Gilbert R 2007 Effectiveness of prenatal treatment for congenital toxoplasmosis: a meta-analysis of individual patients' data. Lancet 369(9556):115–122.

Thulliez P, Remington J S, Santoro F et al 1986 A new agglutination reaction for the diagnosis of the developmental stage of acquired toxoplasmosis. Pathol Biol (Paris) 34(3):173–177.

Valcavi P P, Natali A, Soliani L et al 1995 Prevalence of anti-*Toxoplasma gondii* antibodies in the population of the area of Parma (Italy). Eur J Epidemiol 11(3):333–337.

Velin P, Dupont D, Barbot D et al 1991 Double mother-fetus HIV-1 and *Toxoplasma* contamination. Presse Med 20(20):960.

Wallon M, Liou C, Garner P, Peyron F 1999 Congenital toxoplasmosis: systematic review of evidence of efficacy of treatment in pregnancy. BMJ 318(7197):1511–1514.

Wastling J M, Harkins D, Buxton D 1994 Western blot analysis of the IgG response of sheep vaccinated with S48 *Toxoplasma gondii* (Toxovax). Res Vet Sci 57(3):384–386.

Wilson C B, Remington J S, Stagno S, Reynolds D W 1980 Development of adverse sequelae in children born with subclinical congenital *Toxoplasma* infection. Pediatrics 66(5):767–774.

Zuber P, Jacquier P 1995 Epidemiology of toxoplasmosis: worldwide status. Schweiz Med Wochenschr Suppl 65:19S–22S.

Congenital viral infections and the central nervous system

Guillaume Benoist, J. Nizard, Yves G. Ville

INTRODUCTION

Prenatal ultrasound examination is both a screening and a diagnostic tool for the assessment of fetal congenital infections. Neonatal prognosis of fetal infections is often dependent upon abnormalities visualized during fetal life, because these infectious agents may have devastating long term effects. MRI is a complementary tool for the evaluation of clastic processes secondary to CNS infection that needs to be further studied in order to establish its role in this field of prenatal diagnosis management.

Congenital infections differ from those in adults and children by the fact that their target is a developing organ. The features of brain involvement will depend on the timing of fetal infection. In early pregnancy, the infection will result in abnormal development while later infections will cause clastic lesions. Knowledge of the development process combined with precise dating of maternal infection will help identify brain imaging abnormalities and understand the mechanism and severity of the disease in order to provide prognostic assessment and appropriate counseling.

This chapter aims to review the most important infectious agents affecting the fetal central nervous system (CNS) and to describe the main features of prenatal diagnosis.

CYTOMEGALOVIRUS (CMV)

Virology, pathogenesis, epidemiology

The cytomegalovirus (CMV) or herpesvirus 5 is a member of the Herpetoviridae family. Its size is the largest in this family. Its genome is composed of a double stranded DNA. It is highly species-specific and humans are its only reservoir. Like other members of the herpesvirus group, CMV remains latent in the organism after acute infection. Reactivation can occur during latent infection.

The transmission of the virus occurs by direct or indirect person to person contact, via body secretions or by blood products or organ transplants. Indeed, the CMV is shed for a long time after the primary infection. However, CMV infection is not very contagious and requires intimate contact. The main cells' targets are the endothelial cells and the polymorph nuclear leukocytes (PMLs). The dissemination of the virus is then hematogenous with a viremic phase which can be diagnosed by laboratory testing. After widespread dissemination the CMV replicates mainly in the liver and the spleen.

Seroprevalence ranges from 50 to 85% in the United States and in Western Europe. This rate increases with age and in lower socioeconomic backgrounds.

Incidence of CMV primary infection in pregnancy also varies with socioeconomic conditions and ranges from around 2% per year in developed countries to 6% in developing countries (Stagno et al 1982).

Maternal infection

Most primary infections in immunocompetent hosts are subclinical. Nigro et al (2003) reported fever in 42.1% of primary infection and in 17.1% of recurrent infection ($P > 0.01$), fatigue in 31.4% and 11.4% ($P < 0.001$), myalgia in 21.5% and 6.7% ($P < 0.001$), flu-like syndrome defined as the simultaneous occurrence of fever and at least one of these signs in 24.5% and in 9.5% ($P < 0.001$), lymphocytosis = 40% (39.2% and 5.7%, $P < 0.001$), increased plasma levels of aminotransferases >40 IU/L in 35.3% and in 3.9%, ($P < 0.001$).

The diagnosis of primary infection can be easily confirmed by serologic testings. Seroconversion is the de novo appearance of virus-specific IgG antibodies in a pregnant woman who was seronegative before the onset of pregnancy. It enables the diagnosis of primary infection. Nevertheless, this event is rare as, in most developed countries, non-systematic follow-up of the serologic status is recommended during pregnancy. Serological testing is usually performed when contamination is suspected following maternal clinical symptoms, or when fetal abnormalities are suspected on ultrasound examination.

IgM antibody response begins in the first days after maternal contamination reaching a peak in the first month after maternal contamination. High to medium levels of IgM antibodies can therefore be detected during the first 1 to 3 months after the onset of infection after which the titers start declining. However, IgM can remain positive for more than a year (Revello & Gerna 2002). When dating maternal infection is difficult, evaluation of IgG avidity is useful. Soon after primary infection, antibodies show a low avidity for the antigen, but this increases progressively thereafter. An avidity index (AI) > 70% is considered to reflect a primary infection >3 months, and AI < 30% is highly suggestive of a recent primary infection (<3 months). AI between 30 and 70% is more difficult to interpret. However, standardized methods for measurement of AI are lacking. Furthermore, the efficacy of this method is dependent on gestational age and the IgG titer (Lazzarotto et al 1999, Mace et al 2004, Maine et al 2001). Overall, Mace et al (2004) reported that dating maternal primary infection using IgG AI associated with IgM antibody detection failed to date the onset of infection in only 1% of their cases.

After primary infection, the virus and viral products can be recovered from different body products. However, viral shedding from these sites can occur after recurrences as well. It has also been shown that detection of CMV in blood is diagnostic of primary infection in immunocompetent individuals but not in immunocompromised patients (Revello et al 1998).

Congenital infection

Congenital infection is the result of transplacental transmission. In the United States around 1% of all newborns are found to be infected when screened at birth. Nevertheless, this rate varies greatly among geographic areas and in correlation with seropositivity rates (Stagno et al 1982). The rate of transplacental transmission varies with the type of maternal infection, between 30–50% for primary infections and 2–3% for non-primary infections (Stagno et al 1982, 1986, Yow et al 1988). Although congenital infections are mainly due to primary infections, several reports have shown a possible fetal transmission after reinfection with another strain of the virus or after reactivation of a latent infection (Boppana et al 2001, Schopfer et al 1978, Stagno et al 1977, 1982). Approximately 10% of the congenitally infected newborns are symptomatic at birth. Half of them present the typical cytomegalic inclusion disease (CID) with a high mortality rate. The other half present with atypical symptoms. Symptomatic infected newborns are defined as presenting at least one of these abnormalities: prematurity, hypotrophy, petechiae, jaundice, hepatosplenomegaly, purpura, neurological findings (microcephaly, hypotonia, seizures), elevated alanine aminotransferase levels (>80 UI/L), thrombocytopenia, conjugated hyperbilirubinemia, hemolysis, increased cerebrospinal fluid proteins (Boppana et al 1992). Long term follow-up of these children enabled the establishment of the occurrence of at least one sequela of 90% in this subgroup (psychomotor delay, sensorineural hearing loss, ocular abnormalities). Death consecutive to congenital CMV infection was estimated to be around 6%. In this group, the best predictor for adverse neurodevelopmental outcome is the presence of intracranial computed tomographic (CT) abnormalities within the first month of life (Boppana et al 1997). These abnormalities were also associated with sensorineural hearing loss (SNHL) at birth or with deterioration of audiometric status during the first months of life.

Ninety percent of infected newborns are asymptomatic although infected as shown by the presence of the virus in their urine or their saliva during the first weeks of life. These infants are known to have a better long-term prognosis than symptomatic ones; 10 to 15% will develop sequelae, more often during the first 2 years of life. These sequelae include SNHL in 7%, chorioretinitis in 2%, intellectual deficit in 4% and microcephaly in 2% (Fowler et al 1997, Kumar et al

1973, Melish & Hanshaw 1973, Noyola et al 2000, Saigal et al 1982). SNHL is the most frequent deficit related to congenital CMV infection in asymptomatic neonates. Fowler et al (1997) have reported that 50% of CMV-related audiometric deficits were bilateral, 50% worsened during the first years of life and for 18% of them the audiologic deficit was diagnosed on average only at 27 months. CMV congenital infection could be the cause of one third of all SNHL in childhood.

Prenatal diagnosis

Without screening programs in pregnancy the most frequent circumstance of diagnosis of congenital CMV infection is the fortuitous discovery of abnormal ultrasound findings related to CMV congenital infection. This may explain that severe abnormalities are described more often than subtle findings.

In primary infections around 50% of the infected fetuses can be diagnosed by ultrasound examination. This is more likely to reflect the proportion of papers published on this particular aspect than the performance of ultrasound as a screening test (Ville 1998). It is also important to remember that the correlation between abnormal sonographic findings and evidence of maternal infection is made several weeks apart (Revello & Gerna 2002).

In the literature, ultrasound features of fetal CMV infection are twofold: gross abnormalities leading to the diagnosis of fetal CMV infection (mainly ventriculomegaly or hydrocephalus, microcephaly, posterior fossa cysts, cerebellar hypoplasia, severe intrauterine growth restriction or even hydrops fetalis), and subtle findings discovered after thorough serial ultrasound examination of fetuses at high risk when vertical transmission of the virus has been shown (mainly extracerebral findings or more subtle cerebral abnormalities).

CNS abnormalities can be categorized in both classes of ultrasound findings.

The most characteristic lesions are bilateral periventricular hyperechogenicities (Ghidini et al 1989, Graham et al 1982). These lesions are calcifications and are visualized as hyperechogenic foci, which, despite their high reflectivity, do not cast any acoustic shadow (Fakhry & Khoury 1991, Koga et al 1990). They are the result of a necrotizing inflammation of the periventricular area at the level of the lateral ventricles with subsequent calcification. These calcifications are seen whatever the timing of the infection. However, the lack of specificity does not enable these lesions to be related to the CMV infection.

Tassin et al (1991) reported ring-like areas of the periventricular fluency appearing earlier than calcifications. They could be the earliest stage of brain infection, due to the cellular necrosis consecutive to the cytopathogenic effect of the virus. This effect could ensure edema and local blood effusion. These effusions could be further cleared by the reticuloendothelial system and the calcifications would be the scars of this process (Tassin et al 1991).

Other locations of the calcifications can also be observed in the fetal brain.

Localization of branching linear echogenic areas in the thalami has been described during fetal life and at birth (Estroff et al 1992, Teele et al 1988). These calcifications correspond to the arteries in the basal ganglia and in the thalamus and justify the nickname 'lenticulostrial vasculopathy'. These lesions are due to thickening of the vessels. This abnormality has been observed up to 31 weeks (Estroff et al 1992) (Fig. 31.1).

Calcifications have also been observed inside the parenchyma more often at the convexity of the circumvolutions.

These mineralized necrotized cortical areas are named polymicrogyria.

Differential diagnoses of cerebral calcifications include other infections, intracranial teratomas, tuberous sclerosis, Sturge–Weber syndrome and sagittal or transverse sinus thrombosis. Furthermore, linear areas of the basal ganglia and the thalami have also been described in association with trisomy 13 and 21.

The fetal ventriculitis related to CMV infection is visualized as periventricular cysts. These cysts could be due to ischemia of the subependyma with further necrosis and calcifications (Shaw & Alvord 1974). These cysts are named

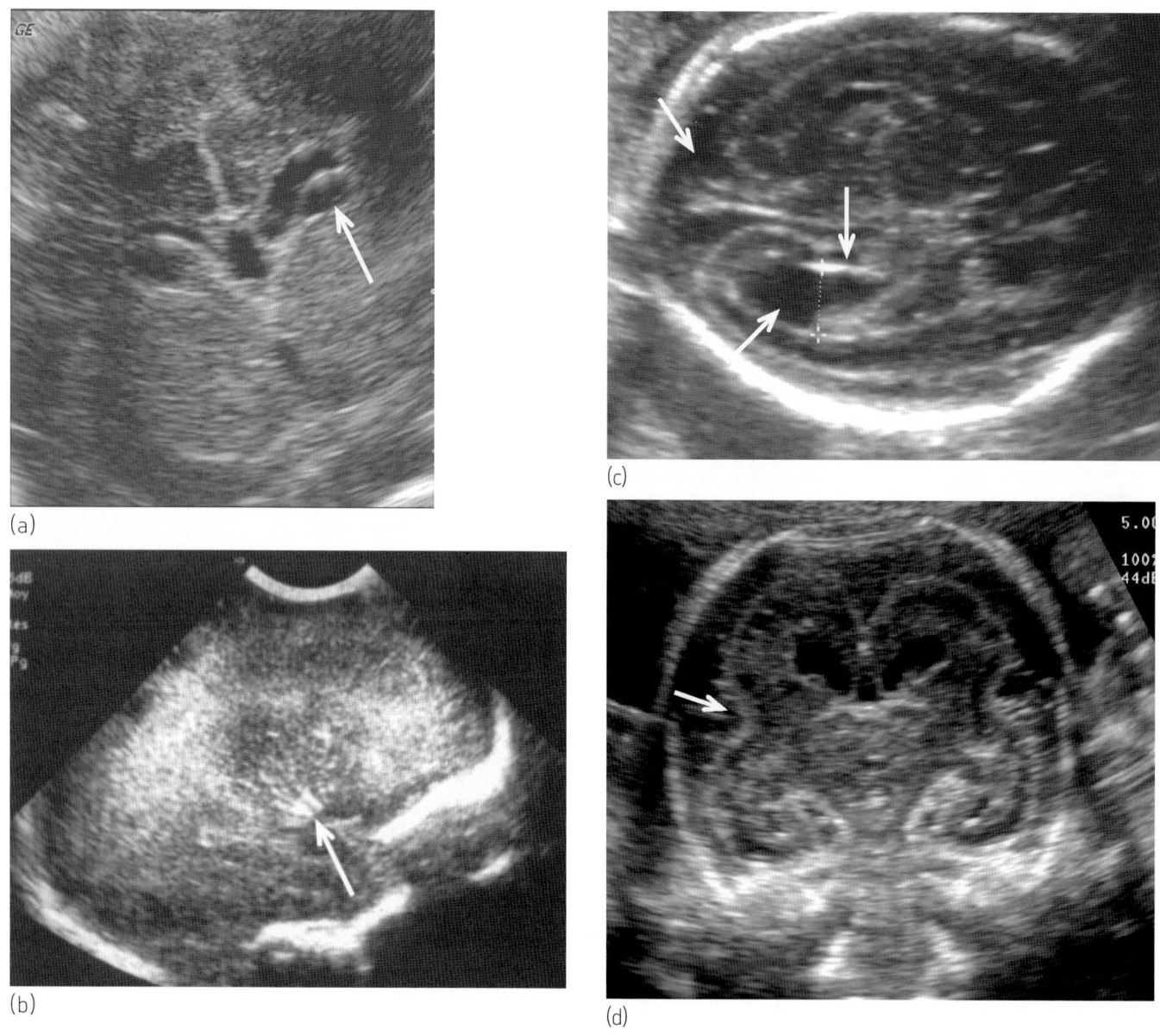

(a)

(b)

(c)

(d)

Figure 31.1 (a) Coronal section. Subependymal germinolysis cysts. (b) Parasagittal section. Linear echogenic areas in the thalami lenticulostriatal vasculopathy. (c) Axial section. Ventriculomegaly, periventricular hyperechogenicities, microencephaly (enlargement of the pericerebral space). (d) Coronal section. Delayed closure of the Sylvian fissure, microencephaly (enlargement of the pericerebral space).

subependymal germinolysis cysts (Shaw & Alvord 1974). They are typically located around the frontal horns of the lateral ventricles (Fig. 31.1).

Inside the ventricular areas intraventricular synechiae or adhesions can also be observed. Ischemic process has also been implicated in the genesis of these lesions.

Other abnormalities related to ischemic phenomenon have also been observed: porencephaly, hydranencephaly and polymicrogyria (Friede & Mikolasek 1978, Marques Dias et al 1984, Tassin et al 1991).

Barkovich and Lindan (1994) have summarized the mechanisms that could explain the development of cerebral lesions due to CMV infection. The lesions of the fetal brain could originate from placentitis causing perfusion insufficiency resulting in ischemia with the consequences described above. They could also be the result of the special affinity of the virus for the immature cells of the germinal matrix (Barkovich & Lindan 1994) that could lead to the loss of brain tissue and abnormalities of the cerebral cortex.

An early infection between 16 and 18 weeks of gestation, occurring at the onset of the neuronal migration, can lead to lissencephaly. Ultrasound features can include microcephaly, ventriculomegaly and absence of normal closure of the sylvian fissure (Barkovich & Lindan 1994, Hayward et al 1991, Twickler et al 1993) (Fig. 31.1).

Cerebellar hypoplasia could also be associated with early infection (Barkovich & Lindan 1994, Steinlin et al 1996). The transverse diameter can be easily measured by ultrasound but examination of the vermis and its measurement are easier by MRI. Precise evaluation of the vermis by prenatal imaging techniques needs further investigations as it is currently difficult to differentiate vermian hypoplasia and partial agenesis of the vermis.

Ventriculomegaly can also be an isolated prenatal finding (Dommergues et al 1996). The severity of the dilatation ranges from mild to severe and up to hydrocephalus (Achiron et al 1994, Sekhsaria et al 1992). Nevertheless, asymmetry between the two occipital horns of the lateral ventricles has also been described without any clinical implications (Achiron et al 1994). The possible etiologies of ventriculomegaly include obstruction of the fourth ventricle or aqueductal stenosis due to ependymitis, or intraventricular hemorrhage but also destructive ventriculomegaly or brain atrophy.

Other exceptional abnormalities have been reported in CMV congenital infections including hemimegalencephaly (Jay et al 1997) and schizencephaly (Iannetti et al 1998, Sener 1998).

Irrespective of the type of injury of the fetal brain during congenital CMV infection, none is specific of this infectious agent. Suspicion of CMV infection is often based on the association of evocative signs such as microcephaly and periventricular calcifications, particularly if they are associated with extra-cerebral lesions.

The development of fetal MRI has become an asset in the assessment of infected fetuses (Barkovich & Lindan 1994, Malinger et al 2003, Soussotte et al 2000). MRI using both T1 and T2 sequences could help define the onset of fetal infection. Sulcation has been precisely described by MRI (Garel et al 2001). Lissencephaly may reflect injury before 16 or 18 weeks whereas polymicrogyria is likely to follow injury of the brain at 18 to 24 weeks and finally cases with normal gyral patterns would have probably been injured during the third trimester showing diffuse heterogeneity in the white matter (Barkovich & Lindan 1994).

The wide spectrum of the extracerebral ultrasound findings illustrates the affinity of CMV for endothelial cells, which explains the large number of organs involved.

Hyperechogenic bowel grade 2 has to be considered often as a transient finding. However, in a series comprising 175 fetuses with hyperechogenic bowel, only one case was related to CMV infection (Al-Kouatly et al 2001). It is recognized to be the expression of viral enterocolitis and is rarely expressed as meconium ileus or peritonitis (Dechelotte et al 1992).

Oligohydramnios is more often reported than polyhydramnios and considering the affinity of CMV for the kidney, it can be seen as the expression of a fetal nephropathy.

The fetal heart can also be affected showing cardiomegaly with a thick myocardium which may contain punctate calcifications. As a functional consequence, Drose et al (1991) have also described tachyarrhythmia. This is a rare finding that could participate in the development of fetal hydrops.

Generalized edema and ascites may also suggest anemia-related hydrops due to the combined effect of liver failure and infection of the bone-marrow. This spectacular presentation has also proven to eventually be transient with both ultrasound and biological normalization at follow-up (Watt-Morse & Hill 1995).

Ultrasound findings are summarized in Table 31.1.

Despite evocative ultrasound findings associated with laboratory diagnosis of maternal infection, confirmation of fetal infection is necessary. It can be done by the recovery of the virus or the viral DNA in the fetal compartment. CMV can be detected in the amniotic fluid by conventional viral isolation, rapid culture or molecular assays. Virus isolation has a high specificity but has a lower sensitivity than polymerase chain reaction (PCR). In recent years, PCR has been established as a reliable technique in reference laboratories. The efficacy of these methods has been evaluated in several studies (Enders et al 2001, Guerra et al 2000, Lazzarotto et al 2000, Liesnard et al 2000, Revello & Gerna 2002). False-negative results could be explained in most cases by inappropriate timing of amniocentesis. Following seroconversion or reactivation, the process leading to CMV excretion in the fetal urine will take an average of 6–8 weeks and this interval should be recognized in order to avoid false negative prenatal diagnosis (Revello & Gerna 2002). Amniocentesis should also be performed once fetal urination is well established and therefore not before 22 weeks. When the conditions of sampling are ideal (Revello et al 1999a), the sensitivity of prenatal diagnosis by PCR in amniotic fluid has been reported to be close to 100%. False positive PCR

Table 31.1 Fetal abnormalities diagnosed in utero by ultrasound examination as reported in 7 series in the literature from 2000 (Guerra et al 2000, Liesnard et al 2000, Azam et al 2001, Enders et al 2001, Gouarin et al 2002, Lipitz et al 2002, Picone et al 2004)

NUMBER OF CASES OF CONGENITAL CMV INFECTION *		277
Overall ultrasound findings		116 (42%)
IUGR**		45 (16%)
Hydrops		8 (3%)
Ascites		20 (7%)
Pericardial effusion		4 (1%)
Pleural effusion		1 (<1%)
Skin edema		2 (<1%)
Hyperechogenic bowel		36 (13%)
Hepatomegaly splenomegaly		8 (3%)
Liver calcifications		2 (<1%)
Placentomegaly		5 (2%)
Oligohydramnios/anhydramnios		15 (5%)
Polyhydramnios		4 (1%)
Other/extra CNS abnormalities	asymmetry of cardiac ventricles	8 (3%)
	cardiomyopathy	
	small lungs	
	hyperechogenic abdominal tumor	
	abnormal head shape	
	no fetal movements	
	short limbs	
Microcephaly		25 (9%)
Hydrocephaly		13 (5%)
Ventriculomegaly		35 (13%)
Other CNS abnormalities	brain calcifications	36 (13%)
	periventricular echogenicity	
	porencephaly	
	lissencephaly	
	subependymal cysts	
	choroid plexus cysts	
	cystic structure in cerebellum	
	agenesis of cerebellar vermis	
	cerebellar hypoplasia	

*Congenital CMV infection proved in urine at birth or after examination of fetuses after termination of pregnancy.
** IUGR: intrauterine growth restriction.

results have also been reported and could be explained by contamination of the AF with infected maternal blood at the time of amniocentesis if the mother had a positive CMV DNAemia at the time of sampling or by laboratory contamination occurring during PCR testing.

Prognostic factors during the prenatal period

Currently, the association of positive DNA detection in amniotic fluid and the presence of ultrasound cerebral abnormalities are considered to be sufficient to accept a woman's request for termination of pregnancy. However, the individual prognostic value of ultrasound findings is very difficult to establish because termination of pregnancy prevents follow-up of these infants. Frequent ultrasound abnormalities such as hyperechogenic bowel or fetal growth restriction do not appear to be associated with a poor outcome. In our experience, the only prognostic factor of a poor outcome during childhood is fetal brain abnormalities on fetal ultrasound examination (unpublished data).

Several studies have suggested that the prognosis could be worse when maternal infection occurred during the first trimester of pregnancy (Ahlfors et al 1983, Liesnard et al 2000, Pass et al 2005, Stagno et al 1986). Fetal infection in the third trimester of pregnancy can also carry a poor neurological outcome (Steinlin et al 1996).

Preconceptional immunity against CMV is only partially protective against intrauterine transmission of the virus. Although vertical transmission rates vary significantly between primary and non-primary infections (30–50% vs. 2–3%) (Stagno et al 1982, 1986, Yow et al 1988), it seems that the prognosis of infected fetuses could be similar in primary and in non-primary maternal infections.

It seems that neither the presence of maternal clinical symptoms during primary infection nor virological parameters in the mother are associated with a higher risk of vertical transmission (Revello et al 1998).

The development of real time PCR allows evaluation of the clinical significance of CMV viral load in amniotic fluid (Gouarin et al 2002, Picone et al 2004, Revello et al 1999b). In three studies the median viral loads were higher in the amniotic fluid of symptomatic fetuses than in the amniotic fluid of asymptomatic fetuses; however this difference reached statistical significance in only one study.

In the fetal blood antigenemia, viremia and DNAemia were found to be higher in fetuses with abnormalities than in asymptomatic fetuses but the difference was significant only for antigenemia (Revello et al 1999). However, negative PCR was only found in asymptomatic patients and very high blood viral loads were recovered only in symptomatic fetuses. The mean values of neonatal blood viral load were statistically higher in newborns that developed sequelae than in those who did not and approximately 70% of sequelae were found in newborns with a qPCR higher than 10000 copies per 10^5 PMNLs (Lanari et al 2006). Further studies are warranted; evaluating the predictive value of fetal blood viral load as well as of non-specific hematological and biochemical parameters on outcome of congenital infection is a topic of current interest but the use of viral sequence information has failed to predict outcome (Rasmussen et al 2003).

In infected fetuses, the proportion of female fetuses with brain abnormalities was statistically higher than that in males (62/258 infected fetuses: 24% vs. 30/251: 12%, P = 0.004). The risk of abnormal brain development in infected fetuses was twice as high in females as in males (OR = 2, [1.26–3.21]) (Picone et al 2005).

Management

Termination of pregnancy is often performed on the basis of a fetal infection alone, despite the absence of ultrasound or MRI signs.

A number of antiviral drugs are active against CMV and the three licensed anti CMV drugs (ganciclovir, cidofovir and foscarnet) are being used successfully in immunocompromised patients. However, their potential teratogenic effects and their well known toxicity do not support their use in pregnancy. Several anti-CMV compounds are at different stages of development; several of these compounds are very promising in term of efficacy and lack of toxicity. To date, preliminary results on treatment of CMV congenital infection during pregnancy are available from two studies with promising results. Nigro et al (2005) have recently published the retrospective results of a non-randomized clinical trial using intravenous CMV hyperimmune globulin (HIG) for CMV maternal primary infection. Jacquemard et al (2005) have recently shown the pharmacological efficacy of valaciclovir (VACV) in a pilot study in 21 cases of CMV congenital infections with ultrasound abnormalities (Jacquemard et al 2005).

RUBELLA

General
Rubella virus is an RNA virus, classified as a togavirus, genus Rubivirus.

It is a worldwide human disease without any animal reservoir. This virus spreads by means of airborne transmission or droplets shed from respiratory secretions from 7 days before to 5–7 days or more after the onset of the cutaneous eruption. The mean incubation time is 2 weeks. Viremia occurs 5–7 days after exposure. Transplacental hematogenous transmission can occur during this phase.

Since the introduction of systematic vaccination in childhood, epidemiologic characteristics have changed, and the number of congenital infections has drastically decreased.

Maternal infection
Rubella is usually a mild disease that develops after an incubation period of 14 to 21 days (mean 17 days) as a rash appearing and lasting for 1 to 5 days, extending from the face passing down through the body to the feet. In adults this rash is often pruriginous, and preceded by fever, headache, conjunctivitis, malaise, coryza, lymphadenopathy and dyspnea. Arthralgia and sometimes frank arthritis may develop after the rash has faded. These symptoms were reported in up to 70% of infected women. Complications are rare including thrombocytopenia, encephalitis, myocarditis, Guillain–Barré syndrome and optic neuritis.

Laboratory diagnosis is essential because the infection is asymptomatic in around half of the cases. The most useful laboratory test is serological testing of maternal blood. Acute rubella is characterized by the appearance of IgG and IgM. When determination of the timing of infection is uncertain, testing avidity of IgG antibodies is helpful. Primary infection is associated with low avidity IgG (Hedman & Seppala 1988). The virus can also be cultured from body samples and its genome can be retrieved by RT-PCR.

Congenital rubella syndrome
The risk of fetal infection and congenital abnormalities decreases with gestation. However, fetal infection can occur at any time during pregnancy. This has been extensively reported by Miller et al (1982). The vertical transmission rate decreases from 81% before 12 weeks' gestation through to 67% between 13 and 14 weeks' gestation and 25% between 23 and 26 weeks' gestation, increasing to 35% between 27 and 30 weeks' gestation, 60% between 31 and 36 weeks' gestation and 100% after 36 weeks' gestation. Periconceptional infection until 11 days after last menstruation period is not associated with any risk of fetal infection (Enders et al 1988).

The rate of defects has been estimated in several studies, and none has been reported after 16–20 weeks of gestation (Ghidini & Lynch 1993, Miller et al 1982, Peckham 1985, Sever et al 1965, 1969) (Table 31.2).

Table 31.2 Risk of defects in children exposed to maternal rubella infection and relation with the term of maternal infection

Reference	Term of maternal infection (weeks of gestation)	Rate of defects
Peckham 1985	<8	75%
	9–12	52%
	13–20	18%
	>20	0
Miller et al 1982	<11	100%
	11–12	50%
	13–14	17%
	15–16	50%
	>16	0

Table 31.3 Extra-CNS defects related to rubella congenital syndrome

Heart defects	patent ductus arteriosus
	pulmonary artery stenosis
	pulmonary valvular stenosis
	coarctation of aortic isthmus
	septal defect
Eye defects	retinopathy
	cataract
	microphthalmia
	glaucoma
	abnormalities of the anterior chamber of the eye
Other systemic involvement	hearing abnormalities
	intrauterine growth retardation
	thrombocytopenia
	hepatosplenomegaly
	obstructive jaundice
	radiographic changes of the long bones
	endocrine dysfunction

Table 31.4 Fetal CNS abnormalities of the congenital rubella syndrome

Microcephaly
Microphthalmia
Polymicrogyria
Cerebellar heterotopy
Calcifications in the central gray nuclei
Calcifications in the white matter
Hydrocephalus by gliosis around the Sylvius aqueductal
Subependymal pseudocysts (Makhoul et al 2001)

Congenital rubella has also been associated with the occurrence of miscarriages and stillbirth. However, rubella congenital infection can also be asymptomatic. Between these two extremes, the spectrum of congenital rubella syndrome has been described since 1941 (Gregg 1941) and includes heart defects, eye defects, hearing abnormalities and extra-CNS involvement (Table 31.3).

The fetal CNS is often involved in congenital rubella syndrome. Microcephaly can be a feature of this syndrome (Cooper et al 1965, Preblud et al 1982, Zinkham & Medearis 1967). Meningoencephalitis may present occasionally in infancy or early childhood but is usually not progressive after infancy. Rubella virus has been recovered from cerebrospinal fluid and pleocytosis and increased protein levels are associated with this meningitis (Desmond et al 1967). Mental retardation and motor impairment are common. Intra-cranial calcifications (Fakhry & Khoury 1991) and subependymal pseudocysts have been found in neonates with congenital rubella (Makhoul et al 2001).

One particular feature of the syndrome is the development of a severe progressive neurologic disease worsening in the second decade of life. This disorder is characterized by progressive cerebellar ataxia, spasticity, increased loss of mental function and seizures. These continue to progress until the patient is in a vegetative state and finally dies. The delayed onset of this rare syndrome is related to the ability of rubella virus to persist inside the organism and reactivate after a long period of latency (Townsend et al 1975, Waxham & Wolinsky 1984, Weil et al 1975, Wolinsky et al 1979).

Late-onset and progressive manifestations of rubella congenital syndrome comprise autism and other behavioral problems. They have been reported in approximately 6% of cases (Cooper 1985).

Sensorineural hearing loss is the most frequent defect associated with congenital rubella and affects around 80% of all infected infants. Its severity is variable and it can be unilateral or more often bilateral. This hearing loss is peripheral and commonly associated with retinopathy. Before the introduction of vaccination programs, rubella was responsible for 16% of hearing loss problems in childhood (Peckham & Marshall 1979).

The organ of Corti is mainly involved in rubella and is vulnerable until 16 weeks of gestation; this is much later than with other defects induced by rubella, such as heart and ocular defects that do not develop when the infection occurs beyond 8 weeks.

Hearing impairment may not manifest for a few years and hearing deficit can worsen over time.

Ocular characteristic signs and symptoms comprise early manifestations such as retinopathy, cataracts (around one half of affected children) and microphthalmia. Nevertheless, some abnormalities may be patent only after several months or years. Glaucoma is one of these delayed manifestations which encompass abnormalities of the anterior chamber (corneal hydrops, keratoconus) and spontaneous lens resorption (Boger 1980, Boger et al 1981a, 1981b).

Main CNS manifestations are summarized in Table 31.4.

Long-term prognosis of congenital rubella syndrome can be estimated from the long-term follow-up studies of Gregg's cohort when 50 patients of the original cohort were reviewed 25 years later (Menser et al 1967). Among these subjects born in Australia between 1939 and 1944, 48 were deaf, 26 had cataracts or retinopathy, 14 had cardiac defects, five were mentally handicapped and one had diabetes mellitus type 2 (Forrest et al 1971).

Prenatal diagnosis

A proven maternal case of rubella during pregnancy does not always lead to vertical transmission, and fetal infection is not always indicative of fetal defects. Fetal infection can be proven by direct isolation of the virus, or its genome, by PCR in the amniotic fluid sampled by amniocentesis at least 6 to 8 weeks after maternal infection to avoid false negative results. This should be done in association with targeted ultrasound examination (Chiba et al 2003, Kobayashi et al 2005).

When rubella infection occurs during the first two months of the pregnancy, ultrasound examination is likely to visualize CNS involvement. Furthermore, CNS involvement rarely occurs in the absence of manifestations involving other systems.

However, during fetal life, the most frequent sonographic findings are cardiac abnormalities (atrial and ventricular septal defects), ocular abnormalities (cataract, microphthalmia), hepatomegaly, splenomegaly and growth restriction. The following anomalies have been reported to occasionally occur with congenital rubella syndrome: glaucoma, peripheral pulmonic stenosis, renal disorders and hypospadias (Benaceraf 1998), meconium peritonitis (Radner et al 1993) and hyperechogenic bowel.

VARICELLA-ZOSTER VIRUS

General

Varicella is caused by VZV (herpesvirus varicellae), and commonly occurs in childhood. Based on serological studies, it appears that less than 25% of adults with no history of chickenpox are susceptible to an acute disease (LaRussa et al 1985). VZV is a member of the Herpesviridae family. The virus is airborne, spread from cutaneous vesicles and by respiratory droplets from patients with varicella or zoster. After the initial replication phase, the virus reaches the local lymph nodes, and spreads by transient moderate viremia towards the viscera. A second replication phase is followed by a second and more intense viremia with a cutaneous rash. Varicella is most contagious at the time of the rash and for the next 2 days. After clinical recovery, the patient is not contagious and the latency phase begins. Zoster occurs in persons who have previously had chickenpox. This vesicular infection is generally confined to the dermatome of the ganglia where the VZV was in latency.

Chickenpox and pregnancy

The incidence of varicella in pregnancy is around 7/10 000 (Balducci et al 1992). Koren (2005) has estimated that with 90% rate seropositivity in childbearing age women in the United States, and 4 million births a year, three out of every 1000 women have varicella, and of these 15 cases a year have congenital varicella syndrome. Hence, 900 cases have occurred in the USA alone since 1947 (the date of the first description of this syndrome).

The incubation period is 10 to 21 days. In adults, the rash is often preceded by prodromal fever by 2 or 3 days and changes from red macules to vesicles, pustules and crusts with all stages of the lesions visualized simultaneously in the same anatomical region. This typically begins on the face or scalp and spreads rapidly to the trunk but sparing the extremities. The overall eruption duration is 5 days. The main risk for infected pregnant women is varicella pneumoniae. This develops in about15% of the cases ranging from isolated radiological signs to severe acute respiratory insufficiency mandating intensive care. Evidence of pneumonia has been found in 16% of a series of 110 cases (Weber & Pellecchia 1965). Dyspnea occurs in 70% of cases, and can be accompanied by cyanosis, pain chest, hemoptysis and bronchial rales. Maternal death has been reported in up to 10% of cases but this includes immunosuppressed patients.

In cases with widespread typical vesicular exanthema and a history of recent exposure, the diagnosis is made clinically. Laboratory diagnosis can be achieved by demonstrating the VZV antigen by immunofluorescence (Rawlinson et al 1989), and VZV DNA by PCR in skin lesions (Koropchak et al 1991, 1992). The virus can also be isolated from vesicular fluid.

VZV infections show at least a fourfold increase in specific antibody titers by using a sensitive test such as FAMA or ELISA. The presence of IgM suggests a recent infection. The persistence of VZV antibodies beyond the age of 8 months is suggestive of intrauterine varicella.

Congenital varicella syndrome

During pregnancy, the virus may be transmitted transplacentally resulting in neonatal or fetal chickenpox and inducing congenital varicella syndrome.

The timing of maternal infection plays a major role in the severity of the fetal damage. Most of the reported cases of congenital varicella syndrome follow maternal infections that occurred during the first trimester or at the onset of the second trimester. Nevertheless, several publications have reported severe defects in fetuses following maternal chickenpox after the 20th week of gestation (Bai & John 1979, Harger et al 2002, Michie et al 1992, Palmer & Pauli 1988). Weeks 7 to 20 are the time of greatest risk (Enders et al 1994).

Enders et al (1994) reported the results of a prospective study of 1373 women with varicella and 366 with zoster during their pregnancy. Among the first group, they reported defects attributable to congenital varicella syndrome in 0.4% for infections between 0 and 12 weeks, 2% between 13 and 20 weeks of gestation. The overall rate of congenital defects was 0.7%.

In another large prospective study performed in the United States comprising 347 cases of maternal varicella, the rate of congenital infection was 1.3% (Harger et al 2002).

However, Tan et al have reviewed nine published cases of infections occurring between 21 and 28 weeks' gestation (Bai & John 1979, Harger et al 2002, Lambert et al 1989, Michie et al 1992, Palmer & Pauli 1988). In eight of these nine cases, there were serious adverse effects on the CNS. The severity of this injury was similar to those consecutive to infections occurring before 20 weeks' gestation.

The incidence of congenital varicella syndrome is significantly higher with varicella than with zoster. In a series of 366 cases of zoster during pregnancy, there was no case of congenital infection syndrome (Enders et al 1994). This probably can be explained by the viremia which is less likely to occur with zoster than with chickenpox. Furthermore, previous immunity acquired with chickenpox probably limits the damage with zoster in the fetus.

The congenital syndrome typically consists of a combination of skin, ocular, limb and neurological abnormalities (Fig. 31.2).

These lesions are summarized in Table 31.5.

Enders and Miller (2000) have reported that skin lesions were present in 72% of cases, neurological lesions in 48%, ocular abnormalities in 44%, limb hypoplasia in 72% and gastrointestinal and genitourinary abnormalities in 20%.

Neurological involvement is about as common as skin and eye abnormalities in infants with this syndrome. The neonatal clinical picture includes cerebral cortical atrophy, diffuse brain involvement, or mental retardation with or without seizures and abnormal electroencephalograms.

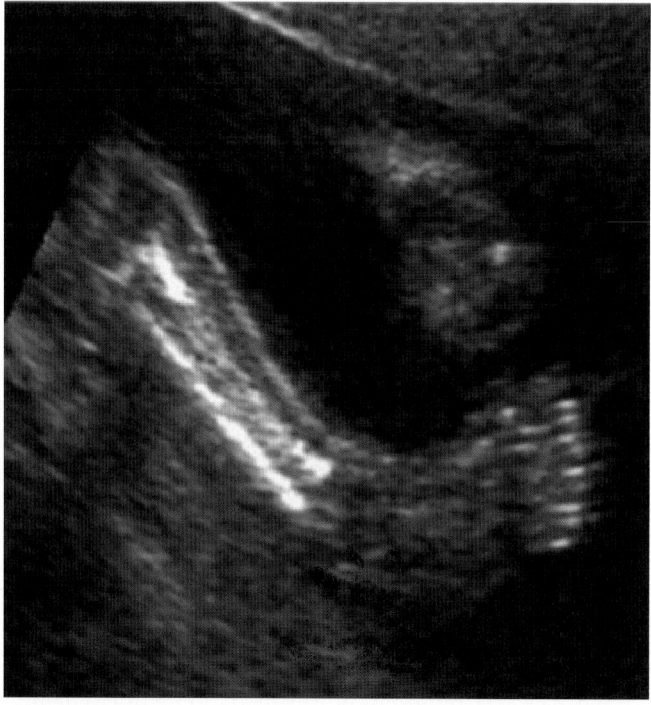

Figure 31.2 Limb malformation: equinovarus clubfoot.

There is an increased level of proteins and leukocytes in the cerebrospinal fluid (Hajdi et al 1986, Rinvik 1969, Savage et al 1973). Deep reflexes are more often diminished or absent (Hammad et al 1989). Sensory deficits have also been reported (Savage et al 1973) as well as vocal cord paralysis (Liang et al 2000, Randel et al 1996). Electromyography can reveal a denervation pattern with loss of motor units (Kotchmar et al 1984). Several features are consistent with the hypothesis that congenital defects result from the viral damage to the neural tissue leading to damage in specific regions. This hypothesis can explain the deformity of the limbs.

When this syndrome is present at birth, the prognosis is poor and around one fourth of these infants will die during the first 14 months of life. Furthermore, one third of the infected fetuses will be born preterm.

Prenatal diagnosis

Prenatal ultrasound examination can identify infected fetuses presenting with marked or specific anomalies. The time interval between maternal infection and an abnormal ultrasound examination was 5 to 19 weeks (Alexander 1979, Cuthbertson et al 1987, Harding & Baumer 1988, Hofmeyr et al 1996, Scharf et al 1990) for abnormalities described in Table 31.6.

Prenatal diagnosis is made by amplification of the VZV genome in amniotic fluid by PCR. Mouly et al (1997) reported the results of amniocentesis and PCR performed in 107 women who had varicella before 24 weeks of pregnancy. Nine of these 107 (8.4%) had positive PCR in amniotic fluid, but only two of these (1.8%) had positive cell culture. Simultaneously fetal blood sampling was performed in 82 cases for anti-varicella zoster virus immunoglobulin M research which was negative in all cases (Enders et al 1994). When varicella develops at the beginning of pregnancy, the indication for amniocentesis is unclear. Targeted ultrasound follow-up is probably sufficient. If prenatal diagnosis is to be offered then amniocentesis should be performed at least 5 weeks after maternal infection to avoid false negative results.

Normal ultrasound examination at 22–24 weeks' suggests that fetal varicella syndrome is unlikely. By contrast, any abnormality at this stage should lead to high suspicion of the syndrome.

Perinatal infection

This is defined by the occurrence of chickenpox in neonates within 10 days of birth. It is due to maternal infection near term where chickenpox develops in 24 to 50% of the neonates within the first 10 days of life (Brunell 1967, Hanngren et al 1985, Meyers 1974, Newman 1965, Pearson 1964, Siegel & Fuerst 1966). The interval between the onset of maternal rash and neonatal infection is 9 to 15 days. When delivery occurs within 10 days of the onset of maternal infection, maternal IgG cannot develop and cross the placenta to protect the fetus/neonate. Neonatal chickenpox can be fatal in up to 30% of cases (Meyers 1974).

Table 31.5 Abnormalities related to varicella congenital syndrome

Cerebral anomalies (Cuthbertson et al 1987, Scharf et al 1990, Hofmeyr et al 1996, Ong & Daniel 1998, Petignat et al 2001)	Cerebral cortical atrophy
	Mental retardation
	Seizures
	Abnormalities of the electroencephalogram
	Increased proteins and leukocytes in the cerebrospinal fluid
	Denervation at the electromyography
	Diminished or abolition of deep reflex
Ophthalmologic anomalies	Congenital cataract
	Microphthalmia
	Chorioretinitis
	Horner syndrome
	Nystagmus
Skin lesions	Cutaneous scars
Musculoskeletal anomalies (Enders et al 1994, Mouly et al 1997)	Limb contractures
	Hypoplasia of a limb
	Hypoplasia or absence of a digit
	Equinovarus position of the foot
	Calcaneovalgus position of the hand
Gastrointestinal tract abnormalities	Reflux
	Duodenal stenosis
	Small bowel dilatation
	Microcolon
	Dysfunction of the anal sphincter
Other findings	Prematurity
	Low birth weight
	Abnormalities of the urinary tract
	Involvement of the spinal cord
	Involvement of the autonomous nervous system

Table 31.6 Prenatal ultrasound abnormalities of the congenital varicella syndrome

Limb deformity, hypoplasia ((Enders et al 1994, Hofmeyr et al 1996)

Microcephaly

Hydrocephalus (Cuthbertson et al 1987, Scharf et al 1990)

Polyhydramnios, oligohydramnios (Hofmeyr et al 1996)

Clubfeet (Scharf et al 1990)

Bullous skin lesion (Alexander 1979)

Chest and abdominal calcifications (myocardium, liver, lungs . . .) (Da Silva et al 1990, Mouly et al 1997)

Intrauterine growth retardation

Cataract

Microphthalmia

Hydrops fetalis

Ventriculomegaly (Hofmeyr et al 1996)

Management options

Antiviral treatment for maternal infection:

Pregnant women who develop varicella should be treated with oral aciclovir, and followed up carefully. Those with pneumonia should be admitted and treated with intravenous antiviral agent. Aciclovir is more effective when administrated within one day after the onset of varicella, and shortens the course of illness by about one day (Dunkle et al 1991).

Passive immunization for infants after possible perinatal infection:

It has been shown that pooled immunoglobulins can attenuate the symptoms when administered to contact persons within 72 hours of exposure (Brunell et al 1969). Its value has also been envisaged to minimize severe illness when administered to mothers who develop chickenpox close to term. For infants born between 2 and 4 days after maternal eruption, the use of zoster immunoglobulins was suggested to decrease the occurrence and severity of the neonatal disease in one uncontrolled study (Hanngren et al 1985). It is also recommended to administer varicella zoster immunoglobulins to infants of mothers who develop varicella within 5 days of delivery (CDC 1996). Doses of 125 IU (1.25 mL or one vial) (Control 1996) have been administered intramuscularly as early as possible after birth.

Infected mothers and infants should be isolated from maternity and neonatal units in order to avoid spreading the infection.

PARVOVIRUS B19

Virology, epidemiology and pathogenesis

Parvovirus B19 is a non-enveloped virus with a single-stranded DNA. The primary targets for B19 parvovirus are the erythroid precursor cells, endothelial cells, fetal myocardial cells, placental cells, mature erythrocytes and megakaryocytes (Chisaka et al 2003).

Seroprevalence of parvovirus B19 infection is estimated to be around 45% in young adults (Koch & Adler 1989). Risk factors for seroconversion in pregnancy are: elementary school workers, contact with 5 to 11 year old children (Cartter et al 1991, Gillespie et al 1990) and women under 30 years of age (Adler et al 1993). Overall 1 to 2% of sero-negative women at the onset of pregnancy would become infected during pregnancy in endemic periods and >10% in epidemic periods (Dembinski et al 2003, Nascimento et al 1990, Trotta et al 2004, Valeur-Jensen et al 1999).

Infection usually occurs through contact with respiratory droplets, but B19 virus can also be transmitted by blood and blood derived products and can be transmitted vertically from mother to fetus (Enders et al 2004). No vertical transmission has been described if the mother is immune at the time of exposure.

Maternal infection

In healthy individuals, infection is usually asymptomatic. Erythema infectiosum (fifth disease) is the most common clinical manifestation during childhood. It is characterized by a rash consisting of maculae that undergo central fading over 1 to 4 days, mainly on the trunk and limbs. Symptoms such as erythema infectiosum, mild fever, arthralgia and headache start approximately 10–14 days after contamination and in about 50% of the infected women. Arthralgia and arthritis are common in the adult form of the disease. Other possible symptoms include: thrombocytopenia, menin-goencephalitis, hepatitis, myocarditis and vasculitis.

The most characteristic symptom is symmetrical arthralgia, sometimes arthritis often involving small joints of the hands, wrists and feet. The proportion of asymptomatic women is around 30%.

Following infection, specific immunoglobulins IgM, IgG and IgA are produced. Specific IgM are the first antibodies to raise around 10 days post infection. Specific IgG rise considerably more slowly about 3 weeks post infection to reach a plateau at around 4 weeks after infection. They probably last for life. Maternal serum should be tested when there is evidence of maternal exposure or clinical symptoms of B19 infection.

The presence of IgM indicates that a recent maternal infection has occurred, regardless of IgG antibody levels.

Congenital infection

Vertical transmission occurs in approximately one third of cases of maternal infections (Gross & Schumann 1990). Fetal infection with parvovirus B19 is associated with intrauterine fetal death (IUFD), non-immune hydrops fetalis (NIHF) and, less often, brain anomalies. Fetal infection can also be asymptomatic (Koch et al 1993).

Fetal manifestations due to parvovirus B19 are summarized in Table 31.7.

The consequences of fetal infection are not univocal throughout the pregnancy. Non-immune hydrops fetalis develops following mainly maternal infection in the first half of the pregnancy. Overall, the risk of adverse fetal outcome when fetal infection is proven is approximately 10% (Chisaka et al 2003, Norbeck et al 2002).

Cases of IUFD have been described mainly at around 20 to 24 weeks' of gestation, but IUFD can occur during the whole pregnancy, and is not always preceded by hydrops fetalis (Gratacos et al 1995, Norbeck et al 2002, Tolfvenstam et al 2001).

Non-immune hydrops fetalis (NIHF) defined by the association of marked ascites, cardiomegaly, pericardial effusion and, in advanced stages, generalized edema and thick hydropic placenta develops in 4% of cases with a maximum of 7.1% when infection occurred between 13 and 20 weeks. It is mainly related to severe anemia, which can also lead to high output heart failure. NIHF is more frequent during

Table 31.7 Ultrasound abnormalities in fetuses infected by parvovirus B19

Cardiac system	Increased cardiac biventricular outer diameter (Sheikh et al 1992)
	Myocarditis
Non-immune hydrops fetalis	Pleural effusion
	Pericardial effusion
	Ascites
	Abdominal wall edema
	Bilateral hydroceles
	Amniotic fluid disorder
Brain abnormalities	Hydrocephalus (Katz et al 1996)
	Microcephaly
	Intracranial calcifications
Gastrointestinal system	Fetal liver calcifications (Simchen et al 2002)
	Meconium peritonitis (Miniero et al 1996, Zerbini et al 1998)
Other findings	Sporadic cases of contractures (Weiner et al 1993)
	Increased nuchal translucency (Smulian et al 1998)
	IUGR (Brandenburg et al 1996)

the hepatic stage (8–20 weeks of gestation) of the hematopoietic activity when the half-life of erythrocytes is shorter rather than later in the bone marrow and splenic hematopoietic stages (Chisaka et al 2003, Enders et al 2004).

The interval between maternal B19 parvovirus infection and the development of NIHF ranges from 2 to 6 weeks (Yaegashi et al 1998). In 539 of the cases reported by Soothill (1990), 30% preceded intrauterine fetal death and 34% resolved spontaneously whereas 29% resolved after intrauterine transfusion, and 6% died despite intrauterine transfusion (Yaegashi et al 1998).

Maternal symptoms of 'mirror-hydrops' or 'Ballantyne syndrome' can develop secondary to lysis of the hydropic placental villi and is responsible for a maternal pre-eclampsia-like syndrome with edema, hypertension, proteinuria and anemia (Proust et al 2006).

The involvement of the fetal heart can be limited to dilatation of the cardiac cavities related to anemia and hydrops, or present as a hypertrophic cardiomyopathy. Myocarditis can also develop autonomously after spontaneous resolution of the NIHF (von Kaisenberg et al 2001).

Fetal B19 infection has also been associated with CNS involvement including ventriculomegaly or hydrocephalus (Fig. 31.3). This could develop as the consequence of prolonged anemia-related hypoxia or secondary to thrombocytopenia-related hemorrhage. Isumi et al (1999) described the neuropathologic changes due to parvovirus B19: multinucleated giant cells of macrophages/microglia lineage and many small calcifications with predilections for areas around the vessels, predominantly in the cerebral white matter, the cerebral cortex, the basal ganglia, the thalamus and the germinal layer. Furthermore, the authors demonstrated the presence of the viral DNA by PCR and in situ hybridization. This neuropathologic approach demonstrates the viral tropism of parvovirus B19 for CNS tissue.

Ocular defects, including retinal folds, microphthalmia, absence of the iris and lens, were associated with myocarditis and mild atrophy of the skeletal muscles (Weiland et al 1987).

During neonatal life, fetal B19 infection has been associated with neurological disorders. Cases of pediatric stroke (Craze et al 1996), neonatal encephalitis/meningitis (Balfour et al 1970, Brass et al 1982, Isumi et al 1999, Tsuji et al 1990), encephalopathy (Breese & Horner 1977) caused by B19 infection have been reported, with perivascular calcifications in the fetal cerebral cortex, basal ganglia, thalamus and germinal layers (Isumi et al 1999). Most of these were isolated cases reported during outbreaks of erythema infectiosum and are old, and serological confirmation was not performed.

Cerebrospinal fluid abnormalities such as pleocytosis and increased levels of proteins have been reported in some patients with meningism or altered levels of consciousness associated with erythema infectiosum (Torok 1990). B19 genome has been retrieved in cerebrospinal fluid by PCR in patients with serologically confirmed B19 infection (Okumura & Ichikawa 1993).

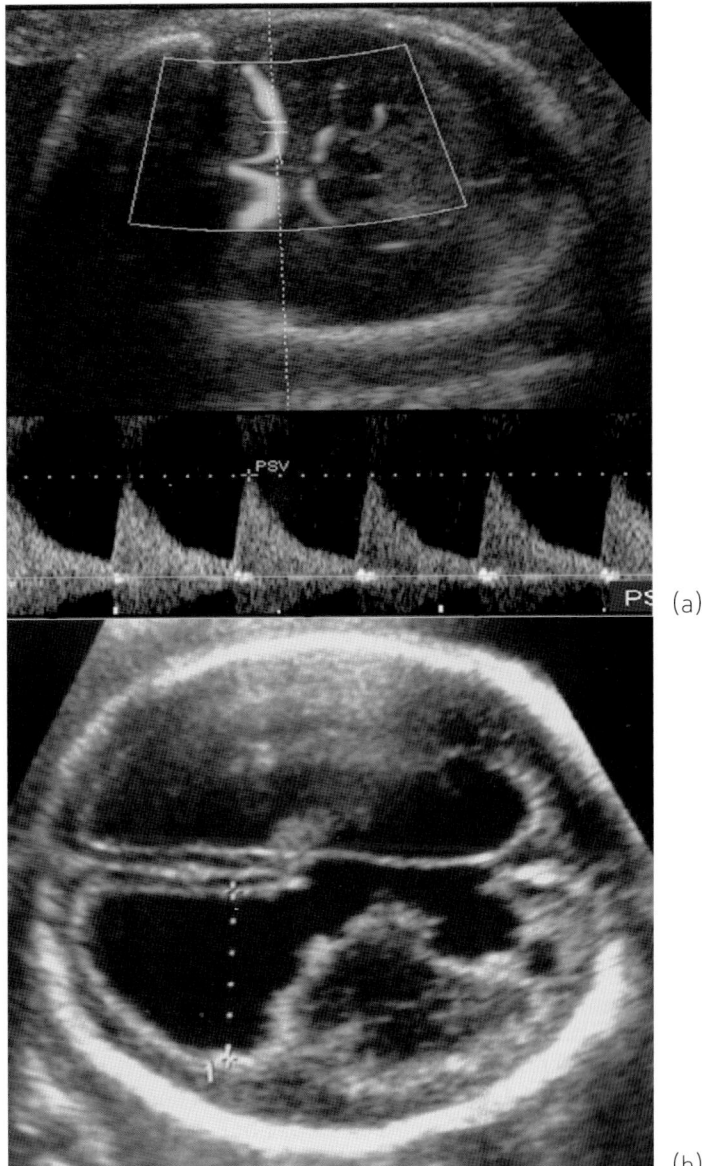

(a)

(b)

Figure 31.3 (a) Median cerebral artery velocity waveform: increased systolic peak velocity. (b) Axial section. Bilateral ventriculomegaly, intraventricular hemorrhage.

Rodis et al (1998) have evaluated the long-term outcomes of children exposed in utero to maternal parvovirus B19 infection. They compared retrospectively the outcomes of pregnancies with serologic evidence of recent parvovirus B19 infection with a group with serologic evidence of ancient infection. There was no increase in the incidence of developmental delays in children in utero exposed to parvovirus.

This was confirmed in a large prospective study of 190 pregnancies with B19 infection. The outcome was good, accounting for a 30% fetal loss rate in the second trimester, without increased risk to babies who survived (Prospective Study of Human Parvovirus (B19) Infection in Pregnancy 1990).

Prenatal diagnosis

Maternal infection is confirmed by an evocative serologic profile. Fetal ultrasound examination should be performed to exclude the presence of fetal anemia and hydrops. In these cases, fetal anemia should be suspected when middle cerebral artery pic-systolic velocities are over 2 MOMs (Cosmi et al 2002, Mari et al 2002) (Fig. 31.3) which is an indication to set up fetal blood sampling and intrauterine transfusion. Severe NIHF together with normal MCA-PSV in B19 infection indicates either spontaneous resolution of fetal anemia or progressive myocarditis.

The virus or its genome can be retrieved from amniotic fluid or fetal blood. Nucleic acid amplification by PCR is extremely sensitive. This can also be applied in pregnant women lacking an adequate antibody-mediated immune response, immunocompromised or immunosuppressed in whom serological testing for B19 parvovirus is unreliable (Jordan et al 2001).

Management options

Pregnant women, who have been exposed to B19 infection, or those developing symptoms compatible with B19 infection, should be assessed by serological testing. Seronegative women should be retested 2 weeks later. They can be reassured in the absence of seroconversion. In cases with primary infection, serial ultrasound examination including MCA-PSV measurements should be performed every fortnight up until 12 weeks after exposure.

Management of B19 parvovirus fetal infection with intrauterine transfusion (IUT) can correct fetal anemia and perinatal mortality. It should be restricted to cases with MCA-PSV >2 MOM in which the levels of hemoglobin are confirmed to be below 9 g/dL by fetal blood sampling. Timely IUT of anemic fetuses with severe hydrops reduces the risk of fetal death (Enders et al 2006, Fairley et al 1995, Rodis et al 1998, Schild et al 1998). In most cases, one transfusion is sufficient to allow for fetal recovery and high reticulocyte levels indicate that anemia is being corrected spontaneously. Hydropic changes can take up to several weeks to resolve (Odibo et al 1998) and MCA-PSV should be used to evaluate the correction of fetal anemia. Children who survived a successful IUT for B19-induced fetal anemia and hydrops fetalis have a good neurodevelopmental prognosis (Dembinski et al 2003). However, severe and prolonged fetal anemia is accompanied by thrombocytopenia that can lead to intraventricular brain hemorrhage and its own prognosis.

HERPES SIMPLEX VIRUS

The herpes simplex viruses are large DNA viruses with double-stranded DNA genome.

Maternal infection

Around 70% of newly acquired HSV infections among pregnant women are asymptomatic or unrecognized (Kulhanjian et al 1992). When clinically apparent, genital herpes shows a wide range of symptoms from minimal lesions and mild discomfort up to painful lesion associated with fever, dysuria, sacral paresthesia and headache. Reactivations are more often unrecognizable. Primary infections and reactivations are undistinguishable by their clinical aspect (Hensleigh et al 1997). Complications of herpes during pregnancy include hepatitis, encephalitis and pneumonia.

In all cases, the diagnosis needs laboratory confirmation. Both culture and PCR are available but the latter has a higher sensitivity (Slomka et al 1998).

Congenital infection

Congenital infection with HSV more commonly occurs during the neonatal period. It is acquired at the time of delivery owing to viral shedding from symptomatic or asymptomatic genital lesions (Whitley et al 1998).

The risk of vertical infection of HSV ranges from 50% for primary maternal infection (defined as a first episode of genital herpes), 33% after non-primary infection (first episode genital herpes with either HSV1 or HSV2 in a patient with pre-existing antibodies to the other viral serotype), down to 3% after recurrences (reactivation of genital herpes) (ACOG 2000).

Intrauterine infection is much less common but several cases are reported in the literature. It can develop through either ascending infection or more rarely by hematogenous transplacental spread. Primary infection causes intrauterine infection more often than other types of maternal infection, probably due to a higher viral load.

Evidence of placental infection and intact membranes at delivery are suggestive of a hematogenous process rather than an ascending route (Chatterjee et al 2001). Funisitis and mesenchymal cell immunostaining of the umbilical cord are consistent with an infection via an ascending route (Heifetz & Bauman 1994, Hyde & Giacoia 1993).

In most cases, the disease was related to HSV2 and caused disseminated forms of severe fetal brain injury (Hutto et al 1987, Johansson et al 2004, Lee et al 2003).

Few authors have demonstrated that neonates infected by HSV2 exhibited more CNS involvement than those infected by HSV1 (Kimura et al 2002, Whitley 1992).

In disseminated forms, liver, spleen and adrenal glands are generally involved. Brain lesions are considered secondary to the cytotoxic effect of the virus or subsequent to ischemia caused by vascular occlusion of cerebellar vessels (Lee et al 2003).

Intrauterine HSV infection may occur at any time during pregnancy.

Ultrasound features of a fetal infection due to HSV are summarized in Table 31.8.

Management

Antiviral therapy is recommended for women with asymptomatic HSV infection during pregnancy. Oral medication (aciclovir 400 mg or valaciclovir 1 g per os for 7 to 14 days for primary infection or first episode) and (aciclovir 400 mg or valaciclovir 500 mg for 5 days in case of symptomatic recurrence) reduces viral shedding and hastens healing of

Table 31.8 Fetal abnormalities related to HSV infection (Lanouette et al 1996, Lee & Major 2001, Diguet et al 2006, Duin et al 2007)

CNS abnormalities	Hydrocephaly
	Cystic encephalomalacia
Other abnormalities	Intrauterine growth restriction
	Non-immune hydrops fetalis
	Intrauterine death
	Thickness of the skin
	Hypechogenicity of the amniotic fluid
	Irregular thickening of membranes and placenta
	Esophageal anomalies
	Limb hypoplasia (Johansson et al 2004)
	Absence of fetal movements
	Pleural of pericardial effusion
	Polyhydramnios, oligoamnios

the lesions. This treatment should be initiated as soon as the diagnosis is suspected. For women with frequent recurrences during pregnancy, daily suppressive treatment can be initiated (aciclovir 400 mg or valaciclovir 500 mg per os from 36 weeks' gestation up until delivery). A registry of neonates exposed to aciclovir during pregnancy found no significant teratogenic effects to the fetus (Stone et al 2004).

For women with genital herpes or prodromal symptoms suggestive of genital herpes, cesarean delivery is recommended to prevent neonatal infection (Brown et al 2000). A cesarean is likely to be more effective if performed before the rupture of the membranes. Clinical examination of the birth canal at admission in labor is the only method to infer the presence of HSV. Nevertheless, this procedure carries a poor sensitivity (Brown et al 1997, 2000).

Women with genital herpes without lesions or symptoms at the time of delivery may proceed with vaginal delivery. However it is recommended to avoid artificial rupture of the membranes, fetal scalp electrodes and to limit assisted extractions to absolute obstetrical indications (Brown et al 2000).

REFERENCES

Achiron R, Pinhas-Hamiel O, Lipitz S et al 1994 Prenatal ultrasonographic diagnosis of fetal cerebral ventriculitis associated with asymptomatic maternal cytomegalovirus infection. Prenat Diagn 14(7):523–526.

ACOG 2000 Practice bulletin. Management of herpes in pregnancy. Number 8 October 1999. Clinical management guidelines for obstetrician-gynecologists. Int J Gynaecol Obstet 68(2):165–173.

Adler S P, Manganello A M, Koch W C et al 1993 Risk of human parvovirus B19 infections among school and hospital employees during endemic periods. J Infect Dis 168(2):361–368.

Ahlfors K, Forsgren M, Ivarsson S A et al 1983 Congenital cytomegalovirus infection: on the relation between type and time of maternal infection and infant's symptoms. Scand J Infect Dis 15(2):129–138.

Alexander I 1979 Congenital varicella. Br Med J 2(6197):1074.

Al-Kouatly H B, Chasen S T, Streltzoff J et al 2001 The clinical significance of fetal echogenic bowel. Am J Obstet Gynecol 185(5):1035–1038.

Azam A Z, Vial Y, Fawer C L et al 2001 Prenatal diagnosis of congenital cytomegalovirus infection. Obstet Gynecol 97(3):443–448.

Bai P V, John T J 1979 Congenital skin ulcers following varicella in late pregnancy. J Pediatr 94(1):65–67.

Balducci J, Rodis J F, Rosengren S et al 1992 Pregnancy outcome following first-trimester varicella infection. Obstet Gynecol 79(1):5–6.

Balfour H H Jr, Schiff G M, Bloom J E 1970 Encephalitis associated with erythema infectiosum. J Pediatr 77(1):133–136.

Barkovich A J, Lindan C E 1994 Congenital cytomegalovirus infection of the brain: imaging analysis and embryologic considerations. AJNR Am J Neuroradiol 15(4):703–715.

Benaceraf B 1998 Rubella — maternal infection. New York.

Boger W P, 3rd 1980 Late ocular complications in congenital rubella syndrome. Ophthalmology 87(12):1244–1252.

Boger W P, 3rd, Petersen R A, Robb R M 1981a Keratoconus and acute hydrops in mentally retarded patients with congenital rubella syndrome. Am J Ophthalmol 91(2):231–233.

Boger W P, 3rd, Petersen R A, Robb R M 1981b Spontaneous absorption of the lens in the congenital rubella syndrome. Arch Ophthalmol 99(3):433–434.

Boppana S B, Fowler K B, Vaid Y et al 1997 Neuroradiographic findings in the newborn period and long-term outcome in children with symptomatic congenital cytomegalovirus infection. Pediatrics 99(3):409–414.

Boppana S B, Pass R F, Britt W J et al 1992 Symptomatic congenital cytomegalovirus infection: neonatal morbidity and mortality. Pediatr Infect Dis J 11(2):93–99.

Boppana S B, Rivera L B, Fowler K B et al 2001 Intrauterine transmission of cytomegalovirus to infants of women with preconceptional immunity. N Engl J Med 344(18):1366–1371.

Brandenburg H, Los F J, Cohen-Overbeek T E 1996 A case of early intrauterine parvovirus B19 infection. Prenat Diagn 16(1):75–77.

Brass C, Elliott L M, Stevens D A 1982 Academy rash. A probable epidemic of erythema infectiosum ('fifth disease'). JAMA 248(5):568–572.

Breese C, Horner F A 1977 Encephalopathy with erythema infectiosum. Am J Dis Child 131(1):65–67.

Brown Z A, Selke S, Zeh J et al 1997 The acquisition of herpes simplex virus during pregnancy. N Engl J Med 337(8):509–515.

Brown Z A, Wald A, Morrow R A et al 2000 Effect of serologic status and cesarean delivery on transmission rates of herpes simplex virus from mother to infant. JAMA 289(2):203–209.

Brunell P A 1967 Varicella-zoster infections in pregnancy. JAMA 199(5):315–317.

Brunell P A, Ross A, Miller L H, Kuo B 1969 Prevention of varicella by zoster immune globulin. N Engl J Med 280(22):1191–1194.

Cartter M L, Farley T A, Rosengren S et al 1991 Occupational risk factors for infection with parvovirus B19 among pregnant women. J Infect Dis 163(2):282–285.

Chatterjee A, Chartrand S A, Harrison C J et al 2001 Severe intrauterine herpes simplex disease with placentitis in a newborn of a mother with recurrent genital infection at delivery. J Perinatol 21(8):559–564.

Chiba M E, Saito M, Suzuki N et al 2003 Measles infection in pregnancy. J Infect 47(1):40–44.

Chisaka H, Morita E, Yaegashi N, Sugamura K 2003 Parvovirus B19 and the pathogenesis of anaemia. Rev Med Virol 13(6):347–359.

Control C 1996 Prevention of varicella: recommendations of the Advisory Committee on Immunization Practices (ACIP). MMWR Morb Mortal Wkly Rep 45:1.

Cooper L Z 1985 The history and medical consequences of rubella. Rev Infect Dis 7 Suppl 1:S2–S10.

Cooper L Z, Green R H, Krugman S et al 1965 Neonatal thrombocytopenic purpura and other manifestations of rubella contracted in utero. Am J Dis Child 110(4):416–427.

Cosmi E, Mari G, Delle Chiaie L et al 2002 Noninvasive diagnosis by Doppler ultrasonography of fetal anemia resulting from parvovirus infection. Am J Obstet Gynecol 187(5):1290–1293.

Craze J L, Salisbury A J, Pike M G 1996 Prenatal stroke associated with maternal parvovirus infection. Dev Med Child Neurol 38(1):84–85.

Cuthbertson G, Weiner C P, Giller R H, Grose C 1987 Prenatal diagnosis of second-trimester congenital varicella syndrome by virus-specific immunoglobulin M. J Pediatr 111(4):592–595.

Da Silva O, Hammerberg O, Chance G W 1990 Fetal varicella syndrome. Pediatr Infect Dis J 9(11):854–855.

Dechelotte P J N M, Bouvier R J , Vanlieferinghen P C, Lemery D J 1992 Pseudo-meconium ileus due to cytomegalovirus infection: a report of three cases. Pediatr Pathol 12(1):73–82.

Dembinski J, Eis-Hubinger A M, Maar J et al 2003 Long term follow up of serostatus after maternofetal parvovirus B19 infection. Arch Dis Child 88(3):219–221.

Desmond M M, Wilson G S, Melnick J L et al 1967 Congenital rubella encephalitis. Course and early sequelae. J Pediatr 71(3):311–331.

Diguet A, Patrier S, Eurin D et al 2006 Prenatal diagnosis of an exceptional intrauterine herpes simplex type 1 infection. Prenat Diagn 26(2):154–157.

Dommergues M, Mahieu-Caputo D, Fallet-Bianco C et al 1996 Fetal serum interferon-alpha suggests viral infection as the aetiology of unexplained lateral cerebral ventriculomegaly. Prenat Diagn 16(10):883–892.

Drose J A, Dennis M A, Thickman D 1991 Infection in utero: US findings in 19 cases. Radiology 178(2):369–374.

Duin L K, Willekes C, Baldewijns M M et al 2007 Major brain lesions by intrauterine herpes simplex virus infection: MRI contribution. Prenat Diagn 27(1):81–84.

Dunkle L M, Arvin A M, Whitley R J et al 1991 A controlled trial of acyclovir for chickenpox in normal children. N Engl J Med 325(22):1539–1544.

Enders G, Bader U, Lindemann L et al 2001 Prenatal diagnosis of congenital cytomegalovirus infection in 189 pregnancies with known outcome. Prenat Diagn 21(5):362–377.

Enders G, Miller E 2000 varicella and herpes zoster in pregnancy and the newborn. In: Arvin A, Gershon A (eds) Varicella-zoster virus virology and clinical management. Cambridge University Press, Cambridge, pp. 317–347.

Enders G, Miller E, Cradock-Watson J et al 1994 Consequences of varicella and herpes zoster in pregnancy: prospective study of 1739 cases. Lancet 343(8912):1548–1551.

Enders G, Nickerl-Pacher U, Miller E, Cradock-Watson J E 1988 Outcome of confirmed periconceptional maternal rubella. Lancet 1(8600):1445–1447.

Enders M, Schalasta G, Baisch C et al 2006 Human parvovirus B19 infection during pregnancy — value of modern molecular and serological diagnostics. J Clin Virol 35(4):400–406.

Enders M, Weidner A, Zoellner I et al 2004 Fetal morbidity and mortality after acute human parvovirus B19 infection in pregnancy: prospective evaluation of 1018 cases. Prenat Diagn 24(7):513–518.

Estroff J A, Parad R B, Teele R L, Benacerraf B R 1992 Echogenic vessels in the fetal thalami and basal ganglia associated with cytomegalovirus infection. J Ultrasound Med 11(12):686–688.

Fairley C K, Smoleniec J S, Caul O E, Miller E 1995 Observational study of effect of intrauterine transfusions on outcome of fetal hydrops after parvovirus B19 infection. Lancet 346(8986):1335–1337.

Fakhry J, Khoury A 1991 Fetal intracranial calcifications. The importance of periventricular hyperechoic foci without shadowing. J Ultrasound Med 10(1):51–54.

Forrest J M, Menser M A, Burgess J A 1971 High frequency of diabetes mellitus in young adults with congenital rubella. Lancet 2(7720):332–334.

Fowler K B, McCollister F P, Dahle A J et al 1997 Progressive and fluctuating sensorineural hearing loss in children with asymptomatic congenital cytomegalovirus infection. J Pediatr 130(4):624–630.

Friede R L, Mikolasek J 1978 Postencephalitic porencephaly, hydranencephaly or polymicrogyria. A review. Acta Neuropathol (Berl) 43(1–2):161–168.

Garel C, Chantrel E, Brisse H et al 2001 Fetal cerebral cortex: normal gestational landmarks identified using prenatal MR imaging. AJNR Am J Neuroradiol 22(1):184–189.

Ghidini A, Lynch L 1993 Prenatal diagnosis and significance of fetal infections. West J Med 159(3):366–373.

Ghidini A, Sirtori M, Vergani P et al 1989 Fetal intracranial calcifications. Am J Obstet Gynecol 160(1):86–87.

Gillespie S M, Cartter M L, Asch S et al 1990 Occupational risk of human parvovirus B19 infection for school and day-care personnel during an outbreak of erythema infectiosum. JAMA 263(15):2061–2065.

Gouarin S, Gault E, Vabret A et al 2002 Real-time PCR quantification of human cytomegalovirus DNA in amniotic fluid samples from mothers with primary infection. J Clin Microbiol 40(5):1767–1772.

Graham D, Guidi S M, Sanders R C 1982 Sonographic features of in utero periventricular calcification due to cytomegalovirus infection. J Ultrasound Med 1(4):171–172.

Gratacos E, Torres P J, Vidal J et al 1995 The incidence of human parvovirus B19 infection during pregnancy and its impact on perinatal outcome. J Infect Dis 171(5):1360–1363.

Gregg N 1941 Congenital cataract following German measles in the mother. Trans Ophthalmol Soc Aust (3):35.

Gross G E, Schumann J 1990 [Herpesvirus infections– indications for chemotherapy in dermato- venereology]. Hautarzt 41(11):591–601.

Guerra B, Lazzarotto T, Quarta S et al 2000 Prenatal diagnosis of symptomatic congenital cytomegalovirus infection. Am J Obstet Gynecol 183(2):476–482.

Hajdi G, Meszner Z, Nyerges G et al 1986 Congenital varicella syndrome. Infection 14(4):177–180.

Hammad E, Helin I, Pacsa A 1989 Early pregnancy varicella and associated congenital anomalies. Acta Paediatr Scand 78(6):963–964.

Hanngren K, Grandien M, Granstrom G 1985 Effect of zoster immunoglobulin for varicella prophylaxis in the newborn. Scand J Infect Dis 17(4):343–347.

Harding B, Baumer J A 1988 Congenital varicella- zoster. A serologically proven case with necrotizing encephalitis and malformation. Acta Neuropathol (Berl) 76(3):311–315.

Harger J H, Ernest J M, Thurnau G R et al 2002 Frequency of congenital varicella syndrome in a prospective cohort of 347 pregnant women. Obstet Gynecol 100(2):260–265.

Hayward J C, Titelbaum D S, Clancy R R, Zimmerman R A 1991 Lissencephaly-pachygyria associated with congenital cytomegalovirus infection. J Child Neurol 6(2):109–114.

Hedman K, Seppala I 1988 Recent rubella virus infection indicated by a low avidity of specific IgG. J Clin Immunol 8(3):214–221.

Heifetz S A, Bauman M 1994 Necrotizing funisitis and herpes simplex infection of placental and decidual tissues: study of four cases. Hum Pathol 25(7):715–722.

Hensleigh P A, Andrews W W, Brown Z et al 1997 Genital herpes during pregnancy: inability to distinguish primary and recurrent infections clinically. Obstet Gynecol 89(6):891–895.

Hofmeyr G J, Moolla S, Lawrie T 1996 Prenatal sonographic diagnosis of congenital varicella infection–a case report. Prenat Diagn 16(12):1148–1151.

Hutto C, Arvin A, Jacobs R et al 1987 Intrauterine herpes simplex virus infections. J Pediatr 110(1):97–101.

Hyde S R, Giacoia G P 1993 Congenital herpes infection: placental and umbilical cord findings. Obstet Gynecol 81(5(Pt 2)):852–855.

Iannetti P, Nigro G, Spalice A et al 1998 Cytomegalovirus infection and schizencephaly: case reports. Ann Neurol 43(1):123–127.

Isumi H, Nunoue T, Nishida A, Takashima S 1999 Fetal brain infection with human parvovirus B19. Pediatr Neurol 21(3):661–663.

Jacquemard F Y M, Picone O, Costa J M et al 2005 Cytomegalovirus intrauterine infection: pharmacokinetics of valacyclovir administration to the mother and changes in DNA viral load in amniotic fluid and fetal blood. Am J Obstet Gynecol S57:191.

Jay V, Otsubo H, Hwang P et al 1997 Coexistence of hemimegalencephaly and chronic encephalitis. Detection of cytomegalovirus by the polymerase chain reaction. Childs Nerv Syst 13(1):35–41.

Johansson A B, Rassart A, Blum D et al 2004 Lower- limb hypoplasia due to intrauterine infection with herpes simplex virus type 2: possible confusion with intrauterine varicella-zoster syndrome. Clin Infect Dis 38(7):e57–e62.

Jordan J A, Huff D, DeLoia J A 2001 Placental cellular immune response in women infected with human parvovirus B19 during pregnancy. Clin Diagn Lab Immunol 8(2):288–292.

Katz V L, McCoy M C, Kuller J A, Hansen W F 1996 An association between fetal parvovirus B19 infection and fetal anomalies: a report of two cases. Am J Perinatol 13(1):43–45.

Kimura H, Ito Y, Futamura M, Ando Y et al 2002 Quantitation of viral load in neonatal herpes simplex virus infection and comparison between type 1 and type 2. J Med Virol 67(3):349–353.

Kobayashi K, Tajima M, Toishi S et al 2005 Fetal growth restriction associated with measles virus infection during pregnancy. J Perinat Med 33(1):67–68.

Koch W C, Adler S P 1989 Human parvovirus B19 infections in women of childbearing age and within families. Pediatr Infect Dis J 8(2):83–87.

Koch W C, Adler S P, Harger J 1993 Intrauterine parvovirus B19 infection may cause an asymptomatic or recurrent postnatal infection. Pediatr Infect Dis J 12(9):747–750.

Koga Y, Mizumoto M, Matsumoto Y et al 1990 Prenatal diagnosis of fetal intracranial calcifications. Am J Obstet Gynecol 163(5 Pt 1):1543–1545.

Koren G 2005 Congenital varicella syndrome in the third trimester. Lancet 366(9497):1591–1592.

Koropchak C M, Graham G, Palmer J et al 1991 Investigation of varicella-zoster virus infection by polymerase chain reaction in the immunocompetent host with acute varicella. J Infect Dis 163(5):1016–1022.

Koropchak C M, Graham G, Palmer J et al 1992 Investigation of varicella-zoster virus infection by polymerase chain reaction in the immunocompetent host with acute varicella. J Infect Dis 165(1):188.

Kotchmar G S Jr, Grose C, Brunell P A 1984 Complete spectrum of the varicella congenital defects syndrome in 5-year-old child. Pediatr Infect Dis 3(2):142–145.

Kulhanjian J A, Soroush V, Au D S et al 1992 Identification of women at unsuspected risk of primary infection with herpes simplex virus type 2 during pregnancy. N Engl J Med 326(14):916–920.

Kumar M L, Nankervis G A, Gold E 1973 Inapparent congenital cytomegalovirus infection. A follow-up study. N Engl J Med 288(26):1370–1372.

Lambert S R, Taylor D, Kriss A et al 1989 Ocular manifestations of the congenital varicella syndrome. Arch Ophthalmol 107(1):52–56.

Lanari M, Lazzarotto T, Venturi V et al 2006 Neonatal cytomegalovirus blood load and risk of sequelae in symptomatic and asymptomatic congenitally infected newborns. Pediatrics 117(1):e76–e83.

Lanouette J M, Duquette D A, Jacques S M et al 1996 Prenatal diagnosis of fetal herpes simplex infection. Fetal Diagn Ther 11(6):414–416.

LaRussa P, Steinberg S P, Seeman M D, Gershon A A 1985 Determination of immunity to varicella-zoster virus by means of an intradermal skin test. J Infect Dis 152(5):869–875.

Lazzarotto T, Spezzacatena P, Varani S et al 1999 Anticytomegalovirus (anti-CMV) immunoglobulin G avidity in identification of pregnant women at risk of transmitting congenital CMV infection. Clin Diagn Lab Immunol 6(1):127–129.

Lazzarotto T, Varani S, Guerra B et al 2000 Prenatal indicators of congenital cytomegalovirus infection. J Pediatr 137(1):90–95.

Lebon P, Lyon G 1974 Letter: Non-congenital rubella encephalitis. Lancet 2(7878):468.

Lee A, Bar-Zeev N, Walker S P, Permezel M 2003 In utero herpes simplex encephalitis. Obstet Gynecol 102(5 Pt 2):1197–1199.

Lee R M, Major C A 2001 Controversial and special situations in the management of preterm premature rupture of membranes. Clin Perinatol 28(4):877–884, viii.

Liang C D, Yu T J, Ko S F 2000 Ipsilateral renal dysplasia with hypertensive heart disease in an infant with cutaneous varicella lesions: an unusual presentation of congenital varicella syndrome. J Am Acad Dermatol 43(5 Pt 1):864–866.

Liesnard C, Donner C, Brancart F et al 2000 Prenatal diagnosis of congenital cytomegalovirus infection: prospective study of 237 pregnancies at risk. Obstet Gynecol 95(6 Pt 1):881–888.

Lipitz S, Achiron R, Zalel Y et al 2002 Outcome of pregnancies with vertical transmission of primary cytomegalovirus infection. Obstet Gynecol 100(3):428–433.

Mace M, Sissoeff L, Rudent A, Grangeot-Keros L 2004 A serological testing algorithm for the diagnosis of primary CMV infection in pregnant women. Prenat Diagn 24(11):861–863.

Maine G T, Lazzarotto T, Landini M P 2001 New developments in the diagnosis of maternal and congenital CMV infection. Expert Rev Mol Diagn 1(1):19–29.

Makhoul I R, Zmora O, Tamir A et al 2001 Congenital subependymal pseudocysts: own data and meta-analysis of the literature. Isr Med Assoc J 3(3):178–183.

Malinger G, Lev D, Zahalka N et al 2003 Fetal cytomegalovirus infection of the brain: the spectrum of sonographic findings. AJNR Am J Neuroradiol 24(1):28–32.

Mari G, Detti L, Oz U, Zimmerman R et al 2002 Accurate prediction of fetal hemoglobin by Doppler ultrasonography. Obstet Gynecol 99(4):589–593.

Marques Dias M J, Harmant-van Rijkevorsel G, Landrieu P, Lyon G 1984 Prenatal cytomegalovirus disease and cerebral microgyria: evidence for perfusion failure, not disturbance of histogenesis, as the major cause of fetal cytomegalovirus encephalopathy. Neuropediatrics 15(1):18–24.

Melish M E, Hanshaw J B 1973 Congenital cytomegalovirus infection. Developmental progress of infants detected by routine screening. Am J Dis Child 126(2):190–194.

Menser M A, Dods L, Harley J D 1967 A twenty-five-year follow-up of congenital rubella. Lancet 2(7530):1347–1350.

Meyers J D 1974 Congenital varicella in term infants: risk reconsidered. J Infect Dis 129(2):215–217.

Michie C A, Acolet D, Charlton R et al 1992 Varicella-zoster contracted in the second trimester of pregnancy. Pediatr Infect Dis J 11(12):1050–1053.

Miller E, Cradock-Watson J E, Pollock T M 1982 Consequences of confirmed maternal rubella at successive stages of pregnancy. Lancet 2(8302):781–784.

Miniero R, Dalponte S, Linari A et al 1996 Severe Shwachman–Diamond syndrome and invasive parvovirus B19 infection. Pediatr Hematol Oncol 13(6):555–561.

Mouly F, Mirlesse V, Meritet J F et al 1997 Prenatal diagnosis of fetal varicella-zoster virus infection with polymerase chain reaction of amniotic fluid in 107 cases. Am J Obstet Gynecol 177(4):894–898.

Nascimento J P, Buckley M M, Brown K E, Cohen B J 1990 The prevalence of antibody to human parvovirus B19 in Rio de Janeiro, Brazil. Rev Inst Med Trop Sao Paulo 32(1):41–45.

Newman C G 1965 Perinatal varicella. Lancet 2(7423):1159–1161.

Nigro G, Adler S P, La Torre R, Best A M 2005 Passive immunization during pregnancy for congenital cytomegalovirus infection. N Engl J Med 353(13):1350–1362.

Nigro G, Anceschi M M, Cosmi E V 2003 Clinical manifestations and abnormal laboratory findings in pregnant women with primary cytomegalovirus infection. BJOG 110(6):572–577.

Norbeck O, Papadogiannakis N, Petersson K et al 2002 Revised clinical presentation of parvovirus B19-associated intrauterine fetal death. Clin Infect Dis 35(9):1032–1038.

Noyola D E, Demmler G J, Williamson W D et al 2000 Cytomegalovirus urinary excretion and long term outcome in children with congenital cytomegalovirus infection. Congenital CMV Longitudinal Study Group. Pediatr Infect Dis J 19(6):505–510.

Odibo A O, Campbell W A, Feldman D et al 1998 Resolution of human parvovirus B19-induced nonimmune hydrops after intrauterine transfusion. J Ultrasound Med 17(9):547–550.

Okumura A, Ichikawa T 1993 Aseptic meningitis caused by human parvovirus B19. Arch Dis Child 68(6):784–785.

Ong C L, Daniel M L 1998 Antenatal diagnosis of a porencephalic cyst in congenital varicella-zoster virus infection. Pediatr Radiol 28(2):94.

Palmer C G, Pauli R M 1988 Intrauterine varicella infection. J Pediatr 112(3):506–507.

Pass R F, Fowler K B, Boppana S B et al 2005 Congenital cytomegalovirus infection following first trimester maternal infection: Symptoms at birth and outcome. J Clin Virol 35(2):216–220.

Pearson H E 1964 Parturition varicella-zoster. Obstet Gynecol 23:21–27.

Peckham C 1985 Congenital rubella in the United Kingdom before 1970: the prevaccine era. Rev Infect Dis 7 Suppl 1:S11–S16.

Peckham C, Marshall W C 1979 Rubella and other virus infections in pregnancy. J Antimicrob Chemother 5 Suppl A:71–80.

Petignat P, Vial Y, Laurini R, Hohlfeld P 2001 Fetal varicella-herpes zoster syndrome in early pregnancy: ultrasonographic and morphological correlation. Prenat Diagn 21(2):121–124.

Picone O, Costa J M, Dejean A, Ville Y 2005 Is fetal gender a risk factor for severe congenital cytomegalovirus infection? Prenat Diagn 25(1):34–38.

Picone O, Costa J M, Leruez-Ville M et al 2004 Cytomegalovirus (CMV) glycoprotein B genotype and

CMV DNA load in the amniotic fluid of infected fetuses. Prenat Diagn 24(12):1001–1006.

Preblud S R, Kushubar R, Friedman H M 1982 Rubella hemaggluttination inhibition titers. JAMA 247(13):1811–1812.

Prospective Study of Human Parvovirus (B19) Infection in Pregnancy 1990 Public Health Laboratory Service Working Party on Fifth Disease. BMJ 300(6733):1166–1170.

Radner M, Vergesslich K A, Weninger M et al 1993 Meconium peritonitis: a new finding in rubella syndrome. J Clin Ultrasound 21(5):346–349.

Randel R C, Kearns D B, Nespeca M P et al 1996 Vocal cord paralysis as a presentation of intrauterine infection with varicella-zoster virus. Pediatrics 97(1):127–128.

Rasmussen L, Geissler A, Winters M 2003 Inter- and intragenic variations complicate the molecular epidemiology of human cytomegalovirus. J Infect Dis 187(5):809–819.

Rawlinson W D, Dwyer D E, Gibbons V L, Cunningham A L 1989 Rapid diagnosis of varicella-zoster virus infection with a monoclonal antibody based direct immunofluorescence technique. J Virol Methods 23(1):13–18.

Revello M G, Gerna G 2002 Diagnosis and management of human cytomegalovirus infection in the mother, fetus, and newborn infant. Clin Microbiol Rev 15(4):680–715.

Revello M G, Zavattoni M, Baldanti F et al 1999a Diagnostic and prognostic value of human cytomegalovirus load and IgM antibody in blood of congenitally infected newborns. J Clin Virol 14(1):57–66.

Revello M G, Zavattoni M, Furione M et al 1999b Quantification of human cytomegalovirus DNA in amniotic fluid of mothers of congenitally infected fetuses. J Clin Microbiol 37(10):3350–3352.

Revello M G, Zavattoni M, Sarasini A et al 1998 Human cytomegalovirus in blood of immunocompetent persons during primary infection: prognostic implications for pregnancy. J Infect Dis 177(5):1170–1175.

RevelloProust S, Philippe H J, Paumier A et al 2006 [Mirror pre-eclampsia: Ballantyne's syndrome. Two cases]. J Gynecol Obstet Biol Reprod (Paris) 35(3):270–274.

Rinvik R 1969 Congenital varicella encephalomyelitis in surviving newborn. Am J Dis Child 117(2):231–235.

Rodis J F, Borgida A F, Wilson M et al 1998 Management of parvovirus infection in pregnancy and outcomes of hydrops: a survey of members of the Society of Perinatal Obstetricians. Am J Obstet Gynecol 179(4):985–988.

Saigal S, Lunyk O, Larke R P, Chernesky M A 1982 The outcome in children with congenital cytomegalovirus infection. A longitudinal follow-up study. Am J Dis Child 136(10):896–901.

Savage M O, Moosa A, Gordon R R 1973 Maternal varicella infection as a cause of fetal malformations. Lancet 1(7799):352–354.

Scharf A, Scherr O, Enders G, Helftenbein E 1990 Virus detection in the fetal tissue of a premature delivery with a congenital varicella syndrome. A case report. J Perinat Med 18(4):317–322.

Schild R L, Plath H, Thomas P et al 1998 Fetal parvovirus B19 infection and meconium peritonitis. Fetal Diagn Ther 13(1):15–18.

Schopfer K, Lauber E, Krech U 1978 Congenital cytomegalovirus infection in newborn infants of mothers infected before pregnancy. Arch Dis Child 53(7):536–539.

Sekhsaria S, Rahbar F, Fomufod A et al 1992 An unusual case of congenital cytomegalovirus infection with glaucoma and communicating hydrocephalus. Clin Pediatr (Phila) 31(8):505–507.

Sener R N 1998 Schizencephaly and congenital cytomegalovirus infection. J Neuroradiol 25(2):151–152.

Sever J L, Hardy J B, Nelson K B, Gilkeson M R 1969 Rubella in the collaborative perinatal research study. II. Clinical and laboratory findings in children through 3 years of age. Am J Dis Child 118(1):123–132.

Sever J L, Nelson K B, Gilkeson M R 1965 Rubella epidemic, 1964: effect on 6000 pregnancies. Am J Dis Child 110(4):395–407.

Shaw C M, Alvord E C Jr 1974 Subependymal germinolysis. Arch Neurol 31(6):374–381.

Sheikh A U, Ernest J M, O'Shea M 1992 Long-term outcome in fetal hydrops from parvovirus B19 infection. Am J Obstet Gynecol 167(2):337–341.

Siegel M, Fuerst H T 1966 Low birth weight and maternal virus diseases. A prospective study of rubella, measles, mumps, chickenpox, and hepatitis. JAMA 197(9):680–684.

Simchen M J, Toi A, Bona M et al 2002 Fetal hepatic calcifications: prenatal diagnosis and outcome. Am J Obstet Gynecol 187(6):1617–1622.

Slomka M J, Emery L, Munday P E et al 1998 A comparison of PCR with virus isolation and direct antigen detection for diagnosis and typing of genital herpes. J Med Virol 55(2):177–183.

Smulian J C, Egan J F, Rodis J F 1998 Fetal hydrops in the first trimester associated with maternal parvovirus infection. J Clin Ultrasound 26(6):314–316.

Soothill P 1990 Intrauterine blood transfusion for non-immune hydrops fetalis due to parvovirus B19 infection. Lancet 336(8707):121–122.

Soussotte C, Maugey-Laulom B, Carles D, Diard F 2000 Contribution of transvaginal ultrasonography and fetal cerebral MRI in a case of congenital cytomegalovirus infection. Fetal Diagn Ther 15(4):219–223.

Stagno S, Pass R F, Cloud G et al 1986 Primary cytomegalovirus infection in pregnancy. Incidence, transmission to fetus, and clinical outcome. JAMA 256(14):1904–1908.

Stagno S, Pass R F, Dworsky M E, Alford C A Jr 1982 Maternal cytomegalovirus infection and perinatal transmission. Clin Obstet Gynecol 25(3):563–576.

Stagno S, Reynolds D W, Huang E S et al 1977 Congenital cytomegalovirus infection. N Engl J Med 296(22):1254–1258.

Steinlin M I, Nadal D, Eich G F et al 1996 Late intrauterine Cytomegalovirus infection: clinical and neuroimaging findings. Pediatr Neurol 15(3):249–253.

Stone K M, Reiff-Eldridge R, White A D et al 2004 Pregnancy outcomes following systemic prenatal acyclovir exposure: Conclusions from the international acyclovir pregnancy registry, 1984–1999. Birth Defects Res A Clin Mol Teratol 70(4):201–207.

Tassin G B, Maklad N F, Stewart R R, Bell M E 1991 Cytomegalic inclusion disease: intrauterine sonographic diagnosis using findings involving the brain. AJNR Am J Neuroradiol 12(1):117–122.

Teele R L, Hernanz-Schulman M, Sotrel A 1988 Echogenic vasculature in the basal ganglia of neonates: a sonographic sign of vasculopathy. Radiology 169(2):423–427.

Tolfvenstam T, Papadogiannakis N, Norbeck O et al 2001 Frequency of human parvovirus B19 infection in intrauterine fetal death. Lancet 357(9267):1494–1497.

Torok T J 1990 Human parvovirus B19 infections in pregnancy. Pediatr Infect Dis J 9(10):772–776.

Townsend J J, Baringer J R, Wolinsky J S et al 1975 Progressive rubella panencephalitis. Late onset after congenital rubella. N Engl J Med 292(19):990–993.

Trotta M, Azzi A, Meli M et al 2004 Intrauterine parvovirus B19 infection: early prenatal diagnosis is possible. Int J Infect Dis 8(2):130–131.

Tsuji A, Uchida N, Asamura S et al 1990 Aseptic meningitis with erythema infectiosum. Eur J Pediatr 149(6):449–450.

Twickler D M, Perlman J, Maberry M C 1993 Congenital cytomegalovirus infection presenting as cerebral ventriculomegaly on antenatal sonography. Am J Perinatol 10(5):404–406.

Valeur-Jensen A K, Pedersen C B, Westergaard T et al 1999 Risk factors for parvovirus B19 infection in pregnancy. JAMA 281(12):1099–1105.

Ville Y 1998 The megalovirus. Ultrasound Obstet Gynecol 12(3):151–153.

von Kaisenberg C S, Bender G, Scheewe J et al 2001 A case of fetal parvovirus B19 myocarditis, terminal cardiac heart failure, and perinatal heart transplantation. Fetal Diagn Ther 16(6):427–432.

Watt-Morse M L L S, Hill L M 1995 The natural history of cytomegalovirus infection as assessed by serial ultrasound and fetal blood sampling: a case report. Prenat Diagn 15(6):567–570.

Waxham M N, Wolinsky J S 1984 Rubella virus and its effects on the central nervous system. Neurol Clin 2(2):367–385.

Weber D M, Pellecchia J A 1965 Varicella pneumonia: study of prevalence in adult men. JAMA 192:572–573.

Weil M L, Itabashi H, Cremer N E et al 1975 Chronic progressive panencephalitis due to rubella virus simulating subacute sclerosing panencephalitis. N Engl J Med 292(19):994–998.

Weiland H T, Vermey-Keers C, Salimans M M et al 1987 Parvovirus B19 associated with fetal abnormality. Lancet 1(8534):682–683.

Weiner C P, Grose C F, Naides S J 1993 Diagnosis of fetal infection in the patient with an ultrasonographically detected abnormality but a negative clinical history. Am J Obstet Gynecol 168(1 Pt 1):6–11.

Whitley R J 1992 Neonatal herpes simplex virus infections: pathogenesis and therapy. Pathol Biol (Paris) 40(7):729–734.

Whitley R J, Kimberlin D W, Roizman B 1998 Herpes simplex viruses. Clin Infect Dis 26(3):541–53, quiz 554–555.

Wolinsky J S, Dau P C, Buimovici-Klein E et al 1979 Progressive rubella panencephalitis: immunovirological studies and results of isoprinosine therapy. Clin Exp Immunol 35(3):397–404.

Yaegashi N, Niinuma T, Chisaka H et al 1998 The incidence of, and factors leading to, parvovirus B19-related hydrops fetalis following maternal infection; report of 10 cases and meta-analysis. J Infect 37(1):28–35.

Yow M D, Williamson D W, Leeds L J et al 1988 Epidemiologic characteristics of cytomegalovirus infection in mothers and their infants. Am J Obstet Gynecol 158(5):1189–1195.

Zerbini M, Gentilomi G A, Gallinella G et al 1998 Intra-uterine parvovirus B19 infection and meconium peritonitis. Prenat Diagn 18(6):599–606.

Zinkham W H, Medearis D N Jr 1967 Osborn J E. Blood and bone-marrow findings in congenital rubella. J Pediatr 71(4):512–524.

Bacterial and fungal infections

Thomas Snelling and David Isaacs

> **Key Points**
>
> - Bacterial meningitis is more common in the first month than at any other age
> - About 10–30% of babies with early-onset septicemia and 10% with late-onset septicemia have meningitis
> - Group B streptococcus is the commonest cause of early-onset meningitis in industrialized countries
> - Gram-negative enteric bacilli are the most common cause of late-onset meningitis
> - Ventriculitis is common in neonatal bacterial meningitis, particularly gram-negative meningitis, and there may be collections of pus in the ventricles and subarachnoid space
> - Vasculitis is common and may lead to venous thrombosis; there may be infarcts and focal necrosis
> - Treatment of early-onset meningitis should be with ampicillin and an aminoglycoside (unless gram-negative bacilli are seen on Gram stain)
> - Treatment of gram-negative meningitis should be with cefotaxime (except for **Pseudomonas** and other resistant organisms) and an aminoglycoside
> - Empirical therapy for neonatal meningitis (organism unknown) should be with ampicillin and cefotaxime
> - Gram-negative meningitis should be treated for at least 3 weeks
> - Bacterial meningitis has a mortality of 10–25%; 20–60% of survivors have major neurodevelopmental sequelae
> - Shunt infections should usually be managed by complete removal of the tubing, external ventricular drain and antibiotics
> - In fungal meningitis, use amphotericin B (±5-flucytosine) or fluconazole as an alternative; treat for at least 4 weeks

INTRODUCTION

Neonatal central nervous system (CNS) infections due to bacteria, viruses or fungi should be considered in the differential diagnosis whenever a clinician is confronted with a sick neonate, even one without neurologic signs or symptoms.

Meningitis in the term neonate is generally a consequence of bloodstream infection and its etiology reflects the pathogens which most commonly cause sepsis in this age group, namely *Streptococcus agalactiacae* (group B streptococcus), *Escherichia coli* and *Listeria monocytogenes*. One advance has been the decrease in the incidence of neonatal group B streptococcal meningitis in industrialized countries with increasing use of intrapartum antibiotics (May et al 2005).

The pathogens responsible for late onset meningitis in neonates who are hospitalized for the complications of prematurity vary from institution to institution. While group B

streptococcus and *E. coli* remain important pathogens in this group, infection with a broad range of gram-negative bacilli and *Candida* species makes the treatment of meningitis in this group especially challenging. The need for invasive monitoring and interventions coupled with the heavy use of broad spectrum antibiotics in neonatal units contribute to the selective pressure which predisposes these neonates to infection with organisms which may have intrinsic or inducible resistance to many of the first-line antibiotics traditionally employed for treatment of neonatal sepsis.

The late neonatal period and early infancy remain periods of high relative risk for meningitis although the organisms more likely to be involved in infancy are *Streptococcus pneumoniae*, *Neisseria meningitidis*, *Salmonella* and in unimmunized populations, *Haemophilus influenzae* type b. Group B streptococcus remains a possible cause in early infancy as do coliform bacteria, especially *E. coli*.

EPIDEMIOLOGY

INCIDENCE

Meningitis is more common in the first month after birth than at any other age and more common in the first week than later. Population-based studies in the United States have consistently shown 0.2–0.5 cases of bacterial meningitis per 1000 live births (Klein et al 1995) (see Table 32.1). The incidence of neonatal bacterial meningitis has remained constant in England and Wales at 0.21–0.32 cases per 1000 live births, from 1969 until 1997 (de Louvois et al 1991, Holt et al 2001, Hristeva et al 1993). In Germany, the incidence remained unchanged at 0.5 per 1000 live births in a group born between 1962 and 1974 compared with those born from 1975 to 1982. The incidence of verified bacterial meningitis decreased from 0.36 to 0.19 per 1000 livebirths in Sweden. The minimum incidence in Australia was reported as 0.17 per 1000 (Francis & Gillbert 1992). In Oxford, the incidence of neonatal bacterial meningitis was 0.25 per 1000; viral meningitis was 0.11 per 1000, and fungal meningitis 0.02 per 1000 live births (Hristeva et al 1993). About 10–30% of cases of early-onset neonatal septicemia and about 10% of late-onset cases are complicated by bacterial meningitis (Palazzi et al 2006). A longitudinal surveillance study of neonatal units in Australia and New Zealand found that the rate of early onset group B streptococcal meninigitis fell significantly between 1992 and 2002 (0.24 to 0.03 per 1000) while rates of early onset *E. coli* meningitis remained unchanged (May et al 2005). The

Table 32.1 Incidence (per 1000 live births) and number of cases of bacterial meningitis in neonates

Country	Incidence	n	GBS	GNR	Predominant organisms	Reference
USA	0.27	257	53% (136)	31% (80)	*E. coli* 16% (42) *L. monocytogenes* 7% (18)	Unhanand et al 1993
England & Wales	0.21	144	48% (69)	30% (43)	*E. coli* 18% (26)	Holt et al 2001
England	0.25	23	47% (7)	40% (6)	*K. oxytoca* 13% (2)	Hristeva et al 1993
England & Wales	0.32	423	38% (118)	34% (106)	*E. coli* 25% (78) *L. monocytogenes* 7% (23)	de Louvois et al 1991
Northern Ireland	0.54	41	7% (2)	62% (18)	*E. coli* 56% (15) *S. aureus* 22% (6)	Bell et al 1989
UK		1846	34% (633)	42% (775)	*E. coli* 29% (526) *L. monocytogenes* 7% (125)	Synnott et al 1994
Australia	0.17	116	35% (41)	36% (42)	*E. coli* 22% (22) *L. monocytogenes* 3% (3)	Francis & Gilbert 1992
Israel	0.5	32	19% (6)	53% (17)	*Klebsiella* + *E. coli* 13% (4) *Proteus* 6% (2)	Greenberg et al 1997
S. Africa	—	60	35% (21)	—	*K. pneumoniae* 28% (17) *E. coli* 17% (10)	Adhikari et al 1995
Nigeria	1.9	36	0	35% (9)	*S. aureus* 42% (11) *Klebsiella* spp. 15% (4)	Airede 1993
Jordan	1.1	53	4% (2)	81% (43)	*K. pneumoniae* 36% (19) *Enterobacter* spp. 19% (10)	Daoud et al 1996
Trinidad	2.9	54	56% (5)	33% (3)	*Enterobacter* 11% (1) *E. coli* 11% (1)	Ali 1995
Thailand		77	12% (9)	51% (39)	*Ps. aeruginosa* 17% (13) *E. coli* 10% (8)	Chotpitayasunondh 1994

Key: GBS = group B streptococcus; GNR = gram-negative rods. Of the positive bacterial isolates, the frequency of GBS, GNR and predominant organisms is given as a percentage and number of positive isolates.

incidence of late onset gram-negative meningitis fell during the same time period (Gordon & Isaacs 2006).

In developing countries, the incidence of neonatal bacterial meningitis is usually higher than that in industrialized countries. The incidence was 1.9 per 1000 in Nigeria (Airede 1993); 2.9 per 1000 in Trinidad, West Indies (Ali 1995), while in Ethiopia, the incidence in preterm neonates over a 10-year period was 3.7 and in term newborns was 1.0 per 1000 live births.

The incidence of neonatal bacterial meningitis is higher in infants of low birthweight, so the reported incidence will vary according to the population being studied. Certain groups of babies are at greatly increased risk of meningitis, irrespective of birthweight. Babies with open myelomeningoceles are particularly likely to develop bacterial meningitis, especially caused by gram-negative enteric bacilli. Cerebrospinal fluid (CSF) shunts are highly likely to become infected with skin organisms, such as coagulase negative staphylococci. Dermal sinuses overlying the CSF anywhere from the bridge of the nose, over the skull, and down the back to the sacrum may penetrate through to the dura and give rise to meningitis. If a dermal sinus is missed (and they can be very small and hidden under the hair), then recurrent meningitis can occur.

ORGANISMS
Group B streptococcus
In most industrialized countries, group B streptococcus (GBS) is the commonest cause of neonatal bacterial meningitis (see Table 32.1). The incidence of early-onset GBS sepsis increased in the UK after the 1970s, but was found in Oxford, UK to have remained steady from 1985 to 1996 with an annual incidence of 0.5 per 1000 live births, of whom 15% had meningitis (Moses et al 1998). In contrast, the incidence was higher in the USA (Platt et al 1999) and Australia, where the peak incidence of early-onset GBS sepsis reached 2.0 per 1000 live births or even greater, of whom 7–10% had meningitis (Isaacs & Royle 1999). However the incidence has fallen substantially to 0.25 cases per 1000 in Australia (Daley et al 2004) and in Boston (Platt et al 1999), almost certainly due to the widespread use of intrapartum antibiotics.

Gram-negative bacilli
After group B streptococcus, gram-negative bacilli are the next most common group of organisms causing neonatal meningitis in industrialized countries (see Table 32.1). Of these, *Escherichia coli* is the most frequently isolated. However, several other enteric gram-negative bacilli can

cause meningitis, including *Pseudomonas, Proteus, Klebsiella* and *Enterobacter. Neisseria meningitidis* and *Haemophilus influenzae* also cause neonatal meningitis occasionally (Shepard et al 2003). An 11 year multicenter study of late onset sepsis in Australia and New Zealand revealed that gram-negative bacilli were a frequent cause of bacteremia and meningitis after 48 hours and that *Pseudomonas aeruginosa* was associated with a particularly poor prognosis (Gordon & Isaacs 2006). A study of 150 neonatal units in the USA found that cases of gram-negative meningitis occurred later and were more commonly associated with antepartum exposure to antibiotics than cases of gram-positive meningitis (Smith et al 2006). Some gram-negative organisms, particularly *Enterobacter sakazakii* and *Serratia marcescens*, have been associated with nursery outbreaks of sepsis and meningoencephalitis (Berger et al 2002). Bizzarro and colleagues (2006) found that sporadic neonatal *Serratia* infections were frequently associated with meningitis and death. In a recent review of 46 cases of invasive *Enterobacter sakazakii* infections in infants, 32 had meningitis and most occurred in term neonates. There was a strong correlation with exposure to contaminated powdered infant formula (Bowen & Braden 2006).

Other organisms

Listeria monocytogenes is an important cause of bacterial meningitis in some industrialized countries, but usually <10% of cases (see Table 32.1). Other causes are various gram-negative and gram-positive cocci (*Streptococcus pneumoniae*, other streptococci including *Streptococcus pyogenes*, and *Enterococcus* species). Anaerobic meningitis is rare. A list of organisms causing bacterial meningitis is given in Table 32.2, based on the studies of de Louvois et al (1991) and Synnott et al (1994), in the approximate order of frequency for the United Kingdom (approximate because bacterial meningitis is under-reported).

The genital mycoplasmas, *Mycoplasma hominis* and *Ureaplasma urealyticum*, have been grown from the CSF of neonates and have been implicated as a cause of indolent meningitis in term and preterm neonates (Waites et al 1990). Because culture requires specialized culture media, the relative contribution of these organisms to neonatal meningitis may have been overlooked.

Rates of coagulase negative staphylococcus meningitis vary considerably in the literature and distinguishing infection from contamination is problematic. A 10 year study found that meningitis accounted for only 5 of 1281 cases of coagulase negative staphylococcus sepsis in Australian nurseries and that mortality from this organism was low (Isaacs 2003).

Developing countries

Typically, the pattern of organisms causing bacterial meningitis in developing countries is very different from those in industrialized countries. For example, group B streptococcal infection is generally rare in developing countries. There were no cases of GBS meningitis over 3 years in Nigeria

Table 32.2 Organisms causing neonatal bacterial meningitis in approximate order of frequency for United Kingdom

Group B streptococcus
Escherichia coli
Listeria monocytogenes
Streptococcus pneumoniae
Enterococci
Other streptococci
Proteus species
Neisseria meningitidis
Staphylococcus aureus
Klebsiella species
Haemophilus influenzae
Pseudomonas species
Enterobacter species
Citrobacter species
Serratia species
Salmonella species
Other gram-negative bacilli
Anaerobes
Mycobacterium tuberculosis
Campylobacter species
Coagulase-negative staphylococci (shunt infections)

Source: From de Louvois & Lambert 1991, Hristeva et al 1993 and Synnott et al 1994.

where the most common causative organisms were *S. aureus* and *Klebsiella* (Airede 1993). GBS caused 11.7% of cases in Thailand (Chotpitayasunondh 1994), the other main organisms being *Pseudomonas aeruginosa* (16.9%), *Klebsiella pneumoniae* (13.0%), *E. coli* (10.4%) and *Enterobacter* species (10.4%). In Mexico 61% of CSF isolates were gram-negative bacilli, and in Ethiopia 67% of isolates were *Klebsiella pneumoniae, E. coli*, or *Enterobacter* species (Rios-Reategui et al 1998). In the 1980s, *Klebsiella* was the commonest cause in Durban, South Africa, followed by *E. coli* and GBS. More recently, in South Africa, GBS has caused more cases (35%) than *Klebsiella* (28%) and *E. coli* (17%), while meningitis was more frequently caused by *E. coli* (46.7%) than GBS (26.7%) or *Klebsiella* (13.3%) in Nairobi (Laving et al 2003). GBS is now the predominant organism in Trinidad, West Indies, with a mean age at presentation of 4 days (Ali 1995), and in Zimbabwe GBS was the predominant organism (61%). Non-typhoidal *Salmonella* infections are common in developing countries (Balaka et al 2004, Totan et al 2002).

High-risk groups

Shunt infections are most commonly due to coagulase-negative staphylococci, but a specimen of CSF should always be obtained in suspected shunt infections because *Staphylococcus aureus*, gram-negative bacilli or fungi are also causes. Meningitis complicating myelomeningocele is usually caused by gram-negative enteric bacilli.

The isolation of certain organisms should alert the physician to special problems. For example, *Citrobacter* meningitis is frequently associated with brain abscess, although abscess may occur with other organisms such as *Proteus*. *Enterobacter sakazakii* has been associated with NICU-based common source outbreaks of meningitis and sepsis with contamination of powdered milk formula commonly implicated (Drudy et al 2006).

Fungal meningitis almost exclusively affects babies <1500 g birthweight and, as their survival increases with improved neonatal care, the incidence of fungal meningitis also increases. It is still extremely rare compared with bacterial meningitis: one-tenth as common in Oxford (Hristeva et al 1993). *Candida* is the most commonly isolated yeast infection, but other fungi such as *Trichosporon beigelii* are rare CNS pathogens.

Summary of epidemiology

- Bacterial meningitis is more common in the first month than at any other age.
- About 10–30% of babies with early-onset septicemia and 10% with late-onset septicemia have meningitis.
- Group B streptococcus has been the commonest cause of early-onset meningitis in industrialized countries, although the incidence is falling.
- Gram-negative enteric bacilli are the commonest cause of late-onset meningitis.

PATHOGENESIS

Organisms reach the subarachnoid space most commonly by bacteremic seeding within the choroid plexus. The magnitude of bacteremia correlates strongly with the probability of meningitis. Less commonly, meningitis can be due to direct spread, either from an infected scalp lesion with spread through skull sutures and thrombosed veins or from otitis media. CSF environmental factors such as pH and osmolality have been shown experimentally to affect bacterial ability to invade brain microvascular endothelial cells.

Low birthweight is the most significant risk factor for meningitis: in a recent prospective study, meningitis was 10 times more common in neonates with a birthweight under 2 Kg than those >2 Kg (de Louvois et al 1991). Other host factors include prematurity (risk ratio 17.8), ventriculo-peritoneal shunts, myelomeningocele, maternal sepsis, multiple pregnancy, prior infant sepsis and invasive procedures on the neonate (Francis & Gilbert 1992). Other risk factors are also associated with sepsis and meningitis such as infants requiring resuscitation, intubation, male sex and socio-economic deprivation (Palazzi et al 2006).

The most common associated site of infection outside the CNS is the lung (pneumonia or empyema). There may also be otitis or omphalitis (which have occasionally been the original source of sepsis), peritonitis, pyelonephritis, enterocolitis, osteomyelitis, septic arthritis and abscesses in other organs (skin, liver, etc.).

VIRULENCE

Escherichia coli

Certain organisms are far more likely to cause bacterial meningitis than others, so that the virulence of the invading organism as well as host factors is important in determining whether or not meningitis occurs. The K1 capsular antigen of *Escherichia coli*, which is similar to the capsular polysaccharide of group B *Neisseria meningitidis*, is important in facilitating bloodstream survival. More than 80% of cases of neonatal *E. coli* meningitis are caused by strains carrying the K1 antigen. The relative pathogenetic importance of predisposing host factors and virulence-associated bacterial characteristics of *E. coli*, such as possession of P-fimbriae, O and K antigens and hemolysins, has been studied. Bacterial factors were more important in neonatal meningitis and UTI, whereas host factors contributed to septicemia or bacteremia. Certain genetic markers have been found to be more common in *E. coli* strains from neonates with meningitis than in *E. coli* in blood or commensals. The specific outer membrane protein (OmpA), which contributes to *E. coli* K1 membrane invasion, has been experimentally shown to be inhibited by wheat-germ agglutinin. Specific gene locations have been identified in the serotype O18:K1:H7 (the most virulent *E. coli* in newborn meningitis), which are associated with its ability to penetrate the blood–brain barrier and invade the brain microvascular endothelial cells. This may allow rapid identification by genotyping organisms, which can be instructive regarding epidemiology. For example, despite concurrent urine and CSF isolation of *E. coli* in one study, the two were proved to be different genotypes.

Group B streptococcus

In a study of neonatal meningitis in Australia (Francis & Gilbert 1992), 80% of neonates with GBS infections had no risk factors for sepsis. This is because late-onset GBS meningitis predominantly affects full-term babies when they are 2–6 weeks old. Risk factors in these babies are virtually confined to having low levels of transplacental antibodies to the type III GBS capsular polysaccharide. Group III GBS strains are disproportionately likely to cause late-onset meningitis (>80% of cases), compared with early-onset sepsis when strains I, II and III are equally common. Thus, early onset GBS meningitis typically involves a high-risk baby who acquires maternal GBS at the time of delivery, develops high-level septicemia and hence meningitis. In contrast, late-onset meningitis usually occurs in an apparently healthy full-term baby whose nasopharynx is colonized (at birth or subsequently) with serotype III GBS and who lacks antibody to the capsule.

Staphylococci

Other organisms that are common causes of neonatal septicemia virtually never cause meningitis. Coagulase-negative staphylococci are one of the commonest causes of late-onset septicemia in industrialized countries, but meningitis virtually only occurs if there is a CSF shunt. *Staphylococcus aureus* is another common cause of septicemia, but a rare cause of meningitis unless there has been surgery, a shunt, or seeding from bacterial endocarditis. A polysaccharide capsule is one characteristic of the organisms causing meningitis that is lacking in staphylococci.

Listeria

Listeria monocytogenes, like GBS, can cause early and late-onset forms of bacterial meningitis. The early form may be acquired transplacentally (granulomatosis infantiseptica) or by inhalation of infected amniotic fluid, whereas the late-onset form follows nasopharyngeal colonization and later invasion of the blood and meninges, usually at 2–6 weeks of age.

PATHOLOGY

Toxic products of the bacterial cell wall, peptidoglycans and teichoic acid from gram-positive and lipopolysaccharide (endotoxin) from gram-negative organisms, cause substantial damage to the endothelial cells of the cerebral capillaries, which form the so-called 'blood–brain barrier'. Disruption of the tight junctions between the endothelial cells increases the permeability and allows entry of bacteria and white cells and leakage of protein (see Fig. 32.1).

The host immune response causes damage to the central nervous system. High levels of tumor necrosis factor (TNF-α) and interleukin-1 and 6 (IL-1β and IL-6) in the CSF have

been correlated with prolonged fever, fits, spasticity and death. These cytokines from mononuclear cells may damage endothelial cells and lead to raised intracranial pressure and cerebral edema. Oxygen free radicals have also been found to be released in association with meningitis-causing strains of *E. coli* in healthy full-term neonates. These could harm surrounding tissue and potentiate the inflammatory process. Arachidonic acid metabolites from platelets are also probably important in pathogenesis. Levels of prostaglandin E_2, a potent vaso-active substance, rise in the CSF in experimental meningitis, and this contributes to cerebral edema; both the increased levels and cerebral edema can be blocked by indometacin. Complement may be important in opsonizing organisms, but can also lyse host cells if bacterial cell-wall products are incorporated into them. Soluble CD14 from intrathecal leucocytes is massively released into the CSF and may play an important role in the pathogenesis of meningitis.

Intracranial pressure (ICP) is always elevated in bacterial meningitis. The possible mechanisms include cerebral edema, vasodilatation of cerebral veins and capillaries, vascular leak, loss of auto-regulation of cerebral blood flow and impaired circulation of CSF. Reduced cerebral blood flow produces regional hypoxemia, increased metabolism of arachidonic acid, and anaerobic glycolysis with increased production of lactate. There is also decreased carrier-mediated transport of glucose into CSF, and this is probably the main cause of the characteristic low CSF glucose (hypoglycorrhachia) seen in bacterial meningitis. Consumption of glucose by bacteria or white cells is unlikely to be a major cause of low CSF glucose, since the CSF sugar can be low, even zero, for weeks after acute bacterial meningitis, without causing any symptoms.

The outcome in neonatal meningitis is generally worse than that in older children. The relatively poor neonatal immune response, permitting rapid bacterial multiplication, is one possible reason. Severe ventriculitis, a hallmark of neonatal meningitis, is rarely seen outside the newborn period. Fever is relatively uncommon in neonatal meningitis, and this may contribute to the poor outcome, since CSF bacterial multiplication in experimental pneumococcal meningitis is far more rapid at normal body temperatures than when animals are febrile.

Summary of pathology

- Ventriculitis is common in neonatal bacterial meningitis, particularly gram-negative meningitis, and there may be collections of pus in the ventricles and subarachnoid space.
- Subdural effusions are rarely of a sufficient size to cause raised intracranial pressure.
- Hydrocephalus may develop secondary to purulent exudate obstructing the arachnoid granulations over the surface of the brain, or as a result of exudate in the ventricles obstructing the foramina of Magendie and Luschka or the aqueduct.

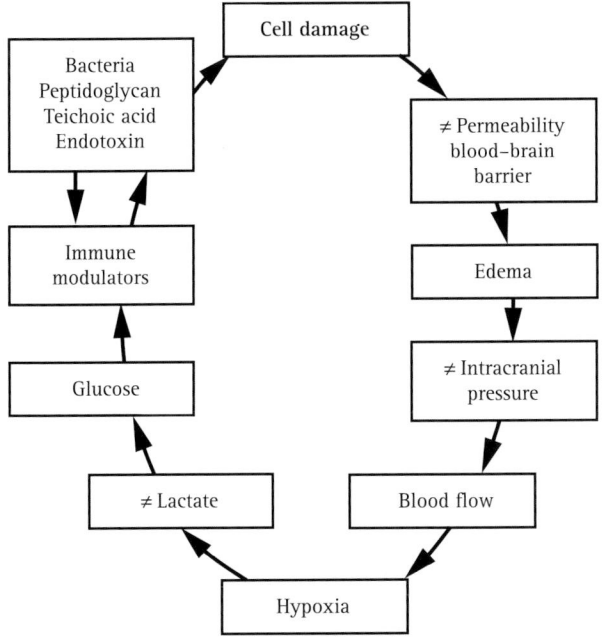

Figure 32.1 Pathophysiology of bacterial meningitis.

- Intraventricular hemorrhage may occur and contribute to hydrocephalus.
- Vasculitis is common and may lead to venous thrombosis; there may be infarcts and focal necrosis.
- Neuronal damage is often widespread in severe cases and leads to necrotic liquefaction or cerebral atrophy.

CLINICAL FEATURES

The classic clinical features of bacterial meningitis are frequently absent and there may be no apparent distinction between the newborn with sepsis with or without meningitis. A body temperature greater than 38°C or less than 36.7°C is an indication for further investigation and consideration of lumbar puncture. However, in one series of 223 proven cases of neonatal bacterial meningitis, only nine cases had a temperature greater than 38°C (de Louvois & Lambert 1991). The neonate may even appear well yet still be found to have meningitis. A bulging fontanelle strongly suggests meningitis but may be absent with dehydration. Group B streptococcal sepsis can present with respiratory distress within a few hours of birth that may be confused with hyaline membrane disease, and will progress rapidly to meningitis if untreated. The majority of gram-negative meningitis associated with obstetric complications occurs in the first 2 weeks. The more premature and the younger the baby, the less specific the symptoms and signs. Palazzi et al (2006) summarized the clinical signs in 255 neonates with bacterial meningitis in six centers (see frequencies in Table 32.3).

LUMBAR PUNCTURE

Indications

Because of the difficulty in making a clinical diagnosis of meningitis, it is vital that if sepsis is suspected, either a lumbar puncture (LP) is performed or, if the LP is delayed because of the baby's unstable condition, blood cultures are taken and antibiotics started that will adequately cover the organisms likely to cause bacterial meningitis. The wide range of possible pathogens makes empiric antimicrobial therapy without a lumbar puncture far more difficult. Up to 40% of cases of neonatal meningitis are associated with negative blood cultures (Garges et al 2006, Visser & Hall 1980), so if antibiotics are started for suspected early-onset sepsis without performing a lumbar puncture, the LP should be done later, particularly if blood cultures are positive. However, occasionally meningitis may be present with normal CSF microscopy, while an intraventricular hemorrhage may complicate the later interpretation of the CSF white-cell count. In a study of 728 LPs performed in the first week of life on babies with early-onset respiratory distress, bacteria were isolated from the CSF of nine, but only one had a clinical course consistent with meningitis.

The indications for lumbar puncture are controversial. They range from inclusion of LP as part of a routine septic work-up in asymptomatic neonates based on maternal risk factors, to restricting LP to those who have signs and symptoms of severe sepsis. A study of 9641 VLBW neonates found that 5% of LPs performed after 72 hours were positive, 34% of which were associated with negative blood cultures (Stoll et al 2004). Visser and Hall (1980) reported that of 21 neonates with late onset bacteremia, 5 also had concurrent meningitis. In one study, 43 cases of meningitis were reviewed retrospectively by application of selective criteria for performing LP only if CNS symptoms or signs were present, and the diagnosis of bacterial meningitis would have been delayed or missed in 37% of them. Of admission lumbar punctures for respiratory distress, only one of over 1700 infants had an organism identified in the CSF that was not isolated in the blood. In Australia, a survey of neonatologists revealed that none performed an LP routinely for a preterm neonate with respiratory distress and 83–85% if the blood culture was positive (Joshi & Barr 1998).

Neonates can decompensate rapidly with handling during lumbar puncture, due to hypoxia and hypercapnia. The LP should be delayed if there is significant respiratory distress or labile blood pressure. Pre-oxygenation can help prevent

Table 32.3 Clinical signs of bacterial meningitis			
Symptoms	Percentage	Signs	Percentage
Lethargy	50	Fever or hypothermia	61
Anorexia		Respiratory distress	47
Vomiting	49	Irritability	32
Diarrhea	14	Jaundice	28
Convulsions	40	Full/bulging fontanelle	28
Apnea	7	Neck stiffness	15
Altered sleep pattern		Hypotonia	
High-pitched cry		Petechiae	
		Hypotension, shock	
		Bradycardia	

Source: Frequencies from Klein et al 1995, Palazzi et al 2006.

desaturation. Local anesthesia decreases the amount of struggling but not physiological changes. The risk of coning of the medulla oblongata into the foramen magnum is low, even with raised intracranial pressure. Topical local anesthetic mixtures reduce pain and are safe in term neonates but cause raised methemoglobin in preterm infants, although this has not been shown to have any clinical consequences. Performing the LP with the neonate in the sitting position has been shown to reduce the degree of hypoxia. The rate of coning in neonates has been reported as 1% (four out of 423 neonates) (de Louvois et al 1991).

Lumbar puncture should be performed with a stiletted needle in preference to a hypodermic needle. This is to prevent the risk of an epidermoid tumor in the spinal canal from a fragment of skin that may not present for many years after neonatal LP. There has been some suggestion that the stylet should be reinserted before the needle is removed to reduce CSF leak. The success rate in 181 neonates using different types of needle has been shown to be the same, and the traumatic taps did not result in pleocytosis on repeat LP. A formula for the depth of insertion of the lumbar puncture needle has been calculated in centimeters as 0.03 × height of child (cm). A sterile technique should be used to prevent introduction of infection and contamination of the specimen. Contamination is particularly important when a shunt is being tapped, as the organisms causing shunt infections are often skin flora. However, iodine containing disinfectants should not be used, because of the risk of transient hypothyroidism. Chlorhexidine is a suitable disinfectant. The opening pressure should be measured. The normal pressure in neonates is 0–5.7 mmHg (7.6 cm water) with the head de-flexed, and the baby horizontal and quiet.

The larger the specimen of CSF, the more chance of isolation of organisms that are present in small numbers such as mycobacteria and fungi. CSF should also be sent for protein and glucose assay with simultaneous blood glucose assay. The measurement of CSF lactate is not routinely useful in meningitis, though it may be of use in the investigation of the neonate with seizures or suspected metabolic abnormality. Further tests may be of use such as latex agglutination test for group B streptococcus, which is commercially available. However, it is possible to have a false-negative result when excess antigen is present (prozone effect) and false positives from skin contamination. Urinary antigen testing is not generally useful because of high false-positive and false-negative rates. Newer methods of ultrasound-enhanced particle agglutination show improved detection rates. The sensitivity of latex agglutination for infants with group B streptococcal meningitis varies from 73–100% for CSF and 75–84% for urine.

If syphilis is suspected, a non-treponemal test such as VDRL should be performed on the CSF. The CSF should be examined by microscopy and a differential cell count. A Gram stain should be performed even if there are no white cells, because meningitis can occur in the absence of pleocytosis. The spun CSF should be cultured on blood agar and chocolate agar routinely. If there is a shunt, this should be brought to the attention of the microbiology laboratory so that the CSF can be cultured in enrichment broth. A viral culture should also be performed when indicated clinically and, if appropriate, specific viral polymerase chain reaction (PCR) for herpes simplex virus (HSV) and enterovirus.

Inflammatory markers can be useful in diagnosing infection. C-reactive protein (CRP) can be measured in the CSF and blood. The result of a meta-analysis suggests that only a negative CRP test is highly informative in the diagnosis of bacterial meningitis. Interleukin-1 receptor antagonist (IL-1ra) and interleukin-6 (IL-6) levels have been found to rise in serum 2 days before clinical manifestation of infection in neonates. However, an LP is effectively a biopsy, giving a rapid diagnosis of the condition and the likely cause, whereas no acute phase reactant will have 100% specificity, nor will it distinguish septicemia from meningitis.

INTERPRETATION OF CSF FINDINGS
CSF white-cell count

In general, CSF white-cell count and protein levels are higher and CSF glucose levels lower in normal neonates than in older children and adults (see Table 32.4). These differences are even more marked in preterm infants. In normal preterm infants, the mean CSF white-cell count is up to 27 μL, about one-half neutrophils, with a range of 0–112. In normal-term infants, the mean white-cell count is lower (5–10 μL) in most studies, but again the range is up to 130 (Ahmed et al 1996). There is no difference in CSF findings between term and preterm infants at high risk of infection but without meningitis. The mean CSF white-cell counts were 8 and 9 μL and the ranges 0–32 and 0–29 for

Table 32.4 Normal CSF combined values from selected studies

	Number of infants	White cells (×10⁶/L)	Protein (g/L)	Glucose (mg/L)
		Mean (range)	Mean (range)	Mean (range)
Preterm	188	12 (0–112)	1.09 (0.31–2.69)	7.1 (2.4–10.6)
Term	409	8.8 (0–130)	0.72 (0.17–1.74)	5.0 (2.6–24.8)

Source: From Klein et al 1995 and Isaacs & Moxon 1999.

term and preterm babies, respectively. Sixteen babies with septicemia without meningitis had a mean CSF white count of 20 µL (range: 0–112). Traumatic taps are common, but interpretation of the ratio of white to red cells is not reliable. A repeat lumbar puncture after a traumatic tap may also be misleading as the blood can cause an inflammatory response or red cells can lyse giving a falsely low RBC count.

Of 21 babies with proven group B streptococcal meningitis and of 98 babies with gram-negative enteric meningitis, 29% and 4%, respectively, had CSF white counts <32 µL. This shows that there is considerable overlap between the CSF white-cell count in babies with and without meningitis. A comparison of 77 cases of gram-positive neonatal meningitis and 86 cases of neonatal meningitis found relatively higher CSF white cell counts in gram-negative cases (Smith et al 2006). Bacteria may sometimes be cultured from the CSF of babies with normal CSF microscopy (no white cells and no organisms seen). Nine per cent of a UK series of 223 neonates with meningitis had less than 10 white cells in the CSF (de Louvois & Lambert 1991). Ahmed et al (1996) closely examined a cohort of 108 full-term neonates and excluded meningitis using the most stringent criteria, including performing PCR for enteroviruses. The mean CSF white-blood-cell count was 7.3 µL (95% confidence interval 6.6–8.0). The SD was 14, so 2SD above the mean would be 35. The median was 4, and most babies had CSF white counts from 0 to 20 (90% had <11). However, there was one baby with a CSF white count of 130 and one with a count of 62. Clearly, this degree of overlap between apparently uninfected babies and babies with meningitis makes interpretation of white counts in the 20–130 range problematic. Leucocyte aggregation is a feature of bacterial meningitis, which distinguishes it from viral or aseptic meningitis.

Because of overlap, a CSF white-cell count alone does not always distinguish the baby with meningitis from the baby without. The CSF white count should always be considered in conjunction with CSF protein and sugar, CSF red-cell count, baby's age, etc. As a useful rule, however, a CSF white-cell count over 20, in the absence of raised red cells, should be considered suggestive of meningitis.

CSF protein

The mean CSF protein in preterm babies without meningitis is about 100 mg/dL (1.0 g/L) with the normal range approximately 50–290 mg/dL (0.5–2.9 g/L). For term babies, the mean is about 60 mg/dL (0.6 g/L) and the range 30–240 mg/dL (0.3–2.4 g/L). The CSF protein is often raised in bacterial meningitis but in one study was within the normal range of 20–170 mg/dL (0.2–1.7 g/L) in 47% of babies with group B streptococcal meningitis and 23% with gram-negative enteric bacillary meningitis. Elevated CSF protein in the absence of pleocytosis may be seen in para-meningeal infections, congenital infections and intracranial hemorrhage. A study of meningitis in 95 neonates in the United States found that elevated CSF protein levels poorly predicted bacterial meningitis (Garges et al 2006).

CSF glucose

Mean absolute CSF glucose concentrations in normal babies have varied from 50 to 80 mg/dL (2.7–4.4 mmol/L) with a range of 24–100 mg/dL (1.5–5.5 mmol/L). The CSF glucose is generally low in bacterial meningitis and may be zero, but in some cases may be higher than the lower limit of the 'normal range'. As CSF and blood glucose concentrations are both lower in healthy newborn infants than in older children, it has been suggested that the ratio of CSF to blood glucose is a useful indicator of neonatal meningitis. In the study by Sarff et al (1976), the mean CSF:blood glucose ratio was 81% (range: 44–248) in preterm infants without meningitis and 74% (range: 55–105) in term infants. However, 45% of infants with group B streptococcal meningitis and 15% with gram-negative bacillary meningitis had CSF:blood glucose ratios >44%, showing that the CSF:blood glucose ratio is relatively poor at discriminating babies with and without meningitis.

In viral meningitis, the CSF glucose level is usually normal, although low glucose levels may occur, the protein level is often elevated, and the mean CSF white cell count is usually <1000 µL, although it may be up to 4500 with a neutrophil predominance. Thus, in the absence of organisms on Gram staining, it can be extremely difficult to distinguish viral from bacterial meningitis.

Gram stain

Of the 117 babies with neonatal meningitis (Sarff et al 1976), only one had completely normal CSF microscopy and biochemistry. The Gram stain reveals organisms in about 80% of cases of meningitis. The CSF white-cell count is generally higher in gram-negative enteric bacillary than in group B streptococcal meningitis; median number more than 2000 µL and less than 100 µL respectively (Palazzi et al 2006). Although neutrophils usually predominate in bacterial meningitis, the same is also true in early viral meningitis.

VENTRICULAR TAP

Ventriculitis is present in most babies with gram-negative enteric meningitis and many with group B streptococcal meningitis. The diagnosis can be made by finding >100 white cells/µL in ventricular CSF obtained by ventricular tap. However, ventricular taps can result in intracerebral cysts, and ventriculitis is so common that it can almost be assumed to be present, particularly in gram-negative bacillary meningitis. Ventriculitis can sometimes be diagnosed on cerebral ultrasound imaging by seeing unusual fibrin strands in the ventricles. Ventricular or cisternal taps may have a role in specific circumstances such as suspected meningitis in a child with spinal bifida or other local contraindication to lumbar puncture. However, they are not justifiable as routine following traumatic lumbar puncture, particularly as the blood from the LP can be seen in the ventricles. Intracranial hemorrhage itself can result in pleocytosis, low CSF glucose and raised CSF protein.

Summary of indication for LP

- Definite sepsis (positive blood culture), early or late onset.
- Suspected severe sepsis, early or late onset.
- Early-onset respiratory distress if associated with signs of sepsis.
- Suspected late-onset sepsis.

MANAGEMENT

CLINICAL ASSESSMENT

When meningitis is 'proven' (organisms seen on CSF Gram stain) or probable (raised CSF white-cell count, but no organisms seen), a careful clinical assessment is the first priority. The baby should be examined for a source of infection, notably otitis, omphalitis, and osteomyelitis of the skull and also for midline CNS anomalies such as congenital dermal sinuses. These can occur anywhere in the midline from the bridge of the nose, on the scalp under the hairline and down the spine to the sacrum.

Skin rashes – erythematous, maculopapular or purpuric – may accompany bacterial meningitis, while a fine, macular rash may occur in enteroviral meningitis. The eyes should be examined for the characteristic retinal or vitreous lesions of fungal meningitis. The head circumference should be measured, both to see if there has been a marked increase from the last measurement and to act as a baseline for serial measurements during treatment.

A full clinical examination is, of course, essential, both to look for other foci of infection and to assess the overall clinical state. The blood pressure should be measured but may be artificially maintained due to raised intracranial pressure and peripheral vasoconstriction. Thus, an assessment for shock should also include an assessment of peripheral perfusion (capillary return and core–peripheral temperature difference), pulse character, heart rate and urinary output.

SUPPORTIVE THERAPY

The same basic principles for supportive therapy apply as for systemic sepsis. The first priority is to support the systemic circulation with fluid. The choice of fluid has been recently reviewed with concerns about human albumin, which is not now recommended as the first line in neonatal hypovolemia. Crystalloid has been shown in randomized controlled trials of hypotensive preterm infants to be as effective as colloid. Fresh frozen plasma (FFP) is not always immediately available, as it needs to be matched and thawed. FFP may raise IgG levels but does not change opsonic activity in neonates with coagulase negative staphylococcal septicemia.

Exchange transfusion with fresh whole blood improves survival in scleremic neonates with sepsis. Immunomodulating drugs may have a role in the future as pentoxifylline has been found to decrease serum levels of tumor necrosis

factor and interleukin-1 and to reduce mortality in a randomized double-blind trial of sepsis in premature infants. Recombinant human granulocyte colony-stimulating factor (G-CSF) in preterm neonates with neutropenia is effective at preventing infection if given prophylactically. However, there are conflicting results regarding its effectiveness if given after the onset of suspected sepsis. A Cochrane review (Ohlsson et al 1998) found that although prophylactic intravenous immunoglobulin (IVIG) has been shown to reduce sepsis in preterm neonates, it did not significantly reduce mortality or other morbidities (NEC, IVH, length of hospital stay). IVIG has been given as therapy for late-onset sepsis, but the numbers studied have been too small to show a significant reduction in mortality, although there is a strong trend to reduced mortality (which was halved). An international randomized controlled trial of IVIG for sepsis (the INIS study) should provide data.

The hypotension associated with sepsis unresponsive to fluids and inotropes has also been improved with the use of methylene blue as an inhibitor of guanylate cyclase, which causes vascular smooth muscle dilation in the presence of excess nitric oxide in septic shock. Although inappropriate secretion of antidiuretic hormone (ADH) and cerebral edema are common in bacterial meningitis, the only prospective randomized trial of fluid restriction versus maintenance fluids with a clinical end point in acute meningitis showed a trend towards lower mortality in the group receiving full maintenance fluids. There is also experimental data from *E. coli* meningitis in rabbits that found that fluid restriction causes higher levels of CSF lactate and lower levels of CSF glucose but has no effect on cerebral edema.

Phenobarbitone is the anticonvulsant of choice for convulsions associated with meningitis in neonates. A loading dose of 15–20 mg/Kg followed by a maintenance dose of 5 mg/Kg once daily is appropriate. The levels of chloramphenicol may be reduced if this antibiotic is being used (as in developing countries), in which case, ampicillin and gentamicin may be a better empiric combination. Diazepam can cause hypotension but is an appropriate first-line anticonvulsant for ongoing seizure activity at a dose of 0.1 mg/Kg, repeated if necessary. While steroids are recommended for older infants and children with bacterial meningitis, they have not been shown to be of benefit for pathogens associated with neonatal meningitis. Furthermore, in animal models of *E. coli* meningitis their use was reportedly detrimental (Spreer et al 2006). A study from Jordan of 52 full-term neonates randomized to receive dexamethasone or not failed to reveal any benefit in mortality or morbidity after 2 years (Daoud et al 1999).

ANTIBIOTIC THERAPY

The choice of antibiotic therapy will depend on which organisms are prevalent in the community, and which are seen on a Gram stain and culture. There may be an initial suggestion from the Gram staining: gram-positive cocci (most probably group B streptococcus, enterococcus or pneumococcus), gram-positive bacilli (*Listeria*) or gram-negative bacilli (most likely *E. coli*, *Pseudomonas*, coliforms or *Haemophilus influenzae*), or no bacteria at all. The situation is completely different for infected ventricular shunts and is considered later in this chapter. However, empiric antibiotic treatment should be continued until the organism is positively identified by culture and sensitivity rather than on Gram stain, which is sometimes misleading.

It is generally acknowledged that all antibiotics should be given parenterally for the entire duration of therapy of neonatal meningitis. Oral absorption of antibiotics is extremely erratic in the neonatal period. Aminoglycosides are sometimes given intramuscularly because intravenous boluses can give rise to high serum peak levels, but recent evidence suggests that high peak levels do not cause toxicity, and i.v. therapy is safe and kinder. All antibiotics used for treating bacterial meningitis should be given intravenously because muscle perfusion may be poor.

For rapid sterilization of the CSF, drug concentrations of at least ten times MIC are required. The entry of hydrophilic antibacterials such as beta-lactams (penicillins and cephalosporins) and glycopeptides (e.g. vancomycin) into the CSF is poor with an intact blood–brain barrier (BBB) but increases with meningeal inflammation. Lipophilic antibacterials such as chloramphenicol or rifampicin penetrate well across the BBB and are not inflammation-dependent.

Developing countries

Third-generation cephalosporins are very expensive in terms of the poorest countries' health budgets. Historically, chloramphenicol was widely used in the United Kingdom. There has been a high rate of side-effects attributed to its use in neonates. In a study of 64 neonates treated with chloramphenicol in ten UK hospitals, five developed 'gray baby syndrome,' four of whom had cardiovascular collapse, one baby became 'very gray' and four more had reversible hematological abnormalities. However, in the treatment of neonates with meningitis, serious toxicity has been associated only with dosages higher than recommended and none if serum levels are kept between 15 and 25 mg/L. Chloramphenicol is bacteriostatic for most gram-negative enteric bacilli. Although glucuronide conjugation is depressed by immaturity, chloramphenicol is metabolized by other pathways.

Streptococci

For Group B streptococcal meningitis, penicillin or ampicillin plus an aminoglycoside is the treatment of choice. GBS has remained sensitive to penicillin G. Recommendations for the dose of penicillin G for treating GBS meningitis vary from 50 000 units/Kg per dose to 240 mg/Kg/day. The dose frequency varies with age (see Table 32.5). There is experimental evidence advocating synergism of an aminoglycoside with the penicillin until the CSF is sterile, although there are no clinical data to suggest that this increases survival.

Isolates of *Streptococcus pneumoniae*, particularly those causing invasive disease, are increasingly being found to be relatively resistant to penicillin and third-generation cephalosporins. In the USA between 1993 and 1996, 12.7% of pneumococci causing meningitis in children had intermediate sensitivity to penicillin, and 6.6% were completely resistant; 4.4% had intermediate resistance to ceftriaxone, and 2.8% were resistant. There have been treatment failures using third-generation cephalosporins to treat pneumococcal meningitis, which has responded to vancomycin. Hence, empiric treatment with vancomycin may be appropriate if *Streptococcus pneumoniae* is suspected from Gram stain or culture from another site. However, vancomycin is not an appropriate first-line empiric therapy in neonates, in whom meningitis is rarely caused by pneumococci.

Enterococci can cause meningitis, sometimes in association with shunt infections. They are resistant to cephalosporins and should be treated with ampicillin, if sensitive, or vancomycin.

Staphylococci

Staphylococcal neonatal meningitis is rare, but occasional cases do occur. Vancomycin may be necessary when there are gram-positive cocci in bunches suggestive of staphylococci seen in the CSF. Local prevalence of methicillin-resistant *Staphylococcus aureus* (MRSA) will determine the choice of flucloxacillin or vancomycin pending sensitivity testing. The true incidence of coagulase negative staphylococcal meningitis in the absence of a foreign body is difficult to determine, as opposed to contamination of CSF culture, which is relatively common. However, if there is a ventriculo-peritoneal shunt in situ, then vancomycin is a reasonable first-line therapy to cover coagulase negative staphylococci.

Vancomycin penetration into the CSF of premature infants with meningitis ranges from 26 to 68% of serum levels, which is a higher proportion than for older infants and children. Serum vancomycin levels should be measured pre-dose (trough) and 30 min after a 1-h infusion (peak). Vancomycin appears safe in neonates, even with vancomycin serum concentrations >40 µg/mL, without causing nephrotoxicity.

Listeria

For meningitis attributable to *Listeria monocytogenes*, ampicillin and an aminoglycoside is the regimen for which there are most data. *Listeria* is susceptible to ampicillin, gentamicin, cotrimoxazole, vancomycin and meropenem in vitro. There is little to choose between penicillin and ampicillin. There have been a few reports of treatment failures using penicillin G and an aminoglycoside, but there are many successes, and ampicillin is not always successful either. The third-generation cephalosporins are inactive against *Listeria*.

Gram-negative bacilli

Cefotaxime is now the preferred antibiotic therapy for most cases of gram-negative bacillary meningitis, although *Pseudomonas* is inherently resistant. Although this choice is that

Table 32.5 Summary of antibiotic therapy

		Dose (mg/Kg/day)	Age (days)	Interval	comment
Group B strep	Penicillin G	240	≤7	12 h	
			>7	6 h	
S. aureus	Flucloxacillin	200	≤7	12 h	
			>7	8 h	
Coagulase neg staph	Vancomycin	20	≤7	Daily	≤1500 g
		30	≤7	12 h	>1500 g
		30	>7	8 h	≤1500 g
		45	>7	8 h	>1500 g
Listeria monocytogenes	Ampicillin	200	≤7	12 h	
		400	>7	8 h	
Gram-negative bacilli	Cefotaxime	150	≤7	12 h	Prem
				8 h	Term
		200	>7	8 h	Prem
				8 h	Term
	Gentamicin	2	≤7	Daily	<800 g
		3	≤7	Daily	800–1499 g
		4	≤7	18 h	1500–2000 g
		5	≤7	12 h	>2000 g
		3–5	>7	Daily	<800 g
		3–5	>7	18 h	800–1499 g
		3–5	>7	12 h	1500–2000 g
		7.5	>7	8 h	>2000 g
Pseudomonas	Ceftazidime	150		8 h	
Anaerobes	Metronidazole	15	≤7	12 h	
		30	>7	12 h	
Candida, Aspergillus	Amphotericin	0.5		Daily	Day 1
		1.0		Daily	Day 2+
	5-Fluorocytosine	100		6–12 h	Prem
		200			Term
Multi-resistant	Meropenem	45–60		8 h	

of the majority of experts polled in the USA in 1992, cefotaxime has never been compared to previous antibiotic regimens, such as ampicillin and gentamicin in controlled trials. However, cefotaxime achieves good CSF levels, whereas aminoglycosides only penetrate inflamed meninges.

Studies from McCracken's group showed that ampicillin and gentamicin sterilized the CSF of most cases of gram-negative meningitis, even when due to ampicillin-resistant E. coli (McCracken et al 1980). Clearance of septicemia plus some CSF penetration of inflamed meninges are the probable mechanisms. Cephalosporins and aminoglycosides act by different mechanisms and synergy might be expected. As prognosis depends on the speed of sterilization of CSF, we recommend using both a third-generation cephalosporin and an aminoglycoside for gram-negative bacillary meningitis, unless the latter is contra-indicated. While it is well established that irreversible ototoxicity and vestibular toxicity can occur with gentamicin use in adults, limited studies

have failed to reveal otovestibular toxicity as a significant problem when gentamicin is used in the neonatal period (Aust & Schneider 2001).

In 1971–1975, the mortality for gram-negative enteric meningitis was 30%, and half the survivors were felt to be normal. In order to improve CSF delivery of antibiotics, McCracken studied intrathecal administration of aminoglycosides, which did not alter the outcome. He then studied intraventricular administration of aminoglycosides, which actually increased the mortality (McCracken et al 1980).

The advent of the third-generation cephalosporins was heralded as solving the problem of CSF penetration of antibiotics. Ceftriaxone has been used in the USA, but caution is needed in the neonatal period because it can displace bilirubin bound to albumin and aggravate hyperbilirubinemia. Trimethoprim-sulfamethoxazole (cotrimoxazole) can be very useful against multi-resistant gram-negative bacilli.

Multi-resistant organisms

One exception to the above antibiotic recommendations is if the baby with meningitis is known to be infected with a cefotaxime-resistant gram-negative bacillus or if there is widespread colonization of other babies with resistant organisms. Some gram-negative organisms have intrinsic resistance to cefotaxime, such as *Pseudomonas aeruginosa* and *Stenotrophomonas maltophilia*. Because the antibiotic susceptibilities of these organisms are variable, treatment should take into consideration the in vitro susceptibility patterns. Optimally, treatment of meningitis caused by these agents should include at least one agent known to have good CSF penetration with the possible addition of an aminoglycoside.

Some other gram-negative organisms, including *Enterobacter*, *Serratia* and *Proteus* species as well as *Citrobacter freundii* and *Morganella morganii*, can produce an inducible AmpC beta-lactamase which degrades most cephalosporins. These organisms not infrequently cause neonatal meningitis, particularly in pre-term infants or in late-onset disease, and treatment complications have been reported when resistance to cefotaxime has arisen whilst on therapy (Sinha et al 2006). *E. coli* rarely expresses inducible beta-lactamase production although early onset *E. coli* meningitis associated with this phenotype has also been reported (Fakioglu et al 2006). More frequently, *E. coli* and *Klebsiella* species may express a plasmid-derived extended spectrum beta lactamase (ESBL) which is broadly resistant to beta lactam antibiotics and which is coinherited with genes for aminoglycoside and other antibiotic-class resistance. Treatment of cefotaxime resistant gram-negative organisms may require carbapenems, fluoroquinolones, or aminoglycosides. Treatment of these organisms should always be in consultation with an infectious diseases physician. Imipenem has good CSF penetration, but lowers the seizure threshold in older children with meningitis, so meropenem should be used in preference. However, either carbapenem should only be used if there are no alternatives. Experience with meropenem is limited but when used to treat 15 neonates (8 preterm) there were no side-effects recorded (Unhanand et al 1993). Although imipenem is more effective in the treatment of multi-resistant gram-positive bacteria, meropenem has good activity against cephalosporin-resistant pneumococci. Multi-resistant *Acinetobacter baumannii* presents a particular challenge in its ability to survive on fomites and develop resistance to carbapenems, but treatment with ampicillin/sulbactam has been successful. Fourth-generation cephalosporins (e.g. cefpirome) have been used in children with bacterial meningitis, and CSF penetration is good, but there are currently no data on neonates.

Duration of therapy

The duration of therapy for neonatal meningitis has not been well studied, is ignored in some textbooks, and is largely empiric. Relapses are not uncommon from gram-negative and, more rarely, gram-positive, meningitis; however, the histories of those babies who have more than one relapse suggest that the relapses are not due to inadequate duration of therapy, but rather to sequestration of organisms.

Ventriculitis is almost invariable in gram-negative enteric meningitis. It may be diagnosed by showing a pleocytosis in CSF obtained by ventricular tap or, less invasively, by showing fibrin strands on a cerebral ultrasound scan. Gram-negative enteric meningitis should be treated for at least 3 weeks because of the difficulty of treating ventriculitis. It is usually stated that GBS meningitis can be treated for 2 weeks. Ventriculitis rarely complicates GBS meningitis, but when it occurs it is associated with a subacute onset and a poor neurological outcome with hydrocephalus a frequent complication (Miyairi et al 2006). We prefer to obtain an ultrasound and treat for at least 3 weeks if fibrin strands are seen.

Summary of treatment

- Empiric treatment of early-onset meningitis should be with penicillin or ampicillin plus cefotaxime until cultures are back.
- Treatment of gram-negative meningitis should be with cefotaxime (except for *Pseudomonas* and other resistant organisms) and an aminoglycoside.
- Gram-negative meningitis should be treated for at least 3 weeks.
- Neither fluid restriction nor steroids have been shown to be of benefit in neonatal meningitis.

COMPLICATIONS

MONITORING

Regular neurological examination is, of course, essential. Close monitoring of vital parameters is essential in order to minimize morbidity and mortality, and newborns with bacterial meningitis should ideally be looked after in a tertiary referral center. For shocked babies, continual monitoring of arterial and central venous pressure allows better fluid balance management. Urine output, urine and serum osmolality, and serum electrolytes should be monitored to permit anticipation of problems with inappropriate ADH secretion. Hematological parameters, including clotting, should be regularly measured. Serial serum CRP measurements can be a useful indicator of progress, low levels showing resolution and elevated levels suggesting continuing infection. Drug levels of antibiotics and anticonvulsants may need to be measured. Head circumference should be measured at least daily, as should the baby's weight.

REPEAT LUMBAR PUNCTURES

Some textbooks recommend daily lumbar puncture, particularly for gram-negative infections, until it is clear that the meningitis is improving. However, others recommend only repeating the lumbar puncture if there is a failure to respond to treatment (de Louvois & Lambert 1991). CSF cultures remain positive in gram-negative bacillary meningitis (mean: 6 days, range: 2–11 days) for longer than in GBS meningitis, in which CSF cultures are usually sterile within 2–3 days of starting treatment. It has not been shown to be useful to do a lumbar puncture just before stopping therapy. Babies with no cells may relapse, while babies with persistent CSF pleocytosis may recover if therapy is stopped. Persisting or recurrent fever may be due to persistence of meningitis, to subdural or intracerebral abscess, to infection in other sites (pleural empyema, septic arthritis and osteomyelitis) or to intercurrent infection.

Recurrences of both gram-positive and gram-negative meningitis may occur after stopping apparently successful treatment. If so, a careful search, both clinical and radiographic, should be made for persisting foci of infection, but these are rarely found. We have seen a baby with two recurrences of *E. coli* meningitis, despite apparently adequate and successful treatment with cefotaxime. No underlying cause was found, and the baby was finally cured using intravenous trimethoprim-sulfamethoxazole. One small study from Australia reported that five (21%) of 24 babies with gram-negative meningitis relapsed when treatment with chloramphenicol and gentamicin (three babies) or cefotaxime (two) was stopped. However, in a national study, only two (5%) of 40 babies with gram-negative and one of 41 with GBS meningitis relapsed (Francis & Gilbert 1992). A relapse rate of 8% was reported in another large study of neonatal meningitis from Sweden.

INTRACRANIAL PRESSURE

Intracranial pressure (ICP) is rarely monitored in the newborn period, but cerebral perfusion pressure (arterial blood pressure minus ICP) may be an important determinant of outcome. The measurement of fontanelle pressure by fontanometer, although non-invasive, is less reliable than invasive ICP monitoring. Invasive monitoring of ICP by subdural catheter or intraventricular catheter is rarely performed in newborns, but might be indicated when there is evidence (e.g. rising blood pressure, falling heart rate) of a significantly raised ICP.

EEG (see also Ch. 12)

Continuous EEG monitoring, particularly of comatose babies and those receiving muscle relaxants, may reveal clinically unrecognized convulsions, which can impair cerebral perfusion. Where this facility is not available, serial EEGs can be helpful. Seizures may be clinically evident; they may present insidiously with apneic attacks or episodes of hypoxia, or may be subclinical and only diagnosed by EEG. In general, the presence of seizures is a poor prognostic feature, particularly if they are not controlled by anticonvulsants. If the EEG appearance is considered in conjunction with the history of seizures and level of consciousness, a reasonably accurate prediction of neurological outcome can be made. A retrospective cohort study of 37 neonates with meningitis found that a moderately or markedly abnormal EEG at baseline

was an accurate predictor of death or poor neurological outcome at 12 months (Klinger et al 2001).

Ultrasound (see also Ch. 6)

Ultrasound detects complications requiring neurosurgical intervention such as empyema, brain abscess or hydrocephalus in infants with bacterial meningitis. Small subdural effusions may be difficult to detect by ultrasound but occur often in bacterial meningitis and very rarely need any intervention. Larger effusions may cause persistent fever and midline shift of the brain with symptoms of raised intracranial pressure. Such effusions may show up on transillumination of the skull. Hydrocephalus is more likely after neonatal meningitis than after meningitis in infancy or in childhood.

CT and MRI (see also Ch. 6)

The role of computed tomography (CT) in detection of the complications of neonatal meningitis is limited when ultrasound has advantages of accessibility and lack of radiation. However, contrast-enhanced CT is useful in diagnosis and follow-up of cerebral candidiasis (see Fig. 32.2). Ring

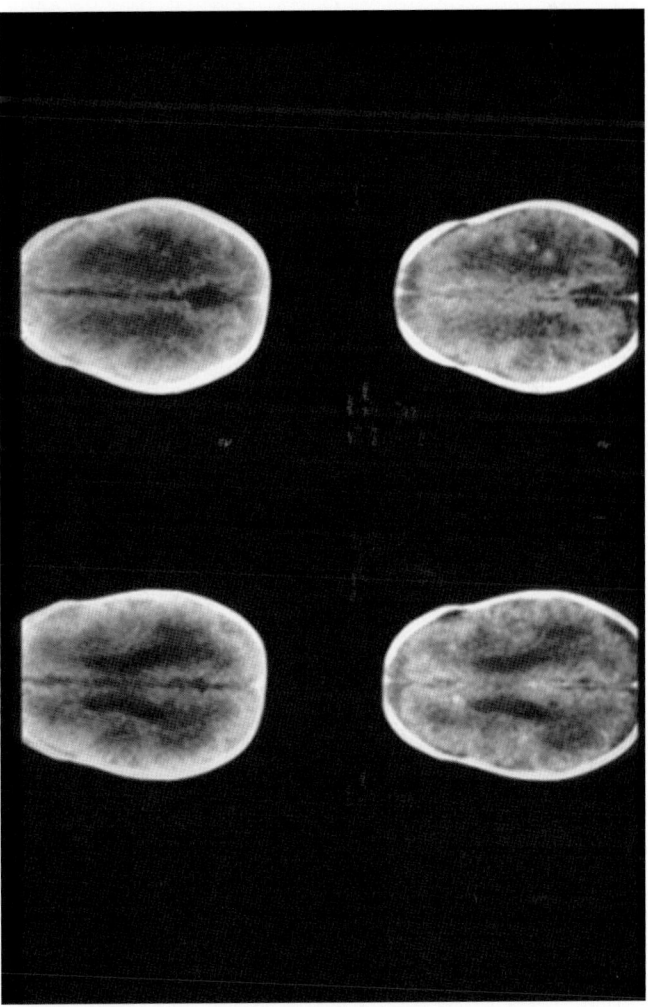

Figure 32.2 CT changes of fungal meningitis.

enhancement seen on CT may be due to infarction as reported with *Enterobacter* mimicking abscess formation. Magnetic resonance imaging (MRI) may rarely have a role in detecting brainstem or spinal-cord complications, but it has not been shown to correlate well with prognosis for seizures. Recurrent meningitis may need investigation with scintigraphic CSF leak studies, particularly if it follows neurosurgery.

BRAIN ABSCESS

Brain abscess, although still rare, is more common in the neonatal period, particularly in association with *Citrobacter* and *Proteus* meningitis (see Fig. 32.3). Other organisms associated with brain abscess include *Serratia marcescens*, *Salmonella enteritidis*, *Morganella morganii*, *Haemophilus influenzae*, *Escherichia coli* and the genital mycoplasmas. *Citrobacter* can be rapidly fatal and has been associated with omphalitis and with the development of pneumocephalus (Alviedo et al 2006, Pooboni et al 2004). *Staphylococcus aureus* brain abscesses have also been reported in term and premature neonates (de Oliveira et al 2006, Vartzelis et al

2005) and may originate from hematogenous dissemination from intravenous cannula sites in premature infants. In brain abscess, there may be a moderate increase in CSF white-cell count, with up to a few hundred cells, mostly mononuclear and raised CSF protein. Organisms are not usually seen on Gram stain nor grown from the CSF. Abscesses are often multiple, which makes surgical drainage more complicated. Ultrasound-guided needle aspiration can be used with local anesthetic to drain single abscesses. They may resolve with medical treatment alone. Brain abscess is associated with a mortality of around 50%. Neurosurgical management of brain abscess is discussed on page 864.

MORTALITY

The mortality of neonatal meningitis still remains high at 20–30%, whether the meningitis is of early or late onset (see Table 32.6). The mortality increases with prematurity and low birthweight. The fatality rate for gram-negative neonatal meningitis has been reported as 17% (of 72) over a 21-year period in the USA (Unhanand et al 1993) to 31% (of 93) in the UK and 33% (of 40) in Australia. The mortality for group B streptococcus in the same studies in the UK was 24% (of 112) and 29% (of 41) in Australia. The number of cases of *Listeria* meningitis was small, and the number of deaths was two out of 19 and one out of three, respectively.

MORBIDITY

Neonatal meningitis results in a high rate of long-term sequelae such as hydrocephalus and neurodevelopmental problems. Although it is not always clear to what extent meningitis and other predisposing factors such as extreme prematurity have contributed to the outcome, significant neurologic sequelae develop in 20–60% of all survivors of neonatal bacterial meningitis caused by any organism

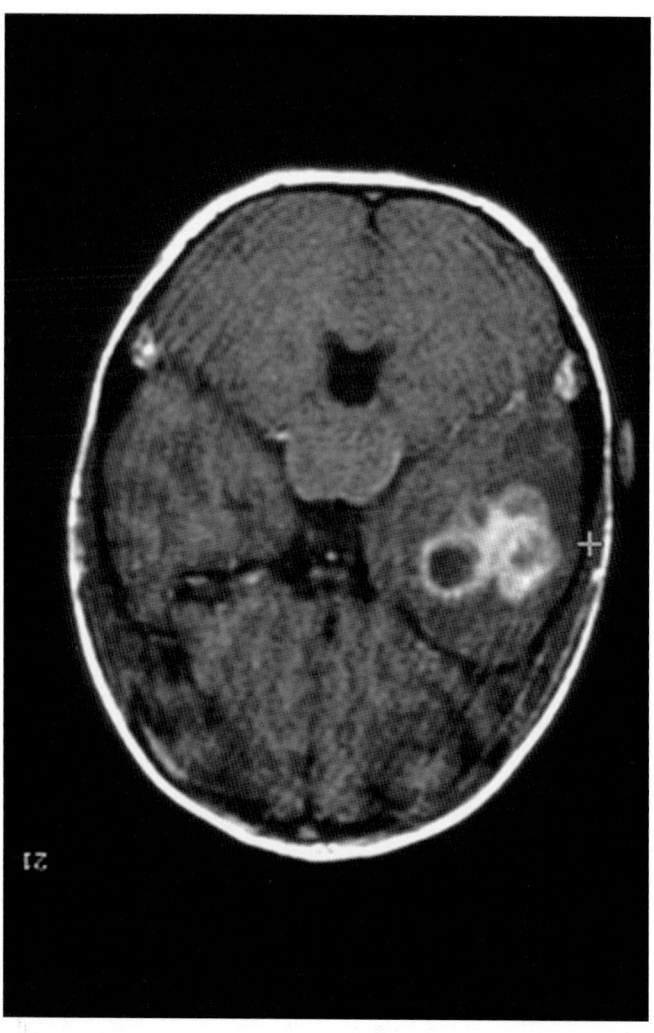

Figure 32.3 MRI showing multifocal brain abscess.

Table 32.6 Mortality rates for neonatal bacterial meningitis				
Years	Country	Cases	Deaths	Reference
1970–1980	USA	26	5 (19%)	Franco et al 1992
1973–1986	N. Ireland	41	20 (49%)	Bell et al 1989
1977–1987	Brazil	109	38 (35%)	Feferbaum et al 1993
1985–1987	UK	423	79 (20%)	de Louvois et al 1991
1987–1989	Australia	116	30 (26%)	Francis & Gilbert 1992
1984–1991	UK	23	6 (26%)	Hristeva et al 1993
1990–1995	Mexico	31	9 (29%)	Rios-Reategui et al 1998

(Palazzi et al 2006, Stevens et al 2003). These sequelae include major neurodevelopmental handicap, hemiparesis, spastic paraparesis, cranial nerve palsies, hydrocephalus, hearing loss, visual handicap, convulsions and speech and hearing disorders.

The rate of hydrocephalus has been reported as 41% (29/71) and gross abnormalities in the neurological examination 62% (44/71) from a study in Brazil. Another study from Brazil of term neonates with meningitis followed up for a mean of 5 years showed neurological sequelae in 64% (35/55), cerebral palsy 58% (severe 24%), hydrocephalus 46% and convulsions 35%. A longitudinal study over 10 years of 111 children with neonatal meningitis from Canada reported 3.6% with sensorineural hearing loss, 2.7% with persistent hydrocephalus and 5.4% with seizures (Stevens et al 2003).

Group B streptococcal meningitis

The risk factors associated with poor outcome in 61 neonates with group B streptococcal meningitis between 1974 and 1979 included presentation comatose or semicomatose, decreased perfusion, total peripheral white-cell count less than 5×10^9/L, absolute neutrophil count less than 1×10^9/L, and CSF protein greater than 3 mg/L. Of 38 survivors followed up for at least 3 years, 29% had severe neurologic sequelae and 21% minor deficits. From another study with follow-up at 3–18 years old, 12% (9/34) had major neurologic sequelae.

Gram-negative meningitis

Of survivors of gram-negative neonatal meningitis, 56% (24/43) had permanent neurologic sequelae (the same percentage in term neonates as preterm neonates): hydrocephalus (13), seizure disorder (13), cerebral palsy (11), developmental delay (14) and hearing loss (7) (Unhanand et al 1993). Significant poor prognostic factors included platelets <100 ($\times 10^9$/L), CSF leucocytes >2000 ($\times 10^6$/L), CSF/blood glucose ratio <0.5, CSF protein 2 (g/L), and positive CSF culture for >48 h after the start of treatment. The rates of sequelae may vary with the organism: the rate for *Escherichia coli* was reported as 43% (13/30) and for *Klebsiella–Enterobacter* species 67% (6/9). Complications are significantly more common in gram-negative, than gram-positive, meningitis (6/10 vs. 13/76; $P = 0.014$; 1987–1989 in Australia) (Francis & Gilbert 1992).

Hearing loss (see also Ch. 38)

Otoacoustic emissions are a useful screening test for hearing loss that can be performed in neonates before discharge from hospital. Auditory brainstem responses (ABR) may be considered the gold standard for testing hearing after meningitis in neonates. However, interpretation of ABR requires expertise, and it can be time-consuming and expensive. Furthermore, young children sometimes require sedation, or even general anesthesia, before ABR can be performed. Insertion of cochlear implants in infancy is possible for profound sensorineural deafness.

Rare neurological sequelae

Reported rare neurologic complications from meningitis include ischemia of the spinal cord resulting from vasculitis associated with *Escherichia coli* meningitis. A transverse myelitis with development of spinal cord cavitation and destruction of the cerebellum developing posterior cysts has been reported in a preterm neonate with group B streptococcal meningitis. Sagittal sinus thrombosis has been reported with *Streptococcus pyogenes* meningitis in a neonate. Central diabetes insipidus as a complication of hypothalamic damage can occur with hemorrhage and hydrocephalus subsequent to group B streptococcal meningitis.

Endophthalmitis

This rare infection of the orbit of the eye has been reported, complicating meningitis in the neonate. It is usually secondary to trauma, such as with face masks or eye pads for phototherapy. However, it can also be hematogenous and may be associated with meningitis. Responsible organisms include *Serratia marcescens* and *Pseudomonas aeruginosa* associated with sepsis and *Escherichia coli* with meningitis. It has also been described congenitally and with *Candida albicans* and *Aspergillus fumigatus*. The diagnosis should be suspected when a hypopyon is seen, and confirmation can be obtained by ultrasound if an anterior uveitis obstructs vision of the retina. The treatment includes urgent intra-ocular antimicrobials, e.g. antibiotics such as vancomycin and intravenous antibiotics such as ceftriaxone that penetrate the globe (more so than cefotaxime). Vitrectomy may also be necessary.

Summary of complications

- Routine lumbar puncture before stopping antibiotics is not necessary.
- Babies with GBS meningitis should have a cerebral ultrasound: treat with at least 2 weeks of antibiotics, but at least 3 weeks if ventriculitis is present.
- Bacterial meningitis has a mortality of 10–25%, and 20–60% of survivors have major neurodevelopmental sequelae.
- Endophthalmitis is often associated with meningitis in neonates and requires urgent intra-ocular antibiotics.

SHUNT INFECTIONS

Infections of ventriculoperitoneal (VP) or ventriculoatrial (VA) shunts should be considered separately from bacterial meningitis. These occur in between 3 and 27% of shunts, with a mean of 11% (Anonymous 1989). Although shunt infections may present like classic bacterial meningitis, they commonly present more insidiously. VP shunt infections cause vomiting, lethargy and irritability with or without fever, whereas VA shunt infections may cause low-grade fever, progressive anemia, and hematuria and hypertension secondary to shunt nephritis. Infection of a newly placed shunt is highly likely if there is significant infection of the skin overlying the reservoir, a situation that readily occurs in small preterm neonates when the skin of the scalp is stretched over the reservoir.

Coagulase-negative staphylococci, such as *Staphylococcus epidermidis*, are the commonest cause of shunt infections, but these may also be caused by *Staphylococcus aureus* and, particularly in babies of low birthweight, by gram-negative bacilli (e.g. *Pseudomonas*), by low-grade pathogens such as diphtheroids and by fungi (see Table 32.7). In a study from Germany, 22 of 28 (79%) were gram-positive cocci and two were gram-negative bacilli. *Staphylococcus epidermidis* produces an extracellular slime that enables it to adhere to implantable devices and resist antibiotic therapy. *Bacillus cereus* has also been reported, causing shunt infections. *Propionibacterium acnes*, a low-grade pathogen, has been associated with 15% of shunt infections (distinguished from being a contaminant by presence in CSF of gram-positive rods and white cells), presenting as gradual shunt malfunction, nausea, headache and malaise, though infrequently fever.

Of 23 cases of gram-negative shunt infections from one center in the USA, 87% (20) occurred within 4 weeks of shunt revision (median 10 days). The most frequent symptoms were fever, lethargy and irritability, but most patients appeared relatively well. *E. coli* was isolated from 52% (12) and *Klebsiella pneumoniae* from five. Four patients had persistence of the bacteria in the CSF despite immediate shunt removal, and all had CSF glucose <1 mmol/L and a positive CSF Gram stain on admission. All were cured with no recurrence.

The first priority in suspected shunt infection is to obtain a specimen of CSF for microscopic examination by tapping the shunt reservoir. Measurement of serum CRP has been helpful in identifying whether babies with non-specific symptoms have shunt infections.

If shunt infection is confirmed, the entire shunt usually needs to be removed. In a review of several trials (Yogev 1985), the success rate of antibiotics alone was 36% (71/195);

antibiotics and immediate replacement with a new shunt had a 65% (75/116) success rate; and antibiotics, shunt removal, external ventricular drain, or repeat ventricular aspirates had a 96% (154/161) success rate. The appropriate antibiotics can be given intravenously. When the protocol was changed in Zagreb to include complete shunt revision and prophylactic antibiotics, the infection rate was reduced from 18% per case to 8%.

Because an intraventricular reservoir or external ventricular drain is usually inserted to drain CSF until the shunt infection is cleared (p. 843), antibiotics can be given directly into the ventricles (e.g. vancomycin, gentamicin) if there is a problem with severe infection or infection with a multiply resistant organism. Intraventricular antibiotics themselves can cause a chemical meningitis, so when the CSF is sterile and organisms are no longer seen, intraventricular antibiotics should not be continued merely because of a raised CSF white-cell count and protein.

Prophylactic antibiotics at the time of shunt insertion have been shown to be associated with a significant reduction in shunt infections in only one study, but when 12 studies were combined in a meta-analysis, on aggregate, the approximate risk reduction was 50%, $P = 0.0002$ (Langley et al 1993). In a prospective study from Italy, a single dose of ceftriaxone was given preoperatively i.v. in 100 cases, and no shunt infections were observed over a 4-year follow-up period.

Although one-half of our isolates of coagulase-negative staphylococci are cloxacillin (methicillin)-resistant, we start empiric antibiotic therapy of shunt infections in which gram-positive cocci are seen on the Gram stain of the CSF, using flucloxacillin and aminoglycoside, rather than vancomycin, because these infections are rarely fulminant, and symptoms often resolve simply with removal of the shunt. Teicoplanin has been used intraventricularly for *Staphylococcus aureus*, *Staphylococcus epidermidis* and *Enterococcus faecalis* shunt infections, though it was not effective given intravenously alone as an alternative to vancomycin for organisms resistant to other penicillins.

Of children with meningomyelocele, 11.5% (20/170) in a study from Italy presented within the first year following shunting with shunt infection. Infections were associated with higher meningomyeloceles, degree of ventricular dilatation, age of meningomyelocele repair, CSF shunting before repair and abnormal CSF values.

In Taiwan, 17% (8/48) of shunt infections were attributed to fungi isolated from the CSF and not thought to be contaminants. All were in infants who had been born prematurely. The presentation was subtle and insidious, and the CSF only showed a mild pleocytosis and raised CSF protein, but only in half was the CSF glucose low.

SUMMARY OF SHUNT INFECTIONS

- Shunt infections should usually be managed by complete removal of the tubing, external ventricular drain and antibiotics.

Table 32.7 CSF shunt infection rates

Year	Country	Case	Procedure	Reference
		Infection rate per		
1978–1983	UK	19% (23/155)	12% (46/380)	Casey et al 1997
1981–1992	Italy	17% (14/81)	7.8% (15/191)	Dallacasa et al 1995
1985–1990	Croatia	18% (36/201)	9.4% (36/382)	Rotim et al 1997
1991–1995	Croatia	8% (6/75)	5.3% (6/112)	Rotim et al 1997
1986–1989	Germany	(25 patients)	8% (28/350)	Kontny et al 1993
1990–1996	USA	13% (20/145)	11% (29/268)	Mancao et al 1998

FUNGAL CNS INFECTIONS

Neonatal central nervous system infection with fungi is a rare, but serious, condition (see Table 32.8). In a retrospective study from Texas, *Candida albicans* accounted for 2% of all positive CSF cultures in neonates. A further review from Texas found that twenty-three of 106 cases of systemic *Candida* infections (0.4% of all NICU admissions) had associated meningitis and that 91% had birth weights less than 1500 g (Fernandez et al 2000). One-third of neonates (three out of nine) in that study and three-quarters (six out of eight) of premature neonates in a retrospective study from Canada with *Candida* meningitis had candidemia. Likewise, a study from the United States found that 37% (7/19) neonates with *Candida* meningitis were fungemic on blood culture and that many had normal CSF parameters (Cohen-Wolkowiez et al 2006). In the Canadian study, of 23 neonates with candidemia, six (26%) had *Candida* meningitis. A similar rate was found in a prospective study from Slovakia, where, of 40 neonates with *Candida* isolated from the blood, eight (20%) had *Candida* meningitis or meningoencephalitis.

Treatment with amphotericin alone in the Texas study resulted in recovery of five out of seven babies with *Candida* meningitis. In Canada, using amphotericin and 5-flucytosine, five out of eight recovered. In Slovakia, using fluconazole alone, four out of eight recovered, and in a study in Italy, five out of six treated with liposomal amphotericin recovered. Beyond the neonatal age group, with an intact blood–brain barrier, the penetration of amphotericin into the CSF is relatively poor, and the addition of 5-flucytosine allows the use of lower doses of amphotericin. This combination is particularly useful for species other than *Candida albicans*. In adults, the starting dose of amphotericin is 0.25 mg/Kg once daily by intravenous infusion. For *Candida albicans*, the dose is increased to 1 mg/Kg/day. Infants tolerate amphotericin better than adults do, and in *Candida* meningitis in neonates, it is appropriate to start at 0.5–1.0 mg/Kg/day. The side-effects of renal toxicity, fever, gastrointestinal upset, bone marrow suppression, anaphylaxis and severe electrolyte disturbances including hypokalemia and hypomagnesemia have been reported in infants. Liposomal amphotericin allows higher doses to be given without increasing toxicity. Because of the ten times greater cost of the liposomal preparation, it is reasonable to reserve it for neonates with renal impairment or those developing side-effects or who are refractory to amphotericin B. Occasional babies with *Candida parapsilosis* do not respond to amphotericin but do respond to fluconazole. Fluconazole is an effective alternative to amphotericin for *Candida albicans* meningitis and has the advantage that can be used orally to complete a course of antifungal therapy if intravenous access is a problem.

The mortality rate in three recent studies (see Table 32.8) was 36% (9/25). Of the five survivors followed up in the Canadian study, three had motor scales >3SD below the mean, two had intelligence scales >3SD below the mean, two had hearing loss and one had vision loss. The mortality rate for *Candida albicans* infection is higher than for *Candida parapsilosis*.

Neonates acquire *Candida albicans* through vertical transmission most commonly, but *Candida parapsilosis* and *Candida lusitaniae* are most often nosocomially acquired infections. The incidence of *Candida parapsilosis* infection is increasing, and it has now been reported as the main cause of candidemia in a NICU in the USA. Contrast-enhanced CT scanning can be useful in the diagnosis of neonatal cerebral candidiasis (see Fig. 32.2).

Apart from *Candida* species, there are other fungal infections, including *Trichosporon beigelii*, reported as causing invasive neonatal infections and shunt infections. This organism can be successfully treated with amphotericin. Other rare case reports of neonatal CNS infections include the fungi *Cryptococcus neoformans*, *Torulopsis glabrata*, *Aspergillus sydowi* and *A. fumigatus*.

SUMMARY OF FUNGAL MENINGITIS

- Use amphotericin B (±5-flucytosine).
- Fluconazole is an acceptable alternative to amphotericin B for *Candida albicans* or *Candida parapsilosis*.
- Fluconazole can be given orally if i.v. access is a problem late in course.
- Treat for at least 4 weeks.

Table 32.8 Fungal CNS infections

Study group	Reference	Country	Total	M:F	Age (days) Mean (range)	CSF WCC Mean (range)	CSF +ve culture	Blood	Died
Candida fungaemia	Huttova et al 1998	Slovakia	8	6:2	27 (15–29)	—	6	8	4
Premature candiasis	Lee et al 1998	Canada	8	—	—	175 (1–529)	5	6	3
CSF *Candida*	Arisoy et al 1994	USA	9	2:7	12 (5–26)	184 (0–1120)	9	3	2

Infantile botulism (see also p. 788)

Infantile botulism is caused by ingestion of spores followed by gut colonization. In a case-control study from the USA of 68 infants with laboratory-confirmed infantile botulism, the main risk factor for infants under 2 months of age was living in a rural area or on a farm. Eleven of the 68 cases had consumed honey.

Clostridium botulinum spores are ubiquitous in the soil. Breast-feeding may generate the optimal conditions for germination of the spores. The organism colonizes the gut and produces a powerful exotoxin. The toxin is absorbed into the bloodstream via the gut and carried hematogenously to cholinergic nerve synapses, particularly neuromuscular junctions. Here, it binds irreversibly to receptors on the presynaptic nerve terminal, blocking acetylcholine release. This explains the atropinic manifestations of the disease such as pupillary dilatation and constipation, as well as the muscular hypotonia and cranial-nerve palsies. The disease is characterized by a descending paralysis of the cranial nerves followed by paralysis of the nerves to the axial and truncal muscles. The presentation can also be acute with a sepsis-like illness and respiratory arrest. Recovery invariably occurs after some days or weeks due to sprouting of new nerve terminals.

The diagnosis is confirmed by intra-peritoneal injection of purified stool from the patient into two mice, one of which is also given the antitoxin. Death of the mouse without the antitoxin and survival of the other confirms the diagnosis. Otherwise, there are commercial assays for type A neurotoxin. Isolation of *Clostridium botulinum* from the stool and the characteristic electromyogram (EMG) also support the clinical diagnosis.

The management of infantile botulism is to protect the airway and support respiration, if necessary, until spontaneous recovery occurs. Tracheostomy prolongs hospitalization. Nasogastric feeds are usually well tolerated and obviate the need for parenteral nutrition. There is no indication for antimicrobial therapy (except for aspiration or hypostatic pneumonia). Penicillin does not speed recovery from infantile botulism, and gentamicin may exacerbate the condition due to its effect on neuromuscular transmission. *Botulinum* immune globulin is available but not in routine use. Equine botulinum immune globulin is more readily available and speeds recovery. The prognosis nowadays is excellent, although relapses can occur. A proposed association between infantile botulism and sudden infant death syndrome is totally unproven. Other species of *Clostridium* including *C. barati* have also been recognized as causing infantile botulism.

SUMMARY OF INFANTILE BOTULISM

- Classic triad of clinical features:
  - bulbar palsies (slow/absent pupil response);
  - alert;
  - absent fever.
- Also commonly presents with constipation, ptosis and poor feeding.

NEONATAL TETANUS

Neonatal tetanus still causes significant mortality in developing countries despite the World Health Organization's goal of global elimination of the disease by the year 2000. The disease is caused by the neurotoxin produced by *Clostridium tetani*, a ubiquitous spore forming bacterium found in high concentrations in soil and animal excrements. The anaerobic conditions of the necrotic cord allow the spores to germinate. The cord becomes contaminated by non-hygienic practices of cutting the cord or traditional practices. In Turkey from 1991 to 1997, 55 babies with neonatal tetanus had all been delivered by untrained birth attendants in rural areas. The cord had been cut with a razor blade (55%), scissors (27%), or knife (18%). In KwaZulu-Natal, cow dung has been used to staunch the blood flow from the severed cord, and in Pakistan, neonatal tetanus has been associated with the practice of bundling, where the infant is wrapped for prolonged periods in a sheepskin cover after dried cow dung is applied.

The incidence in developing countries may not be accurately known, for example, when the infant dies before reaching medical help, and the diagnosis has to be made from care-givers' interviews. In Bangladesh, the sensitivity and specificity of particular combinations of signs are >80% for neonatal tetanus. In 1997, there were an estimated 277 400 deaths world-wide due to neonatal tetanus, but 20 years ago, there were an estimated 800 000 deaths annually. In the USA, there has only been one case from 1989 to 1997. Several studies have shown a male predominance: 78% (161/207) and 76% (42/55).

The mean age of onset of symptoms is 5–6 days (range 1–21 days) with the fatal cases presenting significantly earlier in reviews of cases from 1976 to 1994 and 1991 to 1997. The most common symptoms are spasticity (76%), lack of sucking (71%), trismus (60%), fever (49%), omphalitis (44%), irritability (24%), risus sardonicus (22%) and opisthotonus (15%).

Treatment includes intravenous human tetanus immunoglobulin. The dose required for neonates is not well established. Four thousand international units (IU) are probably appropriate for neonates. The infusion should be started slowly and increased as tolerated (e.g. from 0.1 mL/min for 30 min increased to 0.2 mL/min). If this is not available intramuscular tetanus immune globulin (TIG) should be given. A dose of 500 IU has been effective in neonates, part of the dose traditionally being injected around the umbilicus, though this is not of proven value. If neither is available, equine tetanus antitoxin (TAT) can be given after a test dose because 10–20% develops serum sickness. Ten thousand international units has been found to be an adequate dose. Alternatively intravenous gammaglobulin can be given, though the dose has not been evaluated.

The umbilicus should be débrided if there is necrotic tissue, but wide excision of the umbilical stump is not recommended. Metronidazole (30 mg/Kg/day given at six-hourly intervals) is effective at reducing the number of vegetative forms of *C. tetani* and is the antibiotic of choice. Penicillin G (100000 U/Kg/day) given at 4–6-h intervals is an alternative treatment. The antibiotics should be continued for 10–14 days. High-dose diazepam (40 mg/Kg/day), phenobarbitone and chlorpromazine have been found to lower the mortality significantly compared to less sedation.

The mortality remains high, even when intensive care is available. The mortality rate was 47% in the older study and 40% in the more recent study without any equipment for mechanical ventilation. In Nigeria, a mortality rate of 59% was reported, and in South Africa, where ventilation in a pediatric intensive care setting was available, the mortality rate was 22%. The mean age at death is 9 days and 5 days from admission. In those ventilated, the mean duration of ventilation was 23 days (range 17–60 days) and ICU stay 35 days (range 13–87 days).

The World Health Organization's major strategy for prevention of neonatal tetanus is the administration of at least two properly spaced doses of tetanus toxoid to women of child-bearing age in high-risk areas to passively protect their newborns at birth. Part of the failure to reach the goal of elimination of neonatal tetanus has been subpotent vaccine, as well as a failure to immunize. Other strategies have been the provision of 'safe-birth kits' with a sterile razor blade (or half blade so that it is not taken for use for other purposes!); teaching birth attendants hand washing (OR 0.64 $P = 0.005$); and application of topical antibiotics and disinfectants to the cord.

SUMMARY OF NEONATAL TETANUS

- WHO aims to eliminate neonatal tetanus, but cases still occur, even in industrialized countries.

CONGENITAL NEUROSYPHILIS

A dramatic increase in syphilis, which occurred in the late 1980s and early 1990s in the USA, has subsequently declined. In the UK, there were nine presumptive cases of congenital syphilis reported between 1994 and 1997. Acute syphilitic leptomeningitis usually appears between 3 and 6 months of age. Infants present with symptoms and signs of acute bacterial meningitis, including a stiff neck, progressive vomiting, a positive Kernig sign, bulging of the fontanelles, separation of the sutures and hydrocephalus. The CSF shows a monocytosis, with up to 200 cells/mm^3, a modest increase in protein (0.5–2 g/L) and a normal glucose level. The CSF VDRL is positive. This form of CNS syphilis responds to penicillin.

Late manifestations of involvement of the central nervous system usually occur after 1–2 years of age. Chronic meningovascular syphilis may have a protracted course with progressive communicating hydrocephalus due to obstruction in the basilar cisterns. It may also cause VIIth cranial nerve palsies (occasionally III, IV or VI), optic atrophy and gradual intellectual deterioration. Vascular lesions of the brain have been described, with endarteritis causing convulsions and an acute hemiplegia.

For the diagnosis of neurosyphilis, a raised neonatal CSF protein (>1.8 g/L) and raised CSF white-cell count (>25 × 10^6 WBC/L) in the presence of maternal evidence of inadequately treated syphilis is sufficient for treatment of the infant for neurosyphilis. The CSF white-cell count and protein can be normal in neurosyphilis. The only serological test that should be performed on the CSF is the non-treponemal Venereal Disease Research Laboratory (VDRL) slide test. The other non-treponemal tests such as rapid plasma reagin (RPR) or the automated reagin test (ART) should not be used on the neonatal CSF. The treponemal test such as fluorescent treponemal antibody absorption (FTA-ABS) test or the microhemagglutination test for *T. pallidum* (MHA-TP or TPHA) measure IgG and IgM. IgG can be detected coincidentally in the neonatal CSF after the mother has been successfully treated before pregnancy. IgM detection by immunoblot from CSF of neonates has been found to be positive in two out of six cases of neurosyphilis (defined by Rabbit Infectivity Testing (RIT)). *T. pallidum* DNA PCR was positive in five out of the six cases. A negative CSF VDRL does not exclude neurosyphilis, and the CSF VDRL can be falsely positive by transplacental acquisition of antibody from a mother with high titer. Specific IgM to *T. pallidum* has been found in infants with congenital syphilis and is being evaluated as an alternative diagnostic tool. However, in developing countries where congenital syphilis is most common, the IgM is often not available.

The American Pediatric Association recommends that a lumbar puncture and CSF VDRL, cell count, and protein be performed on the infants of mothers with positive syphilis treponemal tests who have not had appropriate treatment documented or if the treated mother has not had an adequate decrease in non-treponemal antibody titer over 1 month. However, the need for lumbar puncture in asymptomatic infants is debatable, e.g. 329 infants from two Washington hospitals in 1990–1993 met the APA criteria for LP, but the CSF was normal, and CSF protein and glucose were not significantly different from normal controls.

The treatment for neurosyphilis is penicillin G 200000 to 300000 U/Kg/day (50000 U/Kg every 4–6 h) for 10–14 days, possibly followed by benzathine penicillin, 50000 U/Kg/dose in three weekly doses. CSF concentrations of penicillin reach treponemicidal concentrations when given as aqueous penicillin G at 100000 U/Kg/day and were not significantly increased when the dose was raised to 200000 U/Kg/day. They were significantly higher than using procaine penicillin 50000 U/Kg/day, which did not reach treponemicidal levels in CSF in a third of infants.

SUMMARY OF NEUROSYPHILIS

- Consider LP if maternal VDRL is positive and inadequate documentation of maternal treatment.
- LP mandatory if neonate has signs of syphilis.
- CSF dark ground microscopy, WCC and protein.
- CSF VRDL (±*T. pallidum* PCR, IgM if available).

REFERENCES

Adhikari M, Coovadia Y M, Singh D 1995 A 4-year study of neonatal meningitis: clinical and microbiological findings. J Trop Pediatr 41:81–85.

Ahmed A, Hickey S M, Ehrett S et al 1996 Cerebrospinal fluid values in the term neonate. Pediatr Infect Dis J 15:298–303.

Airede A I 1993 Neonatal bacterial meningitis in the middle belt of Nigeria. Dev Med Child Neurol 35:424–430.

Ali Z 1995 Neonatal meningitis: a 3-year retrospective study at the Mount Hope Women's Hospital, Trinidad, West Indies. J Trop Pediatr 41:109–111.

Alviedo J N, Sood B G, Aranda J V, Becker C 2006 Diffuse pneumocephalus in neonatal Citrobacter meningitis. Pediatrics 118: e1576–e1579.

Anonymous 1989 Cerebrospinal fluid shunt infections. Lancet 1:1304–1305.

Arisoy E S, Arisoy A E, Dunne W M Jr 1994 Clinical significance of fungi isolated from cerebrospinal fluid in children. Pediatr Infect Dis J 13:128–133.

Aust G, Schneider D 2001 [Vestibular toxicity of gentamycin in newborn infants]. Laryngorhinootologie 80: 173–176.

Balaka B, Bonkoungou P, Sqalli M et al 2004 [Comparative study of neonatal bacterial meningitis in Lome, Bobo-Dioulasso, Casablanca and Lyon]. Bull Soc Pathol Exot 97:131–134.

Bell A H, Brown D, Halliday H L et al 1989 Meningitis in the newborn — a 14 year review. Arch Dis Childhood 64(6):873–874.

Berger A, Rohrmeister K, Haiden N et al 2002 Serratia marcescens in the neonatal intensive care unit: re-emphasis of the potentially devastating sequelae. Wien Klin Wochenschr 114:1017–1022.

Bizzarro M J, Dembry L M, Baltimore R S, Gallagher P G 2006 Case-control analysis of endemic Serratia marcescens bacteremia in a neonatal intensive care unit. Arch Dis Child Fetal Neonatal Ed 92(2): F120–F126.

Bowen A B, Braden C R 2006 Invasive Enterobacter sakazakii disease in infants. Emerg Infect Dis 12:1185–1189.

Casey A T, Kimmings E J, Kleinlugtebeld A D et al 1997 The long-term outlook for hydrocephalus in childhood. A ten-year cohort study of 155 patients. Pediatr Neurosurg 27:63–70.

Chotpitayasunondh T 1994 Bacterial meningitis in children: etiology and clinical features, an 11-year review of 618 cases. Southeast Asian J Trop Med Public Health 25:107–115.

Cohen-Wolkowiez M, Smith P B, Mangum B et al 2006 Neonatal Candida meningitis: significance of cerebrospinal fluid parameters and blood cultures. J Perinatol (Epub).

Daley A J, Isaacs D, Australasian Study Group for Neonatal Infections 2004 Ten-year study on the effect of intrapartum antibiotic prophylaxis on early onset Group B streptococcal and Escherichia coli neonatal sepsis in Australasia. Pediatr Infect Dis J 23:630–634.

Dallacasa P, Dappozzo A, Galassi E et al 1995 Cerebrospinal fluid shunt infections in infants. Childs Nerv Syst 11:643–648.

Daoud A S, al-Sheyyab M, Abu-Ekteish F et al 1996 Neonatal meningitis in northern Jordan. J Trop Pediatr 42:267–270.

Daoud A S, Batieha A, al-Sheyyab M et al 1999 Lack of effectiveness of dexamethasone in neonatal bacterial meningitis. Eur J Pediatr 158:230–233.

de Louvois J, Blackbourn J, Hurley R et al 1991 Infantile meningitis in England and Wales: a two year study. Arch Dis Childhood 66:603–609.

de Louvois J, Lambert H P (eds) 1991 Infections of the central nervous system. In: Neonatal meningitis. B.C. Decker, Philadelphia, PA, Ch. 13, pp. 161–174.

de Oliveira R S, Pinho V F, Madureira J F, Machado H R 2006 Brain abscess in a neonate: an unusual presentation. Childs Nerv Syst (EPub).

Drudy D, Mullane N R, Quinn T et al 2006 Enterobacter sakazakii: an emerging pathogen in powdered infant formula. Clin Infect Dis 42:996–1002.

Fakioglu E, Queenan A M, Bush K et al 2006 Amp C beta-lactamase-producing Escherichia coli in neonatal meningitis: diagnostic and therapeutic challenge. J Perinatol 26:515–517.

Fernandez M, Moylett E H, Noyola D E, Baker C J 2000 Candidal meningitis in neonates: a 10-year review. Clin Infect Dis 31:458–463.

Francis B M, Gilbert G L 1992 Survey of neonatal meningitis in Australia: 1987–1989. Med J Aust 156:240–243.

Franco S M, Cornelius V E, Andrews B F 1992 Long-term outcome of neonatal meningitis. Am J Dis Children 146:567–571.

Garges H P, Moody M A, Cotten C M et al 2006 Neonatal meningitis: what is the correlation among cerebrospinal fluid cultures, blood cultures, and cerebrospinal fluid parameters? Pediatrics 117:1094–1100.

Gordon A, Isaacs D 2006 Late onset neonatal gram-negative bacillary infection in Australia and New Zealand: 1992–2002. Pediatr Infect Dis J 25:25–29.

Greenberg D, Shinwell E S, Yagupsky P et al 1997 A prospective study of neonatal sepsis and meningitis in southern Israel. Pediatr Infect Dis J 16:768–773.

Holt D E, Halket S, de L J, Harvey D 2001 Neonatal meningitis in England and Wales: 10 years on. Arch Dis Child Fetal Neonatal Ed 84:F85–F89.

Hristeva L, Booy R, Bowler I et al 1993 Prospective surveillance of neonatal meningitis. Arch Dis Childhood 69:14–18.

Huttova M, Hartmanova I, Kralinsky K et al 1998 Candida fungemia in neonates treated with fluconazole: report of forty cases, including eight with meningitis. Pediatr Infect Dis J 17:1012–1015.

Isaacs D 2003 A ten year, multicentre study of coagulase negative staphylococcal infections in Australasian neonatal units. Arch Dis Child Fetal Neonatal Ed 88:F89–F93.

Isaacs D, Moxon E R 1999 Handbook of neonatal infection: a practical guide. WB Saunders, London, Ch. 8, p. 134.

Isaacs D, Royle J 1999 Intrapartum antibiotics and early onset neonatal sepsis caused by group B streptococcus and by other organisms in Australia. Pediatr Infect Dis 18:524–528.

Joshi P, Barr P 1998 The use of lumbar puncture and laboratory tests for sepsis by Australian neonatologists. J Paediatr Child Health 34(1):74–78.

Klein J O, Marcy S M, Remington J S et al (eds) 1995 Infectious diseases of the fetus and newborn infant. In: Bacterial sepsis and meningitis, 4th edn. W.B. Saunders, Philadelphia, PA, Ch. 21, pp. 835–890.

Klinger G, Chin C N, Otsubo H et al 2001 Prognostic value of EEG in neonatal bacterial meningitis. Pediatr Neurol 24:28–31.

Kontny U, Hofling B, Gutjahr P et al 1993 CSF shunt infections in children. Infection 21:89–92.

Langley J M, LeBlanc J C, Drake J et al 1993 Efficacy of antimicrobial prophylaxis in placement of cerebrospinal fluid shunts: meta-analysis. Clin Infect Dis 17:98–103.

Laving A M, Musoke R N, Wasunna A O, Revathi G 2003 Neonatal bacterial meningitis at the newborn unit of Kenyatta National Hospital. East Afr Med J 80:456–462.

Lee B E, Cheung P Y, Robinson J L et al 1998 Comparative study of mortality and morbidity in premature infants (birth weight, <1250 g) with candidemia or candidal meningitis. Clin Infect Dis 27:559–565.

McCracken G H J, Mize S G, Threlkeld N 1980 Intraventricular gentamicin therapy in gram-negative bacillary meningitis of infancy. Report of the Second Neonatal Meningitis Cooperative Study Group. Lancet 1:787–791.

Mancao M, Miller C, Cochrane B et al 1998 Cerebrospinal fluid shunt infections in infants and children in Mobile, Alabama. Acta Paediatr 87:667–670.

May M, Daley A J, Donath S, Isaacs D 2005 Early onset neonatal meningitis in Australia and New Zealand, 1992–2002. Arch Dis Child Fetal Neonatal Ed 90: F324–F327.

Miyairi I, Causey K T, DeVincenzo J P, Buckingham S C 2006 Group B streptococcal ventriculitis: a report of three cases and literature review. Pediatr Neurol 34:395–399.

Moses L M, Heath P T, Wilkinson A R et al 1998 Early onset group B streptococcal neonatal infection in Oxford 1985–96. Arch Dis Childhood Fetal Neonatal Ed 79:F148–F149.

Ohlsson A, Lacy J B, Sinclair J C et al (eds) 1998 Neonatal module of the Cochrane Database of Systematic Reviews. In: Intravenous immunoglobulin for suspected or subsequently proven neonatal infection. The Cochrane Collaboration, Oxford.

Palazzi D L, Klein J O, Baker C J 2006 Bacterial sepsis and meningitis. In: Remington J S, Klein J O, Wilson C B, Baker C J (eds) Infectious diseases of the fetus and newborn infant, 6th edn. Elsevier Saunders, Philadelphia, pp. 247–296.

Platt R, Adleson-Mitty J, Weissman L et al 1999 Resource utilization associated with initial hospital stays complicated by early onset group B streptococcal disease. Pediatr Infect Dis 18:529–533.

Pooboni S K, Mathur S K, Dux A et al 2004 Pneumocephalus in neonatal meningitis: diffuse, necrotizing meningo-encephalitis in Citrobacter meningitis presenting with pneumatosis oculi and pneumocephalus. Pediatr Crit Care Med 5:393–395.

Rios-Reategui E, Ruiz-Gonzalez L, Murguia-de-Sierra T 1998 Neonatal bacterial meningitis in a tertiary treatment center. Revista de Investigacion Clinica 50(1):31–36.

Rotim K, Miklic P, Paladino J et al 1997 Reducing the incidence of infection in pediatric cerebrospinal fluid shunt operations. Childs Nerv Syst 13:584–587.

Sarff L D, Platt L H, McCracken G H Jr 1976 Cerebrospinal fluid evaluation in neonates: comparison of high-risk infants with and without meningitis. J Pediatr 88:473–477.

Shepard C W, Rosenstein N E, Fischer M 2003 Neonatal meningococcal disease in the United States, 1990 to 1999. Pediatr Infect Dis J 22:418–422.

Sinha A K, Kempley S T, Price E et al 2006 Early onset Morganella morganii sepsis in a newborn infant with emergence of cephalosporin resistance caused by depression of AMPC beta-lactamase production. Pediatr Infect Dis J 25:376–377.

Smith P B, Cotten C M, Garges H P et al 2006 A comparison of neonatal gram-negative rod and gram-positive cocci meningitis. J Perinatol 26:111–114.

Spreer A, Gerber J, Hanssen M et al 2006 Dexamethasone increases hippocampal neuronal apoptosis in a rabbit model of *Escherichia coli* meningitis. Pediatr Res 60:210–215.

Stevens J P, Eames M, Kent A et al 2003 Long term outcome of neonatal meningitis. Arch. Dis. Child Fetal Neonatal Ed 88:F179–F184

Stoll B J, Hansen N, Fanaroff A A et al 2004 To tap or not to tap: high likelihood of meningitis without sepsis among very low birth weight infants. Pediatrics 113:1181–1186.

Synnott M B, Morse D L, Hall S M 1994 Neonatal meningitis in England and Wales: a review of routine national data. Arch Dis Childhood 71:F75–F80.

Totan M, Kucukoduk S, Dagdemir A, Dilber C 2002 Meningitis due to *Salmonella* in preterm neonates. Turk J Pediatr 44:45–48.

Unhanand M, Mustafa M M, McCracken G H J et al 1993 Gram-negative enteric bacillary meningitis: a twenty-one-year experience. J Pediatr 122:15–21.

Vartzelis G, Theodoridou M, Daikos G L et al 2005 Brain abscesses complicating *Staphylococcus aureus* sepsis in a premature infant. Infection 33:36–38.

Visser V E, Hall R T 1980 Lumbar puncture in the evaluation of suspected neonatal sepsis. J Pediatr 96:1063–1067.

Waites K B, Duffy L B, Crouse D T et al 1990 Mycoplasmal infections of cerebrospinal fluid in newborn infants from a community hospital population. Pediatr Infect Dis J 9:241–245.

Yatsyk G V 1998 Use of meropenem in the treatment of severe infections in newborns. Antibiotiki i Khimioterapiia 43:32–33.

Yogev R 1985 Cerebrospinal fluid shunt infections: a personal view. Pediatr Infect Dis 4:113–118.

CHAPTER
33

Inborn errors of metabolism presenting with encephalopathy

A. García Cazorla

Key Points

- Inborn errors of metabolism
- Neonatal encephalopathy
- Metabolic intoxication
- Neurologic deterioration
- Neonatal epilepsy
- Neonatal Hypotonia
- Abnormal movements
- Rigid-akinetic syndrome

INTRODUCTION

Neonatal encephalopathies due to metabolic disorders are composed of a group of diverse diseases that combine different aspects of pediatric neurology, neonatology, metabolic medicine and basic neuroscience. Inborn errors of metabolism (IEM) interfere with changes in normal brain neurochemistry and neurophysiology. Some IEM produce the accumulation of a toxic metabolite (for example: ammonia) and, in others, the most significant problem is the lack of a crucial molecule (for example: dopamine). Some other diseases have a more complex pathophysiology and induce abnormal brain morphogenesis in the very early stages of the development of the nervous system through signaling pathway alterations (for example: cholesterol biosynthesis defects) or poor energy-production (for example: mitochondrial disorders). The newborn brain is clearly more vulnerable to different kinds of toxic agents than the brain of an older child or an adult, due to its immature neurobiology. Metabolic processes such as protein synthesis, energetic consumption, brain wiring, synapse formation and all maturation mechanisms are especially active. Therefore disorders of amino acid metabolism, energy production or neurotransmitter defects among others, may result in devastating consequences to the very young brain if appropriate and early treatment is not administered.

Although individually rare, inborn errors of metabolism (IEM) are collectively numerous. Furthermore, it is not uncommon for metabolic diseases to have their first clinical manifestations in the neonatal period. In fact, almost one hundred IEM can start during this period of life. Disorders of small molecules and energetic defects are more likely to exhibit their first signs through the first days of life whereas complex molecule disorders tend to appear later. Amongst all these disorders, only a minority are amenable to treatment.

Metabolic encephalopathies constitute a significant problem in neonatal practice. The majority of such infants will have comparatively common neonatal problems such as systemic infection, neonatal asphyxia or congenital heart disease. Moreover, the predominant clinical manifestations can be non-specific with lethargy, failure to thrive, apneas, etc. An appropriate diagnostic approach is critical and can rely on some basic clinical guidelines together with the proper use of a few screening tests. However, expert laboratory services and interpretation of the results by clinicians specializing in inherited metabolic disease are required. Thus, prompt clinical consultation is important and will generally lead to transfer of the infant to a specialized hospital unit. First line metabolic tests must be readily available in each region but specialized tests are needed in only a small number of reference laboratories (Green & Gray 2001).

Throughout this chapter, a practical approach to the most common causes of neonatal metabolic encephalopathies will be developed. Initially some basic clinical patterns of metabolic encephalopathies will be defined. Nevertheless, these clinical guidelines will need the information given by biochemical and/or neuroimaging studies, in order to reach the proper diagnosis. It is important to consider first those potentially treatable disorders. In the same way, the necessity to schedule emergency treatment as soon as the diagnosis is suspected will be highlighted.

METABOLIC ENCEPHALOPATHIES IN THE NEWBORN: MAIN CHARACTERISTICS

Encephalopathies starting during the neonatal period can be divided into two main groups according to their origin: encephalopathies due to external agents of brain injury in a previously healthy child and encephalopathies caused by inherited disorders. An important part of inherited conditions can be qualified as inborn errors of metabolism (IEM). Some IEM will exhibit abnormal neurological manifestations from the very first hours of life, without a symptom-free interval, revealing a process that has taken place within a variable period of time before birth. Complex molecules and energetic defect disorders may show signs of antenatal brain dysfunction (either anatomic, functional or both). By contrast, metabolic disorders affecting small molecules normally present after a symptom-free period. Therefore, there is no particular incidence during pregnancy, delivery and even the first days of life. There are some exceptions to this general rule. Non-ketotic hyperglycinemia, serine deficiency and neurotransmitter defects can be considered as small molecule disorders. However the exposure to high glycine levels, low serine concentration or low neurotransmitter production may cause severe damage in a prenatal developing brain.

From a morphologic point of view, the newborn brain may be affected by a wide variety of dysgenetic features ranging from migration disorders (peroxisome disorders, cholesterol biosynthesis defects and energetic defects), to white matter abnormalities (acute decompensations of organic acidurias, neonatal adrenoleukodystrophy), basal ganglia involvement (organic acidurias, urea cycle disorders, mitochondrial diseases), brain cysts (Zellweger disease, pyruvate dehydrogenase deficiency and other energetic defect disorders, and Lowe syndrome, all of them with particular differentiating characteristics) or different malformative hallmarks such as agenesis of the corpus callosum (in pyruvate dehydrogenase deficiency) or cerebellum hypoplasia (congenital disorders of glycosylation, purine metabolism defects) among others.

Neurological signs are frequently poorly reported in inborn errors of metabolism. Moreover, the neonate has an apparently limited repertoire of responses to severe illness and the predominant clinical manifestations may appear as non-specific. Probably, this is the reason why the particular neurological manifestations of IEM have been described mainly as gross traits. Nevertheless, expert neonatologists and especially pediatric neurologists may be able to distinguish unusual patterns of clinical signs that in association with special biochemical profiles and the lack of explanation by means of more common diseases, would allow the correct approach to the final diagnosis.

DIAGNOSTIC APPROACH TO NEONATAL ENCEPHALOPATHIES DEPENDING ON CLINICAL MANIFESTATIONS

The main objective of this section is to provide a useful clinical approximation to these disorders. Therefore it seems necessary to divide the whole group of possible neurologic symptoms into some basic types of clinical presentation. However, this classification has some disadvantages. Many IEM presenting with encephalopathy also have multisystem involvement mimicking a generalized infectious process, which means that brain dysfunction signs may be under considered. Moreover, the neonate has a limited repertoire of responses; hence neurologic signs are not always very specific of metabolic disorders and can also be found in many common situations in neonatology, such as hypoxic-ischemic encephalopathy or sepsis. Furthermore, biochemical results are crucial to orientate the diagnosis in neonatal IEM. Thus, although a clinical neurologic approach may be

helpful, it must be considered in conjunction with the general examination of the child and first line metabolic tests.

In general, IEM presenting with encephalopathy may manifest the following neurologic clinical patterns:

1. Neurologic deterioration due to intoxication.
2. Epileptic encephalopathies.
3. Severe hypotonia.
4. Rigid-akinetic syndrome.

It is important to remark that some disorders can eventually be placed in different groups at the same time. For example, peroxisomal disorders give rise to deep global hypotonia but quite frequently refractory epilepsy is also a common trait. In spite of this unavoidable overlapping, they will be classified according to the most representative neurologic presentation. Brain MR and electroencephalographic studies may also provide valuable information. In order to reach the proper diagnosis, these exams should be included in the set of diagnostic tools, as will be exposed later.

Figure 33.1 shows a diagnostic algorithm regarding the predominant neurological manifestations.

IEM GIVING RISE TO NEUROLOGIC DETERIORATION DUE TO INTOXICATION

This group is constituted of inborn errors of intermediary metabolism, which share some common features (Saudubray et al 2002):

- Toxic compounds proximal to the metabolic block accumulate, leading to an acute or progressive intoxication.

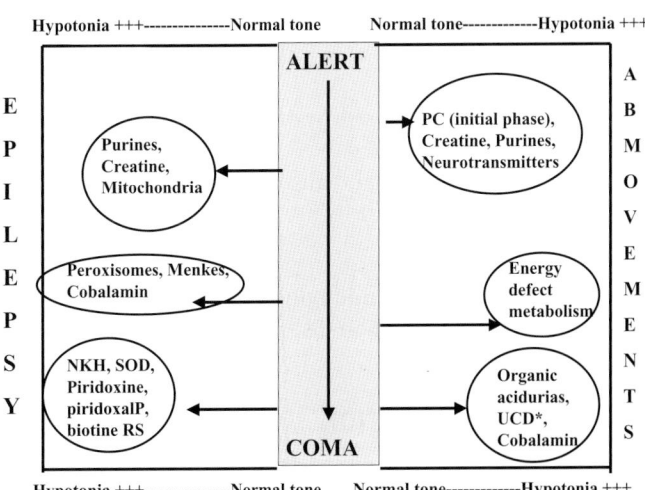

Figure 33.1 Diagnostic algorithm suggesting most likely IEMs based on abnormal neurological signs.
ABMOVEMENTS = abnormal movements. NKH = non-ketotic hyperglycinemia. SOD = sulfite oxidase deficiency.
RS = responsive seizures. *: urea cycle disorders are not associated with abnormal movements except tremor.

- In general, there is a symptom-free interval (ranging from hours to weeks) followed by clinical signs such as poor feeding, vomiting, hypotonia, lethargy and progressive neurologic deterioration. Abnormal movements, seizures and coma are common manifestations of neurologic impairment in the absence of the appropriate treatment.

In most of these IEM, there are signs of extraneurologic involvement (hepatic and hematologic dysfunction occur frequently).

- Basic biochemical analyses give a useful orientation in the differential diagnosis.
- Many of these IEM are treatable. It is important to treat them as early as possible using special diets and/or toxin removal procedures.

In this group we can distinguish the following categories of IEM: aminoacidopathies, organic acidemias and congenital urea cycle defects. Although sugar intolerances (galactosemia, hereditary fructose intolerance) and tyrosinemia also belong to disorders giving rise to intoxication they will not be considered in this chapter because their clinical presentation is dominated by signs of liver failure and cannot be included as neonatal encephalopathies.

BRANCHED-CHAIN ORGANIC ACIDURIAS

These result from inherited conditions affecting specific enzymes that participate in the catabolic pathway of branched amino acids. Figure 33.2 shows biochemical pathways of branched chain amino acid metabolism.

The most common are:

- Maple syrup urine disease (MSUD: caused by branched-chain oxo-acid dehydrogenase deficiency.
- Propionic aciduria: caused by propionyl-CoA carboxylase deficiency, which is a mitochondrial biotin-dependent enzyme.
- Isovaleric aciduria: caused by isovaleryl-CoA dehydrogenase deficiency.
- Methylmalonic academia: caused by methylmalonyl-CoA mutase deficiency, which is a vitamin B_{12}-dependent enzyme.

Furthermore, 3-methylcrotonylglcycinuria and malonic aciduria are very uncommon diseases involving leucine and isoleucine catabolism.

CLINICAL PRESENTATION

The presentation of these disorders in newborns corresponds to types I or II in the classification of the neonatal IEM (Saudubray et al 2002); in other words, they are considered as neurological distress of the intoxication type with either ketosis or ketoacidosis (Ogier de Baulny 2002).

As regards the general characteristics of clinical manifestations, these disorders do not affect fetal development and the child is therefore born after a normal pregnancy and

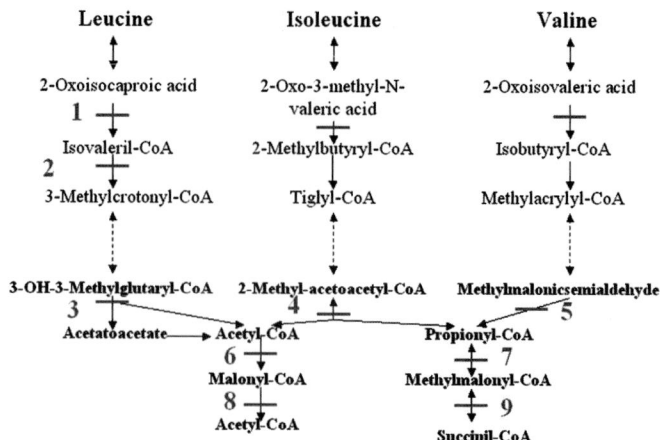

Figure 33.2 Biochemical pathways of branched chain amino acid metabolism. Red bars indicate enzymatic defects. 1: Branched-chain oxo-acid dehydrogenase. This is a common enzyme for leucine, valine and isoleucine. 2: Isovaleryl-coenzyme A dehydrogenase (this is the enzyme responsible for isovaleric aciduria). 3: 3-hydroxy-3-methylglutaryl-CoA lyase. 4: 2-methylacetoacetyl-CoA thiolase. 5: methylmalonylsemialdehyde dehydrogenase. 6: acetyl-CoA deacylase. 7: propionyl-CoA carboxylase (this is the enzyme responsible for propionic aciduria). 8: malonyl-CoA decarboxylase. 9: methylmalonyl-CoA mutase (this enzyme is responsible for methylmalonic aciduria).

delivery. Following an initial symptom-free period, the first reported signs are typically poor sucking and feeding. In some cases the first evoked diagnosis is a gastrointestinal disorder with vomiting, abdominal distension and constipation (Burlina et al 1999, Ogier de Baulny 2002). Later on, neurologic manifestations are the most prominent features.

In respect of neurologic involvement, the main hallmarks can be divided into three main groups of clinical signs:

1. Neurovegetative problems such as apneas, hiccups, alterations of heart rate and temperature regulation.
2. Signs of global neurologic depression, which is progressive. In fact, the newborn initially only has a decreased responses to external stimuli. Then hypotonia and lethargy appear, and finally the child sinks into an unexplained coma. In more advanced stages of the disease, seizures (tonic, myoclonic) may develop, although epilepsy is not a reliable hallmark of these disorders. Electroencephalographic examination (EEG) frequently discloses a burst-suppression pattern (Ohtahara & Yamatogi 2003) even in the absence of clinical convulsions.
3. Movement disorders are also common and poorly reported in the medical literature. It is important to point out that these abnormal movements arise in the comatose state. This specific fact is very characteristic of these disorders. In neonatology, there are other causes of brain injury that may produce coma (hypoxic encephalopathy, birth trauma, infections) but in none

of them does the child manifest these very particular abnormal movements. They have been described as 'pedaling or boxing movements,' which are complex, of large amplitude and sometimes remaining in a fixed position for some seconds. These may be mistaken for post-asphyxial movements of hypoxic–ischemic encephalopathy (HIE) (p. 544). Myoclonic jerks and tremors (either short or large amplitude) without EEG concomitant changes are also very common. In general, these movements may take place spontaneously or upon stimulation (Gascon et al 1994, Ogier de Baulny & Saudubray 2002). In general, these newborns manifest axial hypotonia and limb hypertonia.

NEUROIMAGING STUDIES

There are few reports in the literature concerning neuroimaging examinations in newborn metabolic encephalopathies. Cranial ultrasonography studies in maple syrup urine disease reveal a symmetric increase of echogenicity of periventricular white matter, basal ganglia (mainly pallidi) and thalami in the acute stage. Moreover, these changes seem to have a correlation with the severity of the disease (Fariello et al 1995). By contrast, CT studies disclose hypodensity of cerebral and cerebellar white matter, internal and external capsules, brain stem and the basal ganglia, which appear as high-signal areas on brain MRI (Brismar et al 1990, Kendall 1992, Taccone et al 1992). Increased water content and/or myelination abnormalities may be the origin of these abnormal images. Cerebellar hemorrhage has also been described

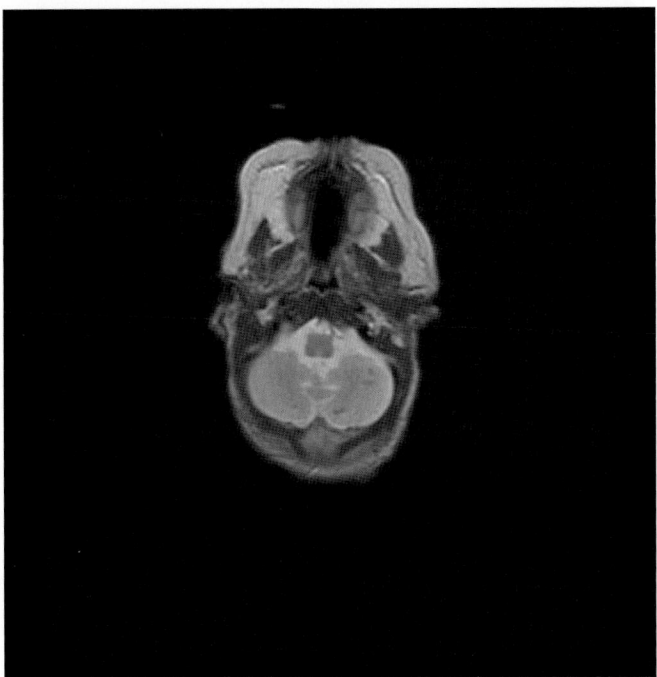

Figure 33.3 Cerebellar hemorrhages in IEM. Axial T2 MRI section. Patchy low intensity images in both cerebellar hemispheres correspond to different bleeding zones in a newborn with propionic aciduria.

(Fig. 33.3). In methylmalonic acidemia it is common to find high-signal T2 images restricted to the globus pallidum whereas in propionic acidemia, putamina and caudate are frequently involved (Andreula et al 1991, Bergman et al 1996). Depending on the severity of the disease and the delay in the application of appropriate treatment, these images can evolve towards atrophy or cystic degeneration.

PATHOPHYSIOLOGY

The etiopathogenesis of neurological symptoms and structural brain abnormalities in organic acidurias is poorly understood and little data has been reported in this respect. It has been postulated that the accumulating organic acids may exert their actions by three neurotoxic pathomechanisms: oxidative stress, energy failure and excitotoxicity. These compounds may induce the generation of reactive oxygen species and reactive nitrogen species and reduce tissue antioxidant defenses, as well as inhibit key enzymatic activities of energy metabolism (Wajner et al 2004).

SPECIFIC CHARACTERISTICS AND BIOCHEMICAL ABNORMALITIES

Clinical, biochemical and other specific features of every type of organic aciduria are shown in Table 33.1.

In maple syrup urine disease, in general there are not pronounced abnormalities in laboratory tests (no metabolic acidosis, no hyperammonemia or only slight elevation, no hyperlactacidemia, no dehydration and normal clinical chemistry), with the exception of 2-oxo acids detected in the DNPH test in urine (2,4-dinitriophenylhydrazine). By contrast, dehydration, metabolic acidosis, ketonuria and hyperammonemia are constant in the other organic acidurias. Mild to moderate hypocalcemia and hyperlactacidemia are also quite common. Glucose can be normal, reduced or increased in blood. Pancytopenia is also a frequent finding. Enzymatic studies performed in cultured fibroblasts or peripheral leukocytes together with genetic tests confirm the diagnosis.

UREA CYCLE DISORDERS (UCD)

The urea cycle is the main pathway for the excretion of ammonium nitrogen (Fig. 33.4). It converts ammonia, which is a brain toxin, into the non-toxic product, urea, which is eliminated by urine. Urea cycle defects (UCD) presenting in the neonatal period are associated with severe hyperammonemia and represent a major emergency (Leonard 2002). The presentation of these disorders in newborns corresponds to type IV (a) in the classification of the neonatal IEM (Saudubray et al 2002). Defects of the mitochondrial ornithine transporter (hyperornithinemia, hyperammonemia, homocitrullinuria syndrome) and ornithine aminotransferase deficiency can also be causes of neonatal hyperammonemia.

CLINICAL PRESENTATION

As in organic acidurias, most babies are initially healthy but after a short symptom-free interval (in UCD it can be less

Table 33.1 Specific clinical and biochemical features of organic acidurias

Disorder	Specific signs	Biochemical signs	Diagnostic tests
Maple syrup urine disease	Maple-syrup odor (caramel-like)	May not display abnormal routine laboratory tests although metabolic acidosis is not rare	Plasma amino acids: high BC AA concentrations, positive urine 2-oxo-acids (DNPH test) Specific acylcarnitine profile (blood, plasma or urine)
Isovaleric aciduria (IVA) Propionic aciduria (PA) Methylmalonic aciduria (MMA)	Dehydration, hepatomegaly, sweaty feet odor in IVA	Metabolic acidosis with increased anion gap, ketonuria, hyperammonemia is not constant Moderate hypocalcemia and hyperlactacidemia Normal, high or low glucose Neutropenia, thrombocytopenia, non-regenerative anemia	Specific organic acid profiles in urine: IVA: high 3-OH-valeric acid and N-isovalerylglycine PA: high 3-OH-propionate, And methylcitrate. MMA: high methylmalonic acid. Specific acylcarnitine profile (blood, plasma or urine) Plasma amino acids may show non-specific hyperglycinemia and hyperalaninemia

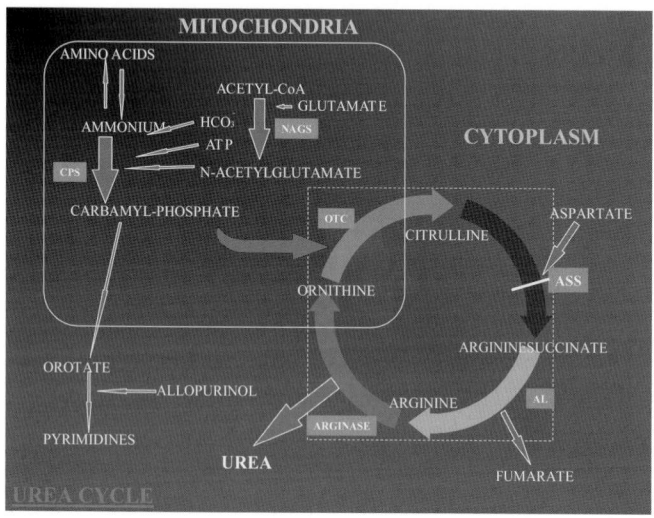

Figure 33.4 Urea cycle. CPS: carbamoyl phosphate synthetase. NAGS: N-acetylglutamate synthetase. OTC: ornithine transcarbamoylase. ASS: argininosuccinic acid synthetase, AL: argininosuccinic lyase.

than 24 hours) they start to manifest poor feeding, vomiting, lethargy and tachypnea that may be associated with respiratory alkalosis. These initial symptoms rapidly evolve towards neurological deterioration characterized by global hypotonia, loss of neonatal reflexes, apnea and other neurovegetative signs (Fernandes 2000, Leonard 2002). No abnormal movements are seen in neonatal UCD disorders, with the exception of jitteriness or tremor in the first non-treated stages of the disease. Liver dysfunction and cerebral or pulmonary hemorrhage can also be present.

Specific biochemical abnormalities of every defect are shown in Table 33.2.

NEUROIMAGING STUDIES

Diffuse severe cerebral edema followed by diffuse atrophy has been reported in newborns with UCD (Choi et al 2001, Takeoka et al 2001). On the other hand, injury to the bilateral lentiform nuclei and the deep sulci of the insular and perirolandic regions have also been documented, reflecting a major susceptibility of these regions to hypoperfusion in the neonate under hyperammonemic condition (Takanashi et al 2003).

PATHOPHYSIOLOGY

The developing brain, and in particular, the neonatal brain is more susceptible to hyperammonemia compared to the adult brain. As the brain has no effective urea cycle, glutamine synthesis through glutamine synthetase is the mechanism that allows removal of the excess ammonia. Glutamine synthetase is predominantly localized in the astrocyte. Neuropathologic studies reveal characteristic alterations of astrocyte morphology ranging from cell swelling in acute hyperammonemia to Alzheimer Type II astrocytosis in chronic hyperammonemia (Felipo et al 2002). Furthermore, exposure of brain to increased ammonia concentrations results in altered expression of key astrocytic proteins including glial fibrillary acidic protein, the glutamate transporter EAAT-2, mitochondrial 'peripheral-type' benzodiazepine receptors as well as glutamine synthetase and the water channel protein aquaporin IV.

Treatment of organic acidurias and urea cycle disorders
A. General initial measures (Ogier de Baulny et al 2000, Zschoke et al 2004)
Once clinical suspicion of intoxication due to an IEM is aroused, there are some common general procedures

Table 33.2 Specific biochemical features and diagnostic tests in urea cycle disorders

Disorder	Plasma amino acid profile	Urine orotic acid	Enzyme diagnosis (tissue)
OTC deficiency	High glutamine and alanine Low citrulline and arginine	High	Liver
CPS deficiency	High glutamine and alanine Low citrulline and arginine	Normal	Liver
Citrullinemia	High citrulline Low arginine	High	Fibroblasts and liver
Argininosuccinic aciduria	High citrulline and argininosuccinic acid Low arginine	High	Fibroblasts, red blood cells and liver
Arginase deficiency	High arginine	High	Red blood cells and liver
NAGS deficiency	High glutamine and alanine	Normal	Liver
HHH syndrome	High ornithine and homocitrulline (plasma and urine)	Normal	Fibroblasts

HHH: hyperammonemia, hyperornithinemia, homocitrullinuria

that should be immediately applied. These routine strategies should be simultaneous to the first line metabolic exams.

1. Stop protein intake: this action should not be extended for more than 48 hours due to the appearance of internal catabolism.
2. Provide hydration and adequate electrolytes: avoid hyperhydration due to the risk of cerebral edema in these children (fluid infusion should be <3 L/m²/day during the first 48 hours). Correct acidosis with i.v. bicarbonate (in some cases, UCD may give rise to some degree of metabolic acidosis that should not be corrected because acidosis protects against NH_4 toxicity) (Ogier de Baulny et al 2000).
3. Nutrition should be based in high caloric intake to stop catabolism: in order to reach this high energy requirement, the insertion of a central venous catheter is necessary in most cases. Due to digestive intolerance, initial parenteral nutrition is quite often necessary. High energetic solutions may provide around 130–150 kcal/Kg/day. These should comprise 65–75% of the total calories supplied by glucose (use fluids with glucose concentration of 15–20%) and the other 25–35% calories furnished by lipids (most available intravenous lipid solutions have a concentration of 20% of lipids). The glucose-lipid mixture should be given as enteral nutrition as early as possible, scheduling the change from parenteral to enteral nutrition in 4–5 days. Osmolarity, electrolytes, micronutrients, minerals and vitamins must be adapted to the recommended dietary allowance (RDA). After 48 hours, protein should be progressively introduced (either parenteral as amino acid solutions or enteral).
4. Intravenous insulin may improve anabolism and control hyperglycemia which is the result of high amounts of glucose administered.

5. Carnitine i.v.: from 100 to 200 mg/Kg/day acts as a toxic remover in both organic acidurias and UCD. However if there is a suspicion of beta oxidation defect carnitine should be avoided.

B. Toxic removal procedures

Peritoneal dialysis, continuous hemofiltration and hemodialysis are the most common detoxifying extracorporeal techniques used in IEM. There is no general consensus about when they should be used. In our practical experience (Hospital Sant Joan de Déu, Barcelona) these procedures are used when:

- The child has refractory unchanging metabolic acidosis continuing for more than 12 hours in spite of appropriate therapy.
- Hyperammonemia higher than 400 µmol/L not responsive to conventional supporting measures and ammonia removers (Na-benzoate, phenylbutyrate, carbamylglutamate).

The type of technique used depends mostly on the clinical expertise of every group. In general, peritoneal dialysis can be performed by most pediatric intensive care units. Continuous hemofiltration (continuous veno-venous filtration is the most suitable technique), although very effective in both organic acidurias and UCD, requires a trained team. Hemodialysis seems to be the most effective method to remove small molecules but it is necessary to request a permanent dialysis team and the results are poor in hyperammonemic newborns (Hiroma et al 2002, Picca et al 2001).

C. Specific therapies

In UCD: use ammonia depurators: Na-benzoate oral or i.v. (250–400 mg/Kg/day divided in 3 doses), Na-phenylbutyrate oral or i.v. (250–400 mg/Kg/day divided in 3 doses), carbamylglutamate (100–300 mg/Kg/day) may also be useful in hyperammonemia due either to *N*-acetylglutamate synthase deficiency or organic acidurias (Guffon et al 2005).

In organic acidurias (other than low natural protein diet, appropriate amino acid free mixture is widely available in the pharmaceutical industry):

- In MSUD: it is important to adjust the branched chain amino acid intake in function of the plasma levels. Leucine requirement is about 300–400 mg/day whereas isoleucine and valine are about 200–250 mg/day. Thiamine (5 mg/Kg/day) may improve protein tolerance although in general it does not work in newborns.
- In propionic acidemia adjust protein administration depending on valine intake although low isoleucine, leucine, methionine and threonine diet will be necessary (amino acid mixture free of these amino acids).
- Methylmalonic aciduria: consider vitamin B_{12} (1–2 mg/day) otherwise management is the same as propionic acidemia.
- Isovaleric aciduria: reduce leucine intake and try L-glycine (150–300 mg/Kg/day).

IEM GIVING RISE TO SEVERE NEONATAL SEIZURES

As a rule, isolated epilepsy is not a reliable hallmark of metabolic diseases. However, there are some IEM that may present as early refractory epilepsy. Consider an IEM in a neonate with refractory epilepsy, mainly early myoclonic encephalopathy (EME) non-responsive to conventional anti-epileptic drugs. EME is characterized by erratic, fragmentary myoclonic jerks often followed by partial seizures, massive myoclonus and infantile spasms and burst-suppression pattern (Tharp 2002). Vitamin-dependent seizures are the first group that must be considered in view of the therapeutic possibilities.

MAIN PATHOPHYSIOLOGICAL GROUPS

1. Energetic defects: pyruvate metabolism disorders and respiratory chain defects. Although they can be very epileptogenic, these will be considered in the group of disorders giving rise to hypotonia as the major features.
2. Amino acid disorders (in some cases with a role in cerebral neurotransmission): non-ketotic hyperglycinemia, serine and sulfite oxidase deficiency are the most representative.
3. Complex molecule disorders: mainly peroxisomal disorders that will also be shown in the group of severe hypotonic.
4. Vitamin-dependent seizures: pyridoxine and pyridoxal phosphate-dependent seizures, biotinidase deficiency and seizures sensitive to folinic acid.
5. Others: copper and purine metabolism defects may also present as refractory epilepsy in newborns.

Glucose transporter deficiency (GLUT-1) will not be considered in this chapter because although epilepsy is a very common hallmark it tends to appear beyond the neonatal period.

AMINO ACID DISORDERS
Non-ketotic hyperglycinemia

This is a disorder of glycine degradation due to a defect in the glycine cleavage system. These babies appear severely hypotonic and lethargic from the very first hours or days of life. Neonatal primitive reflexes are deeply depressed and quite often they present signs of neurovegative dysfunction such as miosis, apneas and hiccupping. Early refractory epilepsy (EME) is a constant feature. Neurologic deterioration and high early mortality are also common. The biochemical diagnostic is based on the absence of ketoacidosis and elevated glycine levels with a CSF/plasma ratio above 0.08 (Applegarth 2001). Enzymatic confirmation requires liver analysis. Genetic studies will be performed depending on which is the defective protein of the cleavage complex (P-protein is the most frequent). Brain MRI may show signs of abnormal white matter, vacuolating myelinopathy or corpus callosum dysgenesis (Mourmans et al 2006). Benzoate (250–750 mg/Kg/day) aims to reduce glycine levels (Van Hove et al 2005) whereas dextromethorphan (5–20 mg/Kg/day) produces NMDA receptor blockage (ketamine, tryptophan, felbamate and benzodiazepines have also been used). In spite of this therapy, prognosis is very poor.

Serine deficiency
Congenital microcephaly, early refractory seizures, bilateral cataracts and hypertonia followed by severe psychomotor retardation make up the typical clinical presentation of 3-phosphoglycerate dehydrogenase deficiency, which is the first step in the biosynthesis of serine. The quantitation of CSF amino acids reveals a marked decrease of serine (de Koning et al 1999) although in some cases it may be present in peripheral fluids. These symptoms respond to a variable degree of L-serine (200–600 mg/Kg/day), sometimes combined with glycine (up to 200 mg/Kg/day) (de Koning 2006).

Sulfite oxidase deficiency and molybdenum cofactor deficiency
These are rare disorders characterized by epileptic encephalopathy, lens dislocation and generalized hypertonia. The neuropathological and MRI findings (Fig. 33.5) mimic the features of hypoxic–ischemic encephalopathy (Hobson et al 2005). Sulfite oxidase catalyses the last step in the oxidation of the sulfur atom of cysteine into inorganic sulfate. Sulfite oxidase is dependent on molybdenum cofactor. Biochemically sulfite can be detected in urine. Cystine plasma levels are very low. Moreover, in molybdenum cofactor deficiency high hypoxanthine in urine and low uric acid in serum are detected.

Vitamin-dependent seizures
Pyridoxine-dependent seizures (p. 705)
This is an autosomal recessive disorder in which seizures usually starts from birth (even recognized in utero) to 3 months (although occasional cases have started at 3 years). The EEG abnormalities are relatively non-specific (Tharp

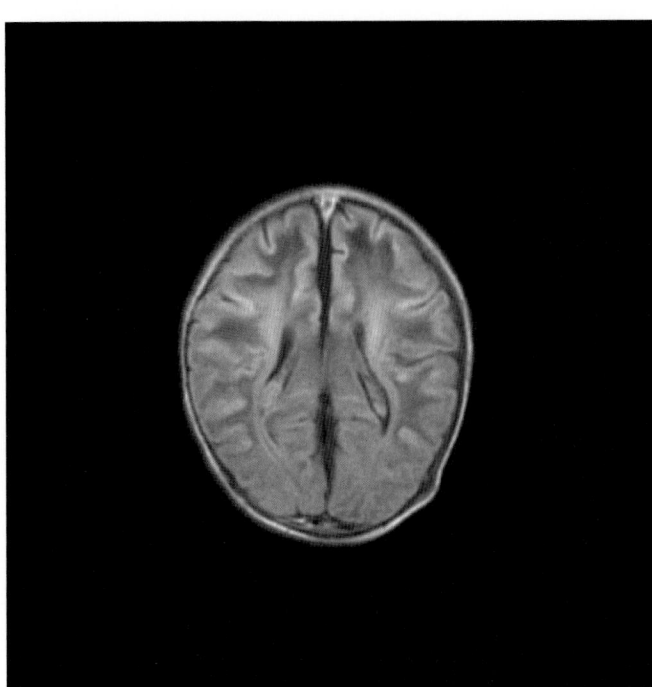

Figure 33.5 Brain MRI of a child with sulfite oxidase deficiency. Axial T1 section. Diffuse cortical and subcortical hypointensities mimicking hypoxic–ischemic lesions in 2 days old boy with sulfite oxidase deficiency.

2002). Intravenous pyridoxine (50–100 mg) leads to rapid cessation of seizures and epileptic activity over the next few hours. Patients usually need lifelong vitamin B_6 therapy (in general from 50 to 100 mg/day) and, despite treatment, some children have psychomotor delay. Recently, it has been demonstrated that a defect of alpha-amino adipic semialdehyde (AASA) dehydrogenase (antiquitin) in the cerebral lysine degradation pathway is responsible for this condition. Both pipecolic acid and AASA are markedly elevated in plasma, urine and cerebrospinal fluid and are biochemical markers of the disease. The study of antiquitin gene confirms the diagnosis (Mills et al 2006, Plecko et al 2006).

Pyridoxal-phosphate-dependent seizures

This is a recently described condition (Mills et al 2005) due to pyridoxamine 5'-phospate oxidase deficiency, which converts pyridoxine into 5-pyridoxal phosphate and, on the other hand, is a cofactor of amino acid decarboxylase (AADC), which regulates the biosynthetic pathways of dopamine and serotonin. This defect gives rise to intractable seizures responding to pyridoxal phosphate (from 30 to 50 mg/Kg/day). Pipecolic acid is elevated in biological fluids. In the CSF, low levels of homovanillic and 5-hydroxyindoleacetic acids, as well as high levels of vanillacetic acid, are also detected.

Biotin responsive seizures

These are associated with one of the two known congenital disorders of biotin metabolism (biotinidase and holocarbox-

ylase synthetase deficiency). Symptoms of both deficiencies may appear during the neonatal period. Refractory seizures, hypotonia, lethargy, feeding difficulties and cutaneous changes such as rash, alopecia, are the most common manifestations. Metabolic acidosis, hyperlactacidemia, ketosis, hyperammonemia and abnormal urine organic acids are characteristic of holocarboxylase synthetase deficiency, whereas in biotinidase deficiency biotin activity in plasma is absent or decreased. A therapy with 10 mg/day of biotin is usually enough to treat these defects. However, in holocarboxylase synthetase deficiency, a few patients have responded only partially even to doses of up to 100 mg/day (Baumgartner et al 1997).

OTHERS

Menkes syndrome

This is an X-linked degenerative condition due to a defect in copper metabolism. Newborns are extremely hypotonic and present refractory seizures. Dysmorphic traits and kinky hair may not be evident in the very first weeks of life. Radiographs may show metaphyseal spurring of the long bones. The evolution includes severe psychomotor delay and refractory seizures. Early onset seizures are mainly characterized by focal status followed later on by myoclonic and multifocal EEG discharges (Bahi-Buisson et al 2006). The biochemical defect is a cell copper transport protein (ATP7A) involved in transport of copper across the gut. Reduced levels of copper and ceruloplasmin are found (Tumer & Horn 1997). The interpretation of these findings may be difficult in this period of life because serum copper and ceruloplasmin concentrations may also be low in normal infants. Copper metabolism studies and DNA analysis confirm the diagnosis. Therapy with copper infusion has been tried with variable success (Sheela et al 2005).

Purines

Adenylosuccinase deficiency (ADSL) is a recessive disorder characterized by biologic fluid accumulation of succinylaminoimidazole carboxamide riboside (SAICAR) and succinyladenosine (S-Ado). There is a considerable clinical variety, but epilepsy is a very common trait (80%) and may be present in the neonatal period (Van den Berghe et al 1998). Burst-suppression pattern may be present and later West syndrome or generalized seizures that are often refractory to conventional antiepileptic therapy (Holder-Espinasse et al 2002).

Therapeutic trials in refractory neonatal seizures

- Pyridoxal phosphate: 30–40 mg/Kg/day in at least three doses. To evaluate efficacy, therapy should be maintained for 5 days. Studies in the CSF/urines should be performed before treatment in order to have a biochemical marker, but should not delay treatment. Genetic studies can be performed as well. Pyridoxal phosphate should also be effective in controlling pyridoxine-dependent seizures.

- If pyridoxal phosphate is not available, pyridoxine should be used first: 100 mg in a neonate (or 30 mg/Kg) either intravenously or orally in a single dose, preferably with EEG monitoring. There is no universal protocol for a pyridoxine trial. The dose of pyridoxine varies according to the physician's approach to the treatment and follow-up of metabolic disorders, but high doses may be necessary to control seizures, at least initially. In classical cases, a starting dose of 100 mg intravenously can be used. If there is no response within 24 hours, the same dose should be repeated (and possibly increased up to 500 mg total) before excluding pyridoxine responsiveness. If there is uncertainty about a partial response, pyridoxine should be continued at 30 mg/Kg/day for seven days before final conclusions are drawn. That does not preclude the introduction of other vitamins/drugs during this period of time if seizures do not stop. Appropriate biochemical tests before therapy are advisable, but treatment should not be delayed by these test, nor should results be waited for.
- Biotin: 10–100 mg/day. Plasma biotinidase/urine organic acids should be analyzed before starting treatment.
- Folinic acid: 10 mg/day. It is recommended to maintain the treatment for at least 1 month to test its efficacy.

IEM GIVING RISE TO SEVERE NEONATAL HYPOTONIA

Hypotonia is a very non-specific sign that is quite common in many sick newborns whatever the origin of the disease. It is defined by the presence of poor muscle tone affecting the limbs, trunk and the cranial-facial musculature. Later on, there is an inability to maintain normal posture during movement and rest (Prasad & Prasad 2003). Genetic causes of neonatal hypotonia may be divided into chromosomal disorders (e.g. Prader–Willi syndrome), neuromuscular diseases (e.g. myotonic dystrophy or spinal muscular atrophy), brain dysgenesis and metabolic disorders. As a rule, isolated hypotonia in a newborn is not a common hallmark for IEM. In fact, only a few IEM present as isolated hypotonia in the neonatal period (Saudubray et al 2002).

MAIN CHARACTERISTICS OF 'NEONATAL METABOLIC HYPOTONIA'

1. *When do we have to suspect a metabolic disorder in a newborn with severe hypotonia?*

In general, all IEM manifesting during the neonatal period may present with global hypotonia reflecting the presence of serious disease in the child. However when severe hypotonia dominates the whole clinical picture, there are some special points that may reinforce the diagnosis of a metabolic disorder:

- *The association of some particular dysmorphic features:* abnormal fat distribution, and inverted nipples in congenital disorders of glycosylation (CDG), prominent forehead and long philtrum in peroxisomal disorders, macroglossia in Pompe disease and different kind of dysmorphic features in cholesterol biosynthesis defects and energy metabolism disorders.
- *The association of visceral involvement* (either visceral enlargement or biochemical dysfunction): mainly peroxisomal, lysosomal, CDG and energy metabolism disorders
- *The association of lethargy or coma, seizures and other neurologic symptoms, pointing out a severe encephalopathy*
- *In the great majority of cases, hypotonia is from central origin.* However spinal atrophy-like features have been described in peroxisomal (Baumgartner et al 1999) and mitochondrial disorders (Rubio-Gozalvo E et al 1999). Peripheral neuropathies are usually due to defects in energy metabolism whereas myopathies are seen in glycogen storage disorders and also in energy metabolism defects.

2. *What kind of metabolic disorders give rise to predominant severe hypotonia?*

Two main groups can be defined:

- Energy metabolism defects: respiratory chain defects, pyruvate dehydrogenase deficiency, pyruvate carboxylase deficiency and fatty acid oxidation disorders.
- Disorders of complex molecules: peroxisomes, glycogen, lysosomes, phosphatidylinositol, cholesterol, congenital disorders of glycosylation.

A very rare organic aciduria, methylcrotonic glycinuria, can also present as a floppy baby.

ENERGY METABOLISM DEFECTS

One of the main causes of severe metabolic hypotonia in the newborn is congenital hyperlactacidemia due to mitochondrial disorders. Brain and muscle are high energy dependent organs. Low ATP production may cause hypotonia, either central or peripheral, although in most cases hypotonia is due to central nervous system dysfunction. The current knowledge about how mitochondria generate energy remains still limited. Three main steps in energy production are recognized (Fig. 33.6):

1. Glucose is broken down by anaerobic glycolysis in the cytoplasm and finally transformed into pyruvate. In anaerobic conditions, lactate dehydrogenase transforms pyruvate into lactate.
2. In aerobic conditions, pyruvate is carried inside the mitochondria and later transformed into acetyl-CoA by the action of the enzymatic complex pyruvate dehydrogenase (PDH). Acetyl-CoA is also a product of fatty acid beta-oxidation. This is incorporated into the Krebs cycle where electrons accumulate in the form of carbonate compounds are transferred to NAD^+

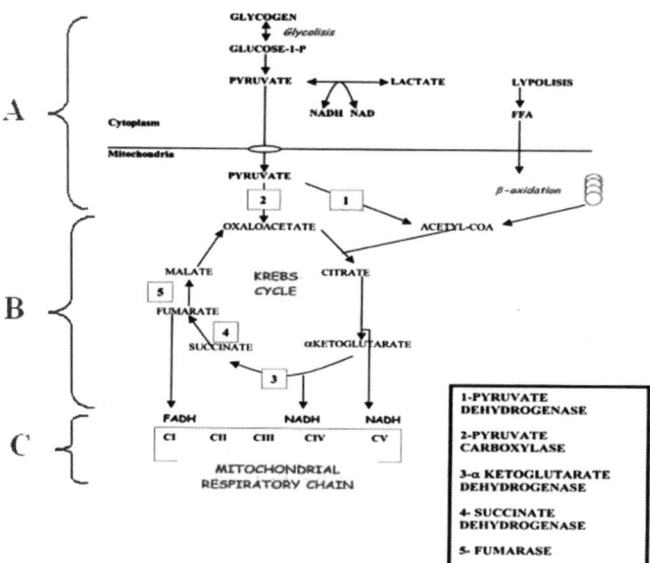

Figure 33.6 Three steps in energy production A: Glucose is broken down by anaerobic glycolysis in the cytoplasm and finally transformed into pyruvate. In anaerobic conditions, lactate dehydrogenase transforms pyruvate into lactate. In aerobic conditions, pyruvate is carried inside the mitochondria and later transformed into acetyl-CoA by the action of the enzymatic complex pyruvate dehydrogenase (PDH). Acetyl-CoA is also a product of fatty acid beta-oxidation. B: This is incorporated into the Krebs cycle, where electrons accumulated in the form of carbonate compounds are transferred to NAD⁺ (nicotinamide adenine dinucleotide) and FAD (flavine adenine dinucleotide). C: Reduced coenzymes, NADH and $FADH_2$ are the substrates for the next step: the mitochondrial oxidative phosphorylation (OXPHOS) by the respiratory chain (complex I to IV) and complex V.

(nicotinamide adenine dinucleotide) and FAD (flavine adenine dinucleotide). Reduced coenzymes, NADH and $FADH_2$ are the substrates for the next step.

3. The mitochondrial oxidative phosphorylation (OXPHOS) by the respiratory chain (complex I to IV) and complex V. Mitochondria have their own DNA (mitochondrial DNA or DNAmt), which is maternally inherited. It codifies 13 subunits belonging to complex I, II, IV and V (Anderson et al 1981). DNAmt regulation is double: nuclear DNA (mendelian inheritance) on one hand and mitochondrial DNA (maternal inheritance) on the other. This rule has an exception: complex II is entirely codified by the nuclear cell (Anderson et al 1981).

Respiratory chain disorders are the most common energy metabolism defect. From a clinical point of view neonates manifest with severe lactic acidosis that normally leads to fatal outcome or initial favorable evolution with progressive impairment from 6 to 12 months (Munnich et al 1996). In a study of 57 newborns affected with diverse respiratory chain disorders, an important proportion of them (36

patients) had severe hypotonia which was associated with lethargy and coma in most of the cases (García-Cazorla et al 2005). Other frequent clinical signs are hepatic failure, hypertrophic myocardiopathy, proximal tubulopathy, intrauterine growth restriction, episodic apnea/tachypnea, feeding difficulties, failure to thrive, nystagmus, cataracts, ptosis and dysmorphic features (Munnich et al 1996). Mitochondrial DNA depletion often presents during the neonatal period as a very severe disease causing fulminant hepatic failure, hepatocerebral disease or mimicking a neuromuscular disorder (severe hypotonia, high CPK and joint contractures). Deoxyguanosine kinase gene (Labarthe et al 2005), thymidine kinase 2 (Wang et al 2005) and POLG mutations (Davidzon et al 2005) have been related to mitochondrial DNA depletion. Whatever the origin of the mitochondrial energetic failure, one of the most common neuroimaging findings is bilateral basal ganglia high intensity signals.

PDH and pyruvate carboxylase deficiency may also present in a similar way, although some differences can be found between them (Table 33.3). Concerning beta oxidation defects, these are associated with hypoketotic hypoglycemia, cardiomyopathy and cardiac arrhythmias (Saudubray et al 1999). Trifunctional protein deficiency may present as severe hypotonia due to its central and peripheral component (neuromyopathy), although this is normally a later-onset phenotype.

PEROXISOMAL DISORDERS

Peroxisomal disorders are rare causes of severe neonatal encephalopathies. Clinically, profound hypotonia, lethargy, seizures, neuronal migration abnormalities together with multisystem involvement (hepatopathy, renal cysts, dysmorphism, calcific stippling of the epiphyses, cataracts, deafness, retinopathy), comprise the spectrum of possible manifestations. They are a group of conditions that have been described by Moser and Goldfischer (1985) in which there is a defect in the functioning of a group of subcellular organelles, termed peroxisomes and first reported in 1969 (DeDuve 1969). Some of these diseases give rise to progressive CNS degeneration in infancy, so it is important to recognize the symptom complexes that may lead to their diagnosis.

Peroxisomal functions include: breakdown of very long-chain fatty acids (VLCFAs), biosynthesis of ether-phospholipids (plasmalogens), biosynthesis of bile acids, catabolism of long- and medium-chain fatty acids, catabolism of phytanic acid, hydrogen peroxide degradation, metabolism of prostaglandins, catabolism of oxalic acid, isoprenoid (cholesterol) biosynthesis, L-pipecolic acid oxidation, biosynthesis of polyunsaturated fatty acids such as DHA (docosahexaenoic acid) (Baumgartner & Saudubray 2002).

At least 21 different disorders of peroxisomal dysfunction have been identified. All of them are clinically and biochemically heterogeneous and most of them present as encephalopathy (Baumgartner & Saudubray 2002). Initially, there were three main clinical descriptions corresponding to the three main early-infantile categories or clinical symptoms of these disorders:

Table 33.3 Main differential characteristics of energy metabolism defects

Disorder	Clinical features	Brain MRI	Diagnostic tests	Treatment
Respiratory chain/ mitDNA depletion	Severe hypotonia, lethargy, joint contractures, hepatic failure, high CPK	High intensity of basal ganglia, white matter cysts, brain dysgenesis	Lactic acidosis, respiratory chain defects in muscle/liver, mitDNA depletion	Vitamins, coenzyme Q10, low efficacy.
Pyruvate dehydrogenase deficiency	Severe hypotonia, optic atrophy, facial dysmorphism	White matter cysts, corpus callosum dysgenesis	Lactic acidosis, high pyruvate, normal or low lactate/ pyruvate/ratio, enzymatic tests in fibroblasts, leukocytes, genetic studies	Test high doses of thiamine (500–2000 mg/day), ketogenic diet
Pyruvate carboxylase deficiency	Severe hypotonia, abnormal ocular movements, rigid-akinetic syndrome	Extensive brain cysts (gray and white matter)	Lactic acidosis. High plasma citrulline, lysine and proline, low glutamine. Mild to moderate hyperammonemia Hypoglycemia	Anaplerotic therapy has been recently introduced (Mochel et al 2005)
Krebs cycle defects	Severe hypotonia, movement disorders, optic atrophy	Progressive brain atrophy (fumarase deficiency)	Lactic acidosis Characteristic organic acid profile in urine: high fumaric acid or 2-oxoglutarate	No known treatment
Fatty acid oxidation defects	Severe hypotonia, heart conduction abnormalities, hepatomegaly, brain, renal dysgenesis, cardiomyopathy, retinopathy, neuropathy	No specific features	Hypoketotic hypoglycemia. Dicarboxylic urine acids. Specific acylcarnitines profile	High dose glucose (>7 mg/Kg/min), no i.v. lipids, no carnitine in decompensations. Riboflavine 100 mg/day
Multiple carboxylase deficiency	Severe hypotonia, seizures, skin rashes	No specific features	Lactic acidosis, mild to moderate hyperammonemia, urine organic acids: high lactate, 3-OH-isovaleric acid, methylcrotonylglycine, methylcitric acids	Biotin 10–100 mg/(day)

- Zellweger syndrome (Opitz et al 1969), predominant with many dysmorphic features;
- neonatal adrenoleukodystrophy (Ulrich et al 1978), predominant neurological presentation;
- infantile Refsum disease (Scotto et al 1982), predominant hepatodigestive features.

As new disorders were described, most of them were classified into these three main categories.

Biochemically, some of these disorders are due to impairment of a single peroxisomal function, and others are due to multiple defects. Those due to a single or dual impairment include X-linked adrenoleukodystrophy, pseudo-Zellweger syndrome, pseudo-neonatal adrenoleukodystrophy, bifunctional protein deficiency, acatalasemia and rhizomelic chondrodysplasia punctata. Those peroxisomal disorders that have multiple defects include Zellweger syndrome, infantile Refsum disease, and neonatal adrenoleukodystrophy and have been found to be due to defects of peroxisomal membrane assembly (Powers & Moser 1998).

For the clinician, the main points that should draw attention are the age of the patient and the predominant clinical features (congenital malformation, neurologic dysfunction, hepatodigestive manifestations). In the neonatal period Zellweger syndrome and rhizomelic chondrodysplasia punctata are the two clinical presentation prototypes.

Zellweger syndrome and related disorders

The main features are severe hypotonia present from birth, depressed level of consciousness, seizures that may be early in onset and refractory, failure to thrive and variable hepatomegaly. The dysmorphic features are subtle, but, as in many syndromes, after seeing a case, they become easier to recognize. They include a high-domed forehead, external ear

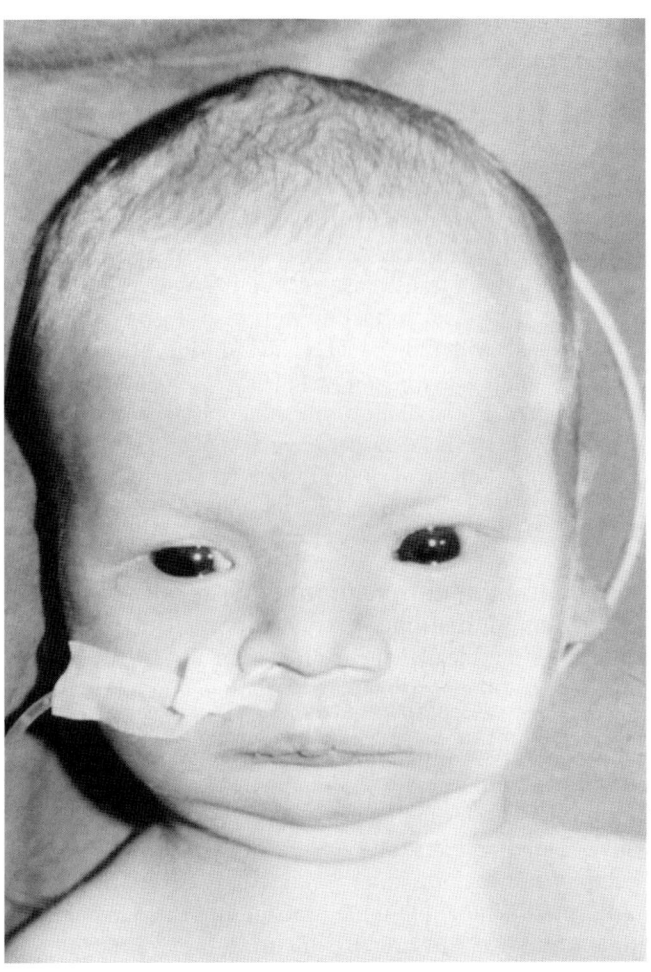
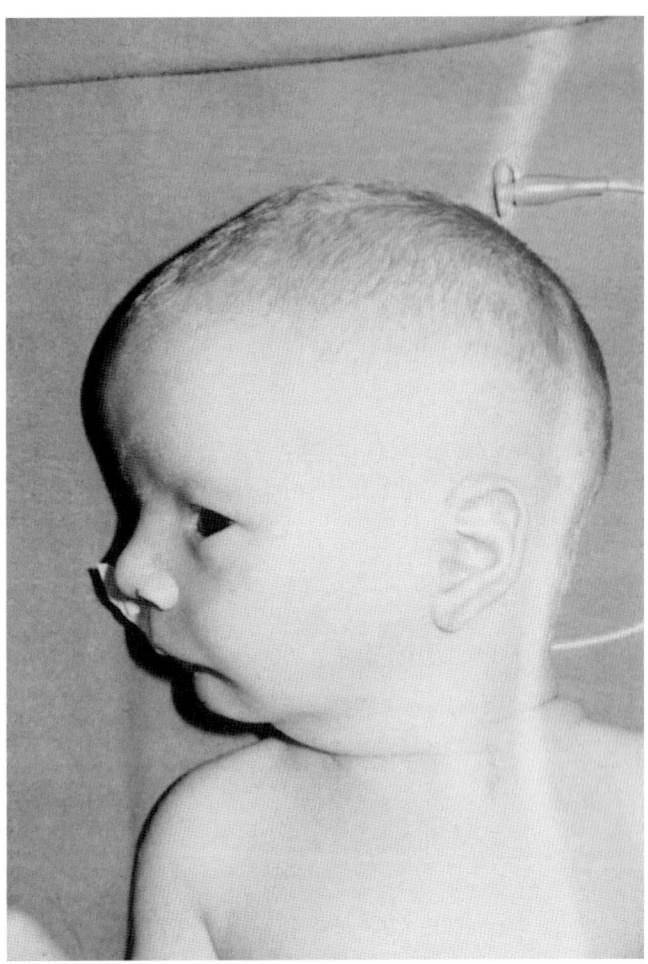

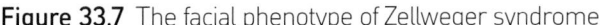

Figure 33.7 The facial phenotype of Zellweger syndrome.

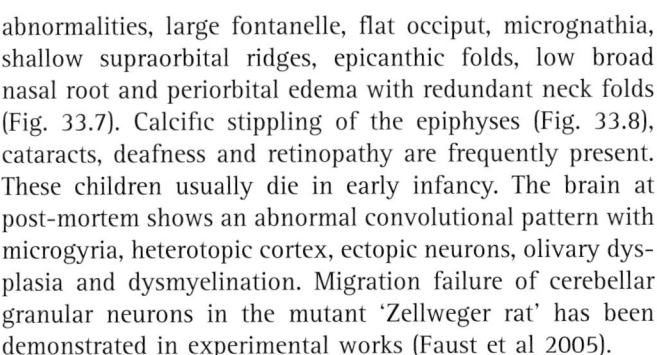

abnormalities, large fontanelle, flat occiput, micrognathia, shallow supraorbital ridges, epicanthic folds, low broad nasal root and periorbital edema with redundant neck folds (Fig. 33.7). Calcific stippling of the epiphyses (Fig. 33.8), cataracts, deafness and retinopathy are frequently present. These children usually die in early infancy. The brain at post-mortem shows an abnormal convolutional pattern with microgyria, heterotopic cortex, ectopic neurons, olivary dysplasia and dysmyelination. Migration failure of cerebellar granular neurons in the mutant 'Zellweger rat' has been demonstrated in experimental works (Faust et al 2005).

Biochemically, the patients show very high concentrations of plasma VLCFAs due to a deficiency of the enzymes of peroxisomal fatty acid β oxidation. Plasma bile acid (cholic and chenodeoxycholic acids) concentrations are often reduced, and intermediates of the bile acid biosynthetic pathway, normally not detectable, are present in greatly increased amounts. The proportion of membrane plasmalogens in erythrocytes and cultured cells is also reduced due to a deficiency of two enzymes involved in the biosynthesis of these ether lipids. In liver tissue, the peroxisomes, as visualized by catalase staining, are absent due to a selective deficiency of peroxisomal catalase.

Infantile Refsum disease (Scotto et al 1982) exhibits the same biochemical abnormalities as Zellweger syndrome but of a milder clinical phenotype. However, at birth, the predominant symptom is also a severe hypotonia without reactivity, disorders of the central and autonomic nervous system, and malformation syndromes (Baumgartner & Saudubray 2002). Retinopathy is often a major feature that may manifest itself as visual dysfunction (a depressed ERG would be a confirmatory finding). There is usually hepatic fibrosis. The plasma phytanic acid concentration is often raised in these children, but usually not until after 6 months of age. Variants of Zellweger syndrome exist with phenotypes intermediate between the classical form and infantile Refsum disease. This is the case with neonatal adrenoleukodystrophy (NALD) that presents with more prominent demyelination but absent or milder craniofacial dysmorphia.

Single peroxisomal oxidation defects

A number of disorders exist that can be clinically identical to the various forms of Zellweger syndrome but only have abnormalities in plasma VLCFAs and/or plasma bile acids. Pseudo-Zellweger syndrome and pseudoneonatal adrenoleu-

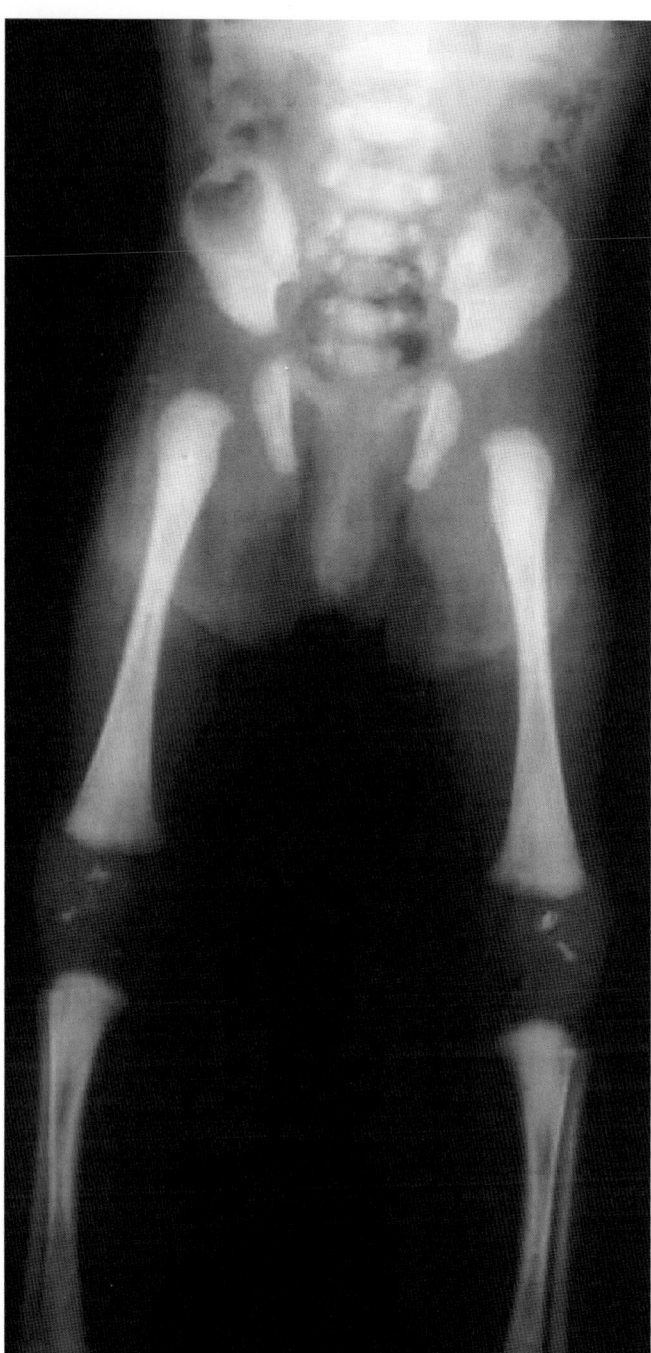

Figure 33.8 Calcific stippling of the epiphyses in a newborn with Zellweger syndrome.

kodystrophy exhibit abnormalities in VLCFAs and bile acids. The patients with a bifunctional protein defect have shown elevated VLCFA but normal bile acid concentrations. In trihydroxycoprostanoic acidemia, only plasma bile acid concentrations are abnormal.

Rhizomelic chondrodysplasia punctata

This is a disorder that presents at birth with rhizomelic limb shortening and punctate calcification of the patella. Calcifications may disappear after the age of 2 years (Gould et al 2001). Growth retardation, failure to thrive, dysmorphic features, coronal clefts of vertebral bodies and psychomotor retardation with truncal hypotonia develop within the first few months. Some patients have ichthyosis (Baumgartner & Saudubray 2002). Variants, however, have been found with no limb-shortening or without marked patellar calcification. In this disorder, there is a deficiency of erythrocyte membrane plasmalogens and in the dihydroxyacetone-phosphate: acyl-CoA transferase enzyme involved in their biosynthesis. In most forms, there is also a gross elevation of the plasma phytanic acid concentration. The primary defect in this disorder is in a gene (*PEX7*) encoding a receptor required for the import of some peroxisomal matrix proteins. Cases of this disorder have also been found without increased phytanic acid and are due to specific defects in gene coding for enzymes of plasmalogen biosynthesis (Braverman et al 1997).

Investigation of peroxisomal disorders

The most useful first-line test for the investigation of these disorders is the measurement of plasma VLCFA concentrations, because they accumulate in most of the peroxisomal disorders with neurologic involvement, although this will not detect rhizomelic chondrodysplasia punctata or trihydroxycoprostanoic acidemia. Impaired biosynthesis of etherphospholipids (plasmalogens) is also associated, therefore assays of plasmalogens in erythrocytes can be also used as a primary test (Baumgartner & Saudubray 2002). Other tests in plasma include phytanic, pristanic acids and PUFAs (polyunsaturated fatty acids). In urine, organic acids and pipecolic acid are also good markers. In a second stage studies in fibroblasts and liver are necessary to complete the investigation of the biochemical phenotype.

Genetics of peroxisomal disorders

All the disorders discussed show an autosomal recessive mode of inheritance. Prenatal diagnosis is available for all the disorders mentioned (enzyme assays in chorion villous samples or amniocytes, analysis of VLCFA in amniotic fluid). Peroxisomal proteins are codified by nuclear genes. Genetic assays have detected numerous *PEX* genes and proteins (peroxins) required for peroxisome biogenesis. Mutations in these genes give rise to different paroxysmal disorders (Steinberg et al 2004).

Therapy

There is no specific therapy for this group of disorders, although it has been suggested that supplementation of docosahexaenoic acid may improve some aspects of peroxisomal biogenesis disorders (Martinez & Vazquez 1998).

LOWE SYNDROME

The oculocerebrorenal syndrome of Lowe (OCRL) is a rare X-linked recessively inherited disease (Lowe et al 1952). The three cardinal clinical features include ocular symptoms (congenital cataracts, glaucoma and micro-ophthalmos), neurological dysfunction (mental retardation, hypotonia, behavior disturbances) and renal Fanconi syndrome. The severity of the clinical phenotype and the age of onset are quite variable (Peveralll et al 2000). In the neonatal period the child presents with severe hypotonia which is axial and peripheral, joint hyperlaxity and areflexia not due to neuropathy but to abnormal connective tissue. Growth retardation and skeletal abnormalities are also present (Kawano et al 1998). Neuroimaging studies disclose white matter cysts that in general are not present in the newborn but may appear over time (Fig. 33.9). Positional cloning in 1992 identified the gene *OCRL1* responsible for the Lowe syndrome and its genomic structure has been known since 1997 (Monnier et al 2000). It is composed of 24 exons and codifies an enzymatic protein that regulates the phosphatidylinositol 4,5-biphosphate intracellular concentration. This enzyme (phosphatidylinositol 4,5-biphosphatase) is localized in the Golgi apparatus (Peveralll et al 2000). Until now at least 58 distinct mutations have been described in the *OCRL1* gene (Monnier et al 2000). The distribution of these mutations is irregular and the majority of them are concentrated in a particular region.

CONGENITAL DISORDERS OF GLYCOSYLATION (CDG)

Congenital disorders of glycosylation (CDG) are recessive multisystemic diseases due to different defects in the biosynthesis or processing of glycan moieties (Jaeken et al 1997). Within *N*-glycosylation defects, CDG-I are disorders of the glycan assembly and/or the transfer to the proteins, while defects in the processing of the oligosaccharide chain attached to the protein are grouped as type II defects (Marquardt et al 2003). CDG-Ia is the most frequent type of CDG with more than 500 patients known worldwide; it is caused by a deficiency of phosphomannomutase (Van Shachtingen et al 1995). This enzyme converts mannose 6-P to mannose 1-P, which is essential for the biosynthesis of GDP-mannose, the donor of mannose for the *N*-glycosylation in the endoplasmic reticulum. The first manifestations of CDG-Ia appear in the neonatal period and infancy. The classic neonatal phenotype is characterized by severe global hypotonia with abnormal fat distribution, inverted nipples (Fig. 33.10) and strabismus. Later on, ataxia and developmental delay are almost constant. Extraneurological manifestations in infancy are frequent and include failure to thrive, enteropathy with vomiting and diarrhea, hepatic dysfunction and coagulopathy. Some patients have a severe systemic illness with hepatic, intestinal, cardiac and renal dysfunction leading to early death (Leonard 2001). A high rate of mortality of approximately 25% has been reported in the first years. Most patients develop the classic neurological form of the disease with mental retardation, severe stable ataxia and progressive peripheral neuropathy. It can be detected by the presence of

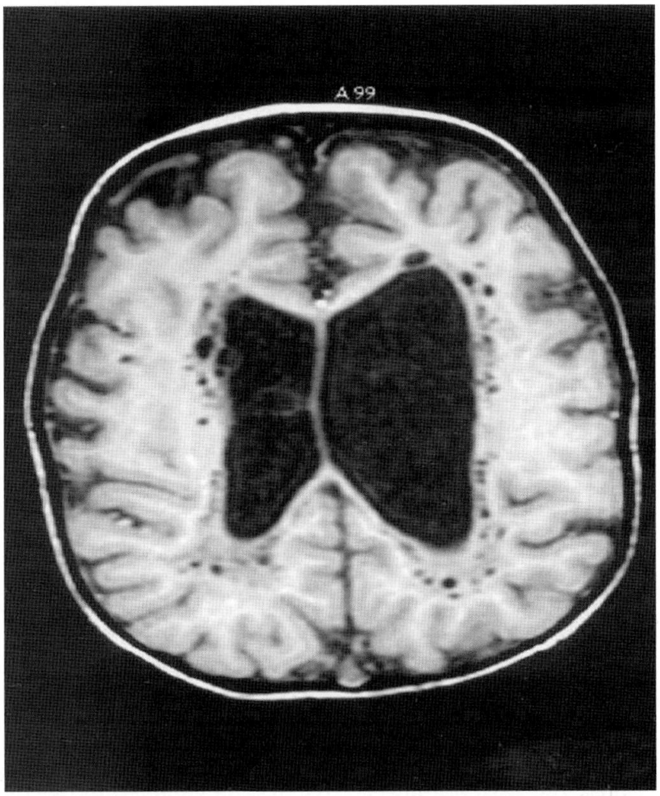

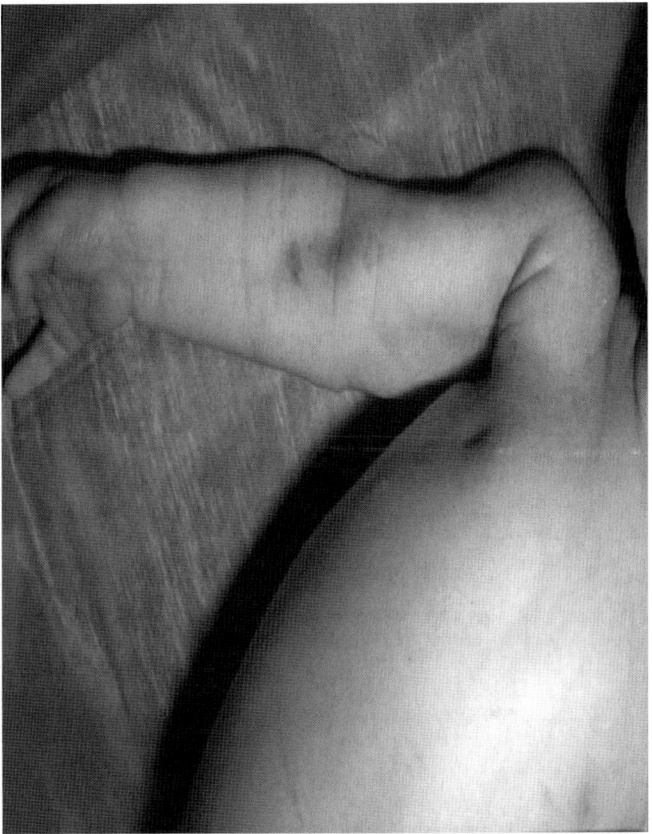

Figure 33.9 Brain MRI of a child with Lowe disease. Cortico-subcortical atrophy, enhanced ventricles and numerous small periventricular cysts.

Figure 33.10 Inverted nipples and abnormal subcutaneous adipose-tissue distribution in a newborn with CDG Ia.

an abnormal pattern of transferrin subtypes on isoelectric focusing or gel electrophoresis of plasma or serum. Enzymatic and genetic tests confirm the diagnosis.

O-glycosylation defects

These are emergent disorders characterized by the abnormal glycosylation of muscle cell proteins that give rise to different congenital muscular dystrophies (Prasad & Prasad 2003). Generalized hypotonia, muscular weakness, joint contractures, microcephaly, eye abnormalities and brain migration disorders are the most common clinical features. Fukuyama muscular dystrophy (p. 797), due to abnormal fukutin protein that modifies cell surface glycoproteins, muscle-eye-brain disease due to defective O-mannosylglycosylation and Walker–Warburg syndrome (p. 234), due to a specific gene mutation in the locus coding for the enzyme O-mannosyltransferase POMT1 (Beltran-Valero et al 2002) have now been identified in patients with these disorders.

DEFECTS OF CHOLESTEROL BIOSYNTHESIS

Neonatal presentation of these disorders gives rise to severe hypotonia in most of the cases. However the clinical hallmark in this group is dysmorphy. In fact, genetic defects in enzymes responsible for cholesterol biosynthesis have recently emerged as important causes of congenital dysmorphology syndromes. Identification of the genetic defect in the Smith–Lemli–Opitz syndrome (Wassif et al 1998) led to the discovery that other similar dysmorphology syndromes were caused by inborn errors of cholesterol biosynthesis: desmosterolosis (Waterham et al 2001), lathosterolosis, CHILD syndrome (Bornholdt et al 2005), CDPX2 (a form of chondrodysplasia punctata), mevalonic aciduria and hydrops-ectopic calcification-moth-eaten skeletal (HEM, also known as Greenberg dysplasia) (Braverman et al 1999). All of these syndromes have been linked to deficiency of the specific enzymes required for the production of cholesterol from lanosterol (Yu & Patel 2005). Patients with these disorders present with complex malformation syndromes involving different organs and systems: cataracts, retinitis pigmentosa, 2,3 syndactyly or postaxial polydactyly, hypoplastic or ambiguous genitalia, major organ or skeletal malformation, failure to thrive, increased creatine kinase, enteropathy, blood disorders such as myelodysplastic syndromes and lymphadenopathy. Variable reduction in serum cholesterol and/or bile acids is found in some of these disorders. High excretion of mevalonic acid is found in the analysis of urine organic acids in mevalonic aciduria. Enzymatic studies in fibroblasts as well as genetic tests in every disease are possible.

LYSOSOMAL DISORDERS

Genetic defects of lysosomal enzymes produce the accumulation of substrates inside the organelle. Clinically, signs of progressive impairment of the affected organs are detected. Nervous system, connective tissue, bone, cartilage and solid organs tend to be involved. However, clinical manifestations

of these disorders during the neonatal period are not frequent. Although hypotonia may be present, the most striking features of the neonatal onset are organomegaly and dysmorphic features. This is the reason why this complex group of disorders will not be discussed in detail in this chapter. Glycosaminoglycans in urine are high in most of the cases and there is a specific urine profile of mucopolysaccharides or oligosaccharides for most of them. Leukocyte enzymes (specific hydrolases) and genetic studies confirm the diagnosis.

POMPE DISEASE (NO ENCEPHALOPATHY, NO SEIZURES)

Pompe disease should be considered as a cause of severe hypotonia during the neonatal period and the first months of life due to a deficiency of alpha-glucosidase that leads to accumulation of glycogen. Muscular weakness, paucity of movements and cardiac problems like heart failure and rhythm disturbances are the main first symptoms (Hannerieke et al 2003). However signs of central nervous system dysfunction such as lethargy or seizures are not present. Therefore this disorder cannot be included in the group of metabolic encephalopathies.

Figure 33.11 provides a diagnostic flow-chart of neonatal hypotonia suspected of metabolic cause.

IEM GIVING RISE TO RIGID-AKINETIC SYNDROME

Rigid-akinetic syndrome is characterized by rigidity of the limbs, hypokinesia or paucity of spontaneous movement and hypomimia. These signs may be difficult to detect in newborns or infants. Depending on the etiology, some abnormal movements such as tremor and dyskinesias may be also associated. There are two main groups of disorders presenting in this manner in the neonatal period: neurotransmitter deficiencies and energetic metabolism defects.

NEUROTRANSMITTER DEFECTS — BIOCHEMICAL PATHWAYS

Biogenic amines are the most representative group amongst neurotransmitters (Blau et al 2001a). They are defects in the biosynthetic and catabolic pathways of the catecholamines (dopamine and norepinephrine) and serotonin. Tyrosine hydroxylase (TH) and tryptophan hydroxylase (TPH) are the rate-limiting steps in the synthetic pathways of serotonin and catecholamines, respectively. These two enzymes require BH_4 (tetrahydrobiopterin), which is synthesized from GTP (guanosine triphosphate). GTPCH (GTP cyclohydroxilase) and sepiapterin reductase (Bonafé et al 2001) are key enzymes contributing to the formation of BH4. Aromatic L-amino acid decarboxylase (AADC) decarboxylates the products of the TH and TPH reactions (L-dopa and 5-hydroxytryptophan, respectively). Deficiencies of the previously mentioned enzymes are the origin of the main pediatric neurotransmitter dis-

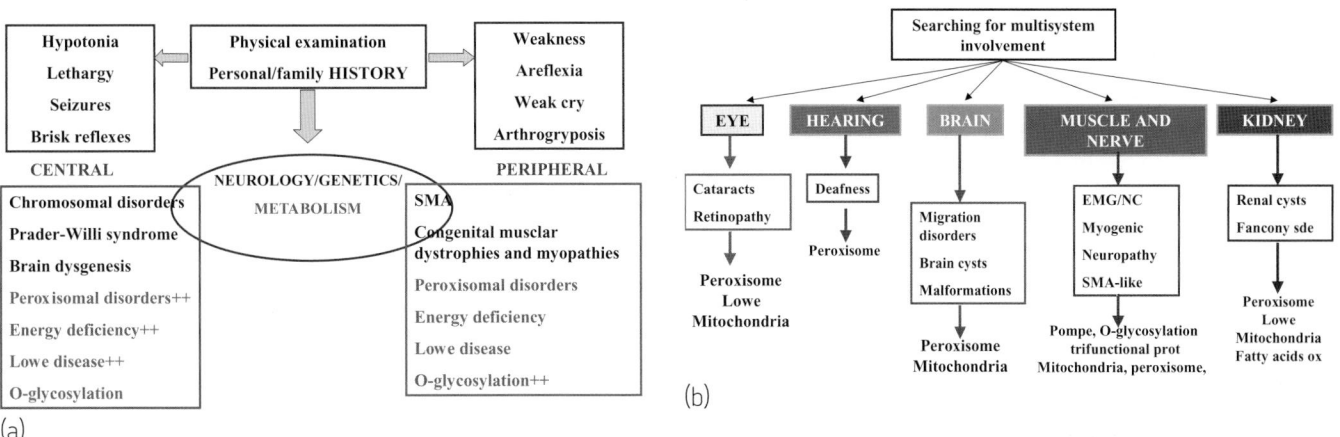

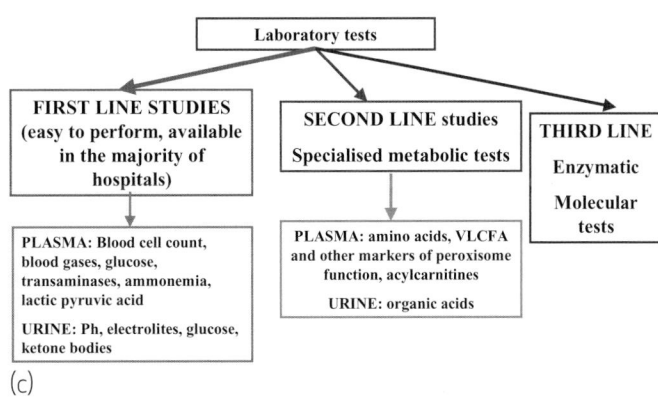

Figure 33.11 Diagnostic flow-chart of neonatal hypotonia. Diagnostic work-up 1: clinical signs found in neurological examination will point towards central or peripheral hypotonia. Metabolic causes of central or peripheral hypotonia are written in red. ++: indicates what kind of hypotonia is more probable in every disease. Diagnostic work-up 2: the presence of some particular extra-neurological signs and symptoms are being very useful to orientate the etiology of hypotonia. Diagnostic work-up 3: First line studies may provide a simple and helpful approach (lactic acidosis, hypoglycemia, high transaminases would point towards energy defects; hypoketotic hypoglycemia is a useful hallmark of beta-oxidation defects; Fanconi renal tubulopathy is characteristic of Lowe disease; blood count abnormalities, high transaminases and renal tubulopathy may appear in congenital forms of CDG syndrome. Second line tests may confirm the diagnosis (example: acylcarnitines in case of beta-oxidation suspicion) or provide additional information if first line tests have not been contributive (e.g. VLCFA in peroxisomal disorders). Third line studies are the final stage and definitely confirm the diagnosis.

eases. The compounds that are measured in the CSF are the end products of catecholamines (mainly homovanillic and 5-hydroxindoleacetic acid) (Ormazábal et al 2005).

NEUROTRANSMITTER DEFECTS — CLINICAL MANIFESTATIONS

Although they may be congenital, they can also appear later, usually during the first two years of life. Any of the following features may be indicative: truncal hypotonia, movement disorders (tremor is especially suggestive in our experience, but dystonia or chorea is also frequent), hypo-

mimia, hypokinesia, rigidity, oculogyric crises and other intermittent ocular movement abnormalities, feeding difficulties and autonomic symptoms (excessive sweating, hypoglycemia and temperature instability) (Chang et al 2004, Grattan-Smith et al 2002). The severe hypotonia associated with poor facial movements may lead to the erroneous diagnosis of congenital muscular disorder. Diurnal variation or fluctuation of symptoms is a very suggestive trait. Aggravation of the clinical manifestations with L-dopa may appear in some cases, particularly if the initial doses are high (De Lonlay et al 2000).

CONDITIONS REQUIRED FOR COLLECTING AND ANALYZING THE CSF

The measurement of lactate, pyruvate, amino acids, biogenic amines, pterins, organic acids and folates is used to identify these disorders. CSF must be collected in a particular well-defined manner for valid information (Ormazábal et al 2005). The patient must be in a fasting state; moreover no drugs should be administered at least 8 hours before the lumbar puncture to avoid interference with the metabolites that are to be analyzed. The same CSF fraction must be measured to be compared to reference values, due to the rostrocaudal concentration gradient of biogenic amines. This is the reason why tubes always have the same collecting order. In our center, the following protocol is used:

The first tube contains 5 drops used to analyze glucose, proteins and cells. The second tube is filled with the next 10 drops of CSF for the study of biogenic amines. The next 10 drops go to the third tube to measure pterins and folates. The fourth tube is filled with the next 10 drops to measure organic acids and amino acids. In, the fifth one needs the same quantity of CSF to analyze lactate and pyruvate. Tubes number 2, 3 and 5 should be immediately put in ice. If the samples are not to be analyzed in the following 20 minutes, they should be stored at −70°C to be measured later.

Plasma concentrations of lactate, pyruvate, glucose, folates and amino acids are measured at the same time (normally before, to avoid the hyperglycemia produced by the lumbar puncture stress). These are necessary to detect NKH, GLUT-1, cerebral folate and serine deficiencies.

HPLC (high-performance liquid chromatography) is used to measure biogenic amines by electrochemistry, whereas pterins are analyzed through fluorescence techniques. A specific profile for every defect allows us to orientate the diagnosis (Table 33.4).

TREATMENT OF BIOGENIC AMINE DEFICIENCIES

In TH deficiency L-dopa + carbidopa should be started at very low doses (0.1 mg/Kg/day) increasing progressively up to 8–10 mg/Kg/day (Wevers et al 1999). It is not rare that these patients present secondary effects to the initial L-dopa therapy: irritability, impairment of movement disorders. These adverse reactions may be avoided with the gradual introduction of the therapy. Some refractory cases have been described (De Lonlay et al 2000, Hoffmann et al 2003).

AADC deficiency has a poorer response to the substitutive therapy than TH deficiency. In general the clinical presentation as well as the outcome is more severe. However some symptoms may improve with some specific drugs. Monoamine oxidase inhibitors avoid dopamine and serotonin degradation leading to a higher concentration of both metabolites. Dopaminergic agonists such as bromocriptine, pergolide and pramipexole improve those symptoms produced by dopamine deficiency (Hyland et al 1992, Swoboda et al 1999). Pyridoxine, which is a cofactor of AADC, may be also used although the clinical and biochemical effect is not optimal. L-dopa + carbidopa has been demonstrated to be effective in some cases (Maller et al 1997).

In sepiapterin reductase deficiency, treatment with L-dopa + carbidopa at low doses (1–2 mg/Kg/day) produces an important clinical improvement whereas 5-hydroxy-tryptophan as serotonin pathway precursor has not been demonstrated to give positive results (Blau et al 2001b).

PYRUVATE CARBOXYLASE DEFICIENCY-ENERGETIC METABOLISM

Pyruvate carboxylase is a biotin-containing mitochondrial enzyme that catalyses the conversion of pyruvate to oxaloacetate. It plays an important role in gluconeogenesis and in energy production through replenishment of the Krebs cycle with oxaloacetate, and in anaplerotic pathways such

Table 33.4 Neurotransmitter defects, clinical and biochemical features

Disorder	CSF studies	Enzyme and genetic tests
Tyrosine hydroxylase deficiency (TH)	HVA and MHPG ↓ 5-HIAA, 5-HTP and pterines Normal	Enzymatic diagnosis is possible only in brain tissue. Genetic study is available
Aromatic L-amino acid decarboxylase deficiency (AADC)	HVA, MHPG and 5-HIAA ↓ 3-OMD, L-dopa and 5-HTP↑	Enzymatic activity in leukocytes and fibroblasts. Genetic study is possible
Sepiapterin reductase deficiency	Biopterins↑ Neopterins Normal HVA and 5-HIAA ↓	Genetic tests
Guanosine triphosphate ciclohydroxylase deficiency (GTPCH)	Biopterins, Neopterins and HVA ↓ Abnormal phenylalanine load	Enzymatic test in fibroblasts

HVA: homovanillic acid, 5-HIAA: 5-hydroxyindoleacetic acid, 5-HTP: 5-hydroxytryptophan, MHPG: 3-methoxy-4-OH-phenylglycol, 3-OMD: 3-orthomethyl-dopa.

as neurotransmitter synthesis and lipogenesis. PC deficiency is a rare autosomal recessive inborn error of metabolism with three different clinical presentations. Robinson et al (1984) defined two forms according to the severity of clinical and biochemical manifestations: The B or 'French' phenotype is a neonatal form with severe biotin unresponsive lactic acidosis, hyperammonemia, hypercitrullinemia and fatal outcome in the first few months of life (Coude et al 1981, Saudubray et al 1976). The A form or 'North American phenotype' is characterized by infantile onset, mild to moderate hyperlactacidemia and longer survival but severe clinical sequelae. Some special neurological signs such as abnormal movements and bizarre ocular behavior may appear during the first days of life (Garcia-Cazorla et al 2006). These findings may be similar to those observed in primary dopamine deficiency. The most common pattern of abnormal movements involves high amplitude tremor of the limbs aggravated by external stimuli, in a child who is otherwise paradoxically hypomimic and shows slow and few spontaneous movements. These groups of manifestations are qualified as hypokinetic-rigid syndrome. Furthermore, pendular nystagmus, rapid conjugated ocular movements and rolling eyes, is usually associated with the previously described uncommon limb movements (Pineda et al 1995).

OTHER DISORDERS

There are other IEM not mentioned in any of the main clinical presentations discussed above due to their more difficult classification. This is the case of disorders of intracellular utilization of cobalamine and creatine defects.

Among disorders of intracellular utilization of cobalamin, cobalamin C deficiency is the most frequent type (Rossenblatt et al 1997). The neonatal onset is characterized by feeding difficulties and hypotonia followed by progressive neurological deterioration that may end up in deep coma associated with abnormal movements (dystonia, tremor) and seizures (Rossenblatt 2000). Multisystem involvement and retinopathy may be present. Macrocytic anemia is frequent. Homocystinuria and methylmalonic acidemia are the biochemical hallmarks of the disease. Fibroblast incorporation of cobalamin and genetic studies are possible. Folic acid, carnitine, betaine and OHCbl are the basis of the treatment.

Creatine is a crucial molecule in energetic metabolism. Disorders of creatine biosynthesis may produce hypotonia, seizures and abnormal movements appearing during the neonatal period although it is more common that the first symptoms arise later on, in general throughout the first year of life. The biochemical markers are: low creatine/creatinine in urine and in MRS brain and high guanidinoacetate in all the biologic fluids in guanidinoacetate methyltransferase deficiency (GAMT), and low guanidinoacetate in plasma and urine, low to normal creatine/creatinine in urine and low creatine in brain MRS in arginine-glycine amidinotransferase deficiency (AGAT). Creatine

supplementation 300–400 mg/Kg/day improves the symptoms.

DIAGNOSTIC STEPS IN A NEWBORN WITH ENCEPHALOPATHY SUSPECTED OF METABOLIC ORIGIN

There are different stages of diagnostic workup for suspected metabolic diseases. In an initial approach, we would perform some basic metabolic investigations that should be undertaken at the same time as general supportive measures are applied. In a second level of investigation, some specific tests will lead to the most accurate diagnosis. In a third stage enzymatic and molecular studies will confirm the disease.

A. Initial investigations: these are simple, available in the great majority of laboratories and in general, the results are obtained in a very short time. In most of the cases these tests give us an idea about what kind of metabolic disorder the child has (intoxication, energetic defect, complex molecules) (Saudubray et al 2002).

   1. In blood: Blood cell count, blood gases and electrolytes, glucose, transaminases, prothrombin time, uric acid, ammonia, lactic, pyruvic acids, ketone bodies (3OH-butyrate, acetoacetate), free fatty acids.

   2. In urine: Abnormal urine odor is characteristic of organic acidurias: maple syrup odor in MSUD and sweaty-feet odor in isovaleric aciduria, pH, electrolytes, urea, creatinine, acetone.

   3. Others: EEG, brain ultrasonography, X-rays, brain MRI, ophthalmologic exam, other neurophysiologic studies.

B. Second line investigations: These will be performed according to the results of the first line tests. In most cases a precise diagnosis will be reached in this stage. Specialized laboratories are required for the great majority of analyses.

   1. In blood: plasma amino acids, free and total carnitine, acylcarnitines (or in blood spots in filter paper), pipecolic acid, VLCFA, phytanic, pristanic acids and PUFAs, isoelectric focusing of transferrin, biotinidase activity, copper, ceruloplasmin, guanidinoacetate, specific leukocyte hydrolases for lysosomal disorders, total cholesterol and triglycerides, precursors of cholesterol.

   2. In urine: organic acids, amino acids, glycosaminoglycans, oligosaccharides, sulfite test, pipecolic acid, vanillacetic acid, copper, guanidinoacetate, creatine/creatinine.

   3. In CSF: glucose, proteins, cells, amino acids, 5-methyltetrahydrofolate, biogenic amine metabolites, creatine.

C. Third line investigations: once the diagnosis is defined as the result of previous tests, specific enzymatic and genetic studies will be performed as indicated.

REFERENCES

Anderson S, Bankier A T, Barrel B G et al 1981 Sequence and organization of the human mitochondrial genome. Nature 290:457–465.

Andreula C F, de Blais R, Carella A 1991 CT and MR studies of methylmalonic acidemia. AJNR Am J Neuroradiol 12:410–412.

Applegarth D A, Toone J R 2001 Non ketotic hyperglycinemia (glycine encephalopathy): laboratory diagnosis. Mol Genet Metab 74:139–146.

Bahi-Buisson N, Kaminska A, Nabbout R et al 2006 Epilepsy in Menkes disease: analysis of clinical stages. Epilepsia 47:380–386.

Baumgartner E R, Suormala T 1997 Multiple carboxylase deficiency: inherited and acquired disorders of biotin metabolism. Int J Vitam Nutr Res 67(5):377–384.

Baumgartner M R, Saudubray J M 2002 Peroxisomal disorders. Semin Neonatol 7:85–94.

Baumgartner M R, Verhoeven N M, Jakobs C et al 1999 Defective peroxisome biogenesis with a neuromuscular disorder resembling Werdnig–Hoffmann disease. Neurology 15(2):383–386.

Beltran-Valero De Bernabe D, Currier S 2002 Mutations in the O-mannosyltransferase gene POMT1 give rise to the severe neuronal migration disorder Walker–Warburg syndrome. Am J Hum Genet 71:1033–1043.

Bergman A J, van der Knaap M S, Smeitink J A et al 1996 Magnetic resonance imaging and spectroscopy of the brain in propionic acidemia: clinical and biochemical considerations. Pediatr Res 40:404–409.

Blau N, Bonafé L, Thony B et al 2001a Tetrahydrobiopterin deficiencies without hyperphenylalaninemia: diagnosis and genetics of dopa-responsive dystonia and sepiaperin reductase deficiency. Mol Genet Metab 74:172–185.

Blau N, Thony B, Cotton R et al 2001b Disorders of tetrahydrobiopterin and relates biogenic amines. In: Scriver, Beaudetal, Sly W S, Valle D (eds) The metabolic and molecular basis of inherited disease. McGraw-Hill, New York, p. 1725.

Bonafé L, Thony B, Penzien J P et al 2001 Mutations in the sepiapterin reductase gene cause a novel tetrahydoropbiopterin-dependent monoamine-neurotransmitter deficient without hyperphenylalaninemia. Am J Hum Genet 69:269–277.

Bornholdt D, Konig A, Happle R et al 2005 Mutational spectrum of NSDHL in CHILD syndrome. J Med Genet 42:e17.

Braverman N, Lin P, Moebius F F et al 1999 Mutations in the gene encoding 3 beta-hydroxysteroid-delta 8, delta 7-isomerase cause X-linked dominant Conradi–Hunermann syndrome. Nat Genet 22:291–294.

Braverman N, Steel G, Obje C et al 1997 Human PEX7 encodes the peroxisomal PTS2 receptor and is responsible for rhizomelic chondrodysplasia punctata. Nat Genet 15:369–370.

Brismar J, Aqeel A, Brismar G et al 1990 Maple syrup urine disease: findings on CT and MR scans of the brain in 10 infants. AJNR Am J Neuroradiol 11:1219–1228.

Burlina A, Bonafé L, Zacchello F 1999 Clinical and biochemical approach to the neonate with a suspected inborn error of amino acid and organic acid metabolism. Semin Perinat 2:162–173.

Chang Y T, Sharma R, Marsh J L et al 2004 Levodopa-responsive aromatic L-amino acid decarboxylase deficiency. Ann Neurol 55:435–438.

Choi C G, Yoo H W 2001 Localized proton MS spectroscopy in infants with urea cycle defect. AJNR Am J Neuroradiol 22:834–837.

Coude FX, Ogier H, Marsac C et al 1981 Secondary citrullinemia with hyperammoniemia in four neonatal cases of pyruvate carboxylase deficiency. Pediatrics 68:914.

Davidzon G, Mancuso M, Ferraris S et al 2005 POLG mutations and Alpers syndrome. Ann Neurol 57:921–923.

De Koning T J 2006 Treatment with amino acids in serine deficiency disorders. J Inherit Metab Dis 29:347–351.

De Koning T J, Poll-The B T, Jaeken J 1999 Continuing education in neurometabolic disorders-serine deficiency disorders. Neuropediatrics 30:1–4.

De Lonlay P, Nassogne MS, van Gennip AJ et al 2000 Tyrosine hydroxylase deficiency with severe clinical course: clinical and biochemical investigations and optimization of therapy. J Pediatr 136:560–562.

DeDuve C 1969 The peroxisome: a new cytoplasmic organelle. Proc Roy Soc Lond (B) 173:71–83.

Fariello G, Dionisi-Vici C, Orazi C et al 1995 Cranial ultrasonography in maple syrup urine disease. AJNR Am J Neuroradiol 17:311–315.

Faust P L, Banka D, Siriratsivawong R et al 2005 Peroxisome biogenesis disorders: the role of peroxisomes and metabolic dysfunction in developing brain. J Inherit Metab Dis 2005;28(3):369–383.

Felipo V, Butterworth R F 2002 Neurobiology of ammonia. Prog in Neurobiol 67:259–279.

Fernandes J, Saudubray J M, van den Berghe G 2000 Inborn metabolic disease. Springer, New York.

García-Cazorla A, De Lonlay P, Nassogne M C et al 2005 Long-term follow-up of neonatal mitochondrial cytopathies: a study of 57 patients. Pediatrics 116(5):1170–1177.

García-Cazorla A, Rabier D, Touati G et al 2006 Pyruvate carboxylase deficiency: metabolic characteristics and new neurological aspects. Ann of Neurol 59:121–127.

Gascon G G, Ozan P T, Brismar J 1994 Movement disorders in childhood organic acidurias, clinical, neuroimaging and biochemical correlations. Brain Dev 16:94–103.

Gould S J, Raymond G V, Valle D 2001 The peroxisome biogenesis disorders. In: Scrive C R, Beaudetal, Valle D, Sly W S (eds) The metabolic and molecular bases of inherited disease. McGraw-Hill, New York, pp. 3181–3217.

Grattan-Smith P J, Wevers R, Steenbergen-Spanjers G C et al 2002 Tyrosine hydroxylase deficiency: clinical manifestations of catecholamine insufficiency in infancy. Mov Dis 17:354–359.

Green S H, Gray R G F 2001 Degenerative disorders of the infant central nervous system. In: Levene M I, Chervenak F A, Martin J Whittle (eds) Fetal and neonatal neurology and neurosurgery, 3rd edn. Churchill Livingstone, Edinburgh.

Guffon N, Schiff M, Cheillan D et al 2005 Neonatal hyperammonemia: the N-carbamoyl-L-glutamic acid test. J Pediatr 147:260–262.

Hannerieke M P, van der Hout, Hop W et al 2003 The natural course of infantile Pompe's disease: 20 original cases compared with 133 cases from the literture. Pediatr 112:332–340.

Hiroma T, Nakamura T, Tamura M et al 2002 Continuous venovenous hemodiafiltration in neonatal onset hyperammonemia. Am J Perinatol 19:221–224.

Hobson E E, Thomas S, Crofton PM et al 2005 Isolated sulphite oxidase deficiency mimics the features of hypoxic ischaemic encephalopathy. Eur J Pediatr 164:655–659.

Hoffmann G F, Assmann B, Brautigam C et al 2003 Tyrosine hydroxylase deficiency causes progressive encephalopathy and dopa-nonresponsive dystonia. Ann Neurol 54 Suppl 6:S56–S65.

Holder-Espinasse M, Marie S, Bourrouillou G et al 2002 Towards a suggestive facial dysmorphism in adenylosuccinate lyase deficiency? J Med Genet 39:440–442.

Hyland K, Surtees R A H, Rodeck C et al 1992 Aromatic L-amino acid decarboxylase deficiency: clinical features, diagnosis, and treatment of a new inborn error of neurotransmitter amine synthesis. Neurology 42:1980–1988.

Jaeken J, Matthijs G, Barone R et al 1997 Carbohydrate deficient glycoprotein (CDG) syndrome type 1. J Med Genet 34:76–83.

Kawano T, Indo Y, Nakazato H et al 1998 Oculocerebrorenal syndrome of Lowe: three mutations in the OCRL1 gene derived from three patients with different phenotypes. Am J Med Gene 77:348–355.

Kendall BE 1992 Disorders of lysosomes, peroxisomes and mitochondrial. AJNR Am J Neuroradiol 13:621–653.

Labarthe F, Dobbelaere D, Devisme L et al 2005 Clinical, biochemical and morphological features of hepatocerebral syndrome with mitochondrial DNA depletion due to deoxyguanosine kinase deficiency. J Hepatol Aug,43(2):333–341.

Leonard J V, Morris A A M 2002 Urea cycle disorders. Semin Neonatol 7:27–36.

Leonard J, Grunewald S, Clayton P 2001 Diversity of congenital disorders of glycosylation. Lancet 357(9266):1382–1383.

Lowe C, Terrey M, Mc Lachlan E A 1952 Organic aciduria, decreased reanal ammonia production, hidrophthalmos and mental retardation: a clinical entity. Am J Dis Child 83:164–184.

Maller A, Hyland K, Milstien S, Biaggioni L et al 1997 Aromatic L-amino acid decarboxylase deficiency: clinical features, diagnosis and treatment of a second family. J Child Neurol 12:349–354.

Marquardt T, Denecke J 2003 Congenital disorders of glycosylation: review of their molecular bases, clinical presentations and specific therapies. Eur J Pediatr 162:359–379.

Martinez M, Vazquez E 1998 MRI evidence that docosahexaenoic acid ethyl ester improves myelination In generalized peroxisomal disorders. Neurology 51:26–32.

Mills P B, Struys E, Jakobs C et al 2006 Mutation in antiquitin in individuals with pyridoxine-dependent seizures. Nat Med 12:307–309.

Mills P B, Surtees R A, Champlon M P et al 2005 Neonatal epileptic encephalopathy caused by mutations in the PNPO gene encoding pyridox(am)ine 5'- phosphate oxidase. Hum Mol Genet 14:1077–1086.

Mochel F, De Lonlay P, Touati G, et al 2005 Pyruvate carboxylase deficiency: clinical and biochemical response to anaplerotic diet therapy. Mol Genet Metabol 84:305–312.

Monnier N, Satre V, Lerouge E et al 2000 OCRL1 Mutation analysis in French Lowe syndrome patients: implications for molecular diagnosis strategy and genetic counseling. Human Mutation 16:157–165.

Moser H W, Goldfischer S L 1985 The peroxisomal disorders. Hosp Prac (office edn) 20:61–70.

Mourmans J, Majoie C B, Barth P G et al 2006 Sequential MR imaging changes in nonketotic hyperglycinemia. AJNR Am J Neuroradiol 27:208–211.

Munnich A, Rotig A, Chretien D et al 1996 Clinical presentation and laboratory investigations in respiratory chain deficiency. Eur J Pediatr 155:262–274.

Ogier de Baulny H, Saudubray J M 2000 Emergency treatments. In: Fernandes J, Saudubray JM, van den Berghe G (eds) Inborn metabolic disease. Springer, New York, pp. 53–61.

Ogier de Baulny H, Saudubray J M 2002 Branched chain organic acidurias. Semin Neontol 7:65–74.

Opitz J M, Zurhein G M, Vitale L 1969 The Zellweger syndrome (cerebrohepatorenal syndrome). Birth defects 5:144.

Ormazábal A, García-Cazorla A, Fernández A et al 2005 HPLC with electrochemical and fluorescence detection procedures for the diagnosis of inborn errors of biogenic amines and pterines. J Neurosc Methods 142:153–158.

Peveralll J, Edkins E, Goldblatt J et al 2000 Identification of a novel deletion of the entire OCRL1 gene detected by FISH analysis in a family with Lowe syndrome. Clin Genet 58:479–482.

Picca S, Dionisi-Vici C, Abeni D et al 2001 Extracorporeal dialysis in neonatal hyperammonemia: modalities and prognostic indicators. Pediatr Nephrol 16:862–867.

Pineda M, Campistol J, Vilaseca M A, Briones P et al 1995 An atypical French form of pyruvate carboxylase deficiency. Brain Dev 17:276–279.

Plecko B, Paul K, Paschke E et al 2006 Biochemical and molecular characterization of 18 patients with pyridoxine-dependent epilepsy and mutations of the antiquitin (ALDH7A1) gene. Hum Mut 26 (Epub ahead of print).

Powers J M, Moser H W 1998 Peroxisomal disorders: genotype, phenotype, major neuropathological lesions and pathogenesis. Brain Pathol 18:101–120.

Prasad A N, Prasad C 2003 The floppy infant: contribution of genetic and metabolic disorders. Brain Dev 27:457–476.

Robinson B H, Oei J, Sherwood W G et al 1984 The molecular basis for the two different clinical presentations of classical pyruvate carboxylase deficiency. Am J Hum Genet 36:283–294.

Rossenblatt D S 2000 Disorders of cobalamin and folate transport and metabolism. In: Fernandes J, Saudubray J M, van den Berghe G (eds) Inborn errors of metabolic diseases. Springer, New York, pp. 285–291.

Rossenblatt D S, Aspler A L, Shevell M I et al 1997 Clinical heterogeneity and prognosis In combined methylmalonic aciduria and homocystinuria (CblC). J Inherit Metab Dis 20:528–538.

Rubio-Gozalbo M E, Smeitink J A, Ruitenbeek W et al 1999 Spinal muscular atrophy-like picture, cardiomyopathy, and cytochrome c oxidase deficiency. Neurology 52(2):383–386.

Saudubray J M, Marsac C, Charpentier L et al 1976 Neonatal congenital lactic acidosis with pyruvate carboxylase deficiency in two siblings. Acta Paediatr Scand 65:717–724.

Saudubray J M, Martin D, de Lonlay et al 1999 Recognition and management of fatty acid oxidation defects: a series of 107 patients. J Inherit metab dis 22:488–502.

Saudubray J M, Nassogne M C, de Lonlay P et al 2002 Clinical approach to inherited metabolic disorders in neonates: an overview. Semin Neontol 7:3–15.

Scotto J M, Hadchouel M, Odievre M 1982 Infantile phytanic acid storage disease, a possible variant of Refsum disease: three cases including ultrastructural studies of the liver. J Inherit Metab Dis 5:83–90.

Sheela S R, Latha M, Liu P et al 2005 Cooper-replacement treatment for symptomatic Menkes disease: ethical considerations. Clin Genet 68:278–283.

Steinberg S, Chen L, Wei L et al 2004 The PEX Gene Screen: molecular diagnosis of peroxisome biogenesis disorders in the Zellweger syndrome spectrum. Mol Genet Metab 83(3):252–263.

Swoboda K W, Hyland K, Goldstein D S et al Clinical and therapeutic observations in aromatic L-amino acid decarboxylase deficiency. Neurology 53:1205–1211.

Taccone A, -Schiaffino M C, Cerone R et al 1992 Computed tomography in maple syrup urine disease. Eur J Radiol 14:207–212.

Takanashi J, Barkovich A J, Cheng SF et al 2003 Brain MR imaging in neonatal hyperammonemic encephalopathy resulting from proximal urea cycle disorders. AJNR Am J Neuroradiol 24:1184–1187.

Takeoka M, Soman T B, Shih et al 2001 Carbamyl phosphate synthetase 1 deficiency: a destructive encephalopathy. Pediatr Neurol 24:193–199.

Tharp B R 2002 Neonatal seizures and syndromes. Epilepsia 43:2–10.

Tumer Z, Horn N 1997 Menkes disease: recent advances and new aspects. J Med Genet 34:265–274.

Ulrich J, Hershkowitz N, Heits P et al 1978 Adrenoleukodystrophy: preliminary report of a connatal case, light-and electron microscopical, immunohistochemical and biochemical findings. Acta Neuropathol (Berl) 43:77–83.

Van den Berghe F, Bosschart A N, Hageman G et al 1998 Adenylosuccinase deficiency with neonatal onset, severe epileptic seizures and sudden death. Neuropediatrics 29:51–53.

Van Hove J L, Vande Kerckhove K, Hennermann J B et al 2005 Benzoate treatment and the glycine index in nonketotic hyperglycinaemia. J Inherit Metab Dis 28(5):651–663.

Van Shachtingen E, Jaeken J 1995 Phosphomannomutase deficiency is a cause of carbohydrate-deficient glycoprotein syndrome type I. FEBS Lett 377:318–320.

Wajner M, Latini A, Wyse A T S et al 2004 The role of oxidative damage in the neuropathology of organic acidurias: insights from animal studies. J Inherit Metab dis 27:427–448.

Wang L, Limongelli A, Vila M R et al 2005 Molecular insight into mitochondrial DNA depletion syndrome in two patients with novel mutations in the deoxyguanosine kinase and thymidine kinase 2 genes. Mol Genet Metab 84:75–82.

Wassif C A, Maslen C, Kachilele-Linjewile S et al 1998 Mutations in the human sterol delta7-reductase gene at 11q12–13 cause Smith–Lemli–Opitz syndrome. Am J Hum Genet 63:55–62.

Waterham H R, Koster J, Romeijn G J et al 2001 Mutations in the 3beta-hydroxysterol delta24-reductase gene cause desmosterolosis, an autosomal recessive disorder of cholesterol biosynthesis. Am J Hum Genet 69:685–694.

Wevers R A, Rijk-Van Adel J F, Bräutigau C et al 1999 A review of biochemical and molecular genetic aspects of tyrosine hydroxylase deficiency including a novel mutation (291delC). J Inher Metab Dis 22:364–373.

Yu H, Patel S B 2005 Recent insights into the Smith–Lemli–Opitz syndrome. Clin Genet 68:383–391.

Zschoke J, Hoffmann G 2004 Diagnosis and management of metabolic disorders. Vademecum metabolicum, 2nd edn. Stuttgart, Germany, Milupa and Schattauer, pp. 58–62.

CHAPTER

34

Seizure disorders of the neonate

Janet M. Rennie and Geraldine B. Boylan

Key Points

- The incidence of neonatal seizure is around 3 per 1000 at term, and around 50 per 1000 in very low birthweight infants
- The immature neuron has a high chloride content, resulting in gamma amino butyric acid (GABA) excitation rather than inhibition; this explains why many antiepileptic drugs (AEDs) which act on the GABA receptor do not work well in the neonate
- There is poor correlation between clinical manifestation of seizure in the newborn and any electrographic signature; this 'electroclinical dissociation' makes the diagnosis and treatment of seizures difficult without EEG
- Lumbar puncture remains an important investigation in neonatal seizure, even in babies with a history of birth depression. CSF with a high white cell count but no organisms on Gram stain suggests herpes infection and aciclovir should be started whilst awaiting the results of polymerase chain reaction (PCR)
- Phenobarbitone remains the standard first line treatment for neonatal seizures, and is effective in about a third of cases. Phenobarbitone is more likely to be effective in babies with a normal background electroencephalogram (EEG), and a relatively low seizure burden
- Babies whose seizures prove refractory to second and third line medication and whose EEG monitoring continues to reveal that more than 50% of the time is spent in seizure have a poor prognosis
- The background EEG activity in a baby with seizures after 12 hours of age is a very useful prognostic indicator, and provides the most precision when combined with clinical examination and the results of magnetic resonance imaging (MRI)
- The outcome of neonatal seizures depends on the etiology, with the worst outcomes in hypoxic–ischemic encephalopathy (HIE), meningitis and cerebral dysplasia and the best outcomes in hypocalcemia, stroke, and benign familial and non-familial neonatal seizures

INTRODUCTION

After many years with little progress, at last basic science research is beginning to provide insight into the conundrum of neonatal seizures, explaining why seizures are so common at this time of life and why antiepileptic drug (AED) treatments which are effective in older individuals do not work in babies. Seizures remain the commonest neonatal neurological emergency, and there is now convincing evidence that seizures can damage the brain and exacerbate pre-existing injury. The physiological changes which accompany many seizures can render intensive care more difficult, or interfere with feeding in babies cared for in the nursery or at home. Continuous EEG monitoring has confirmed the long-held suspicion that clinical diagnosis of neonatal seizures is unreliable, and that the problem of electro-clinical dissociation is worse in this age group and increases after

treatment with AEDs. The availability of digital technology means that EEG machines with the facility to monitor and store huge volumes of data conveniently at the cotside are relatively cheap and widely available. These advances, combined with the great strides which have been made in the laboratory both in genetics and in cell physiology, make this an exciting time to be writing about neonatal seizures. There is real hope that the next decade will finally see an end to the practice of treating babies with multiple potentially toxic and often ineffective AEDs on the basis of clinical impression alone (Rennie & Boylan 2007).

EPIDEMIOLOGY

As yet, there are no population based studies which report the incidence of neonatal seizures diagnosed with EEG, and to perform such a study would be a formidable undertaking. All the published studies are based on clinical recognition of seizure in the first instance, and many report the incidence from high-risk populations cared for in tertiary referral institutions. Clinical diagnosis of subtle seizure is fraught with difficulty and there is poor inter-observer agreement (Malone et al 2006). Further, electrical discharges without clinical manifestations are common, and on occasion babies can exhibit stereotyped movements without an accompanying electrical signature (electro-clinical dissociation). For all these reasons the true incidence of neonatal seizure remains conjectural. Nevertheless, some useful data are available.

A retrospective study of hospital records in Fayette County, Kentucky was carried out for births in the years 1985–1989, yielding an incidence figure for clinically recognized neonatal seizures of 3.5 per 1000 live births (Lanska et al 1995). The risk for babies of very low birthweight was 57.5 per 1000, significantly higher than the risk for heavier babies; for those of birthweight 2.5–4 Kg the risk was 2.8 per 1000. The same authors went on to analyze US national hospital discharge survey information for the years 1980–1991, producing a rather lower incidence figure of 2.84 per 1000 live births (Lanska & Lanska 1996). The US National Collaborative Perinatal Project is now over 40 years old, but because of the large sample size the incidence of 5 per 1000 live births remains of some importance, although the contributing hospitals were all referral centers (Holden et al 1982). A prospective study was carried out in Newfoundland between 1990 and 1994; a nurse coordinator carried out training sessions using video clips before recruitment started and all suspected cases were transported to a single center (Ronen et al 1999). The incidence was 2.6 per 1000 live births (1.9 for = 38 weeks and 8.6 for <38 weeks). Finally, a population based study in Harris County Texas between 1992 and 1994 estimated the incidence of seizure as 1.8 per 1000 live births, 19 per 1000 amongst those weighing less than 1500 g (Saliba et al 1999).

All the epidemiological studies show that most neonatal seizures occur very early in life, with around a third presenting on the first day and a further third on the second (Arpino et al 2001, Ronen et al 1999, Saliba et al 1999). The incidence of early (<48 hours) seizures in term infants has been proposed as an indicator of the quality of perinatal care because the most common cause in this group is hypoxic-ischemic encephalopathy. The incidence of early seizures was 0.87 per 1000 in Dublin between 1980 and 1984 (Curtis et al 1988) and 1.3 per 1000 in Cardiff during 1970–1979 (Minchom et al 1987).

In summary, the incidence of seizure at term is around 3 per 1000, and in very preterm babies estimates vary, but are of the order of 50 per 1000. In many studies almost half the cases are amongst babies born before 37 weeks of gestation and a quarter below 30 weeks.

PATHOPHYSIOLOGY

Neurons function via membrane depolarization and hyperpolarization, which involves ion flux across the neuronal membrane via voltage gated and transmitter gated channels. Membrane depolarization generates an action potential, which releases neurotransmitters and these then bind with the postsynaptic receptors. Neurotransmitters can be excitatory or inhibitory, and normal brain function depends on the maintenance of balance between the two. In the adult brain, glutamate is the primary excitatory neurotransmitter, and gamma amino butyric acid (GABA) is the main inhibitory transmitter. Glutamate receptors are inotropic or metabotropic, and there are three inotropic glutamate sub-receptor types: N-methyl-D-aspartate (NMDA), alpha-amino-3-hydroxy-5-methyl-4-isoxazoleproprionate (AMPA) and kainic acid. Seizures are thought to arise when there is a large and sustained depolarization of neurons without the normal hyperpolarization phase, which is in part achieved by the entry of chloride into the neuron via the GABA and calcium activated potassium channels (Holmes & Ben-Ari 2001).

There is an excess of excitatory synapses in the newborn brain compared with the adult, with a high density of receptors for excitatory neurotransmitters with a relative paucity of inhibitory synapses. Immature neurons have a high chloride content; there are two major chloride transporters which control chloride homeostasis in neurons. The $Na^+K^+2Cl^-$ (NKCCl) co-transporter accumulates chloride in the neuron, whereas the KCC_2 co-transporter exports it. Recently it has been discovered that the neonatal brain expresses the $Na^+K^+2Cl^-$ (NKCCl) co-transporter at birth and for some weeks afterwards, with little KCC_2 expression (Dzhala et al

2005). This contributes to the high intracellular chloride content of the neonatal brain, and opening the chloride permeable $GABA_A$ channel consequently leads to depolarization rather than hyperpolarization (Fig. 34.1). As a result $GABA_A$ is excitatory rather than inhibitory in the neonatal brain (Holmes et al 2002). Further, AMPA receptors are present but not functional, and $GABA_B$ is also underdeveloped and provides little post-synaptic inhibition. For all these reasons, the newborn brain is more susceptible to seizures than the adult brain, and the seizures are more likely to propagate.

Basic science research has shown that, in animals, status epilepticus causes neuronal loss in the hippocampus. Cell death occurs from excessive excitatory neurotransmitter release, which allows calcium to enter the cell and trigger a cascade of biochemical changes including activation of nitric oxide synthase, and enzyme activation. Seizures also activate genes that can lead to abnormal axon growth and synaptic reorganization. This has been seen as 'mossy fiber sprouting' in the hippocampus, and sprouting and neosynapse formation has been seen in other areas of the brain

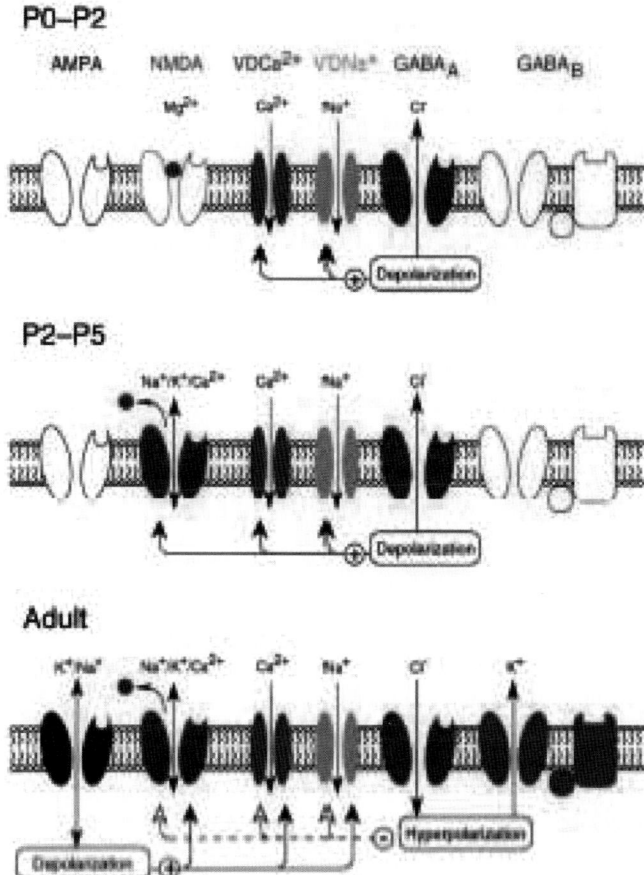

Figure 34.1 Comparison of excitatory and inhibitory channels in neonate and adult. Depol. = depolarization; Hyperpol. = hyperpolarization. (From Holmes et al 2002, with permission.)

(Holmes et al 1999). Holmes' group have also shown alterations of neural pathways in animals subjected to repeated seizures, with early gene activation of *c-fos* (Liu et al 1999), and he has suggested that seizures in early life may modify a wide range of essential processes such as neuronal migration, arborization and synaptogenesis leading to permanent effects on seizure susceptibility, learning and memory (Holmes & Ben-Ari 1998).

CLASSIFICATION, CLINICAL AND EEG FEATURES

The classic generalized tonic-clonic seizure which characterizes epilepsy in later life is rarely seen in the newborn period, and babies rarely exhibit prolonged motor automatisms even if a simultaneous EEG shows that seizure activity is continuing. As a result, there is no internationally agreed definition or classification system for neonatal seizures. Any classification system needs to take account of the fact that babies can manifest motor automatisms which appear seizure-like to many observers and yet have a normal EEG, whereas others have prolonged electrographic seizure discharges without any clinical manifestation whatsoever. This 'electroclinical dissociation' occurs at other times of life but has been identified as a particular problem in the newborn for many years (Weiner et al 1991). We and others have described a small group of healthy term babies who exhibited typical clinical seizure manifestations which were not associated with any electrographic seizure activity and in whom the background EEG was entirely normal ('clinical only' seizures) (Boylan et al 1999). The babies had not been treated with any AEDs and were normal at follow up. In contrast, other babies have very frequent electrographic seizures persisting for hours which are totally clinically silent, and are followed by a very poor neurodevelopmental outcome.

The clinical clue to the diagnosis rests on a high index of suspicion, especially in sick babies in intensive care. A repetitive stereotyped movement of the limbs or face is relatively easy to recognize, but babies with brief periods of repetitive blinking, chewing, staring or eye deviation may also be seizing. Seizures may be associated only with apnea, a rise in blood pressure or change in heart rate. Many babies with seizures exhibit more than one type (Mizrahi & Kellaway 1987, 1998). EEG-video monitoring is not a new tool, but digital technology with cheaper storage means that it is now possible to archive the huge amounts of data which video-EEG telemetry generates at the cotside using a compact laptop computer based system. These advances make prolonged video-EEG monitoring feasible in the nursery, and this technique has given fresh insight into the diagnosis, characterization and quantification of neonatal seizures (Boylan et al 2002, Mizrahi 2005, Mizrahi & Kellaway 1998). In our view, continued reliance on clinical diagnosis alone is increasingly untenable (Rennie & Boylan 2007). Nevertheless, suspicious movement patterns will remain an important

stimulus which should provoke investigation, ideally including some form of continuous or prolonged EEG monitoring. We include a description of the typical abnormal movement patterns in the next section.

CLINICAL SEIZURE TYPES

Tonic

Sustained posturing of the limbs or trunk (opisthotonos), or deviation of the head or eyes are the usual manifestations of tonic seizures in the newborn. Tonic seizures can be focal or generalized in neonates. In focal seizures the EEG background is often abnormal and ictal discharges are relatively common, compared to generalized tonic seizures. Generalized tonic seizures can mimic decerebrate or decorticate posturing. The EEG background activity is almost always severely abnormal. This seizure type is usually associated with a poor prognosis. If seizure activity is seen in the EEG, clinical phenomena are usually associated with autonomic signs.

Clonic

Clonic seizures are rhythmic, rather slow movements (1–3 per second) and can be focal, multifocal (migrating from limb to limb) or rarely hemiconvulsive. These seizures are characterized by repetitive rhythmic contractions of muscle groups in the arms, legs or face but rarely involve a whole side. Clonic seizures can shift rapidly from one part of the body to another; several areas can be involved simultaneously and the migration does not usually occur in a jacksonian, or systematic, fashion. Clonic seizures typically have a rapid flexion phase with a slower relaxation and a relatively slow rate of repetition; they cannot be stopped by restraining the limb. This seizure type is most consistently associated with synchronized EEG discharges.

Myoclonic

These single rapid contractions of muscle groups, myoclonic jerks, can be provoked by stimulation. The movements can be erratic, fragmentary or more generalized and are more rapid than the movements of clonic seizures. They show a predilection for flexor muscle groups. Myoclonic jerks can occur normally in sleep, and if occasional jerks (which are not stimulus sensitive and cease during arousal) are only seen during active sleep in an otherwise healthy baby then a normal EEG should confirm the diagnosis of benign neonatal sleep myoclonus (Coulter & Allen 1982, Egger et al 2003). Myoclonic jerks can also occur in babies who are receiving midazolam for sedation, particularly during weaning. Some babies with serious underlying disorders such as glycine encephalopathy suffer from very troublesome repetitive myoclonic jerking as their only seizure manifestation (Scher 1985). Myoclonus is not the same as hyperexplexia, in which there is a whole body exaggerated startle reflex (Gordon 1993, Tohier et al 1991).

Subtle

Subtle seizures are commonly seen in the neonate, and the wide range of possible manifestations make recognition a challenge (Volpe 2001). Subtle seizures often involve the face, with blinking, eyelid opening, tongue flicking, chewing or sucking movements but apnea (with or without bradycardia), abrupt changes in skin color or level of alertness can all be due to seizure. Distinguishing between the ventilated baby who may be sucking on an endotracheal tube as a reflex comfort activity, from one who is having bursts of eye movements or twitching during active sleep, from the one who is actually fitting is virtually impossible without EEG. Hiccups are usually benign, but excessive hiccupping can be due to seizure induced diaphragmatic contractions. The vast majority of apneas in preterm babies are not due to seizure and the yield of positive EEGs is low in this situation (da Silva et al 1998), but suspicion should be heightened in a term baby with apnea, particularly one who has been given any AED (Boylan et al 2002, Scher et al 2003). Seizures which originate in the temporal lobe have a predilection to cause apnea, usually without bradycardia (Tramonte & Goodkin 2004).

EEG RECOGNITION OF NEONATAL SEIZURES
(see also Ch. 12)

EEG

The most reliable and accurate method of diagnosing neonatal seizures is continuous video-EEG monitoring. This enables the EEG findings to be correlated with the clinical manifestations, and facilitates the prolonged recordings which are necessary to identify short seizures occurring at long intervals. If video-EEG is not available, a conventional routine 40 minute multichannel EEG is certainly worthwhile, although isolated infrequent seizures will be missed (Glauser & Clancy 1992). The interpretation of the neonatal EEG is a highly specialized field, and requires knowledge of the maturational aspects and special features seen at this age. The topic is beyond the scope of this chapter, but several excellent atlases are available and more information can be found in Chapter 12 (Mizrahi et al 2004).

Many seizures in full term neonates arise in the temporo-occipital region, although not all generalize. In contrast to later in life, in the newborn period seizures always have a focal onset and multifocal seizures are common particularly in severe encephalopathies. A reduced montage of 9 electrodes, based on the 10/20 system but focused on the temporal region, detected seizures in all but one of 31 babies, correctly identifying 166/187 seizures (Tekgul et al 2005) (Fig. 34.2). In general, it is agreed that a minimum duration of 10 seconds should distinguish a genuine seizure from a brief non-ictal repetitive epileptic discharge in the newborn (Bye & Flanagan 1995, Clancy & Ledigo 1987, Shewmon 1990). An electrographic seizure is characterized by the sudden appearance of a repetitive, evolving, stereotyped waveform with a definite beginning, middle and end lasting more than 10 seconds (Fig. 34.3) (Patrizi et al 2003). A typical neonatal EEG seizure lasts around 2 minutes (Clancy & Ledigo 1987, Patrizi et al 2003, Scher et al 1993b), but

seizures are often very frequent. The importance of brief ictal (or interictal) rhythmic discharges less than 10 seconds in duration (BIRDS) remains to be established (Oliveira et al 2000). Preterm babies tend to have shorter electrical seizures than those born at term, and are less likely to have sustained or frequent discharges which could be classified as status epilepticus (Scher et al 1993b).

Neonatal status epilepticus

There is no agreed definition for neonatal non-convulsive status epilepticus (NeSSE), and it is clear that definitions suitable for use in older children and adults are not suitable for babies. Neonates rarely sustain clinical or electrographic seizures of more than 30 minutes duration, and conscious level is often difficult to define in sick ventilated babies. Several groups have arbitrarily defined NeSSE as continuous seizure activity for at least 30 minutes or 50% of the recording time (McBride et al 2000, Scher et al 1993b). A further definition, of 'serial seizures' over at least 20 minutes, would imply that status epilepticus was common in the newborn (de Alba et al 1984). Our experience, based on continuous video-EEG monitoring of a large number of high-risk neonates, showed that if a definition of more than 30 minutes electrographic seizure activity in an hour (not continuous) is adopted, about a third of monitored babies met this criterion. Babies who had seizure activity for 15–30 minutes of every hour for many hours with an abnormal background EEG had a poor outcome (Boylan et al 2006). These preliminary data suggest that the incidence of 'status epilepticus' is higher than in later childhood, that there is more likely to be an underlying neurological problem, and that the outcome is worse (Chin et al 2006).

A-EEG diagnosis of neonatal seizures (Ch. 12)

The amplitude integrated EEG (sometimes termed the cerebral function monitor, CFM) is a method for displaying one or two channels of compressed and filtered EEG from one or two channels displayed on a semi-logarithmic scale, chosen to suppress artefact. The method is popular because it is easy to apply, relatively cheap and prolonged recordings can be obtained at the cotside. There has been considerable development in the field following the original descriptions (Viniker et al 1984). In many babies, a-EEG undoubtedly provides useful information about the seizure burden and response to treatment, but the method has significant limitations as a diagnostic tool particularly when interpreted by non-expert observers in the NICU setting (Rennie et al 2004). Short seizures, localized seizures and low voltage seizures occurring against an abnormal background EEG will not be detected by a-EEG. Nevertheless, the technique remains popular because it is easy to use and requires little training for interpretation. Some seizures are easy to spot with a-EEG and in this situation the method is ideal for monitoring the response to treatment (Figs 34.4 and 34.5).

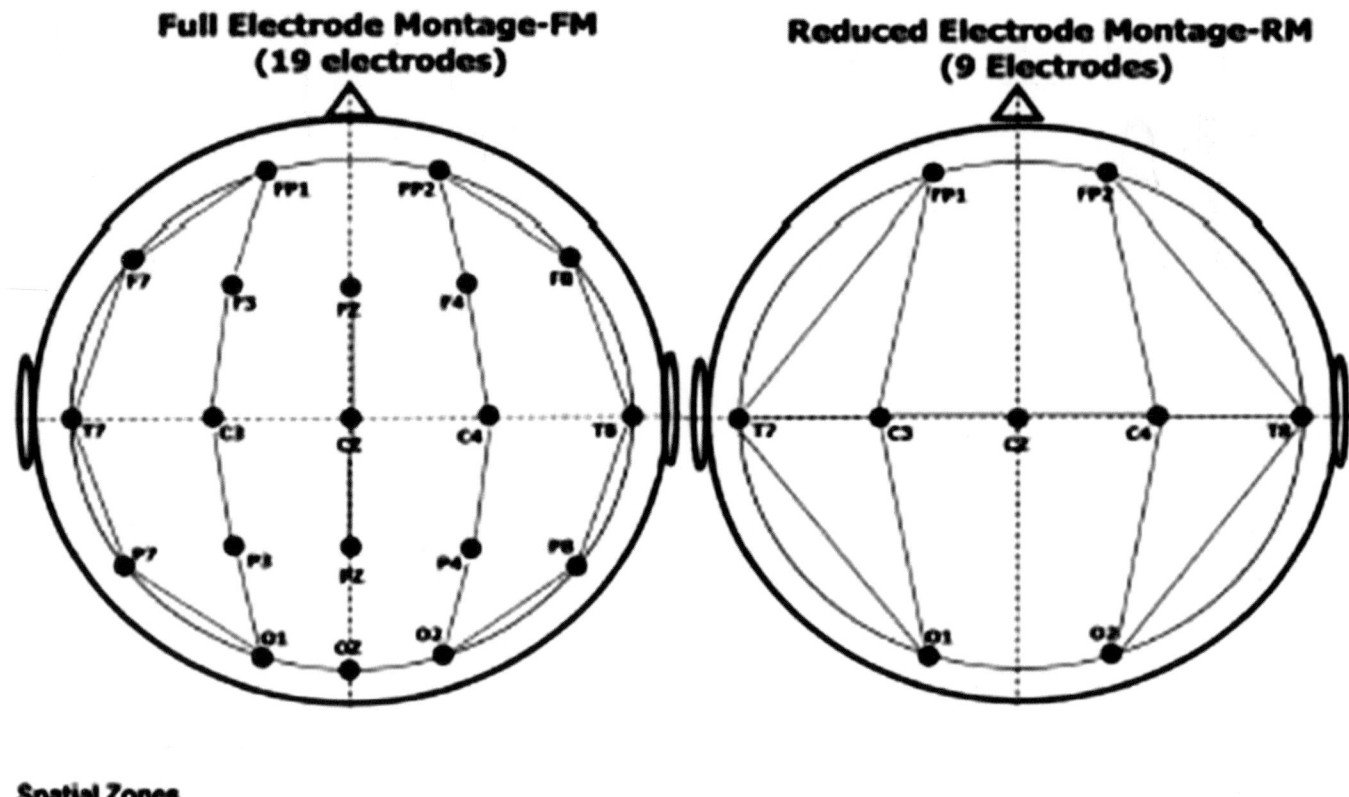

Spatial Zones

1. Left fronto-temporal zone   (LFTZ) : FP1, F7, F3, T7   : FP1, T7
2. Left parieto-occiptal zone   (LPOZ) : P3, P7, O1   : O1
3. Central zone (Cz)   : C3, CZ, C4, FZ, PZ   : C3, CZ, C4
4. Right fronto-occiptal zone   (RFOZ) : FP2, F8, F4, T8   : FP2, T8
5. Right parieto-occiptal zone (RPOZ) : P4, P8, O2   : O2

Figure 34.2 Full electrode montage and reduced electrode montage which proved effective in detection of neonatal seizures (using the 10–20 system). (From Tekgul et al 2005, with permission.)

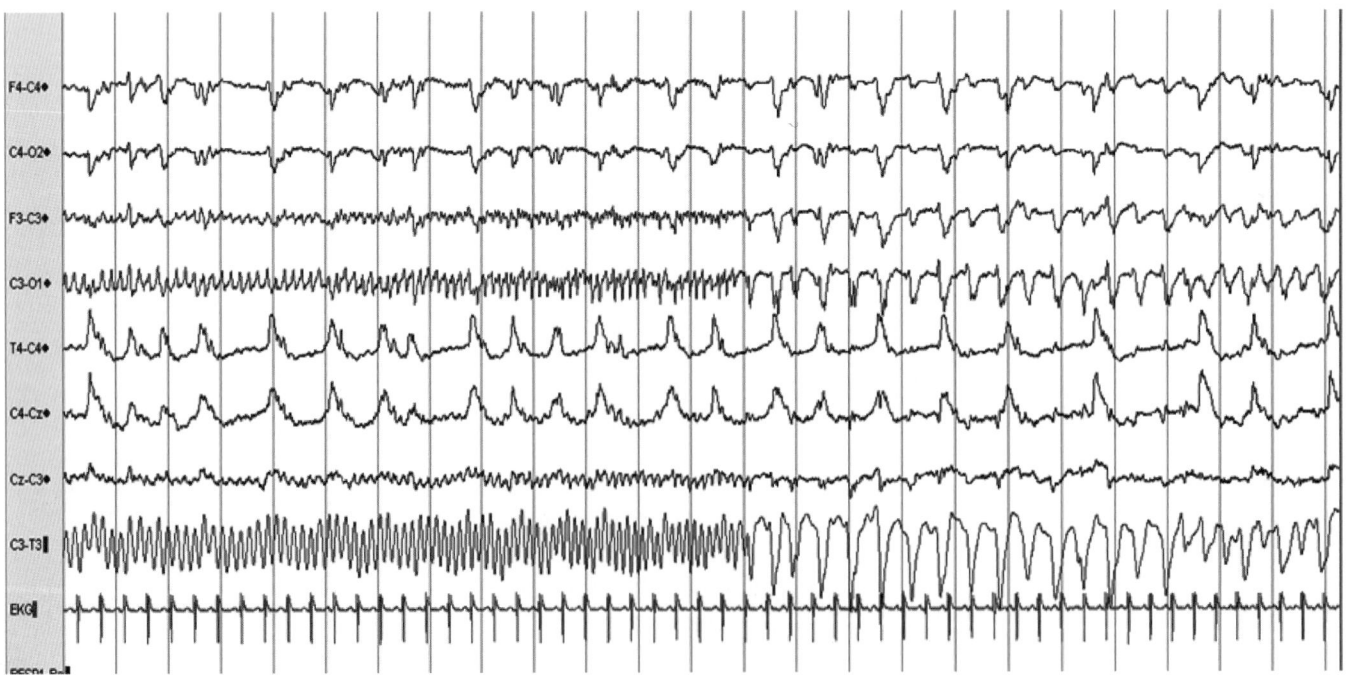

Figure 34.3 Conventional EEG recording showing multifocal seizures in a term baby.

the points marked on the upper trace.

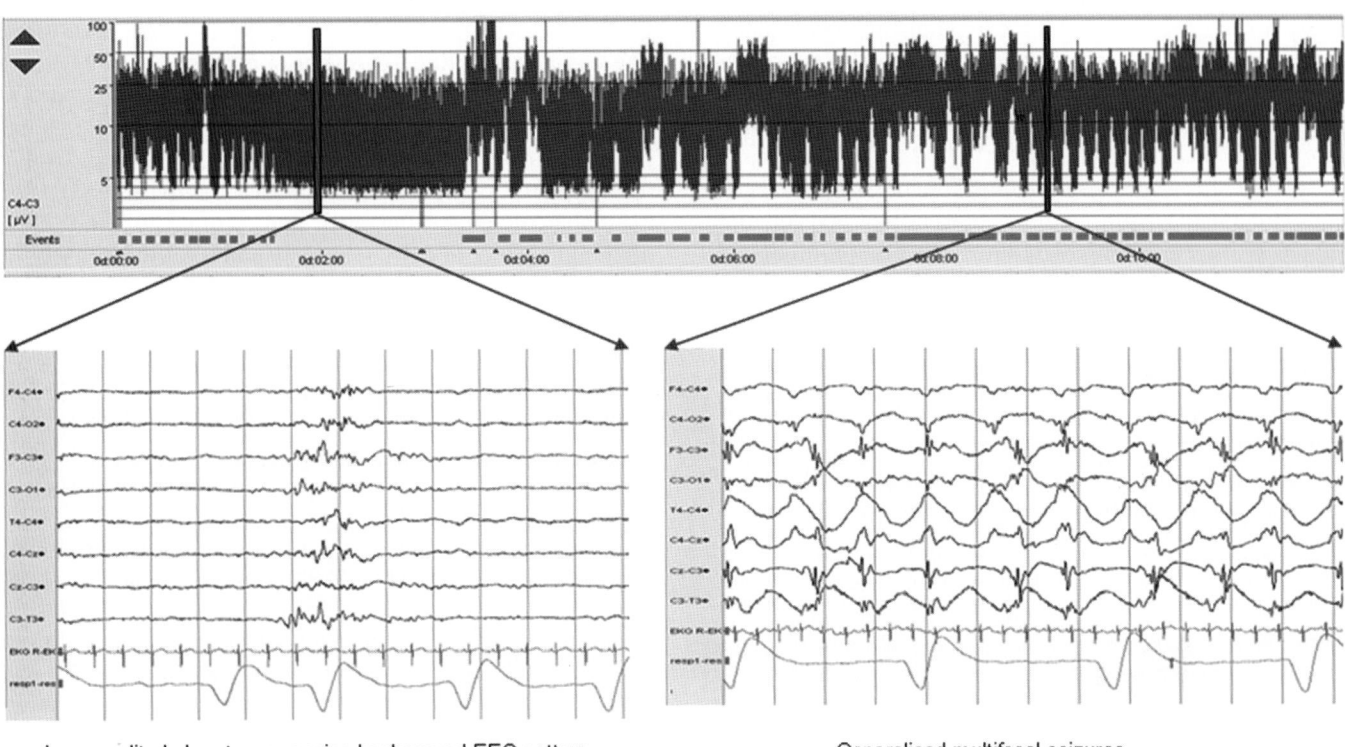

Low amplitude burst suppression background EEG pattern

Generalised multifocal seizures

Figure 34.4 a-EEG recording lasting 2 hours showing seizures (saw-tooth baseline). The lower part of the picture shows a single channel of EEG obtained from the point which is marked on the upper trace.

aEEG

Power

Amplitude envelope

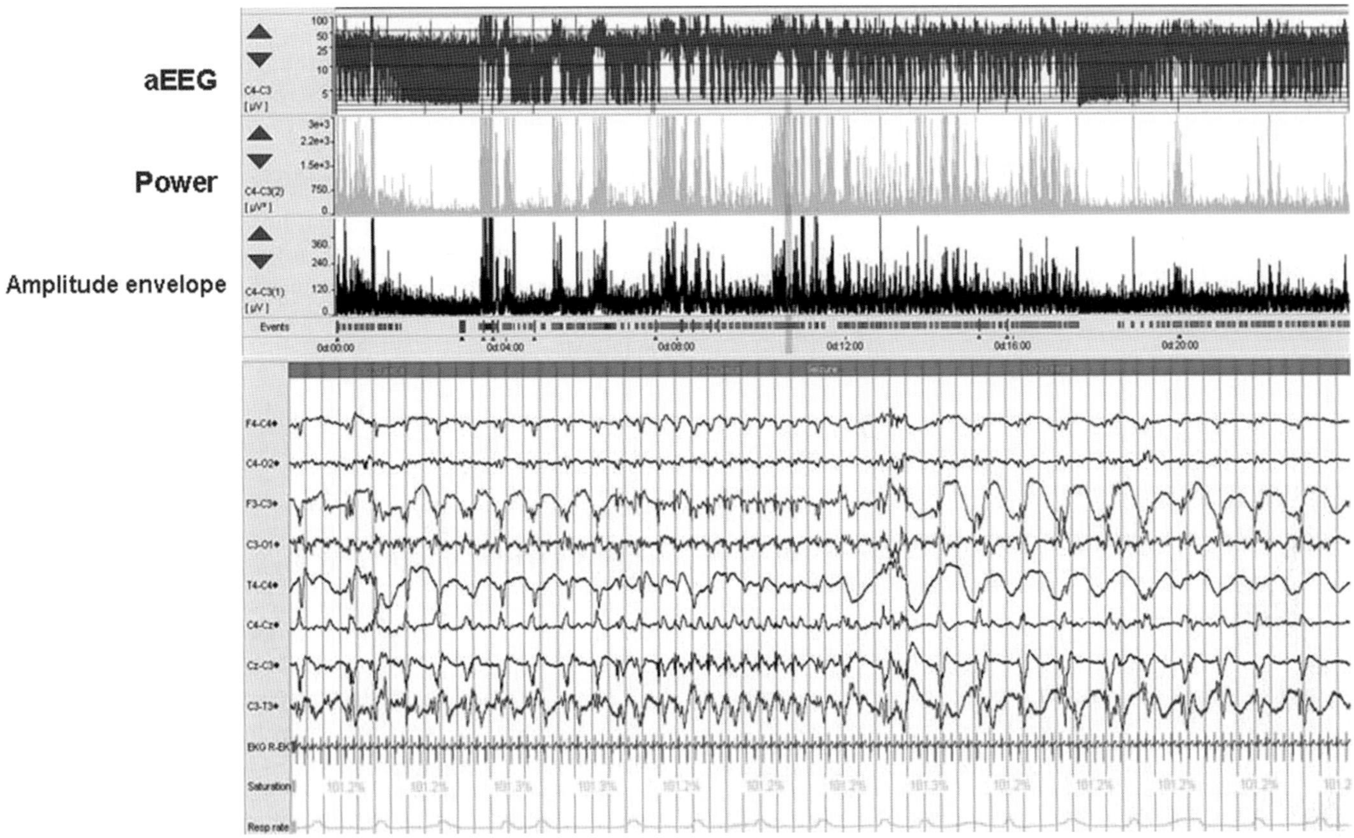

Figure 34.5 Prolonged recording showing seizures over a 24 hour period. Recording obtained from a multichannel EEG, with the a-EEG shown in the top channel. Channels below this show the power and the amplitude envelope of the EEG, then the raw EEG signal obtained from the point marked on the a-EEG trace, about half way along the recording.

ETIOLOGY

There is still no substitute for a careful history and examination as the starting point for determining the most likely cause of a neonatal seizure, backed up by appropriate laboratory tests (not forgetting the importance of lumbar puncture). The main causes are listed in Table 34.1. The commonest causes are HIE, stroke, intracranial hemorrhage, infection and congenital malformations, and initial investigations should be directed along these lines. The proportion of cases for which no cause can be found has fallen considerably since the introduction of neonatal MRI.

HYPOXIC–ISCHEMIC ENCEPHALOPATHY

Hypoxic–ischemic encephalopathy remains the most common cause of early onset seizures at term. However, seizures often remain undetected in babies with HIE and the administration of AEDs can further compound the problem

Table 34.1 Causes of neonatal seizures

Hypoxic–ischemic encephalopathy
Cerebral arterial infarction (stroke)
Cerebral venous sinus thrombosis
Intracranial hemorrhage
  Subarachnoid hemorrhage
  Intraventricular hemorrhage
    Parenchymal hemorrhage
    Cerebellar hemorrhage
    Subdural hematoma
Meningitis or encephalitis, bacterial or viral
Neonatal abstinence syndrome, other drug withdrawal or drug intoxication
Structural cerebral malformations
Metabolic causes
  Hypoglycemia
  Hyponatremia
  Hypernatremia
  Hypocalcemia
  Hypomagnesemia
  Hyperbilirubinemia
Inborn errors of metabolism
  Pyridoxine dependency
  Biotinidase deficiency
  Glucose transporter type 1 deficiency (Glut-1 deficiency, De Vivo syndrome)
  Amino acid, organic acid disorders
Syndromes
  Benign familial neonatal convulsions
  Benign non-familial neonatal convulsions
  Early infantile epileptic encephalopathy (Ohtahara syndrome)
Early myoclonic encephalopathy (neonatal myoclonic encephalopathy)

(Murray et al 2007a). More information on this condition, including the neuroimaging appearances, can be found in Chapter 6. Seizures usually begin within 12 hours of birth. The characteristic time of seizure onset is within 24 hours of birth; seizures often begin in the first 12 hours, but are rare in the first 6 hours unless there has been an antenatal insult (Filan et al 2004). In severe HIE, the EEG can evolve over a period of time. Very suppressed activity is seen for a number of hours after birth and is often followed by a period of seizure activity that, depending on the severity of the insult, can be very difficult to control with anticonvulsants. When seizures resolve, a burst suppression pattern can be seen for a number of days. Our group has recently reported delayed lactate clearance in neonates with HIE and a high EEG seizure burden (Murray et al 2007b).

FOCAL CEREBRAL INFARCTION (STROKE) (see also p. 457)

Seizures in term infants who are not encephalopathic and who remain largely alert between seizures are likely to be due to focal lesions, most commonly middle cerebral artery infarction. Cerebral venous sinus thrombosis, usually in the superior sagittal or transverse sinus, can also trigger seizures. Ultrasound imaging is not reliable for the detection of stroke or sinus venous thrombosis, which often requires magnetic resonance imaging for identification. The background EEG may be normal or show only mild abnormalities. Diagnosis of arterial or venous occlusion in the newborn period should trigger investigations to rule out an underlying thrombotic tendency. EEG is useful for prognosis and should ideally be performed within 24 hours of signs; some neonates will have seizures early in the postnatal period (Estan & Hope 1997).

INTRACRANIAL HEMORRHAGE (Ch. 20)

Intraventricular hemorrhage continues to be the most important cause of seizures in preterm babies, but babies of any gestation can seize because of bleeding into the subarachnoid space, the dural space, the cerebellum or cortex. A diagnosis of intracranial bleeding in a term baby should lead to a search for a coagulation disorder, including vitamin K deficiency and testing for hemophilia in boys. MR imaging has shown that a small amount of subarachnoid or subdural bleeding is common in the newborn period, and these collections usually resolve without sequelae.

MENINGITIS, ENCEPHALITIS (see also Ch. 32)

Every baby who develops seizures deserves a thorough investigation aimed at diagnosing infection, including viral infection. Aciclovir treatment should be started if the lumbar puncture reveals a high white cell count in the CSF yet no organisms are seen on Gram stain in a baby who has not been treated with antibiotics, whilst awaiting the results of PCR for herpes virus. The risks of starting treatment in this situation are minimal, whereas delay will worsen the prognosis.

NEONATAL ABSTINENCE SYNDROME AND OTHER DRUG RELATED CAUSES OF NEONATAL SEIZURE

Withdrawal seizures can occur for the first time at any age up to three weeks, with a median time of onset of 10 days. They can persist for several months. EEG abnormalities are present in 50% of cocaine exposed neonates, persist up to one year, and are associated with an adverse neurodevelopmental outcome. Maternal methadone addiction is more likely to be associated with neonatal withdrawal seizures than heroin (Herzlinger et al 1977). Tremors have been noted in children who received prolonged infusions of narcotics for analgesia (French & Nocera 1994), and there has been concern about the effects of midazolam for sedation in preterm babies (Montenegro et al 2001).

CONGENITAL MALFORMATIONS OF THE BRAIN
(see also Ch. 13)

Malformations such as lissencephaly or schizencephaly can present with neonatal seizures. Barkovich has suggested that these disorders should be broadly classified into four groups; those due to abnormal neuronal/glial proliferation, malformations due to abnormal neuronal migration, malformations due to abnormal cortical organization and other unspecified malformations (Barkovich et al 2001). Diagnosis has been facilitated with the advent of magnetic resonance imaging but is sometimes possible with ultrasound (see Ch. 6). Accurate diagnosis is important because there may be genetic implications (Gressens 2000, 2006).

METABOLIC CAUSES

Hypoglycemia (see also Ch. 35)
Screening of high risk babies should minimize the incidence of hypoglycemic seizures, but a seizure can be the presenting sign of hyperinsulinism in a baby of normal weight who had established feeding. Prolonged symptomatic hypoglycemia carries a risk of permanent brain injury. Although the classic diagnostic 'triad' states that seizures due to hypoglycemia resolve after the serum glucose level is restored, we have seen babies who develop an encephalopathy in the ensuing days.

Hyponatremia, hypernatremia
Breast milk insufficiency is the commonest cause of hypernatremia, and seizures can occur at the time of the high serum sodium or because of a rapidly falling serum sodium level. The brain adapts to a slowly changing serum sodium level, and it is recommended that the level be reduced at a rate not exceeding 0.5–1 mmol/L/h when rehydrating hypernatremic babies. In hypernatremia the brain manufactures intracellular osmolytes which protect against the adverse effects of high extracellular osmolarity, and the presence of these has been confirmed with MRS (Hee Lee et al 1994). These intracellular osmolytes persist after rehydration begins, hence the need for a slow correction. Babies have also developed hyponatremic seizures after being given excess solute-free water in intravenous solutions, or orally in the form of cheap alternatives to correctly balanced oral rehydration solutions.

Hypocalcemia, hypomagnesemia
Hypocalcemia was a common cause of neonatal seizure until the 1970s (because of the high phosphate content of cow's milk based formula feeds) but is now rare (Lynch & Rust 1994). A diagnosis of hypocalcemia should lead to consideration of CATCH-22 (22q11.2 deletion syndrome), which can be diagnosed with fluorescent in situ hybridization genetic studies. Another important cause is maternal vitamin D deficiency, particularly common amongst the infants of Asian mothers who have immigrated to countries with limited sunlight. A diagnosis of neonatal hypocalcemia should lead to estimation of the mother's serum calcium and alkaline phosphatase. Less often there is congenital hypoparathyroidism or calcium-sensing receptor defects.

Familial hypomagnesemia with secondary hypocalcemia is a rare autosomal recessive disease which can present with tremor, tetany and seizures shortly after birth. In this disorder, as with other causes of hypocalcemia and hypomagnesemia, magnesium should be replaced together with calcium or the seizures will continue.

Hyperbilirubinemia (see also Ch. 36)

INBORN ERRORS OF METABOLISM (see also Ch. 33)
A wide variety of inborn errors can present in the neonatal period with encephalopathy and seizures. The diagnosis and management of these conditions are beyond the scope of this book, but can include urea cycle defects, organic acidurias and aminoacidopathies. The first clue lies in the presence of a persisting metabolic acidosis and a high ammonia is also suspicious. Other rare causes of neonatal seizures are disorders of biotin metabolism, molybdenum cofactor deficiency, sulfite oxidase deficiency or disorders of fructose metabolism.

PYRIDOXINE DEPENDENCY (p. 684)
The seizures of pyridoxine dependency can begin during intra-uterine life (mothers describe 'hammering' movements lasting 15–20 minutes several times a day) and are very resistant to conventional anticonvulsant treatment, yet often cease within minutes of parenteral pyridoxine (50–100 mg) and return within days of withdrawal. This therapeutic trial can cause hypotonia requiring ventilatory support and should be carried out in an intensive care unit (Kroll 1985). There is no other way to make the diagnosis although characteristic EEG abnormalities have recently been recognized (Nabbout et al 1999). The EEG shows a suppression-burst pattern with bursts or runs of high voltage, bilateral synchronous sharp and slow wave activity alternating with periods of suppression. Other abnormal EEG activity such as generalized epileptiform activity may be observed. Atypical cases who respond more slowly and who have late-onset seizures requiring unusually high doses of pyridoxine (up to

500 mg) have been described (Baxter 2001, Gospe 1998), and yet others respond to very small doses. Gospe suggests that a trial of pyridoxine should involve 100 mg intravenously every 10 minutes until the seizures stop or a total of 500 mg is reached.

The underlying defect is probably defective binding of the pyridoxal phosphate co-enzyme with glutamic acid decarboxylase (GAD), a step which is necessary for GABA synthesis (Gospe 2002). The condition is autosomal recessive. Supplementation of the diet with pyridoxine (vitamin B_6) 20–100 mg twice daily is required for life, and the dose may need to be increased with age (Baxter 2001). Unfortunately many of these children are retarded despite early diagnosis and treatment. Recently, a better outcome has been achieved with bigger doses of pyridoxine, leading to the suggestion that sufficient pyridoxine should be given to restore the CSF glutamate levels to normal. Too much pyridoxine may not be a good thing either; a dorsal root ganglionopathy has been described in adults taking 2 g daily for months or years.

Glycine encephalopathy (non-ketotic hyperglycinemia) (p. 684)

Non-ketotic hyperglycinemia is a rare inborn error of metabolism in which there is a defect in cleavage of the excitatory amino acid glycine, hence large amounts of glycine accumulate and cause intractable seizures (p. 684). Hiccups can be troublesome. Levels of glycine in blood, urine and cerebrospinal fluid are very high. The EEG shows unusual periodic discharges on a near silent background. Dextromethorphan monotherapy (35 mg/Kg/day) was associated with cessation of seizures and normalization of the EEG in a single case, but this regimen is not always successful (Schmitt et al 1993).

Glucose transporter type 1 deficiency (GLUT-1 deficiency; De Vivo syndrome)

Glucose transport across the blood–brain barrier is mediated by the facilitative glucose transporter isoform 1 (GLUT-1). A deficiency of this transporter results in impaired energy supply to the brain, and was recognized by De Vivo in 1991 (De Vivo et al 1991). This rare disorder is important because treatment has the potential to lead to a normal neurological outcome, and because the inheritance is autosomal dominant (Fishman 1991). Babies have a low CSF glucose concentration, with low to normal CSF lactate levels despite normal blood glucose concentrations. Elevated lactate levels would suggest a mitochondrial disorder. The diagnosis should be suspected if the CSF glucose is less than a third of the blood glucose level, and GLUT-1 deficiency can be confirmed with an assay that measures the uptake of 14C-O-methyl-D-glucose in erythrocytes. Treatment is with a ketogenic diet, which is usually successful in controlling the seizures but does always prevent the microcephaly, developmental delay and ataxia. There may be a transient form of the disorder which does not require long term treatment, but the three cases so far described may have had alternative explanations for the low CSF glucose levels such as low-grade meningitis or subarachnoid hemorrhage (Klepper et al 2003).

Biotinidase deficiency (p. 685)

This is one of the few treatable causes of resistant neonatal seizures, hence the importance of considering this rare autosomal recessive condition. There is usually a skin rash, similar in appearance to seborrheic dermatitis, and as the condition progresses there is ataxia and developmental delay. Screening using the neonatal blood spot is possible but is not currently carried out in the UK.

SYNDROMIC NEONATAL SEIZURES

Benign familial neonatal convulsions

Seizures usually begin in the first week of life, and the baby is normal between the seizures. The seizures ceased after 6 weeks of age in 68% of the largest kindred reported, and rarely persist beyond 6 months (Ronen et al 1993).

This rare condition has an autosomal dominant inheritance with 85% penetrance, and mutations have been found in the genes situated on chromosomes 20q and 8q which code for a family of voltage gated potassium channels (M (for muscarine) channels). Benign familial neonatal convulsions (BFNC) are thus an example of a 'channelopathy'. M channels can be kept open with a new AED, retigabine, and it has been suggested that this drug might hold promise for other types of neonatal seizure apart from those in BFNC.

Benign non-familial neonatal convulsions ('fifth-day fits')

The seizures in this rare condition begin between days 3–5 and last for up to two weeks. The cause remains a mystery, although low cerebrospinal fluid zinc was found in a few cases (Goldberg 1982). The interictal neurologic state and EEG remain normal and the prognosis is good. Recently we cared for a baby with this condition who had marked tonic-clonic seizures which are otherwise very unusual in the newborn period; she has thrived (Guerra et al 2002).

Early myoclonic epilepsy

This rare syndrome, originally described by Aicardi, presents with erratic, fragmentary myoclonus in the first month of life, evolving into focal seizures and infantile spasms. Seizure manifestations include partial or fragmented myoclonus; massive myoclonias; partial motor seizures; tonic spasms. Myoclonias may shift from one part of the body to another and usually persist in sleep. Normal background activity is absent. The background EEG shows a burst-suppression pattern with complex bursts of spikes, sharp waves and slow waves lasting for 1–5 seconds in both waking and sleep. The fragmented myoclonias usually have no EEG correlate, whereas massive myoclonias may be synchronous with the bursts. The underlying cause is often an inborn error of metabolism such as non-ketotic hyperglycinemia, but some have cerebral malformations and in others no cause can be found.

Ohtahara syndrome (early infantile epileptic encephalopathy)

This disorder presents with intractable tonic seizures beginning in the neonatal period or early infancy, and is one of the age-dependent epileptic encephalopathies (the others being West syndrome and Lennox–Gastaut syndrome). Seizures are usually accompanied by a severe encephalopathy and are resistant to treatment. The EEG is characterized by a burst suppression pattern both in sleep and waking which may be asymmetric, asynchronous or even unilateral (Ohtahara 1978). During seizures, desynchronization of the pattern is seen. The prognosis is very poor. Vigabatrin has been tried in a few cases (Baxter et al 1995).

TREATMENT

Phenobarbitone remains the current first line treatment of neonatal seizures, worldwide, in spite of evidence that it is effective in only about a third of cases and concern about the effects of this drug on brain development, including apoptosis (Bittigau et al 2002, Kaindl et al 2006, Painter et al 1999). In our experience, phenobarbitone is more likely to be effective when the background EEG is normal and the seizure burden is low. Phenytoin is our current second line choice, although this drug needs to be used with caution (and given slowly i.v.) in babies with hypoxic–ischemia who often have cardiac depression. About a third of babies fail to respond to a combination of phenobarbitone and phenytoin; they are usually suffering from severe hypoxic-ischemic encephalopathy and their prognosis is poor. The choice of third line anticonvulsant varies, but one of the benzodiazepines is often chosen. Doses of commonly used anticonvulsant drugs are given in Table 34.2.

We recently evaluated midazolam in an open comparison with lidocaine as a second line treatment in babies whose seizures failed to respond to phenobarbitone; seizures were monitored with continuous video-EEG (Boylan et al 2004). Six babies received either clonazepam or midazolam, but none responded. Others have had better success with midazolam, one study using very high doses of 1000 microg/Kg/hour (Castro Conde et al 2005, Van Leuven et al 2004). Lorazepam is more popular in the US (Maytal et al 1991, Riviello 2004). Paraldehyde, formerly given rectally, can work well intravenously but is currently difficult to obtain in Europe and is not available in the US. Those who have used intravenous paraldehyde as a third line report success in over 80% of cases with 200 mg/Kg i.v. as a single slow infusion repeated 12 hourly if required (Armstrong & Battin 2001). The problem with many of the studies which evaluate AED treatments in babies is that the outcome measure is clinical seizure control, which can be very misleading.

Lidocaine has a very narrow therapeutic range and accumulates in the blood, so that it can only be given as an infusion for 48 hours. There are reports of success with this agent, mainly from Scandinavia (Hellstrom-Westas et al 1988, Kobayashi et al 1999). Three of the five babies who received lidocaine as second line in our open study responded, but much more information is required before this drug can be recommended for routine use. A baby who has been given phenytoin already should not receive lidocaine because of the risk of cardiac toxicity; the drugs act on the same sodium channels (Table 34.3). The newborn have yet to benefit from the recent explosion of new AEDs (lamotrigine, gabapentin, topiramate, tiagabine, levetiracetam) and because of the mode of action (Table 34.3) these drugs may be no more effective than those which have been

Table 34.2 AED doses used in the newborn, with usual therapeutic levels. Compiled from various sources, including the Neonatal Formulary 5th edn. 2007, Blackwell

Drug	Loading dose	Maintenance dose	Therapeutic level	Comment
Phenobarbitone	40 mg/Kg i.v. in two divided doses	5 mg/Kg orally or i.v. daily	20–40 mg/L (1 mg/L = 4.42 micromol/L)	
Phenytoin	20 mg/Kg i.v.	3–4 mg/Kg i.v. or orally three times a day	10–20 mg/L (1 mg/L = 3.96 micromol/L)	Not suitable for maintenance treatment in the newborn
Clonazepam	100 microg/Kg as a slow bolus	No benefit from infusions, repeat load 24 hourly if required	30–100 microg/L	Long half-life, no need for an infusion
Midazolam	60 microg/Kg i.v.	150 microg/Kg/h, possible increase to 300		
Lorazepam	100 microg/Kg i.v.	Repeat dose every 8–12 h		Long half-life, no need for an infusion
Lidocaine (lignocaine)	2 mg/Kg i.v.	2–4 mg/Kg/hour i.v. infusion; 6 mg/Kg/hour maximum	3–10 mg/L	Accumulates. Do not use for more than 48 h

Table 34.3 Molecular targets of antiepileptic drugs

Drug	GABA system	Glutamate receptor	Sodium channels	Calcium channels	Chloride channels
Phenobarbitone	+	+		+	
Phenytoin			+		
Benzodiazepines	+				
Vigabatrin	+				
Valproate	+				
Topiramate	+	+	+	+	
Lamotrigine			+	+	
Levetiracetam	+			+	
Bumetanide?					+
Gabapentin	+			+	

in the pharmacopeia for longer. The recent work already referred to, showing that the neonatal brain expresses the $Na^+K^+2Cl^-$ (NKCCl) co-transporter at birth and for some weeks afterwards, has led to the intriguing possibility that bumetanide might work well as an AED in the newborn, and the rat experiments look promising (Fukuda 2005).

Any concern about the effects of anticonvulsant treatment on the developing brain (Kaindl et al 2006) means that most UK and European neonatologists would only discharge a baby on maintenance phenobarbitone if the neurological examination was abnormal and the baby was continuing to seize. Only two of 55 Swedish infants discharged without medication relapsed (Hellström-Westas et al 1995). Some would perform an EEG at a month and continue anticonvulsants only if this were abnormal. In contrast, only 3% of US neonatologists discontinued treatment prior to discharge (Massingale & Boutross 1993). If babies are discharged on anticonvulsants we recommend discontinuation of treatment if they remain seizure-free at nine months.

PROGNOSIS

The prognosis depends largely on the cause of the seizures, being worse for those with HIE, meningitis and cerebral malformations than hypocalcemia, benign familial neonatal seizures, subarachnoid hemorrhage or stroke (Tekgul et al 2006). Mortality and morbidity are greater in preterm babies

(Scher et al 1993a). The background EEG can be helpful, and a normal background EEG with well organized sleep stages has consistently been shown to be associated with an 80% chance of normal development (Holmes & Lombroso 1993, Rose & Lombroso 1970, Tekgul et al 2006). The background EEG features of encephalopathy evolve over time, and it is important not to prognosticate from a recording made too early; both we and others have shown that a low voltage trace seen in the first 6 hours of life can recover (Pressler et al 2001, Toet et al 1999). The number of electrographic seizures is not in general an indicator of prognosis, nor is the clinical seizure type. Some have suggested that the outcome is worse for babies with a large number of independent electrographic seizure foci, but this work requires confirmation (Bye et al 1997). There is increasing consensus that seizures (including electrographic seizures which are clinically silent) which persist despite third line AEDs carry a poor prognosis (McBride et al 2000). The adverse outcomes seen include cerebral palsy and microcephaly with significant learning difficulties.

The risk of subsequent epilepsy after neonatal seizures also depends on the etiology, and is more likely if spike and sharp wave activity persists on the EEG at 3 months (Clancy & Legido 1991). The later seizure type includes infantile spasms, minor motor seizures, complex partial and tonic-clonic seizures, which often only emerge after a year or so.

REFERENCES

Armstrong D L, Battin M R 2001 Pervasive seizures caused by hypoxic-ischemic encephalopathy: treatment with intravenous paraldehyde. J Child Neurol 16:915–917.

Arpino C, Domizio S, Carrieri M P et al 2001 Prenatal and perinatal determinants of neonatal seizures occurring in the first week of life. J Child Neurol 16:651–656.

Barkovich A J, Kuzniecky R I, Jackson G D et al 2001 Classification system for malformations of cortical development. Neurology 57:21168–22178.

Baxter P 2001 Pyridoxine-dependent and pyridoxine-responsive seizures. Dev Med Child Neurol 43:416–420.

Baxter P S, Gardner-Medwin D, Barwick D D et al 1995 Vigabatrin monotherapy in resistant neonatal seizures. Seizure 4:57–59.

Bittigau P. Sifringer M. Genz K et al 2002 Antiepileptic drugs and apoptotic neurodegeneration in the developing brain. P Natl Acad Sci USA 99:15089–15094.

Boylan G B, Murray D M, Greene B R et al 2006 What is neonatal status epilepepticus? Clin Neurophysiol 117: S1;1.

Boylan G B, Pressler R M, Rennie J M et al 1999 Outcome of electroclinical, electrographic, and clinical seizures in the newborn infant. Dev Med Child Neurol 41:819–825.

Boylan G B, Rennie J M, Pressler R M et al 2002 Phenobarbitone, neonatal seizures and video-EEG. Arch Dis Child.

Boylan G, Rennie J M, Chorley G et al 2004 Second line anticonvulsant treatment of neonatal seizures: a video-EEG monitoring study. Neurology 62:486–488.

Bye A M E, Cunningham C A, Chee K Y, Flanagan D 1997 Outcome of neonates with electrographically identified seizures, or at risk of seizures. Pediatr Neurol 16:225–231.

Bye A M E, Flanagan D 1995 Spatial and temporal characteristics of neonatal seizures. Epilepsia 36:1009–1016.

Castro Conde J R, Borges A A H, Martinez E D et al 2005 Midazolam in neonatal seizures with no response to phenobarbital. Neurology 64:876–879.

Chin R F M, Neville B G R, Peckham C et al 2006 Incidence, cause and short-term outcome of convulsive status epilepticus in childhood: prospective population-based study. Lancet 368:222–229.

Clancy R R, Ledigo A 1987 The exact ictal and interictal duration of electroencephalographic neonatal seizures. Epilepsia 28:537–541.

Clancy R R, Legido A 1991 Postnatal epilepsy after EEG-confirmed neonatal seizures. Epilepsia 32(1):69–76.

Coulter D L, Allen R J 1982 Benign neonatal sleep myoclonus. Arch Neurol 39:191–192.

Curtis P D, Matthews T G, Clarke T A et al 1988 Neonatal seizures. Arch Dis Child 63:1065–1067.

da Silva O, Guzman G M C, Young G B 1998 The value of standard electroencephalograms in the evaluation of the newborn with recurrent apneas. J Perinatol 18(5):377–380.

de Alba G O, Mora E U, Valdez J M et al 1984 Neonatal status epilepticus 11: electroencephalographic aspects. Clin Electroencephal 15(4):197–200.

De Vivo D, Garcia-Alvarez M, Ronen G, Trifiletti R 1991 Defective glucose transport across the blood-brain barrier as a cause of persistent hypoglycorrhachia, seizures and developmental delay. New Engl J Med 325:703–709.

Dzhala V I, Talos D M, Sdrulla D A et al 2005 NKCC1 transporter facilitates seizures in the developing brain. Nat Med 11:1205–1213.

Egger J, Grossmann G, Auchterlonie I A 2003 Benign sleep myoclonus in infancy mistaken for epilepsy. Brit Med J 326:975–976.

Estan J, Hope PL 1997 Unilateral neonatal cerebral infarction in full term infants. Arch Dis Child 76: F88–F93.

Filan P, Boylan G, Chorley G et al 2004 The relationship between the onset of electrographic seizure activity after birth and the time of cerebral injury in utero. Brit J Obstet Gynaecol 112:504–507.

Fishman R A 1991 The glucose transporter protein and gluconeogenic brain injury. New Engl J Med 325:731–732.

French J P, Nocera M 1994 Drug withdrawal symptoms in children after continuous infusions of fentanyl. J Ped Nurs 9:107–113.

Fukuda A 2005 Diuretic soothes seizures in newborns. Nat Med 11:1153–1154.

Glauser T A, Clancy R R 1992 Adequacy of routine EEG examinations in neonates with clinically suspected seizures. J Child Neurol 7:215–220.

Goldberg H J 1982 Fifth day fits — an acute zinc deficiency syndrome? Arch Dis Child 57:633–635.

Gordon N 1993 Startle disease or hyperexplexia. Dev Med Child Neurol 35:1015–1024.

Gospe S M 1998 Current perspectives on pyridoxine-dependent seizures. J Pediatr 132:919–923.

Gospe S M 2002 Pyridoxine-dependent seizures: findings from recent studies pose new questions. Pediatr Neurol 26:181–185.

Gressens P 2000 The developing nervous system: mechanisms and disturbances of neuronal migration. Pediatr Res 48(6):725–730.

Gressens P 2006 Pathogenesis of migration disorders. Curr Opin Neurol. 19:135–140.

Guerra M P, Wilson G A, Boylan G B, Rennie J M 2002 An unusual presentation of fifth-day fits in the newborn. Pediatr Neurol 26:398–401.

Hee Lee J, Arcinue E, Ross B D 1994 Brief report: organic osmolytes in the brain of an infant with hypernatremia. New Engl J Med 331:439–442.

Hellstrom-Westas L, Blennow G, Lindroth M et al 1995 Low risk of seizure recurrence after early withdrawal of antiepileptic treatment in the neonatal period. Arch Dis Child 72:f97–f101.

Hellstrom-Westas L, Westgren U, Rosen I, Svenningsen N W 1988 Lidocaine for treatment of severe seizures in newborn infants. Acta Paediatr Scand 77:79–84.

Herzlinger R A, Kandall S R, Freeman J M 1977 Neonatal seizures association with drug withdrawal. J Pediatr 91:638–641.

Holden K R, Mellits E D, Freeman J M 1982 Neonatal seizures 1: correlation of prenatal and perinatal events with outcomes. Pediatrics 70:165–176.

Holmes G L, Ben-Ari Y 1998 Seizures in the developing brain: perhaps no so benign after all. Neuron 21:1231–1234.

Holmes G L, Ben-Ari Y 2001 The neurobiology and consequences of epilepsy in the developing brain. Pediatr Res 49(3):320–325.

Holmes G L, Khazipov R, Ben-Ari Y 2002 New concepts in neonatal seizures. Neuroreport 13:A3–A8.

Holmes G L, Lombroso C T 1993 Prognostic value of background patterns in the neonatal EEG. J Clin Neurophysiol 10(3)323–352.

Holmes G L, Sarkisian M, Ben-Ari Y, Chevassus-Au-Louis N 1999 Mossy fiber sprouting after recurrent seizures during early development in rats. J Compar Neurol 404:537–553.

Kaindl A M, Asimiadou S, Manthey D et al 2006 Antiepileptic drugs and the developing brain. Cell and Molecular Life Sciences 63:399–413.

Klepper J, De Vivo D, Webb D W et al 2003 Reversible infantile hypoglycorrhachia: possible transient disturbance in glucose transport? Pediatr Neurol 29:321–325.

Kobayashi K, Ito M, Miyajima T et al 1999 Successful management of intractable epilepsy with intravenous lidocaine and lidocaine tapes. Pediatr Neurol 21:476–480.

Kroll J 1985 Pyridoxine for neonatal seizures: an unexpected hazard. Dev Med Child Neurol 27:369–382.

Lanska M J, Lanska D J 1996 Neonatal seizures in the United States: Results of the national hospital discharge survey, 1980–1991. Neuroepidemiology 15:117–125.

Lanska M J, Lanska D J, Baumann R J, Kryscio R J 1995 A population-based study of neonatal seizures in Fayette county, Kentucky. Neurology 45:724–732.

Liu Z, Yang Y, Silveira D C et al 1999 Consequences of recurrent seizures during early brain development. Neuroscience 92(4):1443–1454.

Lynch B J, Rust R S 1994 Natural history and outcome of neonatal hypocalcemic and hypomagnesemic seizures. Pediatr Neurol 11:23–27.

McBride M C, Laroia N, Guillet R 2000 Electrographic seizures in neonates correlate with poor neurodevelopmental outcome. Neurology 55:506–513.

Malone A, Boylan G, Ryan C A, Connolly S 2006 Ability of medical personnel to accurately differentiate neonatal seizures from non-seizure movements. Clinical Neurophysiol 117: S1.

Massingale T W, Boutross S 1993 Survey of treatment practices for neonatal seizures. J Perinatol 13:107–110.

Maytal J, Novak G P, King K C 1991 Lorazepam in the treatment of refractory neonatal seizures. J Child Neurol 6:319–323.

Minchom P, Niswander K, Chalmers I et al 1987 Antecedents and outcome of very early neonatal seizures. Brit J Obstet Gynaec 94:431–439.

Mizrahi E M 2005 Electroencephalographic-video monitoring in neonates, infants, and children. J Child Neurol 9:S46–S56.

Mizrahi E M, Hrachovy R A, Kellaway P 2004 Atlas of neonatal electroencephalography, 3rd edn. Lippincott, Williams and Wilkins, Philadelphia.

Mizrahi E M, Kellaway P 1987 Characterization and classification of neonatal seizures. Neurology 37:1837–1844.

Mizrahi E M, Kellaway P 1998 Diagnosis and management of neonatal seizures, 1st edn. Lippincott-Raven, Philadelphia.

Montenegro M A, Guerreiro M M, Caldas J P S et al 2001 Epileptic manifestations induced by midazolam in the neonatal period. Arq Neuro-Psiquiat 59(2-A):242–243.

Murray D M, Boylan G B, Ali I et al 2007a Clinical seizure expression in neonates: the tip of the iceberg. Arch Dis Child (in press).

Murray D M, Boylan G B, Fitzgerald A P et al 2007b Persistent lactic acidosis in neonatal hypoxic ischaemic encephalopathy correlates wtih EEG grade and electrographic seizure burden. Arch Dis Child, Fetal and Neonatal Edition 93:F183–F186.

Nabbout R, Soufflet C, Plouin P, Dulac O 1999 Pyridoxine dependent epilepsy: a suggestive electroclinical pattern. Arch Dis Child 81:F125–F129.

Ohtahara S 1978 Clinico-electrical delineation of epileptic encephalopathies in childhood. Asian Medicine 21:7–17.

Oliveira A J, Nunes M L, Haertel L M et al 2000 Duration of rhythmic EEG patterns in neonates: new evidence for clinical and prognostic significance of brief rhythmic discharges. Clin Neurophysiol 111:1646–1653.

Painter M J, Scher M S, Stein A D et al 1999 Phenobarbital compared with phenytoin for the treatment of neonatal seizures. New Engl J Med 341:485–489.

Patrizi S, Holmes G L, Orzalesi M, Allemand F 2003 Neonatal seizures: characteristics of EEG ictal activity in preterm and fulterm infants. Brain Dev 25:427–437.

Pressler R M, Boylan G B, Morton M et al 2001 Early serial EEG in hypoxic ischaemic encephalopathy. Clin Neurophysiol 112:31–37.

Rennie J M, Boylan G B 2007 Treatment of neonatal seizures. Arch Dis Child 92:F148–F150.

Rennie J M, Chorley G, Boylan G B et al 2004 Non-expert use of the cerebral function monitor for neonatal seizure detection. Arch Dis Child 89(1):37–40.

Riviello J J 2004 Drug therapy for neonatal seizures: part 1. Neoreviews 5(5):e215–e220.

Ronen G M, Penney S, Andrews W 1999 The epidemiology of clinical neonatal seizures in Newfoundland: a population based study. J Pediatr 134:71–75.

Ronen G M, Rosales T O, Connolly M et al 1993 Seizure characteristics in chromosome 20 benign familial neonatal convulsions. Neurology 43:1355–1360.

Rose A, Lombroso C T 1970 Neonatal seizure states: a study of clinical, pathological, and electroencephalographic features in 137 full-term babies with a long-term follow-up. Pediatrics 45:404–425.

Saliba R M, Annegers J F, Waller D K et al 1999 Incidence of neonatal seizures in Harris County, Texas, 1992–1994. Am J Epid 150:763–769.

Scher M S 1985 Pathologic myoclonus of the newborn: electrographic and clinical correlations. Pediatr Neurol 1:342–348.

Scher M S, Alvin J, Gaus L et al 2003 Uncoupling of EEG-clinical neonatal seizures after antiepileptic drug use. Pediatr Neurol 28:277–280.

Scher M S, Aso K, Beggarly M E et al 1993a Electrographic seizures in preterm and full-term neonates: clinical correlates, associated brain lesions, and risk for neurologic sequelae. Pediatrics 91:128–134.

Scher M S, Hamid M Y, Steppe D A et al 1993b Ictal and interictal electrographic seizure durations in preterm and term neonates. Epilepsia 34:284–288.

Schmitt B, Steinmann B, Gitzelman R et al 1993 Non-ketotic hyperglycinaemia: clinical and electrical effects of dextromethorphan, an antagonist of the NMDA receptor. Neurology 43:421–424.

Shewmon D A 1990 What is a neonatal seizure? Problems in definition and qualification for investigative and clinical purposes. J Clin Neurophysiol 7:315–368.

Tekgul H, Bourgeois B F D, Gauvreau K, Bergin A M 2005 Electroencephalography in neonatal seizures: comparison of a reduced and a full 10/20 montage. Pediatr Neurol 32(3):155–161.

Tekgul H, Gaubreau K, Soul J et al 2006 The current etiologic profile and neurodevelopmental outcome of seizures in term newborn infants. Pediatrics 117(4):1270–1280.

Toet M G, Hellstrom-Westas L, Groenendaal F et al 1999 Amplitude integrated EEG 3 and 6 hours after birth in full term neonates with hypoxic–ischaemic encephalopathy. Arch Dis Child 81:F19–F23.

Tohier C, Roze J C, David A et al 1991 Hyperexplexia or stiff baby syndrome. Arch Dis Child 66:460–461.

Tramonte J J, Goodkin H P 2004 Temporal lobe hemorrhage in the full-term neonate presenting as apneic seizures. J Perinataology 24:726–729.

Van Leuven K, Toet M C, Schobben A F A M et al 2004 Midazolam and amplitude-integrated EEG in asphyxiated full-term neonates. Acta Paediatris 93:1221–1227.

Viniker D A, Maynard D E, Scott D F 1984 Cerebral function monitor studies in neonates. Clinical Electroencephalogy 15:185–192.

Volpe J J 2001 Neonatal seizures. In: Volpe J J (ed.) Neurology of the newborn, 4th edn. WB Saunders, Philadelphia, pp. 178–214.

Weiner S P, Painter M J, Geva D et al 1991 Neonatal seizures: electroclinical dissociation. Pediatr Neurol 7:363–368.

CHAPTER 35

Hypoglycemia and brain injury — when neonatal metabolic adaptation fails

Jane M. Hawdon

INTRODUCTION

At birth, the newborn baby undergoes many adaptive changes to independent extrauterine life. The most immediate, and the most commonly taught in the medical education curriculum, are those relating to the respiratory and cardiovascular systems to ensure gas exchange and oxygenation of body systems. These must be rapidly followed by the changes of metabolic adaptation, equally essential to ensure energy provision to vital organs and then to sustain growth and further development, but upon which less emphasis is placed in standard teaching programs.

The changes of neonatal metabolic adaptation must be understood prior to reflecting upon the conditions whereby metabolic adaptation fails. These conditions are often erro-

neously bundled into the single diagnostic term 'neonatal hypoglycemia'. However, as will be illustrated within this chapter, it is not appropriate to ascribe neonatal hypoglycemia as a diagnostic term, first, because glucose is not the only fuel in the neonate's fuel economy and, second, because hypoglycemia is the consequence of a number of various underlying disorders and thus does not in itself warrant a diagnostic label. Failure of metabolic adaptation results in the insufficient supply of fuels (including glucose), that are most important to the neonatal brain. Understanding the totality of the metabolic changes and adaptive responses when blood glucose fails provides information regarding when the brain is most vulnerable.

There have been extensive studies of metabolic adaptation and of the mechanisms of brain injury when metabolic adaptation fails in neonatal non-human mammals. These studies have identified those mammals most similar to humans in terms of metabolic adaptation, and sought to compare nutritionally comparable time frames, e.g. suckling versus weaning periods. While the processes of metabolic adaptation are well described in term and preterm human neonates, there are few, if any, clinical studies in human neonates of sufficient rigor to provide evidence for the circumstances in which brain injury may occur, and thus it is not possible to provide evidence based guidelines for the prevention and management of clinically significant hypoglycemia. Therefore recommendations in this chapter, and in the referenced review articles by recognized experts, remain pragmatic urging clinicians to individualize management for each baby, placing heavy emphasis on careful clinical evaluation and avoiding single numerical definitions of brain-injuring hypoglycemia (Cornblath & Ichord 2000, Cornblath et al 2000, Hawdon 2006, Rozance & Hay 2006, Vannucci & Vannucci 2001, Williams 2005).

The facts that 'neonatal hypoglycemia' can cause injury when sufficiently prolonged and severe, and its status as a putative insult in many medicolegal claims, are inescapable. The late and highly respected Marvin Cornblath has likened the effect of his seminal paper of 1959 (Cornblath et al 1959) on hypoglycemia to that of the legendary Helen of Troy — 'the face that launched a thousand ships — the paper that launched a thousand lawsuits' (personal communication). Cornblath and other experts have long recognized and resisted the temptation to attribute poor neurodevelopmental outcomes to single low blood glucose levels in the neonatal period, and have urged experts to take a more informed approach. It is to be hoped that this chapter will guide the sensible application of current knowledge of metabolic adaptation in the neonate to allow these cases to be evaluated impartially.

FETAL METABOLISM AND METABOLIC CHANGES AT BIRTH

During intrauterine life, the fetus receives via the placenta a constant supply of nutrients, initially for growth but in the third trimester also for storage. Glucose crosses the healthy placenta at a rate approximately 5 mg/Kg/min. In addition to that required for basal fetal metabolism, glucose is converted to glycogen which is stored in the liver, cardiac muscle and central nervous system. In the third trimester excess glucose is converted to triglycerides which are stored in adipose tissue. Insulin is an important hormone to ensure glucose and other substrates are utilized for growth and storage, but in normal circumstances insulin is not required for fetal glucose control.

In the infant of the mother with poorly controlled diabetes, transfer of glucose across the placenta is at a higher rate driven by the maternal-fetal concentration gradient; this results in increased insulin secretion, excess growth, and increased storage of glycogen and adipose tissue (macrosomia), along with increased risk of intracellular hypoxia. These factors influence the perinatal complications experienced by some babies where maternal diabetic control has not been good and are factors contributing to adverse long term outcome after poor control of maternal diabetes.

Conversely, in the fetus affected by severe placental insufficiency, transfer of glucose and other nutrients across the placenta is at a lower rate, and the fetus is required to metabolize first its own fuel stores and then structural proteins (e.g. in muscle) to ensure energy delivery to the vital organs, assisted by the redistribution of blood flow to these organs. Should placental function deteriorate further, these adaptive responses fail. Fetal hypoglycemia has been described in these circumstances, although it has not been possible to determine whether this alone influences long term outcome given the many other risk factors for adverse outcome in severe placental insufficiency (Hawdon et al 1992b, Soothill et al 1987).

When placental nutrition abruptly ceases at birth, the healthy neonate is dependent first upon endocrine changes to initiate metabolic adaptation. Insulin levels fall steadily and the action of any residual circulating insulin is overcome by the surge of the counterregulatory hormones, glucagon and the catecholamines. This change in the balance of glucoregulatory hormones induces the activity of key enzymes for glycogenolysis (release of glucose from glycogen stores), gluconeogenesis (production of glucose from precursors including glycerol and amino acids), lipolysis (release of free fatty acids and glycerol from adipose tissue stores), and beta oxidation of fatty acids to produce ketone bodies (Deshpande et al 1999, Ward Platt 2005). If fasting is prolonged, structural protein is broken down to release gluconeogenic amino acids. Other than lipolysis and proteolysis, all of these processes take place in the liver. Glycogenolysis also takes place in cardiac muscle and the central nervous system providing immediate energy (in the form of glucose or lactate) at this crucial time (Eyre et al 1994, Rozance & Hay 2006). Clearly, during this catabolic phase of immediate postnatal nutrition, prior to the establishment of suckling feeds, provision of energy for vital organ function is at the expense of growth and fuel storage.

These key metabolic processes are summarized in Table 35.1.

'TRANSITIONAL HYPOGLYCEMIA' AND PROTECTIVE RESPONSES

In the majority of neonates, an uncomplicated transition to the extrauterine environment occurs. This transition is characterized by low circulating blood glucose concentrations, compared to those of older infants and children, often for a number of days (Hawdon et al 1992a). This is almost always of no pathological significance for a number of reasons, which are summarized in Table 35.2.

First, it is likely that the neurons are protected from fluctuating blood glucose levels by the storage of glycogen within the astrocytes and the metabolic function of the astrocytes in processing fuels (Eyre et al 1994, Forsyth et al 1996).

Table 35.1 Fetal metabolism and metabolic changes at birth — key hormones and metabolic processes

	Fetal metabolism *Anabolic*	Immediate postnatal metabolism *Catabolic*
Hormones	Insulin	Glucagon Catecholamines (Cortisol — weak effect)
Processes	Glycolysis	Glycolysis Gluconeogenesis
	Glycogen synthesis	Glycogenolysis
	Lipogenesis	Lipolysis Beta oxidation (ketogenesis)
	Protein deposition	Proteolysis

Table 35.2 Protective factors during neonatal hypoglycemia

Brain astrocyte fuel storage and processing
Low cerebral metabolic rate for glucose
Alternative fuel utilization — lactate, ketone bodies
Increased cerebral blood flow

Second, the cerebral metabolic rate for glucose (the rate at which the brain takes up and metabolizes glucose) is lower in the neonate than in the older child and adult (Kinnala et al 1996, Nehlig 1993). Increases in cerebral metabolic rate for glucose vary by region of the brain and parallel the neurodevelopmental changes, and with a distinct step up at weaning to a carbohydrate based diet (Table 35.3).

Third, it has been demonstrated that the cerebral metabolic rate for oxygen is preserved during hypoglycemia, although at the same time the cerebral metabolic rate for glucose falls (Auer & Siesjo 1993). This indicates that fuels other than glucose are taken up and utilized to maintain cerebral function during hypoglycemia.

There is extensive and enduring evidence to indicate that the physiological postnatal fall in blood glucose level is accompanied by the generation of ketone bodies, which have been identified as alternative fuels to glucose, and this provision protects the neonatal brain from the effects of hypoglycemia (Hawdon 1999, Hawdon et al 1994, Massieu et al 2003, Yamada et al 2005). Studies, now dating back many years, have demonstrated the marked potential for ketogenesis in the neonate (Hawdon et al 1992a, Vannucci & Vannucci 2001). Studies of non-human neonatal mammals have shown that circulating ketone bodies are taken up and metabolized by the brain, often providing more energy than cerebral glucose metabolism and in addition providing substrate for structural molecules within the brain (Nehlig 2004).

It has been demonstrated that in non-human neonatal mammals and in adult humans ketone bodies restore brain function during symptomatic hypoglycemia (Thurston et al 1986, Veneman et al 1994). It is clearly very difficult to carry out such clinical studies in the human neonate. However, as long ago as the 1970s increased cerebral ketone body uptake in the neonate, as compared to the child and adult, was demonstrated (Kraus et al 1974). A more recent study of infants with hyperinsulinism confirmed that there was effective uptake of orally administered beta-hydroxy-butyrate across the blood–brain barrier (Plecko et al 2002). It is noteworthy, and of clinical relevance to those caring for mothers and babies, that in all groups of infants studied to date those who are breast fed have higher circulating ketone body levels than those who are formula fed, even after correcting for blood glucose levels (de Rooy & Hawdon 2002, Hawdon et al 2000, Ward Platt & Deshpande 2005).

There are now emerging data that ketone bodies have protective roles in neuroprotection in conditions other than neonatal hypoglycemia, for example in preservation of energy metabolism and reduction of area of injury after hypoxic–ischemic injury (Dardzinski et al 2000, Suzuki et al 2002, Yager et al 1992). This will be an area of great interest for future research, and it should be anticipated that future editions of this book will carry ever increasing sections on the wider aspect of neurometabolism.

Finally, animal studies have identified additional protective responses – the availability of lactate and amino acids as alternative fuels, and increase in cerebral blood flow (Anwar & Vannucci 1988, Hernandez et al 1980, Rozance & Hay 2006, Vannucci & Vannucci 2001, Vannucci et al 1981). The role of lactate as an alternative fuel has been confirmed in humans when studying children with hypoglycemia secondary to glycogen storage disorders (Fernandes et al 1984).

It is to be hoped that this section has illustrated both the physiological postnatal fall in blood glucose and the evidence for protective responses when blood glucose levels are lower than those of older subjects. It is hoped that this also demonstrates that to define the potential insult to the brain simply in terms of a circulating blood glucose level is erroneous. To view the cerebral fuel economy in such terms could be likened to a child counting only 1 pence pieces in his money box, ignoring all other denominations of coin. It is essential that the pathology is defined as a deficiency or failure of metabolic adaptation, but unfortunately this concept is not yet widely recognized.

WHEN NEONATAL METABOLIC ADAPTATION FAILS — THE PATHOLOGICAL SEQUELAE OF HYPOGLYCEMIA

There are circumstances when profound and/or prolonged hypoglycemia occurs and at the same time the protective metabolic responses fail. Underlying etiological factors vary and may be related to reduced body fuel stores, failure of the normal endocrine changes at birth, or systemic illnesses which impede function of the liver, where the key metabolic processes occur (Table 35.4). Infants who have been born preterm even some months later may not develop the fully mature metabolic pathways, but the clinical implications of this are not known (Hume et al 2005).

Given the wide variations in fuel availabilities within these 'at risk' groups of infants and the additional confounding risk factors for adverse sequelae, it is not surprising that

Table 35.3 Local cerebral metabolic rate for glucose in rat and human brain (Nehlig 1993, Kinnala et al 1996)

Human		Rat	
PCA weeks	LCMRgluc μmol/100g/min	Age days	LCMRgluc μmol/100g/min
32–36	5.5	Birth	2–4
38–42	7.2	10	17–24
43–48	7.4	20–21*	40–53
49–56	12.2	35	64
>56	18.7	Adult	67

*weaning.

Table 35.4 Conditions in which neonatal hypoglycemia may be clinically significant, associated risk factors for adverse neurodevelopmental sequelae

Etiology	Risk factors
Intrauterine growth restriction	Blood glucose low
	Alternative fuels variable
	Hypoxia–ischemia
	Genetic syndrome
	Congenital infection
Hypoxic–ischemic encephalopathy	High glucose requirement
	Fluid restricted, low glucose provision
	Liver enzyme dysfunction
	Alternative fuels variable
	Hypoxia–ischemia
Extreme prematurity	Immature liver metabolism
	Alternative fuels absent
	Hypoxia–ischemia
	Infection
Systemic illness (e.g. septicemia)	Increased glucose requirements
	Blood glucose variable
	Alternative fuels variable
	Liver enzyme dysfunction
	Tissue underperfusion
	Cellular hypoxia
Infant of diabetic mother	Blood glucose variable
	Alternative fuels variable
	Abnormal intrauterine metabolic environment
	Hypoxia–ischemia
Neonatal hyperinsulinism (persistent hyperinsulinemic hypoglycemia of infancy, Beckwith–Weidemann syndrome	Blood glucose low
	High glucose requirement
	Alternative fuels absent
Inborn error of metabolism (e.g. glycogen storage disease, beta-oxidation defect)	Blood glucose variable
	Alternative fuels variable
	Accumulation toxic metabolites
Endocrine insufficiency (rare, e.g. pituitary, adrenal insufficiency)	Blood glucose variable
	Alternative fuels variable
	Electrolyte imbalance
	Associated brain abnormalities

reported outcomes vary (see below). However, it must be recognized that at highest risk of all are the infants with hyperinsulinism as this condition, if undiagnosed, results in prolonged and profound hypoglycemia with no protective ketogenic response (Hussain 2005).

There have been detailed studies in animal models, documenting the acute neurophysiological and pathological affects of neonatal hypoglycemia, usually using the model of hyperinsulinemia which is an effective proxy for total failure of metabolic adaptation as lipolysis is suppressed in addition to gluconeogenesis so there is no protective ketogenic response (Auer & Siesjo 1993, Hawdon 1999). These studies are informative in that they use a 'pure' model of hypoglycemia, with no additional confounding factors. However, they are of course open to the criticism that the findings may not be directly applicable to the human neonate.

Therefore, there have been extensive efforts to use data from clinical studies of the human neonate to determine the significance of neonatal hypoglycemia in terms of neurophysiological, neurodevelopmental and neuroradiological sequelae. However, there are major difficulties in interpreting these clinical studies which have, to date, been flawed by confounding factors, such as immaturity, placental insufficiency and co-existing complications, by heterogeneity of subjects, and by failure to take into account protective mechanisms.

a) IN VITRO AND NEUROPATHOLOGICAL STUDIES

In vitro studies have indicated a number of possible mechanisms for brain injury during hypoglycemia. These include increased cellular calcium influx, excitotoxic amino acid (aspartate and glutamate) release, reactive oxygen species within mitochondria, and cysteine-induced brain injury (Auer & Siesjo 1993, Gazit et al 2003, 2004, McGowan et al 2006). Injury is likely to be via N-methyl-D-aspartate (NMDA) receptors as injury is reduced by pre-treatment with NMDA receptor antagonists.

The excitotoxic amino acid mediated damage commences in the neuronal dendrites ('neuron specific' and 'axon-sparing dendritic lesions') and is associated with swelling of the dendritic mitochondria. These pathological appearances have been described in rat brain after 10 minutes of EEG silence induced by profound (<1 mmol/L) hypoglycemia (Auer & Siesjo 1993). Neuronal necrosis did not occur, even at comparable blood glucose levels, if the EEG was slowed but still active. Studies in piglets have confirmed evidence of injury (release of excitatory amino acids) only when hypoglycemia was sufficiently prolonged (below 0.6 mmol/L) and severe to cause iso-electric EEG (Ichord et al 1999).

Animal studies have demonstrated widespread neuronal necrosis after profound hypoglycemia associated with iso-electric EEG, with the most affected areas being the cerebral cortex, dentate gyrus, hippocampus and caudate nucleus (Auer & Siesjo 1993). There is sparing of the brainstem and cerebellum. This pattern may be differentiated from the patterns seen after experimental hypoxia–ischemia, and reflects the differing mechanisms of injury. Unlike hypoxic-ischemic brain injury, the majority of damage occurs early once the excitotoxic process has started, there is no evidence of delayed neuronal loss as occurs with hypoxia–ischemia induced apoptosis. This theoretically limits strategies for treatment or neuroprotection once the injurious processes have commenced in profound hypoglycemia associated with iso-electric EEG.

Pathological studies of the human brain after neonatal hypoglycemia are fortunately rare, and results must be interpreted in the light of possible co-morbidities. However, on the whole the pattern described is of damage to the gray matter, and of a different appearance at both distribution and cellular level to the injury caused by hypoxia–ischemia (Vannucci & Vannucci 2001). It has been suggested that white matter injury may also occur, but this is less commonly reported and may be caused by other brain insults or co-morbidities. Take, for example, the scenario of mid trimester fetal hypoxia–ischemia resulting in brain injury such that the baby when born at full term is not neurologically normal. This in turn results in poor feeding and secondarily low blood glucose levels, but the brain injury is all too easily ascribed to hypoglycemia.

b) NEUROPHYSIOLOGICAL STUDIES AND ACUTE CLINICAL SIGNS

Studies of neonatal animals have demonstrated the neurophysiological effects of profound hypoglycemia (Auer & Siesjo 1993). First there is slowing of the EEG associated with 'stupor' but with no evidence of energy failure or neuronal injury. This is followed by iso-electric EEG and coma, during which neuronal injury rapidly occurs.

Vannucci and colleagues have carried out a large series of studies investigating the effect of insulin-induced (hypoketonemic) hypoglycemia on newborn dogs (Vannucci & Vannucci 2001). They noted increased cerebral blood flow when blood glucose levels averaged 0.9 mmol/L. Despite changes in glucose flux within the brain and in EEG at low blood glucose levels, high-energy phosphate reserves were conserved, even at extreme hypoglycemia. The group demonstrated increased lactate uptake and proposed this was the predominant alternative fuel to glucose. Vannucci stated, 'The newborn animal brain cannot be damaged by even profound hypoglycemia.'

There are few neurophysiological data relating to the human neonate. A much quoted study is that of Koh et al (1988). The latencies of brain stem evoked potentials were noted to be prolonged at low blood glucose levels in a number of pediatric subjects (including 5 neonates) who were being investigated for possible inborn error of metabolism. However, the blood glucose threshold at which these changes occurred varied markedly between subjects and ketone body levels (in the few subjects in whom these were measured) were low. For some subjects the brainstem evoked potentials remained normal at very low blood glucose levels. However, as the highest blood glucose level at which brain stem evoked potential became abnormal was 2.5 mmol/L, the authors recommended that a blood glucose level of 2.6 mmol/L and above should be adopted as a safe level. There are a number of reasons why it is inadvisable to adopt this recommendation – this was a selected group of subjects, with only 5 neonates, the role of alternative fuels was not investigated, the threshold for abnormality of brain stem evoked potential varied widely, and the long term significance of the increased latency in brain stem evoked potential is not known.

Another group conducted a similar study, this time in neonates only, but could not replicate the findings. It was postulated that an increase in cerebral blood flow was the protective mechanism by which hypoglycemia did not cause neurophysiological changes in these subjects (Pryds et al 1988).

More recent studies have identified differences in EEG patterns in hypoglycemic babies when compared to those who are normoglycemic (Nunes et al 2000). However, in this study almost all of the hypoglycemic infants had additional pathology. As with the study of Koh et al (1988) the long-term implications of the described persistence of frontal sharp transients are not known.

In the clinical setting, it is well known that significant neuroglycopenia will result in reduced level of consciousness and/or fits. However, many authorities have cautioned against jumping to cause and effect conclusions as there may be an underlying pathology such that abnormal signs and hypoglycemia are co-morbidities (for example a primary neurological problem causing both abnormal signs and hypoglycemia secondary to poor feeding), or there may be reverse causation (fits in themselves being a direct cause of reduced blood glucose level) (Cornblath et al 2000, Williams 2005).

It has been demonstrated that co-existing hypoxia-ischemia and hypoglycemia are more damaging than either insult alone (Vannucci & Vannucci 2001). This is of potential clinical relevance to the growth restricted fetus (Hawdon et al 1992b, Soothill et al 1987), or on the rare occasions that postnatal hypoglycemic collapse is not recognized and treatment not urgently commenced.

Conversely, in studies of non-human neonatal mammals when hypoxia-ischemia is followed by hypoglycemia, the outcome is favorable when compared to subjects who are hyperglycemic after the insult (Park et al 2001). This may be related to the neuroprotective effect of ketone bodies, which is an emerging concept described above.

c) NEURORADIOLOGICAL STUDIES

There are emerging studies relating to putative neuroradiological findings after neonatal hypoglycemia. However, existing case reports are of computed tomography (CT) or magnetic resonance imaging (MRI) of infants after prolonged (at least 12 hours), severe, untreated or treatment-resistant hypoglycemia associated with fits or coma. Thus, hypoglycemic injury may be compounded by hypoxia-ischemia co-existing with hypoglycemia (see above). These studies describe generalized thinning of the cerebral cortex throughout the brain but particularly affecting the occipital cortex (Alkalay et al 2005, Barkovich et al 1998, Spar et al 1994, Traill et al 1998).

A case series is reported of findings on both MRI and ultrasound imaging of 18 full term infants who were admitted to a neonatal unit with hypoglycemia (blood glucose <2.6 mmol/L) but who were reported to be free of other disease (Kinnala et al 1999). However, there are insufficient antenatal and perinatal clinical data to rule out prenatal and perinatal insults which may have resulted in both hypoglycemia and neuroradiological/neurological sequelae. Seven babies in this series were reported to have MRI or ultrasound abnormalities. There was great variation in the nature and distribution of the early lesions but occipital lobes were affected in four. It is of interest that despite the apparent clinical severity of hypoglycemia, the MRI lesions resolved completely in 4 infants, and 2 had very minor residual abnormalities. One of the 18 infants had marked residual MRI abnormalities and neurological sequelae. This infant (an infant of a diabetic mother) had a very low initial blood glucose concentration but rapid resolution of hypoglycemia, and the authors considered that in his case damage was caused by prenatal vascular insult. Despite their considering that their cohort was not affected by other disease, they postulated a pre-existing condition for the cause of injury in the only subject with longstanding sequelae.

Two studies have examined the possible association of white matter injury with neonatal hypoglycemia. In a paper by Yokochi, 13 cases of white matter injury are described, 3 of whom had neonatal hypoglycemia (Yokochi 1998). Two of these three babies were severely small for gestational age and one had hyperinsulinism. The hypoglycemic babies had truncal instability on follow up, but did not have spastic quadriplegia. A paper by Murakami et al (1999) suggests that white matter damage, if it occurs in association with neonatal hypoglycemia, is in the parieto-occipital region. Of the eight cases in this series, four were markedly small for gestational age. In this series, no patient had spastic cerebral palsy in association with the white matter changes. As with other studies reviewing neuroradiological and neurodevelopmental outcomes after neonatal hypoglycemia, it is unlikely that hypoglycemia was the only potential insult and there is no adjustment for other confounding pathologies.

Finally, although neuroradiology does not often conclusively prove that neonatal hypoglycemia is the cause of brain injury, there is an additional important role for neuroradiology in the investigation of primary brain malformations, for example midline defects, which may be associated with pituitary insufficiency and therefore risk of hypoglycemia.

d) NEURODEVELOPMENTAL OUTCOME STUDIES

There are abundant published studies and case reports purporting to describe the long-term sequelae of neonatal hypoglycemia in terms of major handicap or intellectual deficit. However, no study is controlled and prospective, and none satisfactorily takes into account other exacerbating factors (Cornblath et al 2000, Hawdon 1999, 2006, Rozance & Hay 2006, Vannucci & Vannucci 2001). Older studies report the outcomes of babies who were cared for in an era when hypoglycemia was more common and more likely to be severe and prolonged, and when other co-existing complications may not have been detected or treated. Therefore, it is to be hoped that these findings seldom apply to our present generation of at-risk infants in whom hypoglycemia is usually prevented by close observation and early and adequate provision of energy. Consistent in all studies is the finding that there is more likely to be an adverse outcome when there have been clinical signs, usually fits, in association with hypoglycemia. Studies that have extended follow up into childhood have noted a progressive reduction with advancing age in the apparent impact of neonatal hypoglycemia (Rozance & Hay 2006).

Follow up studies of infants with congenital hyperinsulinism over many years have characteristically demonstrated the favorable prognostic significance of early identification and expert management of hypoglycemia, as compared to when early treatment was not achieved and severe mental retardation and epilepsy ensued (Cherian & Abduljabbar 2005, Hussain 2005, Menni et al 2001).

Three of the published outcome studies will be discussed in detail to demonstrate the difficulties in interpreting such data.

A widely quoted study which has suggested that neonatal hypoglycemia affects neurodevelopmental outcome is that of Lucas et al (1988). Retrospective data were obtained for a group of preterm babies who had been enrolled in a multi-center feeding study (the primary aim of the study was not to examine the long term effects of hypoglycemia). Many factors were associated with adverse neurodevelopmental outcome (as assessed by presence of cerebral palsy, and using Bayley motor and developmental scales). The following remained significant after entry into multiple regression analysis — number of days of hypoglycemia (defined as blood glucose below 2.6 mmol/L), clinical complications, and family, social and educational factors. Hypoglycemia for at least 5 days was associated with a significant increased risk of impairment, a risk (after adjustment for other factors) of 3.5 times that of infants who were never found to be hypoglycemic.

Despite this study (along with that of Koh et al 1988) being a major influence on working definitions of hypoglycemia in the 1990s, these findings cannot be extrapolated to all neonates because the study was of preterm infants only, and in fact perhaps the findings cannot even be applied to current day preterm neonates. Those currently working on neonatal units will recognize the rarity of babies, managed according to standard policies, having low blood glucose levels for 5 or more consecutive days. This raises questions regarding possible confounding factors, including variations in feed and fluid administration, which were omitted from the regression analysis. In addition, the study was limited by the lack of matched controls.

A more recent retrospective analysis of preterm infants with birthweights <10th centile for gestational age, has also suggested that hypoglycemia (blood glucose <2.6 mmol/L) is associated with adverse neurodevelopmental sequelae (Duvanel et al 1999). Applying a significance limit of <0.01 (for caution see below), infants with 7 or more episodes of hypoglycemia had lower head circumference than controls at 18 months (but not at 5 years). The only neuropsychological outcome significantly ($P < 0.01$) associated with hypoglycemia was perception index at 3.5 years. This actually suggests a relatively good outcome even after severe or prolonged hypoglycemia. The study carried out comparisons between many subdivided risk groups (e.g. by severity of hypoglycemia and numbers of episodes) and used 7 different outcome measures at 5 follow-up points. When such multiple comparisons are made, a rigorous level of statistical significance must be defined. In addition, the potential confounding factors of severity of placental dysfunction, antenatal or intrapartum hypoxia–ischemia, congenital infection, and socio-economic status were not adequately considered, and there was potential bias in that the sickest infants would have undergone more frequent blood glucose estimations. These and other points were discussed in an accompanying editorial advising caution in extrapolating these data to full term babies, even those who are small for gestational age (Cowett 1999).

These studies have sought to conclude that moderate hypoglycemia is associated with neurodevelopmental impairment. However, there are no similar studies of normally grown, full term neonates. Prospective controlled study of different groups of neonates, should this be practicable, is the only method of confirming these suspicions.

It is often stated that hypoglycemia in infants of diabetic mothers is associated with an adverse outcome. However, most studies investigating this association use early, and often single, blood glucose levels alone as the independent variable and, in common with the studies described above, do not take into account potential antenatal and perinatal confounding factors. A recent study comparing infants of diabetic mothers and control babies reported deficits at 6 months in recognition memory, which was thought to be mediated via hippocampal damage. However there were no other differences in neurodevelopmental outcome. The authors recognized that many factors may be implicated, including chronic fetal hypoxia, neonatal hypoglycemia and fetal iron deficiency, and they were unable to predict whether the findings at 6 months would translate to longer term deficits (Nelson et al 2000).

A final caution in the analysis of clinical studies described above, is that very few have used accurate methods of glucose measurement. It is well recognized that near-patient methods of blood glucose testing are not sufficiently accurate to allow discrimination between blood glucose concentrations at the decimal point level (Hawdon 2005, Hussain & Sharief 2000, Rozance & Hay 2006). Therefore, studies that have divided babies between groups according to such methods of measurement will have inherent inaccuracies.

The conclusions drawn from the above analysis and the many expert commentaries that have been referred to in this chapter are that rigorous prospective, controlled study of infants at risk for or experiencing neonatal hypoglycemia are required. These analyses indicate that such studies should have the following characteristics:

- Prospective study.
- Specific study groups — e.g. intrauterine growth restriction/intrauterine growth retardation (IUGR).
- Correct/control for confounders — antenatal and perinatal insults, social.
- Avoid selection bias by applying consistent screening policy.
- Accurate method of blood glucose measurement.
- Measurement of alternative fuels.
- Detailed recording by experienced clinicians of acute clinical status and clinical signs associated with low blood glucose levels and change in these when blood glucose is restored.
- Measurement of cerebral blood flow during normoglycemia and hypoglycemia, each baby being its own control.
- Studies of acute neurophysiological function during normoglycemia and hypoglycemia, each baby being its own control.
- MRS/MRI studies of acute and long term brain injury.
- Large numbers.
- Ethical approval to continue to study babies with low blood glucose levels but no clinical signs.

The reality is that it is unlikely that clinical studies will be conducted to meet all these standards. In the absence of a satisfactory prospective study of human neonates, we must again return to studies of non-human neonatal mammals.

A study of Rhesus monkeys investigated the effects of perinatal insulin-induced hypoglycemia of varying duration on performance in psychometric tests at 8 months age (Schrier et al 1990). Any protective ketogenic response would have been abolished by insulin. Monkeys who had been hypoglycemic for 10 hours (compared to normoglycemic controls and monkeys with hypoglycemia of shorter duration) required more alterations of procedure and additional help from the tutor during the pre-training period. These differences were perceived to reflect difficulties in adaptability and motivation. However, with this extra attention there were no differences between any of the groups in terms of ability to complete the tasks, personality characteristics or neurological findings. The authors concluded that even prolonged hypoglycemia did not affect later neurodevelopmental outcome, although problems of adaptability and motivation were identified.

These problems are reminiscent of those of children who have attention deficit disorder. It is of interest that hyperactivity and attention deficit are features found in follow-up studies of small for gestational age (SGA) babies (Hawdon et al 1990). Although there have been no prospective or even retrospective studies of the association between neonatal hypoglycemia and attention deficit disorder, it could be speculated that prolonged (antenatal or postnatal) hypoglycemia in babies with intrauterine restriction is a factor contributing to attention deficit disorder and its associated specific learning difficulties.

The evidence from both animal and human studies suggests 'pure' hypoglycemic brain injury is rare, and for hypoglycemic brain injury to occur there must be co-existing failure of metabolic adaptation such that alternative fuels are not available, that the overall fuel insufficiency must be prolonged and associated with clinical signs, and that simultaneous hypoxia–ischemia and hypoglycemia have additive effects. There is no evidence that 'transitional' hypoglycemia in the healthy neonate is associated with acute or long term sequelae, and indeed, for many babies in the at risk groups protective factors will prevail.

APPLICATION TO CLINICAL PRACTICE

The current state of knowledge is succinctly summarized by leading experts:

> The newborn animal brain cannot be damaged by even profound hypoglycemia.
>
> *Vannucci & Vannucci (2001)*

> Although transiently low plasma glucose concentrations are a frequent occurrence in the neonatal nursery, significant hypoglycemia leading to cerebral injury is rare.
>
> *Williams (2005)*

Neonatal hypoglycemia is a common diagnosis, most often based on a single blood glucose level and using inaccurate methods of measurement, and with disregard for the presence or absence of associated clinical signs. However, no characteristic neurological, developmental or neuroradiological sequelae have yet been described in human neonates who have had hypoglycemia that is uncomplicated by other risk factors for brain injury. This is undoubtedly because there are many underlying causes of hypoglycemia which vary with respect to the resulting duration and severity of hypoglycemia and the ability to mount protective metabolic responses (Table 35.4). In addition, some of these disorders have associated neurological abnormalities, independent of the effect of hypoglycemia, and some are associated with additional neurological risk, e.g. hypoxia–ischemia.

It appears that prolonged hypoglycemia, sufficiently severe to cause clinical signs, is most likely to be associated with long-term sequelae. Therefore, it is essential in clinical practice to identify babies at risk of significant hypoglycemia and manage them in such a way as to prevent prolonged, severe hypoglycemia but at the same time avoiding overly invasive practices which cause parental anxiety, separate mother and baby, disrupt breastfeeding, and even impair protective metabolic responses (Cornblath et al 2000, de Rooy & Hawdon 2002, Hawdon et al 2000). Detailed neurodevelopmental follow up of affected individuals is essential but appropriate prospective controlled studies, controlling for other adverse factors and measuring protective responses, is the only way to determine the specific long-term risk posed by hypoglycemia.

There is thus a 'gray area' between the many healthy babies with low blood glucose concentrations and those whose low blood glucose levels present a threat to neurological function and development, this risk being affected by underlying cause of hypoglycemia, coexisting clinical complications and presence or absence of protective mechanisms (Table 35.1). This has resulted in much controversy and confusion around the diagnosis and management of neonatal hypoglycemia. A recent review by a multinational group of experts has attempted to examine critically the evidence on which clinical recommendations should be made (Cornblath et al 2000). Following detailed analysis, the authors considered it impossible to define hypoglycemia as a single blood glucose level. They concluded that low blood glucose levels accompanied by neurological signs should be investigated and treated regardless of the absolute blood glucose level and it is suggested that for sick or very low birth weight babies there should be a 'therapeutic goal' to maintain blood glucose levels above 2.5 mmol/L.

These authors, and others, also highlight that the commonly used reagent strips are insufficiently accurate to diagnose hypoglycemia and monitor at risk infants (Cornblath et al 2000, Deshpande & Ward Platt 2005, Hawdon 2005, Hussain & Sharief 2000). Fortunately, many neonatal units now incorporate benchtop instruments in their neonatal unit laboratory to enable them to determine immediate and accurate blood glucose levels.

SUMMARY

Much controversy and confusion surrounds neonatal hypoglycemia, particularly with respect to potential neuropsychological sequelae. Studies to date are flawed by many factors including retrospective data collection, inability to control for coexisting clinical complications, and failure to take into account protective mechanisms. There is evidence from studies of humans and other animals to suggest that long term sequelae do occur after prolonged hypoglycemia which is sufficiently severe to cause neurological signs and profound EEG abnormalities. Such situations should be avoided by close clinical observation of vulnerable infants whilst avoiding excessively invasive management (namely unnecessary separation of mother and baby, routine or excessive formula milk supplementation, or intravenous glucose administration) which themselves inhibit protective metabolic responses and impede successful establishment of breastfeeding.

REFERENCES

Alkalay A L, Flores-Sarnat L et al 2005 Brain imaging findings in neonatal hypoglycaemia: case report and review of 23 cases. Clin Paediatr 44:783–790.

Anwar M, Vannucci R C 1988 Autoradiographic determination of regional cerebral blood flow during hypoglycemia in newborn dogs. Ped Res 24:41–45.

Auer R N, Siesjo B K 1993 Brain neurochemistry and neuropathology. Clin End Metab 7.3:611–626.

Barkovich J A, Al Ali F et al 1998 Imaging patterns of neonatal hypoglycemia. Am J Neuroradiol 19:523–528.

Cherian M P, Abduljabbar M A 2005 Persistent hyperinsulinemic hypoglycemia of infancy (PHHI): long term outcome following 95% pancreatectomy. J Pediatr Endocrinol Metab 18:1441e–1448e.

Cornblath M, Hawdon J M et al 2000 Controversies regarding definition of neonatal hypoglycemia: suggested operational thresholds. Pediatrics 105:1141–1145.

Cornblath M, Ichord R 2000 Hypoglycemia in the neonate. Semin Perinatol 24:136–149.

Cornblath M, Odell G B, Levin E Y 1959 Symptomatic hypoglycemia associated with toxemia of pregnancy. J Pediatr 55:545–562.

Cowett R M 1999 Neonatal hypoglycemia: a little goes a long way. J Pediatr 134:389–391.

Dardzinski B J, Smith S L et al 2000 Increased plasma beta-hydroxybutyrate, preserved cerebral energy metabolism, and amelioration of brain damage during neonatal hypoxia–ischemia with dexamethasone pre-treatment. Pediatr Res 48:248–255.

de Rooy L, Hawdon J M 2002 Nutritional factors that affect the postnatal metabolic adaptation of full-term small- and large-for gestational age infants. Pediatrics 109:e42.

Deshpande S, Hawdon J M, Rodeck C et al 1999 Adaptation to extrauterine life. In: Rodeck and Whittle (eds) Fetal medicine: basic science and clinical practice. Churchill Livingstone, Edinburgh.

Deshpande S, Ward Platt M P 2005 The investigation and management of neonatal hypoglycaemia. Sem Fetal Neonatal Med 10:351–361.

Duvanel C B, Fawer C-L et al 1999 Long-term effects of neonatal hypoglycemia on brain growth and psychomotor development in small-for gestational-age preterm infants. J Pediatr 134:492–498.

Eyre J A, Stuart A G et al 1994 Glucose export from the brain in man: evidence for a role for astrocytic glycogen as a reservoir of glucose for neural metabolism. Brain Res 28:349–352.

Fernandes J, Berger R et al 1984 Lactate as a cerebral metabolic fuel for glucose-6-phosphate deficient children. Ped Res 18:335–339.

Forsyth R, Fray A et al 1996 A role for astrocytes in glucose delivery to neurons? Dev Neurosci 18:360–370.

Gazit V, Ben-Abraham R et al 2003 Long term neurobehavioural and histological damage in brain of mice induced by L-cysteine. Pharmacol Biochem Behav 75:795–799.

Gazit V, Ben-Abraham R et al 2004 Cysteine-induced hypoglycaemic brain damage: an alternative mechanism to excitotoxicity. Amino Acids 26:163–168.

Hawdon J M 1999 Hypoglycaemia and the neonatal brain. Eur J Paediatr 158(11):S9–S12.

Hawdon J M 2005 Disorders of blood glucose homeostasis in the neonate. In: Rennie J (ed.). Roberton's textbook of neonatology, 4th edn. Churchill Livingstone, Edinburgh.

Hawdon J M 2006 Hypoglycaemia in newborn infants: defining the features associated with adverse

outcomes — a challenging remit. Biol Neonate 90:87–88.

Hawdon J M, Hey E et al 1990 Born too small: is outcome still affected? Dev Med Child Neurol 32:943–953.

Hawdon J M, Ward Platt M P et al 1992a Patterns of metabolic adaptation for preterm and term infants in the first neonatal week. Arch Dis Child 67:357–365.

Hawdon J M, Ward Platt M P et al 1992b Prediction of impaired metabolic adaptation by antenatal Doppler studies in small for gestational age fetuses. Arch Dis Child 67:787–792.

Hawdon J M, Ward Platt M P et al 1994 Controversy. Prevention and management of neonatal hypoglycaemia. Arch Dis Child 70:60–65.

Hawdon J M, Williams A F et al 2000 Formula supplements given to healthy breastfed preterm babies inhibit postnatal metabolic adaptation: results of a randomized controlled trial. Arch Dis Child 82:A30.

Hernandez M J, Vannucci R C et al 1980 Cerebral blood flow and metabolism during hypoglycemia in newborn dogs. J Neurochem 35:622–628.

Hume R, Burchell A et al 2005 Glucose homeostasis in the newborn. Early Human Dev 81:95–101.

Hussain K 2005 Congenital hyperinsulinism. Semin Fetal Neonatal Med 10:369–376.

Hussain K, Sharief N 2000 The inaccuracy of venous and capillary blood glucose measurement using reagent strips in the newborn period and the effect of haematocrit. Early Hum Dev 57:111–121.

Ichord R N, Northington F J et al 1999 Brain O_2 consumption and glutamate release during hypoglycemic coma in piglets are temperature sensitive. Am J Neurophysiol 276:H2053–H2062.

Kinnala A, Rikalainen H et al 1999 Cerebral magnetic resonance imaging and ultrasonography findings after neonatal hypoglycaemia. Pediatrics 103:724–729.

Kinnala A, Suhone-Polvi H et al 1996 Cerebral metabolic rate for glucose during the first six months of life: an FDG positron emission tomography study. Arch Dis Child 74:F153–F157.

Koh T H H G, Aynsley Green A et al 1988 Neural dysfunction during hypoglycaemia. Arch Dis Child 63:1353–1358.

Kraus H, Schenkler S et al 1974 Developmental changes of cerebral ketone body utilisation in human infants. Hoppe-Seyler's Z Physiol Chem 355:164–170.

Lucas A, Morley R et al 1988 Adverse neurodevelopmental outcome of moderate neonatal hypoglycaemia. BMJ 297:1304–1308.

McGowan J E, Chen L et al 2006 Increased mitochondrial reactive oxygen species production in newborn brain during hypoglycaemia. Neurosci Lett 399:111–114.

Massieu L, Haces M L et al 2003 Acetoacetate protects hippocampal neurons against glutamate-mediated neuronal damage during glycolysis inhibition. Neuroscience 120:365–378.

Menni F, de Lonlay P et al 2001 Neurologic outcomes of 90 neonates and infants with persistent hyperinsulinemic hypoglycemia. Pediatrics 107:476–479.

Murakami Y, Yamashita et al 1999 Cranial MRI of neurologically impaired children suffering from neonatal hypoglycaemia. Pediatr Radiol 29:23–27.

Nehlig A 1993 Imaging and the ontogeny of brain metabolism. Clin End Metab 7.3:627–642.

Nehlig A 2004 Brain uptake and metabolism of ketone bodies in animal models. Prostaglandins Leukot Essent Fatty Acids 70:265–275.

Nelson C A, Wewerka S et al 2000 Neurocognitive sequelae of infants of diabetic mothers. Behav Neurosci 5:950–956.

Nunes M L, Perula M M et al 2000 Differences in the dynamics of frontal sharp transients in normal and hypoglycaemic newborns. Clin Neurophysiol 111:305–310.

Park W S, Chang Y S et al 2001 Effects of hyperglycaemia or hypoglycaemia on brain cell membrane function and energy metabolism during the immediate reoxygenation-reperfusion period after acute transient global hypoxia–ischaemia in the newborn piglet. Brain Res 901:102–108.

Plecko B, Stoeckler-Ipsiroglu S et al 2002 Oral beta-hydroxybutyrate supplementation in two patients with hyperinsulinemic hypoglycemia: monitoring of beta-hydroxybutyrate levels in blood and cerebrospinal fluid, and in the brain by in vivo magnetic resonance spectroscopy. Pediatr Res 52:301–306.

Pryds O, Greisen G et al 1988 Compensatory increase of CBF in preterm infants during hypoglycaemia. Acta Paediatr Scand 77:632–637.

Rozance P J, Hay W W 2006 Hypoglycaemia in newborn infants: features associated with adverse outcomes. Biol Neonate 90:74–86.

Schrier A M, Wilhelm P B et al 1990 Neonatal hypoglycaemia in the Rhesus monkey: effect on development and behaviour. Inf Behav Dev 13:189–297.

Soothill P W, Nicolaides K H et al 1987 Prenatal asphyxia, hyperlacticaemia, hypoglycaemia and erythroblastosis in growth retarded fetuses. BMJ 294:1051–1053.

Spar J A, Lewine J D et al 1994 Neonatal hypoglycaemia: CT and MR findings. Am J Neuroradiol 15:1477–1478.

Suzuki M, Suzuki M et al 2002 Beta-hydoxybutyrate, a cerebral function improving agent, protects rat brain against ischaemic damage caused by permanent and transient focal cerebral ischaemia. Jpn J Pharmacol 89:36–43.

Thurston J H, Hawhart R E et al 1986 β-hydroxybutyrate reverse insulin-induced hypoglycaemic coma in suckling-weanling mice despite low blood and brain glucose levels. Metab Brain Dis 1:63–82.

Traill Z, Squier M et al 1998 Brain imaging in neonatal hypoglycaemia. Arch Dis Child 79:145–147.

Vannucci R C, Nardis E E et al 1981 Cerebral carbohydrate and energy metabolism during hypoglycemia in newborn dogs. Am J Physiol 256:H1659–H1666.

Vannucci R C, Vannucci S J 2001 Hypoglycaemic brain injury. Semin Neonatol 6:147–155.

Veneman T, Mitrakou A et al 1994 Effect of hyperketonaemia and hyperlacticacidaemia on symptoms, cognitive dysfunction, and counterregulatory hormone responses during hypoglycaemia in normal humans. Diabetes 43:1311–1317.

Ward Platt M, Deshpande S 2005 Metabolic adaptation at birth. Sem Fetal Neonatal Med 10:341–350.

Williams A F 2005 Neonatal hypoglycaemia: clinical and legal aspects. Semin Fetal Neonatal Med 10:363–368.

Yager J Y, Heitjan et al 1992 Effect of insulin-induced and fasting hypoglycemia on perinatal hypoxic-ischemic brain damage. Pediatr Res 31:138–142.

Yamada K A, Rensing N et al 2005 Ketogenic diet reduces hypoglycaemia-induced neuronal death in young rats. Neurosci Lett 385:210–214.

Yokochi K 1998 Clinical profiles of subjects with subcortical leukomalacia and borderzone infarction revealed by MR. Acta Paediatr 87:879–883.

CHAPTER
36

Kernicterus
Charles E. Ahlfors

INTRODUCTION: KERNICTERUS THEN AND NOW

Kernicterus is a generic term referring to specific pathological and clinical patterns of central nervous system injury that follow exposure to high levels of the orange-yellow 4Z,15Z isomer of bilirubin-IXα (Fig. 36.1). This isomer is produced when heme (ferriprotoporphyrin IX), derived mostly from senescent red blood cells, is catabolized. Most kernicterus occurs in newborns during the early postpartum period when bilirubin levels are transiently elevated and visible jaundice is present, but it can also occur in jaundiced children and adults with a rare disorder of bilirubin metabo-

lism known as Crigler–Najjar syndrome (Crigler & Najjar 1952, Strauss et al 2006). A similar disorder in the jaundiced Gunn rat has provided an invaluable animal model for investigating the pathogenesis of kernicterus (Blanc & Johnson 1959, Johnson et al 1959, Menken et al 1966).

KERNICTERUS THEN: KERNICTERUS AND HEMOLYTIC DISEASE OF THE NEWBORN

In the 19th century yellow (bilirubin) staining of various brain nuclei was noted at autopsy in babies dying with severe neonatal jaundice, referred to at the time as icterus gravis neonatorum (Hansen 2000). Schmorl (1903), a pathologist, coined the term 'kernikterus' to describe these lesions, kern from the German for nucleus and ikterus from the Greek for jaundice. Case reports of neurological symptoms and sequelae compatible with damage to these nuclei subsequently appeared (e.g. Claireaux 1950, Gerrard 1952, Zimmerman & Yannet 1935).

A remarkable body of clinical and basic research determined that icterus gravis neonatorum and kernicterus resulted from excessive neonatal hemolysis caused by maternal isoimmunization to fetal red blood cell antigens (typically the Rh antigen). In this condition, hemolysis in the fetus often produces severe anemia (erythroblastosis fetalis) with heart failure and edema (hydrops fetalis) leading to fetal demise. Fetal jaundice is absent, however, as the placenta clears the excess bilirubin produced (Lester et al 1963). About 15% of newborns with this condition, now referred to as hemolytic disease of the newborn (HDN), accumulate bilirubin in amounts sufficient to produce kernicterus (Claireaux 1950, Gerrard 1952, Richards 1951, Vaughan et al 1950).

Treatment of affected newborns with exchange transfusion (ET) was described as early as 1925 (Hart 1925), but it was not considered in earnest (Diamond 1948, Wallerstein 1946) or proven effective until the etiology of the condition was clarified (Allen et al 1950, Mollison & Walker 1952). The rough correlation between serum total bilirubin concentration (TBC) prompted the suggestion that ET be used when the TBC reached 'about' 20 mg/dL (342 μmol/L) (Hsia et al 1952). Without further study the 20 mg/dL (342 μmol/L) ET criterion was widely adopted for all jaundiced newborns and remains a contentious point to this day (Brown & Zuelzer 1957, Newman & Maisels 1992, Newns & Norton 1958, Stern & Denton 1965, Valaes et al 1992, Watchko & Oski 1983, Watchko 2005).

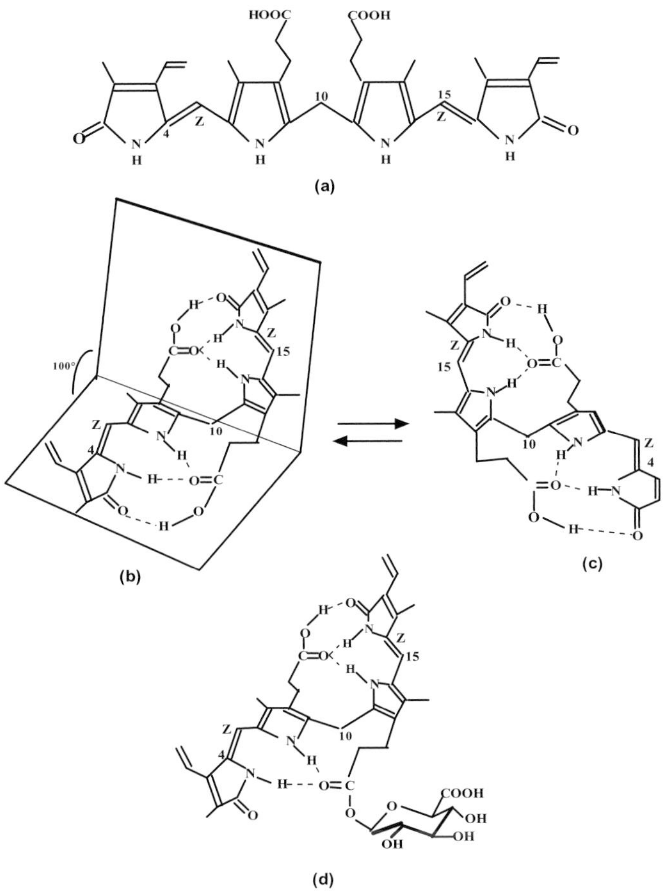

Figure 36.1 Planar (a) and 3-dimensional representations (b and c) of the bilirubin IX-a 4Z,15Z enantiomers (non-superimposable mirror images) that rapidly interconvert in solution. The 'ridge tile' conformation indicated in (b) is favored by bilirubin in crystalline form and in solution. Intramolecular hydrogen bonds are indicated by the dashed lines. Bilirubin conjugated with a single glucuronic acid is shown in (d).

Brain bilirubin staining was initially considered by many a pathological epiphenomenon (Gerrard 1952, Zimmerman & Yannet 1935), but kernicterus associated with non-hemolytic jaundice (Crigler & Najjar 1952) and the in vitro demonstration of bilirubin toxicity by Day (1954) indicated that bilirubin itself was neurotoxic. Bilirubin may on occasion cause incidental, non-specific staining of the brain (Ahdab-Barmada 1987, Ahdab-Barmada & Moossy J 1984, Turkel 1990, Turkel et al 1982).

ET and newer therapeutic modalities (Liley 1963, Pollack et al 1968, Rubo et al 1992) have virtually eliminated kernicterus caused by HDN, once the most prevalent cause of kernicterus. Its dispatch, however, was accompanied by the emergence of the premature newborn as another population of babies at significant risk for kernicterus (Aiden et al 1950, Zuelzer & Mudgett 1950).

KERNICTERUS THEN AND NOW: KERNICTERUS AND THE PREMATURE NEWBORN

Between 1 and 3% of the premature newborns cared for in the developing special care nurseries of the late 1940s and 1950s developed kernicterus (Crosse et al 1955, 1958, Rapmund et al 1960). This kernicterus was remarkable in that it often occurred in the absence of hemolysis (Aiden et al 1950) and at surprisingly low TBCs (Ackerman et al 1970, Gartner et al 1970, Harris et al 1958, Silverman et al 1956, Stern & Denton 1965). The poor TBC/kernicterus correlation coupled with the substantial risks of ET (Crosse et al 1958, Forfar et al 1958) prompted renewed efforts to understand normal bilirubin metabolism (Billing 1978) and the underlying pathophysiological and clinical factors associated with kernicterus. The goal was (and remains) to develop diagnostic and intervention criteria that eliminate kernicterus while minimizing unnecessary treatment (Blanc & Johnson et al 1959, Hugh-Jones et al 1960, Johnson et al 1959, Koch et al 1959, Meyer 1956, Mores et al 1959, Odell 1959).

Unfortunately, prospective establishment of ET criteria proved elusive (Ackerman et al 1970, Gartner et al 1970, Stern & Denton 1965, Wishingrad et al 1965). Instead, guidelines for ET in premature newborns were gradually lowered from the 20 mg/dL (342 µmol/L) TBC 'standard' mainly through trial and error usually reflecting local experience, expertise and biases (Gartner et al 1970, Pearlman et al 1978). Remarkably, kernicterus at most (but not all) centers began to disappear (Gartner et al 1970, 1985, Pearlman et al 1978, Ritter et al 1982), and the introduction of phototherapy (PT) provided a non-invasive means for lowering the TBC without resorting to ET (Cremer et al 1958, Kalpoyiannis et al 1982, Lee et al 1977).

While authorities continued to argue over the pathophysiology of bilirubin neurotoxicity and intervention criteria (Levine 1979, Lucey 1982, Wennberg et al 1979), by the early 1980s kernicterus was probably encountered legally more often than clinically (Maisels & Newman 1995). At least so it seemed. In retrospect, subtle, unrecognized bilirubin-induced neuropathy was occurring (Johnson & Boggs 1974, Odell et al 1970) as evidenced by later reports (Bhutani et al 2004, de Vries et al 1987, Govaert et al 2003, Hansen et al 1991, Oh et al 2003, Salamy et al 1989, Stein et al 1996).

The 'disappearance' of kernicterus associated with hemolytic disease and prematurity produced a waning concern about newborn jaundice and a waxing concern that the ET intervention guidelines (Pearlman et al 1978) were too strict (Eberhard & Drew 1994, Newman & Maisels 1992, Watchko & Claassen 1994). However, a sudden reappearance of kernicterus, often in otherwise well term newborns, revealed the rumored demise of kernicterus to be premature and tragically exposed the still ongoing shortcomings in our clinical management of newborn jaundice (Ahlfors & Herbsman 2003, Brown & Johnson 1996, JCAHO 2001, Merhar & Gilbert 2005, Mollen et al 2004, Palmer et al 2004,

Penn et al 1994, Perlman et al 1997, Ross 2003, Stanley 1997, Stevenson et al 2005, Wennberg et al 2006).

KERNICTERUS NOW: KERNICTERUS AND THE TERM NEWBORN

Kernicterus in newborns born after 35 weeks of gestation probably occurs in less than 1 per 30 000 (Trolle 1961), leading some to question whether it occurred at all (Newman & Maisels 1990, Watchko 2005). Unfortunately, a TBC of 20 mg/dL (342 µmol/L) is not infrequent (Newman et al 2003, 2006), and an otherwise healthy term baby with a TBC of 20 mg/dL (342 µmol/L) receiving an ET is far more likely to be injured by the procedure than to develop kernicterus if the procedure were withheld (Ahlfors & Wennberg 2004, Jackson 1997). The understandable arguments for relaxing the TBC 20 mg/dL (342 µmol/L) guideline (Eberhard & Drew 1994, Newman & Maisels 1992), however, were criticized for, among other things, recommending changes in practice without appropriate studies (Valaes et al 1992). Regardless, these arguments supported the increasingly lackadaisical approach to newborn jaundice, which coupled with the increasing interest in breast feeding and financially driven shortened postpartum hospital stays (American Academy of Pediatrics Committee on Fetus and Newborn 2004), set the stage for the reappearance of kernicterus. While the kernicterus was frequently associated with undiagnosed glucose-6-phosphate dehydrogenase (G6PD) deficiency (Ahlfors & Herbsman 2003, Penn et al 1994, Stanley 1997, Worley et al 1996), many cases occurred in previously healthy newborns (Ebbesen 2000, Hansen 2000a, 2002, Johnson et al 2002, Maisels & Newman 1995, Sentinel Event Alert 2001). It is now painfully clear that *all* jaundiced newborns are at risk and an overhaul of the clinical management of newborn jaundice is required (Johnson et al 2002, Stevenson et al 2005, Wennberg et al 2006).

Minimizing the social and financial costs of sorting through the 20 million or so babies that each year become visibly jaundiced and identifying *without fail* the 400 or so babies that might develop kernicterus is a daunting task indeed (Ahlfors & Wennberg 2004, American Academy of Pediatrics Subcommittee on Hyperbilirubinemia 2004, Bhutani & Johnson 2003, Blackmon et al 2004, Hansen 2002, Holtzman 2004, Ip et al 2004, Johnson et al 2002, Newman et al 2006, Palmer et al 2004, Stevenson et al 2005, Suresh et al 2004). The lack of evidence-based support for current clinical practices and reliable laboratory testing also seriously complicate matters (American Academy of Pediatrics Subcommittee on Hyperbilirubinemia 2004, Bhutani & Johnson 2003, 2004, Blackmon et al 2004, Hansen 2001, Ip et al 2004, Stevenson et al 2005, Wennberg et al 2006).

It is with this brief history of kernicterus in mind that the following are reviewed in this chapter: the molecular bases of bilirubin metabolism and neurotoxicity, their relationship to clinical kernicterus, the clinical features of newborn jaundice and kernicterus, and the current and possible future strategies for preventing kernicterus in the jaundiced newborn.

BILIRUBIN CHEMISTRY, METABOLISM AND NEWBORN JAUNDICE

NOMENCLATURE

Bilirubin nomenclature has been described as bizarre and, at the very least, confusing (McDonagh & Lightner 1985). Herein the terms *bilirubin* and *unconjugated bilirubin* refer to bilirubin IX-α 4Z,15Z (Fig. 36.1). One or both carboxyl groups may be conjugated with glucuronic acid to form non-neurotoxic *conjugated bilirubin* (Fig. 36.1). The older terms *direct bilirubin* (mostly conjugated bilirubin) and *indirect bilirubin* (unconjugated bilirubin) are specific to the diazo test used by clinical laboratories to fractionate plasma bilirubin into its conjugated and unconjugated components (Ahlfors 2000). The plasma *TBC* is the sum of the concentrations of conjugated and unconjugated (direct + indirect) bilirubin, and the plasma unbound or free bilirubin (B_f) is the concentration of conjugated and unconjugated bilirubin not bound to proteins (albumin) (Ahlfors 2000). Conjugated bilirubin in jaundiced newborns is typically low and therefore TBC is considered as all unconjugated bilirubin unless clinical circumstances suggest otherwise (American Academy of Pediatrics Subcommittee on Hyperbilirubinemia 2004).

The two carboxylic acid groups are variably ionized in solution (Ostrow et al 1994), making bilirubin a mixture of molecules with no (BH_2), one (BH^-), or two ($B^=$) carboxylate anion(s) (Figs 36.1 and 36.2).

$$[\text{Bilirubin}] = [BH_2] + [BH^-] + [B^=]$$

Plasma from newborns undergoing PT contains the bilirubin configurational photoisomer *4Z,15E bilirubin IXα* and structural photoisomer *lumirubin* (Fig. 36.3) (McDonagh & Lightner 1985, McDonagh 2006).

BILIRUBIN CHEMISTRY

The behavior of bilirubin at physiologic pH is complex. Its limited solubility, tendency to aggregate, interaction with proteins and lipids, and light sensitivity all have potentially significant clinical implications for kernicterus. The chemical properties of bilirubin are also important in gallstone formation (Ostrow & Celic 1984, Tiribelli & Ostrow 1996).

Bilirubin solubility

The pathophysiology of kernicterus has long centered on bilirubin solubility (Brodersen 1972, Brodersen & Stern 1990, Ostrow et al 1994, 2004). Bilirubin is amphipathic, meaning it has both hydrophilic and hydrophobic ('lipophilic') regions that influence its chemical behavior. Its two chemically equivalent carboxyl groups (Boiadjiev et al 2004, Hahm et al 1992) are pivotal in its 'hydrophilic' behavior and therefore water solubility (Fig. 36.2). Intramolecular hydrogen bonds make BH_2 nearly insoluble in water (Bonnett et al 1976, Overbeek et al 1955), while the negatively charged BH^- and $B^=$ are much more hydrophilic and water soluble (Fig. 36.2).

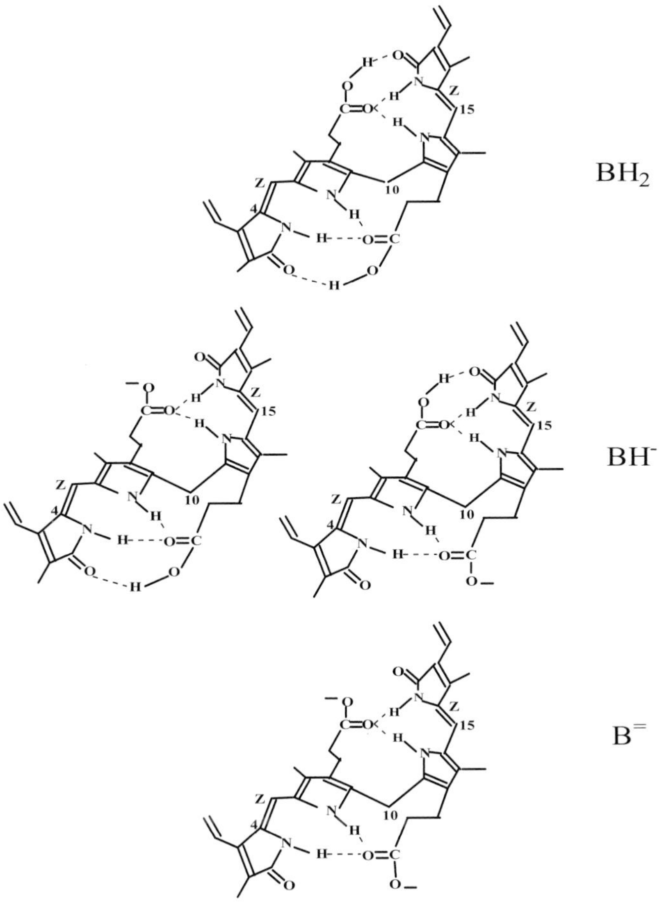

BH_2

BH^-

$B^=$

Figure 36.2 The three ionic species of bilirubin IX-a 4Z,15Z. Neither carboxyl group is ionized in the top figure (BH_2), both are ionized in the bottom figure ($B^=$), and the two chemically equivalent singly ionized forms are shown between (BH^-).

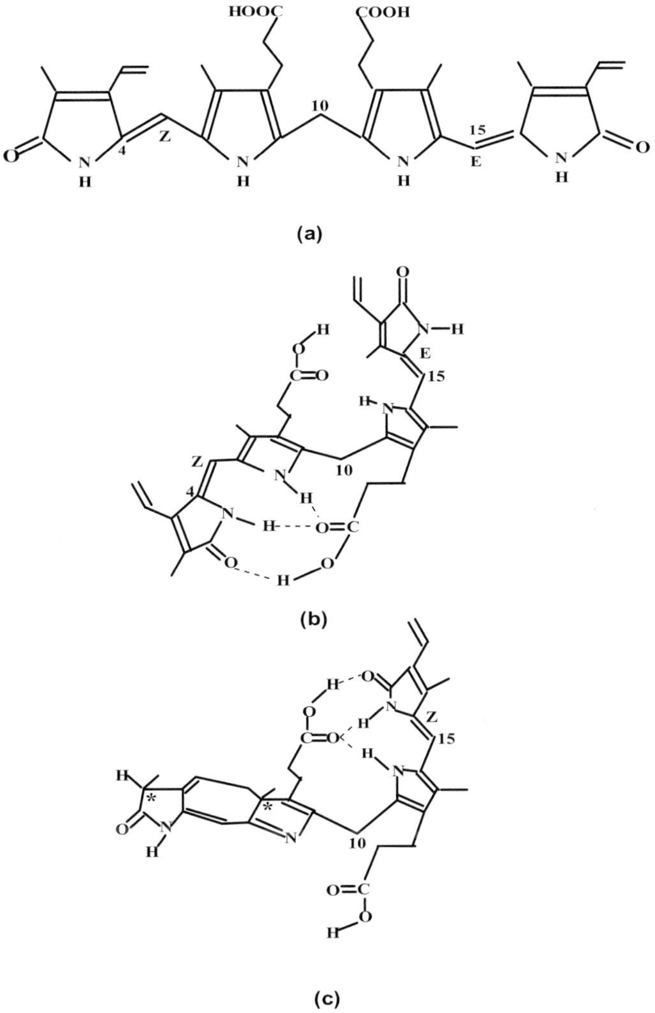

(a)

(b)

(c)

Figure 36.3 Planar (a) and 3 dimensional (b) representations of the 4Z,15E configurational photoisomer of bilirubin IX-a. The structural photoisomer lumirubin is the lowest figure (c).

The relative concentrations of BH_2, BH^-, and $B^=$ depend on the pH and carboxyl group ionization constant, K_a, which for carboxylic acids typically ranges between 10^{-4} and 10^{-5} mol/L (Boiadjiev et al 2004).

$$(precipitate \leftarrow)BH_2 \xleftrightarrow{K_a} BH^- \xleftrightarrow{K_a} B^=.$$

If K_a and the bilirubin concentration (i.e. BH_2 + BH^- + $B^=$) are known, BH_2 can be obtained from the BH^-/BH_2 and $B^=/BH^-$ ratios calculated using the Henderson–Hasselbalch equation, where pK_a is the negative logarithm of K_a.

$$pH = pK_a + \log\left(\frac{Salt(BH^-)}{Acid(BH_2)}\right) = pK_a + \log\left(\frac{Salt(B^=)}{Acid(BH^-)}\right)$$

Unfortunately, experimentally determined K_a values differ by three orders of magnitude ranging from a high of 10^{-5} mols/L ($pK_a \approx 5$) (Boiadjiev et al 2004, Hansen 1979, Lightner et al 1996, Overbeek et al 1955) to a low of 10^{-8} mol/L ($pK_a \approx 8$) (Hahm et al 1992, Mukerjee et al 2002). These vastly different K_a values lead to very different conclusions about bilirubin ionization and solubility. At pH 7.4, if $K_a \approx 10^{-5}$ mol/L over 99% of the bilirubin is $B^=$ and the

BH_2 solubility limit is 0.03 nmol/L (Overbeek et al 1955), giving an overall bilirubin solubility limit (BH_2 + BH^- + $B^=$) of 2000 nmol/L. However, if $K_a \approx 10^{-8}$ mol/L, 75% of the bilirubin is BH_2, the BH_2 solubility limit is 66 nmol/L (Hahm et al 1992), bilirubin solubility is 87 nmol/L. Both K_a values were obtained by competent, experienced researchers; yet they cannot both be correct.

$K_a \approx 10^{-5}$ mol/L seems more likely (Broiadjiev 2004, Trull et al 1997), particularly given the predicted solubility limit of 87 nmol/L at $K_a \approx 10^{-8}$ mol/L. In vitro bilirubin toxicity has been estimated to occur between 71 and 770 nmol/L (Ostrow et al 2003), which is not 'modestly above' 87 nmol/L as argued by some (Ostrow et al 2004). The calculated 95% CI for mean brain B_f in asymptomatic Gunn rats is 556 to 1110 nmol/L (Daood & Watchko 2006), and B_f in sick but non-kernicteric premature newborns regularly exceeds 90 nmol/L without evidence of bilirubin insolubility or toxicity (Ahlfors et al 2006). If fact, kernicterus in the latter is unlikely until B_f, adjusted for plasma dilution (Ahlfors 1981), exceeds 200 nmol/L *per kg* (Ahlfors & Herbsman 2003, Cashore & Oh 1982, Nakamura et al 1992, Ritter et al 1982). These data make the 87 nmol/L solubility estimate for bilirubin seem unlikely.

The appeal of $K_a \approx 10^{-8}$ mol/L is that BH_2 predominates at pH 7.4 and its 'lipophilic' behavior seems positioned to explain the normal and toxic interactions of bilirubin with lipid membranes (Mustafa & King 1970, Ostrow et al 1994, 2003a, 2004, Tiribelli & Ostrow 1996). However, $K_a \approx 10^{-5}$ mol/L does not preclude BH_2-lipid interactions. For example, if $K_a \approx 10^{-5}$ mol/L, at the intracellular pH of 7, bilirubin becomes insoluble at about 300 nmol/L, which is consistent with the toxicity data cited above as well as the observation that tissue bilirubin uptake increases as pH decreases (Nelson et al 1974). Regardless, the unresolved and hotly contested K_a issue is made more problematic and perhaps moot by the tendency of bilirubin to aggregate (Brodersen 1966, Ostrow & Celic 1984). In addition, its local behavior in the complex anatomical and chemical (e.g. pH) microenvironments of lipid membranes and cellular organelles may be more relevant to kernicterus than the solubility of bilirubin at the pH of the surrounding environment (Nagaoka & Cowger 1978, Wennberg 1988, 1991).

Bilirubin aggregation

$B^=$ reversibly forms soluble dimers ($B^= + B^= \leftrightarrow B_2^{4-}$), more so at higher pH, with about half being dimers at pH 10 and 25% at pH 8 (Brodersen 1966, Carey & Koretsky 1979).

$$\text{(Precipitation} \leftarrow)BH_2 \leftrightarrow BH^- \leftrightarrow B^= \leftrightarrow \text{Dimers}$$

A significant concentration of B_2^{4-} may be present at physiologic pH, but its impact on the chemical behavior or toxicity of bilirubin is unknown.

In vitro, bilirubin aggregates into multimers of varying solubility depending on its concentration, the temperature, pH, and ionic strength (Boiadjiev et al 2004, Brodersen & Theilgaard 1969, Brodesen 1966). At pH 7.4, fairly stable colloidal suspensions, often invisible to the naked eye, may occur at bilirubin levels as low as 100 nmol/L (Brodersen & Theilgaard 1969).

$$\text{(Precipitation} \leftarrow)BH_2 \leftrightarrow BH^- \leftrightarrow B^= \leftrightarrow \text{Dimers} \rightarrow \text{Multimers}$$
$$\text{(Colloids)}$$

The insoluble colloidal particles are composed of BH_2 surrounded by a layer of bilirubin anions keeping them dispersed (Brodersen & Theilgaard 1969). Colloid formation can be reversed by alkalinization and will not occur if albumin is present when bilirubin is added. However, once formed, albumin cannot re-dissolve them and bilirubin-albumin crystals may form (Brodersen & Theilgaard 1969, Brodersen et al 1972).

Bilirubin also aggregates in lipid suspensions in a concentration (and lipid) dependent fashion (Brodersen 1979, Eriksen et al 1981, Nagaoka & Cowger 1978). These aggregates are soluble in chloroform (Boiadjiev et al 2004) indicating that they are composed of BH_2 or that anion charges are directed inward. Prior to aggregation, bilirubin–lipid interaction is reversible with binding constants approximating that of bilirubin-albumin binding and the likely involvement of BH_2, BH^-, and $B^=$ (Eriksen et al 1981, Nagaoka & Cowger 1978, Ostrow et al 1994, Wennberg 1988, 1991, Zucker et al 1999, 2001). It appears that $B^=$ binds at the membrane surface (Ostrow et al 1994, Zucker et al 2001), and depending on local ionization (i.e. generation of BH^- or BH_2) bilirubin either passes into and through or dissociates from the membrane (Wennberg 1988, 1991, Zucker et al 1999, 2001). While membrane dysfunction caused by bilirubin aggregation has been posited as the likely triggering event for kernicterus (Brodersen & Stern 1990, Brodersen 1972, 1979, Eriksen et al 1981, Nagaoka & Cowger 1978), it is just as plausible that prior to bilirubin aggregation, bilirubin saturates the membrane sufficiently to disrupt its function (Ahlfors 2001a). This, in fact, seems more likely given the apparent reversibility of bilirubin neurotoxicity with ET (Brown & Zuelzer 1957, Johnson et al 2002, Wennberg et al 1982).

Nature, as will be discussed below, exposes a baby to bilirubin far differently than the way experiments expose animals, cells, organelles and molecules to bilirubin. The disparate K_a values reveal that, even in the best of hands and under the best of circumstances, bilirubin is extremely difficult to study (Brodersen & Stern 1987, McDonagh & Assisi 1971). Suffice it to say that theories of kernicterus centered on bilirubin solubility and/or aggregation as the necessary or triggering events often test the limits of the data on which they are based (Brodersen & Stern 1990, Brodersen 1972, Ostrow et al 1994, 2003a, Tiribelli & Ostrow 1996, 2005, Volpe 2001).

Bilirubin interaction with proteins and lipids

Bilirubin binds avidly but reversibly to plasma proteins (mostly albumin) without which it would precipitate at its concentration of 17 000 nmol/L in adults. Protein binding is important in normal bilirubin metabolism (e.g. Litwack et al 1971, Pascolo et al 1996, Stollman et al 1983), and compromised binding was recognized very early as a factor in kernicterus (Johnson et al 1959, Odell 1959, Silverman et al 1956). Only $B^=$ binds to albumin (Brodersen 1979, 1979a) but hydrophobic interactions in the albumin binding domains determine the spectral properties of the complex (Brodersen 1979a) and influence drug interference with bilirubin binding (Robertson et al 1991).

In plasma, the TBC, B_f, and albumin are related by the law of mass action where K is the equilibrium association constant (Ahlfors & Parker 2005).

$$K = \frac{TBC - B_f}{B_f \cdot (\text{albumin} - TBC + B_f)}$$

K in undiluted plasma is about 5 L/μmol (Ahlfors et al 2006, Weisiger et al 2001), and B_f in *undiluted plasma* under normal circumstances may reach levels as high as 100 nmol/L *per kg* (Ahlfors et al 2006).

Bilirubin binding may interfere directly with protein function, or it may disrupt membrane factors regulating protein function (Conlee et al 2000, Gennuso et al 2004, Karp 1979, Mustafa & King 1970, Mustafa et al 1969, Shapiro et al 2006, Spencer et al 2002). The latter appears more germane to bilirubin toxicity.

As noted previously bilirubin in vitro reversibly binds to and eventually aggregates with suspensions of lipids, including red blood cell membranes (Alexandra-Brito et al 2006, Bratlid 1972, Oski & Naiman 1963). In its normal metabolism it must also move across the polar surfaces and hydrophobic interiors of lipid membranes, a process as noted above that possibly requires all three species. Passive diffusion occurs in vitro (Zucker et al 1999) and facilitated and active transport also appear likely (Ostrow et al 2004, Watchko 2006) (Fig. 36.4). Once in the cell, protein and lipid membrane binding play important roles in its normal metabolism and most likely its neurotoxicity as well, as discussed below.

Bilirubin and light

Bilirubin, especially when exposed to intense blue light, undergoes oxidization into to smaller, water soluble compounds (Lightner et al 1984, 1984a, Ostrow & Branham 1970). Blue light also converts bilirubin to several water soluble photoisomers that are (presumably) non-toxic and rapidly excreted (Onishi et al 1979). The two of relevance in

humans are shown in Figure 36.3 (Ennever et al 1987, McDonagh & Lightner 1985, McDonagh 2006).

BILIRUBIN PRODUCTION

In the tissues of the reticuloendothelial system (primarily the spleen) heme oxygenase catalyzes the degradation of heme to iron, carbon monoxide (CO) and biliverdin. Biliverdin reductase then catalyzes the reduction of biliverdin to bilirubin.

$$\text{Heme} \xrightarrow[\text{Oxygenase}]{\text{Heme}} Fe^{2+} + CO + \text{Biliverdin} \xrightarrow[\text{reductase}]{\text{Biliverdin}} \text{Bilirubin}$$

Bilirubin diffuses into the blood where it binds to plasma albumin, other proteins (Goessling & Zucker 2000), and red blood cell membranes (Bratlid 1972, Oski & Naiman 1963).

BILIRUBIN EXCRETION

On reaching the liver, blood plasma filters through fenestrated capillaries into the space of Disse and bathes the hepatocytes. Free bilirubin (B_f) (Pascolo et al 1996, Stollman et al 1983) crosses the hepatocyte plasma membrane by an incompletely understood combination of passive, facilitated, and active transport (Berk et al 1996, Pascolo et al 1996, Passamonti et al 2005). Binding to cytosol proteins prevents efflux (Litwack et al 1971), and conjugation in the endoplasmic reticulum with glucuronic acid catalyzed by uridine diphosphate glucuronosyltransferase (UGT1A1) renders bilirubin water soluble (Fig. 36.1). Conjugated bilirubin is actively transported into the bile canaliculus (Kamisako et al 2000) through which it travels and ultimately enters the intestines. There bacterial enzymes (minimal in newborns) may degrade it further before it is excreted in the stool. Hydrolysis of conjugated bilirubin in the intestine can result in bilirubin reuptake into the portal blood, referred to as enterohepatic circulation of bilirubin (Lester et al 1961). Enzymatic oxidation (bilirubin oxidase) may aid bilirubin excretion and possibly protect neurons from bilirubin toxicity (Hansen 2000b, Hansen et al 1997, Yokosuka & Billing 1987).

NEWBORN JAUNDICE (UNCONJUGATED HYPERBILIRUBINEMIA)

Newborn bilirubin production is 2–3 times greater than that of adults (Maisels et al 1971), mostly due to the shortened life span of fetal red blood cells. In addition, hepatic UGT1A1 activity and perhaps liver B_f uptake are transiently decreased (Grimmer et al 1978, Levi & Sauve 1970). The imbalance produces a temporary, usually benign, and perhaps helpful (Kaplan et al 2002, McDonagh 1990, Vitek 2005) bilirubin accumulation (see below). Visible jaundice occurs in ⅔ of term newborns, resolving within 10 days except in about 10% of breast fed infants. In these babies maternal milk appears to contain factors interfering with bilirubin excretion (Gartner & Herschel et al 2001, Leung & Sauve 1989, Monaghan et al 1999, Tazawa et al 1991). Formula feeding is associated with less and faster resolution of jaundice (Gourley et al 2005, Maisels & Gifford 1986).

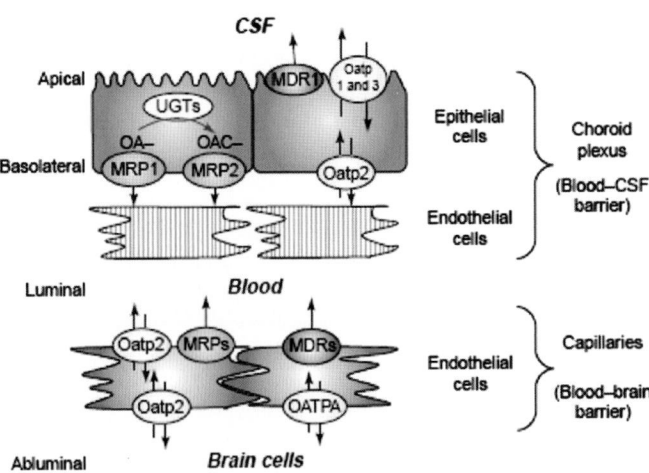

Figure 36.4 Schematic of the CNS transporting mechanisms available for regulating bilirubin movement between blood and brain across the choroid plexus (CP) and blood–brain barrier (BBB). Organic anion transport proteins (OATP) move substrates in either direction, and the ATP cassette binding (ABC) multidrug resistance P-glycoproteins (MDRs) and multidrug resistance-associated proteins (MRPs) export substrates utilizing ATP. UGT is a bilirubin conjugating enzyme. Luminal/apical and basolateral/abluminal are interchangeable terms. (Reprinted from Trends in Molecular Medicine Volume 10, Ostrow J D, Pascolo L, Brites D, Tiribelli C 2002 Molecular basis of bilirubin-induced neurotoxicity, 65–70, with permission.)

NEWBORN BILIRUBIN ACCUMULATION AND THE MISCIBLE BILIRUBIN POOL

The gradual accumulation of bilirubin over hours or days has always been the linchpin in human kernicterus that separates it from experimental models of bilirubin neurotoxicity (Brodersen 1980, Kaplan et al 2002, Wennberg et al 1979). As blood levels of TBC and B_f gradually increase, the protein bound bilirubin (TBC − B_f), which is nearly all the bilirubin in the blood (TBC − $B_f ≈$ TBC), cannot escape from the vascular space (Ahlfors 2001a). The tiny B_f fraction, however, is free to cross endothelial cell membranes and does so. Bilirubin therefore begins to slowly accumulate in the tissues, including the brain. The rate of accumulation depends on the imbalance between bilirubin production and excretion as well as the relative affinities of blood and tissues (e.g. skin, fat, brain, etc.) for bilirubin as indicated below (Berk et al 1969, Brown & Zuelzer 1957a, Diamond & Schmid 1966, Schmid & Hammaker 1963, Valaes 1963, Wennberg et al 1979). The accumulated pool of bilirubin in the blood and tissues is referred to as the 'bilirubin load' and also, to emphasize the dynamic reversible movement of bilirubin between tissues and blood, the 'miscible bilirubin pool' (Berk et al 1969, Schmid & Hammaker 1963).

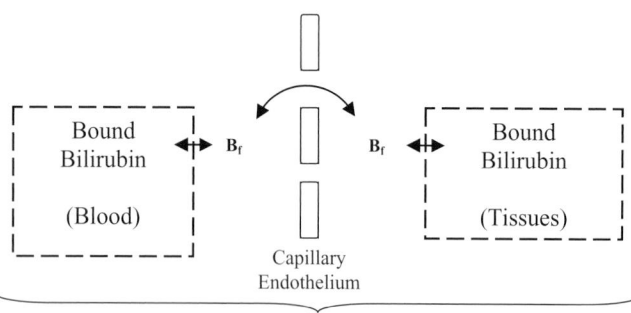

Miscible Bilirubin Pool

About 60% of the pool in humans resides in the blood (Schmid & Hammaker 1963), and although the brain is a small percentage of the overall pool size, the accumulated brain bilirubin is the critical factor underlying the development of kernicterus (Ahlfors & Parker 2005, Brodersen 1972a, Daood & Watchko 2006, Davis & Yeary 1975). Since the bilirubin-albumin mass action binding constant K (see above) varies considerably in newborns (Ahlfors & Parker 2005, Ahlfors et al 2006, Jacobsen & Wennberg 1974), the TBC and B_f together provide a better indication of the likelihood of bilirubin neurotoxicity than TBC alone (Ahlfors & Parker 2005, Ahlfors & Shapiro 2001, Ahlfors 1994, 2001a, Amin et al 2001, Cashore & Oh 1982, Funato et al 1994, Nakamura et al 1992, Ritter et al 1982, Silverman et al 1956, Wennberg et al 2006).

BILIRUBIN AND KERNICTERUS

The spectrum of neurological sequelae associated with bilirubin neurotoxicity is increasing (Shapiro et al 2006). For unknown reasons the areas of the brain injured, which overlap with those damaged by hypoxia–ischemia (Ahdab-Barmada & Moossy 1984, Ferriero et al 1988), are variably targeted (Gerrard 1952, Hansen et al 2001, Johnston & Hoon 2000, Shapiro et al 2006, Watchko 2006). However, the sequelae are thought to be at least partly modulated by the accompanying clinical circumstances (Ackerman et al 1970, de Vries et al 1987, Oh et al 2003, Pearlman et al 1980, Perlman et al 1997, Perlstein 1961, Shapiro 2003, Shapiro et al 2006, Silverman et al 1956, Watchko 2006).

NOMENCLATURE

The American Academy of Pediatrics Committee on Fetus and Newborn (2004) recommends 'acute bilirubin encephalopathy' (ABE) be used for the acute symptoms and 'kernicterus' be reserved for the 'classical' chronic neurological sequelae outlined below. The acronym BIND (bilirubin-induced neurological dysfunction) refers to a variety of subtle neurological sequelae thought secondary to bilirubin injury (Shapiro 2005, Shapiro et al 2006) and a scoring system (Table 36.1) proposed for assessing the severity and likely reversibility of ABE (Bhutani & Johnson 2005, Johnson et al 1999).

BILIRUBIN ENTRY INTO THE CNS

The large size of bilirubin along with its protein binding and ionization make it, like many xenobiotics, a poor candidate for penetrating the blood–brain barrier (BBB) (Ahlfors &

Table 36.1 A scoring system for estimating severity of acute bilirubin encephalopathy (ABE) according to Johnson et al 1999. Any score above 0 requires urgent bilirubin reduction by PT/ET regardless of the condition of the infant. Recovery may be incomplete at scores above 6			
Score	Mental status	Muscle tone	Cry pattern
0	Normal	Normal	Normal
1	Sleepy Poor feeding	Neck stiffness Mild hypertonia Mild hypotonia	High pitched
2	Lethargic Irritable	Arching neck Retrocollis Arching trunk	Shrill
3	Stupor Seizures Coma	Bowing of trunk Opisthotonus	Inconsolable

Score 1–3: Mild ABE
Score 4–6: Moderate ABE
Score 7–9: Severe ABE

Parker 2005, Ostrow et al 2004). Nonetheless, it crosses the choroid plexus (CP) and BBB (Ahlfors & Parker 2005, Diamond & Schmid 1966, Hansen et al 1989) at a net rate that may depend in part on local membrane transport mechanisms (Ostrow et al 2004) (Fig. 36.4). B_f typically moves across the CP and BBB (Diamond & Schmid 1966, Hansen et al 1989, Jacobsen et al 1982, Møllgård & Saunders 1986, Ohsugi et al 1992, Wennberg 2000), but experimental disruption of the BBB allows albumin-bound bilirubin to enter the brain (Levine & et al 1982). This produces acute EEG and energy metabolism changes (Wennberg 2000, Wennberg & Hance 1986, Wennberg et al 1991), but the toxic responses correlate with B_f better than the TBC at the site of the injury (Wennberg & Hance 1986). Bilirubin rapidly exits the brain by diffusion and perhaps active transport following reversible disruption of the BBB without obvious brain injury (Levine & et al 1985). BBB disruption could account for the occasional non-specific brain bilirubin staining seen post mortem that must be distinguished from kernicterus (Ahdab-Barmada 1983, 1987, Ahdab-Barmada & Moossy 1984, Turkel 1983, 1990, Turkel et al 1980, 1982).

BILIRUBIN AND THE CHOROID PLEXUS

CSF bilirubin levels in jaundiced newborns are lower than but proportional to TBC (Kulkarni et al 1989, Nasralla et al 1958), even in the presence of kernicterus (Kulkarni et al 1989). The positioning of organic anion (OA) and ATP binding cassette (ABC) proteins in the choroid plexus epithelial cells (Fig. 36.4) support bilirubin efflux from the CSF (Ostrow et al 2004) but require $B^=$ or BH^- as substrates. CP function appears unaltered in the presence of toxic bilirubin levels (Kulkarni et al 1989).

BILIRUBIN AND THE BLOOD–BRAIN BARRIER

B_f diffuses across artificial lipid membranes (Zucker et al 1999) and moves readily across the intact BBB (Diamond & Schmid 1966, Hansen et al 1989, Wennberg et al 1991). Experimental data suggests that its net uptake is restricted by transport proteins located on endothelial cell plasma membranes (Fig. 36.4) (Ostrow et al 2004, Watchko 2006, Watchko et al 2001) using $B^=$ or BH^- as substrates (Wennberg 1988, 1991). Bilirubin appeared 'lipophilic' in a rat BBB model (Ives & Gardiner 1990) suggesting that simple diffusion of BH_2 might account for brain bilirubin uptake, but the bilirubin brain distribution in that study was not typical of kernicterus.

The bilirubin gradient across the BBB decreases with decreasing nervous system maturity (Lee et al 1995, Roger et al 1995), which is consistent with the onset of ABE at lower TBC levels as gestation decreases (Gartner et al 1970, Pearlman et al 1978, Stern & Denton 1965). Maturing neurons are thought to have 'windows of vulnerability' when they are especially sensitive to bilirubin toxicity, which may explain some of the variability in sequelae (Falcao et al 2006, Keino et al 1985, Notter & Kendig 1986, Shapiro 2003, Wennberg 1991). It is unknown whether

variation in BBB structure (cf. the circumventricular organs) or BBB-neuronal links (Bauer & Bauer 2000) play a role in the selective pattern of neuronal injury seen with kernicterus. More likely intrinsic cell type, maturity, activity and sensitivity are the major determinants (Falcao et al 2006, Hansen et al 2001, Ives et al 1988, Johnston & Hoon 2000, Notter & Kendig 1986, Roger et al 1995). Whether BBB bilirubin transport per se is altered during conditions such as acidosis, hypercarbia, hypoglycemia, infection, or asphyxia, which are associated with kernicterus, is unknown (Ives et al 1988, Roger et al 1995, Wennberg 2000).

BILIRUBIN-INDUCED NEURONAL AND/OR GLIAL INJURY

Once across the BBB, bilirubin will encounter interstitial fluid (ISF) and the astrocytes foot processes that envelope the BBB endothelium. The ISF pH is lower in that of blood (Gilboe et al 1998), which may alter the bilirubin ionic species present. Variation in net ISF flow (Abbott 2004) might also enhance or initiate damage by changing the local ISF bilirubin concentration and/or time of neuronal exposure (Hanko et al 2006, Johnson & Boggs 1974, Spector et al 1977, Szentistvanyi et al 1984).

Bilirubin interference with plasma and intracellular membrane function appears a likely trigger of bilirubin neurotoxicity (Hansen et al 2001, Ostrow et al 2003, Shapiro et al 2006, Watchko 2006). Although a myriad of toxic effects may follow (Fernandes et al 2006, Karp 1979, Ostrow et al 2004, Rodrigues et al 2002, 2002a, Silva et al 1999, 2001, Spencer et al 2002, Watchko 2006), interference with calcium regulation is a common underlying theme (Shapiro et al 2006, Watchko 2006). The contention that bilirubin has a predilection for neurons (Volpe 2001) is not supported by recent evidence (Falcao et al 2006, Fernandez 2006, Gennuso et al 2004, Gordo et al 2006, Silva et al 1999, 2002). Interference with astrocyte calcium ion and glutamate metabolism regulation (Padmashri & Sikdar 2006, Silva et al 1999) could induce excitotoxic neuronal damage (see below). Active cellular efflux of bilirubin and intracellular bilirubin oxidation may help prevent neuronal injury (Dallas et al 2006, Gennuso et al 2004, Hansen 2000b, Hansen et al 1997, Ostrow et al 2004).

Excitotoxicity, disruption of energy metabolism, and calcium regulation have emerged as the likely causes of bilirubin induced neuronal cell death by necrosis or apoptosis (Shapiro et al 2006, Watchko 2006). Excitotoxicity results when excess glutamate at the synaptic junction causes overstimulation of neuronal N-methyl-D-aspartate (NMDA) receptors often resulting in neuronal necrosis and apoptosis (Johnston 2005). Although bilirubin, like hypoxia (Ferriero et al 1988), induces excitotoxicity injury in vitro (Grojean et al 2000, 2001, Hanko et al 2006, Silva et al 1999) and in the Gunn rat (Conlee et al 2000, McDonald et al 1998), there is some evidence to the contrary (Tiribelli & Ostrow 2005, Warr et al 2000). Radiological data showing elevated glutamate levels in the globus pallidus of newborns with kernicterus (Oakden et al 2005) suggests that excito-toxicity may be occurring in humans.

Bilirubin interference with brain respiration (Day 1954) due to uncoupling of mitochondrial oxidative phosphorylation (Ernster & Zetterstom 1956, Mustafa et al 1969) was the first toxic bilirubin effect linked to membrane function (Karp 1979, Mustafa & King 1970). Recent in vitro data documents severe bilirubin-induced changes in mitochondrial membrane structure and function (Rodrigues et al 2000a) and induction of the mitochondrial apoptosis pathway (Rodrigues et al 2002). Mitochondrial damage may not be a necessary condition for kernicterus, however, as bilirubin induces only minor changes in oxidative phosphorylation in the Gunn rat (Schenker et al 1966), and Purkinje cell mitochondrial damage (Shutta 1970, 1971) may be secondary to cytoplasmic disruptions (Schutta & Johnson 1971). Brann et al (1987) were unable to demonstrate changes in oxidative metabolism in piglets despite symptoms consistent with bilirubin toxicity, and rats or rat neurons (Grosjean 2001, Roger et al 1995) exposed to bilirubin have impeded brain glucose uptake rather than the increased glucose uptake expected with impaired oxidative phosphorylation. Notably, however, high lactate resonance demonstrated by proton magnetic resonance spectroscopy in a newborn with kernicterus (Groenendaal et al 2004) is suggestive of impaired energy metabolism.

Bilirubin, like global ischemia (Churn et al 1990), may ultimately cause neuronal toxicity through increased intracellular calcium levels that trigger second messenger pathways (Conlee et al 2000, Shapiro et al 2006, Spencer et al 2002, Watchko 2006). How these events cause cell necrosis and/or apoptosis and alter clinical outcome are areas of active and needed research (Mattson 2003, Shapiro 2003, 2005, Shapiro et al 2006, Watchko 2006).

Bilirubin begins to alter neurological function well before it reaches levels where aggregation is likely (Lenhardt et al 1984). Changes in behavior and cry (Mansi et al 2003, Paludetto et al 002, Vohr et al 1989), the brainstem auditory response (ABR) (Lenhardt et al 1984, Nwsasei 1984, Perlman et al 1983, Wennberg et al 1982, Fig. 36.5), and the visual evoked response (Chen & Wong 2006, Chin et al 1985) all may occur at TBC levels well below those typically seen with kernicterus.

ABR changes begin at TBC levels near 10 mg/dL (Lenhardt et al 1984, Perlman et al 1983) and deteriorate as TBC and particularly B_f levels rise (Ahlfors & Shapiro 2001, Ahlfors et al 1986, Amin et al 2001, Funato et al 1992, Wennberg et al 1982). ABR changes reverse when the miscible bilirubin pool is reduced by ET (Ahlfors 1986, Brown & Zuelzer 1957, Nwsasei 1984, Valaes 1963, Wennberg et al 1982) suggesting that the ABR changes are not caused by bilirubin insolubility or aggregation; however, they may eventually become irreversible (Chisin et al 1979, Kaga et al 1979). Animal studies suggest the ABR changes result from bilirubin interference with synaptic transmission (Zhang et al 2003).

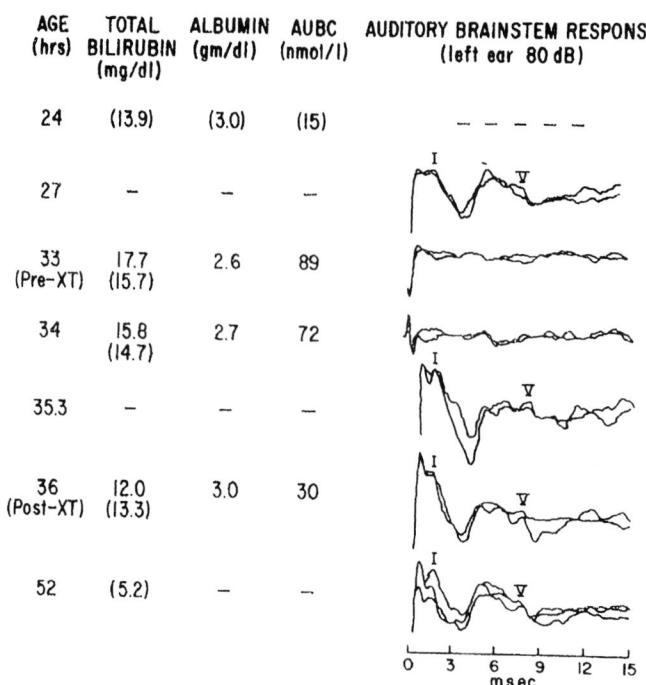

AGE (hrs)	TOTAL BILIRUBIN (mg/dl)	ALBUMIN (gm/dl)	AUBC (nmol/l)	AUDITORY BRAINSTEM RESPONSE (left ear 80 dB)
24	(13.9)	(3.0)	(15)	
27	–	–	–	
33 (Pre-XT)	17.7 (15.7)	2.6	89	
34	15.8 (14.7)	2.7	72	
35.3	–	–	–	
36 (Post-XT)	12.0 (13.3)	3.0	30	
52	(5.2)	–	–	

Figure 36.5 Bilirubin-albumin binding and changes in auditory brainstem response in a newborn with HDN. AUBC (apparent unbound bilirubin concentration), pre-XT (pre-exchange transfusion), post-XT (post-exchange transfusion). The data in parentheses are clinical laboratory measurements at a 42-fold plasma dilution, while the others are research laboratory measurements at a 2-fold plasma dilution. The ABR, present at 27 hours of age is absent by 33 hours of age. The exchange transfusion produces a much greater reduction in AUBC (75%) than total bilirubin (32%) (Arkans & Cassidy 1978), and the corresponding reduction in the size of the miscible bilirubin pool is associated with a restoration of the ABR as bilirubin exits the neural tissues. (From Wennberg R P, Ahlfors C E, Bickers R et al 1982 Abnormal auditory brainstem response in a newborn infant with hyperbilirubinemia: Improvement with exchange transfusion. J Pediatr 100:624–626, with permission.)

PATHOLOGY

The pathological findings in kernicterus were originally described in hemolytic disease of the newborn (HDN), which is frequently complicated by the accompanying anemia (Becker & Vogel 1948, Claireaux 1950, Claireaux et al 1953, Haymaker et al 1961). More recently, studies in the Gunn rat (Conlee et al 2000, Spencer et al 2002) and kernicteric premature newborns (Ahdab-Barmada 1982, 1987, Ahdab-Barmada & Moossy 1984, Turkel 1983, Turkel et al 1982) have clarified the pathological changes specific to bilirubin.

Gross bilirubin staining (Fig. 36.6) is best seen on fresh cut specimens (Turkel 1990) and microscopically in neurons in frozen sections (Dublin 1951). Persistence of yellow color

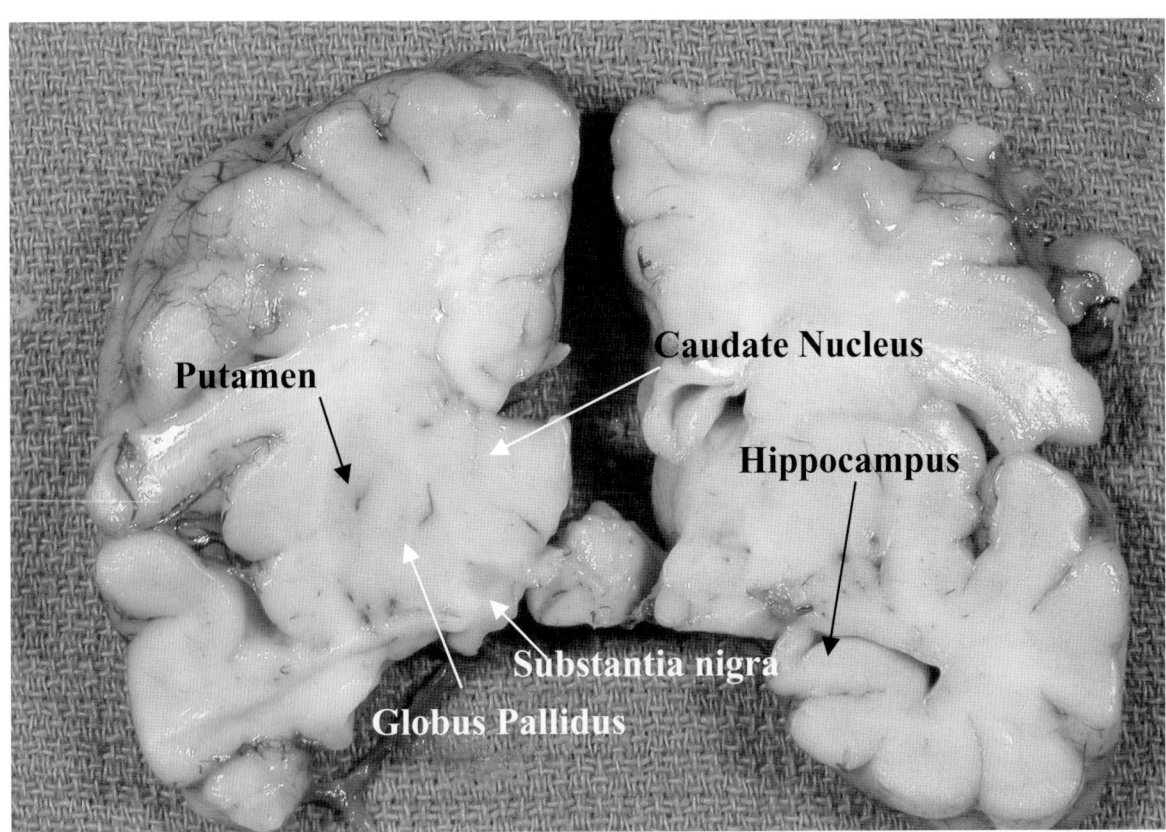

Subcortical

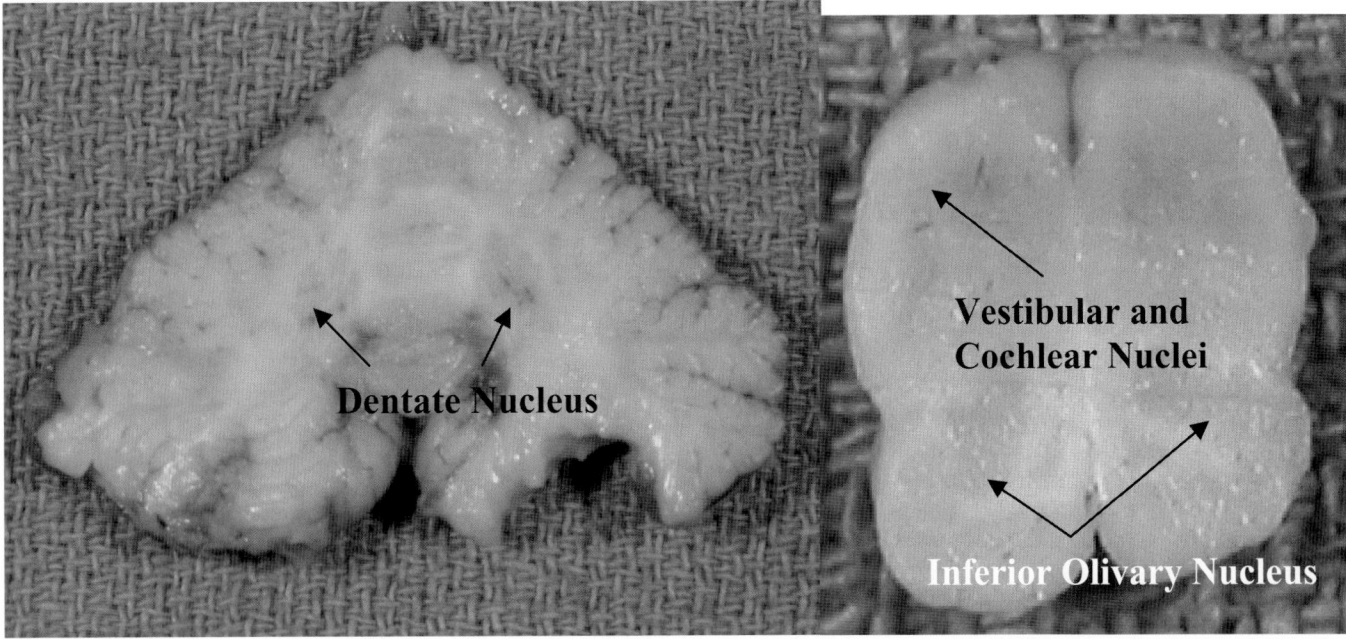

Cerbellum

Brainstem

Figure 36.6 Bilirubin staining in various areas of the brain in a term newborn with kernicterus (see Ahlfors & Herbsman 2003 for clinical details).

after fixation differentiates incidental bilirubin staining from kernicterus (Ahdab-Barmada 1987, Ahdab-Barmada & Moossy 1984, Turkel 1990). Staining may be seen in subcortical nuclei (caudate nucleus, putamen, globus pallidus, subthalamic nucleus, substantia nigra), hippocampus (dentate gyrus, Ammon horn), brainstem nuclei (inferior olivary nucleus, the oculomotor nucleus (III), vestibular nucleus (VII), and cochlear nucleus VIII among others), and in the cerebellum (roof nuclei, dentate nucleus) (Ahdab-Barmada 1987, Ahdab-Barmada & Moossy 1984, Becker & Vogel 1948, Claireaux 1950, Claireaux et al 1953, Dublin 1951, Gerrard 1952, Haymaker et al 1961, Malamud 1961, Turkel 1990). The pattern is similar in term and premature human newborns as well as the Gunn rat (Ahdab-Barmada 1987).

Microscopic changes (Fig. 36.7) will depend on the fixation as well as the time between injury and death (Ahdab-Barmada & Moossy 1984, Becker & Vogel 1948, Gerrard 1950, Turkel 1990). Early changes include vacuolated spongy neuropil (Turkel 1983), neuronal cytoplasmic microvascuolization, loss of Nissl substance, and alterations of cytoplasmic and nuclear membrane (Ahdab-Barmada & Moossy 1984). Certain neurons (e.g. Purkinje cells) may be swollen and contain periodic acid–schiff-positive granules, cytoplasmic vacuoles sometimes containing yellow granules, and yellow cytoplasm which is seen in better preserved cells (Ahdab-Barmada & Moossy 1984). Irreversible damage is indicated by focal cytoplasmic alterations with cellular dissolution or hyperchromasia, increased nuclear density,

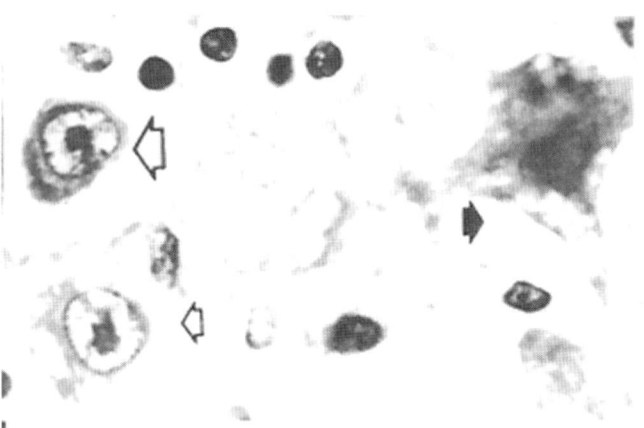

Figure 36.7 Microscopic changes in neurons of the oculomotor nerve nucleus (hematoxylin-eosin, oil immersion × 1600). The large arrow indicates a relatively well preserved neuron. The small arrow indicates a neuron with early vacuolization and loss of Nissl substance. The dark arrow indicates a neuron with increased nuclear density and an irregular nuclear membrane. (From Ahdab-Barmada M 1983 Neonatal kernicterus: Neuropathologic diagnosis. In: Levine R L, Maisels M J (eds) Hyperbilirubinemia in the newborn. Report of the eighty-fifth Ross conference on pediatric research. Ross Laboratories, Columbus, Ohio, pp. 11–16, with permission).

membrane (nuclear and cytoplasmic) fragmentation (Ahdab-Barmada & Moossy 1984). Granular mineralization, neuronal loss, astrocytosis and gliosis are late findings (Ahdab-Barmada & Moossy 1984, Malamud 1961). Bilirubin associated with hypoxia–ischemia injury may result in overlap that may be impossible to apportion (Ahdab-Barmada 1987, Turkel 1990).

CLINICAL ASPECTS OF KERNICTERUS

RISK FACTORS

Gestation, genetics, concurrent illness, and difficulties in extra-uterine transition and adaptation may predispose jaundiced newborns to ABE.

Gestation

Kernicterus occurs at lower TBCs as gestation decreases (Gartner et al 1970, Govaert et al 2003, Harris et al 1958, Oh et al 2003, Pearlman 1978, Stern & Denton 1965) (Table 36.2). This is partly explained by the correspondingly lower albumin levels (Ahlfors 1994, Hyvarinen et al 1973) and the transient impairment of bilirubin-albumin binding following birth (Kapitulnik et al 1975, Ritter & Kenny 1986), which may be further compromised by concurrent illness (Cashore 1980, Ebbesen et al 1986, Reynolds & Cluff 1960). Premature newborns are more likely to receive drugs that interfere with bilirubin-albumin binding, which may cause kernicterus (Ahlfors 2001b, 2004, Ritter et al 1982, Robertson et al 1991, Silverman et al 1956). Their reduced body fat may also deprive them of a tissue bilirubin 'buffer' causing a higher percentage of the miscible bilirubin pool to reside in the brain.

Genetics

The role of genetics in HDN and Crigler–Najjar syndrome is well documented, but additional genetic factors may also increase the risk of kernicterus (Hansen et al 1997, Kaplan et al 1998, 2003, Watchko 2006, Watchko et al 2002).

Increased bilirubin production (hemolysis) caused by G6PD deficiency figured heavily in the recent spate of kernicterus (Ahlfors & Herbsman 2003, Frank 2005, Penn et al 1994, Slusher et al 1995). Other red cell defects causing increased bilirubin production are pyruvate kinase deficiency (Zanella et al 2005), hereditary spherocytosis (Berardi et al 2006) and hereditary elliptocytosis (Delauney 2006). Elevated bilirubin production has also been reported with Down syndrome (Kaplan et al 1999).

Although less recognized, genetics also affects bilirubin-albumin binding. Genetically determined variation in plasma albumin levels (Ahlfors 1994, Hyvarinen et al 1973) and albumin polymorphism (Lorey et al 1985) causes highly variable bilirubin binding in newborn plasma (Ahlfors & Parker 2005, Ahlfors et al 2006). This is a major contributor to the poor correlation between the TBC and kernicterus (Ahlfors 2001a, Ahlfors & Herbsman 2003).

Genetic polymorphism is common in UGT 1A1, the hepatic enzyme that conjugates bilirubin (Kaplan et al 2003,

Monaghan et al 1999). The enzyme is missing in Crigler–Najjar syndrome (Strauss et al 2006) and low but inducible with barbiturates in Crigler–Najjar Type II (Petit et al 2006). The hepatic isoform associated with Gilbert syndrome is associated with increased delay in bilirubin excretion and larger bilirubin loads (Kaplan et al 2003). Similar UGT1A1 polymorphisms in the Asian population may explain their higher TBC levels (Yoshihiro et al 2000).

Incidental conditions

Hypoxia–ischemia as noted above (Ebbesen & Knudsen 1992) and impaired albumin binding with illness (Ebbesen et al 1986, Reynolds & Cluff 1960) may predispose to bilirubin neurotoxicity. Infection in general (Ebbesen & Knudsen 1993, Hamilton & Sass-Kortsak 1963, Ng & Rawstron 1971, Pearlman et al 1980) and specifically with the TORCH group (cytomegalovirus, toxoplasmosis, syphilis, herpes, or rubella) (Epps et al 1995) may be associated with excessive jaundice. Maternal diabetes (Bucalo et al 1984), and polycythemia, bruising, or cephalohematoma may lead to excessive bilirubin production and increased risk of kernicterus (Johnson et al 2002, Maisels & Newman 1995). Acidosis does not alter plasma bilirubin-albumin binding at bilirubin/albumin molar ratios less than one (Nelson et al 1974, Yeung & Wong 1992), but in vitro (Nelson et al 1974, Wennberg 1988) and animal data (Hansen et al 1989, Wennberg et al 1991) suggest acidosis (particularly hypercarbia) increases susceptibility of neural tissues to bilirubin toxicity.

Poor transition/adaptation

Difficulty with breast feeding has been associated with the recent resurgence of kernicterus (Bhutani & Johnson 2003, Maisels & Newman 1995). Delayed passage of meconium, enhanced enterohepatic circulation (Hansen 1997) and inhibition of bilirubin conjugation are likely contributors (Gartner & Herschel et al 2001, Yoshihiro et al 2000). Kernicterus prevention clearly includes ongoing support and monitoring of nursing mothers and their newborns, particularly when discharged early (American Academy of Pediatrics Committee on Fetus and Newborn 2004).

CLINICAL MANIFESTATIONS OF BILIRUBIN TOXICITY

TERM NEWBORN

Symptoms and sequelae vary depending on the specific brain areas targeted and associated conditions. The clinical findings presented below are 'typical' but the clinical presentation may be quite varied (Volpe 2001). ABE usually begins in a previously healthy but jaundiced newborn as a prodrome of increasing lethargy accompanied by poor feeding, drowsiness and hypotonia (Ahlfors & Herbsman 2003, Gerrard 1952, Mollen et al 2004, Volpe 2001). A shrill or high pitched cry may be noted (Vohr et al 1989), which worsens as the baby becomes more irritable and displays intermittent hyper- and hypotonic changes in tone often

accompanied by retrocollis or opisthotonus. Stupor or coma, paralysis of upward gaze ('setting sun' sign), fever, hemorrhage (often pulmonary), and seizures are all signs of severe toxicity (Table 36.1). Cardio-respiratory collapse heralds the baby's demise (Ahlfors & Herbsman 2003, Mollen 2004), often accompanied by a rapid fall in TBC (Ahlfors & Herbsman 2003, Harris et al 1958). The 'low' TBC may cause kernicterus to be overlooked in the differential diagnosis despite suggestive symptoms.

ABE is a clinical diagnosis, and imaging is being used increasingly to aid in the diagnosis (Coskun et al 2004, Govaert et al 2003, Harris et al 2001, Ives et al 1988, Oakden et al 2005, 2006, Paksoy et al 2004, Penn et al 1994) (Fig. 36.8). Bilirubin-induced MRI changes may lessen over time (Okumura et al 2006), but this should not be construed as evidence that kernicterus did not occur (Newman 2000). ABR (Fig. 36.5) and visual evoked potentials may also be helpful (Ahlfors 1985, AlOtaibi et al 2005, Amin et al 2001, Chen & Wong 2006, Chin et al 1985, Chisin et al 1979, de Vries et al 1987, Funato et al 1994, Kaga et al 1979, Nakamura et al 1992, Nwaesei et al 1984, 1985, Shapiro et al 2006, Wennberg et al 1982).

Subtle BIND, particularly auditory neuropathy/dyssynchrony (AN/AD), has emerged to complicate matters (Berg et al 2005, de Vries et al 1987, Govaert et al 2003, Johnson & Boggs 1974, Odell et al 1970, Oh et al 2003, Salamy et al 1989, Shapiro 2003, 2005, Shapiro et al 2006, Stein et al 1996). AN/AD is characterized by normal otoacoustic emissions but abnormal or absent ABR (Chisin et al 1979, Kaga et al 1979, Stein et al 1996). Undiagnosed sequelae secondary to BIND may emerge as our ability to detect subtle neurological deficits improves (Shapiro 2005, Shapiro et al 2006).

Neurological sequelae of ABE correspond to the areas of the brain stained yellow at autopsy (Claireaux 1950, Gerrard 1952, Merhar & Gilbert 2005, Perlstein 1960, Van Praagh 1961). The classic 'tetrad' includes athetosis or choreoathetosis, paralysis of upward gaze, deafness or high pitch hearing loss and linear staining of deciduous teeth (Perlstein 1960). However, given variable sequelae and advances in treatment, it may be more relevant to classify them as movement (extrapyramidal), perceptual (e.g. auditory, visual) and functional (e.g. gastrointestinal, emotional) sequelae (Shapiro 2003, 2005, Shapiro et al 2006). The movement disorders may improve with age (Gerrard 1952, Perlstein 1961).

PREMATURE NEWBORNS

Symptoms of ABE are usually non-specific or absent. Lethargy, seizures, apnea, oxygen desaturation, and unstable vital signs associated with kernicterus are also common with hypoxia–ischemia, metabolic or respiratory acidosis, or infection. A high degree of suspicion, comprehensive laboratory assessment, and close follow-up of hearing and development are needed. Auditory sequelae are particularly common and often the only bilirubin sequelae found with prematurity (de Vries et al 1987, Oh et al 2003, Salamy et al 1989, Volpe 2001). Bilirubin neurotoxicity may also

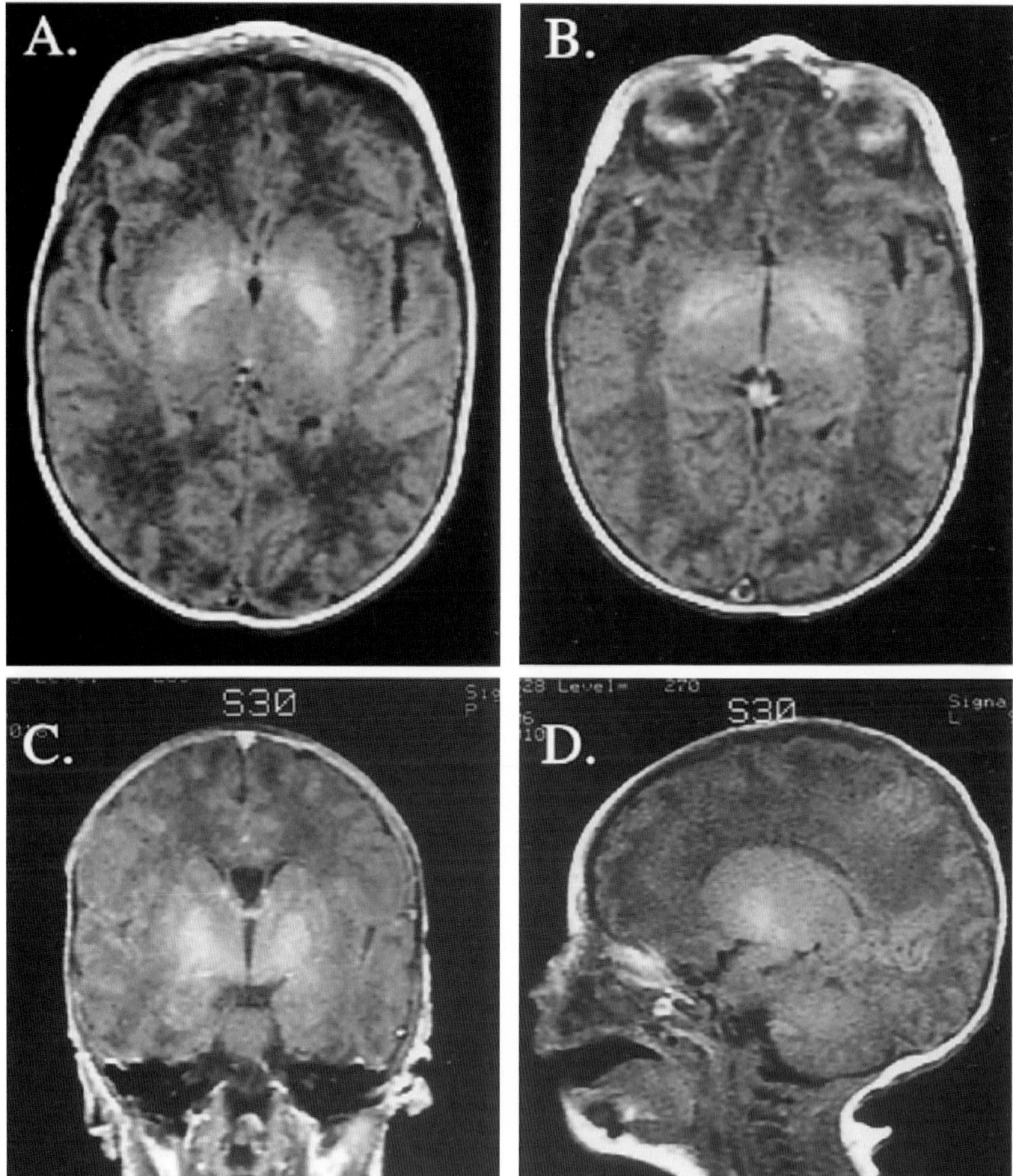

Figure 36.8 Magnetic resonance imaging in a 6 day old 37 week gestation male with kernicterus (peak TBC 36 mg/dL). A and B are axial T₁-weighted images (TR = 500, TE = 12); C is coronal (TR = 600,TE = 34), and D is sagittal (TR = 450, TE = 12). Note the bilateral increase in intensity of the globus pallidus. (From Shapiro S M 2003 Bilirubin toxicity in the developing nervous system. Pediatr Neurol 29:410–421, with permission.)

contribute to the spastic diplegia that accompanies anoxic brain injury in the premature infant (Perlstein 1960).

EVALUATION OF THE JAUNDICED NEWBORN

ABE may be reversible with timely intervention (Table 36.1) after the onset of symptoms up to a point (Bhutani et al 2006, Harris et al 2001, Johnson et al 2002). However, as symptoms progress, recovery with treatment is less likely (Table 36.1), and efforts should be directed at interrupting the progression of jaundice before potentially toxic levels of bilirubin occur (Table 36.2).

The medical history may provide important clues about the likelihood of excessive jaundice, and note should be taken of previous siblings or genetic conditions associated with jaundice. Pregnancy complications, maternal medications (Forna et al 2006), or maternal illnesses (Bucalo et al 1984) may also predispose to kernicterus. Difficulties with labor and delivery, low Apgar scores, and the need for resuscitation may lead to bruising, cephalohematomas, lethargy and poor breast feeding, all of which may place the baby at increased risk for kernicterus (Johnson et al 2002, Maisels & Newman 1995).

Haphazard nursery protocols for managing newborn jaundice add to the likelihood a jaundiced newborn may 'fall through the cracks' (Bhutani et al 2006). Visual assessment of jaundice or clinical risk scores correlate poorly with the TBC (Keren et al 2005, Moyer et al 2000, Riskin et al 2003). However, a screening TBC or transcutaneous bilirubin measurement (Yamanouchi et al 1980) early in life (Bhutani et al 1999, 2000) may be reliable and cost effective (Eggert et al 2006). The screening TBC is compared with the hour-specific TBC nomogram (Bhutani et al 1999) shown in Figure 36.9 to assess the likelihood of subsequent 'hyperbilirubinemia'. The drawbacks are: (1) the sensitivity and specificity of the hour-specific TBC as a predictor of subsequent 'hyperbilirubinemia' are not particularly robust (Keren et al 2005) and (2) variability in bilirubin-albumin binding confounds the correlation between TBC and the size of the miscible bilirubin pool (Ahlfors 2001a, 2004).

Laboratory blood tests

The TBC is the standard laboratory blood test used to evaluate jaundiced newborns. The American Academy of Pediatrics guidelines (American Academy of Pediatrics Committee on Fetus and Newborn 2004) recommend that the TBC and albumin be used to guide treatment decisions (Fig. 36.10). Elevated conjugated bilirubin levels usually indicate disorders of the liver and biliary tree but do not preclude the development of kernicterus (Bertini et al 2005, Kaplan et al 1998, Poláček 1966, Smith et al 2004). The lack of precision and accuracy in clinical laboratory bilirubin measurements

Table 36.2 Exchange transfusion criteria for jaundiced newborns. For the total bilirubin and bilirubin/albumin ratio, the lower of the two numbers separated by the semicolon (;) is used if any of the indicated risk factors are present. For B_f, the two numbers represent the range of values occurring over the corresponding weight range. The B_f criteria for an individual baby is the weight in kg multiplied by 13 or 100 depending on whether B_f is measured at a 42-fold or 2-fold ('undiluted') plasma dilution. Exchange transfusion should be considered as soon as any of the criteria are met. A commercially available device measures B_f at a 42-fold sample dilution (Ahlfors et al 2007). (Adapted from Ahlfors 1994 Criteria for exchange transfusion in jaundiced newborns. Pediatrics 93:488–494, with permission.)

Birth weight (Kg)	Total bilirubin mg/dL (µmol/L)	Bilirubin/albumin ratio mg/g (molar ratio)	B_f nmol/L Range	
			42-fold Plasma dilution	2-fold Plasma dilution
<1	10 (171)	4 (0.45)	22	100
1–1.249	10;13* (171;222)	4;5.2* (0.45;0.59)	22–27**	100–125**
1.25–1.499	13;15 (222;256)	5.2;6.0 (0.59;0.68)	27–33	125–150
1.5–1.999	15;17 (256;291)	6.0,6.8 (0.68–0.77)	33–44	150–200
2–2.499	17;18 (291;308)	6.8,7.2 (0.77–0.81)	44–55	200–250
>2.5 and >35 weeks gestation	18;25 or 30 (308;427 or 513)	7.2–8.0 (0.81–0.90)	55–70	250–350

*Use the lower number when any of the following risk factors are present.
Risk factors: Apgar <3 at 5 minutes; PaO_2 < 40 torr ≥2 h; pH ≤ 7.15 for ≥1 h; hemolysis; clinical or central nervous system deterioration
**Range of B_f values over the corresponding weight range. The individual Bf criterion is the weight in Kg multiplied by 22 nmol/L (42-fold plasma dilution) or 100 (2-fold plasma dilution) up to a maximum of 70 or 350 nmol/L, respectively (Ahlfors & Herbsman 2003).

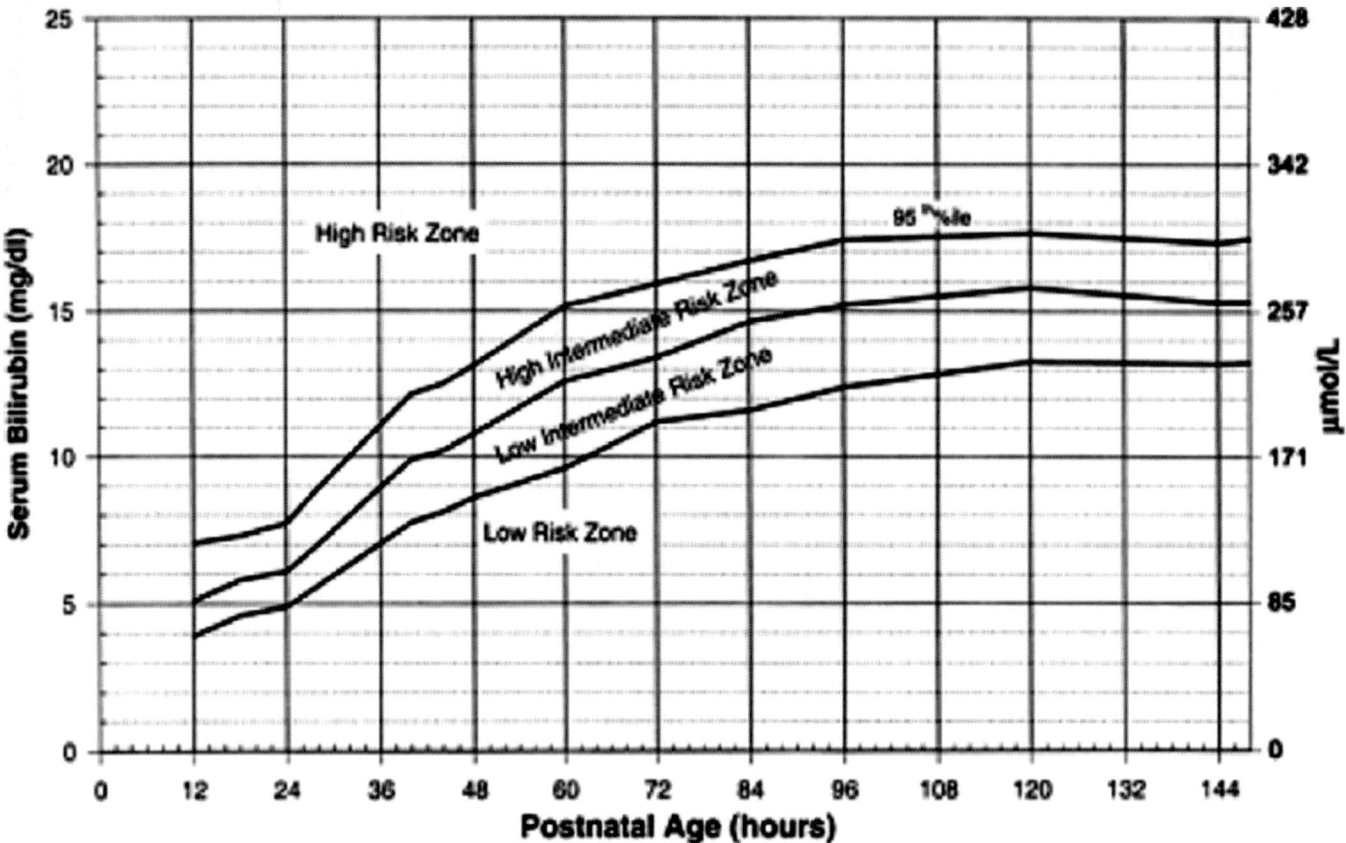

Figure 36.9 Bhutani hour-specific nomogram for bilirubin levels in term and near term newborns. Newborns with hour-specific TBC values in the higher percentiles are more likely to develop 'hyperbilirubinemia' (From Bhutani V K, Johnson L, Sivieri E M 1999 Predictive ability of a predischarge hour-specific serum bilirubin for subsequent significant hyperbilirubinemia in healthy term and near-term newborns. Pediatrics 103:6–14, with permission.)

remains a concern (Bhutani & Johnson 2004), and the presence of bilirubin photoisomers generated during PT may further confound TBC measurements (McDonagh 2006).

The TBC/albumin ratio, a surrogate measure of bilirubin-albumin binding (Ahlfors 1994, American Academy of Pediatrics Committee on Fetus and Newborn 2004, Amin et al 2001, Govaert et al 2003) is being used increasingly as an adjunct when evaluating jaundiced newborns (Fig. 36.10). A commercially available device for measuring TBC and B_f is available (Shimabuku & Nakamura 1982), but B_f, although potentially very useful (Ahlfors & Herbsman 2003), is not routinely measured by clinical laboratories. B_f measurements by the peroxidase method have recently been validated for use in organelle or tissue culture studies of bilirubin toxicity (Burgos et al 2006).

Table 36.2 provides an internally consistent and integrated approach for using TBC, albumin, and B_f when assessing jaundice. It should be noted that because bilirubin-albumin binding changes with dilution (Ahlfors 1982) the B_f values in Table 36.2 are substantially lower if plasma is diluted prior to B_f measurement (Ahlfors 1982, Ahlfors et al 2006). Establishing population norms for B_f and K would help make the use of routine B_f measurements feasible (Ahlfors 2004, Wennberg et al 2006).

For reasons previously stated, the direct antiglobulin test (DAT or Coombs test), G6PD screening, hematocrit/hemoglobin, reticulocyte count, and blood smear are commonly used tests in the evaluation of newborn jaundice.

Non-invasive tests

Transcutaneous bilirubinometry (Bhutani et al 2000, Yamanouchi et al 1980) uses skin light reflectance to estimate the TBC and is better than visual assessment of jaundice (Moyer et al 2000, Riskin et al 2003). It correlates fairly well with TBCs to at least 11 and perhaps as high as 18 mg/dL (Bhutani et al 2000, Nanjundaswamy et al 2004). It also reduces the total number of blood draws in premature newborns (De Luca et al 2006).

CO in exhaled gases correlates with the bilirubin production in newborns (Stevenson et al 2001). A commercial device developed for this measurement is no longer available but the measurement appears clinically useful (Herschel et al 2002).

The ABR has evolved from a sophisticated research tool (Chisin et al 1979, Kaga et al 1979) to a widely used screening test for newborn hearing (Korres et al 2006). This technology has been used to study the toxic effects of bilirubin

Phototherapy

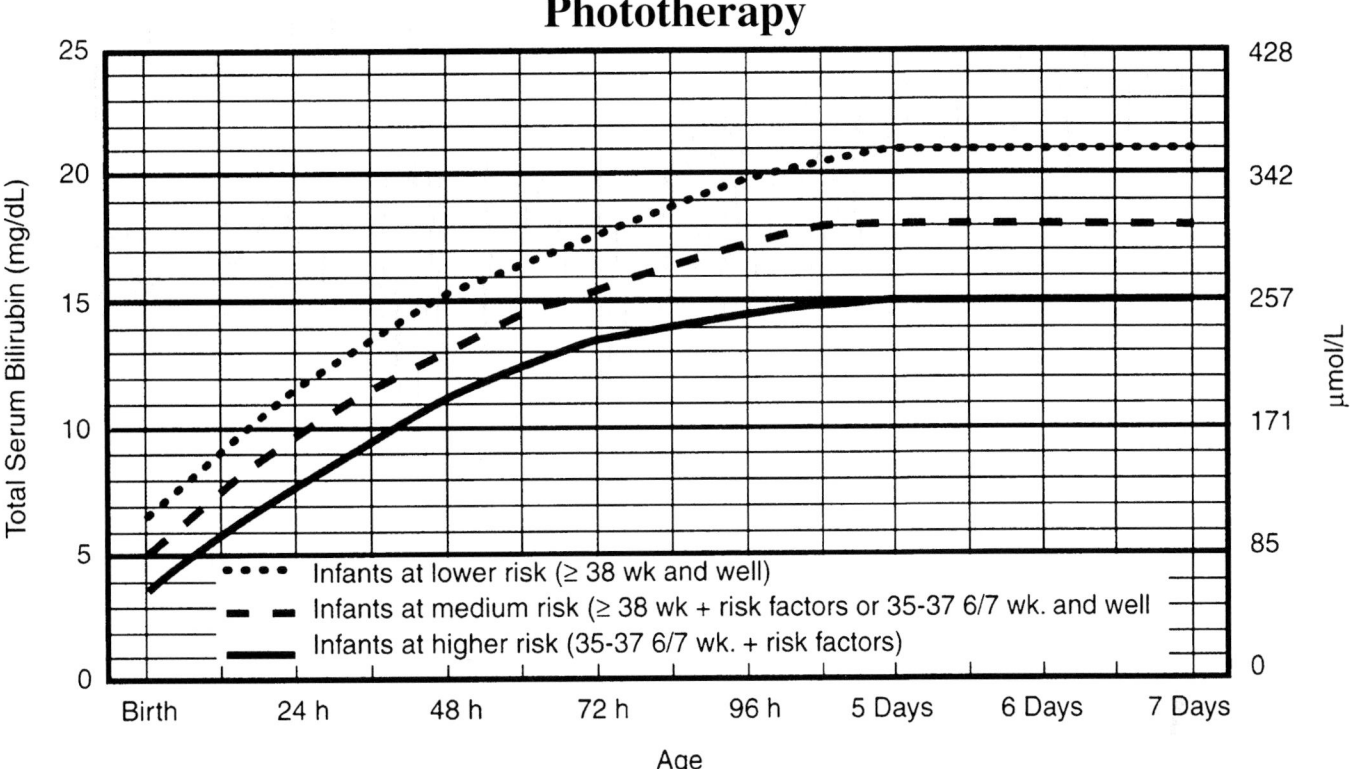

- Use total bilirubin. Do not subtract direct reacting or conjugated bilirubin.
- Risk factors = isoimmune hemolytic disease, G6PD deficiency, asphyxia, significant lethargy, temperature instability, sepsis, acidosis, or albumin < 3.0g/dL (if measured)
- For well infants 35-37 6/7 wk can adjust TSB levels for intervention around the medium risk line. It is an option to intervene at lower TSB levels for infants closer to 35 wks and at higher TSB levels for those closer to 37 6/7 wk.
- It is an option to provide conventional phototherapy in hospital or at home at TSB levels 2-3 mg/dL (35-50mmol/L) below those shown but home phototherapy should not be used in any infant with risk factors.

Figure 36.10 American Academy of Pediatrics guideline for intervention with phototherapy in term and near term newborns based on age in hours. (From American Academy of Pediatrics Subcommittee on Hyperbilirubinemia 2004 Management of hyperbilirubinemia in the newborn infant 35 or more weeks of gestation. Pediatrics 114:297–316, with permission)

on the auditory system (Chisin et al 1979, Wennberg et al 1982) (Fig. 36.5) and has exposed AN/AD as a previously unappreciated sequela of BIND (Shapiro 2005). Bilirubin induced ABR changes have been used to support the hypothesis that B_f improves the diagnosis of bilirubin neurotoxicity (Amin et al 2001, Funato et al 1994). The beneficial effects of ET have been documented with ABR (Bhandari et al 1993, Deliac et al 1990, Kuriyama et al 1986, Nwaesei et al 1984, Wennberg et al 1982). Behavioral changes (Brazelton Test) correlate with ABR changes occurring in jaundiced newborns (Vohr et al 1990), and ABR may be useful in detecting bilirubin toxicity in the presence of high level conjugated bilirubin (Smith et al 2004). It is conceivable that the automated ABR used for hearing screening could be adapted for dedicated use in evaluating jaundiced newborns (Ahlfors & Parker 2008, Shapiro et al 2006).

Magnetic resonance imaging has substantiated injury to the globus pallidus and subthalamic nucleus during acute bilirubin encephalopathy (Coskun et al 2004, Govaert et al 2003, Harris et al 2001, Merhar & Gilbert 2005, Penn et al 1994, Yilmaz & Ekinci 2002) (Fig. 36.8). Advances in this area are likely to further improve the detection of ABE (Groenendaal et al 2004, Oakden et al 2005, Okumura et al 2006, Paksoy et al 2004), although some continue to question the use of either magnetic resonance imaging or ABR in the diagnosis of acute or impending bilirubin encephalopathy (Newman & Maisels 2002).

TREATMENT OF NEWBORN JAUNDICE

ET is an effective, invasive and inherently risky procedure (Jackson 1997). The lack of agreement as to when it should be used underscores the poor correlation between TBC and kernicterus (Gartner et al 1998). Even when the TBC reaches levels where ET is recommended, PT and other less invasive interventions are often used to try to circumvent the need for ET (Hansen et al 1997). ET is particularly difficult in the tiny premature baby, and even at excessive TBC levels is often withheld with encouragement to do so from the literature (Watchko & Claassen 1994). Valaes (1963) has described in detail the mechanics, dynamics and technique of ET and its impact on the miscible bilirubin pool. ET has been shown to significantly lower B_f (Arkans & Cassidy 1978).

Phototherapy

PT significantly reduces the TBC when light with an action spectrum in the 400 to 520 nm wavelength range and intensity near 35 $\mu W/cm^2$ per nm at the skin is used (Maisels 1996). It is primarily used to prevent the TBC from reaching levels of concern and as a temporizing measure while preparing for ET (American Academy of Pediatrics Committee on Fetus and Newborn 2004, Hansen 1997).

PT works primarily by converting bilirubin in the skin to configurational and structural isomers (Fig. 36.3) that are readily excreted through the liver and kidneys. Lumirubin is most important in TBC reduction in humans (Ennever et al 1987) while the configurational isomers appear more important in the Gunn rat. In the latter, PT is enhanced by oral agents that trap the configurational isomers in the gut (Hafkamp et al 2006), but this approach might be less beneficial in humans. Although up to 30% of the plasma TBC may be photoisomers, their contribution to the composition of B_f is unknown (McDonagh 2006).

Barbiturates have been used pre- or postpartum with mixed results to try to up-regulate UGT1A1 and increase bilirubin excretion (Arya et al 2004, Kumar et al 2002, Murki et al 2005). Albumin infusion prior to ET to extract bilirubin from the tissue fraction of the miscible bilirubin pool does not improve the efficiency of the ET (Valaes 1963). Attention should be paid to stabilizing vital signs and reversing acidosis, shock, or hypoxia–ischemia when present.

SUMMARY

The relationship between kernicterus and bilirubin chemistry and metabolism is complex and poorly understood. The exact levels of bilirubin that cause kernicterus and why only selected areas of the brain are injured are also unknown. Many genetic and other clinical factors impact on whether a baby will develop kernicterus, and care is best directed at preventing excessive bilirubin loads. The TBC, which is the standard laboratory test used to assess newborn jaundice, is not a particularly specific indicator of risk. Measurements of B_f, albumin, CO and ABR as well as MRI images may be helpful in detecting kernicterus when the diagnosis is in doubt. Treatment of jaundice is usually precautionary and almost always unnecessary in otherwise healthy term newborns (Newman et al 2006). However, even non-invasive PT may have negative and lasting social impacts on the family (Hansen et al 1991, 2001, Willis et al 2002). All jaundiced newborns are at risk for kernicterus. We are in the process of discovering why in hopes of finding innovative and creative ways to prevent it (Ross 2003, Wennberg et al 2006), much like our colleagues who faced the tragedy of icterus gravis neonatorum over 100 years ago.

REFERENCES

Abbott N J 2004 Evidence for bulk flow of brain interstitial fluid: significance for physiology and pathology. Neurochem Int 45:545–552.

Ackerman B D, Dyer G Y, Leydorf M M 1970 Hyperbilirubinemia and kernicterus in small premature infants. Pediatrics 45:918–925.

Ahdab-Barmada M 1983 Neonatal kernicterus: Neuropathologic diagnosis. In: Levine R L, Maisels M J (eds) Hyperbilirubinemia in the newborn. Report of the eighty-fifth Ross conference on pediatric research. Ross Laboratories, Columbus, Ohio, pp. 11–16.

Ahdab-Barmada M 1987 Kernicterus in the premature neonate. J Perinatol 7:149–152.

Ahdab-Barmada M, Moossy J 1984 The neuropathology of kernicterus in the premature neonate: diagnostic problems. J Neuropathol Exp Neurol 43:45–56.

Ahdab-Barmada M, Moosy J 1983 Kernicterus reexamined. Pediatrics 71:463–464.

Ahlfors C E 1982 Effect of serum dilution on apparent unbound bilirubin concentration as measured by the peroxidase method. Clin Chem 27:692–696.

Ahlfors C E 1986 Changes in the auditory brainstem response associated with unconjugated hyperbilirubinemia in the newborn. J Perinatol 6:193–196.

Ahlfors C E 1994 Criteria for exchange transfusion in jaundiced newborns. Pediatrics 93:488–494.

Ahlfors C E 2000 Measurement of plasma unbound unconjugated bilirubin. Anal Biochem 279:130–135.

Ahlfors C E 2001a Bilirubin-albumin binding and free bilirubin. J Perinatol 21:S40–S42.

Ahlfors C E 2001b Benzyl alcohol, kernicterus, and unbound bilirubin. J Pediatr 139:317–319.

Ahlfors C E 2004 Effect of ibuprofen on bilirubin-albumin binding. J Pediatr 144:386–388.

Ahlfors C E, Bennett S H, Shoemaker C T et al 1986 Changes in the auditory brainstem response associated with intravenous infusion of unconjugated bilirubin into infant rhesus monkeys. Pediatr Res 20:511–515.

Ahlfors C E, Herbsman O 2003 Unbound bilirubin in a term newborn with kernicterus. Pediatrics 111:1110–1112.

Ahlfors C E, Parker A E 2005 Evaluation of a model for brain bilirubin uptake in jaundiced newborns. Pediatr Res 58:1175–1179.

Ahlfors C E, Parker A E 2008 unbound bilirubin is associated with abnormal automated auditory brainstem response to jaundiced newborns. Pediatrics 121:976–978.

Ahlfors C E, Shapiro S M 2001 Auditory brainstem response and unbound bilirubin in jaundiced (jj) Gunn rat pups. Biol Neonate 80:158–162.

Ahlfors C E, Shwer M L, Wennberg R P 1982 Absence of bilirubin binding competitors during phototherapy for neonatal jaundice. Early Hum Dev 6:125–130.

Ahlfors C E, Vreman H J, Wong R J et al 2007 Effects of sample dilution, peroxidase concentration, and chloride ion on the measurement of unbound bilirubin in premature newborns. Clin Biochem 40:261–267.

Ahlfors C E, Wennberg R P 2004 Bilirubin-albumin binding and neonatal jaundice. Semin Perinatol 28:334–339.

Aiden R, Corner B, Tove G 1950 Kernicterus and prematurity. Lancet 1:1153–1154.

Alexandra Brito M, Silva R F, Brites D 2006 Bilirubin toxicity to human erythrocytes: A review. Clin Chim Acta 374:46–56.

Allen F H, Diamond L K, Vaughn V C 1950 Erythroblastosis fetalis VI. Prevention of kernicterus. Am J Dis Child 80:779–791.

AlOtaibi S F, Blaser S, MacGregor D L 2005 Neurological complications of kernicterus. Can J Neurol Sci 32:311–315.

American Academy of Pediatrics Committee on Fetus and Newborn 2004 Hospital stay for healthy newborns. Pediatrics 113:1434–1436.

American Academy of Pediatrics Subcommittee on Hyperbilirubinemia 2004 Management of Hyperbilirubinemia in the Newborn Infant 35 or More Weeks of Gestation. Pediatrics 114:297–316.

Amin S B, Ahlfors C, Orlando M S et al 2001 Bilirubin and serial auditory brainstem responses in premature infants. Pediatrics 107:664–670.

Arkans H D, Cassidy G 1978 Estimation of unbound serum bilirubin by the peroxidase assay method:

Effect of exchange transfusion on unbound bilirubin and serum bindings. J Pediatr 92:1001–1005.

Arya V B, Agarwal R, Paul V K, Deorari A K 2004 Efficacy of oral phenobarbitone in term 'at risk' neonates in decreasing neonatal hyperbilirubinemia: a randomized double-blinded, placebo controlled trial. Indian Pediatr 41:327–332.

Bauer H C, Bauer H 2000 Neural induction of the blood-brain barrier: still an enigma. Cell Mol Neurobiol 20:13–28.

Becker P F L, Vogel P 1948 Kernicterus. A review with a report of the findings in a study of seven cases. J Neuropathol Exp Neurol 7:190–215.

Berardi A, Lugli L, Ferrari F et al 2006 Kernicterus associated with hereditary spherocytosis and UGT1A1 promoter polymorphism. Biol Neonate 3090:243–246.

Berg A L, Spitzer J B, Towers H M et al 2005 Newborn hearing screening in the NICU: profile of failed auditory brainstem response/passed otoacoustic emission. Pediatrics 116:933–938.

Berk P D, Bradbury M, Zhou S L et al 1996 Characterization of membrane transport processes: lessons from the study of BSP, bilirubin, and fatty acid uptake. Semin Liver Dis 16:107–120.

Berk P D, Howe R B, Bloomer J R, Berlin N I 1969 Studies of bilirubin kinetics in normal adults. J Clin Invest 48:2176–2190.

Bertini G, Dani C, Fonda C et al 2005 Bronze baby syndrome and the risk of kernicterus. Acta Paediatr 94:968–971.

Bhandari V, Narang A, Mann S B et al 1993 Brain stem electric response audiometry in neonates with hyperbilirubinemia. Indian J Pediatr 60:409–413.

Bhutani V K, Gourley G R, Adler S et al 2000 Noninvasive measurement of total serum bilirubin in a multiracial predischarge newborn population to assess the risk of severe hyperbilirubinemia. Pediatrics 106:e17.

Bhutani V K, Johnson L 2005 Kernicterus: a preventable neonatal brain injury. J Arab Neonatal Forum 2:12–24.

Bhutani V K, Johnson L H 2003 Newborn jaundice and kernicterus–health and societal perspectives. Indian J Pediatr 70:407–416.

Bhutani V K, Johnson L H 2004a Urgent clinical need for accurate and precise bilirubin measurements in the United States to prevent kernicterus. Clin Chem 50:477–480.

Bhutani V K, Johnson L H, Schwoebel A, Gennaro S 2006 A systems approach for neonatal hyperbilirubinemia in term and near-term newborns. J Obstet Gynecol Neonatal Nurs 35:444–455.

Bhutani V K, Johnson L H, Shapiro S M 2004 Kernicterus in sick and preterm infants 1999–2002): A need for an effective preventive approach. Semin Perinatol 28:319–325.

Bhutani V K, Johnson L, Sivieri E M 1999 Predictive ability of a predischarge hour-specific serum bilirubin for subsequent significant hyperbilirubinemia in healthy term and near-term newborns. Pediatrics 103:6–14.

Billing B H 1978 Twenty-five years of progress in bilirubin metabolism (1952–77). Gut 19:481–491.

Blackmon L R, Fanaroff A A, Raju T N, National Institute of Child Health and Human Development 2004 Research on prevention of bilirubin-induced brain injury and kernicterus: National Institute of Child Health and Human Development conference executive summary. Pediatrics 114:229–233.

Blanc W A, Johnson L 1959 Studies on kernicterus; relationship with sulfonamide intoxication, report on kernicterus in rats with glucuronyl transferase

deficiency and review of pathogenesis. J Neuropathol Exp Neurol 18:165–187.

Boiadjiev S, Watters K, Wolf S et al 2004 pK$_a$ and aggregation of bilirubin: Titrimetric and ultracentrifugation studies on water-soluble pegylated conjugates of bilirubin and fatty acids. Biochemistry 43:15617–15632.

Bonnett R, Davies J E, Hursthouse M B 1976 Structure of bilirubin. Nature 262:327–328.

Brann B S 4th, Stonestreet B S, Oh W, Cashore W J 1987 The in vivo effect of bilirubin and sulfisoxazole on cerebral oxygen, glucose, and lactate metabolism in newborn piglets. Pediatr Res 22:135–140.

Bratlid D 1972 Bilirubin binding by human erythrocytes. Scand J Clin Lab Invest 29:91–97.

Brodersen R 1966 Dimerisation of bilirubin anion in aqueous solution. Acta Chem Scand 20:2895–2896.

Brodersen R 1972 Supersaturation with bilirubin followed by colloid formation and disposition, with a hypothesis on the etiology of kernicterus. J Clin Lab Invest 29:447–452.

Brodersen R 1972a Localization of the bilirubin pools in the non-jaundiced rat with a note on bilirubin dynamics in normal human adults and in Gilbert's syndrome. Scand J clin Lab Invest 30:95–106.

Brodersen R 1979 Bilirubin. Solubility and interaction with albumin and phospholipid. J Biol Chem 254:2364–2369.

Brodersen R 1979a Binding of bilirubin to albumin: implications for prevention of bilirubin encephalopathy in the newborn. CRC Crit Rev Clin Lab Sci 11:305–399.

Brodersen R 1980 Bilirubin transport in the newborn infant, reviewed with relation to kernicterus. J Pediatr 96:349–356.

Brodersen R, Funding A, Perdersen A O, Röigaard-Pertersen H 1972 Binding of bilirubin to low-affinity sites of human serum albumin in vitro followed by co-crystallization. Scand J Clin Lab Invest 29:443–446.

Brodersen R, Stern L 1987 Aggregation of bilirubin in injectates and incubation media: its significance in experimental studies of CNS toxicity. Neuropediatrics 18:24–36.

Brodersen R, Stern L 1990 Deposition of bilirubin acid in the central nervous system–a hypothesis for the development of kernicterus. Acta Paediatr Scand 79:12–19.

Brodersen R, Theilgaard J 1969 Bilirubin colloid formation in neutral aqueous solution. Scand J Clin Lab Invest 24:395–398.

Brown A K, Johnson L L 1996 Loss of concern about jaundice and the re-emergence of kernicterus in full-term infants in the era of managed care. In: Fanaroff A A, Klaus M H (eds) The yearbook of neonatal and perinatal medicine. Mosby: St. Louis, Mo, pp. 17–28.

Brown A K, Zuelzer W W 1957 Studies in hyperbilirubinemia, I: hyperbilirubinemia of the newborn unrelated to isoimmunization. Am J Dis Child 93:263–273.

Brown A K, Zuelzer W W, Robinson A R 1957a Studies in hyperbilirubinemia. II. Clearance of bilirubin from plasma and extravascular space in newborn infants during exchange transfusion. AMA J Dis Child 93:274–286.

Bucalo L R, Cohen R S, Ostrander C R et al 1984 Pulmonary excretion of carbon monoxide in the human infant as an index of bilirubin production. IIc. Evidence for the possible association of cord blood erythropoietin levels and postnatal bilirubin production in infants of mothers with abnormalities of gestational glucose metabolism. Am J Perinatol 1:177–181.

Burgos L R, Calligaris S, Wennberg R P et al 2006 Factors affecting the binding of bilirubin to serum albumins: validation and application of the peroxidase method. Pediatr Res 60:1–5.

Carey M C, Koretsky A P 1979 Self-association of unconjugated bilirubin-IX alpha in aqueous solution at pH 10.0 and physical-chemical interactions with bile salt monomers and micelles. Biochem J 179:675–689.

Cashore W J 1980 Free bilirubin concentrations and bilirubin-binding affinity in term and preterm infants. J Pediatr 96:521–527.

Cashore W J, Oh W 1982 Unbound bilirubin and kernicterus in low-birth-weight infants. Pediatrics 69:481–485.

Chen W X, Wong V 2006 Visual evoked potentials in neonatal hyperbilirubinemia. J Child Neurol 21:58–62.

Chin K C, Taylor M J, Perlman M 1985 Improvement in auditory and visual evoked potentials in jaundiced preterm infants after exchange transfusion. Arch Dis Child 60:714–717.

Chisin R, Perlman M, Sohmer H 1979 Cochlear and brain stem responses in hearing loss following neonatal hyperbilirubinemia. Ann Otol Rhinol Laryngol 88:352–357.

Churn S B, Taft W C, DeLorenzo R J 1990 Effects of ischemia on multifunctional calcium/calmodulin-dependent protein kinase type II in the gerbil. Stroke 21(Suppl):III112–III116.

Claireaux A 1950 Haemolytic disease of the newborn: A pathological study of 157 cases. Arch Dis Child 25:61–80.

Claireaux A E, Cole P G, Lathe G H 1953 Icterus of the brain in the newborn. Lancet 1:1226–1230.

Conlee J W, Shapiro S M, Churn S B 2000 Expression of the alpha and beta subunits of Ca2+/calmodulin kinase II in the cerebellum of jaundiced Gunn rats during development: a quantitative light microscopic analysis. Acta Neuropathol (Berl) 99:393–401.

Coskun A, Yikilmaz A, Kumandas S et al 2004 Hyperintense globus pallidus on T1-weighted MR imaging in acute kernicterus: is it common or rare? Eur Radiol 15:1263–1267.

Cremer R J, Perryman P W, Richards D H 1958 Influence of light on the hyperbilirubinaemia of infants. Lancet 1:1094–1097.

Crigler J F, Najjar V A 1952 Congenital familial nonhemolytic jaundice with kernicterus. Pediatrics 10:169–180.

Crosse V M, Meyer T C, Gerrard J W 1955 Kernicterus and prematurity. Arch Dis Childh 30:501–508.

Crosse V M, Wallis P G, Walsh A 1958 Replacement transfusion as a means of preventing kernicterus of prematurity. Arch Dis Child 33:403–408.

Dallas S, Miller D S, Bendayan R 2006 Multidrug resistance-associated proteins: expression and function in the central nervous system Pharmacol Rev 58:140–161.

Daood M J, Watchko J F 2006 Calculated in vivo free bilirubin levels in the central nervous system of Gunn rat pups. Pediatr Res 60:44–49.

Davis D R, Yeary R A 1975 Effects of sulfadimethoxine on tissue distribution of (14C)bilirubin in the newborn and adult hyperbilirubinemic Gunn rat. Pediatr Res 9:846–850.

Day R L 1954 Inhibition of brain respiration in vitro by bilirubin; reversal of inhibition by various means. Proc Soc Exp Biol Med 85:261–164.

De Luca D, Zecca E, de Turris P et al 2006 Using Bilicheck® for preterm neonates in a sub-intensive unit: Diagnostic usefulness and suitability. Early Hum Dev Aug 31, [Epub ahead of print].

de Vries L S, Lary S, Whitelaw A G, Dubowitz L M 1987 Relationship of serum bilirubin levels and hearing impairment in newborn infants. Early Hum Dev 15:269–277.

Delaunay J 2006 The molecular basis of hereditary red cell membrane disorders. Blood Rev 25, [Epub ahead of print].

Deliac P, Demarquez J L, Barberot J P et al 1990 Brainstem auditory evoked potentials in icteric fullterm newborns: alterations after exchange transfusion. Neuropediatrics 21:115–118.

Diamond I, Schmid R 1966 Experimental bilirubin encephalopathy. The mode of entry of bilirubin-14C into the central nervous system. J Clin Invest 45:678–689.

Diamond L K 1948 Replacement transfusion as a treatment for erythroblastosis fetalis. Pediatrics 2:520–524.

Dublin W B 1951 Neurologic lesions of erythroblastosis fetalis in relation to nuclear deafness. Am J Clin Pathol 21:935–939.

Ebbesen F 2000 Recurrence of kernicterus in term and near-term infants in Denmark. Acta Paediatr 89:1213–1217.

Ebbesen F, Foged N, Brodersen R 1986 Reduced albumin binding of MADDS–a measure for bilirubin binding–in sick children. Acta Paediatr Scand 75:550–554.

Ebbesen F, Knudsen A 1992 The possible risk of bilirubin encephalopathy as predicted by plasma parameters in neonates with previous severe asphyxia. Eur J Pediatr 151:910–912.

Ebbesen F, Knudsen A 1993 The risk of bilirubin encephalopathy, as estimated by plasma parameters, in neonates strongly suspected of having sepsis. Acta Paediatr 82:26–29.

Eberhard B A, Drew J H 1994 Perhaps vigintiphobia should only apply to infants with Rhesus erythroblastosis. J Paediatr Child Health 30:341–344.

Eggert L D, Wiedmeier S E, Wilson J, Christensen R D 2006 The effect of instituting a prehospital-discharge newborn bilirubin screening program in an 18-hospital health system. Pediatrics 117:e855–e862.

Ennever J F, Costarino A T, Polin R A, Speck W T 1987 Rapid clearance of a structural isomer of bilirubin during phototherapy. J Clin Invest 79:1674–1678.

Epps R E, Pittelkow M R, Su W P 1995 TORCH syndrome. Semin Dermatol 14:179–186.

Eriksen E F, Danielsen H, Brodersen R 1981 Bilirubin-liposome interaction. J Biol Chem 256:4269–4274.

Ernster L, Zetterstrom R 1956 Bilirubin, an uncoupler of oxidative phosphorylation in isolated mitchondria. Nature 178:1335–1337.

Falcao A S, Fernandes A, Brito M A et al 2006 Bilirubin-induced immunostimulant effects and toxicity vary with neural cell type and maturation state. Acta Neuropathol (Berl) 112:95–105.

Fernandes A, Falcao A S, Silva R F et al 2006 Inflammatory signalling pathways involved in astroglial activation by unconjugated bilirubin. J Neurochem 96:1667–1679.

Ferriero D M, Arcavi L J, Sagar S M et al 1988 Selective sparing of NADPH-diaphorase neurons in neonatal hypoxia-ischemia. Ann Neurol 24:670–676.

Forfar J O, Keay A J, Elliott W D, Cumming R H 1958 Exchange transfusion in neonatal hyperbilirubinemia. Lancet 2:1131–1137.

Forna F, McConnell M, Kitabire F N et al 2006 Systematic review of the safety of trimethoprim-sulfamethoxazole for prophylaxis in HIV-infected pregnant women: implications for resource-limited settings. AIDS Rev 8:24–36.

Frank J E 2005 Diagnosis and management of G6PD deficiency. Am Fam Physician 72:1277–1282.

Funato M, Tamai H, Shimada S, Nakamura H 1994 Vigintiphobia, unbound bilirubin, and auditory brainstem responses. Pediatrics 93:50–53.

Gartner L M, Herrarias C T, Sebring R H 1998 Practice patterns in neonatal hyperbilirubinemia. Pediatrics 101:25–31.

Gartner L M, Herschel M 2001 Jaundice and breastfeeding. Pediatr Clin North Am 48:389–399.

Gartner L M, Lee K, Keenan W J et al 1985 Effect of phototherapy on albumin binding of bilirubin. Pediatrics 75:401–441.

Gartner L M, Snyder R N, Chabon R S, Bernstein J 1970 Kernicterus: high incidence in premature infants with low serum bilirubin concentrations. Pediatrics 45:906–917.

Gennuso F, Fernetti C, Tirolo C et al 2004 Bilirubin protects astrocytes from its own toxicity by inducing up-regulation and translocation of multidrug resistance-associated protein 1 (Mrp1). Proc Natl Acad Sci U S A 101:2470–2475.

Gerrard J 1952 Kernicterus. Brain 75:526–570.

Gilboe D D, Kintner D B, Anderson M E, Fitzpatrick J H Jr 1998 NMR-based identification of intra- and extracellular compartments of the brain Pi peak. J Neurochem 71:2542–2548.

Goessling W, Zucker SD 2000 Role of apolipoprotein D in the transport of bilirubin in plasma. Am J Physiol Gastrointest Liver Physiol 279:G356–G365.

Gordo A C, Falcao A S, Fernandes A et al 2006 Unconjugated bilirubin activates and damages microglia. J Neurosci Res 84:194–201.

Gourley G R, Li Z, Kreamer B L, Kosorok M R 2005 A controlled, randomized, double-blind trial of prophylaxis against jaundice among breastfed newborns. Pediatrics 16:385–391.

Govaert P, Lequin M, Swarte R et al 2003 Changes in globus pallidus with (pre)term kernicterus. Pediatrics 112:1256–1263.

Grimmer I, Moller R, Gmyrek D, Gross J 1978 Bilirubin UDP-glucuronyltransferase activity in human fetal liver homogenates. Acta Biol Med Ger 37:131–135.

Groenendaal F, van der Grond J, de Vries L S 2004 Cerebral metabolism in severe neonatal hyperbilirubinemia. Pediatrics 114:291–294.

Grojean S, Koziel V, Vert P, Daval J L 2000 Bilirubin induces apoptosis via activation of NMDA receptors in ceveloping rat brain neurons. Exp Neurol 166:334–341.

Grojean S, Lievre V, Koziel V et al 2001 Bilirubin exerts additional toxic effects in hypoxic cultured neurons from the developing rat brain by the recruitment of glutamate neurotoxicity. Pediatr Res 49:507–513.

Hafkamp A M, Havinga R, Ostrow J D et al 2006 Novel kinetic insights into treatment of unconjugated hyperbilirubinemia: phototherapy and orlistat treatment in Gunn rats. Pediatr Res 59:506–512.

Hahm J, Ostrow J D, Mukerjee P, Celic L 1992 Ionization and self-association of unconjugated bilirubin, determined by rapid solvent partition from chloroform, with further studies of bilirubin solubility. J Lipid Res 33:1123–1137.

Hamilton J R, Sass-Kortsak A 1963 Jaundice associated with severe bacterial infection in young infants. J Pediatr 63:121–132.

Hanko E, Hansen T W, Almaas R, Rootwelt T 2006 Recovery after short-term bilirubin exposure in human NT2-N neurons. Brain Res 1103:56–64.

Hannon P R, Willis S K, Scrimshaw S C 2001 Persistence of maternal concerns surrounding neonatal jaundice: an exploratory study. Arch Pediatr Adolesc Med 155:1357–1363.

Hansen P E, Thiessen H, Brodersen R 1979 Bilirubin acidity. Titrimetric and 13C NMR studies. Acta Chem Scand B 33:281–293.

Hansen R L, Hughes G G, Ahlfors C E 1991 Neonatal bilirubin exposure and psychoeducational outcome. J Dev Behav Pediatr 12:287–293.

Hansen T W 1997 Acute management of extreme neonatal jaundice–the potential benefits of intensified phototherapy and interruption of enterohepatic bilirubin circulation. Acta Paediatr 86:843–846.

Hansen T W 2000a Kernicterus in term and near-term infants–the specter walks again. Acta Paediatr 89:1155–1157.

Hansen T W 2000b Bilirubin oxidation in brain. Mol Genet Metab 71:411–417.

Hansen T W 2002 Kernicterus: an international perspective. Semin Neonatol 7:103–109.

Hansen T W R 2000 Pioneers in the scientific study of neonatal jaundice and kernicterus. Pediatrics 106:e15.

Hansen T W R 2001 Guidelines for treatment of neonatal jaundice. Is there a place for evidence-based medicine? Acta Paediatr 90:239–241.

Hansen T W, Oyasaeter S, Stiris T, Bratlid D 1989 Effects of sulfisoxazole, hypercarbia, and hyperosmolality on entry of bilirubin and albumin into brain regions in young rats. Biol Neonate 56:22–30.

Hansen T W, Tommarello S, Allen J 2001 Subcellular localization of bilirubin in rat brain after in vivo i.v. administration of [3H] bilirubin. Pediatr Res 49:203–207.

Hansen T W, Tommarello S, Allen J W 1997 Oxidation of bilirubin by rat brain mitochondrial membranes-genetic variability. Biochem Mol Med 62:128–131.

Harris M C, Bernbaum J C, Polin J R et al 2001 Developmental follow-up of breastfed term and near-term infants with marked hyperbilirubinemia. Pediatrics 107:1075–1080.

Harris R C, Lucey J F, MacClean J R 1958 Kernicterus in premature infants associated with low concentrations of bilirubin in the plasma. Pediatrics 21:875–884.

Hart A P 1925 Can Med Assoc J 15:1008.

Haymaker W, Margolis C, Pentschew A et al 1961 Pathology of kernicterus and posticteric encephalopathy. In: Swingard C A (ed.) Kernicterus and its importance in cerebral palsy. Charles C Thomas, Springfield, IL, pp. 21–228.

Herschel M, Karrison T, Wen M et al 2002 Evaluation of the direct antiglobulin (Coombs') test for identifying newborns at risk for hemolysis as determined by end-tidal carbon monoxide concentration (ETCOc); and comparison of the Coombs' test with ETCOc for detecting significant jaundice. J Perinatol 22:341–347.

Holtzman N A 2004 Management of hyperbilirubinemia: quality of evidence and cost. Pediatrics 114:1086–1088.

Hsia D Y, Allen F H, Gellis S S, Diamond L K 1952 Erythroblastosis fetalis VII: Studies of serum bilirubin in relation to kernicterus. N Engl J Med 247:668–671.

Hugh-Jones K, Slack J, Simpson K et al 1960 Clinical course of hyperbilirubinemia in premature infants. A preliminary report. N Engl J Med 263:1223–1229.

Hyvarinen M, Zeltzer P, Oh W, Stiehm E R 1973 Influence of gestational age on serum levels of alpha-1 fetoprotein, IgG globulin, and albumin in newborn infants. J Pediatr 82:430–437.

Ip S, Chung M, Kulig J et al 2004 An evidence-based review of important issues concerning neonatal hyperbilirubinemia. Pediatrics 114:e130–e153.

Ives N K, Cox D W, Gardiner R M, Bachelard H S 1988 The effects of bilirubin on brain energy metabolism during normoxia and hypoxia: an in vitro study using 31P nuclear magnetic resonance spectroscopy. Pediatr Res 23:569–573.

Ives N K, Gardiner R M 1990 Blood-brain barrier permeability to bilirubin in the rat studied using intracarotid bolus injection and in situ brain perfusion techniques. Pediatr Res 27:436–441.

Jackson J C 1997 Adverse events associated with exchange transfusion in healthy and ill newborns. Pediatrics 99:E7.

Jacobsen J, Wennberg R P 1974 Determination of unbound bilirubin in the serum of newborns. Clin Chem 20:783–789.

Jacobsen M, Clausen P P, Jacobsen G K et al 1982 Intracellular plasma proteins in human fetal choroid plexus during development. I. Developmental stages in relation to the number of epithelial cells which contain albumin in telencephalic, diencephalic and myelencephalic choroid plexus. Brain Res 255:239–250.

JCAHO issues warning on kernicterus danger 2001 Hosp Peer Rev 26:100–101.

Johnson L H, Bhutani V K, Brown A K 2002 System-based approach to management of neonatal jaundice and prevention of kernicterus. J Pediatr 140:396–403.

Johnson L, Boggs T 1974 Bilirubin-dependent brain damage: incidence and indications for treatment. In: Odell G E, Simopoulos A P, Shaffer R (eds) Phototherapy in the newborn: an overview. National Academy of Sciences, Washington, DC, pp. 122–149.

Johnson L, Brown A K, Bhutani V K 1999 BIND–A clinical score for biliruibn induced neurological dysfunction in newborns. Pediatrics 104:746–747 (Abstract).

Johnson L, Sarmiento F, Blanc W A, Day R 1959 Kernicterus in rats with an inherited deficiency of glucuronyl transferase. AMA J Dis Child 97:591–608.

Johnston M V 2005 Excitotoxicity in perinatal brain injury. Brain Pathol 15:234–240.

Johnston M V, Hoon A H Jr 2000 Possible mechanisms in infants for selective basal ganglia damage from asphyxia, kernicterus, or mitochondrial encephalopathies. J Child Neurol 15:588–591.

Kaga K, Kitazumi E, Kodama K 1979 Auditory brain stem responses of kernicterus infants. Int J Pediatr Otorhinolaryngol 1:255–264.

Kalpoyiannis N, Androulakis N, Hadjigerorgiou E et al 1982 Efficacy of phototherapy and/or exchange transfusions in neonatal jaundice. Clin Pediatr (Phila) 21:602–606.

Kamisako T, Kobayashi Y, Takeuchi K et al 2000 Recent advances in bilirubin metabolism research: the molecular mechanism of hepatocyte bilirubin transport and its clinical relevance. J Gastroenterol 35:659–664.

Kapitulnik J, Horner-Mibashan R, Blondheim S H et al 1975 Increase in bilirubin-binding affinity of serum with age of infant. J Pediatr 86:442–445.

Kaplan M, Hammerman C, Maisels M J 2003 Bilirubin genetics for the nongeneticist: Hereditary defects of neonatal bilirubin conjugation. Pediatrics 111:886–893.

Kaplan M, Muraca M, Hammerman C et al 1998 Bilirubin conjugation, reflected by conjugated bilirubin fractions, in glucose-6-phosphate dehydrogenase-deficient neonates: a determining factor in the pathogenesis of hyperbilirubinemia. Pediatrics 102:E37.

Kaplan M, Muraca M, Hammerman C et al 2002 Imbalance between production and conjugation of bilirubin: a fundamental concept in the mechanism of neonatal jaundice. Pediatrics 110:e47.

Kaplan M, Vreman H J, Hammerman C, Stevenson D K 1999 Neonatal bilirubin production, reflected by carboxyhaemoglobin concentrations, in Down's syndrome. Arch Dis Child Fetal Neonatal Ed 81:F56–F60.

Karp WB 1979 Biochemical alterations in neonatal hyperbilirubinemia and bilirubin encephalopathy: a review. Pediatrics 64:361–368.

Keino H, Sato H, Semba R et al 1985 Mode of prevention by phototherapy of cerebellar hypoplasia in a new Sprague-Dawley strain of jaundiced Gunn rats. Pediatr Neurosci 12:145–150.

Keren R, Bhutani V K, Luan X et al 2005 Identifying newborns at risk of significant hyperbilirubinaemia: a comparison of two recommended approaches. Arch Dis Child 90:415–421.

Koch C A, Jones D V, Dine M S, Wagner E A 1959 Hyperbilirubinemia in premature infants; a follow-up study. J Pediatr 55:23–29.

Korres S G, Balatsouras D G, Lyra C et al 2006 A comparison of automated auditory brainstem responses and transiently evoked otoacoustic emissions for universal newborn hearing screening. Med Sci Monit 12:CR260–CR263.

Kulkarni S V, Merchant R H, Gupte S C, Divekar R M 1989 Clinical significance of serum and cerebrospinal fluid bilirubin indices in neonatal jaundice. Indian Pediatr 26:1202–1208.

Kumar R, Narang A, Kumar P, Garewal G 2002 Phenobarbitone prophylaxis for neonatal jaundice in babies with birth weight 1000–1499 grams. Indian Pediatr 39:945–951.

Kuriyama M, Tomiwa K, Konishi Y, Mikawa H 1986 Improvement in auditory brainstem response of hyperbilirubinemic infants after exchange transfusions. Pediatr Neurol 2:127–132.

Lee C, Stonestreet B S, Oh W et al 1995 Postnatal maturation of the blood-brain barrier for unbound bilirubin in newborn piglets. Brain Res 689:233–238.

Lee K, Gartner L M, Eidelman A I, Ezhuthachan S 1977 Unconjugated hyperbilirubinemia in very low birth weight infants. Clin Perinatol 4:305–320.

Lenhardt M L, McArtor R, Bryant B 1984 Effects of neonatal hyperbilirubinemia on the brainstem electric response. J Pediatr 104:281–284.

Lester R, Behrman R E, Lucey J F 1963 Transfer of bilirubin-C14 across monkey placenta. Pediatrics 32:416–419.

Lester R, Ostrow J D, Schmid R 1961 Enterohepatic circulation of bilirubin. Nature 192:372.

Leung A K, Sauve R S 1989 Breastfeeding and breast milk jaundice. J R Soc Health 109:213–217.

Levi A J, Gatmaitan Z, Arias I M 1970 Deficiency of hepatic organic anion-binding protein, impaired organic amnion uptake by liver and 'physiologic' jaundice in newborn monkeys. N Engl J Med 283:1136–1139.

Levine R L 1979 Bilirubin: worked out years ago? Pediatrics 64:380–385.

Levine R L, Fredericks W R, Rapoport S I 1982 Entry of bilirubin into the brain due to opening of the blood-brain barrier. Pediatrics 69:255–259.

Levine R L, Fredericks W R, Rapoport S I 1985 Clearance of bilirubin from rat brain after reversible osmotic opening of the blood-brain barrier. Pediatr Res 19:1040–1043.

Lightner D A, Holmes D L, McDonagh A F 1996 On the acid dissociation constants of bilirubin and biliverdin. pKa values from 13C NMR spectroscopy. J Biol Chem 71:2397–2405.

Lightner D A, Linnane W P 3rd, Ahlfors C E 1984 Bilirubin photooxidation products in the urine of jaundiced neonates receiving phototherapy. Pediatr Res 18:696–700.

Lightner D A, McDonagh A F 1984a Molecular mechanisms of phototherapy for neonatal jaundice. Acc Chem Res 17:417–424.

Liley A W 1963 Intrauterine transfusion of foetus in haemolytic disease. Br Med J 2:1107–1109.

Litwack G, Ketterer B, Arias I M 1971 Ligandin: a hepatic protein which binds steroids, bilirubin, carcinogens and a number of exogenous organic anions. Nature 234:466–467.

Lorey F W, Ahlfors C E, Smith D G, Neel J V 1984 Bilirubin binding by variant albumins in Yanomama Indians. Am J Hum Genet 36:1112–1120.

Lucey J F 1982 Bilirubin and brain damage — a real mess. Pediatrics 69:381–382.

McDonagh A F 1990 Is bilirubin good for you? Clin Perinatol 17:359–369.

McDonagh A F 2006 Ex uno plures: the concealed complexity of bilirubin species in neonatal blood samples. Pediatrics 118:1185–1187.

McDonagh A F, Assisi F 1971 Commercial bilirubin: A trinity of isomers. FEBS Lett 18:315–317.

McDonagh A F, Lightner D A 1985 'Like a shrivelled blood orange'–bilirubin, jaundice, and phototherapy. Pediatrics 75:443–555.

McDonald J W, Shapiro S M, Silverstein F S, Johnston M V 1998 Role of glutamate receptor-mediated excitotoxicity in bilirubin-induced brain injury in the Gunn rat model. Exp Neurol 150:21–29.

Maisels M J 1996 Why use homeopathic doses of phototherapy? Pediatrics 98:283–287.

Maisels M J, Gifford K 1986 Normal serum bilirubin levels in the newborn and the effect of breast-feeding. Pediatrics 78:837–843.

Maisels M J, Newman T B 1995 Kernicterus in otherwise healthy, breast-fed term newborns. Pediatrics 96:730–733.

Maisels M J, Pathak A, Nelson N M et al 1971 Endogenous production of carbon monoxide in normal and erythroblastotic newborn infants. J Clin Invest 50:1–8.

Malamud N 1961 Pathogenesis of kernicterus in the light of its sequelae. In: Swingard CA (ed.) Kernicterus and its importance in cerebral palsy. Charles C Thomas, Springfield, IL, pp. 21–228.

Mansi G, De Maio C, Araimo G et al 2003 'Safe' hyperbilirubinemia is associated with altered neonatal behavior. Biol Neonate 83:19–21.

Mattson M P 2003 Excitotoxic and excitoprotective mechanisms: abundant targets for the prevention and treatment of neurodegenerative disorders. Neuromolecular Med 3:65–94.

Menken M, Barrett P V D, Swarm R L, Berlin N I 1966 Kernicterus: Development of an experimental model using bilirubin 14C. Arch Neurol 15:68–73.

Merhar S L, Gilbert D L 2005 Clinical (video) findings and cerebrospinal fluid neurotransmitters in 2 children with severe chronic bilirubin encephalopathy, including a former preterm infant without marked hyperbilirubinemia. Pediatrics 116:1226–1229.

Meyer T C 1956 A study of serum bilirubin levels in relation to kernicterus and prematurity. Arch Dis Child 31:75–80.

Mollen T J, Scarfone R, Harris M C 2004 Acute, severe bilirubin encephalopathy in a newborn. Pediatr Emerg Care 20:599–601.

Møllgård K, Saunders N R 1986 The development of the human blood-brain and blood-CSF barriers. Neuropathol Appl Neurobiol 12:337–358.

Mollison P L, Walker W 1952 Controlled trials of the treatment of hemolytic disease of the newborn. Lancet 1:429–433.

Monaghan G, McLellan A, McGeehan A et al 1999 Gilbert's syndrome is a contributory factor in prolonged unconjugated hyperbilirubinemia of the newborn. J Pediatr134:441–446.

Mores A, Fargašová I, Minariková E 1959 The relation of hyperbilirubinemia in newborns without isoimmunization to kernicterus. Acta Paediatr 48:590–602.

Moyer V A, Ahn C, Sneed S 2000 Accuracy of clinical judgment in neonatal jaundice. Arch Pediatr Adolesc Med 154:391–394.

Mukerjee P, Ostrow J D, Tiribelli C 2002 Low solubility of unconjugated bilirubin in dimethylsulfoxide-water systems: implications for pKa determinations. BMC Biochem 3:17.

Murki S, Dutta S, Narang A et al 2005 A randomized, triple-blind, placebo-controlled trial of prophylactic oral phenobarbital to reduce the need for phototherapy in G6PD-deficient neonates. J Perinatol 25:325–330.

Mustafa M G, Cowger M L, King T E 1969 Effects of bilirubin on mitochondrial reactions. J Biol Chem 244:6403–6414.

Mustafa M G, King T E 1970 Binding of bilirubin with lipid. A possible mechanism of its toxic reactions in mitochondria. J Biol Chem 245:1084–1089.

Nagaoka S, Cowger M L 1978 Interaction of biliruibn with lipids studied by fluorescence quenching method. J Biol Chem 2005–2011.

Nakamura H, Takada S, Shimabuku R et al 1985 Auditory nerve and brainstem responses in newborn infants with hyperbilirubinemia. Pediatrics 75:703–708.

Nakamura H, Yonetani M, Uetani Y et al 1992 Determination of serum unbound bilirubin for prediction of kernicterus in low birth weight infants. Acta Paediatr Jpn 34:642–647.

Nanjundaswamy S, Petrova A, Mehta R et al 2004 The accuracy of transcutaneous bilirubin measurements in neonates: a correlation study. Biol Neonate 85:21–25.

Nasralla M, Gawronska E, Hsia D Y 1958 Studies on the relation between serum and spinal fluid bilirubin during early infancy. J Clin Invest 37:1403–1412.

Nelson T, Jacobsen J, Wennberg R P 1974 Effect of pH on the interaction of bilirubin with albumin and tissue culture cells. Pediatr Res 8:963–967.

Neurobiol 20:97–109.

Newman T B, Liljestrand P, Escobar G 2003 Infants with bilirubin levels of 30 mg/dL or more in a large managed care organization. Pediatrics 111:1303–1311.

Newman T B, Liljestrand P, Jeremy R J et al 2006 Outcomes among newborns with total serum bilirubin levels of 25 mg per deciliter or more. N Engl J Med 354:1889–1900.

Newman T B, Maisels M J 1990 Does hyperbilirubinemia damage the brain of healthy full-term infants? Clin Perinatol 17:331–358.

Newman T B, Maisels M J 1992 Evaluation and treatment of jaundice in the term newborn: a kinder, gentler approach. Pediatrics 89:809–818.

Newman T B, Maisels M J 2002 Magnetic resonance imaging and kernicterus. Pediatrics 109:555.

Newns G H, Norton K R 1958 Hyperbilirubinemia in prematurity. Lancet 2:1138–1140.

Ng S H, Rawstron J R 1971 Urinary tract infections presenting with jaundice. Arch Dis Child 46:173–176.

Notter M F, Kendig J W 1986 Differential sensitivity of neural cells to bilirubin toxicity. Exp Neurol 94:670–682.

Nwaesei C G, Van Aerde J, Boyden M, Perlman M 1984 Changes in auditory brainstem responses in hyperbilirubinemic infants before and after exchange transfusion. Pediatrics 74:800–803.

Oakden W K, Moore A M, Blaser S, Noseworthy M D 2005 1H MR spectroscopic characteristics of kernicterus: a possible metabolic signature. AJNR Am J Neuroradiol 26:1571–1574.

Odell G B 1959 Studies in kernicterus. I. The protein binding of bilirubin. J Clin Invest 38:823–833.

Odell G B, Storey G N, Rosenberg L A 1970 Studies in kernicterus. 3. The saturation of serum proteins with bilirubin during neonatal life and its relationship to brain damage at five years. J Pediatr 76:12–21.

Oh W, Tyson J E, Fanaroff A A et al 2003 National Institute of Child Health and Human Development Neonatal Research Network. Association between peak serum bilirubin and neurodevelopmental outcomes in extremely low birth weight infants. Pediatrics 112:773–779.

Ohsugi M, Sato H, Yamamura H 1992 Transfer of bilirubin covalently bound to 125I–albumin from blood to brain in the Gunn rat newborn. Biol Neonate 62:416–423.

Okumura A, Hayakawa F, Maruyama K et al 2006 Single photon emission computed tomography and serial MRI in preterm infants with kernicterus. Brain Dev 28:348–352.

Onishi S, Itoh S, Kawade N et al 1979 The separation of configurational isomers of bilirubin by high pressure liquid chromatography and the mechanism of jaundice phototherapy. Biochem Biophys Res Commun 90:890–896.

Oski F A, Naiman J L 1963 Red cell binding of bilirubin. J Pediatr 63:1034–1037.

Ostrow J D, Branham R V 1970 Photodecomposition of bilirubin and biliverdin in vitro. Gastroenterology 58:15–25.

Ostrow J D, Celic L 1984 Bilirubin chemistry, ionization and solubilization by bile salts. Hepatology 4(5 Suppl):38S–45S.

Ostrow J D, Mukerjee P, Tiribelli C 1994 Structure and binding of unconjugated bilirubin: relevance for physiological and pathophysiological function. J Lipid Res 35:1715–1737.

Ostrow J D, Pascolo L, Brites D, Tiribelli C 2004 Molecular basis of bilirubin-induced neurotoxicity. Trends in Molecular Medicine 10:65–70.

Ostrow J D, Pascolo L, Shapiro S M, Tiribelli C 2003a. New concepts in bilirubin encephalopathy. Eur J Clin Invest 33:988–997.

Ostrow J D, Pascolo L, Tiribelli 2002 Mechanisms of bilirubin neurotoxicity. Hepatology 35:1277–1280.

Ostrow J D, Pascolo L, Tiribelli C 2003 Reassessment of the unbound concentrations of unconjugated bilirubin in relation to neurotoxicity in vitro. Pediatr Res 54:98–104.

Overbeek J T G, Vink C L F, Deenstra H 1955 The solubility of bilirubin. Recl Trav Chim Pays-Bas Belg 74:81–84.

Padmashri R, Sikdar S K 2006 Glutamate pretreatment affects Ca(2+) signaling in processes of astrocyte pairs. J Neurochem 24(100):105–117.

Paksoy Y, Koc H, Genc B O 2004 Bilateral mesial temporal sclerosis and kernicterus. J Comput Assist Tomogr 28:269–272.

Palmer R H, Keren R, Maisels M J, Yeargin-Allsopp M 2004 National Institute of Child Health and Human Development (NICHD) conference on kernicterus: a population perspective on prevention of kernicterus. J Perinatol Nov, 24(11):723–725.

Paludetto R, Mansi G, Raimondi F et al 2002 Moderate hyperbilirubinemia induces a transient alteration of neonatal behavior. Pediatrics 110:e50.

Pascolo L, Del Vecchio S, Koehler R K et al 1996 Albumin binding of unconjugated [3H]bilirubin and its uptake by rat liver basolateral membrane vesicles. Biochem J 316:999–1004.

Passamonti S, Terdoslavich M, Margon A et al 2005 Uptake of bilirubin into HepG2 cells assayed by thermal lens spectroscopy. Function of bilitranslocase. FEBS J 272:5522–5535.

Pearlman M A, Gartner L M, Lee K et al 1978 Absence of kernicterus in low-birth weight infants from 1971

through 1976: comparison with findings in 1966 and 1967. Pediatrics 62:460–464.

Pearlman M A, Gartner L M, Lee K et al 1980 The association of kernicterus with bacterial infection in the newborn. Pediatrics 65:26–29.

Penn A A, Enzmann D R, Hahn J S, Stevenson D K 1994 Kernicterus in a full term infant. Pediatrics 93:1003–1006.

Perlman J M, Rogers B B, Burns D 1997 Kernicteric findings at autopsy in two sick near term infants. Pediatrics 99:612–615.

Perlman M, Fainmesser P, Sohmer H et al 1983 Auditory nerve-brainstem evoked responses in hyperbilirubinemic neonates. Pediatrics 72:658–664.

Perlstein M A 1960 The late clinical syndrome of posticteric encephalopathy. Pediatr Clin North Am 7:665–687.

Petit F, Gajdos V, Capel L et al 2006 Crigler-Najjar type II syndrome may result from several types and combinations of mutations in the UGT1A1 gene. Clin Genet 69:525–527.

Polácek K 1966 Risk of kernicterus in newborn infants with a high level of conjugated bilirubin. Acta Paediatr Scand 55:401–404.

Pollack W, Gorman J G, Freda V J et al 1968 Results of clinical trials of RhoGAM in women. Transfusion 8:151–153.

Rapmund G, Bowman J M, Harris R C 1960 Bilirubinemia in non-erythroblastotic premature infants. Am J Dis Child 99:604–616.

Reynolds R C, Cluff L E 1960 Interaction of serum and sodium salicylate: changes during acute infection and its influence on pharmacological activity. Bull Johns Hopkins Hosp 107:278–290.

Richards B W 1951 Kernicterus. Am J Ment Defic 55:529–534.

Riskin A, Kugelman A, Abend-Weinger M et al 2003 In the eye of the beholder: how accurate is clinical estimation of jaundice in newborns? Acta Paediatr 92:574–576.

Ritter D A, Kenny J D 1986 Bilirubin binding in premature infants from birth to 3 months. Arch Dis Child 61:352–356.

Ritter D A, Kenny J D, Norton H J, Rudolph A J 1982 A prospective study of free bilirubin and other risk factors in the development of kernicterus in premature infants. Pediatrics 69:260–266.

Robertson A, Karp W, Brodersen R 1991 Bilirubin displacing effect of drugs used in neonatology. Acta Paediatr Scand 80:1119–1127.

Rodrigues C M, Sola S, Brites D 2002 Bilirubin induces apoptosis via the mitochondrial pathway in developing rat brain neurons. Hepatology 35:1186–1195.

Rodrigues C M, Sola S, Brito M A et al 2002a Bilirubin directly disrupts membrane lipid polarity and fluidity, protein order, and redox status in rat mitochondria. J Hepatol 36:335–341.

Roger C, Koziel V, Vert P, Nehlig A 1995 A mapping of the consequences of bilirubin exposure in the immature rat: local cerebral metabolic rates for glucose during moderate and severe hyperbilirubinemia. Early Hum Dev 43:133–144.

Ross G 2003 Hyperbilirubinemia in the 2000s: What should we do next? Am J Perinatol 20:415–424.

Rubo J, Albrecht K, Lasch P et al 1992 High–dose intravenous immune globulin therapy for hyperbilirubinemia caused by Rh hemolytic disease. J Pediatr 121:93–97.

Salamy A, Eldredge L, Tooley W H 1989 Neonatal status and hearing loss in high-risk infants. J Pediatr 114:847–852.

Schenker S, McCandless D W, Zollman P E 1966 Studies of cellular toxicity of unconjugated bilirubin in kernicteric brain. J Clin Invest 45:1213–1220.

Schmid R, Hammaker L 1963 Metabolism and disposition of C14-bilirubin in congenital nonhemolytic jaundice. J Clin Invest 42:1720–1734.

Schmorl G 1903 Zur kenntniss des ikterus neonatorum insbesondere der dabei auftretenden gehirnveranderungen. Verhandlung Deutsche Pathologische Gesellschaft 6:109–115.

Schutta H S, Johnson L 1971 Electron microscopic observations on acute bilirubin encephalopathy in Gunn rats induced by sulfadimethoxine. Lab Invest 24:82–89.

Schutta H S, Johnson L, Neville H E 1970 Mitochondrial abnormalities in bilirubin encephalopathy. J Neuropathol Exp Neurol 29:296–305.

Sentinel event alert 2001 Kernicterus threatens healthy newborns. Jt Comm Perspect 21:10–11.

Shapiro S M 2003 Bilirubin toxicity in the developing nervous system. Pediatr Neurol 29:410–421.

Shapiro S M 2005 Definition of the clinical spectrum of kernicterus and bilirubin-induced neurologic dysfunction (BIND). J Perinatol 25:54–59.

Shapiro S M, Bhutani V K, Johnson L 2006 Hyperbilirubinemia and kernicterus. Clin Perinatol 33:387–410.

Shimabuku R, Nakamura H 1982 Total and unbound bilirubin determined using an automated peroxidase micromethod. Kobe J Med Sci 28:91–104.

Silva R F, Mata L M, Gulbenkian S, Brites D 2001 Endocytosis in rat cultured astrocytes is inhibited by unconjugated bilirubin. Neurochem Res 26:793–800.

Silva R F, Rodrigues C M, Brites D 2002 Rat cultured neuronal and glial cells respond differently to toxicity of unconjugated bilirubin. Pediatr Res 51:535–541.

Silva R, Mata L R, Gulbenkian S et al 1999 Inhibition of glutamate uptake by unconjugated bilirubin in cultured cortical rat astrocytes: role of concentration and pH. Biochem Biophys Res Commun 265:67–72.

Silverman W A, Andersen D H, Blanc W A, Crozier D N 1956 A difference in mortality rate and incidence of kernicterus among prematures allotted to two prophylactic antibacterial regimens. Pediatrics 1956, 18:614–625.

Slusher T M, Vreman H J, McLaren D W et al 1995 Glucose-6-phosphate dehydrogenase deficiency and carboxyhemoglobin concentrations associated with bilirubin-related morbidity and death in Nigerian infants. J Pediatr 126:102–108.

Smith C M, Barnes G P, Jacobson C A, Oelberg D G 2004 Auditory brainstem response detects early bilirubin neurotoxicity at low indirect bilirubin values. J Perinatol 24:730–732.

Spector R, Spector A Z, Snodgrass S R 1977 Model for transport in the central nervous system. Am J Physiol 232:R73–R79.

Spencer R F, Shaia W T, Gleason A T et al 2002 Changes in calcium-binding protein expression in the auditory brainstem nuclei of the jaundiced Gunn rat. Hear Res 171:129–141.

Stanley T V 1997 A case of kernicterus in New Zealand: a predictable tragedy? J Paediatr Child Health 33:451–453.

Stein L, Tremblay K, Pasternak J et al 1996 Brainstem abnormalities in neonates with normal otoacoustic emissions. Sem Hear 17:197–213.

Stern L, Denton R L 1965 Kernicterus in small premature infants. Pediarics 35:483–485.

Stevenson D K, Fanaroff A A, Maisels M J et al 2001 Prediction of hyperbilirubinemia in near-term and term infants. Pediatrics 108:31–39.

Stevenson D K, Wong R J, Vreman H J et al 2005 NICHD Conference on Kernicterus: Research on prevention of bilirubin-induced brain injury and kernicterus: bench-to-bedside-diagnostic methods

and prevention and treatment strategies. J Perinatol 24:521–525.

Stollman Y R, Gartner U, Theilmann L et al 1983 Hepatic bilirubin uptake in the isolated perfused rat liver is not facilitated by albumin binding. J Clin Invest 72:718–723.

Strauss K A, Robinson D L, Vreman H J et al 2006 Management of hyperbilirubinemia and prevention of kernicterus in 20 patients with Crigler–Najjar disease. Eur J Pediatr 165:306–319.

Suresh G K, Clark R E 2004 Cost-effectiveness of strategies that are intended to prevent kernicterus in newborn infants. Pediatrics 114:917–924.

Szentistvanyi I, Patlak C S, Ellis R A, Cserr H F 1984 Drainage of interstitial fluid from different regions of rat brain. Am J Physiol 246:F835–F844.

Tazawa Y, Abukawa D, Watabe M et al 1991 Abnormal results of biochemical liver function tests in breast-fed infants with prolonged indirect hyperbilirubinaemia. Eur J Pediatr 150:310–313.

Tiribelli C, Ostrow J D 1996 New concepts in bilirubin and jaundice: Report of the third international bilirubin workshop, April 6–8, 1995, Trieste, Italy. Hepatology 24:1296–1311.

Tiribelli C, Ostrow J D 2005 The molecular basis of bilirubin encephalopathy and toxicity: report of an EASL Single Topic Conference, Trieste, Italy, 1–2 October, 2004. J Hepatol 43:156–166.

Trolle D 1961 Discussion on the advisability of performing exchange transfusion in neonatal jaundice of unknown aetiology. Acta Paediatr 50:392–398.

Trull F R, Boiadjiev S, Lightner D A, McDonagh A F 1997 Aqueous dissociation constants of bile pigments and sparingly soluble carboxylic acids by 13C NMR in aqueous dimethyl sulfoxide: effects of hydrogen bonding. J Lipid Res 38:1178–1188.

Turkel S B 1983 Clinical and pathological correlations with kernicterus and yellow pulmonary hyaline membranes. In: Levine R L, Maisels M J (eds) Hyperbilirubinemia in the newborn. report of the eighty-fifth Ross conference on pediatric research. Ross Labaratories, Columbus, Ohio, pp. 11–16.

Turkel S B 1990 Autopsy findings associated with neonatal hyperbilirubinemia. Clin Perinatol 17:381–396.

Turkel S B, Guttenberg M E, Moynes D R, Hodgman J E 1980 Lack of identifiable risk factors for kernicterus. Pediatrics 66:502–506.

Turkel S B, Miller C A, Guttenberg M E et al 1982 A clinical pathologic reappraisal of kernicterus. Pediatrics 69:267–272.

Valaes T 1963 Bilirubin distribution and dynamics of bilirubin removal by exchange transfusion. Acta Paediatr 52 Suppl 149:1–117.

Valaes T, Wennberg R P, Merenstein G B et al 1992 Commentaries regarding: Evaluation and treatment of jaundice in the term newborn: A kinder, gentler approach. Pediatrics 89:819–831.

Van Praagh R 1961 Diagnosis of kernicterus in the neonatal period. Pediatrics 28:870–876.

Vaughan V C, Allen F H, Diamond L K 1950 Erythroblastosis fetalis I. Problems in the interpretation of changing mortality in erythroblastosis fetalis. Pediatrics 6:173–182.

Vítek, L 2005 Impact of serum bilirubin on human diseases. Pediatrics 115:1411–1412.

Vohr B R, Karp D, O'Dea C et al 1990 Behavioral changes correlated with brain-stem auditory evoked responses in term infants with moderate hyperbilirubinemia. J Pediatr 117:288–291.

Vohr B R, Lester B, Rapisardi G et al 1989 Abnormal brain-stem function (brain-stem auditory evoked

response) correlates with acoustic cry features in term infants with hyperbilirubinemia. J Pediatr 115:303–308.

Volpe J J 2001 Bilirubin and brain injury. In: Neurology of the newborn, 4th edn. WB Saunders, Philadelphia, PA, pp. 521–546.

Wallerstein H 1946 Treatment of severe erythroblastosis by simultaneous removal and replacement of the blood of the newborn infant. Science103:583–584.

Warr O, Mort D, Attwell D 2000 Bilirubin does not modulate ionotropic glutamate receptors or glutamate transporters. Brain Res 879:13–16.

Watchko J F 2005 Vigintiphobia revisted. Pediatrics 115:1747–1753.

Watchko J F 2006 Kernicterus and the molecular mechanisms of bilirubin-induced CNS injury in newborns. Neuromolecular Med 8:513–530.

Watchko J F, Claassen D 1994 Kernicterus in premature infants: current prevalence and relationship to NICHD Phototherapy Study exchange criteria. Pediatrics 93:996–999.

Watchko J F, Daood M J, Biniwale M 2002 Understanding neonatal hyperbilirubinaemia in the era of genomics. Semin Neonatol 7:143–152.

Watchko J F, Daood M J, Mahmood B et al 2001 P-glycoprotein and bilirubin disposition. J Perinatol 21: S43–S47.

Watchko J F, Oski FA 1983 Bilirubin 20 mg/dL = vigintiphobia. Pediatrics 71:660–663.

Weisiger R A, Ostrow J D, Koehler R K et al 2001 Affinity of human serum albumin for bilirubin varies with albumin concentration and buffer composition: results of a novel ultrafiltration method. J Biol Chem 276:29953–299560.

Wennberg R P 1988 The importance of free bilirubin acid salt in bilirubin uptake by erythrocytes and mitochondria. Pediatr Res 23:443–447.

Wennberg R P 1991 Cellular basis of bilirubin toxicity. N Y State J Med 91:493–496.

Wennberg R P 2000 The blood-brain barrier and bilirubin encephalopathy. Cell Mol

Wennberg R P, Ahlfors C E, Bhutani V K et al 2006 Toward understanding kernicterus: a challenge to improve the management of jaundiced newborns. Pediatrics 117:474–485.

Wennberg R P, Ahlfors C E, Bickers R et al 1982 Abnormal auditory brainstem response in a newborn infant with hyperbilirubinemia: improvement with exchange transfusion. J Pediatr 100:624–626.

Wennberg R P, Ahlfors C E, Rasmussen L F 1979 The pathochemistry of kernicterus. Early Hum Dev 3:353–372.

Wennberg R P, Gospe S M Jr, Rhine W D et al 1993 Brainstem bilirubin toxicity in the newborn primate may be promoted and reversed by modulating PCO_2. Pediatr Res 34:6–9.

Wennberg R P, Hance A J 1986 Experimental bilirubin encephalopathy: importance of total bilirubin, protein binding, and blood-brain barrier. Pediatr Res 20:789–792.

Wennberg R P, Johansson B B, Folbergrova J, Siesjo B K 1991 Bilirubin-induced changes in brain energy metabolism after osmotic opening of the blood-brain barrier. Pediatr Res 30:473–478.

Willis S K, Hannon P R, Scrimshaw S C 2002 The impact of the maternal experience with a jaundiced newborn on the breastfeeding relationship. J Fam Pract 51:465.

Wishingrad L, Cornblath M, Takakuwa T et al 1965 Studies of non-hemolytic hyperbilirubinemia in premature infants: I. prospective randomized selection for exchange transfusion with observations on the levels of serum bilirubin with and without exchange transfusion and neurologic evaluations one year after birth. Pediatrics 36:162–172.

Worley G, Erwin C W, Goldstein R F et al 1996 Delayed development of sensorineural hearing loss after neonatal hyperbilirubinemia: a case report with brain magnetic resonance imaging. Dev Med Child Neurol 38:271–277.

Yamanouchi I, Yamauchi Y, Igarashi I 1980 Transcutaneous bilirubinometry: preliminary studies of noninvasive transcutaneous bilirubin meter in the Okayama National Hospital. Pediatrics 65:195–202.

Yeung C Y, Wong H N 1992 Effect of serum pH on bilirubin-protein binding. Acta Paediatr Jpn 34:23–27.

Yilmaz Y, Ekinci G 2002 Thalamic involvement in a patient with kernicterus. Eur Radiol 12:1837–1839.

Yokosuka O, Billing B 1987 Enzymatic oxidation of bilirubin by intestinal mucosa. Biochim Biophys Acta. 923:268–274.

Yoshihiro M, Nishizawa K, Sato H et al 2000 Prolonged unconjugated hyperbilirubinemia associated with breast milk and mutations of the bilirubin uridine diphosphate-glucuronosyltransferase gene. Pediatrics 106:e59.

Zanella A, Fermo E, Bianchi P, Valentini G 2005 Red cell pyruvate kinase deficiency: molecular and clinical aspects. Br J Haematol 130:11–25.

Zhang L, Liu W, Tanswell A K, Luo X 2003 The effects of bilirubin on evoked potentials and long-term potentiation in rat hippocampus in vivo. Pediatr Res 53:939–944.

Zimmerman H M, Yannet H 1935 Cerebral sequelae of icterus gravis neonatorum and their relation to kernicterus. Am J Dis Child 49:418–430.

Zucker S D, Goessling W, Bootle E J, Sterritt C 2001 Localization of bilirubin in phospholipid bilayers by parallax analysis of fluorescence quenching. J Lipid Res 42:1377–1388.

Zucker S D, Goessling W, Hoppin A G 1999 Unconjugated bilirubin exhibits spontaneous diffusion through model lipid bilayers and native hepatocyte membranes. J Biol Chem 274:10852–10862.

Zuelzer W W, Mudgett 1950 Kernicterus; etiologic study based on an analysis of 55 cases. Pediatrics 6:452–474.

CHAPTER
37

Disorders of vision
Alistair R. Fielder and Laura A. Crawley

Key Points

- Differentiating normal and abnormal eye movements in the neonatal period can be very difficult
- Eye movement disorders are subdivided into nuclear/infranuclear, supranuclear or nystagmus-related oscillations
- The presence of nystagmus occurs in disorders of the anterior but not posterior visual pathway
- The timing of the insult during fetal life influences optic nerve morphology
- There are many patterns of visual development and the predictive value of a single measure is limited and multiple assessments are essential for this

INTRODUCTION

This chapter is primarily concerned with the neuro-ophthalmology of the first 6 months of life. Thus, ocular disorders such as infantile cataract, glaucoma or retinopathy of prematurity are not considered here. Thus, we will not discuss the clinical or molecular biological details of individual retinal conditions. In view of the rapid maturation occurring during infancy, various aspects of normal development are reviewed before considering the abnormal. Individual conditions are covered only briefly and referencing commences with a bibliography of major texts, followed by a list of the cited articles.

EYE MOVEMENTS

NORMAL EYE MOVEMENTS

In this section a brief description of the various types of eye movements is given. For more detailed accounts there are several reviews (Boothe et al 1985, Cassidy et al 2000, Fielder 1985, Garbutt and Leigh 2005, Hertle 2005, Hoyt et al 1982).

Embryology of the extraocular muscles

The extraocular muscles are formed as condensations of mesoderm which commence differentiation at 6 weeks of gestation and are fully formed by 12 weeks. By this time the ocular motor nerves have reached their destination. The supranuclear eye movement system, which is responsible for feeding information to the brainstem ocular motor nuclei, is not fully developed until after full-term.

Fetal eye movements

Eye movements can be detected, using ultrasonography, from 16 weeks of gestation (Birnholz 1981, Inoue et al 1986, Prechtl & Nijhuis 1983). These are discussed in detail in Chapter 7. Eye movements commence as slow changes of eye position, but these later become faster. Rapid eye movements are seen between 30 and 33 weeks of gestational age (GA) and are organized into periods of activity, which after 36 weeks GA are related to fetal behavioral state.

TYPES OF EYE MOVEMENT

Conjugate eye movements are movements of both eyes in the same direction and are also called versions. In disjugate movements the two eyes move in opposite directions, and these are called vergence movements. Conjugate movements include pursuit, saccadic, optokinetic and vestibulo-ocular eye movements. Pursuit movements enable the eyes to follow a relatively slow-moving target and hold the image on the fovea of the retina so that the target is seen clearly. If the object moves too fast for the pursuit system, a catch-up saccade is required to refixate the image back on to the fovea. Saccades are fast movements which allow us to change our direction of visual interest and direct the object of interest on to the fovea. Both optokinetic and vestibulo-ocular movements coordinate head and eye movements during body movements. Each type of eye movement is subserved by a separate supranuclear system, but all share a final common infranuclear pathway from the ocular motor nuclei to the eye muscles.

Finally, eye movement control requires a neural integrator which enables a chosen and eccentric eye position (gaze) to be maintained, even in the dark (absence of vision). The neural substrates include brain stem and cerebellar components (Hertle 2005).

Eye movements in infancy

The distinction between normal and abnormal eye movements in the neonatal period is not always easy to determine.

Ocular alignment and excursion

The eyes of neonates commonly appear divergent (Fig. 37.1), particularly if they are born prematurely (Rethy 1969). This has been studied by Nixon et al (1985) and Archer et al (1989), and while most neonates appear to be divergent, by 3 and 6 months of age 75 and 97%, respectively, had no deviation. The suggestion that normally the eyes are initially divergent but this diminishes over time has been challenged

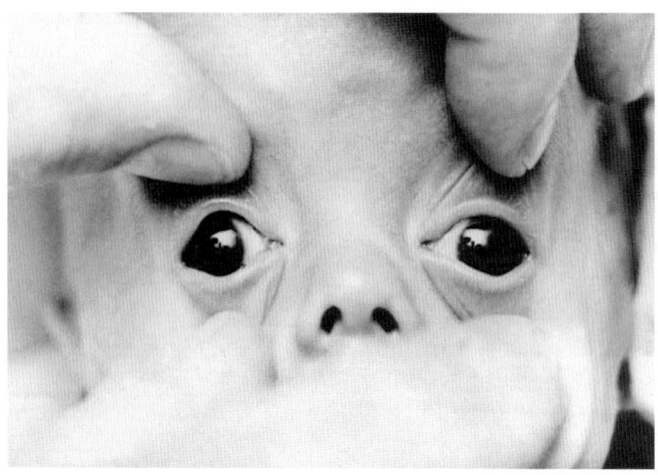

Figure 37.1 The divergent appearance of the eyes of a preterm neonate.

by Thorn et al (1994) and Horwood (1993) who say that mostly the divergent appearance is due, in part, to the shape of the neonatal eye (large angle κ) and absence of convergence until around 3 months of age. Slater and Findlay (1975) showed that the mean empirical angle kappa of neonates is 8°.

Horwood (2003) coined the term 'neonatal misalignments' distinguishing brief periods of intermittent squinting in the early neonatal period from true pathological strabismus. Transient esodeviations are common up to 4 months (73.2% transient misalignments within the first month.) These transient neonatal misalignments are thought to represent early inaccurate attempts at convergence.

Horizontal gaze probably develops before vertical (Jones, quoted by McGinnis 1930), and rotation generates full excursion.

Pursuit movements

The pursuit system enables the eyes to follow a moving target accurately and smoothly while maintaining foveal fixation, so that during a pursuit movement clear vision is maintained. Pursuit movements have been demonstrated in the first week of life and mature with age. The neonate can only make slow smooth eye and head movements (Hertle 2005, Kremenitzer et al 1979, Lengyel et al 1998, Roucoux et al 1983). Time to maturation to adult form is not wholly proven but does not occur before 6 months of age (Jacobs et al 1997) and may occur as late as adolescence (Katsanis et al 1998).

Tests of pursuit involve following a slow-moving target or the slow phase of optokinetic nystagmus (see later).

Saccadic movements

The saccadic system allows us to change our direction of visual interest and place the new object of regard on to the fovea so that it can be seen distinctly. An everyday example

is the shifting of gaze from the end of one line to the beginning of the next whilst reading. Saccades are rapid movements and the example given is a voluntary movement, but saccades also include reflex changes of fixation and the fast phases of all forms of nystagmus (vestibular and optokinetic nystagmus). In contrast to pursuit, vision is partially suppressed during a saccade. For instance, the reader is not aware of background movement when gaze switches from the end of one line to the beginning of the next line of text.

The infant achieves refixation by means of multiple hypometric saccades (Aslin & Salapatek 1975, Harris et al 1993, Regal et al 1983, Roucoux et al 1983). Infants rely more on coordinated head and eye movements than do adults when shifting gaze. By the age of 1 year the saccadic system has developed, enabling a change of fixation on to an eccentric target to be achieved by using a single saccade: *normometria*. Clinically these changes are easily observed: for example, it takes much longer to attract the visual interest of a neonate to a novel stimulus in the periphery of the visual field compared with a 9-month-old infant.

It had been suggested that infant saccades to simple geometric forms were slower than adult saccades to the same stimuli (Hainline et al 1984). Garbutt et al (2006) challenged this and demonstrated comparable and sometimes faster saccades in infants compared to adults.

Persistent slow saccades are a common finding in spinocerebellar ataxias and mitochondrial disorders, while multiple hypometric saccades occur in cerebellar disease, saccade initiation failure (congenital ocular motor apraxia) and basal ganglia disorders.

Tests of saccadic function involve inducing refixation eye movements, and voluntary and command movements.

Optokinetic nystagmus

This response is elicited by moving a striped tape or drum across the field of vision. It is characterized by a slow (following) phase in the direction of the moving stripe followed by a fast corrective phase which returns the eye to its original position. The amplitude of the optokinetic nystagmus (OKN) response is about 15°. Functionally, OKN is part of the vestibulo-ocular reflex (VOR) and coordinates head and eye movements, ensuring clear vision during body movements. OKN can be elicited from the first day of life in the full-term infant (Gorman et al 1957, McGinnis 1930).

Before the age of 3 months an OKN response can be obtained when the tape is moved in a temporal-to-nasal (TN) direction but not in a nasal-to-temporal (NT) direction when each eye is tested separately. In early infancy vision may be subserved largely at a subcortical level (Atkinson 1992, Mercuri et al 1997) and this OKN asymmetry for moderate stimulus speeds declines after 3 months due to the establishment of cortical vision (Braddick & Atkinson 1983); specifically the maturation of projections from the retina through the visual cortex to the pretectum (Katsanis et al 1998,

Valmaggia et al 2003). Fully symmetrical and adult like TN and NT OKN responses using high velocity stimuli are achieved at 10–11 months (Valmaggia et al 2004). For the preterm infant the transition from asymmetrical to symmetrical OKN occurs later postnatally, corresponding to about 3 months of corrected age (van Hof-van Duin & Mohn 1984a). Persistence of monocular OKN asymmetry beyond this age may be associated with strabismus and an absence of binocular function.

The pathways involved in the OKN response are poorly understood (Braddick & Atkinson 1983, van Hof-van Duin & Mohn 1983). The temporal-to-nasal response is probably mediated to a large extent subcortically via the contralateral nucleus of the optic tract and the dorsal terminal nucleus (Hoffman 1982), whereas the nasal-to-temporal response requires a functioning cortex (Simson 1988). Responses have been obtained in cortical blindness (van Hof-van Duin & Mohn 1983), while more recently OKN could not be elicited in the absence of a cortex (Braddick et al 1992).

Tests of OKN. The OKN tape or drum should be moved slowly in both horizontal and vertical directions, the responses being recorded separately in each direction, graded 0 to ++++. Its clinical uses include:

1. Vision assessment. A valuable but crude indication that vision is present. However, this is a test of visibility, not resolution (see later). Be aware of the extremely rare possibility of a positive response in severe visual cortical damage (van Hof-van Duin & Mohn 1983).
2. Eye movements. OKN is a test of both pursuit (slow phase) and saccadic (fast phase) systems, and binocular eye movements. This is also a simple means of detecting subtle slowness of the adducting eye in internuclear ophthalmoplegia.
3. Nystagmus. In infantile (congenital) nystagmus the OKN responses along the horizontal meridian are characteristically inverted (see later) but normal when the stripes are presented vertically. This is a useful diagnostic aid and helps to differentiate infantile nystagmus from the variable nystagmus associated with reduced vision. In the latter OKN response cannot be elicited in any direction.
4. The OKN test procedure may permit the best close-up, hands-off view of the infant's eye and its movements.

Vestibulo-ocular reflexes

The VOR ensures that the image remains stationary on the retina during head and body movements. Acceleration induces a movement of endolymph in the semicircular canals from which impulses are conveyed by the vestibular nerve to the brainstem and via the medial longitudinal fasciculus to the ocular motor nuclei. The VOR is vital for everyday activities, but can be modified by vision except under extreme 'fairground' conditions.

Tests of the VOR. There are three clinical tests: the doll's head maneuver, rotation of the infant and caloric testing.

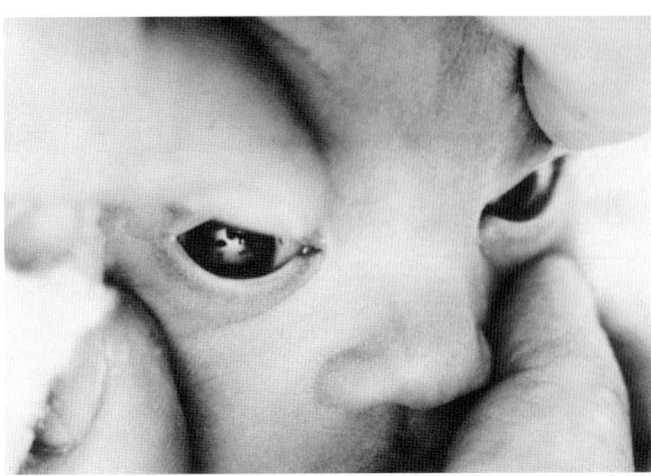

Figure 37.2 Doll's head maneuver: head turn to the left induces a deviation of the eyes to the right.

1. *Doll's head maneuver.* In the unconscious adult and conscious infant, head rotation induces a conjugate ocular deviation towards the opposite side; *head to the left, eyes to the right* (Fig. 37.2) — the doll's head movement. This is only observed in infancy before vision has developed sufficiently to suppress this response, or in the comatose adult patient. A normal response indicates an intact vestibular apparatus and ocular motor system — including the nuclei and peripheral nerves. The doll's head maneuver can therefore be used to detect limitation of ocular movements due to a gaze or cranial nerve palsy. This test is not informative about the pursuit or saccadic systems.
2. *Rotational tests.* These fall into two groups which induce different responses:
   a. Barany chair rotation. In this laboratory technique the infant is held upright and is rotated about his or her own vertical axis. This induces an ocular deviation in the direction opposite to the direction of rotation, as in the doll's head maneuver (Eviatar et al 1974). In the premature infant only a slow tonic deviation is induced, but with increasing gestational age a recovery fast phase develops, thereby inducing nystagmus.
   b. Rotation at arm's length. For this method the infant is held upright at arm's length with the head inclined slightly forward and then rotated. This procedure, commonly used in clinical practice, induces a tonic ocular deviation in the direction of the movement (as if the infant is looking ahead of the movement), i.e. rotation to the right, eyes deviate to the right (Fig. 37.3); in the older infant nystagmus also occurs. This response using a different axis of rotation induces a movement in the opposite direction to that seen using the Barany method.

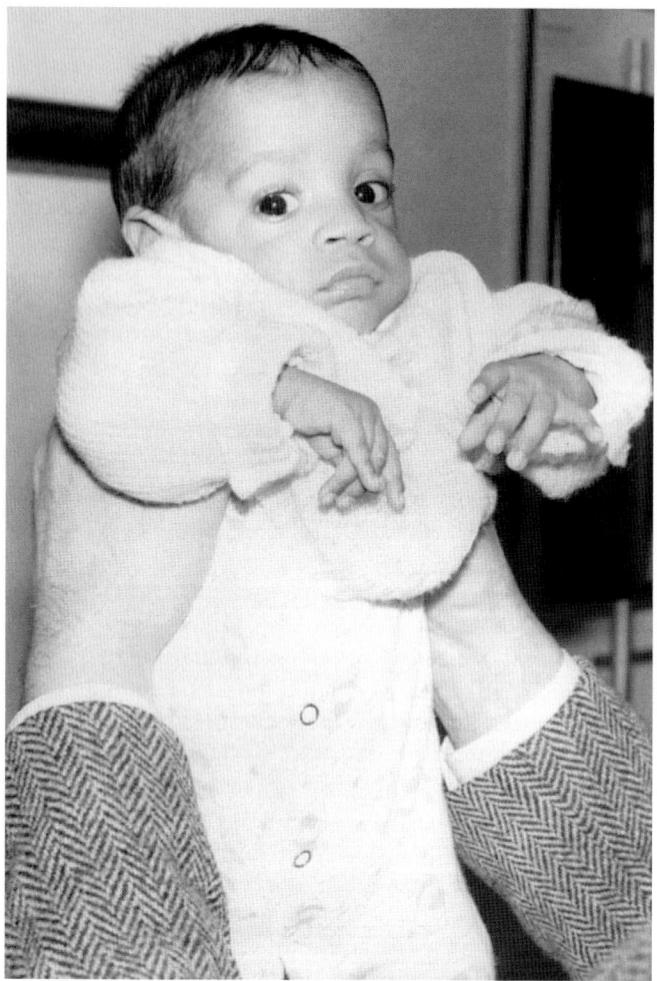

Figure 37.3 Rotation at arm's length. This baby is being rotated to his right, and his eyes deviate to the right — the opposite direction to that seen in the doll's head maneuver.

Whichever method is used, rotation of the premature infant induces a tonic deviation alone, and the fast phase (nystagmus) does not develop until about 45 weeks postmenstrual age (PMA) (Cordero et al 1983, Donat et al 1980, Eviatar et al 1979, Mitchell & Cambon 1969, Ornitz et al 1979, Rossi et al 1979). Behavioral state can influence this test: a fast phase elicited when the infant is awake may not be present when drowsy.

Once the age at which nystagmus occurs has been reached, post-rotatory nystagmus, in the opposite direction to that occurring during rotation, is seen. Its duration depends upon PMA, behavioral state, whether the test is performed in the dark, and the stage of visual development (Cordero et al 1983, Mitchell & Cambon 1969, Ornitz et al 1979), but in the alert sighted infant post-rotational nystagmus should cease within 5 seconds. Persistence of post rotational nystagmus beyond this is abnormal and may indicate severe visual impairment or an abnormality of smooth pursuit.

Rotation at arm's length is simple to perform and provides a great deal of clinically useful information on vision, the saccadic system, the vestibular system, ocular motor nuclei and infranuclear pathways.

Thus, rotation of the premature infant induces a full ocular deviation, because at this age vision is not sufficiently developed to modify the VOR. Later, vision dampens the VOR and hence the per-rotational excursion decreases — these maturational changes are very simple to demonstrate. In clinical terms, severely reduced vision can be suspected if rotation after 3 months of age induces an inordinately large rotational excursion and post-rotatory nystagmus persists for more than 5 seconds. This test is also a simple method of evaluating the range of eye movements in infancy and enables a sixth nerve palsy to be differentiated from a concomitant convergent squint.

3. *Caloric tests.* Donat et al (1980) confirmed the observation that the preterm infant cannot generate the fast phase of nystagmus. They observed, on caloric testing, an internuclear ophthalmoplegia in some normal premature infants, indicating immaturity of the medial longitudinal fasciculus, i.e. the brainstem communication between the vestibular apparatus and the ocular motor nuclei. As the doll's head maneuver always induced complete excursion they considered caloric testing to be a sensitive test of brainstem interconnections.

Vergence movements

The eye movements considered so far have all been conjugate. Convergence to near targets is clearly disjugate and cannot be consistently demonstrated until between 2 and 4 months of age (Aslin 1977, 1993, Hainline 1998, Horwood 2003, Ling 1942, Thorn et al 1994) and accommodation and convergence are both inaccurate before about 4 months of age (Aslin 1993). Fusion, the response to a base-out prism, is not established until 6 months (Aslin 1977). The onset of sensory (fusion and stereopsis) and motor binocularity (convergence) at the same time indicates the development of cortical function (Thorn et al 1994).

Tests of vergence observe convergence and divergence when an object is brought nearer or taken further away.

ABNORMAL EYE MOVEMENTS

Many of these conditions have important neurological or ophthalmological associations. Some of these disorders persist throughout life, but the emphasis will be directed towards those aspects relating particularly to the neonatal period and early infancy. Details of examination are adequately covered in other texts. Eye movement disorders can be divided into three groups: nuclear and infranuclear disorders, supranuclear disorders, nystagmus and related oscillations.

Nuclear and infranuclear disorders

These disorders limit the movement of one eye, whereas supranuclear abnormalities affect the movement of both eyes. Conditions involving the peripheral nerves, the cavernous sinus, orbit, and the extraocular muscles, as in myasthenia, are all included in this category. This section focuses on strabismus.

Strabismus

Strabismus (squint) may be the first sign of a serious ocular or systemic disorder and this possibility must always be borne in mind.

It has already been noted that neonates are, or appear to be divergent (see Fig. 37.1) (Archer et al 1989, Nixon et al 1985, Rethy 1969, Thorn et al 1994) or exhibit transient eso misalignments (Horwood 2003). With time this appearance resolves.

So-called congenital esotropia (concomitant convergent strabismus) is rarely, if ever, present at birth (Nixon et al 1985) but develops within the first 6 months of life and is therefore more appropriately called infantile esotropia. Abduction is often initially considered to be limited, but by rotation full excursions are generated, so differentiating infantile esotropia from a sixth nerve palsy.

Paralytic squints, either congenital or acquired, are not frequent in early infancy. Congenital palsies may be due to maldevelopment of the cranial nerve nuclei or nerves, or prenatal infection, although in most the etiology is unknown. The role of birth trauma as a cause of nerve palsy has been greatly overemphasized. A sixth nerve palsy can rarely present at birth as a very large-angle esotropia. If an isolated anomaly, as it usually is, it characteristically resolves spontaneously over a few weeks. While third or sixth nerve palsies are relatively obvious, a congenital fourth nerve palsy, which may have no systemic connotations, can easily be missed for some years until a compensatory head tilt is noted. Holmes et al (1999) reported 36 cases of paralytic squint over a 15 year period. The most commonly affected nerve was fourth nerve (36%) followed by sixth nerve (33%) the third (22%) and multiple nerve palsies (9%). Only 4 cases presented under the age of 1 and only one case of congenital sixth nerve palsy was found, presenting in an infant aged 2 weeks. It had resolved by four months.

In contrast, an acquired cranial nerve palsy frequently denotes a significant neurological disorder such as hydrocephalus, intracranial inflammation, tumor, neurodegenerative disorder and trauma, and as such may develop at any age (Fielder 1989).

- Squint may be the presenting feature of an infant with severe neurological or ophthalmic pathology. A blind eye may diverge or, less commonly, converge (Fig. 37.4), although this usually becomes apparent later in childhood.

The prevalence of concomitant squint in the general population is about 2–3%, but occurs more commonly in children who have suffered brain damage (von Noorden 1990), or are experiencing neurodevelopmental problems (Bankes 1974). Preterm birth is also associated with an increased incidence

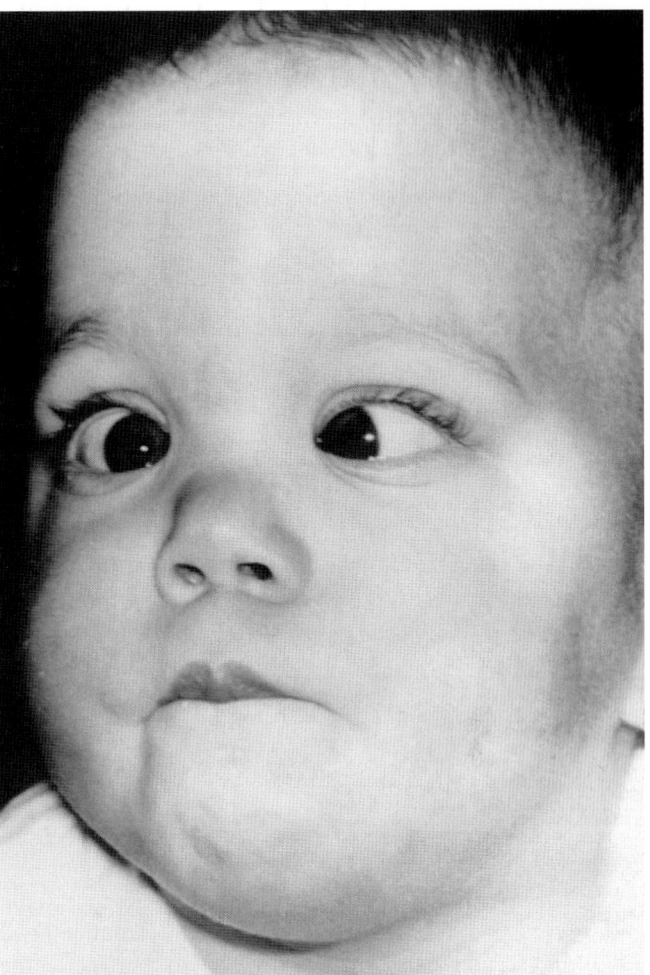

Figure 37.4 Left convergent squint due to ocular pathology. Cicatricial retinopathy of prematurity has severely affected the vision of the left eye.

of squint from 11 to >30% (Bremer et al 1998, Burgess & Johnson 1991, Holmstrom et al 1999, 2006, Laws et al 1992, McGinnity & Bryars 1992, Page et al 1993). O'Connor et al (2002) looked at the prevalence of strabismus in low birth weight children of <1701 g at age 10–12 years and reported a significant difference of 20.1% vs. 3% prevalence in a matched school cohort. Multivariate analysis showed that independent risk factors for strabismus were ROP, refractive error (greatest risk >+3.00 DS) low birth weight (<1500 g and <1000 g), anisometropia and cerebral palsy. They also looked at the relationship between abnormalities in cranial ultrasound and strabismus in this low birth weight cohort and found strabismus prevalence was 70.6% in those neonates with severe abnormalities on ultrasound imaging compared with 19.8% and 19.7% in the normal and mild abnormality groups respectively. In the most severe group with strabismus cystic periventricular leukomalacia was found in 70%, parenchymal ventricular hemorrhage in 100% and persistent ventricular dilatation in 71%. Gibson et al (1990) in a follow-up of infants of 1500 g birth weight and below reported strabismus in 50% of those with cystic periventricular leukomalacia and 70% of those with posterior cysts while Pike et al (1994) reported an incidence of 49%.

- Because of the possibility of coexistent or causative neurological or ophthalmic pathology every infant with a squint should have a detailed ophthalmic assessment and neurological work-up as indicated (Fielder 1989).

Supranuclear disorders

The reader is referred to the excellent review of supranuclear eye movements by Cassidy et al (2000). The supranuclear eye movement system governs the movements of both eyes in unison: pursuit, saccadic, vestibulo-ocular, OKN and vergence movements. According to the site of the lesion the various types of movement are affected differentially, but retention of some infranuclear movement and bilaterality which characterize the supranuclear disorder differentiates it from a lesion of the infranuclear pathways. Currently it is impossible to fully differentiate the possible influences on the development of strabismus of: prematurity per se, ROP, or neurological insults. Indeed in many infants more than one of these is present.

Saccadic palsy

This is not uncommon in infancy and is usually the result of an intracranial hemorrhage in the neonatal period affecting either the frontal cortex or the frontomesencephalic pathway as this descends to the brainstem (Trounce et al 1985). In saccadic palsy the eyes deviate to the side of the lesion (Fig. 37.5); thus ipsilateral, but not contralateral sac-

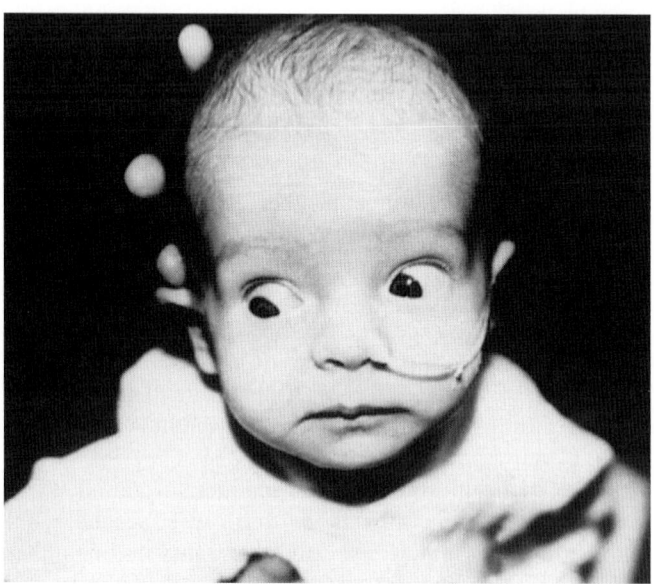

Figure 37.5 Neonatal thalamic hemorrhage (see p. 420). Ocular signs include 'sunsetting', skew deviation (left eye is higher than the right), and a tonic deviation of the eyes to the right (saccadic paresis).

cades can be elicited. Pursuit and the slow phase of the VOR are both unaffected if the lesion is above the brainstem.

Pursuit disorders

Isolated abnormalities of pursuit that do not also involve saccades are exceptionally rare.

Disorders of OKN

OKN can be affected by disorders of pursuit, saccades, brainstem connections (internuclear ophthalmoplegia) or a muscle paresis. OKN is often abnormal in parietal lobe lesions with a hemianopia. OKN is often abnormal in infantile nystagmus and neurological lesions affecting the brain stem, cerebellum or cortex.

Gaze palsy

In gaze paresis both saccadic and pursuit functions are affected and, depending on the site of the lesion, also the VOR. Most gaze palsies are caused by brainstem pathology where the various supranuclear eye movement pathways are close together. Horizontal gaze palsy may be congenital, as an isolated anomaly (Hoyt et al 1977), or in association with other abnormalities, e.g. in the Klippel–Feil or Möbius syndromes. Syndromes such as horizontal gaze palsy and progressive scoliosis (HGPPS) are genetic in origin with mutations in the human *ROBO3* gene located on chromosome 11q (Bosley et al 2005). In this syndrome there is usually a distinctive malformation of the inferior pons and medulla on MRI, namely anterior and posterior midline clefts and hypoplasia of the pons and cerebellar peduncles. The resultant impaired decussation of pontine oculomotor pathways is thought to explain the absence of horizontal eye movements. Brainstem glioma may produce an acquired palsy. In neonates, vertical gaze palsies are more common than horizontal. Up-gaze is usually affected more than down-gaze, and the eyes may deviate down – 'sunsetting' sign (Fig. 37.5). Eyelid retraction is common, although occasionally ptosis is present. Transient downward deviation of the eyes can occur in healthy neonates (Hoyt et al 1980) but an up-gaze gaze abnormality is usually indicative of a midbrain lesion, e.g. tumor, neurodegenerative disorder, encephalitis or hydrocephalus. Paroxysmal tonic upgaze which lasts a few months has also been described (Campistol et al 1993). Up-gaze palsy has been reported in preterm infants who sustained intraventricular hemorrhages (Tamura & Hoyt 1987). These infants showed tonic downward ocular deviations and convergent squints due to hemorrhage in thalamic and mesencephalic structures. Unilateral congenital vertical gaze palsy (double-elevator palsy) was observed affecting the left eye of identical prematurely born twins (Bell et al 1990). Rarely, a periodic alternating gaze deviation has been reported in infants in association with hindbrain anomalies (Legge et al 1992).

Congenital ocular motor apraxia

In congenital ocular motor apraxia (COMA), horizontal saccades to command are defective, hence the alternative term saccadic initiation failure. The affected child cannot shift gaze to either side voluntarily, and in order to look from one object to another has to insert a jerky head thrust characteristic of COMA (Cogan 1952, 1966). The head thrust, which is in the direction of the target, uses the VOR to drive the eyes to the opposite side of the orbit. This head movement carries on past the target, dragging the eyes with it until they are aligned on the target; the head then moves slowly back as the eyes remain fixed on the object of interest. While COMA is a defect of saccades, slow pursuit and the VOR are also affected, especially in early infancy as at this age no eye movements at all can be elicited along the horizontal meridian. In COMA vertical movements are unaffected.

Before the head thrust develops around 5 months of age, when adequate head control is achieved, the infant may be suspected to be blind as he or she will not show any visual interest in objects placed to one side, and no horizontal following movements can be demonstrated. At this early age the diagnosis can be suspected if the OKN response is absent horizontally but normal vertically. Also, rotation induces nystagmus if performed in the vertical but not in the horizontal meridian. After the head thrust has developed, the diagnosis is obvious, although over the years signs subside considerably. A degree of asymmetry is common.

In COMA, motor delay is probably universal in infancy and lessens, but does not necessarily completely resolve, with time. Delay in other spheres, particularly with speech, is common (Fielder et al 1986a, Hertle 2005, Rappaport 1987). Recently, Marr et al (2005) found that COMA without demonstrable structural abnormality on MRI scanning was associated with more severe developmental delay than previous reports have suggested.

Structural CNS malformations are common and may involve the cerebrum, cerebellar vermis, brainstem, rostral interstitial nucleus of the medial longitudinal fasciculus and basal ganglia (Harris et al 1996, Fielder et al 1986, Sargent et al 1997). In particular, agenesis of the corpus callosum and cerebellar hypoplasia have been repeatedly reported in association with COMA (Jan et al 1998, Marr et al 2005, Riva & Georgi 2000). Soo Kim et al (2003) reported cerebellar hypoplasia in a patient with both COMA and spasmus nutans. The range of neurological associations with COMA is now extensive including the aforementioned developmental abnormalities, neurodegenerative disorders (e.g. infantile Gaucher disease), acquired disease such as posterior fossa tumors and herpetic encephalitis (Hertle 2005).

Neonatal eye movements

As mentioned, eye movements, which would be considered abnormal and even warrant urgent neuro-ophthalmic investigation in the older child, are quite common in the neonate, particularly if preterm. Bursts of eye movements may be seen through closed eyelids but are most commonly seen when the infant is turned or disturbed. Tonic downward deviation, up- or down-beat nystagmus and nystagmus in other directions are commonly observed. Ocular flutter, opsoclonus (bursts of saccades) and skew deviations are less commonly seen. There is essentially no information on the prevalence and possible significance of these neonatal eye movements, or indeed whether they should even be considered abnormal. Dubowitz et al (1981) reported a strong correlation between intraventricular hemorrhage and roving eye movements. Hoyt et al (1980) examined 242 full-term neonates, without neurological abnormalities, and observed downward deviations (five infants), opsoclonus (nine) and skew deviation (22). Five of those with a skew deviation later developed a squint. Archer and Helveston (1994) commented on the rarity of skew deviation as they had not observed it once in 2271 examinations.

Clinicians should have a low threshold for investigating an abnormal eye movement if it persists more than a 'few weeks,' especially if associated with other signs.

Nystagmus

The reader is referred to the reviews of nystagmus by Gottlob (2001), Maybodi (2003) and Garbutt and Leigh (2005).

Physiological nystagmus

The various types of physiological nystagmus, including rotational, caloric and optokinetic nystagmus, have already been discussed.

CNS conditions — neurological nystagmus

Nystagmus can occur in many CNS conditions such as cerebellar, brainstem and vestibular lesions. In the adult these often produce predictable specific types of nystagmus which point to a particular anatomical location, whereas in the infant features tend to be more variable and have less diagnostic value (Dell'Osso et al 1990). Clearly nystagmus due to a CNS cause may be apparent at any age, in contrast to the so-called congenital nystagmus (see later). Thus, nystagmus observed within the first week or so of life is more likely to have a CNS basis. Dubowitz et al (1981) observed roving eye movements some time after the development of germinal matrix hemorrhage-intraventricular hemorrhage in preterm infants.

Sensory deprivation nystagmus

Bilaterally reduced vision in infancy and early childhood leads to nystagmus, but only if the lesion involves the anterior visual pathway. Consequently, nystagmus is not a feature of cortical blindness (Fielder & Evans 1988, Whiting et al 1985). Any condition of the anterior visual pathway sufficient to preclude normal visual development will cause sensory deprivation nystagmus. These conditions include: corneal scarring, albinism, achromatopsia, aniridia, congenital cataracts and optic nerve pathology, including atrophy and hypoplasia. Occasionally bilateral nystagmus may result from a uniocular condition (Good et al 1997).

Nystagmus due to a visual deficit does not develop until about 3 months of age, and presents clinically in two forms:

1. Wandering eye movements associated with blindness.
2. Nystagmus which is clinically indistinguishable from or very similar to congenital nystagmus.

It should be recognized that these may simply represent different ends of a single spectrum and not two distinct entities (Fielder & Evans 1988).

Blindness. As mentioned, severe visual deprivation before the age of 2 years, and sometimes later, results in nystagmus. As a very crude guide, the better the vision the faster the oscillation. In complete blindness the eye movements are slow, large in amplitude and variable in direction – nystagmoid movements of the blind.

Nystagmus indistinguishable from congenital nystagmus. Conditions such as albinism, achromatopsia and aniridia cause a visual defect, but not blindness, and result in nystagmus which is either similar or identical to that seen in congenital nystagmus. As mentioned, the oscillation usually starts at about 3 months. Occasionally the movement may be vertical on presentation (Fielder & Evans 1988, Hoyt & Gelbart 1984), but this subsequently becomes horizontally directed, as is the rule in congenital nystagmus. The ocular findings in many of these conditions are subtle and easily missed, thus, it is essential that congenital nystagmus is a diagnosis of exclusion, made only after all other possibilities have been excluded (see later). The clinical severity of certain conditions may vary between patients: thus, Leber congenital amaurosis or optic nerve hypoplasia may both cause either blindness or nystagmus of the blind or, if less severe, reduced vision and a congenital nystagmus picture. Two conditions deserve special mention: albinism and achromatopsia.

Albinism. A straightforward diagnosis to make in most instances but can sometimes be difficult early on, especially in the infant from a blond family or the X-linked ocular form. Albinism may present in early infancy with reduced vision, which subsequently improves (delayed visual maturation), around the time that the nystagmus commences. Slit-lamp examination reveals iris transillumination, and the foveal reflex is absent. The finding of the typical carrier retinal picture in the mother or sister of a suspected ocular albino is diagnostic. The definitive test for albinism is the visually evoked potential (VEP) by which visual pathway misrouting at the optic chiasm, characteristic of this condition, is identified (Apkarian & Tijssen 1992). Albinism is a complex genetic disease with varying degrees of severity in the phenotype. Those who have obvious nystagmus have poorer visual acuity and a higher incidence of strabismus (Wolf et al 2005). The precise explanation for this variability is unclear but is thought to be due to differences in ocular pigmentation and/or the degree of optic pathway misrouting.

Achromatopsia. This is a congenital absence of retinal cones and is inherited as an autosomal recessive trait.

Retinal cones function optimally in bright light and subserve fine discrimination (acuity) and color vision, thus the infant with achromatopsia (complete color blindness) presents with photosensitivity and poor vision, particularly under conditions of bright illumination. Visual function is reduced especially in sunlight, and color vision is absent. Nystagmus in achromatopsia closely resembles congenital nystagmus but its amplitude is less (Yee et al 1981). Ocular examination is essentially negative in infancy except for two subtle clues: a paradoxical pupil response and significant refractive error (Evans et al 1989). Neither of these is diagnostic, as both signs are also seen in Leber congenital amaurosis. Color vision testing is impossible at this age and the diagnosis can only be established definitively by electroretinography at 30 Hz (Figs 37.6 and 37.7). Unsurprisingly achromatopsia is rarely diagnosed correctly in the first year of life.

Infantile (congenital) nystagmus

The term 'infantile nystagmus' should be reserved for nystagmus presenting in infancy which is not associated with any other ocular abnormality (Dell'Osso et al 1990). The words 'congenital' and 'infantile' are used interchangeably with reference to nystagmus. The term 'motor nystagmus' is sometimes used to avoid confusion with nystagmus due to a sensory defect. The condition may be inherited as a domi-

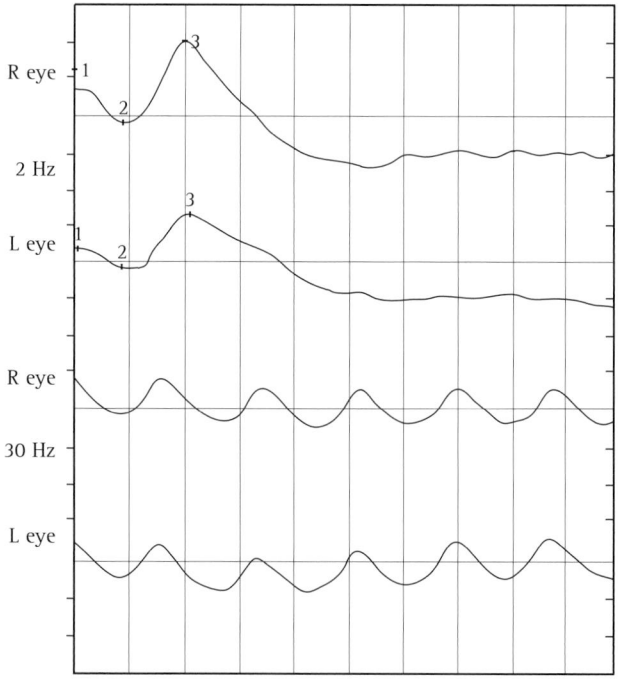

Figure 37.6 Electroretinogram (ERG) traces at 2 Hz (rod and cone response) and 30 Hz (cone response alone). These are normal responses obtained from a 2-year-old child without sedation using skin electrodes.

nant, recessive or X-linked disorder. While familial congenital nystagmus is free of neurodevelopmental problems, this is often not so for non-familial types (Jan et al 1992). Infantile is preferred to congenital as the onset is usually at about 6 weeks of age, although very occasionally it is observed immediately after birth. Sometimes, if associated with delayed visual maturation (see later), it does not develop for a few months, until around the time when vision develops.

In infantile nystagmus the oscillation is binocular, symmetrical and horizontally directed in all positions of gaze, except for the rare vertical variant (Chaudry et al 1996). In early infancy the oscillation is slow and of large amplitude, and may be horizontal, vertical or rotatory, but with increasing age the movement becomes more rapid, fine and horizontal (Hertle et al 2002, Reinecke 1997, Reinecke et al 1988). This waveform progression from infancy to toddler age from predominantly pendular to more jerk type reflects modification of the nystagmus by growth and development of the visual sensory system (Maybodi 2003). The movement is dampened by convergence and often increases on lateral gaze. Vertical OKN is normal but horizontal OKN is commonly absent. As these children are often initially thought to be blind, demonstration of intact vertical OKN responses reassures the parents that vision is present. Compensatory head nodding, the null position and the compensatory head posture will not be covered here as they develop after infancy.

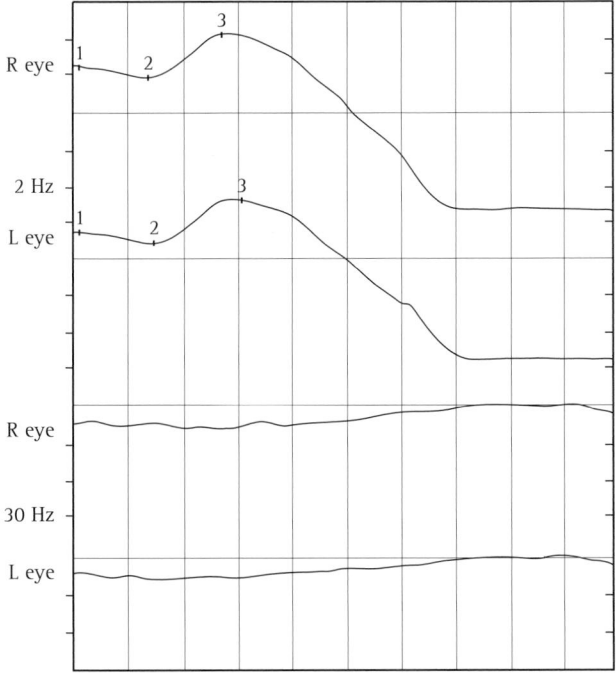

Figure 37.7 ERG traces from a child with achromatopsia. A response is obtained at 2 Hz, indicating the presence of rod photoreceptors, but not at 30 Hz, due to an absence of retinal cones.

On an anatomical level we now know that there are structural abnormalities of the extraocular muscle tendons as they insert into the scleral fibers thus leading to altered proprioception (Hertle et al 2002).

Making a diagnosis of infantile nystagmus can be difficult, particularly as during early infancy it may be variable and the aforementioned characteristics may not be apparent. Furthermore, as many other forms of nystagmus with ocular or neurological associations mimic this condition to the extent that they are clinically indistinguishable, the diagnosis of infantile nystagmus must be one of exclusion (Weiss & Biersdorf 1989).

Spasmus nutans

This syndrome consists of the triad nystagmus, head nodding and torticollis, and commences between 4 and 18 months of age. Not all features are present at one time; thus, the head nod may be present before the nystagmus and vice versa. Although the nystagmus is usually bilateral, it can be grossly asymmetrical and may be either horizontal or vertical. Like congenital nystagmus, spasmus nutans is a diagnosis of exclusion. Infants with these signs can harbor intracranial tumors (Antony et al 1980, Arnoldi & Tycheson 1995). Full neurological assessment is mandatory, all the more important because there are no clinical features which distinguish those infants with and without CNS lesions (Gottlob et al 1990, 1992). Spasmus nutans resolves spontaneously usually within 1–2 years and with good outcome, but there have been reports of increased incidence of strabismus in these patients (Gottlob et al 1995). Wizov et al (2002) reported new findings on the demographics and socioeconomic differences in patients with spasmus nutans and idiopathic infantile strabismus. They found that low socioeconomic status was an independent risk factor for the development of spasmus nutans.

Asymmetric nystagmus

Nystagmus which is either totally monocular or significantly asymmetric between the two eyes may be seen in infancy, as in spasmus nutans. Farmer and Hoyt (1984) emphasized the frequency of monocular nystagmus in infants with chiasmal tumors. Monocular blindness can cause monocular nystagmus, but the latter usually develops after infancy. Unfortunately, as there are no clinical features which distinguish absolutely infants with spasmus nutans from those with chiasmal tumors, full neurological and neuroradiological investigations are necessary (Gottlob et al 1990). Conversely, occasionally monocular visual defects can be associated with binocular nystagmus (Good et al 1997).

Special nystagmus types

Many other types of nystagmus not considered here may have important neurological implications – such as downbeat, upbeat, see-saw, dissociated (e.g. in internuclear ophthalmoplegia), ocular bobbing, and retraction nystagmus (Dell'Osso et al 1990, Hertle 2005).

The investigation of nystagmus

Nystagmus must always be taken seriously as it may signify a serious neurological or ocular disorder. The pattern of eye movement must be carefully evaluated, in each eye individually, by recording the direction (convention dictates this to be in the direction of the fast phase), amplitude and frequency of the nystagmus in the nine positions of gaze. The distinction between pendular and jerk nystagmus is not diagnostically helpful as both may exist in the same patient in different positions of gaze. Accurate diagnosis is rarely possible from the observation of the pattern of nystagmus alone. Because the incidence of neurological and visual pathway disorders is high and these cannot always be differentiated on a clinical basis (Jan et al 1992. Weiss & Biersdorf 1989), all infants with nystagmus should have a full ophthalmic and pediatric-neurological assessment which includes electrophysiological investigations. The latter may be performed simply without sedation in most infants and the stimulus frequencies should be 2 Hz (which elicits a combined rod and cone response) and 30 Hz (cone response alone) (Figs 37.6 and 37.7).

VISION

NORMAL DEVELOPMENT

The rapid development of vision in the first few months of life is one of the most rewarding features of infancy, although its quantitative assessment remains a major clinical challenge. In this section only brief mention is made of the qualitative assessment of visual function, emphasis being on the quantitative measurement of visual acuity, particularly the adaptation of the preferential looking technique – the acuity card procedure.

As described by Slater (1998) infants exhibit 'natural' preferences for:

- Patterned rather than unpatterned visual stimuli.
- Horizontal rather than vertical stripes.
- Moving compared to stationary targets.
- 3-dimensional rather than 2-dimensional stimuli.
- Curvilinear rather than rectilinear patterns.
- Objects in the fronto-parallel plane rather than at an angle.
- High contrast rather than low contrast stimuli.
- Optimally sized objects.
- Face-like stimuli.

Qualitative aspects of visual development

Many infants' responses have a visual basis and consequently provide a useful, qualitative indication of visual development (Isenberg 1994, Slater 1998, Taylor 2005, van Hof-van Duin & Mohn 1984a, Vital-Durand et al 1996).

Blink reflex

The blink reflex to a bright light is said to be present from 28 weeks PMA (Robinson 1966) and in almost all full-term and preterm babies at 40 weeks PMA (Kurtzberg et al 1979). This contrasts with the tactile corneal reflex which is present in only 10% of newborns 35–40 weeks GA, increasing to 100% at 12 weeks GA (Snir et al 2002). A response does not invariably indicate the presence of vision, as a blink reflex has been observed in hydranencephaly with absence of the visual cortex (Aylward et al 1978).

Eyelid opening

Eyelid opening is a function of PMA. Thus babies have their eyes shut for over 90% of the time at 28 weeks PMA, but by 34 weeks they are open for 40% (Robinson et al 1989). The development of 4D sonography in recent years demonstrates spontaneous blinking in utero in third trimester (Yigiter et al 2006). Spontaneous blinking increases with age (Zametkin et al 1979). Bacher and Smotherman (2004) found that spontaneous blinking in 10–12 week old babies is also influenced by environmental surroundings, increasing during feeding and following the introduction of new visual stimuli.

Awareness and fixation

From 30 weeks PMA there are periods of awareness during which visual fixation occurs, and these periods naturally increase with increasing age (Hack et al 1981).

Visual attention is not considered here, but it is pertinent to many of the behavioral tests currently used to measure a range of visual functions. Before about 54 weeks PMA the latency of phasic orientation (attention getting) is stable, but decreases thereafter. Similarly the duration of tonic orientation (attention holding) exhibits a plateau until around 54 weeks PMA and then decreases (Foreman et al 1991). These alterations of attention getting and holding with age are obvious during all tests of preferential looking (see later), both as the speed of response by the neonate compared to the older infant to a peripherally located stimulus, and the duration of looking at the stimulus respectively. Indeed, understanding of these changes is required to prevent misinterpretation. Infants at 1 month, compared to those of 3 months of age, are more disrupted by, and respond slower to, a competitive stimulus consisting of two stimuli (Atkinson et al 1992). It has also been suggested that in certain neurological impairments, attention may be selectively affected compared to VEP measures (Hood & Atkinson 1990).

Orientation

Head turning to a diffuse light can be demonstrated from about 32 weeks PMA (Robinson 1966) and is elicited in most by full-term (Goldie & Hopkins 1964). After 36 weeks PMA there is no significant difference between preterm and full-term infants (Robinson 1966), although Ferrari et al (1983) have reported that preterm infants examined around 40 weeks PMA are significantly poorer in orientation. Anderson et al (1989) noted poor orientation in some infants with intraventricular hemorrhage.

Following

Using a red ball, Brazelton et al (1966) detected following in 57% of normal infants at full-term. Dubowitz et al (1980) found a red woollen ball to be a better stimulus and were able to elicit following from 31 weeks PMA. Vehrs and Baum (1970), in testing preterm and full-term neonates around full-term, considered a flashing light to be a more effective stimulus than either a red ball or diffuse light.

Optokinetic nystagmus

Responsiveness to an OKN stimulus can be elicited at full-term (Kremenitzer et al 1979).

Visual threat response

Eyelid closure to an approaching threatening object does not develop until about 16 weeks of corrected age for full-term and preterm infants and is thought to be a cortical response. When performing this test it is important to avoid tactile stimulation, e.g. a rush of air (van Hof-van Duin & Mohn 1984a).

Reaching

Visually directed reaching with one hand is first seen from about 2 months (Cavanagh 1997, White et al 1964).

Smiling

Vision can be an important component of this response, thus failure to smile by 6 weeks of age may signify a serious visual defect.

Other visual functions

Pupil reactions

The onset of the pupillary response to light is between 30 and 34 weeks GA (Robinson & Fielder 1990). These reactions are clinically difficult to assess in infants and care must be taken to ensure that light and near reactions are not also active.

The pupillary response to light is one of the best known reflexes; however that the pupil reacts to other visual stimuli such as its spatial structure, color and movement, is less well known. Thus, the subtle pupillary constriction to a grating stimulus, the pupil grating response (PGR) measured by infrared pupillometry, can be used to quantify visual acuity (Cocker et al 1994). The PGR in contrast to the pupil light response (PLR) is cortically mediated and is not present until one month of age, by which age behavioral responses have been obtainable for several weeks (Fig. 37.8).

Color vision

At 1 month of age infants do not discriminate between colors (Hainline 1998), but this has developed by 2 months and by 3 months color vision is similar to that in adults (Adams & Courage 1995, Boothe et al 1985, Mercer et al 1991, Teller 1998). Infants are probably more sensitive to brightness than color cues (Hainline 1998) and the size of the stimulus is also important (Adams & Courage 1995).

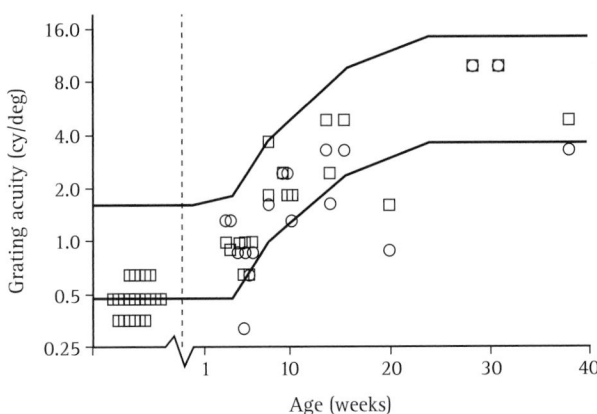

Figure 37.8 Visual acuities obtained by pupillometry and behavioral (ACP) methods. Binocular age norms are indicated by the solid lines. Open squares: behavioral acuities. Open circles: pupil acuities. No pupil acuities were measurable during the neonatal period, following which, they correlated well with ACP values.

Visual field

At birth the visual field is approximately 30° on either side of the horizontal, and this reaches adult proportions after 3 years of age (Dobson et al 1998, Mohn et al 1986). Premature infants with white matter damage have been shown to have varying degrees of abnormality in their visual fields. These abnormalities are more pronounced in the inferior rather than superior visual field (Jacobsen et al 2006). Lewis and Maurer (1992) have also studied the development of the visual field and discuss the relative merits of kinetic (stimulus location moves, intensity constant) and static (stimulus stationary, its intensity increases) perimetry. The application of perimetry to the infants and young children has been reviewed by Mayer and Fulton (1993).

DEVELOPMENT OF VISUAL ACUITY — METHODS OF MEASUREMENT

Resolution, recognition and visibility — types of visual acuity

A prerequisite to evaluating a patient's history or tests of visual function is an understanding of the parameter being measured. This topic bewilders clinicians of all disciplines, particularly those who attempt to correlate measurements obtained by different methods. No clinician would dream of equating X-ray, CT and MRI scans as they so obviously measure different parameters. So it is with the various stimuli used to assess vision. There are three stimulus types in common usage:

Visibility: the assessment of vision using a single object containing no detail, such as a sweet or white ball. Tests include the Catford drum, Stycar balls or sweets.

Resolution acuity: the ability to distinguish two separate points such as stripes in a grating or the squares of a checker board. Tests include preferential-based tests and the visually evoked potential.

Recognition acuity: the ability to distinguish the detail of letters or pictures. For the older child and adult these are the tests used in everyday clinical practice. Tests include the Snellen, Sheridan and Gardiner letter tests, Cardiff cards, Kays pictures and today's gold standard – the logMAR chart.

In infancy, resolution and visibility tests are used, but as the figure shows (Fig. 37.9) the correlation between the two is poor (Atkinson et al 1981, van Hof-van Duin 1989). Tests of visibility seriously overestimate vision when compared with resolution acuities (Atkinson et al 1981, van Hof-van Duin 1989). Thus, a parent's observation that a child can see a very small sweet is merely a comment on visibility and does not preclude a serious defect of resolution visual acuity, to the extent that in our opinion, visibility tests are so misleading that they should not be used.

BEHAVIORAL METHODS — PREFERENTIAL LOOKING-BASED TESTS

Parents are rewarded by their infant's visually directed look or smile; and in the absence of accurate methods of measuring visual acuity this has been the mainstay of clinical assessment of visual performance. Fantz in the 1950s transferred this subjective response to a test of visual acuity based on the infant's preference to look at a patterned rather than a non-patterned stimulus. In the 1970s this was taken further, and forced-choice preferential looking was developed, mainly by Teller and associates. Techniques based on the preferential looking (PL) (Dobson 1994, Pearson et al 1989) are too tedious and time-consuming for routine clinical use, but they have added greatly to our knowledge of normal and abnormal visual development (Teller 1997) and led to a simplified modification – the acuity card procedure (ACP) (McDonald et al 1985) (and a similar test used by Dubowitz et al 1980, Morante et al 1982). This is suitable for use in everyday practice and permits the quantitative evaluation of infants and children who could not be previously be assessed (e.g. Fielder et al 1992) (Figs 37.10 and 37.11).

With ACP the following issues can be problematic: judging looking patterns in the presence of nystagmus, congenital ocular motor apraxia, a field defect, or strabismus. In these situations holding the cards vertically rather than horizontally is helpful. All preferential looking-based tests including ACP depend on the behavioral response of the infant and thus their state of alertness at the time of testing. Thus, a poor response may be caused by an inability or reluctance to generate the behavioral response on that occasion rather than poor visual acuity.

PL-based studies indicate that vision develops at a rate of one cycle per degree per month and does not reach adult levels of 30 cycles until 3–5 years of age (Atkinson & Braddick 1983, Boothe et al 1985, Teller et al 1986). Grating acuities are measured in cycles per degree, i.e. the number of pairs of black and white stripes per degree of visual angle. Thus the infant whose vision is developing normally sees 3 cycles/degree (6/60) at 3 months, 6 cycles/degree (6/30) at 6 months and 12 cycles/degree (6/18) at 1 year of age. It is interesting to note that PL-based tests enable the effect of dietary intake on visual development to be quantified. Birch et al (1993) observed significantly better acuities in infants fed ω-3 fatty acids (human milk) compared to those fed a corn oil-based formula low in these substances. Auestad et al reported (2003) that both docosahexanoic acid and arachidonic acid promote visual, cognitive and language development (for review see Fleith & Clandinin 2005).

The success rate for binocular testing by ACP is around 95% in the first 2 years of life (Chandna et al 1988, Courage & Adams 1990, Fielder & Moseley 1988, Salomao & Ventura 1995, Sebris et al 1987, Teller et al 1986), but falls to around 80% between 2 and 3 years of age in clinical settings (Fielder & Moseley 1988). Success rates for monocular testing range from 66 to 96% under 3 (Chandna et al 1988, Mayer et al 1995) and 5 years (Sebris et al 1987) of age. The acuity difference between the two eyes in the normal infant is within 0.5 octaves (Chandna 1991, Raye et al 1992).

Optokinetic nystagmus

This response has been used to measure visual acuity (Gorman et al 1957), although in recent years this technique has attracted relatively little interest.

Visual evoked potentials

This is discussed in Chapter 12, but a few aspects need to be mentioned here. Both the flash (Fielder et al 1983) and pattern VEP (Moskowitz & Sokol 1983) reflect visual pathway maturation (Birch & Petrig 1996, Crognale et al 1997). However, only the latter, as it contains an edge, can be used to measure acuity. Pattern reversal VEP estimates of infant visual acuity indicate that adult levels are reached by about 6–12 months (Marg et al 1976, Sokol 1978). However, in a study by de Vries-Khoe and Spekreijse (1982), using a pattern onset stimulus, this level was not achieved until about 4 years of age. It is interesting to note that maturation of the pattern reversal VEP occurs faster in female infants than males (Malcolm et al 2002). This gender difference persists into adulthood and is not fully explained by head circumference or brain size alone. Apkarian et al (1991) have shown that behavioral state dramatically affects all VEP components, resulting in considerable intra- and intersubject variability. Recently, the sweep visually evoked potential has been introduced to measure resolution acuity in infants. This technique employs a rapidly reversing sinusoidal grating (steady-state VEP) that changes its spatial frequency every 5–10 seconds. This enables a range of spatial frequencies to be 'swept' in a short time, and an acuity estimate derived (Norcia 1994, Norcia et al 1987, Thompson & Liasis 2005).

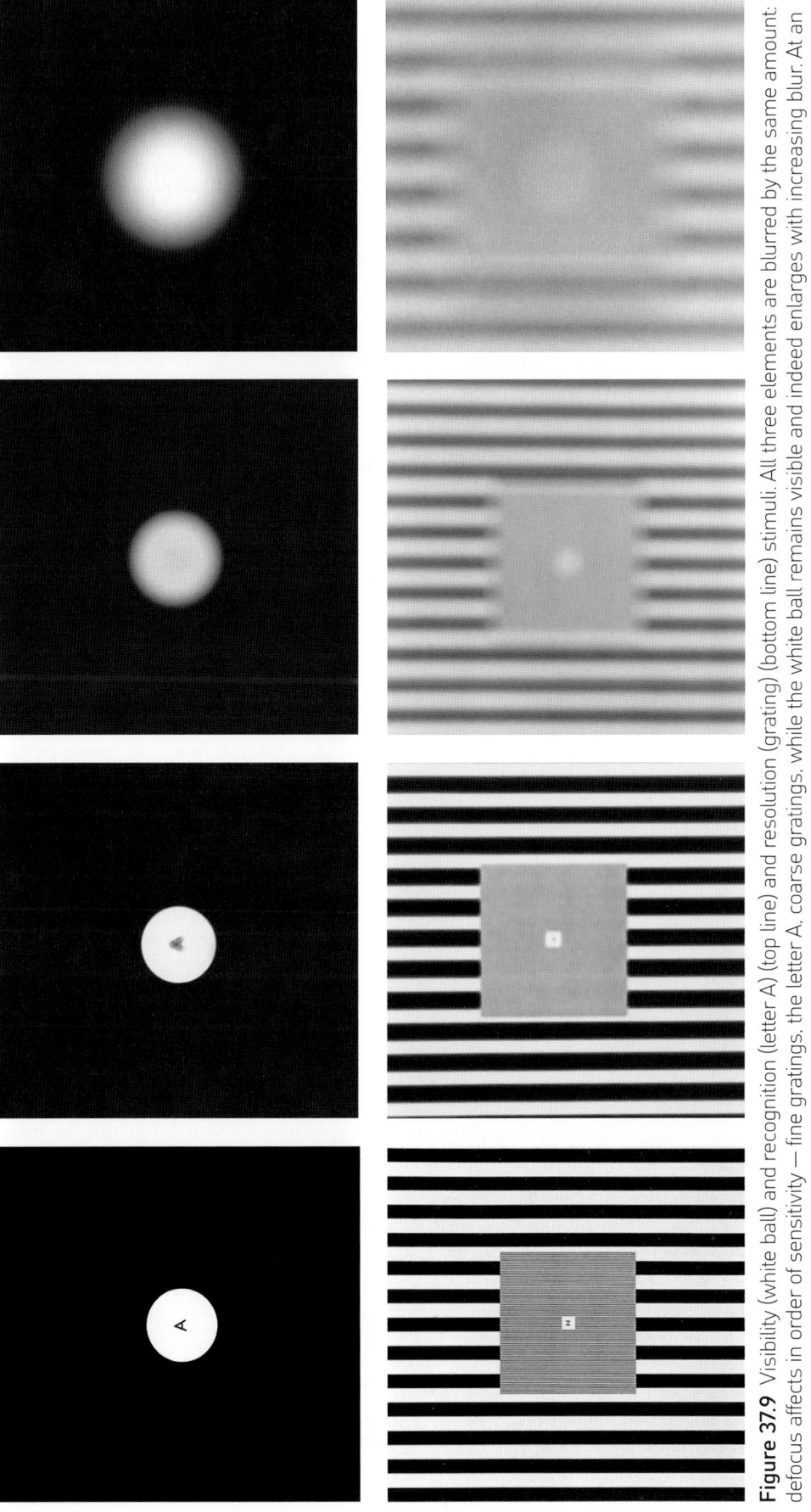

Figure 37.9 Visibility (white ball) and recognition (letter A) (top line) and resolution (grating) (bottom line) stimuli. All three elements are blurred by the same amount: defocus affects in order of sensitivity — fine gratings, the letter A, coarse gratings, while the white ball remains visible and indeed enlarges with increasing blur. At an early stage of blur, the fine gratings are invisible as such, while the letter A, although indistinct, remains recognizable as either an A or an upside down V. This figure provides the explanation for how a severely visually impaired child can still see a sweet! PL* will be used here to cover all tests based on the preferential looking principle, although ACP will be used specifically for the acuity card procedure.

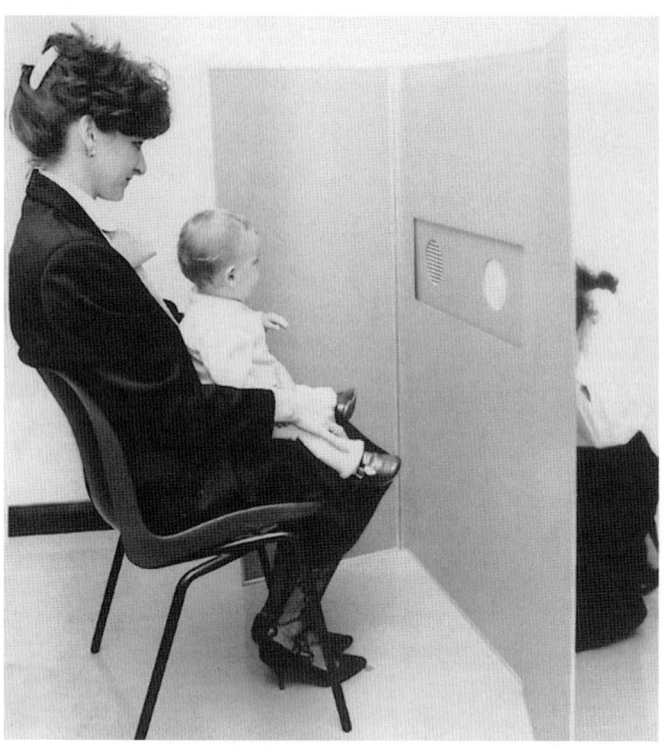 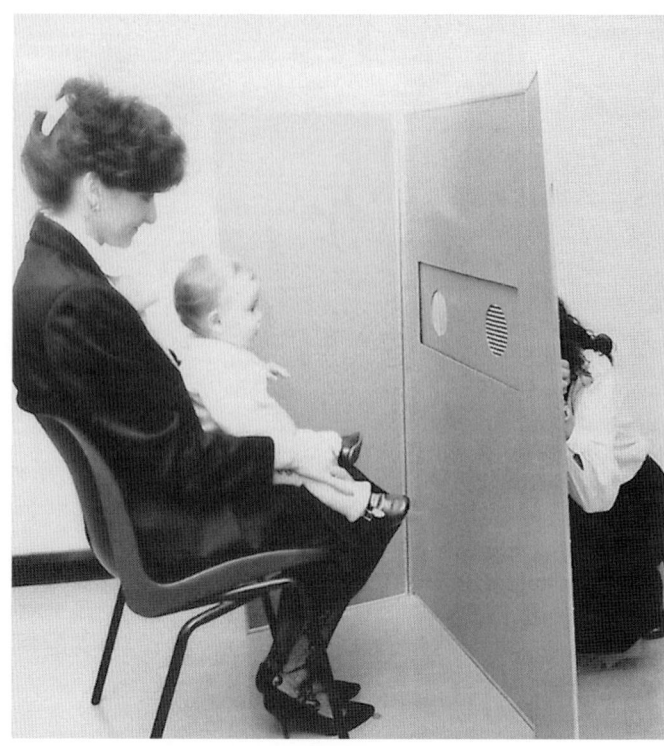

Figure 37.10 Acuity card procedure. The infant is clearly looking towards the grating (the near-side panel has been turned sideways for the photograph).

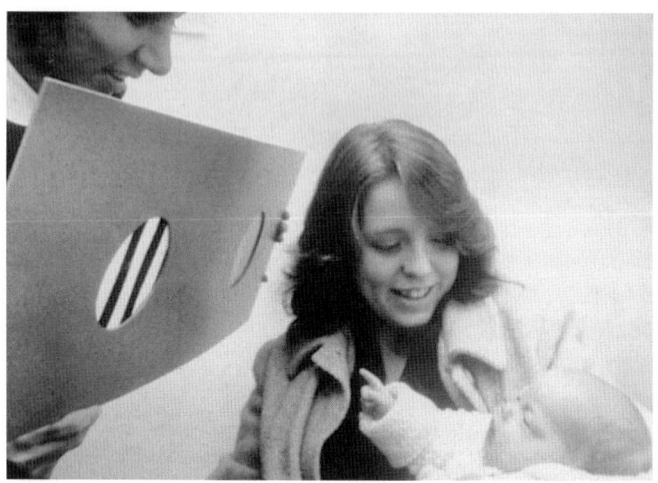

Figure 37.11 Acuity card procedure. In certain circumstances, the stimulus cards may be used without the surrounding apparatus.

The VEP : PL-based test discrepancy

Using standard pattern reversal and flash techniques, VEP acuity estimates tend to be higher than those obtained by PL. The basis of this discrepancy has not been fully resolved, but it is interesting to note that foveal development takes much longer than originally thought, maturity not being reached until between 15 and 45 months after birth (Hendrickson & Yuodelis 1984), corresponding closer to PL than VEP results. One exception is the VEP study of de Vries-Khoe and Spekreijse (1982), which correlates with both anatomical and PL data. In 1992 Sokol et al reported a smaller discrepancy if phase-alternating gratings were used to estimate both VEP and PL, compared to the usual method which employs phase-alternating gratings to estimate the VEP and stationary gratings to estimate PL. Prager et al (1999) compared the test-retest variability of the 3 main testing modalities of visual function in infants: card procedure (ACP), sweep VEPs and pattern VEPs. They found the test-retest results of all 3 methods to be reliable for group testing; however there was poorer agreement in testing an individual infant. They concluded that each test, while valid, is probably evaluating a different aspect of vision a point emphasized by Madan et al (2005). In summary, PL-based test results correlate quite closely with the sweep VEP.

The PL : Snellen acuity discrepancy

The clinician, already confused by the discrepancy between behavioral (ACP) and evoked potential acuity estimates, is now confronted with another discrepancy: that between PL and Snellen estimates. Acuities obtained by PL are not always directly comparable to those obtained by Snellen or other recognition targets. Thus, PL grating acuities may be significantly better than Snellen acuities in certain clinical conditions, particularly amblyopia (Mayer et al 1984). This difference is not fully understood (Fielder et al 1992) but may be due partly to methodological differences in measuring PL and Snellen acuities (Moseley et al 1988). While it does not negate the value of PL it does reduce its value as a method of determining the precise magnitude of amblyopia. Despite these problems it should not be forgotten that the ACP is the only quantitative test of vision which can be used simply and rapidly in the clinical situation and gives far more information than existing qualitative tests. Its value in recording visual development and assessing the infant who appears not to see well is not in question (Fielder et al 1992).

Pupil grating response

The subtle pupillary constriction to sinusoidal gratings of varying frequency can be used to measure visual acuity and correlates well with levels obtained by behavioral methods by 4–6 weeks after birth (Cocker et al 1994). The use of pupillometry is currently confined to clinical research.

Visual development of preterm infants

It is now pertinent to consider the effect of preterm birth on the visual system (Fielder et al 1988, 1993, van Hof-van Duin & Mohn 1986). What is the effect of removal from the protective milieu of the uterus and early exposure to the harsh neonatal environment? Does additional time in the extrauterine environment accelerate visual maturation? Central retinal photoreceptor cells although formed by 24 weeks gestation have only rudimentary outer segments (Johnson et al 1985, Provis et al 1985). Rod photoreceptors are still developing at 40 weeks (Hollenberg et al 1972). The preterm infant brain blood supply also differs significantly from that of the term infant (Madan et al 2005). With this background it is pertinent to consider whether visual development is hastened, retarded or unaffected by premature exteriorization (Fielder & Moseley 2000).

This is not the place to consider retinopathy of prematurity, but it should be borne in mind that most neonates with a birth weight below 1000 g will have developed at least minor stages of this condition.

The ERG can be recorded from around 32 weeks PMA (Mactier et al 2000) and Kennedy et al (1997) did not detect any effect with light reduction by goggling.

At full-term, the vision of the preterm infant is lower than that of his or her full-term counterpart (Morante et al 1982), and remains so until about 30 weeks, if postnatal age is used as the parameter (van Hof-van Duin & Mohn 1984a, van Hof-van Duin et al 1983). However, when corrected for the degree of prematurity, preterm and full-term infants develop similarly as assessed by behavioral techniques (Brown & Yamamoto 1986, Dobson et al 1980, Kos-Pietro et al 1997, Morante et al 1982, Roy et al 1995, van Hof-van Duin & Mohn 1984a, van Hof-van Duin et al 1983, Weinacht et al 1999). In con-

trast to the above, some VEP studies show mild hastening of acuity development (Norcia et al 1987, Sokol & Jones 1978), although, more recently (Mirabella et al 2006), all showed that preterm birth had no effect on VEP development. All these results show that, very broadly speaking, premature birth neither hastens nor retards visual development in infancy, i.e. the visual maturation is controlled predominantly by innate rather than environmental processes.

Neurologically abnormal preterm infants may show a delay in visual acuity maturation (Dubowitz et al 1983, Groenendaal et al 1989, Norcia et al 1987, Placzek et al 1985). Controversy still exists as to whether the flash VEP (within days to 3 weeks of birth) is a reliable prognostic tool in predicting neurological outcome in preterm infants. Shepherd et al (1999), Pike and Marlow (2000) and Kato et al (2000) and Kato and Watanabe (2006) showed that the flash VEP in preterm neonates has some predictive value for both survival and cerebral palsy. This contrasts with Beverley et al (1990) and Ekert et al (1997) who did not find any prognostic value of the flash VEP in predicting neurological outcome. Harvey et al (1997a) reported that grating acuity is affected by IVH, but this is not related to its grade or presence of PVL, and visual field development is reduced only before 17 months. For children with bronchopulmonary dysplasia, uncomplicated by neurological problems, their grating and field development is normal, but recognition acuity may be affected (Harvey 1997b). The predictive value of a single measure in early infancy is limited as the slope of visual development (whatever function is assessed) may differ and multiple assessments are essential so that this slope can be calculated (O'Connor et al 2007).

ABNORMALITIES OF VISION — GENERAL

One of the most difficult clinical problems is the assessment of the infant or child who might be harboring a visual deficit. A carefully taken history can be more informative than the subsequent clinical examination. Concern voluntarily expressed by a parent must always be taken seriously as this is rarely unfounded and usually more reliable than most qualitative tests of vision. Seeming lack of concern must, however, be treated with caution as it does not necessarily indicate that all is well. This attitude can be adopted for a number of reasons. First, a low expectancy is generally held for vision in very early infancy. Second, anxiety may be hidden until the parent's fear that their baby has defective vision is either allayed or confirmed by medical staff, following which they may pour out a detailed account accurately describing reduced vision dating back to very early infancy. Third, information may be withheld for fear of biasing the professional towards an unfavorable verdict.

The visual pathway abnormalities to be considered in this section are divided into those affecting the anterior (eye to optic chiasm) and posterior (optic tracts to visual cortex) portions. Only neuro-ophthalmic conditions are considered, and problems such as cataract and retinopathy of prematurity are omitted.

While the above two paragraphs represent the current situation, the situation is changing rapidly. Thus, we are now aware of certain patterns of acuity development (Fielder et al 1992) which are shown in a stylized form in Figs 37.12–37.14. This information has introduced a degree of complexity hitherto unsuspected, but it does offer the clinician insight into fundamental mechanisms and provides valuable information for patient care and for counseling.

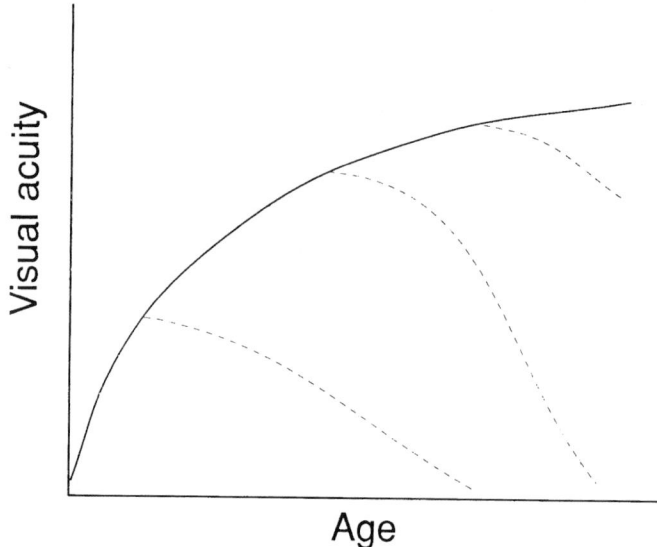

Figure 37.14 Regression. This may occur in a large range of progressive ophthalmic or neuro-ophthalmic disorders.

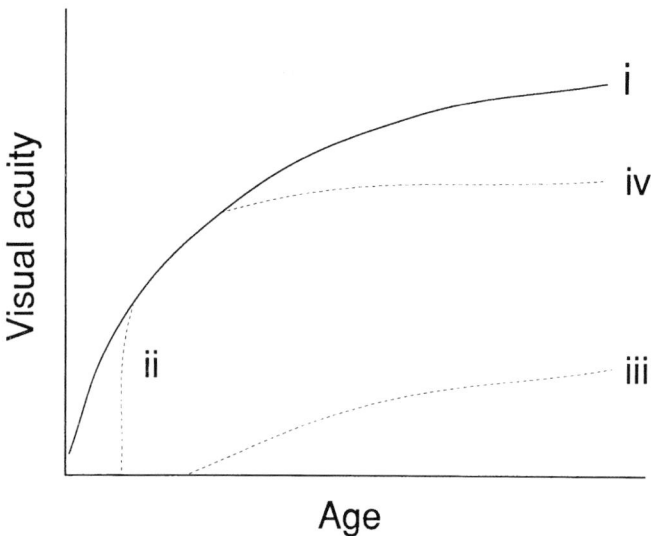

Figure 37.12 Normal visual development is shown by line (i). Early delayed visual development may be followed by rapid (ii) or slow (iii) improvement. These patterns are seen in delayed visual maturation types 1 and 4 (see later). Following normal or delayed development, acuity may plateau or become asymptotic (iv). The level at which this occurs depends on the severity of the visual pathway abnormality, but is seen in infantile nystagmus.

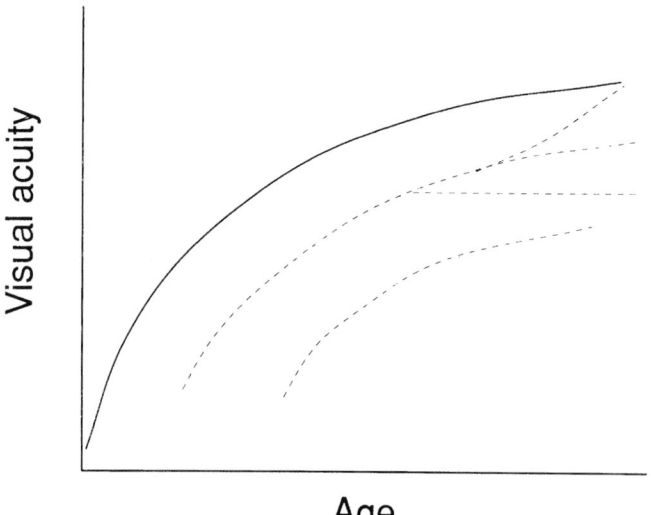

Figure 37.13 Parallel visual development. This is seen after surgery for congenital cataract surgery or severe retinopathy of prematurity. Late catch-up does not always occur.

DISORDERS OF THE ANTERIOR VISUAL PATHWAY

Lesions of the anterior visual pathway (i.e. eye to the optic chiasm) sufficient to reduce vision bilaterally in early life lead to nystagmus and afferent pupillary defects. The latter can be difficult to test clinically in infants and children.

Electroretinography in infancy

For several conditions ophthalmoscopic signs are either minimal or absent. In this situation an ERG is essential to distinguish retinal pathology from that elsewhere in the visual pathway (Weleber & Palmer 1991). Clinicians must have a low threshold for arranging this test. As a general rule it should be performed on all infants and children with unexplained low vision, nystagmus, myopia or optic atrophy, i.e. where there is a possibility of retinal disease.

As mentioned, an ERG can be obtained without sedation, using lid, fiber, gold foil or, even, contact lens electrodes. Stimulus rates of 2 Hz (generating both rod and cone responses) and 30 Hz (generating only a cone response) (see Fig. 37.6). Performed this way it is probably advisable to consider the ERG obtained as qualitative rather than quantitative, but in most clinical instances this is adequate.

Retinal disorders

Many retinal disorders produce a severe visual defect. Some of these are ophthalmoscopically obvious such as retinopathy of prematurity or chorioretinal scarring. Other conditions such as achromatopsia (see p. 750) and the tapetoretinal degenerations (including Leber congenital amaurosis) frequently do not have significant ophthalmoscopically visible signs, at least in early infancy, so an ERG is essential to make a diagnosis.

The cherry-red spot

This classic, but rarely seen sign, results from storage of abnormal substances in the retinal ganglion cells. As these cells are abundant around the macula but are absent from the very centre, the fovea is red and its surround white. This subtle sign, which fades with time, is seen in a number of conditions, including Tay–Sachs, Sandhoff, Niemann–Pick and Farber diseases, metachromatic leukodystrophy and the mucolipidoses.

Optic nerve disorders

Optic atrophy

Optic atrophy is a sign and not a diagnosis, which can be difficult to identify if mild. The appearance of the optic disc alone does not indicate the amount of visual function. Optic atrophy (particularly if associated with retinal arteriolar attenuation) may be the only visible sign of serious retinal disease, for instance in Leber congenital amaurosis or the Laurence–Moon–Biedl (Biedl–Bardet) syndrome. Only by an ERG can retinal involvement be confirmed or eliminated.

Optic nerve damage secondary to retinal disease is termed consecutive or ascending atrophy.

Damage to the optic radiation and visual cortex can cause trans-synaptic degeneration and a descending type of optic atrophy, but this response is confined to visual pathway insults before and during early infancy.

Hereditary optic atrophy. Behr optic atrophy is an autosomal recessive condition in which optic atrophy is associated with mild mental retardation, hypertonia and ataxia. Onset may be within the first year of life. Whether isolated recessive optic atrophy is a true entity is uncertain.

Other hereditary optic atrophies such as Leber optic neuropathy, dominant optic atrophy and the DIDMOAD syndrome all present after the first year of life and are not considered here.

Retinal disease. Tapetoretinal degenerations such as Leber's congenital amaurosis, and Laurence–Moon–Biedl (Biedl–Bardet) and Zellweger syndromes, may all cause optic atrophy.

Intrauterine disease. Optic atrophy may occur following intrauterine infections, asphyxia and cerebral malformations (described elsewhere).

Perinatal damage. It is well established that optic atrophy can result from neonatal events, but even following very premature birth is infrequent. The mechanism(s) by which this occurs is poorly understood. Birth trauma very rarely leads to unilateral nerve damage. Birth asphyxia is sometimes associated with optic atrophy which may be trans-synaptic, resulting from damage to the postgeniculate pathway (Hellström et al 1997). This is a feature of the immature visual system alone and may result from perinatal brain asphyxia or malformation, e.g. holoprosencephaly, porencephaly and hydranencephaly. It is generally thought that damage between 24 and 28 weeks is associated with small optic disc (optic nerve hypoplasia) while damage after this time but before 34 weeks may cause optic discs with large cups (pseudoglaucomatous) (Dutton & Jacobson 2001). Optic atrophy may follow damage to both the visual cortex and subcortex, although with cortical damage the discs are frequently normal. Subcortical damage is frequently associated with optic nerve hypoplasia (Brodsky et al 2002). It is likely that the timing of the insult influences optic nerve morphology (Brodsky 2003, Jacobson et al 2003), although a recent study (McLoone et al 2006) could not detect such an relationship.

Inflammatory. Severe meningoencephalitis in infancy may cause optic atrophy.

Compression. Hydrocephalus, by stretching or compression, can lead to optic atrophy. Tumors may compress the chiasm or nerve (e.g. craniopharyngioma) or involve the anterior visual pathway (glioma).

Metabolic. This includes the lipid storage diseases (e.g. Tay–Sachs disease), Leigh subacute necrotizing encephalopathy and osteopetrosis.

Optic nerve hypoplasia

This is a congenital anomaly of the optic nerve (Brodsky 1991, 2005) whose incidence may be increasing (Robinson & Jan 1987). Typically, the optic disc is small, surrounded by a peripapillary pigmented ring (Fig. 37.15), the retinal vessels are slightly tortuous and the nerve fiber layer is thinned (Frisen & Holmegaard 1978, Skarf & Hoyt 1984). As none of these signs are pathognomonic, mild optic nerve hypoplasia (ONH) may be difficult to diagnose – the disc may be of normal size and examination of the nerve fiber layer is not feasible in infancy. To add to this difficulty the double-ring sign is quite common in the 'normal' premature infant.

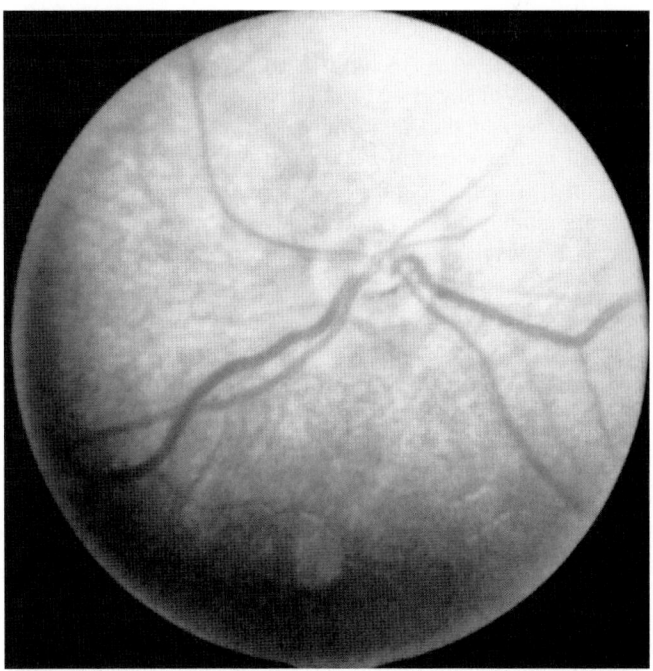

Figure 37.15 Optic-nerve hypoplasia.

The pathogenesis of optic nerve hypoplasia is not known but it may represent a non-specific manifestation of damage to the developing visual system (Frisen & Holmegaard 1978). Not surprisingly, therefore, a degree of optic atrophy often coexists (Brodsky et al 2002). Thus, optic nerve hypoplasia (ONH) may be associated, particularly if bilateral, with a large variety of ocular or systemic abnormalities (Margalith et al 1984, Skarf & Hoyt 1984). Optic nerve hypoplasia is more common in areas with higher unemployment and teenage pregnancy rates (Patel et al 2006) and also can be associated with preterm birth, fetal alcohol syndrome, maternal diabetes and endocrine abnormalities (Garcia et al 2006).

Structural CNS abnormalities associated with ONH include absence of the septum pellucidum, hydranencephaly, porencephaly, holoprosencephaly, cerebral atrophy and cystic subcortical leukomalacia, and may therefore be occasionally detected on routine examination of neurologically abnormal neonates (Fielder et al 1986b). Optic nerve hypoplasia has been described in infants exposed to cocaine in utero (Good et al 1992).

Neuroendocrine dysfunction occurs in 20–30% of cases of optic nerve hypoplasia, with or without a structural neurological anomaly. As this often does not become apparent until about 2–5 years of age, continued surveillance is necessary. Growth, thyroid and gonadotropin hormones may all be affected, and diabetes insipidus has been reported (Costin & Murphree 1985, Margalith et al 1984, 1985, Skarf & Hoyt 1984). Transient neonatal cholestatic jaundice and hypoglycemia are reported associations (Stanhope et al 1984), but it is not known whether these are the patients liable to develop other neuroendocrine problems later. Absence of a septum pellucidum is not in itself associated with intellectual, behavioral or neurological deficits (Williams et al 1993). Finally it is important to note that sudden death during a febrile illness has been reported in children with ONH and corticotropin deficiency (Brodsky et al 1997). Because of this possibility it is recommended that all children with ONH should have a detailed neuroendocrine workup.

CT or ultrasound scanning may determine the extent of, and anticipate, possible future neurodevelopmental problems. Also, MRI spectroscopy may predict neuroendocrine problems (Brodsky & Glasier 1993). It is important for clinicians to recognize that while neurological and neuroendocrine abnormalities are more frequent in bilateral they do occur in unilateral ONH (Garcia et al 2006).

Other congenital abnormalities of the optic disc
Abnormalities such as coloboma, the morning glory syndrome and pits are not considered here.

DISORDERS OF THE POSTERIOR VISUAL PATHWAY

Disorders of the posterior visual pathway, in contrast to those of the anterior visual pathway, do not affect the pupil responses and nystagmus is not a feature. As a caveat to the last comment, many posterior visual pathway disorders are the consequence of widespread neurological damage. Thus, a few jerks of nystagmus may be present, but this is not the sustained oscillation in the straight ahead position which is due to the visual deficit per se.

Delayed visual maturation
Parents and clinicians have known for years that the sight of a blind infant may later improve. First described by Beauvieux in 1926, the term 'delayed visual maturation' (DVM) was introduced by Illingworth (1961). This is probably the most common cause of a severe bilateral visual defect in early infancy and, at its simplest, DVM is an isolated defect with subsequent complete and permanent visual improvement. Unfortunately, as Beauvieux (1947) recognized, not all infants with DVM do so well. Although a degree of visual improvement by definition occurs in all, some with associated ocular and/or neurological problems behave differently clinically and suffer a permanent visual defect, the extent being dependent upon the underlying pathology.

Expanding upon Beauvieux's observations, DVM has been classified by Uemera et al (1981), Fielder et al (1985) and by Fielder and Mayer (1991):

Type 1. DVM as an isolated anomaly:
  A. Normal perinatal period.
  B. With perinatal problems.
Type 2. DVM associated with obvious and persistent neurodevelopmental problems.
Type 3. DVM associated with nystagmus and albinism.
Type 4. DVM with severe congenital, bilateral structural ocular abnormalities.

The spectrum is becoming increasingly broad. As Russell-Eggitt et al stated (1998), DVM is not a single condition but a feature common to neurological abnormalities affecting several areas of the brain. In practice many reserve the term to DVM as an isolated anomaly.

DVM as an isolated anomaly – types 1A and 1B. In this type of DVM the infant presents with severely reduced or absent vision. There are no abnormal signs on examination, other than those attributable to the visual defect (e.g. ocular divergence). Nystagmus is never present. The ERG is always normal, and the flash VEP may range from absent to normal. The time of visual improvement ranges from about 10 to 18 weeks for type 1A, although for type 1B this may not occur for up to 24 weeks. Characteristically this change is rapid, often occurring over only a few days or a week or so, and the subsequent visual acuity development is normal (Fig. 37.16). Although DVM is considered the sole abnormality in this group, a significant number are either born prematurely or suffer perinatal problems (type 1B), on occasion resulting in permanent, usually mild, neurological sequelae including squint (Tresidder et al 1990).

DVM associated with obvious and persistent neurodevelopmental problems – type 2. That blind infants with severe

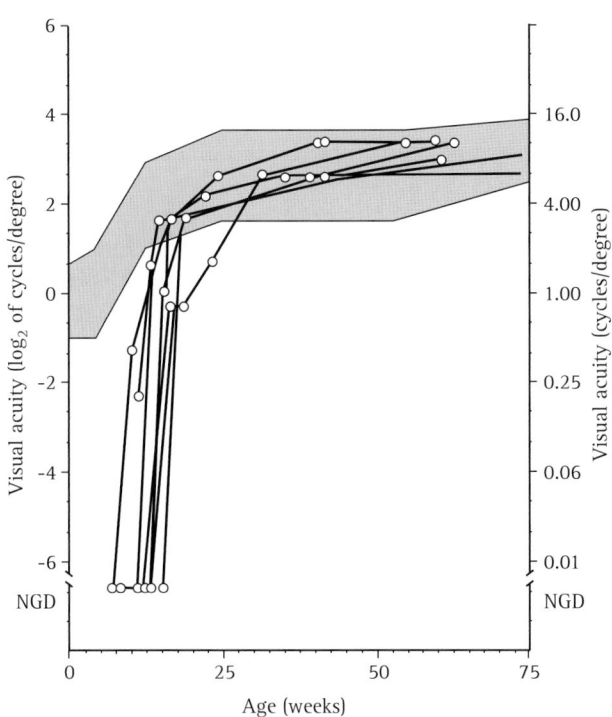

Figure 37.16 Delayed visual maturation type 1A. Visual acuities recorded by the ACP. (Reprinted, with permission, from Tresidder et al 1990.)

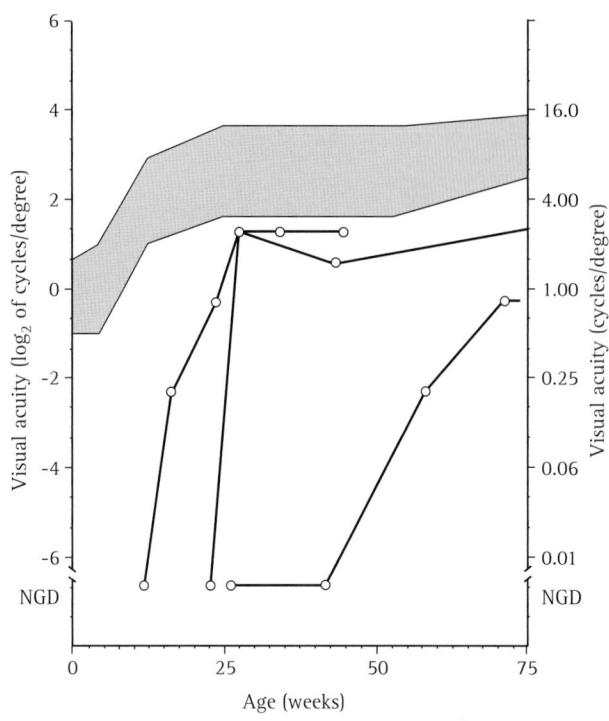

Figure 37.17 Delayed visual maturation type 2. No infant achieved normal acuity. (Reprinted, with permission, from Tresidder et al 1990.)

neurodevelopmental problems may later improve visually is well known. However, in contrast to the first type of DVM the improvement is often slow, occurring over weeks and months rather than days (Fig. 37.17). The eventual level of vision achieved is obviously governed by the amount of visual pathway damage but does not reach normal levels. Nystagmus, consequent upon associated neurological damage, may be present in this group, but this is rarely sustained. Again the ERG is always normal and the VEP variably affected, and may be normal during the period of amaurosis (Lambert et al 1989).

DVM associated with infantile nystagmus and albinism – type 3. For over a century it has been known that infants with albinism may be blind in early infancy and then subsequently improve. This also occurs in congenital/infantile nystagmus. It is interesting to note that during the period of blindness nystagmus is not a feature, and this oscillation commences around the time of (or slightly before) the development of vision (see earlier that nystagmus rarely commences at birth). Vision improves in this group between 13 and 21 weeks (Tresidder et al 1990) (Fig. 37.18), and the pattern of change is quite different from that seen in type 4 DVM, which is slow and extremely limited.

Delayed visual maturation with severe congenital, bilateral structural ocular abnormalities (excluding albinism) – type 4. Clinicians have known for years that some infants who are blind due to severe ocular abnormalities may exhibit a degree of improvement (Fielder & Mayer 1991) (Fig. 37.19). Type 4 DVM is seen in optic nerve hypoplasia, Leber's con-

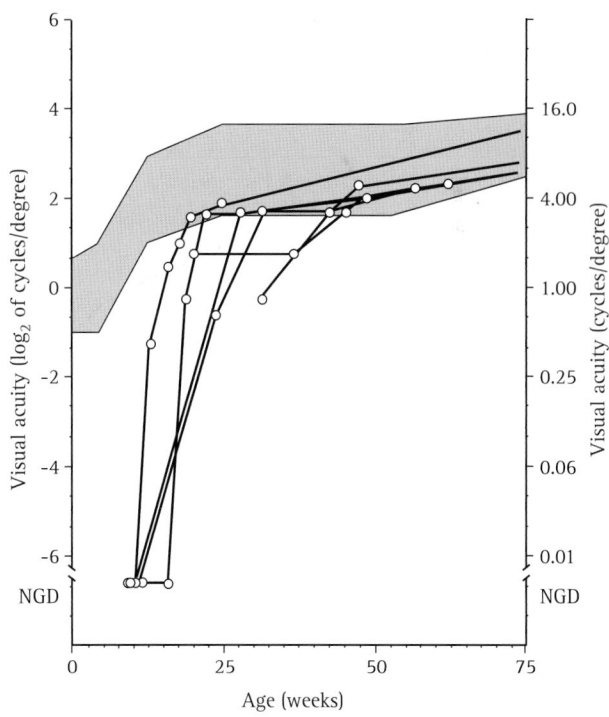

Figure 37.18 Delayed visual maturation type 3. Although normal acuity (ACP data) was achieved during infancy, if the measurements had continued, plateauing would have become apparent in early childhood as children with nystagmus have subnormal acuity (see Fig. 33.10). (Reprinted, with permission, from Tresidder et al 1990.)

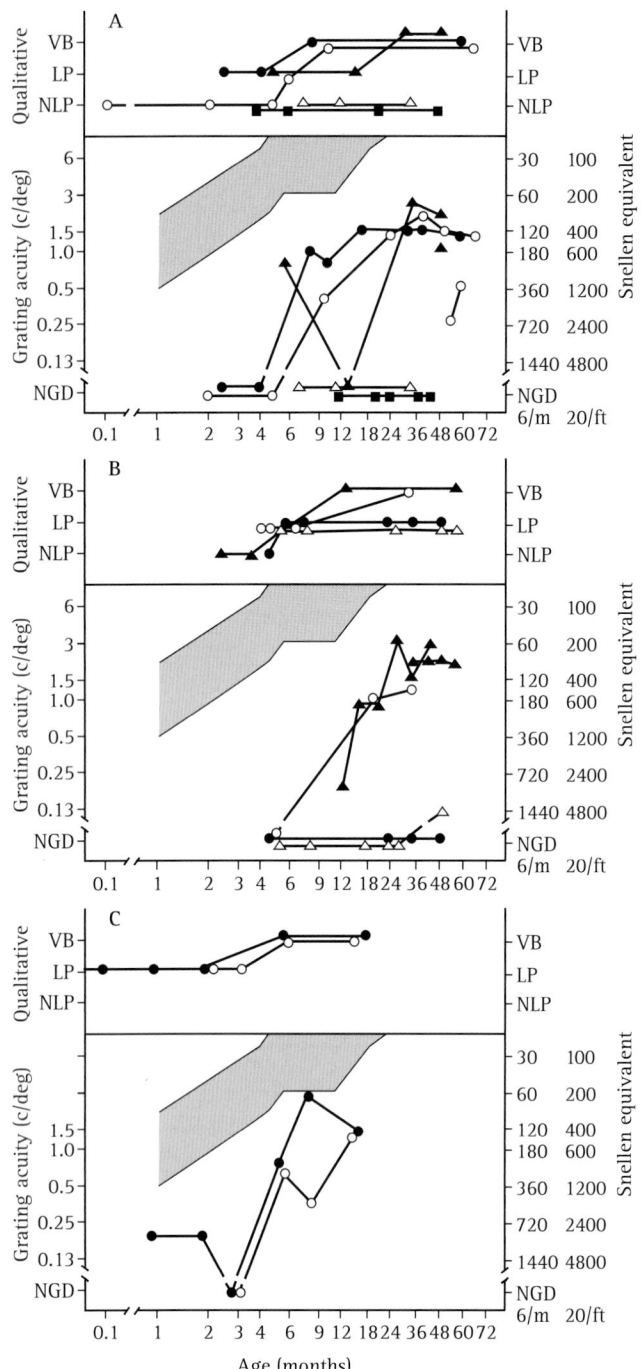

Figure 37.19 Delayed visual maturation type 4. Qualitative visual responses (upper) and ACP acuities (lower). (A) Five patients with Leber's congenital amaurosis. (B) Four with optic nerve hypoplasia and (C) two infants with bilateral colobomata. NLP = no light perception; VB = visually guided behavior; NGD = no grating detection. (Redrawn, from Fielder et al 1991. Copyright 1991, with permission from Elsevier Science.)

genital amaurosis and coloboma (Fielder et al 1991, Good et al 1992). While the functional importance of this improvement must not be underestimated, it is nevertheless limited, and all children remain visually impaired and probably legally blind. Initially confusing, in clinical practice differentiating types 3 and 4 is not a problem. In type 3, DVM dominates the clinical picture, whereas in type 4 the ocular abnormality is the major feature and the improvement is relatively modest, but functionally very useful.

Summary of the clinical features of DVM

All infants show reduced or absent visual responsiveness from birth which subsequently improves. The degree of improvement is governed by any coexisting visual pathway or CNS pathology, but in the absence of these is complete. Nystagmus is not a feature during the period of blindness, but becomes apparent in type 3 around the time of visual improvement. The possible exception to the last comments is type 4, in which the early natural history is unknown.

Pathogenesis of DVM. This cannot be discussed in detail here (Fielder & Mayer 1991, Hoyt & Good 1993, Russell-Eggitt et al 1998, Tresidder et al 1990). With a normal ERG a retinal origin is improbable, and a defect in myelination is unlikely to be the whole story. During the period of visual inattentiveness the flash VEP has been reported as normal (Lambert et al 1989) or abnormal (Kraemer & Sjöström 1999), while the pattern VEP and vernier acuity have been shown to be normal (Good & Hou 2004). This provides good evidence that the afferent visual pathway and some cortical functions are operational. The evidence at present therefore points either to a cortical and/or subcortical defect; the latter is currently favored as vision in early infancy may be subserved on a subcortical basis (Atkinson 1992), and the onset of vision coincides with the emergence of cortical vision (Cocker et al 1998). In connection with the latter it is interesting to note the suggestion that the VEP in early infancy may have a subcortical origin (Dubowitz et al 1986). As a number of these infants have experienced problems in the neonatal period there is a possibility that a subtle neurological insult may be a factor in some cases of DVM and it is pertinent to recall the observation that neurologically abnormal preterm infants may show delayed acuity maturation (Placzek et al 1985). It is unlikely that the full spectrum of DVM, ranging from DVM as an isolated anomaly to associated involvement with other ocular and neurological conditions, has the same basis. For DVM type 1 with its tight clinical course we have postulated a discrete rather than a widespread structural abnormality (Cocker et al 1998), which may cause an attentional deficit which may impinge on parietal cortex function (Harris et al 1996, Russell-Eggitt et al 1998). Hoyt recently made a plea for the term delayed visual maturation to be replaced by 'temporary visual inattention' (Hoyt 2004).

Periventricular leukomalacia (see Ch. 21)

This ischemic neurological lesion which may complicate birth at term or before is dealt with in detail elsewhere in this book. A frequent cause of cerebral vision impairment, it is considered separately first to cover aspects other than the visual acuity deficit, which will be dealt with below. Visual pathway involvement is probably frequent in periventricular leukomalacia (PVL), particularly if the lesion is located posteriorly (Gibson et al 1990). Involvement includes low acuity, delayed visual field and acuity development, visuoperceptual problems, optic disc abnormalities (Jacobson et al 2003), strabismus and supranuclear disorders of eye movement (Calvert et al 1986, Cioni et al 1992, de Vries et al 1987, Dutton & Jacobson 2001, Gibson et al 1990, Jacobson & Dutton 2000, Lambert et al 1987, Pike et al 1994, Scher et al 1989). The mechanism of visual pathway involvement is not known, but it is interesting to note that infants who experience recurrent hypoxia (bronchopulmonary dysplasia) but who do not have PVL show normal development of both grating acuity and visual field (Luna et al 1992). As mentioned subtle optic nerve abnormalities that may represent transsynaptic degeneration have been reported (Hellström et al 1997).

Cerebral visual impairment

Over the past decade or so the term cortical blindness has evolved to cortical visual impairment to the currently preferred 'cerebral visual impairment' (CVI). The most common cause of severe vision impairment in high income communities (Rahi & Cable 2003), CVI denotes a patient with reduced vision or even blind but with a normal ocular examination including preservation of the pupillary responses. A reported 40–75% children with CVI show improvement (Huo et al 1999, Matsuba & Jan 2006, Watson et al 2007), this wide range reflecting selection bias, the severity of the neurological insult and also neurological plasticity (Edmond & Foroozan 2006). The location of the lesion also influences the propensity for improvement, being less frequent when PVL is the cause. The child with CVI has often suffered widespread brain damage and may exhibit many diverse CNS and ocular signs (Cioni et al 1996, Dutton et al 1999, Good et al 1994, Jan & Wong 1991, Lambert 1997, Whiting et al 1985).

Causes of CVI include:

- *Prenatal*: malformations, intrauterine infection and toxemia.
- *Perinatal*: hypoxic–ischemic episodes as in neonatal asphyxia and intracerebral hemorrhage, hypoglycemia, meningitis and encephalitis. It is important to differentiate the effect of neurological damage on the preterm and term brain (Brodsky et al 2002, Dutton & Jacobson 2001). In the term baby, ischemia affects the watershed areas between the cortex and subcortex which are between the anterior and middle, and also between the middle and posterior cerebral arteries. If severe the injury may also affect the thalami and basal ganglia. For the preterm baby the hypoxic injury involves the subcortex, mainly the periventricular white matter — the germinal matrix — with periventricular

leukomalacia (PVL) as the outcome. Because the optic radiations and other tracts traverse the periventricular white matter, cerebral vision impairment and cerebral palsy are frequent associations in preterm with brain damage (Edmond & Foroozon 2006, Hoyt 2003). In addition to these specific and focal neurological lesions in which effects on motor function are prominent, recent MRI work has shown that being born early 'disrupts the coordinated growth of the whole brain' (Kapellou et al 2006). This may be related to neurocognitive developmental rather than neuromotor deficits, and also other visual pathway functions.

- *Acquired*: meningitis, encephalitis, cardiac arrest, neurodegenerative disorders, trauma, cortical vein thrombosis and shunt failure.

Clinical assessment of these infants is often difficult, and as many have suffered diffuse brain damage, coexistent ophthalmic and neurological signs are common (Huo et al 1999, van Hof-van Duin & Mohn 1984b, Whiting et al 1985). The absence of nystagmus is an important clue to cortical involvement, with the qualification that in the presence of multiple pathology poorly sustained CNS nystagmus may be present.

The role of the VEP in the evaluation of CVI has long been disputed. It was abnormal in less than half of the children reported by Whiting et al (1985) and because of these and other findings the value of the VEP in this situation has been questioned. However, it is becoming apparent that the rigorously performed sweep VEP is of value in evaluation of CVI and correlates well with grating acuities obtained by acuity cards (Good & Hou 2006). In addition, the presence of a normal VEP is helpful in predicting those infants and children who may subsequently improve.

The clinical course of cortical blindness is extremely variable, as mentioned, and is determined to a certain extent by its etiology. Neither Hoyt (1986b) nor Watson et al (2007) were able to establish any correlation between the duration of the blindness and the extent of the visual recovery. However, total recovery within a few hours has been observed in children who suffered 'trivial' head trauma (Griffith & Dodge 1968). Visual improvement is obviously not anticipated in patients with neurodegenerative disorders, and the prognosis following bacterial meningitis is worse than for other causes (Ackroyd 1984), and may be very limited in PVL. Thus, complete recovery has been reported following head injury (Griffith & Dodge 1968) and cardiac arrest (Weinberger et al 1962) but in only 50% of patients with bacterial meningitis (Ackroyd 1984). Chen et al (1992) reported lack of improvement only with hypoxia. Martin and Barkovich (1995) reported a good correlation between the MRI signs taken within three days of the insult and subsequent outcome.

Complete blindness is rarely permanent in CVI (Good et al 1994, Jan & Wong 1991, Lambert et al 1987), although it should be emphasized that the degree of improvement is

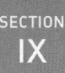
often incomplete (Hoyt 1986b); for this reason the current designation cerebral visual impairment (CVI) is more appropriate (Whiting et al 1985). The relationship between CVI and DVM needs to be clarified, as almost by definition DVM type 2 falls into this complex of CVI. It is possible that in many instances the distinction is one of timing and degree rather than the site of the lesion. Improvement in CVI is very common (Khetpal & Donahue 2007, Lim et al 2005, Schenk-Rootlieb et al 1992). Visual improvement may take from a few hours to more than 2 years, and begins first with light perception and then the ability to follow objects. Eye-to-eye contact is often lacking and visual function may vary from hour to hour. Most children achieve at least navigational vision, although severe visual-perceptual difficulties frequently persist (Dutton & Jacobson 2001, Dutton et al 1999, Edmond & Forozoon 2006).

Investigation and management of the visually inattentive infant

Each infant should have a detailed ophthalmic and pediatric assessment, the extent of which is governed by clinical findings. Nowadays this should include both qualitative and quantitative assessment of visual functions. In view of the varied natural history of many of these disorders and the absence in many conditions of ophthalmoscopically visible signs, the clinician should have a very low threshold to undertake electrophysiological investigations, particularly the ERG. Excepting the vision deficit, should the infant be normal in all respects, the likelihood of some improvement of vision occurring is very high and should be conveyed to parents. In general however, caution is recommended in counseling, for misplaced optimism results in considerable and unnecessary parental anxiety and turmoil.

REFERENCES

Ackroyd R S 1984 Cortical blindness following bacterial meningitis: a case report with reassessment of prognosis and aetiology. Dev Med Child Neurol 26:227–230.

Adams R J, Courage M L 1995 Development of chromatic discrimination in early infancy. Behavioural Brain Research 67:99–101.

Anderson L T, Coll C G, Vohr B R et al 1989 Behavioral characteristics and early temperature of premature infants with intracranial haemorrhage. Early Hum Dev 18:273–283.

Antony J H, Ouvrier R A, Wise G 1980 Spasmus nutans: a mistaken identity. Arch Neurol 37:373–375.

Apkarian P, Mirmian M, Tijssen R 1991 Effects of behavioural state on visual processing in neonates. Neuropediatrics 22:85–91.

Apkarian P, Tijssen R 1992 Detection and maturation of VEP albino asymmetry: an overview and a longitudinal study from birth to 54 weeks. Behav Brain Res 49:57–67.

Archer S M, Helveston E M 1994 Strabismus and eye movement disorders. In: Isenberg I (ed.) The eye in infancy, 2nd edn. Mosby, St Louis, MO, pp. 254–274.

Archer S M, Sondhi N, Helveston E M 1989 Strabismus in infancy. Ophthalmology 96:133–137.

Arnoldi K A, Tycheson L 1995 Prevalence of intracranial lesions in children initially diagnosed awith disconjugate nystagmus (spasmus nutans). J Pediatr Ophthalmol Strabismus 32:296–301.

Aslin R 1993 Infant accommodation and convergence. In: Simons K (ed.) Early visual development: normal and abnormal. Oxford University Press, Oxford, pp. 30–38.

Aslin R N 1977 Development of binocular fixation in human infants. J Exp Psychol 23:133–150.

Aslin R, Salapatek P 1975 Saccadic localization of visual targets by the very young human infant. Percept Psychophys 17:293–302.

Atkinson J 1992 Early visual development: differential functioning of parvocellular and magnocellular pathways. Eye 6:129–135.

Atkinson J, Braddick O 1983 Assessment of visual acuity in infancy and early childhood. Acta Ophthalmol (Copenhagen) 157(suppl):18–26.

Atkinson J, Braddick O J, Pimm-Smith E et al 1981 Does the Catford drum give an accurate assessment of acuity? Br J Ophthalmol 66:652–656.

Atkinson J, Hood B, Wattam-Bell J et al 1992 Changes in infants' ability to switch visual attention in the first three months of life. Perception 21:643–653.

Auestad N, Scott D T, Janowsky J S et al 2003 Visual, cognitive, and language assessments at 39 months: a follow-up study of children fed formulas containing long-chain polyunsaturated fatty acids to 1 year of age. Pediatrics 112:e177–e183.

Aylward G P, Lazzara A, Meyer J 1978 Behavioural characteristics of a hydranencephalic infant. Dev Med Child Neurol 20:211–217.

Bacher L F, Smotherman W P 2004 Systematic temporal variation in the rate of spontaneous eye blinking in human infants. Dev Psychobiol 44:140–145.

Bankes J L K 1974 Eye defects of mentally handicapped children. BMJ ii:533–535.

Beauvieux J 1926 La pseudo-atrophie optique des nouveaux-nes (dysgenesie myelinique des voies optiques). Annales d'Oculistique 163:881–921.

Beauvieux M 1947 La cecite apparente chez le nouveau-ne la pseudoatrophie grise du nerf optique. Archives Ophthalmologie (Paris) 7:241–249.

Bell J A, Fielder A R, Viney S A 1990 Congenital double elevator palsy in identical twins. J Clin Neuro-ophthalmol 10:32–34.

Beverley D W, Smith I S, Beesley P et al 1990 Relationship of cranial ultrasonography, visual and auditory evoked responses with neurodevelopmental outcome. Dev Med Child Neurol 32:210–322.

Birch E E, Birch D, Hoffman D et al 1993 Breast-feeding and optimal visual development. J Pediatr Ophthalmol Strabismus 30:33–38.

Birch E E, Stager D R 1988 Prevalence of good visual acuity following surgery for congenital unilateral cataract. Arch Ophthalmol 106:40–43.

Birch E, Petrig B 1996 FPL and VEP measures of fusion, stereopsis and stereoacuity in normal infants. Vis Res 36:1321–1327.

Birnholz J C 1981 The development of human fetal eye movement patterns. Science 213:679–681.

Boothe R G, Dobson V, Teller D Y 1985 Postnatal development of vision in human and nonhuman primates. Ann Rev Neurosci 8:495–545.

Bosley T M, Salih M A M, Jen J C et al 2005 Neurologic features of horizontal gaze palsy and progressive scoliosis with mutations in ROBO3. Neurology 64:1196–1203.

Braddick O, Atkinson J 1983 Some recent findings on the development of human binocularity: a review. Behav Brain Res 10:141–150.

Braddick O, Atkinson J, Hood B et al 1992 Possible blindsight in infants lacking one cerebral hemisphere. Nature 360:461–463.

Brazelton T B, Scholl M L, Robey J S 1966 Visual responses in the newborn. Pediatrics 37:284–290.

Bremer D L, Palmer E A, Fellows R R et al 1998 Arch Ophthalmol 116:329–333.

Brodsky M C 1991 Septo-optic dysplasia: a reappraisal. Semin Ophthalmol 6:227–232.

Brodsky M C 2003 Semiology of periventricular leucomalacia and its optic disc morphology. Br J Ophthalmol 87:1309–1310.

Brodsky M C 2005 Congenital optic disc anomalies. In: Taylor D, Hoyt C S (eds) Pediatric ophthalmology and strabismus, 3rd edn. Elsevier, Edinburgh, pp. 625–645.

Brodsky M C, Conte F A, Taylor D et al 1997 Sudden death in septo-optic dysplasia. Report of 5 cases. Arch Ophthalmol 115:66–70.

Brodsky M C, Fray K J, Glasier C M 2002 Perinatal cortical and subcortical visual loss: mechanisms of injury and associated ophthalmologic signs. Ophthalmology 109:85–94.

Brodsky M, Glasier C 1993 Optic nerve hypoplasia: clinical significance of associated central nervous system abnormalities in magnetic resonance imaging. Arch Ophthalmol 111:66–74.

Brown A M, Yamamoto M 1986 Visual acuity in newborn and preterm infants measured with grating acuity cards. Am J Ophthalmol 102:245–253.

Burgess P, Johnson A 1991 Ocular defects in infants of extremely low birthweight and low gestational age. Br J Ophthalmol 75:84–87.

Calvert S A, Hoskins E M, Fong K W et al 1986 Periventricular leukomalacia: ultrasound diagnosis and neurological outcome. Acta Paediatr Scand 75:489–496.

Campistol J, Prats J M, Garaizar C 1993 Benign paroxysmal tonic upgaze of childhood with ataxia. A neuro-ophthalmological syndrome of familial origin. Dev Med Child Neurol 35:436–438.

Cassidy L, Taylor D, Harris C 2000 Abnormal supranuclear eye movements in the child: A practical guide to examination and interpretation. Surv Ophthalmol 44:479–506.

Cavanagh N 1997 Normal child development. In: Taylor D (ed.) 1997 Paediatric ophthalmology, 2nd edn. Blackwell Science, Oxford, pp. 33–37.

Chandna A 1991 Natural history of the development of visual acuity in infants. Eye 5:20–26.

Chandna A, Pearson C M, Doran R M L 1988 Preferential looking in clinical practice: a year's experience. Eye 2:488–495.

Chen T C, Weinberg M H, Catalano R A et al 1992 Development of object vision in infants with permanent cortical visual impairment. Am J Ophthalmol 114:575–578.

Cioni G, Bartalena L, Biagioni E et al 1992 Neuroimaging and functional outcome of neonatal leukomalacia. Behav Brain Res 49:7–19.

Cioni G, Ipata A E, Canapicchi R et al 1996 MRI findings in children with cerebral visual impairment. In: Vital-Durand F, Atkinson J, Braddick O J (eds) Infant vision. Oxford University Press, Oxford, pp. 373–382.

Coakes R L, Clothier C, Wilson A 1979 Binocular reflexes in the first 6 months of life: preliminary results of a study of normal infants. Child Care, Health Dev 5:405–408.

Cocker K D, Moseley M J, Bissenden J G et al 1994 Visual acuity and pupillary responses to spatial structure in infants. Invest Ophthalmol Vis Sci 35:2620–2625.

Cocker K D, Moseley M J, Stirling H F et al 1998 Delayed visual maturation: pupillary responses implicate subcortical and cortical visual systems. Dev Med Child Neurol 40:160–162.

Cogan D G 1952 A type of congenital ocular motor apraxia presenting jerky head movements. Trans Am Acad Ophthalmol Otolaryngol 56:853–862.

Cogan D G 1966 Congenital ocular motor apraxia. Can J Ophthalmol 1:253–260.

Cordero L, Clark D L, Urrutia J G 1983 Postrotatory nystagmus in the full-term and premature infant. Int J Pediat Otorhinolaryngol 5:47–57.

Costin G, Murphree A L 1985 Hypothalamic-pituitary function in children with optic nerve hypoplasia. Am J Dis Children 139:249–254.

Courage M L, Adams R J 1990 Visual acuity assessment from birth to three years using the acuity card procedure: cross-sectional and longitudinal samples. Optometry Vis Sci 67:713–718.

Crognale M A, Kelly J P, Chang S et al 1997 Development of pattern visual evoked potentials: longitudinal measurements in human infants. Optometry Vis Sci 74:808–815.

de Vries L S, Connell J A, Dubowitz L M S et al 1987 Neurological electrophysiological and MRI abnormalities in infants with extensive cystic leukomalacia. Neuropediatrics 18:61–66.

de Vries-Khoe L H, Spekreijse H 1982 Maturation of luminance and pattern EPs in man. In: Niemayer G (ed.) Documenta Opthalmologica Proceedings Series 31:461–475.

Dell'Osso L F, Daroff R B, Todd Troost B 1990 Nystagmus and saccadic intrusions and oscillations. In: Glaser J S (ed.) Neuro-ophthalmology. Harper and Row, Hagerstown, pp. 325–356.

Dobson V 1994 Visual acuity testing by preferential looking techniques. In: Isenberg I (ed.) The eye in infancy, 2nd edn. Mosby, St Louis, MO, pp. 131–156.

Dobson V, Brown A M, Harvey E M et al 1998 Visual field extent in children 3.5–30 months of life tested with a double-arc LED perimeter. Vis Res 38:2743–2760.

Dobson V, Mayer D L, Lee C P 1980 Visual acuity screening of preterm infants. Invest Ophthalmol Vis Sci 19:1498–1504.

Dobson V, Schwartz T L, Sandstrom D J et al 1987 Binocular visual acuity of neonates: the acuity card procedure. Dev Med Child Neurol 29:199–206.

Donat J F, Donat J R, Lay K S 1980 Changing response to caloric stimulation with gestational age in infants. Neurology 30:776–778.

Dubowitz L M S, Dubowitz V, Morante A et al 1980 Visual function in the preterm and fullterm newborn infant. Dev Med Child Neurol 22:465–475.

Dubowitz L M S, Levene M I, Morante A et al 1981 Neurologic signs in neonatal intraventricular hemorrhage: a correlation with real-time ultrasound. J Pediatr 99:127–133.

Dubowitz L M S, Mushin J, de Vries L et al 1986 Visual function in the newborn infant: is it cortically mediated? Lancet i:1139–1141.

Dubowitz L M S, Mushin J, Morante A et al 1983 The maturation of visual acuity in neurologically normal and abnormal newborn infants. Behav Brain Res 10:39–45.

Dutton G N, Day R E, McCulloch D M 1999 Who is a visually impaired child? A model is needed to address this question for children with cerebral visual impairment. Dev Med Child Neurol 41:211–213.

Dutton G N, Jacobson L K 2001 Cerebral visual impairment in children. Semin Neonatol 6:477–485.

Edmond J C, Foroozan R 2006 Cortical visual impairment in children. Curr Opin Ophthalmol 17:509–512.

Ekert PG, Keenan NK, Whyte HE et al 1997 Visual evoked potentials for prediction of neurodevelopmental outcome in preterm infants. Biology of the Neonate 71:148–155.

Evans N M, Fielder A R, Mayer D L 1989 Ametropia in congenital cone deficiency — achromatopsia: a defect of emmetropisation? Clin Vis Sci 4:129–136.

Eviatar L, Eviatar A, Naray 1974 Maturation of neurovestibular responses in infants. Dev Med Child Neurol 16:435–446.

Eviatar L, Miranda S, Eviatar A et al 1979 Development of nystagmus in response to vestibular stimulation in infants. Ann Neurol 5:508–514.

Farmer J, Hoyt C S 1984 Monocular nystagmus in infancy and early childhood. Am J Ophthalmol 98:504–509.

Ferrari F, Grosoli M V, Fontana G et al 1983 Neurobehavioural comparison of low-risk preterm and fullterm infants at term conceptual age. Dev Med Child Neurol 25:450–458.

Fielder A R 1985 Neonatal eye movements: normal and abnormal. B Orthop J 42:10–15.

Fielder A R 1989 The management of squint. Arch Dis Childhood 64:413–418.

Fielder A R, Dobson V, Moseley M J et al 1992 Preferential looking — clinical lessons. Ophthal Paediatr Genet 13:101–110.

Fielder A R, Evans N M 1988 Is the geniculostriate system a prerequisite for nystagmus? Eye 2:628–635.

Fielder A R, Foreman N, Moseley M J et al 1993 Prematurity and visual development. In: Simons K (ed.) Early visual development: normal and abnormal. Oxford University Press, New York, pp. 485–504.

Fielder A R, Fulton A B, Mayer D L 1991 Visual development of infants with severe ocular disorders. Ophthalmology 98:1306–1309.

Fielder A R, Gresty M A, Dodd K L et al 1986a Congenital ocular motor apraxia. Trans Ophthalmol Soc UK 105:589–598.

Fielder A R, Harper M W, Higgins J E et al 1983 The reliability of the VEP in infancy. Ophth Paediatr Genet 3:73–82.

Fielder A R, Levene M I, Trounce J Q et al 1986b Optic nerve hypoplasia in infancy. J Roy Soc Med 79:25–29.

Fielder A R, Mayer D L 1991 Delayed visual maturation. Semin Ophthalmol 6:182–193.

Fielder A R, Moseley M J 1988 Do we need to measure the vision of children? J Roy Soc Med 81:380–383.

Fielder A R, Moseley M J 2000 Environmental light and the preterm infant. Semin Perinatol 24:291–298.

Fielder A R, Moseley M J, Ng Y K 1988 The immature visual system and premature birth. Br Med Bull 44:1093–1118.

Fielder A R, Russell-Eggitt I R, Dodd K L et al 1985 Delayed visual maturation. Trans Ophthalmol Soc UK 104:653–661.

Fleith M, Clandinin M T 2005 Dietary PUFA for preterm and term infants: review of clinical studies. Crit Rev Food Sci Nutr 45:205–229.

Foreman N, Fielder A, Price et al 1991 Tonic and phasic orientation in full-term and preterm infants. J Exp Child Psychol 51:407–422.

Frank Y, Torres F 1979 Visual evoked potentials in the evaluation of 'cortical blindness' in children. Ann Neurol 6:126–129.

Frisen L, Holmegaard L 1978 Spectrum of optic nerve hypoplasia. Br J Ophthalmol 62:7–15.

Garbutt S, Harwood M, Harris C 2006 Infant saccades are not slow. Dev Med Child Neurol 48:662–667.

Garbutt S, Leigh R J 2005 Infantile nystagmus syndrome (congenital nystagmus. In: Taylor D, Hoyt C S (eds) Pediatric ophthalmology and strabismus, 3rd edn. Elsevier, Edinburgh, pp. 812–820.

Garcia M L, Ty E B, Taban M et al 2006 Systemic and ocular findings in 100 patients with optic nerve hypoplasia. J Child Neurol 21:949–945.

Gibson N A, Fielder A R, Trounce J Q et al 1990 Ophthalmic findings in infants of very low birthweight. Dev Med Child Neurol 32:7–13.

Goldie L, Hopkins I J 1964 Head turning towards diffuse light in the neurological examination of newborn infants. Brain 87:665–672.

Good W V, Ferriero D M, Golabi M et al 1992 Abnormalities of the visual system in infants exposed to cocaine. Ophthalmology 99:341–346.

Good W V, Hou C 2004 Normal vernier acuity in infants with delayed visual maturation. Am J Ophthalmol 138:140–142.

Good W V, Hou C 2006 Sweep visual evoked potential grating acuity thresholds paradoxically improve in low-luminance conditions in children with cortical visual impairment. Invest Ophthalmol Vis Sci 47:3220–3224.

Good W V, Jan J E, DeSa L et al 1994 Cortical visual impairment in children. Surv Ophthalmol 38:351–364.

Good W V, Jan J E, Hoyt C S et al 1997 Monocular vision loss can cause bilateral nystagmus in young children. Dev Med Child Neurol 39:421–424.

Gorman J J, Cogan D G, Gellis S S 1957 An apparatus for grading the visual acuity of infants on the basis of opticokinetic nystagmus. Pediatrics 19:1088–1092.

Gottlob I 2001 Nystagmus. Curr Opin Ophthalmol 12:378–383.

Gottlob I, Wizov SS, Reinecke RD 1995 Spasmus nutans. A longterm follow up. Investigative Ophthalmology & Visual Science 36:2768–2771.

Gottlob I, Zubcov A A, Wizow S S et al 1992 Head nodding is compensatory in spasmus nutans. Ophthalmology 99:1024–1031.

Gottlob I, Zubcov A, Catalano R A et al 1990 Signs distinguishing spasmus nutans (with and without central nervous system lesions) from infantile nystagmus. Ophthalmology 97:1166–1175.

Griffith J G, Dodge P R 1968 Transient blindness following head injury in children. N Engl J Med 278:648–651.

Groenendaal F, van Hof-van Duin J, Baerts W et al 1989 Effects of perinatal hypoxia on visual development during the first year of (corrected) age. Early Hum Dev 20:267–279.

Hack M, Muszynski S Y, Miranda S B 1981 State of awakeness during visual fixation in preterm infants. Pediatrics 68:87–92.

Hainline L 1998 The development of basic visual abilities. In: Slater A (ed.) Perceptual development: visual, auditory and speech perception in infancy. Psychology Press, Hove, pp. 5–50.

Hainline L, Turkel J, Abramov I, Lemerise E, Harris C M 1984 Characteristics of saccades in human infants. Vis Res 24:1771–1780.

Harris C M, Jacobs M, Shawkat F et al 1993 The development of saccadic accuracy in the first 7 months. Clin Vis Sci 8:85–96.

Harris CM, Shawkat F, Russell-Eggitt I et al 1996 Intermittent horizontal saccade failure in children. Br J Ophthalmol 80:151–158.

Harvey E M, Dobson V, Luna B 1997b Long-term grating acuity and visual-field development in preterm children who experienced bronchopulmonary dysplasia. Dev Med Child Neurol 39:167–173.

Harvey E M, Dobson V, Luna B et al 1997a Grating acuity and visual-field development in children with intraventricular hemorrhage. Dev Med Child Neurol 39:305–312.

Hellström A, Chen Y H, Svenson E 1997 Optic disc size and retinal vessel characteristics in healthy children. Arch Ophthalmol 115:1263–1269.

Hendrickson A E, Youdelis C 1984 The morphological development of the human fovea. Ophthalmology 91:603–612.

Hertle R W 2005 Supranuclear eye movement disorders, acquired and neurological nystagmus. In: Taylor D, Hoyt C S (eds). Pediatric ophthalmology and strabismus, 3rd edn. Elsevier, Edinburgh, pp. 790–811.

Hertle R W, Chan C C, Galita D A 2002 Neuroanatomy of the extraocular muscle tendon enthesis in macaque, normal human and patients with congenital nystagmus. JAAPOS 6:319–327.

Hollenberg MJ, Spira AW 1972 Early development of the human retina. Canadian Journal of Ophthalmology 7:472–491.

Holmes J M, Mutyala S, Maus T et al 1999 Pediatric third, fourth and sixth nerve palsies: A population-based study. Am J Ophthalmol 127:388–392.

Holmstrom G, el-Azazi M, Kugelberg U 1999 Ophthalmological follow up of preterm infants: a population based, prospective study of visual acuity and strabismus. Br J Ophthalmol 83:143–150.

Holmstrom G, Rydberg A, Larsson E 2006 Prevalence of development of strabismus in 10 year old premature children. J Paediatr Ophthalmol Strabismus 43:348–352.

Hood B, Atkinson J 1990 Sensory visual loss and cognitive deficits in the selective attentional system of normal infants and neurologically impaired children. Dev Med Child Neurol 32:1067–1077.

Horwood A M 1993 Maternal observations of ocular alignment in infants. J Paediatr Ophthalmol Strabismus 30:100–105.

Horwood A M 2003 Neonatal ocular misalignments reflect vergence development but rarely become esotropia. Br J Ophthalmol 87:1146–1150.

Hoyt C S 1986a Objective techniques of visual acuity assessment in infancy. In: Pediatric ophthalmology and strabismus: Transactions of the New Orleans Academy of Ophthalmology. Raven, New York, NY, pp. 7–13.

Hoyt C S 1986b Cortical blindness in infancy. In: Pediatric ophthalmology and strabismus: Transactions of the New Orleans Academy of Ophthalmology. Raven, New York, NY, pp. 235–243.

Hoyt C S 2004 Delayed visual maturation: The apparently blind infant. J Am Ass Pediatric Ophthalmol & Strabismus 8:215–219.

Hoyt C S, Billson F A, Taylor H 1977 Isolated unilateral gaze palsy. J Pediat Ophthalmol 14:343–345.

Hoyt C S, Gelbart S S 1984 Vertical nystagmus in infants with congenital ocular abnormalities. Ophthal Paediatr Genet 4:155–162.

Hoyt C S, Good W V 1993 Visual factors in developmental delay and neurological disorders in infants. In: Simons K (ed.) Early visual development: normal and abnormal. Oxford University Press, New York, pp. 505–512.

Hoyt C S, Mousel D K, Weber A A 1980 Transient supranuclear disturbances of gaze in healthy neonates. Am J Ophthalmol 89:708–713.

Hoyt C S, Nickel B L, Billson F A 1982 Ophthalmological examination of the infant: developmental aspects. Surv Ophthalmol 26:177–189.

Hoyt CS 2003 Visual function in the brain-damaged child. Eye 17:369–384.

Huo R, Burden S K, Hoyt C S et al 1999 Chronic cortical visual impairment in children: aetiology, prognosis, and associated neurological deficits. Br J Ophthalmol 83:670–675.

Illingworth R S 1961 Delayed visual maturation. Arch Dis Childhood 36:407–409.

Inoue M, Koyanagi T, Nakahara H et al 1986 Functional development of human eye movement in utero assessed quantitatively with real-time ultrasound. Am J Obstet Gynecol 155:170–174.

Isenberg I (ed.) 1994 The eye in infancy, 2nd edn. Mosby, St Louis, MO.

Jacobs M, Harris CM, Shawat F, Taylor D 1997 Smooth pursuit development in infants. Aust NZ J Ophthalmol 25:199–206.

Jacobsen L, Flodmark O, Martin L 2006 Visual field defects in prematurely born patients with white matter damage of immaturity: a multiple case study. Acta Ophthalmol Scand 84:357–362.

Jacobson L K, Dutton G N 2000 Periventricular leukomalacia: an important cause of visual and ocular motility dysfunction in children. Surv Ophthalmol 45:1–13.

Jacobson L, Hard A L, Svensson E et al 2003 Optic disc morphology may reveal timing of insult in children with periventricular leucomalacia and/or periventricular haemorrhage. Br J Ophthalmol 87:1345–1349.

Jan J E, Carruthers J D, Tillson G 1992 Neurodevelopmental criteria in the classification of congenital nystagmus. Can J Neurosci 19:76–79.

Jan J E, Kearney S, Groenveld M et al 1998 Speech, cognition and imaging studies in congenital motor apraxia. Dev Med Child Neurol 40:95–99.

Jan J E, Wong P K H 1991 The child with cortical visual impairment. Semin Ophthalmol 6:194–200.

Johnson A T, Kretzer F L, Hittner H M et al 1985 Development of the subretinal space in the preterm human eye: ultrastructural and immunocytochemical analysis. J Comp Neurol 233:497–505.

Kapellou O, Counsell S J, Kennea N et al 2006 Abnormal cortical development after premature birth shown by altered allometric scaling of brain growth. PLoS Medicine 3:e265.

Kato T, Hayakawa F, Okumura A et al 2000 Flash visual evoked potentials in preterm infants, Correlation with neurodevelopmental outcome. J Jap Soc Perinatal Neonatal Med 36:248.

Kato T, Watanabe K 2006 Visual evoked potential in the newborn: Does it have predictive value? Semin Fetal Neonatal Med 11:459–463.

Katsanis J, Iacono W G, Harris M 1998 Development of oculomotor functioning in preadolescence, adolescence, adulthood. Psychophysiol 35:64–72.

Kennedy K A, Ipson M A, Birch D G et al 1997 Light reduction and the electroretinogram of preterm infants. Arch Dis Childhood 76:F168–F173.

Khetpal V, Donahue S P 2007 Cortical visual impairment: etiology, associated findings, and prognosis in a tertiary care setting. J AAPOS 11:235–239.

Kos-Pietro S, Towle V L, Cakmur R et al 1997 Maturation of human visual evoked potentials: 27 weeks conceptional age to 2 years. Neuropediatrics 28:318–323.

Kraemer M, Sjöström A 1999 Lack of short-latency-potentials in the VEP reflects immature extrageniculate visual function in delayed visual maturation (DCM). Doc Ophthalmol 97:189–201.

Kremenitzer J P, Vaughan H G, Kurtzberg D et al 1979 Smooth-pursuit eye movements in the newborn infant. Child Dev 50:442–448.

Kurtzberg D, Vaughan H G Jr, Daum C et al 1979 Neurobehavioral performance of low-birthweight infants at 40 weeks conceptional age: comparison with normal fullterm infants. Dev Med Child Neurol 5:590–607.

Lambert S R 1997 Brain problems. In: Taylor D (ed.) 1997 Paediatric ophthalmology, 2nd edn. Blackwell Science, Oxford, pp. 740–750.

Lambert S R, Hoyt C S, Jan J E et al 1987 Visual recovery from hypoxic cortical blindness during childhood: computed tomographic and magnetic resonance imaging predictors. Arch Ophthalmol 105:1371–1377.

Lambert S R, Kriss A, Taylor D 1989 Delayed visual maturation in infancy: a longitudinal study — clinical and electrophysiological assessment. Ophthalmology 96:524–528.

Laws D, Shaw D E, Robinson J et al 1992 Retinopathy of prematurity: a prospective study. Review at six months. Eye 6:477–483.

Legge R H, Weiss H S, Hedges T R et al 1992 Periodic alternating gaze deviation in infancy. Neurology 42:1740–1743.

Lengyel D, Weinacht S, Charlier J et al 1998 The development of visual pursuit during the first month of life. Graefe's Arch Clin Exp Ophthalmol 236:440–444.

Lewis T L, Maurer D 1992 The development of the temporal and nasal visual fields during infancy. Vis Res 32:903–911.

Lim M, Soul J S, Hansen R M et al 2005 Development of visual acuity in children with cerebral visual impairment. Arch Ophthalmol 123:1215–1220.

Ling B-C 1942 A genetic study of sustained visual fixation and associated behaviour in the human infant from birth to six months. J Genet Psychol 61:227–277.

Luna B, Dobson V, Guthrie R D 1992 Grating acuity and visual field development of infants with bronchopulmonary dysplasia. Dev Med Child Neurol 34:813–821.

McDonald M A, Dobson V, Sebris S L et al 1985 The acuity card procedure: a rapid test of infant acuity. Invest Ophthalmol Vis Sci 26:1158–1162.

McGinnis J M 1930 Eye-movements and optic nystagmus in early infancy. Genet Psychol Monogr 8:321–427.

McGinnity F G, Bryars J H 1992 Controlled study of ocular morbidity in school children born preterm. Br J Ophthalmol 76:520–524.

McLoone E, O'Keefe M, Donoghue V et al 2006 RetCam image analysis of optic disc morhpology in premature infants and its relation to ischaemic brain injury. Br J Ophthalmol 90:465–471.

Mactier H, Hamilton R, Bradnam M S et al 2000 Contact lens electroretinography in preterm infants from 32 weeks after conception: a development in current technology. Arch Dis Childhood 82:F233–F236.

Madan A, Jan J E, Good W 2005 Visual development in preterm infants. Dev Med Child Neurol 47:276–280.

Malcolm C A, McCulloch D L, Shepherd A J 2002 Pattern reversal visual evoked potentials in infants: gender differences during early visual maturation. Dev Med Child Neurol 44:345–351.

Marg E, Freeman D N, Peltzman P et al 1976 Visual acuity development in human infants: evoked potential measurements. Invest Ophthalmol 15:150–153.

Margalith D, Jan J E, McCormick A Q et al 1984 Clinical spectrum of congenital optic nerve hypoplasia: a review of 51 patients. Dev Med Child Neurol 26:311–322.

Margalith D, Tze W J, Jan J E 1985 Congenital optic nerve hypoplasia with hypothalamic-pituitary dysplasia. Am J Dis Children 139:361–366.

Marr J E, Green S H, Willshaw H E 2005 Neurodevelopmental implications of ocular motor apraxia. Dev Med Child Neurol 47:815–819.

Martin E, Barkovich A J 1995 Magnetic resonance imaging in perinatal asphyxia. Arch Dis Childhood 72:62–70.

Matsuba C A, Jan J E 2006 Long-term outcome of children with cortical visual impairment. Dev Med Child Neurol 48:508–512.

Maybodi M 2003 Infantile onset nystagmus. Curr Opin Ophthalmol 14:276–285.

Mayer D L, Beiser A S, Warner A F et al 1995 Monocular acuity norms for the Teller Acuity Cards between ages one month and four years. Invest Ophthalmol Vis Sci 36:671–685.

Mayer D L, Fulton A B 1993 Development of the visual field. In: Simons K (ed.) Early visual development: normal and abnormal. Oxford University Press, New York, pp. 117–129.

Mayer D L, Fulton A B, Rodier D 1984 Grating and recognition acuities of pediatric patients. Ophthalmology 91:947–953.

Mayer D L, Moore B, Robb R M 1989 Assessment of vision and amblyopia by preferential looking tests after early surgery for unilateral cataracts. J Pediatr Ophthalmol Strabismus 26:61–67.

Mercer M E, Courage M L, Adams R J 1991 Contrast/color card procedure: a new test of young infants' color vision. Optometry Vis Sci 68:522–532.

Mercuri E, Atkinson J, Braddick O et al 1997 Visual function in full-term infants with hypoxic-ischaemic encephalopathy. Neuropaediatrics 28:155–161.

Mirabella G, Kjaer P, Norcia A et al 2006 Visual development in very low birth weight infants. Pediatric Research 60:435–439.

Mitchell T, Cambon K 1969 Vestibular response in the neonate and infant. Arch Otolaryngol 90:40–41.

Mohn G, Dobson V, Schwartz T et al 1986 The visual field of human infants: kinetic perimetry. Behav Brain Res 20:122.

Morante A, Dubowitz L M S, Levene M I et al 1982 The development of visual function in normal and neurologically abnormal preterm and fullterm infants. Dev Med Child Neurol 24:771–784.

Moseley M J, Fielder A R, Thompson J R et al 1988 Grating and recognition acuities of young amblyopes. Br J Ophthalmol 72:50–54.

Moskowitz A, Sokol S 1983 Developmental changes in the human visual system as reflected by the latency of the pattern reversal VEP. Electroencephalogr Clin Neurophysiol 56:1–15.

Nixon R B, Helveston E M, Miller K et al 1985 Incidence of strabismus in neonates. Am J Ophthalmol 100:798–801.

Norcia A M 1994 Vision testing by visual evoked potential techniques. In: Isenberg I (ed.) The eye in infancy, 2nd edn. Mosby, Chicago, pp. 157–173.

Norcia A M, Tyler C W, Piecuch R et al 1987 Visual acuity development in normal and abnormal preterm human infants. J Pediatr Ophthalmol Strabismus 24:70–74.

O'Connor A R, Spencer R, Birch E E 2007 Predicting long-term visual outcome in children with birth weight under 1001 g. JAAPOS 11:541–545.

O'Connor AR, Stephenson TJ, Johnson A et al 2002 Strabismus in children of birth weight less than 1701g. Arch Ophthalmol 120:767–773.

Ornitz E M, Atwell C W, Walter D O et al 1979 The maturation of vestibular nystagmus in infancy and childhood. Acta Otolaryngol 88:244–256.

Page J M, Schneeweiss S, Whyte H E A et al 1993 Ocular sequelae in premature infants. Pediatrics 92:787–790.

Patel L, McNally R J, Harrison E et al 2006 Geographical distribution of optic nerve hypoplasia and septo-optic dysplasia in Northwest England. J Pediatr 148:85–88.

Pearson C M, Chandna A, Doran R M L 1989 Preferential looking: the state of the art. Br Orthop J 46:66–72.

Pike A A, Marlow N 2000 The role of cortical evoked responses in predicting neuromotor outcome in very preterm infants. Early Hum Dev 57:123–135.

Pike M G, Holmstrom G, de-Vries L S et al 1994 Patterns of visual impairment associated with lesions of the preterm infant brain. Dev Med Child Neurol 36:849–862.

Placzek M, Mushin J, Dubowitz L M S 1985 Maturation of the visual evoked response and its correlation with visual acuity in preterm infants. Dev Med Child Neurol 27:448–454.

Prager T C, Zou Y L, Jensen C L et al 1999 Evaluation of methods for assessing visual function in infants. JAAPOS 3:275–282.

Prechtl H F R, Nijhuis J G 1983 Eye movements in the human fetus and newborn. Behav Brain Res 10:119–124.

Provis JM, Van Driel D, Billson FA, Russell P 1985 Development of the human retina: patterns of cell distribution and redistribution in the ganglion cell layer. J Comparative Neurol 233:429–451.

Rahi J S, Cable N 2003 British Childhood Visual Impairment Study Group. Severe visual impairment and blindness in children in the UK. Lancet 362:1359–1365.

Rappaport L, Urion D, Strand K et al 1987 Concurrence of congenital ocular motor apraxia and other motor problems: an expanded syndrome. Dev Med Child Neurol 29:85–90.

Raye K, Pratt E, Beiser A et al 1992 Normative Teller acuity card study: II. Test-retest reliability. Invest Ophthalmol Vis Sci 33(suppl):717.

Regal D M, Ashmead D H, Salapatek P 1983 The coordination of eye and head movements during early infancy: a selective review. Behav Brain Res 10:125–132.

Reinecke R D 1997 Idiopathic infantile nystagmus: diagnosis and treatment. Costenbader Lecture. JAAPOS 1:67–82.

Reinecke R D, Guo S, Goldstein H P 1988 Waveform evolution in infantile nystagmus: an electro-oculographic study of 35 cases. Binoc Vis 3:191–202.

Rethy I 1969 Development of the simultaneous fixation from the divergent anatomic eye-position of the neonate. J Pediatr Ophthalmol 6:92–96.

Riva D, Georgi C 2000 The cerebellum contributes to higher functions during development. Evidence from a series of children surgically treated for posterior fossa tumours. Brain 123:1051–1061.

Robinson G C, Jan J E 1987 Congenital ocular blindness in children, 1945 to 1984. Am J Dis Children 141:1321–1324.

Robinson J, Fielder A R 1990 Pupillary diameter and reaction to light in preterm neonates. Arch Dis Childhood 65:35–38.

Robinson J, Moseley M J, Thompson J R et al 1989 Eyelid opening in preterm neonates. Arch Dis Childhood 64:943–948.

Robinson R J 1966 Assessment of gestational age by neurological examination. Arch Dis Childhood 41:437–447.

Rossi L N, Pignataro O, Nino L M et al 1979 Maturation of vestibular responses: preliminary report. Dev Med Child Neurol 21:217–224.

Roucoux A, Culee C, Roucoux M 1983 Development of fixation and pursuit eye movements in human infants. Behav Brain Res 10:133–140.

Roy M S, Barsoum-Homsy M, Orquin J et al 1995 Maturation of binocular pattern visual evoked potentials in normal full-term and preterm infants from 1 to 6 months of age. Pediatr Res 37:140–144.

Russell-Eggitt J, Harris C M, Kriss A 1998 Delayed visual maturation: an update. Dev Med Child Neurol 40:130–136.

Salomao S R, Ventura D F 1995 Large sample population age norms for visual acuities obtained with Vistech-Teller Acuity Cards. Invest Ophthalmol Vis Sci 36:657–670.

Sargent M A, Poskitt K J, Jan J E 1997 Congenital motor apraxia: imaging findings. Am J Neuroradiol 18:1915–1922.

Schenk-Rootlieb A J F, van Nieuwenhuizen O, van der Graff Y et al 1992 The prevalence of cerebral visual disturbance in children with cerebral palsy. Dev Med Child Neurol 34:473–480.

Scher M S, Dobson V, Carpenter N A et al 1989 Visual and neurological outcome of infants with periventricular leukomalacia. Dev Med Child Neurol 31:353–365.

Sebris S L, Dobson V, McDonald M A et al 1987 Acuity cards for visual acuity assessments of infants and children in clinical settings. Clin Vis Sci 2:45–58.

Shepherd A J, Saunders K J, McCulloch D L et al 1999 Prognostic value of flash visual evoked potentials in preterm infants. Dev Med Child Neurol 41:9–15.

Simons K (ed.) 1993 Early visual development: normal and abnormal. Oxford University Press, Oxford.

Simson J, Giolli R, Blanks R 1988 The pretectal nuclear complex and the accessory optic system. In: Buttner-Ennever J (ed.) Neuroanatomy of the Oculomotor System. Elsevier, New York, pp. 355–364.

Skarf B, Hoyt C S 1984 Optic nerve hypoplasia in children. Arch Ophthalmol 102:62–67.

Slater A 1998 The competent infant: innate organisation and early learning in infant visual perception. In: Slater A (ed.) Perceptual development: visual, auditory and speech perception in infancy. Psychology Press, Hove, pp. 105–130.

Snir M, Axer-Siegel R, Bourla D et al 2002 Tactile corneal reflex development in full-term babies. Ophthalmology 109:526–529.

Sokol S 1978 Measurement of infant visual acuity from pattern reversal evoked potentials. Vis Res 18:33–39.

Sokol S, Jones K 1978 Implicit time of pattern evoked potentials in infants: an index of maturation of spatial vision. Vis Res 19:747–755.

Sokol S, Moskowitz A, McCormack G 1992 Infant VEP and preferential looking acuity measured with phase alternating gratings. Invest Ophthalmol Vis Sci 33:3156–3161.

Soo Kim J, Park S H, Lee K W 2003 Spasmus nutans and congenital ocular motor apraxia with cerebellar vermian hypoplasia. Arch Neurol 60:1621–1624.

Stanhope R, Preece M A, Brooke C G D 1984 Hypoplastic optic nerves and pituitary dysfunction. Arch Dis Childhood 59:111–114.

Tamura E E, Hoyt C S 1987 Oculomotor consequences of intraventricular hemorrhages in premature infants. Arch Ophthalmol 105:533–535.

Taylor D, Hoyt C S (eds) 2005 Pediatric ophthalmology and strabismus 3rd edn. Elsevier, Edinburgh.

Taylor D, Scott A 1997 Optic nerve: congenital abnormalities. In: Taylor D (ed.) Paediatric ophthalmology, 2nd edn. Blackwell Science, Oxford, pp. 660–700.

Teller D Y 1997 First glances: the vision of infants: the Friedenwald lecture. Invest Ophthalmol Vis Sci 38:2183–2203.

Teller D Y 1998 Spatial and temporal aspects of infant color vision. Vis Res 38:3275–3282.

Teller D Y, McDonald M A, Preston K et al 1986 Assessment of visual acuity in infants and children: the acuity card procedure. Dev Med Child Neurol 28:779–789.

Thompson D, Liasis A 2005 In: Taylor D, Hoyt C S (eds) Pediatric ophthalmology and strabismus, 3rd edn. Elsevier, Edinburgh, pp. 87–96.

Thorn F, Gwiazda J, Cruz A A V et al 1994 The development of eye alignment, convergence, and sensory binocularity in young infants. Invest Ophthalmol Vis Sci 35:544–553.

Tresidder J, Fielder A R, Nicholson J 1990 Delayed visual maturation: ophthalmic and neurodevelopmental aspects. Dev Med Child Neurol 32:872–881.

Trounce J Q, Dodd K L, Fawer C-L et al 1985 Primary thalamic haemorrhage in the newborn: a new clinical entity. Lancet i:190–192.

Uemera Y, Oguchi Y, Katsumi O 1981 Visual developmental delay. Ophthal Paediatr Genet 1:49–58.

Valmaggia C, Proudlock F, Gottlob I 2003 Optokinetic nystagmus in strabismus: are asymmetries related to binocularity? Invest Ophthalmol Vis Sci 44:5142–5150.

Valmaggia C, Rütsche A, Baumann A et al 2004 Age related change of optokinetic nystagmus in healthy subjects: a study from infancy to senescence. Br J Ophthalmol 88:1577–1581.

Van Hof-van Duin J 1989 The development and study of visual acuity. Dev Med Child Neurol 31:543–552.

Van Hof-van Duin J, Heersema D J, Groenendaal F et al 1992 Visual field and grating acuity development in low-risk preterm infants during the first 2½ years after term. Behav Brain Res 49:115–122.

Van Hof-van Duin J, Mohn G 1983 Optokinetic and spontaneous nystagmus in children with neurological disorders. Behav Brain Res 10:163–176.

Van Hof-van Duin J, Mohn G 1984a Vision in the preterm infant. Clin Dev Med 94:93–114.

Van Hof-van Duin J, Mohn G 1984b Visual defects in children after cerebral hypoxia. Behav Brain Res 14:147–155.

Van Hof-van Duin J, Mohn G 1986 The development of visual acuity in normal fullterm and preterm infants. Vis Res 26:909–916.

Van Hof-van Duin J, Mohn G, Petter W P F et al 1983 Preferential looking in preterm infants. Behav Brain Res 10:47–50.

Vehrs S, Baum D 1970 A test of visual responses in the newborn. Dev Med Child Neurol 12:772–774.

Vital-Durand F, Atkinson J, Braddick O J (eds) 1996 Infant vision. Oxford University Press, Oxford.

Von Noorden G K 1990 Burian von Noorden's binocular vision and ocular motility: theory and management of strabismus. C V Mosby, St Louis, MO.

Watson T, Orel-Bixler D, Haegerstrom-Portnoy G 2007 Longitudinal quantitative assessment of vision function in children with cortical visual impairment. Optom Vis Sci 84:471–480.

Weinacht S, Kind C, Monting J S et al 1999 Visual development in preterm and full-term infants: a prospective masked study. Invest Ophthalmol Vis Sci 40:346–353.

Weinberger H A, Van der Woude R, Maier H C 1962 Prognosis of cortical blindness following cardiac arrest in children. JAMA 179:126–129.

Weindling A M, Rochefort M J, Calvert S A et al 1985 Development of cerebral palsy after ultrasonographic detection of periventricular cysts in the newborn. Dev Med Child Neurol 27:800–806.

Weiss A H, Biersdorf W R 1989 Visual sensory disorders in congenital nystagmus. Ophthalmology 96:517–523.

Weleber R G, Palmer E A 1991 Electrophysiological evaluation of children with visual impairment. Semin Ophthalmol 6:161–168.

White B L, Castle P, Held R 1964 Observations on the development of visually-directed reaching. Child Dev 35:349–364.

Whiting S, Jan J E, Wong F K H et al 1985 Permanent cortical visual impairment in children. Dev Med Child Neurol 27:730–739.

Williams J, Brodsky M C, Griebel C M et al 1993 Septo-optic dysplasia: the clinical significance of an absent septum pellucidum. Dev Med Child Neurol 35:490–501.

Wizov S S, Reinecke R D, Bocarnea M 2002 A comparative demographic and socioeconomic study of spasmus nutans and infantile nystagmus. Am J Ophthalmol 133:256–262.

Wolf A B, Rubin S E, Kodsi S 2005 Comparison of clinical findings in pediatric patients with albinism and different amplitudes of nystagmus. JAAPOS 9:363–368.

Yee R D, Baloh R W, Honrubia V 1981 Eye movement abnormalities in rod monochromacy. Ophthalmology 88:1010–1018.

Yigiter A B, Kavak Z N 2006 Normal standards of fetal behaviour assessed by four dimensional sonography. J Matern Fetal Neonatal Med 19:707–721.

Zametkin A J, Stevens J R, Pittman R 1979 Ontogeny of spontaneous blinking and of habituation of the blink reflex. Ann Neurol 5:453–457.

CHAPTER

38

Hearing disorders

K. S. Sirimanna

INTRODUCTION

Incidence of congenital permanent hearing loss (CPHL) is estimated to be 1 per 1000 live births in the developed world (Davis et al 1997). This increases to 1.7 per 1000 by 10 years of age (Fortnum et al 2001). Of the CPHL approximately 50% is due to genetic causes while the rest is acquired either during the pregnancy or at birth. Incidence of hearing loss is higher in certain communities or countries. Vanniasegaram et al (1993) found 3–4 times higher incidence of CPHL in predominantly Bangladeshi population in Tower Hamlets (a district in east London, UK) while a recent study by Attias et al (2004) found 7 times higher incidence of hearing loss in Jordanian infants compared to those from Israel.

In addition, permanent sensorineural hearing loss (SNHL) results from various causes during infancy including neonatal infections, head injury, ototoxic medication, noise exposure and genetic etiologies. Babies during the first year of life are susceptible to middle ear infections and also 'glue ear' (synonyms: middle ear effusions (MEE), otitis media with effusion (OME) that cause temporary conductive hearing loss (hearing loss due to a poor sound conduction through the middle ear). This chapter deals mainly with the causes of hearing loss in the fetus and infant.

Until recently average age of identification of congenital hearing loss was over 18 months with those who are diagnosed soon after birth having had a hearing screen through a targeted hearing screening program because of the presence of a 'risk factor'. The opportunities for determining the etiology of hearing loss in this population have been poor with less than 50% ending up with an etiological diagnosis (Morzaria et al 2004). However, more recently, since the establishment of universal newborn hearing screening programs, there has been a significantly better yield leading to better understanding of the causes of congenital hearing loss. Further, our own experience at Great Ormond Street Hospital, London has been different with etiology of deafness identified in 60–70% of children with hearing loss, with the use of a comprehensive protocol for etiological investigations as a routine.

DEVELOPMENT OF THE EAR

Development of the human ear starts around the third gestational week and is normally complete by 24 weeks. Adverse environmental factors especially during the first 24 weeks of gestation can therefore affect this process leading to various forms and degrees of permanent hearing loss.

Thickening of the ectoderm dorsal to the second brachial cleft invaginates to form the otic pit around the third week of gestation marking the beginning of the development of the inner ear. The otic pit deepens and subsequently separates off from the surface to form the otic capsule or otic placode, close to the hind brain part of the neural tube, around the fifth week. Otic placode then differentiates into the endolymphatic sac, utricle and the saccule. Around the same time cochlear and vestibular ganglion cells develop from the medial aspect of the otic capsule. Cochlear duct develops from the saccule and forms the cochlea while the cochlear vestibular nerve develops laterally from the hindbrain part of the neural tube towards the cochlear vestibular ganglion cells. The mesoderm of the otic capsule starts to ossify around the fifth month forming a hard shell around the membranous part of the inner ear, i.e. membranous labyrinth.

The middle ear cleft develops from a dorsolateral evagination from the first pharyngeal pouch (pharyngo-tympanic tube) to meet an invagination between the first and second pharyngeal arches. At the same time cartilage from the first pharyngeal arch differentiates to become malleus, incus and the head of the stapes, while the second pharyngeal arch forms the crura and the footplate of the stapes. These form the three ossicles in the middle ear conducting sounds from the eardrum (tympanic membrane) to the inner ear. The endoderm of the pharyngotympanic tube drapes these bones within the middle ear, while the distal part develops into the mastoid antrum and subsequently the air cells. The ectodermal invagination forms the external ear canal and the outer stratified squamous epithelial layer of the tympanic membrane (TM) while the inner layer of the TM is formed by the endoderm of the pharyngotympanic tube with mesoderm sandwiched between the two. The middle ear ossicles start to ossify from the eleventh week of gestation and by the eighth embryonic month the ossicles have reached the full adult size (Bowden 1977, Freeman et al 1999, Hall 2000, Torres & Giraldez 1998).

From the embryonic point of view it is the first trimester that is most important with regard to the formation of the ear. Any significant insult to this process can lead to abnormalities in the development of the ear resulting in a hearing loss that may be significant.

The following section deals with those conditions that may lead to a hearing loss in the fetus.

MATERNAL DIABETES AND DEAFNESS

This is a form of maternally inherited non-insulin dependant diabetes usually appearing before the age of 40 years associated with a sensorineural deafness, that is due to a mutation in mitochondrial DNA (3243 tRNA). As in other mitochondrial disease, transmission is from mother to the child and can present with features involving other organs and tissues (Guillausseau et al 2001, Kountakis et al 2002). Further, auricular abnormalities and hearing loss can be associated with insulin dependent diabetes as a part of oculo-auriculo-vertebral spectrum (Wang et al 2002).

MATERNAL INFECTIONS AND DEAFNESS

Deafness from congenital rubella, a pleomorphic RNA virus, was frequent in the past, but a rarity in most developed or developing countries currently, due to mass immunization (Batnavala & Brown 2004, Kadoya et al 1998, Upfold & Oong 2004). However it may still be an important cause of deafness in the newborn where there are no such coordinated immunization policies (Chakravarti & Jain 2006). When it occurs the hearing loss is normally severe to profound, progressive and is sensorineural. It also could be asymmetric and is often associated with learning difficulties and other neurological involvement (Kayan & Bellman 1990).

OTHER INFECTIONS CAUSING HEARING LOSS

Measles and mumps in the infant can lead to deafness occasionally, from viral labyrinthitis. Measles usually causes a mild to moderate sensorineural hearing loss while mumps leads to unilateral or asymmetric hearing loss of a severe degree (Kayan & Bellman 1990). There are a number of reports of mumps, measles and rubella (MMR) vaccination causing sensorineural hearing loss. These are mostly individual case reports but in the absence of good quality evidence the debate continues (Stewart & Prabhu 1993).

Herpes zoster is not usually associated with congenital hearing loss but may cause acquired hearing loss in the first year of life. It may occur with viral encephalitis, Ramsay Hunt syndrome and may present with sudden loss of hearing (Ohtani et al 2006). Some authors have argued that early diagnosis and treatment of herpes zoster infections may lead to prevention or recovery of hearing loss (Murakami et al 1997).

Currently the commonest maternal infection causing deafness in the newborn is cytomegalovirus (p. 640), a pleomorphic RNA virus in the Togaviridae family of the genus *Rubivirus* (Lagasse et al 2000). This is usually asymptomatic in the mother and the infection could be transferred to the baby through the placenta. The incidence of congenital CMV infection can be as high as 2.5% but only about 10–20% of these are symptomatic. These include intrauterine growth retardation, microcephaly, hepatosplenomegaly and jaundice, mental retardation and sensorineural hearing loss that can be progressive. There is no evidence of postnatally acquired cytomegalovirus causing hearing loss in the newborn (Iwasaki et al 2007, Vollmer et al 2004). However, a proportion of congenitally infected babies will develop sensorineural hearing loss that can be progressive and fluctuating (Fowler et al 1997, Williamson et al 1992). Dahle et al (2000) described 860 children with congenital CMV and found that of those who had a hearing loss about 50% had a profound hearing loss and the rest had mild to severe hearing loss. In this group there were 651 asymptomatic children and 209 who were symptomatic. Of the asymptomatic group 7.4% developed SNHL (including approximately 50% with unilateral SNHL) and 40.7% of the symptomatic group either had or developed SNHL with 50% showing a progressive hearing loss. Delayed onset of hearing loss was most common in the asymptomatic group and was detectable by 2 years of age, with a steady increase in the percentage of SNHL in this group up to about 6 years. In the University Hospital of Alabama universal hearing-screening program, Fowler and Boppana (2006) showed that about 75% of the children with a hearing loss due to congenital CMV were detected at or soon after birth and the rest later. They also stated that it is not possible to predict who would develop a hearing loss postnatally. It is therefore recommended that children with congenital CMV with normal hearing at or soon after birth are followed up until they are at least 6 years of age.

Other infections that may cause deafness are toxoplasma, herpes and syphilis (Pickering 1985). Infection during pregnancy with *Toxoplasma gondii*, which is a protozoal organism, can lead to deafness occasionally. McLeod et al (2006) reviewed children who have been treated for congenital toxoplasmosis and suggested that treatment can lead to reduced neurological sequelae including deafness. Acquired and congenital syphilis can occasionally cause sensorineural hearing loss (Dobbin & Perkins 1983) and therefore need to be kept in mind especially with the increase in reported incidence of syphilis lately.

DRUGS DURING PREGNANCY AND DEAFNESS

In addition those drugs known to cause hearing loss, indulgence in alcohol and other drugs such as cocaine during pregnancy can lead to hearing loss in the baby (Church & Abel 1998, Cone-Wesson 2005) in addition to speech and language development.

GENETIC CONDITIONS AFFECTING HEARING

About 50% of congenital permanent hearing loss (CPHL) is due to genetic causes (the other 50% is acquired either during the pregnancy or at birth). Of the genetic hearing loss about 70–80% is autosomal recessive (AR) with most of the remainder due to autosomal dominant (AD) causes (Fig. 38.1). A small percentage is chromosomal with occasional mitochondrial and X-linked deafness (Samanich et al 2007).

Some patients with genetic hearing loss have a syndrome although the majority is non-syndromic (NS). Of the non-syndromic autosomal recessive group, most hearing losses are due to mutations in the *GJB2* (connexin 26) gene that accounts for 40–50% of all autosomal recessive non-syndromic hearing loss (ARNSHL) in the Caucasian population. Connexin is a protein that is responsible for the gap junctions that exist between cells and therefore allows transfer of intracellular signaling ions to adjacent cells. As with other AR conditions consanguinity increases the risk of having a child with hearing loss with a recurrence risk of 1:4. A large number of recessive and a very few dominant *Cx26* mutations responsible for deafness have been identified while significant polymorphism and nonsense mutations also have been identified with often unknown pathological significance. Of the main mutations *35delG* is responsible for ARNS hearing loss while in Ashkenazi population *167delT* and in Indian subcontinent *W24X* are the commonest, although the incidence may depend on the ethnic group (Samanich et al 2007). Hearing loss can be from mild to profound (Apps et al 2007) and also can be progressive (Pagarkar et al 2006).

About 25 mutations causing ARNSHL have been identified and it is assumed that there are more unidentified recessive mutations responsible for hearing loss (see Hereditary Hearing Loss Homepage www.webh01.uc.ac.be/hhh/).

Over 20 mutations responsible for autosomal dominant non-syndromic autosomal recessive hearing loss including connexin 30 have been recognized but these produce less severe deafness that is usually progressive and usually appears later in life. Increased susceptibility to aminoglycoside antibiotics can be inherited as a mitochondrial mutation (see under ototoxicity).

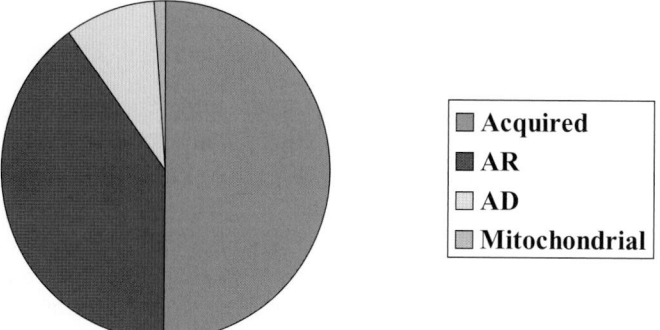

Figure 38.1 Causes of congenital permanent hearing loss showing genetic inheritance patterns (AR, autosomal recessive; AD, autosomal dominant).

- Acquired
- AR
- AD
- Mitochondrial

SYNDROMIC DEAFNESS INCLUDE THE FOLLOWING CONDITIONS

Usher syndrome is an autosomal recessive condition with deafness and retinitis pigmentosa. In these patients there may not be obvious abnormalities at birth or infancy except the hearing loss, and the other features such as retinitis pigmentosa leading to blindness develop later and are progressive (Sadeghi et al 2006). Early diagnosis by electroretinography can be vital in order to better manage these patients. Variability of the phenotype is well known in Usher syndrome with those with profound hearing loss also having bilateral vestibular failure that may manifest in the first year with significantly delayed motor milestones (Cohen et al 2007).

Jervell–Lange–Nielsen syndrome, another AR syndromic hearing loss, is a rare condition with profound sensorineural hearing loss and vestibular dysfunction with prolonged QT interval that may lead to syncope and death if not diagnosed early and treated (Neyroud et al 1997).

Pendred syndrome is also transmitted autosomal recessively and usually has a severe to profound, progressive sensorineural hearing loss with cochlear abnormalities such as Mondini defect and large vestibular aqueduct (Glaser 2003, Luxon et al 2003). It is caused by mutations in the *PDS* (*SLC26A4*) gene encoding anion transfer pendrin, thought to enable efflux of iodide into the thyroid follicle lumen (Taylor et al 2002). These patients also have a defect in organification of iodine and may develop goiter, usually during the peri-pubertal age. MRI of the inner ear helps to identify these patients very early (Sharghi et al 2007). Progressive hearing loss with head injury is common in patients with enlarged endolymphatic sac especially when it occurs with Pendred syndrome, and early diagnosis will therefore provide an opportunity to prevent or minimize further deterioration by providing parents with better advice (Colvin et al 2006). This is different from congenital hypothyroidism that can be associated with sensorineural hearing loss (Vandersschueren-Lodeweyckx et al 1983) but these early studies may well have included cases of Pendred syndrome. In some countries congenital hypothyroidism is diagnosed soon after birth using heel prick blood spot samples (Kaye 2006) and these children must undergo a hearing assessment in order to detect and manage permanent sensorineural hearing loss early.

Waardenburg syndrome is characterized by pigmentary abnormalities such as heterochromia irides, white forelock and depigmented skin patches with increased inner canthal distance (dystopia canthorum) and sensorineural hearing loss (Newton 2002, Read & Newton 1997). Genetic heterogeneity is seen in Waardenburg syndrome although mutations in *PAX3* gene have been identified and the hearing loss can be progressive, asymmetrical and vary from moderate to profound.

Alport syndrome is characterized by glomerular basement membrane abnormalities (thickening and splitting) leading to hematuria and eventually renal failure, usually with X-linked inheritance and sensorineural hearing loss. Being an X-linked condition, it leads to severe hearing loss in the male, while in the female there is a wide variation in the presentation from normal to severely affected individuals due to X-chromosome inactivation. Hematuria may only be occasionally detected in infancy and therefore it is important for suspected children to have repeated urine examinations. The diagnosis can be confirmed by a renal biopsy that will show the typical electron microscopic picture (Sirimanna 1993). Mutations seen in Alport syndrome are in type IV collagen genes (e.g. *COL4A5*) and therefore other tissues can be affected, especially the eyes, showing abnormalities such as lenticonus and cataracts (Wilson et al 2006).

Branchio-oto-renal syndrome (BOR) is inherited as an autosomal dominant condition, with a variable phenotypic presentation. Babies affected may have preauricular pits or tags, or branchial sinuses. In a proportion of these patients there will be renal abnormalities that can be detected usually by an ultrasound examination. The hearing loss can vary from mild to profound and can be conductive, sensorineural or mixed. Inner ear scans may show ossicular abnormalities and/or inner ear abnormalities that usually include hypoplastic or absent semicircular canals and wide vestibular aqueduct. Mutations in the *EYA1* gene are often associated with the syndrome (Misra & Nolph 1998, Rodriguez & Soriano 2003).

Craniosynostosis syndromes such as Apert, Crouzon and Pfeiffer are also associated with various forms of hearing loss (Sirimanna 2004). These conditions are usually due to mutations in fibroblast growth factor receptor genes (*FGFR2*, *FGFR3*). In Apert syndrome the hearing loss is almost always conductive and due to middle ear effusions or sometimes from congenital ossicular fixation (Rajendrakumar et al 2005). Congenital ossicular fixation leading to a conductive hearing loss is common in both Crouzon and Pfeiffer syndromes where a few patients will have atresia of the external ear canal (especially in Crouzon) and also sometimes sensorineural hearing loss.

Treacher Collins syndrome is associated with second arch abnormalities that lead to a conductive hearing loss in about 50% of cases, from either external meatal atresia or ossicular abnormalities, or a combination of the two (Dixon 1996, Marres 2002).

Cleft palate including submucous cleft is associated with, normally conductive hearing loss (Goudy et al 2006, Sheahan et al 2004) when it is non-syndromic. Syndromic cleft palate can be associated with a sensory neural hearing loss in addition to above depending on individual syndromes, e.g. Pierre Robin. It therefore important for any baby with cleft palate or submucous cleft (often missed unless the palate is carefully examined) to have a hearing assessment. Cleft lip is, on the other hand, not associated with increased incidence of hearing loss.

There are a number of other syndromes that are occasionally associated with hearing loss and it would be impossible to cover all these in this chapter, and therefore the reader is advised to refer to other texts on this topic.

PERINATAL CONDITIONS AFFECTING BABIES' HEARING

Hypoxia: The general belief has been that hypoxia alone is not a cause of hearing loss (Borg 1997) but Ferber-Viart et al (1996) have argued otherwise and shown that there is no difference in the hearing loss due to hypoxia, with or without other risk factors. There is some evidence that hypoxia causes cochlear (sensory) as well as neural hearing loss and in at least some hypoxic babies the hearing loss may improve during the immediate post hypoxic period (Jiang-Ze et al 2004, Makishima et al 1976). In a postmortem study of inner ears of 4 asphyxiated preterm neonates and in a case of severe neonatal asphyxia Koyama et al (2005) found 'degeneration and disappearance of outer hair cells of the organ of Corti and edematous changes in the stria vascularis' (Koyama et al 2005) suggesting post-hypoxic damage to the inner ear. On the other hand Mazurek et al (2003) using hypoxic–ischemic newborn rats showed that inner hair cells are more susceptible to oxygen deprivation than the outer hair cells. Jiang et al (2005) using distortion product otoacoustic emissions in 46 term infants who suffered perinatal hypoxia–ischemia showed that hypoxic hearing loss is mainly in the frequency range of 1–5 kHz. Interesting research carried out by Sohmer et al (1994) showed that preterm fetal threshold to sound stimulation in utero improves with maternal inhalation of oxygen that leads to better fetal oxygenation. However, as this is a behavioral response it may well be that it is the responsiveness rather than the hearing threshold that improves.

Hyperbilirubinemia: Hyperbilirubinemia is a recognized cause of hearing loss in the newborn (see Ch. 36). Lima et al (2006) examined automated auditory brainstem response hearing test (AABR) results of 979 newborn babies admitted to the Intensive and Intermediate Care unit and found a 10.2% prevalence of hearing loss of more than 35 dBNA. Using multivariate analysis they further examined the risk factor for hearing loss and found hyperbilirubinemia ($P = 0.002$) in addition to asphyxia ($P < 0.001$), low birth weight less than 1000 g ($P = <0.001$) and craniofacial deformity ($P = <0.001$). Al Otabi et al (2005) reviewed 9776 admissions to Toronto Sick Children's Hospital and identified 12 neonates with bilirubin levels of more than 400 μmol/L and no evidence of hypoxic–ischemic encephalopathy. Bilirubin levels in these babies ranged from 405 to 825 μmol/L. Seven out of ten of these patients had abnormal brainstem auditory evoked potentials. In a retrospective study of 1032 children with hearing loss, Oysu-Cagatay et al (2002) found that 67 cases had hearing loss due to hyperbilirubinemia and of these 30 had no other identifiable factor. They also found that both cochlear and auditory neural pathways could be affected in hyperbilirubinemia.

Prematurity: Prematurity has been associated with increased incidence of hearing loss in the neonate, especially when the gestational age is less than 32 weeks (Jiang et al 2001). Often these babies have other factors that make them more prone to have a hearing loss, such as hypoxia, being treated with ototoxic antibiotics and hyperbilirubinemia and therefore it is often difficult to identify the exact cause of their hearing loss. Further, these factors act synergistically and therefore one factor, at a level that may not cause a hearing loss acting on its own, may lead to cochlear damage in the presence of other factors as evident from animal experiments (Alles & Pye 1993).

Ototoxic medication: There are a number of drugs that may cause hearing loss when given to the mother during the pregnancy or to the newborn. These mainly include aminoglycosides (e.g. gentamicin, streptomycin, neomycin, amikacin, tobramycin, kanamycin), loop diuretics and platinum drugs (cisplatin and carboplatin) but other drugs such as salicylates less frequently cause sensorineural hearing loss. Vancomycin, although it can be ototoxic, is not an aminoglycoside but a glycopeptide. Anti-malarials such as quinine may still be in use in the developing world and can lead to deafness. When used in combination these drugs may show a potentiating effect with regard to ototoxicity (Huang & Schacht 1989). Henley and Rybak (1993) reviewed the literature and found that ototoxicity varied with the drug used, its dosage, duration and the age of the patient. They also noted that combining ototoxic drugs is likely to increase their ototoxicity by acting synergistically. Therefore ototoxicity may occur even when the serum levels of individual ototoxic agent are within recommended levels if other ototoxic agents are administered simultaneously. Histological studies of temporal bones of patients who have had aminoglycoside antibiotics have shown that outer hair cells in the high frequency region are affected before the inner hair cells are damaged (Huizing & de Groot 1987). High trough levels (pre-dose) of these agents appear to lead to more frequent ototoxicity compared to peak or post-dose blood levels. Systematic review of randomized controlled trials of gentamicin treatment regimens by Rao et al (2006) showed that although no difference in ototoxicity was noted in these studies, once a day dose of gentamicin was superior to multiple doses per day regimen in achieving high peak levels of the drug while avoiding toxic trough levels, in treating neonatal sepsis.

Increased susceptibility to aminoglycosides has also been reported in some families with mitochondrial mutations such as A1555G or C1494T (Fischel-Ghodsian et al 1993, Min-Xin 2006, Prezant et al 1993). In these families there may be a history of hearing loss from 30–40 years of age even without any previous exposure to aminoglycosides while ototoxicity occurs with blood levels that are within recommended levels. The hearing loss is dose dependent and will progress with repeated doses of aminoglycosides and should therefore be detected early to prevent further deterioration of hearing.

It is also important to remember that renal failure can lead to rapid increase in blood levels of these ototoxic drugs that may produce inner ear damage within a short period, especially in a pre-term baby. Regular audiological monitoring of babies who receive ototoxic antibiotics is therefore extremely important (Fausti et al 1992). Ototoxic drugs affect both vestibular and cochlear end organs and for example gentamicin is twice as vestibulotoxic as cochlear toxic (Sande & Mandell 1990). In a neonate vestibular toxicity may manifest as delay in sitting up and walking and can be easily overlooked. Platinum based drugs include carboplatin and cisplatin that are commonly used anti-tumor agents. Cisplatin causes hearing loss in over 50% of patients treated with this drug while carboplatin is much less ototoxic, and the hearing loss can be progressive (Bertolini et al 2004). In animal studies carboplatin has been shown to be toxic to inner hair cells initially but this has not been a common observation in humans. Hearing loss appears to start in the extended high frequency range and therefore distortion product otoacoustic emission screen (DPOAE) to include higher frequencies up to 8 kHz is more useful than the conventional transient evoked otoacoustic emissions (TEOAE) screen in this group of patients (Dhooge et al 2006). There has been some discussion recently on preventing ototoxicity from platinum drugs by using antioxidant drugs (Husain et al 2005, Skinner 2006).

Another group of drugs that has been reported to cause SNHL is loop diuretics, e.g. furosemide (Brown et al 1991, Shine & Coates 2005) although this has been questioned more recently (Bagshaw et al 2007).

Noise exposure – Incubator noise and noisy toys have been linked to hearing loss in babies and children in the past (Kent et al 2002). However, there is little supporting evidence from other studies.

CONDITIONS IN THE NEONATE AND INFANT AFFECTING HEARING

Infections: Of the infections the commonest is congenital cytomegalovirus infection and this, and hearing loss due to mumps and measles have been discussed earlier in this chapter.

Bacterial meningitis is probably the next common infection in the infant to cause permanent sensorineural hearing loss (see Ch. 32). The three main bacteria to cause SNHL are pneumococcus (*Streptococcus pneumoniae*), meningococcal (*Neisseria meningitidis*) and haemophilus (*Haemophilus influenzae*). The reported incidence of hearing loss in bacterial meningitis varies from 3.5% to as high as 37.2% with an incidence of bilateral profound SNHL between 1% and 4% (Fortnum 1992). Since the introduction in the UK of *Haemophilus influenzae* (HiB) vaccination in 1992 the incidence of *Haemophilus* meningitis has dropped significantly. Of the three responsible bacteria, pneumococcus causesa a high incidence of hearing loss that can vary from 21% to 50% (Fortnum 1992). There is a general view that hearing loss in bacterial meningitis occurs very early in the course of illness and can be reversible or progressive (Richardson et al 1997). Early diagnosis and appropriate treatment can prevent hearing loss or minimize its severity. Cochlear obliteration due to new bone formation is common in post-meningitic hearing loss and therefore these children should be referred for audiological assessment as a matter of urgency. Viral meningitis does not normally cause cochlear hearing loss although there have been isolated case reports in the literature but these are most likely to be following viral encephalitis.

Middle ear infections are not uncommon in infants and may lead to, or on top of, non-suppurative otitis media (synonyms: 'glue ear,' otitis media with effusion – OME). Often, in otherwise healthy infants, OME resolves spontaneously (Burton & Rosenfield 2006). However, there is emerging evidence from USA newborn hearing screening programs suggesting that these children may be at risk of developing OME over the next few years of life and therefore should be included in a surveillance program. Children with head and neck abnormalities are more likely to have a hearing loss (both permanent and temporary) and therefore require hearing assessments.

Other causes of hearing loss include head injury and this is usually associated with a temporal bone fracture (Ishman & Friedland 2004). Some of these patients have a progressive hearing loss due to perilymph leak that should to be identified early for repairing the leak so that further deterioration can be prevented.

ASSESSING HEARING IN THE NEWBORN AND INFANT, AND FOLLOW-UP

It is now possible to assess hearing in a child of any age. Most developed countries (e.g. UK, USA, Canada and Australia) have established or are establishing universal newborn hearing screening programs (UNHSP) leading to identification of significant hearing loss very early so that appropriate interventions including amplification can be provided to optimize the child's speech and language, and intellectual development and educational achievements. Other countries have used targeted newborn hearing screens (TNHSP) by screening those babies who are at a higher risk of having a hearing loss. While UNHSP can detect almost 100% of babies with permanent congenital hearing loss TNHSP detects only 40% of the same.

It is important to remember that 7 children per 10 000 will acquire permanent deafness over the first 10 years of life (Fortnum et al 2001) and therefore it is important for professionals to be vigilant as parents may go away with a false sense of security after their child passes the newborn hearing screen.

NHSP in the UK use automated otoacoustic emissions (AOAE) and automated auditory brainstem response (AABR) systems to screen babies for hearing loss (Fig. 38.2). Those babies who do not pass the screen are referred for a hearing assessment using a combination of high frequency tympanometry (middle ear function test), otoacoustic emissions (a test of outer hair cell function), and auditory brainstem responses for establishing frequency specific hearing thresholds. Amplification is provided if appropriate, often using digital hearing aids, as early as a few weeks of age (depending on the clinical situation). Tools are being developed to objectively assess the benefit of early hearing aid fitting in babies under six months of age.

Children over six months of age have their hearing tested using behavioral techniques such as visual reinforcement audiometry or distraction test. The former has the ability to determine ear specific hearing thresholds and bone conduction thresholds by using insert earphones and bone transducers to deliver sound stimuli. Babies with a significant hearing loss enter into a rehabilitative program that delivers not only amplification (Fig. 38.3) and medical assessment to determine the etiology of deafness, but also support to the parents, early support to children, with the involvement of peripatetic teacher of the deaf and where necessary specialist speech and language therapist and social services including support from voluntary organizations (e.g. National Deaf Children's Society in the UK).

SPECIFIC CONDITIONS

Auditory neuropathy/auditory dyssynchrony (AN/AD): In the majority of those who have a sensorineural hearing loss the cochlea is affected. They show absent outer hair cell (OHC) function and the inner hair cells are also damaged. However, a small percentage (about 1%) of cases of SNHL are due to neural involvement (compared to sensory organ involvement). The lesion could be due to absent or damaged inner hair cells (IHC), abnormality in the synapse (between the IHC and auditory nerve) function, pathology involving the auditory nerve or cochlear nucleus and second order neurons in the brainstem. The diagnosis of this group of patients is based on normal OHC function as shown by evoked otoacoustic emissions and absent or disordered auditory brainstem responses. Madden et al (2002) reported the etiology of 22 children with auditory neuropathy/dyssynchrony that included hyperbilirubinemia (50%), prematurity (45%), ototoxic drug exposure (41%), are neonatal ventilator dependency (36%). In some children an autosomal recessive mutation (otoferlin) is responsible for auditory dyssynchrony, caused by IHC (inner hair cell) dysfunction (Rodriguez-Ballesteros et al 2003, Varga et al 2003). In some cases it can also be due to delayed maturation (myelination) of the peripheral auditory pathways (Aldosari et al 2003). The dyssynchronous firing of the peripheral auditory pathways means that these babies hear very 'garbled' speech and, therefore, may not develop speech themselves if the degree of dyssynchrony is severe. The clinical picture varies from difficulty in hearing when there is background noise to the picture of the typically 'deaf'. Further, true neuropathy of the auditory nerve can be a part of a generalized peripheral

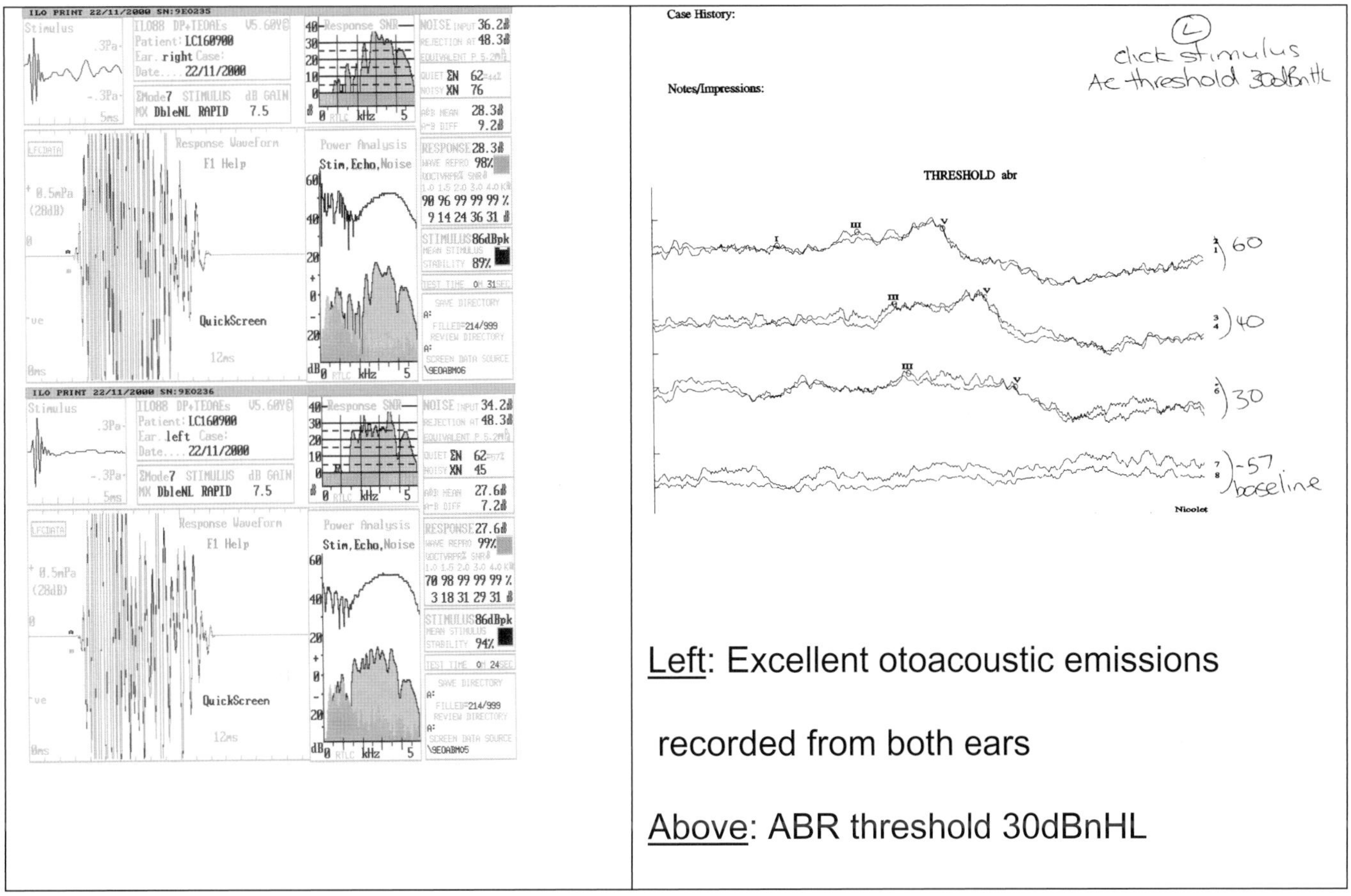

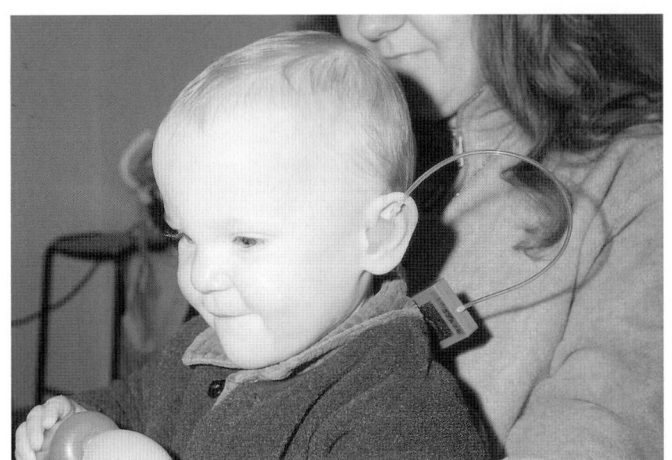

Figure 38.2 Otoacoustic emissions (OAE) and ABR recording from a baby with normal hearing.

Figure 38.3 Child with insert earphones ready for visual reinforcement audiometry.

neuropathy and, therefore, require a full neurological examination. When diagnosed these babies should be managed in tertiary centers with appropriate expertise. The prevalence of AD/AN is not exactly known but is estimated to be 2–3% (Tang et al 2004) with most having had significant perinatal problems including hypoxia and hyperbilirubinemia. The management varies from environmental modifications and using some form of signing to, in some cases, cochlear implantation (Madden et al 2002).

SUMMARY

About 50% of congenital hearing loss is due to genetic causes while the other 50% is acquired. The acquired causes include infections and drug abuse during the pregnancy. Perinatal problems including asphyxia, hyperbilirubinemia, prematurity and ototoxicity can cause deafness either acting on their own or together. In addition to the above, head and neck abnormalities increase the risk of a baby having a hearing loss and, therefore, should be referred for a hearing assessment. Most developed countries have set up or are setting up universal newborn hearing screening with the intention of detecting children with hearing loss very early. This enables early intervention and provision of appropriate support to the child and also to the family leading to much better outcome. Congenital cytomegalovirus infection is becoming an important cause of not only permanent congenital hearing loss but also progressive hearing loss in a child who may have passed the neonatal hearing screen. In addition, there are other reasons for developing permanent sensorineural hearing loss postnatally and, therefore, a program of surveillance is required to detect these children early.

REFERENCES

Al Otabi S F, Blaser S, MacGregor D L 2005 Neurological complications of kernicterus. Can J Neurol Sci 32(3):311–315.

Aldosari M, Mabie A, Husain A M 2003 Delayed visual maturation associated with auditory neuropathy/dyssynchrony. J Child Neurol 18(5):358–361.

Alles R M, Pye A 1993 Cochlear damage in guinea pigs following contralateral sound stimulation with and without gentamicin. Br K Audiol 27(3):183–193.

Apps S A, Rankin W A, Kurmis A P 2007 Connexin 26 mutations in autosomal recessive deafness disorders: A review. Int J Audiology 46(2):75–81.

Attias J, Al-Masri M, Abukader L et al 2006 The prevalence of congenital and early onset hearing loss in Jordanian and Israeli infants. Int J Audiol 45(9):528–536.

Bagshaw S M, Delaney A, Hasse M et al 2007 Loop diuretic in the management of acute renal failure: a systematic review and meta-analysis. Crit Care Resusc 9(1):68.

Batnavala J E, Brown D W 2004 Rubella. Lancet 363(9415):1127–1137.

Bertolini P, Lassalle M, Mercier G et al 2004 Platinum compound related hearing loss in children: long-term follow-up reveals continuous worsening of hearing loss. J Paediatr Haematol Oncol 26(10):649–655.

Borg E 1997 Perinatal asphyxia, hypoxia, ischemia and hearing loss. An overview. Scand Audiol 26(2):77–91.

Bowden R E M 1977 Development of the middle and external ear in the man. Proc R Soc Med 70(11):807–815.

Brown D R, Watchko J E, Sabo D 1991 Neonatal sensorineural hearing loss associated with furosemide: a case controlled study. Dev Med Child Neurol 33(9):816–823.

Burton M J, Rosenfield R M 2006 Grommets (ventilation tubes) for hearing loss associated with otitis media with effusion in children. Otolaryngol Head Neck Surg 135(4):507–510.

Chakravarti A, Jain M 2006 Rubella prevalence and its transmission in children. Indian J Pathol Microbiol 49(1):54–56.

Church M W, Abel E L 1998 Fetal alcohol syndrome. Hearing, speech, language, and vestibular disorders. Obstet Gynaecol Clin North Am 25(1):85–97.

Cohen M, Bitner-Glindzicz M, Luxon L 2007 The changing face of Usher syndrome: Clinical implications. Int J Audiology 46(2):82–93.

Colvin I B, Beale T, Harrop-Griffiths K 2006 Long-term follow up of hearing loss in children and young adults with enlarged vestibular aqueducts: relationship to radiological findings and Pendred syndrome diagnosis. Laryngoscope 116(11):2007–2036.

Cone-Wesson B 2005 Prenatal alcohol and cocaine exposure: influences on cognition, speech, language, and hearing. J Commun Disord 38(4):279–302.

Dahle A J, Fowler K B, Wright J D et al 2000 Longitudinal investigation of hearing disorders in children with congenital cytomegalovirus. J Am Acad Audiol 11:283–290.

Davis A, Bamford J, Wilson I et al 1997 Critical review of the role of neonatal hearing screening in the detection of congenital hearing impairment. Health Technology Assessment. Health Technol Assessment 1997 1(10).

Dhooge I, Dhooge C, Geukens S et al 2006 Distortion product otoacoustic emissions: an objective technique for screening of hearing loss in children treated with platinum derivatives. Int J Audiol 45(6):337–343.

Dixon M J 1996 Treacher Collins syndrome. Hum Mol Genet 5 Spec No:1391–1396.

Dobbin J M, Perkins J H 1983 Otosyphilis and hearing loss: response to penicillin and steroid therapy. Laryngoscope 93(12):1540–1543.

Edlich R F, Winters K L, Long W B 3rd et al 2005 Rubella and congenital rubella (German measles). J Long Term Eff Med Implants 15(3):319–328.

Fausti S A, Henry J A, Schaffer H I et al 1992 High-frequency audiometric monitoring for early detection of aminoglycoside ototoxicity. J Infect Dis 165(6):1026–1032.

Ferber-Viart C, Morlet T, Maison S et al 1996 Type of initial brainstem auditory evoked potentials (BAEP) impairment and risk factors in premature infants. Brain Dev 18(4):287–293.

Fischel-Ghodsian N, Prezant T R, Bu X et al 1993 Mitochondrial ribosomal RNA gene mutation in a patient with sporadic aminoglycoside ototoxicity. Am J Otolaryngol 14(6):399–403.

Fortnum H M 1992 Hearing impairment after bacterial meningitis: A review. Arch Dis Child 67(9):1128–1133.

Fortnum H M, Summerfield Q, Marshall D H et al 2001 Prevalence of permanent childhood hearing impairment in the United Kingdom and implications for universal neonatal hearing screening: questionnaire based ascertainment study. BMJ 323(7312):536.

Fowler K B, Boppana S B 2006 Congenital cytomegalovirus (CMV) infection and hearing deficit. J Clin Virol 35(2):226–231.

Fowler K B, McCollister F P, Dahle A J et al 1997 Progressive and fluctuating sensorineural hearing loss in children with asymptomatic congenital cytomegalovirus infection. J Pediatr 130(4):624–630.

Freeman S, Geal-Dor M, Sohmer H 1999 Development of inner ear (cochlear and vestibular) function in the fetus-neonate. J Basic Clin Physiol Pharmacol 10(3):173–189.

Glaser B 2003 Pendred syndrome. Paediatr Endocrinology Rev Suppl 2:199–204.

Goudy S, Lott D, Canady J, Smith R J 2006 Conductive hearing loss and otopathology in cleft palate patients. Otolaryngol Head Neck Surg 134(6):946–948.

Guillausseau P J, Massin P, Dubois-LaForgue D et al 2001 Maternally inherited diabetes and deafness: A multi-centre study. Ann Intern Med 134(9):721–728.

Hall J W 3rd 2000 Development of the ear and hearing. J Perinatol 20(8 pt 2):512–520.

Henley C M, Rybak L P 1993 Developmental ototoxicity. [Review] Otolaryngologic Clinics of North America 26(5):857–871.

Huang M Y, Schacht J 1989 Drug-induced ototoxicity. Pathogenesis and prevention. Med Toxicol Adverse Drug Exp 4(6):452–467.

Huizing E H, de Groot J C 1987 Human cochlear pathology in aminoglycoside ototoxicity — a review. Acta Oto Laryngol — Supplement 436:117–125.

Husain K, Whitworth C, Somani S M et al 2005 Partial protection by lipoic acid against carboplatin induced ototoxicity in rats. Biomed Environ Sci 18(3):198–206.

Ishman S L, Friedland D R 2004 Temporal bone fractures: traditional classification and clinical relevance. Laryngoscope 114(10):1734–1741.

Iwasaki S, Yamashita M, Maeda M et al 2007 Audiological outcome of infants with congenital cytomegalovirus infection in a prospective study. Audiol Neurotol 12:31–36.

Jiang Z D, Brosi D M, Wilkinson A R 2001 Hearing impairment in preterm very low birth-weight babies detected at term by brainstem auditory evoked responses. Acta Paediatr 90(12):1411–1415.

Jiang Z D, Zhang Z, Wilkinson A D 2005 Distortion product otoacoustic emissions in term infants after hypoxia–ischaemia. Eur J Pediatr 164(2):84–87.

Jiang-Ze D, Xu-Xiu, Yin-Rong et al 2004 Differential changes in peripheral and central components of the brain stem auditory evoked potentials during the neonatal period in term infants after perinatal hypoxia–ischemia. Ann Otol Rhinol Laryngol 113(7):571–576.

Kadoya R, Ueda K, Miyazaki C et al 1998 Incidence of congenital rubella syndrome and influence of the rubella vaccination program for schoolgirls in Japan, 1981–1989. Am J Epidemiol 148(3):263–268.

Kayan A, Bellman H 1990 Bilateral senosorineural hearing loss due to mumps. Br J Clin Pract 44(12):757–759.

Kaye C I 2006 Newborn screening fact sheets. Paediatrics 118(3):1304–1312.

Kent W D, Tan A K, Clarke M C et al 2002 Excessive noise levels in the neonatal ICU: potential effects on auditory system development. J Otolaryngol 31(6)355–360.

Kountakis S E, Skoulas I, Phillips D et al 2002 Risk factors for hearing loss in neonates: A prospective study. Am J Otolaryngol — Head and Neck Med Surg 23(3):133–137.

Koyama S, Kaga K, Sakata H et al 2005 Pathological findings in the temporal bone of newborn infants with neonatal asphyxia. Acta Otolaryngol 125(10):1028–1032.

Lagasse N, Dhooge I, Govaert P 2000 Congenital CMV-infection and hearing loss. Acta Otorhinolaryngol Belg 54(4):431–436.

Lima G M L, Marba S T M, Santos M F C 2006 Hearing screening in a neonatal intensive care unit. J Pediatr 82(2):110–114.

Luxon L M, Cohen M, Coffey R A et al 2003 Neuro-otological findings in Pendred syndrome. Int J Audiology 42(2):82–88.

McLeod R, Boyer K, Karrison T et al 2006 Outcome of treatment for congenital toxoplasmosis, 1981–2004: the National Collaborative Chicago-Based, Congenital Toxoplasmosis Study. Clin Infect Dis 42(10):1383–1394.

Madden C, Hilbert L, Rutter M et al 2002 Paediatric cochlear implantation in auditory neuropathy. Otol Neurotol 23(2):163–168.

Madden C, Rutter M, Hilbert L et al 2002 Clinical and audiological features in auditory neuropathy. Arch Otolaryngol Head Neck Surg 128(9):1026–1030.

Makishima K, Katz R B, Snow J B Jr. 1976 Hearing loss of a central type secondary to anoxic anoxia. Ann Otol Rhinol Laryngol 85(6 Pt 1):826–832.

Marres H A 2002 Hearing loss in Treacher Collins syndrome. Adv Otorhinolaryngol 61:209–215.

Mazurek B, Winter E, Fuchs J et al 2003 Susceptibility of the hair cells of the newborn rat cochlea to hypoxia and ischemia. Hear Res 182(1–2):2–8.

Min-Xin G 2006 Mitochondrial DNA mutations associated with aminoglycoside ototoxicity. Audiological Medicine 4:170–178.

Misra A, Nolph K D 1998 Renal failure and deafness: branchio-oto-renal syndrome. Am J Kidney Dis 32(2):334–337.

Morzaria S, Westerberg B D, Kozak F K 2004 Systematic review of the etiology of bilateral sensorineural hearing loss in children. Int J Pediatric Otorhinolaryngol 68(9):1193–1198.

Murakami S, Hato N, Horiuchi J et al 1997 Treatment of Ramsay Hunt syndrome with acyclovir-prednisone: Significance of early diagnosis and treatment. Ann Neurol 41(3):353–357.

Newton V E 2002 Clinical features of the Waardenburg syndromes. Adv Otorhinolaryngol 61:201–208.

Neyroud N, Tesson F, Denjoy I et al 1997 A novel mutation in the potassium channel gene *KVLQT1* causes the Jervell and Lange–Nielsen cardioauditory syndrome. Nat Genet 15(2):113–115.

Ohtani F, Furuta Y, Aizawa H et al 2006 Varicella-zoster virus load and cochleovestibular symptoms in Ramsay Hunt syndrome. Ann Otol Rhinol Laryngol 115(3):233–238.

Oysu-Cagatay, Aslan-Ismet, Ulubil-Arif et al 2002 Incidence of cochlear involvement in hyperbilirubinemic deafness. Ann Otol Rhinol Laryngol 111(11):1021–1025.

Pagarkar W, Bitner-Glindzicz M, Knight J et al 2006 Late postnatal onset of hearing loss due to GJB2 mutations. Int J Paed Otolangology 70(6):1119–1124.

Pickering L K 1985 Diagnosis and therapy of patients with congenital and primary syphilis. Pediatr Infect Dis 4(5):602–605.

Prezant T R, Agapian J V, Bohlman M C et al 1993 Mitochondrial ribosomal RNA mutation associated with both antibiotic-induced and non-syndromic deafness. Nat Genet 4(3):289–294.

Rajendrakumar D, Bamiou D E, Sirimanna T 2005 Audiological profile in Apert syndrome. Arch Dis Child 90(6):592–593.

Rao S C, Ahmed M, Hagan R 2006 One dose per day compared to multiple doses per day of gentamicin for treatment of suspected or proven sepsis in neonates. Cochrane Database Syst Rev 25(1):CD005091.

Read A, Newton V E 1997 Waardenburg syndrome. J Med Genetic 34(8):656–665.

Richardson M P, Reid A, Tarlow M J et al 1997 Hearing loss due to bacterial meningitis. Arch Dis Child 76(2):134–138.

Rodriguez, Soriano J 2003 Branchio-oto-renal syndrome. J Nephrol 16(4):603–605.

Rodriguez-Ballesteros M, del Castillo F J, Martin Y et al 2003 Auditory neuropathy in patients carrying mutations in the otoferlin gene (OTOF). Hum Mutat 22(6):451–456.

Sadeghi A M, Eriksson K, Kimberling W J et al 2006 Long-term visual prognosis in Usher syndrome types 1 and 2. Acta Ophthalmol Scand 84(4):537–44.

Samanich J, Lowes C, Burk R et al 2007 Mutations in GJB2, GJB6, and mitochondrial DNA are rare in African American and Caribbean Hispanic individuals with hearing impairment. Am J Med Genet A Mar (electronic publication ahead of print)

Sande M A, Mandell G L 1990 Antimicrobial agents. In: Gilman A G, Rall T W, Nies A S, Taylor (eds) Goodman and Goldman's the pharmacological basis of therapeutics, 8th edn. Pergamon, Elmsford, NY, pp. 1103–1121.

Sharghi S, Haghpanah V, Heshmat R et al 2007 Comparison of MRI findings with traditional criteria in diagnosis of Pendred syndrome. Int J Audiol 46(2):69–74.

Sheahan P, Miller I, Earley M J et al 2004 Middle ear disease in children with congenital velopharyngeal insufficiency. Cleft palate Craniofac J 41(4):364–367.

Shine N P, Coates H 2005 Systemic ototoxicity: a review. East Afr Med J 82(10):536–539.

Sirimanna K S 1993 Detection of carriers in Alport syndrome. MSc Thesis. University of Manchester, UK.

Sirimanna T 2004 Hearing problems in children with craniosynostosis. In: Hayward R, Jones B, Dunaway D, Evans R (eds) The clinical management craniosynostosis. Mac Keith, Cambridge University Press, Cambridge.

Skinner R 2006 Preventing platinum induced ototoxicity in children: Is there a potential role for sodium thiosulphate. Paediatr Blood Cancer 47(2):120–122.

Sohmer H, Geal-Dor M, Weinstein D 1994 Human fetal auditory threshold improvement during maternal oxygen respiration. Hear Res 75(1–2):145–150.

Stewart B J, Prabhu P U 1993 Reported sensorineural deafness after measles, mumps, and rubella immunisation. Arch Dis Child 69(1):153–154.

Tang T P, McPherson B, Yuen K C et al 2004 Auditory neuropathy/auditory dys-synchrony in school children with hearing loss: frequency of occurrence. Int J Pediatr Otorhinolaryngol 68(2):175–183.

Taylor J P, Mecalfe R A, Watson P F et al 2002 Mutations of the *PDS* gene, encoding pendrin, are associated with protein mislocalization and loss of iodide efflux: implications for thyroid dysfunction in Pendred syndrome. J Clin Endocrinol Metab 87(4):1778–1784.

Torres M, Giraldez F 1998 Development of vertebrate ear (Review). Mech Dev 71(1–2):5–21.

Upfold L, Oong-R 2004 Maternal rubella, vaccination, and congenital hearing impairment in Australia. Aust New Zealand J Audiol 26(2):133–138.

Vandersschueren-Lodeweyckx M, Debruyne F, Dooms L et al 1983 Sensorineural hearing loss in sporadic congenital hypothyroidism. Arch Dis Child 58(6):419–422.

Vanniasegaram I, Tungland O P, Bellman S C 1993 A 5 year review of children with deafness in a multiethnic community. J Audiol Med 2:9–19.

Varga R, Kelley P M, Kesats B J et al 2003 Non-syndromic recessive auditory neuropathy is the results of mutations in the otoferlin (*OTOF*) gene. J Med Genet 40(1):45–50.

Vollmer B, Seibold-Weiger K, Schmitz-Salue C et al 2004 Postnatally acquired cytomegalovirus infection via breast milk: Effects on hearing and development in preterm infants. Pediatr Infect Dis J 23(4):322–327.

Wang R, Martínez-Frías M L, Graham Jr J M 2002 Infants of diabetic mothers are at increased risk for the oculo-auriculo-vertebral sequence: A case-based and case-control approach. J Paediatr 41(5):611–617.

Williamson W D, Demmler G J, Percy A K et al 1992 Progressive hearing loss in infants with asymptomatic congenital cytomegalovirus infection. Pediatrics 90(6):862–866.

Wilson M E Jr, Trivedi R H, Biber J M et al 2006 Anterior capsule rupture and subsequent cataract in Alport syndrome. J Am Assoc Paed Ophthal Strabis 10(2):182–183.

Disorders of the spinal cord, cranial and peripheral nerves

Malcolm I. Levene

Key Points

- Facial palsy recovers spontaneously in 90% of cases and surgical exploration is rarely necessary
- Spinal cord injury is rare but must always be considered as a cause of impoverished spontaneous limb movement
- Trauma to the cervical cord as well as focal vascular insults are the commonest cause of acute cord lesions
- Prognosis after brachial plexus injury is generally good. If complete recovery has not occurred by 3–4 months, eventual recovery is very unlikely
- At present, there are no definite indications for surgery in the absence of evidence for direct or indirect root avulsion

---

INTRODUCTION

As a group of disorders, those affecting the spine, cranial and peripheral nerves are not common but are important because of the risk of severe sequelae in terms of permanent neurologic disability. Although trauma is the commonest underlying pathology, it is clear that, in a minority, other poorly understood mechanisms are important in their etiology.

CRANIAL NERVES

The seventh cranial nerve is most commonly recognized to be abnormal in the newborn period because its dysfunction is most obvious in its effect on facial symmetry. Although congenital or acquired abnormalities of other cranial nerves occur, they may not be recognized as such in the neonatal period because loss of function is less obvious or, if present, may be part of a much more severe neurologic disturbance as the result of massive injury such as birth asphyxia. An example of this is bulbar palsy in the presence of a grossly neurologically abnormal infant. Involvement of cranial nerves, other than VII, is rarely described in the literature as a pure entity. Multiple cranial nerve involvement is generally considered in the diagnostic category of the Möbius sequence (see below).

FACIAL PALSY

Facial palsy has been reported to occur with an incidence of 0.23% (McHugh et al 1969), but more recent figures are not available.

Etiology

The etiology of facial palsy can be considered as either developmental or acquired (Table 39.1). It may be difficult to distinguish between these two major categories in the neonatal period, but the developmental problems tend not to improve, unlike traumatic facial palsy (Toelle & Boltshauser 2001). Congenital facial nerve palsy due to a developmental disorder is often associated with other features, including the Möbius sequence (see below) and may be due to dysplasia of central nuclei. Rarely has bilateral facial palsy together with other developmental problems been related to abnormalities occurring very early in pregnancy such as bilateral infarction of the anterior operculum (Gropman et al 1997). Disease in and around the middle ear may cause congenital facial palsy including otitis media (Rizk et al 2005), tuberculosis (Pejham et al 2002) and very rarely middle ear teratoma (Navarro Cunchillos et al 1996). Facial palsy is also reported as part of unilateral CHARGE syndrome (Trip et al 2002) and in association with deletion of chromosome 22q11 (Punal et al 2001).

The role of trauma in facial nerve palsy is controversial; Smith et al (1981) reported trauma to account for 78% of all cases. The extracranial course of the facial nerve is very superficial as it leaves the stylomastoid foramen and is reported to be particularly liable to neurapraxia as a result of pressure either from impaction of the head against the pelvic outlet or as the result of forceps application. Forceps delivery was reported to be associated with facial palsy in 75% of cases (Smith et al 1981). In distinction to this, there was no statistically increased risk of facial nerve palsy in a large study of 53 children with permanent facial palsy when delivery by forceps was compared with the normal population (Laing et al 1996). They suggest that cases of long-standing facial palsy are due to prenatal factors. An alternative cause of acquired 'traumatic' injury is as the result of pressure from the maternal sacrum on the facial nerve. To support this, Hepner (1951) showed that those babies with transient facial palsy who were born without forceps had a left-sided palsy if they were delivered from a left occipitoanterior position and vice versa for those presenting right occipitoanteriorly. Supranuclear facial palsy is also rarely associated with intracranial hemorrhage (Paine 1997).

Clinical features

The lesion is most obvious when the baby cries. The baby's lower lip fails to move downward and outward on the

Table 39.1 Classification of causes of facial nerve palsy

Developmental
Agenesis/dysplasia of the facial nerve nuclei
  Primary
  Associated with other defects
    Möbius sequence
    Hemifacial microsomia
    Oculoauriculovertebral dysplasia
    Cardiofacial syndrome
    Poland syndrome
Degeneration of the facial nerve nuclei
  Ischemia and infarction
  Brainstem hemorrhage
Teratogenesis
  Thalidomide embryopathy
  Viruses (rubella)
Dystrophia myotonica
Acquired
  Birth trauma
    Forceps injury
    Maternal sacral compression
    Intracranial hemorrhage
Otitis media
  Meningitis
  Viral infections
    Congenital varicella
    Infectious mononucleosis
    Poliomyelitis

Source: Adapted from Harris et al (1983) © American Medical Society.

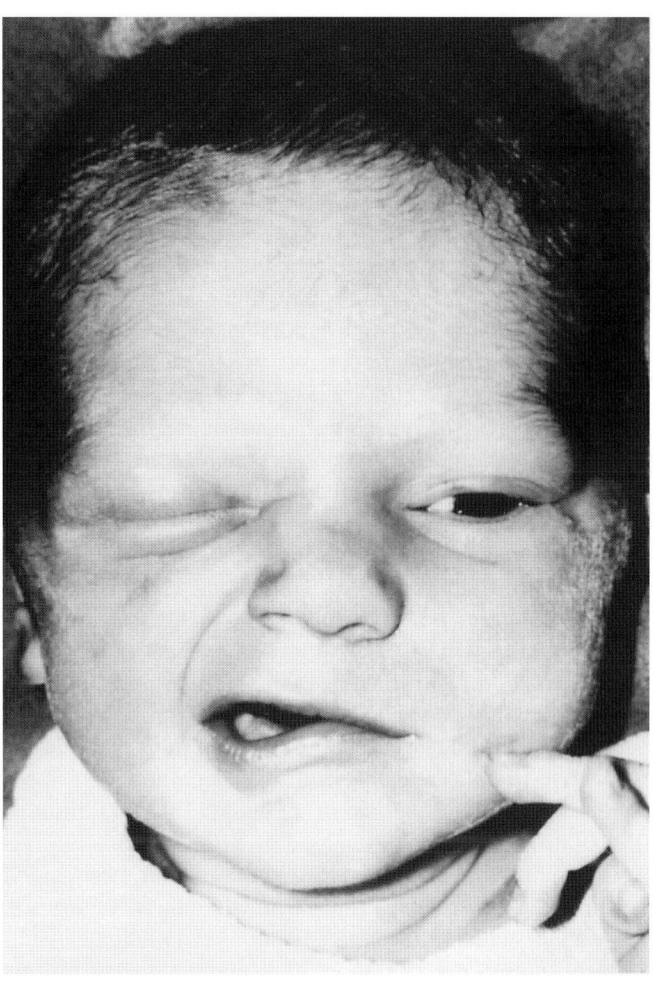

Figure 39.1 Left-sided facial nerve palsy. On crying, the baby is unable to close the left eye or open the mouth normally on the left side.

affected side and there may be an inability to close the eye on the ipsilateral side (Fig. 39.1). This condition must be distinguished from asymmetric crying facies (see below). The child should be carefully examined for evidence of abnormalities in other cranial nerves or other congenital malformations/deformations. Examination of the ear may reveal a hematotympanum that supports a traumatic origin (Harris et al 1983).

Investigations

Neurophysiologic assessment may help in determining whether the lesion is congenital or acquired. Investigations include a maximal stimulation test as well as evoked and standard electromyograms (EMGs). If the nerve is non-stimulatable on maximum impulse and has a silent EMG, then it is very likely that there is a developmental cause (Harris et al 1983). Auditory brainstem responses (see Ch. 12) may be useful as the auditory pathways lie close to the facial nerve nuclei in the brainstem and abnormalities may indicate a more widespread dysplastic process involving these structures.

Management

Ninety percent of facial nerve palsies show signs of spontaneous recovery within 4 weeks of birth (Smith et al 1981). Surgical exploration is therefore unwarranted in the majority of cases. Indications for surgical decompression of the nerve (Bergman et al 1986) include:

1. hematotympanum with a displaced fracture of the petrous bone;
2. no recovery of function either clinically or electrophysiologically at 5 weeks of age.

It is suggested that the initial surgical approach should be directed towards the intraparotid portion of the nerve in the stylomastoid region. Inability to locate the nerve suggests agenesis and further surgery is unwarranted (Narcy et al 1982).

Prognosis

A follow-up study of 12 children with isolated congenital unilateral facial nerve palsy reported a poor spontaneous recovery rate with incomplete functional recovery (Toelle & Bolthauser 2001). The majority of cases were thought to be non-traumatic and in this group no case recovered.

Möbius sequence

The first report of an abnormality of multiple cranial nerves was by Graefe in 1880, and further cases were reported by Möbius in 1888 and 1892 (for a review, see Pitner et al 1965). The sequence is best described by the minimum combination of facial palsy (usually bilateral) together with involvement of at least one cranial nerve controlling eye movement. The abducent nerve (VI) is reported to be affected in 68–85% of cases (Abramson et al 1998, Carr et al 1997) and involvement of other cranial motor nerves (including III, IV, V, IX, X and XII) is more variable. Other associated malformations are seen in about one-third of cases (Smith 1982). These involve the lower limb (talipes equinovarus), upper limbs, facial structures (microtia, micrognathia and microphthalmia) and chest-wall anomalies, as seen in Poland anomaly (Sugarman & Stark 1973). Familial cases have been reported and a variety of gene loci have been identified on chromosome 3 and 10 (Verzijl et al 1999), as well as a 1; 2 reciprocal translocation (Nishikawa et al 1997). It has also been reported to occur as the result of an autosomal dominant gene (Baraitser 1997). In a Swedish study 7/25 cases were associated with autism or an autistic-like condition as the children got older (Stromland et al 2002).

The underlying pathologic abnormality has been much debated and still remains unclear. In the majority of cases, the Möbius sequence is not due to any one pathologic insult, and it is to be expected that multiple etiologies exist for this sequence of abnormalities. Degenerative and dysplastic causes have both been described. Calcification of the brainstem, pons and medulla has been reported at autopsy (Thakkar et al 1977) and on computerized tomography (CT) (Govaert et al 1989), supporting a prenatal ischemic brainstem insult hypothesis. The associated non-cranial abnormalities seen in this condition also support a more systemic circulatory insult. Other studies where there has been careful inspection of the brain, facial nerves and involved muscles have not revealed any evidence of acquired disorders. A peripheral muscular dysplastic disorder with secondary atrophy of brainstem nuclei has been suggested to be one cause (Pitner et al 1965).

Recently, it has been shown that in Brazil, the use of misoprostol as an attempted abortifacient in early pregnancy increased the risk of the baby being born with the Möbius sequence by almost 30-fold (Pastuszak et al 1998). Others have suggested that induction of uterine contractions with drugs such as misoprostol or ergotamine at 6–7 weeks of pregnancy induces this abnormality as the result of vasoconstriction (Graf & Shepard 1997).

Asymmetric crying facies

This condition may be easily confused with facial nerve palsy. The term 'asymmetric crying facies,' which describes the condition well, was coined by Pape and Pickering (1972),

but is also known by the term 'congenital unilateral lower lip palsy' (CULLP) (Kobayashi 1979). Its incidence is estimated at 1 in 160 live births (Sapin et al 2005). It causes a relatively minor cosmetic disorder with a unilateral abnormality of the muscle, which draws down the lower lip. It affects the left side more commonly than the right (Kobayashi 1979, Pape & Pickering 1972). When the child cries, the normal side of the mouth is pulled down and the abnormal side remains horizontal. This is the opposite of facial nerve palsy.

Approximately 40% have other abnormalities, of which minor ear anomalies were the most common; 7% had associated cardiac defects (Kobayashi 1979). Mandibular asymmetry and maxillary-mandibular asynclitism are often present but may be overlooked (Sapin et al 2005). The cause is unknown, but there are reported cases of familial grouping (Perlman & Reisner 1973). The disorder causes no disability and no treatment is necessary. The asymmetry appears to improve with age.

RECURRENT LARYNGEAL NERVE INJURY

The recurrent laryngeal nerve is a branch of the vagus and, on the left side, loops under the aortic arch and behind the ductus arteriosus at its junction with the aorta. It innervates the larynx. Its anatomic proximity to the ductus arteriosus renders it very vulnerable to accidental transection during ductal ligation or coarctation repair. Left laryngeal palsy has been reported to occur in 4% of cases following this operation in children and 8% in infants with a birthweight below 1500 g (Fan et al 1989). A recent study found left vocal cord paralysis in 9% of infants having undergone a Norwood procedure and in 25% of neonates after biventricular repair with aortic arch reconstruction (Skinner et al 2005). A large ductus arteriosus aneurysm has been reported to cause recurrent laryngeal nerve and phrenic nerve palsy, which was reversible after resolution of the aneurysm following surgery (Hornung et al 1999). Persisting symptoms include stridor and hoarseness, and spontaneous recovery of laryngeal nerve paresis is rare.

Bilateral vocal cord palsy

This interesting group of babies presenting in the newborn period with stridor and bilateral vocal cord palsy includes babies with a variety of underlying causes (Table 39.2). The commonest cause was Arnold–Chiari malformation or where no cause was found. Associated neurological abnormalities were noted including generalized hypotonia and developmental delay.

In one study of 22 patients, 68% required tracheostomy and of these, 10 of the 15 could be eventually decannulated. Of those not requiring tracheostomy most spontaneously recovered vocal cord function (Miyamoto et al 2005).

HYPOGLOSSAL NERVE INJURY

This may be associated with the Möbius sequence (see above). Damage to the hypoglossal nerve has rarely been

Table 39.2 Classification of abnormalities of the spinal cord presenting within the neonatal period

Malformations
    Neural tube defects
        Meningocele
        Myelomeningocele
        Spina bifida occulta
        Diastematomyelia
    Segmental spinal dysgenesis
    Caudal regression syndrome
    Split notochord syndrome
    Anterior sacral meningocele
Intraspinal tumor
    Ependymoma
    Teratoma
    Histiocytosis-X
    Neuroblastoma
    Ganglioneuroma
    Hamartoma
    Neurenteric cyst
Trauma
    Cord transection
    Extradural hemorrhage and compression
Vascular injury
Watershed insult
    Focal ischemic damage secondary to trauma
    Emboli

Table 39.3 Causes of bilateral vocal cord palsy

Arnold–Chiari malformation
Idiopathic
Hydrocephalus
Holoprosencephaly
Severe hypoxic–ischemic brain injury
Agenesis of the corpus callosum
Neurofibromatosis
Pena Shokeir II syndrome
Peripheral neurological disease

reported as the result of birth injury (Greenberg et al 1987, Haenggeli & Lacourt 1989). It results from excessive lateral flexion of the neck with torsion affecting the brainstem. Brachial plexus is usually the major clinical feature. Hypoglossal nerve injury causes ipsilateral paralysis of the tongue with immobility and bulging on the affected side. When the tongue is extended, it curves towards the affected side, and this is associated with difficulties in sucking. Swallowing remains normal. Spontaneous recovery is reported in affected cases.

THE SPINAL CORD

The embryologic development of the spinal cord is discussed in detail in Chapter 2, and some inherited disorders of the spinal cord such as spinal muscular atrophy, which may cause confusion with other neuromuscular problems, are discussed in Chapter 40. Abnormalities of the spinal cord may be classified as either malformations or deformations, acquired as the result of an insult occurring after a stage of normal development. Pathology affecting the spinal cord can be classified, as is shown in Table 39.3. By far the most common abnormalities involving the spinal cord involve disorders of the neural tube, and many of these are discussed in detail in Chapter 13. Spinal-cord pathology in the neo-

natal period is usually overt and presents with either major clinical neurologic signs such as paresis, or associated with obvious anatomic maldevelopment. Less obvious neural tube disorders may have a cutaneous marker of spinal abnormality such as spina bifida occulta (p. 224). Other congenital anomalies of the spine or spinal cord rarely present in the neonatal period, and diagnosis may be delayed until growth and neurologic development unmask the functional effects of the abnormality (see below). The most important in this respect are lipomatous infiltration of the cord, tethered cord, diastematomyelia, hemangiolipomata, dermoid cysts and enterogenous cysts. Very rarely, tumors of the cord may cause neurologic problems in the neonate.

DEVELOPMENTAL DISORDERS

CAUDAL REGRESSION SYNDROME (CRS)

This acquired anomaly is due to an insult occurring in the first 6–8 weeks of intrauterine life and usually involves the lower spinal cord. Its incidence is 0.01–0.05 per 1000 births and 16% of cases are seen in association with maternal diabetes (Egelhoff 1999). An inherited form of partial sacral agenesis has been described (Say & Coldwell 1975). CRS may be ischemic in nature, and the timing and nature of the insult may cause associated abnormalities in other organs that develop rapidly at that time. The baby presents with a neurogenic bladder and anal flaccidity, possibly paraplegia depending on the level of cord involvement with arthrogryposis. The lumbar spine is abnormal in about 25% of cases and can be best evaluated by MR imaging. Sirenomelia is considered to be an extreme form of CRS.

Segmental spinal dysgenesis

Segmental spinal dysgenesis (SSD) is a very rare disorder with localized agenesis or dysgenesis of the lumbar or thoracolumbar cord and associated spinal column disruption. This usually includes severe congenital kyphosis or kyphoscoliosis of the thoracolumbar, lumbar, or lumbosacral spine present at birth. Rarely, complete aplasia of the cord below the affected level may be seen. It has been suggested that the caudal regression syndrome is a variant of SSD affecting the lower caudal segments (Tortori-Donati et al 1999).

MR imaging shows a normal upper cord, a markedly abnormal section (thinned or apparently absent) with a bulky, thickened and low-lying lower cord (Tortori-Donati et al 1999). Clinically, the infant shows severe flaccid paralysis below the level of the affected spinal cord with orthopedic abnormalities of the lower limbs.

Surgery is indicated if there is compression of the remaining cord from the abnormally formed bony elements of the spine.

Split notochord syndrome

This rare condition may present either with spina bifida in its posterior-anterior form or with intact skin and underlying posterior structures, but visceral malformations (neurenteric cyst). In this latter case, there is a posterior cyst that can be either mediastinal or abdominal and extends into the spinal canal causing anterior cord compression. It may be associated with diastematomyelia (partial or complete clefting of the spinal cord). Cord compression requires neurosurgical treatment.

Anterior sacral meningocele

In this condition, there is anterior herniation of a dural sac through a bony sacral or coccygeal defect. Presentation may be with neurologic disruption of bladder and/or bowel function or a pelvic mass. The diagnosis is confirmed on MR scanning, which shows a CSF filled pelvic mass in continuity with the distal thecal sac through a narrow neck (Egelhoff 1999). Neurosurgical excision is required.

INTRASPINAL TUMORS (see also p. 865)

Tumors are individually rare, but an important cause of spinal paresis. Those reported to occur in infancy are listed in Table 39.3. The baby may present with swelling over the spine or with more insidious progression of neurologic signs with bladder distension or reduced movement of the lower limbs. Tumors arising from non-spinal origins such as teratoma, neuroblastoma and hamartoma are rarely associated with neurologic complications, and this will only occur if there is infiltration into the spinal canal with cord compression.

TRAUMATIC CORD LESIONS

The incidence of trauma to the cord is unknown, particularly when it is not severe enough to cause persisting neurologic abnormalities. It is certainly less common now than it was before modern intrapartum care became of a consistently high standard in developed countries. Trauma to the spinal cord resulting in permanent disability is now a rare, but devastating, condition.

Etiology

The neonatal spine is particularly vulnerable to stretching, and Towbin (1969) reported that autopsy studies found that the spinal cord can only be stretched by 6 mm before tearing occurs, whereas the vertebral column can be stretched to 5 cm without disruption. This explains why major cord disruption may occur in the absence of bony damage or dislocation. Traction due to excessive neck rotation over 90° from occipito-posterior or occipito-transverse (Menticoglou et al 1995) may damage higher cervical structures and breech delivery with excessive rotation, flexion or hyperextension of the spine may cause cervico-thoracic or thoracolumbar damage.

Bony damage is rare, but has been reported in cases of cord trauma, with fractures of the odontoid peg and dislocation of the atlas vertebra (Schulman et al 1971). Severe overextension of the neck may also cause occipito-osteodiastasis (see p. 415), which has been reported to cause medullary transection and tearing of the tentorium (Pape & Wigglesworth 1979). The asphyxiated infant appears to be particularly prone to cord injury. It is suggested that asphyxia-induced hypotonia predisposes the baby to greater tractional and rotational forces to the unprotected neck (Clancy et al 1989).

Case reports of infants with major cord trauma describe functional damage either in the upper cervical cord (above C4) or lower in the region of the cervico-thoracic or thoracolumbar spine. MacKinnon et al (1993) describe 22 babies who had sustained spinal cord injury at birth from five Canadian centers. Fourteen had upper cervical lesions and all were delivered cephalically after attempted forceps rotation of the head. All the babies with lesions below C4 were born by the breech.

The fetus presenting by the breech with hyperextension of the head (the 'stargazing' or 'flying' fetus) is at particular risk of cord damage after vaginal delivery (Abroms et al 1973, Bhagwanani et al 1973, Maekawa et al 1976). Abroms et al (1973) estimate that 25% of fetuses delivered vaginally in this position will have permanent neurologic deficit, and cesarean section may not protect the fetus fully from permanent spinal cord injury (Maekawa et al 1976). In these cases, the cord lesion is probably of prenatal onset due to vascular compromise (Maekawa et al 1976).

Pathology

Towbin (1969) examined the spinal cord in a large number of neonatal deaths and found that 10% had evidence of trauma to the cord or adjacent structures. Pathology included:

1. meningeal damage, the commonest form of injury, with bleeding into the subarachnoid and epidural spaces;
2. nerve root laceration or avulsion (see brachial plexus injury);
3. cord injury ranging from relatively minor lacerations to complete transection;
4. dislocation or fracture of vertebral bodies.

The pattern of pathologic findings relates to the duration of time from injury to pathologic examinations. Early changes include hemorrhage, which may lead to severe hematomyelia with blood filling the dura at the site of laceration, cord edema and acute neuronal damage. Bleeding and edema may lead to progressive neuronal necrosis due to compression. If death does not occur in the first few days following the injury, then severe cord atrophy develops at the level of the injury, with cystic degeneration, loss of axons, myelin and gliosis. Proliferation of Schwann cells in the remaining cord tissue has been described (Babyn et al 1988). The 'dying back' phenomenon is associated with degeneration of descending corticospinal tracts and ascending spinothalamic tracts above the level of cord transection, which extends up into the pons.

Clinical features

Loss of spontaneous movement of the upper and/or lower limbs may take some days to be clinically apparent, particularly when the infant is ill and consequently, the diagnosis of spinal cord injury is often delayed. Bladder distension is usually present and should alert the clinician to the need for a more careful neurologic inspection. Concurrent asphyxia with severe hypoxic–ischemic encephalopathy is reported in 64% of babies with high cervical lesions (MacKinnon et al 1993), and this may obscure the neurologic signs of associated cord damage.

The infant with an acute cord injury will initially show 'spinal shock' with hypotonia and reduced or absent tendon reflexes. The baby will often not breathe spontaneously for several days, even in the absence of a high cervical cord lesion (MacKinnon et al 1993). Signs of recovery within the first few days of life indicate less severe neurologic damage. Regular reassessment is necessary in the first week of life. Neurologic evaluation of a motor and sensory level should be documented, although this may initially be patchy and asymmetric. Flexion withdrawal of the lower limbs to painful stimuli may represent a spinal reflex and should not be confused with spontaneous recovery. In one study, five of six babies with lower cord lesions breathed spontaneously by 20 days of age (MacKinnon et al 1993), but babies with high cervical lesions will remain dependent on mechanical ventilation indefinitely.

Some infants with early features of lower limb paralysis may show progressive signs of ascending involvement, with paresis of the upper limbs within 24 hours due to hemorrhage or edema of the cord. Similarly, babies who initially breathe spontaneously may show ascending involvement of respiratory muscles with progressive hypoventilation and respiratory arrest. A markedly asymmetric motor level may be seen, which is most likely to be due to a relatively low spinal lesion with unilateral brachial plexus injury.

A sensory level is usually detected on careful clinical examination, but this may not necessarily correlate with the level of motor involvement. An asymmetric sensory level is not uncommon. A neurogenic bladder with distension and urine dribbling from the urethra is usually seen in severe cord trauma together with paralysis of the anal sphincter. Tendon and grasp reflexes are lost, but touch or painful stimuli to the limbs or body may elicit vigorous withdrawal reflexes, which may be confused with spontaneous move-ment. Horner syndrome may be present (see p. 787). Diaphragmatic paralysis may also be present.

Differential diagnosis includes spinal muscular atrophy (see p. 804), HIE (see p. 552), bilateral brachial plexus injury (see p. 785) and respiratory disease.

Investigations

Plain X-ray of the spine should be performed in all suspected cases to assess evidence of bony damage or vertebral instability. Imaging the cord in the acute phase is important to establish the level of injury and the extent of associated hemorrhage and edema. High frequency ultrasound examination of the spinal canal and cord is possible up to the age of 6 months due to poor ossification of the vertebral spines and serial real-time scanning at the cotside appears to be the most sensitive modality in the acute phase of cord injury. Demonstration of acute cord injury, echogenic hematomyelia and hemorrhage around the cord has been reported (Babyn 1988, de Vries et al 1995, Jequier et al 1984, MacKinnon et al 1993, Simon et al 1999). It has been suggested that serial ultrasound scanning is the most accurate imaging technique for diagnostic purposes (MacKinnon et al 1993). In the later stages of recovery when atrophy has developed, ultrasound examination may demonstrate myelomalacia and a decrease in cord diameter. Ultrasound is reported to be poor at differentiating edema from hemorrhage within the cord (Mills et al 2001).

Magnetic resonance is becoming widely used to image the spine but appears to be more sensitive after the acute phase of spinal cord injury for localizing the site and type of damage (Lanska et al 1990, Mills et al 2001). False-negative findings with MR have been reported in the acute stages of cord injury (MacKinnon et al 1993, Simon et al 1999). There is no place for myelography and CT scanning is the least useful of the imaging techniques.

Electrophysiologic assessment may also help confirm the diagnosis and determine the level of cord trauma. Motor and sensory nerve conduction times will be normal for peripheral nerves. Electromyography may reveal changes of acute denervation, which include no spontaneous electrical activity, polyphasic motor unit potentials of small amplitude and short duration, and spontaneously occurring fibrillation potentials. These may be intermixed with larger-amplitude, longer-duration motor unit potentials (Clancy et al 1989). Somatosensory evoked potentials have also been used to confirm the level of the cord injury (Bell & Dykstra 1985).

Prognosis

In general, the prognosis both for survival and functional outcome is very poor (MacKinnon et al 1993, Simon et al 1999) but is dependent on the level of the cord lesion and the rate of clinical recovery over the first few weeks of life. MacKinnon et al (1993) have reported that all infants with an upper cervical lesion had a very poor prognosis. Fifty percent died early, and all but one of the survivors remained partially or wholly dependent on mechanical ventilation. The child who came off the ventilator showed rapid signs of neurologic recovery and was weaned from the ventilator at 19 days. In patients with lesions lower than C4 (MacKinnon et al 1993), all but one showed some spontaneous breathing activity on day 1 (the other commenced breathing on day 8). In fact, only two children in this group survived, both of whom were described as having paraplegia on follow-up and one required mechanical ventilation at night. MacKinnon et al (1993) recommend withdrawal of mechanical ventilation if there has been no spontaneous respiratory activity by 3 weeks after birth. Koch and Eng (1979) reported that in surviving infants, flaccidity in the neonatal period led to spastic paraplegia in the majority of cases. In contrast to this, others have found that neonatal flaccidity and areflexia persisted into infancy and childhood in one-half of survivors (Burcher et al 1979). Imaging may help to distinguish those with more severe cord lesions and the presence of intra-cord hemorrhage is particularly ominous (Mills et al 2001).

Management

Damage to the bony vertebral structures rarely requires surgical stabilization. If a fracture occurs, it is usually through the epiphyseal plate of the vertebral body, and management by positioning in extension is all that is required. Extradural hemorrhage may cause compression or spinal block, but there is little evidence that neurosurgical drainage improves outcome. Management of the nerve injury of the spine is expectant.

VASCULAR ACCIDENTS OF THE CORD

Etiology

It is proposed that some neonates with paraplegia without an obvious traumatic etiology have sustained hypoxic–ischemic injury to the spinal cord (Clancy et al 1989, Singer et al 1991). Ruggieri et al (1999) suggested that in about half of babies with perinatal spinal cord injury the cause was vascular in origin. The anterior horn cells of the spinal cord may be particularly susceptible to hypoxic–ischemic insult, which causes marked transient weakness, flaccidity and areflexia in affected babies. This may be confused with, or be a major part of, signs of severe hypoxic–ischemic encephalopathy (Clancy et al 1989).

The spinal cord has a rich anastomotic blood supply from both extraspinal and intraspinal sources. The extraspinal vessels arise from the aorta or vertebral arteries via the anterior spinal artery (Fig. 39.2) supplying segments C1–T3, the dorsal radicular artery supplying segments T4–T8 and the artery of Adamkiewicz, which is the main branch of the lower anterior spinal artery supplying T9–L1. There is some inconstancy as to the precise levels of origin of these three arteries. There is therefore a potentially vulnerable watershed area between these vascular territories, which may predispose to focal spinal cord infarction. Ebinger et al (2003) reported three cases of infants with myelomalacia and marked thinning of the cord on imaging to be due to ischemic infarction.

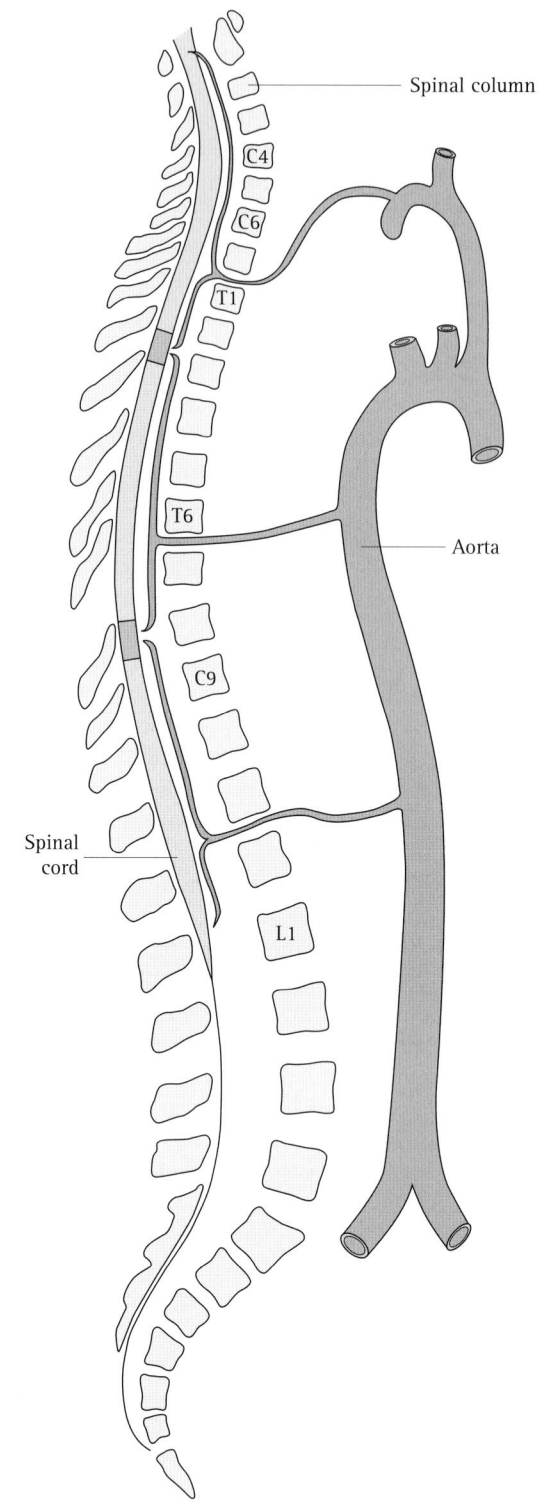

Figure 39.2 Arterial supply of the spinal cord. The shaded areas within the spinal cord represent watershed regions susceptible to potential underperfusion.

Sladky and Rorke (1986) have described two distinct sites for cord damage as the result of vascular injury. The commonest type involved injury to the lumbosacral region. In these cases, there was more severe damage to central, rather than peripheral, regions, suggesting a radial artery watershed distribution. Another study has shown a selective vulnerability of some cellular elements in the lumbar cord but not suggestive of a vascular distribution (DeGirolami & Zivin 1982). Less commonly, Sladky and Rorke (1986) found infarction to be limited to dorsal gray matter in the mid- and upper-thoracic regions, and this may correspond to the thoracic watershed territory.

Jacobs et al (1987) have shown that ligation of the abdominal aorta in an animal model caused complete hind limb paralysis with functional recovery 4 hours after release of the ligature. From 12 to 18 hours following the ischemic insult, a secondary and permanent loss of hind-limb function occurred, and it has been suggested that this is due to a secondary impairment of blood flow to the spinal cord. Infarction of the cord may occur as a result of obstruction to flow through the feeding vessels arising from the aorta by an umbilical artery catheter placed in the aorta.

The spinal cord appears to be a more resistant structure to ischemic insults than the brain and consequently, global ischemia or asphyxia is more likely to damage the brain than the spinal cord alone. Ischemic lesions of the spinal cord alone therefore are most likely to have a more focal etiology such as local impairment of blood flow in the aorta or emboli from an arterial catheter placed in the lower aorta.

Four major etiological factors for ischemic cord lesions have been reported.

1. Acute spinal cord infarction as a complication of generalized hypoxic/ischemic lesions. This has been described as occurring after cardiac arrest or severe asphyxial insults (Schneider et al 1975, Sladky & Rorke 1986). Basal ganglia and brainstem abnormalities occur commonly in association with spinal cord damage (Schneider et al 1975) similar to that which has been described after acute total asphyxial insult (p. 544). This was the most commonly described form of spinal infarction in a group of neonates who came to autopsy examination (Sladky & Rorke 1986).
2. Localized infarction of the spinal cord secondary to a traumatic lesion such as transection or extradural spinal hemorrhage in which regional blood supply is compromised (Sladky & Rorke 1986). Focal infarction has also been reported to occur prenatally (Darwish et al 1981, Farrell & McGillivray 1983, Young et al 1983).
3. Embolic infarction associated with the placement of an umbilical artery catheter in the descending aorta (Aziz & Robertson 1973, Dulac & Aicardi 1975, Krishnamoorthy et al 1976). A catheter tip position between T10 and L2 may predispose to embolic damage to the lower cord through the artery of Adamkiewicz. An alternative mechanism for irreversible spinal injury is catheter-induced, prolonged spinal-artery spasm. Cardiac surgery requiring prolonged clamping of the descending aorta has been reported to cause spinal cord injury in infants but rarely in the neonate.

4. Extravasation of parenteral nutrition fluid into the spinal canal causing cord compression and paresis has been reported (Knobel et al 2001, Lavandosky et al 1996). Placement of a Silastic intravenous feeding line in the inferior vena cava may cause extravasation of fluid into the epidural venous plexus via the ascending lumbar vein and then into the spinal canal. Careful checking of the position of such lines should be made radiographically prior to the commencement of parenteral nutrition.

BRACHIAL PLEXUS PALSY

The brachial plexus is a web of nerves emerging from the lower cervical and upper thoracic roots. These may be damaged by stretching during delivery, but there is increasing evidence that, in some, the injury to the brachial plexus may predate the birth process. Although the majority of babies with brachial plexus injury recover spontaneously, surgical intervention may improve the functional outcome of some of the more severe cases.

CLASSIFICATION

The brachial plexus comprises the merging and subsequent demerging of spinal nerves from C4–C8 and T1. Combinations of these spinal nerves unite to form the major nerves of the upper limb (Fig. 39.3). Tearing or damage to these spinal nerves will cause functional disability to the arm

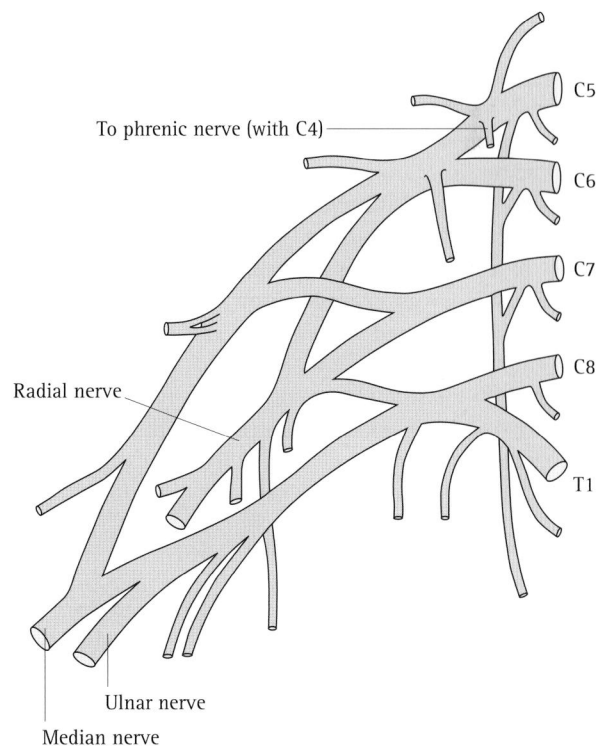

Figure 39.3 The components of the brachial plexus showing the formation of the major nerves of the arm.

depending on the level at which the damage has occurred. Clinically, two main types of brachial plexus lesions are recognized:

1. upper (C5–7) and described as Erb palsy;
2. upper and lower (C5–T1) and described as Klumpke palsy.

Incidence

The incidence of congenital brachial palsy (flaccid paralysis of one arm) in the United Kingdom and Republic of Ireland in 1998–1999 was 0.42 per 1000 live births (Evans-Jones et al 2003). The incidence of brachial plexus injury in 11 centers was reviewed by Gherman et al (1998). He describes an overall incidence from these studies of 1.8 per 1000 live-born births. There have been two large geographically based cohorts from the state of California (1994–1995) and the whole of Sweden (1980–1989) (Bager 1997). The reported incidence from these studies was 1.5 and 1.6 per 1000, respectively.

Prospectively collected Swedish data show that there has been a statistically significant increase in the incidence of this condition in a 10-year period from 1980 (1.3/1000) to 1994 (2.2/1000) (Bager 1997). Data from the USA (Graham et al 1997) show no significant increase over a 30-year period in one institution when the period 1954–1959 (1.2/1000) was compared with 1987–1991 (1.0/1000), although there had been a fourfold increase in cesarean section rates over this same period of time.

Etiology

In a large national study 64% of cases of congenital brachial plexus were associated with shoulder dystocia (Evans-Jones et al 2003) and although shoulder dystocia and macrosomia are the two most commonly recognized risk factors for this condition, there are increasing numbers of reports of cases due to factors other than severe neck traction at delivery. In a large British study only 9% of infants had no identifiable unusual traction forces during the course of delivery (Evans-Jones et al 2003). The classic insult reported to cause brachial plexus palsy is excessive downward traction on the neck during attempted delivery of the anterior shoulder during vaginal delivery. Fetal macrosomia is an important risk factor for shoulder dystocia, which is the underlying cause for excessive neck traction resulting in damage to the anterior plexus. Gherman et al (1998) have estimated from their data that 18% of patients with shoulder dystocia requiring the McRoberts maneuver to facilitate delivery resulted in brachial plexus injury. In Sweden, half the infants with brachial plexus lesions were large for gestational age, and for those of birthweight >4500 g, the incidence was 45 times higher than for those with birthweight <3500 g (Bager 1997).

A second group at risk of obstetric trauma at delivery is those born by the breech where the posterior arm is used to rotate the baby. Geutjens et al (1996) reviewed 36 babies with brachial plexus injury who had been born by the breech. They had a different pattern of injury, with 81% having avulsion of the upper cervical roots with poor prognosis for complete recovery.

It is now well recognized that brachial plexus injury occurs in the absence of shoulder dystocia and is estimated to not be associated with shoulder dystocia in 49 (15%) of 329 cases of brachial plexus palsy at Johns Hopkins 1993–2004 (Gurewitsch et al 2006). In other much smaller studies, almost 50% of cases occur without a history of difficult delivery (Dunn & Engle 1985, Gherman et al 1998, Graham et al 1997, Jennett et al 1992, Koenigsberger 1980, Ouzounian et al 1997 for a review), and these babies have a significantly lower birthweight than the dystocic group and a worse prognosis for full recovery. Alexander et al (2006) reported brachial plexus palsy in 0.02% of cesarean section births. In one report, fracture of the clavicle was only seen with Erb palsy occurring in the absence of shoulder dystocia (Gherman et al 1998). Interestingly, the posterior shoulder was more likely to be affected when the baby was born without shoulder dystocia compared with the anterior shoulder in dystocic deliveries (Gherman et al 1998). It is suggested that in these cases of brachial plexus injury without shoulder dystocia, there is an intrapartum etiology, possibly pressure of the shoulder against the sacral promontory, or symphysis pubis. Cases of Erb palsy with transient facial palsy have been cited to add weight to this hypothesis (Gherman et al 1998). A study of infants with 'obstetrical brachial palsy' found that 4.4% of all babies with this condition also had ipsilateral deformations of chest, arm or leg. These babies also had excessive traction forces at delivery and the authors hypothesize that these babies were predisposed to brachial plexus injury as a result of earlier compressive forces (Alfonso et al 2006). A case has been reported of proven prenatal onset of brachial plexus injury associated with a bicornuate uterus (Dunn & Engle 1985).

Right-sided palsy occurs more commonly than lesions on the left (Gilbert et al 1991), and this appears to be due to the more common cephalic left occipital anterior presentation, which predisposes the right shoulder to a higher risk of impaction. Bilateral brachial plexus palsy is more commonly seen following difficult breech extraction.

Rarely families have been reported with brachial plexus palsy in multiply affected children (Al-Qattan & al-Kharfy 1996, Brett 1991, Gordon et al 1973). Other reported causes include neonatal hemangiomatosis (Lucas et al 1995) and osteomyelitis with late-onset group-B streptococcal infection (Estienne et al 2005, Sadleir & Connolly 1998).

Pathology

The injury involves a number of the brachial plexus roots comprising C_5–T_1. The roots may be stretched, totally ruptured, or avulsed from the spinal cord. Avulsion rarely occurs in the region of C_5 and C_6 and is much more common at the level of C_8 and T_1. Lesions confined to the lower roots are rare. Traumatic meningoceles may develop at the site of root avulsion.

Clinical assessment

The clinical diagnosis of brachial plexus injury is made by observing loss of active movement of the upper limb together with a full range of passive movements. Attention must be given to the diagnosis of Horner syndrome (see below), phrenic nerve involvement (chest X-ray may show an elevated diaphragm) and associated fracture of the ipsilateral humerus or clavicle. A full neurologic examination should evaluate spontaneous movement of all limbs to exclude a cerebral (hemiplegia) or spinal (tetraplegia) cause for loss of spontaneous movement.

Erb palsy

The arm is adducted and internally rotated at the shoulder and the elbow is extended with pronation of the forearm. The wrist and fingers are flexed. This produces the classic 'waiter's tip' position (Fig. 39.4). Involvement of C_7 causes the elbow to be slightly flexed. Tendon reflexes (biceps, triceps, brachioradialis) are usually absent or markedly reduced in the affected limbs.

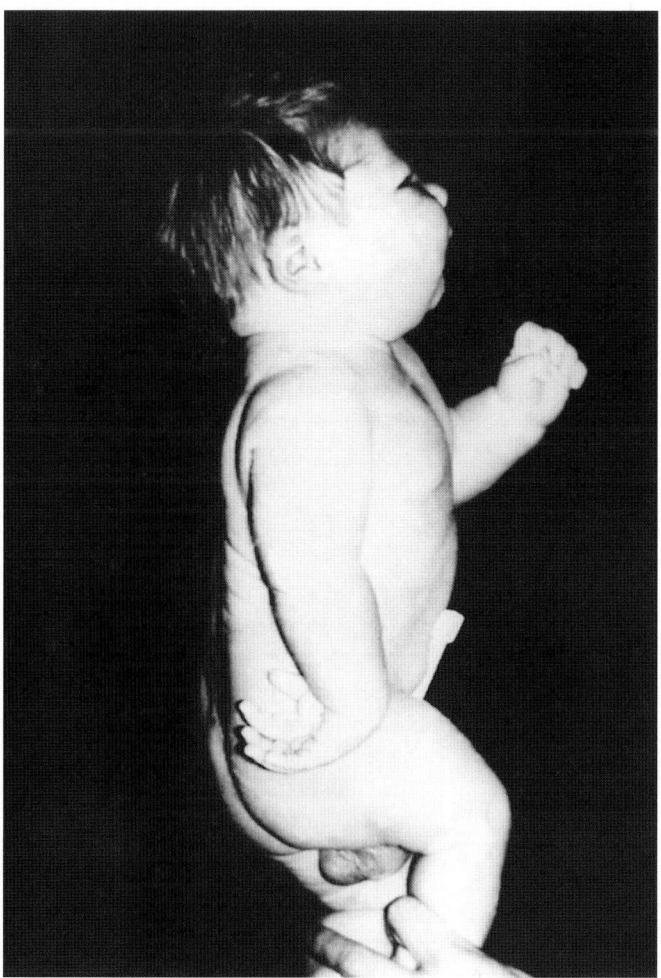

Figure 39.4 Erb palsy. The infant's right arm is adducted and internally rotated with the elbow extended and pronated. The wrist and fingers are flexed.

Klumpke palsy

There is damage to all nerve roots and the arm is flail with a claw hand. There is often vasomotor disturbance with mottling of the arm. Diaphragmatic palsy may occur and a Horner syndrome (see below) may be a variable finding. Although the majority of cases of Klumpke palsy are apparent immediately after birth, Rossi et al (1982) reported that five of 36 cases were not diagnosed until some weeks after birth. It is not clear whether these children were entirely asymptomatic prior to diagnosis.

If improvement occurs, it starts distally, and a total paralysis may regress to involve only the upper roots over a number of weeks. In patients who improve to a complete recovery, the biceps and deltoid muscle are the first to show contraction, and this has been found to occur by 1 month with normal contractions by 2 months (Gilbert et al 1991). Incomplete, but adequate, recovery of the shoulder musculature was seen if the biceps and deltoid muscles started to show spontaneous contractions by 3 months. If there was no recovery in biceps or triceps by 3 months, then the prognosis for adequate recovery was poor.

Horner syndrome

This is due to a lesion of the cervical sympathetic nerve fibers. Preganglionic fibers emerge from the spinal cord in the upper thoracic roots and travel superiorly in the paravertebral sympathetic chain to the superior cervical ganglion. This long course makes them particularly vulnerable to traumatic forces similar to those that produce brachial plexus injury. Rarely, congenital neuroblastoma of the neck can cause Horner syndrome.

Horner syndrome involves abnormalities in motor and sweating function over the face. The most obvious features are ptosis due to weakness of the levator palpebrae muscles of the eye, pupillary constriction and absence of sweating over the affected side of the face (Fig. 39.5). If the lesion occurs as the result of a prenatal lesion or birth insult, then

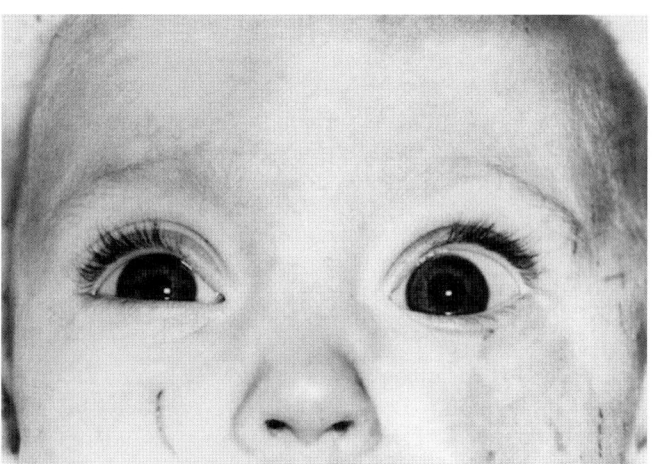

Figure 39.5 Horner syndrome. Note the ptosis and pupillary constriction on the affected right side.

enophthalmos and heterochromia may result due to lack of sympathetic innervation of the pupil, which affects pigmentation.

Investigations

EMG and nerve-conduction studies may be useful in determining the timing of the brachial plexus injury (see below) and for determining the need for and timing of surgery but are unlikely to be of clinical value in the first few weeks of the injury.

Imaging with MR or intrathecally enhanced CT myelography has been described (Medlock & Hanigan 1997), but there are very few indications for this in the majority of cases. MRI has been shown to be useful in delineation of nerve-root avulsion with development of pseudomeningocele (Popovich et al 1989).

Prognosis

The prognosis of brachial plexus injury is generally good and the following general points can be made with regard to the eventual outcome of brachial plexus lesion:

1. If complete recovery has not occurred by 3–4 months, eventual full recovery is very unlikely.
2. Complete recovery is much more likely in lesions involving C_5 and C_6.
3. Full recovery in lesions involving the lower roots is unlikely.

In a large British study, 52% of babies with brachial plexus palsy and a flaccid arm had a full recovery and only 2% had no recovery (Evans-Jones et al 2003). Prognosis for recovery is better in babies without shoulder dystocia. Two studies from Sweden have carefully evaluated the neurologic and functional outcome in groups of children with perinatal brachial plexus injury. Bager (1997) reported 41 children born in 1980–1989. Forty-nine percent had no long-term impairment and 22% were judged to have severe impairment. Sundholm et al (1998) reviewed the progress of 105 children examined at 5 years of age. In this study, 34% were considered to show no residual symptoms and 23% had severe impairment involving both arm and hand function. A recent meta-analysis of outcome data suggests that methodological problems with follow-up studies may overestimate the reported good prognosis (Pondaag et al 2004).

Sundholm et al (1998) describe the extensive variation in disability despite apparently similar neuroanatomic lesions. Hand function was remarkably good, even in children with residual weakness around the shoulder, although approximately half of these children were shown to have some reduction in hand-grip strength on formal testing with a vigorimeter (Bager 1997, Sundholm et al 1998). Sensation was preserved in almost all the children. In one study of overall functional ability, children were generally not seriously limited in their day-to-day activities (Sundholm et al 1998), but in another study, Bager (1997) reported that 22% had a severe functional impairment. Shoulder weakness was associated with difficulties in inserting the arm into a sleeve

and reaching the handle-bars of a bike. Reduced grip strength made activities requiring both hands such as doing up buttons, zips and putting on gloves difficult. A longer-term follow-up study showed that after 5 years of age shoulder and hand function continued to show slight improvement, but elbow function showed significant deterioration (Strombeck et al 2007).

Surprisingly, almost all reports on children with less than optimal recovery from perinatal brachial plexus injury suggest that additional disability due to cerebral palsy or mental retardation is very uncommon (Bager 1997, Gordon et al 1973, Sjoberg et al 1988).

It has been suggested that phrenic nerve palsy in association with Erb palsy is a marker of adverse outcome, but a recent report (Al-Qattan et al 1998) has shown that diaphragmatic palsy poorly predicts adverse outcome in motor power of the affected limb with a sensitivity of only 2% and a positive predictive value of 13%.

Management

The initial management is expectant as spontaneous recovery almost always occurs to some extent. Physiotherapy is important to prevent contractures, particularly of the shoulder. Splinting of the affected arm is not recommended.

Recently, the role of microsurgical reconstruction of the brachial plexus has been reassessed. The role of surgery has been well reviewed by Kay (1998) and remains controversial. To date, no randomized controlled trials have been undertaken. In general, there is reasonable consensus that surgery for the majority of lesions should not be undertaken prior to 3–4 months from birth as significant spontaneous recovery is likely to occur during this time. Those infants with signs of a lower root injury (C5–T1 with Horner syndrome) may benefit from surgery at about 2 months of age. Studies from Sweden do not report that nerve reconstruction surgery improves outcome compared with non-operated children (Strombeck et al 2000, 2007). Kay (1998) concludes that 'the present justification for surgery is based on the comparison of surgical outcomes with studies of the natural history and at present there are no incontrovertible indicators for surgery in the absence of direct or indirect evidence of root avulsion'.

PERIPHERAL NERVE PALSIES

Sporadic injuries to peripheral nerves usually arise as the result of trauma, which is often avoidable. Peripheral nerve injury may occur as the result of prenatal compression of which amniotic bands are most commonly reported. Rarely, fetal embolic phenomenon may cause extensive tissue necrosis (aplasia cutis congenita) with the involvement of peripheral nerves. In general, the earlier in pregnancy the insult occurred, the poorer the prognosis.

INFANT BOTULISM (see also p. 674)

This condition is due to swallowed spores of botulin toxin producing clostridia which colonize the bowel. Most cases are due to botulinum toxin types A and B although F has also been rarely reported to cause paralysis. Recently *C. baratii* and *C. butyricum* have also been recognized to cause toxin release with similar clinical effects (Fox et al 2005). The toxin is absorbed through the gut mucosa and binds irreversibly with cholinergic synapses, causing peripheral neuromuscular paralysis. Recovery requires regeneration of new motor end plates in the nerve endings.

Infant botulism was first reported in 1976 and, since then, over 900 cases have been described in the literature (see Cochrane & Appleton 1995 for a review). The vast majority of these are from the USA, where the spores may be more endemic in the soil. The major etiological factors are breast feeding (almost universal), and consumption of honey and corn syrup contaminated with botulinum spores. The observation that breast feeding is highly associated with the condition is interesting. This may be because breast milk actually confers some protection on the baby, thereby delaying the speed of onset and progression of the disease so that the child is recognized to be unwell and admitted to hospital. Sudden infant death syndrome due to infant botulinum toxin is well described in non-breastfed infants.

Clinical features

The presenting features are usually insidious and remarkably constant (Cochrane & Appleton 1995). These include weakness (90%), poor feeding (88%) and constipation (75%). On physical examination, the baby is found to be hypotonic, often with a bulbar palsy, decreased gag reflex and dilated, poorly constricting pupils. The condition may progress to respiratory failure requiring mechanical ventilation. Autonomic dysfunction may be present with urinary retention, labile blood pressure and flushing.

The diagnosis depends on demonstrating *C. botulinum* in the stool and abnormal electrodiagnostic tests. Many of the children are severely constipated due to a loss of bowel motility and rectal washout may be required to obtain a stool specimen for bacteriology. Electrodiagnostic tests include repetitive nerve stimulation and electromyography and may show presynaptic dysfunction. Graf et al (1992) suggest that these tests may remain negative in affected children, but this is not the experience of others in a review of 57 cases from the Children's Hospital of Philadelphia (Schreiner et al 1991).

The differential diagnosis includes sepsis, dehydration, Werdnig–Hoffman disease (p. 804), Guillain–Barré syndrome, myasthenia gravis, metabolic disorders, meningoencephalitis, myelitis and poliomyelitis. Infant botulism must be considered in young infants presenting with catastrophic collapse (Mitchell & Tseng-Ong 2005).

Management

The management of infant botulism has been vastly improved with the recent introduction of human botulism immune globulin (BIG-IV) which neutralizes botulinum toxin. A randomized double-blind controlled trial showed that BIG-IV given within 3 days of admission significantly reduced the mean length of mechanical ventilation by 2.6 weeks,

the mean duration of intensive care by 3.2 weeks and the mean hospital stay from 5.7 weeks to 2.6 weeks when compared with controls (Arnon et al 2006). Severe cases require mechanical ventilation and this may need to be prolonged. Oral feeding may not be possible for many weeks. Antibiotics do not hasten the resolution of the condition. With careful supportive management, the prognosis is excellent.

RADIAL NERVE PALSY

Radial nerve palsy is rare and is usually associated with prolonged labor or complicated delivery (for a review, see Ross et al 1983). The infants present with isolated flaccid paralysis of wrist and finger extensor muscles, and this may be easily confused with brachial plexus injury. It is often not present in the first few days of life and develops following local trauma. It is associated with localized subcutaneous fat necrosis overlying the course of the radial nerve proximal to the radial epicondyle. Radial nerve palsy has also been caused by constriction of the upper arm with damage to the nerve as it winds around the humerus. This has been reported to be due to intermittent blood pressure monitoring by a tight cuff (Tollner et al 1980) and tight splinting of the arm to maintain an intravenous cannula in situ (Goel et al 1989). Swelling of the shoulder due to bacterial sepsis may cause radial nerve palsy with recovery after aspiration of pus (Lejman et al 1995). The prognosis for most causes is good and spontaneous recovery occurs in the majority of cases.

MEDIAN NERVE PALSY

Damage to the median nerve has been described as the result of repeated needle sampling of the brachial artery in the antecubital fossa (Pape et al 1978). They reviewed 139 infants with a birth weight of 1500 g and below and found that 13% showed persistent median nerve damage. Anatomic dissection of the antecubital fossa showed varying degrees of perineural sheath hemorrhage and Wallerian degeneration of the median nerve. The affected infants were found to have mild to moderate impairment of pincer grasp at 18 months. There was also a reduction in flexion of the lateral two or three fingers when the hand was held in the 'position of rest'. Spontaneous recovery occurs in some cases, although a persisting disability at 3 years has been reported (Pape et al 1978).

SCIATIC NERVE PALSY

The sciatic nerve is most commonly damaged either by intragluteal injection or as a result of an errantly placed umbilical artery catheter, although in one study of 21 cases no apparent cause was found in the majority (Ramos-Fernandez et al 1998). The common peroneal division of the sciatic nerve is most frequently involved. Palsy rarely arises as a result of direct trauma from the needle to the nerve but more commonly as the result of inflammation associated with the injected substance (Gilles & Matson 1970). Others have suggested that sciatic nerve damage occurs through thrombosis of the inferior gluteal artery, which supplies the nerve following injection of a hypertonic solution into the buttock. These lesions are entirely avoidable by giving intramuscular injections into the anterior thigh.

Misplacement of an aortic catheter into the internal iliac artery may cause ischemic infarction of the structures supplied by this artery, including the sciatic nerve (Cumming & Burchfield 1994). The inferior gluteal artery has also been reported to have been thrombosed following injection of a hypertonic solution (50% glucose) into the umbilical artery. This caused extensive deep and superficial damage to the buttock as well as severe sciatic nerve involvement secondary to the thrombosis (San Agustin et al 1962).

Prognosis is uncertain. In one study full recovery was not seen in any of the 13 patients with peroneal nerve (a branch of the sciatic nerve) palsy as a result of drug injection into the umbilical vessel (de Sanctis et al 1995). In contrast Ramos-Fernandez et al (1998) reviewed 21 cases of neonatal sciatic nerve palsy and in 76% of cases, there was spontaneous recovery with independent ambulation by 14 months of age. They suggested that the outcome is better after umbilical artery cannulation than for drug-injection-induced inflammation.

REFERENCES

Abramson D L, Cohen M M, Mulliken J B 1998 Mobius syndrome: classification and grading system. Plastic Reconstruct Surg 102:961–967.

Abroms I F, Bresnan M J, Zuckerman J E et al 1973 Cervical cord injuries secondary to hyperextension of the head in breech presentations. Obstet Gynecol 41:369–378.

Alexander J M, Leveno K J, Hauth J et al 2006 Fetal injury associated with caesarean delivery. Obstet Gynecol 108(4):885–890.

Alfonso I, Diaz-Arca G, Alfonso D T et al 2006 Fetal deformations: a risk factor for obstetrical brachial plexus palsy? Pediatr Neurol 35(4):246–249.

Al-Qattan M M, al-Kharfy T M 1996 Obstetric brachial plexus injury in subsequent deliveries. Ann Plastic Surg 37:545–548.

Al-Qattan M M, Clarke H M, Curtis C G 1998 The prognostic value of concurrent phrenic nerve palsy in newborn children with Erb's palsy. J Hand Surg (Br Eur Vol) 23B:225.

Arnon S S, Schechter R, Maslanka S E et al 2006 Human botulism immune globulin for the treatment of infant botulism. N Eng J Med 354(5):462–471.

Aziz E M, Robertson A F 1973 Paraplegia: A complication of umbilical artery catheterization. J Pediatr 82:1051–1052.

Babyn P S, Chuang S H, Daneman A et al 1988 Sonographic evaluation of spinal cord birth trauma with pathologic correlation. Am J Roentgenol 151:763–766.

Bager B 1997 Perinatally acquired brachial plexus palsy — a persisting challenge. Acta Paediatr 86:1214–1219.

Baraitser M, Stewart F, Winter R M et al 1997 A syndrome of brachyphalangy, polydactyly and absent tibiae. Clin Dysmorphol 6:111–121.

Bell H J, Dykstra D D (1985 Somatosensory evoked potentials as an adjunct to diagnosis of neonatal spinal cord injury. J Pediatr 106:298–301.

Bergman I, May M, Wessel H B et al 1986 Management of facial palsy caused by birth trauma. Laryngoscope 96:381–384.

Bhagwanani S G, Price H V, Laurence K M et al 1973 Risks and prevention of cervical cord injury in the management of breech presentation with hyperextension of the fetal head. Am J Obstet Gynecol 115:1159–1162.

Brett E M (ed.) 1991 Paediatric Neurology, 2nd edn. Churchill Livingstone, Edinburgh.

Burcher H U, Bolthauser E, Friderich J et al 1979 Birth injury to the spinal cord. Helv Paediatr Acta 34:517–527.

Carr M M, Ross D A, Zuker R M 1997 Cranial nerve defects in congenital facial palsy. J Otolaryngol 26:80–87.

Clancy R R, Sladky J T, Rorke L B 1989 Hypoxic-ischemic spinal cord injury following perinatal asphyxia. Ann Neurol 25:185–189.

Cochrane D P, Appleton R E 1995 Infant botulism — is it that rare? Dev Med Child Neurol 37:274–278.

Cumming W A, Burchfield D J 1994 Accidental catheterization of internal iliac artery branches: a serious complication of umbilical artery catheterization. J Perinatol 14:304–309.

Darwish H, Sarnat H, Archer C et al 1981 Congenital cervical spinal atrophy. Muscle Nerve 4:106–110.

De Sanctis N, Cardillo G, Nunziata Rega A 1995 Gluteoperineal gangrene and sciatic nerve palsy after umbilical vessel injection. Clin Orthopaed Relat Res 316:180–184.

De Vries E, Robben S G, van den Anker J N 1995 Radiologic imaging of severe cervical spinal cord birth trauma. Eur J Pediatr 154:230–232.

DeGirolami U, Zivin J A 1982 Neuropathology of experimental spinal cord ischemia in the rabbit. J Neuropathol Exp Neurol 41:129–149.

Dulac O, Aicardi J 1975 Paraplegia complicating umbilical artery catheterization. Archives Francaises de Pediatrie 32:659–664.

Dunn D W, Engle W A 1985 Brachial plexus palsy: intrauterine onset. Pediatr Neurol 1:367–369.

Ebinger F, Boor R, Bruhl K et al 2003 Cervical spinal cord atrophy in the atraumatically born neonate: one form of prenatal or perinatal ischaemic insult? Neuropediatr 34:45–51.

Egelhoff J C 1999 MR imaging of congenital anomalies of the pediatric spine. MRI Clin N Am 7:459–479.

Estienne M, Scaioli V, Zibordi F et al 2005 Enigmatic osteomyelitis and bilateral upper limb palsy in a neonate. Ped Neurol 32(1):56–59.

Evans-Jones G, Kay S P J, Weindling A M et al 2003 Congenital brachial palsy: incidence, causes, and outcome in the United Kingdom and Republic of Ireland. Arch Dis Child Fetal Neonatal Ed 88: F185–F189.

Fan L L, Campbell D N, Clarke D R et al 1989 Paralyzed left vocal cord associated with ligation of patent ductus arteriosus. J Thorac Cardiovasc Surg 98:611–613.

Farrell K, McGillivray B C 1983 Arthrogryposis following maternal hypotension. Dev Med Child Neurol 25:648–650.

Fox C K, Keet C A, Strober J B 2005 Recent advances in infant botulism. Pediatr Neurol 32(3):149–154.

Geutjens G, Gilbert A, Helsen K 1996 Obstetric brachial plexus palsy associated with breech delivery. A different pattern of injury. J Bone Joint Surg (Br Vol) 78:303–306.

Gherman R B, Ouzounian J G, Miller D A et al 1998 Spontaneous vaginal delivery: a risk factor for Erb's palsy? Am J Obstet Gynaecol 178:423–427.

Gilbert A, Brockman R, Carlioz H 1991 Surgical treatment of brachial plexus birth palsy. Clin Orthopaed Relat Res 264:39–47.

Gilles F H, Matson D D 1970 Sciatic nerve injury following misplaced gluteal injection. J Pediatr 76:247–254.

Goel S P, Agarwal R P, Garg B K et al 1989 Nerve injuries in neonates. J Ind Med Assoc 87:132–134.

Gordon M, Rich H, Deutschberger J et al 1973 The immediate and long-term outcome of obstetric birth trauma. I. Brachial plexus paralysis. Am J Obstet Gynecol 117:51–56.

Govaert P, Vanhaesebrouck P, De Praeter C et al 1989 Moebius sequence and prenatal brainstem ischemia. Pediatrics 84:570–573.

Graf W D, Hays R M, Astley S J et al 1992 Electrodiagnosis reliability in the diagnosis of infant botulism. J Pediatr 120:747–749.

Graf W D, Shepard T H 1997 Uterine contraction in the development of Mobius syndrome. J Child Neurol 12:225–227.

Graham E M, Forouzan I, Morgan M A 1997 A retrospective analysis of Erb's palsy cases and their relation to birth. J Maternal-Fetal Med 6:1–5.

Greenberg S J, Kandt R S, D'Souza B J 1987 Birth injury-induced glossolaryngeal paresis. Neurology 37:533–535.

Gropman A L, Barkovich A J, Vezina L G et al 1997 Pediatric congenital bilateral perisylvian syndrome: clinical and MRI features in 12 patients. NeuroPediatrics 28:198–203.

Gurewitsch E D, Johnson E, Hamzehzadeh S et al 2006 Risk factors for brachial plexus injury with and without shoulder dystocia. Am J Obstet Gynecol 194(2):486–492.

Haenggeli C A, Lacourt G 1989 Brachial plexus injury and hypoglossal paralysis. Pediatr Neurol 5:197–198.

Harris J P, Davidson T M, May M et al 1983 Evaluation and treatment of congenital facial paralysis. Arch Otolaryngol 109:145–151.

Hepner W R 1951 Some observations on facial paresis in the newborn infant. Etiology and incidence. Pediatrics 8:494–497.

Hornung T S, Nicholson I A, Nunn G A et al 1999 Neonatal ductus arteriosus aneurysm causing nerve palsies and airway compression: surgical treatment by decompression without excision. Pediatr Cardiol 20:158–160.

Jacobs T P, Shohami E, Baze W et al 1987 Deteriorating stroke model: histopathology, edema, and eicosanoid changes following spinal cord ischemia in rabbits. Stroke 18:741–750.

Jennett R J, Tarby T J, Kreinick C J 1992 Brachial plexus palsy: an old problem revisited. Am J Obstet Gynecol 166:1673–1677.

Jequier S, Cramer B, O'Gorman A M 1984 Ultrasound of the spinal cord in neonates and infants. Annales de Radiologie 28:225–231.

Kay S P J 1998 Obstetrical brachial palsy. Br J Plastic Surg 51:43–50.

Knobel R B, Meetze W, Cummings J 2001 Case Report: Total parenteral nutrition extravasation associated with spinal cord compression and necrosis. J Perinatol 21:68–71.

Kobayashi T 1979 Congenital unilateral lower lip palsy. Acta Otolaryngol 88:303–309.

Koch B M, Eng G M 1979 Neonatal spinal cord injury. Arch Phys Med Rehab 60:378–381.

Koenigsberger M R 1980 Brachial plexus palsy at birth: intrauterine or due to delivery trauma? Ann Neurol 8:228.

Krishnamoorthy K S, Fernandez R J, Todres I D et al 1976 Paraplegia associated with umbilical artery catheterization in the newborn. Pediatrics 58:443–445.

Laing J H E, Harrison D H, Jones B M et al 1996 Is permanent congenital facial palsy caused by birth trauma? Arch Dis Childhood 74:56–58.

Lanska M J, Roessmann U, Wiznitzer M 1990 Magnetic resonance imaging in cervical cord birth injury. Pediatrics 85:760–764.

Lavandosky G, Gomez R, Montes J 1996 Potentially lethal misplacement of femoral central venous catheters. Crit Care Med 24, 893–896.

Lejman T, Strong M, Michno P 1995 Radial-nerve palsy associated with septic shoulder in neonates. J Pediatr Orthop 15:169–171.

Lucas J W, Holden K R, Purohit D M et al 1995 Neonatal hemangiomatosis associated with brachial polexus palsy. J Child Neurol 10:411–413.

McHugh H, Sowaen K A, Levitt M N 1969 Facial paralysis and muscle agenesis in the newborn. Arch Otolaryngol 89:157–168.

MacKinnon J A, Perlman M, Kirpalani H et al 1993 Spinal cord injury at birth: Diagnostic and prognostic data in twenty-two patients. J Pediatr 122:431–437.

Maekawa K, Masaki T, Kokubun Y 1976 Fetal spinal cord injury secondary to hyperextension of the neck: no effect of caesarean section. Dev Med Child Neurol 18:229–238.

Medlock M D, Hanigan W C 1997 Neurologic birth trauma. Clin Perinatol 24:845–857.

Menticoglou M, Perlman M, Manning A 1995 High cervical spinal cord injury in neonates delivered with forceps: report of 15 cases. Obstet Gynecol 86(4):589–594.

Mills J F, Dargaville P A, Coleman L T et al 2001 Upper cervical spinal cord injury in neonates: the use of magnetic resonance imaging. J Ped 138:105–108.

Mitchell W G, Tseng-Ong L 2005 Catastrophic presentation of infant botulism may obscure or delay diagnosis. Pediatrics 116(3):e436–438.

Miyamoto R C, Parikh S R, Gellad W et al 2005 Bilateral congenital vocal cord paralysis: a 16-year institutional review. Otolaryngol Head Neck Surg 133(2):241–245.

Narcy P, Tran-Ba-Huy E, Margoloff B et al 1982 Indications therapeutiques dans les paralysies faciales du nouveau-ne. A propos de 9 observations. Annales d'Otolaryngologie 99:377–382.

Navarro Cunchillos M, Bonachera M D, Navarro Cunchillos M et al 1996 Middle ear teratoma in a newborn. J Laryng Otology 110(9):875–877.

Nishikawa M, Ichiyama T, Hayashi T, Furukawa S 1997 Mobius-like syndrome associated with a 1;2 chromosome translocation. Clin Genet 51:122–123.

Ouzounian J G, Korst L M, Phelan J P 1997 Permanent Erb palsy: A traction-related injury? Obstet Gynaecol 89:139–141.

Paine R S 1997 Facial paralysis in children. J Pediatr 19:303–315.

Pape K E, Armstrong D L, Fitzhardinge P M 1978 Peripheral median nerve damage secondary to brachial arterial blood gas sampling. J Pediatr 93:852–856.

Pape K E, Pickering D 1972 Asymmetric crying facies: an index of other congenital anomalies. J Pediatr 81:21–24.

Pape K E, Wigglesworth J S 1979 Haemorrhage, ischaemia and the neonatal brain. Clin Dev Med 69/70:85–99.

Pastuszak A L, Schuler L, Speck-Martins C E et al 1998 Use of misoprostol during pregnancy and Mobius' syndrome in infants. N Engl J Med 338:1881–1885.

Pejham S, Altman R, Li K I et al 2002 Congenital tuberculosis with facial nerve palsy. Ped Inf Disease J 21(11):1085–1086.

Perlman M, Reisner S H 1973 Asymmetric crying facies and congenital anomalies. Arch Dis Childhood 48:627–630.

Pitner S E, Edwards J E, McCormick W F 1965 Observations on the pathology of the Mobius syndrome. J Neurol Neurosurg Psychiatr 28:362–374.

Pondaag W, Malessy M J A, Gert van Dijk J et al 2004 Natural history of obstetric brachial plexus palsy: a systematic review. Dev Med Child Neurol 46:138–144.

Popovich M J, Taylor F C, Helmer E 1989 MR imaging of birth-related brachial plexus avulsion. Am J Neurol Res 10:S98.

Punal J E, Siebert M F, Angueira F B et al 2001 Three new patients with congenital unilateral facial nerve palsy due to chromosome 22q11 deletion. J Child Neurol 16(6):450–452.

Ramos-Fernandez J M, Oliete-Garcia F M, Roldan-Aparicio S et al 1998 Neonatal sciatic palsy: etiology and outcome of 21 cases. Revista de Neurologia 26:752–755.

Rizk E B, El-Bitar M A, Matae G M et al 2005 Facial nerve palsy with acute otitis media during the first 2 weeks of life. J Child Neurol 20(5):452–454.

Ross D, Royden Jones H, Fisher J et al 1983 Isolated radial nerve lesion in the newborn. Neurology 33:1354–1356.

Rossi L N, Vassella F, Mumenthaler M 1982 Obstetrical lesions of the brachial plexus. Natural history in 34 cases. Eur Neurol 21:1–7.

Ruggieri M, Smarason A K, Pike M 1999 Spinal cord insults in the prenatal, perinatal, and neonatal periods. Dev Med Child Neurol 41:311–317.

Sadleir L G, Connolly M B 1998 Acquired brachial-plexus neuropathy in the neonate: a rare presentation of late onset group-B streptococcal osteomyelitis. Dev Med Child Neurol 40:496–499.

San Agustin M, Nitowsky H M, Borden J N 1962 Neonatal sciatic palsy after umbilical vessel injection. J Pediatr 60:408–413.

Sapin S O, Miller A A, Bass H N 2005 Neonatal asymmetric crying facies: a new look at an old problem. Clin Ped 44(2):109–119.

Say B, Coldwell J G 1975 Heriditary defect of the sacrum. Humangenetik 27:231–234.

Schneider H, Ballowitz L, Schachinger H 1975 Anoxic encephalopathy with predominant involvement of basal ganglia, brainstem and spinal cord in the perinatal period. Acta Neuropathol 32:287–238.

Schreiner M S, Field F, Ruddy R 1991 Infant botulism: A review of 12 years experience at the Children's Hospital of Philadelphia. Pediatrics 87:159–165.

Schulman S T, Madden J D, Esterly J R et al 1971 Transection of spinal cord. A rare obstetrical complication of cephalic delivery. Arch Dis Childhood 46:291–294.

Simon L, Perreaux F, Devictor D et al 1999 Clinical and radiological diagnosis of spinal cord birth injury. Arch Dis Childhood Neonatal Ed 81: F235–F236.

Singer R, Joseph K, Gilai A N et al 1991 Nontraumatic, acute neonatal paraplegia. J Pediatr Orthoped 11:588–593.

Sjoberg I, Erichs K, Bjerre I 1988 Cause and effect of obstetric (neonatal) brachial plexus palsy. Acta Paediatr Scand 77:357–364.

Skinner M L, Halstead L A, Rubinstein C S et al 2005 Laryngopharyngeal dysfunction after the Norwood procedure. J Thoracic Cardiovascular Surgery 130(5):1293–1301.

Sladky J T, Rorke L B 1986 Perinatal hypoxic/ischemic spinal cord injury. Pediatr Pathol 6:87–101.

Smith D W 1982 Recognizable patterns of human malformation, 3rd edn. W B Saunders, Philadelphia, PA, pp. 168–169.

Smith J D, Crumley R C, Harker L A 1981 Facial paralysis in the newborn. Otolaryngol Head Neck Surg 89:1021–1024.

Strombeck C, Krumlinde-Sundholm L, Forssberg H 2000 Functional outcome at 5 years in children with obstetrical brachial plexus palsy with and without microsurgical reconstruction. Dev Med Child Neurol 42:148–157.

Strombeck C, Krumlinde-Sundholm L, Remahl S et al 2007 Long-term follow-up of children with obstetric brachial plexus palsy I: functional aspects. Dev Med Child Neurol 49:198–203.

Stromland K, Sjogreen L, Miller M et al 2002 Mobius sequence — a Swedish multidiscipline study. Europ J Ped Neurol 6(1):35–45.

Sugarman G I, Stark H H 1973 Mobius syndrome with Poland's anomaly. J Med Genet 10:192–196.

Sundholm L K, Eliasson A C, Forssberg H 1998 Obstetric brachial plexus injuries: assessment protocol and functional outcome at age 5 years. Dev Med Child Neurol 40:4–11.

Suri S, Salfield S, Baxter P 1999 Congenital paraplegia following maternal hypotension. Dev Med Child Neurol 41:273–274.

Thakkar N, O'Neil W, Duvally J 1977 Mobius syndrome due to brainstem tegmental necrosis. Arch Neurol 34:124–126.

Toelle S P, Boltshauser E 2001 Long-term outcome in children with congenital unilateral facial nerve palsy. NeuroPediatrics 32:130–135.

Tollner U, Bechinger D, Pohlandt F 1980 Radial nerve palsy in a premature infant following long-term measurement of blood pressure. J Pediatr 96:921–922.

Tortori-Donati P, Fondelli M P, Rossi A et al 1999 Segmental spinal dysgenesis: neuroradiologic findings with clinical and embryologic correlation. Am J Neuroradiol 20:445–456.

Towbin A 1969 Latent spinal cord and brain stem injury in newborn infants. Dev Med Child Neurol 11:54–60.

Trip J, van Stuijvenberg M, Dikkers F G et al 2002 Unilateral CHARGE association. Europ J Ped 161(2):78–80.

Verzijl H T, van den Helm B, Veldman B et al 1999 A second gene for autosomal dominant Mobius syndrome is localized to chromosome 10q, in a Dutch family. Am J Hum Genet 65:752–756.

Young R K, Towgighi J, Marks K H 1983 Focal necrosis of the spinal cord in utero. Arch Neurol 40:654–655.

CHAPTER

40 Neuromuscular disorders

Eugenio Mercuri and Victor Dubowitz

Although the neuromuscular disorders in infancy and childhood have had extensive coverage (Dubowitz 1980, 1985, 1995), the recent improvement in understanding of the genetic basis of neuromuscular disorders has allowed a better definition of the clinical phenotypes associated with the individual forms. This chapter concentrates on the neuromuscular disorders specific to the neonatal period, and provides a problem-oriented approach as well as dealing with each disorder individually.

CLINICAL PRESENTATION

A neuromuscular disorder should be suspected when the infant has a problem, such as weakness, hypotonia, contractures, feeding difficulty or persistent ventilatory failure. Neonatal hypotonia is a constant feature in infants with neuromuscular disorders, but it is a non-specific sign as it can also be found in infants with central nervous system involvement, genetic or metabolic diseases (Dubowitz 1980, Vasta et al 2005). The observation of difficulty with antigravity movements is one of the key elements to detect *weakness*. Movements should be judged at peak of activity, such as when crying or stimulated. Weak children, such as those with neuromuscular involvement, will show few movements, even in response to stimulation. Contractures are also frequent and may be localized to a few joints or involve several joints and in a newborn they are often the result of reduced motility in utero.

Other important clues are: (1) delayed quickening and poor fetal movements throughout the pregnancy or normal movements initially but reduction later, (2) polyhydramnios suggesting involvement of the muscles of swallowing, (3) a family history of neonatal death and stillbirth, (4) a history of possible or definite neuromuscular disease in the mother and other members of the family, and (5) thin ribs on the chest radiograph, suggesting poor respiratory muscle movement in utero. Feeding abnormalities and respiratory impairment are also frequent.

In a recent study we have retrospectively assessed the main clinical features that present in infancy associated with hypotonia, establishing their sensitivity and specificity in identifying neuromuscular disorders (Table 40.1). The results of our study suggest that marked weakness, with absent or extremely reduced antigravity movements and contractures are the two signs that can more reliably identify infants with neuromuscular disorders.

THE TIMING OF THE CLINICAL ONSET

Some disorders may already have an antenatal onset, others present in the immediate newborn period and others are delayed for hours or days after birth. For example, myotonic dystrophy is associated with an antenatal onset while neonatal myasthenia usually presents a few hours after birth, and the mitochondrial myopathies present a few days or weeks after birth. Spinal muscular atrophy (Werdnig–Hoffmann disease) may be present at birth or after a period of normality before the onset of weakness.

THE FAMILY

Most neuromuscular disorders are genetic, and establishing a pattern of inheritance is important in the differential diagnosis. There may be subclinical manifestations in dominant and X-linked disorders. For example, myotonic dystrophy is inherited as an autosomal dominant trait. In many cases the mother, who is always affected, and other affected family members may only have mild involvement and are unaware they have the disease. It is therefore important to inquire about any family history that would indicate myotonic dystrophy, in particular presenile cataract, muscle stiffness, progressive weakness, frontal baldness and early death from cardiorespiratory disease. In addition, family members should be examined personally for abnormal physical signs, such as facial weakness (which may consist only of inability to bury the eyelashes), wasting of the facial muscles (especially the temporalis and the sternomastoids), percussion myotonia of the tongue and hands, and relaxation myotonia of the hands. It is important to alert all affected persons to the risk of anesthesia.

Severe centronuclear myopathy, which is characterized by a similar clinical presentation to myotonic dystrophy in the newborn, is X-linked recessive, and there may be a family history of stillbirth and neonatal death stretching back several generations.

The other neuromuscular disorder that should be excluded in the mother is myasthenia gravis, which may lead to transient neonatal myasthenia due to passive transfer of antibody across the placenta.

CLINICAL EXAMINATION

On examination of the baby there are often clinical features, such as the distribution of weakness that may help to suspect specific neuromuscular disorders.

Overt *facial weakness* is characteristic of myotonic dystrophy and centronuclear myopathy, but also often occurs

Table 40.1 Sensitivity, specificity, positive predictive value (PPV) and negative predictive value (NPV) of neonatal clinical features in floppy infants (modified by Vasta et al 2005)

	Sensitivity (%)	Specificity (%)	PPV (%)	NPV (%)
Extremely reduced/absent antigravity movements	97.4	75.0	77.5	97.0
Partial range antigravity movements	2.5	61.3	5.5	41.5
Contractures	69.2	61.3	61.3	69.2
Reduced fetal movements	46.1	88.6	78.2	65.0
Oligopolydramnios	38.4	75.0	57.6	57.8
Apgar <5	43.5	61.3	50.0	55.1
Resp. problems at birth	69.2	31.8	47.3	53.8
Feeding difficulties	87.1	6.8	45.3	37.5
Poor alertness	15.3	43.1	19.3	36.5
Seizures	5.1	70.4	13.3	45.5
Dysmorphism	25.6	43.1	28.5	39.5

in other congenital myopathies such as nemaline myopathy and in some forms of congenital muscular dystrophy. External *ophthalmoplegia* is a feature of centronuclear myopathy. In the severe type of spinal muscular atrophy, the facies is usually normal and the infant is likely to be quite bright and able to follow with the eyes, despite being very weak generally. *Tongue fasciculation* at rest is a characteristic feature of spinal muscular atrophy. While spinal muscular atrophy is highly likely to be associated with severe paralysis, other neuromuscular disorders such as myotonic dystrophy and congenital muscular dystrophy are more variable.

The distribution of the *respiratory muscle weakness* is important. Diaphragmatic weakness with paradoxical movement of the abdominal muscles with respiration occurs in congenital muscular dystrophy, some of the congenital myopathies such as myotubular, nemaline and mini-core, and in congenital myasthenia. In contrast, in spinal muscular atrophy the weakness is mainly intercostal, the breathing pattern is abdominal and the rib cage moves paradoxically with the abdomen.

Fixed bilateral *talipes* is associated with congenital myotonic dystrophy and myotubular myopathy. *Arthrogryposis* (i.e. contractures of several joints) is associated with congenital dystrophy and certain neurogenic disorders. Fixed joint contractures are not a feature of severe spinal muscular atrophy.

These physical signs may be difficult to assess on one single occasion if the baby is severely ill (e.g. on a ventilator) and repeated examination is often useful. It is not always easy to differentiate a CNS from a neuromuscular disorder, especially as the baby may have overt CNS involvement (e.g. seizures, hydrocephalus, intraventricular hemorrhage/periventricular leukomalacia) in association with a neuromuscular disorder, and this may not always relate to severe birth asphyxia. Furthermore, a baby with neuromuscular disease may have reasonable power in the limbs and still have severe respiratory muscle weakness.

INVESTIGATIONS

The serum creatine kinase (CK) activity is normally increased in cord blood up to 1000 units (normal levels for adults <200 IU/L). This increased activity reflects muscle damage during labour and usually comes down in the first 10 days of life. Measurement of serum CK activity is likely to be of most value in preclinical Duchenne muscular dystrophy, where it will be markedly elevated (several thousand units); in congenital muscular dystrophy the elevation is moderate and variable and only occurs in about half the patients. A motor nerve conduction study will reveal an absent motor action potential in spinal muscular atrophy due to the extensive denervation. If myasthenia gravis is suspected, then repetitive stimulation of the peripheral nerve may show decrement in the motor action potential. A slow nerve conduction velocity may point to a hereditary motor neuropathy which may rarely present in early infancy.

An electromyogram (EMG) can be useful in diagnosis and differential diagnosis of neuromuscular disorders in later infancy. However, in the neonatal period interpretation can be difficult as the severely weak baby often makes little spontaneous movement. If there is any suggestion that the infant may have myotonic dystrophy, then one should obtain EMGs from both parents (and particularly the mother), looking for myotonic discharges. The favored site for this is the first dorsal interosseus muscle of the hand.

Ultrasound imaging of muscle can help to demonstrate striking selective involvement, such as sparing of the rectus femoris and marked involvement of the vasti within the quadriceps muscle (Heckmatt et al 1987). This is of considerable practical importance when taking a biopsy. Muscle biopsy is done using a 4 mm Bergstrom needle. The success rate is as high as in older children, despite the small size of the patient. This is because there has been no time for muscle atrophy, nor extensive replacement of muscle by fat and connective tissue to occur, and also because the size of the individual muscle fibers is small and only a relatively small sample is needed. Needle muscle biopsy is done under local anesthetic in the cot or incubator, and the critically sick newborn can readily have the investigation with minimal disturbance. A detailed description of the technique is given in Heckmatt et al (1984).

It is important to be aware of the value and limitations of muscle biopsy in the newborn period. Muscle biopsy is always needed when congenital myopathies, congenital muscular dystrophies or, more generally, when muscle diseases are suspected. The exceptions are in infants with suspected congenital myotonic dystrophy or spinal muscular atrophy, in whom the genetic tests can reliably lead to a diagnosis without the need for muscle biopsy. Brain imaging, cranial ultrasound and/or brain magnetic resonance imaging (MRI) can help to identify intracranial abnormalities, such as structural brain lesions, hemorrhage and/or ischemic lesions or ventricular dilatation, which is a common associated feature in myotonic dystrophy and centronuclear myopathy. In the last few years there has been increasing evidence of a number of disorders in which muscle involvement is associated with structural brain changes, such as the various forms of congenital muscular dystrophy secondary to alpha glycosylation disorder (see below).

MANAGEMENT

The major problem of management presented by these disorders is that of ventilatory failure and deciding a prognosis and how long to continue giving ventilatory support. It will be necessary to take into account any CNS complication, such as progressive ventricular dilatation. In myotonic dystrophy, there is a trend for improvement in muscle power and a reasonable chance of the infant becoming independent of the ventilator (see later). The respiratory failure may be compounded by premature delivery, which is more common in these cases. If an infant with spinal muscular atrophy is put on a ventilator, it may be extremely difficult to wean him or her off, but most infants with this disorder have sufficient diaphragm function to cope without ventilatory support. The other disorders are more variable, but in myotubular myopathy and congenital muscular dystrophy there is a trend for improvement although it is slow, and a tracheostomy may be necessary for long-term respiratory management.

There now follows a systematic description of the various neuromuscular disorders that may affect the neonate, including muscular dystrophies, congenital myopathies, myasthenia and motoneuron diseases.

THE MUSCULAR DYSTROPHIES

CONGENITAL MYOTONIC DYSTROPHY

The first description of congenital myotonic dystrophy was by Vanier (1960) of six children between the ages of 9 months and 13 years, all of whom had presented as floppy infants; four had had feeding difficulty and three had bilat-

eral talipes. Vanier pointed out the severe facial muscle weakness and wasting (particularly of the sternomastoids leading to a long 'swan-like' neck), nasal speech and mental retardation. The mothers in all the cases were affected but only had minimal signs of the disease. In two families the maternal uncles were severely affected and in one family both the mother and maternal grandmother had presenile cataracts.

Another important early report was that by Dodge et al (1965) of five definite cases. The bilateral facial weakness had led to severe feeding difficulties in infancy, and this was accompanied by marked generalized weakness and hypotonia. One girl had an affected 4-year-old brother who had been admitted at the age of 2 months for eventration of the diaphragm associated with partial collapse of the right lung; he had been cyanosed as an infant but had sucked better than his sister and had good limb strength and reflex activity.

Harper (1975a, 1975b) reported an extensive survey of all available cases in Britain. He emphasized the polyhydramnios and reduced fetal movements and suggested a high incidence of missed cases as there was an elevated neonatal mortality (16%) in liveborn siblings. Of the 70 cases in his study, the mean intelligence quotient was only 66. However, there was no correlation with respiratory problems, suggesting a prenatal cause for the mental deficiency. In all cases the mother was affected, and Harper postulated that an intrauterine factor must be operating, in addition to the gene that has to be present to have the disease.

Outside the neonatal period, most cases with the congenital type survive but few become independent. Of 46 congenital cases followed up retrospectively, only four had died, but of the 42 survivors only two were in normal education, and only one was gainfully employed. Testicular atrophy was evident in all affected males at puberty (O'Brien & Harper 1984).

Table 40.2 summarizes our experience of ten patients who presented in the neonatal period. In general these were more severely affected than previously reported cases, which perhaps reflects selective referral to our neonatal intensive care unit. The extent of the weakness was variable but most had some antigravity power in the limbs. There was no direct relationship between limb power and degree of respiratory muscle involvement, and the baby with the best limb power spent the longest time on the ventilator (112 days) because of elevation of the diaphragm, which required plication. The eight infants who had cranial ultrasound showed ventricular dilatation. In three of these this was present on the first day of life, without evidence for intraventricular hemorrhage, suggesting an antenatal cause (Regev et al 1987). Three of the infants had gastrointestinal stasis, with bile-stained aspirate, requiring a period of intravenous feeding (duration 2–7 weeks). A typical case is illustrated in Figure 40.1.

Percussion myotonia of the tongue, facial weakness and myotonic discharge on the EMG were demonstrated in all ten mothers. Clinical myotonia of the hands was more vari-

Table 40.2 Congenital myotonic dystrophy: presenting features

Patient	Gestation (weeks)	Birth weight (Kg)	Fetal movements	Hydramnios	Apgar score (1/5/10 min)	IPPV[a]	Talipes
1	32	1.8	?	–		–	–
2	34	1.7	Reduced	+	4/5	31	+
3	34	1.8	?	+		16	+
4	34	2.2	?	+	1/5/10	1	+
5	35	1.3	Reduced	–	2/4	112	–
6	35	2.3	Reduced	+	4/5/5	12	–
7	36	1.9	Reduced	+	6/7/8	>49	+
8	38	2.7	Reduced	–	0/3/4	1	–
9	40	2.7	?	–	1/7/5	–	–
10	40	4.0	Reduced	+	1/7/4	–	+

[a]IPPV = intermittent positive-pressure ventilation.

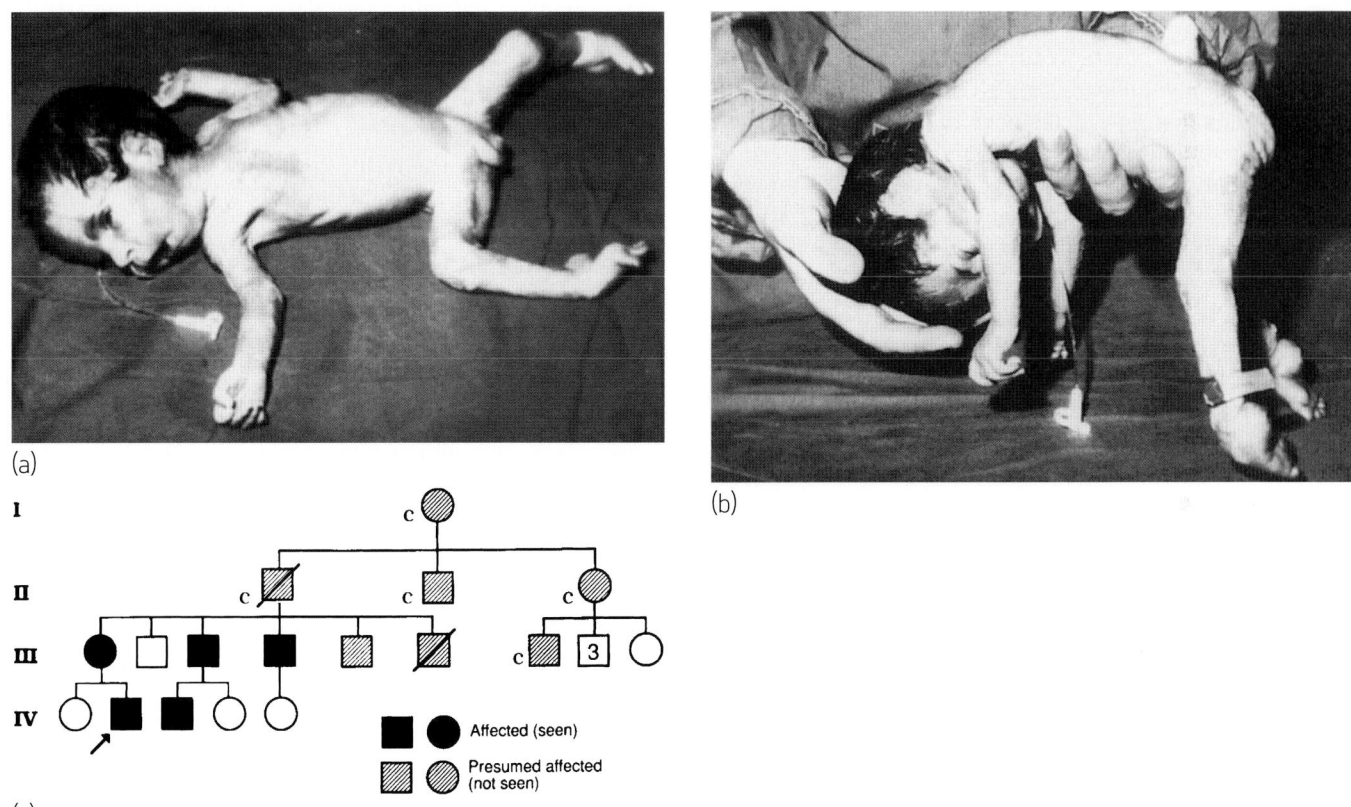

(a)

(b)

(c)

Affected (seen)

Presumed affected
(not seen)

Figure 40.1 (a,b) Infant with congenital myotonic dystrophy admitted at the age of 20 days, having been ventilator-dependent from birth till 15 days without overt lung problem. He was born at 34 weeks of gestation (birth weight 1.8 Kg), by elective cesarean section for breech presentation. On examination, he was generally hypotonic with fixed bilateral talipes equinovarus. He had a large head with wide open fontanelles and parted sutures, and ultrasound scan showed bilateral ventricular dilatation. The mother had definite signs of the disease although she had not been previously diagnosed. (c) On investigation of the family, two maternal uncles (III 3 and 4) and one cousin (IV 3) were affected with facial weakness, myotonia and a positive EMG. Two uncles (III 5 and 6) were not available, but one was said to have frontal baldness and the other to have some stiffness of the hands. One of these uncles subsequently died following dental anesthesia, possibly due to undue sensitivity to muscle relaxants and an unsuspecting anesthetist. There was a history of presenile cataract in several relatives on the maternal grandfather's side of the family.

able. Three mothers had been previously diagnosed, two on the basis of an affected baby, one born to the same mother and one to an aunt. In only one case had the mother previously presented with symptoms of myotonia, and this had led to the diagnosis in other members of her family. In all cases there was a strongly suggestive family history, apart from evidence of disease in the mother. In these ten families, we were personally able to confirm the diagnosis beyond doubt in seven previously undiagnosed adults, apart from the mothers, and were suspicious about a further five, either on the basis of presenile cataract (three cases), or frontal baldness with probable facial muscle wasting (two cases) but without other physical signs, or abnormality on the EMG.

MOLECULAR GENETICS

The abnormality of the gene in myotonic dystrophy on chromosome 19 has been shown to be an expansion of the DNA with an increase in the number of CTG trinucleotide repeats. In normal people there may be up to 30 or so of these repeats, but in affected patients it usually seems to be beyond about 50, and some may have several thousand repeats. The cases of congenital myotonic dystrophy have in general had a much bigger expansion of the gene than other members of the family with later onset (Buxton et al 1992).

This new advance provides an additional method for confirming the diagnosis in an individual case and also in identifying subclinical cases within a family. It also provides the opportunity for prenatal diagnosis on chorionic villus biopsy early in pregnancy (Aslanidis et al 1992).

CONGENITAL MUSCULAR DYSTROPHIES

This is an important group of neuromuscular disorders characterized by weakness, usually from birth, and a muscle biopsy showing striking pathological changes similar to other muscular dystrophies (Dubowitz 1995). The classification of congenital muscular dystrophies (CMD) has become increasingly complicated due to the ever growing number of genes and proteins identified (Mercuri & Longman 2005, Muntoni & Voit 2005). Until recently the classification of CMD was mainly based on the involvement of the central nervous system (CNS) and on the presence or absence of merosin, an extracellular matrix protein found to be missing in approximately half of the cases with CMD. In the last few years however this classification has proved to be inadequate as both groups with normal and reduced merosin have been found to be heterogeneous groups including various forms which have been identified as genetically distinct entities. The most recent classification includes 9 forms of CMD for which the genetic defect has been identified (Mercuri & Longman 2005). From a practical point of view, for the clinician it is useful to separate forms with central nervous system involvement from those in which CNS involvement is absent or rare. We will describe the most frequent forms of CMD observable in the neonatal period, providing clinical, pathological and imaging details to help their identification.

CLINICAL PRESENTATION

With the exception of the forms of CMD with structural brain changes in which signs of involvement of the central nervous system can predominate, most of the other forms of CMD have similar onset and neonatal clinical signs.

Generalized weakness and hypotonia are usually present at birth. Facial weakness is frequently present but not as severe or striking as that in congenital myotonic dystrophy (Fig. 40.2). Many will have contractures at birth, sometimes extensive arthrogryposis (see later), and will show a tendency to develop contractures during infancy. It is particularly important to recognize these patients and start a program of active treatment of the contractures in infancy to try and improve the range of joint mobility. A few patients have respiratory involvement at birth. A feature of this condition is that the disease process may pick out certain muscles, including those of respiration, leaving others relatively spared (Fig. 40.3). A further group presents later in the first or second years of life with motor delay, having not apparently had any recognized problem in infancy.

MEROSIN-NEGATIVE CONGENITAL MUSCULAR DYSTROPHY

The reported incidence of this form ranges between 30–40% of all the forms of CMD (Muntoni & Voit 2005). Children with merosin deficiency have in general a more severe clinical course than the children with merosin positive congenital muscular dystrophy. They are usually symptomatic at birth or in the first few weeks of life with hypotonia and muscle weakness, weak cry and, in 10–30% of cases, with contractures.

Children with merosin negative CMD (Helbling-Leclerc et al 1995) generally do not show structural brain changes but diffuse white matter changes on MRI are a constant feature in these children. These changes are not obvious on the conventional scans performed in the first months of life, and become more evident around 6 months (Mercuri et al 1996, 2001). Despite their dramatic appearance on imaging, these changes are not usually associated with clinical signs of CNS involvement. The only sign of the involvement of the central nervous system is epilepsy, which has been observed in 10–30% of children (Voit 1998). Other patterns of brain lesions, such as cerebellar hypoplasia and/or cortical dysplasia, can be observed in a small proportion of these patients.

FORMS OF CONGENITAL MUSCULAR DYSTROPHY WITH STRUCTURAL BRAIN CHANGES AND EYE INVOLVEMENT

There are three forms of CMD associated with structural brain changes and ocular abnormalities.

Walker–Warburg syndrome

This is the most severe of the conditions with CNS involvement. There is neonatal onset with a combination of weakness and severe hypotonia suggestive of muscle involvement

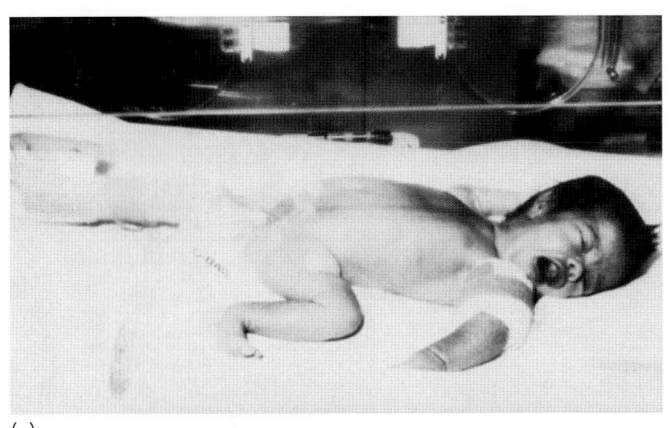

(a)

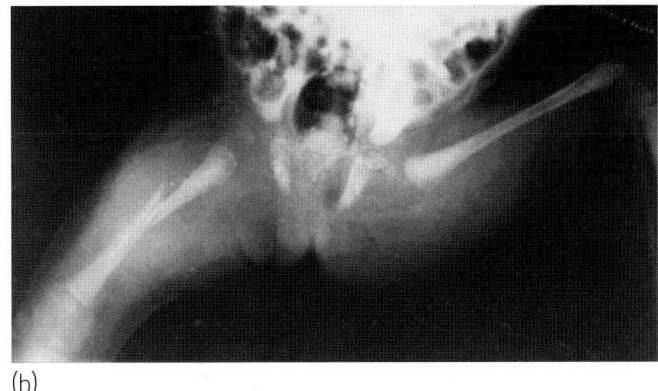

(b)

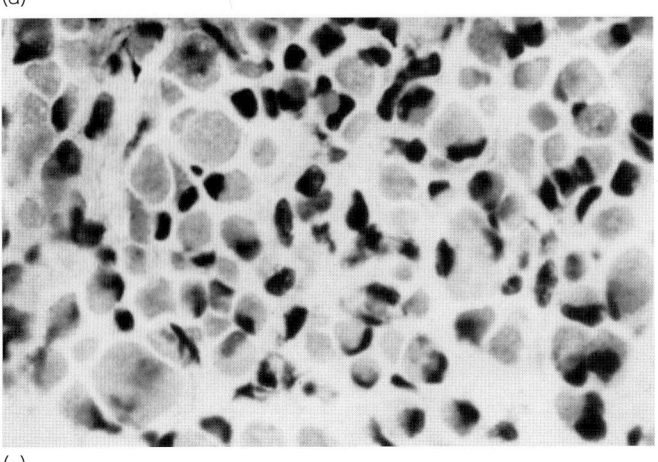

(c)

Figure 40.2 (a) A 5-day-old girl with congenital muscular dystrophy. She was born by elective cesarean section at 39 weeks of gestation and sustained a fracture of the femur during delivery (birth weight 2.3 Kg), and subsequently a fracture of the left humerus during normal nursing care. On examination she had mild facial weakness and no antigravity power in the limbs. A brother had also been affected, had been born with fractures of all four limbs and had died on the first day of life of intracranial hemorrhage. He had been suspected of having osteogenesis imperfecta. (b) The girl's radiograph shows slender bones but only minimal osteoporosis. Her serum CK level was normal (28 IU/L). (c) Needle muscle biopsy at 5 days of age showed unequivocal pathological change with variability in fiber size, proliferation of endomysium and some cellular infiltration. The poor bone development was presumably secondary to the weak muscles. Following an intensive program of regular passive stretching of all joints and early mobilization in a standing frame, she was walking independently by the age of 4 years in light-weight knee-ankle-foot orthoses, and subsequently unaided, and there were no further fractures.

and signs of central nervous system involvement, such as poor visual attention and decreased alertness, associated with ocular abnormalities including retinal dysgenesis, microphthalmia or anterior chamber malformations (Dobyns et al 1989).

Brain MRI shows a type II lissencephaly with the typical micropolygyric cobblestone cortex and the white matter is also severely abnormal. Other structural changes include cerebellar and brainstem hypoplasia, Dandy–Walker syndrome or encephaloceles. Progressive hydrocephalus is often present (Dobyns et al 1989).

The presence of a muscular dystrophy, suggested by a combination of clinical signs and often by elevated CK levels, is confirmed on muscle biopsy.

• *Muscle-eye-brain disease*

This is a form of CMD, initially identified in Finland but is now recognized to occur worldwide. Clinical signs are usually present at birth or in the first months of life with hypotonia and weakness. Ocular abnormalities may become evident only after the first years of life. These children invariably develop severe mental retardation and, often, epilepsy; but approximately 25% of children eventually learn to walk (Muntoni & Voit 2005).

Brain MRI shows extensive abnormalities of neuronal migration, such as pachygyria and polymicrogyria and often brainstem and cerebellar hypoplasia and periventricular white matter changes.

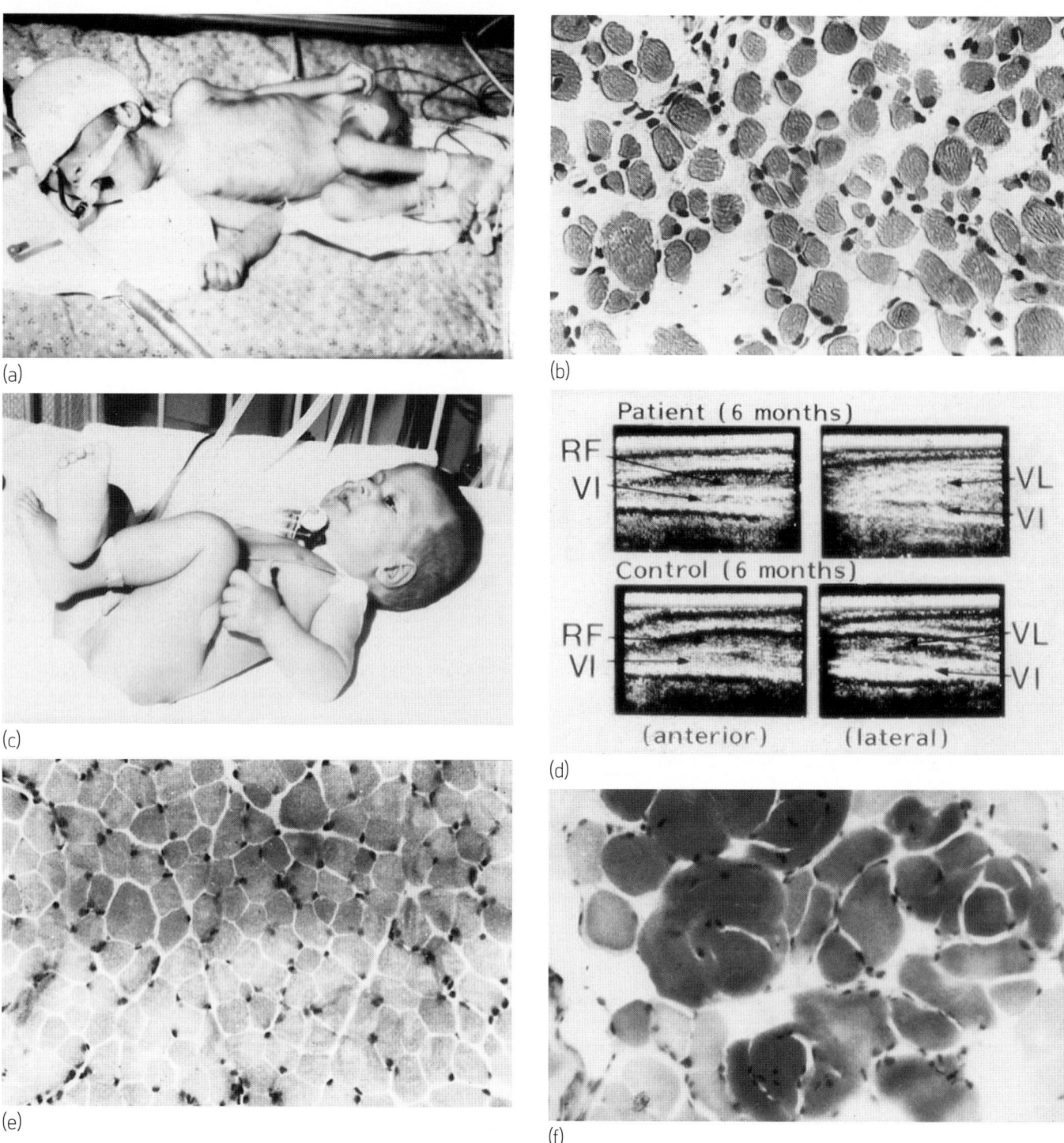

Figure 40.3 (a) An 8-day-old boy with congenital muscular dystrophy presenting with persistent ventilatory failure. Pregnancy was complicated by polyhydramnios and reduced fetal movements. He was born at 34 weeks of gestation (birth weight 1.6 Kg). He was severely asphyxiated and needed immediate intubation and intermittent positive-pressure ventilation. His serum CK level was normal (66 IU/L). (b) Needle muscle biopsy (vastus lateralis) at 8 days of age showed variability in fiber size and proliferation of connective tissue. (c) There was a marked improvement in limb power by 6 months of age but he still needed ventilation and had had a tracheostomy. (d) Real-time ultrasound scans of the thigh (longitudinal views) at that time showed a normal appearance of the rectus femoris (RF) and marked echogenicity of the vastus lateralis (VL) and of the vastus intermedius (VI). A second needle muscle biopsy was performed, taking a piece concurrently from the rectus femoris and the vastus lateralis. This showed that (e) the rectus was normal while (f) the vastus was abnormal, with adipose and connective tissue proliferation and variability in fiber size, including some large whorled fibers with multiple internal nuclei (hematoxylin and eosin staining, H and E). This suggested that the respiratory muscles were selectively affected in the same way as the vastus lateralis. By 13 months he only needed ventilatory support at night, could sit unsupported and stand with support, and vocalize with a speaking tube in situ. At 15 months of age he had a sudden respiratory and cardiac arrest while having tracheostomy care, suffering irreversible brain damage, and died the following day.

• *Fukuyama congenital muscular dystrophy*

This form is exceptional outside Japan (Fukuyama et al 1981). The gene responsible for Fukuyama congenital muscular dystrophy is another glycosyltransferase, named fukutin (Kondo et al 1999). The clinical features of the Fukuyama congenital muscular dystrophy are mild to moderate hypotonia at birth and a progressive course with increasing weakness, joint contractures, high CK levels, moderate to severe mental retardation and frequent association with epilepsy. Ocular abnormalities occur in approximately 70% of these children but are rarely severe.

Brain MRI shows structural changes consisting of pachygyria and polymicrogyria and low density white matter areas (Yoshioka et al 1991).

Until recently it was suggested that each of these forms was due to mutations in different genes, namely fukutin for *FCMD*, *POMT1* for Walker–Waburg and *POMGnT1* for MEB (Balci et al 2005, Beltran Valero et al 2002), but it has become obvious that Walker–Waburg syndrome and MEB can be associated with mutations in all the genes involved in the glycosylation of the alpha dystroglycan, such as fukutin-related protein (FKRP), fukutin, *POMT1*, *POMT2* and *POMGnT1* (Beltran Valero et al 2003, 2004, Currier et al 2005). Conversely, mutations in some of these genes have been found to be associated with different brain MRI findings. Mutations in the FKRP gene for example were originally found in patients with normal MRI (Brockington et al 2001) but have subsequently been found in patients with various patterns of structural brain changes ranging from cerebellar cysts to Walker–Waburg-like findings (see Mercuri et al 2003, 2005 for a review). In patients affected by these forms of congenital dystrophy, all these genes should therefore be screened for mutations.

THE CONGENITAL MYOPATHIES

The congenital myopathies are a heterogeneous group of disorders associated with a structural abnormality within the muscle fiber. They can all present in the neonatal period as a floppy infant. Centronuclear and nemaline myopathy are described here because of their propensity to severe respiratory problems.

MYOTUBULAR (CENTRONUCLEAR) MYOPATHY

There are three clinical and genetic subtypes: (1) a severe X-linked type, presenting in the neonatal period; (2) a less severe infantile type, which is probably autosomal recessive; and (3) a mild juvenile or adult type, which is autosomal dominant in some cases.

The X-linked type is the most severe and has the earliest onset with severe hypotonia and weakness at birth, associated with persistent ventilatory failure and often with feeding difficulties (Fig. 40.4). It closely mimics congenital myotonic dystrophy. These infants usually have an antenatal history of polyhydramnios (Dubowitz 1995, Heckmatt et al 1985, Wallgren-Petterson & Thomas 1994). The majority of these infants die within the first days or weeks of life and only few survive into adulthood (Dubowitz 1995, Wallgren-Petterson et al 1995). Intracranial ventricular dilatation was a feature in these infants, as it is in congenital myotonic dystrophy. The autosomal dominant and recessive types of myotubular myopathy show a milder course and their onset is generally after the neonatal period.

The principal pathological feature (irrespective of the genetics) is the presence of large central nuclei in fibers of both types. Only a proportion of the fibers show the central nuclei in transverse section because they are spaced out along the fibers with gaps in between them. The central area of the fibers is devoid of myofibrils but occupied by mitochondria and glycogen. Histochemical stains show a large proportion of fibers with central aggregation of stain with the NADH-TR and periodic acid–Schiff (PAS) reactions and 'holes' in the center of the fibers on the ATPase reaction due to the absence of myofibers.

Molecular genetics

The gene for the severe X-linked form of congenital myotubular myopathy has been localized on Xq28 (Thomas et al 1990) and numerous mutations have been identified. The gene encodes the tyrosine phosphatase myotubularin and has been called *MTM1*. This has allowed not only to confirm the diagnosis but also to perform prenatal diagnosis (Tanner et al 1998).

NEMALINE MYOPATHY

This congenital myopathy is of variable severity and inheritance and may present in the neonatal period. The ENMC international consortium on nemaline myopathy, formed in 1996, has agreed on the following, broad definition: 'nemaline myopathy is a neuromuscular disorder characterized by muscle weakness and the presence in the muscle fibers of nemaline (rod) bodies, in the absence of other known conditions sometimes associated with nemaline bodies' (Wallgren-Petterson & Laing 1996). The rods are easily overlooked on the hematoxylin and eosin section and readily demonstrated with the Gomori trichrome stain, being a striking red color in contrast to the blue-green of the muscle fibers. There may be two populations of fibers, one hypertrophic and the other atrophic, and the rods are mainly in the atrophic fibers.

The most common mode of inheritance is autosomal recessive and the spectrum of clinical phenotypes within the autosomal recessive nemaline myopathy is quite wide (Wallgren-Petterson 1998, Wallgren-Petterson & Laing 1996). The most common form is the so-called 'typical' form, with onset generally in infancy and pronounced facial and proximal weakness.

A severe perinatal form has also been described and is often fatal. The first severe infantile case was reported by Shafiq et al (1967) in a 15-week-old male infant, who presented with generalized hypotonia and difficulty in feeding. The infant's main problem was the accumulation of

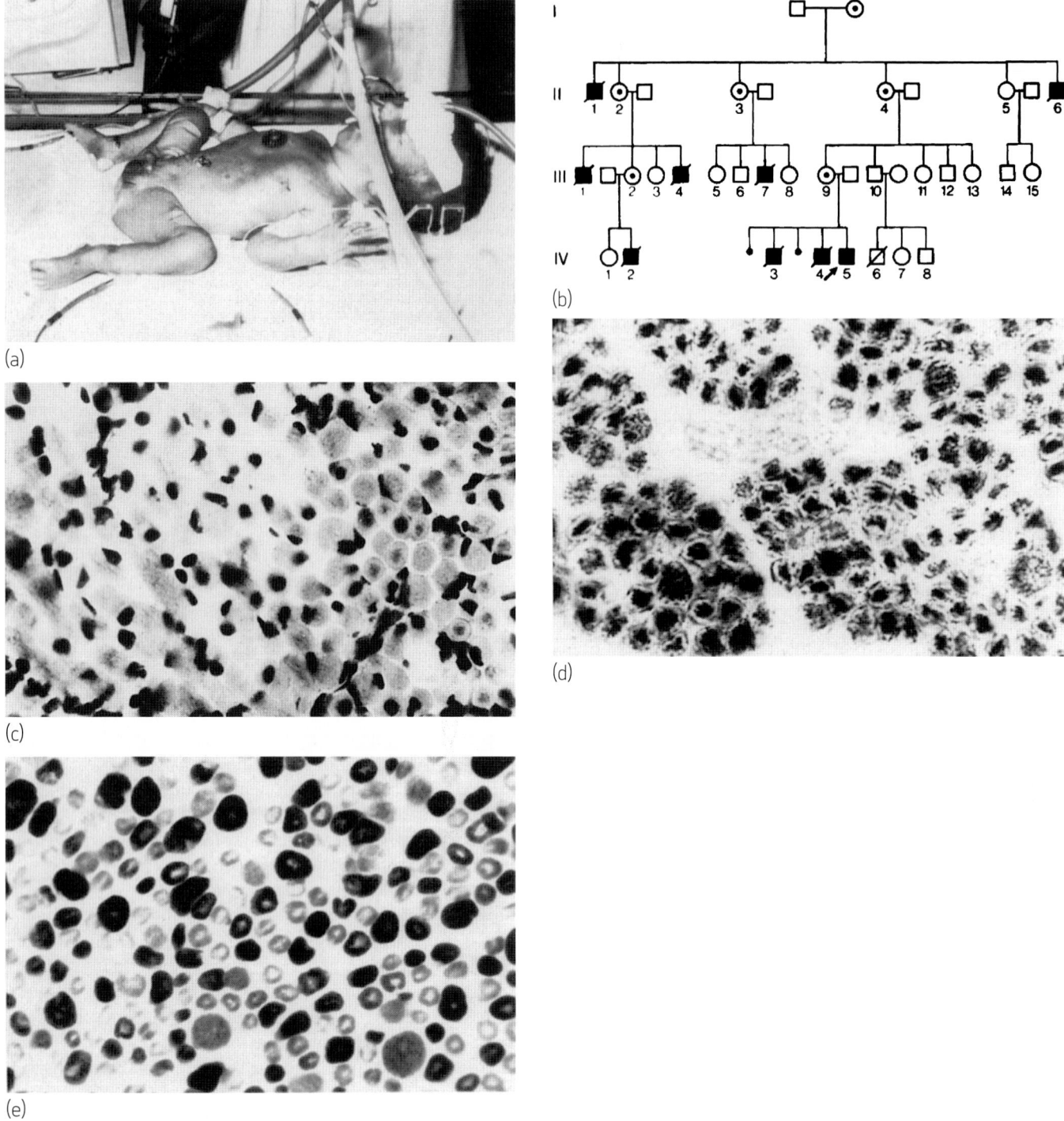

Figure 40.4 (a) A 10-day-old male infant with X-linked centronuclear myopathy who presented with persistent ventilatory failure from birth and poor limb movements. The pregnancy was complicated by polyhydramnios and poor fetal movements. (b) The mother was an obligate carrier, and there were eight other affected males in three generations, all of whom were either stillborn or had died in the neonatal period. She had mild facial weakness with difficulty in burying her eyelashes, but she had no evidence of myotonia (Heckmatt et al 1985). (c) Needle muscle biopsy (quadriceps) from the patient at 10 days of age showed prominent central nuclei in about 40% of fibers (H and E). (d) The NADH-TR reaction showed central aggregation of stain in virtually all fibers. (e) The ATPase 9.5 showed a clear zone in the center of many fibers.

secretions, which tended to obstruct and compromise his airway. His face was expressionless but moved symmetrically on crying. He had had multiple episodes of pneumonitis and atelectasias, and at 4 months a feeding gastrostomy was performed. Subsequently his muscle power improved but he died at the age of 10 months from a fulminating pneumonia. Post-mortem examination showed involvement of the tongue, diaphragm and pharynx, in addition to variable involvement of the skeletal muscles.

Kuitunen et al (1972) described two unrelated children who had been weak from birth with sucking difficulty – both improved and had eventually became ambulant. Neustein (1973) reported three affected siblings who had been floppy from birth. The first had died at 3 months of age, the second at 2 days, and the third at 11 months, probably from respiratory causes in each case. All had reduced fetal movements in utero. The third sibling had a detailed autopsy and involvement of skeletal muscle was widespread.

There have also been reports of nemaline myopathy presenting as ventilatory failure in the newborn. Norton et al (1983) reported two infants, one a girl born at 35 weeks of gestation who had persistent ventilatory failure with no improvement, and ventilatory support was discontinued after 3 months. Tsujihata et al (1983) reported a female infant, born at 37 weeks of gestation, who was hypotonic from birth, failed to establish effective respiration and required ventilatory support, and subsequently died at the age of 3 months. Autopsy again revealed widespread involvement of skeletal muscles, particularly the diaphragm.

Molecular genetics

Our understanding of the genetic aspects of nemaline myopathy has advanced dramatically over the last few years.

It has been demonstrated that there are at least 5 genes involved in the different types of nemaline myopathy (Wallgren-Petterson et al 2004, Wallgren-Petterson & Laign 2006). In the neonatal forms, de-novo dominant mutations in the ACTA1 gene account for a significant proportion of the severe form, while the rest are due to mutations in an, as yet, unidentified gene. Mutations in the gene for tropomyosin, TPM3 on chromosome 1q21 have been found in both dominant and recessive nemaline myopathies (Tan et al 1998, Wallgren-Petterson 1998) while mutations localized on chromosome 2q22, in a region harboring the gene for the muscle protein nebulin have been found in most of the classic milder, non-progressive or slowly progressive forms (Wallgren-Petterson 2004).

MYASTHENIA GRAVIS

AUTOIMMUNE

Neonatal myasthenia gravis is a transient disorder occurring in about 12% of the offspring of myasthenic mothers. Namba et al (1970) did a detailed review of 82 cases from the literature and included two of their own. The infants presented usually within a few hours of birth, or at the very latest the

first 72 hours, with feeding difficulty, generalized weakness, poor respiratory effort and inability to handle pharyngeal secretions (Fig. 40.5). At least half had facial weakness characterized by 'mask-like' facies and infrequent blinking and staring; 15% had ptosis, and 8% decreased ocular movements. Virtually all cases reviewed responded to anticholinesterases. Some of the patients had repetitive stimulation, at 5–20 Hz, which showed a decrement in the amplitude of the motor action potential. Nine died and in six who came to autopsy the cause was respiratory failure, with atelectasis and pneumonia. The mean duration of illness was 18 days, with a maximum of 7 weeks.

Neonatal myasthenia cannot be related to duration or severity of maternal disease, to any alteration in the maternal symptoms during pregnancy, or to thymectomy. It is associated with acetylcholine receptor (ACHR) antibody, which is passively transferred across the placenta in both affected and unaffected babies but is more persistent in the serum of affected babies. Exchange transfusion is said to be of no value in the management of the baby (Lefvert & Osterman 1983), which is contrary to what might be expected, considering the undoubted response to plasma exchange in most adults.

NON-AUTOIMMUNE

The term 'congenital myasthenic syndromes' includes a heterogeneous group of hereditary disorders affecting the neuromuscular junction. Conomy et al (1975) reported an 18-month-old boy with familial infantile myasthenia who had recurrent episodes of choking from the age of 2 weeks, who responded dramatically to edrophonium, and whose sister had had delayed motor milestones and 'bedroom eyes' and had died suddenly during a respiratory infection at the age of 15 months. Robertson et al (1980) reported a 14-year-old boy who had had repeated episodes of severe apnea from the neonatal period which resolved at around the age of 2 years. Marked fatigability had persisted and there was mild proximal weakness. He had responded to prostigmin, which was first tried at the age of 4 years. An older brother had had similar episodes of apnea which also ceased at the age of 2 years. On repetitive stimulation, there was a marked decrement in the size of the motor action potential in the biceps. Albers et al (1984) reported a clinically atypical infant who had to be ventilated from 1 week of age and who failed to respond to anticholinesterase but showed a striking decrement in the motor action potential on repetitive stimulation at 2 Hz. The baby died at the age of 8 months of pneumonia. The authors suggested a failure of resynthesis, mobilization or storage of acetylcholine.

Vincent et al (1981) reported five male patients, including two brothers, aged 13–25 years with congenital myasthenia gravis. Three had an onset at birth with feeding difficulty, ptosis and facial involvement and two had an onset before 2 years. Four had oculomotor paralysis but none had major respiratory involvement. The response to anticholinesterases was variable but three showed a definite improvement. The

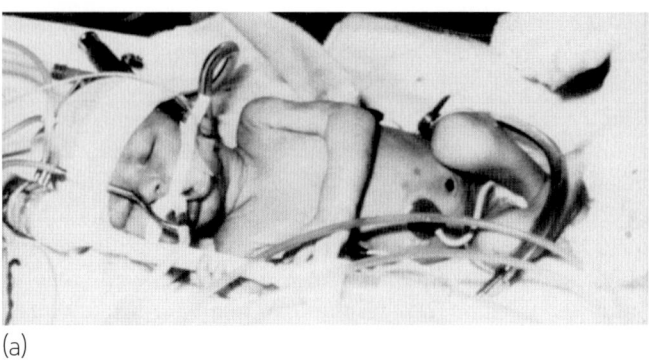

(a)

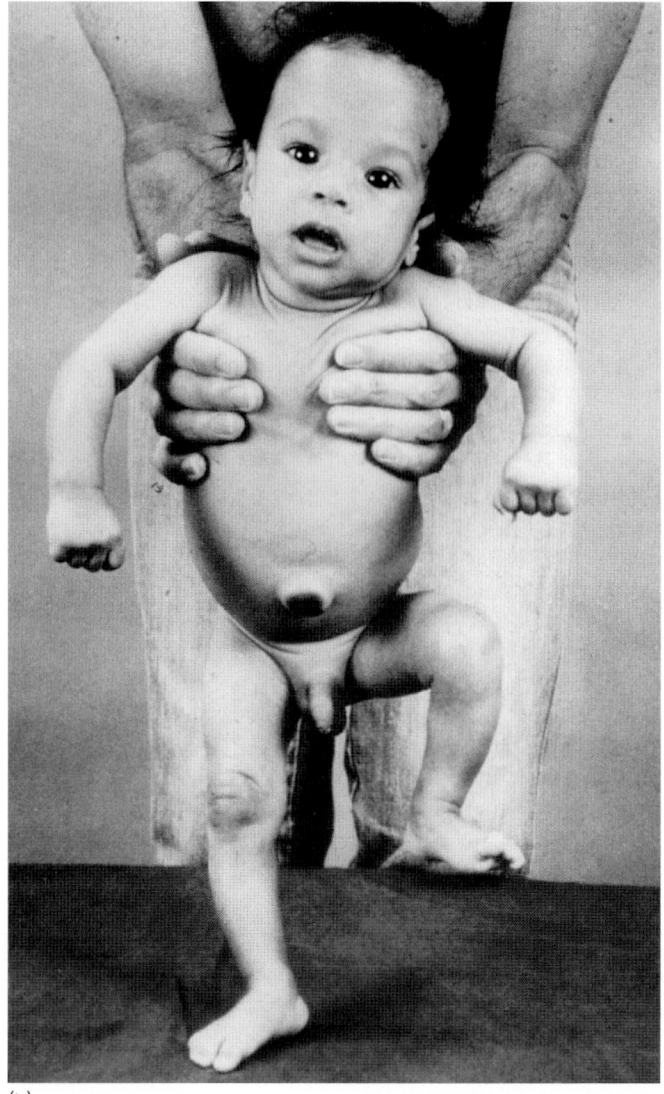

Figure 40.5 (a) A 10-day-old boy with transient neonatal myasthenia. Atypical presentation at birth with diaphragmatic and pharyngeal paralysis in the presence of normal limb and facial movements. The mother had a similar pattern of muscle involvement and developed ventilatory failure postpartum, due to severe diaphragm weakness, responding eventually to plasma exchange and immunosuppressive medication. The baby presented at birth because the mother was not on anticholinesterase medication; this is transferred passively across the placenta and has some transient protective effect. Magnetometry of the rib cage and abdomen, and repetitive stimulation of the peripheral nerve, were both suggestive of muscle fatigue (Heckmatt et al 1987). By 6 weeks of age the baby had made a complete recovery. (b) The infant attempting to stand at the age of 6 months.

(b)

authors performed end-plate electrophysiology on intercostal muscle biopsies and found a variety of pre- and post-synaptic defects, suggesting that congenital myasthenia is a heterogeneous condition.

Historically, two clinical types of non-autoimmune myasthenia, so-called 'familial' and 'congenital' forms, have been described (Vincent et al 1981). The familial infantile type is characterized by episodes of severe respiratory and feeding difficulties at birth or during infancy and normal extraocular movements. Patients show a good response to anticholinesterase treatment and a high remission rate. The disease occurs frequently in siblings and inheritance is probably autosomal recessive. Congenital myasthenia usually develops before the age of 2 years, and in many cases symptoms have been present at birth or in utero. Males tend to be affected more than females and affected siblings are frequently encountered, which also suggests autosomal recessive inheritance. Ocular muscles are the most commonly affected but severe weakness of bulbar, trunk and limb muscles can occur. The symptoms tend to be non-progressive and, in contrast to the familial type, anticholinesterase is not always beneficial and remission is unusual. It is occasionally associated with congenital arthrogryposis (Smit & Barth 1980, Teyssier et al 1982).

This distinction however was somehow confusing as congenital myasthenia is also familial. An ENMC international workshop on congenital myasthenic syndromes in 1995 suggested a new classification based on the mode of inheritance, with type i including the autosomal recessive forms, type ii the autosomal dominant and type iii the sporadic cases. Each type was further subdivided into further subtypes (Middleton 1995). According to this classification the form classically called familial is a subtype of the type i congenital myasthenic syndromes (Ia) and this has created some confusion between the old and new terminology (Deymeer et al 1999). In a new approach to classification the forms have been re-classified according to whether the defect is present at a presynaptic, synaptic or postsynaptic level. Recent studies have been able to demonstrate the defect at the molecular level, identifying several mutations in the gene encoding the collagenic tail subunit of the end-plate species of acetylcholinesterase (Donger et al 1998) and from mutations in acetylcholine receptor (AChR) subunit genes (Engel et al 1998).

OTHER NEUROMUSCULAR DISORDERS
ARTHROGRYPOSIS

This disorder is defined as congenital non-progressive limitation of movement in two or more joints in different body areas (Hageman & Willemse 1983). It is not a diagnosis as such but a symptom complex and the potential and result of several different types of pathological process. There is general agreement that the final mechanism is immobility in utero. This might be produced by restriction of the fetus, or inability of the fetus to move due to some failure of the motor system.

Hall (1985) stated that affected limbs are, on average, 20% shorter than expected for gestational age, while the trunk and head are of normal size, which suggests part of normal limb growth relates to forces engendered by use. Catch-up may occur during vigorous use of limbs and also a return to normal size of lungs, and cranial-facial structures. Hall (1985) states that return of range of motion could occur up to 1 year (in our experience this is a conservative estimate) and relative increases in strength of the muscle for many years.

Prolonged oligohydramnios or a bicornute uterus might be a cause in some cases (Fig. 40.6). It has been generally assumed that very few are due to primary muscle disease. After an extensive review of the literature, Swinyard (1982) estimated that the proportion was only 10–15%. In a study of the spinal cord of 11 infants with arthrogryposis, Clauren and Hall (1983) found a reduction in the number of a motor neurons and an increase in the numbers of small neurons in all but one, and CNS involvement in three. These results cannot be applied to all arthrogryposis patients, as those who die may be a selected population. The Pena–Shokeir syndrome of multiple ankyloses, facial abnormalities, pulmonary hypoplasia and cryptorchidism has been associated with problems in brain formation and loss of anterior horn cells in the spinal cord, but a primary muscle disorder could also have the same clinical end-result (Moerman et al 1983).

There have been relatively few reports of EMG and muscle studies done systematically in arthrogryposis, particularly with modern histochemical techniques. One such study was by Strehl and Vanasse (1985) in 22 patients, and they found ten with a neurogenic cause (five with a spinal origin, two of cerebral origin and three mixed), and nine myopathic (three congenital muscular dystrophy, three congenital myo-

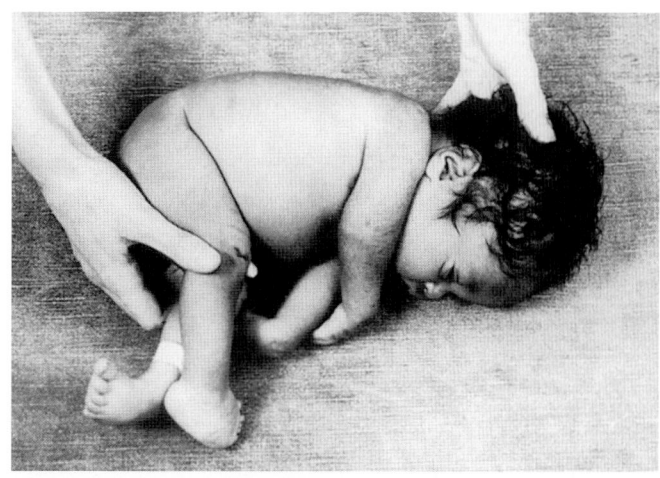

(a)

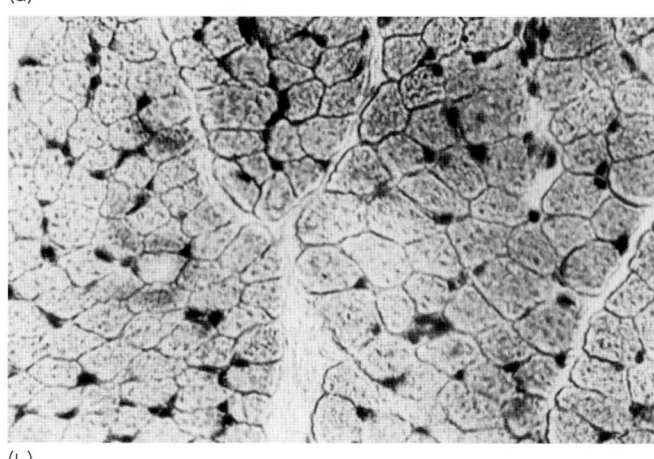

(b)

Figure 40.6 (a) A 2-day-old boy, born at full term with arthrogryposis. Continuous drainage of liquor occurred from the sixth month of pregnancy and fetal movements diminished from that time. He was delivered at full-term. Note the flexion deformities of the fingers and wrists and equinus deformities of the feet but no hip and knee contractures. Shoulder abduction was limited and elbows were held in extension. The muscles of the shoulders were atrophic but there seemed to be reasonable power of the hip and thigh muscles. The trunk seemed normal but there was excessive head lag. The facies was normal. (b) Needle muscle biopsy at 2 days of age (quadriceps) was normal. The arthrogryposis was thought to be due to intrauterine restriction secondary to the oligohydramnios.

tonic dystrophy, one fiber-type disproportion and two non-specific myopathy). One had an inherited malformation syndrome and in two the cause was unknown. They stated that precise diagnosis would have been impossible without needle muscle biopsy. This is more in accord with our own experience, where the most common associated neuromuscular disorder is congenital muscular dystrophy (Fig. 40.7).

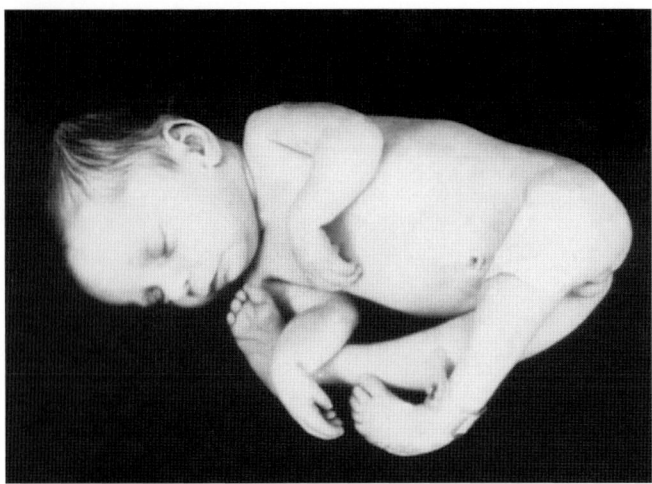

(a)

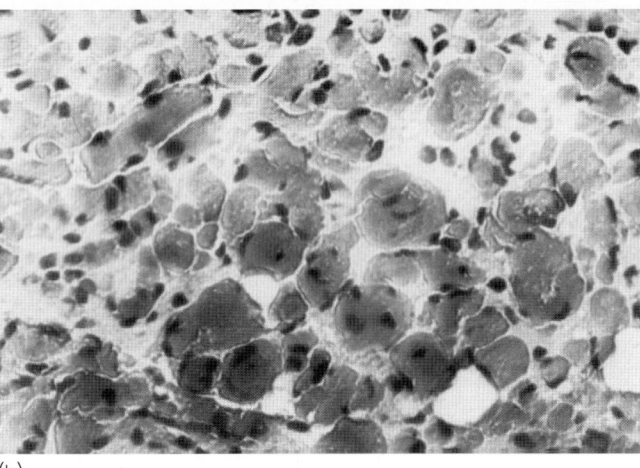

(b)

Figure 40.7 (a) A 2-week-old girl with arthrogryposis and generalized hypotonia. Fetal movements were reduced throughout pregnancy; there was oligohydramnios and poor fetal growth. The baby was delivered at full-term (birth weight 2 Kg) and adopted a 'fetal' position with the arms tucked under the chin and the legs flexed at the hips, the left against the chest and the right along the trunk behind the arm. There were no spontaneous movements of the limbs. She sucked well, however, and there were no breathing difficulties. She had fixed flexion contractures of both elbows, 30° flexion contractures of both wrists, dislocated right hip, right genu recurvatum and severe bilateral talipes. Her serum CK was normal (107 IU/L). (b) Needle muscle biopsy at 2 weeks of age (quadriceps) showed dystrophic change. She had bilateral talectomy to correct the talipes at the age of 19 months and is now standing regularly in a frame.

SPINAL MUSCULAR ATROPHY

Although there is a broad range of severity in classic spinal muscular atrophy, cases presenting in the newborn period usually have the severe infantile form (SMA 1; 'Werdnig–Hoffmann disease') (Dubowitz 1995, 1999). Weakness may already be present at birth or may develop in the first weeks

of life. These infants show a very consistent phenotype characterized by general hypotonia, with axial and limb weakness. The legs are more affected than the arms and proximal muscles more than distal. There is little spontaneous activity, mainly limited to the feet and hands. Facial muscles are spared and the infants show a normal bright expression (Fig. 40.8). The intercostal muscles are always affected but the diaphragm is spared. This is a cardinal feature of spinal muscular atrophy, and indeed the only neuromuscular disorder with paralysis of the intercostals and sparing of the diaphragm. In addition to the extensive paralysis of the limbs and distinctive breathing pattern, other useful pointers to the diagnosis are the characteristic 'jug-handle' posturing of the upper limbs with internal rotation of the shoulders and pronation of the forearms, tongue fasciculation and the bright alert facies (Fig. 40.8). McLeod et al have recently documented some cases of prenatal onset spinal muscular atrophy with reduced fetal movements, severe weakness and asphyxia at birth and short survival time (McLeod et al 1999). Dubowitz (1999) suggested this very severe form of SMA be designated SMA0 on the numerical classification.

When there is a short history of weakness and the muscle biopsy is normal or shows only universal atrophy, the nerve conduction study is useful because it will show an absent or greatly diminished amplitude of the motor action potential, whereas in the myopathies the motor action potential is usually of reasonable size (>0.5 mV). The EMG may show some fibrillation potentials at rest, and isolated motor units of normal size and configuration on volition, but will not show the classic changes of reinnervation (i.e. large isolated motor units).

Spinal muscular atrophy is autosomal recessive, and the severity in affected siblings is usually similar, but occasionally there may be marked discordance in severity.

Infants with Werdnig–Hoffmann disease generally do not show central nervous system involvement, but non-specific changes such as cerebral atrophy or other ischemic changes have been observed in some of these children, mainly associated with prematurity or birth asphyxia (Rudnick-Schoneborn et al 1996).

Management

The median age of survival in infants with SMA 1 is reported to be around 9 months. In the last few years there has been increasing evidence that infants with SMA type 1 may benefit from non-invasive ventilation (Bach et al 2000, 2002, Bush et al 2005). Although there are no systematic double blind studies to establish the long term effect of these procedures on survival, these have become part of the routine in many centers and there is evidence that the combined use of non-invasive ventilation and of other tools that reduce the accumulation of secretions, such as the insufflator-exsufflator machine can increase the chance of survival during acute respiratory infections and the overall management of these children.

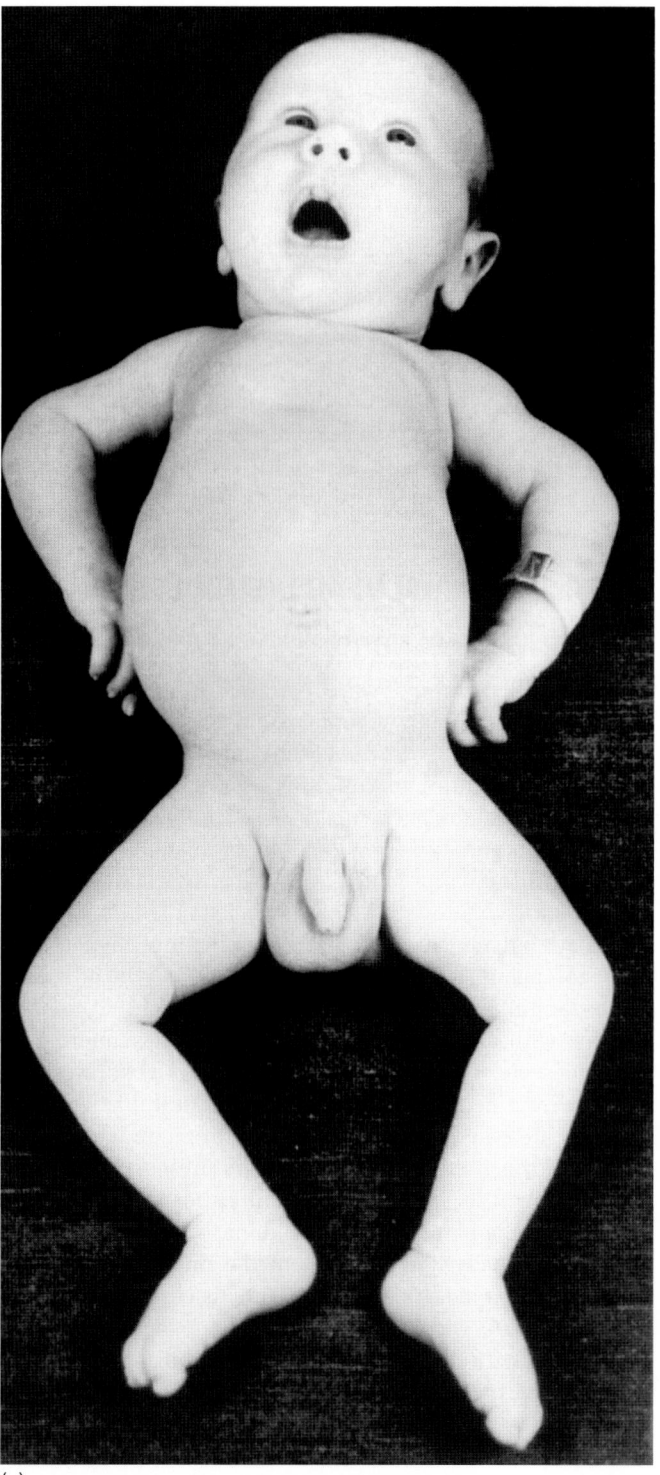

(a)

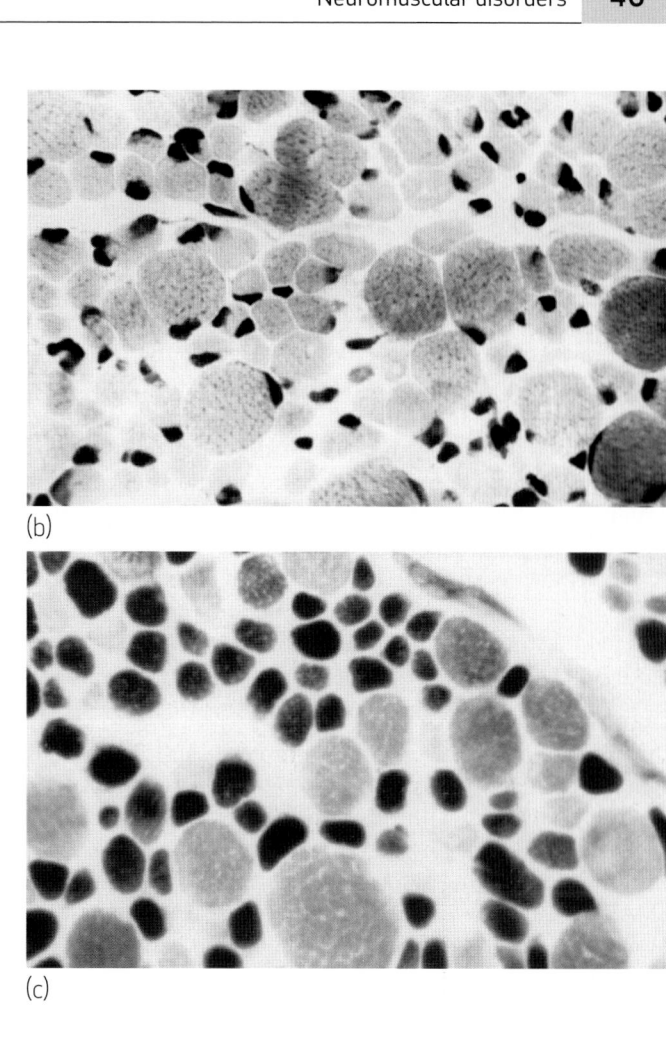

(b)

(c)

Figure 40.8 (a) A 4-week-old boy with severe spinal muscular atrophy. There was insidious onset of weakness with poor limb movement and internal rotation of the arms. Fetal movements were normal, and movements seemed normal at birth. Note the typical frog posture, together with the jug-handle posture of the arms and internal rotation at the shoulders, and the alert facies. There is also a narrow chest with poor intercostal movement and a distended abdomen, reflecting the well-preserved diaphragmatic function. With inspiration there is further expansion of the abdomen and costal retraction. Tongue fasciculation was present. Motor nerve conduction (peroneal nerve) showed a markedly reduced motor action potential at 0.05 mV (normal >0.5 mV). Electromyography of the quadriceps showed fasciculation potentials at rest but no activity on volition. (b) Needle muscle biopsy (quadriceps) at 4 weeks of age showed variability in fiber size (H and E) (c) The larger fibers were all type 1, suggestive of some reinnervation (ATPase 9.5).

It has recently also been suggested that other measures such as gastrostomy at the onset of swallowing problems or even before their onset may also help not only to prolong survival but also to improve management and quality of life, reducing the risk of choking episodes and aspiration pneumonia.

Molecular genetics

The gene for the autosomal recessive, proximal symmetrical spinal muscular atrophies was localized to chromosome 5q11-q13 in 1990 (Melki et al 1990a, 1990b), but it took another 5 years before the molecular defect, was identified by Lefevbre et al (1995) because of the duplication of this part of chromosome 5. The hitherto unknown gene was designated survival motor neuron gene (SMN) and in over 95% of classic cases there was a deletion of exon 7 in the active telomeric copy of the SMN gene, now designated SMN1. This has provided a very useful and rapid diagnostic tool, and also opened the possibility for prenatal diagnosis of chorionic villus biopsy.

Diaphragmatic SMA

Diaphragmatic spinal muscular atrophy, also known as spinal muscular atrophy with respiratory distress (SMARD), is another disorder with onset in infancy characterized by spinal muscular atrophy and diaphragmatic weakness, with early life-threatening respiratory failure. The prevalence of SMARD is unknown, but it has been estimated that diaphragmatic paralysis could comprise about 1% of patients with early-onset SMA (Rudnik-Schöneborn et al 1996).

In contrast to the typical spinal muscular atrophy (SMA) with proximal limb involvement, the distal muscles are predominantly involved in SMARD. Another striking clinical difference is that in SMARD respiratory distress results from severe diaphragmatic paralysis with an elevation of both hemidiaphragms on chest X-ray, while in typical SMA the diaphragm is spared and the respiratory pattern is mainly diaphragmatic and the intercostal muscles are more severely affected, showing costal recession with inspiration.

SMARD is a clinically and genetically heterogeneous condition. SMARD1 results from mutations in the gene encoding the immunoglobulin-binding protein 2 (IGHMBP2) on chromosome 11q13.

Pontocerebellar hypoplasia type 1

In the condition called pontocerebellar hypoplasia type 1, spinal muscular atrophy is associated with hypoplasia of the cerebellar vermis and, often also of the cerebellar hemispheres, associated with a thin brainstem and pons (Barth 1993). Infants affected by this form show a combination of clinical signs related to both spinal and central nervous system involvement. The clinical course is progressive, and respiratory and feeding difficulties, already present at birth or in early infancy, become more severe.

Molecular genetics

This form is not allelic to SMA (Dubowitz et al 1995) and the gene responsible for this form has not yet been identified.

The differential diagnosis is with other forms, such as the *carbohydrate-deficient glycoconjugate* syndromes which show cerebellar and brainstem hypoplasia and peripheral nerve involvement. The *carbohydrate-deficient glycoconjugate* syndromes include a group of genetic disorders characterized by a deficiency of the carbohydrate moiety of glycoconjugates (Jaeken et al 1991, 1997). Type 1 is the most common and has been related to a deficit in phosphomannomutase. Infants present with dysmorphic features, hypotonia and hyporeflexia, abnormal eye movements and poor feeding. Other signs, such as skeletal abnormalities, hepatomegaly, proteinuria and cardiomyopathy, are also frequent. The involvement of the peripheral nerves is shown by abnormal motor and sensory nerve conduction velocity. Brain MRI shows brainstem and cerebellar hypoplasia (Akaboshi et al 1995, Jaeken 1991, 1997).

NON-NEUROMUSCULAR DISORDERS

PRADER–WILLI SYNDROME

Prader–Willi syndrome usually presents in the newborn period with profound hypotonia associated with sucking and swallowing difficulty, without any associated respiratory problems, in contrast to conditions such as myotonic dystrophy or myotubular myopathy, which have both. With time the hypotonia resolves, and all these children become ambulant, but then problems with hyperphagia and obesity usually start.

It is a relatively common disorder with an estimated incidence of about 1 in 10 000 births. It occurs in all races. It was originally described by Prader et al (1956), in five patients with adiposity, short stature, mental subnormality and undescended testes in the males. There is a characteristic facies, with a high forehead, narrow bifrontal diameter, upslanting almond-shaped palpebral fissures, and triangular mouth with a thin upper lip. Squint is present in approximately two-thirds, and there are small hands and feet, which may be more apparent in later childhood. The facies may be more distinctively abnormal when the infant is crying, as these infants tend to screw up the face in a particular way (Fig. 40.9). The striking feature about these infants, in comparison with those with neuromuscular disorders, is that the severity of the hypotonia is disproportionate to the intermittently good antigravity movements which may be observed.

There is no neuromuscular involvement; the EMG, nerve conduction velocity and muscle biopsy are normal. Diagnosis is primarily clinical. Routine chromosome analysis is usually normal in these patients, but with high-resolution techniques a deletion may be demonstrated on the long arm of chromosome 15 (15q12) (Fear et al 1985, Ledbetter et al 1982). A further important observation was that the deletion appears to be of paternal origin (Butler & Palmer 1983). Recent advances with molecular genetic techniques have shown that those cases without an overt deletion usually

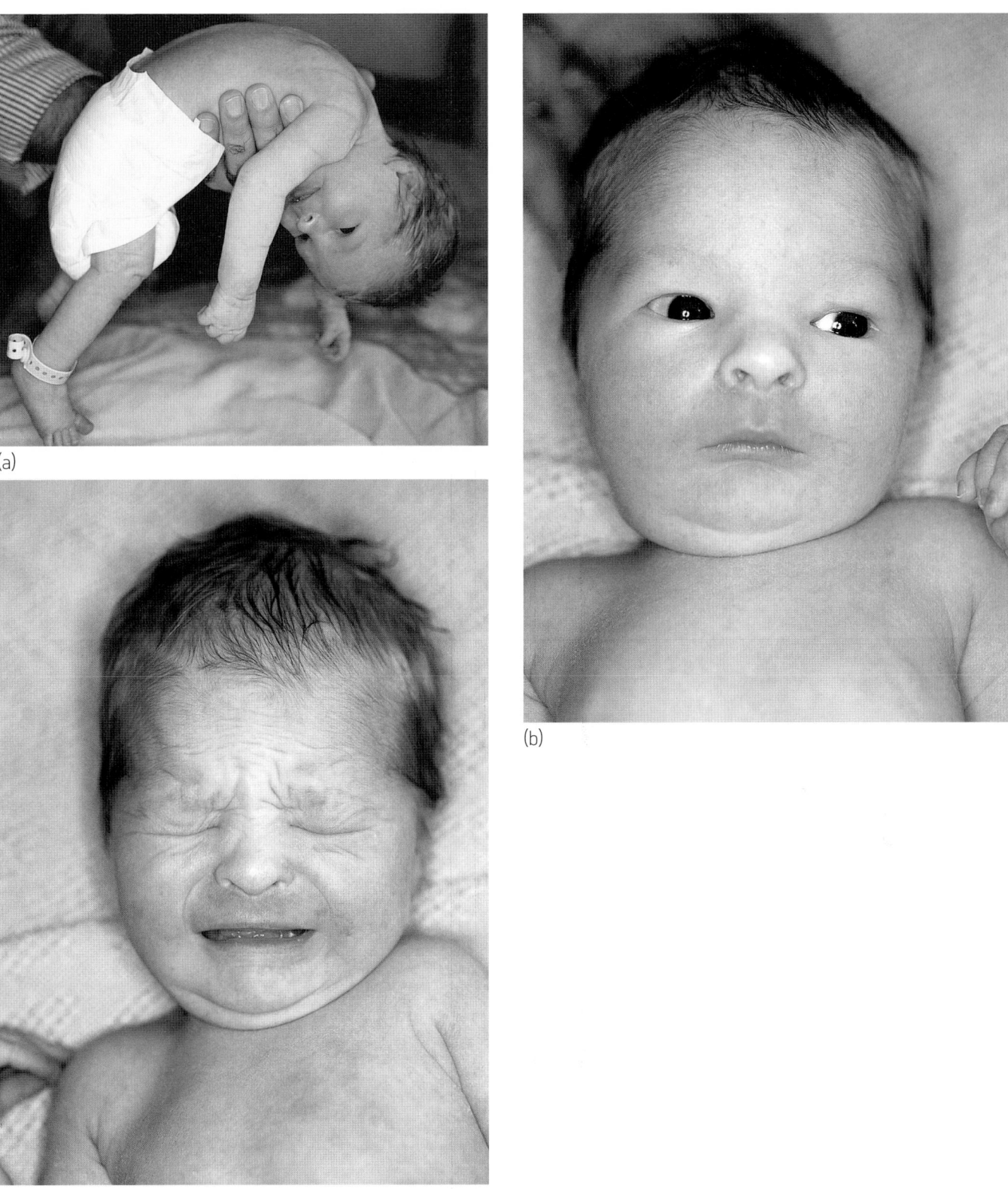

(a)

(b)

(c)

Figure 40.9 Male infant with Prader–Willi syndrome. (a) The baby was clearly hypotonic on day 4. (b) The facies show dysmorphic features at rest. (c) There is excessive wrinkling of the forehead when crying.

have maternal disomy, with two copies of the maternal chromosome and a corresponding absence of the paternal contribution. This is an example of genetic imprinting.

CONCLUSION

Hopefully this comprehensive description will alert the clinician to the wide range of neuromuscular and non-neuromuscular disorders that may present in the neonatal period with hypotonia and associated problems. A good clinical assessment of the baby and of the mother remains the first important step towards a provisional clinical diagnosis, and giving guidance as to the appropriate investigations to establish a definitive diagnosis. Inappropriate and unnecessary investigations often delay the diagnosis in these cases.

REFERENCES

Akaboshi S, Ohno K, Takeshita K 1995 Neuroradiological findings in the carbohydrate-deficient glycoprotein syndrome. Neuroradiology 37:491–495.

Albers J W, Faulkner J A, Dorovini-Zis K et al 1984 Abnormal neuromuscular transmission in an infantile myasthenic syndrome. Ann Neuro 16:28–34.

Aslanidis C, Jansen G, Amemiya C et al 1992 Cloning of the essential myotonic dystrophy region and mapping the putative defect. Nature 355:1253–1255.

Bach J R, Baird J S, Plosky D et al 2002 Spinal muscular atrophy type 1: management and outcomes. Pediatr Pulmonol 34:16–22.

Bach J R, Niranjan V, Weaver B 2000 Spinal muscular atrophy type 1: A noninvasive respiratory management approach. Chest 117:1100–1105.

Balci B, Uyanik G, Dincer P et al 2005 An autosomal recessive limb girdle muscular dystrophy (LGMD2) with mild mental retardation is allelic to Walker–Warburg syndrome (WWS) caused by a mutation in the POMT1 gene. Neuromuscul Disord 15:271–275.

Barth P G 1993 Pontocerebellar hypoplasia. An overview of a group of inherited neurodegenerative disorders with fetal onset. Brain Dev 15:411–422.

Beltran-Valero de Bernabe D, Currier S, Steinbrecher A et al 2002 Mutations in the O-mannosyltransferase gene POMT1 give rise to the severe neuronal migration disorder Walker–Warburg syndrome. Am J Hum Genet 71:1033–1043.

Beltran-Valero de Bernabe D, van Bokhoven H, van Beusekom E et al 2003 A homozygous nonsense mutation in the Fukutin gene causes a Walker–Warburg syndrome phenotype. J Med Genet 40:845–848.

Beltran-Valero de Bernabe D, Voit T, Longman C et al 2004 Mutations in the FKRP gene can cause muscle-eye-brain disease and Walker–Warburg syndrome. J Med Genet 41:e61.

Brockington M, Blake DJ, Prandini P et al 2001 Mutations in the fukutin-related protein gene (FKRP) cause a form of congenital muscular dystrophy with secondary laminin alpha2 deficiency and abnormal glycosylation of alpha-dystroglycan. Am J Hum Genet 69:1198–1209.

Bush A, Fraser J, Jardine E et al 2005 Respiratory management of the infant with type 1 spinal muscular atrophy. Arch Dis Child 90:709–711.

Butler M G, Palmer C G 1983 Parental origin of chromosome 15 deletion in Prader–Willi syndrome. Lancet i:1285–1286.

Buxton J, Shelbourne P, Davies J et al 1992 Detection of an unstable DNA specific to individuals with myotonic dystrophy. Nature 355:547–548.

Clauren S K, Hall J G 1983 Neuropathological findings in the spinal cords of 10 infants with arthrogryposis. J Neurol Sci 58:89–102.

Conomy J P, Levinsohn M, Fanaroff A 1975 Familial infantile myasthenia gravis: a cause of sudden death in young children. J Pediatr 87:428–430.

Currier S C, Lee C K, Chang B S et al 2005 Mutations in POMT1 are found in a minority of patients with Walker–Warburg syndrome. Am J Med Genet A 133:53–57.

Deymeer F, Serdaroglu P, Ozdemir C 1999 Familial infantile myasthenia: confusion in terminology. Neuromusc Disord 9:129–130.

Dobyns W B, Pagon R A, Armstrong D et al 1989 Diagnostic criteria for Walker–Warburg syndrome. Am J Med Genet 32:195–210.

Dodge P R, Gamstorp I, Byers R K et al 1965 Myotonic dystrophy in infancy and childhood. Pediatrics 35:3–19.

Donger C, Krejci E, Pou Serradell, A et al 1998 Mutation in the human acetylcholinesterase-associated collagen gene, COLQ, is responsible for congenital myasthenic syndrome with end-plate acetylcholinesterase deficiency (Type Ic). Am J Hum Genet 63:967–975.

Dubowitz V 1980 The floppy infant, 2nd edn. Heinemann, London.

Dubowitz V 1985 Muscle biopsy, a practical approach. Baillière Tindall, London.

Dubowitz V 1995 Muscle disorders in childhood, 2nd edn. Saunders, London.

Dubowitz V 1999 Very severe spinal muscular atrophy (SMA type 0): an expanding clinical phenotype. Eur J Paediatr Neurol 3:49–52.

Dubowitz V, Daniels R J, Davies K E 1995 Olivopontocerebellar hypoplasia with anterior horn cell involvement (SMA) does not localize to chromosome 5q. Neuromusc Disord 5:25–29.

Engel A G, Ohno K, Milone M, Sine S M 1998 Congenital myasthenic syndromes. New insights from molecular genetic and patch-clamp studies. Ann N Y Acad Sci 13(841):140–156.

Fear C N, Mutton D E, Berry A C et al 1985 Chromosome 15 in Prader–Willi syndrome. Dev Med Child Neurol 27:305–311.

Fukuyama Y, Osawa M, Suzuki H 1981 Congenital progressive muscular dystrophy of the Fukuyama type — clinical, genetic and pathological considerations. Brain Dev 3:1–29.

Hageman G, Willemse J 1983 Arthrogryposis multiplex congenita. Neuropediatrics 14:6–11.

Hall J G 1985 In utero movement and use of limbs are necessary for normal growth: a study of individuals with arthrogryposis. Prog Clin Biol Res 200:155–162.

Harper P S 1975a Congenital myotonic dystrophy in Britain. 11. Genetic basis. Arch Dis Childhood 50:514–521.

Harper P S 1975b Congenital myotonic dystrophy in Britain. 1. Clinical aspects. Arch Dis Childhood 50:505–513.

Heckmatt J Z, Dubowitz V 1987 Ultrasound imaging and directed needle biopsy in the diagnosis of selective involvement in neuromuscular disease. J Child Neurol 2:205–213.

Heckmatt J Z, Moosa A, Hutson C et al 1984 Diagnostic needle muscle biopsy, a practical and reliable alternative to open biopsy. Arch Dis Childhood 59:528–532.

Heckmatt J Z, Sewry C A, Hodes D et al 1985 Congenital centronuclear (myotubular) myopathy: a clinical and genetic study in eight children. Brain 108:941–964.

Helbling-Leclerc A, Zhang X, Topaloglu H et al 1995 Mutations in the laminin alpha 2-chain gene (LAMA2) cause merosin-deficient congenital muscular dystrophy. Nat Genet 11:216–218.

Jaeken J, Casaer P 1997 Carbohydrate-deficient glyconjugate (CDG) syndromes: a new chapter of neuropaediatrics. Eur J Paediatr Neurol 2/3:61–66.

Jaeken J, Stibler H, Hagberg B 1991 The carbohydrate-deficient glycoprotein syndrome: a new inherited multisystemic disease with severe nervous system involvement. Acta Paediatr Scand Suppl 375: monograph.

Kondo-Iida E, Kobayashi K, Watanabe M et al 1999 Novel mutations and genotype-phenotype relationships in 107 families with Fukuyama-type congenital muscular dystrophy (FCMD). Hum Mol Genet 8:2303–2309.

Kuitunen P, Rapola J, Noponen A L et al 1972 Nemaline myopathy. Acta Paediatr Scand 61:353–361.

Ledbetter D H, Mascarello J T, Riccardi V M et al 1982 Chromosome 15 abnormalities and the Prader–Willi syndrome: follow-up report of 40 cases. Am J Hum Genet 34:278–285.

Lefebvre S, Bürglen L, Reboullet S et al 1995 Identification and characterization of a spinal muscular atrophy-determining gene. Cell 13(80):1–5.

Lefvert A K, Osterman P O 1983 Newborn infants to myasthenic mothers: a clinical study and an investigation of acetylcholine receptor antibodies in 17 children. Neurology 33:133–138.

MacLeod M J, Taylor J E, Lunt P W et al 1999 Prenatal onset spinal muscular atrophy. Eur J Paediatr Neurol 3:65–72.

Melki J, Abdelhak S, Sheth P et al 1990a Gene for chronic proximal spinal muscular atrophies maps to chromosome 5q. Nature 344:767–768.

Melki J, Sheth P, Abdelhak S et al 1990b Mapping of acute (type 1) spinal muscular atrophy to chromosome 5q12–q14. Lancet 336:271–273.

Mercuri E, Brockington M, Straub V et al 2003 Phenotypic spectrum associated with mutations in the fukutin-related protein gene. Ann Neurol 53:537–542.

Mercuri E, Longman C 2005 Congenital muscular dystrophy. Pediatr Ann 34:564–568.

Mercuri E, Pennock J, Goodwin F et al 1996 Sequential study of central and peripheral nervous system involvement in an infant with merosin-deficient CMD. Neuromusc Disord 6:425–429.

Mercuri E, Rutherford M, De Vile C et al 2001 Early white matter changes on brain magnetic resonance imaging in a newborn affected by merosin-deficient congenital muscular dystrophy. Neuromuscul Disord 11:297–299.

Middleton L T 1995Report on the 34th ENMC International workshop — congenital myasthenia syndromes. Neuromusc Disord 6:133–136.

Moerman P H, Fryns J P, Goddeeris P et al 1983 Multiple ankyloses, facial anomalies, and pulmonary hypoplasia associated with severe antenatal spinal muscular atrophy. J Pediatr 103:238–241.

Muntoni F, Voit T 2005 133rd ENMC International Workshop on Congenital Muscular Dystrophy (IXth International CMD Workshop) 21–23 January 2005, Naarden, The Netherlands. Neuromuscul Disord 15:794–801.

Namba T, Brown S B, Grob D 1970 Neonatal myasthenia gravis: report of two cases and review of the literature. Pediatrics 45:488–504.

Neustein H B 1973 Nemaline myopathy, a family study with three autopsied cases. Arch Pathol 96:192–195.

Norton P, Ellison P, Sulaiman A R et al 1983 Nemaline myopathy in the neonate. Neurology 33:351–356.

O'Brien J A, Harper P S 1984 Course prognosis and complications of childhood onset myotonic dystrophy. Dev Med Child Neurol 26:62–67.

Ohno K, Anlar B, Engel A G 1999 Congenital myasthenic syndrome caused by a mutation in the Ets binding site of the promoter region of the acetylcoline receptor ε subunit gene. Neuromusc Disord 9:131–135.

Prader A, Labhart A, Willi H 1956 Ein Syndrom von Adipositas, Kleinwuchs, Kryptorchismus und Oligophrenie nach Myatonieartigm zustand im Neugeborenenatter. Schweizerische Medizinische Wochenschrift 86:1260–1261.

Regev R, de Vries L S, Heckmatt J Z et al 1987 Cerebral ventricular dilation in congenital myotonic dystrophy. J Pediatr 111:372–376.

Robertson W C, Chun R W M, Kornguth S E 1980 Familial infantile myasthenia. Arch Neurol 37:117–119.

Rudnick-Schöneborn, Forkert R, Hahnen E et al 1996 Clinical spectrum and diagnostic criteria of infantile spinal muscular atrophy: further delineation on the basis of SMN deletion findings. Neuropediatrics 27:8–15.

Shafiq S A, Dubowitz V, Hart de C Peterson et al 1967 Nematine myopathy: report of a fatal case, with histochemical and electron microscopic studies. Brain 90:817–828.

Smit L M E, Barth P G 1980 Arthrogryposis multiplex congenita due to congenital myasthenia. Dev Med Child Neurol 22:371–373.

Strehl E, Vanasse M 1985 EMG and needle muscle biopsy studies in arthrogryposis multiplex congenita. Neuropediatrics 16:225–227.

Swinyard C A 1982 Concepts of multiple congenital contractures in man and animals. Teratology 25:247–258.

Tan P, Briner J, Bolthauser E et al 1998 Homozygosity for a nonsense mutation in the alpha-tropomyosin gene TPM3 in a patient with severe congenital nemaline myopathy. Neuromuscular Disord 9:573–579.

Tanner S M, Laporte J, Guiraud-Chaumeil C et al 1998 Confirmation of prenatal diagnosis results of X-linked recessive myotubular myopathy by mutational screening and description of three new mutations in the MTM1 gene. Hum Mutat 11:62–68.

Teyssier G, Damon G, Bertheas M F et al 1982 Congenital myasthenia and arthrogryposis: apropos of 2 cases manifesting at birth. Pediatrie 37:295–298.

Thomas N S T, Williams H, Cole G et al 1990 X-linked neonatal centronuclear/myotubular myopathy: evidence for linkage to Xq28 DNA marker loci. J Med Genet 27:284–287.

Tsujihata M, Shimomura C, Yoshimura T et al 1983 Fatal neonatal myopathy; a case report. J Neurosurg Psychiatry 46:856–859.

Vanier T M 1960 Dystrophia myotonica in childhood. Br Med J ii:1284–1288.

Vasta I, Kinali M, Messina S et al 2005 Can clinical signs identify newborns with neuromuscular disorders? J Pediatr 146:73–79.

Vincent A, Cull-Candy S Q, Newsom-Davis J et al 1981 Congenital myasthenia: end plate acetylcholine receptors and electrophysiology in five cases. Muscle and Nerve 4:306–318.

Voit T 1998 Congenital muscular dystrophies: 1997 update. Brain Dev 20:65–74.

Wallgreen-Petterson C, Avela K, Marchmand S et al 1995 A gene for autosomal recessive nemaline myopathy assigned to chromosome 2q by linkage analysis. Neuromusc Disord 5:441–443.

Wallgreen-Petterson C, Laing N G 1996 Nemaline myopathy. Neuromusc Disord 6:389–391.

Wallgreen-Pettersson C, Thomas N S T 1994 A report on the 20th ENMC sponsored workshop: myotubular/centronuclear myopathy. Neuromusc Disord 4:71–74.

Wallgren-Petterson C 1998 Genetics of the nemaline myopathies and the myotubular myopathies. Neuromuscul Disord 8:401–404.

Wallgren-Petterson C, Laign N G 2006 138th ENMC Workshop: nemaline myopathy, 20–22 May 2005, Naarden, The Netherlands. Neuromuscul Disord 16:54–60.

Wallgren-Petterson C, Pelin K, Nowack K J et al 2004 ENMC International Consortium On Nemaline Myopathy. Genotype-phenotype correlations in nemaline myopathy caused by mutations in the genes for nebulin and skeletal muscle alpha-actin. Neuromuscul Disord 14:461–470.

Yoshioka M, Saiwai S, Kuroki S, Nigami H 1991 MR imaging of the brain in Fukuyama-type congenital muscular dystrophy. AJNR Am J Neuroradiol 12:63–65.

CHAPTER

41

Fetal neurosurgical interventions

Lan T. Vu, Russell W. Jennings, Robert H. Ball and Hanmin Lee

---

Key Points

- Fetal surgery can now be considered if: prenatal diagnostic methods can accurately identify fetuses that would most benefit, the pathophysiology and natural history of the disease are well understood, the natural history can be altered by intervention and the risk to the mother is small
- The successful treatment of neonatal hydrocephalus with postnatal CSF shunting generated considerable enthusiasm to attempt prenatal treatment of fetal hydrocephalus, but results to date have not been encouraging
- Approximately 25% of MMCs can be prevented by adequate dietary folic acid intake during pregnancy; a significant number will still develop despite adequate replacement
- With widespread maternal serum alpha-fetoprotein screening and the use of high-resolution ultrasonography, over 80% of the cases of fetal MMC are now detectable in the mid-second trimester of pregnancy
- Despite early detection, management options have been limited to either termination or continuation of the pregnancy with neonatal therapy
- Open fetal surgery for myelomeningocele has emerged as a viable solution to prevent neurological dysfunction in the newborn
- Fetal surgery remains an innovative treatment strategy and is not currently the standard of care for any neurological anomalies
- The principal obstacle still encountered in fetal surgery is maternal morbidity and fetal morbidity and mortality from preterm labor
- Ultimately, the decision to widely apply in utero surgical techniques for neurological anomalies as well as for other organ system anomalies will depend on the long-term effectiveness of the treatment protocols and their ethical acceptability in terms of safety for the mother and quality of life for the affected infant

---

INTRODUCTION

Fetal neurosurgical intervention is the natural sequela of advances in sonography and invasive diagnostic procedures that have dramatically changed the understanding and management of many congenital neurological anomalies. Prenatal sonographic detection and serial examinations have made it possible not only to define their natural history, but also to determine the features that most affect clinical outcome. Sonography can now identify a growing number of disorders at a stage of development early enough to plan management strategies to improve prognosis. Fetal surgery can now be considered if: (1) prenatal diagnostic methods can accurately identify fetuses that would most benefit; (2) the pathophysiology and natural history of the disease are well understood; (3) the natural history can be altered by intervention; and (4) the risk to the mother is small (Harrison 1993). From the fetus' perspective, the risk

of the procedure is weighed against the benefit of correcting a fatal or debilitating defect. The risks and benefits for a mother are more difficult to assess. She must incur the risk of surgery and preterm labor while not deriving any direct health benefits. If the uterus is opened, the mother may require a cesarean section for all subsequent births to prevent the possibility of uterine rupture. It still remains unknown whether in utero intervention for hydrocephalus and myelomeningocele potentially offers better outcomes than management by medical and surgical therapy after term delivery.

TREATMENT OF FETAL HYDROCEPHALUS

ANIMAL STUDIES

The successful treatment of neonatal hydrocephalus with postnatal CSF shunting generated considerable enthusiasm in attempting prenatal treatment of fetal hydrocephalus. Experimentally, Michejda and Hodgen (1981) created a fetal rhesus monkey model of fetal hydrocephalus by administering the teratogen triamcinolone acetonide to pregnant females during the first several weeks of gestation resulting in hydrocephalus and neural tube defects in 90% of fetuses. They followed the neural tube defects and development of hydrocephalus using ultrasonography, alpha-fetoprotein levels and fetoscopy. Untreated hydrocephalic monkeys developed severe, progressive ventricular enlargement, marked growth retardation, poor coordination and frequent seizures; most died within 2 weeks of delivery. The monkeys that received antenatal CSF shunts at the beginning of the third trimester not only survived, but also demonstrated markedly superior postnatal development of motor skills and grew at near-normal rates (Michejda & Hodgen 1981). Glick and Harrison, working with fetal lambs and monkeys, created animal models of hydrocephalus uncomplicated by concomitant neurological abnormalities by injecting kaolin into the cisterna magna during the third trimester (Glick et al 1984). They reported that shunting, 21–25 days later, improved gross ventriculomegaly and overall survival.

HUMAN STUDIES

Birnholz and Frigoletto (1981) described the first human trial of in utero treatment of hydrocephalus in a fetus with progressive hydrocephalus diagnosed at 24 weeks. Six serial, atraumatic, cephalocenteses were performed between weeks 25 and 32 under ultrasound guidance (Fig. 41.1a–d). After

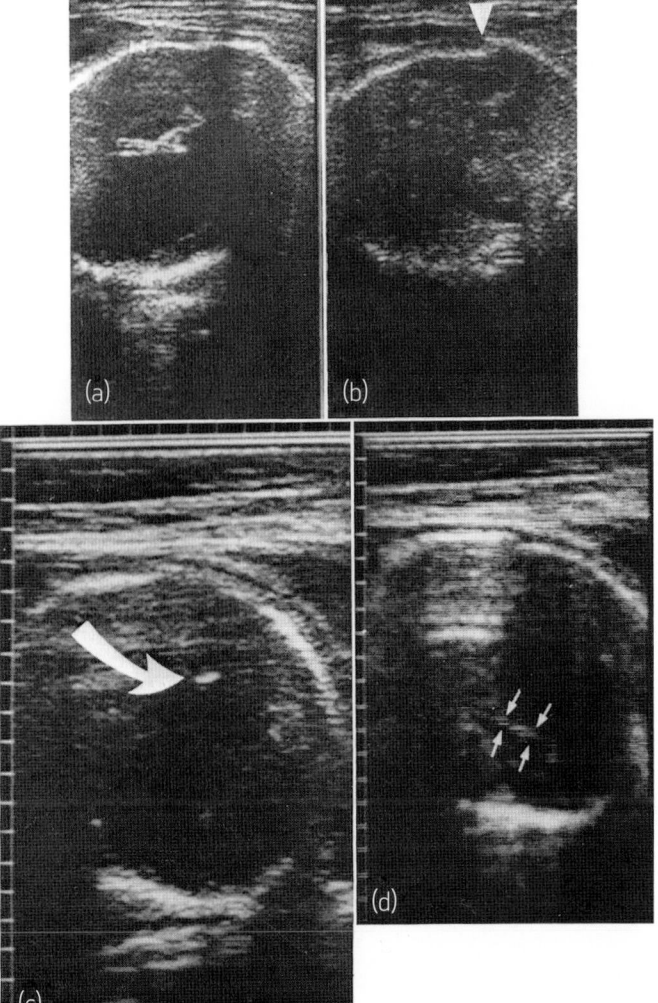

Figure 41.1 (a) Sonogram of fetal head prior to cephalocentesis. (b) Sonogram of fetal head after cephalocentesis with arrow pointing to overlapping cranial sutures. (c) Sonogram of fetal head with arrow pointing to tip of 18-gauge needle in dilated ventricle. (d) Sonogram of fetal head after cephalocentesis, with arrows outlining stream of blood.

the 28th week, cranial puncture became increasingly difficult because of advanced ossification. Delivered at 35 weeks of gestation, the infant received a postnatal ventricular-peritoneal shunt; however, at 16 months of age, the infant remained severely developmentally retarded. It was later discovered that the infant had Becker muscular dystrophy and unrecognized intracranial abnormalities (Cromblehome 1994). Nevertheless, it was felt that intermittent serial cephalocentesis would not be able to deliver consistent ventricular decompression (Lorber & Grainger 1983, Milhorat 1978).

This led to the development of experimental ventriculo-amniotic shunt systems. Clewell et al (1982) described the first ventriculo-amniotic shunt placement for hydrocephalus

in a human fetus in 1982 (Fig. 41.2a–c). The fetus carried a diagnosis of X-linked aqueductal stenosis, and the treatment plan was conceived and performed by a multispecialty team of perinatologists, radiologists, a neurosurgeon, a bioengineer and a geneticist. After the procedure, there was a decrease in the ventricular size, lateral ventricle width to hemisphere width ratio and biparietal diameter, with a concomitant increase in cortical mantle thickness. The infant was delivered at 32 weeks of gestation, and a standard ventriculo-peritoneal shunt was placed postnatally. Several other groups reported similar decreases in ventricular size after shunt placement (Depp et al 1983, Duncan et al 1982, Frigoletto et al 1982).

The following guidelines for fetal hydrocephalus patient selection were recommended by Frigoletto et al 1981 (Birnholz & Frigoletto 1981).

1. The hydrocephalus should be detected sufficiently early that delivery and postnatal shunting are not realistic options.
2. The hydrocephalus should appear as a simple obstructive variety without associated major dysmorphic brain development.
3. The hydrocephalus should not be associated with other major malformations that are incompatible with survival or that indicate an irremediable malformation syndrome.
4. Each pregnancy should be evaluated for chromosomal abnormalities and associated neural tube defects during initial work-up.
5. The ventricular dilatation should be progressive.
6. Pretreatment evaluation should include a multidisciplinary team's consultation with physicians in perinatology, neonatology, ultrasonography, neurosurgery and genetics.

The consensus in the early 1980s was that the ideal patient for intervention was one with progressive ventriculomegaly that was isolated from any concomitant congenital anomalies. Subsequently, the international Fetal Surgery Registry was established in 1982 with the dual goal of (1) providing updated information on cumulative results to all inquiring institutions and (2) accumulating data to assess treatment efficacy and safety (Clewell et al 1982, Manning et al 1986). In 1986, the results of 44 procedures for obstructive hydrocephalus reported to the registry over the preceding 3 years were published (Table 41.1) (Manning et al 1986). These cases were drawn from a large number of centers but had no consistent selection criteria for intervention. In this series of patients, the survival after in utero shunt placement was 83%. However, the overall mortality was 19%, over half of which were procedure-related (10.25%) (Fig. 41.3a–c). Even more troubling was that 53% of survivors were left with moderate to serious neurological handicaps and only 12% developed normally (Manning et al 1986). Although these shunt systems had sparked considerable enthusiasm, it became clear that the results were poor (Cromblehome 1994).

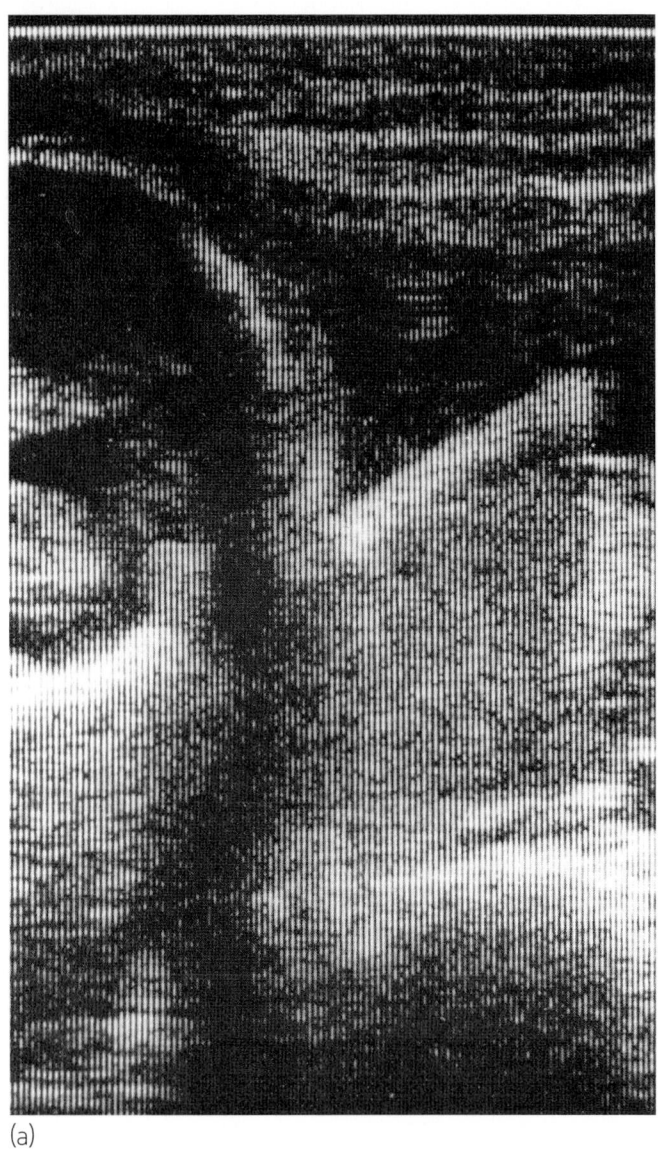

(a)

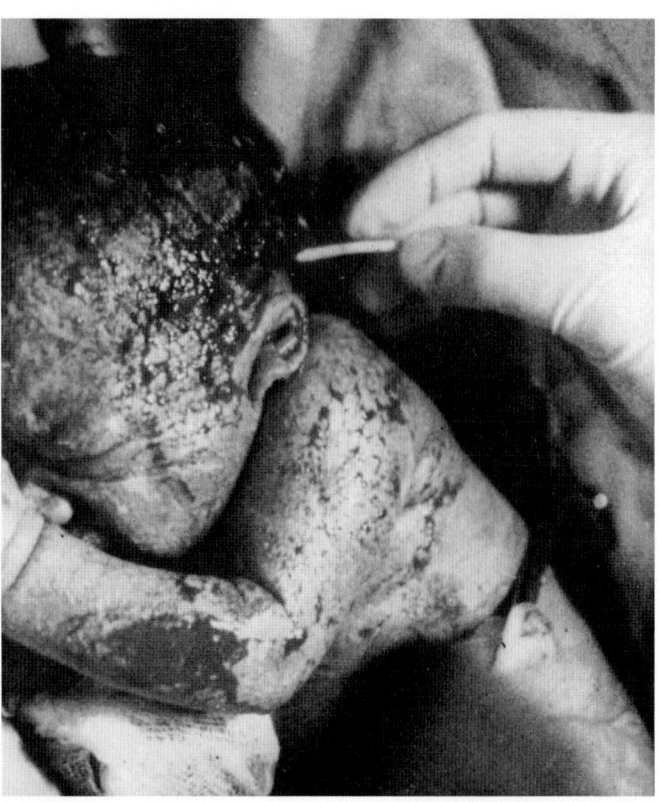

(b)

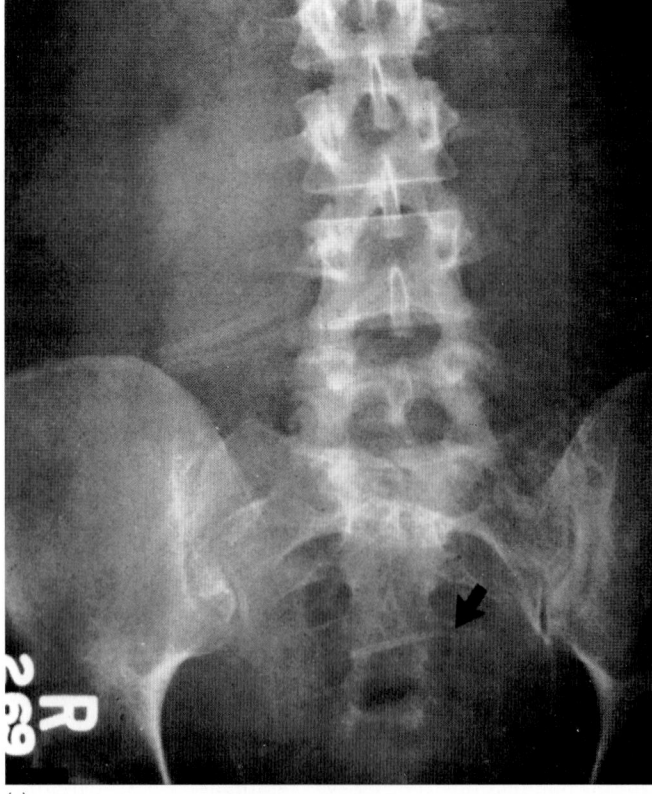

(c)

Figure 41.2 (a) Cranial sonogram demonstrating ventriculoamniotic shunt protruding from fetal skull. (b) Ventriculoamniotic shunt protruding from skull of newborn infant. (c) Radiograph demonstrating ventriculoamniotic shunt entering fetal skull (arrow).

Table 41.1 Fetal obstructive hydrocephalus: distribution by primary diagnosis and survival in 41 treated cases

Primary diagnosis (postnatal)	No of cases	Percentage of total cases diagnosis	No of deaths	Percentage mortality by	No of survivors	Percentage survival by diagnosis
Aqueductal stenosis	32	76.9	4	13.3	28	87.5
Associated anomalies	5	12.7	2	40	3	60
Holoprosencephaly	1	2.6	0	0	1	100
Dandy–Walker syndrome	1	2.6	0	0	1	100
Parencephalic cyst	1	2.6	0	0	1	100
Arnold–Chiari syndrome	1	2.6	0	0	1	100
Total	41	100	17	17	34	83

Source: Adapted from Manning et al (1986).

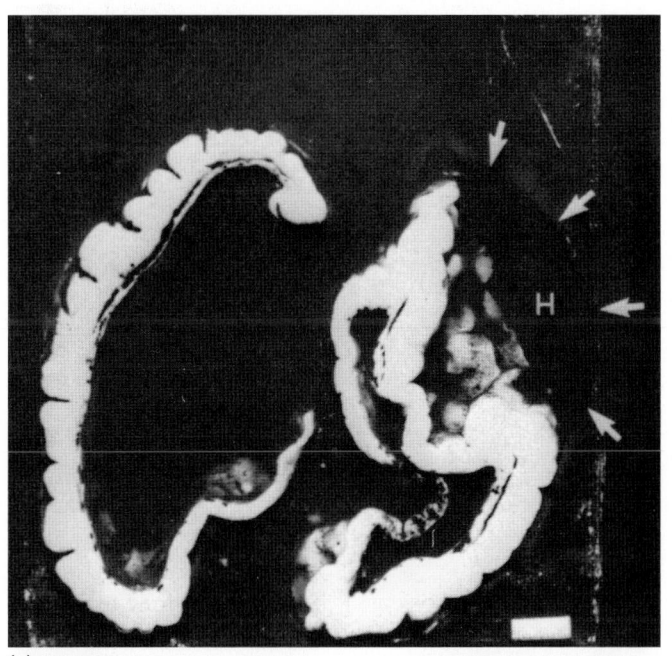

(a)

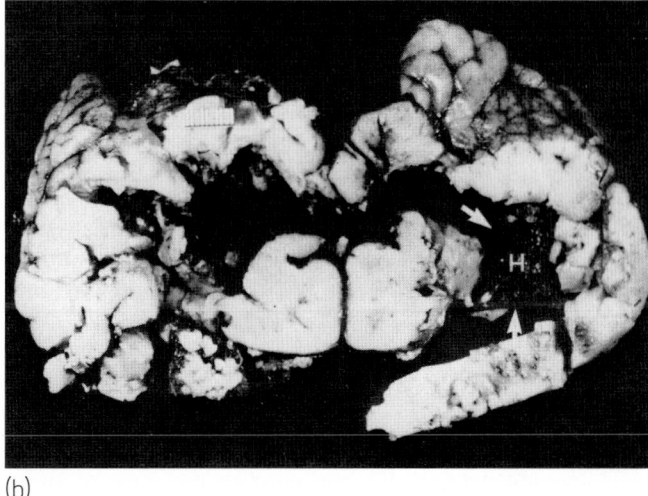

(b)

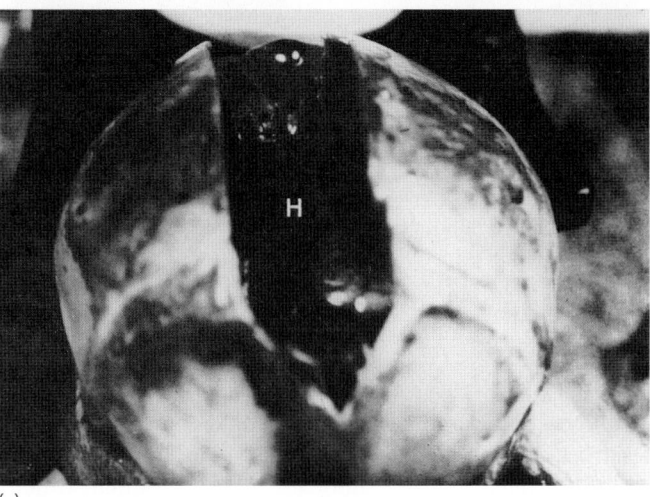

(c)

Figure 41.3 (a) Coronal section of brain demonstrating a large subarachnoid hemorrhage (H) resulting from cephalocentesis. (Modified from Isaacson 1984). (b) Section of brain demonstrating intraventricular hemorrhage (H) resulting from cephalocentesis. (c) Subdural hematoma (H) resulting from cephalocentesis.

This was primarily because many of these patients had CNS and non-CNS anomalies that went undetected. In fact, the associated comorbidities, rather than the degree of ventriculomegaly, overwhelmingly determined prognosis. Furthermore, the shunts failed to deliver consistent ventricular decompression due to clogging and migration (Manning et al 1986). As a result of this 1986 report and the inadequacies in diagnosis and shunting technique, the Fetal Medicine and Surgery Society recommended that intrauterine treatment of obstructive hydrocephalus be considered of unproven efficacy and an experimental procedure to be attempted only at highly specialized centers (Adzick & Harrison 1994, Manning 1986).

The introduction of open fetal surgery for the treatment of hydrocephalus had initially renewed public interest in the possibility of fetal treatment for hydrocephalus in the late 1900s. From 1999 to 2003, Bruner and colleagues placed ventriculoamniotic shunts through a hysterotomy during the second trimester of pregnancy on four cases of isolated aqueductal stenosis. Even though the cases were technically successful, there was no improved neurological function in any of the infants, whose neonatal course was also complicated by prematurity and infection (Bruner et al 2006). Despite advances in fetal imaging studies, appropriate case selection still remains the main limitation to fetal shunting and, currently, this intervention has failed to improve perinatal outcomes.

TREATMENT OF MYELOMENINGOCELE AND THE CHIARI II MALFORMATION (see also p. 224)

Myelomeningocele (MMC), the most severe form of spina bifida, is defined as a herniation of the meninges, spinal cord, and nerve roots through a cleft in the spinal column (Harrison et al 1980, Longaker et al 1991, Reigel 1982). All children born with MMC develop an associated Chiari II malformation that is characterized by a low-lying tentorium, small posterior fossa and abnormal cerebellum with downward displacement of the vermis through the foramen magnum (Coltran et al 1999, Guin 1999) (see Table 41.2).

ANIMAL STUDIES

Although it is accepted that the congenital defect of MMC contributes significantly to neurological dysfunction, growing experimental evidence suggests major damage to the exposed spinal cord as a result of environmental factors occurring during gestation. Drewek et al (1997) showed that after 34 weeks of gestation, the amniotic fluid became toxic to cultured rat spinal cord tissue. Studies of surgically induced neural tube defects in fetal animals have demonstrated that prenatal repair of the lesion may preserve neurological function (Heffez et al 1990). Mueli et al (1995a, 1995b) created a spina bifida-type defect at 75 days of gestation in fetal lambs. Four weeks later, the developing MMC lesions were repaired in utero. Unrepaired lambs were characterized by complete sensorimotor paraplegia and urinary

Table 41.2 Chiari classification of hindbrain hernias

Chiari class	Pathologic changes
Chiari I	Caudal movement of the cerebellar tonsils
	Impaction of the tonsils through the foramen magnum (usually >3 mm)
	Tip of the tonsils is rarely below C-2
	Commonly associated with syringohydromyelia
Chiari II	Caudal movement of the cerebellar vermis through the foramen magnum
	Commonly, the lower brainstem and 4th ventricle migrate caudally as well
	Seen almost exclusively in association with MMC
Chiari III	Displacement of the cerebellum and brainstem into a high cervical pouch
	Patients generally have a guarded prognosis with regard to eventual level of function

Source: Adapted from Guin (1999).

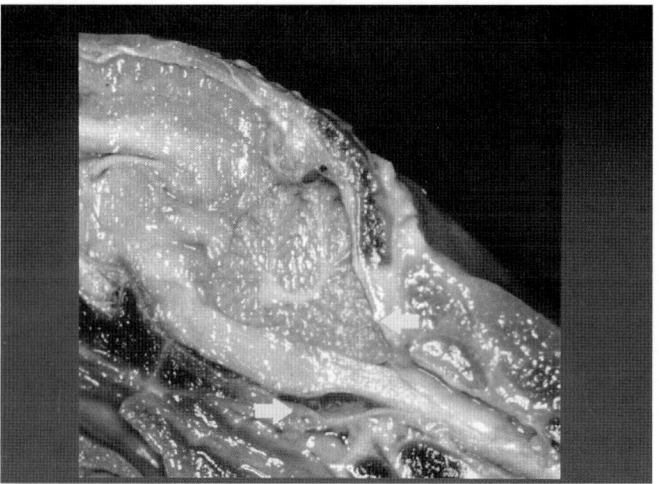

Figure 41.4 Development of the Chiari II malformation in the unrepaired myelomeningocele-type lesion.

and stool incontinence. Evaluation of the sagittal brain sections revealed that lambs undergoing the creation of a myelomeningocele-type lesion developed distinct signs of the Chiari II malformation (Fig. 41.4). Repaired lambs, however, demonstrated near-normal neurological function with only mild paraparesis and no signs of incontinence. Additionally, all animals that had undergone repair of the lesion either by coverage with Alloderm or by primary neurosurgical repair did not show any signs of a Chiari II malformation (Fig. 41.5a–c). The posterior fossa was of normal size, and the medulla and vermis of the cerebellum were located well above the foramen magnum.

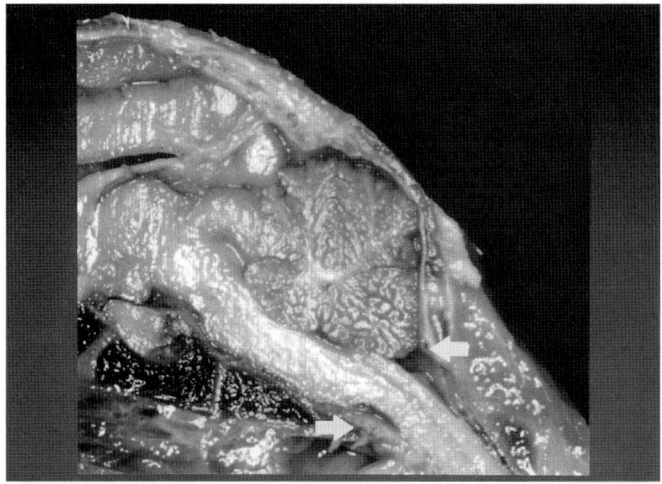

(a)

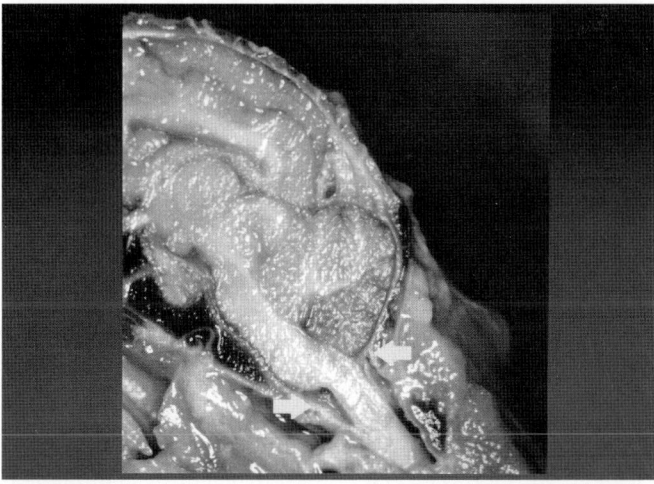

(b)

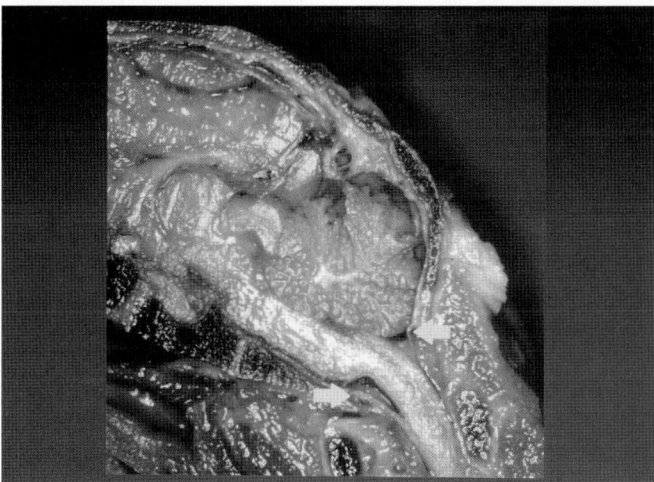

(c)

Figure 41.5 Absence of Chiari II malformation. Arrows indicate level of foramen magnum. (a) Control lamb without creation of a surgical myelomeningocele-type lesion. (b) Lamb with standard neurosurgical repair. (c) Lamb with synthetic Alloderm used as coverage.

Similarly, Michejda (1984) created a spina bifida-like lesion in eight *Macaca mulatta* fetuses by performing intrauterine lumbar laminectomies and displacing the spinal cords from the central canals. In five monkeys, this condition was repaired in utero. At delivery, the five repaired animals developed normally, while those with open lesions were paraplegic with lower extremity somatosensory loss and incontinence. Heffez et al (1990) reproduced similar results in a rat model. In addition, Julia et al (2006) showed that, even though there was no difference in the gross motor function, the somatosensory-evoked potentials of the hind limbs were absent in the group of rabbits who did not have in utero repair of their defects. Therefore, from these animal studies, it is hypothesized that the neurological defects seen in children with MMC result from both congenital myelodysplasia and progressive intrauterine spinal cord injury (Hoffman et al 1987).

The mechanism of injury, physical and/or chemical trauma, to exposed neural elements is unknown. The milieu of amniotic fluid can be caustic to exposed spinal cord. One study showed that meconium exposure increases spinal cord necrosis in fetal rats. In the control group, after laminectomy, amniotic fluid was restored with saline solution, while a solution of human meconium diluted in saline (10%) was used in the experimental group. All liveborn pups had severe paralysis of hind limbs and tail. However, histologic examination of spinal cords at site of surgical exposure showed increased necrosis and delay in repair processes in those that were exposed to meconium (Correia-Pinto et al 2002).

PATHOGENESIS

The development of the fetal brain and calvaria are interlinked and exquisitely dependent on fluid pressures. In the normally developing fetal CNS, the CSF develops in the lateral and third ventricles and passes through the aqueduct into the fourth ventricle. From here, the fluid flows through the lateral recesses into the posterior fossa to bathe the developing fetal cerebellum. This gentle fluid distention enlarges the size of the fetal posterior fossa as the fluid works its way around the tentorium, separating the cerebellum from the cranial fossa. Upon reaching the vein of Galen, the fluid is reabsorbed. Of note, the CSF also flows around the developing spinal cord. However, within the central spinal canal, the CSF is essentially stagnant. The fluid access to the spinal canal is via the obex located on the anterior surface of the fourth ventricle.

Early views suggested that the Chiari II malformation was a result of a tethered spinal cord pulling the posterior fossa structures downward (Fig. 41.6). In the 1960s, Gardner proposed the hydrodynamic hypothesis in which alteration in CSF dynamics at the craniospinal junction arises from a failure of the primitive rhombic roof to be permeable during fetal development (Caban & Bentson 1982). Accordingly, obstruction of the foramen of Magendie results in hydrocephalus and caudal displacement of the tentorium and hindbrain (Carmel 1982).

An alternative hypothesis is that fluid drainage from the posterior fossa creates a low-pressure situation so that the posterior cranial fossa is not induced to increase its capacity (Fig. 41.7). This leakage of low-pressure fluid can occur through an open MMC. In such a case, CSF in the fourth ventricle flows into the obex, down the central canal and out into the amniotic fluid. This creates a low-pressure circuit with concomitant lower posterior fossa distention pressures. Because of this low-resistance circuit, there is little fluid accumulation in the posterior fossa. As the fetal cerebellum develops, it is forced to fill a smaller volume, resulting in a higher resistance to flow around the cerebellum in order to get the outside of the cerebellum into the posterior fossa.

Due to the unique anatomy of the fetal brain, even when the cerebellum essentially obstructs fluid flow around and into the posterior fossa, the fluid still flows out through the obex and down the central canal into the amniotic fluid. It is only later in the development of the brain that fluid egress is inhibited to create the hydrocephalus that results from increased fluid build-up within the ventricles. In this theory, hydrocephalus is a consequence of hindbrain herniation, rather than the cause. Based on this relatively simple hydrodynamic theory of fetal brain development, correction of the MMC lesion may prevent some or all elements of impending Chiari II malformation.

CURRENT PREVENTION AND TREATMENT

Although approximately 25% of MMCs can be prevented by adequate dietary folic acid intake during pregnancy (see Ch. 14), a significant number will still develop despite adequate replacement. With widespread maternal serum α-fetoprotein screening and the use of high-resolution ultrasonography, over 80% of the cases of fetal MMC are now detectable in the mid-second trimester of pregnancy. Nevertheless, despite early detection, management options have been limited to either termination or continuation of the pregnancy with neonatal therapy. In light of this, the concept of in utero surgery to correct the defect of MMC before the open spinal cord can be damaged remains extremely attractive.

PROSPECTS FOR FETAL SURGERY

Early results from endoscopic in utero repair of myelomeningocele, where operating ports were inserted directly into the uterine wall after maternal laparotomy, showed a high incidence of mortality and no improvement of neurological function. The 50% mortality in four fetuses that underwent endoscopic coverage of the defect with a maternal split-thickness skin graft halted further use of this technique.

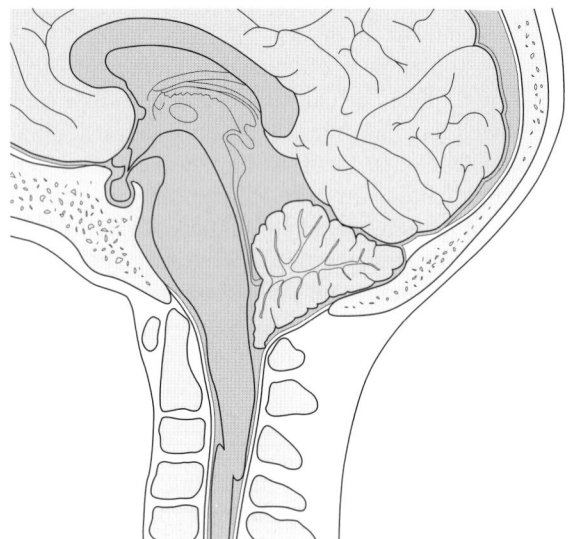

Figure 41.6 Chiari II malformation.

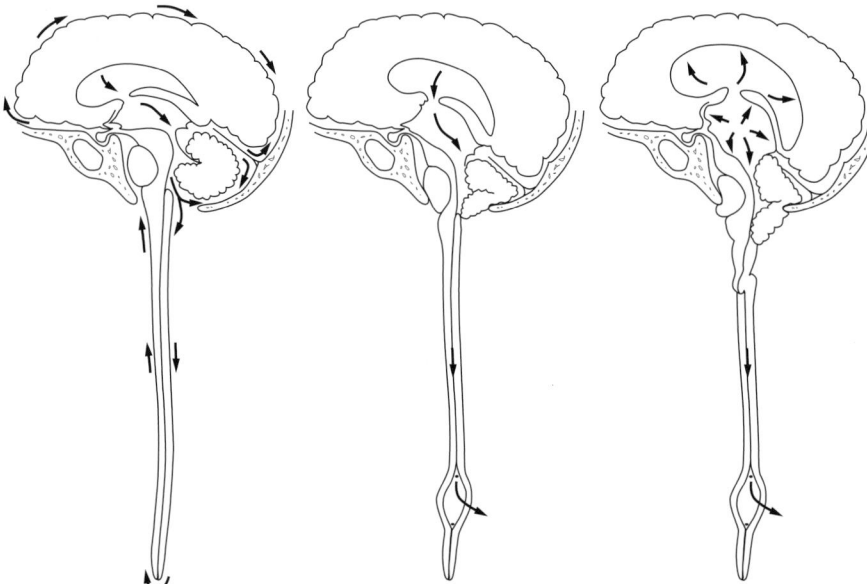

Figure 41.7 Development of the Chiari II malformation. Normal development of the brain and the skull, in particular the posterior fossa, is thought to be dependent upon gentle distention of the embryonic ventricles. Decrease of pressure due to loss of spinal fluid through a myelomeningocele lesion induces the development of an abnormally small posterior fossa. This malformation causes the herniation of brainstem and cerebellum through the foramen magnum and tentorium. As the cerebellum herniates through the foramen magnum, the normal circulation of CSF is obstructed. Hydrocephalus subsequently develops.

Furthermore, endoscopic patching was only a temporary solution since the graft degraded and the infants needed definitive postnatal repair (Bruner et al 1999a). Farmer et al (2003) also reported limited success with the fetoscopic approach (FETENDO), which did not require maternal laparotomy. One case was converted to open fetal repair, and two other repairs were noted to be leaking CSF at birth and required definitive neonatal closure.

Open fetal surgery for myelomeningocele has emerged as a viable solution to prevent neurological dysfunction in the newborn. Adzick et al (1998) reported the first clinical case of fetal surgery for MMC in a 23-week infant who later demonstrated improved distal neurological function. Subsequently, Tulipan and Bruner have shown that, despite a significant risk of preterm labor and preterm delivery, patients treated with in utero repair had a significantly decreased need for ventriculo-peritoneal (VP) shunting and hindbrain herniation compared to cohort controls (Tulipan & Bruner 1998, Tulipan et al 1998). They initially published a single-institution, observational study comparing 29 patients with isolated fetal MMC repaired between 24 and 30 weeks to 23 historical controls (Bruner et al 1999b). Cases were matched for diagnosis, level of lesion, practice parameters and calendar time, and all infants were followed up for a minimum of 6 months after delivery. They noted that older median age at shunt placement (50 vs. 5 days) as well as a 35% reduction in the need for VP shunting after in utero repair. The results might be explained by a 60% reduction in the incidence of hindbrain herniation among study infants. However, the patients were at a significantly higher risk of oligohydramnios and preterm labor compared to controls. Concurrently, Adzick et al reported on a series of ten patients undergoing MMC closure between 22 and 25 weeks (Sutton et al 1999). No controls were utilized. Using serial MRI scans at 19–24 weeks (prior to fetal surgery) and 3 and 6 weeks after fetal surgery, they demonstrated serial improvement in hindbrain herniation. Recently, Tulipan et al (2003) published an observational study comparing 104 patients with isolated fetal MMC repaired between 24 and 30 weeks at two institutions to 189 historical controls (Tulipan et al 2003). There was an overall absolute 30% reduction in the need for VP shunting after in utero repair; this difference, when stratified by level of lesion, was only statistically significant for lesions below L2. In addition, the benefit of in utero repair was seen only in fetuses younger than 25 weeks of gestation.

Even though case series have demonstrated improvement in surrogate markers of neurological function, e.g. need for VP shunting and radiographic reduction of hindbrain herniation, improvement in long-term function, such as lower extremity gross motor function, neurocognitive development and urinary continence has yet to be proven. Tubbs et al (2003) showed no difference in lower extremity function between the group of 37 consecutive patients who had fetal surgery for myelomeningocele and the group of 40 controls who had traditional postnatal repair. The neurode-

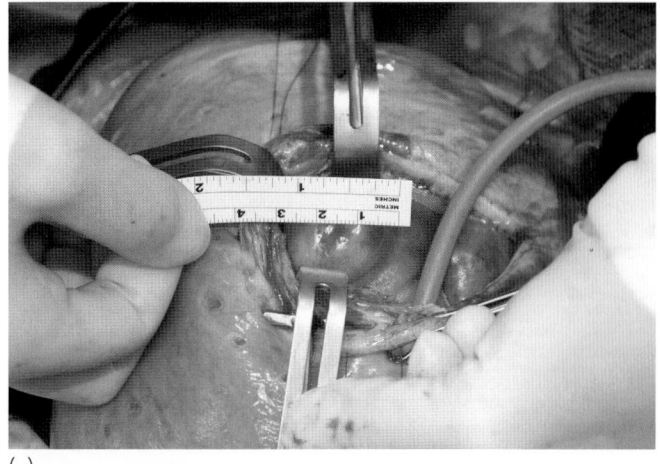

(a)

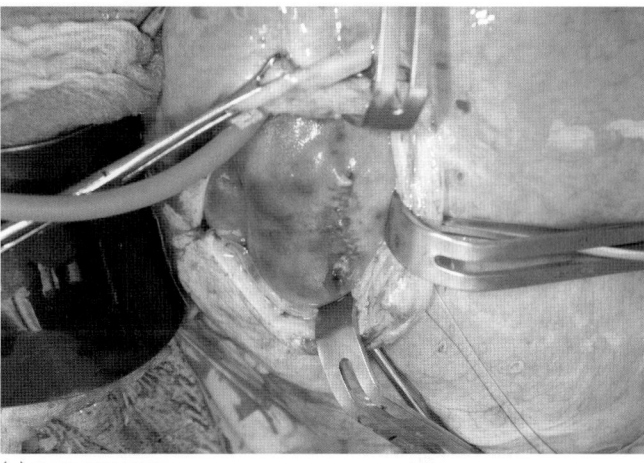

(b)

Figure 41.8 Open fetal repair of myelomeningocele. (a) Fetus at 22 weeks of gestation with myelomeningocele sac at level S1. Only the defect is exposed through the hysterotomy. (b) The same defect after primary closure.

velopmental outcomes at two years of age were assessed in 30 patients who had fetal closure of myelomeningocele and compared to the published reports in patients who had postnatal closure. Even though the incidence of shunting was lower, the overall cognitive and developmental scores were similar in both groups (Johnson et al 2006). In addition, both Holmes et al (2001) and Holzbeierlein et al (2000) showed no difference in the short-term urodynamic profiles. They hypothesized that in utero repair had the potential to reverse the detrimental effects on somatic neurons, but the damage on the sensory neurons that control urinary function was irreversible.

The role of fetal surgery for myelomeningocele is currently under investigation in a prospective randomized clinical trial involving three centers in United States. Eligible cases include fetal myelomeningocele at level T1 through S1 with hindbrain herniation. Open fetal surgery occurs between 19 and 26 weeks of gestation and involves a single layer closure (Fig. 41.8a, b). The results of this study will hopefully answer the question of whether the possible neurological benefit to the infant justifies the risk of fetal surgery to mother and fetus.

HORIZONS IN FETAL NEUROSURGERY

Fetal surgery remains an innovative treatment strategy and is not currently the standard of care for any neurological anomalies. The principal obstacle still encountered in fetal surgery is maternal morbidity and fetal morbidity and mortality from preterm labor. Ultimately, however, the decision to apply in utero surgical techniques widely for neurological anomalies as well as for other organ system anomalies will depend on the long-term effectiveness of the treatment protocols and their ethical acceptability in terms of safety for the mother and quality of life for the affected infant (Wilberg & Baghai 1983).

REFERENCES

Adzick N S, Harrison M R 1994 Fetal surgical therapy. Lancet 343:897–902.

Adzick N S, Sutton L N, Crombleholme T M et al 1998 Successful fetal surgery for spina bifida [letter]. Lancet 352(9141):1675–1676.

Birnholz J C, Frigoletto F D 1981 Antenatal treatment of hydrocephalus. N Engl J Med 303:1021–1023.

Bruner J P, Davis G, Tulipan N 2006 Intrauterine shunt for obstructive hydrocephalus — still not ready. Fetal Diagn Ther 21:532–539.

Bruner J P, Tulipan N, Pachal R L et al 1999a Fetal surgery for myelomeningocele and the incidence of shunt-dependent hydrocephalus. JAMA 282:1819–1825.

Bruner J P, Tulipan N, Reed G et al 2004 Intrauterine repair of spina bifida: preoperative predictors of shunt-dependent hydrocephalus. Am J Obstet Gynecol 190:1305–1312.

Bruner J P, Tulipan N, Richards W O et al 1999b In utero repair of myelomeningocele: a comparison of endoscopy and hysterotomy. Fetal Diagn Ther 15:83–88.

Caban L, Bentson J 1982 Considerations in the diagnosis and treatment of syringomyelia and the Chiari malformation. J Neurosurg 57:24–31.

Carmel P 1982 The Arnold–Chiari malformation. Pediatric neurosurgery of the developing nervous system. Grune & Stratton, New York, NY, pp. 61–77.

Clewell W H, Johnson M L, Meier P R et al 1982 A surgical approach to the treatment of hydrocephalus. N Engl J Med 306:1320–1325.

Coltran R S, Kumars V, Collins T 1999 Robbins pathologic basis of disease, 6th edn. WB Saunders, Philadelphia, PA, pp. 1301–1302.

Correia-Pinto J, Reis J L, Hutchins G M et al 2002 J Pediatr Surg 37:488–492.

Cromblehome T M 1994 Invasive fetal therapy: Current status and future directions. Semin Perinatol 18:385–391.

Depp R, Sabbagha R E, Brown J T et al 1983 Fetal surgery for hydrocephalus: successful in utero ventriculoamniotic shunt for Dandy–Walker syndrome. Obstet Gynecol 61:710–714.

Drewek M J, Bruner J P, Whetfell W O et al 1997 Pediatr Neuro Surg 27:190–193.

Duncan C C, Berkowitz R L, Hobbins J C 1982 Fetal hydrocephalus: An approach to management.

Presented at the 32nd Annual Meeting of the Congress of Neurological Surgeons. Toronto, Canada, October 3–8.

Farmer D L, von Koch C S, Peacock W J et al 2003 In utero repair of myelomeningocele. Arch Surg 138:872–878.

Frigoletto F D, Birnholz J C, Greene M F 1982 Antenatal treatment of hydrocephalus by ventriculoamniotic shunting. N Engl J Med 248:2496–2497.

Glick P L, Harrison M R, Halks-Miller M et al 1984 Correction of congenital hydrocephalus in utero. II. Efficacy of in utero shunting. J Pediatr Surg 19:870–881.

Guin P R 1999 Arnold–Chiari malformation. A closer look. World Arnold–Chiari Association,.

Harrison M 1993 Fetal surgery. West J Med 159:341–349.

Harrison M R, Jester J A, Ross N A 1980 Correction of congenital diaphragmatic hernia in utero. The model: intrathoracic balloon produces fetal pulmonary hypoplasia. Surgery 88:174–182.

Heffez D S, Aryanpur J, Hutchins G M et al 1990 The paralysis associated with myelomeningocele: clinical and experimental data implicating a preventable spinal cord injury. Neurosurgery 26:987–992.

Hoffman H J, Neill J, Crone K R et al 1987 Hydrosyringomyelia and its management in childhood. Neurosurgery 21:347–351.

Holmes N M, Nguyen H T, Harrison M R et al 2001 Fetal intervention for myelomeningocele: Effect on postnatal bladder function. J Urol 166:2383–2386.

Holzbeierlein J, Pope J C, Adams M C et al 2000 The urodynamic profile of myelodysplasia in childhood with spinal closure during gestation. J Urol 164:1336–1339.

Johnson M P, Gerdes M, Rintoul N et al 2006 Maternal-fetal surgery for myelomeningocele: Neurodevelopmental outcomes at 2 years of age. Am J Obstet Gynecol 194:1145–1154.

Julia V, Sancho M A, Albert A et al 2006 Prental covering of the spinal cord decreases neurologic sequelae in a myelomeningocele model. J Pediatr Surg 41:1125–1129.

Longaker M T, Golbus M S, Filly R A et al 1991 Maternal outcome after open fetal surgery. A review of the first 17 human cases. JAMA 265:737–741.

Lorber J, Grainger R G 1983 Cerebral cavities following ventricular puncture in infants. Clin Radiol 14:98–109.

Manning F A 1986 International fetal surgery registry: 1985 update. Clin Obstet Gynecol 29:551–557.

Manning F A, Harrison M R, Rodeck C et al 1986 Catheter shunts for fetal hydronephrosis and hydrocephalus. Report of the International Fetal Surgery Registry. N Engl J Med 315:336–340.

Michejda M 1984 Intrauterine treatment of spina bifida: primate model. Z Kinderchir 39:259–261.

Michejda M, Hodgen G D 1981 In utero diagnosis and treatment of non-human primate fetal skeletal anomalies. I. Hydrocephalus. JAMA 246:1093–1097.

Milhorat T H 1978 Pediatric neurosurgery. FA Davis, Philadelphia, PA, p. 112–121.

Mueli M, Meuli-Simmen C, Hutchins G M et al 1995b In utero surgery rescues neurological function at birth in sheep with spina bifida. Nat Med 1:342–347.

Mueli M, Meuli-Simmen C, Yingling C D et al 1995a Creation of myelomeningocele in utero: A model of functional damage from spinal cord exposure in fetal sheep. J Pediatr Surg 30:1028–1032.

Reigel D H 1982 Spina bifida in pediatric neurosurgery, surgery of the developing nervous system. Section of Pediatric Neurosurgery of the American Association of Neurological Surgeons. Grune & Stratton, New York, NY, Ch. 2, pp. 23–47.

Sutton L N, Adzick N S, Bilaniuk L T et al 1999 Improvement in hindbrain herniation demonstrated by serial fetal magnetic resonance imaging following fetal surgery for myelomeningocele. JAMA 282:1826–1831.

Tubbs R S, Chambers M R, Smyth M D et al 2003 Late gestational intrauterine myelomeningocele repair does not improve lower extremity function. Pediatr Neurosurg 38:128–132.

Tulipan N, Bruner J P 1998 Myelomeningocele repair in utero: a report of three cases. Pediatr Neurosurg 28:177–180.

Tulipan N, Hernanz-Shulman M, Bruner J P 1998 Reduced hindbrain hernation after intrauterine myelomeningocele repair: a report of 4 cases. Pediatr Neurosurg 29:274–278.

Tulipan N, Sutton L N, Bruner J P et al 2003 The effect of intrauterine myelomeningocele repair on the incidence of shunt-dependent hydrocephalus. Pediatr Neurosurg 38:27–33.

Wilberg J E, Baghai P 1983 Fetal neurosurgery. Neurosurgery 13:596–600.

Neonatal hydrocephalus — clinical assessment and non-surgical treatment

Andrew Whitelaw and Kristian Aquilina

Key Points

- Use recognized diagnostic criteria, e.g. 4 mm over 97th centile for ventricular width
- Differentiate cerebral atrophy or leukomalacia from CSF-driven ventricular enlargement
- Note the presence, location and extent of any parenchymal cerebral lesions
- Do a neurologic examination and assess the rate of head enlargement and ICP effects
- If there is symptomatic raised pressure or rapid enlargement averaging 2 mm/day, the pressure should be normalized (to <7 mmHg) and the effects on neurologic signs and physiologic parameters documented. This may be achieved by lumbar puncture/ ventricular reservoir or external ventricular drain depending on local expertise and availability of a neurosurgeon. We favor repeated tapping of a ventricular reservoir as a safe and effective way to control pressure and enlargement.
- If there is no evidence of signs or symptoms from raised ICP, observe without intervention
- Progressive and persistent enlargement of the ventricles together with accelerated head enlargement (8–14 mm/week) without obvious symptoms over 4 weeks should prompt careful assessment for neurologic and physiologic deterioration, and this may shift the baby into the symptomatic group
- Progressive and persistent enlargement of ventricles and accelerated head growth over 6 weeks, even without symptoms, should prompt evaluation for shunt surgery. The surgeon may wish to defer if the CSF is still blood-stained or has a protein content over 1.5 g/L, if there is infection, or if the baby's cardiorespiratory condition is poor
- Elective use of early repeated lumbar punctures is not recommended
- Acetazolamide and furosemide are not recommended

DEFINITION

Hydrocephalus is defined as excessive accumulation of cerebrospinal fluid (CSF) accompanied by excessive growth of the head. Ventricular dilatation occurs before head enlargement, as the first stage of hydrocephalus, but not all ventricular dilatation progresses to hydrocephalus. Ventricular dilatation can be reversible, may become static without accelerated enlargement, and may be due to cerebral atrophy and not to CSF accumulation.

CSF CIRCULATION AND ABSORPTION

The mechanism of hydrocephalus is nearly always obstruction somewhere along the pathways to CSF absorption. The choroid plexus in the lateral and third ventricles is the major site of CSF production. The fluid then has to flow through the aqueduct of Sylvius to the fourth ventricle. From here, the fluid leaves through the foramina of Luschka and Magendie into the cisterna magna, from whence it flows through the subarachnoid space around the cerebral hemispheres to be reabsorbed into the blood via the cranial venous sinuses (Fig. 42.1).

In adults and in children, there is good evidence that reabsorption occurs through the arachnoid granulations with their microscopic villi projecting into the venous sinus (Davson et al 1987). Four mechanisms for CSF reabsorption have been proposed: (1) passage through pores on the arachnoid villi; (2) an energy-consuming pinocytotic process by which intracytoplasmic vacuoles are transported from one side of the arachnoid membrane to the other; (3) transport via olfactory nerves, cribriform plate and nasal lymphatics (Johnston et al 2004) and (4) absorption across brain tissue into blood vessels (Greitz & Hannerz 1996). The principal advantage of the growth of arachnoid granulations and villi is thought to be the greatly increased surface area available for reabsorption. However, newborn infants do not have visible arachnoid granulations, and microscopic examination has not yet demonstrated any structure corresponding to arachnoid villi in the neonate. The absence of such structures may mean that CSF is absorbed by different mechanisms in the neonate or that the maximum capacity for reabsorption is less than in the adult.

ETIOLOGY

The overall incidence of infantile hydrocephalus is given as three per 1000 live births. As an isolated congenital disorder, the incidence was 0.9–1.5 per 1000 births, and when associated with myelomeningocele, was 1.3–2.9 per 1000 births in 1961 (Myrianthopoulos & Kurland 1961). Over the last 40 years, congenital hydrocephalus has decreased as a consequence of folate supplementation and acquired hydrocephalus has increased as a consequence of improved survival of very low birth weight infants.

A classification into those cases due to, or associated with, a cerebral malformation, as opposed to those cases due to an acquired lesion, is given in Table 42.1. Hydrocephalus has been noted in a larger number of syndromes (see p. 268), but a genetic etiology for this condition is uncommon. The etiology of the acquired lesions is usually self-evident.

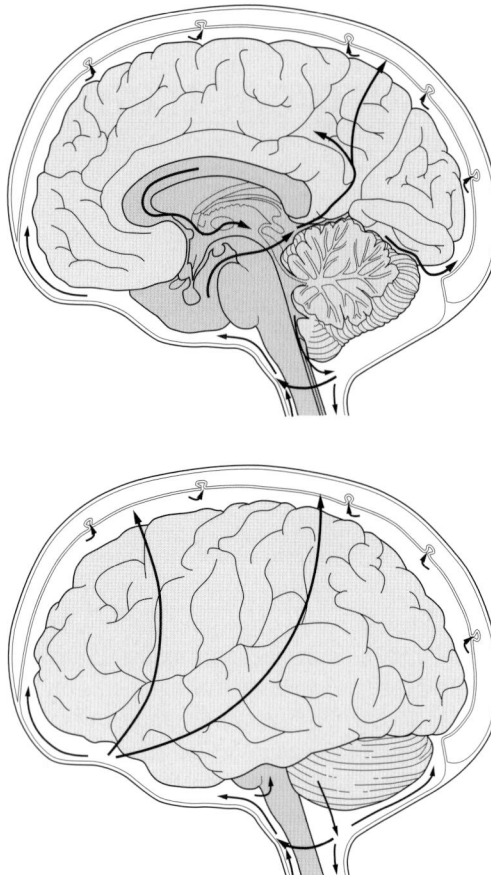

Figure 42.1 Pathways of CSF flow. (Reproduced, with permission, from Milhorat 1972.)

Table 42.1 Causes of neonatal hydrocephalus

1. Congenital malformation
   Aqueduct stenosis:
      Gliosis
      Forking of the aqueduct
      Aqueductal septum
      'True' narrowing of the aqueduct
      X-linked aqueductal stenosis
   Arnold–Chiari malformation type 2 (hydrocephalus and
      meningomyelocele)
   Atresia of the foramina of Luschka and Magendie (Dandy–
      Walker malformation)
   As part of a major cerebral malformation, e.g.
      encephalocele and holoprosencephaly
   As part of an inherited metabolic disease, e.g.
      achondroplasia or Hurler disease
2. Posthemorrhagic
   Intraventricular hemorrhage:
      Intrauterine bleeding because of thrombocytopenia or
         coagulation factor deficiency
      Respiratory distress syndrome after preterm birth
   Birth trauma:
      Subdural hemorrhage
      Subarachnoid hemorrhage
3. Postinfection
   Neonatal ventriculitis/meningitis, especially when due to
      gram-negative bacilli
   Intrauterine virus infection, e.g. cytomegalovirus
   Intrauterine *Toxoplasma gondii*
4. Tumor or vascular malformations
5. Benign external hydrocephalus
6. Overproduction of CSF
   Choroid plexus papilloma
7. Others
   Craniofacial dysmorphisms
   Platybasia
   Osteogenesis imperfecta

CONGENITAL OBSTRUCTION OF THE VENTRICULAR SYSTEM

The majority of cases of congenital hydrocephalus are due to narrowing of the aqueduct of Sylvius. Aqueductal stenosis may be due to gliosis, forking of the aqueduct, a septum across the aqueduct or true narrowing. A small minority of cases of aqueduct stenosis have an X-linked inheritance and this has been associated with mutations in the gene encoding the neural cell-adhesion molecule L1 (Jouet et al 1995). Such cases have more widespread abnormalities of brain development than just aqueduct stenosis and carry a worse prognosis for development than other causes of hydrocephalus. Congenital obstruction of the foramina of Luschka and Magendie leads to gross enlargement of the fourth ventricles into the cisterna magna. The Dandy–Walker malformation is described on page 253. Rarely hydrocephalus in the neonatal period may be due to a tumor such as a medulloblastoma obstructing the fourth ventricle (Fig. 42.2).

The majority of cases of meningomyelocele have hydrocephalus with an associated malformation of the brain. This is referred to as the type 2 Chiari malformation (Carmel 1982). The features are caudal dislocation of the medulla oblongata and cerebellar vermis, and the majority has a kink in the medulla. The disturbed anatomy of the fourth ventri-

cle and cisterna magna is thought to be the main reason for hydrocephalus. Arachnoid cysts, congenital tumors, and vascular malformations may produce hydrocephalus by expanding to the extent that they distort and obstruct the aqueduct or fourth ventricle.

ACQUIRED HYDROCEPHALUS AFTER HEMORRHAGE OR INFECTION

Hydrocephalus may follow either intraventricular or subarachnoid hemorrhage into the CSF (Fig. 42.3). Multiple small clots may obstruct the ventricular system or the channels of reabsorption initially but lead to a chronic arachnoiditis of the basal cisterns involving the deposition of

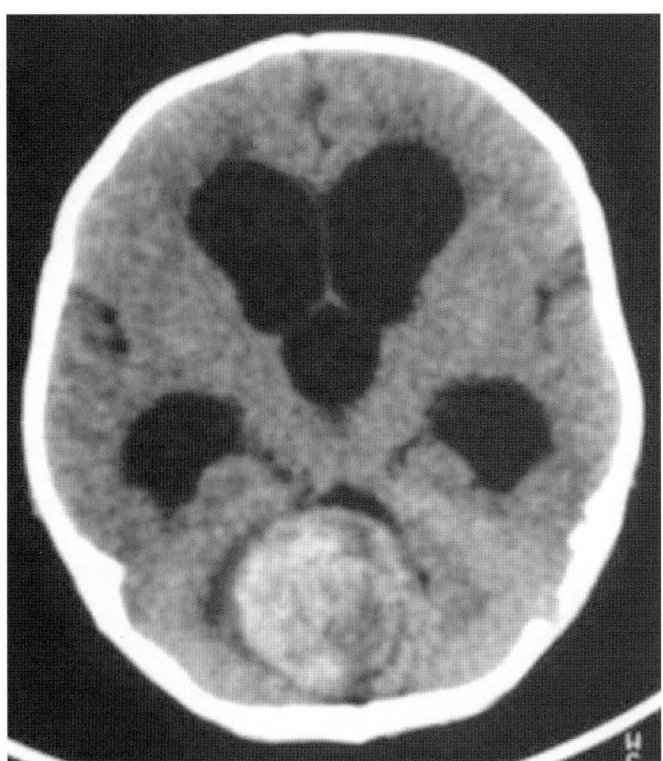

Figure 42.2 CT scan of an infant with hydrocephalus from obstruction of the fourth ventricle by a medulloblastoma.

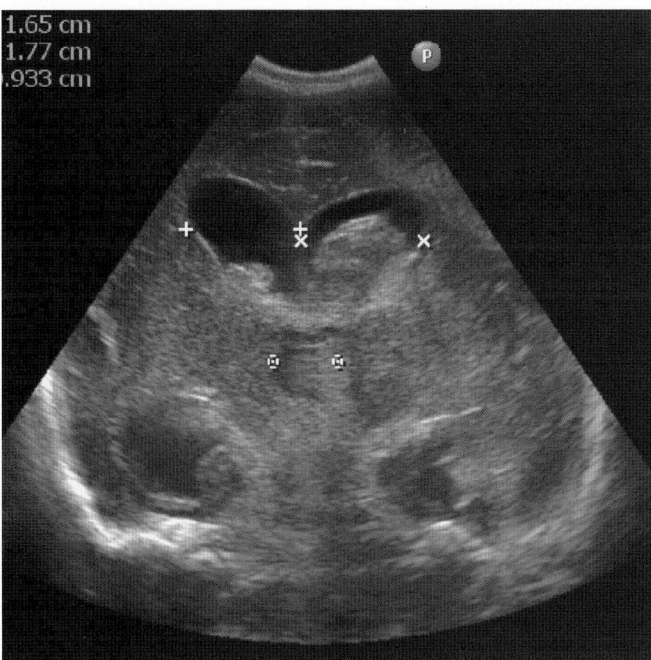

Figure 42.3 Cerebral ultrasound (coronal view) showing a large intraventricular hemorrhage in the right ventricle. The contralateral ventricle has begun to dilate, and there is CSF visible above the clot. Two caliper marks indicate where the ventricle width was from the midline to the lateral border of the lateral ventricle. The width of the third ventricle in the midline is also indicated by calipers.

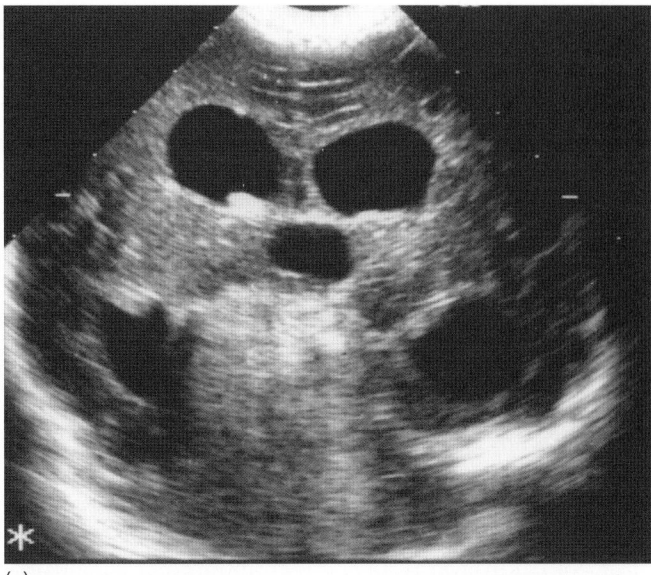

(a)

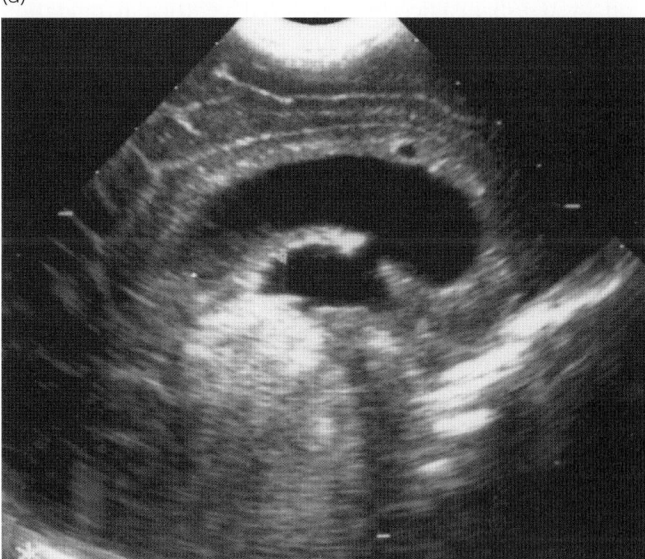

(b)

Figure 42.4 (a) Cerebral ultrasound (coronal view) showing marked dilatation of both lateral ventricles and the third ventricle with a hemorrhage just below the third ventricle obstructing the aqueduct. (b) Cerebral ultrasound scan (sagittal view) of the same infant as in (A) showing the dilated third ventricle with a hemorrhage below it. The hemorrhage was due to birth trauma.

extracellular matrix proteins and obstruction of the foramina of the fourth ventricles or the subarachnoid space over the cerebral hemispheres (Larroche 1972).

Traumatic hemorrhage into the tentorium or falx may also lead to hydrocephalus by displacement of the aqueduct (Fig. 42.4).

Ventriculitis can give rise to hydrocephalus by inflammatory obstruction of the aqueduct or foramina, and meningitis can produce chronic thickening of the leptomeninges with fibrin deposition (Stewart 1964).

TRANSFORMING GROWTH FACTOR-β1 AND POSTHEMORRHAGIC HYDROCEPHALUS

There is mounting evidence that transforming growth factor-β1 (TGF-β1) is involved in the pathogenesis of posthemorrhagic hydrocephalus. TGF-β1 is a cytokine that is chemotactic for fibroblasts and upregulates the expression of genes encoding fibronectin, collagen and other extracellular matrix proteins. TGF-β1 is involved in wound healing, scar formation, and a variety of pathologic processes including fibrosis in the lung, liver cirrhosis and glomerulonephritis. TGF-β1 is synthesized by leptomeningeal cells and is stored in granules of platelets, and these mechanisms may explain how the cytokine could have gained access to the CSF following IVH. It has been shown that lysis of blood clot in vitro releases TGF-β1. TGF-β1 has been demonstrated in the CSF of adults with subarachnoid hemorrhage, and those with elevated levels went on to hydrocephalus (Flood et al 2001, Kitisawa & Tada 1994). Intrathecal administration of TGF-β in mice has produced ventricular dilatation and reduced the number of cilia on the ependyma (Tada et al 1994). Whitelaw et al (1999) showed that TGF-β1 is detectable at very low concentrations in neonatal CSF, infants with transient PHVD have increased CSF concentrations of TGF-β1, and infants who later develop permanent hydrocephalus have even higher CSF concentrations of TGF-β1. An animal model of posthemorrhagic hydrocephalus in rat pups has shown expression of TGFβ and products of TGFβ such as laminin and vitronectin (Cherian et al 2004). In addition, transgenic mice who over-express TGF β1 are born with hydrocephalus (Wyss-Coray et al 1995).

TGFβ has not been investigated in post-meningitic hydrocephalus but it is found in the CSF in bacterial meningitis (Huang et al 1997). The cytokine, vascular endothelial growth factor (VEGF) opens the blood–brain barrier and tends to increase cerebral edema. It is elevated in the CSF of children with tuberculous meningitis (van der Flier et al 2004) and posthemorrhagic hydrocephalus (Heep et al 2004).

BENIGN EXTERNAL HYDROCEPHALUS

Ment et al (1981) described 18 infants with transient enlargement of the subarachnoid space without any evidence of subarachnoid hemorrhage. The prognosis is good, but the cause is not understood. A transient disturbance in CSF reabsorption has been postulated. It is important to distinguish the condition from subdural effusion and posthemorrhagic hydrocephalus. There is initially excessive head growth and CSF pressure may be moderately raised. These two features distinguish it from cerebral atrophy. We have seen seven infants with this condition, and all had a good outcome without surgery (Fig. 42.5).

OVERPRODUCTION OF CSF

Since the choroid plexus is the main site of CSF production, it is not surprising that enlargement of the plexus (choroid

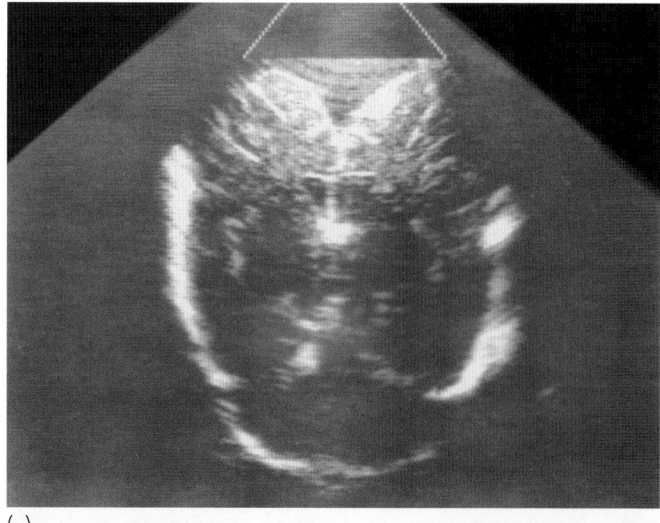

(a)

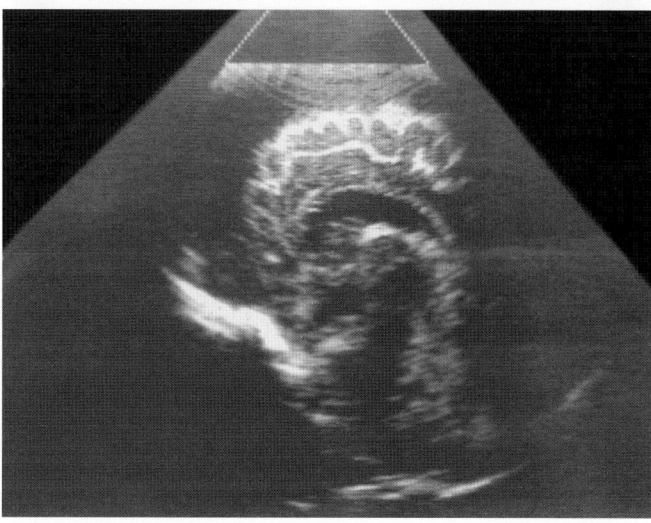

(b)

Figure 42.5 (a) Cerebral ultrasound scan (coronal view) showing external hydrocephalus. The subarachnoid space is enlarged over the cerebral hemispheres. (b) Cerebral ultrasound scan (parasagittal view) of the same infant as in (a). The subarachnoid space over the cerebral hemisphere is enlarged.

plexus papilloma: Fig. 42.6) can overproduce CSF to a greater extent than it can be absorbed (Milhorat 1982).

COMMUNICATING AND NON-COMMUNICATING HYDROCEPHALUS

It is conventional to classify hydrocephalus according to whether there is normal communication between the ventricular system and the subarachnoid space. In non-communicating hydrocephalus, a lumbar puncture yields only a few drops of CSF, usually less than 2 mL. In communicating hydrocephalus, a lumbar puncture usually produces at least 5 mL of CSF and can produce much more. Non-communicating hydrocephalus tends to give a higher CSF pressure

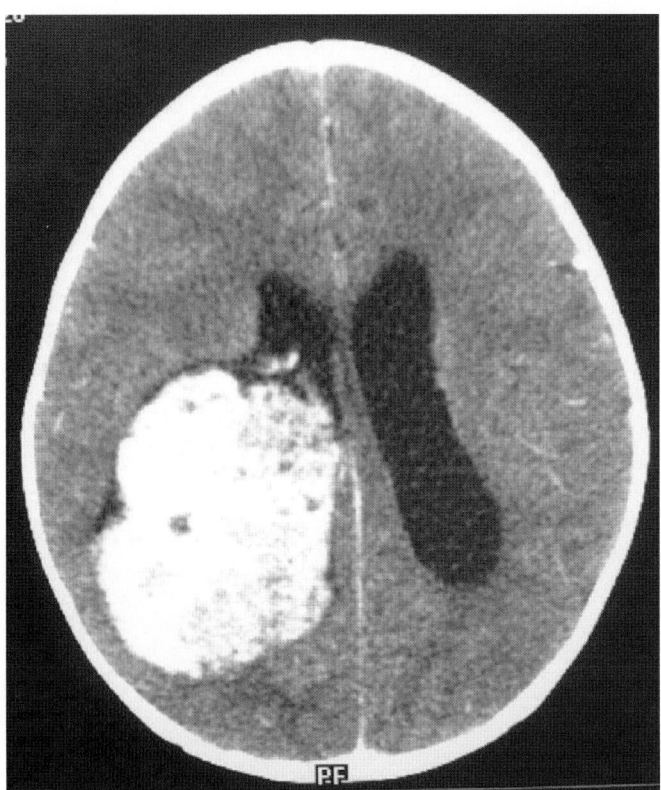

Figure 42.6 A CT scan of an infant with a right-sided choroid plexus papilloma and dilated ventricles.

posthemorrhagic CSF (Savman et al 2002), as have free iron and hypoxanthine, both of which can generate highly reactive radicals (Bejar et al 1983, Savman et al 2001). Such periventricular damage would be likely to lead to motor deficits, but mental and sensory functions of the brain might also be damaged and epileptic foci initiated if the effects of edema and pressure were more widespread in the small immature brain.

DIAGNOSIS

Hydrocephalus may be considered at birth on the basis of a disproportionately large head with bulging fontanelles, wide sutures and congested scalp veins. In many other cases, hydrocephalus becomes gradually apparent weeks or months after birth. The presence of spina bifida or evidence of previous intracranial hemorrhage or infection further increases the index of suspicion. The confirmation of hydrocephalus requires (1) the demonstration of enlargement of the ventricular system and (2) the demonstration that excessive head enlargement has occurred.

HEAD CIRCUMFERENCE

Head circumference should be measured with a paper tape measure around the largest part of the occiput and the mid-frontal area of the brow without exerting enough pressure to actually compress the head. The head circumference must be plotted on a centile chart that is appropriate for the gestational and postnatal age, sex and ethnic group of the infant but a modern one is available online (Fenton 2003). Head circumference enlarges by approximately 1 mm per day between 26 weeks of gestation and 32 weeks, and about 0.7 mm per day between 32 and 40 weeks. We regard a persistent increase of 2 mm per day as excessive. A difference of 2 mm from one day to the next may be difficult to measure accurately but an increase of 4 mm over 2 days is easier to ascertain.

CRANIAL ULTRASOUND

Cranial ultrasound is by far the quickest, cheapest and most convenient method of demonstrating ventricular enlargement. Ventricular width measured from the midline to the lateral border of the lateral ventricle in the mid-coronal view is the measurement with the least interobserver variability, and centiles for postmenstrual (gestational) age have been compiled (Levene 1981). We have found 4 mm over the 97th centile (Fig. 42.7) to be a useful criterion for defining genuinely pathologic ventricular enlargement. The frequency of PHVD using this definition is 1 in 2500–3000 births among residents of Bristol, UK. However, ventricular enlargement is not always sideways and sometimes the most marked changes are enlargement posteriorly or a change from thin slit to round balloon. With this in mind, Davies et al (2000) published reference ranges for anterior horn width (to capture the change in shape to balloon) (95th centile approximately 3 mm) (Fig. 42.8a), thalamo-occipital (to capture

and a more rapid rate of ventricular enlargement and therefore requires more urgent investigation and treatment. Communicating hydrocephalus tends to be less rapid in its course, and some cases may be appropriately managed by non-surgical treatment. Isotope cisternography, by which an isotope is injected into the lumbar CSF and its spread to the ventricular or cisternal spaces is followed by gamma camera imaging, is rarely used in infants to determine management. Posthemorrhagic and postinfectious hydrocephalus may begin as communicating and then become non-communicating after several months.

HYDROCEPHALUS PRODUCES NEUROPATHOLOGIC CHANGES

Animal models of hydrocephalus have demonstrated that progressive ventricular dilatation driven by raised CSF pressure produces flattening and destruction of the ependymal lining, as well as edema and necrosis of the periventricular white matter (Weller et al 1971). There is evidence from neuropathologic studies that a similar process occurs in the developing brain of the human infant (Weller & Shulman 1972). In addition to the physical effects of pressure, edema and distortion, there is evidence that inflammation and free radical attack may contribute to white matter injury in posthemorrhagic hydrocephalus. High concentrations of pro-inflammatory cytokines have been demonstrated in

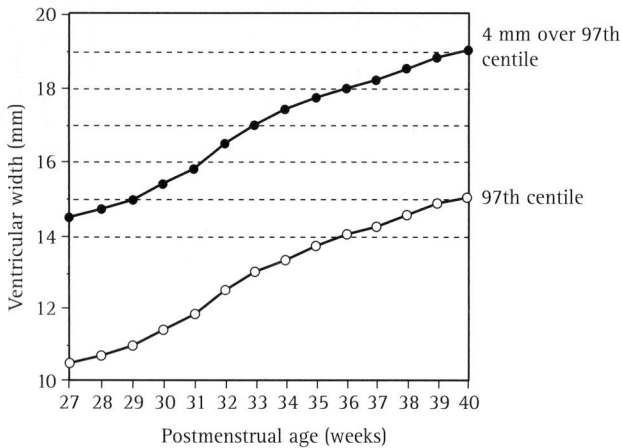

Figure 42.7 The lower line is the 97th centile for ventricular width of Levene (1981). The upper line defines ventricular dilatation severe enough to be treated (Kaiser & Whitelaw 1985).

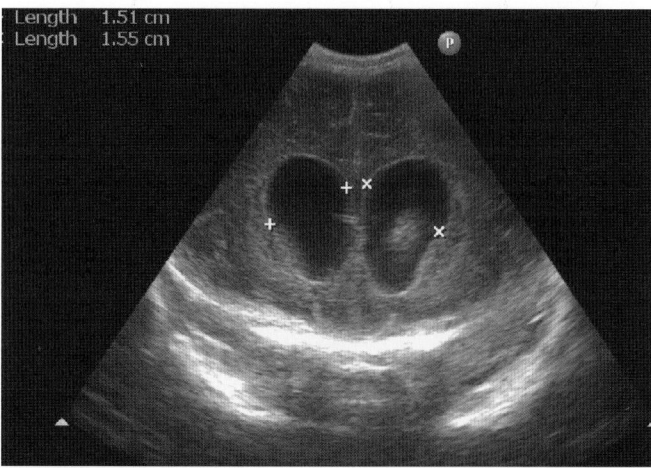

(a)

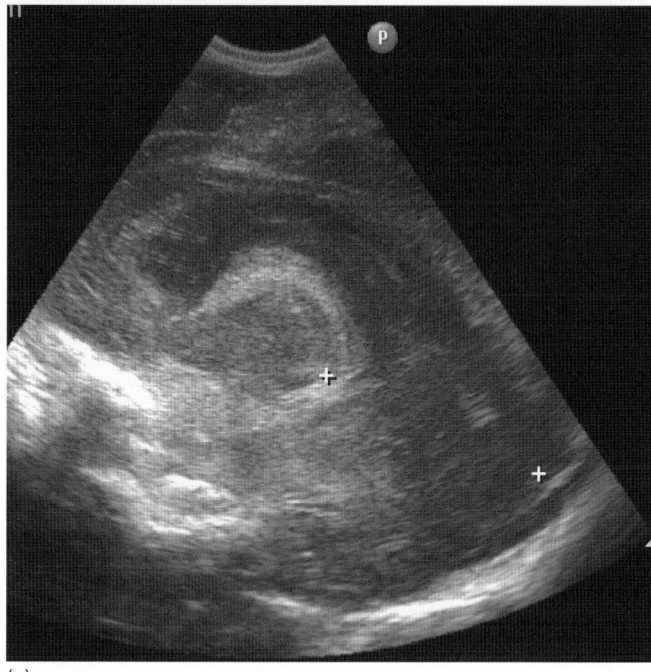

(b)

Figure 42.8 (a) Coronal view of anterior horns with calipers indicating the diagonal anterior width. (b) Parasagittal view of a dilated lateral ventricle with calipers indicating the thalamo-occipital dimension.

posterior enlargement) (95th centile approximately 25 mm) (Fig 42.8b), third ventricular width (95th centile approximately 2 mm) (Fig 42.3) and fourth ventricular width. We have found the anterior horn width, thalamo-occipital and third ventricular width to be practical and useful but with greater interobserver variation. We have used all three measurements since 2003, requiring all three measurements (bilaterally) to be 1 mm over the 95th centile as criteria for PHVD. Fourth ventricular width we have found too challenging to achieve reproducible measurements and we do not use this routinely.

Ultrasound has the enormous advantages of portable equipment, brief examination time without sedation and no irradiation, and remains the first choice for imaging in preference to computerized tomography (CT) or magnetic resonance imaging (MRI).

Ultrasound can demonstrate abnormalities such as a third ventricle clot (Fig. 42.9), and intracerebral calcification or intraventricular fibrin strands after ventriculitis (Fig. 42.10).

CT or MR may be needed to better define atypical cases or to show a tumor or subdural hematoma. The role of different imaging techniques is discussed in Chapter 6.

WHEN IS VENTRICULAR DILATATION DUE TO ATROPHY OR MALFORMATION?

It is important to distinguish ventricular dilatation due to atrophy from hydrocephalus due to excessive CSF under pressure. Cerebral atrophy can result in enlargement of the ventricles, but the ventricular outline is usually irregular, and there may be other features of cerebral atrophy such as widening of the interhemispheric fissure. Observation over time will show whether the head is growing excessively or not. In pure cerebral atrophy, the head growth is usually slower than normal and certainly does not grow excessively. Loss of cerebral substance following hemorrhagic infarction

or periventricular leukomalacia may coexist with progressive hydrocephalus. Some infants with midline cerebral defects such as agenesis of the corpus callosum or holoprosencephaly have dilated cerebral ventricles without raised CSF pressure or excessive head growth.

NEUROLOGIC EXAMINATION

As well as establishing the diagnosis, it is important to document the infant's neurologic state (Ch. 9). Raised intracranial pressure (ICP) may be associated with irritability, vomiting and increased extensor tone in the limbs with increased tendon reflexes. However, some infants with defi-

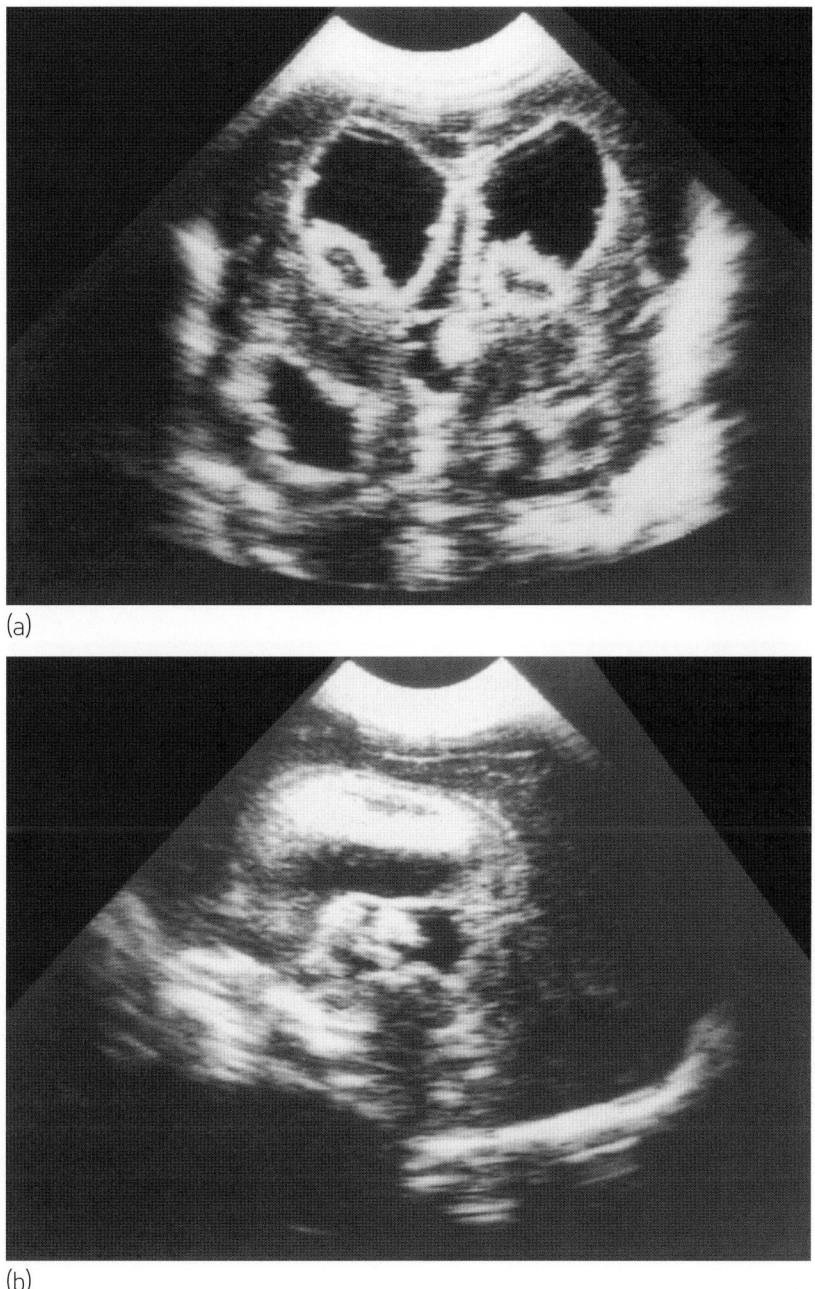

(a)

(b)

Figure 42.9 (a) Cerebral ultrasound scan (coronal view) showing large clots in both lateral ventricles. In addition, the third ventricle is dilated and contains several clots. (b) Cerebral ultrasound scan (sagittal view) showing the dilated third ventricle containing several clots in addition to the normal massa intermedia.

nite hydrocephalus exhibit no such signs. The hydrocephalus may have developed slowly, and the splaying of the sutures may have prevented the ICP from rising considerably. Some infants with hydrocephalus after intraventricular hemorrhage may show hypotonia with a disproportionately tight popliteal angle. Asymmetry is unusual. In neonates, visual fixation to a target may be impaired, but the hearing response is usually normal. Eye movements may be abnormal with failure of upward gaze, but sunsetting is uncommon. An objective means of recording the neurologic

examination is helpful in comparing examinations (Dubowitz et al 2000).

After a full review of the pregnancy, delivery, and immediate neonatal period, together with a clinical examination and a careful ultrasound examination, it is usually possible to classify the baby into one of the etiological groups above. If no obvious explanation for the hydrocephalus can be given, intrauterine infection should be investigated, and a careful family history should be taken. Coagulation factor deficiency as well as thrombocytopenia should be excluded

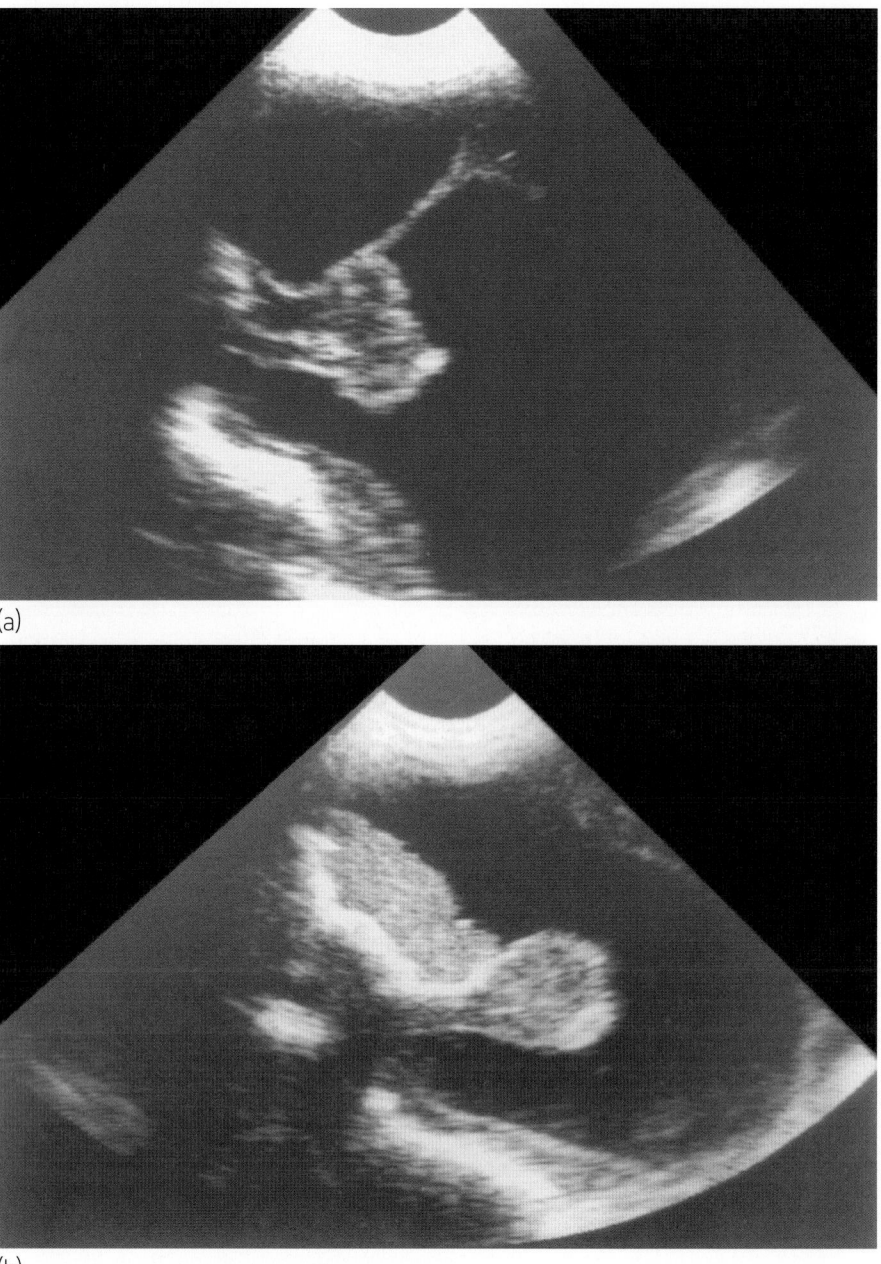

(a)

(b)

Figure 42.10 (a) Cerebral ultrasound scan (sagittal view) showing marked ventricular dilatation with a fibrinous septum across the ventricle. The infant had chronic bacterial ventriculitis. (b) The same infant as in (a) with chronic ventriculitis. Parasagittal view of one dilated ventricle showing necrotic material on a layer of calcification.

before any surgery is undertaken. Isoimmune thrombocytopenia and coagulation factor V deficiency can present as congenital hydrocephalus resulting from antenatal intraventricular hemorrhage (see Ch. 20).

CSF PRESSURE MEASUREMENT

Technique of CSF pressure measurement

CSF pressure measurement can be helpful in distinguishing hydrocephalus from other causes of ventricular dilatation, in assessing the acuteness of the process and in deciding treatment. We have not found non-invasive measurement

of ICP by a fontanometer to correlate well with directly measured ventricular pressure (Kaiser & Whitelaw 1987). Changes in ICP appeared to be well represented, but the absolute values in millimeters of mercury (mmHg) were disappointingly inaccurate. CSF pressure can be measured with a conventional fluid-filled manometer, but an electronic pressure transducer gives a trace on the monitor screen that is useful for demonstrating that the measurement is stable and can also demonstrate the CSF pulse pressure (Kaiser & Whitelaw 1986). The transducer must be carefully zeroed before the measurement, and the position of the transducer during the measurement should be level with the middle of the head. The infant should be horizontal and not forcefully restrained during the measurement. A wide pulse pressure is a sign that the limits of cranial compliance have been reached and the inflow of blood with each contraction of the heart is enough to increase ICP.

CSF pressure in normal neonates and infants with posthemorrhagic ventricular dilatation

Kaiser and Whitelaw (1986) studied CSF in neonates undergoing lumbar puncture to exclude sepsis and who were retrospectively classified as neurologically normal. When the infant was horizontal, at rest, and had no pressure on the abdomen, neck or head, the lumbar CSF pressure had a mean of 2.8 mmHg, and the upper limit was 6 mmHg. Kaiser and Whitelaw (1985) studied CSF pressure in a group of infants with progressive posthemorrhagic ventricular dilatation. Many of the infants had communicating ventricular dilatation and could be studied with lumbar puncture. In cases of non-communicating ventricular dilatation, the CSF pressure was measured at the time of ventricular puncture. Infants who were actively expanding their ventricles after intraventricular hemorrhage had a mean CSF pressure of 8.8 mmHg (three times the normal) but with a wide scatter. Some preterm infants could dilate their lateral ventricles and expand their heads at pressures that were still within the normal range, whereas few generated pressures over 15 mmHg. Probably because infants with communicating hydrocephalus rarely generate dangerously high pressures, we have never encountered acute herniation of the brainstem (coning), despite having lumbar punctured many infants with CSF pressures considerably above the normal range. It has not been easy to define the level of CSF pressure at which action should be taken to lower pressure, but 12 mmHg has been used as the trigger pressure (Ventriculomegaly Trial Group 1990).

NEUROPHYSIOLOGIC ASSESSMENT IN HYDROCEPHALUS

De Vries et al (1990) have shown that the latency of somatosensory evoked potentials (SEPs) in infants with hydrocephalus correlates well with CSF pressure and improved when treatment lowered pressure. As clinical neurologic examination correlates poorly with CSF pressure measurement, SEPs (see Ch. 12) may prove to be a valuable way of demonstrating the effect of pressure on cerebral function and thus help in prognosis and treatment decisions.

CEREBRAL BLOOD FLOW VELOCITY WAVEFORMS IN HYDROCEPHALUS

Resistance index = (*systolic* velocity − *diastolic* velocity)/ systolic velocity

Blood flow velocity measurement by Doppler on the middle cerebral artery or anterior cerebral artery enables us to calculate Resistance Index (RI) which is independent of the angle of the beam to the vessel (p. 167). This tends to

increase as ICP increases. In other words, the diastolic part of the pulse becomes reduced in relative terms. Absent end-diastolic velocities (Resistance Index 1.0) are a definite sign of impaired cerebral perfusion and indicate raised ICP, left to right ductal shunting or hypotension (Fig. 42. 11). However, Hanlo et al (1995) have made simultaneous long-term transcranial Doppler and invasive ICP recordings. Although pulsatility and resistance indices tended to go down after successful shunt surgery, there was much variability between the Doppler and ICP measurements, and they concluded that Doppler indices are inadequate for monitoring dynamic changes in patients with raised ICP. Taylor and Madsen (1996) confirmed the poor correlation between baseline resistive index and ICP but found that fontanelle compression (which increased ICP) changed the Doppler measurement in an informative way. A large change in Doppler resistive index had a 0.8 correlation with elevated ICP.

PROGNOSIS

PROGNOSIS OF UNCOMPLICATED HYDROCEPHALUS

Eighty survivors of 'pure' hydrocephalus operated on between 1956 and 1976 in Cleveland were reviewed by Nulsen and Rekate (1982). These were infants with hydrocephalus not complicated by primary brain disease or spina bifida. Of these, 43 had aqueduct stenosis, 13 had blockage at the fourth ventricle outlets and 24 had communicating hydrocephalus. There was a good correlation between intelligence quotient (IQ) and the thickness of the frontal cerebral mantle (determined at follow-up). Normally, the cerebral mantle is 5.0–5.5 cm. The children with a cerebral mantle of 3.0 cm or more had an IQ distribution approaching normal. All eight patients failing to achieve a cerebral mantle of 2.0 cm

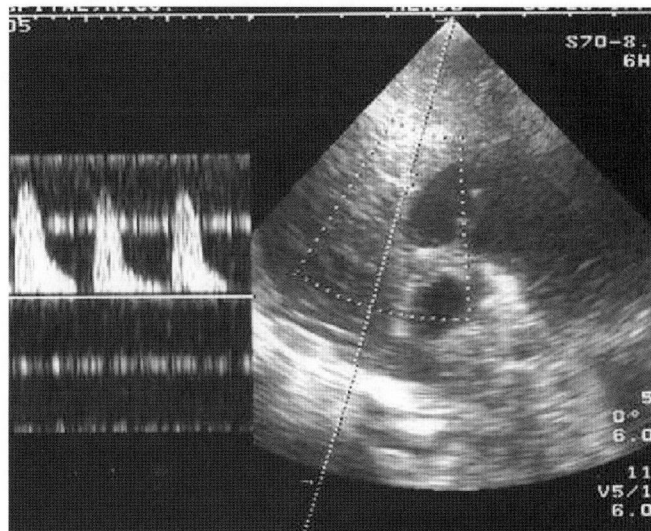

Figure 42.11 Doppler blood flow velocities from the anterior cerebral artery. Absent end-diastolic velocities because of raised intracranial pressure.

were not adequately shunted until after 6 months of age. Six cases with a final mantle of 2.0–3.0 cm (IQ 63–95) were all first adequately shunted after 5 months of age. All cases adequately shunted before 5 months had a mantle measurement over 3.0 cm, including nine cases with initial mantles of less than 1.0 cm. No increase in mantle size occurred in any of the five children first operated after age 18 months. The authors concluded that if infantile hydrocephalus is severe with a frontal mantle of less than 2.0 cm, the opportunity for a good developmental result diminishes with time. The benefit of early shunting in severe hydrocephalus is supported by experimental work. Rat pups with inherited hydrocephalus were shunted at 4–5 days or 10–11 days; this early shunting greatly reduced neuronal injury in the visual cortex (Boillat et al 1997). The outcome for fetal ventriculomegaly is discussed in Chapter 41.

PROGNOSIS OF HYDROCEPHALUS WITH MYELOMENINGOCELE

The relationship between frontal cerebral mantle thickness and IQ is much less predictable than in 'pure' hydrocephalus. These children are identified at birth because of the myelomeningocele, and hydrocephalus is to be expected. Very few are operated on late because of a delay in diagnosis. Thus, it is relatively unusual to fail to develop at least a 3 cm-thick frontal mantle. The IQ distribution in the Cleveland series of hydrocephalus and spina bifida was much lower than for the corresponding group of children with pure hydrocephalus and a 3-cm-thick mantle (Nulsen & Rekate 1982). Over 50% had an IQ below 80 (versus 15%), and only 15% were above 100 (versus 51%). Clearly, some children in this group have a considerable degree of paraplegia that affects many of their activities and this, plus the frequency of CSF infection, may have an adverse effect on development and thus IQ.

PROGNOSIS OF POSTHEMORRHAGIC VENTRICULAR DILATATION

Preterm infants who develop a large intraventricular hemorrhage are at risk of developing progressive ventricular dilatation leading to hydrocephalus. This condition has a worse prognosis than congenital hydrocephalus.

Epidemiologic surveillance of neurologic disabilities in south-west Sweden has shown a disturbing increase in the numbers of preterm infants surviving with posthemorrhagic hydrocephalus and multiple severe disabilities. Of these infants requiring shunt surgery, 78% subsequently developed cerebral palsy, 72% had a developmental quotient or IQ below 70, and 56% had epilepsy (Fernell et al 1990). In a group of 33 infants with posthemorrhagic ventricular dilatation (PHVD) followed to a mean age of 50 months, 58% had delayed motor development and 52% had delayed mental development (Shankaran et al 1989).

The Ventriculomegaly Trial Group (1990, 1994) studied 157 infants with PHVD: 32 infants died after entry to the study using the entry criterion of ventricular width 4 mm

over the 97th centile, 13 were lost to follow-up and 112 survivors were examined by one neurodevelopmental pediatrician at 30 months post-term. Overall, 54% scored below 70 on the Griffith developmental scales, 90% had neuromotor impairment and 76% had marked disability. Fifty-six percent had multiple impairments. Vision was severely affected in 9% and 27% had a field defect. Six percent had a sensorineural hearing loss and 14% were taking regular anticonvulsants. An important factor affecting prognosis in PHVD was the presence or absence of parenchymal cerebral lesions in the neonatal period. Periventricular leukomalacia or parenchymal hemorrhagic infarction with subsequent formation of a porencephalic cyst substantially worsened the prognosis.

An important study by Fletcher et al (1997) compared the outcome at an average age of 8.5 years of a group of prematurely born children with and without hydrocephalus. Four groups were studied: preterm no hydrocephalus, preterm arrested hydrocephalus, preterm shunted hydrocephalus and term children. Those born preterm who developed hydrocephalus had an equal severity of underlying parenchymal involvement. The only significant difference in these groups on later performance was that the shunted preterm group was significantly poorer in motor performance and visual-spatial tests, but not language tests. This study adds further weight to the independent adverse effect of hydrocephalus on non-verbal cognitive skills.

NON-SURGICAL TREATMENT OF HYDROCEPHALUS

REPEATED TAPPING OF CSF

The experimental hydrocephalus findings and the moderately elevated CSF pressure suggested that early CSF tapping by lumbar puncture or ventricular puncture might benefit babies with PHVD by (1) reducing pressure, thus reducing periventricular tissue damage and (2) removing excess protein and blood in the CSF, thus preventing permanent blockage of the CSF pathways. Mantovani et al (1980) and Anwar et al (1985) carried out randomized trials of serial lumbar punctures in babies with a large intraventricular hemorrhage. Both studies concluded that these measures did not reduce the progression to hydrocephalus and eventual surgical shunting. Dykes et al (1989) carried out a randomized trial of repeated lumbar puncture in infants with asymptomatic large IVH and found that there was no significant reduction in the numbers of infants shunted, the mortality, or single or multiple disabilities.

The hypothesis that early tapping of infants with PHVD by either the lumbar or ventricular route might reduce neurodevelopmental impairment and disability was tested in the Ventriculomegaly Trial Group's (1990) multicenter trial, which recruited 157 infants in England, Ireland and Switzerland from 1984 to 1987. Infants fulfilling the diagnostic criteria described above were randomized to either early CSF tapping to prevent further ventricular enlargement or conservative management. The survivors were examined at 12 and 30 months post-term by one developmental pediatrician. The mean CSF pressure was 9 mmHg in both treatment groups, and early tapping did succeed in reducing the rate of ventricular and head expansion. The mean gestational age in the infants randomized was 28 weeks, and the mean birth weight was just over 1200 g. Of the survivors, 62% received ventriculoperitoneal shunts, the same percentage in each treatment group.

At 12 months past term, 85% of survivors had abnormal neuromotor signs and 77% had disability, with no difference between the treatment groups (Ventriculomegaly Trial Group 1990). The proportion of children with neuromotor impairment plus other types of disability, such as mental retardation and visual or hearing loss, was not significantly different between the two treatment groups. There was a suggestion that infants who had already had a parenchymal cerebral lesion at the time of entry to the trial had a lower proportion of multisystem impairments at the 12-month follow-up examination, but the level of significance was only 5% (39), and this finding was not confirmed at the 30-month examination (Ventriculomegaly Trial Group 1994). The high frequencies of single and multiple impairments were the same for both treatment groups. Repeated CSF tapping was followed by CSF infection (ventriculitis) in 11 infants (7%). An additional complication of repeated ventricular tapping is the production of needle track lesions through the cerebral hemisphere (Fig. 42.12).

The Cochrane Collaboration has published a systematic review of repeated lumbar or ventricular puncture after IVH, and the meta-analysis (in Table 42.2) shows that there is no significant effect on shunt surgery, disability or multiple disability (Whitelaw 1998).

Because of the lack of any consistent neurodevelopmental benefit, the absence of any reduction in surgical shunt dependence, and the significant risk of serious infection, early treatment by CSF tapping cannot be recommended for PHVD.

We reserve CSF tapping for relief of symptoms associated with excessive pressure or excessive head expansion. We consider 12 mmHg to be an excessive CSF pressure. This is four times the normal mean and 100% over the upper limit of normal. This pressure is not necessarily associated with specific signs, but we have often noted irritability and a tense fontanelle at this level. If tapping is carried out, then CSF should be allowed to drip out without suction as rapid suction with a syringe usually causes discomfort in the baby and may precipitate fresh intraventricular bleeding. Fluid can be removed until the normal mean of 3 mmHg is reached. The volume we have found to be effective is 10–20 mL CSF/Kg. If more than two therapeutic lumbar punctures are required or if more than one ventricular tap is required, we consider the surgical insertion of a ventricular access device, such as an Ommaya reservoir, to facilitate tapping (de Vries et al 2002). This allows the infant to be sent back to the referring hospital where tapping can be continued.

DRUGS TO REDUCE CSF PRODUCTION

Because of the risks and lack of benefit from repeated tapping, non-invasive treatment to reduce the production of CSF was an attractive alternative.

ACETAZOLAMIDE

Acetazolamide (Diamox) reduces CSF production by inhibiting the enzyme carbonic anhydrase and has been used in

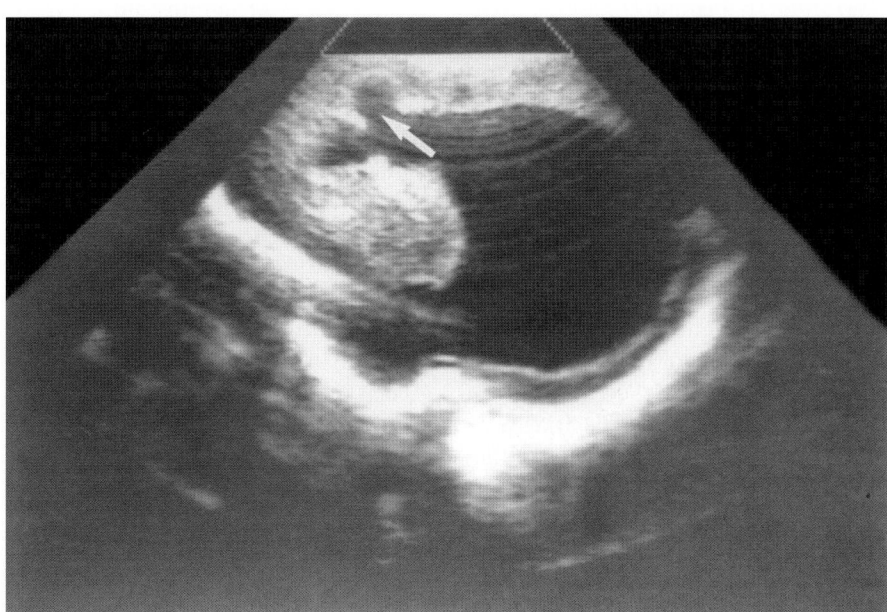

Figure 42.12 Cerebral ultrasound (parasagittal view) showing a needle track lesion (arrow) in the roof of the lateral ventricle after repeated ventricle taps.

Table 42.2 Comparison: repeated lumbar or ventricular punctures (Expt) vs. conservative management (Cont) for PHVD

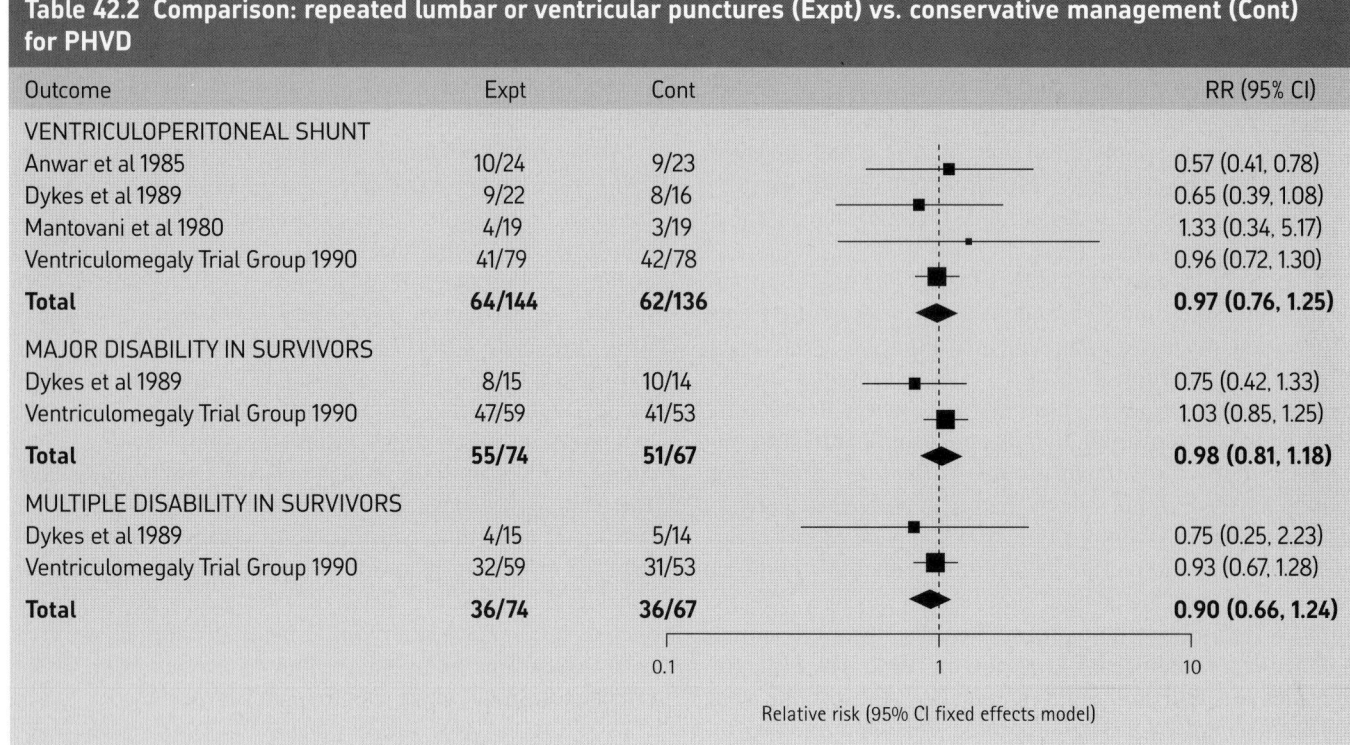

Outcome	Expt	Cont		RR (95% CI)
VENTRICULOPERITONEAL SHUNT				
Anwar et al 1985	10/24	9/23		0.57 (0.41, 0.78)
Dykes et al 1989	9/22	8/16		0.65 (0.39, 1.08)
Mantovani et al 1980	4/19	3/19		1.33 (0.34, 5.17)
Ventriculomegaly Trial Group 1990	41/79	42/78		0.96 (0.72, 1.30)
Total	**64/144**	**62/136**		**0.97 (0.76, 1.25)**
MAJOR DISABILITY IN SURVIVORS				
Dykes et al 1989	8/15	10/14		0.75 (0.42, 1.33)
Ventriculomegaly Trial Group 1990	47/59	41/53		1.03 (0.85, 1.25)
Total	**55/74**	**51/67**		**0.98 (0.81, 1.18)**
MULTIPLE DISABILITY IN SURVIVORS				
Dykes et al 1989	4/15	5/14		0.75 (0.25, 2.23)
Ventriculomegaly Trial Group 1990	32/59	31/53		0.93 (0.67, 1.28)
Total	**36/74**	**36/67**		**0.90 (0.66, 1.24)**

0.1   1   10

Relative risk (95% CI fixed effects model)

Source: Adapted from a systematic review (Whitelaw 1998).

many centers for treatment of PHVD. Furosemide has an inhibitory effect on CSF production in experimental animals. Shinnar et al (1985) described a selected uncontrolled group of infants with hydrocephalus, some of whom were below 1500 g, in whom 100 mg/Kg/day of acetazolamide was combined with 1 mg/Kg/day of furosemide. The authors concluded that they avoided shunt insertion in 50% of the babies who would otherwise have been candidates for surgery.

The International PHVD Drug Trial Group (1998) reported the results of a randomized controlled trial of acetazolamide 100 mg/Kg/day and furosemide 1 mg/Kg/day in infants with posthemorrhagic ventricular dilatation using identical eligibility criteria to the Ventriculomegaly Trial. Forty-nine out of 75 (65%) infants receiving drug treatment died or required shunt insertion and 35 out of 76 (46%) infants in the control group died or required shunt insertion (relative risk 1.42, confidence interval 1.06–1.9). Twenty-one out of 151 (14%) infants developed CNS infections with no difference between the two treatment groups. Thirty-eight out of 48 (79%) infants in the drug treatment group were impaired or disabled at 1 year, whereas 30 out of 57 (53%) in the control group were impaired or disabled at 1 year. The trial was stopped by the data-monitoring committee before the planned completion, as the results clearly showed a worse outcome in the drug-treated infants. These findings could not be explained by differences between the groups of infants at trial entry, delays in shunt surgery, or an increase in infections in the drug-treated group.

Acetazolamide has a number of effects on important physiologic systems that may be relevant to the findings of this trial. Cerebral blood flow is increased substantially for several hours following 50 mg/Kg of acetazolamide. Blood pressure does not change, but the cerebral vasodilatation can give a transient rise in intracranial pressure before the reduced production of CSF has time to reduce the intracranial pressure (Cowan & Whitelaw 1991). These effects on the cerebral circulation are not thought to increase the risk of intraventricular hemorrhage in stable infants who are several weeks or months old.

The effects on PCO_2 can be clinically significant. Carbonic anhydrase is necessary for the rapid conversion of circulating bicarbonate to carbon dioxide, which is exhaled as blood flows through the alveolar capillaries of the lungs. Acetazolamide inhibits pulmonary carbon dioxide elimination. In newborn piglets which had been tracheostomized, ventilated and paralyzed to hold the PCO_2 constant, intravenous acetazolamide produced an immediate reduction in end-tidal PCO_2 measured by tracheal catheter and a rise in arterial PCO_2 of 1.5 kPa within 10 min (Thoresen & Whitelaw 1990).

This inhibition of CO_2 elimination is not a clinical problem in infants with normal lungs as they can compensate by breathing faster, thus holding PCO_2 constant. However, infants who are ventilator-dependent or who have significant bronchopulmonary dysplasia cannot compensate (Cowan & Whitelaw 1991). In four such infants, acetazolamide produced a median increase of 2.0 kPa (range 0.6–3.4 kPa) with a corresponding reduction in pH such that acetazolamide had to be discontinued and mechanical ventilation increased.

Many preterm infants with PHVD are also likely to have chronic lung disease. Acetazolamide also has a mild diuretic effect and increases urinary excretion of bicarbonate. Thus, it is normally necessary to give 4 mmol/Kg/day of sodium bicarbonate and, if furosemide is used as well, 1 mmol/Kg/day of potassium chloride, as replacement for urinary losses. A considerable proportion of infants under 1500 g with PHVD is also likely to have chronic lung disease and immature renal function and may therefore be at risk of acid–base, blood-gas and electrolyte disturbances. Aplastic anemia has been associated with acetazolamide therapy (Keisu et al 1990).

ISOSORBIDE

Isosorbide reduces CSF production by an osmotic effect, but a high incidence of side-effects such as vomiting has been reported (Liptak et al 1992).

GLYCEROL

Glycerol is another osmotic agent that has been used for control of hydrocephalus. There is no published experience with small preterm infants.

For all of the above reasons, drug therapy to reduce CSF production cannot be recommended.

VENTRICULAR RESERVOIR

If there is persistent intracranial hypertension and excessive head growth, despite attempts at medical management, surgical treatment becomes the only option. Excessive head growth is arbitrarily defined as an average of 2 mm/day or crossing from below the 50th centile to 2 cm over the 90th centile. A ventricular catheter can be inserted through a burr hole and connected to a subcutaneous reservoir (Fig. 42.13). Such a reservoir can be used to measure CSF pressure and remove CSF as often as is necessary to control pressure and head growth. This can be done even in the presence of blood-stained, protein-rich or infected CSF. Such CSF tapping does require sterile technique, and there is a small risk of introducing infection, but it is considerably easier than ventricular or lumbar puncture. Another possible advantage is that fresh needle tracks are not made through the brain every time CSF is removed. Thus, a ventricular reservoir is an alternative to repeated ventricular punctures. The surgical procedure is shorter and simpler than a full shunt, and many infants below 1000 g have been treated in this way (Anwar et al 1986). A ventricular reservoir provides temporary control in hospital while waiting for (1) the PHVD to resolve spontaneously, (2) protein and blood to clear from the CSF and (3) growth and recovery of the infant from lung disease before insertion of a permanent shunt. The details of shunt surgery and its complications are discussed in Chapter 43.

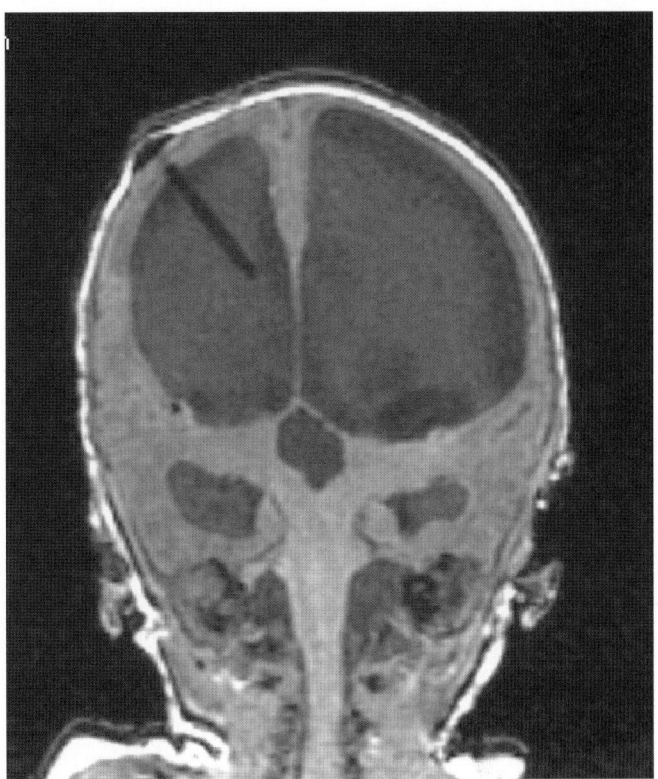

Figure 42.13 MRI coronal view showing a ventricular catheter connected to an Ommaya reservoir.

INTRAVENTRICULAR FIBRINOLYTIC THERAPY

Urokinase and streptokinase in hydrocephalus after ventriculitis

Fibrin deposition can also lead to hydrocephalus after ventriculitis and streptokinase and urokinase have been given intraventricularly to infants with ventriculitis to prevent hydrocephalus (Stewart 1964). The effectiveness of this approach cannot be judged as no controlled trials have been carried out.

INTRAVENTRICULAR THROMBOLYTIC THERAPY IN POSTHEMORRHAGIC HYDROCEPHALUS

Obstruction of the ventricular foramina by multiple small blood clots is part of the mechanism of PHVD, and the presence of X oligomer (a fibrin degradation product) in the CSF of infants with PHVD is evidence of endogenous fibrinolysis in the CSF (Whitelaw et al 1991). We have also been able to demonstrate fibrinolytic activity in the CSF of infants with PHVD by a fibrin plate assay. It seemed logical to try to augment the natural fibrinolysis with a plasminogen activator in the CSF. A controlled trial in dogs showed that intraventricular urokinase given after intraventricular injection of blood significantly reduced the risk of hydrocephalus (Pang et al 1986). An open study of six adult patients with intraventricular hemorrhage showed that repeated intraventricular injections of urokinase gave a lower incidence of hydrocephalus than a group of historical control patients (Todo et al 1991). In a pilot, non-randomized study, nine infants with PHVD (with the same diagnostic criteria as described above: ventricular width 4 mm over the 97th centile) received intraventricular infusions of streptokinase at 1000 units/h for about 48 h via a ventricular catheter inserted percutaneously through the lambdoid suture. They were nearly all very-low-birthweight preterm infants and were treated between 7 and 28 days of age. Secondary bleeding occurred in only one infant and the proportion of infants subsequently requiring shunt surgery was much lower than expected (Whitelaw et al 1992). Intraventricular streptokinase increases fibrin degradation products in the CSF. Luciano et al (1997) carried out a randomized trial of intraventricular streptokinase in 12 infants developing post-hemorrhagic ventricular dilatation. Twenty thousand units of streptokinase/day were given for 4 days via a ventricular reservoir. Three out of six infants in each group had to be shunted, and one died in each group. One of the infants in the streptokinase group developed secondary intraventricular hemorrhage and meningitis.

Recombinant human tissue plasminogen activator (rtPA) activates all the available plasminogen to plasmin and has the additional advantage of not being antigenic. Many adult patients with subarachnoid or intraventricular hemorrhage have been treated with intrathecal or intraventricular rtPA. The overall conclusion of these uncontrolled observations was that intrathecal fibrinolytic therapy had helped to reduce vasospasm and clear blood from the CSF. A phase 1 open trial of intraventricular tPA (0.5 mg for infants below 1000 g and 1.0 mg for infants 1000 g or more) in 22 infants with PHVD used the same inclusion criteria as the Ventriculo-megaly and PHVD Drug trials. The tPA was given by bolus injection, and the median number of doses was two. Twelve of the 22 infants survived without shunt surgery, nine infants required shunts and one infant died with hydro-cephalus. One definite case of secondary intraventricular hemorrhage was observed. There was no secondary infection (Whitelaw et al 1996). These results were only marginally better than historical controls, and, taken with the negative results from the randomized trial of Luciano et al (1997), mean that intraventricular thrombolytic therapy cannot be recommended.

Drainage, irrigation and fibrinolytic therapy (DRIFT)

We have evaluated a procedure that involves insertion of two intraventricular catheters, one frontal on the right, and one occipital on the left. tPA (0.5 mg) is given intraventricu-larly and after 8 hours, the ventricular system is irrigated with isotonic artificial CSF (without protein) at 20 mL/h for 72 hours. The second catheter is attached to a drainage system that can be positioned to increase or decrease the rate of drainage (usually at least 20 mL/h), and a pressure transducer on the infusion line provides continuous ICP monitoring. The objectives are to remove old blood, cyto-kines, free iron and hypoxanthine before permanent hydro-cephalus is established. Of 25 infants with PHVD treated with this protocol, eighteen survived without a shunt (Whitelaw et al 2003). This highly invasive and experimental intervention has been tested in a multicenter randomized trial. There was an excess of secondary intraventricular hemorrhage in the DRIFT group and no significant reduction in the primary outcome, shunt or death (Whitelaw et al 2007).

SUMMARY OF MANAGEMENT OF PHVD

There are few randomized controlled trials to guide the best management of PHVD, but the current advice on the prin-ciples of management is summarized in the Key Points.

REFERENCES

Anwar M, Dolye A J, Kadam S et al 1986 Management of posthemorrhagic hydrocephalus in the preterm infant. J Pediatr Surg 21:334–337.

Anwar M, Kadam S, Hiatt I M et al 1985 Serial lumbar punctures in prevention of posthemorrhagic hydrocephalus in preterm infants. J Pediatr 107:446–449.

Bejar R, Saugstad O D, James H, Gluck L 1983 Increased hypoxanthine concentrations in cerebrospinal fluid of infants with hydrocephalus. J Pediatr 103:44–48.

Boillat C A, Jones H C, Kaiser G L, Harris N G 1997 Ultrastructural changes in the deep cortical pyramidal cells of infant rats with inherited hydrocephalus and the effect of shunt treatment. Exp Neurol 147:377–388.

Carmel P W 1982 The Arnold–Chiari malformation. In: Pediatric neurosurgery. Section of Pediatric Neurosurgery of the American Association of Neurological Surgeons. Grune and Stratton, New York, NY.

Cherian S, Thoresen M, Silver I A et al 2004 Transforming growth factor-betas in a rat model of neonatal posthaemorrhagic hydrocephalus. Neuropathol Appl Neurobiol 30:585–600.

Cowan F, Whitelaw A 1991 Acute effects of acetazolamide on cerebral blood flow velocity and PCO_2 in the newborn infant. Acta Paediatr Scand 80:22–27.

Davies M W, Swaminathan M, Chuang S L et al 2000 Reference ranges for linear dimensions of intracranial ventricles in preterm neonates. Arch Dis Child 82:F218–F23.

Davson H, Welch K, Segal M B 1987 The physiology and pathophysiology of the cerebrospinal fluid. Churchill Livingstone, Edinburgh.

De Vries L S, Liem K D, van Dijk K et al 2002 Early versus late treatment of posthaemorrhagic ventricular dilatation: results of a retrospective study from five neonatal intensive care units in The Netherlands. Acta Paediatrica 91(2):212–217.

De Vries L S, Pierrat V, Minami T et al 1990 The role of short latency somatosensory evoked responses in infants with rapidly progressive ventricular dilatation. Neuropediatrics 21:136–139.

Dubovitz L, Dubowitz V, Mercuri E 2000 The neurological assessment of the preterm and full-term newborn infant. Mac Keith, London.

Dykes F D, Dunbar B, Lazarra A et al 1989 Posthemorrhagic hydrocephalus in high risk infants: Natural history, management and long term outcome. J Pediatr 114:611–618.

Fenton T R 2003 A new growth chart for preterm babies: Babson and Benda's chart updated with recent data and a new format. BMC Pediatrics 3:13 doi:10.1186/1471-2431-3-13 http://www.biomedcentral.com/1471-2431/3/13.

Fernell E, Hagberg G, Hagberg B 1990 Infantile hydrocephalus — the impact of enhanced preterm survival. Acta Paediatr Scand 79:1080–1086.

Fletcher J M, Landry S H, Bohan T P et al 1997 Effects of intraventricular hemorrhage and hydrocephalus on the long-term neurobehavioural development of preterm very-low-birthweight infants. Dev Med Child Neurol 39:596–606.

Flood C, Akinwunmi J, Lagord C et al 2001 Transforming growth factor-beta1 in the cerebrospinal fluid of patients with subarachnoid hemorrhage: titers derived from exogenous and endogenous sources. J Cereb Blood Flow Metab 21:157–162.

Greitz D, Hannerz J 1996 A proposed model of cerebrospinal fluid circulation: observations with radionuclide cisternography. AJNR 17:431–438.

Hanlo P W, Gooskens R H, Nijhuis I J et al 1995 Value of transcranial Doppler indices in predicting raised ICP in infantile hydrocephalus. Childs Nerv Syst 11:595–603.

Heep A, Stoffel-Wagner B, Bartmann P et al 2004 Vascular endothelial growth factor and transforming growth factor-beta1 are highly expressed in the cerebrospinal fluid of premature infants with posthemorrhagic hydrocephalus. Pediatr Res 56:768–774.

Huang C C, Chang Y C, Chow N H, Wang S T 1997 Level of transforming growth factor beta 1 is elevated in cerebrospinal fluid of children with acute bacterial meningitis. J Neurol 244:634–638.

International PHVD Drug Trial Group 1998 International randomised controlled trial of acetazolamide and furosemide in posthaemorrhagic ventricular dilatation in infancy. Lancet 352:433–440.

Johnston M, Zakharov A, Papaiconomou C et al Evidence of connections between cerebrospinal fluid and nasal lymphatic vessels in humans, non-human primates and other mammalian species. Cerebrospinal Fluid Res 10:2.

Jouet M, Moncla A, Paterson J et al 1995 New domains of neural cell-adhesion molecule L1 implicated in X -linked hydrocephalus and MASA syndrome. Am J Hum Genet 56:1304–1314.

Kaiser A, Whitelaw A 1985 Cerebrospinal fluid pressure in infants with post-haemorrhagic ventricular dilatation. Arch Dis Childhood 60:920–924.

Kaiser A, Whitelaw A 1986 Normal cerebrospinal fluid pressure in the newborn. Neuropediatrics 17:100–102.

Kaiser A, Whitelaw A 1987 Non-invasive measurement of intracranial pressure. Fact or fancy. Dev Med Child Neurol 29:320–326.

Keisu M, Wiholm B E, Öst A et al 1990 Acetazolamide-associated aplastic anaemia. J Intern Med 228:627–632.

Kitisawa K, Tada T 1994 Elevation of transforming growth factor-β-1 level in cerebrospinal fluid of patients with communicating hydrocephalus after subarachnoid hemorrhage. Stroke 25:1400–1404.

Larroche J C 1972 Posthaemorrhagic hydrocephalus in infancy. Biologia Neonatorum 20:287–299.

Levene M I 1981 Measurement of the growth of the lateral ventricles in pretem infants with real time ultrasound. Arch Dis Childhood 56:900–940.

Liptak G S, Gellerstedt M E, Klionsky N 1992 Isosorbide in the medical management of hydrocephalus in children with myelodysplasia. Dev Med Child Neurol 34:150–154.

Luciano R, Velardi F, Romagnoli C et al 1997 Failure of fibrinolytic endoventricular treatment to prevent neonatal post-haemorrhagic hydrocephalus. Childs Nerv System 13:73–76.

Mantovani J F, Pasternak J F, Mathew O P et al 1980 Failure of daily lumbar punctures to prevent the development of hydrocephalus following intraventricular hemorrhage. J Pediatr 97:278–281.

Ment L R, Duncan C C, Geehr R 1981 Benign enlargement of the subarachnoid spaces in the infant. J Neurosurg 54:504–508.

Milhorat T H 1972 Hydrocephalus and the cerebrospinal fluid. Williams & Wilkins, Baltimore, MD.

Milhorat T H 1982 Hydrocephalus: historical notes, etiology and clinical diagnosis. In: Pediatric neurosurgery. Section of Pediatric Neurosurgery of the American Association of Neurological Surgeons. Grune and Stratton, New York, NY.

Myrianthopoulos N C, Kurland L T 1961 Present concepts of the epidemiology and genetics of hydrocephalus. In: Fields W J, Demond M M (eds) Disorders of the developing nervous system. Charles C Thomas, Springfield, IL, pp. 187–702.

Nulsen F E, Rekate H L 1982 Results of treatment for hydrocephalus as a guide to future management. In: Pediatric neurosurgery. Section of Pediatric Neurosurgery of the American Association of Neurological Surgeons. Grune and Stratton, New York, NY.

Pang D, Sclabassi R J, Horton J A 1986 Lysis of intraventricular blood clot with urokinase in a canine model: part 3. Neurosurgery 19:553–572.

Savman K, Blennow M, Hagberg H et al 2002 Cytokine response in cerebrospinal fluid from preterm infants with posthaemorrhagic ventricular dilatation. Acta Paediatr 91:1357–1363.

Savman K, Nilsson U A, Blennow M et al 2001 Non-protein-bound iron is elevated in cerebrospinal fluid from preterm infants with posthemorrhagic ventricular dilatation. Pediatr Res 49(2):208–212.

Shankaran S, Koepke T, Woldte E et al 1989 Outcome after posthemorrhagic ventriculomegaly in comparison with mild hemorrhage without ventriculomegaly. J Pediatr 114:109–114.

Shinnar S, Gammon K, Bergman E W et al 1985 Management of hydrocephalus in infancy: use of acetazolamide and furosemide to avoid cerebrospinal fluid shunts. J Pediatr 107:31–63.

Stewart G T 1964 Fibrinolytic therapy in meningitis and ventriculitis. J Clin Pathol 17:355–359.

Tada T, Kanaji M, Kobayashi S 1994 Induction of communicating hydrocephalus in mice by intrathecal injection of human recombinant transforming growth factor-β-1. J Neuroimmunol 50:153–158.

Taylor G A, Madsen J R 1996 Neonatal hydrocephalus: hemodynamic response to fontanelle compression — correlation with intracranial pressure and need for shunt placement. Radiology 201:685–689.

Thoresen M, Whitelaw A 1990 Effect of acetazolamide on cerebral blood flow velocity and CO, elimination in normotensive and hypotensive newborn piglets. Biol Neonate 58:200–207.

Todo T, Usui M, Takakura K 1991 Treatment of severe intraventricular hemorrhage by intraventricular infusion of urokinase. J Neurosurg 74:81–86.

Van der Flier M, Hoppenreijs S, van Rensburg A J et al 2004 Vascular endothelial growth factor and blood-brain barrier disruption in tuberculous meningitis. Pediatr Infect Dis J 23:608–613.

Ventriculomegaly Trial Group 1990 Randomised trial of early tapping in neonatal posthaemorrhagic ventricular dilatation. Arch Dis Childhood 65:3–10.

Ventriculomegaly Trial Group 1994 Randomised trial of early tapping in neonatal posthaemorrhagic ventricular dilatation: results at 30 months. Arch Dis Childhood 70:F129–F136.

Weller R, Shulman K 1972 Infantile hydrocephalus: clinical, histological, and ultrastructural study of brain damage. J Neurosurg 36:255–265.

Weller R, Wisnieski H, Shulman K et al 1971 Experimental hydrocephalus in young dogs: histological and ultrastructural study of the brain tissue damage. Neuropathol Exp Neurol 30:613–627.

Whitelaw A 1998 Repeated lumbar or ventricular punctures in newborns with intraventricular haemorrhage. Oxford: The Cochrane Library, Update Software. Disk Issue 4.

Whitelaw A, Christie S, Pople I 1999 Transforming growth factor beta: a possible signal molecule for post-hemorrhagic hydrocephalus. Pediatr Res 46:576–580.

Whitelaw A, Creighton L, Gaffney P 1991 Fibrinolytic activity in cerebrospinal fluid after intraventricular haemorrhage. Arch Dis Childhood 66:808–809.

Whitelaw A, Evans D, Carter M et al 2007 Randomized clinical trial of prevention of hydrocephalus after intraventricular hemorrhage in premature infants: brain-washing versus tapping fluid. Pediatrics 119: e1071–1078.

Whitelaw A, Pople I, Cherian S et al 2003 Phase 1 trial of prevention of hydrocephalus after intraventricular hemorrhage in newborn infants by drainage, irrigation, and fibrinolytic therapy. Pediatrics 111(4 Pt 1):759–65.

Whitelaw A, Rivers R, Creighton L et al 1992 Low dose intraventricular fibrinolytic therapy to prevent posthaemorrhagic hydrocephalus. Arch Dis Childhood 67:12–14.

Whitelaw A, Suliba E, Fellman V et al 1996 Phase 1 study of intraventricular recombinant tissue plasminogen activator for treatment of post haemorrhagic hydrocephalus. Arch Dis Child 75: F20–26.

Wyss-Coray T, Feng L, Masliah E et al 1995 Increased central nervous system production of extracellular matrix components and development of hydrocephalus in transgenic mice overexpressing transforming growth factor-beta 1. Am J Pathol 147:53–67.

CHAPTER

43

Neurosurgical management of hydrocephalus

Guirish A. Solanki and Anthony D. Hockley

> **Key Points**
>
> - Hydrocephalus is a common birth defect, affecting more than 10 000 babies each year. One birth in 2000 results in the condition
> - In children under 2 years of age the first sign is the abnormally large head
> - Treatment of hydrocephalus includes physiological methods, for example, endoscopic third ventriculostomy (ETV). This is not a 'cure,' and children need to be followed up by MR imaging
> - The mainstay of treatment for infantile hydrocephalus remains ventricular shunting procedures, usually ventriculo-peritoneal (VP) shunts
> - The problems with shunts are their complications, occurring in approximately 46% of cases

INTRODUCTION

Hydrocephalus is the most common disorder treated by pediatric neurosurgeons. It is a condition in which there is a pathological increase in the amount of cerebrospinal fluid (CSF) within the ventricular system (Fig. 43.1) and subarachnoid space. Theoretically this may arise in three ways, namely: from oversecretion of CSF, from obstruction of the CSF pathways or from impaired venous absorption of the fluid. Of these, only obstruction of the CSF pathways due to congenital or acquired lesions is a proven cause.

Hydrocephalus has been recognized for a long time. Galen noted the thin brain and skull associated with excess water in the ventricles. In 1504 Leonardo da Vinci produced a wax cast of the ventricles. The first accurate description of hydrocephalus was by Vesalius in the sixteenth century (Whytt 1768). Attempts to relieve the condition were made by the ancient Greeks, Hippocrates being credited with having first punctured the dilated ventricles. External removal of ventricular fluid was practiced in the eighteenth century, but such interventions were followed almost invariably by death. In order to provide continuous drainage of CSF, whilst at the same time avoiding infection or too rapid removal of the fluid, the next logical development was to introduce internal drainage of CSF with or without the use of implanted materials, the principles upon which modern methods of treatment have been developed.

PATHOLOGY

Under normal circumstances the rate of CSF formation in man is approximately 0.35 mL/minute, or 500 mL/day (Cutler et al 1968). The classic observations by Dandy and Blackfan (1914) indicated that CSF is produced by the choroid plexus in the lateral ventricles. Modern evidence supports this origin for 60% of the fluid, the remaining 40% being produced by ependymal cells and probably elsewhere in the subarachnoid space. CSF then circulates from the lateral ventricles, through the paired intra-ventricular foramina of Monro to reach the third ventricle (Fig. 43.2). It then flows through the aqueduct of Sylvius into the fourth ventricle, where it passes into the subarachnoid space through the paired lateral foramina of Luschka and the midline foramen of Magendie. It then circulates over the surface of the brain and spinal cord, where it is absorbed into the bloodstream through the arachnoid villi, mainly situated over the cerebral convexities. A number of other sites of absorption, including the ventricle wall, the meninges themselves, and the lymphatics of the spinal and cranial nerves, provide compensatory sites in pathological states such as hydrocephalus. Since the total CSF volume in children varies from 50–150 mL, it is evident that this fluid is renewed at least every eight hours.

In clinical practice, virtually all cases of hydrocephalus are due to an obstructive lesion (Russell 1949). Rare exceptions include choroid plexus hyperplasia or papilloma (Fig. 43.3), where in some cases there may be excess CSF production. The term 'non-communicating' hydrocephalus has been used where the obstructive lesion prevents a free communication between the ventricular system and the subarachnoid space. The term 'communicating' hydrocephalus describes those conditions in which the obstructive lesion is outside the brain, thus allowing communication between the cerebral ventricles and at least part of the subarachnoid spaces. Communicating hydrocephalus is often an accompaniment of severe prematurity where the absorptive arachnoid villi may not have developed fully or in sufficient numbers, much akin to surfactant failure seen in the lungs. Similarly failure of CSF absorption by arachnoid villi, leading to hydrocephalus, can occur after meningeal infections including bacterial, fungal and tuberculosis (TB). Subarachnoid hemorrhage, which may be spontaneous, traumatic or post-operative, and diffuse carcinomatous meningitis can also adversely affect absorption.

Finally a rare but striking form of communicating hydrocephalus is hydranencephaly or anencephaly (p. 257), a post-neurulation defect that results in total or near total absence of the cerebral tissue. This is usually due to bilateral internal carotid artery infarcts resulting in massive hydrocephalus with just a brainstem nodule consisting of the basal

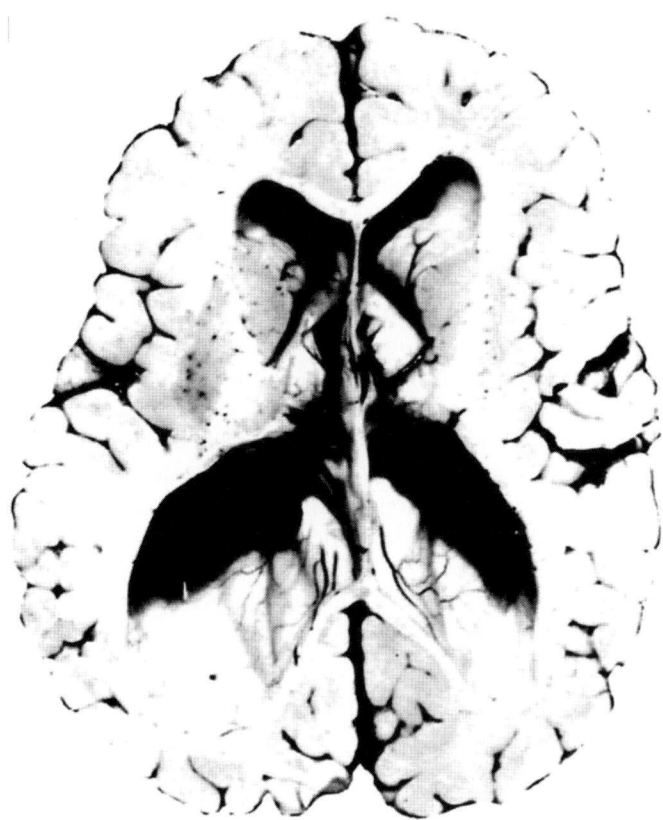

Figure 43.1 Appearance of brain with enlarged ventricles due to communicating hydrocephalus.

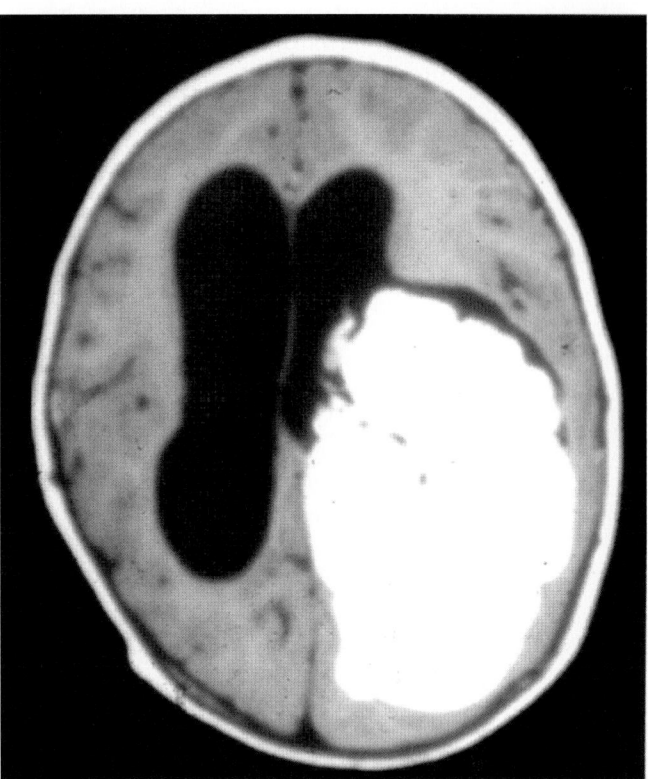

Figure 43.3 MRI scan showing the typical appearance of a choroid plexus papilloma which can be responsible for excess CSF production. There is associated hydrocephalus.

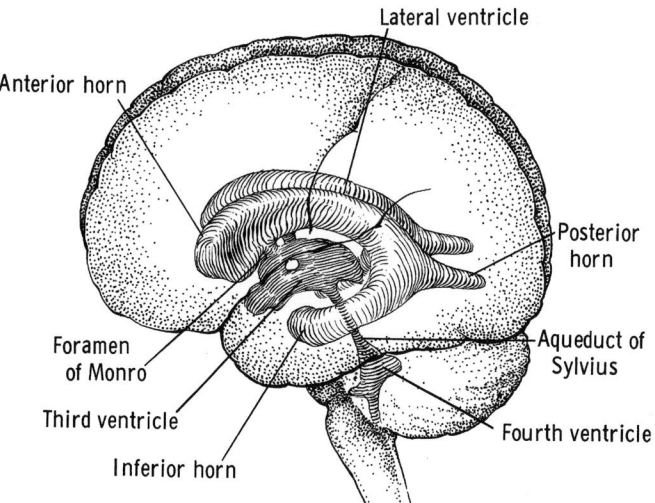

Figure 43.2 Diagram to demonstrate the anatomy of the ventricular system.

ganglia medial parts of occipital cortex and structures caudal to it. Other organic brain malformations such as agenesis of corpus callosum and alobar holoprosencephaly may also be associated with hydrocephalus.

Numerous classifications of hydrocephalus exist, with confusing terminology. A simple and easily understandable classification is based on the location of the CSF block (Table 43.1) and its pathogenesis in relation to birth. During the neonatal to late infancy period (0–2 years) hydrocephalus is usually caused by a developmental abnormality, aqueduct stenosis being the most common. The hydrocephalus found in babies with spina bifida usually results from an associated Arnold–Chiari malformation where there is downward herniation of the cerebellum through the foramen magnum. Perinatal hemorrhage and meningitis are other possible causes in this age group. An inheritable form of aqueduct stenosis has been described which occurs only in males and is transmitted by a female carrier. This so-called 'X-linked hydrocephalus' (p. 269) is extremely rare, accounting for less than 2% of all cases of congenital hydrocephalus. In early to late childhood (2–10 years) the most common causes of hydrocephalus are posterior fossa tumors and aqueduct stenosis.

Hydrocephalus is one of the most common 'birth defects' and afflicts in excess of 10 000 babies each year. Studies by the World Health Organization show that one birth in every 2000 results in hydrocephalus. In the United States, a little over 1 in 1000 births is affected by hydrocephalus. The incidence of infantile hydrocephalus recognized from the first three months of life is approximately 3–4 per 1000 births. Occurring as a single congenital disorder, the incidence of hydrocephalus is 0.9–1.5 per 1000 births and

835

Table 43.1 Common causes of hydrocephalus by location of obstruction

Site of block	Cause
Lateral ventricle	Perinatal ventricular hemorrhage
	Ventriculitis
	Choroid plexus cyst
Foramen of Monro	Ventriculitis
	Colloid cyst
	Glioma
Third ventricle	Glioma
	Suprasellar cyst/tumor
Aqueduct of Sylvius	Developmental stenosis
	Tumor
	Arteriovenous malformation
Fourth ventricle	Cerebellar tumor
	Meningitis
	Ependymal/arachnoid cyst
	Dandy–Walker syndrome
Subarachnoid spaces	Arnold–Chiari malformation
	Meningitis
	Subarachnoid hemorrhage
	Subdural hematoma
	Craniosynostosis syndromes

occurring with spina bifida it varies from 1.3–2.9 per 1000 births (Milhorat 1972).

CLINICAL FEATURES

With the current advances in ante-natal monitoring, the vast majority of congenital cases of hydrocephalus are diagnosed early allowing for planned cesarean delivery in the moderate to severe cases where cephalo-pelvic disproportion is expected.

The clinical features of hydrocephalus depend on the time of onset in relation to closure of the cranial sutures and the nature of the obstruction. *In children under two years of age*, the first clinical indication is the abnormally large head. In a minority of cases this is present at birth. In most however the hydrocephalus only gradually becomes obvious. The onset may be so insidious that the condition is overlooked for several weeks. The baby usually continues in good general health, alert and feeding normally (Kirkpatrick et al 1989). When the intracranial pressure becomes significantly raised, there may be vomiting after feeds, a palpable tense anterior fontanelle and limitation of upward gaze ('sun setting' sign).

Only in the older baby, over the age of six months, are abnormal neurological signs such as limb spasticity likely to be found. Papilledema with or without consecutive optic atrophy is not usually seen in the neonatal period. Epileptic seizures are very rarely seen as a result of hydrocephalus alone.

When making a diagnosis of hydrocephalus in *neonates* or *infants*, it is essential to establish there is a truly abnormal rate of skull growth. The head circumference needs to be recorded with a patient's exact age and plotted on an accepted growth curve chart. In newborns and infants, soon after birth an examination of the anterior fontanelle will reveal a widened fontanelle and sutural diastasis. The fontanelle may become tense or bulge out. The head circumference is likely to be in the 98th percentile or above rather than on the 50th percentile. These babies have a disproportionately large head to their body size. In advanced cases, clinical examination reveals a significant craniofacial disproportion with expansion of the dome and low-set ears and eyes. The skull is often thin and forehead veins distended. Palpable separation of the cranial sutures and a hollow or 'cracked-pot' percussion note (Macewen sign) may be found. In very severe cases, where the cerebral cortex is thinned, trans-illumination of the head may be possible.

The differential diagnosis of an enlarged head includes subdural hematomas or effusions (hygromas), considered to be related to birth trauma. In such cases the head and facial appearance are typically square in shape, in contrast to the disproportionate head in hydrocephalus. Certain metabolic and degenerative disorders such as glycogen storage and Alexander disease can cause macrocephaly. There may be an innocent explanation such as a family history of large heads. Finally, some brain tumors of infancy may reach enormous size, producing a large head quite apart from whether there is any associated hydrocephalus. Radiological imaging will resolve the issue.

The term 'benign external hydrocephalus' is applied to infants and children with enlarged subarachnoid spaces, accompanied by increasing head circumference and with normal or mildly dilated ventricles. This benign form implies lack of any neurological deficits. The condition is also known as 'benign subdural collections of infancy' or 'pericerebral CSF collections'. Some postulate that this is a variant of communicating hydrocephalus (Barlow 1984). It tends to run a benign course and stabilizes by 12 to 18 months of age (Ment et al 1981). Close serial monitoring of head circumference and CT or MR imaging to monitor for ventriculomegaly is recommended. Shunting is rarely, if ever, required.

In older children (2–10 years), patients may be divided into two groups. In the first group are those children with pre-existing (infantile) but unrecognized progressive hydrocephalus, which may or may not be partially compensated. Neurological development may be normal, borderline or retarded. The head may be enlarged and an erroneous diagnosis of 'arrested hydrocephalus' may be used. These patients may later deteriorate after a head injury or a viral infection. There may also be endocrine changes resulting in poor growth, obesity, gigantism, precocious or delayed puberty, diabetes insipidus or menstrual irregularities. Such hormonal changes are probably due to abnormal hypothalamic function secondary to increased intracranial pressure or dilatation of the third ventricle. Spasticity and reduced intellectual function are common. These patients may reach adulthood before the diagnosis is suspected.

The second group consists of children who develop hydrocephalus after closure of the cranial sutures, so that the head circumference usually remains within normal limits. Headaches and vomiting are common, and the clinical features are those of any lesion producing increased intracranial pressure.

INVESTIGATIONS

The majority of cases can be diagnosed immediately and simply by ultrasound scanning through the anterior fontanelle. This easy and safe investigation is very helpful for babies with enlarged heads or failure to thrive associated with vomiting, for which there is no other immediately obvious cause. Improved anatomical detail is provided by computerized tomography (CT) scanning or magnetic resonance imaging (MRI). MRI scanning is particularly helpful in assessing the feasibility of third ventriculostomy as treatment for the hydrocephalus in an individual patient. It helps to plan the surgical approach and exclude mass or cystic lesions.

Computed tomography (CT) scan has a lesser role as a diagnostic tool and goes against the 'ALARA' (as low as reasonably achievable) principles for avoiding radiation (Suess & Chen 2002). However, although not ideal, it remains the usual investigation for serial follow-up given its widespread availability out of hours. This is covered in detail in Chapter 6 of this book.

MANAGEMENT

Several studies have demonstrated that untreated hydrocephalus results in brain damage to the surrounding white matter and cortical thinning. Ultrastructural changes in the periventricular tissues leading to gliotic scarring and neuron destruction is a late consequence of hydrocephalus (Weller et al 1971, Wozniak et al 1975).

Any baby with progressive hydrocephalus will, if untreated, reach a condition of stability where no further enlargement of the ventricle or skull will take place. When this stage is reached, the child may be of normal intelligence but is more likely to be seriously handicapped. The aim of surgical treatment is to prevent brain damage over a period of time until a stage of equilibrium or 'arrest' concerning the CSF circulation is reached.

Medical management is discussed in Chapter 42.

SURGICAL TREATMENT OF HYDROCEPHALUS

Dandy in 1918 wrote:

> No form of treatment, either medical or surgical, has yet a valid claim to the cure of a single case of hydrocephalus, accept in those cases caused by tumor and relieved by tumor extirpation.

This position remains the same.

The multiplicity of operations devised for the treatment of hydrocephalus is evidence of the unsatisfactory nature of most of them. Essentially the various methods of treatment fall into two main groups, firstly, the so-called '*physiological*' operations not requiring the use of implanted materials and second '*non-physiological*' operations employing mechanical tubes and valves (shunts) to bypass the obstruction in the ventricular system.

PHYSIOLOGICAL PROCEDURES

The physiological procedures include coagulation or removal of the choroid plexus (choroid-plexectomy) and the surgical re-canalization of occluded pathways such as endoscopic aqueductoplasty or creation of an additional pathway through the floor of the third ventricle, namely endoscopic third ventriculostomy (ETV).

Choroid-plexectomy, removal or destruction of the choroid plexus and hence reduction of CSF formation, was first described in 1918 by Dandy as an open procedure but this proved dangerous and unsuccessful. Endoscopic coagulation was pursued in the pre-shunt era (Putnam 1934, Scarff 1970). With the advent of modern neuro-endoscopy there has been some revival of interest in this approach. In a series of 71 patients treated by endoscopic choroid-plexectomy between 1972 and 1983, the overall success rate was 49% (there was only one operative death) (Griffith 1986). The same team, in a later report, described a high rate of infection which was probably attributable to a regimen of postoperative ventricular irrigation (Griffith & Jamjoom 1990). Currently despite the improved technology of endoscopy, choroid plexus coagulation is mainly confined to a very small number of patients with genuine hypersecretion of CSF or an occasional neonate in whom there are desperate reasons, such as intra-abdominal sepsis, for postponing insertion of a ventriculo-peritoneal shunt (Bucholz & Pittman 1991).

Endoscopic third ventriculostomy (ETV) aims to restore the CSF circulation when hydrocephalus involves an obstructed third ventricle (Fig. 43.4). An opening is made surgically in the floor of the third ventricle, anterior to the mamillary bodies, to allow drainage of CSF into the basal cisterns and subarachnoid space. Although the first endoscopic third ventriculostomy was performed in 1920 (Mixter 1923) and was actively pursued by a few neurosurgeons, notably Scarff (Scarff 1936), the technique was generally abandoned when ventricular shunts were introduced. However, stimulated by a revival of interest (Vries 1978), and the frequent problems with shunt complications, ETV has been reintroduced.

Stimulated by a long and broadly favorable experience in Sydney, Australia, and aided by advances in endoscope design, the technique has undergone a renaissance. The largest series with long follow-up is that accumulated in Sydney and extends back to 1978 with an overall success rate of 61% in a mixed series of 103 children and adults (Jones et al 1994). Much smaller series have reported bigger

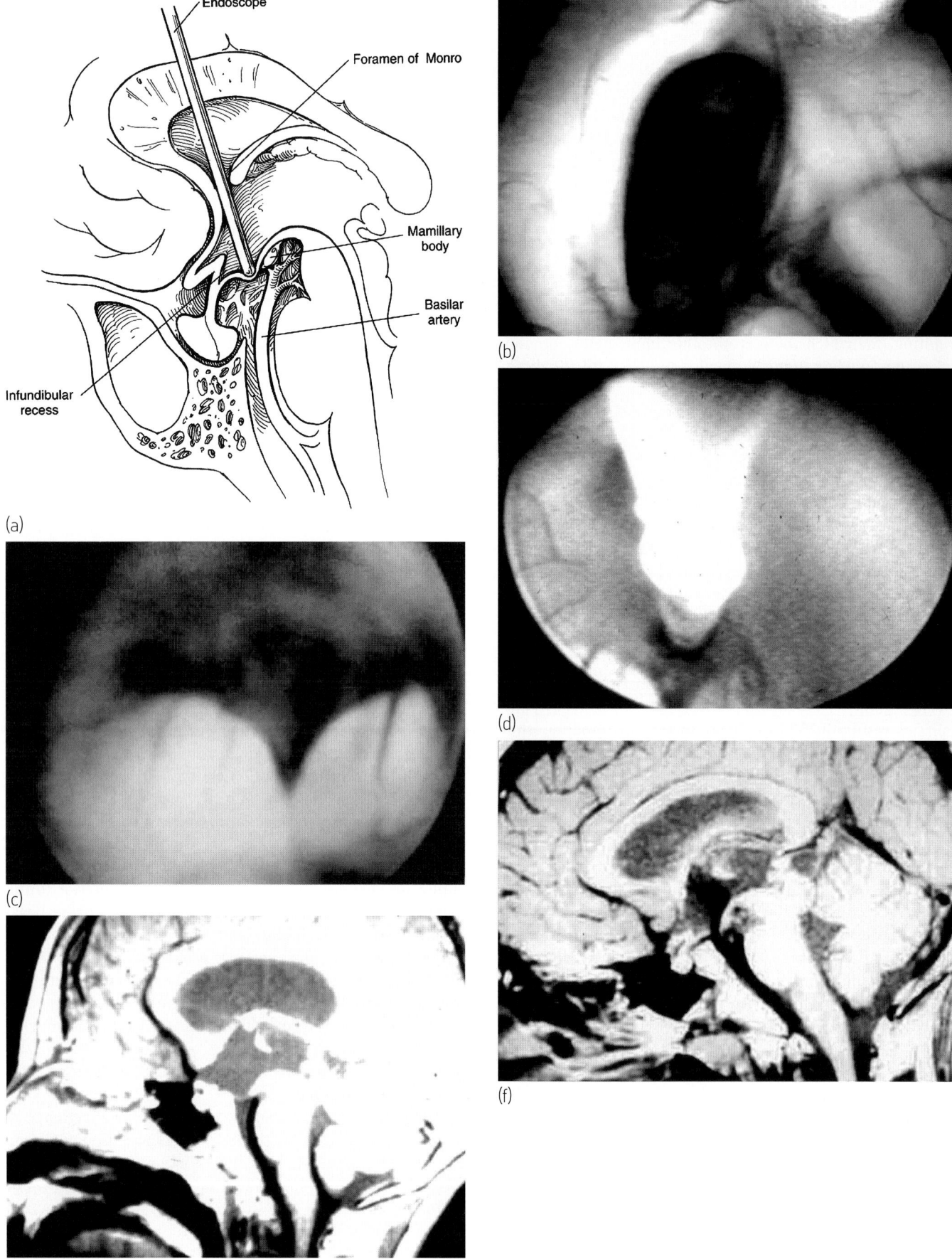

(a)

(b)

(c)

(d)

(e)

(f)

success rates but in highly selected cases: for example, an American center recorded 8 successes in 10 patients followed for up to 3 years (Cohen 1994) and a French center reported 33 successes in 35 previously untreated cases of aqueduct stenosis or posterior third ventricle tumor (Decq et al 1994). Another group reported that 42 of 69 patients, of median age 16 months, were asymptomatic and shunt-free at a median interval of 20 months' follow-up (Punt & Vloeberghs 1998). A more recent pediatric prospective series with a mean follow-up of 19 months described 550 cases of infectious, non-infectious and myelomeningocele infants with a mortality of 1.3% and an infection rate of less than 1% (Warf 2005a).

It is generally stated that ETV is less successful in neonates. In one series specifically examining the very young, only six out of 27 children of median age 3.7 months had a successful outcome (Buxton & Punt 1998). In a further group of 19 babies born at a mean of 32 weeks' gestational age and all operated upon in the first year of life (mean 9 weeks), ETV was successful in six (Buxton & Punt 1998). Although this was a low overall rate of success, the benefit of a shunt-free existence in the successful cases is not to be underrated. ETV is therefore a reasonable approach in the first year of life, especially in patients with obstructive hydrocephalus, providing that morbidity is low. This is particularly the case in underdeveloped or developing countries where dependence on shunts may be dangerous (Warf 2005b).

The success of ETV depends on patient selection. Two specific conditions are required:

1. The hydrocephalus should be of the non-communicating type.
2. There should be preservation of CSF pathways between the subarachnoid spaces and the venous system, meaning no evidence of communicating hydrocephalus.

Results are best in patients with late-onset or 'non-infantile' acquired aqueduct stenosis. In infants the subarachnoid spaces including the basal cisterns may not have opened, and there may be concomitant communicating hydrocephalus. Pre-operative MRI imaging will define the nature of the aqueduct obstruction and the position of the basilar artery. It should optimally demonstrate enlargement of the third ventricle with its floor bowed downwards.

In older children who present with shunt malfunction, ETV may offer an alternative and has been successful in

allowing removal of the shunt. However, it must be stressed that ETV is not a 'cure' (Walker et al 1992). There have been recent and increasing reports of children presenting with an acute and rapidly progressive history of raised intracranial pressure and even death (Javadpour et al 2003), who have had a previous ETV. This is considered to be due to closure of the ventriculostomy presumably due to fibrosis, and subsequent acute hydrocephalus. Surgical relief by revisional ETV or insertion of a shunt is required. This issue undermines the need to clinically monitor children with ETV as one would children with shunts. Some neurosurgeons now place a Rickham reservoir at the site of the endoscopy to allow for rapid aspiration of fluid in case of emergency.

NON-PHYSIOLOGICAL (BY-PASS) SHUNTS

The mainstay of treatment for infantile hydrocephalus remains a ventricular shunting procedure. These shunting procedures include both *intracranial* operations, with the obstruction by-passed within the ventricular system, and the more frequent and preferred *extra-cranial* operations with CSF diverted into other areas for absorption.

Of the *intracranial* shunts, the most successful historically has been *Torkildsen ventriculo-cisternostomy*, with CSF diverted by a catheter from one lateral ventricle into the cisterna magna (Torkildsen 1939).

This is of value in the treatment of hydrocephalus due to obstruction of the third ventricle, and once diversion is established the incidence of late complications is much lower than with extra-cranial procedures. Both ends of the catheter are bathed in CSF, and its function is generally unaffected by the growth of the patient. It is however a major operation and rarely used today. However some surgeons leave such a catheter in place at the time of posterior fossa tumor surgery.

Extra-cranial diversion of CSF into the blood stream or body cavities however remains the most frequent method of treating hydrocephalus. Historically the first device was the *ventriculo-atrial shunt* or VA shunt (Fig. 43.5). Early experience made it clear that artificial drainage of CSF from ventricle to venous system would succeed only if it incorporated a mechanical device that would control the flow of fluid and prevent a reverse flow of blood. The invention of such a valve is credited to Holter, an engineer, and the operative technique for its insertion of Nulsen and Spitz (1952). Although there have been subsequent modifications of their technique and the tubing and valve materials, the operation

Figure 43.4 (a) Diagram to illustrate the principle of endoscopic third ventriculostomy. The endoscope is introduced through the foramen of Monro into the third ventricle. A surgical opening is then made into the floor of the third ventricle. (b) Endoscopic view of the foramen of Monro with choroid plexus present. (c) Endoscopic view of the floor of the third ventricle, showing the mamillary bodies, and area for the ventriculostomy. (d) Balloon catheter introduced to enlarge the opening in the floor of the third ventricle. (e) Pre-operative sagittal MRI image demonstrating the floor of the third ventricle. The black 'flow void' in front of the pons represents the basilar artery. (f) Post-operative sagittal MRI image demonstrating a black 'flow void' beneath the ventriculostomy site, suggesting satisfactory flow of CSF out from the third ventricle. This is anterior to the black flow void from the basilar artery.

has remained substantially the same. A curved scalp incision is made behind and above the ear (on either side) with reflection of the scalp and pericranium. A burr hole is placed and a suitably long silicone ventricular catheter inserted into the ventricle with the aid of a stilette. The right internal jugular vein is exposed in the neck through a transverse incision, and a silicone atrial catheter pushed down into the right atrium, its position being assessed by measurement, X-ray or changes in the ECG wave using the saline-filled catheter as an electrode. The upper end of this atrial catheter is connected to the lower nozzle of the Holter valve, which is positioned in a subcutaneous tunnel between the two incisions. The upper nozzle of the Holter valve is attached to the ventricular catheter. An alternative drainage arrangement was introduced, as animal experiments found that reflux of blood into the open end of the atrial catheter might occur. A slit in the cardiac termination of the catheter was incorporated to prevent this problem (Pudenz et al 1957).

Diversion of CSF into the peritoneal cavity (*ventriculo-peritoneal* or VP shunt) has increasingly been preferred as an alternative method (Fig. 43.6). Since a longer tube can be put into the peritoneum to allow for an infant's growth, some surgeons prefer this method initially. The same shunt devices are used, with a lower catheter passed subcutaneously to a small abdominal incision and then introduced into the peritoneal cavity. As seen below, complications occur from both types of shunt, but the complications after VA shunts are more serious. Hence in current practice VP shunts are the more frequent, with VA shunts reserved for when the peritoneum is unable to absorb the fluid or there are other intra-abdominal surgical problems.

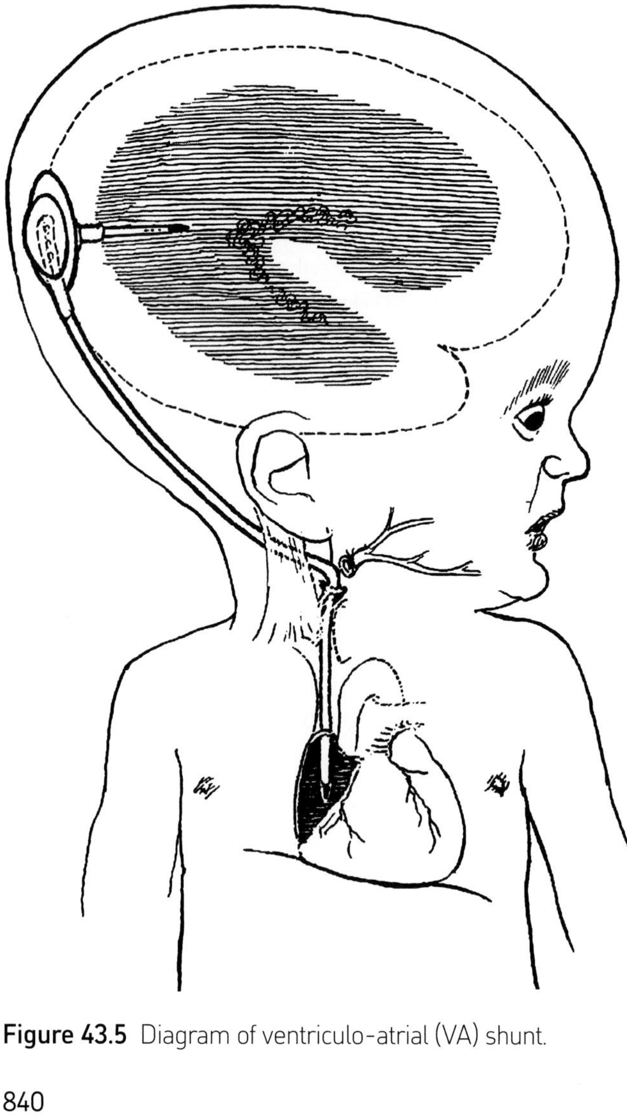

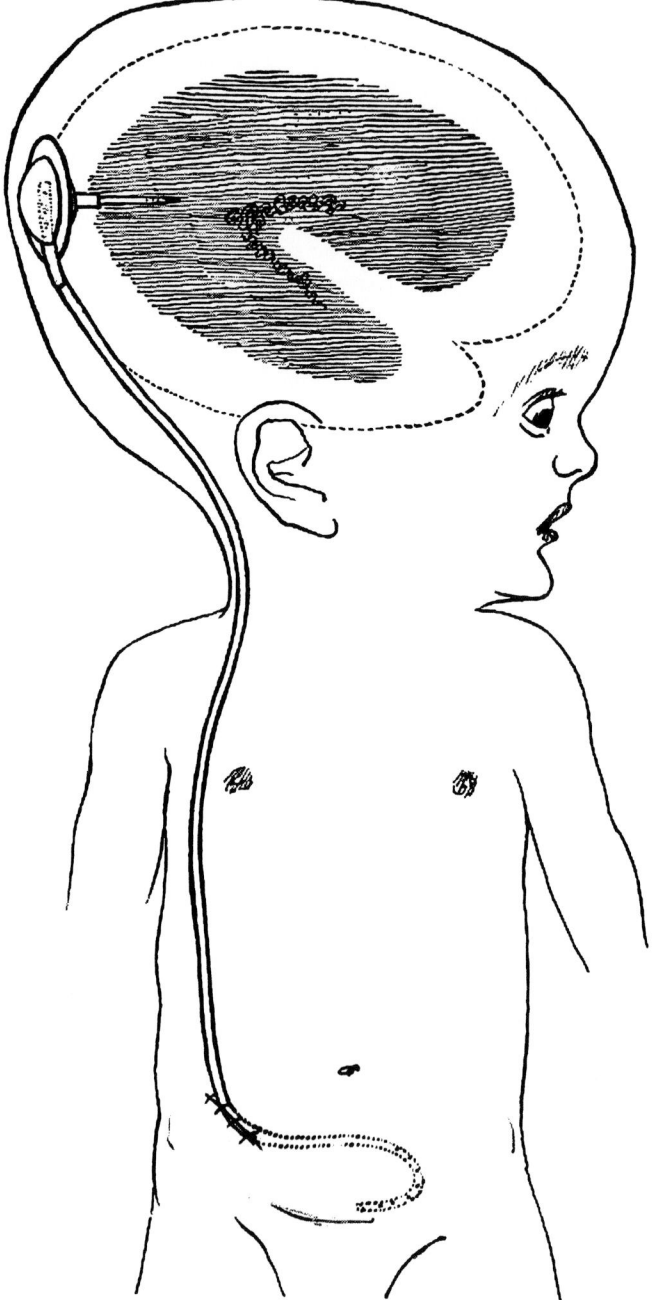

Figure 43.5 Diagram of ventriculo-atrial (VA) shunt.

Figure 43.6 Diagram of ventriculo-peritoneal (VP) shunt.

Shunting CSF into the pleural cavity or gall-bladder may be used when, for technical reasons, it may be impossible to use the peritoneal route or internal jugular veins. A direct insertion of the lower catheter into the right atrium or azygos vein may also be used but each route requires a thoracotomy.

Lumbo-peritoneal shunting has been suggested as treatment for children with communicating hydrocephalus (Hoffman et al 1976). Early complications are relatively few, but there are potentially serious late complications which include spinal deformity, arachnoiditis, slit ventricles and hindbrain herniation (Chumas et al 1993).

EXTERNAL VENTRICULAR DRAINAGE

There are situations where temporary external ventricular drainage is required. Most frequently this is needed to relieve raised intracranial pressure when there is a problem with the shunt such as after a ventricular hemorrhage or where there is infection necessitating removal of the shunt. When an *external ventricular drain* (EVD) is inserted, it should be tunneled as far as possible to an exit point at a distance from the incision used to insert the device so as to reduce the risk of infection. Incisions should be made with careful consideration to avoid potential future shunt sites. The volume of CSF lost externally should be replaced by oral or intravenous routes as normal saline. With care, tunneled drains can be maintained in neonates for a few weeks with low rates of secondary infection (Berger et al 2000, Cornips et al 1997) before a new shunt is placed. In the case of an infection affecting the lower end of the peritoneal catheter, which typically becomes blocked from the formation of an inflammatory pseudo-cyst inside the peritoneal cavity, an alternative to an EVD is to exteriorize the existing catheter or shunt system above the problem. Once the infection has been treated the original shunt and tubing are removed and replaced.

POSTOPERATIVE CARE

Postoperatively, the child is handled and fed normally. Some premature babies who have only recently become independent of ventilatory support may require a period of assisted ventilation. Indeed, it is a sound practice to plan to ventilate these babies electively, if only for a few hours. This also makes transport between the operating room and the neonatal unit safer. The shunt track is examined daily for the first week; some bruising is permissible, but any inflammation indicates an acute infection, and only immediate removal will prevent ascending infection and damaging ventriculitis. Malnourished premature babies should be provided with protection for several weeks when lying on the side of the shunt, and prolonged pressure on the cranial end should be avoided, otherwise decubitus ulceration may result with inevitable shunt infection. Routine follow-up imaging is not required if the child remains well and without signs of recurrent intracranial hypertension.

FOLLOW-UP

The initial shunt operation is only the beginning in the care of a hydrocephalic child. Routine clinic follow-up continues with regular measurements of the head circumference. Symptoms or signs of increased intracranial pressure may indicate shunt dysfunction and the need for surgical revision.

Prophylactic elective shunt revision procedures, mainly for lengthening of the atrial catheter in a growing child, are favored by some surgeons. The authors' preference is to re-operate on shunts only when there are symptoms of shunt malfunction.

Follow-up should continue by both neurosurgeon and pediatrician. Specific serial neuro-developmental evaluation is likely to be required and the need for special educational provision considered. In cases where multiple handicaps are envisaged, enrolment in a child development clinic is advisable. The family should be instructed throughout on the probable symptoms of shunt malfunction that might be expected as the child develops and matures. In the first 2 years of life, symptoms may be non-specific, but a combination of irritability, vomiting and reduced responsiveness is very suggestive. Head circumference should be charted, as chronic shunt failure in the first 5 years of life may well manifest itself simply as progressive disproportionate head growth. There is of course nothing about a shunt that protects a child from the usual childhood upper respiratory tract and gastro-intestinal illnesses, or the acute specific fevers. There is a natural tendency to attribute all symptoms to the shunt, however improbable. A useful guideline is that illnesses that are predominantly febrile, or in which repeated vomiting is the principal feature, are unlikely to be shunt-related.

For every new 'shunt family,' there is always an element of learning what is, and what is unlikely to be, a symptom of shunt malfunction. It is mutually advantageous for all involved in the child's care to learn together. Particular problems may arise with those children who have severe neuro-developmental handicaps and, for these children especially, it is sensible to be guided by the family and other carers as to what represents unusual patterns of behavior. Certain children with a regular shunt malfunction develop stereotyped patterns of presentation, and it is a foolish doctor who ignores the family's observations. '*Whatever mother says*' (Hendrick 1986) is usually more reliable than 'what the CT scan shows,' and should not be underestimated. Shunt revision is only undertaken for symptomatic malfunction. Routine digital pumping by carers and attendants is unnecessary and undesirable as it provides no reliable information and is potentially hazardous in terms of promoting overdrainage and aspirating brain of choroid plexus into the ventricular catheter.

Ideally follow-up should be for life so that guidance can be given to the child, the family and relevant parties as to the effects of hydrocephalus on everyday activities and social aspects. Families should be offered contact with a support group such as the UK Association of Spina Bifida and Hydrocephalus (ASBAH). Some families find written information of value.

Although some surgeons have questioned the need for regular neurosurgical review at intervals of less than 2 years (Colak et al 1997) and others have suggested that it may not be needed at all for non-tumoral cases (Kimmings et al 1996), it is more generally accepted that there is a responsibility incumbent upon the neurosurgeon to continue follow-up (Hayden et al 1983, Rekate 1991). This is important if the risks of additional disabilities, especially visual loss, are to be avoided.

Failure of follow-up may have expensive medico-legal consequences (Hockley 1999) and may cause otherwise avoidable deaths (Buxton & Punt 1998). In one study of 28 children with shunts who died of shunt-related causes, at least ten had experienced typical symptoms of shunt malfunction for days or weeks prior to presentation; five of these ten had not had adequate follow-up (Iskandar et al 1998a). Furthermore, complications continue into adult life, with 16% of revisions occurring after the age of 16 years in one institutional series (Sgouros et al 1995).

The purpose of follow-up is, however, not just concerned with chance detection of shunt malfunction; the likelihood of detecting this at a routine annual appointment is improbable. It is the need to care for the child rather than just the condition that is one of the hallmarks and ambitions of pediatric neurosurgery (James 1998). Whatever arrangements are made for follow-up, it is crucial that the carers, and later the child, are afforded a rapid and effective route of return to specialist care. Families must have 24 hour open access to their neurosurgical unit for emergency advice. Deteriorating conscious level, with or without headaches and vomiting, visual symptoms or bradycardia implies dangerous intracranial hypertension and constitutes a neurosurgical emergency. Urgent medical advice must be sought in this situation; this may mean that the child will be seen at their local hospital initially where doctors can stabilize the child's condition and seek advice form the neurosurgical team prior to emergency transfer.

Pediatricians and adult physicians seeing patients with shunts should appreciate that the diagnosis of shunt malfunction relies heavily on careful attention to the clinical features as neither CT nor MR can reliably confirm or negate a diagnosis of shunt malfunction (Iskandar et al 1998b). There can be normal shunt malfunction with dilated ventricles, and conversely symptomatic raised intracranial pressure with small ventricles. Helpful clues include poor position of the ventricular catheter, obliterated basal cisterns and cortical sulci, and extravasation of CSF along the track of the ventricular catheter. If the shunt is functioning, the ventricle containing the catheter is typically smaller than the contralateral ventricle. Despite a variety of tests proposed from time to time (Howman-Giles et al 1984), shunt independence cannot always be assumed, and life-threaten-

ing problems may occur (Hemmer & Boehm 1976, Punt 1993, Vaishnav & Mackinnon 1986).

COMPLICATIONS OF SHUNTS

Despite a very low operative mortality, the problems with shunts are their numerous and frequent complications. McLaurin (1982) used to say *'the history of the evolution of ventricular shunting for hydrocephalus is largely a history to prevent the complications of shunting'*. It has been estimated that up to 80% of shunts develop mechanical complications at some stage (Drake & Sainte-Rose 1995). One third of shunt complications occur in the first year of life, and a significant number occur in childhood. Complications after a ventriculo-atrial or ventriculo-peritoneal shunt occur in approximately 46% of patients.

There are complications common to all shunts, and special complications related to VA and VP shunts. The most common complication is shunt malfunction, infection and overdrainage.

Shunt malfunction is usually due to obstruction of the ventricular or distal catheter, but can also result from fractures, disconnections in the tubing or failure of the valve itself.

Infection may occur on the external surface of the shunt tubing, with signs of acute inflammation and sometimes scalp or skin erosion.

Alternatively, infection may occur within the shunt tubing and ventricular fluid ('ventriculitis'), usually due to a less virulent organism, typically *Staphylococcus epidermidis*, introduced at the time of the initial operation. Usually this causes a 'ventriculitis,' an acute illness with malaise, fever and sometimes fits. In patients with a ventriculo-peritoneal shunt, infection often presents as a lower end shunt obstruction due to a localized peritonitis or pseudocyst formation.

In the case of a ventriculo-atrial shunt, infection can produce a more serious and sometimes chronic bacteremia with endocarditis and shunt nephritis. The endocarditis may damage the heart valves, requiring their surgical replacement. Shunt nephritis can lead to renal failure, dialysis and even kidney transplantation. Recurrent thrombo-embolic disease may lead to pulmonary hypertension and cor pulmonale, which can be severe enough for a pulmonary and/or cardiac transplant to be considered. Hence it is not surprising that VA shunts are not the first choice, but a reserve option when the peritoneal cavity for whatever reason cannot be used. One such example is the neonate who has had complicated abdominal surgery for necrotizing enterocolitis.

Overdrainage may lead to subdural effusions or hematomas, 'slit ventricle' syndrome or secondary craniosynostosis.

There are specific, but less serious, complications from VP shunts that include ascites, intestinal obstruction, bowel and other visceral perforation.

A rare but not to be forgotten complication for patients with shunts undergoing surgery, and in particular shunt revision, is an anaphylactic collapse associated with latex allergy. It has been estimated that a severe intra-operative allergic reaction occurs in approximately 1 in 5000 cases (Beard 1985). This has happened in 2 cases, treated by one of the authors. This is more likely to happen in patients having multiple and repeated procedures, such as children with shunts and spina bifida. Typically the reaction happens well into the operation, usually after 30 minutes with a sudden loss of blood pressure and pulse irregularity for no apparent reason. The collapse can be quickly reversed with intravenous epinephrine (adrenaline) and steroid by an astute anesthetist. Subsequent investigations will confirm an allergic reaction and the finding of an elevated specific antibody is diagnostic for latex allergy. This will assist patients, their families and their doctors to adopt avoidance strategies in the future.

MANAGEMENT OF SHUNT COMPLICATIONS

OBSTRUCTION

Obstruction usually results from occlusion of the ventricular catheter with choroid plexus, or ependymal tissue (Collins et al 1978) and also from occlusion of the lower peritoneal catheter. In some patients this does not result in clinical symptoms. These so-called 'shunt independent' patients may no longer require a shunt, or somehow a small amount of fluid can occasionally flow through or around the shunt tubing to maintain a normal balance. In the majority of 'shunt dependent' patients, shunt malfunction produces raised intracranial pressure that is clinically manifest either with a short history ('acute shunt failure') or sometimes with a more insidious, intermittent illness.

Acute shunt failure is a surgical emergency and can present with headache, vomiting, fits and drowsiness which may lead to coma, respiratory arrest and death. When suspected it is necessary to identify and rectify the cause. There may not always be time for a CT scan to assess ventricular size or X-rays to show the integrity of the shunt tubing, before the patient is taken to the operating theatre. If the patient presents in a critical condition with deep coma or respiratory arrest, needle aspiration, before definitive corrective treatment, from the shunt apparatus or ventricle may be life-saving. It is recognized that the history may be so short that death occurs before access to medical help is possible.

Patients with shunt malfunction may present with more subtle symptoms that include personality change, lack of interest at school and visual problems. Some patients may develop double vision or squint from unilateral or bilateral sixth nerve palsy. Of special importance is loss of visual acuity. Affecting one or both eyes, loss of visual acuity even to the point of blindness may very easily be missed by doctors, including pediatricians and neurosurgeons. Even some ophthalmologists may not always appreciate shunt malfunction as a potential cause and give an alternative diagnosis. There have been and will continue to be medico-legal claims where the main disability for compensation is the visual loss due to failed or delayed diagnosis of shunt malfunction (Hockley 1999). If recognized early enough, shunt revision can rescue visual function, partially or even completely.

Under normal circumstances investigations of a suspected shunt malfunction should include plain X-rays of trunk and abdomen to check the position of the shunt tubing and its continuity. A skull X-ray may not be required if a CT scan of the head has been done which can show the integrity of the valve and ventricular catheter. Specific imaging can be by ultrasound if the anterior fontanelle is still open, or by CT or MRI. The purpose is to assess ventricular size, the position of the ventricular catheter and to exclude other pathology such as subdural effusion or, for example, recurrent tumor (Fig. 43.7).

When there is symptomatic shunt malfunction, revision and/or replacement of the defective part in the shunt system is normally required, unless there is a possibility of an ETV which may allow the patient to no longer be shunt-dependent. It has been known for some time that an initial 'communicating' hydrocephalus can become 'non-communicating' with aqueductal obstruction after shunting (Foltz & Shurtleff 1966). Hence it is not surprising that ETV has increasingly been found to be helpful in such circumstances (Cinalli et al 1998, Mallucci et al 1997).

INFECTION

This is the most serious complication encountered in infancy, as it relates to poor ultimate intellect (McLone et al 1982). In premature and very young babies the risk is in the order of 25%. Considerable attention to surgical technique and peri-operative care has resulted in significant reduction of this problem in some specialized pediatric neurosurgical centers (Choux et al 1992). It is recognized that shunt infection occurs at the time of shunt insertion, so any measures which can successfully reduce this complication are to be strongly supported. Recently the value of antibiotic-impregnated shunts is being examined as a prophylactic measure against shunt infection (Bayston et al 1989, Joseph et al 2006).

The clinical presentation of shunt infection has been described above. Internal shunt infection or ventriculitis is confirmed by microbiological examination of the CSF that can be aspirated from the shunt reservoir or by ventricular puncture. The typical appearance of an external shunt tubing infection with a red line of inflammation, tenderness and swelling overlying the tube is diagnostic.

When there is a shunt infection, debate continues as to whether this can be cured without removing the shunt. Although there have been some successes with antibiotics alone (Ward & McLaurin 1980), most agree that either removal or exteriorization of the shunt, with temporary external drainage of the CSF, is necessary before the infection can be controlled and a new shunt can be inserted.

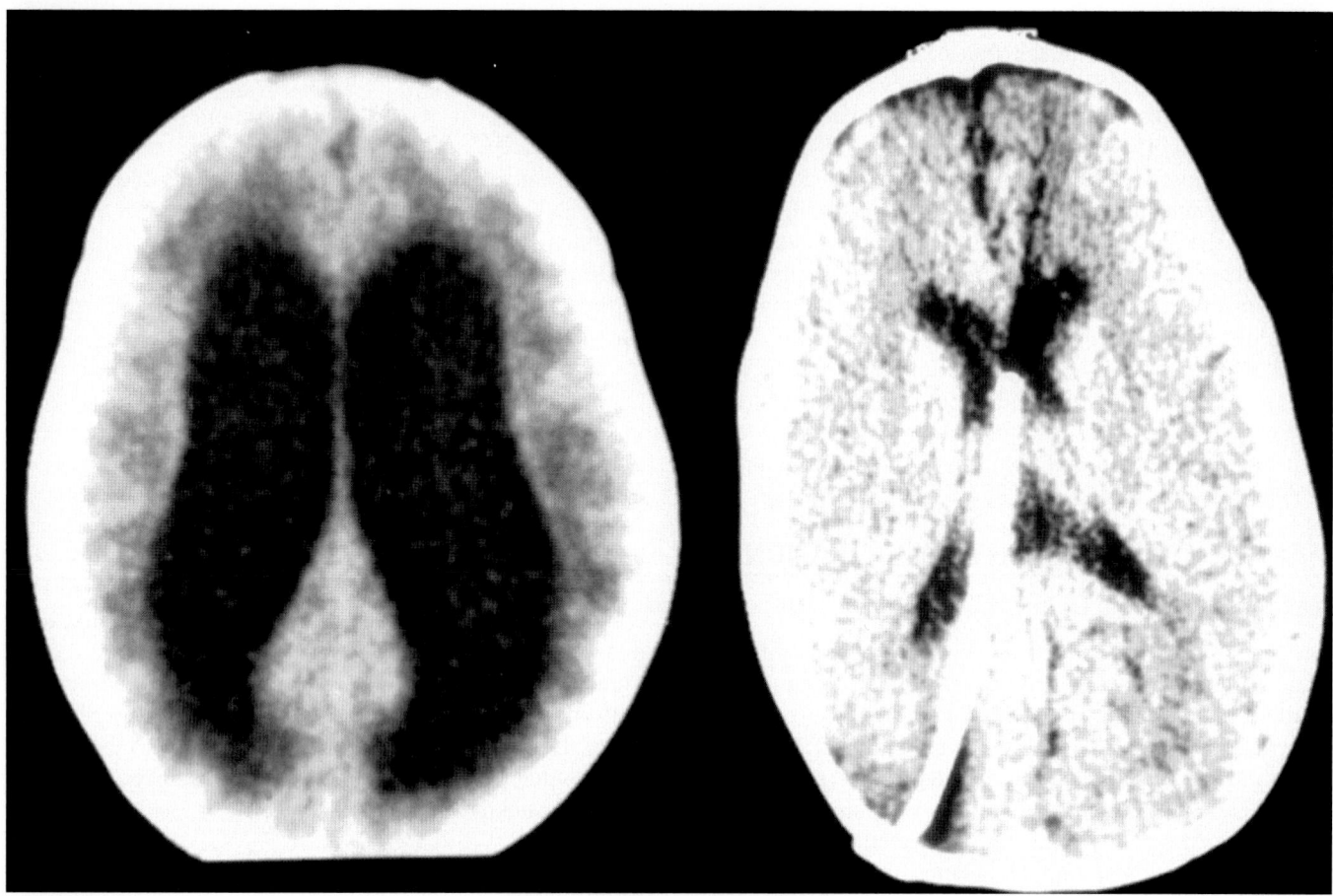

Figure 43.7 CT scan images before and after shunting for hydrocephalus. The post-operative scan demonstrates reduction in ventricular size and the position of the ventricular catheter.

OVERDRAINAGE

The third most frequent complication from shunts is overdrainage, which produces 'slit ventricle' syndrome, subdural fluid accumulations and craniosynostosis. These patients may develop symptoms of raised intracranial pressure from shunt malfunction, but without enlargement of the ventricles and this may lead to difficult technical problems. Fortunately true slit ventricle syndrome only affects about 5% of children. They present with recurrent episodes of intermittently raised intracranial pressure that may be of such frequency that they erode the quality of life and interfere with education. They may deteriorate acutely and vision may be lost.

One treatment approach is to change the shunt. Sophisticated modifications in valve manufacture, including externally programmable valves and anti-siphon devices, have been introduced to overcome this problem. There are now over 127 different types of valve available (Aschoff 2001). An alternative technique, favored by the authors, is to carry out a subtemporal craniectomy with opening of the dura which allows the ventricles to enlarge (Epstein et al 1974).

In the shunt-dependent patient this not only relieves intracranial pressure, but facilitates ventricular catheter replacement and also provides a palpable 'fontanelle' which allows the clinical assessment of intracranial pressure. Another maneuver is to replace the shunt with an external ventricular drain, and then promote expansion of the ventricles by progressively raising the level of the drain, until they are large enough to allow an ETV to be attempted.

OUTCOME

For any treatment to be worthwhile, it must convincingly improve on the natural history of the disorder. Before the advent of shunts the outcome for children with hydrocephalus was poor. There was an approximately 20% chance of reaching adulthood and a 50% chance of brain damage. With the introduction of shunts, and comparing results from the literature after allowing for differences in case selection, two conclusions may be drawn. Firstly, the natural mortality of hydrocephalus is reduced by half after surgical treatment (Laurence & Coates 1962). Secondly, the number of educable survivors is double in the operated as opposed to the non-operated group (Milhorat 1972). The present position is that now 70–80% of children with shunts survive long term. The majority attend normal schools and can achieve social independence.

The differences in outcome depend on the cause of hydrocephalus. Children with aqueduct stenosis have an excellent prognosis. While there are major physical deficits from other aspects of their condition, children with spina bifida have a better intellectual outcome than children whose hydrocephalus is the result of previous meningitis or neonatal intraventricular hemorrhage (Sgouros et al 1995).

SUMMARY

From a neurosurgical point of view, there is no satisfactory 'cure' for most cases of hydrocephalus, except where an identified cause can be removed. While medical treatment (discussed in other chapters) may be of temporary benefit, surgery is currently still the mainstay of treatment. The main options continue to be shunts or third ventriculostomy. This situation is likely to remain until a pharmacological agent to reduce CSF formation by 25–30% is found.

REFERENCES

Aschoff A, Hashemi B et al 2001 Gentlemen, it is no humbug: the eradication of shunt overdrainage. Abstract from 3rd International Hydrocephalus Workshop, 17–20th May 2001, Kos, Greece.

Barlow C F 1984 CSF dynamics in hydrocephalus–with special attention to external hydrocephalus. Brain Dev 6(2):119–127.

Bayston R, Grove N, Siegel J et al 1989 Prevention of hydrocephalus shunt catheter colonization in vitro by impregnation with antimicrobials. J Neurol Neurosurg Psych 52:605–609.

Beard K, Jick H 1985 Cardiac arrest and anaphylaxis with anaesthetic agents. JAMA 254:2742.

Berger A,Weninger M, Reinprecht A et al 2000 Long-term experience with subcutaneous tunnelled external ventricular drainage in preterm infants. Child's Nerv Syst 16:103–110.

Bucholz R D, Pittman T 1991 Endoscopic coagulation of the choroids plexus using the Nd:YAG laser: initial experience and proposal for management. Neurosurgery 28:421–427.

Buxton N, Punt J 1998 Failure to follow patients with hydrocephalus shunts causes deaths. Br J Neurosurg 12:399–401.

Choux M, Genitori L, Lang D, Lena G 1992 Shunt implantation: reducing the incidence of shunt infection. J Neurosurg 77:875–880.

Chumas P D, Kulkarni A V, Drake J M et al 1993 Lumboperitoneal shunting: a retrospective study in the pediatric population. Neurosurgery 32:376–383.

Cinalli G, Salazar C, Mallucci C et al 1998 The role of endoscopic third ventriculostomy in the management of shunt malfunction. Neurosurgery 43:1323–1329.

Cohen A R 1994 Ventriculoscopic surgery. Clin Neurosurg 41:546–562.

Colak A, Albright L, Pollak I F 1997 Follow-up of children with shunted hydrocephalus. Pediatr Neurosurg 27:208–210.

Collins P, Hockley A D, Woollam D H M 1978 Surface ultrastructure of tissues occluding ventricular catheters. J Neurosurg 48:609–613.

Cornips E, Van Calenbergh F, Plets C et al 1997 Use of external drainage for posthaemorrhagic hydrocephalus in very low birth weight premature infants. Child's Nerv Syst 13:368–374.

Cutler R W P, Page L, Galicich J, Watters G V 1968 Formation and absorption of cerebrospinal fluid in man. Brain 91:707–717.

Dandy W E 1918 Extirpation of the choroid plexus of the lateral ventricles in communicating hydrocephalus. Ann Surg 68:569–579.

Dandy W E, Blackfan K D 1914 Internal hydrocephalus: an experimental, clinical and pathological study. Am J Dis Children 8:406–482.

Decq P, Yepes C, Anno Y et al 1994 L'endoscopie neurochirurgicale. Indications diagnostiques et therapeutiques. Neurochirurgie 40:313–321.

Drake J M, Sainte-Rose C 1995 The shunt book. Blackwell Science, Cambridge, MA.

Epstein F J, Fleischer A S, Hochwald G M, Ransohoff J 1974 Subtemporal craniectomy for recurrent shunt obstruction secondary to small ventricles. J Neurosurg 41:29–31.

Foltz E L, Shurtleff D B 1966 Conversion of communicating hydrocephalus to stenosis or occlusion of the aqueduct during ventricular shunt. J Neurosurg 24:520–524.

Griffith H B 1986 Endoneurosurgery: endoscopic intracranial surgery. In: Griffith H B, Symon L (eds) Advances and technical standards in neurosurgery. Springer, New York.

Griffith H B, Jamjoon A B 1990 The treatment of hydrocephalus by choroid plexus coagulation and artificial cerebrospinal fluid perfusion. Br J Neurosurg 4:95–100.

Hayden P W, Shurtleff D B, Stuntz T J 1983 A longitudinal study of shunt function in 36 patients with hydrocephalus. Dev Med Child Neurol 25:334–337.

Hemmer R, Boehm B 1976 Once a shunt, always a shunt? Dev Med Child Neurol 18 (suppl 37):69–73.

Hendrick E B 1986 Whatever mother says. Pediatr Neurosci 12:193.

Hippocrates 1768 De Morbis. Cited by Whytt R: Observations on the dropsy in the brain. Balfour, Edinburgh, p. 4.

Hockley A D 1999 Congenital anomalies of the central nervous system. In: Garfiel J, Earl C (eds) Medical negligence. The cranium and spine. Blackwell Science, Oxford.

Hoffman H J, Hendrick E B, Humphreys R P 1976 New lumboperitoneal shunt for communicating hydrocephalus (technical note). J Neurosurg 44:258–261.

Howman-Giles R, McLaughlin A, Johnston I et al 1984 A radionucleotide method of evaluating shunt function and CSF circulation in hydrocephalus. A technical note. J Neurosurg 61:604–605.

Iskandar B J, McLaughlin C, Mapstone T B et al 1988b Pitfalls in the diagnosis of ventricular shunt dysfunction: Radiology reports and ventricular size. Pediatrics 101:1031–1036.

Iskandar B J, Tubbs S, Mapstone T B et al 1998a Death in shunted hydrocephalic children in the 1990's. Pediatr Neurosurg 28:173–176.

James H 1998 Follow-up of children with shunted hydrocephalus. Pediatr Neurosurg 28:327.

Javadpour M, May P, Mallucci C 2003 Sudden death secondary to delayed closure of endoscopic third ventriculostomy. Brit J Neurosurg 17:266–269.

Jones R F, Kwok B C, Stening W A et al 1994 Neuroendoscopic third ventriculostomy. A practical alternative to extracranial shunts in non-communicating hydrocephalus. Acta Neurochir Suppl 61:79–83.

Joseph R, Walsh A R, Kay A et al 2006 Inclusion of antibiotic-impregnated (Bactiseal) catheters into shunt systems for the treatment of hydrocephalus in children: Does it make a difference? Childs Nerv Syst 22:212.

Kimmings E, Kleinlugtebied A, Casey T H et al 1996 Does the child with shunted hydrocephalus require long-term neurosurgical follow-up? Brit J Neurosurg 10:77–81.

Kirkpatrick M, Engelman H, Minns R A 1989 Symptoms and signs of progressive hydrocephalus. Arch Dis Childhood 64:124–128.

Laurence K M, Coates S 1962 The natural history of hydrocephalus. Arch Dis Childhood 37:345–362.

McLaurin R L 1982 Shunt complications. In: McLaurin R L (ed.) Pediatric neurosurgery: surgery of the developing nervous system. Grune & Stratton, New York.

Mallucci C L, Vloeberghs M, Punt J 1997 Neuroendoscopic III ventricolostomy: the first-line treatment for blocked ventriculo-peritoneal shunts? Child's Nerv Syst 13:498.

Ment L R, Duncan C C, Geehr R 1981 Benign enlargement of the subarachnoid spaces in the infant. J Neurosurg 54(4):504–508.

Milhorat T H 1972 Hydrocephalus and the cerebrospinal fluid. Williams & Wilkins, Baltimore.

Mixter W J 1923 Ventriculoscopy and puncture of the floor of the third ventricle. Boston Med Surg J 188:277–278.

Nulsen F E, Spitz E B 1952 Treatment of hydrocephalus by direct shunt from ventricle to jugular vein. Surg Forum 2:399–403.

Pudenz R H, Russell F E, Hurd A H, Shelden C H 1957 Ventriculo-auriculostomy. A technique for shunting cerebrospinal fluid into the right auricle: a preliminary report. J Neurosurg 14:171–179.

Punt J 1993 Principles of CSF diversion and alternative treatments. In: Schurr P H, Polkey C E (eds) Hydrocephalus. Medical Publications, Oxford.

Punt J, Vloeburghs M 1998 Endoscopy in neurosurgery. Min Invas Ther Allied Technol 7:159–170.

Putnam T J 1934 Treatment of hydrocephalus by endoscopic coagulation of the choroid plexus. N Engl J Med 210:1373–1376.

Rekate H L 1991 Shunt revision: Complications and their prevention. Pediatr Neurosurg 17:155–162.

Russell D S 1949 Observations on the pathology of hydrocephalus. Special reports and services of the Medical Research Council, No. 265. HMSO, London.

Scarff J E 1936 Endoscopic treatment of hydrocephalus. Description of a ventriculoscope and preliminary report of cases. Arch Neurol Psychiatr 35:853–861.

Scarff J E 1970 The treatment of non-obstructive (communicating) hydrocephalus by endoscopic cauterization of the choroids plexuses. J Neurosurg 33:1–18.

Sgouros S, Mallucci C, Walsh A R, Hockley A D 1995 Long term complications of hydrocephalus. Paed Neurosurg 23:127–132.

Suess C, Chen X 2002 Dose optimization in pediatric CT: current technology and future innovations. Pediatr Radiol 32:729–734.

Torkildsen A 1939 A new palliative operation in cases of inoperable occlusion of the Sylvian aqueduct. Acta Chir Scandinav 82:117–124.

Vaishnav A, MacKinnon A E 1986 Progressive hydrocephalus in teenage spina bifida patients. Zeitschrift fur Kinderchirurgie 41(suppl 1):36–37.

Vesalius, cited by Whytt R 1768 Observations on the dropsy of the brain. Balfour, Auld and Smellie, Edinburgh.

Vries J K 1978 An endoscopic technique for third ventriculostomy. Surg Neurol 9:165–168.

Walker M L, MacDonald J, Wright L C 1992 The history of ventriculoscopy: where do we go from here? Pediatr Neurosurg 18:218–223.

Ward S L, McLaurin R L 1980 Cerebrospinal fluid antibiotic levels during treatment of shunt infections. J Neurosurg 52:41–46.

Warf B C 2005a Hydrocephalus in Uganda: the predominance of infectious origin and primary management with endoscopic third ventriculostomy. J Neurosurg (Suppl Pediatrics) 102:1–15.

Warf B C 2005b Comparison of endoscopic third ventriculostomy alone and combined with choroid plexus cauterization in infants younger than 1 year of age, prospective study in 550 African children. J Neurosurg (Suppl Pediatrics) 103:475–481.

Weller R O, Wisniewski H, Shulman K et al 1971 Experimental hydrocephalus in young dogs: histological and ultrastructural study of the brain tissue damage. J Neuropathol Exp Neurol 30:613–627.

Wozniak M, McLone D G, Raimondi A J 1975 Micro- and macrovascular changes as the direct cause of parenchymal destruction in congenital murine hydrocephalus. J Neurosurg 43:535–545.

CHAPTER
44

Surgical management of neural tube defects

Anthony D. Hockley and Guirish A. Solanki

Key Points

- Neural tube defects (NTDs) are the most common congenital abnormalities of the central nervous system
- Encephaloceles occur 1 in 8, compared with spinal defects
- Myelomeningoceles can be diagnosed antenatally by maternal serum alpha-protein (AFP), ultrasound and amniocentesis
- Occult spinal dysraphism includes different neural tube defects, usually with normal skin cover. Progressive neurological deficits can occur
- A dermal sinus needs investigation and surgical treatment to prevent potentially serious infective complications
- Diastamatomyelia and a congenitally tight filum terminalae justify prophylactic surgical treatment
- Lipomas (lipomyelomeningoceles) may produce progressive deficit, in addition to the cosmetic problem. The role of prophylactic surgery remains controversial

---

INTRODUCTION

Neural tube defects (NTD) are the most common congenital abnormalities of the central nervous system and overall second after congenital heart disease. Neural tube defects are important because of their significant morbidity and mortality in children and adults. Patients may present to different specialties, including neurology, dermatology, orthopedic, renal and psychiatry. Many of the lesions are surgically treatable, and there are also medico-legal issues. An understanding of the potential implications, probable outcome and the range of possible surgical management is essential knowledge for colleagues, who may be in a position to identify these lesions during infancy. These include the obstetrician, radiologist, neonatologist, pediatrician, nurse and health visitor.

EMBRYOLOGY

Embryologically the central nervous system develops from the outer of three cell layers with a special part (neuro-ectoderm) forming a 'neural tube'. On the 17th day of gestation an area of thickening appears in the ectoderm overlying the notochord, which becomes the neuro-ectoderm or neural plate. On day 18 the neural plate invaginates along the midline, forming a neural groove with neural folds on either side. The neural folds fuse ('primary neurulation') between 18 and 27 days with formation of the neural tube. This process of closure, like a zip, is also called 'raphism'. The cranial end of the neural tube closes by 24 days and the caudal by 25–26 days. Then the neural tube is covered dorsally by mesenchyme that forms the vertebral arches and skull. Closure of the vertebral arches is completed at 11 weeks of gestation.

A spectrum of anomalies ('*neural tube defects*') occurs when there is a fault in this closure ('*dysraphism*'). Neural tube defects may involve the skull (cranial dysraphism) and include encephaloceles and anencephaly. Involving the spine, the defects are referred to as spinal dysraphism or spina bifida. These anomalies vary from major external lesions with neurological deficit and associated abnormalities, such as hydrocephalus, to intermediate and more minor forms. Open neural tube defects can be detected by the elevation of the alpha-protein (AFP) and acetyl cholinesterase in the amniotic fluid and maternal blood.

EPIDEMIOLOGY

The prevalence of NTD varies according to geography and race. Higher rates have been reported in Northern Ireland, Egypt, India and China (more than 8 per 1000 live births). In the UK there was a peak in 1954–1955, followed by a substantial decline in the early 1970s. This was not due entirely to prenatal screening, and it pre-dated the widespread use of folic acid (FA) supplementation in pregnancy. By 1994, the prevalence of NTD in England and Wales was just under 0.8 per 1000 total births. There is an increased (genetic) risk if one member of a family has been affected. For parents who have given birth to one affected child the recurrence risk is 3%. With two previously affected pregnancies, this figure rises to 6%.

ETIOLOGY

Most neural tube defects result from a complex interaction between several genes and environmental factors. Major genes have been identified in the mouse, but their relevance to human defects is still not clear. Neural tube defects occur in different syndromes and chromosomal disorders, but if an NTD is the only anomaly karyotyping is not indicated.

With regard to environmental factors, vitamin supplements containing folic acid (FA) during pregnancy have been shown to reduce the incidence of NTD. In England it is currently recommended that women, who are planning pregnancy, should take folic acid daily before conception and during the first 12 weeks of pregnancy.

Some drugs taken during pregnancy may increase the risk of NTD in the fetus, including sodium valproate, folic acid antagonists such as trimethoprim, carbamazepine and other anti-convulsants.

ENCEPHALOCELES (p. 233)

Encephaloceles arise as congenital developmental defects affecting the calvarium and skull base. These are congenital hernias that may contain meninges, cerebrospinal fluid and sometimes brain tissue. Usually midline they occur 1 in 8 compared with spinal defects, with an estimated incidence of 1–3 per 10 000 live births (Warrell et al 2003). The most widely accepted classification is based on the anatomical studies at post mortem by Suwanwela and Suwanwela (1972). Occipital lesions are the most common and account for 60–70% in the western world, with females twice as affected as males. Geographical differences exist however with anterior lesions more common in Asians and both sexes equally affected (Table 44.1).

The diagnosis of an encephalocele is usually made at birth, although larger lesions may be recognized by antenatal ultrasound examination from around 16 weeks of gestation.

The indications for surgery are usually elective (Table 44.2), but in some instances may be urgent and life saving (Table 44.3). A thin skin covering or a ruptured lesion, like spina bifida, has loss of cerebrospinal fluid (CSF), hemorrhage or infection as major threats. An obstructed airway from an intranasal encephalocele can affect both breathing and feeding. Eyeball displacement or obstruction to the normal development of vision is another urgent indication. Recurrent meningitis or cerebrospinal fluid leakage after an inappropriate biopsy of a so-called nasal glioma or polyp, which in fact is a nasal encephalocele, similarly indicates the need for surgical repair.

The objectives of surgery are removal or replacement of the herniated cranial contents, water tight closure of the dura and repair of major bone defects with adequate and cosmetically acceptable skin cover (Hockley et al 1990). For occipital lesions, these aims can usually be achieved with a single procedure, although large skull defects may have to await further growth of the skull and secondary repair by bone grafting taken from elsewhere on the cranial vault. It is best to wait until the child's skull growth will allow split calvarial grafts to be harvested usually from the parietal regions. An intact cranium can often therefore be achieved during the early primary school years.

Anterior encephaloceles may be associated with complex skull bone defects and resulting major cosmetic deformity, but usually mental development is normal whatever the contents of the lesion (Nakamura et al 1974). Detailed radiological assessment, including CT and MRI imaging, is required for these lesions and sometimes staged multiple surgical procedures may be necessary. Ideally these cases should be referred to pediatric neurosurgical centers with a multidisciplinary craniofacial surgical team.

The decision to surgically repair an encephalocele is based on prognosis, which depends on the location of the lesion, its contents, size and associated anomalies. From the literature it is known that occipital lesions do less well compared to anterior lesions (Matson 1969). There are also significant differences between those lesions that do not contain brain tissue ('meningoceles') and those with brain tissue ('encephaloceles'), both with respect to mortality and intellectual outcome. Hydrocephalus complicates 50% of occipital encephaloceles that contain cerebellar tissue. Of children with no brain tissue in the sac, 60–80% will develop normally, in contrast to those infants, with brain tissue present in the sac, in whom only 10–25% will have normal development (Guthkelch 1970, Lorber 1967). Only 30% of those infants with hydrocephalus but no herniated brain tissue will have normal intellect (Mealey et al 1970). Some infants will have defective brain growth, their head circumference remaining below the 10th centile ('microcephaly'). These infants virtually all show developmental delay (Guthkelch 1970, Lorber 1967).

Table 44.1 Anterior encephaloceles in African and Asian populations

Nigeria	Odeku	1967
South Africa	Lipschitz et al	1969
India	Tandon	1970
Thailand	Suwanwela and Suwanwela	1972
Burma	Whatmore	1973
Pakistan	Rahman	1979

Table 44.2 Encephaloceles. Indications for elective surgery

Protect brain
Facilitate nursing
Prevent infection
Improve function (airway, speech, vision)
Associated anomalies (hydrocephalus, hypertelorism)
Cosmetic and psychological

Table 44.3 Encephaloceles. Indications for urgent surgery

Absence of skin cover
Hemorrhage
Airway obstruction
Impairment of vision

ANENCEPHALY (p. 235)

This lethal defect results from failure of rostral neural tube closure between 18 and 25 days of gestation. The cranial vault is absent, and an angiomatous mass lies on the floor of the skull. The eyes are protuberant because of shallow orbits, and there is variable involvement of the spinal cord. When identified by antenatal ultrasound an increasing number of such pregnancies are terminated. In liveborn anencephalic babies the initial neurological examination may be surprisingly normal if brainstem structures are intact, and seizures may occur despite the absent cerebral hemispheres. However babies usually die within hours or days.

SPINA BIFIDA (p. 225)

The term 'spina bifida' literally means a double or unfused spinous process as a result of failure of closure of the vertebral arches. It incudes 'spina bifida occulta' ('occult spinal dysraphism'), without an external lesion and 'spina bifida cystica' in which there is a cystic lesion on the back. The lesion may be either a 'meningocele' without neural tissue or a 'myelomeningocele' in which the spinal cord is a component of the cyst wall. The term 'rachischisis' is used for the most severe defect in which there is a wide opening of the spine, often with anencephaly.

MYELOMENINGOCELE

Myelomeningocele has been called '*the most complex, treatable, congenital anomaly consistent with life*' (Bunch et al 1972). In its most severe form, this neural tube defect may be open with an elevated alpha-fetoprotein level in maternal serum and amniotic fluid allowing antenatal diagnosis, in addition to diagnostic ultrasound imaging. The real incidence is steadily falling in most parts of the world, for example in the UK there has been a reduction by one-third over a twenty year period (Cuckle et al 1985).

PRENATAL DIAGNOSIS (see p. 292)

Maternal serum alpha-protein (AFP) levels are usually elevated when the fetus has an open neural tube defect. The fetal liver is the main source of AFP, which leaks through open defects into the amniotic fluid and then into the maternal blood. An elevated AFP can also be caused by ventral wall defects, multiple gestation, fetal death or inaccurate gestational age. Screening is best done at 15–18 weeks' gestation.

Ultrasonography (U/S) is recommended for all at-risk women, particularly for those with positive AFP screening, a previous history of an affected child, or exposure to cause-related drugs. Anencephaly can be detected by U/S from the 12th week of gestation, and spina bifida from 16–20 weeks.

Amniocentesis in the management of spina bifida has largely been replaced by detailed U/S imaging. If in doubt, amniocentesis allows the measurement of AFP and acetylcholinesterase.

It is helpful for the parents to be given an opportunity of consultation with a pediatric neurosurgeon, in addition to advice from the obstetrician or pediatrician. It is important that the parents understand that the condition is for life, and that as complications can arise throughout childhood and adult life there will be a permanent need for their child to receive medical care. Cases have occurred where the obstetrical team either did not follow up appropriately or inform the parents of a positive antenatal diagnostic result. This has led to later claims for 'wrongful life' because the parents in such circumstances would have opted for a termination of pregnancy (see also Ch. 48). Alternatively for those pregnancies that proceed, there are obvious advantages to all involved if the various issues can be discussed antenatally when emotions are more collected and there are no great pressures of time.

Unless there is an issue with rapidly progressive hydrocephalus, there is not usually an indication for early delivery. Vaginal delivery is perfectly acceptable and ideally the baby should be born near to the neonatal neurosurgery facility so that prolonged separation of mother from baby can be avoided.

The possibility of intra-uterine surgery (Ch. 41) has been recently proposed in the hope that such surgery may reduce the incidence of hydrocephalus or Chiari malformation (Tullipan 1999). Currently evidence for a major benefit from in-utero closure of the spinal lesion has not been convincing. Such surgery is not without risk both to mother and baby (Harrison 1993). It does involve two cesarean operations for the mother. Currently the results from a limited number of centers need to be analyzed with appropriate controls to make sure that there are definite benefits that exceed the risks (Dias 1999).

POSTNATAL MANAGEMENT

Once delivered, there are a number of problems for the baby with myelomeningocele (Fig. 44.1). Treatment is not just a question of repairing the defective skin cover over the exposed spinal cord. There will likely be significant neurological deficit below the level of the lesion which will affect limb function and sphincter control. Orthopedic, urological and other colleagues from several disciplines will be involved in the patient's later management. The majority of infants will develop hydrocephalus with all its problems. A so-called Chiari II malformation or hindbrain hernia is present in over 90% of cases of myelomeningocele (Curnes et al 1989). The most common of the 4 types of Arnold–Chiari malformation, it consists of downward protrusion of the medulla below the foramen magnum to overlap the spinal cord. The medulla is kinked and the cerebellar vermis indented by the posterior lip of the foramen magnum. The fourth ventricle is elongated and the midbrain distorted, which can cause early or late problems. These include lower cranial nerve palsies, central apnea and limb weakness.

Left alone at birth, the infant with myelomeningocele will probably not die. Although some spontaneous epithelialization of the lesion will occur, the development in later years of a spontaneous and fatal squamous cell carcinoma has been increasingly reported at the site of a previous

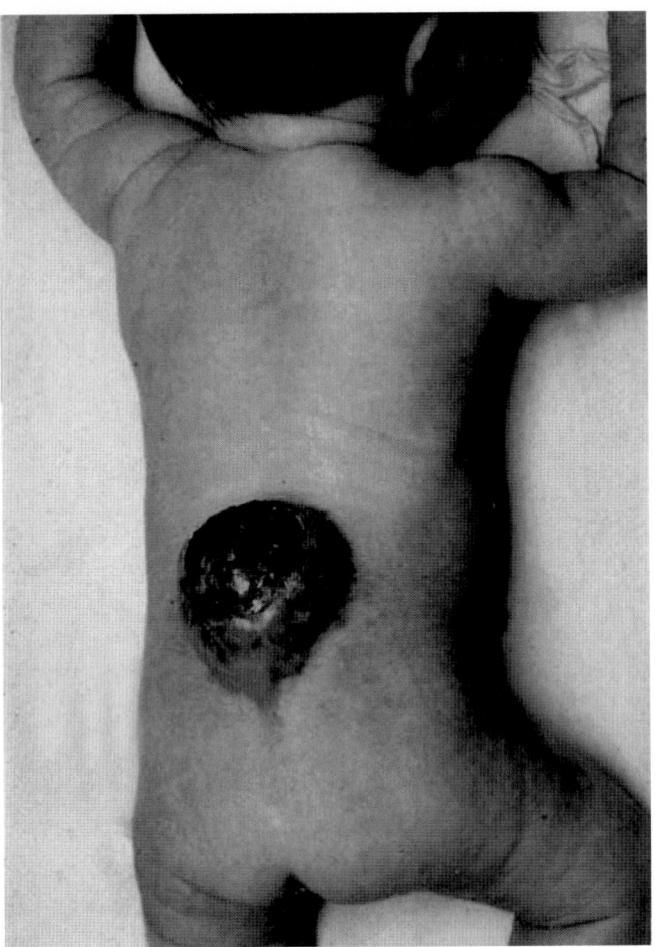

Figure 44.1 Newborn infant with myelomeningocele. The pink spinal cord ('placode') is exposed and the skin is defective.

unrepaired myelomeningocele. Generally, it is now policy in most pediatric neurosurgical departments to operate on the majority of myelomeningocele babies. In a very small number however the lesion may be so severe that survival for more than a few days is unlikely, and surgery is deferred.

Effective surgical treatments only became possible for children with spina bifida with the development of shunts for hydrocephalus in the late 1950s. In 1971, Lorber, a pediatrician, published the results of surgical treatment in 524 cases from Sheffield and described his 'adverse criteria,' correlating morbidity and handicap with more serious spina bifida lesions.

Lorber's 'adverse criteria' noted at birth were as follows:

1. Paraplegia (below the level of the lesion).
2. Hydrocephalus.
3. Kyphosis.
4. Thoraco-lumbar lesion.
5. Other anomalies.

Lorber and colleagues undertook a trial of no treatment in 25 infants with these criteria, and all but two died within 6 months, the remainder by 9 months. This had a profound

effect on medical management in the UK, where 'selection' became the standard policy. Later the issue was reopened when several centers reported cases where the early decision not to operate had been reversed when the children survived. An important study from Dublin showed that babies being treated 'expectantly,' who were going to die, did so in the first 3 months (Guiney & Surana 1994). The view at that time was that early surgery perhaps was not always necessary, and a policy of immediate back closure became reserved for the good prognosis group. Initial conservative treatment was advocated for the more severe cases and, providing the hydrocephalus was effectively treated, surgery to the back could be safely delayed.

The current position, bearing in mind the reduced incidence of myelomeningocele, both real and from terminations of pregnancy, has been back towards active treatment. Unless there are special circumstances, active treatment consists of closure of the lesion within the first 24 hours of birth to reduce the risk of serious infection of the central nervous system, to obtain watertight closure of the dura and to provide good skin cover.

Under general anesthesia in the prone position, the myelomeningocele sac is opened directly into the subarachnoid space through an incision between the epithelialized part of the sac and the arachnoid membrane. The neural placode is mobilized, and dural flaps raised from either side before bringing them over the placode in a watertight fashion to create as capacious a sac as possible and so reduce the risk of later re-tethering. The fascia, subcutaneous layers and skin are then closed with sutures and a tight dressing applied. Most pediatric neurosurgeons advocate a period of prophylactic antibiotics.

In the neonatal period, hydrocephalus usually becomes apparent within the first 2–4 weeks, evident by head circumference measurements and ultrasound or CT imaging. Insertion of a ventriculo-peritoneal shunt or, in some cases endoscopic third ventriculostomy is required.

The associated hindbrain hernia or Chiari II malformation can produce a bulbar palsy or quadriparesis in the neonatal period even in the presence of a functioning shunt. Fortunately, this is a rare clinical problem, and when a hindbrain hernia becomes symptomatic soon after birth there is a high mortality and persisting deficit. The results from surgical decompression have been disappointing (Hoffman et al 1975, Rauzzino & Oakes 1995).

Following surgical closure of the myelomeningocele and treatment of the hydrocephalus, continuing orthopedic and urological management is required in addition to continuing pediatric and neurosurgical follow-up. Genetic counseling is suggested in view of the 2–4% recurrence risk of neural tube defects in subsequent siblings.

With regard to outcome the prognosis for children with myelomeningocele varies. Earlier studies in the UK documented a five year survival rate for these children of around 50%, but these would appear to have been improved to figures of over 80% in North America.

The quality of survival however has been disappointing. According to a large unselected series from Sheffield by Lorber in 1971, only 1% of the total and 4% of the survivors were without handicap. Fifteen percent had a moderate handicap and 49% were severely disabled. Only 40% of the handicapped survivors could attend ordinary schools and barely 7% were expected to become independent. Hunt (1990) reviewed the outcome 16–20 years after treatment of a cohort of 117 cases treated in Cambridge between 1963 and 1970. From this group 48 patients died before the age of 16 years, leaving 69 survivors. The most frequent cause of death was cardio-respiratory problems associated with the spinal scoliosis and chest deformity that these patients develop, narrowly followed by renal causes, subsequent to their chronic neuropathic bladder. The next frequent causes of death were related to infection within the central nervous system or complications related to the shunt and hydrocephalus.

Of the 69 survivors, 60 patients had a shunt for hydrocephalus, 22 were mentally retarded (IQ less than 80), 35 were wheelchair dependent and 52 were incontinent. Approximately half (33) were unable to live without help and 17 were unemployed.

MENINGOCELE

Spinal meningoceles by definition are protrusions of the dura mater and arachnoid membrane through defects in the spinal column, with the spinal cord remaining within the spinal canal. These are much less frequent than myelomeningoceles, usually posterior, but can occur anteriorly in association with 'sacral agenesis,' or in an antero-lateral position at lumbar, thoracic or cervical levels.

POSTERIOR MENINGOCELES

Most posterior meningoceles are not 'pure' in that they contain aberrant nerve roots adherent to the inner wall, occasional ganglion cells or even a glial nodule that may represent a diverticulum of the central canal of the spinal cord. Even though these fragmentary neural elements are outside the spinal canal, the spinal cord is not (McComb 1999).

The newborn with a posterior, usually *lumbo-sacral*, meningocele is recognizable because of the obvious lesion. The lesion may be pedunculated, is usually reducible, can vary in size, transilluminates well and is fully covered with skin. Sometimes part of the skin covering may be dysplastic, but rupture of the sac is very rare.

Because the lesion is covered with skin surgical correction can be done electively, although in many instances the defect is repaired before the newborn leaves hospital. At operation the sac usually constricts to a neck, where it enters the spinal canal. The spinal cord should be visualized and freed from any tethering fibrous or glial tissue. Excess dura is trimmed and closed with absorbable sutures. As there is normally redundant skin present, a tension-free closure can

be easily achieved. The prognosis for these babies with a 'closed' NTD is generally excellent.

At cervical level, posterior meningoceles may be associated with a midline attachment to the cord, described by some as a 'limited dorsal myeloschisis,' an additional embryological fault (Pang & Dias 1993). The attachment may comprise a dorsal band of connective tissue, nodules within the sac, an ependymal-lined cavity, or a split cord malformation (Steinbok & Cochrane 1995). In all cases the spinal cord lies within the spinal canal. Sometimes cervical meningoceles are associated with anterior vertebral column anomalies such as the Klippel–Feil syndrome. The importance of these lesions is that there may be cervical cord tethering with progressive neurological deficit in the limbs, acquired symptomatic Chiari-type problems and hydrocephalus. In surgical repair it is essential to fully explore the contents of the sac, and 'untether' the cervical spinal cord. Pre-operative imaging (particularly MRI) will help determine the extent of surgical exploration needed.

ANTERIOR SACRAL MENINGOCELES (SACRAL AGENESIS)

Anterior sacral meningoceles are really occult, and much less common than posterior lesions. These are often associated with rectal anomalies, malformation of the uterus and vagina, duplication of the renal pelvis and ureter, bony anomalies, dermoids and teratomas or hamartomas associated with the cyst (Currarino et al 1981). The bony deficiency (sacral agenesis) allows herniation of the dura to produce an anterior sacral meningocele. It is considered as a form of 'caudal regression' syndrome, probably due to an ischemic injury to the developing spine (Barkovitch et al 1989). Approximately 16% of affected infants are born to mothers with diabetes mellitus (Passage & Lenz 1966).

Clinically these lesions are discovered because of the mass effect, giving rise to bladder and bowel symptoms. While small in infancy, these lesions progressively grow secondary to hydrostatic pressure and CSF (cerebrospinal fluid) pulsations. X-rays of the spine show the characteristic crescent or 'scimitar' sacral deficiency. When symptomatic the lesion needs to be surgically corrected, and where possible the posterior approach is preferred with identification and ligation of the fistula. The collapsed cyst is left in place. With more complex lesions, an anterior approach may also be necessary, including removal of associated tumor masses. This condition may be associated with a tethered spinal cord, diastematomyelia, syringomyelia or lipomyelomeningocele. Progressive neurological deterioration can occur and these associated lesions may require neurosurgical treatment as described below.

ANTEROLATERAL MENINGOCELES

Meningoceles can arise through an intervertebral foramen or coalesced foramina. Usually at thoracic level, rarely cervical, this lesion occurs in neurofibromatosis (NF) and other conditions such as Marfan syndrome. It is usually discovered as an incidental finding on chest X-rays, but up to a third of patients have symptoms of back or chest pain. Larger lesions can cause respiratory or swallowing difficulties.

MRI imaging is the investigation of choice with CT scanning added for details of bony anatomy if required. When symptomatic, surgery to deflate the sac and ligate its pedicle may be necessary.

OCCULT SPINAL DYSRAPHISM

In contrast to myelomeningocele, there are a variety of different conditions in which there has been disordered closure of the neural tube but in which the resultant lesion is still skin covered. The traditional term 'spina bifida occulta' is inappropriate because some 10–20% of the population may have a single deficient lamina in the lumbosacral spine and a similar number of people have a totally innocent skin dimple overlying the tip of the coccyx which is of no sinister significance.

The importance of this group of lesions is that they can produce progressive neurological, sphincter and orthopedic problems later in childhood or even adult life as a result of cord tethering (James & Lassman 1972, Park 1992, Till 1969). Most infants and young children are neurologically normal at birth, and it is the finding of a cutaneous blemish that alerts the pediatricians or parents as to their presence. All neonates must have the midline of their spine properly examined for the presence of skin-covered meningoceles, subcutaneous fatty pads, and hemangiomas or vascular abnormalities in the skin, hairy tufts, unusual scars, appendages or dermal sinuses.

The important clinical varieties of occult spinal dysraphism include the dermal sinuses (with or without an intradural dermoid cyst), diastematomyelia, congenitally tight filum terminale and spinal lipoma (or more correctly called lipomyelomeningocele).

DERMAL SINUS

A dimple usually in the midline above the level of the buttocks may be the external opening of a congenital dermal sinus. These vary from a simple epithelial tube which ends blindly in the soft tissues to an elongated tract which ends intraspinally as a port of entry for infection. At any point along the tract, usually at its termination, the sinus may expand into a dermoid cyst (Fig. 44.2). Although occasionally diagnosed in asymptomatic patients, the most frequent presentation is infection with meningitis, that may be recurrent or the development of a spinal abscess within the dermoid cyst. *Meningitis* not infrequently is caused by a pneumococcus infection, and when this is found a search for a fistula (such as a dermal sinus) is important.

A *spinal abscess* typically presents with symptoms referable to a spinal mass or tethered cord in association with back pain, scoliosis, or progressive neurological and sphincter deficit. In the diagnosis of dermal sinus and its complications, ordinary spine X-rays are of limited value, but MRI

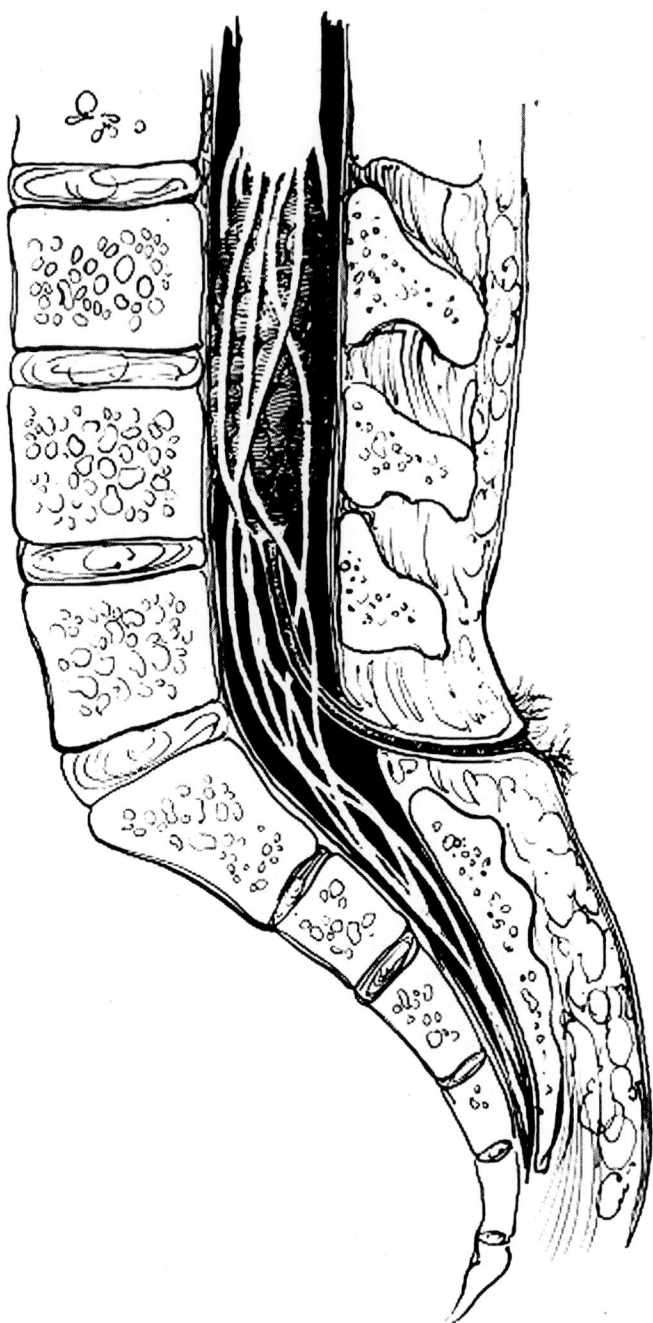

Figure 44.2 Diagram of a lumbar dermal sinus communicating with an intradural dermoid cyst, surrounded by nerve roots of the cauda equina.

scanning has now replaced invasive contrast radiology in demonstrating the extent of these lesions. The aim of treatment is to prevent recurrent infection by totally excising the tract up to and including its termination (Fig. 44.3), which may be as high as the conus medullaris.

While most lesions of this nature occur in the lower lumbar region, the same can occur elsewhere in the spine up to and including the cervical spine, over the calvarium and down the midline anteriorly to the tip of the nose.

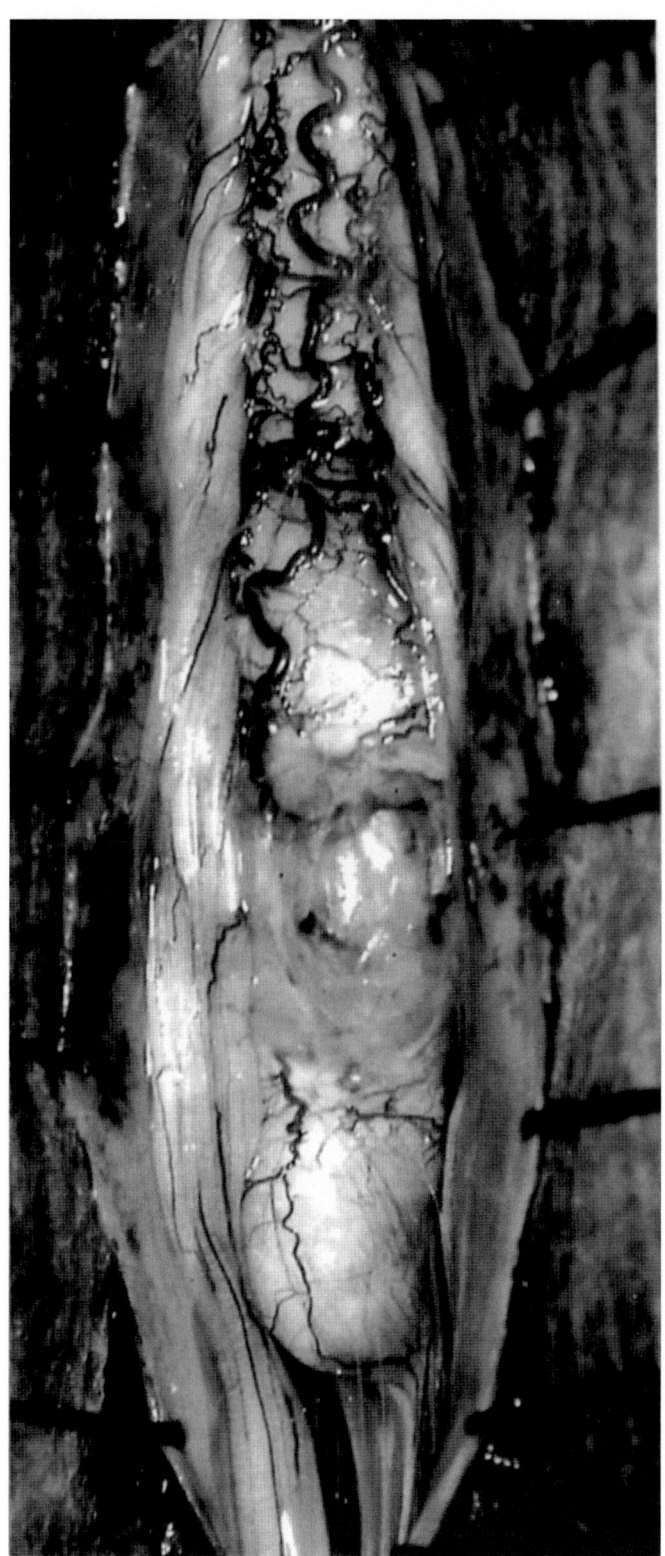

Figure 44.3 Intra-operative photograph of intradural dermoid cyst situated at the termination of the spinal cord amongst nerve roots (with kind permission from Mr John Garfield).

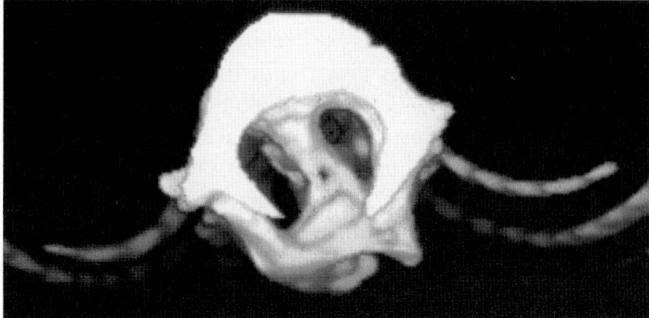

Figure 44.4 CT scan showing bony diastematomyelia at thoracic level. Note the bifid spinous process.

Despite this knowledge, well described in medical and pediatric textbooks, failure to diagnose the true nature of this lesion may result in permanent deficit. This can also be a problem when surgery has to be undertaken in the acute phase for an infected dermoid cyst, when the normal anatomical appearances may be obscured.

The dermal sinus is an important lesion but it needs to be stressed that the very common skin dimple found between the buttocks immediately overlying the coccyx is innocent. Its intact skin base can be demonstrated and it is not a surgical problem. The large number of children with dimples, now sent to pediatric neurosurgical clinics, indicates the increased awareness by GPs and pediatricians concerning the diagnosis of potential communicating sinuses. If a sinus is suspected, referral to the pediatric neurosurgical clinic is recommended. Appropriate investigation by MRI scan will allow prophylactic and appropriate surgical treatment to prevent recurrent infection and persisting neurological deficit.

DIASTEMATOMYELIA

Usually asymptomatic in small infants, the presence of a split spinal cord in association with a fibrous or bony septum ('diastematomyelia') is often associated with a hairy patch in the skin overlying the spinal abnormality (Fig. 44.4). Untreated these children may develop progressive spinal symptoms that include scoliosis, pain and neurological deficit. Surgical excision of the offending bone peg and reconstituting a single dural tube may prevent progressive neurological symptoms, including the development of later scoliosis. When scoliosis is diagnosed later in childhood or adolescence and corrective spinal surgery is being considered, most pediatric neurosurgeons would advocate surgical treatment of the diastematomyelia either as a preliminary or synchronous procedure.

TIGHT FILUM TERMINALE

Described in 1953 by Garceau, the condition of a tight filum terminale is a form of occult spinal dysraphism in which the spinal cord is tethered by an abnormally thick and shortened filum terminale without other pathology. There may or may not be any cutaneous clue. MRI scanning demonstrates the spinal cord comes lower down with the conus well below its normal L1-2 level. Children or adolescents may develop low back pain with restriction of spinal flexion in addition to neurological symptoms and signs in the legs and disturbance of bladder control. These children benefit from release (division) of the filum terminale.

LIPOMA (LIPOMYELOMENINGOCELE)

Congenital lumbosacral lipomas or lipomyelomeningoceles are the most frequent form of occult spinal dysraphism. Treatment remains controversial as there remains uncertainty concerning their natural history in addition to the risks of surgery and the quality of post-operative long-term outcome. Apart from the obvious cosmetic effect, most newborn infants have no neurological deficit. Problems may arise with growth of the infant due to tethering of the lower spinal cord.

Unlike diastematomyelia and tight filum terminale, where the surgery is safe and technically simple, operative treatment of spinal lipomas can be extremely difficult. In many there is no easy plane of cleavage between the lipoma and lower cord or nerve roots (Fig. 44.5). There are postoperative neurological risks and there remain differences of opinion in whether these lesions should or should not be treated prophylactically. If apart from the fatty lump there are no neurological symptoms, many pediatric neurosurgeons adopt a conservative attitude. In the presence of progressive neurological symptoms or signs surgery would then be undertaken. Such a view has been supported in the literature by the pediatric neurosurgery group in Paris (Pierre-Kahn et al 1997). By contrast another group of pediatric neurosurgeons, notably led by colleagues in Chicago (McLone et al 1983), take the view that all spinal lipomas should undergo prophylactic untethering surgery. It therefore remains controversial as to when and whether spinal lipomas should undergo surgical exploration. The issue really concerns the question of untethering. When the fatty lipoma constitutes a significant cosmetic problem it is accepted that the mass should be reduced. Collaboration with colleagues

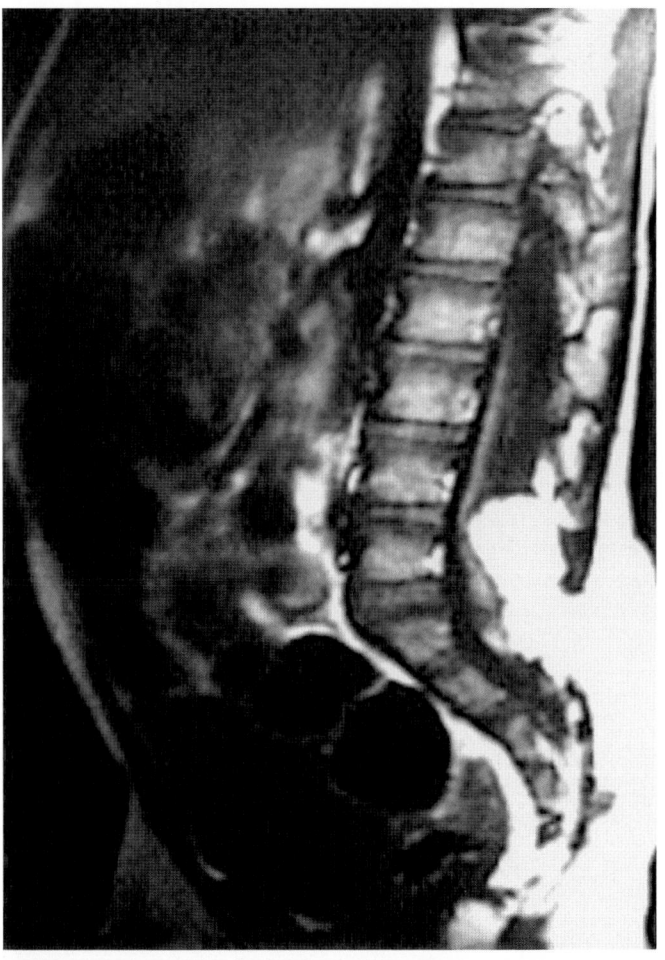

Figure 44.5 T2 sagittal MRI scan showing lipomyelomeningocele. The fatty lump enters the spinal canal and is intimately involved with the lower spinal cord.

in plastic surgery is helpful in achieving a satisfactory contour, whether by liposuction or open surgery. Clearly if a decision has been made to explore a lipoma with a view to untethering the cord, this is a sensible time to also deal with its cosmetic aspect.

REFERENCES

Barkovitch A J, Raghavan N, Chuang et al 1989 The wedge-shaped cord terminus: a radiographic sign of caudal regression. Am J Neuroradiol 10:1223–1231.

Bunch W H, Cass A S, Benson A S et al 1972 Modern management of myelomeningocele. Warren H Green, St Louis, MO.

Cuckle H S, Wald N J, Cuckle P M 1985 Prenatal screening and diagnosis of neural tube defects in England and Wales in 1985. Prenatal Diag 9:393–400.

Curnes J T, Oakes W J, Boyko O B 1989 MR imaging of hindbrain deformity in Chiari II patients with and without symptoms of brainstem compression. Am J Neuroradiol 10:293–302.

Currarino G, Coln D, Votteler T 1981 Triad of anorectal, sacral and presacral anomalies. Am J Radiol 137:395–398.

Dias M S 1999 Myelomeningocele in utero. Pediatr Neurosurg 30:108.

Garceau G J 1953 The filum terminale syndrome. J Bone Joint Surg 35A:711–716.

Guiney E G, Surana R 1994 Selective treatment of spina bifida. Arch Dis Child 56:822–830.

Guthkelch A N 1970 Occipital cranium bifidum. Arch Dis Childhood 45:104–109.

Harrison M R, Adzick N S, Flake A W et al 1993 Correction of diaphragmatic hernia in utero VI. Hard-learned lessons. J Pediatr Surg 28:1411–1418.

Hockley A D, Goldin J H, Wake M J C 1990 Management of anterior encephalocele. Child Nerv Syst 6:444–446.

Hoffman H J, Hendrick E B, Humphreys R P 1975 Manifestations and management of Arnold–Chiari malformations in patients with myelomeningocele. Child's Brain 1:255–259.

Hunt G M 1990 Open spina bifida: outcome for a complete cohort treated unselectively and followed into adulthood. Dev Med Child Neurol 32:108–118.

James C C M, Lassman L P 1972 Spinal dysraphism: spina bifida occulta. Butterworth, London.

Lipschitz R, Beck J M, Froman C 1969 An assessment of the treatment of encephalo-meningoceles. S Afr Med J 43:609–610.

Lorber J 1967 The prognosis of occipital encephalocele. Dev Med Child Neurol 9(Suppl 13):75–86.

Lorber J 1971 Results of treatment of myelomeningocele: an analysis of 524 unselected cases with special reference to possible selection for treatment. Dev Med Child Neurol 13:279–303.

McComb J G 1999 Spinal meningoceles. In: Albright L, Pollack I, Adelson D (eds) Principles and practice of pediatric neurosurgery. Thieme Medical, New York.

McLone D G, Mutluer S, Naidich T P 1983 Lipomyelomeningoceles of the conus medullaris. In: Raimondi A J (ed.) Concepts in pediatric neurosurgery. Karger, Basel, pp. 170–177.

Matson D D 1969 Neurosurgery of infancy and childhood, 2nd edn. Charles Thomas, Springfield, Illinois.

Mealey J Jr, Dzenitis A J, Hackey A A 1970 The prognosis of encephaloceles. J Neurosurg 22:209–218.

Nakamura T, Grant J A, Hubbard R F 1974 Nasoethmoidal meningoencephalocele. Arch Otolaryngol 100:62–64.

Odeku E L 1967 Congenital malformations of the cerebro-spinal axis seen in Western Nigeria. The African child with 'encephalocele'. Int Surg 48:52–62.

Pang D, Dias M S 1993 Cervical myelomeningoceles. Neurosurg 33:363–373.

Park T S (ed.) 1992 Contemporary issues in neurological surgery: Spinal dysraphism. Blackwell, Boston, MA.

Passage E, Lenz 1966 Syndrome of caudal regression in infants of diabetic mothers: observations of further cases. Pediatrics 37:672–675.

Pierre-Kahn A, Zerah M, Renier et al 1997 Congenital lumbosacral lipomas. Child's Nerv Syst 13:298–334.

Rahman N U 1979 Nasal encephalocele: treatment by transcranial operation. J Neurol Sci 42:73–85.

Rauzzino M, Oakes W J 1995 Chiari II malformation and syringomyelia. Neurosurg Clin N Amer 6:293–308.

Steinbok P, Cochrane D D 1995 Cervical meningoceles and myelocystoceles: a unifying hypothesis. Pediatr Neurosurg 23:363–373.

Suwanwela C, Suwanwela N 1972 A morphological classification of sincipital encephalo-meningoceles. J Neurosurg 36:201–211.

Tandon P N 1970 Meningo-encephaloceles. Acta Neurol Scand 46:369–383.

Till K 1969 Spinal dysraphism in a study of congenital malformations of the lower back. J Bone Joint Surg (Br) 51:415–422.

Tullipan N, Bruner J P, Hernanz-Schulman et al 1999 Intrauterine myelomeningocele repair reverses pre-existing hindbrain hernia. Pediatr Neurosurg 31:137–142.

Warrell D A, Cox T M, Firth J D, Benz E J Jr 2003 Oxford textbook of medicine, 4th edn. Oxford University Press, Oxford.

Whatmore W J 1973 Sincipital encephaloceles. Br J Surg 60:261–270.

Congenital defects, vascular malformations and other lesions

Hiroshi Nishikawa and Anthony D. Hockley

Key Points

- Congenital defects affecting the head and neck involve the brain and skull, the brain and face, and defects of the skull
- Aplasia cutis congenita is a scalp and skull defect in the midline, which may require corrective surgery
- Cranial dermal sinuses are epithelial tracts, usually occipital (85%) but can occur anteriorly. As with spinal dermal sinuses, surgery is required to prevent infection. It is necessary to excise the epithelial tract completely and, if present, the associated intracranial dermoid cyst
- Craniosynostosis occurs in 1 in 2000 per head of population, and may cause skull deformity, raised intracranial pressure, and associated anomalies. It may occur alone ('simple') or with complex facial deformities ('syndromic'), frequently with a genetic basis. These cases are best managed by a multi-disciplinary cranio-facial team

---

INTRODUCTION

A useful classification of congenital defects and lesions affecting the head and neck has been proposed by Van der Meulen based on the embryology of the brain, cranium and face (Van Der Meulen et al 1990). Such defects can be explained by dysplasia or 'failure of development' of brain structures, the eyes and the fusion of facial processes (clefts). Abnormal formation of bone, with delayed or more frequently premature fusion of skull sutures, along with muscle and connective tissue abnormalities completes the picture. On the basis of chronological events in brain and facial growth, Van der Meulen classified craniofacial malformations and defects in four major groups:

Group 1. Cerebrocranial dysplasia.
Group 2. Cerebrofacial dysplasia.
Group 3. Craniofacial dysplasia (craniosynostosis, associated syndromes and clefts).
Group 4. Craniofacial dysplasia of other origin.

This chapter describes the management of some of these defects, and also other malformations and neurosurgical lesions which are of importance during the neonatal period.

GROUP 1. CEREBROCRANIAL DYSPLASIA (BRAIN AND SKULL DEFECTS)

ANENCEPHALY

In this group, failure of brain formation gives rise to anencephaly, congenital skull defects and microcephaly. Anencephaly is a lethal condition. The vault of the skull is missing and the anterior brain structures are replaced by a spongy vascular mass (pseudencephaly). The presence of a brain stem and a face suggests that this condition may be due to a vascular disruption of the territories supplied by the internal carotid arteries.

APLASIA CUTIS CONGENITA

Scalp and skull defects centered on the vertex are referred to as aplasia cutis congenita. This condition can range from a patch of alopecia of the scalp to total lack of scalp, calvarium and dura with exposure of pia mater and brain. Aplasia cutis congenita can be associated with epidermolysis bullosa, limb abnormalities (Adams–Oliver syndrome), herpes simplex infection and chromosomal defects such as trisomy 13 (Patau syndrome) and 4p- (Wolf-Hirschhorn syndrome). Isolated skin defects on the limbs can also occur. There is a reported 50% surgical mortality with severe forms of the condition, especially if attempts are made to close defects with injudicious rotation scalp flaps at the neonatal stage. Meningitis, hemorrhage, occlusion of the superior sagittal sinus and cortical damage are the potential complications.

The management of choice is the application of non-adherent occlusive dressings to keep the area moist enough for healthy granulation tissue to form and eventually epithelialize (Lahiri & Nishikawa 2005). The successful use of cultured skin grafts has been reported instead of dressings. In later childhood, the cranial defect can be closed either with autologous calvarial bone grafts or a custom-made titanium plate. The scalp can be reconstructed using a balloon tissue expander technique.

PARIETAL FORAMINA

The term 'parietal foramina' refers to the anomalous enlargement of the osseous foramina which surround the paired parasagittal emissary veins as they pass through the skull. These circular skull defects present as an incidental finding on a skull X-ray, or occasionally as bilateral soft scalp swellings. Very rarely these defects may be large enough to put the underlying brain at risk from mechanical injury and cranioplasty may be indicated. It is best to wait until the child is 4–5 years of age when skull growth is nearly complete.

SPHENOID DYSPLASIA

Neurofibromatosis (type 1) may be associated with a congenital and progressive skull deficiency involving the walls of the orbit, referred to as 'sphenoid dysplasia'. It may be associated with intracranial arachnoid cysts and plexiform neurofibromas of the orbit. In cases with pulsatile exophthalmos later surgical reconstruction may be necessary. The surgery is complex and needs a combined craniofacial team approach.

CRANIAL DERMAL SINUSES

Congenital midline cranial dermoid sinuses are epithelial tracts which, like the spinal lesions, vary in their depth of extension. The tract can expand anywhere along its length to form dermoid cysts. The majority are occipital (85%) but can occur anteriorly. Most are diagnosed before the age of 5 years and present as skin dimples, sometimes mass lesions or recurrent meningitis. The best method of demonstrating the tract is by a combination of MRI and CT imaging. As with spinal dermal sinuses, the surgical principle is that the tract and associated dermoid cyst must be prophylactically removed following diagnosis. Such excision must include the full extra- and intra-dural extensions.

GROUP 2. CEREBROFACIAL DYSPLASIA (BRAIN AND FACE DEFECTS)

RHINENCEPHALIC DYSPLASIA

These deformities are linked with failure or defects in the formation of forebrain, eye and facial midline structures and consist of a group of severe facial defects presenting as a single central orbit with one eye (cyclopia), fused orbits with two eyes (synophthalmus), or orbits too close together (hypotelorism) with or without a premaxilla, which is the central part of the upper jaw (ethmocephaly, cebocephaly, median cleft). Neonates with a combination of facial dysmorphism, hypotelorism and absence of a premaxilla almost always have severe mental deficiency and usually die shortly after birth. Those however with a premaxilla present have a better prognosis and will benefit from future reconstructive surgery.

OCULO-ORBITAL DYSPLASIA

These rare defects result from a failure of the primary optic vesicle to develop from the neuroectoderm of the anterior neural plate. Failure of ocular development leads to a lack of orbital growth as well as hypoplastic eyelids. In microorbitism the orbit is small and contains a very small malformed globe. Complete absence of the globe is seen in anophthalmia. These conditions are usually idiopathic but can be caused by maternal infections during pregnancy with toxoplasmosis or rubella or associated with chromosome deletion in band 14q22-23 and trisomy 13–15. Anophthalmia can occur in other craniofacial conditions such as Goldenhar syndrome.

Management is difficult and directed at orbital and eyelid expansion. Treatment should commence as early as possible. Unless this is achieved, the facial and occlusal asymmetry that occurs in later childhood is very deforming.

GROUP 3. CRANIOFACIAL DYSPLASIA (SKULL AND FACIAL DEFECTS)

CRANIOSYNOSTOSIS

Craniosynostosis is the premature closure of skull sutures causing fusion of the calvarial growth plates. The term was introduced by Virchow in 1851 when he described the classic mechanism. This can involve single or multiple sutures alone ('simple') or in association with deformities involving the orbits and face (complex or 'syndromic'). Most often a primary congenital disorder of skull growth, craniosynostosis can also be secondary to metabolic disease such as rickets or hyperthyroidism, vitamin D deficiency, renal osteodystrophy and hypercalcemia. It is also seen from inadequate brain growth due to over shunted hydrocephalus or microcephaly.

The incidence of craniosynostosis is 1 in 2000 per head of population (Anderson 1977). In 18% of cases there is premature fusion of both coronal sutures, half of them as part of a complex or syndromic cranio-facial anomaly (Mohr et al 1978, Simmons & Peyton 1947).

In recent years there have been major advances identifying a genetic basis for both syndromic but also some nonsyndromic cases. The role of the dura in determining fusion of the sutures is considered critical (Opperman et al 1993) and under genetic control, principally through fibroblast growth factors (FGF) (Alden et al 1999). FGFs are a family of at least 22 known molecules that regulate cell proliferation. Mutations in the FGF receptor gene *FGFR2* are found in Crouzon and Apert syndromes (Besnick & Schnendel 1995, 1998, Wilkie et al 1995). A recurrent point mutation in the *FGFR3* gene is found in 73% of familial and 12% of sporadic cases of coronal synostosis. The mutation converts proline 250 into arginine, and is associated with lower IQ and less satisfactory results from surgical correction (Renier et al 2000). The clinical features of craniosynostosis are: (1) *the skull deformity*, (2), *raised intracranial pressure* and (3) *associated abnormalities*.

(1) *The skull deformity* is anatomically related to the number and type of suture fusion. Restriction across one suture reduces the skull dimension perpendicular to the fused suture, while compensatory growth occurs across patent sutures. As a result in simple craniosynostosis, characteristic deformities are produced (Fig. 45.1). Premature fusion of the sagittal suture is the most commonly affected with an incidence of about 1 : 5000, with boys affected in approximately 80% of cases. A positive family history is present in 6%. Sagittal synostosis causes restriction of biparietal brain growth, resulting in a characteristically narrow, long head with frontal bossing known as *scaphocephaly* (Fig. 45.1a). There is rarely cerebral compression, and surgery is usually advocated for cosmetic reasons.

Premature fusion of both coronal sutures produces a shortened anterior fossa and flattened forehead, the condition referred to as *brachycephaly* (Fig. 45.1d). This may occur as an isolated feature (simple) or in association with midface and orbital anomalies as part of a syndrome, mentioned below.

If only one of the coronal sutures is involved, then a complex unilateral calvarial and orbital deformity results called *anterior synostotic plagiocephaly* or *unicoronal synostosis*. It occurs approximately as 1 : 10 000 live births. The ear on the side of the synostosis is pulled forwards with ipsilateral flattening of the forehead. The nasal root is also deviated towards the side of the synostosis and the orbital shape is distorted on one side due to asymmetry of the cranial base (Fig. 45.1c). This also results in the abnormal insertion of the extraocular muscles resulting in squints and ocular torticollis. The baby has to tilt its head to gain horizontal vision and this accentuates the cranial and orbital deformity. It is now recognized that unilateral anterior plagiocephaly can be syndromic (Cassileth et al 2001).

The term 'plagiocephaly' (Gk. *plagios* meaning oblique or slant), literally meaning an asymmetric head shape, is more frequently used in describing unilateral flattening at the back of the head. This may be due to an extremely rare premature fusion of one or both lambdoid sutures. Much more frequent is *posterior deformational plagiocephaly* (PDP), otherwise known as *postural moulding*.

The incidence of PDP has increased significantly from 1992 onwards as a result of the recommendation by the American Academy of Pediatrics to nurse neonates on their backs to prevent sudden infant death syndrome ('SIDS'). Although not a malformation, PDP is included in this chapter because it is a condition that will be encountered by all neonatologists. At present, there is controversy concerning its management possibly with moulding helmets. It is also important not to misdiagnose this condition with unilateral lambdoid synostosis, the management of which is completely different. The most reliable diagnosis is by clinical examination. In PDP, the unilateral flattening of the occiput is associated with ipsilateral frontal bossing in 85% of babies, and 95% have contralateral occipital bossing producing a 'parallelogram' head shape. The ipsilateral ear is usually pushed forwards. In contrast, babies with unilateral lambdoid synostosis have the ipsilateral ear pulled inferiorly and posteriorly.

The management of PDP is non-surgical. The majority improve with conservative measures such as postural advice during sleep with periods of prone posture during the day along with physiotherapy for torticollis if present. The use of moulding helmets to restrict calvarial growth opposite to the occipital flattening is controversial, and so far there have been no controlled studies. Management of unilateral lambdoid synostosis, like all single suture synostoses, depends on esthetic considerations and concerns regarding possible raised intracranial pressure.

Premature fusion of the metopic suture gives rise to a keel-like, triangular-shaped forehead known as *trigonocephaly* or *metopic synostosis* (Fig 45.1b). The prevalence is 1 : 15 000, although worldwide the incidence appears to be increasing. There is a positive family history in 6% of cases and there is a link with maternal administration of sodium valproate (Lajeunie et al 1998). Language or developmental delay and, more rarely, structural abnormalities of the brain such as agenesis of the corpus callosum are associated with metopic synostosis (Becker et al 2005).

(2) *Raised intracranial pressure* may arise in craniosynostosis because the cranial volume becomes too small for the growing brain. There can also be associated hydrocephalus, as especially occurs in Crouzon and other syndromes. Renier measured the intracranial pressure of 92 infants with craniosynostosis, and found that 14% had raised intracranial pressure with only single suture involvement (>15 mmHg); compared to 42% when more than one suture was affected (Renier et al 1982). The incidence of raised intracranial pressure is higher in syndromic cases.

(3) *Associated abnormalities*. Premature fusion of the skull usually involves the cranial base, and this may modify the growth of the facial skeleton producing certain deformities and syndromes, of which Apert and Crouzon are the best known examples.

CRANIOSYNOSTOSIS SYNDROMES

A syndrome can be defined as congenital malformations occurring in two or more embryologically unrelated areas. A few important syndromes, which are part of the FGFR-related craniosynostosis spectrum, are described below.

APERT SYNDROME

Apert syndrome has a prevalence of 15.5 per million or 1 per 160 000 live births (Bergsma 1973). A baby with Apert syndrome will have bicoronal synostosis and a widely patent midline defect, corresponding to the open sagittal suture, which allows some anterior growth (Fig. 45.1d). Other cranial sutures such as the lambdoids may be involved (Cohen &

Figure 45.1 The three dimensional CT scans on the left correspond to the clinical appearance of the craniosynostosis depicted on the right. (a) shows the scaphocephalic skull shape of a baby with sagittal craniosynostosis. The CT scan demonstrates fusion of the sagittal suture. (b) is a case of metopic craniosynostosis. The skull base is triangular in form and the forehead is typically keel-shaped (trigonocephaly) with a midline ridge. There is relative hypotelorism of the orbits. (c) illustrates right-sided unilateral coronal synostosis (anterior plagiocephaly). The nasal root is deviated towards the side of the flattened forehead and the ear on this affected side is pulled forwards. The orbital shape is different due to skull base distortion and in this case there is a degree of orbital dystopia. (d) is a baby with Apert syndrome. The CT scan shows bicoronal craniosynostosis as well as the wide open enlarged sagittal suture, typically seen in neonates with Apert syndrome. The skull shape is brachycephalic, the canthi are downward slanting, and there is midface hypoplasia. The open mouth is a sign of airway compromise.

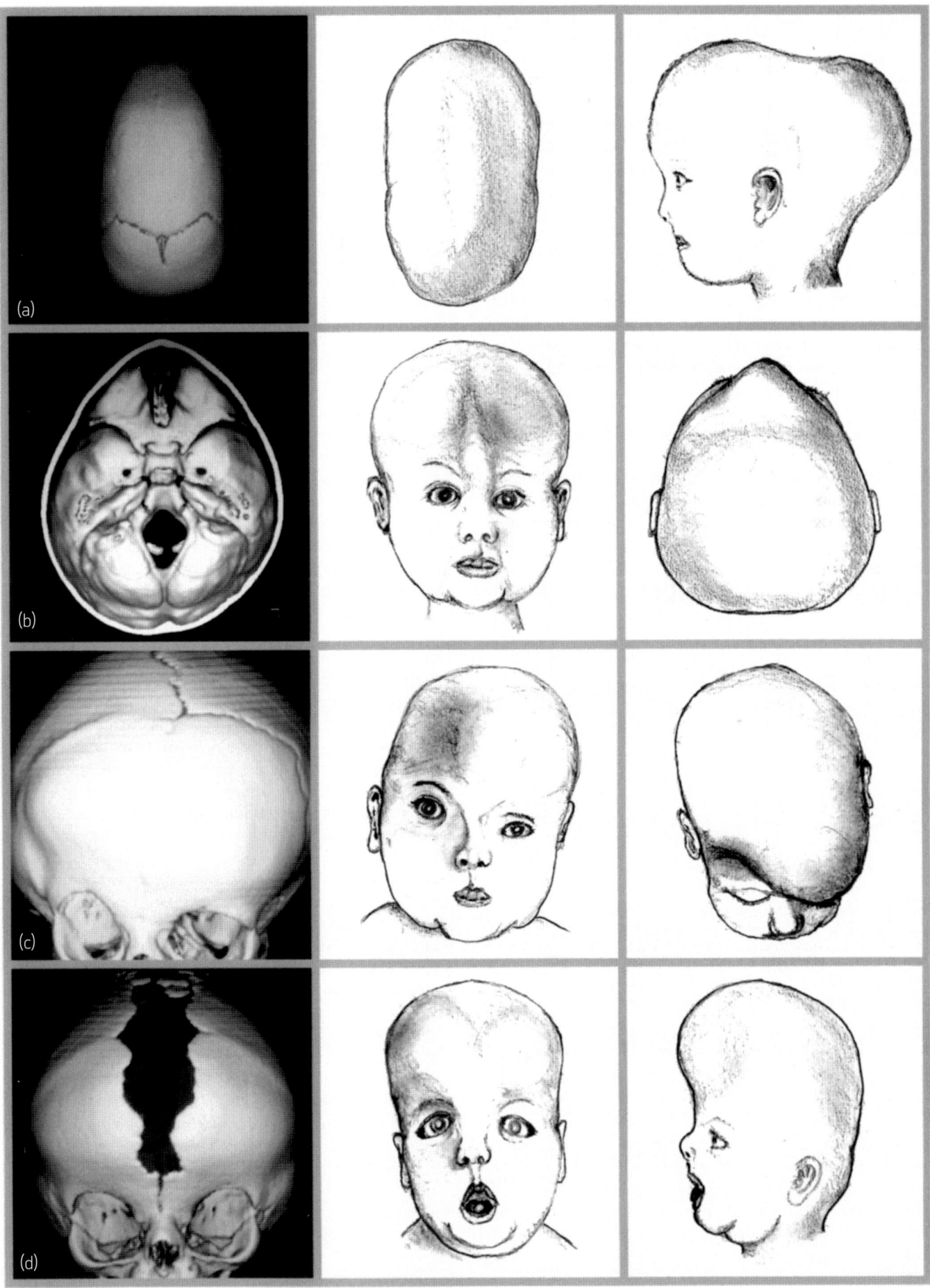

Kreiborg 1993). There is constriction of the cranial base and approximately 5 to 10% has hydrocephalus with diminished venous outflow. An associated Chiari malformation is a frequent finding on MRI. Bony and soft tissue abnormalities are also present such as complex bilateral syndactyly of the hands and feet. There is a high incidence of cleft palate and all have characteristic downward-sloping canthi with varying degrees of midface hypoplasia. Sometimes the midface constriction is so severe that the airways are significantly impaired. Deafness occurs in 30% of cases and developmental delay is common (Renier et al 1996).

CROUZON SYNDROME

Crouzon syndrome is associated with craniosynostosis of the coronal, but also sagittal, metopic and lambdoid sutures, which can be involved singly or multiply. Crouzon syndrome occurs in 1 in 25 000 live births and follows an autosomal dominant mode of transmission, although 30–60% of cases are sporadic (Al-Qattan & Phillips 1997). Hydrocephalus affects 10% of neonates. The orbits are hypoplastic so that in severe cases extreme proptosis can occur endangering the eyes due to exposure. As in Apert, Crouzon babies have mid face hypoplasia and can have severe airway compromise. Conductive hearing deficits are also common.

PFEIFFER SYNDROME

Pfeiffer syndrome has heterogeneous characteristics and consists of craniosynostosis, orbital dystopia (uneven position of the eye sockets), variable midface hypoplasia and broad, medially deviated thumbs. Syndactyly can also occur along with brachydactyly, elbow ankylosis and visceral abnormalities. Inheritance is autosomal dominant and Cohen (1986) described 3 types. Type 1 usually presents with bicoronal synostosis with severe to mild midface hypoplasia. The prognosis is good and intelligence can be normal. Type 2 Pfeiffer syndrome has cloverleaf skull deformity ('Kleeblattschädel'), and the midface deficiency is severe. Hydrocephalus is present and the life span is usually limited. Type 3 is the rarest. These cases present with turricephalic (tower-shaped) skulls, extreme proptosis, hydrocephalus, choanal atresia and laryngotracheal abnormalities. Their prognosis is poor.

MANAGEMENT OF CRANIOSYNOSTOSIS: SYNDROMIC AND NON-SYNDROMIC

Management of craniosynostosis should be under a multi-disciplinary team in a center regularly dealing with craniofacial conditions (Posnick & Ruiz 2000). Diagnosis is made on clinical grounds, with skull X-rays and CT scans confirming the nature of the synostosis. MRI is helpful in recognizing the type of hydrocephalus if present and the presence of a Chiari malformation.

The indications for surgery in craniosynostosis are to relieve raised intracranial pressure, improve functions (ocular, nasal, phonetic, dental), cosmetic and psychological.

The aim is to correct established deformity, prevent complications and redirect growth towards normality (Hockley et al 1988).

In simple craniosynostosis when only one suture is affected and the deformity mild then expectant treatment may be appropriate. The decision on what constitutes an unacceptable deformity is not easy, and one must take into consideration the feelings of the parents, society and the natural history of that particular craniosynostosis.

When surgery is advocated the next issue is timing. Under normal conditions the infant's skull enlarges in response to the growing brain, which reaches 50% of adult size by the age of 6 months and 80% by the age of 2 years. The traditional method of excising the prematurely fused suture ('linear craniectomy'), using the brain growth or 'drive' to relieve pressure and correct deformity, can be regarded as 'passive surgery'. With modern 'active' surgical techniques, based on the pioneering work of Dr. Paul Tessier in the 1960s (Tessier 1967), corrective repositioning of bony structures is possible.

For most cases of simple craniosynostosis surgery at the age of 1 year is considered a good compromise between brain drive and the easier surgical handling of maturing neonatal bone. The exception is scaphocephaly where earlier calvarial remodeling at three months of age has been shown to produce superior esthetic results. The use of the limited linear craniectomy of the sagittal suture before the age of 6 months has been found to be unpredictable (Panchal et al 1999). Minimally invasive techniques involving endoscopic strip craniectomy with postoperative moulding helmet therapy are under evaluation.

Established surgical methods for syndromic synostosis involve exposure of the skull and orbits using craniofacial approaches. The aim of surgery is to increase intracranial volume as well as improve the esthetic appearance of the calvarium, forehead and upper orbits (Fig. 45.2).

The timing of intervention depends upon the threat of raised intracranial pressure and exposure of the eyes, which occur in severe syndromic cases such as Apert and Crouzon syndromes. Sometimes an emergency tarsorrhaphy may be necessary to achieve corneal protection. Ventricular shunts or posterior calvarial decompression (Sgouros et al 1996), within the first few months of life, may be necessary to relieve the raised intracranial pressure from associated hydrocephalus or the craniosynostosis. A Chiari malformation is a frequent finding in multi-sutural and syndromic craniosynostosis. It has been reported in 70% of patients with Crouzon syndrome, 50% with Pfeiffer syndrome and 100% with Kleeblattschädel deformity (Cinalli et al 2005).

The definitive procedure for most craniosynostosis involves a fronto-orbital advancement, which can be done primarily or at a second stage following a posterior skull decompression or shunt. In severe Apert and Crouzon cases it may also be necessary to address airway problems and sleep apnea due to midface hypoplasia. Early tracheostomy may be necessary.

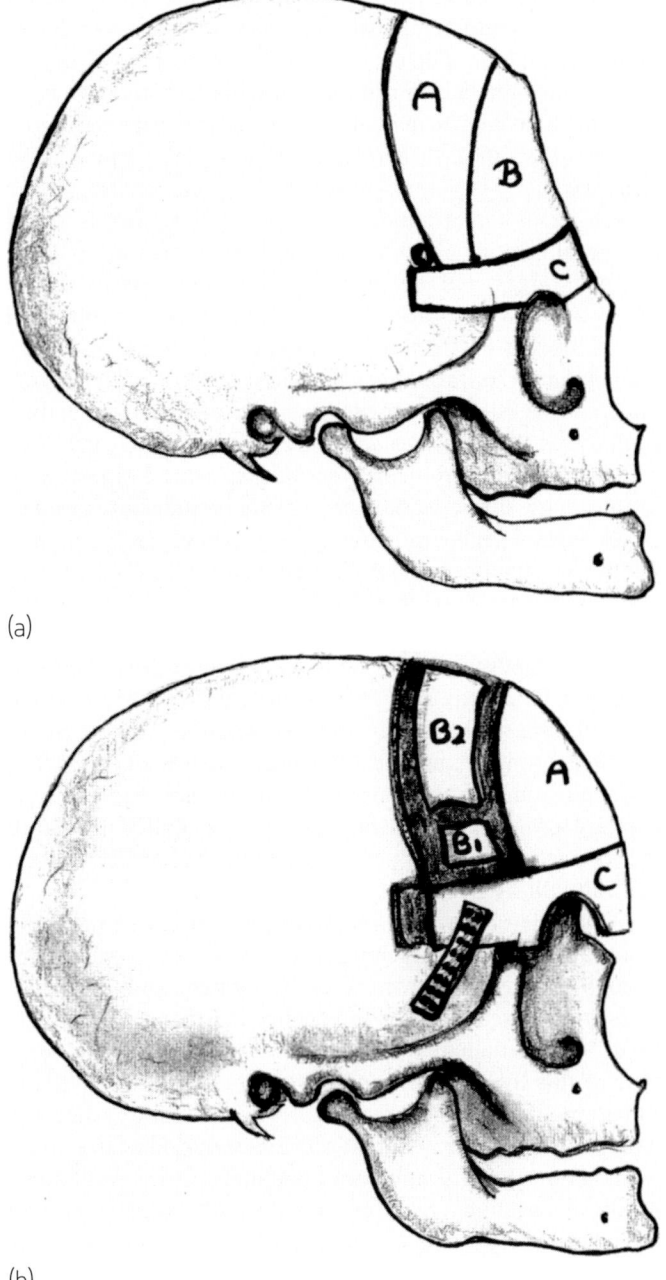

(a)

(b)

Figure 45.2 Fronto-orbital advancement and cranial remodeling as carried out for coronal and metopic synostosis is schematically shown in (a) and (b). The deformed frontal bone B is swapped with the more normal contoured bone flap A, whilst the orbital bar C is reshaped and moved forward. This allows improved forehead shape and an increase in intracranial volume. Absorbable plates are used for fixation.

The use of a technique called 'monoblock distraction' advancement is currently becoming established to treat raised ICP, ocular exposure and midface hypoplasia at the same time. The frontal bone, the orbits and the bones of the mid face are advanced, using internal or external distraction

devices. This increases the intracranial, orbital and airway passage volumes in one stage (Mathijssen et al 2006). It is possible now to carry this out before one year of age but these babies will need long-term observation for raised ICP, ocular and airway difficulties. Inevitably they all have inherent midface hypoplasia and will require further surgery to address this in early adulthood.

CRANIOFACIAL DYSPLASIA WITH CLEFTING
HYPERTELORISM

Hypertelorism is the increase of the apparent distance between the orbits. This is not a syndrome but is a clinical sign of several pathologies affecting the craniofacial skeleton and soft tissues, including those that fall into this category of craniofacial dysplasia with clefting.

CRANIOFACIAL CLEFTS

Craniofacial clefts are rare but form an important group of deformities. Tessier has classified these clefts on a clinical and observational basis (Tessier 1976). They are numbered from 0 to 14 and follow predictable paths through the soft tissues of the lips, nose, cheeks, eyelids, as well as the underlying craniofacial skeleton. The clefts are orbitocentric in that the clefts numbered from 0 to 7 lie below the orbit. Cleft 8 runs lateral to the orbit, while clefts 9 to 14 are above the orbit. These clefts generally run in a north–south direction and those above and below the orbit can occur in combination.

FRONTONASAL DYSPLASIA

Frontonasal dysplasia is a midline facial clefting that encompasses several anomalies, with clinical features including orbital hypertelorism, a broadened nasal root, a grooved or deficient nasal tip, a widow's peak and occult cranium bifidum. Frontonasal dysplasia is also associated with agenesis of the corpus callosum and basal encephaloceles. Developmental delay can be present but is not pathognomonic. The degree of clefting and hypertelorism is variable. The management of frontonasal dysplasia is multidisciplinary and should be carried out in a craniofacial center in order to correct the hypertelorism, and the deformities of the nose and lips caused by the midline cleft.

GROUP 4. CRANIOFACIAL DYSPLASIA OF OTHER ORIGIN

This group consists of defects which do not fit well with the sequential embryology of the brain or the timing of facial fusion processes.

VASCULAR ANOMALIES

Vascular anomalies may be either high flow or low flow and are classified as either hemangiomas or vascular malformations (Mulliken & Glowaki 1982). They can occur anywhere on the body and the majority can be diagnosed by history and examination alone. The management of major vascular

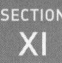
anomalies should be multidisciplinary as they can affect any part of the body and treatment can involve several medical disciplines.

HEMANGIOMA

Seventy percent of hemangiomas (formerly called strawberry nevi) arise on the head and neck, but they can also involve bone, liver or the viscera. These are high flow vascular tumors and usually present shortly after birth. They rapidly expand over a period of months. They are usually solitary but it is not unusual for several to be present. Multiple hemangiomas were thought to cause the consumptive coagulopathy of the Kasabach–Merrit syndrome. However this is now known to be caused by Kaposiform hemangio-endothelioma and tufted angiomas, which are very rare vascular tumors (Enjrolas & Wassef et al 1997). Diffuse hemangiomas of the face can be associated with Dandy–Walker malformations, which are characterized by agenesis or hypoplasia of the cerebellar vermis and cystic dilatation of the fourth ventricle with enlargement of the posterior fossa. Approximately 70–80% of these patients develop hydrocephalus postnatally (Reese et al 1993).

Hemangiomas, which ulcerate and bleed, can be managed with non-adherent dressings and topical antibiotic steroid preparations (Terra-Cortril®). Hemangiomas affecting the face cause distressing esthetic deformity but they should be treated conservatively during the growth phase. The exceptions to this are hemangiomas which obscure vision which, if untreated can cause amblyopia; hemangiomas affecting the airways; and multiple hemangiomas causing high output cardiac failure. Steroid, injected directly into an isolated hemangioma or given orally at a dose of up to 4 mg/Kg/d, is the first-line treatment. Other agents have been used to treat hemangiomas such as interferon alpha-2a (Spiller et al 1992) and vincristine. Its anti-angiogenic affects have been demonstrated to be very effective in steroid resistant hemangiomas (Enjrolas et al 2004).

After this growth phase, which can last for a period of 12 months or more, they all involute. Most regress totally and most have disappeared by the age of 10 years with little or no scarring. However larger hemangiomas, or those which have ulcerated, can leave permanent fibrofatty skin remnants, which require surgical treatment. Extensive, subcutaneous hemangiomas can also lead to differential bony growth and facial asymmetry requiring specialized plastic and maxillofacial treatment in later childhood (Enjrolas & Mulliken 1997).

VASCULAR MALFORMATIONS: EXTRACRANIAL

Vascular malformations, unlike hemangiomas, are present at birth and do not have a proliferative or regressive phase. They will grow in proportion with the baby and are classified according to the dominant vessel type they contain.

Capillary malformations (port-wine stains) are cutaneous malformations and if located in the distribution of the trigeminal nerve, Sturge-Weber syndrome should be considered (Comi 2003). The associated abnormal blood vessels in the brain (leptomeningeal angioma) can lead on to developmental delays, epilepsy and eye problems (glaucoma).

The management of capillary vascular malformations is not indicated in the neonate and in later childhood lasers and plastic surgical techniques with tissue expansion can be employed.

Venous malformations are slow flow lesions consisting of abnormal ectatic collections of veins. These can affect large or small areas and encroach upon several tissue planes. There are few indications for treatment in the neonatal period, except if affecting the airway or feeding.

Lymphatic malformations (formerly called cystic hygromas) can be either macrocystic or microcystic in structure. Both types, if extensive and large enough, can cause significant airway problems for the neonate. Macrocystic lesions tend not to affect the oropharyngeal airways but cause mass effects from the surface. They can be treated with sclerotherapy in later childhood.

Extensive lesions affecting tongue, oral cavity and the neck are among the most difficult vascular malformations to treat. Usually not amenable to sclerotherapy, they can pose serious airway and feeding problems for the neonate necessitating tracheostomy and feeding tubes. Microcysts in the cheek, tongue and neck can cause macroglossia leading to facial and jaw deformity and permanent open bite or occlusal problems. Multistage surgery involving debulking and correction of facial ptosis as well as orthognathic intervention will be necessary.

An *arterio-venous malformation* (AV *fistula*) of the scalp is a rare lesion, characterized by abnormal arterial and venous connections with grossly dilated and expansile masses of vessels that can predispose to dramatic complications. The so-called 'cirsoid aneurysm' is a rare but florid type of this lesion seen in neonates. These lesions may be a threat to life due to high-output cardiac failure, disseminated intravascular coagulation and septicemia secondary to infection. Such lesions are also at risk from local complications such as recurrent hemorrhage, ulceration and infection. There are a large number of treatment methods for arterio-venous malformations of the scalp which include embolization, selective ligation of feeding vessels and surgical excision (Taylor et al 1990).

VASCULAR MALFORMATIONS: INTRACRANIAL

Intracranial aneurysms and intracranial arterio-venous malformations do occur in childhood, but rarely in the neonatal period.

Intracranial aneurysms in children usually present with spontaneous intracranial hemorrhage, producing irritability and seizures. In the young infant other features are a bulging fontanelle, retinal hemorrhages, low hemoglobin level and blood stained CSF obtained at lumbar puncture that has been performed to exclude meningitis. These features may suggest non-accidental injury, but the pattern of the intracranial hemorrhage on CT scan is more suggestive of a spontaneous rather than traumatic origin (McLellan et al 1986).

The general principles of diagnosis and treatment for aneurysms in childhood are basically the same as for adults. After the causative aneurysm has been demonstrated by angiography (either by MR angiography or arterial catheterization), and the child is in a stable state, treatment to exclude the aneurysm from the circulation is undertaken. Such treatment may be by craniotomy with clipping of the aneurysm, or increasingly now by interventional radiology methods, using detachable metal coils or balloons.

Aneurysms in young children are frequently large and occur in the posterior circulation three times more commonly than in adults, even more so during the first two years of life. It should be remembered that children with coarctation of the aorta, polycystic kidney disease and Ehlers–Danlos syndrome are at increased risk of developing intracerebral aneurysms and should undergo screening studies. So-called 'infectious' or 'mycotic' aneurysms can arise within two days from septic emboli in children (Khoo & Levy 1999).

Intracranial arterio-venous malformations are twice as common as aneurysms as a cause of spontaneous intracranial hemorrhage in childhood (Humphreys 1982). Only 4% of childhood arterio-venous malformations occur in infancy (Shapiro 1985), and virtually none of these occur in the neonatal period. Intracranial arterio-venous malformations may present with congestive cardiac failure or spontaneous intracranial hemorrhage that may be intraventricular, intracerebral or subdural (Wakai et al 1990). Raised intracranial pressure from hydrocephalus may be the presentation, when the arterio-venous malformation is within the ventricular system or there is a secondary dilation of the vein of Galen obstructing the aqueduct. Epilepsy, presumably from gliosis of the brain due to ischemia adjacent to the arterio-venous malformation, can occur as a presenting symptom in 20–67% of adult patients, but in contrast less than 15% of children present with a chronic seizure disturbance. Spontaneous intracranial hemorrhage is the means by which 80% of children declare their malformations. While modern radiology techniques have revolutionized the ability to diagnose and treat vascular malformations of the central nervous system, surgical excision remains the most common treatment for localized intracranial arterio-venous malformations.

Endovascular embolization may be helpful as a prelude to surgical excision. The advent of stereotactic radiotherapy ('radiosurgery') has been successful for smaller lesions, either in strategic locations such as the thalamus or motor cortex, or for small residual lesions after operative removal of their hematoma and major malformation components.

Venous angiomas are the most common of all the vascular malformations of the brain, yet are the least likely to cause symptoms. The current view is held that a venous angioma represents an anomalous but competent venous drainage pattern.

Cavernous malformations account for 8–16% of all cerebral vascular malformations and occur most frequently in the cerebral hemispheres. The appearance on CT and MRI scanning is of a well circumscribed mass, with the surrounding brain frequently stained by old hemorrhage (hemosiderin). The cavernous malformation (or 'cavernoma') typically comes to attention because of hemorrhage, seizures or progressive neurological deficit. With the exception of those lesions in the brainstem, most episodes of bleeding are minor and may be undetected. The majority of cavernous malformations do not demonstrate abnormal vasculature, and MRI scanning is now the investigation of choice. Once there has been a clinical hemorrhage, and it is technically possible, surgical excision is the treatment of choice. If seizures are well controlled medically excision may be kept in reserve. Perhaps the most challenging cavernoma is the brainstem lesion which has bled. While there are significant neurological risks from surgery, the presence of a surrounding hematoma can facilitate surgery and neurological recovery when the bleed has caused profound deficit.

VEIN OF GALEN AND DURAL MALFORMATIONS IN CHILDHOOD

A rare group of vascular lesions in infancy and childhood are the vein of Galen and dural malformations, which have a high vascular flow and characteristic clinical presentation.

Vein of Galen malformations are thought to result from fistulous connections that develop near the embryonic choroid plexus. The consequent high-flow arterio-venous shunt between branches of the anterior, middle, posterior cerebral and superior cerebellar arteries and the vein of Galen, leads to progressive aneurysmal dilation of the vein, whose wall becomes thick and tough.

Vein of Galen malformations can be classified clinically (Gold 1964), or angiographically. These lesions tend to be age dependent and can be placed in three categories

1. Neonates present with severe congestive heart failure.
2. Infants with hydrocephalus and/or seizures.
3. Older children or adults with subarachnoid hemorrhage, or hydrocephalus.

Angiographically, there are two types of malformation. In one type there is a primary vein of Galen malformation in which large arteries feed directly into the aneurysmal sac. In the other type a secondary vein of Galen aneurysmal dilation, in which an adjacent arterio-venous malformation in the cerebral or cerebellar hemispheres, brainstem or tentorium drains via the Galenic vein, which becomes dilated.

Until the advent of interventional radiology, the morbidity and mortality for this lesion when symptomatic were unacceptably high. The mortality related to the intractable neonatal heart failure and intra-operative hemorrhage. In addition there was a high incidence of severe neurodevelopmental deficits in the survivors after surgery. Occasionally spontaneous obliteration with calcification has been reported (Chapman & Hockley 1989).

With increasing experience from multidisciplinary teams involving interventional radiologists and neurosurgeons, results are improving in specialized centers. With early aggressive trans-arterial or trans-venous embolization employing N-butyl cyanoacrylate (Berenstein & Lasjaunias 1992) it is possible to reverse neonatal cardiac failure.

In children who can be stabilized and who do not have severe cerebral damage, there is a therapeutic 'window of opportunity' that, if missed, will lead to progressive loss of brain tissue with inevitable neuro-developmental deficits. It is now known that ventricular shunting for the frequent associated hydrocephalus is to be avoided, because there are major complications and a poor neurological outcome. A shunting procedure does not solve the complex hemodynamic problems that exist in these babies (Zerah et al 1992).

Dural malformations in childhood are very rare and less frequent than vein of Galen aneurysms. They generally have a more benign course than intra-parenchymal AVMs, presenting with hemorrhage in only 10% of cases. These high flow shunts usually involve a major dural sinus at the base, but usually involve more posteriorly placed sinuses, in particular the transverse and sagittal sinuses and torcula.

Clinically these lesions present by causing increased intracranial pressure from hydrocephalus, seizures, spontaneous subarachnoid hemorrhage and in neonates high output cardiac failure.

The arterial supply of these lesions consists of dural vessels from the external carotid, vertebral and internal carotid arteries. Venous drainage occurs through either virtually normal sinuses or abnormal sinuses that may be duplicated or stenosed.

Treatment in these rare lesions has mainly concerned neonates with cardiac failure, and these have been treated by embolization methods similar to those used with vein of Galen malformations. Both trans-venous and trans-arterial therapies are effective and surgical resection of the involved sinus is not usually required.

OTHER NEUROSURGICAL LESIONS IN THE NEONATAL PERIOD

INTRACRANIAL INFECTION

The major aspects of neonatal central nervous system infections have been covered in Chapters 30–32. There are aspects of neonatal meningitis or intracranial suppuration where neurosurgical intervention is required.

CONSEQUENCES OF NEONATAL MENINGITIS

There are really two complications of neonatal meningitis that may require neurosurgical assistance, namely hydrocephalus and subdural effusions.

A degree of usually temporary *hydrocephalus* occurs at some stage in 30% of cases of neonatal meningitis (Karan 1986). When suspected clinically by a tense anterior fontanelle, increased head circumference or a poor neurological condition, further investigation is indicated with ultrasound, CT or MRI imaging. Diagnostic and therapeutic ventricular punctures can assist both the management of the infection and the temporary hydrocephalus. When repeated ventricular CSF samples are needed or intraventricular therapy, surgical implantation of a ventriculostomy reservoir or an external ventricular drain can be extremely helpful.

At a later stage even if the meningitis has been successfully treated, a progressive hydrocephalus, usually of the communicating type, may result from the leptomeningeal fibrosis. Endoscopic third ventriculostomy has been uniformly unsuccessful, so that treatment is by insertion of a ventricular shunt (Buxton et al 1998). So-called 'post-meningitic' hydrocephalus occurs particularly with certain forms of meningitis, including listeria, pneumococcal and tuberculosis. The prognosis in terms of neuro-developmental sequelae relates to the extent of brain damage (cerebral infarction) rather than to the occurrence of hydrocephalus. The management of hydrocephalus in this group of children can be complicated by the development of multiloculated ventricles, requiring additional surgical procedures.

Subdural effusions are seen on imaging in the convalescent phase of neonatal pyogenic meningitis in up to 50% of cases. Usually such effusions are asymptomatic, but occasionally in about 5% of cases (Milhorat 1978) can cause symptoms. These comprise persistent fever, irritability, seizures or signs of raised intracranial pressure. A subdural needle aspiration, with the needle inserted through the lateral corner of the anterior fontanelle (on each side) will provide a sample for microbiological investigations as well as relieving intracranial pressure. Most symptomatic subdural effusions will resolve with or without repeated subdural taps. However, occasionally a sizeable subdural effusion may re-accumulate. If this happens and the subdural fluid is sterile, a subdural shunt into the peritoneal cavity may be required (Till 1968).

INTRACRANIAL SUPPURATION

There are two types of intracranial purulent collection, a subdural empyema and intracerebral abscess, whose management requires surgical drainage along the same principles as for adult intracranial infection.

In neonates the presence of an anterior fontanelle may allow drainage of a *subdural empyema* in its early stage when the fluid is thin. When the pus is too thick to be drained in this way it can only be evacuated adequately by burr holes or craniotomy.

Intracerebral or *brain abscesses* (p. 670) in neonates are the result of bacteremia occurring during or shortly after birth. They are predominantly due to gram-negative organisms and the abscess may reach a large size, associated with thin walls and extensive surrounding cerebral edema. Any neonate who displays features that are atypical for meningitis should undergo cranial imaging. While ultrasound will exclude any large parenchymal abscess, a CT or preferably MRI scan will give more detailed information. Most abscesses are frontal in location and not usually multiple (Renier et al 1988).

The principles of treatment are the same as for cerebral abscess whatever the patient's age, namely accurate microbiological diagnosis from the pus, relief of raised intracranial pressure by aspiration of pus from the abscess, control of the sepsis by appropriate antibiotics in high intravenous dosage, and suppression of fits with anticonvulsant drugs (Hockley & George 1982).

In the neonate, the abscess may be aspirated by needle aspirations through the anterior fontanelle, through a diastased suture or through a burr hole. Aspirations should be repeated until the abscess cavity has collapsed, and surgical excision of the acute abscess can usually be avoided.

INTRACRANIAL TUMORS

Intracranial tumors very rarely present at birth or produce symptoms within the first few months of life. According to the literature, they account for 0.5–1.9% of all childhood brain tumors (Jooma & Kendall 1982, Sato et al 1964), an incidence of 0.34 per million live births. Unlike older children, 70% of neonatal brain tumors are supratentorial and only 30% infratentorial. Presentation is with symptoms of raised intracranial pressure. Macrocephaly may be severe enough to cause disproportion and dystocia. Babies may be stillborn or premature, with teratoma as the most frequent tumor type.

Neonatal brain tumors are frequently very large and vascular, with surgical excision a major challenge to the neurosurgeon and anesthetist. The use of chemotherapy may enable safer and more complete excision as seen in the case of malignant choroid plexus tumors (Greenberg 1999), and such a strategy might apply to other tumor types.

SPINAL TUMORS

Spinal tumors are exceptionally rare in the neonatal period, but should be suspected in an infant with paraplegia who does not have features of spinal dysraphism or other abnormalities. The majorities are neuroblastomas (Punt et al 1980) but other tumor types occur. After appropriate imaging, surgical decompression is indicated to prevent neurological deterioration and obtain tissue for histological diagnosis. In the case of neuroblastoma, without progressive neurological deterioration, treatment is initially with chemotherapy, surgical excision being reserved for any residuum. The outcome is dependent upon the nature of the tumor and the neurological condition at presentation. For infants with neuroblastoma, the prospects of survival are excellent. Late spinal deformity may require corrective surgery.

REFERENCES

Alden T D, Lin K Y, Jane J A 1999 Mechanisms of premature closure of cranial sutures. Child's Nerv Syst 15:670–675.

Al-Qattan M M, Phillips J H 1997 Clinical features of Crouzon's syndrome patients with positive family history of Crouzon's syndrome. J Craniofac Surg 8(1):11–13.

Anderson H 1977 Craniosynostosis. In Vinken P J, Bruyn G W (eds) Handbook of clinical neurology. Congenital malformations of the brain and skull. Elsevier, Amsterdam, vol 30, part 1, pp. 19–233.

Becker D B, Petersen J D, Kane A A et al 2005 Speech, cognitive and behavioural outcomes in nonsyndromic craniosynostosis. Plast Reconstr Surg 116(2):400–407.

Berenstein A, Lasjaunias P 1992 Surgical neuroangiography volume 4: Endovascular treatment of cerebral intravascular lesions. Springer, Berlin.

Bergsma 1973 Birth defects. Atlas and compendium. Williams and Williams, Baltimore.

Besnick S, Schnendel S 1995 Crouzon's disease correlates with low fibroblast growth factor receptor activity in stenosed cranial sutures. J Craniofacial Surg 6:245–248.

Besnick S, Schnendel S 1998 Apert's syndrome correlates with low fibroblast growth factor receptor activity in stenosed cranial sutures. J Craniofacial Surg 9:92–95.

Buxton N, Macarthur D, Malluci C et al 1998 Neuroendoscopic third ventriculostomy in patients less than one year old. Pediatr Neurosurg 29:73–76.

Cassileth L B, Bartlett S P, Glat P M et al 2001 Clinical characteristics of patients with unicoronal synostosis

and mutations of fibroblast growth factor receptor 3: a preliminary report. Plast Reconstr Surg 108(7):1849–1854.

Chapman S, Hockley A D 1989 Calcification of an aneurysm of the vein of Galen. Ped Radiol 19:541–542.

Cinalli G, Spennato P, Sainte-Rose C et al 2005 Chiari malformations in craniosynostosis. Childs Nerv Syst 21(10):889–901.

Cohen M M 1986 Craniosynostosis diagnosis, evaluation, and management. Raven, New York.

Cohen M M, Kreiborg S 1993 An updated pediatric perspective on Apert syndrome. Am J Dis Child 147(9):989–993.

Comi A M 2003 Pathophysiology of Sturge–Weber syndrome. J Child Neurol 18(8):509–616.

Enjrolas O, Breviere G M, Roger G et al 2004 Vincristine treatment for the function- and life-threatening infantile hemangioma. Arch Pediatr 11(2):99–107.

Enjrolas O, Mulliken J B 1997 Vascular tumours and vascular malformations (new issues). Adv Dermatol 13:375–423.

Enjrolas O, Wassef M, Mazoyez E et al 1997 Infants with Kasabach–Merritt syndrome do not have 'true' hemangiomas. J Pediatr 130(4):631–640.

Gold A P, Ransohoff J R, Carter S 1964 Vein of Galen malformation. Acta Neuro Scand 40 (suppl 11):5.

Greenberg M 1999 Chemotherapy of choroid plexus carcinoma. Child's Nerv Syst 15:571–577.

Hockley A D, George R 1982 Brain abscess. In: Current therapy (the nervous system). WB Saunders, Philadelphia.

Hockley A D, Wake M J, Goldin J H 1988 Surgical management of craniosynostosis. Br J Neurosurg 2:307–314.

Humphreys R P 1982 Arteriovenous malformations of the brain and spinal cord. Pediatric neurosurgery: surgery of the developing nervous system. Grune and Stratton, New York.

Jooma R, Kendall B E 1982 Intracranial tumours in the first year of life. Neuroradiology 23:267–274.

Karan S 1986 Purulent meningitis in the newborn. Child's Nerv Syst 2:26–31.

Khoo L T, Levy M L 1999 Intracerebral aneurysms. In: Albright A L, Pollack I F, Adelson P D (eds) Principles and practice of pediatric neurosurgery. Thieme, New York.

Lahiri A, Nishikawa H 2005 A nonadherent dressing for aplasia cutis congenita. J Plast Reconstr Surg 59(7):781–782.

Lajeunie E, Le Merrer M, Marchac M et al 1998 Syndromal and nonsyndromal trigonocephaly: analysis of a series of 237 patients. Am J Med Genet 13,75(2):211–215.

McLellan N H, Prasad R, Punt J 1986 Spontaneous subhyaloid and retinal haemorrhages in an infant. Arch Dis Childhood 61:1130–1132.

Mathijssen I, Arnaud E, Marchac D et al 2006 Respiratory outcome of midface advancement with distraction: a comparison between Le Fort III and frontofacial monoblock. J Craniofac Surg 17(5):880–882.

Milhorat T 1978 Pediatric neurosurgery. Davis, Philadelphia, PA.

Mohr G, Hoffman H J, Munro I R et al 1978 Surgical management of unilateral and bilateral coronal craniosynostosis. Neurosurgery 2:83–92.

Mulliken J B, Glowaki J 1982 Haemangiomas and vascular malformations in infants and children: a classification based on endothelial characteristics. Plast Reconstr Surg 69:412.

Opperman L A, Sweeney T M, Redman J et al 1993 Tissue interactions with underlying dura mater inhibit osseous obliteration of developing cranial sutures. Dev Dynam 198:312–322.

Panchal J, Marsh J L, Park T S et al 1999 Sagittal craniosynostosis outcome assessment for two methods and timings of intervention. Plast Reconstr Surg 103(6):1574–1584.

Posnick J C, Ruiz R L 2000 The craniofacial dysostosis syndromes: current surgical thinking and future directions. Cleft Palate Craniofac J 37(5):433.

Punt J, Pritchard J, Pincott J et al 1980 Neuroblastoma: a review of 21 cases presenting with spinal cord compression. Cancer 45:3095–3102.

Reese V, Frieden I J, Paller AS et al 1993 Association of facial hemanigiomas with Dandy–Walker and other posterior fossa malformations. J Pediatr 122(3):379–384.

Renier D, Arnaud E, Cinalli et al 1996 Prognosis for mental function Apert syndrome. J Neurosurg 85:66.

Renier D, El Ghouzi V, Bonaventure et al 2000 Fibroblast growth factor receptor 3 mutation in nonsyndromic coronal synostosis: clinical spectrum, prevalence, and surgical outcome. J Neurosurg 92:631–636.

Renier D, Flandin C, Hirsch E et al 1988 Brain abscesses in neonates. A study of 20 cases. J Neurosurg 69:877–882.

Renier D, Saint–Rose C, Marchac D et al 1982 Intracranial pressure in craniosynostosis. J Neurosurg 57(3):370–377.

Sato O, Tumura A, Sano K 1964 Brain tumours of early infants. Child's Brain 1:121–125.

Sgouros S, Goldin J H, Hockley A D, Wake M J C 1996 Posterior skull surgery in craniosynostosis. Child's Nerv Syst 12:727–733.

Shapiro K 1985 Subarachnoid haemorrhages in children. In: Fein J M, Flamm E S (eds) Cerebrovascular surgery. Springer, New York.

Simmons D R, Peyton W T 1947 Premature closure of the cranial sutures. J Pediatr 31:528–547.

Spiller J C, Sharma V, Woods G M et al 1992 Diffuse neonatal hemangiomatosis treated successfully with interferon alfa-2a. J Am Acad Dermatol 27:102–104.

Taylor J L, Hockley A D, Downing R 1990 Vascular anomalies of the scalp. Child's Nerv Syst 6:356–359.

Tessier P 1967 Osteotomies totales de la face. Syndrome de Crouzon, syndrome d'Apert: Oxycephalies, scaphocephalies, turricephalies. Ann Chir Plast 12:173–186.

Tessier P 1976 Anatomical classification of facial, cranio-facial and latero-facial clefts. J Maxillofacial Surg 4(2):69–92.

Till K 1968 Subdural haematoma and effusion in infancy. BMJ ii:400–402.

Van Der Meulen J C, Mazolla R, Stricker M et al 1990 Classification of craniofacial malformations. In: Stricker M, Van Der Meulen J C, Raphael B et al (eds) Craniofacial malformations. Churchill Livingstone, Edinburgh.

Virchow R 1851 Uber den Cathismus, namentlich in Franken, und uber pathologische. Schadeljormen Verk Phys-Med Ges Wurzberg 2:230–270.

Wakai S, Andon Y, Nagai M et al 1990 Choroid plexus arteriovenous malformation in a full-term neonate. Case report. J Neurosurg 72:127–129.

Wilkie A O, Slaney S F, Oldridge M et al 1995 Apert syndrome results from localized mutations of FGFR2 and is allelic with Crouzon syndrome. Nat Genet 9(2):165–172.

Zerah M, Garcia-Monaco, Rodesch G et al 1992 Hydrodynamics in vein of Galen malformation in 43 cases. Child's Nerv Syst 8:111–117.

The epidemiology of the cerebral palsies

Eve Blair and Fiona Stanley

Key Points

- Cerebral palsy is defined as motor impairment resulting from a non-progressive brain lesion or anomaly acquired early in life
- It is a clinical description, not a diagnosis
- Since it cannot be applied until the motor impairment becomes apparent, only neonatal survivors are at risk
- Despite considerable efforts, inter-center agreement of sub-classification remains elusive
- The effect on function ranges from imperceptible to total incapacitation
- Motor impairment may be accompanied by other impairments, which may additionally limit functional attainment
- Its causes are heterogeneous and may be multifactorial
- Risk factors include preterm birth, restricted intra-uterine growth, multiple gestation, male gender, several antenatal factors, sentinel intrapartum events, poor condition at birth or neonatally and post neonatal cerebral infection or trauma
- With the exception of post neonatal events, the relationships between risk factors and causes are often poorly understood and no risk factor is an accurate predictor
- Birth prevalence has changed little in the latter half of the twentieth century, but an increasing proportion are born very prematurely, concurrent with the increasing survival of premature infants associated with the increasing sophistication of neonatal intensive care

---

DEFINITION: A REAL CHALLENGE FOR EPIDEMIOLOGISTS

Cerebral palsy is an umbrella term (Mutch et al 1992) covering a group of clinical descriptions that have four criteria common to the many proposed definitions (Bax et al 2005, Stanley et al 2000): (1) a disorder of movement or posture, (2) resulting from some developmental or acquired abnormality in the brain (3) that is acquired early in life and (4) static by the time the motor disorder is recognized.

It is an unusual medical definition that provides a real challenge for epidemiologists. There is no diagnostic test for cerebral palsy. Although the cerebral pathology can now be visualized in some cases, these images cannot tell us whether the four defining criteria will be met. Instead cerebral palsy can be identified only by following clinical description over time. If the clinical symptoms disappear or the condition proves to be progressive, it is the description of cerebral palsy that is withdrawn, rather than amending the natural history of cerebral palsy, hence, to assess whether the criteria are met the person must be followed over time.

However, the four criteria above are not sufficiently specific to ensure that the classification of cerebral palsy is sufficiently reliable to allow valid comparisons between

different observers (Blair & Love 2005). The criteria do not specify: (a) how severe the movement disorder must be, (b) how to ensure that the cerebral abnormality is static, (c) the age by which the cerebral abnormality must be acquired or (d) the age before which cerebral palsy cannot be reliably recognized. In practice the four criteria are interpreted variously, and the limits of (a) to (d) defined differently by different individuals. In addition, a number of conditions that do meet the four criteria may not necessarily be included, depending on the purpose of classifying and local conditions and customs (Badawi et al 1998). Therefore, given that the cerebral palsies are heterogeneous with respect to etiology, pathology and to clinical description, we suggest that a label of cerebral palsy is not useful for communicating the cause, severity or prognosis of a child's condition. Since the term also appears to have limited reliability, it is reasonable to ask whether 'cerebral palsy' is a term worth retaining.

The term 'cerebral palsy' refers to a group of disorders with clinical similarities, which is useful for service providers. With decreasing perinatal mortality, the prevalence of cerebral palsy has been used as a measure of pregnancy outcome to evaluate obstetric and neonatal care. This is of dubious validity for term infants for whom the quality of medical care has been reported as either not (Niswander 1985) or only weakly (Blair 1994, Gaffney et al 1994, Richmond et al 1994) associated with the likelihood of cerebral palsy. It may be a more reasonable measure of the care of infants born extremely preterm, though the evidence for separating motor from other central nervous system impairments is weak (Stanley et al 2000). There are better grounds for using it together with other adverse pregnancy outcomes to assess the general health of a population and for using the incidence of post-neonatally acquired cerebral palsy as a measure of preventable social risks (Stanley et al 2000), similar to the use of perinatal and post neonatal deaths respectively.

A major reason for retaining the term is not medical. It identifies a group at risk of severe disability and handicap in a non-pejorative manner which is now familiar to policy-makers and to the public. Additionally, in this era of information technology the term is short and unique. A keyword of cerebral palsy or even of palsy will give references almost exclusively related to non-progressive motor impairments of central origin recognized in childhood or infancy. It conveys considerable information and yet it is flexible. However, the term can be most useful if it conveys the same information to everyone. This could be achieved by increasing the specificity of the four generally accepted criteria for cerebral palsy by:

(1) defining the lower limit of severity using a recognized and validated measure; e.g. defining the degree of functional impairment required (now usually assessed with the Gross Motor Function Classification System (GMFCS) (Palisano et al 1997) or whether neurological signs alone are sufficient;

(2) specifying the upper age limit of acquired brain injury; e.g. this has varied between birth and 13 years. If post neonatally acquired cases are included, this limit usually lies between 2 and 10 years;

(3) specifying the inclusion status of known syndromes (see Badawi et al 1998);

(4) defining the age at which the possibility of progression or resolution can be rejected and cerebral palsy (CP) status confirmed; in current registers this varies between 2 and 8 years, the majority choosing 5 years of age; and

(5) defining the minimum age of inclusion and the criteria to be met should the child die before the age of confirmation. Several registers accept a description of cerebral palsy from a reliable source at any age; for others this criterion is set between 1 and 3 years of age. A higher minimum age will make the prediction of cerebral palsy more secure, but risks excluding the most severe cases, since severity of impairment correlates with mortality, which drops exponentially over time (Blair et al 2001). Compared with including cases at first description of CP, delaying the minimum age to 2 years would exclude 7% of Western Australian cases who would not achieve independent ambulation, and they would be the most severely impaired in this category.

Agreement on these further criteria may not be necessary, but they should be specified when describing CP samples. Maximum flexibility is achieved with the most inclusive criteria, together with clinical descriptions and age of acquisition and/or death where applicable, so that appropriate comparisons may be made with collections which have different inclusion criteria.

The only impairment necessary to meet the criteria for CP is a disorder of movement or posture, but CP is frequently associated with cognitive and learning disabilities, seizure and behavioral disorders and sensory defects which can very significantly affect functional prognosis. The likelihood and severity of associated impairments increase with increasing severity of motor impairment (see Table 46.1).

DIFFERENTIAL DESCRIPTIONS: IMPORTANT FOR BOTH EPIDEMIOLOGISTS AND SERVICE PROVIDERS

Sub-classification of cerebral palsy may logically be based on clinical description, etiology or pathology. Etiology is an

Table 46.1 Percentage of persons with CP born in Western Australia 1975–1999 with severe associated impairments, by severity of motor impairment

| | | Severity of motor impairment | | | |
		Minimal	Mild	Moderate	Severe
	N	221	522	439	412
		%	%	%	%
ASSOCIATED IMPAIRMENT					
Current epilepsy		17.7	19.4	27.6	61.9
IQ/DQ	>70	83.7	74.5	62.2	18.9
	50–69	10.0	14.6	16.2	9.0
	35–49	3.6	7.5	12.8	19.9
	<35	2.7	3.5	8.9	52.2
Blind		1.4	1.9	3.6	23.1
Deaf		0.5	1.2	1.6	4.1

unsatisfactory basis for classification at present as it is unknown or uncertain in many cases. Progress with cerebral imaging is making the classification on the basis of pathology a reality (see Bax et al 2006, De Vries et al 2004, Woodward et al 2006, Wu et al 2006) but appropriate imaging studies are not always available. Clinical description is the most universally available and has been the traditional basis of sub-classification. However, the heterogeneity of clinical descriptions included under the cerebral palsy umbrella has thus far defied standardized sub-classification. Many sub-classification schemes have been suggested, but inter-observer reliability tends to be poor (Blair & Stanley 1985, Evans & Alberman 1985, Love 2007, SCPE 2000). This poses a problem not only when interpreting the literature but also when conducting research, given the current tendency towards the globalization of cerebral palsy research to create samples of greater size and homogeneity (ACPR 2006, Scher et al 2002, SCPE 2000).

Traditionally, cases have been differentiated by type, distribution and severity of motor impairment, often without consideration of associated impairments. Nevertheless, the term cerebral palsy is not an umbrella to a few discrete clinical entities but to several continua of clinical characteristics, and thus does not lend itself to division into groups with discrete labels (Blair et al 2007a). Some clinical characteristics tend to cluster, which has given rise to traditional labels such as spastic diplegia, athetoid cerebral palsy, etc. However, these labels have no standardized definitions and their interpretations vary so widely that they cannot be used as a reliable basis of classification (Love 2007) and it may not be appropriate that they should be. The epidemiological response has been to seek agreement on clinical observations rather than on classification category. The Surveillance of Cerebral Palsy in Europe (SCPE) considers only a small number of clinical characteristics, such as the lateral symmetry and type of motor impairment (SCPE 2000), while the Australian Register proposes to seek clinical agreement on a wide variety of primary clinical observations (Love 2007). This has the advantage of flexibility, allowing classifications to be made according to any criteria appropriate to the task at hand (Blair et al 2007a).

HETEROGENEITY AND MULTIFACTORIALITY OF CAUSE: THE IMPORTANCE OF CAUSAL PATHWAY THINKING

It is clear from the definition that any circumstances that can affect the integrity of motor areas of the brain at any time between conception and early childhood are possible causes of cerebral palsy. While there are many conceivable causes, for many cases no cause is readily apparent though they may have many risk factors that could contribute to a causal pathway (Blair & Stanley 1993a). This suggests heterogeneity of cause and the possibility of multifactorial causes (Blair & Stanley 1993b). There are some confirmed causes of cerebral palsy, many of which are now largely confined to developing countries, such as maternal methyl mercury exposure (Amin-Zaki et al 1979, Takeuchi & Matsumoto 1969), maternal rubella (Stanley et al 1986) or cytomegalovirus infection (Hagberg et al 1996), neonatal kernicterus secondary to maternal Rhesus iso-immunization and genetically acquired defects (Hughes & Newton 1992) responsible for an association between cerebral palsy and consanguineous marriage (Al-Rajeh et al 1991, Gustavson et al 1969).

There are a far greater number of risk factors. These factors are associated with the occurrence of cerebral palsy, but their role in its causation, if any, is often poorly understood. Because there may be a significant delay between the occurrence of the irreversible brain damage and clinical recognition of cerebral palsy in early childhood, factors following the occurrence of the irreversible cerebral damage may well appear as risk factors. If these are the result of the brain damage, they may more properly be considered early manifestations of cerebral palsy. Such factors will of course be strongly associated with cerebral palsy with a tendency to be more strongly associated than are causal factors, because, given the heterogeneity of etiology, each causal factor may only be associated with a small proportion of all cerebral palsy. These post hoc risk factors, which may include neonatal encephalopathic signs such as seizures and cerebral imaging abnormalities, are of considerable clinical interest as they are the strongest predictors of cerebral palsy, but this strength of association must not be confused with causation.

THE FREQUENCY OF CEREBRAL PALSY: THE NEED FOR CAREFUL INTERPRETATION

Frequency can be measured as either prevalence or incidence. Prevalence, the proportion of the population with a condition at a given point in time, is useful for planning services and can be measured by simple, if labor-intensive, surveys. Incidence, the proportion of the population acquiring the condition, is useful when studying causal pathways to the responsible pathology. In this situation it is reasonable to consider the incidence of relevant types of brain damage whether or not the child dies before any motor impairment is recognized. Although many forms of cerebral damage can now be recognized in vivo with cerebral imaging and many have been associated with cerebral palsy, the sensitivity and specificity of these images are dependent on the imaging modality and the age at which imaging is performed. Abnormalities identified by the more easily available modality in the neonatal nursery (e.g. cranial ultrasound) or in infancy are less accurate in predicting cerebral palsy than less easily available modalities (MRI, CT) used after infancy (Bax et al 2006, De Vries et al 2004, Paneth et al 1994, Woodward et al 2006). Specificity may be limited by cortical plasticity following developmentally early injury (Krageloh-Mann 2004), but even the more accurate imaging modalities used in childhood demonstrate limited sensitivity. In a proportion of cases of cerebral palsy no cerebral abnormality can be identified particularly for milder cases (Bax et al 2006, Krageloh-Mann et al 1995, Wu et al 2006). In a study of retrospective data concerning infants born at term collected by a health care program, 273 (72%) of the 377 term infants described as having cerebral palsy had had cerebral MRI or CT studies, and they tended to be the more severely impaired. Of the 271, 85 (31%) had no cerebral abnormality identified (Wu et al 2006). Even with hemiplegia, where visualizable cerebral abnormalities might be most expected, 18% had no imaging abnormalities (Wu et al 2006). Since children with less severe forms of cerebral palsy are both less likely to undergo appropriate cerebral imaging and less likely to have visualizable cerebral abnormalities, the sensitivity of MRI and CT images for cerebral palsy may generally be over-estimated.

Cerebral palsy cannot therefore be reliably predicted from cerebral imaging, particularly imaging in infancy. This complicates the classification of perinatal deaths, as it cannot be known with certainty whether a child dying perinatally would have met the criteria for cerebral palsy had they survived. Therefore, the true incidence of the relevant brain damage cannot be measured. A quasi prevalence is its most usual surrogate and for a given rate of relevant brain damage, this quasi prevalence will vary with the proportion dying perinatally. The numerator is the number of children in a birth cohort described as cerebral palsy according to criteria chosen concerning the minimum duration of survival and age of confirmation. Logically the denominator should be the number of children in the birth cohort surviving to the age at which the cerebral palsy is identified in the cases. Statistics on survival to such as age, particularly if it is variable, are not easily available. In practice total births, livebirths or neonatal survivors are usually used as the denominator. Where perinatal mortality is low, estimated rates vary little between these denominators, but where it is high, as with extremely preterm born infants, rates may be artifactually suppressed by the use of total births or livebirths (see Fig. 46.1), and the number of neonatal survivors is the preferred denominator, particularly since the majority of early deaths of extremely preterm born children occur in the neonatal period. This quasi prevalence maybe somewhat inaccurately called the 'incidence' or 'birth prevalence;' hereafter it will be referred to as the 'rate' and the denominator specified.

Comparisons of estimates of frequency, whether over time or between populations, are the mainstay of cerebral palsy epidemiology, so it is unfortunate that so many factors need to be taken into account when comparing reported estimates of rates of cerebral palsy.

TRENDS IN FREQUENCY OVER TIME

It is therefore often invalid to make direct comparisons between reported rates. The most reliable trends will be obtained from longitudinal studies that have maintained consistent methods over time in populations with sufficient numbers of births to minimize random variation. There are now registers of cerebral palsy in at least 22 geographically defined populations, all in the developed world (Stanley et al 2000). However, only two (Western Sweden and Western Australia) commenced before 1960, both with annual birth cohorts of the order of 20 000. Two further registers commenced in the decade of the 1960s. Trends observed by these four registers are in agreement that although there has been little change in overall rate in CP throughout this period, there was a rising tendency throughout the 1970s and 1980s (Blair & Watson 2006).

Data from Western Australia are shown in Figure 46.2 for all cerebral palsy, for cerebral palsy excluding those post neonatally acquired, and for cerebral palsy excluding both the post neonatally acquired and cases with neurological signs but without readily discernible motor impairment (minimal).

It can be seen that the increasing tendency over the last two decades is due primarily to an increase in those regis-

tered with minimal motor impairment. At least part of this increase is due to an increased willingness to include children under the cerebral palsy umbrella in order to access botulinum toxin-A therapy for mild hypertonia or spasticity in the lower limbs. The overall rate for those with discernible motor functional impairment rose during the 1970s, but has not changed in the 1980s and 1990s.

However the rates associated with some risk factors, particularly gestation of delivery, have changed significantly.

RISK FACTORS FOR CEREBRAL PALSY

GESTATIONAL AGE

The risk of cerebral palsy increases dramatically with decreasing gestational age at delivery. In Western Australia during the period 1980–1999 the rate was 38 times higher in children born before 28 weeks of gestation than among those born 37–41 weeks. Post-term birth is also a risk factor with the rate of cerebral palsy among births of more than 41 completed weeks of gestation being three times that of births at term. For the 1980–1999 birth cohort in Western Australia, preterm births (<37 completed weeks) accounted for 36% of cases of cerebral palsy, but only 7.3% of neonatal survivors and births before 32 weeks accounted for 22.1% of cerebral palsy but only 0.9% of neonatal survivors. Very preterm survival is a relatively new phenomenon resulting from technological progress in neonatal intensive care and so is restricted to developed countries where its rate mirrors developments in neonatal intensive care. The Western Australian gestation specific cerebral palsy rates per neonatal survivor by birth cohort (Fig. 46.3) suggest that the gestation specific rate of cerebral palsy increases initially as survival increases, peaks and then decreases after survival is relatively assured. Gestational duration has been available

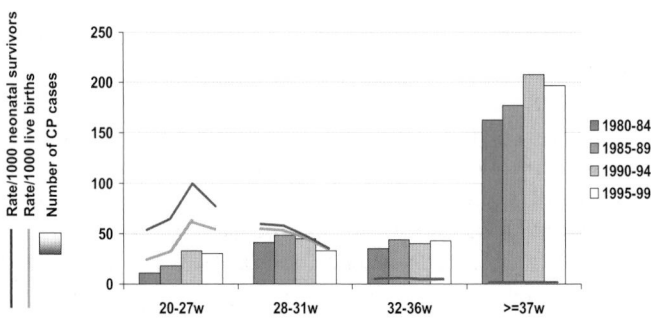

1 Excluding cerebral palsy due to postneonatal causes

Figure 46.1 Cerebral palsy[1] numbers and rates by gestational age in Western Australia, 1980–1999.

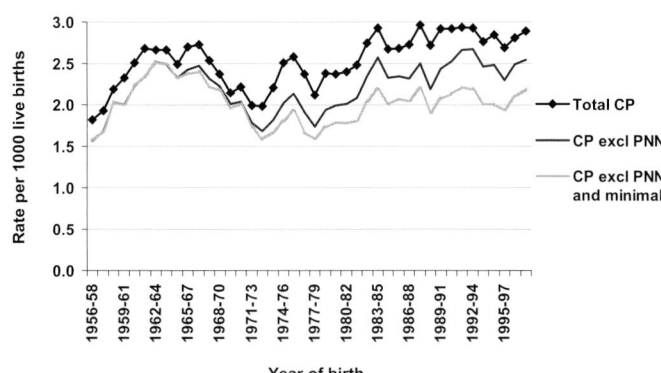

Figure 46.2 Rates (3-year moving averages) for total cerebral palsy (CP), CP excluding postneonatal causes (PNN), and CP excluding both PNN and minimal CP (note: 'minimal' CP included in the 'mild' category prior to 1966).
(From Watson L, Blair E, Stanley F. Report of the Western Australian Cerebral Palsy Register to Birth Year 1999. Perth: Telethon Institute for Child Health Research, 2006.)

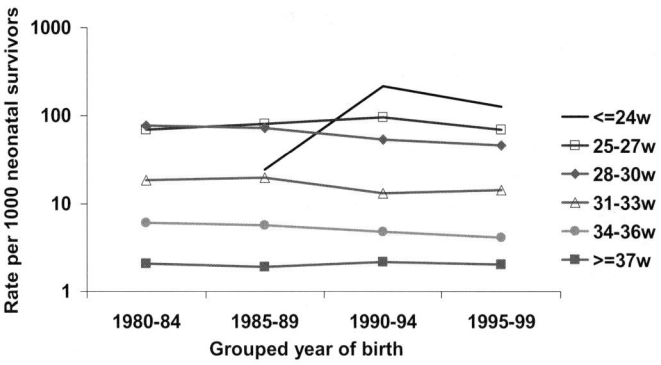

Figure 46.3 Gestational age specific cerebral palsy[1] rates per 1000 neonatal survivors, Western Australia, 1980–1999.

1 Excludes cerebral palsy due to postneonatal causes

in Western Australian statutory data only since 1980. From 1980–1999 survival has been the norm for infants born at more than 30 weeks gestation for whom there has been little consistent variation in cerebral palsy rates. The trends in rates for more preterm born infants vary according to gestation. Among births 28–30 weeks, rates have decreased consistently since 1980, before which they had the highest rate. The rate increased gradually over time in 25–27 week infants and increased sharply in <25 week infants, peaking in the early 1990s and then declining in the late 1990s. These data suggest that the ability of Western Australian neonatal intensive care to enable survival for very preterm births of any particular gestational age preceded its ability to enable intact survival. Reports from other locations (see Himmelmann et al 2005, Topp et al 2001) are compatible with this suggestion, though few are stratified sufficiently finely by gestational duration and year of birth to definitively demonstrate or refute the pattern, the existence of which may well depend on local or individual policies governing the degree of aggression with which extremely preterm survival is pursued (Lorenz et al 2001).

Among very preterm infants, cerebral palsy is closely associated with intraparenchymal hemorrhage/leukomalacia. When present, this cerebral pathology can be considered the organic basis for the movement disorder and cannot therefore be considered a cause of the cerebral palsy; it *is* the cerebral palsy. The cause of the cerebral palsy is therefore the cause of the cerebral lesions, and it is these precursors of the cerebral pathology that must be understood in order to prevent the cerebral palsy. However, not all very preterm children with cerebral palsy have parenchymal involvement, and not all very preterm born children with parenchymal involvement have cerebral palsy (Stanley et al 2000), though those with parenchymal involvement are likely to represent a more etiologically homogeneous group of cases. While all very preterm born children with cerebral palsy without obvious postneonatal causes (see below) are grouped with cases likely to be of antepartum or intrapartum origin, it is quite likely that at least some

proportion acquire a responsible brain lesion postnatally or even post neonatally due to post natal complications associated with their prematurity.

APPROPRIATENESS OF INTRAUTERINE GROWTH

Appropriateness of growth is usually inferred from birthweight for gestational age, though the increasing use of serial ultrasound and Doppler flow studies provides more direct means of assessment for those fetuses considered at risk for growth restriction (Kingdom et al 2000). For infants born after 33 weeks of gestation, there is a strong and consistent association between measures of growth restriction and cerebral palsy (Blair & Stanley 1990, Jarvis et al 2006, Kyllerman et al 1982, Palmer et al 1994, Uvebrant & Hagberg 1992), with the risk increasing with decreasing proportion of expected birthweight (Jarvis et al 2006) and with evidence of long-standing restriction (Blair & Stanley 1992).

Since very preterm birth is always associated with pathology, it is not possible to measure a similar association in infants born before 33 weeks of gestation because there is no satisfactory (normal) control group with which to compare very preterm infants who are also growth-restricted. The associations with cerebral palsy measured by comparing very preterm infants considered small for gestational age (SGA) with equally preterm infants who are not SGA are not consistent (Blair & Stanley 1990, Murphy et al 1995, Topp et al 1996, Uvebrant & Hagberg 1992). This may be because the distribution of pathologies associated with very preterm birth in the comparison groups varies between studies. Using European data and a fetal standard for intrauterine growth, in which the weight of a preterm born infant is compared with the fetometrically estimated weight of fetuses of the same gestational age who subsequently deliver at term, indicated that being inappropriately small was also associated with cerebral palsy in infants born before 33 weeks, but the relative risks are not as elevated as for moderately preterm born infants (Jarvis et al 2006).

There is less agreement as to whether relatively accelerated intrauterine growth increases the risk of cerebral palsy (Jarvis et al 2006). In Western Australian data, cases of cerebral palsy with inappropriately high birthweights were hydropic rather than well grown. In studies where additional data are not considered, the high birth weights of hydropic infants could be misinterpreted as indicating accelerated growth.

There are many causes of intrauterine growth restriction. It is not clear whether associated pathologic outcomes are associated more closely with the cause of the restriction or with characteristics of the restriction. These characteristics, such as the gestational age at onset, duration and severity of restriction, are themselves associated with the cause (Blair 2000).

MULTIPLE BIRTH (see also Ch. 18)

Multiple birth is a strong risk factor for cerebral palsy and the risk increases with increasing number of fetuses (Stanley et al 2000). Multiple birth is a cause of both intrauterine growth restriction and preterm birth, but these are not the only factors increasing the risk of cerebral palsy in children resulting from multiple pregnancies. Combining the relevant studies published by 1998, the relative risk (and 95% confidence interval) of cerebral palsy was 4.5 (3.9–5.2) for each twin and 18.2 (10.4–31.9) for each triplet (Stanley et al 2000). The relative risk of cerebral palsy was therefore of the order of 9 for a twin and 50 for a triplet pregnancy. Comparing twin pregnancies with singletons born at the same gestational ages, the relative risk of cerebral palsy in a twin pregnancy is most elevated for term infants 3.0 (1.9–4.9), followed by twins of 33–36 weeks' gestation, 2.3 (1.3–3.7), extremely preterm twins (<29 weeks), 1.9 (1.2–3.2) and very preterm twins (29–32 weeks) 1.0 (0.7–1.6) (Stanley et al 2000). This was confirmed in a collaborative population based study with a combined cohort of 1.14 million births, including 24 115 twin births, that compared gestation specific rates of cerebral palsy (described by 1 year) in twins with that in singletons (Scher et al 2002). The excess of cerebral palsy in twins born at term demonstrates that while the prematurity associated with twinning contributes to the excess risk of cerebral palsy in twins, it is not entirely responsible for it. The risk of cerebral palsy in twins is not associated with zygosity, or, in the absence of information on zygosity, with like-sex, rather than unlike-sex twins or, in recent studies, with birth order (Grether et al 1993, Petterson et al 1993, Scher et al 2002), but is associated with growth discordance, though the increased risk applies to both smaller and larger twin (Scher et al 2002). Among multiple births, antenatal fetal death of one fetus is a strong risk factor for cerebral palsy in surviving fetuses, with the survivor of a twin pregnancy in whom one fetus died antenatally being at 11 times the risk of cerebral palsy as a twin whose co-twin survived the neonatal period. Fetal death of a co-twin is biologically a very plausible cause of brain damage in the surviving twin for monochorionic twins with placental anastomoses. It is less likely to account for the increased risk in dizygotic twins. However, as the antenatal death of one and only one twin after 20 weeks' gestation is reasonably uncommon, fetal death of a co-twin is responsible for only a small proportion of the risk of cerebral palsy associated with multiple pregnancy. Intrapartum factors were previously thought to put the second-born twin at greater risk. The lack of association with birth order threw doubt on this hypothesis. However, of a twin pair with one live and one stillbirth, it is usually the liveborn twin that is born first (Grether et al 1993, Petterson et al 1993). Thus, birth order is sometimes determined by factors that are themselves determinants of death or cerebral palsy and should not be considered simply as a marker for intrapartum difficulties. The role of intrapartum difficulties in twin deliveries may need re-assessment.

The proportion of cerebral palsy arising from multiple pregnancies is increasing with the increasing rate of multiple birth in developed countries, which is a result of both an increase in mean maternal age and the increasing use of reproductive technologies. The association between in vitro fertilization and cerebral palsy has been attributed entirely to the increased rates of multiple pregnancy and preterm birth associated with the technique, rather than to the underlying infertility or to teratogenic or toxic effects of the technology itself (Hvidtjorn et al 2006). However since the higher risks of cerebral palsy (and other poor outcomes) are incontrovertible, the ethics of pursuing this entirely elective intervention have been questioned (Bellieni & Buonocore 2006).

GENDER

There is a tendency for males to be at somewhat greater risk of cerebral palsy. For example, the ratio of males to females on the Western Australian Cerebral Palsy Register born in 1960–1999 was 1.34 (Watson et al 2006). This ratio varies over time more than might be expected from random variation alone, but has almost always been greater than the male proportion of all births. There are a few exceptions to this general rule. In the SW Swedish 1983–1986 birth cohort, the ratio of males to females was 0.9, whereas in 1987–1990, it was 1.1. The origin of the male excess is not understood: the few identified X-linked causes of cerebral palsy are not sufficiently numerous to be responsible.

ANTEPARTUM FACTORS

Several maternal factors such as menstrual abnormalities (Nelson & Ellenberg 1986), seizure disorders (Nelson & Ellenberg 1982), advanced maternal age (Freud 1968), parity (first births and births after the third) (Blair 1996) and low social class (Dolk et al 1996, Dowding & Barry 1990) have been associated with cerebral palsy.

In addition to the association with reduced intrauterine growth, consistent evidence of a strong association with suboptimal antepartum events comes from the association with birth defects, since the events themselves are frequently unrecorded and perhaps even unobserved. While the very strong association with central nervous system anomalies is to be expected, associations with malformations outside the central nervous system are also often (Coorssen et al 1991, Fletcher & Foley 1993, Miller 1991, Palmer et al 1995) though not universally (Croen et al 2001) reported. A study investigating the origins of this discrepancy suggested that ascertainment bias was responsible for only a small part of an observed association with non-cerebral defects, failure to detect associated cerebral defects could be responsible for a greater proportion and that non-cerebral defects, particularly cardiac defects, were responsible for a proportion of post-neonatally acquired cerebral palsy (Blair et al 2007b). The antenatal insults may consist of congenital infections, particularly those of the TORCH group (Gilbert 1996), infections of the fetal membranes (Wu & Colford 2000, Wu et al 2003), maternal thyroid abnormalities (Badawi et al 2000, Blair & Stanley 1993a), iodine deficiency, which, if sufficiently severe, results in cretinism (spastic diplegia and deaf mutism) (Hetzel 1994), toxic exposures, which may include alcohol (Olegård et al 1979) and even mechanical trauma (Gilles et al 1996). The role of the inflammatory effects of infection, that is of infection per se rather than any specific infection, is coming under increasing scrutiny and suspicion as a causal factor for cerebral palsy in births of all gestational ages and the effects of inflammation may be exacerbated by co-existing asphyxia (Hermansen & Hermansen 2006) (see also Ch. 19). Alternatively, or perhaps additionally, hyperthermia, which frequently accompanies maternal infection, has been suggested as a potent agent of central nervous system disruption, the precise outcome depending on the gestation, duration and degree of hyperthermia experienced by the fetus as well as constitutional factors (Edwards 2006).

INTRAPARTUM FACTORS

In the middle of the 19th century, Little described 'the forms of abnormal parturition that he had observed to precede certain mental and physical derangements' (Little 1958). From that time to the beginning of the 1990s, intrapartum factors, particularly asphyxia, were believed to be the primary initiators of the pathway to cerebral palsy. This occurred despite both Little's paper suggesting that intrapartum factors were only one of several possible causes and could represent the final step in a multicausal pathway and Freud's suggestions in 1897 (Freud 1968) that antepartum factors may play an important role. In developed countries, during the intervening 140 years, obstetric practices and public-health measures have largely abolished the risks associated with intrapartum factors that Little mentioned as antecedents of cerebral palsy, yet an association continues to be observed between cerebral palsy and the intrapartum and neonatal observations from which damaging asphyxia is inferred. How often do these signs represent de-novo damaging asphyxia, how often are they the final straw in a multicausal pathway and how often the first readily observable clinical signs of cerebral malformation or damage occurring earlier in pregnancy (Blair & Stanley 2002)? Recently reviewed (Perlman 2006), available evidence suggests that intrapartum factors contribute only a small proportion of all cerebral palsy yet the concept is increasingly responsible for a crippling volume of medical litigation. In response, relevant medical fraternities have created guidelines for determining conditions under which intrapartum factors are likely to be causal (American College of Obstetricians and Gynecologists 2003, MacLennan et al 1999, Society of Obstetricians and Gynaecologists of Canada 1996).

Determining precisely which children have experienced de novo damaging asphyxia during labor became more important with the understanding from animal studies that there is a period of about 6 hours between an acute asphyxial event and the secondary cell death responsible for much of the cerebral damage. Several suggestions have been made as to how to take advantage of this 'window of opportunity'

for neuronal rescue, the least unpromising to date being hypothermia (p. 569). Two recent trials considering longer term outcomes using either head cooling with mild systemic hypothermia (rectal temperature 34–35°C) (Gluckman et al 2005) or whole body cooling to 33.5°C (Shankaran et al 2005) found significant reductions in disability for those initially moderately affected by the asphyxia, but not in those initially severely affected.

POSTNEONATAL FACTORS

A proportion of all cerebral palsy is acquired in infancy or childhood as the result of a variety of brain damaging events, traditionally cerebral infection or traumatic head injury. Whichever upper age limit of acquisition is chosen, most postneonatally acquired cerebral palsy is acquired before 1 year of age and the resulting disabilities are at least as severe as those acquired earlier. These cases, termed 'postneonatally acquired,' are often considered separately to those acquired earlier, because the immediate causes are well understood, they may have systematic differences in their response to cerebral pathology (Carr 1996) and are traditionally considered to be independent of events during pregnancy and delivery. Its strong association with social disadvantage suggests it may often be the result of poverty and ignorance combining to create barriers to effective parenting. With increasing economic development, the profile of immediate causes changes with cerebral infection and febrile convulsions becoming less prominent and head injuries, which may previously have been fatal, becoming more prominent (Stanley et al 2000). However as the frequencies of cerebral infections and head trauma decrease as a result of vaccinations and an increasing awareness of the risks of head trauma in infancy and the overall rate of post neonatally acquired cerebral palsy decreases, the relative contribution of antenatal factors such as congenital vascular anomalies (Badawi et al 1998, Himmelmann et al 2005) and metabolic abnormalities (Morton et al 1991) increases. Cerebro-vascular accidents during infant surgery for congenital cardiac defects now account for 1% of all cerebral palsy in Western Australia (Blair et al 2007b).

As with hypothermic treatment for acutely asphyxiated neonates, the surgical correction of major cardiac anomalies represents an intervention very late in the causal path, when some biological damage is already in place. By increasing survival, both interventions risk creating some, as well as avoiding other, long term disability, so efforts should also be directed to identifying and preventing the primary causes of these problems.

CONCLUSION

Decreasing rates of perinatal mortality initiated by changes in public health status have been maintained in recent decades by changes in obstetric and neonatal service provision. While these changes may have resulted in a net gain in unimpaired survival, the high rate of cerebral palsy among surviving very premature infants and other neonatal intensive care graduates is of considerable concern. These observations should temper our enthusiasm for pushing the new perinatal technologies to their limits without equal enthusiasm for investigating causal pathways leading to compromised births and identifying the most effective and acceptable means of interrupting them.

ACKNOWLEDGMENTS

We are grateful for the support of the NH&MRC who fund cerebral palsy studies in Western Australia, also to Linda Watson, who maintains the WA Cerebral Palsy Register, and provided the figures, and to the many health professionals who provide information to the Register.

REFERENCES

ACPR 2006 Proposed new definition of cerebral palsy does not solve any of the problems of existing definitions. Dev Med Child Neurol 48:78.

Al-Rajeh S, Bademosi O, Awada A et al 1991 Cerebral palsy in Saudi Arabia: A case-control study of risk factors. Dev Med Child Neurol 33:1048–1052.

American College of Obstetricians and Gynecologists 2003 Task force on neonatal encephalopathy and cerebral palsy. American College of Obstetricians and Gynecologists, Washington, DC.

Amin-Zaki L, Majeed M A, Elhassani S B et al 1979 Prenatal methylmercury poisoning. Clinical observations over five years. Am J Dis Child 133:172–177.

Badawi N, Kurinczuk J, MacKenzie C et al 2000 Newborn encephalopathy: an association with maternal thyroid disease. Br Med J 107:798–801.

Badawi N, Watson L, Petterson B et al 1998 What constitutes cerebral palsy? Dev Med Child Neurol 40:520–527.

Bax M, Goldstein M, Rosenbaum P et al 2005 Proposed definition and classification of cerebral palsy, April 2005. Dev Med Child Neurol 47:571–576.

Bax M, Tydeman C, Flodmark O 2006 Clinical and MRI correlates of cerebral palsy: the European cerebral palsy study. J Am Med Assoc 296(13):1602–1608.

Bellieni C, Buonocore G 2006 Assisted procreation: too little consideration for the babies? Ethics Med 22(2):93–98.

Blair E 1994 Cerebral palsy and intrapartum care: Wrong denominator used (letter). Br Med J 309:1229.

Blair E 1996 Obstetric antecedents of cerebral palsy. Fetal Matern Med Rev 8:199–215.

Blair E 2000 Paediatric implications of intrauterine growth restriction with special reference to cerebral palsy. In: Kingdom J, Baker P (eds) Intrauterine growth restriction: aetiology and management. Springer-Verlag, London, pp. 351–366.

Blair E, Al Asedy F, Badawi N, Bower C 2007a Is cerebral palsy associated with birth defects other than cerebral defects? Dev Med Child Neurol 49:252–258.

Blair E, Badawi N, Watson L 2007b The definition and classification of cerebral palsy: the Australian view. Dev Med Child Neurol 49:33–34.

Blair E, Love S 2005 Definition and classification of cerebral palsy — invited commentary. Dev Med Child Neurol 47:510.

Blair E, Stanley F 2002 Causal pathways to cerebral palsy. Cur Paediatr 12:179–185.

Blair E, Stanley F J 1985 Interobserver agreement in the classification of cerebral palsy. Dev Med Child Neurol 27:615–622.

Blair E, Stanley F J 1990 Intrauterine growth and spastic cerebral palsy I. Association with birth weight for gestational age. Am J Obstet Gynecol 162:229–237.

Blair E, Stanley F J 1992 Intrauterine growth and spastic cerebral palsy II. The association with morphology at birth. Early Hum Dev 28:91–103.

Blair E, Stanley F J 1993a When can cerebral palsy be prevented? The generation of causal hypotheses by multivariate analysis of a case-control study. Paediatr Perinat Epidemiol 7:272–301.

Blair E, Stanley F J 1993b Aetiological pathways to spastic cerebral palsy. Paediatr Perinatal Epidemiol 7:302–317.

Blair E, Watson L 2006 Epidemiology of cerebral palsy. Sem Fetal Neonatal Med 11(2):117–125.

Blair E, Watson L, Badawi N, Stanley F J 2001 Life expectancy among people with cerebral palsy in Western Australia. Dev Med Child Neurol 43:508–515.

Carr L J 1996 Development and reorganization of descending motor pathways in children with hemiplegic cerebral palsy. Acta Paediatrica 85 Suppl 416:53–57.

Coorssen E A, Msall M E, Duffy L C 1991 Multiple minor malformations as a marker for prenatal etiology of cerebral palsy. Dev Med Child Neurol 33:730–736.

Croen L A, Grether J K, Curry C J, Nelson K B 2001 Congenital abnormalities among children with cerebral palsy: More evidence for prenatal antecedents. J Pediatr 138:804–810.

De Vries L S, Van Haastert I L, Rademaker K J et al 2004 Ultrasound abnormalities preceding cerebral palsy in high-risk preterm infants. J Pediatr 144(6):815–820.

Dolk H, Parkes K, Hill A E 1996 Cerebral palsy prevalence in relation to socio-economic deprivation in Northern Ireland. Paediatr Perinat Epidemiol 10: A4.

Dowding V M, Barry C 1990 Cerebral palsy: social class differences in prevalence in relation to birthweight and severity of disability. J Epidemiol Com Health 44:191–195.

Edwards M 2006 Review: Hyperthermia and fever during pregnancy. Birth Defects Res (Part A) 76:507–516.

Evans P, Alberman E 1985 Recording motor defects of children with cerebral palsy. Dev Med Child Neurol 27:404–406.

Fletcher N A, Foley J 1993 Parental age, genetic mutation, and cerebral palsy. J Med Genet 30:44–46.

Freud S 1968 Infantile cerebral paralysis (translation by Russin L A of: Die infantile Cerebrallahmung. Vienna: A. Holder, 1897). University of Miami Press, Coral Gables, Florida.

Gaffney G, Sellers S, Flavell V et al 1994 Case-control study of intrapartum care, cerebral palsy, and perinatal death. Br Med J 308:743–750.

Gilbert G L 1996 Congenital fetal infections. Sem Neonatol 1:91–105.

Gilles M T, Blair E, Watson L et al 1996 Maternal trauma in pregnancy and cerebral palsy — Is there a link? Med J Aust 164:500–501.

Gluckman P, Wyatt J, Azzopardi D et al 2005 Selective head cooling with mild systemic hypothermia after neonatal encephalopathy: multicentre randomised trial. Lancet 365(9460):663–670.

Grether J K, Nelson K B, Cummins S K 1993 Twinning and cerebral palsy: Experience in four nothern California counties, births 1983 through 1985. Pediatrics 92:854–858.

Gustavson K-H, Hagberg B, Sanner G 1969 Identical syndromes of cerebral palsy in the same family. Acta Paediatrica Scand 58:330–340.

Hagberg B, Hagberg G, Olow I, von Wendt L 1996 The changing panorama of cerebral palsy in Sweden. VII. Prevalence and origin in the birth year period 1987–90. Acta Paediatrica 85:954–960.

Hermansen M, Hermansen M 2006 Perinatal infections and cerebral palsy. Clin Perinatol 33:315–333.

Hetzel B S 1994 Iodine deficiency and fetal brain damage. N Eng J Med 331:1770–1771.

Himmelmann K, Hagberg G, Beckung B et al 2005 The changing panorama of cerebral palsy in Sweden. IX. Prevalence and origin in the birth-year period 1995–1998. Acta Paediatrica 2005 94:287–294.

Hughes I, Newton R 1992 Genetic aspects of cerebral palsy. Dev Med Child Neurol 34:80–86.

Hvidtjorn D, Grove J, Schendel D E et al 2006 Cerebral palsy among children born after in vitro fertilization: the role of preterm delivery — a population-based, cohort study. Pediatrics 118(2):475–482.

Jarvis S, Glinianaia S, Blair E 2006 Cerebral palsy and intrauterine growth. Clin Perinatol 33:285–300.

Kingdom J, Baker P, Blair E 2000 Definitions of intrauterine growth restriction. In: Kingdom J, Baker P (eds) Intrauterine growth restriction: aetiology and management. Springer-Verlag, London, pp. 1–4.

Krageloh-Mann I 2004 Imaging of early brain injury and cortical plasticity. Exp Neurol 190 Suppl 1:S84–S90.

Krageloh-Mann I, Petersen D, Hagberg G et al 1995 Bilateral spastic cerebral palsy — MRI pathology and origin, analysis from a representative series of 56 cases. Dev Med Child Neurol 37:379–397.

Kyllerman M, Bager B, Bensch J et al 1982 Dyskinetic cerebral palsy I. clinical categories, associated neurological abnormalities and incidences. Acta P<ae>diatrica Scand 71:543–550.

Little W J 1958 On the influence of abnormal parturition, difficult labors, premature birth, and asphyxia neonatorum, on the mental and physical condition of the child, especially in relation to deformities. Cereb Palsy Bul 1:5–36.

Lorenz J, Paneth N, Jetton J et al 2001 Comparison of management strategies for extreme prematurity in New Jersey and the Netherlands: Outcomes and resource expenditure. Pediatrics 108:1269–1274.

Love S 2007 Better description of spastic cerebral palsy for reliable classification. Dev Med Child Neurol 49(suppl 109):24–25.

MacLennan A, Badawi N, Bennet L et al 1999 A template for defining a causal relation between acute intrapartum events and cerebral palsy: international consensus statement. BMJ 319:1054–1059.

Miller G 1991 Cerebral palsy and minor congenital anomalies. Clin Pediatr 30:97–98.

Morton D H, Bennett M J, Seargeant L E et al 1991 Glutaric aciduria type I: common cause of episodic encephalopathy and spastic paralysis in the Amish of Lancaster County, Pennsylvania. Am J Med Genet 41:89–95.

Murphy D J, Sellers S, MacKenzie I Z et al 1995 Case-control study of antenatal and intrapartum risk factors for cerebral palsy in very preterm singleton babies. Lancet 346:1449–1454.

Mutch L W, Alberman E, Hagberg B et al 1992 Cerebral palsy epidemiology: where are we now and where are we going? Dev Med Child Neurol 34:547–555.

Nelson K B, Ellenberg J H 1982 Maternal seizure disorder, outcome of pregnancy, and neurologic abnormalities in the children. Neurology 32:1247–1254.

Nelson K B, Ellenberg J H 1986 Antecedents of cerebral palsy. Multivariate analysis of risk. N Eng J Med 315:81–86.

Niswander K R 1985 Quality of obstetric care and occurrence of fetal asphyxia and cerebral palsy: Is there a relationship? Postgrad Med 78:57–60, 62, 64.

Olegård R, Sabel K-G, Aronsson M et al 1979 Effects on the child of alcohol abuse during pregnancy: retrospective and prospective studies. Acta P<ae>diatrica Scand (Suppl 275):112–121.

Palisano R, Rosenbaum P, Walter S et al 1997 Development and reliability of a system to classify gross motor function in children with cerebral palsy. Dev Med Child Neurol 39:214–223.

Palmer L, Blair E, Petterson B, Burton P 1995 Antenatal antecedents of moderate and severe cerebral palsy. Paediatr Perinat Epidemiol 9:171–184.

Palmer L, Petterson B, Blair E, Burton P 1994 Family patterns of gestational age at delivery and growth in utero in moderate and severe cerebral palsy. Dev Med Child Neurol 36:1108–1119.

Paneth N, Rudelli R, Kazam E, Monte W 1994 Prognosis. In: Brain damage in the preterm infant. McKeith, London, pp. 171–185.

Perlman J 2006 Intrapartum asphyxia and cerebral palsy: is there a link? Clin Perinatol 33(2):335–353.

Petterson B, Nelson K B, Watson L, Stanley F J 1993 Twins, triplets, and cerebral palsy at birth in Western Australia in the 1980s. Br Med J 307:1239–1243.

Richmond S, Niswander K, Snodgrass C A, Wagstaff I 1994 The obstetric management of fetal distress and its association with cerebral palsy. Obstet Gynecol 83:643–646.

Scher A I, Petterson B, Blair E et al 2002 The risk of mortality or cerebral palsy in twins: a collaborative population-based study. Pediatr Res 52:671–681.

SCPE 2000 Surveillance of cerebral palsy in Europe: a European collaboration of cerebral palsy surveys and registers. Dev Med Child Neurol 42(12):816–824.

Shankaran S, Laptook A, Ehrenkranz R et al 2005 Reduction in death or moderate/severe disability by whole body hypothermia for hypoxic–ischaemic encephalopathy (HIE). PAS 57:1548.

Society of Obstetricians and Gynaecologists of Canada 1996 Policy Statement: Task Force on Cerebral Palsy and Neonatal Asphyxia (Part I). J Soc Obstetr Gynaecol Can 18:1267–1279.

Stanley F J, Blair E, Alberman E 2000 The cerebral palsies: epidemiology and causal pathways. MacKeith, Oxford.

Stanley F J, Sim M, Wilson G, Worthington S 1986 The decline in congenital rubella syndrome in Western Australia: an impact of the school girl vaccination program? Am J Pub Health 76:35–39.

Takeuchi T, Matsumoto H 1969 Minamata disease of human fetuses. In: Mishimura H, Miller J R (eds) Methods for teratological studies in experimental animals and man. Igatsu Shoin, Tokyo, pp. 280–282.

Topp M, Langhoff-Roos J, Uldall P, Kristensen J 1996 Intrauterine growth and gestational age in preterm infants with cerebral palsy. Early Hum Dev 44:27–36.

Topp M, Uldall P, Greisen G 2001 Cerebral palsy births in eastern Denmark, 1987–90: implications for neonatal care. Paediatr Perinat Epidemiol 15:271–277.

Uvebrant P, Hagberg G 1992 Intrauterine growth in children with cerebral palsy. Acta Paediatrica 81:407–412.

Watson L, Blair E, Stanley F 2006 Report of the Western Australian Cerebral Palsy Register to birth year 1999. Telethon Institute for Child Health Research, Perth.

Woodward L, Anderson P, Austin N et al 2006 Neonatal MRI to predict neourodevelopmental outcomes in preterm infants. N Eng J Med 355(7):685–694.

Wu Y, Colford J 2000 Chorioamnionitis as a risk factor for cerebral palsy: a meta-analysis. J Am Med Assoc 284(11):1417–1424.

Wu Y, Croen L, Shah S, Newman T, Najjar D 2006 Cerebral palsy in a term population: risk factors and neuroimaging findings. Pediatrics 118:690–697.

Wu Y, Escobar G, Grether J et al 2003 Chorioamnionitis and cerebral palsy in term and near-term infants. J Am Med Assoc 290(20):2677–2684.

Wu Y, Lindan C, Henning L, Yoshida C et al 2006 Neuroimaging abnormalities in infants with congenital hemiparesis. Pediatr Neurol 35:191–196.

CHAPTER
47

The epidemiology of intellectual disabilities

Kim Van Naarden Braun and Marshalyn Yeargin-Allsopp

Key Points

- Intellectual disabilities (ID) are among the most prevalent serious developmental conditions of childhood, affecting approximately 1.5% of school-aged children and one of the most costly, estimating $51.2 billion in lifetime costs
- Since the early 1980s, studies in developed countries have reported a range of prevalence estimates for ID overall from 5 to 42 per 1000
- Severity is a crucial factor for understanding the epidemiology of ID, commonly defined as mild ID (IQ 50–55 to 70–75) and moderate to profound ID (IQ less than 50–55)
- The prevalence of ID varies by several social and demographic characteristics, most notably age, gender, race and ethnicity and socioeconomic status
- Although there are many recognized causes of ID, they collectively account for less than half of all cases. Prenatal causes remain most prevalent overall
  - Genetic factors account for most known prenatal etiology, yet non-genetic risk factors that are modifiable and/or preventable have also been identified including: maternal smoking, alcohol exposure, maternal medical conditions, certain medications, intrauterine infections, nutritional deficiencies, environmental toxins and birth defects
  - Well-documented and accepted perinatal risk factors for ID include low birth weight, perinatal asphyxia, infection such as group B streptococcus and human immunodeficiency virus, newborn endocrine and metabolic disorders and multiple births
  - Postnatal factors shown to be associated with ID include postnatally acquired infections, injuries and environmental lead exposure
- The acquisition of normative adult social roles is particularly difficult for young adults with ID, therefore it is important to understand the experiences of individuals with ID as they transition from adolescence to adulthood

INTRODUCTION

Intellectual disabilities (ID) are among the most prevalent serious developmental conditions of childhood, affecting approximately 1.5% of school-aged children (ADDM Network, in preparation). It is also one of the most costly with an estimate of $51.2 billion in lifetime costs (Honeycutt et al 2004). In addition to significant psychosocial implications, there are both direct and indirect lifetime costs associated with ID such as costs of special education, physician visits, prescription medications, therapy and rehabilitation and long-term care as well as limitations in an individual's ability to perform in the workplace. Data from the 2001–2004 National Health Interview Survey (NHIS) Sample Child File show that children ages 3–17 whose parents were told by a doctor or health professional that their child had an ID

were more likely to have seen a medical specialist as well as have seen a mental health provider or a therapist in the past 12 months. Children with ID were also significantly more likely than their peers without a developmental disability to have more than five office visits, to have more than one emergency room visit, to have surgery or a medical procedure in the past 12 months and to have taken prescription medication regularly for at least 3 months (Boulet in preparation). The high prevalence of ID coupled with its lifelong impact on the individual and society underscore the significance of furthering our understanding of this condition.

The terms used to describe ID have evolved and will continue to evolve, as our understanding of ID increases. Historically in epidemiologic research, the term 'mental retardation' has been used to refer to this condition yet in accordance with the recent decision by the American Association on Intellectual and Developmental Disabilities (AAIDD), formerly the American Association on Mental Retardation (AAMR) – the world's oldest organization representing professionals of developmental disabilities – this chapter will use the term 'intellectual disabilities' rather than 'mental retardation' to reflect society's efforts to appropriately address individuals with cognitive disabilities (AAIDD 2006). In addition to new terminology, new classifications for intellectual disabilities have been established and these are built upon the concept of greater reliance on measures of adaptive functioning as important complements to results of IQ testing in determining whether an individual has ID and if so, their level of functioning (Table 47.1).

The prevalence and descriptive characteristics of ID continue to be areas of epidemiologic investigation. Prevalence is affected by many factors, including case definition, methods of case ascertainment and size and characteristics of the population studied. However, despite differences among studies, the prevalence of ID has remained relatively stable over time, which may be due to a balance between decreased numbers (through elective termination) of pregnancies affected by chromosomal disorders associated with severe to profound ID and increased survival of preterm and medically compromised infants that previously would not have survived. Any potential decrease in the number of children with ID has to be balanced with increased improvements in the survival of low birth weight, medically affected infants and increases in the numbers of children with disability secondary to interventions such as artificial reproductive technology (Leonard & Wen 2002).

Table 47.1 Definitions of intellectual disabilities

Source	Definition
American Psychiatric Association (APA) Diagnostic and Statistical Manual of Mental Disorders, fourth edition (DSM-IV)[a]	Significantly subaverage general intellectual functioning (Criterion A) that is accompanied by significant limitations in adaptive functioning in at least two of the following skill areas: communication, self-care, home living, social/interpersonal skills, use of community resources, self-direction, functional academic skills, work, leisure, health, and safety (Criterion B). The onset must occur before 18 years (Criterion C)
American Association on Intellectual and Developmental Disabilities (AAIDD)/American Association on Mental Retardation (AAMR)[b]	A disability characterized by significant limitations in both intellectual functioning and adaptive behavior as expressed in conceptual, social, and practical adaptive skills. The disability originates before age 18
World Health Organization (WHO)	
International Classification of Diseases, Ninth Revision, Clinical Modification (ICD-9-CM)[c]	Subnormal intellectual functioning that originates during the developmental period
International Classification of Diseases, Tenth Revision (ICD-10)[d]	A condition of arrested or incomplete development of the mind, which is especially characterized by impairment of skills manifested during the developmental period, skills which contribute to the overall level of intelligence, i.e. cognitive, language, motor and social abilities
International Classification of Functioning, Disability and Health (ICF)[e,*]	Classified with intellectual growth, intellectual retardation and dementia under Intellectual Functions: 'General mental functions, required to understand and constructively integrate the various mental functions, including all cognitive functions and their development over the life span.'

[a] American Psychiatric Association 1994.
[b] Luckasson R et al 2002.
[c] International Classification of Diseases 1988.
[d] WHO 1992.
[e] WHO 2001.
*IQ is not a construct in ICF. All three components classified in ICF-Body Functions and Structures; Activities and Participation; and Environmental Factors are quantified using the same generic scale, from 'no problem' to 'complete problem'.

Although there are many recognized causes of ID, they collectively account for less than half of all cases. Prenatal causes remain most prevalent overall, with genetic conditions such as Down syndrome accounting for approximately two-thirds or more of all known genetic causes of ID (Cans et al 1999, Fernell 1998, Hou et al 1998, Stromme & Hagberg 2000, Yeargin-Allsopp et al 1997). In all studies, perinatal and postnatal causes occur less frequently than prenatal causes (Yeargin-Allsopp et al 1997). However, new genetic techniques such as fluorescence in situ hybridization, methylation DNA studies and studies to look for microdeletions and subtle rearrangements that disrupt genes in the subtelomeric regions hold much promise for helping to identify more underlying causes of ID. The growing field of genetic epidemiology can also help us understand underlying causes of ID by providing for example, information on the risk of recurrence of ID. From an individual family and larger societal perspective, this is an extremely important practical application of epidemiology of ID.

From changes in terminology applied to epidemiologic studies to the description of risk factors according to timing of their insult, to the identification of newly discovered genes that are associated with ID, the epidemiology of ID is continually changing. This chapter reflects much of what is new. Taking a life stage perspective, both genetic and non-genetic influences that occur early in life often have a lasting effect on ultimate functioning of the individual. Recognizing that ID affects individuals across life stages, this chapter also presents information about the functioning of young adults with ID, in support of the idea that fetal and early-life influences may have life-long consequences.

DEFINITION AND CLASSIFICATION

The terminology and definition of intellectual disabilities have changed many times in an attempt to provide both an accurate and reliable measure and a more acceptable and less socially stigmatizing label of the condition. As previously described, this chapter uses the term 'intellectual disabilities' rather than 'mental retardation' to reflect the recent terminology change by the AAIDD. While more than one definition is currently in use, there is general agreement that the core feature of ID is significantly subaverage general intellectual functioning accompanied by significant limitations in adaptive functioning.

Three organizations have produced the most common definitions and subclassification schemes for ID: (1) the American Psychiatric Association in its Diagnostic and Statistical Manual of Mental Disorders, 4th edn (DSM-IV); (2) the American Association of Intellectual and Developmental Disabilities (AAIDD) – formerly the American Association of Mental Retardation (AAMR); and (3) the World Health Organization (WHO) in its International Statistical Classification of Diseases and Related Health Problems (ICD) and the International Classification of Functioning, Disability and Health (ICF) (Tables 47.1 and 47.2). The DSM-IV and AAIDD definitions are similar in that they both emphasize significant limitations in intellectual and adaptive functioning and specify the age of onset as before 18 years of age. The AAIDD definition describes the interaction between the capabilities of the individual in terms of intellectual and adaptive skills, the structure and expectations of the individual's personal and social environment and the intensities of supports needed to improve functioning with respect to independence, relationships, societal contributions, participation in school and community and personal wellbeing (Luckasson et al 2002). The third set of definitions for ID reflects a 'family' of international classifications established by the WHO, which uses the International Statistical Classification of Diseases and Related Health Problems, most recently published as ICD-10 (WHO 1992). While the ICD-10 was ratified by the WHO more than a decade ago it has been used for reporting mortality; it is the clinical modification of the previous version, the ICD-9CM, that is used for reporting morbidity and assigning of diagnoses in clinical settings. Therefore, the ICD-9CM is frequently used for epidemiologic purposes to identify individuals with various disorders, including ID. In contrast to the ICD, the ICF provides a conceptual framework and taxonomy for functioning, disability and health. The ICF health and health-related domains are described from the perspective of the body, individual and society and include two parts: (1) functioning and disability and (2) contextual factors. Each part has two components. Functioning and disability includes: (a) body functions and structures and (b) activities and participation. Contextual factors includes: (a) environmental factors and (b) personal factors. Unlike the other classification schemes, the ICF provides for specific measurement of environmental factors. ID is classified within the body functions and structures component as part of a more specific group of intellectual functions (WHO 2001a). Different from the DSM-IV and AAIDD definitions, the WHO classification schemes (ICD-9, ICD-10 or ICF) do not specify an age cutoff for defining ID. The ICF is being modified to capture the experiences of children and young adults specifically.

Because there are few disorders for which there is a one-to-one relationship with ID, the prevailing approach to further defining and classifying ID is by severity rather than etiology. ID has traditionally been divided into various levels of severity based on results from standardized psychometric testing, more specifically the normal statistical distribution of intelligence quotient (IQ) scores. The cutoff points for these levels are based on the number of standard deviations (1 SD = 15 points) below the accepted statistical population

Table 47.2 Subclassifications of intellectual disabilities by IQ

Level of retardation	DSM-IV[a]	AAIDD/AAMR[b] intensity of support	ICD-9CM[c]	ICD-10[d]	ICF[e]*
Mild	50–55 to 70	Intermittent	50–70	50–69	Mild problem (slight, low –5%–24%)
Moderate	35–40 to 50–55	Limited	35–49	35–49	Moderate problem (medium, fair –25%–49%)
Severe	20–25 to 35–40	Extensive	20–34	20–34	Severe problem (high, extreme –50%–95%)
Profound	Below 20–25	Pervasive	0–19	0–19	Complete problem (total –96%–100%)

[a]American Psychiatric Association 1994.
[b]Luckasson et al 2002.
[c]International Classification of Diseases 1988.
[d]WHO 1992.
[e]WHO 2001.
*IQ is not a construct in ICF. All three components classified in ICF-Body Functions and Structures; Activities and Participation; and Environmental Factors are quantified using the same generic scale, from 'no problem' to 'complete problem'.

mean IQ of 100, taking into consideration the concept of standard error, which is approximately 5 points on either side of the cutoff score but can vary according to the type of psychometric test administered. The American Psychiatric Association (APA) has retained the conventional severity levels of intellectual impairment based on IQ scores and maintained an IQ cutoff point of 70 or below as defining ID (APA 1994). Both the ICD-9 and ICD-10 use IQ cutoff scores for subclassifications of mild, moderate, severe, and profound ID. The AAIDD, on the other hand, has replaced the previous classification of severity by IQ with a three-step approach that includes 'intensity of needed levels of support' (Luckasson et al 1992). This change is believed to be more relevant to the provision of services and improved functioning (Leonard & Wen 2002, Luckasson et al 1992). Likewise, in the ICF, IQ is not a construct. Rather severity of ID is quantified using a generic scale, from 'no problem' to 'complete problem' (Table 47.2).

Both the AAIDD definition of severity and ICF framework incorporate the role of environmental factors, which has implications for epidemiologic research. Although adaptive functioning has generally been accepted as a necessary component of the ID definition for clinical and service provision purposes, it has not been considered in the case definition for most epidemiologic studies which typically rely on retrospective collection of administrative data. Because it is important in epidemiologic studies that the measure for case definition is both valid and reliable, most studies have used standardized IQ scores to define ID. Operationalizing the new AAIDD definition, which uses non-standardized evaluation of the intensity of supports, raises potential issues about the completeness of information in available administrative data as well as the reliability and validity of data that are present. Likewise, the new ICF paradigm, while useful from a consumer and services perspective, will likely be challenging to use for most epidemiologic research. Historically issues have been raised as to racial and ethnic bias in IQ testing which warrants consideration when interpreting results.

Despite the recognition of the importance of adaptive functioning and social participation, and their interaction with an individual's environment, the vast majority of epidemiologic research in ID has continued to measure ID by IQ scores and focus exclusively on prevalence and etiology.

PREVALENCE

For the majority of children with ID, the cause of their condition is considered to be of prenatal origin (i.e. children are born with the disorder). However, the presence of ID, particularly more mild forms, may not be apparent until months or years after the causal event. As a result, prevalence, the proportion of individuals with ID in a given population at a specified point or period in time, is the epidemiologic measure of choice used to determine the frequency of ID in the population. While incidence is often thought to be the appropriate epidemiologic measure of frequency of a condition, it is not feasible for ID because of mortality (spontaneous abortion, fetal and neonatal deaths) and out-migration before establishing a diagnosis which is often based on psychometric testing at school age.

Most epidemiologic studies examining the prevalence of ID rely exclusively on the results of IQ testing to determine case status. Relatively recent improvements in standardization of adaptive functioning testing have made it more feasible to systematically incorporate adaptive functioning into case definitions for epidemiologic purposes; however, this is still not common in population-based epidemiologic investigations. Interestingly, Hansen et al (1980) reported that when adaptive functioning has been used, the prevalence of ID has declined.

Dating back to the early 1960s, the range of prevalence estimates for ID generated from epidemiologic studies has varied greatly from 2 to 79 per 1000 (Roeleveld et al 1997). Since the early 1980s, studies in developed countries have reported a slightly narrower range of prevalence estimates for ID overall, ranging from 5 to 42 per 1000; in developing countries, however, some estimates are as high as 65 per 1000 (Table 47.3). This variation is attributable to a number of issues in obtaining numerator data. These include differences in case definition and methodologies used for case ascertainment across studies, quality of data available when using administrative data sources both within and across studies, characteristics of the populations studied (e.g. developed vs. developing country, age, sex, race, ethnicity, socio-economic status), and revisions in definitions and classification schemes for ID over time that have a direct influence on data collection. The largest recent epidemiologic study of one age cohort in the United States is the Autism and Developmental Disabilities Monitoring (ADDM) Network which uses multiple health and education data sources for case ascertainment and a common methodology. The 2002 surveillance year of the ADDM Network, which included a population of 150 795 8-year-old children across five communities in the United States, reported a weighted average period prevalence of 15 per 1000 with a range of 8 to 21 per 1000 (Table 47.3, ADDM Network, personnel communication, K. Van Naarden Braun, November, 20, 2006).

The source of denominator data must also be considered when comparing prevalence estimates. The majority of studies measure period or point prevalence using the population denominator for the defined geographic area under study, but birth prevalence estimates are also commonly calculated to evaluate child and parental birth characteristics. In contrast to period and point prevalence, birth prevalence estimates use the number of births in the defined geographic area as the denominator and often yield lower prevalence estimates due to factors related to in and out migration.

Table 47.3 Select studies of the prevalence of intellectual disabilities conducted from 1980 to present

Study year(s)	Reference	Location	Source(s) for case ascertainment	Age (years)	Overall prevalence per 1000	Prevalence MID per 1000	Prevalence MPID per 1000
1980	McQueen et al 1986	Maritime region, Canada	School records and agencies	7–10	NR	NR	3.7
1980–81	McDermott 1994	South Carolina, USA	School placement	3–21	41.7	37.4	4.4
1983	Diaz-Fernandez 1988	Galicia, Spain	Registry	5–14	5.0	NR	3.4
1984	Hagberg et al 1987	Gothenburg, Sweden	National register	8–12, 14–18	NR	3.7, 3.9	3.0, 3.3
1984	Wellesley et al 1992	Western Australia	State register and agencies	6–16	7.6	3.0	3.9
1985–87	Murphy et al 1995	Atlanta, USA	School and health service record review	10	12.0	8.4	3.6
1987–99	Croen et al 2001	California, USA	Statewide diagnostic and service agency	Birth–12	5.2	NR	NR
1987–88	Islam et al 1993	Bangladesh*	Household survey, evaluations	2–9	NR	14.4	5.9
1988–89	Durkin et al 1998	Karachi, Pakistan*	Household survey, evaluations	2–9	NR	65.3	19.0
1991–96	Hou et al 1998	Taiwan	Special schools and institutions	6–18	28.0	NR	NR
1992	Cans et al 1999	3 regions in France	Medical records	7–16	NR	NR	3.5
1993	Stromme & Valvatne 1998	Akershus County, Norway	Multiple sources including schools and birth registry	8–13	6.2	3.5	2.7
1995	Fernell et al 1996, 1998	Stockholm, Sweden	Medical records, registry for ID services	9–15	NR	12.8	4.5
1996, 2000	Karapurkar Bhasin et al 2006	Atlanta, USA	School and health service provision record review	8	15.5 (1996) 12.0 (2000)	10.0 (1996) 7.3 (2000)	4.3 (1996) 3.3 (2000)
1999	Leonard et al 2003	Western Australia	Multiple sources, registry for educational support	6–15	14.3	10.6	1.4
2002	ADDM Network, 2002 surveillance year	5 sites in USA: Arkansas (AR) Georgia (GA), North Carolina (NC), South Carolina (SC), Utah (UT)	School and health service provision record review	8	Weighted average: 15.4 (5 sites)	Weighted average: 12.1 (4 sites)	Weighted average: 3.2 (4 sites)

MID = Mild intellectual disability, MPID = moderate to profound intellectual disability, NR = Not reported.
*Represents developing country, the remainder represent developed countries.

SEVERITY

A crucial factor for understanding the epidemiology of ID is examining level of severity. For epidemiologic study purposes, the prevalence of ID is commonly examined using two IQ levels, with an IQ 50–55 to 70–75 being considered mild intellectual disabilities (MID) and an IQ less than 50–55 being considered moderate to profound ID (MPID) which historically had been referred to as severe mental retardation or intellectual disability (Kiely 1987, Roeleveld et al 1997). Most studies have shown that the majority of individuals have MID (75%–80%) (Murphy et al 1998); however studies of MID prevalence since the 1980s have shown great variability, ranging from 3 to 37 per 1000 in developed countries and as high as 65 per 1000 in developing countries (Table 47.3). These inconsistencies likely result from the methodologic issues described earlier.

Unlike estimates for MID, estimates of MPID prevalence are less variable across studies. Studies conducted since 1980 report the prevalence of MPID ranging from 1.4 to 4.5 per 1000 in developed countries and as high as 19 per 1000 in developing countries (Table 47.3). Leonard et al (2003) reported a prevalence of 1.4 per 1000 for MPID, but the nature of their data necessitated that they define MPID as IQ less than 35 or 40 rather than IQ less than 50–55, which would be more comparable to the other studies described in Table 47.3. Therefore, the prevalence of MPID from this study may not be the most appropriate lower bound estimate of the range of prevalence of MPID as defined for these purposes. Data from the ADDM Network (2002) surveillance year found a weighted average period prevalence among 8-year-olds of 12.1 per 1000 for MMR and 3.2 per 1000 for SMR (Table 47.3).

In addition to measuring severity of ID by IQ, severity can also be considered with respect to the presence of co-morbidities. About one fifth of children with ID have another developmental disability, most frequently cerebral palsy or epilepsy (Boyle et al 1996, Murphy et al 1995). The likelihood of a co-existing developmental disability is greater for children with MPID than for those with MID (45% vs. 12%) and, therefore, has also been used as a proxy for severity.

SOCIAL AND DEMOGRAPHIC CHARACTERISTICS

The prevalence of ID varies by several social and demographic characteristics, most notably age, gender, race and ethnicity and socioeconomic status. Sociodemographic differences in prevalence are further modified by severity of ID. Therefore it is important to consider each of these factors in tandem with severity when evaluating prevalence estimates.

Age

Studies have shown variation in the prevalence of ID by age, ranging from 1 per 1000 in children 4 years of age or younger to 97 per 1000 in children 10–14 years of age (Kiely 1987, Murphy et al 1995, Roeleveld et al 1997). Studies support a peak in ID administrative prevalence at age 10–14

years, slight declines among adolescents, and marked declines thereafter (Wen 1997). The age range for peak prevalence is driven largely by the differential in age of identification by severity of ID. Typically, children with MPID are diagnosed at younger ages and children with MID are identified more often once they reach school age. The peak in overall prevalence at 10–14 years of age reflects the significant impact of the education system on identification of children with ID, more specifically children with MID through standardized psychometric evaluations.

Understanding the prevalence of MID in adults is challenging for a number of reasons. As children with developmental disabilities reach young adulthood, their specialized pediatric, rehabilitation and special education services often cease. As they exit these various administrative service systems it is difficult to measure the prevalence of the condition. In addition, individuals with MID, particularly those with good adaptive functioning skills may experience successful integration into the community and, therefore, are no longer identified as having MID. Since IQ scores are a reflection of performance on a standardized test at a given point in time, not innate intellectual capacity, changes may occur over time, particularly for individuals with MID whose functional skills may increase with age. Finally, another factor contributing to the decline in ID prevalence into adulthood may be the reported higher mortality rates for individuals with ID (Decoufle & Autry 2002). By comparing data from two large population-based studies on mortality rates among individuals with ID with USA life table rates, Honeycutt et al (2003) estimated that the cumulative probability of survival from birth to age 65 for all ID is 64% that of the general population (Decoufle & Autry 2002, Strauss & Eyeman 1996).

Gender

Most studies have reported a slightly higher prevalence of ID among males than among females, with the male-to-female ratio of approximately 1.5:1 (Leonard & Wen 2002). Although it has been suggested that this gender difference is driven by MID, data from the ADDM Network found similar male-to-female ratios for both MID and MPID (ADDM Network, K. Van Naarden Braun, November 15, 2006). The reported higher prevalence of MID among males is thought to be highly associated with social factors. For example, boys might exhibit behaviors that elicit greater attention and result in earlier concern and evaluation than girls. Gissler et al (1999), studied gender differences in a range of childhood morbidities, including ID and found an increased risk for ID among males. In addition, males are twice as likely to have delayed development and to require special education services after adjusting for other health-related variables (Leonard & Wen 2002). This finding speaks to the role of the education system both in identifying children with ID and in potentially offering intervention. The overall preponderance of ID among males may also be driven, in part, by X-linked genetic conditions such as fragile X

(Partington et al 2000). Chelly and Mandel (2001) reported that an estimated 13%–21% of ID in males is caused by X-linked mutations. A recent review identified 178 X-linked conditions associated with ID (Chiurazzi et al 2000, Lubs et al 1999).

Race and ethnicity

Differences in the prevalence of ID have been reported in various racial and ethnic subgroups. Yeargin-Allsopp et al (1995) and Murphy et al (1995) reported a higher prevalence of ID among black 10-year-old children in metropolitan Atlanta than among their white counterparts. This association remained significant after controlling for select demographic and socioeconomic factors including sex, maternal age and education, birth order and economic status. Croen et al (2001) found an increased risk for both MID and MPID among children born to black mothers compared to white mothers and an increased risk for MPID among Hispanic and Asian mothers, but a decreased risk for MID among Asian mothers. In addition, a study from Australia found a higher rate of ID among Australian indigenous (ethnic minority) children (Leonard & Wen 2002). Despite the reported lack of effect of economic status on ID prevalence in the Atlanta study, confounding by socioeconomic factors is assumed to contribute to these racial and ethnic differences. More studies are needed in order to better determine the impact and meaning of racial and ethnic differences in ID prevalence.

Socioeconomic factors

Extensive literature supports an inverse association between socioeconomic status and the prevalence of MID defined by IQ of approximately 50–70 (Birch et al 1970, Broman et al 1987, Decoufle & Boyle 1995, Drews et al 1995, Kiely 1987, Mercer 1973, Munro 1986, Rutter et al 1970, Stein & Susser 1963, Stromme & Magnus 2000, Yeargin-Allsopp et al 1995). Many studies have consistently shown that MID is highly correlated with lower socioeconomic status and that a greater proportion of cases of MPID have been reported to have a biologic basis (Leonard & Wen 2002, McLaren & Bryson 1987). Older studies have further suggested that MID is rarely found among children in families of high socioeconomic status unless accompanied by evidence of organic damage (Birch et al 1970, Stein & Susser 1960, 1963). By contrast, this association with lower socioeconomic status has not been consistently found for children with MPID, rather a greater proportion of cases of MPID have been reported to have a biological etiology. More recent work conducted in metropolitan Atlanta by Drews et al (1995) supported an increased association between MID and low economic status (OR = 1.6) as well as maternal education of less than high school (OR = 4.1) with no significant associations reported for MPID. Interestingly, even in a developing country such as Bangladesh, a similar trend was found in that the association with low socioeconomic status was stronger for MID than for MPID (Islam et al 1993). Although the majority of epidemiologic data support this inverse

association, the large population-based study in California, mentioned previously, which differentiated between ID with or without an identified cause subclassified by IQ level of severity found an increased risk associated with increasing maternal age and decreasing maternal education for both MID and MPID among children with ID of unknown etiology (Croen et al 2001).

To further clarify the relationship between selected socioeconomic and demographic factors and subgroups of ID, Drews et al (1995) attempted to create more homogeneous subgroups of ID by categorizing children with ID based on the presence of other developmental disabilities or neurological conditions and the level of severity as measured by IQ. Using these categories the authors hypothesized that the risk factors for ID may be different for children with these types of co-morbidities than for children with isolated ID. They found that markers for lower socioeconomic status were associated with MID and that trends for isolated MID were similar to isolated MPID whereas patterns for MID with other neurological conditions were similar to those with MPID and other neurological conditions suggesting that classification by the presence of other neurological conditions may be more informative than by level of ID severity. Both categorizations by IQ distribution and the presence of other neurological conditions have provided support to the theory posited by Zigler et al (1984) of a dichotomy in terms of biologic causation associated with level of functioning in that ID can be subclassified into two different types; i.e. the 'two group theory' of intellectual disabilities, with a smaller IQ curve shifted to the left for 'organic damage' superimposed on the normal gaussian curve for overall intelligence.

ETIOLOGY AND RISK FACTORS

Given the significant etiologic heterogeneity among individuals with ID, it is challenging from an epidemiologic perspective to establish a comprehensive understanding of the causes of ID in the population. A universally accepted, consistently applied etiological classification system that can accommodate our rapidly growing knowledge of primarily genetic causes does not exist (Leonard & Wen 2002). The proportion of ID cases with a known etiology has been reported to range from 22% in Georgia (USA) to 80% in Norway (Table 47.4). The proportion of cases with a known etiology has consistently been higher among those with MPID, ranging from 25% to 96%, than among those with MID ranging from 12% to 68% (Table 47.4). Rapid progress with improved diagnostic capabilities, such as fluorescence in situ hybridization, DNA testing and testing to identify submicroscopic deletions in the subtelomeric chromosomal regions, suggests that these may be underestimates of known etiology for individuals with ID (Rauch et al 2006, Skellern et al 2000).

The wide range in the proportion of cases with a known etiology is likely influenced by methodologic differences

Table 47.4 Epidemiologic studies of etiology of intellectual disabilities[a]

Reference	Location, source of case ascertainment	Number of cases total/MID/MPID	Method for determining etiology	Prevalence per 1000 children total/MID/MPID	Etiology % total/MID/MPID	% Genetic total/MID/MPID % specific etiology[a]
Yeargin-Allsopp et al 1997	Atlanta, GA, USA. Metropolitan Atlanta Developmental Disabilities Study	715/509/206	Education and medical administrative records from multiple sources	10.3/7.4/3.0	Any: 22/12/43 Prenatal: 12/7/25 Perinatal: 6/4/11 Postnatal: 4/2/7 Unknown: 78/87/57	Genetic: 7/3/17 Down syndrome: 5 Fragile X: 0.1 Prader-Willi syndrome: 0.1
Fernell, 1998	Stockholm, Sweden Hospital, outpatient pediatric clinics and local center for ID	NR/NR/64	Medical records	NR/NR/4.5	Any: NR/NR/77 Prenatal: NR/NR/66 Perinatal: NR/NR/6 Postnatal: NR/NR/5 Unknown: NR/NR/23	Genetic: NR/NR/NR Down syndrome: 20
Hou et al 1998[b]	Taiwan Special schools and institutions	11,892/7492/4400	Medical records, parental interview, cytogenetic and molecular testing	28.0/NR/NR	Any: 68/58/86 Prenatal: 55/47/70 Perinatal: 10/9/11 Postnatal: 3/2/5 Unknown: 32/43/14	Genetic: 39/32/50 Down syndrome: 13 Fragile X: 2 Prader-Willi syndrome: 0.5 Angelman syndrome: 0.3 Williams syndrome: 0.04
Stromme & Hagberg 2000	Akershus County, Norway Multiple sources	185/NR/NR 178/NR/NR for etiologic analyses	Parental interview, chromosomal analysis (i.e. karyotyping, metabolic screening), FISH, physical and neurological exam, psychometric testing	6.2/3.5/2.7	Any[c]: 80/68/96 Prenatal: 59/51/70 Perinatal: 4.5/5/4 Postnatal: 3/1/5 Unknown: 20/32/4	Genetic: 35/25/48 Down syndrome: 10 Fragile X: 2 Williams syndrome: 2 Prader-Willi syndrome: 1 Angelman syndrome: 1
Cans et al 1999	France: 3 regions Departmental Commission for Special Education	NR/NR/1,150	Medical records	NR/NR/3.5	Any: NR/NR/25 Prenatal: NR/NR/NR Perinatal: NR/NR/NR Postnatal:NR/NR/NR Unknown:NR/NR/NR	Genetic: NR/NR/18 Down syndrome: 16
Partington et al 2000	New South Wales, Australia Australian Child and Adolescent Study	429/114/280	Diagnostic exam, genetic evaluation, parent interview	NR/NR/NR	Any: 45/NR/NR Prenatal: 32/NR/NR Perinatal: 8/NR/NR Postnatal: 5/NR/NR Unknown: 56/NR/NR	Genetic: 29/NR/NR Down syndrome: 15 Prader-Willi syndrome: 0.7 Angelman syndrome: 0.7 Williams syndrome: 0.5

MID = mild intellectual disability, MPID = moderate to profound intellectual disability, NR = not reported.

[a] Few studies delineated specific etiologies by level of severity, therefore only the total is reported. This is the proportion of all ID cases.

[b] Children without a specified etiology and a family history of ID were classified as having prenatal etiology. If these children are classified as having an unknown etiology rather than a prenatal etiology, the results would be as follows using the presentation format above: Any: 50/37/73; Prenatal: 37/26/57; Perinatal: 10/9/11; Postnatal: 3/2/5; Unknown: 50/63/27.

[c] Includes children with a known etiology for which the timing is unknown. 14 % for total ID, 11% for MID and 18% for MPID.

across studies, including the definition of 'known etiology,' completeness of case ascertainment and methods used to obtain etiologic information. With respect to definition, more stringent criteria for what constitutes a 'cause' lead to a larger proportion of ID cases of undetermined etiology (McLaren & Bryson 1987, Yeargin-Allsopp et al 1997). Most studies rely on multiple sources to identify cases, which increase the completeness of case ascertainment. The use of traditional medical or social service providers may yield more complete ascertainment for MPID, while use of education sources is necessary to identify children with MID. Therefore, studies that have included education sources in conjunction with traditional medical and social service provider sources have greatly reduced differential ascertainment by severity.

As seen in Table 47.4, widely varying methods have been used to determine etiology. In general, studies that relied exclusively on existing medical record review had lower proportions with known etiologies. Those that used multiple types of evaluations including medical records, interviews of parents to obtain a medical and family history, and selected cytogenetic and molecular analyses, to identify specific genetic etiologies found higher proportions with known etiologies. Hou et al (1998) differed from the other studies in how they defined their cases with unknown etiology. ID cases with an unknown etiology and a family history of ID were classified as having a known prenatal etiology. Had these children been classified as having an unknown etiology as in other studies, the proportion of ID cases with a known etiology would have been substantially lower: 50% of ID cases overall would have had a known etiology compared with the reported 68% using the former categorization (Table 47.4). Nevertheless, this study was the most comprehensive in the characteristics of ID etiology reported from a large, population-based sample using multiple methods for both ascertainment and etiologic information.

Many investigators have classified the etiology of ID by the probable timing of the presumed insult: prenatal (arising before birth); perinatal (arising between birth and the first month of life); postnatal (occurring after the first month of life and before 18 years of age); and unknown (Table 47.4). Interestingly, while the proportion of cases with a known etiology across studies varied widely, the patterns are similar within these timing categories such that the majority of children have a prenatal etiology and, as previously mentioned, a higher proportion of those with MPID have a known etiology.

GENETIC

On a population level, epidemiology plays an important role by characterizing risk factors and the range of phenotypic expressions associated with specific genetic disorders, determining prevalence of individual mutations, providing useful information for genetic counseling purposes, and identifying subgroups of the population for which genetic factors may be of particular concern. That said, the majority of specific genetic causes of ID have not been identified from epidemiologic studies, but rather from genetic and molecular studies of clinical populations with similar phenotypes or from family studies (Couvert et al 2001, Crawford et al 2002).

Although more than 500 genetic diseases are known to cause ID, and more than 1300 entries for ID appeared on the Online Mendelian Inheritance in Man in November, 2006, the prevalence estimates of each of these diseases is low and individually do not contribute substantially to the overall prevalence of ID (Flint & Wilkie 1996, Murphy et al 1998, NIH 2006). Chromosomal anomalies are the predominant cause of MPID and may be structural or numerical in nature. Structural chromosomal anomalies occur as duplications, deletions, translocations, insertions or inversions of chromosome parts or as rings on selected chromosomes. Numerical anomalies happen through non-disjunction during meiosis or mitosis or through lagging of chromosomes at anaphase of cell division (Durkin et al 2002). The majority of chromosomal abnormalities result in fetal death rather than live-births (and subsequent ID) which supports the necessity to measure prevalence of ID rather than incidence. Kline et al (1989) reported that approximately 40% of miscarriages are chromosomally aberrant (including autosomal trisomies, trisomies of sex chromosomes, monosomy X, triploidy and tetraploidy) and that within 6 weeks post conception the proportion of chromosomal anomalies lost by miscarriage exceeds 70% for all but trisomies of sex chromosomes including Klinefelter syndrome (XXY), XXX and XYY (Kline et al 1989). After 6 weeks post conception it appears that about 6% of surviving conceptuses have chromosomal abnormalities. Among surviving pregnancies in developing countries, chromosomal abnormalities account for more than 30% of MPID (Durkin et al 2002, Hagberg 1987).

The most common genetic cause of ID among live births in the United States continues to be Down syndrome, with a prevalence of about 1 per 800 live births (National Center on Birth Defects and Developmental Disabilities 2004a). Down syndrome is the most common etiology across all studies in Table 47.4, with a range of approximately 5% in metropolitan Atlanta to about 20% in Sweden with the majority of studies clustering between 10–16%. Down syndrome has been shown to account consistently for about two-thirds or more of all known genetic causes of ID (Cans et al 1999, Fernell 1998, Hou et al 1998, Stromme & Hagberg 2000, Yeargin-Allsopp et al 1997).

Epidemiologic evidence has shown an exponential increased risk for Down syndrome after a mother reaches 35 years of age (Morris et al 2003). This finding was the impetus for the previous recommendation that pregnant women aged 35 and older should be offered amniocentesis to diagnostically evaluate the presence of chromosomal abnormalities, biochemical disorders and a number of single gene disorders (Cunniff & Committee on Genetics 2004). In January, 2007, the American College of Obstetricians and Gynecologists

(ACOG 2007) released its most recent recommendation that screening and invasive diagnostic testing for aneuploidy should be available to all women who present for prenatal care before 20 weeks gestation regardless of maternal age (ACOG 2007). Prenatal screening for Down syndrome in the first and second trimesters uses results from various combinations of measurements of serum alpha-fetoprotein, unconjugated estriol, human chorionic gonadotropin, inhibin A, serum pregnancy-associated plasma protein A and nuchal translucency obtained by ultrasonography depending on the level of the screen (i.e. double, triple, quadruple, combined or integrated). Data from the FASTER (First- and Second-Trimester Evaluation of Risk) trial which compared various screening test protocols demonstrated the highest detection rate of 94–96% for Down syndrome at a 5% screen-positive rate for the integrated screen which includes all measurements noted above (Malone et al 2005). Similar results were achieved in the SURUSS (Serum, Urine, and Ultrasound Screening Study) trial (Wald et al 2003). Early identification of Down syndrome which presents the option for termination of the pregnancy has begun to change the epidemiology of the prevalence of Down syndrome among live births (Siffel et al 2004).

The second leading cause of ID in the United States is fragile X syndrome, with a prevalence of 1 per 4000 males and 1 per 8000 females (Turner et al 1996). Fragile X is considered the most common form of inherited ID and accounts for a range of 0.1%–2% of ID cases (Table 47.4). Other genetic conditions include Prader–Willi (0.1%–1.0%), Angelman (0.3%–1.0%) Williams (0.04%–2%) and Cornelia de Lange (0.2%) syndromes. Nevertheless, as shown by the respective percentages these genetic disorders still contribute a very low proportion of ID cases (Table 47.4).

Advances in the genetics of ID have greatly increased our knowledge of the molecular basis of this condition. Improved specificity in diagnosis through fluorescence in situ hybridization, subtelomeric screening, extended banding chromosome analysis, and other techniques provides a greater number of individuals and families with accurate information about prognosis, treatment, management and the risk for recurrence (Rauch et al 2006, Skellern et al 2000). In addition, newer techniques such as microarray based comparative genomic hybridization provide promise in improving diagnosis of ID (UK Genetic Testing Network Working Party 2006). The phenomenon known as genetic imprinting was recognized in Prader–Willi and Angelman syndromes and provides interesting insight into these syndromes. While both syndromes usually arise from deletions in the same chromosome region of 15q11.2–13, their phenotypic expression is different with respect to ID such that individuals with Prader–Willi often have mild to moderate ID while Angelman is accompanied by MPID. Moreover, if the 15q deletion occurred on the paternally inherited chromosome, the phenotype is Prader–Willi and if the deletion is on the maternally inherited chromosome, the expression is Angelman syndrome (Flint & Wilkie 1996, Nicholls & Knepper 2001).

These findings suggest that for imprinted genes, genes from both parents are needed to ensure normal intelligence. In addition, these results underscore the complexity and lack of one common pathway or mechanism for intellectual processing.

Genetic epidemiology

When the cause of a child's ID is known or the pattern of inheritance is apparent, genetic counseling for parents who have a child with ID and are planning another pregnancy is often straightforward. For parents with a child whose ID is of unknown cause, genetic counselors must rely on empirical recurrence risk estimates. Most recurrence risk estimates for ID are based on studies conducted on clinical samples more than 10 years ago and therefore include a proportion of children for whom we now have the ability to identify their specific genetic etiology. Since the majority of studies were based on hospital or clinic populations, the resultant recurrence risk estimates are likely overestimates of the risk of recurrence in the general population as families with a history of ID or those already experiencing recurrence have a greater likelihood of visiting a medical provider. In addition, family size plays a role in calculation of recurrence risk estimates and reproductive decisions may be influenced by the presence of a child with ID. In most research on recurrence risks, regardless of the data source, it is not possible to know a couple's true family planning intentions. Nevertheless, in a recent population-based study on recurrence risk of developmental disabilities (DD), Van Naarden Braun et al (2005) found that families with more than one child with a DD, which included ID, were more likely to have subsequent children than those families with only one child with a DD. This suggests that having a child with DD might not have influenced the parents' decision to not have more children. Despite the existing methodologic limitations, there is utility in presenting the existing literature on recurrence risks for ID.

Recurrence risk estimates have little meaning without comparison to the baseline prevalence of the disorder in the study population. A high recurrence risk may reflect a high prevalence in the population in which the recurrence risk is comparable to the risk of having one child with ID. Herbst and Baird (1982), reported that the risk of ID among subsequent siblings of the first affected child was 3.7%, about 8 times their reported birth prevalence. Similarly, the Metropolitan Atlanta Developmental Disabilities Surveillance Program (MADDSP) reported the recurrence risk for ID to be 8.3%, also about 8 times the ID birth prevalence (Van Naarden Braun et al 2005).

Previous studies have examined recurrence risk for ID by gender, severity and the presence of co-morbidities. While ID is more prevalent in males, there is conflicting evidence as to whether boys with ID are more likely to have affected siblings. More specifically, it is hypothesized that, due to X-linked ID, brothers of males with ID may be at higher risk than sisters for ID (Bundey et al 1989, Herbst & Baird 1982,

Turner et al 1971). Herbst and Baird (1982) found that there was no increased risk for brothers of males with ID, but the risk of recurrence was greater for subsequent siblings of individuals with MID.

Many studies have shown a higher risk for recurrence for MID than for MPID and that the presence of co-morbidities decreases the chance for recurrence (Costeff & Weller 1987, Herbst & Baird 1982, Van Naarden Braun et al 2005). Studies have reported recurrence risk estimates of 2.4%–26.0% for idiopathic MID (Bundey et al 1989, Turner et al 1971) and 2.2%–14.0% for idiopathic MPID, but these studies have not taken into account the presence of multiple DDs (Bundey & Carter 1974, Opitz et al 1978). Recurrence risk estimates from the MADDSP data were within these ranges for isolated MID (7.1%) and isolated MPID (4.7%). These recurrence risk estimates are approximately 13 times greater than the birth prevalence for isolated MID and about 24 times greater for isolated MPID (Van Naarden Braun et al 2005). These findings are consistent with a handful of non-population-based studies that have reported the recurrence risk for MPID, while lower than the absolute risk for MID, to be higher when compared with the baseline prevalence.

Traditional and recent innovative epidemiologic methods provide exciting opportunities for genetic epidemiology and investigation of gene–environment interactions. Associations between genetic variants (exposure) and specific disorders have been examined through the use of case control studies. Yet, the use of this epidemiologic study design to assess potential genetic associations raises the problem of population stratification bias, defined by confounding attributable to differences in genetic backgrounds between cases and controls (Khoury 1994). While adjustment for factors possibly related to differing allelic distributions is possible using information on ethnicity, social background and geographical origin of the parents, these factors are also often related to the disorder under study for other reasons (Wacholder et al 2002). Some argue that such bias does not pose a major threat to the validity of results from case-control studies, but without adequate adjustment of these systematic differences between cases and controls, it may obscure identification of a weak association of genes with modest effects (August et al 1981).

Three alternative study designs have been suggested. The case-parent triad uses biological family members of cases as controls matching the cases and controls on their genetic descent and controlling for a number of non-genetic factors (e.g. socioeconomic status). The case-cohort study conceptualizes and samples the case-parent triad as a case-cohort study producing an exposure odds measure of effect that is generalizable to the source population from which the cases and controls were drawn (Ahsan et al 2002). Newschaffer et al (2002) proposed the case-parent/control-parent design, which is an expansion of the case-parent triad design, to include controls and their parents. This study design, while more complex, might be best suited to estimating and testing the full combination of genetic and non-genetic effects of

interest in developmental disabilities research because it allows for estimations at both parent and child levels as well as all estimations of possible interactions. The overriding challenge in understanding the etiology of ID, which permeates methodologic and resource issues across all proposed study designs, is that of conceptualizing and operationalizing specific hypotheses for testing interactions between genetic and non-genetic factors using population-based data and epidemiologic methods.

NON-GENETIC
Prenatal risk factors
As shown in Table 47.4, insults experienced during the prenatal period contribute the most to the etiology of ID. While genetic factors account for most known prenatal etiology, non-genetic risk factors that are modifiable and/or preventable have also been identified. Such factors for ID include maternal smoking (Drews et al 1996, Rantakallio & Koiranen 1987, Roeleveld et al 1992); alcohol exposure (Abel 1995, Streissguth et al 1990, 1991); maternal medical conditions, most notably thyroid disease (Haddow et al 1999, Qian et al 2000), urinary tract infections (McDermott et al 2001), maternal phenylketonuria (PKU) (Lenke & Levy 1980, Waisbren et al 1997); certain medications, such as hydantoins (Adams et al 1990, Hanson 1986, Holmes et al 2005, Scolnik et al 1994); intrauterine infections (Murphy et al 1998); nutritional deficiencies (Hetzel 1983); and environmental toxins such as polychlorinated biphenyls (PCBs) and mercury (Mendola et al 2002). Birth defects other than chromosomal abnormalities have also been shown to be an important risk factor for intellectual disabilities (Decoufle et al 2001).

Behavioral risk factors
While maternal smoking during pregnancy has been linked to low birth weight and less severe cognitive and achievement deficits, its association with ID has been less conclusive. Of the four main studies that have examined the association between maternal smoking during pregnancy and ID, three found no significant effect (Broman et al 1987, Rantakallio & Koiranen 1987, Roelveld 1992). The one study with a positive finding reported that the prevalence of idiopathic ID was increased by slightly more than 40% in children whose mothers smoked during pregnancy, after controlling for sociodemographic risk factors and low birth weight, and that the prevalence of ID increased with the number of packs smoked per day (Drews at al 1996). It is important to note that the mechanism by which maternal smoking may increase the risk of ID is unclear.

Chronic maternal alcohol exposure during pregnancy has been consistently shown to be a risk factor for ID. Cognitive deficits together with physical malformations, especially of the face, stunted growth and delayed psychomotor development describe fetal alcohol syndrome (FAS) which has been reported to affect a range of 0.2–1.5 per 1000 live births (Bertrand et al 2005, National Center on Birth Defects and

Developmental Disabilities 2004b). Approximately one fourth of individuals who receive a diagnosis of FAS perform at two standard deviations below the mean on standardized measures of cognition (Streissguth et al 1996). In a 10 year follow-up study of persons diagnosed with FAS in infancy or childhood, Spohr et al (1993) found a strong association with ID and suggested that environmental and educational factors do not have strong compensatory effects on cognitive development.

Maternal health conditions

Select maternal medical conditions have been documented to be associated with ID mainly attributable to lack of identification or poor compliance with treatment. Using data from the Collaborative Perinatal Project (CPP), McDermott et al (2001) found that urinary tract infections (UTI) in the third trimester had an increased relative risk of 1.4 for ID or developmental delay in the children. Although there were no data on treatment in the CPP, Medicaid data from South Carolina during 1994–1996 found similar outcomes among women who did not have treatment following the UTI diagnosis and no association among women who received treatment (McDermott et al 2001). Untreated, often unrecognized, thyroid deficiency during pregnancy is an important, recognized risk factor for ID and an important contributor to lowered IQs and ID in children. Klein (2005) reported that children born to mothers with subclinical hypothyroidism comprise approximately 1.5% of all children with IQs < 70 (Haddow et al 1999, LaFranchi et al 2005, Qian et al 2000). Another risk factor for ID is maternal PKU. In the 1970s, physicians began seeing women of childbearing age who had been successfully treated with PKU diets since birth and, hence avoided developing ID. As these young women aged, the PKU diets had been discontinued. Waisbren et al (2003) reported that 47% of children born to women with PKU whose metabolic control was reached either after 20 weeks gestation or never during the index pregnancy had ID (IQ ≤ 70). This study also found that women with PKU who kept their blood phenylalanine levels within the recommended range of 2–6 mg % during pregnancy have the same probability of having a normal infant as women without PKU (Waisbren et al 2003).

Medication use

Although epidemiologic data on the relationship between ID and prenatal exposure to maternal medications are limited, some maternal medications have been shown to be teratogenic and associated with ID in the offspring. Among them are antiepileptics (AEDs) and antipsychotics including hydantoins, carbamazepine, phenobarbital, trimethadione and valproate, as well as other medications such as warfarin and retinoic acid (Adams et al 1990, Drane & Meador 1996, Hanson 1986, Holmes et al 2005, Jones 1997, Jones et al 2001, Scolnik et al 1994, Stevenson et al 1980). One study that examined the presence of developmental delay defined by presence of speech and/or motor delays among children of mothers who took AEDs during pregnancy found that

children whose mothers took carbamazepine or valproate were significantly more likely to have a developmental delay than were children whose mothers were not exposed to either drug (Dean et al 2002). Recent data suggest that the risk of serious adverse outcomes such as birth defects may be lower in newer AEDs and antipsychotic medications than in older generations of these types of medications, but it could be that these drugs have been in use a shorter length of time and adverse events have yet to be reported. For example, the North American Antiepileptic Drug (NAAED) Pregnancy Registry recently reported an increased risk of non-syndromic oral clefts associated with maternal lamotrigine exposure during pregnancy over the reference population; until then lamotrigine had been considered among the safest of the AEDs to be taken during pregnancy (Holmes et al 2006, Meador et al 2006). Data on the long-term neurodevelopment of children exposed to these newer drugs in utero is even more limited (Drane & Meador 1996, Meador et al 2006). Other studies have shown increased risk of ID among children of mothers who used retinoic acid as well as other synthetic vitamin A derivatives (Jones et al 2001) and who took the anticoagulant warfarin during the first eight weeks of pregnancy (Stevenson et al 1980). It is important to note that, while it is optimal to abstain from medication during pregnancy to eliminate the risk of adverse effects on the developing fetus, women with seizure and/or psychiatric disorders who must take medications to control their condition should work with their health care provider to use the drug with the least likelihood of teratogenic effects.

Intrauterine infections

In the 1970s, intrauterine infections were the cause of ID in 8%–35% of children with ID (Hagberg & Kyllerman 1983). Today that percentage continues to decrease because of immunizations and better recognition and practice of prevention measures. Nevertheless, as a group, the STORCH (syphilis, toxoplasmosis, other agents, rubella, cytomegalovirus and herpes simplex) intrauterine infections continue to be an important cause of fetal and perinatal morbidity and mortality. Yeargin-Allsopp et al (1997) found that among 10-year-old children with ID with a known etiology 4% of cases were caused by congenital infections, the most common being neonatal human cytomegalovirus (CMV).

CMV has consistently been shown to be the most common congenital infectious cause of ID (Fowler et al 1992, CDC 2002). Neonatal CMV occurs in only 0.3%–1% of all live births, 85% to 90% of these infections are not apparent, and 15%–25% of those infants will have neurologic sequelae, including ID (Fowler et al 1992). The greatest risk of congenital CMV infection is for infants born to women who are infected with CMV for the first time during pregnancy (1%–3%) (CDC 2002). In a follow-up study of children 5 years of age or younger, 13% of children born to mothers who seroconverted during pregnancy developed ID (Fowler et al 1992). There is controversy around prenatal screening for congenital CMV infection (Demmler 2005, Naessens et al

2005) because CMV infects 50%–85% of adults in the United States by 40 years of age, and for the vast majority of people, CMV infection is not a serious problem. Additionally, safe treatments are not available for use during pregnancy (CDC 2002).

Congenital toxoplasmosis occurs in approximately 1 per 1000 live births (Sever et al 1988). A follow-up study of children who were born to mothers infected with toxoplasmosis showed a 30% increase in the prevalence of ID (Sever et al 1988). Treatment is available for women who are infected during pregnancy, and for both the mother and infant if the infant is shown to be infected. However, there have been no randomized controlled trials to evaluate the effectiveness of treatment in preventing the long-term developmental sequelae of congenital toxoplasmosis in children (Gilbert et al 2001). Although routine screening of pregnant women and screening of newborns are equally controversial (Boyer et al 2005), two states screen for toxoplasmosis in the newborn period.

With the near elimination of rubella in the United States, congenital rubella, with a prevalence of less than 1 per 100 000 live births in the United States, is no longer considered a contributor to ID during childhood (National Center for Infectious Diseases 2000, 2005a). From 2001 through 2004, there were only 4 cases of congenital rubella syndrome reported to the CDC, and 3 of the 4 mothers were born outside the United States.

Similarly, sexually transmitted diseases are also decreasing in their importance as causes of ID in the United States. The US rate of congenital syphilis continues to decline: from 2003 to 2004, it decreased 18% from 10.7 to 8.8 per 100 000 live births (CDC 2001, 2005b). ID occurs in about one-third of children with congenital syphilis (Rozien & Johnson 1996). Neonatal herpes simplex virus (HSV) infection occurs in 1 in 3000–20 000 live births; however, congenital HSV infection is often severe, with high mortality rates (AAP 2003a). In 2-year survivors of HSV encephalitis, as many as 50% have permanent neurological impairment, including ID (Rozien & Johnson 1996).

Nutrient deficiencies

In developing countries where iodine deficiency is endemic, it is the leading preventable cause of ID (Hetzel 1989). Rectification of iodine deficiency in women prior to conception is crucial to prevent ID, and the most efficient and effective intervention in developing countries is through universal iodine dietary supplementation. Salt and drinking water iodination are two viable public health measures to implement supplementation, but they have been difficult to implement in some developing countries. As this preventable cause of ID continues to be a major international concern, it has been identified as a priority by the World Health Organization (Durkin et al 2002, WHO 2001b).

Prenatal environmental toxins

The dose–response relationship of prenatal PCB exposure and childhood neurodevelopmental outcomes has been studied extensively. When pregnant women were exposed to very high levels of PCBs, with the majority of exposure occurring through maternal consumption of PCB-contaminated fish, ID and other deficits occurred in their offspring (Chen et al 1992, Jacobson & Jacobson 1996, 1997, Lonky et al 1996, Mendola et al 2002, Yu et al 1991).

Mercury, a powerful neurotoxin, has caused ID at very high levels of prenatal exposure resulting from acute poisonings (Davidson et al 2004, Harada 1968, Marsh et al 1987, Mendola et al 2002). Data about the associations between ID and low-level mercury exposure are limited and conflicting. Exposure to monomethyl mercury, found in fish, the most common source of mercury for humans, has been studied most and documented to be of greatest concern (Davidson et al 2004).

Birth defects

Some birth defects are known risk factors for ID. Data from metropolitan Atlanta found that 6.3% of children with a major birth defect had ID compared with 0.7% of children with no major birth defect for a prevalence ratio of 8.9 (Decoufle et al 2001). When children with a known isolated chromosomal birth defect were removed from the calculations, 5.4% of children with a major birth defect had ID yielding a prevalence ratio of 7.7. More specifically, these data showed that children with neural tube defects (NTDs) were 20 times more likely to have ID than those without an NTD. It is estimated that folate supplementation, when initiated before conception or very early in pregnancy, can prevent between 50%–70% of NTDs (Czeizel & Dudas 1992, MRC Vitamin Study Group 1991). While folic acid supplementation may not eliminate the occurrence of NTDs entirely, increasing compliance with the public health recommendation that all woman of childbearing age who are capable of becoming pregnant should consume 400 micrograms (400 µg or 0.4 mg) of folic acid daily will undoubtedly decrease the portion of ID prevalence attributable to NTDs. Data from 24 population-based birth defects surveillance systems in the USA found that the prevalence of spina bifida, which is highly associated with ID, decreased 31% from the pre-January 1995–December 1996 to mandatory October 1998–December 1999 fortification period (Williams et al 2002).

Perinatal risk factors

Well-documented and accepted perinatal risk factors for ID include low birth weight (LBW) (Cooke 1994, Hack et al 1994, Mervis et al 1995); perinatal asphyxia (Paneth & Stark 1983, Yeargin-Allsopp et al 1997); infection such as group B streptococcus (GBS) and human immunodeficiency virus (HIV) (CDC 1997); newborn endocrine and metabolic disorders (CDC 1999, Van Naarden Braun et al 2003) and multiple births (Boyle et al 1997, Croen et al 2001). Of the spectrum of developmental disabilities, cerebral palsy (CP) has the closest association with adverse perinatal events. Nevertheless, the high co-morbidity between CP and ID and the documented risk for ID in isolation warrant discussion.

Low birth weight and prematurity

Improvements in neonatal care in the past 3 decades have resulted in drastic increases in survival of lower birth weight and premature newborns. For example, before the 1980s, few newborns weighing less than 750 grams were treated and now intervention is accepted practice for most newborns weighing at least 500 grams (Hack et al 1994). Since low birth weight (<2500 grams) and preterm delivery (<37 weeks gestation) are widely accepted risk factors for ID, the impact of these birth characteristics is of concern. The majority of studies in the United States on the cognitive outcome of premature infants have been examined primarily in terms of birth weight due to poor completeness and reliability of data on gestational age obtained from birth certificates. In a nationwide study of very preterm and/or small for gestational age infants (<32 weeks and/or <1500 grams) born in the Netherlands, cognitive outcome at age 5 years was significantly worse for SGA infants than those of appropriate weight for gestational age and at 9 years significantly more SGA infants needed special education services (Kok et al 1998). Work by Goldenberg et al (1996) supported these findings in that both term SGA infants and those born at less than 34 weeks had significantly lower IQs and SGA infants had increased risk for ID at age 5 years.

Studies that have used birth weight as a metric have consistently shown an inverse relationship between birth weight and ID. That is, as birth weight increases, risk for ID decreases. Mervis et al (1995) found that in metropolitan Atlanta, LBW (<2500 grams) children had nearly 3 times the risk of ID as children of normal birth weight. The risk varied, however, between children with very low birth weight (VLBW) (<1500 grams) and children with moderately low birth weight (1500–2499 grams), with the highest risk among VLBW children. The risk was also greater for MPID than for MID. Children with normal birth weight (≥2500 grams) who were born preterm were also at increased risk of ID. Similar to the findings by Mervis et al (1995), Camp et al (1998) found that as many as 16.5% of infants with a birth weight of <2000 grams had ID at 7 years of age. Hack et al (1994) reported 21% of school-aged children born under 750 g had an IQ less than 70. At 5 years of age, Californian children who had been LBW had a more than threefold risk for MID (McDermott et al 1993). In the very large population-based study of Croen et al (2001), LBW was the strongest predictive factor for both MID and MPID of unknown cause. Most recently, Collier and Hogue (2007) estimated that in Georgia, 13% of cases of ID were attributable to low birth weight.

Perinatal asphyxia

Dating back to the late 1970s, perinatal asphyxia was thought to be a major contributor to ID and CP (Beard & Rivers 1979, Quilligan & Paul 1976). Difficulties with consistency in defining birth asphyxia, time interval between birth and establishment of spontaneous respiration or alternatively use of Apgar scores, have made epidemiologic comparison of the proportion of ID attributable to oxygen deprivation a challenge. Based on review of medical records in a population-based sample, Yeargin-Allsopp et al (1997) found that birth asphyxia accounted for about 5% of all ID. Infants who do experience ID as a result of perinatal asphyxia were likely to have had prolonged and severe asphyxia, and they are more likely to have had clinical evidence of moderate to severe neonatal encephalopathy (Murphy et al 1998, Nelson & Emery 1993, Paneth & Stark 1983, Robertson & Finer 1985).

Perinatal infection

The contribution of perinatal infections, including group B strep (GBS), HSV (described under prenatal infections), and HIV, to the prevalence of ID is small. In the 1970s, GBS was the leading cause of sepsis in newborns, but the Centers for Disease Control and Prevention (CDC) recommendation for GBS screening at 35–37 weeks gestation has dramatically reduced the incidence of this newborn infection. According to the Active Bacterial Core (ABC) Surveillance Report produced by the Emerging Infection Program Network of CDC, the rate of GBS infection has decreased from 1.2 cases per 1000 live-births in 1997 to 0.7 cases per 1000 live-births in 2004 (CDC 1997). Although HSV is transmitted during the perinatal period, it remains a low incidence condition and, therefore, is not a major contributor to the prevalence of ID (AAP 2003a).

The devastating HIV pandemic, particularly in developing countries, the high and increasing seroprevalence of HIV in women of childbearing age in high risk populations (20%–30%) and the association of central nervous system damage with HIV exposure in utero have caused HIV to emerge as an important cause of neurodevelopmental impairment in high risk populations (Chadwick & Yogev 1995, Wachtel & Conlon 1996). As newborn screening for HIV in some US states is mandatory, surveillance of pediatric HIV is becoming more systematic. Oleske (1994) reported that 5% of women delivering at major urban hospitals (such as hospitals in New York City) tested positive for HIV.

In 1994, antiretroviral therapy was proven effective when given to the mother during the last trimester and during labor and delivery and to the newborn for the first few weeks of life. Since then, the risk of vertical HIV transmission (from mother to child) has been reduced from 25% to less than 10% in developed countries; when combined with cesarean delivery the risk has dropped to as low as 2% (Durkin et al 2002). Unfortunately, in developing countries where prenatal services aren't available the risk remains much greater at 30%–40% (Durkin et al 2002). The advent of antiretroviral treatments for children with HIV necessitates further study on long-term developmental functioning and on the effect of antiretroviral treatment on the developing nervous system (Pearson et al 2000).

Metabolic and endocrine disorders

Newborns are routinely screened for metabolic and endocrine disorders. These disorders are primarily genetic disorders which would imply they are of prenatal origin. Yet, for many infants failure to identify and treat these disorders in the early neonatal period can result in ID. If identified and appropriate nutritional intervention is made and sustained, ID can be prevented. Therefore, metabolic and endocrine disorders such as phenylketonuria, homocystinuria, maple syrup urine disease, tyrosinemia, congenital hypothyroidism and galactosemia are discussed in the context of the perinatal period.

Epidemiologic data on the neurodevelopmental status of children who test positive on newborn screening for a metabolic or endocrine disorder are limited. Waisbren et al (2003) reported that children with biochemical disorders (including metabolic and endocrine) who are identified by newborn screening may experience fewer developmental problems and function significantly better in aspects of daily living than children identified clinically. In that study, 42% of children identified clinically had a score of less than 71 on the Mental Development Index of the Bayley Scale of Infant Development compared with 2% of children identified by newborn screening. Van Naarden Braun et al (2003) linked data from the Georgia newborn metabolic screening program with population-based surveillance data on school-age children with ID and found that newborn screening was effective in preventing ID associated with phenylketonuria, maple syrup urine disease, congenital hypothyroidism and galactosemia. These data underscored the effectiveness of the newborn screening program and the need for continued monitoring of the neurodevelopmental status of children who screen positive for a metabolic or endocrine disorder to maximize identification and intervention of this preventable cause of ID. It is unclear whether the increasing use of tandem mass spectrometry and the growing number of metabolic and endocrine disorders being added to the screening panel in the USA will result in a decrease in the prevalence of ID or more mild learning disorders because the neurodevelopmental outcomes associated with many of these newly added disorders is unknown.

Multiple births

Children born as multiples have been reported to have lower IQ than children born as singletons and are at an estimated two-fold risk of having ID. (Boyle et al 1997, Ronalds et al 2005). This increased risk appears to be due in large part to the shorter gestation and decreased birth weight of multiple births (Croen et al 2001). Recent studies have shown that the dramatic rise in use of assisted reproductive technology (ART) has increased the prevalence of multiple births (Wright et al 2007) which may contribute to a higher prevalence of ID. Bernasko et al (1997) reported no differences in the risk for obstetric complications or perinatal morbidity between twins conceived spontaneously compared with those conceived by ART. A meta-analysis by Bower and Hansen (2005) supported this finding among twins. However, they found an approximate twofold increase risk of perinatal mortality, low birth weight, and preterm birth; a 50% increase in small for gestational age; and 30%–35% increase

in birth defects among singletons conceived using ART compared with singletons conceived spontaneously. Schieve et al (2002) also found that among singleton infants born at 37 weeks or later, those conceived with ART had a 2.6 times higher risk of low birth weight (≤2500 grams) than the general population. Olson et al (2005) found a significantly higher risk of birth defects among children born to infertile couples conceived through in vitro fertilization and a non-significant increase among children conceived with the use of intrauterine insemination. Researchers have also found that unexplained infertility itself increases the risk for some obstetric complications such as intrauterine growth restriction during pregnancy (Isaksson et al 2002).

Postnatal etiology

Given our current understanding of etiology, ID is least likely to be caused by insult occurring in the postnatal period, but these causes are often preventable. Postnatal factors shown to be associated with ID include postnatally acquired infections (CDC 1996, Yeargin-Allsopp et al 1997), injuries (CDC 1996, Yeargin-Allsopp et al 1997), and environmental lead exposure (Mendola et al 2002, Needleman 1992a, 1992b).

Postnatal infection

Postnatally acquired meningitis is a known cause of ID in children and is associated with a number of infectious organisms, the three most common being *Haemophilus influenzae* type b (Hib), *Streptococcus pneumoniae* and *Neisseria meningitidis* (Baraff et al 1993). Hib used to be the leading cause of bacterial meningitis in children, but the conjugate Hib vaccine made available in 1988, and the recommendation by CDC in 1991 that all infants be vaccinated starting at age 2 months, caused a more than 99% decline in the incidence of Hib invasive disease among children younger than 5 years of age (CDC 2002). Because bacterial meningitis may be caused by a variety of organisms, this drop in Hib infection does not ensure a drastic reduction in ID caused by bacterial meningitis. Baraff et al (1993) examined studies of outcomes from bacterial meningitis in children 2 months of age or older caused by one of the three most common organisms and found that ID occurred among 2.1% of children with *Neisseria*; 6.1% of children with Hib; and 17% of children infected with *Streptococcus pneumoniae*. In a study examining developmental disabilities in children aged 3–10 years in 1991 in metropolitan Atlanta, bacterial meningitis accounted for 30% of cases of postnatally acquired ID (CDC 1996). Pneumococcal vaccine is now also recommended for all children 23 months of age and younger (CDC 2000b). The incidence of *Streptococcus pneumoniae* infections in young children is decreasing; however, there have been outbreaks of the disease in childcare settings (CDC *Streptococcus pneumoniae* Disease Fact Sheet, 2003).

Injury

Head injury is another major, preventable postnatal cause of ID. Data on 10-year-old children with ID in metropolitan

Atlanta in 1985–1987 showed that of those with a known etiology, 17% had a postnatal cause; of those, 23% had a head injury as the cause of their ID (Yeargin-Allsopp et al 1997). A subsequent study in metropolitan Atlanta on 3 to 10-year-old children in 1991 found that 56% of postnatally acquired ID was caused by injuries, making injuries the largest contributor, greater than infectious and chronic diseases (CDC 1996). Of the injuries reported in this subsequent Atlanta study, child battering was the most frequent cause (18%), followed by being hit by a motor vehicle (9%) and falls (8%). Bacterial meningitis, stroke (primarily related to sickle cell disease), near drownings, motor vehicle crashes and brain tumors accounted for 30%, 7%, 4%, 4% and 1% respectively (CDC 1996). Ashley-Koch et al (2001) reported a statistically significant association between sickle cell disease and ID in a population of metropolitan Atlanta school children, which was attributable almost entirely to the occurrence of stroke. Sickle cell disease contributed to 0.4% of ID in black children in that population (Ashley-Koch et al 2001).

Postnatal environmental toxins

Exposure to an environmental agent such as lead in the postnatal period has neurotoxic effects on the developing central nervous system (CDC 2003b, Mendola et al 2002). ID is recognized as one of the most devastating long-term and irreversible outcomes of high blood lead levels ($\geq$60 micrograms per deciliter (μg/dL)) in childhood. A series of prospective studies in communities in a wide spectrum of geographic locations and socioeconomic and ethnic backgrounds have consistently shown that, depending on the age under study, low levels of lead exposure (increase of 10–30 μg/dL) are associated with a 4 to 7-point decrease in IQ scores after adjusting for confounding sociodemographic factors (Baghurst et al 1992, Bellinger et al 1992, Dietrich et al 1993, McMichael et al 1985, Wasserman et al 2000). Although the number of children with confirmed elevated blood lead levels ($\geq$10 μg/dL) has steadily declined significantly over the last 50 years, this preventable cause of ID remains a serious public health concern. The proportion of children aged 6 years and younger with confirmed blood lead levels greater than the current cutoff for defining lead toxicity ($\geq$10 μg/dL) was 3.1% in 2001 across 44 states in the United States, the District of Columbia and New York City (Meyer et al 2003). It is important to note that the rate of decline in childhood blood levels has been disproportionately lower among minority, often urban, lower socioeconomic subgroups of the population, which highlights the need for targeted intervention in these populations (Durkin et al 2002).

The relationship between cognitive deficits and postnatal exposure to PCBs has also been examined. Stewart et al (2003) found differences in cognitive development among children exposed to PCBs at age 38 months; however when reassessed 1.5 years later, children with high PCB exposure caught up to those with lower levels of exposure by 54 months. Jacobson and Jacobson (1996) studied 11-year-olds who had postnatal exposure to PCBs through breastfeeding or through usual environmental levels during childhood and did not find PCB exposure to be significantly associated with poor IQ, achievement measures or ID.

There are concerns that ID and other developmental disabilities are associated with postnatal organic mercury exposure (methyl and ethylmercury). The concern about postnatal methylmercury exposure has been primarily related to fish consumption while that of postnatal ethylmercury exposure has been related to vaccinations preserved with small amounts of thimerosal which is composed of 49% ethylmercury (Davidson et al 2004). Further investigations on the range of developmental effects, if any, associated with postnatal mercury exposure are needed (Myers & Davidson 2000).

TRANSITION INTO ADULTHOOD

The majority of epidemiologic research on ID has focused on prevalence, risk factors and etiology with limited population-based data on the consequences of ID in adulthood. It is clear from the data we have presented in this chapter that genetic and non-genetic influences in the early stages of life, from the prenatal period through school-age, can have a significant and lasting impact on an individual's cognitive functioning. Nevertheless, the assumption that there is a one-to-one correlation with negative outcomes as these children reach young adulthood may not be valid. By examining the epidemiology of ID within the conceptual framework of a life stages approach we can attempt to evaluate this assumption and identify modifiable factors to help individuals with ID in reaching their full potential in society. Therefore, we feel that it is crucial to discuss the epidemiology of the consequences of ID as children transition to young adulthood.

Transition from adolescence to adulthood is a gradual process of assuming new and different adult social roles that can be challenging for all young adults. The acquisition of normative adult social roles is particularly difficult for young adults with a history of developmental disabilities, specifically ID (Affleck et al 1990, Blackorby & Wagner 1996, Cooper & Lackus 1984, Haring & Lovett 1990, Rantakallio 1987, Richardson & Koller 1996). While the types of adult roles differ across various countries and cultures, in the United States, being competitively employed, attending postsecondary education, and being a caregiver are considered the three normative social roles of young adulthood (Arnett 1997, Cohen et al 2003, Greene et al 1992).

Two major population-based studies conducted in the United States have examined attainment of various markers of transition: the National Longitudinal Transition Study of Special Education Students (NLTS) and the Metropolitan Atlanta Developmental Disabilities Study Follow-up of Young Adults (MADDS Follow-Up). The NLTS consisting of more than 8000 students ages 13–21 receiving special education services in secondary school in 1985 used a two-wave longitudinal design (data collection in 1987 and 1990) to examine the characteristics of youth and their educational experiences, social activities, post-school employment, independence and use of adult services. Changes in four main outcome areas – employment, wages, post-secondary schooling, and residential living – were examined at the two time periods in a subset of this cohort that had left secondary school at the time of the first wave of data collection. Using data from the NLTS, Blackorby and Wagner (1996) reported that among young adults whose primary disability category was ID 25% were competitively employed 3–5 years after high school (second follow-up time period), 10% were earning more than $6/hour, 8% were attending postsecondary school, and 4% were living independently compared with 57%, 40%, 27% and 37%, respectively, among all young adults receiving special education. Although slight improvements were seen across these outcomes between the two follow-up periods for young adults with ID, the only statistically significant finding was the increase in the proportion of young adults with ID who were living independently which rose from 4% to 24%. The MADDS Follow-Up Study was conducted with young adults aged 21–25 years ($n = 635$) who were identified as having one of five developmental disabilities, including ID, at age 10 in the metropolitan Atlanta area in 1985–1987. This study captured similar adult social role outcomes including competitive employment and post-secondary education as well as caregiving and other types of vocational or educational activities specific to young adults with ID. All young adults with ID in this study had an IQ of 70 or less at age 10 years, and subsequent analyses examined these young adults in three subgroups: MPID (IQ < 50) with other developmental disabilities (DDs), isolated MPID (no other developmental disabilities identified by MADDS), and isolated MID (IQ 50–70). Researchers found that 3% of young adults with MPID with other DDs, 14% of those with isolated MPID, and 49% with isolated MID were competitively employed compared with 46% of young adults with any DD identified by the MADDS FU and 86% of those without a DD (Van Naarden Braun et al 2006a). These data emphasize the importance of considering the presence of co-existing DDs as well as severity of ID. Fewer than 2% of young adults with any type of ID were attending post-secondary school and fewer than 4% of those with MPID with or without another DD reported being caregivers. After controlling for social and demographic factors, young adults with ID regardless of severity or the presence of co-existing DDs were significantly less likely than young adults without a DD to acquire one of the three measured normative adult social roles. The MADDS Follow-Up Study showed some encouraging data. A sizable proportion of the young adults with MPID (33% for isolated MPID and 37% for MPID with other DDs) who had not acquired one of the three adult social roles were participating in a DD-related vocational or educational program, such as supported employment, a sheltered workshop or a day activity program (Van Naarden Braun et al 2006a). In addition to examining the frequency of attaining these transition outcomes, Van Naarden Braun et al (2006a) tested the mediating effects of daily functioning and found that prevention of limitations in activities of daily living (ADLs) and instrumental activities of daily living (IADLs) for young adults with ID may increase the probability of being competitively employed, attending post-secondary school or being a caregiver. This finding was most pronounced among young adults with MPID, but it was significant for young adults with isolated MID. While accounting for activity limitations lessened the strength of association between MPID and these negative outcomes, the likelihood of young adults with MPID not attaining a normative adult social role remained high.

Obtaining a complete understanding of the epidemiology of ID throughout the life stages is crucial not only to improving education and vocational opportunities for young adults with ID, but also in addressing factors that affect quality of life. Participation in leisure activity is an important measure of quality of life and commonly reflects social interaction (Dattilo & Schleien 1994). Because an individual's free time is not valued as highly as time devoted to employment, little epidemiologic data are available on the characteristics and factors influencing a wide range of leisure activities. Previous data from the MADDS Follow-Up Study demonstrated that young adults with MPID, regardless of the presence of co-existing DDs, were significantly less likely to acquire an adult social role and that young adults with isolated MID were more similar in their transition outcomes to those with other isolated types of DDs (Van Naarden Braun et al 2006a). Based on the notion that the acquisition of markers of young adulthood is positively correlated with a wider range and number of leisure activities, the authors expected to find a similar severity gradient with participation in leisure activities among young adults with ID (Van Naarden Braun et al 2006b). Instead, data from the MADDS Follow-Up Study supported that it is the presence of co-existing DDs that exacerbates restrictions in leisure activity rather than the presence of MPID.

Healthy lifestyles and indicators greatly contribute to an individual's quality of life. Several studies have reported a high prevalence of overweight and obesity among adults with ID (Bell & Bhate 1992, Fernhall 1993, Horwitz et al 2000, Rimmer et al 1993, Suzuki et al 1991). Rimmer et al (1993) and Rurangirwa et al (2006) specifically found this association among adults with MPID. Individuals with ID have also been reported to be more likely to lead sedentary lifestyles and to have poorer muscular fitness and muscular strength than their counterparts without developmental disabilities (Bandini et al 1991, Bell & Bhate 1992, Pitetti et al 1993, Rimmer et al 1993, Stallings et al 1995, 1996, Suzuki et al 1991, Van den Berg-Emons et al 1995, 1998). Rurangirwa et al (2006) reported that young adults with isolated ID were significantly more likely to have been attacked or beaten in the past 12 months and less likely to have used tobacco or alcohol than young adults without a history of DD.

CONCLUSION

The field of epidemiology has contributed significantly to our understanding of ID. Monitoring of the prevalence and characteristics of ID has identified subgroups of the population at greater risk for ID for further investigation into specific etiologies. Surveillance of ID continues to be a necessary activity as standardized data on functioning become increasingly systematically available in administrative records, the frequency of prenatal identification of syndromes associated with ID and subsequent terminations increases, molecular and biomedical advances continue, and genetic etiologies are identified. In addition, the development and refinement of methods to examine gene–environment interactions provide new opportunities to apply epidemiology to this area. All of these factors, and others discussed in this chapter, may change the landscape and provide a better understanding of the epidemiology of ID which, in turn, may result in better prevention strategies and guidance for providing effective medical and education services for individuals with ID.

As environmental and societal influences for individuals with ID change, epidemiologic research needs to explore the current status of children with ID as they transition into adulthood, giving analytic consideration of the severity of ID and the presence of co-existing conditions. In addition, further epidemiologic analyses are needed to understand education and health care use among individuals with ID so that the most appropriate services and programs can be established. As these surveillance and research activities are developed, the methodologic issues raised in this chapter need to be carefully considered and addressed, but not deemed prohibitive in order for progress in understanding the epidemiology of ID to continue on its current encouraging trajectory.

REFERENCES

AAIDD (American Association of Intellectual and Developmental Disabilities) 2007 Retrieved on March 13, 2007 from: http://www.aamr.org/About_AAIDD/MR_name_change.htm

AAP (American Academy of Pediatrics) 2003a *Haemophilus influenzae* infections. In: Pickering L K (ed.) Redbook: 2003 Report of the Committee on Infectious Diseases, 26th edn. American Academy of Pediatrics, Elk Grove Village, IL.

AAP (American Academy of Pediatrics) 2003b Herpes simplex. In: Pickering L K (ed.) Redbook: 2003 Report of the Committee on Infectious Diseases, 26th edn. American Academy of Pediatrics, Elk Grove Village, IL, pp. 344–345.

AAP (American Academy of Pediatrics) 2003c Group B streptococcal infections. In: Pickering L K (ed.) Redbook: 2003 Report of the Committee on Infectious Diseases, 26th edn. American.

Abel E L 1995 An update on incidence of FAS: FAS is not an equal opportunity birth defect. Neurotoxicol Teratol 17:437–443. Academy of Pediatrics, Elk Grove Village, IL.

ACOG (American College of Obstetrics and Gynecology) 2007 Screening for fetal chromosomal abnormalities. ACOG Practice Bulletin. Obs Gynecol 109:217–227.

Adams J, Voorhees C V, Middaugh L D 1990 Developmental neurotoxicity of anticonvulsants: human and animal evidence on phenytoin. Neurotox Teratol 12:203–214.

Affleck J Q, Edgar E, Levine P, Kortering L 1990 Postschool status of students classified as mildly mentally retarded, learning disabled, or nonhandicapped: Does it get better with time? Education and Training of the Mentally Retarded 25:315–324.

Ahsan H, Hodge S E, Heiman G A et al Relative risk for genetic associations: The case-parent triad as a variant of case-cohort design. Inter J Epidemiol 31(3):669–678.

APA (American Psychiatric Association) 1980 Diagnostic and statistical manual of mental disorder, 3rd edn. American Psychiatric Association, Washington, DC.

APA (American Psychiatric Association) 1987 Diagnostic and statistical manual of mental disorder, 3rd edn.(rev) (DSM II-IV). American Psychiatric Association, Washington, DC.

APA (American Psychiatric Association) 1994 Diagnostic and statistical manual of mental disorders, (DSM-IV), 4th edn. American Psychiatric Association, Washington, DC.

Arnett J J 1997 Young people's conceptions of the transition into adulthood. Youth Society 29:1–23.

Ashley-Koch A, Murphy C C, Khoury M J, Boyle C A 2001 Contribution of sickle cell disease to the occurrence of developmental disabilities: A population-based study. Genetics in Medicine 3:181–186.

August G J, Stewart M A, Tsai L 1981 The incidence of cognitive disabilities in the siblings of autistic children. Br J Psych 138:416–442.

Autism and Developmental Disabilities Monitoring Network-2002 Surveillance Year. Multiple-Source Surveillance of Intellectual Disability in 5 U.S. States, in preparation.

Baghurst P A, McMichael A J, Wigg N R et al 1992 Environmental exposure to lead and children's intelligence at the age of seven years. The Port Pirir Cohort Study. New Eng J Med 327:1279–1284.

Bandini L G, Schoeller D A, Fukagawa N K et al 1991 Body composition and energy expenditure in adolescents with cerebral palsy or myelodysplasia. Pediatric Research 29(1):70–77.

Baraff L J, Lee S I, Schriger D L 1993 Outcomes of bacterial meningitis in children: a meta-analysis. Pediat Infect Dis J 12:389–394.

Beard R W, Rivers R P 1979 Fetal asphyxia in labor. Lancet 2:1117.

Bell A J, Bhate M S 1992 Prevalence of overweight and obesity in Down's syndrome and other mentally handicapped adults living in the community. J Intell Dis Res 36(Pt 4):359–364.

Bellinger D C, Stiles K M, Needleman H L 1992 Low-level lead exposure, intelligence and academic achievement: A long-term follow-up study. Pediatrics 90:855–861.

Bernasko J, Lynch L, Lapinski R, Berkowitz R L 1997 Twin pregnancies conceived by assisted reproductive techniques: Maternal and neonatal outcomes. Obstet Gynecol 89:368–372.

Bertrand J, Floyd R L, Weber M K 2005 Guidelines for identifying and referring persons with fetal alcohol syndrome. Morbidity and Mortality Weekly Report 54(RR11):1–10.

Birch H G, Richardson S A, Baird D, Horobin G 1970 Illsley. Mental subnormality in the community. Williams & Wilkins, Baltimore.

Blackorby J, Wagner M 1996 Longitudinal postschool outcomes of youth with disabilities: Findings from the National Longitudinal Transition Study. Exceptional Children 62:399–413.

Boulet S, Schieve L, Boyle C. Trends in health care utilization and health impact of developmental disabilities in US children, 1997–2005. (in preparation.)

Bower C, Hansen M 2005 Assisted reproductive technologies and birth outcomes: overview of recent systematic reviews. Reprod Fertil Dev 17:329–333.

Boyer K M, Holfels E, Rozien N et al 2005 Risk factors for *Toxoplasma gondii* infection in mothers of infants with congenital toxoplasmosis: Implication for prenatal management and screening. Am J Obs Gyn 192:564–571.

Boyle C A, Keddie A, Holmgreen P 1997 The risk of mental retardation in twins. Paed Perinatal Epidemiol 11:A10.

Boyle C A, Yeargin-Allsopp M, Doernberg N et al 1996 Prevalence of selected developmental disabilities in children aged 3–10 years: The Metropolitan Atlanta Developmental Disabilities Surveillance Program, 1991. MMWR Surveillance Summary 45(No. SS-2):1–14.

Broman S, Nichols P L, Shaughnessy P, Kennedy W 1987 Retardation in young children: a developmental study of cognitive development. Lawrence Erlbaum Associates, Hillsdale, NJ.

Bundey S, Carter C O 1974 Recurrence risks in severe undiagnosed mental deficiency. J Ment Defic Res 18:115–134.

Bundey S, Thake A, Todd J 1989 The recurrence risks for mild idiopathic mental retardation.

Camp B W, Borman S H, Nichols P L 1998 Maternal and neonatal risk factors for mental retardation: defining the 'at risk' child. Early Hum Develop 50:159–173.

Cans C, Wilhelm L, Baille M F et al 1999 Aetiological findings and associated factors in children with severe mental retardation. Develop Med Child Neurol 41:233–239.

CDC (Centers for Disease Control and Prevention) 1996 Postnatal causes of developmental disabilities in children aged 3–10 years–Atlanta, Georgia, 1991. Morbidity and Mortality Weekly Report, 45, 130–134.

CDC (Centers for Disease Control and Prevention) 1997 Decreasing incidence of perinatal group B streptococcal disease. United States, 1993–1995. Morbidity and Mortality Weekly Report 46:473–477.

CDC (Centers for Disease Control and Prevention) 1999 Mental retardation following diagnosis of a metabolic disorder in children aged 3–10 years–metropolitan Atlanta, Georgia, 1991–1994. Morbidity and Mortality Weekly Report 48:353–356.

CDC (Centers for Disease Control and Prevention) 2000a Measles, rubella, and congenital rubella syndrome–United States and Mexico, 1997–1999. Morbidity and Mortality Weekly Report 49:1048–1050.

CDC (Centers for Disease Control and Prevention) 2000b Preventing pneumococcal disease among infants and young children: recommendations of the Advisory Committee on Immunization Practices (ACIP). Morbidity and Mortality Weekly Report, 49:1–35.

CDC (Centers for Disease Control and Prevention) 2001 Congenital syphilis — United States, 2000. Morbidity and Mortality Weekly Report, 50:573–577.

CDC (Centers for Disease Control and Prevention) 2002 Progress toward elimination of Haemophilus influenzae type B invasive disease among infants and children–United States 1998–2000. Morbidity and Mortality Weekly Report 51(11):234–237.

CDC (Centers for Disease Control and Prevention) 2003a Division of Bacterial and Mycotic Disease Information. Streptococcus pneumoniae disease. Retrieved March 5, 2005, from http://www.cdc.gov/ncidod/dbmd/diseaseinfo/streppneum_t.htm

CDC (Centers for Disease Control and Prevention) 2003b Surveillance Summaries: Surveillance for elevated blood lead levels among children — United States, 1997–2001. Morbidity and Mortality Weekly Report,, 52. No. SS-10.

CDC (Centers for Disease Control and Prevention) 2005a Achievements in public health: Elimination of rubella and congenital rubella syndrome–United States, 1969–2004, Morbidity and Mortality Weekly Report 54(11):279–282.

CDC (Centers for Disease Control and Prevention) 2005b Sexually Transmitted Disease Surveillance 2004 Supplement, syphilis surveillance report. Retrieved [November 15, 2006], from http://www.cdc.gov/std/Syphilis2004/SyphSurvSupp2004.pdf

Chadwick E G, Yogev R 1995 Pediatric AIDS. Ped Clin N Am 42:969–992.

Chelly J, Mandel J L 2001 Monogenic causes of X-linked mental retardation. Nature Rev: Gen 2:669–680.

Chen Y-C J, Guo Y-L, Hsu C-C 1992 Cognitive development of Yu-Cheng ('Oil Disease') children prenatally exposed to heat-degraded PCBs. J Am Med Ass 268:3213–3218.

Chiurazzi P, Hamel B C, Neri G 2000 XLMR genes: Update 2000. Euro J Human Gen 9:71–81.

Cohen P, Kasen S, Chen H et al 2003 Variations in patterns of developmental transitions in the emerging adulthood period. Develop Psychol 39:657–659.

Collier S A, Hogue C J R 2007 Modifiable risk factors for low birth weight and their effect on cerebral palsy and mental retardation. Maternal and Child Health J 11:65–71.

Cooke R W I 1994 Factors affecting survival and outcome at 3 years in extremely preterm infants. Arch Dis Child 71 F28–F31.

Cooper B, Lackus B 1984 The social class background of mentally retarded children: A study in Mannheim. Soc Psych 19:3–12.

Costeff H, Weller L 1987 The risk of having a second retarded child. Am J Med Gen 27:753–766.

Couvert P, Bienvenu T, Aquaviva C et al 2001 MECP2 is highly mutated in X-linked mental retardation. Hum Mol Genet 10:941–946.

Crawford D C, Meadows K L, Newman J L et al 2002 Prevalence of the fragile X syndrome in African-Americans. Am J Med Genet 110:226–233.

Croen L A, Grether J K, Selvin S 2001 The epidemiology of mental retardation of unknown cause. Pediatrics 107:E86.

Cunniff C, Committee on Genetics 2004 Prenatal screening and diagnosis for pediatricians. Pediatrics 114:889–894.

Czeizel A E, Dudas I 1992 Prevention of first occurrence of neural tube defects by peri-conceptional vitamin supplementation. New Eng J Med 327:1832–1835.

Dattilo J, Schleien S J 1994 Understanding leisure services for individuals with mental retardation. Mental Retardation 32:53–59.

Davidson P W, Myers J, Weiss B 2004 Mercury exposure and child development outcomes. Pediatrics 113(4):1023–1027.

Dean J C S, Hailey H, Moore S J et al 2002 Long term health and neurodevelopment in children exposed to antiepileptic drugs before birth. J Med Genet 39:251–259.

Decoufle P, Autry A 2002 Increased mortality in children and adolescents with developmental disabilities. Paed Perinatal Epidemiol 16(4):375–382.

Decoufle P, Boyle C A 1995 The relationship between maternal education and mental retardation in 10-year old children. Ann Epidemiol 5:347–353.

Decoufle P, Boyle C A, Paulozzi L, Lary J 2001 Increased risk for developmental disabilities in children who have major birth defects: A population-based study. Pediatrics 108:728–734.

Demmler G J 2005 Screening for congenital cytomegalovirus infection: A tapestry of controversies. J Pediatrics 146:162–164.

Diaz-Fernandez F 1988 Descriptive epidemiology of registered mentally retarded persons in.

Dietrich K N, Berger O, Succop P 1993 Lead exposure and the motor developmental status of urban six year old children in the Cincinnati Prospective Study. Pediatrics 91:301–307.

Drane D L, Meador K J 1996 Epilepsy, anticonvulsant drugs and cognition. Baillieres Clin Neurol 5:877–885.

Drews C D, Murphy C C, Yeargin-Allsopp M, Decoufle P 1996 The relationship between idiopathic mental retardation and maternal smoking during pregnancy. Pediatrics 97:547–553.

Drews C D, Yeargin-Allsopp M, Decoufle P, Murphy C C 1995 Variation in the influence of selected sociodemographic risk factors for mental retardation. Am J Pub Health 85:329–334.

Durkin M S, Schupf N, Stein Z A, Susser M W 2002 Epidemiology of mental retardation. In: Levene M I, Chervenak F A, Whittle M (eds) Fetal and Neonatal Neurology and Neurosurgery, 3rd edn. Churchill Livingstone, Edinburgh.

Fernell E 1998 Aetiological factors and prevalence of severe mental retardation in children in a Swedish municipality: The possible role of consanguinity. Develop Med Child Neurol 40:608–611.

Fernhall B 1993 Physical fitness and exercise training of individuals with mental retardation. Medicine Science Sports Exercise 25(4):442–450.

Flint J, Wilkie A O M 1996 The genetics of mental retardation. Br Med Bull 52:453–464.

Fowler K B, Stagnos S, Paas R F et al 1992 The outcome of congenital cytomegalovirus infection in relation to maternal antibody status. New Eng J Med 326:663–667.

Galicia (northwest Spain). Am J Mental Retard 92:385–392.

Gilbert R, Dunn D, Wallon M et al 2001 Ecological comparison of the risks of mother-to-child transmission and clinical manifestations of congenital toxoplasmosis according to prenatal treatment period. Epidemiol Infect 127:113–120.

Gissler M, Jarvelin M R, Louhiala P 1999 Boys have more health problems in childhood than girls: Follow-up of the 1987 Finnish birth cohort. Acta Paediatrica 88:310–314.

Goldenberg R L, DuBard M B, Cliver S P et al 1996 Pregnancy outcome and intelligence at age five years. Am J Obstet Gynecol 175:1511–1515.

Greene A L, Wheatley S M, Aldava J F 1992 Stages on life's way: Adolescents' implicit theories of life course. J Adolescent Res 7:364–381.

Hack M, Taylor H G, Klein N et al 1994 School-age outcomes in children with birth weights under 750 g. New Eng J Med 331:753–759.

Haddow J E, Palomaki G E, Allan W C et al 1999 Maternal thyroid deficiency during pregnancy and subsequent neuropsychological development of the child. New Eng J Med 341:549–555.

Hagberg B 1987 Pre- and perinatal environmental origin of mild mental retardation. Uppsala J Med Sci 44(Suppl):178–182.

Hagberg B, Kyllerman M 1983 Epidemiology of mental retardation–A Swedish survey. Brain Develop 5:441–449.

Hansen H, Belmont L, Stein Z 1980 Epidemiology. Mental Retard Develop Dis 11:21–54.

Hanson J W 1986 Teratogen update: Fetal hydantoin effects. Teratol 33(3):349–353.

Harada Y 1968 Congenital (or fetal) Minamata disease. In: Study Group of Minamata Disease (eds) Minamata disease. Kumamoto University, Kumamoto, Japan, pp. 93–118.

Haring K A, Lovett D L 1990 A follow-up study of special education graduates. J Special Edu 23:463–477.

Herbst D S, Baird P A 1982 Sib risks for nonspecific mental retardation in British Columbia. Am J Med Gen 13:197–208.

Hetzel B S 1983 Iodine deficiency disorders (IDD) and their eradication. Lancet 2:1126–1128.

Hetzel B S 1989 The story of iodine deficiency: An international challenge in nutrition. Oxford University Press, Oxford.

Holmes L B, Coull B A, Dorfman J, Rosenberger P 2005 The correlation of deficits in IQ with midface and digit hypoplasia in children exposed in utero to anticonvulsant drugs. J Pediat 146(1):118–122.

Holmes L B, Wyszynski D F, Baldwin E J et al 2006 Increased risk for non-syndromic cleft palate among infants exposed to lamotrigine during pregnancy (abstract). Birth Defects Research Part A: Clin Molecular Teratol 76(5):318.

Honeycutt A, Dunlap L, Chen H et al 2004 Economic costs associated with mental retardation, cerebral palsy, hearing loss and vision impairment–United States, 2003. Morbidity and Mortality Weekly Report 53(3):57–59.

Horwitz S M, Kerker B D, Owens P L, Zigler E 2000 Physical health conditions contributing to morbidity and mortality of individuals with mental retardation. In: Health status and needs of individuals with mental retardation. Special Olympics Inc. 29–57. Retrieved March 16, 2007, from http://www.specialolympics.org/NR/rdonlyres/e5lq5czkjv5vwulp5lx5tmny4mcwhyj5vq6euizrooqcaekeuvmkg75fd6wnj62nhlsprlb7tg4gwqtu4xffauxzsge/healthstatus_needs.pdf

Hou J W, Wang T R, Chuang S M 1998 An epidemiological and aetiological study of children with intellectual disability in Taiwan. J Intel Dis Res 42:137–143. http://www.who.int/nutrition/publications/en/idd_assessment_monitoring_eliminination.pdf

International Classification of Diseases 1988 Clinical Modification (ICD-9CM), 9th edn. (rev.). Public Health Service, US. Dept of Health and Human Service, Washington, DC.

Isaksson R, Gissler M, Tiitinen A 2002 Obstetric outcome among women with unexplained fertility after IVF: A matched case control study. Human Repro 17:1755–1761.

Islam S, Durkin M S, Zaman S S 1993 Socioeconomic status and the prevalence of mental retardation in Bangladesh. Ment Retard 31(6):412–417. J Med Gen 26:260–266.

Jacobson J L, Jacobson S W 1996 Intellectual impairment in children exposed to polychlorinated biphenyls in utero. New Eng J Med 333:783–789.

Jacobson J L, Jacobson S W 1997 Teratogen update: Polychlorinated biphenyls. Teratology 55:338–347.

Jones K I 1997 Smith's recognizable patterns of human malformation, 5th edn. WB Saunders, Philadelphia.

Jones K L, Adams J, Chambers C D et al 2001 Isotretinoin and pregnancy. J Am Med Ass 285:2079–2081.

Karapurkar Bhasin T, Brockson S, Nonkin Avchen R, Van Naarden Braun K 2006 Prevalence of four developmental disabilities in 8-year-old children: Metropolitan Atlanta Developmental Disabilities Surveillance Program, 1996 and 2000. Morbidity and Mortality Weekly Report 55(SS1):1–9.

Khoury M J 1994 Case-parental control methods in the search for disease susceptibility genes. Am J Human Gen 55:414–415.

Kiely M 1987 The prevalence of mental retardation. Epidemiol Rev 9:194–218.

Klein R Z, Mitchell ML 2002 Maternal hypothyroidism and cognitive development of the offspring. Current Opinion in Pediatrics. 14:443–446.

Kline J, Stein Z, Susser M 1989 Conception to birth: Epidemiology of prenatal development. Oxford University Press, New York.

Kok J H, den Ouden A L, Verloove-Vanhorick S P, Brand R 1998 Outcome of very preterm small for gestational age infants: The first nine years of life. Br J Obst Gynaecol 105:162–168.

LaFranchi S H, Haddow J E, Hollowell J G 2005 Is thyroid inadequacy during gestation a risk factors for adverse pregnancy and developmental outcomes? Thyroid 15:60–71.

Lenke R R, Levy H L 1980 Maternal phenylketonuria and hyperphenylalaninemia. An international survey of the outcome of untreated and treated pregnancies. New Eng J Med 303(21):1202–1208.

Leonard H, Petterson B, Bower C, Sanders R 2003 Prevalence of intellectual disability in Western Australia. Paed Perinatal Epidemiol 17:58–67.

Leonard H, Wen X 2002 The epidemiology of mental retardation: Challenges and opportunities in the new millennium. In: Yeargin-Allsopp M, Boyle C (eds) The epidemiology of neurodevelopmental Disabilities. Mental Retardation and Developmental

Disabilities Research Reviews, 8(117–134) Wiley Liss, New York.

Lonky E, Reihman J, Darvill T et al 1996 Neonatal Behavioral Assessment Scale performance in humans influenced by maternal consumption of environmentally contaminated Lake Ontario fish. J Great Lakes Research 22:198–212.

Lubs H, Chiurazzi P, Arena J et al 1999 XLMR genes: Update 1998. Am J Med Gen 83:237–247.

Luckasson R, Coulter D L, Polloway E A et al 1992 Mental retardation: Definition, classification and levels of supports. American Association on Mental Retardation, Washington, DC.

Luckasson R, Coulter D L, Polloway E A et al 2002 Mental retardation: Definition, classification and systems of supports. American Association on Mental Retardation, Washington, DC.

McDermott S, Cokert A L, McKeown R E 1993 Low birthweight and risk of mild mental retardation by ages 5 and 9 to 11. Paed Perinatal Epidemiol 7:195–204.

McDermott S, Daguise V, Mann H et al 2001 Perinatal risk for mortality and mental retardation associated with maternal urinary tract infections. J Fam Pract 50:433–437.

McLaren J, Bryson S E 1987 Review of recent epidemiological studies of mental retardation: prevalence, associated disorders, and etiology. Am J Ment Retard 92:243–254.

McMichael A J, Baghurst P A, Robertson E F et al 1985 The Port Pirie cohort study: Blood lead concentrations in early childhood. Med J Australia 143:499–503.

Malone F, Canick J A, Ball RH et al 2005 First trimester or second trimester screening, or both, for Down's syndrome. New Eng J Med 353:2001–2011.

Marsh D O, Clarkson T W, Cox C et al 1987 Fetal methylmercury poisoning: Relationship between concentration in single strands of maternal hair and child effects. Arch Neurol 44:1017–1022.

Meador K J, Baker G A, Finnell R H et al (for the NEAD Study Group) 2006 In utero antiepileptic drug exposure: Fetal death and malformations. Neurology 67:407–412.

Mendola P, Selevan S, Gutter S, Rice D 2002 Environmental factors associated with a spectrum of neurodevelopmental deficits. In: Yeargin-Allsopp M, Boyle C (eds) The epidemiology of neurodevelopmental disabilities. Mental Retardation and Developmental Disabilities Research Reviews, 8. Wiley Liss, New York, 3, pp. 188–197.

Mercer J R 1973 Labeling the mentally retarded. University of California Press, Berkeley.

Mervis C A, Decoufle P, Murphy C C, Yeargin-Allsopp M 1995 Low birthweight and the risk for mental retardation later in childhood. Paed Perinatal Epidemiol 9:455–468.

Meyer P A, Pivetz T, Dignam T A et al 2003 Surveillance for elevated blood lead levels among children–United States, 1997–2001. Morbidity and Mortality Weekly Report 52:1–21.

Morris J K, Wald N J, Mutton D E, Alberman E 2003 Comparison of models of maternal age-specific risk for Down syndrome live-births. Prenatal Diagnosis 23:252–258.

MRC Vitamin Study Group 1991 Prevention of neural tube defects: results from the Medical Research Council vitamin study. Lancet 338:1–137.

Munro J D 1986 Epidemiology and the extent of mental retardation. Psych Persp Men Retard 9(4):591–624.

Murphy C C, Boyle C, Schendel D et al 1998 Epidemiology of mental retardation in children.

Murphy C C, Yeargin-Allsopp M, Decoufle P, Drews C 1995 The administrative prevalence of mental

retardation in 10-year-old children in metropolitan Atlanta, 1985 through 1987. Am J Public Health, 5(85):319–323.

Myers G J, Davidson P W 2000 Does methylmercury have a role in causing developmental disabilities in children? Environmental Health Perspectives Supplements 108(3):413–419.

Naessens A, Casteels A, Decatte L, Foulon W 2005 A serologic strategy for detecting neonates at risk for congenital cytomegalovirus infection. J Pediatrics 146(2):194–203.

National Center for Infectious Diseases 2002 Cytomegalovirus (CMV) infection. Retrieved November 21, 2006, from http://www.cdc.gov/ncidod/diseases/cmv.htm

National Center on Birth Defects and Developmental Disabilities 2004a Risk factors for Down syndrome. Retrieved November 21, 2006, from http://www.cdc.gov/ncbddd/bd/ds.htm.

National Center on Birth Defects and Developmental Disabilities 2004b How common is fetal alcohol syndrome? Retrieved November 21, 2006 from website, from Atlanta, GA: Centers for Disease Control and Prevention. Website: http://www.cdc.gov/ncbddd/fas/fasask.htm#how

Needleman H (ed.) 1992a Low level lead exposure: the clinical implications of current research. Raven Press, New York.

Needleman H 1992b Human lead exposure. CRC, Boca Raton.

Nelson K B, Emery E S 1993 Birth asphyxia and the neonatal brain: What do we know and when do we know it? Clin Perinatol 20:327–344.

Newschaffer C J, Fallin D, Lee N L 2002 Heritable and nonheritable risk factors for autism spectrum disorders. Epidemiol Rev 24:137–153.

Nicholls R D, Knepper J L 2001 Genome organization, function and imprinting in Prader–Willi and Angelman syndromes. Ann Rev Genomics Human Gen 2:153–175.

NIH (National Institutes of Health) 2006 Online Mendelian Inheritance in Man. Retrieved November 2006, from http://www.ncbi.nlm.nih.gov/entrez/query.fcgi?CMD=search&DB=OMIM.

Oleske J M 1994 The many needs of the HIV-infected child. Hosp Pract 29:63–69.

Olson C K, Keppler-Noreuil K M, Romitti P A et al 2005 In vitro fertilization is associated with an increase in major birth defects. Fertil Steril 84:1308–1315.

Opitz J M, Kaveggia E G, Durkin-Stamm M V, Pendleton E 1978 Diagnostic/genetic studies in severe mental retardation. Birth Defects 14:1–38.

Paneth N, Stark R I 1983 Cerebral palsy and mental retardation in relation to the indicators of perinatal asphyxia. Am J Obst Gynecol 147:960–966.

Partington M, Mowat D, Einfeld S et al 2000 Genes on the X chromosome are important in undiagnosed mental retardation. Am J Med Gen 92:57–61.

Pearson D, Mcgrath N, Nozyce M et al 2000 Predicting HIV disease progression in children using measures of neuropsychological and neurological functioning. Pediatrics 106(6):E76.

Pitetti K H, Rimmer J H, Fernhall B 1993 Physical fitness and adults with mental retardation. An overview of current research and future directions. Sports Medicine 16(1):23–56.

Qian M, Wang D, Chen Z 2000 A preliminary meta-analysis of 36 studies on impairment of intelligence development induced by iodine deficiency. J Prevent Med 24(2):75–77.

Quilligan E, Paul R H 1976 Fetal monitoring: Is it worth it? Obst Gynecol 45:96.

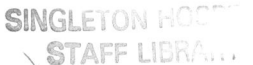

Rantakallio P 1987 Social class differences in mental retardation and subnormality. Scandanavia J Soc Med 15:63–66.

Rantakallio P, Koiranen M 1987 Neurologic handicaps among children whose mothers smoked during pregnancy. Prevent Med 16:597–606.

Rauch A, Hoyer J, Guth S et al 2006 Diagnostic yield of various genetic approaches in patients with unexplained developmental delay or mental retardation. Am J Med Gen Part A, 140A:2063–2074.

Richardson S A, Koller H 1996 Twenty-two years: causes and consequences of mental retardation. Harvard University Press, Cambridge, MA.

Rimmer J H, Braddock D, Fujiura G 1993 Prevalence of obesity in adults with mental retardation: Implications for health promotion and disease prevention. Mental Retardation 31(2):105–110.

Robertson C, Finer N 1985 Term infants with hypoxic-ischemic encephalopathy: Outcome at 3–5 years. Develop Med Child Neurol 27:473–484.

Roeleveld N, Vingerhoets E, Zielhius G A, Gabreels F 1992 Mental retardation associated with parental smoking and alcohol consumption before, during, and after pregnancy. Prevent Med 21:110–119.

Roeleveld N, Zielhuis G A, Gabreels F 1997 The prevalence of mental retardation: A critical review of recent literature. Develop Med Child Neurol 39:125–132.

Ronalds G A, De Stavola B L, Leon D A 2005 The cognitive cost of being a twin: Evidence from comparisons within families in the Aberdeen children of the 1950s cohort study. Br Med J 331:1306.

Rozien N J, Johnson D 1996 Congenital infections. In: Capute A J, Accardo P J (eds) Developmental disabilities in infancy and childhood: Vol. 1. Neurodevelopmental diagnosis and treatment 2nd edn. Paul H. Brookes, Baltimore, MD.

Rurangirwa J K, Van Naarden Braun K, Schendel D E, Yeargin-Allsopp M 2006 Healthy behaviors and lifestyles in young adults with a history of developmental disabilities. Res Develop Dis 27(4):381–399.

Rutter M, Tizard J, Whitmore K 1970 Education, health and behavior: psychological and medical study of childhood development. John Wiley, New York.

Schieve L A, Meikle S F, Ferre C et al 2002 Low and very low birth weight in infants conceived with use of assisted reproductive technology. New Eng J Med 346:731–737.

Scolnik D, Nulman I, Rovet J et al 1994 Neurodevelopment of children exposed in utero to phenytoin and carbamazepine monotherapy. J Am Med Ass 271:767–770.

Sever J L, Ellenberg J H, Ley A C et al 1988 Toxoplasmosis: Maternal and pediatric findings in 23 000 pregnancies. Pediatrics 82:181–192.

Siffel C, Correa A, Cragan J, Alverson C J 2004 Prenatal diagnosis, pregnancy terminations and prevalence of Down Syndrome in Atlanta. Birth Defects Research (Part A) 70:565–571.

Skellern C, Lennox N, Glass I 2000 New insights into the genetic basis of intellectual disabilities. Australian Fam Physic 29:41–45.

Spohr H L, Willms J, Steinhausen H C 1993 Prenatal alcohol exposure and long-term developmental consequences. Lancet 342:907–910.

Stallings V A, Cronk C E, Zemel B S, Charney E B 1995 Body composition in children with spastic quadriplegic cerebral palsy. J Pediatrics 126(5):833–839.

Stallings V A, Zemel B S, Davies J C et al 1996 Energy expenditure of children and adolescents with severe disabilities: a cerebral palsy model. Am J Clin Nutrition 64(4):627–634.

Stein Z, Susser M 1960 The families of dull children and classification for predicting careers. Br J Prevent Soc Med 14:83–88.

Stein Z, Susser M 1963 The social distribution of mental retardation. Am J Ment Defic Res 67:811–821.

Stevenson R E, Burton O M, Ferlauto G J, Taylor 1980 Hazards of oral anticoagulants during pregnancy. JAMA 243:1549–1551.

Stewart P W, Reihman J, Lonky E I et al 2003 Cognitive developmental in preschool children prenatally exposed to PCBs and MeHg. Neurotox Teratol 25:11–22.

Strauss D, Eyman R K 1996 Mortality of people with mental retardation in California with and without Down syndrome, 1986–1991. Am J Mental Retard 100:643–653.

Streissguth A P, Aase J M, Clarren S K et al 1991 Fetal alcohol syndrome in adolescents and adults. J Am Med Ass 265:1961–1967.

Streissguth A P, Barr H M, Kogan J, Bookstein F L 1996 Understanding the occurrence of secondary disabilities in clients with fetal alcohol syndrome (FAS) and fetal alcohol effects (FAE): final report. University of Washington Publication Services, Seattle, WA.

Streissguth A P, Barr H M, Sampson P D 1990 Moderate prenatal alcohol exposure: Effects on child IQ and learning problems at age 7½ years. Alcoholism, Clinical and Experimental Research 14:662–669.

Stromme P, Hagberg G 2000 Aetiology in severe and mild mental retardation: A population-based study of Norwegian children. Develop Med Child Neurol 42:76–86.

Stromme P, Magnus P 2000 Correlations between socioeconomic status, IQ and aetiology in mental retardation: A population-based study of Norwegian children. Soc Psych Psych Epidemiol 35(1):12–18.

Stromme P, Valvatne K 1998 Mental retardation in Norway: Prevalence and subclassification in a cohort of 30 037 children born between 1980 and 1985. Acta Paediatrica 87:291–296.

Suzuki M, Saitoh S, Tasaki Y et al 1991 Nutritional status and daily physical activity of handicapped students in Tokyo metropolitan schools for deaf, blind, mentally retarded, and physically handicapped individuals. Am J Clin Nutrition 54(6):1101–1111.

Turner G, Collins E, Turner B 1971 Recurrence risk of mental retardation in sibs. Med J Australia 1:1165–1167.

Turner G, Webb T, Wake S, Robinson H 1996 Prevalence of fragile X syndrome. Am J Med Gen 64:196–197.

UK Genetic Testing Network Working Party 2006 Evaluation of the use of array comparative genomic hybridization in the diagnosis of learning disability. Pub Health Gen 1:1–86.

Van den Berg-Emons H J, Saris W H, de Barbanson D C et al 1995 Daily physical activity of schoolchildren with spastic diplegia and of healthy control subjects. J Pediatrics 127(4):578–584.

Van den Berg-Emons R J, Van Baak M A, Speth L, Saris W H 1998 Physical training of school children with spastic cerebral palsy: Effects on daily activity, fat mass and fitness. Inter J Rehab Res 21(2):179–194.

Van Naarden Braun K, Autry A, Boyle C 2005 A population-based study of the recurrence of developmental disabilities–Metropolitan Atlanta Developmental Disabilities Surveillance Program, 1991–1994. Paed Perinatal Epidemiol 19(1):69–79.

Van Naarden Braun K, Yeargin-Allsopp M, Lollar D 2006a A multi-dimensional approach to the transition of children with developmental disabilities into young adulthood: The acquisition of adult social roles. Disability and Rehabilitation 28(15):915–928.

Van Naarden Braun K, Yeargin-Allsopp M, Lollar D 2006b Factors associated with leisure activity among young adults with developmental disabilities. Research in Developmental Disabilities, 2005; Nov. 6th. Epub. ahead of print.

Van Naarden Braun K, Yeargin-Allsopp M, Schendel D, Fernhoff P 2003 Long-term developmental outcomes of children identified through a newborn screening program with a metabolic or endocrine disorder: A population-based approach. J Pediatrics 143:236–242.

Wacholder S, Rothman N, Caporaso N 2002 Counterpoint: Bias from population stratification is not a major threat to the validity of conclusions from epidemiological studies of polymorphisms and cancer. Cancer Epidemiology Biomarkers Prev 11:505–512.

Wachtel R C, Conlon C J 1996 Pediatric, Neuro-AIDS. In: Capute A J, Accardo P J (eds), Developmental disabilities in infancy and childhood: (Vol. 1). Neurodevelopmental diagnosis and treatment, 2nd edn. Paul H Brookes, Baltimore, MD, pp. 195–213.

Waisbren S E, Albers S, Amato S et al 2003 Effect of expanded newborn screening for biochemical genetic disorders on child outcomes and parental stress. J Am Med Ass 290(19):2564–2572.

Waisbren S E, Azen C 2003 Cognitive and behavioral development in maternal phenylketonuria offspring. Pediatrics 112:1544–1547.

Waisbren S E, Rokni H, Bailey I et al 1997 Social factors and the meaning of food in adherence to medical diets: Results of a maternal phenylketonuria summer camp. J Inher Metab Dis 20(1):21–27.

Wald N J, Rodeck C, Hackshaw A K et al 2003 First and second trimester antenatal screening for Down's syndrome: the results of the Serum, Urine and Ultrasound Screening Study (SURUSS). Journal Medical Screen 10:56–104 (Level II-2).

Wasserman G A, Liu X, Popovac D et al 2000 The Yugoslavia Prospective Lead Study: Contributions of prenatal and postnatal lead exposure to early intelligence. Neurotoxicol Teratol 22:811–818.

Wellesley D G, Hockey K A, Montgomery P D, Stanley F J 1992 Prevalence of intellectual handicap in Western Australia: a community study. Med J Australia 156:94–96, 100, 102.

Wen X 1997 The definition and prevalence of intellectual disability in Australia. Australian Institute of Health and Welfare, Canberra.

WHO (World Health Organization) 1980 International classification of impairments, disabilities, and handicaps. WHO, Geneva.

WHO (World Health Organization) 1992 International statistical classification of diseases and related health problems: (10th rev, vol 1). WHO, Geneva.

WHO (World Health Organization) 2001a International classification of functioning, disability and health. WHO, Geneva.

WHO (World Health Organization) 2001b Assessment of iodine deficiency disorders and monitoring their elimination. Retrieved [November 20, 2006].

Williams L J, Mai C T, Edmonds L D et al 2002 Prevalence of spina bifida and anencephaly during the transition to mandatory folic acid fortification in the United States. Teratology 66:33–39.

Wright V C, Chang J, Jeng G, Chen M, Macaluso M 2007 Assisted reproductive technology surveillance — United States, 2004. Morbidity and Mortality Weekly Report 56(SS06):1–22.

Yeargin-Allsopp M, Drews C D, Decoufle P, Murphy C C 1995 Mild mental retardation in black and white children in metropolitan Atlanta: A case-control study. Am J Pub Health 85:324–328.

Yeargin-Allsopp M, Murphy C C, Cordero J F et al 1997 Reported biomedical causes and associated medical conditions for mental retardation among 10-year-old children, metropolitan Atlanta, 1985 to 1987. Develop Med Child Neurol 39:142–149.

Yu M-L, Hsu C-C, Gladen B, Rogan W J 1991 In-utero PCB/PCDF exposure: Relation of developmental delay and dysmorphology and dose. Neurotoxicol Teratol 13:95–202.

Zigler E, Balla D, Hodapp R 1984 On the definition and classification of mental retardation. Am J Ment Defic 89:215–230.

The findings and conclusions in this report are those of the authors and do not necessarily represent the views of the Centers for Disease Control and Prevention.

CHAPTER

48

Issues for the obstetrician

Frank A. Chervenak and Laurence B. McCullough

Key Points

- Ethics is an essential dimension of fetal neurology and neurosurgery
- The concept of the fetus as a patient is basic to fetal medicine
- The previable fetus is a patient solely as a function of the pregnant woman's decision to confer this status
- The viable fetus is a patient when (a) it is presented to the physician and (b) there exist clinical interventions that are reliably expected to be efficacious
- Before viability counseling about the management of pregnancy complicated by CNS anomalies should be non-directive
- After viability aggressive management for fetal benefit is the ethical standard of care, with three possible exceptions, each of which must be ethically justified: Termination of pregnancy; Non-aggressive management; Cephalocentesis

INTRODUCTION

Ethics is an essential dimension of fetal neurology, as it is of other specialty and subspecialty aspects of medical practice. In this chapter, we provide an account of obstetric ethics and address the important clinical concept of the fetus as a patient. With this background, we then consider the ethical and clinical dimensions of the obstetric management options for pregnancies complicated by fetal neurologic anomalies and disorders. These management options include aggressive management, abortion, termination of pregnancy during the third trimester, and non-aggressive management. We close with a consideration of cephalocentesis with its complex ethical dimensions.

OBSTETRICS ETHICS

ETHICS

Ethics as an intellectual discipline can be distinguished from morals or morality. Ethics is the disciplined study of morality. Morality concerns both right and wrong behavior and good and bad character. The basic question that ethics addresses is, 'What ought morality to be?' This question entails two further questions, 'What ought our behavior to be?', and 'What virtues ought to be cultivated in our moral lives?' Ethics in obstetric practice addresses these same questions, focusing on what morality ought to be for obstetricians (McCullough & Chervenak 1994).

The bedrock for what morality ought to be in clinical practice for centuries has been the physician's obligation to protect and promote the interests of the patient (Beauchamp & Childress 2001). This is a fairly general ethical obligation. It therefore needs to be made more specific if it is to be clinically useful. This specification can be accomplished by attending to two perspectives in terms of which the patient's interests can be understood: that of the physician and that of the patient (McCullough & Chervenak 1994).

BENEFICENCE AND RESPECT FOR AUTONOMY

In the history of Western medical ethics, the older of these two perspectives on the interests of patients is a rigorous clinical perspective. On the basis of scientific knowledge, shared clinical experience, and a careful, unbiased evaluation of the patient, the physician should identify clinical strategies that will most likely serve the health-related interests of the patient and those that should not be expected to do so. The health-related interests of the patient include preventing premature death and preventing, curing, or at least managing disease, injury, disability, or unnecessary pain and suffering. This is because these matters are constitutive of any patient's health-related interests; they are functions of the competencies of medicine as a social institution. The identification of a patient's health-related interests should not be a function of the personal or subjective outlook of a particular physician but rather of rigorous clinical judgment about the fetal patient's condition.

The ethical principle of beneficence structures obstetric clinical judgment about the interests of the patient in that it obliges the physician to seek the greater balance of clinical goods over clinical harms for the health of both the pregnant woman and the fetal patient. On the basis of rigorous clinical judgment, the obstetrician should identify those clinical strategies that are reliably expected to result in the greater balance of clinical goods, i.e. the protection and promotion of health-related interests, over clinical harms, i.e. impairments of those interests.

The principle of beneficence in obstetrics should be clearly distinguished from the ethical principles of non-maleficence, commonly known as Primum non nocere or First, do no harm (Beauchamp & Childress 2001). Contrary to the common belief among physicians, Primum non nocere does not appear in the Hippocratic Oath or in the texts that accompany the Oath. The principle of beneficence was the primary consideration of the Hippocratic writers (Hippocrates 1923).

There are good reasons to be skeptical about the adequacy of Primum non nocere as a basic principle of obstetric ethics.

If Primum non nocere were to become the basic principle of obstetric ethics, virtually all of obstetric practice would be unethical because virtually all medical interventions involve unavoidable risks of harm. Primum non nocere is therefore superseded in obstetric ethics by the principle of beneficence. The latter is sufficient to alert the physician to those circumstances in which a clinical intervention has the potential on balance to harm a patient: when a clinical intervention is on balance clinically harmful to a patient, it should not be employed. That is, Primum non nocere, as a corollary of beneficence, makes it obligatory not to act in a way that is only harmful. In particular, as Strong (1987) puts it, there is a powerful beneficence-based prohibition against killing. This is obviously of direct relevance to the ethical evaluation of cephalocentesis in beneficence-based clinical judgment, as we shall see below.

The physician's perspective on the interests of the patient is only one of two legitimate perspectives on those interests. The perspective of the patient on the patient's interests is at least equally worthy of consideration by the physician (McCullough & Chervenak 1994). Each patient has developed a set of values and beliefs according to which she is to be presumed capable of making judgments about what will and will not protect and promote her interests. It is commonplace that in other aspects of her life, the patient regularly makes such judgments concerning matters of considerable complexity, e.g. choosing a professional calling, rearing and educating children, purchasing property, and writing a will of property. Despite the complexity of these and many other decisions of daily life, she is rightly assumed to be competent to make them, with the burden of proof on anyone who would challenge her competence.

The same is true about health-care decisions made by the pregnant woman. She should be assumed by her obstetrician to be competent to determine which clinical strategies serve her health-related and other interests and which do not. In making such judgments, it is important to note that the pregnant woman will utilize values and beliefs that can range beyond the scope of health-related interests, e.g. religious beliefs or beliefs about how many children she wants to have. Beneficence-based clinical judgment, because it rests on the competencies of medicine, provides no authoritative basis for assessing the worth or meaning to the patient of the patient's non-health-related interests. These are matters for the patient alone to determine. Those values and beliefs help shape the patient's perspective on her interests.

The ethical significance of this perspective is expressed by the ethical principle of respect for autonomy. This ethical principle obligates the physician to respect the integrity of the patient's values and beliefs, to respect her perspective on her interests, and to implement only those clinical strategies authorized by her as the result of the informed consent process unless there is some overriding, well-established objection to doing so. Respect for autonomy is put into clinical practice by the informed consent process, which is usually understood to have three elements: (1) disclosure by the physician to the patient of adequate information about the patient's condition and its management; (2) understanding of that information by the patient; (3) a voluntary decision by the patient to authorize or refuse clinical management (Faden & Beauchamp 1986).

The physician obviously has both beneficence-based and autonomy-based obligations to the pregnant patient (McCullough & Chervenak 1994). The physician's perspective on the pregnant woman's interests provides the basis for beneficence-based obligations owed to her. Her own perspective on those interests provides the basis for autonomy-based obligations owed to her. Because of an insufficiently developed central nervous system, the fetus cannot meaningfully be said to possess values and beliefs. There is therefore no biological or conceptual basis for saying that a fetus has a perspective on its interests. There can therefore be no autonomy-based obligations to any fetus (Chervenak & McCullough 1985, 1990, McCullough & Chervenak 1994). Hence, the language of fetal rights has no meaning in obstetric ethics, despite its popularity in public and political discourse. This point cannot be overemphasized in obstetric ethics. This chapter, therefore, makes no further reference to fetal rights. Obviously, the physician has a perspective on the fetus's health-related interests, and the physician can have beneficence-based obligations to the fetus, but only when the fetus is a patient. Because of its importance for obstetric ethics generally and the ethics of destructive procedures in obstetrics, the concept of the fetus as a patient requires detailed consideration.

THE CONCEPT OF THE FETUS AS A PATIENT

The concept of 'the fetus as a patient' has recently developed largely as a consequence of developments in fetal diagnosis and management strategies to optimize fetal outcome (McCullough & Chervenak 1994), including those discussed elsewhere in this volume, and has become widely accepted (Chervenak & McCullough 1991, Fletcher 1981, Harrison et al 1984). This obstetric-ethics concept has considerable clinical significance because, when the fetus is a patient, directive counseling, i.e. recommending a form of management, for fetal benefit would seem to be appropriate and, when the fetus is not a patient, non-directive counseling, i.e. offering, but not recommending, a form of management, would seem to be appropriate. However, these apparently straightforward roles for directive and non-directive counseling are often difficult to apply in clinical practice because of uncertainty about when the fetus is a patient. One approach to resolving this uncertainty would be to argue that the fetus is or is not a patient in virtue of personhood (Engelhardt 1986, Strong 1987), or some other form of independent moral status (Dunstan 1984, Elias & Annas 1987, Evans et al 1988). We will show that this approach fails to resolve the uncertainty, and we will therefore defend an alternative approach that does resolve the uncertainty.

THE INDEPENDENT MORAL STATUS OF THE FETUS

One fairly prominent approach for establishing whether or not the fetus is a patient has involved attempts over many centuries to show whether or not the fetus has independent moral status. The concept of the independent moral status for the fetus means that one or more characteristics that the fetus is thought to possess in and of itself and, therefore, independently of the pregnant woman or any other factor generate and therefore ground obligations to the fetus on the part of the pregnant woman and her physician.

A wide variety of characteristics have been nominated for this role in the history of the debate on the moral status of the fetus. These include the 'moment' of conception, implantation, central nervous system development, quickening, and the 'moment' of birth (Chervenak & McCullough 1985, Curran 1978, Hellegers 1970). Given the variability of proposed characteristics, there have been, and are, markedly varied views about when the fetus acquires independent moral status. Some take the view that the fetus has independent moral status from the moment of conception or implantation (Noonan 1979, Bopp 1984). Others believe that independent moral status is acquired in degrees, thus resulting in 'graded' moral status (Dunstan 1984, Evans et al 1988, Strong 1987). Still others hold, at least by implication, that the fetus never has independent moral status so long as it is in utero (Elias & Annas 1987).

Despite a continuing and enormous theologic and philosophical literature on this subject, stretching over more than 2000 years, there has been no closure on a single, intellectually authoritative account of the independent moral status of the fetus (Callahan & Callahan 1984, Roe v. Wade 1973). This is not a surprising outcome: given the absence of a single methodology that would be authoritative for all of the markedly diverse theologic and philosophical schools of thought involved in this endless debate, closure is impossible. For closure ever to be possible, debates about such a final intellectual authority within and between theologic and philosophical traditions would have to be resolved in a way satisfactory to all. Because this is an inconceivable event, it is best to abandon futile attempts to understand the fetus as a patient in terms of independent moral status of the fetus and turn to an alternative approach that identifies ethically distinct senses of the fetus as a patient and their clinical implications for obstetric practice.

BENEFICENCE-BASED OBLIGATIONS TO THE FETUS

This alternative approach starts with the recognition that being a patient does not require that one possesses independent moral status. Rather, being a patient means that one can benefit from the applications of the clinical skills of the physician. Put more precisely, a human being (with or without independent moral status) is properly regarded as a patient when two conditions are met: that (a) a human being

is presented to the physician, and (b) there exist clinical interventions that are reliably expected to be efficacious, in that they are reliably expected to result in a greater balance of goods over harms for the human being in question. (Of course, if the woman's body is a necessary condition, then her consent is necessary) (Chervenak & McCullough 1991, McCullough & Chervenak 1994).

The authors have argued elsewhere that beneficence-based obligations to the fetus exist when the fetus can later achieve independent moral status (McCullough & Chervenak 1994). That is, the fetus is a patient when the fetus is presented to the physician, and there exist medical interventions, whether diagnostic or therapeutic that reasonably can be expected to result in a greater balance of goods over harms for the fetus now and/or in its future. The moral status of the fetus as a patient depends on links that can be established between the fetus in utero and its being reliably expected to achieve independent moral status.

One such link is viability, introducing the first application of the concept of the fetus as a patient. Viability should not be understood as an intrinsic property of the fetus because viability must be understood in terms of both biologic and technologic factors (Fletcher 1981, Fost et al 1980, Roe v. Wade 1973). Both factors result in a viable fetus that can exist ex utero and then achieve independent moral status. It is important to note that these two factors do not exist as a function of the autonomy of the pregnant woman. When a fetus is viable, i.e. when it is of sufficient maturity so that it can survive into the neonatal period and later achieve independent moral status, given the availability of the requisite technologic support, and when it is presented to the physician, the fetus is a patient. The fetus at term is a patient when the pregnant woman presents herself to a physician or a hospital or clinic for obstetric services.

Viability exists as a function of biomedical and technologic capacities, which are different in different parts of the world. As a consequence, there is, at the present time, no world-wide, uniform gestational age to define viability. In the United States, the authors believe, viability presently occurs at approximately 24 weeks of gestational age (Chervenak & McCullough 1997, Chervenak et al 2007). It follows directly from this sense of the fetus as a patient that destructive procedures on the at-term fetal patient, cephalocentesis in particular, must be ethically justified, a task to which we turn in the next section.

The only possible link between the previable fetus and the child it can become is the pregnant woman's autonomy, introducing the second clinical application of the concept of the fetus as a patient. This is because technologic factors cannot result in the previable fetus becoming a child. This is simply what previable means. The link, therefore, between a fetus and the child it can become, when the fetus is previable, can be established only by the pregnant woman's decision to confer the status of being a patient on her previable fetus. The previable fetus, therefore, has no claim to the status of being a patient independently of the pregnant woman's autonomy. The pregnant woman is free to with-hold, confer, or, having once conferred, withdraw the status of being a patient on or from her previable fetus according to her own values and beliefs. The previable fetus is presented to the physician solely as a function of the pregnant woman's autonomy. This has important ethical implications for a range of ethical issues in obstetrics, including antenatal diagnosis and abortion (Hellegers 1970).

MANAGEMENT OPTIONS FOR PREGNANCIES COMPLICATED BY FETAL NEUROLOGIC ANOMALIES AND DISORDERS

Before viability, the management of a pregnancy complicated by fetal neurologic anomalies and disorders is ethically straightforward. The pregnant woman is free to withhold or withdraw the moral status of being a patient from any previable fetus including that with such anomalies or disorders. When such an anomaly is detected, counseling should therefore be rigorously directive. The woman should be given the choice between abortion and continuing her pregnancy to viability and thus to term. If the woman elects an abortion, it should be performed or an appropriate referral made. If the woman elects to continue her pregnancy, she should be apprised about decisions that will need to be made later, such as cesarean delivery for fetal indications (McCullough & Chervenak 1994).

After viability, aggressive management is the ethical standard of care. By aggressive management, we mean optimizing perinatal outcome by utilizing effective antepartum and intrapartum diagnostic and therapeutic modalities.

One important exception to aggressive management is termination of pregnancy after the usual gestational age of fetal viability. This exception applies when there is: (1) certainty of diagnosis and either (2a) certainty of death as an outcome of the anomaly diagnosed or (2b) in some cases of short-term survival, certainty of the absence of cognitive developmental capacity as an outcome of the anomaly diagnosed (McCullough & Chervenak 1994). When these criteria are satisfied, recommending a choice between non-aggressive management and termination of pregnancy is justified. Anencephaly is a classic example of a fetal neurologic anomaly that satisfies these criteria.

A second exception to aggressive management is non-aggressive management. This exception applies when there is: (1) a very high probability but sometimes less than complete certainty about the diagnosis and either (2a) a very high probability of death as an outcome of the anomaly diagnosed or (2b) survival with a very high probability of severe and irreversible deficit of cognitive developmental capacity as a result of the anomaly diagnosed (Beauchamp & Childress 2001). When these two criteria apply both aggressive and non-aggressive management can be justified, from which it follows that a choice between aggressive or non-aggressive management, but not termination, can be recommended. Encephalocele is a classic example of a fetal neurologic anomaly that satisfies these criteria.

A third important and ethically complex exception to aggressive management is cephalocentesis.

CEPHALOCENTESIS FOR INTRAPARTUM MANAGEMENT OF HYDROCEPHALUS

Cephalocentesis is the drainage of an enlarged fetal head, secondary to hydrocephalus (Chervenak & Romero 1984). Fetal hydrocephalus is caused by obstruction of cerebrospinal flow and is diagnosed by such sonographic signs as dilatation of the atrium or body of the lateral ventricles (Chervenak et al 1993). In the third trimester, macrocephaly often accompanies the ventriculomegaly. In addition, sonography can diagnose hydrocephalus in association with gross abnormalities suggestive of poor prognosis, for example, hydranencephaly, microcephaly, encephalocele, alobar holoprosencephaly, or thanatophoric dysplasia with cloverleaf skull (Chervenak et al 1993). (See chapters in Section 1 of this volume.) In the absence of defined anatomical abnormalities, however, diagnostic imaging is, at the present time, unable to predict the outcome. Although cortical mantle thickness can be measured with ultrasound, its value as a prognostic index is not established (Chervenak et al 1993).

Cephalocentesis should be performed under simultaneous ultrasound guidance so that needle placement into the cerebrospinal fluid is facilitated. An 18-gauge needle is used with collapse of the cranial bones, the endpoint for this procedure. Enough fluid is drained to permit reduction of the skull diameters so that passage through the birth canal is possible (Chasen et al 2001, Chervenak et al 1985, Clark et al 1985).

Cephalocentesis is a potentially destructive procedure. Perinatal death following cephalocentesis has been reported in over 90% of cases (Chervenak & Romero 1984). The sonographic visualization of intracranial bleeding during cephalocentesis, and the demonstration of this hemorrhage at autopsy, further emphasizes the morbid nature of the procedure. However, if decompression is performed in a controlled manner, the mortality may be reduced (Birnholz & Frigoletto 1981).

Because fetal hydrocephalus is the product of varied etiologies having varied outcomes, ethical analysis must be carried out by respecting the heterogeneity of this condition (Chervenak et al 1993). Therefore, we consider clinical management strategies for two extremes of the continuum between isolated fetal hydrocephalus and fetal hydrocephalus with severe associated abnormalities (those incompatible with postnatal survival or those characterized by the virtual absence of cognitive function). We then consider fetal hydrocephalus with milder associated abnormalities as a middle ground on the continuum. The proposed analysis of each of these situations takes place in the following steps. First, we identify the beneficence-based and autonomy-based obligations of the physician to the pregnant woman and the fetal patient. Second, we identify the conflicts that can occur among these obligations. Third, we weigh these obligations against each other in an attempt to arrive at a balance among conflicting obligations to guide clinical judgement and intervention.

ISOLATED FETAL HYDROCEPHALUS

We begin the clinical and ethical analysis of isolated fetal hydrocephalus by noting that there is considerable potential for normal, sometimes superior, intellectual function for fetuses with even extreme, isolated hydrocephalus (Lorber 1968, McCullough & Balzer-Martin 1982, Raimondi & Soare 1974, Sutton et al 1980). However, as a group, infants with isolated hydrocephalus experience a greater incidence of mental retardation and early death than the general population. In addition, associated anomalies may go undetected, and a fetus may be incorrectly diagnosed as having isolated hydrocephalus (Chervenak et al 1985, Nyberg et al 1987). One thing is clear in obstetric ethics: a viable at-term fetus with isolated hydrocephalus is a fetal patient, because neither of the two exceptions described above apply, given the variable outcomes of isolated hydrocephalus.

There are compelling, beneficence-based ethical reasons for concluding that continuing existence of fetuses with isolated hydrocephalus is in their interests. Beneficence directs the physician to prevent mortality and morbidity for the fetal patient. Beneficence also directs the physician to undertake interventions that ameliorate handicapping conditions such as mental retardation. The probability of mental retardation does not diminish the interests of the fetal patient with isolated hydrocephalus in continuing existence because (1) it is impossible to predict which fetuses with isolated hydrocephalus will have mental retardation and (2) the degree of mental retardation cannot be predicted in advance.

In light of this ethical analysis of the at-term fetal patient's interests, the beneficence-based obligation of the physician caring for the fetus is to recommend strongly, and to attain, the woman's consent to perform a cesarean delivery because this clinical intervention clearly involves the least risk of mortality, morbidity, and handicap for the fetus compared with cephalocentesis to permit subsequent vaginal delivery. Even when performed under maximal therapeutic conditions (i.e. under sonographic guidance), cephalocentesis cannot reasonably be regarded as protecting or promoting the interests of the fetal patient with isolated hydrocephalus. This procedure is followed by a high rate of perinatal mortality, fetal heart rate deceleration, and pathologic evidence of intracranial bleeding (Chervenak et al 1985, Nyberg et al 1987). As a consequence, cephalocentesis cannot reasonably be construed as an ethically justifiable mode of management, in so far as it is inconsistent with beneficence-based obligations to avoid increased mortality and morbidity risks for the fetal patient. Cephalocentesis, employed with a destructive intent, is altogether antithetical to this beneficence-based prohibition against killing.

It is essential in obstetric ethics that beneficence-based obligations to the fetal patient be balanced against beneficence-based and autonomy-based obligations to the preg-

nant woman. First, the physician has a beneficence-based obligation to avoid performing a cesarean delivery because the possibility of morbidity and mortality for the woman is higher than that associated with vaginal delivery. Respect for autonomy obligates the physician to undertake only those interventions or forms of treatment to which the woman has given voluntary, informed consent. Informed consent is grounded in an autonomy-based right of the pregnant woman to control what happens to her body. In particular, the woman has the right to authorize or refuse operative intervention – those that are, as well as those that are not, consistent with the physician's beneficence-based obligations (McCullough & Chervenak 1994).

We are now in a position to consider the full complexity of the management of the fetal patient with isolated hydrocephalus: beneficence-based and autonomy-based obligations to the pregnant woman, as well as beneficence-based obligations to her fetus, must all be considered for clinical ethical judgment to be complete and therefore reliable. If, with informed consent, the woman authorizes cesarean delivery, there is no conflict among these obligations. The autonomy-based obligation to act on informed consent overrides the beneficence-based obligations to the pregnant woman that were identified earlier.

By contrast, her physician faces a significant and challenging ethical conflict if the woman refuses cesarean delivery. Two clinical interventions, each with substantial ethical justification in beneficence-based and autonomy-based clinical judgment, can be employed in intrapartum management. On the one hand, the physician has an autonomy-based obligation to the pregnant woman to perform cephalocentesis followed by vaginal delivery. On the other hand, cephalocentesis violates beneficence-based obligations to the fetal at-term patient. This conflict should be resolved in favor of the beneficence-based obligations to the fetal patient. These obligations properly override beneficence-based and autonomy-based obligations to the woman because the harm to the fetal patient is final, namely, death, and will occur with high probability. Moreover, if the fetal patient survives (death is not guaranteed by cephalocentesis), it is likely to be more damaged due to intracranial hemorrhage than if cesarean delivery is performed. Morbidity and mortality of the pregnant woman are both minimal and therefore risks that she ought to accept to protect the fetal patient's interest (McCullough & Chervenak 1994). Such ethical conflict should be prevented by employing the preventive ethics strategies of informed consent as an ongoing dialogue, negotiation, respectful persuasion and the proper use of ethics committees (Chervenak & McCullough 1990a, McCullough & Chervenak 1994).

If these preventive ethics strategies do not succeed and the pregnant woman continues to refuse cesarean delivery, the physician confronts tragic circumstances. If neither cesarean delivery nor cephalocentesis is performed, the woman is at risk for uterine rupture and death, and the fetal patient is at risk for death. This logic of beneficence-based obligations is to prevent such total and irreversible harm. Therefore, we believe that because of the grave nature of possible consequences for the woman and her fetus, because of the dangers for the woman of performing a surgical procedure on a resistant patient, and because of the pitfalls of attempted legal coercion, the physician should act on beneficence-based obligations to the woman in such an extreme circumstance. In addition, failure to respect an unwavering, voluntary, and informed refusal of a cesarean delivery would count as a fundamental assault on the woman's autonomy. The fetal patient is at high risk for death under either alternative. The woman's death, at least, can be avoided. Serious beneficence-based obligations to the fetal patient on the part of both the physician and the pregnant woman will probably be violated, and a needless death will most probably result, however, by performing a cephalocentesis. Herein lies the tragedy of these circumstances. To avoid this tragedy, redoubled efforts of preventive ethics should be undertaken. In one author's (F.A.C.) experience, carefully explaining the fact that cephalocentesis does not guarantee death and may produce a worse outcome is very powerfully persuasive. In those rare cases in which this effort at respectful persuasion fails, cephalocentesis should be performed in the least destructive way possible or an appropriate referral made.

HYDROCEPHALUS WITH SEVERE ASSOCIATED ABNORMALITIES

Some abnormalities that occur in association with fetal hydrocephalus are severe in nature for the child afflicted with them. We define 'severe' abnormalities as those that are either (1) incompatible with continued existence, e.g. bilateral renal agenesis or thanatophoric dysplasia with cloverleaf skull or (2) compatible with survival in some cases but result in virtual absence of cognitive function, e.g. trisomy 18 or alobar holoprosencephaly (Chervenak & McCullough 1990b, Chervenak et al 1985). Because there is no available intervention to prevent postnatal death in the first group, beneficence-based obligations of the physician and the pregnant woman to attempt to prolong the life of the fetal patient are non-existent. No ethical theory and no version of obstetric ethics based on beneficence and respect for autonomy obligate the physician to attempt the impossible. For the second group, beneficence-based obligations of the physician and the pregnant woman to sustain the life of the fetal patient are minimal because the handicap imposed by the abnormality is severe. In these cases, the potential for cognitive development – and therefore the achievement of other 'good' for the child, e.g. relationships with others – are virtually absent. Such fetuses are fetal patients to which there are owed only minimal beneficence-based obligations.

In these circumstances, the woman is therefore released from her beneficence-based obligations to the at-term fetal patient to place herself at risk, because no significant good can be achieved by cesarean delivery for the fetal patient or the child it will become. There remain only the autonomy-

based and beneficence-based obligations of the physician to the pregnant woman. After the preceding analysis of these obligations, we conclude that the physician's overriding moral obligations are to the pregnant woman's voluntary and informed decision about employment of cephalocentesis.

Because there are no weighty beneficence-based obligations to the fetus in such clinical and ethical circumstances, the physician may justifiably recommend a choice between cesarean delivery and cephalocentesis to enable vaginal delivery. Cesarean delivery permits women who wish to do so to have a live birth and satisfy religious convictions or help with the grieving process. A cesarean delivery performed in this clinical setting is best viewed as an autonomy-based maternal indication. The strategy of offering a choice also avoids the potential negative consequences for maternal health of cesarean delivery. Because the prognosis for infants with hydrocephalus associated with severe anomalies is poor, we believe that intrapartum fetal death resulting from cephalocentesis would not be a tragic outcome as it might be in the death of a fetal patient with isolated hydrocephalus.

HYDROCEPHALUS WITH OTHER ASSOCIATED ANOMALIES

On the continuum between the extreme cases of isolated hydrocephalus and hydrocephalus with severe associated abnormalities, there is a variety of cases of hydrocephalus associated with other abnormalities with varying degrees of impairment of cognitive physical function. They range from hypoplastic distal phalanges to spina bifida to encephalocele (Chervenak et al 1998, Lorber & Zachary 1968). Because these conditions have varying prognoses, it would be clinically inappropriate and, therefore, ethically misleading to treat this third category as homogeneous. Therefore, we propose a working distinction between different kinds of prognoses. The first we call 'probably promising,' by which we mean that there is a significant possibility that the child will experience cognitive development with learning disabilities and physical handicaps that perhaps can be ameliorated to some extent. The second we call 'probably poor'. By this phrase, we mean that there is only a limited possibility for cognitive development because of learning disabilities and physical handicaps that cannot be ameliorated to a significant extent. We propose these definitions as tentative, so they are subject to revision as clinical and ethical investigations of such associated anomalies continue. As a consequence, our ethical analysis of these two categories cannot be carried out as extensively as those in the previous two sections. In essence, we propose that the clinical continuum in these cases is paralleled by an ethical continuum or progressively less weighty, beneficence-based obligations to the fetus. Such at-term fetuses are indeed fetal patients.

When the prognosis is probably promising, e.g. isolated arachnoid cyst, there are serious beneficence-based obligations to the fetal patient. However, they are not necessarily on the same order as those that occur in cases of isolated hydrocephalus. (It has been suggested that any associated anomaly may increase the possibility of a poor outcome (Chervenak et al 1985.)) Therefore, in such cases with a prognosis of probably promising, we propose that the physician recommend cesarean delivery, although perhaps not as vigorously as in cases of isolated hydrocephalus. A pregnant woman's informed refusal of cesarean delivery should therefore be respected.

In cases when the prognosis, even though uncertain, is probably poor, e.g. encephalocele, beneficence-based obligations to the fetal patient are less weighty than those owed to the fetal patient with a promising prognosis. These cases, then, resemble ethically those of hydrocephalus with severe anomalies, with the proviso that some, albeit limited, benefits can be achieved for the fetal patient by cesarean delivery and aggressive perinatal treatment. None the less, the physician may in these cases justifiably accept an informed voluntary decision by the woman for cephalocentesis followed by vaginal delivery. However, the physician cannot assume an advocacy role for such a decision with the same level of ethical confidence that he or she can in cases of hydrocephalus associated with severe anomalies.

CONCLUSION

Ethics is an essential dimension of the obstetric management of pregnancies complicated by fetal neurologic anomalies and disorders. This chapter has provided an ethical framework for obstetric ethics and practical guidance, based on that framework, for the management of pregnancies complicated by such fetal anomalies and disorders. In the authors' view, managing pregnancies complicated by fetal neurologic anomalies without careful attention to their ethical dimension is clinically inappropriate.

REFERENCES

Beauchamp T L, Childress J F 2001 Principles of biomedical ethics. 5th edn. Oxford University Press, New York.

Birnholz J C, Frigoletto F D 1981 Antenatal treatment of hydrocephalus. N Engl J Med 104:1021.

Bopp J 1984 Restoring the right to life: the human life amendment. Brigham Young University, Provo.

Callahan S, Callahan D 1984 Abortion: understanding differences. Plenum, New York.

Chasen S T, Chervenak F A, McCullough L B 2001 The role of cephalocentesis in modern obstetrics. Am J Obstet Gynecol 185:734–736.

Chervenak F A, Berkowitz R L, Tortora M et al 1985 Management of fetal hydrocephalus. Am J Obstet Gynecol 151:933–937.

Chervenak F A, Isaacson G, Campbell S 1993 Anomalies of the cranium and its contents. Textbook of ultrasound in obstetrics and gynecology. Little Brown, Boston, p 825–852.

Chervenak F A, McCullough L B 1985 Perinatal ethics: A practical method of analysis of obligations to mother and fetus. Obstet Gynecol 66:442–446.

Chervenak F A, McCullough L B 1990 Does obstetric ethics have any role in the obstetrician's response to the abortion controversy? Am J Obstet Gynecol 163:1425–1429.

Chervenak F A, McCullough L B 1990a Clinical guides to preventing ethical conflicts between pregnant women and their physicians. Am J Obstet Gynecol 162:303–307.

Chervenak F A, McCullough L B 1990b An ethically justified.clinically comprehensive management strategy for third-trimester pregnancies complicated by fetal anomalies. Obstet Gynecol 75:311–316.

Chervenak F A, McCullough L B 1991 The fetus as patient: implications for directive versus nondirective counseling for fetal benefit. Fetal Diagn Ther 6:93–100.

Chervenak F A, McCullough L B 1997 The limits of viability. J Perinat Med 25:418–420.

Chervenak F A, Romero R 1984 Is there a role for fetal cephalocentesis in modern obstetrics? Am J Perinatol 1:170–173.

Chervenak FA, McCullough LB, Levene MI 2007 An ethically justified, clinically comprehensive approach to peri-viability: Gynaecological, obstetric, perinatal and neonatal dimensions. J Obstet Gynaecol 27:3–7.

Clark S L, DeVore G R, Platt L D 1985 The role of ultrasound in the aggressive management of obstructed labor secondary to fetal malformations. Am J Obstet Gynecol 152:1042–1044.

Curran C E 1978 Abortion: Contemporary debate in philosophical and religious ethics. In: Reich.W T (ed) Encyclopedia of Bioethics. Macmillan, New York, pp. 17–26.

Dunstan G R 1984 The moral status of the human embryo. A tradition recalled. J Med Ethics 10: 38–44.

Elias S, Annas G J 1987 Reproductive genetics and the law. Year Book Medical, Chicago.

Engelhardt H T Jr 1986 The foundations of bioethics. Oxford University Press, New York.

Evans M I, Fletcher J C, Zador I E et al 1988 Selective first-trimester termination in octuplet and quadruplet pregnancies: Clinical and ethical issues. Obstet Gynecol 71:289–296.

Faden R R, Beauchamp T L 1986 A history and theory of informed consent. Oxford University Press, New York.

Fletcher J C 1981 The fetus as patient: ethical issues. JAMA 246:772–773.

Fost N, Chudwin D, Wikker D 1980 The limited moral significance of fetal viability. Hastings Cent Rep 10:10–13.

Harrison M R, Golbus M S, Filly R A 1984 The unborn patient. Grune & Stratton, New York.

Hellegers A E 1970 Fetal development. Theological Studies 31:3–9.

Jones W H S (trans) 1923 Hippocrates. Epidemics i: xi. Loeb Classical Library.vol. 147. Harvard University Press, Cambridge.

Lorber J 1968 The results of early treatment on extreme hydrocephalus. Med Child Neurol (Suppl) 16: 21.

Lorber J, Zachary R B 1968 Primary congenital hydrocephalus: long-term results of controlled therapeutic trial. Arch Dis Child 43: 516.

McCullough D C, Balzer-Martin L A 1982 Current prognosis in overt neonatal hydrocephalus. J Neurosurg 57:378.

McCullough L B, Chervenak F A 1994 Obstetric ethics. Oxford University Press, New York.

Noonan J T 1979 A Private Choice. Abortion in America in the Seventies. The Free Press, New York.

Nyberg DA, Mack LA, Hirsch J et al 1987 Fetal hydrocephalus: sonographic detection and clinical significance of associated anomalies. Radiology 163:187.

Raimondi A J, Soare P 1974 Intellectual development in shunted hydrocephalic children. Am J Dis Child 127:664.

Roe v. Wade, 410 US 113 1973.

Strong C 1987 Ethical conflicts between mother and fetus in obstetrics. Clin in Perinatology Perinat 14:313–328.

Sutton L N, Bruce D A, Schut L 1980 Hydranencephaly versus maximal hydrocephalus: an important clinical distinction. Neurosurgery 6:35.

CHAPTER
49

Issues for the neonatologist
Terence Stephenson

Key Points

- There are five situations where the withholding or withdrawal of life-prolonging treatment might be considered:
  - The brain dead child
  - The persistent vegetative state
  - The 'no-chance' situation
  - The 'no-purpose' situation
  - The 'unbearable' situation
- In infants below 37 weeks gestation, the concept of brain stem death is not appropriate
- Withdrawal of treatment is a misnomer; the aims of treatment are changed from cure to care rather than total withdrawal of treatment
- Where there is reasonable uncertainty about the benefits of treatment, there should be a presumption in favor of initiating it. Clinical intervention can be discontinued later after reflection and discussion with parents
- It is important that a single senior doctor takes overall responsibility for orchestrating the actions of the whole team involved with the family
- If the parents' views are at odds with those of the team caring for the child the doctor should ask the following five questions:
  - Do the parents understand the prognosis?
  - Should they consult with others?
  - Do they require more time?
  - Is their decision in the interests of the child?
  - Is their decision so unreasonable in terms of benefit to the child as to request them to seek a second opinion or for the doctor to seek the advice of the courts?
- The clinician must always act in the best interest of the child

---

INTRODUCTION

When faced with ethical decisions in the management of newborn babies (Anonymous 1986, Bissenden 1986, Campbell 1982, Kennedy 1981, Rhein 1992, Stinson & Stinson 1981), the actions of doctors will be directed by the wishes of the parents, the doctor's conscience, the advice of the medical protection societies and the law of the country in which they practise (in this chapter, all references are to United Kingdom law). There are three important moral philosophical points (Kuhse & Singer 1985).

THE PRINCIPLE OF THE SANCTITY OF LIFE

Most of us think it is wrong to kill people. Some think it is wrong in all circumstances, while others think that in special circumstances (say, in a just war or in self defence) some killing may be justified. The assumption is that killing can at best only be justified to avoid a greater evil (Glover 1977).

Doctors practising 'conviction medicine' feel that not only is it wrong to take life but it is equally wrong to withhold maximal treatment. Doctors practising 'consensus medicine' may feel that their actions are influenced by parental wishes and prognosis, and that withdrawing maximal treatment can be seen as justified in order to avoid the 'greater evil' of an unacceptable quality of life.

QUALITY OF LIFE

In our view the most important medical criterion is the degree of abnormality of the central nervous system. If there is little or no prospect of brain function sufficient to allow a personal life of meaning and quality or no potential for development in harmony with Fletcher's indicators of humanhood, non-treatment seems the prudent course of action (Duff & Campbell 1973).

Fletcher's 'tentative profile of man' suggests that positive criteria for humanhood would include minimal intelligence, self-awareness, self-control, a sense of time, a sense of futurity and a sense of the past, the capability to relate to others, concern for others, communication, control of existence, and curiosity (Fletcher 1972). Baby J was born very preterm and was severely brain-damaged (Re J 1990). The court held that to continue invasive treatments would not be in his best interests because he 'suffered from physical disabilities so grave that his life would from his point of view be so intolerable' that if he were able to make a sound judgement, he would not choose treatment. The Court of Appeal ruled that baby J should not be put back on a ventilator if he fell critically ill.

When faced with this kind of dilemma, some doctors take a paternalistic attitude. They would argue that the child's parents, perhaps two young lay people with no previous experience of such situations, can never be sufficiently well informed to take such a difficult decision at a time when they are deeply emotionally upset. The doctor has the experience and knowledge to take this burden (Schultz 1992). Others argue for a more democratic process.

ACTS OF COMMISSION AND OMISSION

Switching off a ventilator when a baby has very severe brain damage may result in the death of the baby. The baby's death is hastened (i.e. the timing of death) as a result of an act of omission (Autton 1985). There is a doctrine within moral philosophy, known as the 'acts and omissions doctrine,' which states that there is a moral difference between causing death to happen through an action, and allowing the same thing to happen by failing to act. Intuitively, it seems right that causing death is a greater offence than letting someone die through inaction. The strongest demand on us is that we do not harm others (the duty of non-maleficence), whereas the duty to actively help others (the duty of beneficence) is usually recognized to be weaker (Farsides 1992). Doctors may decide not to treat a child and view this as different from deciding to end the child's life actively by a lethal injection (Byrne 1990), although the intention and consequences are equivalent (Glover 1977). It has been argued that, assuming the death is morally justifiable, then this should be done in the most humane way possible, irrespective of whether this involves killing the child or letting him or her die (Rachels 1975). However, the law rarely takes such an equal view of active and passive euthanasia. The legal formalization of euthanasia is most advanced in Holland (Hellema 1992).

> Clinicians engaged in terminal care would argue that they do not withhold treatment, they change treatment. They change it from a treatment for the living, to a treatment for the dying. The doctor has the moral tool of the double effect. Although his primary intention is to relieve suffering, it may be that death will predictably follow from the course of treatment adopted.
>
> *Autton 1985*

The aims of treatment are changed from cure to care. Care involves controlling pain, distress, and suffering of the patient. Morphine controls pain but may also expedite death. It cannot be emphasized enough that the withdrawal of treatment does not equate with the withdrawal of care (Winter & Cohen, 1999). In a case involving an adult in a 'permanent vegetative state' (Tresch et al 1991), the court took the view that nasogastric feeding constituted a medical treatment, and therefore it was lawful to withdraw this treatment. If the patient could manage to swallow food, it is likely that the legal view would be that withdrawal of food would amount to starvation (Lennard-Jones 1999). The use of enteral tube feeding for preterm infants is regarded by some as analogous to a bottle feed and thus a part of basic care (McHaffie & Fowlie 1997), but this has not been tested in a UK court. UK courts have never considered a case of withdrawing artificial nutrition or hydration from patients who are not in PVS.

Withdrawal of treatment is not an unusual situation on a neonatal intensive care unit, and the doctors involved rarely seek the advice of the courts, although the Leonard Arthur case (Anonymous 1981a) and the baby Doe case (Kopelman et al 1988) drew attention to the risks of such action. Practice in the neonatal setting may be different because defining brain death criteria (Pallis 1983) and 'persistent vegetative state' (Tresch et al 1991) is more difficult. For children older than 2 months, the recommendations are similar to those

for adults (British Paediatric Association 1991). The guidelines apply only to children who are comatose, totally apneic and requiring ventilation, the cause of brain damage is known, and the coma cannot be explained by drugs, hypothermia, or endocrine or metabolic disturbance. For children between 37 weeks' gestation and 2 months of age, the working party concluded that it would be rarely possible to diagnose brainstem death. In infants below 37 weeks' gestation, the working party concluded that the concept of brainstem death was inappropriate, and electrophysiologic assessment had little to offer over clinical assessment.

In summary, most doctors who care for newborn babies feel that there are occasions when a baby has a right to die (Anonymous 1981b). Doctors will often claim that 'every case is different'. 'It is one thing to justify an act; it is another to justify general practice' (Beauchamp & Childress 1989). There are five situations where the withholding or withdrawal of life-prolonging treatment might be considered (Royal College of Paediatrics and Child Health 1997):

- the brain dead child;
- the persistent vegetative state;
- the 'no chance' situation;
- the 'no purpose' situation;
- the 'unbearable situation'.

DIAGNOSIS OF NEUROLOGIC AND NEUROSURGICAL PROBLEMS IMMEDIATELY AFTER DELIVERY

Where there is reasonable uncertainty about the benefits of treatment, there should be a presumption in favor of initiating it (British Medical Association Medical Ethics Committee 1999). Clinical intervention can be discontinued later after reflection and discussion with parents, although it is often easier to withhold a treatment than to withdraw it (Winter & Cohen 1999). Misperceptions may have arisen as a result of society's acceptance of abortion for serious handicap (Leigh 1990). Some doctors and some parents believe that late termination of pregnancy because of serious handicap means that more leeway should be allowed regarding withholding or withdrawing life-prolonging treatment from handicapped newborns (British Medical Association Medical Ethics Committee 1999).

The experience of managing neural-tube defects illustrates the dilemmas for clinicians. The follow-up of a policy of operating on all children with spina bifida showed that half died (Lorber 1972). Of the 424 survivors, six had no handicap, 73 had a moderate degree of handicap, and 345 had severe physical handicaps. If selective criteria had been used for intervention (see below), not a single moderately handicapped child or one with no handicap would have been lost. One great difficulty is that some babies with the severest physical handicaps had normal intelligence. The formal criteria put forward by Lorber were: severe paraplegia, gross enlargement of the head, kyphosis, and associated gross congenital anomalies or major birth injuries. If one or more of these adverse criteria are present, the position is discussed in detail with both parents together.

Once the decision is made, whether it is to treat or to allow to die, much support will be needed in the hospital and home (Forest et al 1982). It appears that withdrawal of care is perceived as easier if there is a central nervous system problem than chronic lung disease or damaged bowel (Anonymous 1981b). Distress can be caused to the family if the professional staff are unaware of their religious customs, particularly as an approach will often be made to the family for a post-mortem (Green 1989).

The question of organ donation should be handled by a professional who is outside the team caring for the infant so that it is clear to the family that there is no conflict of interests. Tests for brainstem death are not appropriate for neonates, and therefore, organs are rarely obtained from living donors. The corneas and heart valves can be obtained up to 12 hours after death. A request for organ donation or post-mortem should never be made until it has been agreed with the parents that treatment has failed, and withdrawal of treatment is imminent (Working Party of the Health Department of Great Britain and Northern Ireland 1983).

DIAGNOSIS OF NEUROLOGIC AND NEUROSURGICAL PROBLEMS AFTER PROLONGED INTENSIVE CARE

The high-technology medicine that is practised in neonatal units runs a risk of being 'disease-oriented'. Each problem as it arises is attacked with all the skill and technology that is available (Duff & Campbell 1976). There is also the danger when multiple specialists are involved. Each specialist may give the utmost attention to a particular area of expertise, but a baby is not a constellation of separate organs but is a child in his or her own right. It is important that a single senior doctor takes overall responsibility for orchestrating the actions of the several specialists involved and liaising with the family (Brahams 1988). When caring for a baby at the very limits of viability, the parents must be given realistic information about the chances of mortality and morbidity (Chiswick 1990). Of babies born at less than 26 weeks' gestation and offered intensive care, survival rates to discharge are 2, 21, 33 and 52% at 22, 23, 24 and 25 weeks, respectively (Costeloe 1998). At 2 years, half have recognized disabilities.

It has been estimated that two-thirds of all deaths in a neonatal unit result from withdrawal of therapy (Balfour Lynn & Tasker 1996). Ultrasound examination of the neonatal brain helps in making these decisions, but there remain gray areas where the long-term outcome remains unclear (Levene 1990). Moreover, doctors use words such as 'probably,' 'possible,' or 'likely,' but the lay public's interpretation of such concepts of statistical probability is not the same as that of the physician (Shaw & Dear 1990).

If a decision is made with the parents to allow the child to die, all the equipment is disconnected at a time of the parents' choosing. The child is placed in the parents' arms in a quiet room where freedom from interruption can be guaranteed. An alternative is to elect not to resuscitate the infant when he or she next deteriorates, but this is a less satisfactory strategy for both family and staff. The ethics of making decisions not to resuscitate have been well reviewed (Davies & Reynolds 1992a, 1992b, Lloyd 1993). It is very important that parents are encouraged to see and hold their child after death (Finlay & Dallimore 1991). Palliative care should be continued until the child dies.

A difficult situation arises if the parents' views are at odds with those of the doctors or nurses caring for the child. In the author's experience, this is very rare provided the parents are involved in all discussions and given time to reach a view (McCall Smith 1992). When this does happen, the doctor should ask five questions (Dunn 1990):

- Do the parents understand the prognosis?
- Should they consult with others?
- Do they require more time?
- Is their decision in the interests of the child?
- Is their decision so unreasonable in terms of benefit to the child as to request them to seek a second opinion or for the doctor to seek the advice of the courts?

Conflict may also arise within the clinical team or between the two parents (Royal College of Paediatrics and Child Health, 1997). Those with parental responsibility for a baby are, in general, legally and morally entitled to give or withhold consent to treatment. Their decision will usually be determinative unless they conflict seriously with the views of the clinical team on the child's best interests (British Medical Association Medical Ethics Committee, 1999). However, parents cannot insist on enforcing decisions based solely on their own preferences where these conflict with good medical evidence. For desperate parents to expose fatally ill children to painful, unproven, or futile treatments breaches the child's rights. The doctor's first duty is to the patient. If a conflict cannot be resolved after a reasonable time period, a court may provide guidance on whether life-prolonging treatment would benefit the child, taking into account the 1989 Children Act (Hendrick Elton et al 1995, Kurtz 1995). In Re R (1993), the court invoked the Children Act to authorize blood transfusion to treat a child, against the parents' religious beliefs. However, each case is different. The High Court in the UK has both endorsed a doctor's decision to withhold ventilation and refrain from resuscitating a child against the parents' wishes (Re C 1998) and also upheld the parents' refusal to consent to surgery against the advice of doctors (Re T 1997). Two babies with apparently similar medical conditions may have different decisions made about them (Sherlock 1979) because of other factors related to parental wishes and beliefs.

Finally, it is very important that a senior member of staff writes to the family after the child's death and offers to see them in privacy away from the place where the child died. By this time, the full results of the post-mortem will be available, and the intervening period also allows the parents time to decide about any issues they would like to discuss.

interests of the child. Potential conflicts with this guiding principle include:

CONCLUSION

In tackling the ethical dilemmas of lifesaving intervention in the newborn, the clinician must always act in the best

- the interests of the child versus those of the parents or the state;
- ethics versus economics;
- heroic management versus humanitarianism.

REFERENCES

Anonymous 1981a Dr. Leonard Arthur: his trial and its implications. BMJ 283:1340–1341.

Anonymous 1981b The right to live and the right to die. BMJ 283:569–570.

Anonymous 1986 In the rear and limping a little: ethics and law in medicine. BMJ 292:1028.

Autton N 1985 Doctors talking. A R Mowbray, Oxford.

Balfour-Lynn I M, Tasker R C 1996 Futility and death in paediatric medical intensive care. J Med Ethics 22:279–281.

Beauchamp T L, Childress J F 1989 Principles of biomedical ethics. Oxford University Press, Oxford, pp. 120–183.

Bissenden J G 1986 Ethical aspects of neonatal care. Arch Dis Childh 61:639–641.

Brahams D 1988 No obligation to resuscitate a non-viable infancy. Lancet i:1176.

British Medical Association Medical Ethics Committee 1999 Witholding or withdrawing life-prolonging medical treatment — Guidance for decision making. BMJ Books, London.

British Paediatric Association 1991 Criteria for the diagnosis of brain death in infants and children that could be recommended for use by the medical profession as a whole. BMA, London.

Byrne P 1990 The BMA on euthanasia: the philosopher versus the doctor. In: Byrne P (ed.) Medicine, medical ethics and the value of life. Wiley, Chichester.

Campbell A G M 1982 Which infants should not receive intensive care? Arch Dis Childh 57:569–571.

Chiswick M 1990 Withdrawal of life support in babies: deceptive signals. Arch Dis Childh 65:1096–1097.

Costeloe K 1998 EPICure: Survival and morbidity of extremely preterm infants at discharge from hospital. Ped Res 43:211A.

Davies J M, Reynolds B M 1992a The ethics of cardiopulmonary resuscitation. I. Background to decision making. Arch Dis Childh 67:1498–1501.

Davies J M, Reynolds B M 1992b The ethics of cardiopulmonary resuscitation. II. Medical logistics and the potential for a good response. Arch Dis Childh 67:1498–1501.

Duff R S, Campbell A G M 1973 Moral and ethical dilemmas in the special care nursery. N Engl J Med 289:890–894.

Duff R S, Campbell A G M 1976 On deciding the care of severely handicapped or dying persons; with particular reference to infants. Paediatrics 57:487–493.

Dunn P M 1990 Life saving intervention in the neonatal period: dilemmas and decisions. Arch Dis Childh 65:557–558.

Elton A, Honig P, Bentovim A et al 1995 Withholding consent to lifesaving treatment: three cases. BMJ 310:373–377.

Farsides C 1992 Act of impassive euthanasia — is there a distinction? Care Crit Ill 8(3):126–128.

Finlay I, Dallimore D 1991 Your child is dead. BMJ 302:1524–1525.

Fletcher J 1972 Indicators of humanhood: a tentative profile of man. Hastings Centre Report 2:1–4.

Forest G C, Standish E, Baum J D 1982 Support after a perinatal death: a study of support and counselling after perinatal bereavement. BMJ 285:1475–1479.

Glover J 1977 Causing death and saving lives. Penguin, London.

Green J 1989 Death with dignity series. Islam, 1 Feb: 56–57 Hinduism, 8 Feb: 50–51. Sikhism, 15 Feb: 56–57. Judaism, 22 Feb: 64–75. Nursing Times, London.

Hellema H 1992 Dutch issue guidelines on handicapped babies. BMJ 305:1312–1313.

Kennedy I 1981 Unmasking medicine (Reith Lectures). Allen and Unwin, London.

Kopelman L M, Irons T G, Kopelman A E 1988 Neonatologists judge the 'baby Doe' regulations. N Engl J Med 318:677–683.

Kuhse H, Singer P 1985 Should the baby live? Oxford University Press, Oxford.

Kurtz Z 1995 Do children's rights to health care in the UK ensure their best interests? J Royal College Physicians London 29:508–516.

Leigh M A M S 1990 Capable of being born alive. J Med Defence Union Spring:3.

Lennard-Jones J E 1999 Giving or witholding fluid and nutrients: ethical and legal aspects. J Royal College Physicians London 33:39–45.

Levene M I 1990 Cerebral ultrasound and neurological impairment: telling the future. Arch Dis Childh 65:469–471.

Lloyd A 1993 'Do not resuscitate' orders. Br J Intensive Care February: 58–62.

Lorber J 1972 Spina bifida cystica. Arch Dis Childh 47:854.

McCall Smith A 1992 Consent to treatment in childhood. Arch Dis Childh 67(10):1247.

McHaffie H E, Fowlie P W 1997 Life, death and decisions: doctors and nurses reflect on neonatal practice. Hochland and Hochland, Hale.

Pallis C 1983 ABC of brain death. The Devonshire Press, London.

Rachels J 1975 Active and passive euthanasia. N Engl J Med 292:78–80.

Re C (Medical Treatment) [1998] 1 FLR 384.

Re J (A Minor) (Wardship: Medical Treatment) [1990] 3 All ER 930.

Re R (A Minor) (Medical Treatment) [1993] 2 FCR 544.

Re T (A Minor) (Wardship: Medical Treatment); sub nom Re C (A Minor) (Parents' Consent to surgery) [1997] 1 All ER 906.

Rhein R 1992 California says no to euthanasia. BMJ 305:1175.

Royal College of Paediatrics and Child Health 1997 Withholding or withdrawing life saving treatment in children: a framework for practice. RCPCH, London.

Schultz K 1992 Treating defective neonates in Hungary. Bull Med Ethics May:20–21.

Shaw N J, Dear P R F 1990 How do parents of babies interpret qualitative expressions of probability? Arch Dis Childh 65:520–523.

Sherlock R 1979 Selective non-treatment of newborns. J Med Ethics 5:139–142.

Stinson R, Stinson P 1981 On the death of a baby. J Med Ethics 7:5–18.

Tresch D D, Sims F H, Duthie E H, et al 1991 Clinical characteristics of patients in the persistent vegetative state. Arch Intern Med 151:930–932.

Winter B, Cohen S 1999 ABC of intensive care — withdrawal of treatment. BMJ 319:306–308.

Working Party of the Health Department of Great Britain and Northern Ireland 1983 Cadaveric organs for transplantation. A code of practice including the diagnosis of brain death. London: DHSS.

Index

Please note that page references relating to non-textual content such as Figures or Tables are in *italic* print